Comprehensive
Clinical Nephrology

Comprehensive Clinical Nephrology

2nd Edition

EDITED BY

Richard J Johnson MD FACP

Professor and Chief, Renal Section, Baylor College of Medicine, Houston, Texas, USA

John Feehally MA DM FRCP

Professor of Renal Medicine, University of Leicester; and
Consultant Nephrologist, Leicester General Hospital, Leicester, UK

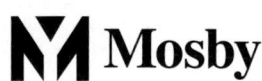 Mosby

Edinburgh   London   New York   Oxford   Philadelphia   St Louis   Sydney   Toronto   2003

First edition 2000
Second edition 2003

ISBN 0723432589

British Library Cataloguing in Publication Data
A catalogue record for this book is available from the British Library

Library of Congress Cataloging in Publication Data
A catalog record for this book is available from the Library of Congress

Notice
Medical knowledge is constantly changing. Standard safety precautions must be followed, but as new research and clinical experience broaden our knowledge, changes in treatment and drug therapy may become necessary or appropriate. Readers are advised to check the most current product information provided by the manufacturer of each drug to be administered to verify the recommended dose, the method and duration of administration, and contraindications. It is the responsibility of the practitioner, relying on experience and knowledge of the patient, to determine dosages and the best treatment for each individual patient. Neither the Publisher nor the Editor assumes any liability for any injury and/or damage to persons or property arising from this publication.
The Publisher

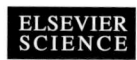

your source for books,
journals and multimedia
in the health sciences
www.elsevierhealth.com

Printed in Spain

Commissioning Editor:	Susan Pioli
Project Development Manager:	Tim Kimber
Project Manager:	Jess Thompson
Illustration Manager:	Mick Ruddy
Design Manager:	Jayne Jones
Illustrator:	First edition, Read Creative; Second edition, Antbit Illustrations
Page Layout:	Alan Palfreyman (PTU Elsevier)

Cover: Rat kidney fluorescently labeled with lens culinaris agglutinin (brown) and anti-WT-1 (green). Image captured on a two-photon microscope and rendered with Voxx. Photograph provided by Carrie Phillips, Indiana Center for Biological Microscopy, with support from INGEN, a grant from the Lilly Endowment to Indiana University School of Medicine.

The publisher's policy is to use paper manufactured from sustainable forests

Contents

Contents

SECTION 17
Drugs and the Kidney

Contributors

Magdalena Adeva Andany MD
Nephrology Division
Hospital Juan Canalejo
La Coruña
Spain

Horacio J Adrogué MD
Professor of Medicine
Veterans Affairs Medical Center
Houston, Texas
USA

Suhail Ahmad MB BS
Associate Professor and Medical Director
University of Washington
Seattle, WA
USA

Robert J Alpern
Professor of Internal Medicine
Dean, University of Texas
Southwestern Medical School
Department of Internal Medicine
Dallas, TX
USA

Charles E Alpers MD
Professor of Pathology and Adjunct
Professor of Medicine
University of Washington
Seattle, WA
USA

Hisham Alrefai MD
Department of Internal Medicine
University Health Center
Detroit, MI
USA

John Amerena MB BS FRACP FACC
Senior Lecturer (Cardiology)
Department of Cardiology
Geelong Hospital
Geelong, Victoria
Australia

Sharon Anderson MD
Professor of Medicine
Division of Nephrology and Hypertension
Oregon Health and Science University
Portland, OR
USA

Thomas E Andreoli MD MACP FRCP
Nolan Professor and Chairman
Department of Internal Medicine
University of Arkansas College of
Medicine
Little Rock, AR
USA

Pierre Aucouturier PhD
Associate Professor of Immunology
Hôpital Necker
Paris
France

**Arvind Bagga MD Diplomate
National Board**
Associate Professor of Paediatric
Nephrology
Department of Pediatrics
All India Institute of Medical Sciences
New Delhi
India

George L Bakris MD
Associate Professor of Preventive and
Internal Medicine
Vice Chairman, Department of
Preventative Medicine
Rush-Presbyterian St. Lukes Medical
Center
Chicago, IL
USA

**Ramasamy Bakthavatsalam MD,
FRCS(G)**
Acting Assistant Professor of Surgery
Transplant Services
University of Washington Medical Center
Seattle, WA
USA

Rashad S Barsoum MD FRCP FRCPE
Professor of Medicine, Cairo University
Chairman, Cairo Kidney Center
Barb-el-Louk
Egypt

Chris Baylis PhD
Professor of Physiology
West Virginia University
Morgantown, WV
USA

Yolanda Becker MD
Assistant Professor of Surgery
Division of Transplantation
University of Wisconsin School of
Medicine
Madison, WI
USA

William M Bennett MD
Medical Director
Transplant Services
Legacy Good Samaritan Hospital
Portland, OR
USA

Tomas Berl MD
Professor of Medicine
Head of Division of Renal Diseases
University of Colorado Health Sciences
Center
Denver, CO
USA

Suresh Bhat MBBS MS MCh
Assistant Professor of Genitourinary
Surgery
Trivandrum Medical College
Kerala
India

Gemma Bircher BSc(Hons), SRD
Dietetic Manager
Dietetic Department
Leicester General Hospital
Leicester
UK

Michael Boulton-Jones MA MB FRCP
Consultant Nephrologist
Renal Unit
Glasgow Royal Infirmary
Glasgow
UK

**Lucy Bowyer BMedSci MB BS
MRCOG**
Research Fellow
St George Hospital
Kogaragh
New South Wales
Australia

Hugh Brady MD PhD FRCPI
Professor of Medicine and Therapeutics
Mater Misericordiae Hospital
Dublin
Ireland

William E Braun MD
Consultant in Organ Transplantation
Department of Nephrology and
Hypertension
Cleveland Clinic
Cleveland, OH
USA

Mark A Brown MB BS FRACP MD
Professor of Medicine and Senior Staff
Nephrologist
Department of Renal Medicine
St George Hospital
Sydney
New South Wales
Australia

Emmanuel A Burdmann MD PhD
Associate Professor of Medicine
São José do Rio Preto Medical School
São José do Rio Preto
Brazil

David A Bushinsky MD
Professor of Medicine and of
Pharmacology and Physiology
University of Rochester Medical Center
Rochester, NY
USA

J Stewart Cameron CBE MD FRCP
Emeritus Professor of Renal Medicine
Guy's, King's and St Thomas' Medical
School
King's College
London
UK

Giovambattista Capasso MD
Associate Professor of Nephrology,
Chair of Nephrology
Second University of Naples
Naples
Italy

Susan J Carr MD FRCP
Consultant Nephrologist/Honorary
Senior Lecturer
Department of Nephrology
Leicester General Hospital
Leicester
UK

Praveen N Chander MD
Professor of Medicine
New York Medical College
Valhalla, NY
USA

Dinesh K Chatoth MD
Assistant Professor of Medicine
University of Arkansas for Medical
Sciences
Little Rock, AR
USA

Ignatius KP Cheng MBBS, PhD
Honorary Associate Professor of
Medicine
University of Hong Kong
Hong Kong

Glenn Chertow MD
Assistant Professor in Residence
Division of Nephrology
University of California
San Francisco, CA
USA

Peter J Conlon FRCPI
Consultant Nephrologist
Department of Nephrology
Beaumont Hospital
Dublin
Ireland

Mark E Cooper MD PhD
Professor of Medicine
Division of Diabetes, Lipoproteins and
Metabolism
Baker Medical Research Institute
Victoria
Australia

William G Couser MD
Belding H Scribner Professor of
Medicine
Division of Nephrology
University of Washington
Seattle, WA
USA

Simon J Davies
Consultant Nephrologist
Renal Unit
North Staffordshire Hospital
Stoke on Trent
UK

Connie I Davis MD
Medical Director
Kidney and Pancreas Transplant Program
Professor of Medicine
University of Washington Medical Center
Seattle, WA
USA

John M Davison MD
Professor of Obstetric Medicine
Consultant Obstetrician
Department of Obstetrics and
Gynaecology
University of Newcastle upon Tyne
Newcastle-upon-Tyne
UK

Paul E de Jong MD PhD
Head, Division of Nephrology
Department of Medicine
University Hospital Groningen
The Netherlands

Angelo M de Mattos MD
Division of Nephrology, Hypertension
and Clinical Pharmacology
Oregon Health Sciences University
Portland, OR
USA

Gerald DiBona MD
Professor of Medicine
Department of Internal Medicine
University of Iowa College of Medicine
Iowa City, IA
USA

Michael J Dillon FRCP FRCPCH
Professor of Pediatric Nephrology
Great Ormond Street Hospital for
Children
London
UK

Tilman B Drüeke MD
Director of Research, INSERM
Division of Nephrology
Hôpital Necker
Paris
France

Marlies Elgar MD
Abt. Nephrologie
Forschungszentrum der Medizinischen
Hochschule am Oststadtkrankenhaus
Hannover
Germany

Renee Ellis MD
c/o George L Bakris
Department of Preventative Medicine
Rush-Presbyterian St Lukes Medical
Center
Chicago, IL
USA

Meguid El Nahas PhD FRCP
Professor of Nephrology
Sheffield Kidney Institute
Northern General Hospital
Sheffield
UK

Joseph W Eschbach MD
Senior Research Advisor
Northwest Kidney Centers
700 Broadway
Seattle, WA
USA

Kenneth F Fairley MD FRCP
Physician and Nephrologist
Epworth Medical Centre
Victoria
Australia

Ronald J Falk MD
Professor of Medicine
Division of Nephrology and
Hypertension
University of North Carolina
Chapel Hill, NC
USA

Kenneth Farrington BSc MD FRCP
Consultant Nephrologist
Lister Hospital
Stevenage
UK

John Feehally MA DM FRCP
Professor of Renal Medicine
University of Leicester
Consultant Nephrologist
Leicester General Hospital
Leicester
UK

Leon Fernando Ferder MD FAHA
Professor and Chairman
Physiology Department
Ponce School of Medicine
Ponce, PR
USA

Evelyne A Fischer MD PhD
Assistant Professor of Nephrology
Department of Nephrology
University Hospital of Strasbourg
Strasbourg
France

John M Flack MD MPH
Professor and Associate Chairman for
Academic Affairs and Chief Quality
Officer
Department of Internal Medicine
Wayne State University Health Center
Detroit, MI
USA

Jürgen Floege MD
Professor of Medicine
Medizinische Klinik II
University of Aachen
Aachen
Germany

Giovanni B Fogazzi MD
Director, Renal Laboratory
Divisione di Nefrologia
Ospedale Maggiore
Milano
Italy

John W Foreman MD
Professor of Pediatrics
Chief, Division of Pediatric Nephrology
Duke University Medical Center
Durham, NC
USA

Megumu Fukunaga MD PhD
Assistant Professor/Lecturer
Department of Integrated Medicine
Kawaga Medical University Hospital
Kawaga-ken
Japan

Reinold Gans MD, PhD
Professor of Internal Medicine
University Hospital Groningen
Groningen
The Netherlands

Jay Garg MD
c/o George L Bakris
Department of Preventative Medicine
Rush-Presbyterian St Lukes Medical
Center
Chicago, IL
USA

F John Gennari MD
Professor of Medicine, Director,
Nephrology Unit
Department of Medicine
University of Vermont
Burlington, VT
USA

Louise Giblin MD MRCPI
Specialist Registrar in Nephrology
Beaumont Hospital
Dublin
Ireland

Richard E Gilbert MB BS PhD FRACP
Associate Professor of Medicine
Department of Medicine
St Vincent's Hospital
Victoria
Australia

Richard J Glassock MD MACP
Emeritus Professor
The David Getten School of Medicine
UCLA
Laguna Niguel, CA
USA

Thomas A Golper MD
Professor of Medicine
Vanderbilt University Medical Center
Nashville, TN
USA

Esther A González MD FACP
Associate Professor of Internal Medicine
Division of Nephrology
St. Louis University Hospital
St. Louis, MO
USA

Barbara Ann Greco MD
Western New England Renal Transplant
Associates,
Springfield, MA
USA

Roger N Greenwood MSc MD FRCP
Consultant Nephrologist
Department of Renal Medicine
Lister Hospital
Stevenage
UK

Lisa Guay-Woodford MD
Professor of Medicine
University of Alabama at Birmingham
Birmingham, AL
USA

Philip Halloran MD
Professor of Medicine
Division of Nephrology and Immunology
University of Alberta
Edmonton, Alberta
Canada

Kevin P G Harris MA MD FRCP
Reader in Nephrology
Leicester General Hospital
Leicester
UK

Lukas Hilbrands MD
Senior Lecturer in Nephrology
University Hospital Nijmegen
Nijmegen
The Netherlands

Luis G Hidalgo BSc
Division of Nephrology and Immunology
University of Alberta
Edmonton, Alberta
Canada

Andries J Hoitsma MD
Assistant Professor of Nephrology
University Hospital Nijmegen
Nijmegen
The Netherlands

Thomas M Hooton MD
Professor of Medicine
Harborview Medical Center
Seattle, WA
USA

Masaru Horio MD PhD
Associate Professor of Clinical
Laboratory Sciences
School of Allied Health Sciences Faculty
of Medicine
Osaka-fu
Japan

Jeremy Hughes MA MRCP PhD
Wellcome Trust Senior Research Fellow
in Clinical Science
Honorary Consultant Physician at Royal
Infirmary
MRC Centre for Inflammation Research
Edinburgh
UK

Hisham A A Ibrahim MB ChB MRCP (UK)
Research Fellow in Diabetes and
Endocrinology
Royal Liverpool University Hospital
Liverpool
UK

Munawar Izhar MD
Department of Preventative Medicine
Rush-Presbyterian St Lukes Medical
Center
Chicago, IL
USA

Bertrand L Jaber MD
Assistant Professor of Medicine,
Tufts University School of Medicine
Division of Nephrology
Boston, MA
USA

Ashley Jefferson MD MRCP
Assistant Professor
Division of Nephrology
University of Washington
Seattle, WA
USA

J Charles Jennette MD
Brinkhous Distinguished Professor and
Chair of Pathology and Laboratory
Medicine
University of North Carolina
Chapel Hill, NC
USA

Richard J Johnson MD FACP
Professor and Chief
Renal Section
Baylor College of Medicine
Houston, TX
USA

Stevo Julius MD
Professor of Medicine and Physiology
Department of Internal Medicine
Division of Hypertension
University of Michigan Medical Center
Ann Arbor, MI
USA

John Kanellis MBBS FRACP PhD
Nephrologist
The Austin Hospital
Melbourne
Australia

Clifford E Kashtan MD
Associate Professor of Pediatrics
University of Minnesota Medical School
Minneapolis, MN
USA

Bertram L Kasiske MD
Professor of Medicine
University of Minnesota
Department of Medicine
Hennepin County Medical Center
Minneapolis, MN
USA

Niamh Kieran MB BCh BAO MRCPI
Lecturer in Medicine
Department of Medicine and
Therapeutics
University College Dublin
Dublin 7
Ireland

Priscilla Kincaid-Smith DSc MD FRCP FRACP FRCPA
Director of Nephrology
Epworth Hospital
University of Melbourne
Parkville
Victoria
Australia

Wilhelm Kriz MD
Professor
Institute for Anatomy and Cell Biology
Heidelberg
Germany

Sumit Kumar MD
Clinical Assistant Professor of Medicine
Indiana University School of Medicine
Indianapolis, IN
USA

Kiyoshi Kurokawa MD MACP
Dean and Professor of Medicine
Tokai University School of Medicine
Kanagawa
Japan

Bernard Lacour PhD
Chief, Division of Biochemistry
Hôpital Necker
Paris
France

Anthony J Langone MD
Assistant Professor of Medicine
Division of Nephrology
Department of Internal Medicine
Vanderbilt University Medical Center
Nashville, TN
USA

William J Lawton MD
Associate Professor
Department of Internal Medicine
University of Iowa Hospitals
Iowa City, IA
USA

Jeremy Levy MA PhD MRCP
Consultant Nephrologist
Renal Section, Division of Medicine
Hammersmith Hospital
London
UK

Julia Lewis MD
Professor of Medicine
Vanderbilt University Medical Center
Nashville, TN
USA

Stuart L Linas MD
Professor of Medicine
University of Colorado School of
Medicine
Denver, CO
USA

Kelvin Lynn MB ChB FRACP
Associate Professor of Medicine
Department of Nephrology
Christchurch Hospital
Christchurch
New Zealand

Nicolaos E Madias MD
Professor of Medicine
Tufts University School of Medicine
Chief, Division of Nephrology
New England Medical Center
Boston, MA
USA

Colm Magee MD MPH
Instructor in Medicine
Renal Division
Brigham and Women's Hospital
Boston, MA
USA

Christopher Marsh MD
Associate Professor of Surgery and
Urology
University of Washington Medical
Center
Seattle, WA
USA

Mark Marshall MD
Consultant Nephrologist
Middlemore Hospital
Auckland
New Zealand

Kevin J Martin MB BCh FACP
Professor of Internal Medicine
St Louis University
St Louis, MO
USA

Philip D Mason BSc PhD MBBS FRCP
Consultant Nephrologist
Churchill Hospital
Oxford
UK

Anette Melk MD
Post-doctorate Fellow
University of Heidelberg
Heidelberg
Germany

John Kilian Mellon MD FRCS
Professor of Urology
Clinical Sciences Unit
Leicester General Hospital
Leicester
UK

Edgar L Milford MD
Associate Professor of Medicine
Harvard Medical School
Brigham and Women's Hospital
Boston, MA
USA

Rebeca D Monk MD
Assistant Professor of Medicine
University of Rochester School of
Medicine
Rochester, NY
USA

Bruno Moulin MD
Professor of Nephrology
Hôpital Universitaire de Strasbourg
Strasbourg
France

**Guy H Neild MBBS MD FRCP
FRCPath**
Professor of Nephrology
The Middlesex Hospital
London
UK

**Gary Nicholls MBChB MD FRACP
FRCP FACC**
Professor of Medicine
The Christchurch School of Medicine
Christchurch
New Zealand

Deidre A O'Sullivan MD
Associate Consultant in Nephrology
Park Nicollet Medical Center
Minneapolis, MN
USA

Ali Olyaei Pharm D
Assistant Professor of Medicine
Division of Nephrology, Hypertension
and Clinical Pharmacology
Oregon Health Sciences University
Portland, OR
USA

Vuddhidej Ophascharensuk MD
Associate Professor of Medicine
Renal Division, Department of Medicine
Chiang Mai University
Chiang Mai
Thailand

Yoshimasa Orita MD PhD
Dean of College of Nutrition,
Koshieu University
Takarazuka
Japan

**David K Packham MBBS MD FRCP
FRACP**
Consultant Nephrologist
The Royal Melbourne Hospital
Victoria
Australia

Biff F Palmer MD
Professor of Internal Medicine
Division of Nephrology
University of Texas Southwestern
Medical Center
Dallas, TX
USA

Chirag Parikh MD
Associate Professor
Division of Nephrology
University of Colorado Health Sciences
Center
Denver, CO
USA

Rosaleen B Parsons MD
Chairman of Diagnostic Imaging
Department of Diagnostic Imaging
Fox Chase Cancer Center
Philadelphia, PA
USA

Brian J G Pereira MD
Professor of Medicine
Tufts University School of Medicine
Boston, MA
USA

Richard Phelps MB BChir PhD MRCP
Senior Lecturer in Nephrology
Renal Autoimmunity Group
Centre for Inflammation Research
University of Edinburgh
Edinburgh
UK

Roberto Pisoni MD
Clinical Research Center for Rare
Diseases
Ranica
Italy

**Charles D Pusey DSc FRCP FRCPath
FMedSci**
Professor of Renal Medicine
Imperial College School of Medicine
London
UK

Venkat Ramanathan MD
Department of Medicine
Division of Nephrology
Vanderbilt University Medical Center
Nashville, TN
USA

T K Sreepada Rao MD
Professor of Medicine
Renal Diseases Division
State University of New York
Brooklyn, NY
USA

**Hugh C Rayner MA MB BS(Hons) MD
FRCP DipMedEd**
Consultant Nephrologist
Department of Renal Medicine
Birmingham Heartlands Hospital
Birmingham
UK

Giuseppe Remuzzi MD
Professor of Medicine
Director, Mario Negri Institute for
Pharmacological Research
Bergamo
Italy

Helmut Rennke
Professor of Pathology
Harvard Medical School
Brigham and Women's Hospital
Boston, MA
USA

**Mark Richards MB ChB MD PhD DSc
FRACP FAHA FRSNZ**
Professor of Medicine
Department of Medicine
Christchurch School of Medicine and
Health Sciences
Christchurch
New Zealand

Bernardo Rodriguez-Iturbe
Professor of Medicine
Nephrologia
Hospital Universitario de Maracaibo
Maracaibo
Venezuela

Pierre M Ronco MD PhD
Professor of Renal Medicine
Service de Nephrologie
Pierre et Marie Curie University
Hôpital Tenon
Paris
France

John Ross MD PA
Access Connections, LLC
Bamberg, SC
USA

Jérôme Rossert MD PhD
Professor of Nephrology
Hôpital Tenon
Paris
France

Piero Ruggenenti MD
Assistant Professor of Nephrology
Mario Negri Institute for
Pharmacological Research
Bergamo
Italy

Michael J Ryan MD
Assistant Professor of Medicine
Harborview Medical Center
Seattle, WA
USA

F Paolo Schena MD
Professor of Nephrology
University of Bari
Bari
Italy

John E Scoble MD
Consultant Nephrologist
Guy's Hospital
London
UK

Stuart J Shankland MD
Associate Professor of Medicine
Division of Nephrology
University of Washington Medical Center
Seattle, WA
USA

David Shirley BSc, PhD
Research Fellow/Honorary Senior
Lecturer
Centre for Nephrology
Royal Free and University College
Medical School
London
UK

William Simpson MD
Assistant Professor of Radiology
Mount Sinai Medical Center
New York, NY
USA

James A Sloand MD FACP
Associate Professor of Medicine
Highland Hospital
Rochester, NY
USA

Jack D Sobel MD
Professor of Medicine
Chief, Division of Infectious Diseases
Department of Internal Medicine
Harper Hospital
Detroit, MI
USA

Hans Sollinger MD PhD
Folkert O. Belzer Professor
Chairman, Division of Organ
Transplantation
University of Wisconsin Medical School
Madison, WI
USA

Jan C ter Maaten MD PhD
Consultant of Internal Medicine
University Hospital Groningen
Groningen
The Netherlands

Stephen C Textor MD
Professor of Medicine
Divisions of Hypertension and
Nephrology
Mayo Clinic
Rochester, MN
USA

**Charles R V Tomson MA BM BCh DM
(Oxon) FRCP**
Consultant Nephrologist
Southmead Hospital
Bristol
UK

Vicente E Torres MD
Professor of Medicine
Mayo Clinic/Mayo Foundation
Rochester, MN
USA

A Neil Turner PhD FRCP
Professor of Nephrology
Medical Renal Unit
The Royal Infirmary of Edinburgh
Edinburgh
UK

Robert J Unwin BM PhD FRCP
Professor of Nephrology and Physiology
Middlesex Hospital
London
UK

Jose Vazquez MD
Associate Professor of Medicine
Division of Infectious Diseases
Wayne State University School of
Medicine
Detroit, MI
USA

**R Kasi Visweswaran MBBS MD DM
MNAMS**
Professor of Nephrology and formerly
Vice Principal Trivandrum Medical
College
Kerala
India

Jiten Vora MA MD FRCP
Consultant Endocrinologist
Royal Liverpool Hospital
Liverpool
UK

Rowan G Walker MBBS FRACP MD
Professor of Medicine
Department of Nephrology
Royal Melbourne Hospital
Parkville
Victoria
Australia

Myron H Weinberger MD
Professor of Medicine
Director, Hypertension Research Center
Indiana University School of Medicine
Indianapolis, IN
USA

I David Weiner MD
Associate Professor of Medicine and
Physiology
University of Florida College of
Medicine
Gainesville, FL
USA

John D Williams MD FRCP
Professor of Nephrology
University of Wales College of Medicine
Cardiff
Wales
UK

**Christopher G Winearls MBChB,
DPhil, FRCP (London)**
Consultant Nephrologist
Renal Unit
Churchill Hospital
Oxford
UK

Charles S Wingo MD
Professor, University of Florida
Chief, Nephrology Section
Veterans Affairs Medical Center
Gainesville, FL
USA

Richard A Zager MD FHCRC
Professor of Medicine
Fred Hutchinson Cancer Center
Seattle, WA
USA

Preface

We have been encouraged by the success of the first edition of *Comprehensive Clinical Nephrology*, and in this second edition, we have sought to improve the text further in response to the advice and comments we have received from many readers and colleagues. All chapters have been extensively revised and we have provided new chapters on Aging and the Kidney, Interventional Nephrology, and Urological Issues for the Nephrologist. The number of references for each chapter has been increased to improve access to further in-depth reading. We have also improved the pagination and indexing to make the book more rapidly accessible.

The tables, figures and images proved to be a well liked feature of the first edition, which we have seen reproduced in lectures and seminars around the world over the last three years. Wherever possible we have improved these further in the second edition, and we are providing readers with a CD-Rom of these images to ensure their wide use.

We continue to offer a text for fellows, practicing nephrologists and internists that covers all aspects of the clinical work of the nephrologist including fluid and electrolytes, hypertension, diabetes, dialysis and transplantation. We recognize that this single volume does not compete with multivolume, highly referenced texts, and it remains our goal to provide 'comprehensive' coverage of clinical nephrology yet also ensure that the enquiring nephrologist can find the scientific issues and pathophysiology that underlie their clinical work.

RJJ and JF 2003

Dedication

We dedicate this book to:

Our mentors in nephrology – especially Bill Couser and Stewart Cameron

Our colleagues and collaborators as well as others whose research continues to light the way

Our wives and families who have once again endured the preparation of this second edition with unfailing patience and support, and to J Richard Johnson, clinician teacher, whose love of academic medicine was a major stimulus for one of us (RJJ) to pursue this career

Our patients with renal disease for whom it is a privilege to care

RJJ and JF 2003

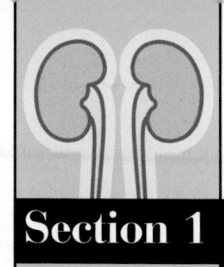

Chapter 1

Renal Anatomy

Wilhelm Kriz and Marlies Elgar

INTRODUCTION

The complex structure of the mammalian kidney is best understood in the unipapillary form that is common to all small species. Figure 1.1 is a schematic coronal section through such a kidney with a cortex enclosing a pyramid-shaped medulla the tip of which protrudes into the renal pelvis. The medulla is divided into an outer and an inner medulla; the outer medulla is further subdivided into an outer and an inner stripe.

STRUCTURE OF THE KIDNEY

The specific components of the kidney are the nephrons, the collecting ducts, and a unique microvasculature[1]. The multipapillary kidney of humans contains roughly one million nephrons. This number is already established during prenatal development; after birth new nephrons cannot be developed, a lost nephron cannot be replaced.

Nephrons

A nephron consists of a renal corpuscle (glomerulus) connected to a complicated and twisted tubule that finally drains into a collecting duct (see Fig. 1.2 and Table 1.1). Based on the

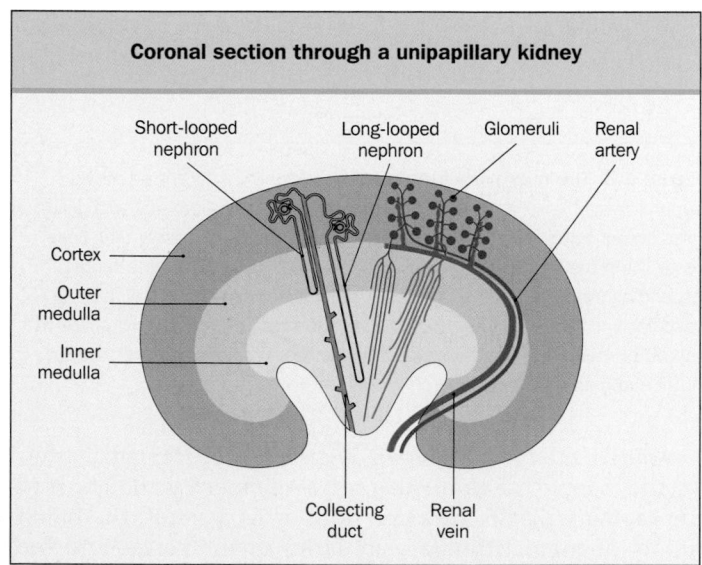

Figure 1.1 Coronal section through a unipapillary kidney.

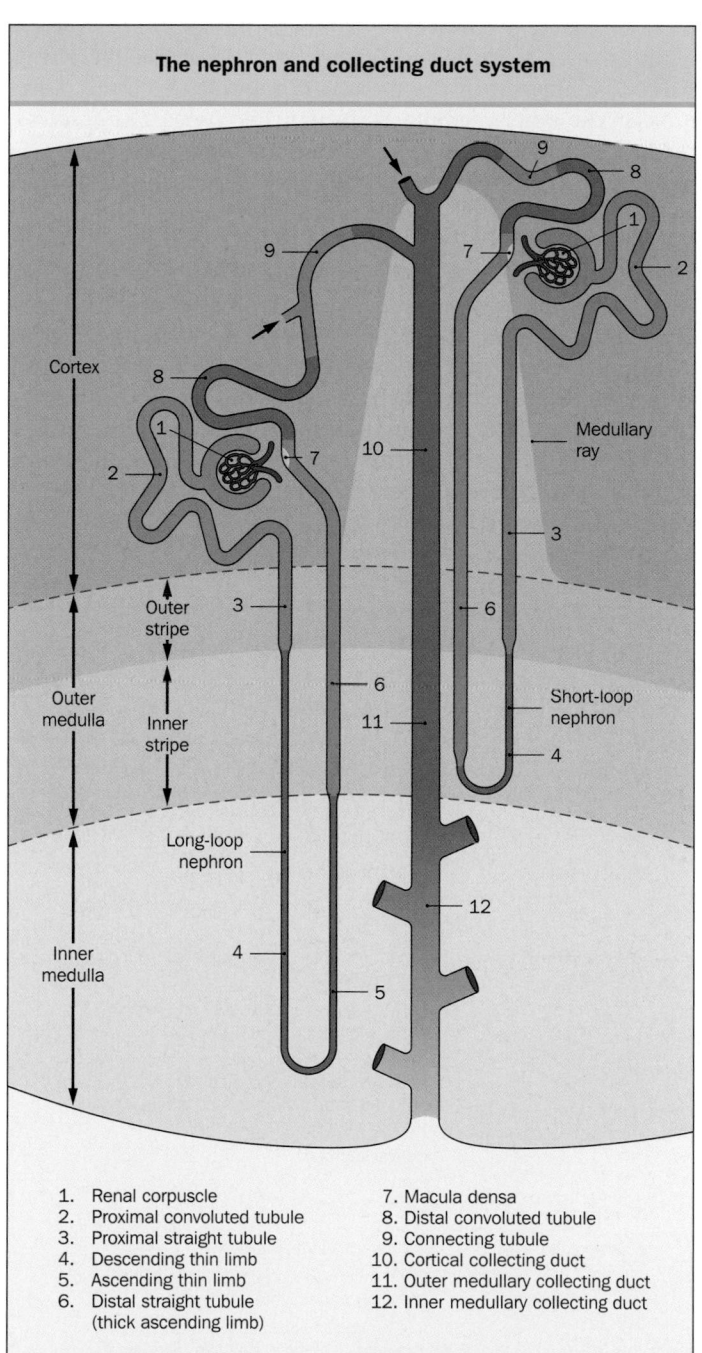

The nephron and collecting duct system

1. Renal corpuscle
2. Proximal convoluted tubule
3. Proximal straight tubule
4. Descending thin limb
5. Ascending thin limb
6. Distal straight tubule (thick ascending limb)
7. Macula densa
8. Distal convoluted tubule
9. Connecting tubule
10. Cortical collecting duct
11. Outer medullary collecting duct
12. Inner medullary collecting duct

Figure 1.2 Nephrons and the collecting duct system. Shown are a short-looped and a long-looped nephron, together with a collecting duct (not drawn to scale). Arrows denote confluence of further nephrons.

location of renal corpuscles within the cortex, three types of nephron can be distinguished: superficial, midcortical, and juxtamedullary nephrons. The tubular part of the nephron consists of a proximal tubule and a distal tubule connected by a loop of Henle (see below). There are two types of nephron, those with long loops of Henle and those with short loops. Short loops turn back in the outer medulla or even in the cortex (cortical loops). Long loops turn back at successive levels of the inner medulla.

Collecting ducts

A collecting duct is formed in the renal cortex when several nephrons join. A connecting tubule is interposed between a nephron and a cortical collecting duct. Cortical collecting ducts descend within the medullary rays of the cortex. They traverse the outer medulla as unbranched tubes. On entering the inner medulla they fuse successively and open finally as papillary ducts into the renal pelvis (see Fig. 1.2 and Table 1.1).

Microvasculature

The microvascular pattern of the kidney (see Figs 1.1 and 1.3) is also similarly organized in mammalian species[1]. The renal artery after entering the renal sinus finally divides into the interlobar arteries, which extend towards the cortex in the space between the wall of the pelvis (or calyx) and the adjacent cortical tissue. At the junction between cortex and medulla they divide and pass over into the arcuate arteries, which also branch. They give rise to the cortical radial arteries (interlobular arteries) that ascend radially through the cortex. No arteries penetrate the medulla.

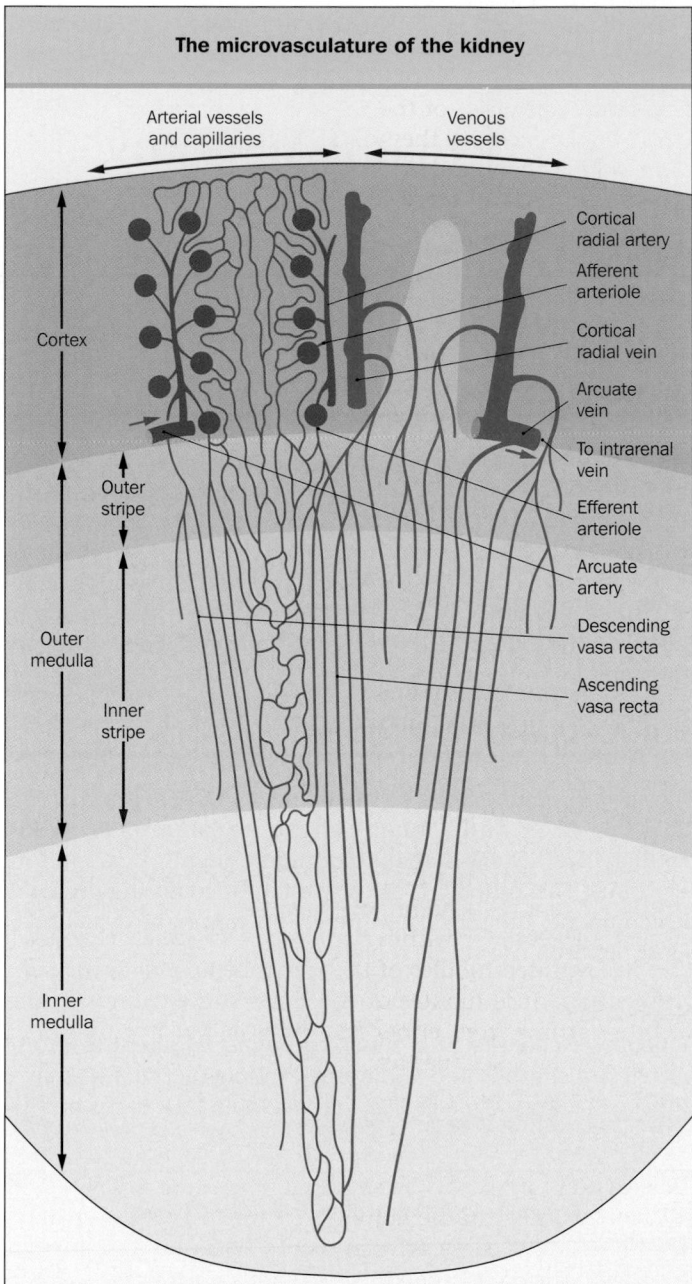

Figure 1.3 The microvasculature of the kidney. Afferent arterioles supply the glomeruli and efferent arterioles leave the glomeruli and divide into the descending vasa recta, which, together with the ascending vasa recta, form the vascular bundles of the renal medulla. The vasa recta ascending from the inner medulla all traverse the inner stripe within the vascular bundles, whereas most of the vasa recta from the inner stripe of the outer medulla ascend outside the bundles. Both types traverse the outer stripe as wide, tortuous channels.

Afferent arterioles generally arise from cortical radial arteries; they supply the glomerular tufts. Aglomerular tributaries to the capillary plexus are rarely found. As a result, the blood supply of the peritubular capillaries of the cortex and the medulla is exclusively postglomerular. Glomeruli are drained by efferent arterioles. Two basic types can be distinguished: cortical and juxtamedullary efferent arterioles. Cortical efferent

The nephron and collecting duct system	
Section	**Subsections**
Nephron	
Renal corpuscle	Glomerulus: the term used most frequently to refer to the entire renal corpuscle
	Bowman's capsule
Proximal tubule	Convoluted part
	Straight part (pars recta) or thick descending limb of Henle's loop
Intermediate tubule	Descending part or thin descending limb of Henle's loop
	Ascending part or thin ascending limb of Henle's loop
Distal tubule	Straight part or thick ascending limb of Henle's loop: subdivided into a medullary and a cortical part; the latter contains in its terminal portion the macula densa
	Convoluted part
Collecting duct system	
Connecting tubule	Includes the arcades in most species
Collecting duct	Cortical collecting duct
	Outer medullary collecting duct subdivided into an outer- and an inner-stripe portion
	Inner medullary collecting duct subdivided into a basal, middle, and papillary portion

Table 1.1 The subdivisions of the nephron and collecting duct system

arterioles, which derive from superficial and midcortical glomeruli, supply the capillary plexus of the cortex.

The efferent arterioles of juxtamedullary glomeruli represent the supplying vessels of the renal medulla. Within the outer stripe of the medulla they divide into the descending vasa recta, which then penetrate the inner stripe in cone-shaped vascular bundles. At intervals, individual vessels leave the bundles to supply the capillary plexus at the adjacent medullary level.

Ascending vasa recta drain the renal medulla. In the inner medulla they arise at every level, ascending as unbranched vessels. They traverse the inner stripe within the vascular bundles. The ascending vasa recta that drain the inner stripe may either join the vascular bundles or may ascend directly to the outer stripe between the bundles. All the ascending vasa recta traverse the outer stripe as individual wavy vessels with wide lumina interspersed among the tubules. Since true capillaries derived from direct branches of efferent arterioles are relatively scarce, it is the ascending vasa recta that form the capillary plexus of the outer stripe. Finally the ascending vasa recta empty into arcuate veins.

The vascular bundles represent a countercurrent exchanger between the blood entering and that leaving the medulla. In addition, the organization of the vascular bundles results in a separation of the blood flow to the inner stripe from that to the inner medulla. Descending vasa recta supplying the inner medulla traverse the inner stripe within the vascular bundles. Therefore, blood flowing to the inner medulla has not been exposed previously to tubules of the inner or outer stripe. All ascending vasa recta originating from the inner medulla traverse the inner stripe within the vascular bundles, thus blood that has perfused tubules of the inner medulla does not subsequently perfuse tubules of the inner stripe. However, the blood returning from either the inner medulla or the inner stripe afterwards does perfuse the tubules of the outer stripe. It has been suggested that this arrangement in the outer stripe functions as the ultimate trap to prevent solute loss from the medulla.

The intrarenal veins accompany the arteries. Central to the renal drainage of the kidney are the arcuate veins, which, in contrast to arcuate arteries, do form real anastomosing arches at the corticomedullary border. They accept the veins from the cortex and from the renal medulla. The arcuate veins join to form interlobar veins, which run alongside the corresponding arteries.

The intrarenal arteries and the afferent and efferent arterioles are accompanied by sympathetic nerve fibers and terminal axons representing the efferent nerves of the kidney[1]. Tubules have direct contact to terminal axons only when they are located around the arteries or the arterioles. As stated by Barajas, 'the tubular innervation consists of occasional fibers adjacent to perivascular tubules'[4]. The density of nerve contacts to convoluted proximal tubules is low; contacts to straight proximal tubules, thick ascending loops of the limbs of Henle, and to collecting ducts (located in the medullary rays and the outer medulla) have never been encountered. The vast majority of tubular portions have no direct relationships to nerve terminals. Afferent nerves of the kidney are commonly believed to be sparse[5].

THE NEPHRON

The renal glomerulus (renal corpuscle)

The glomerulus comprises a tuft of specialized capillaries attached to the mesangium, both of which are enclosed in a pouch-like extension of the tubule, i.e., Bowman's capsule (Figs 1.4 and 1.5). The capillaries together with the mesangium are covered by epithelial cells (podocytes), forming the visceral epithelium of Bowman's capsule. At the vascular pole, this is reflected to become the parietal epithelium of Bowman's capsule. At the interface between the glomerular capillaries and the mesangium on one side and the podocyte layer on the other side, the glomerular basement membrane (GBM) is developed. The space between both layers of Bowman's capsule represents the urinary space, which at the urinary pole continues as the tubule lumen.

When entering the tuft, the afferent arteriole immediately divides into several (two to five) primary capillary branches, each of which gives rise to an anastomosing capillary network representing a glomerular lobule. In contrast to the afferent arteriole, the efferent arteriole is already established inside the

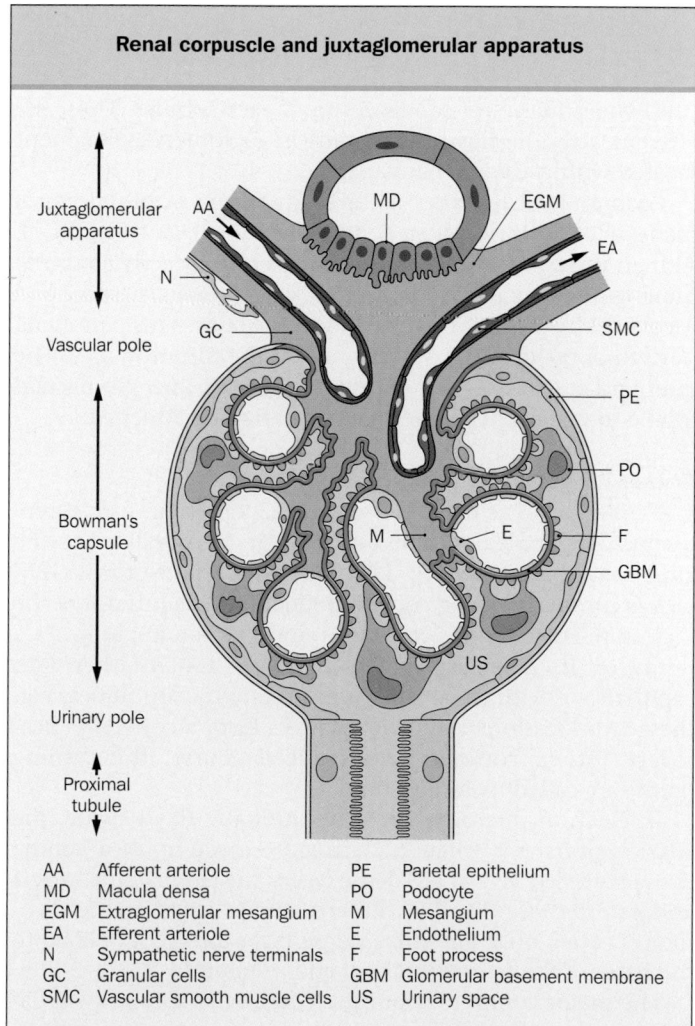

Renal corpuscle and juxtaglomerular apparatus

AA	Afferent arteriole	PE	Parietal epithelium
MD	Macula densa	PO	Podocyte
EGM	Extraglomerular mesangium	M	Mesangium
EA	Efferent arteriole	E	Endothelium
N	Sympathetic nerve terminals	F	Foot process
GC	Granular cells	GBM	Glomerular basement membrane
SMC	Vascular smooth muscle cells	US	Urinary space

Figure 1.4 Renal corpuscle and juxtaglomerular apparatus (JGA).
(Adapted with permission from Kriz and Kaissling[1].)

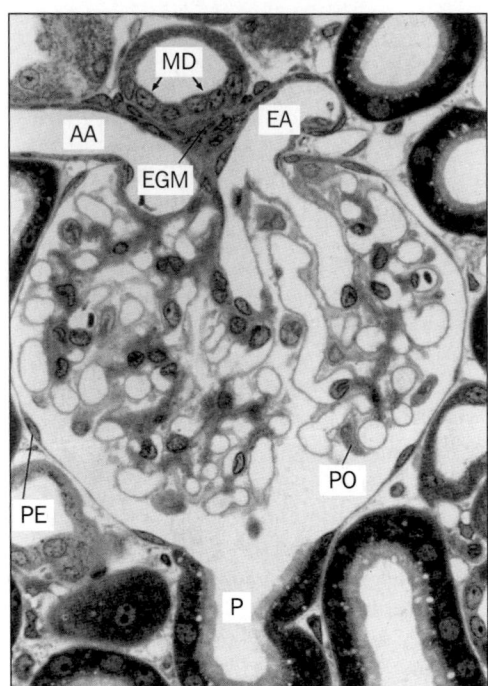

Figure 1.5 Longitudinal section through a glomerulus (rat). At the vascular pole the afferent arteriole (AA), the efferent arteriole (EA), the extraglomerular mesangium (EGM), and the macula densa (MD) are seen. At the urinary pole the parietal epithelium (PE) transforms into the proximal tubule (P). PO, podocyte; PE, parietal epithelial cell (light microscopy: ×390).

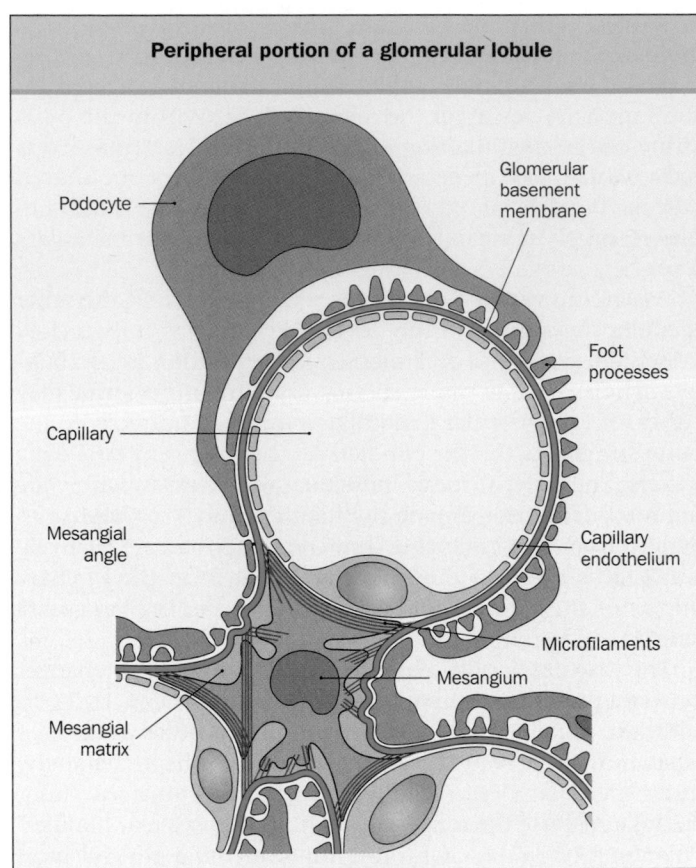

Figure 1.6 The peripheral portion of a glomerular lobule. This shows a capillary, the axial position of the mesangium, and the visceral epithelium (podocytes). At the capillary–mesangial interface the capillary endothelium directly abuts the mesangium.

tuft by confluence of capillaries from each lobule[6]. Thus, the efferent arteriole has a significant intraglomerular segment located within the glomerular stalk.

Glomerular capillaries are a unique type of blood vessel made up of nothing but an endothelial tube (Figs 1.6 and 1.7). A small stripe of the outer aspect of this tube directly abuts the mesangium; a major part bulges towards the urinary space and is covered by the GBM and the podocyte layer. This peripheral portion of the capillary wall represents the filtration area. The glomerular mesangium represents the axis of a glomerular lobule to which the glomerular capillaries are attached.

Glomerular basement membrane

The GBM serves as the skeleton of the glomerular tuft. It represents a complexly folded sack with an opening at the glomerular hilum (see Fig. 1.4). The outer aspect of this GBM sack is completely covered with podocytes. The interior of the sack is filled with the capillaries and the mesangium. As a result, on its inner aspect the GBM is in touch either with capillaries or with the mesangium. At any transition between these two locations the GBM changes from a convex pericapillary into a concave perimesangial course; the turning points are called mesangial angles.

In electron micrographs of traditionally fixed tissue, the GBM appears as a trilaminar structure made up of a lamina densa bounded by two less dense layers: the lamina rara interna and externa (see Fig. 1.7). Recent studies using freeze techniques reveal only one thick dense layer directly attached to the bases of the epithelium and endothelium[7].

The major components of the GBM include type IV collagen and laminin, heparan sulfate proteoglycans, as in basement membranes at other sites. Type V and VI collagen and nidogen have also been demonstrated. However, the GBM has

several unique properties, notably a distinct spectrum of type IV collagen and laminin isoforms. The mature GBM is made up of collagen IV consisting of α_3, α_4 and α_5 chains (instead of α_1 and α_2 chains of most other basement membranes) and of laminin-11 consisting of α_5, β_2 and γ_1 chains[8]. Type IV collagen is the antigenic target in Goodpasture's disease (see Chapter 25), and mutations in the genes of the α_3, α_4 and α_5 chains of type IV collagen are responsible for Alport's Syndrome (see Chapter 48).

Current models depict the basic structure of the basement membrane as a three-dimensional network of collagen type IV[7]. The type IV collagen monomer consists of a triple helix of length 400 nm that has a large noncollagenous globular domain at its C-terminal end called NC1. At the N terminus, the helix possesses a triple helical rod of length 60 nm: the 7S domain. Interactions between the 7S domains of two triple helices or the NC1 domains of four triple helices allow collagen type IV monomers to form dimers and tetramers. In addition, triple helical strands interconnect by lateral associations via binding of NC1 domains to sites along the collagenous region. These interactions between type IV collagen triple helices result in a flexible, nonfibrillar polygonal assembly that is considered to provide mechanical strength to the basement membrane and to serve as a scaffold for alignment of other matrix components.

The electronegative charge of the GBM mainly results from the presence of polyanionic proteoglycans. The major proteoglycans of the GBM are heparan sulfate proteoglycans, among them perlecan and agrin. Proteoglycan molecules aggregate to form a meshwork that is kept highly hydrated by water molecules trapped in the interstices of the matrix.

Mesangium

Three cell types occur within the glomerular tuft, all of which are in close contact with the GBM: mesangial cells, endothelial cells, and podocytes. In the rat, the numerical ratio has been calculated to be 2 : 3 : 1. The mesangial cells, together with the mesangial matrix, establish the glomerular mesangium.

Mesangial cells

Mesangial cells are quite irregular in shape with many processes extending from the cell body towards the GBM (see Figs 1.6 and 1.7). In these processes, dense assemblies of microfilaments are found that contain actin, myosin, and α-actinin[9]. The processes are attached to the GBM either directly or through the interposition of microfibrils (see below). The GBM represents the effector structure of mesangial contractility. Mesangial cell–GBM connections are especially prominent alongside the capillaries, interconnecting the two opposing mesangial angles of the GBM.

Mesangial matrix

The mesangial matrix fills the highly irregular spaces between the mesangial cells and the perimesangial GBM, anchoring the mesangial cells to the GBM[6]. The ultrastructural organization of this matrix is incompletely understood. In specimens prepared by a technique that avoids osmium tetroxide and uses tannic acid for staining a dense network of elastic microfibrils is seen. A large number of common extracellular matrix proteins have been demonstrated within the mesangial matrix, including several types of collagens (IV, V, and VI) and several components of microfibrillar proteins (fibrillin, and the 31-kDa microfibril-associated glycoprotein (MAGP)). The matrix also contains several glycoproteins (fibronectin is most abundant) as well as several types of proteoglycan.

Endothelium

Glomerular endothelial cells consist of cell bodies and peripherally located, attenuated, and highly fenestrated cytoplasmic sheets (see Figs 1.6 and 1.7). Glomerular endothelial pores lack diaphragms, which are only encountered in the endothelium of the final tributaries to the efferent arteriole[6]. The round-to-oval pores have a diameter of 50–100 nm. The luminal membrane of endothelial cells is negatively charged because of its cell coat of several polyanionic glycoproteins, including podocalyxin. In addition the endothelial pores are filled with 'sieve plugs' probably made up of sialoglycoproteins[10].

Visceral epithelium (podocytes)

The visceral epithelium of Bowman's capsule comprises highly differentiated cells, the podocytes (see Figs 1.6 and 1.8). In the developing glomerulus, podocytes have a simple polygonal shape. In rat, mitotic activity of these cells is completed soon after birth together with the cessation of the

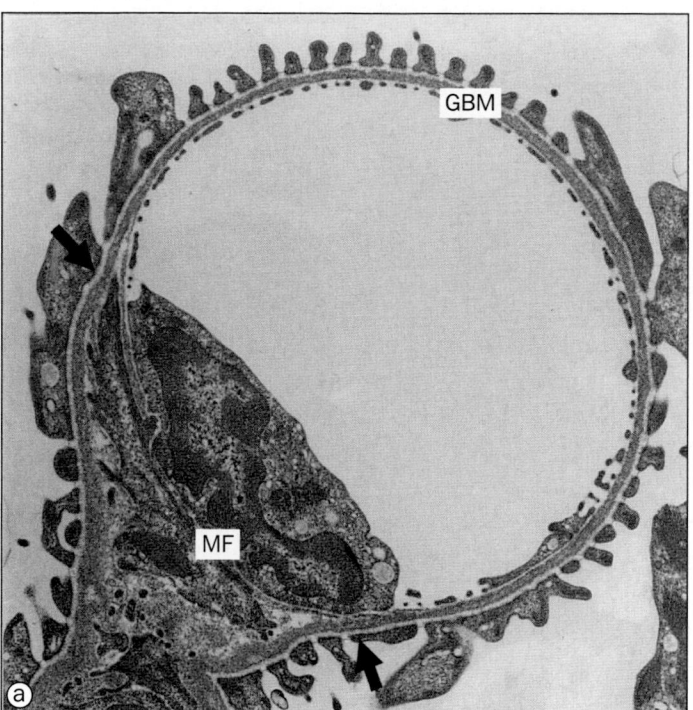

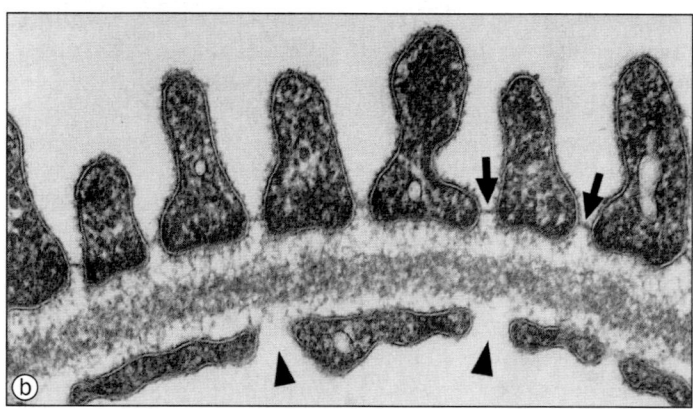

Figure 1.7 Glomerular capillary. (a) The layer of interdigitating podocyte processes and the glomerular basement membrane (GBM) do not completely encircle the capillary. At the mesangial angles (arrows) both deviate from a pericapillary course and cover the mesangium. Mesangial cell processes, containing dense bundles of microfilaments (MF), interconnect the GBM and bridge the distance between the two mesangial angles. (b) Filtration barrier. The peripheral part of the glomerular capillary wall comprises the endothelium with open pores (arrowheads), the GBM, and the interdigitating foot processes. The GBM shows a lamina densa bounded by the lamina rara interna and externa. The foot processes are separated by filtration slits bridged by thin diaphragms (arrows). (Transmission electron microscopy: (a) ×8770; (b) ×50440.)

formation of new nephron anlagen. In humans, this point is already reached during prenatal life. The differentiation of the adult podocyte phenotype with the characteristic cell process pattern (see below) is associated with the appearance of several podocyte-specific proteins, including podocalyxin, nephrin, podocin, synaptopodin and GLEPP-1[11]. Differentiated podocytes are unable to replicate; therefore, in the adult, degenerated podocytes cannot be replaced. In response to

Essential Renal Anatomy and Physiology

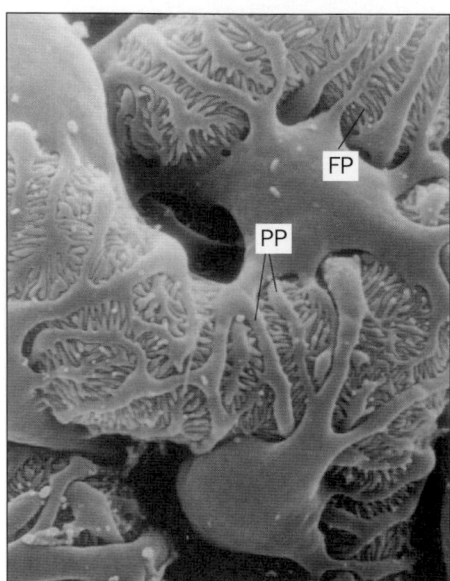

**Figure 1.8
Glomerular
capillaries in the rat.**
The urinary side of the
capillary is covered by
the highly branched
podocytes. The
interdigitating system
of primary processes
(PP) and foot
processes (FP) lines
the entire surface of
the tuft extending also
beneath the cell
bodies. The foot
processes of
neighboring cells
interdigitate but spare
the filtration slits in
between. (Scanning
electron microscopy,
×2200.)

an extreme mitogenic stimulation (e.g., by basic fibroblast growth factor, FGF-2), these cells may undergo mitotic nuclear division; however, the cells are unable to complete cell division, resulting in bi- or multinucleated cells[12].

Podocytes have a voluminous cell body that floats within the urinary space. The cell bodies give rise to long primary processes that extend towards the capillaries, to which they affix by their most distal portions and by an extensive array of foot processes. The foot processes of neighboring podocytes regularly interdigitate with each other, leaving between them meandering slits (filtration slits) that are bridged by an extracellular structure, the slit diaphragm (see Figs 1.6–1.8). Podocytes are polarized epithelial cells with a luminal and a basal cell membrane domain; the latter corresponds to the sole plates of the foot processes that are embedded into the GBM. The border between basal and luminal membrane is represented by the slit diaphragm[13].

The luminal membrane and the slit diaphragm are covered by a thick surface coat that is rich in sialoglycoproteins (including podocalyxin and podoendin) and is responsible for the high negative surface charge of the podocytes. By comparison, the abluminal membrane (i.e., the soles of podocyte processes) contains specific transmembrane proteins which connect the cytoskeleton to the GBM. Two systems are known; first, $\alpha_3\beta_1$ integrin dimers that interconnect the cytoplasmic focal adhesion proteins vinculin, paxillin and talin with the α_3, α_4 and α_5 chains of collagen type IV and second, β-α-dystroglycans that interconnect the cytoplasmic adapter protein utrophin with agrin and laminin a_5 chains in the GBM[11]. Other membrane proteins, such as the C3b receptor and gp330/megalin, are present over the entire surface of podocytes[12].

In contrast to the cell body (harboring a prominent Golgi system), the cell processes contain only a few organelles. A well-developed cytoskeleton accounts for the complex shape of the cells. In the cell body and the primary processes, microtubules and intermediate filaments (vimentin, desmin) dominate.

Microfilaments form prominent bundles arranged in the longitudinal axis of the foot processes. Peripherally they are linked to the GBM by integrins and dystroglycans (see above).

The filtration slits are the site of convective fluid flow through the visceral epithelium. They have a constant width of about 30 to 40 nm. The structure and biochemical composition of the slit membrane are insufficiently understood. Chemically fixed and tannic acid-treated tissue reveals a zipper-like structure with a row of 'pores' approximately 14 nm square on either side of a central bar. At present four proteins are known to participate in the molecular organization of the slit membrane: nephrin, NEPH1, p-cadherin and FAT. However, how these molecules interact with each other to establish a size selective porous membrane is unknown[11].

Parietal epithelium

The parietal epithelium of Bowman's capsule consists of squamous epithelial cells resting on a basement membrane (see Figs 1.4 and 1.5). The flat cells are filled with bundles of actin filaments running in all directions. The parietal basement membrane differs from the GBM in that it comprises several dense layers that, in addition to type IV, contain type XIV collagen. The predominant proteoglycan of the parietal basement membrane is a chondroitin sulfate proteoglycan[1].

Filtration barrier

Filtration through the glomerular capillary wall occurs along an extracellular pathway including the endothelial pores, the GBM, and the slit diaphragm (see Fig. 1.7b). All these components are quite permeable for water; the high permeability for water, small solutes, and ions results from the fact that no cell membranes are interposed. The hydraulic conductance of the individual layers of the filtration barrier is difficult to study. In a mathematical model of glomerular filtration, the hydraulic resistance of the endothelium was predicted to be small, whereas the GBM and filtration slits contribute roughly one half each to the total hydraulic resistance of the capillary wall[14].

The barrier function of the glomerular capillary wall for macromolecules is selective for size, shape, and charge[12]. The charge selectivity of the barrier results from the dense accumulation of negatively charged molecules throughout the entire depth of the filtration barrier, including the surface coat of endothelial cells, and the high content of negatively charged heparan sulfate proteoglycans in the GBM. Polyanionic macromolecules, such as plasma proteins, are repelled by the 'electronegative shield' originating from these dense assemblies of negative charges.

The size selectivity of the filtration barrier is in part established by the dense network of the GBM. The most restrictive structure, however, appears to be the slit diaphragm[14]. Uncharged macromolecules up to an effective radius of 1.8 nm pass freely through the filter. Larger components are more and more restricted (indicated by their fractional clearances, which progressively decrease) and are totally restricted at effective radii > 4.0 nm. Plasma albumin has an effective radius of 3.6 nm; without the repulsion from the negative charge, plasma albumin would pass through the filter in considerable amounts.

Stability of the glomerular tuft

The main challenge for the glomerular capillaries is to combine selective leakiness with stability. The walls of capillaries do not appear to be capable of resisting high transmural pressure gradients. Several structures/mechanisms are involved in counteracting the distending forces to which the capillary wall is constantly exposed. The locus of action of all these forces is the GBM.

Two systems appear to be responsible for the development of stabilizing forces. A basic system consists of the GBM and the mesangium. Cylinders of the GBM, in fact, largely define the shape of glomerular capillaries. These cylinders, however, do not completely encircle the capillary tube; they are open towards the mesangium. Mechanically, they are completed by contractile mesangial cell processes that bridge the gaps of the GBM by interconnecting the opposing mesangial angles[9].

Podocytes act as a second structure-stabilizing system. Two mechanisms appear to be involved. First, podocytes stabilize the folding pattern of glomerular capillaries by fixing the turning points of the GBM between neighboring capillaries[10]. Second, podocytes may contribute to structural stability of glomerular capillaries by a mechanism similar to that of pericytes elsewhere in the body. Podocytes are attached to the GBM by foot processes that cover almost entirely the outer aspect of the GBM. The foot processes possess a well-developed contractile system connected to the GBM. Since the foot processes are attached in various angles on the GBM, they may function as numerous small, stabilizing patches on the GBM, counteracting locally the elastic distension of the GBM[12].

The renal tubule

The renal tubule is subdivided into several distinct segments: a proximal tubule, an intermediate tubule, a distal tubule, a connecting tubule, and the collecting duct (see Fig. 1.1 and Table 1.1)[1]. The loop of Henle comprises the straight part of the proximal tubule (representing the thick descending limb), the thin descending and the thin ascending limb (both thin limbs together represent the intermediate tubule), and the thick ascending limb (representing the straight portion of the distal tubule), which includes the macula densa. The connecting tubule and the various collecting duct segments form the collecting duct system.

The renal tubules are outlined by a single-layered epithelium anchored to a basement membrane. The epithelium is a transporting epithelium consisting of flat or cuboidal epithelial cells connected apically by a junctional complex consisting of a tight junction (zonula occludens), an adherens junction, and, rarely, a desmosome. As a result of this organization, two different pathways through the epithelium exist (Fig. 1.9): a transcellular pathway, including the transport across the luminal and the basolateral cell membrane and through the cytoplasm, and a paracellular pathway through the junctional complex and the lateral intercellular spaces. The functional characteristics of the paracellular transport are determined by the tight junction, which differs markedly in its elaboration in the various tubular segments. The transcellular transport is determined by the specific channels, carriers, and transporters included in the apical and basolateral cell membranes. The various nephron segments differ markedly in function, distribution of important transport proteins, and responsiveness to drugs such as diuretics.

The proximal tubule

The proximal tubule reabsorbs the bulk of filtered water and solutes (Fig. 1.10). The epithelium shows numerous structural

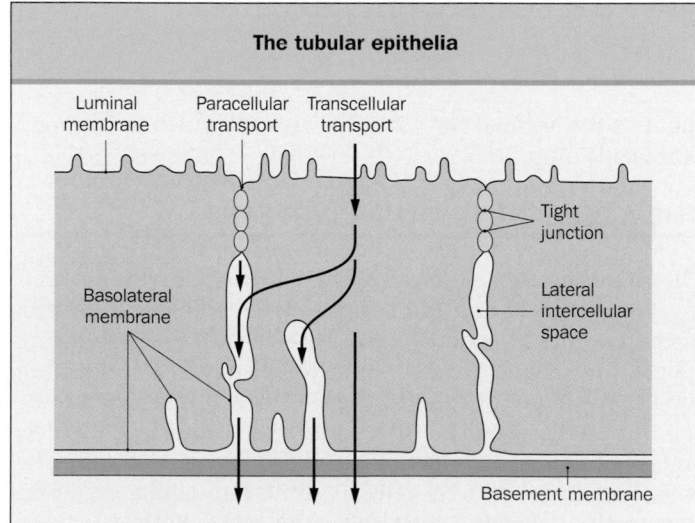

Figure 1.9 The tubular epithelia. Transport across the epithelium may follow two routes: transcellular across luminal and basolateral membranes and paracellular through the tight junction and intercellular spaces.

The tubular epithelia

Luminal membrane / Paracellular transport / Transcellular transport / Tight junction / Basolateral membrane / Lateral intercellular space / Basement membrane

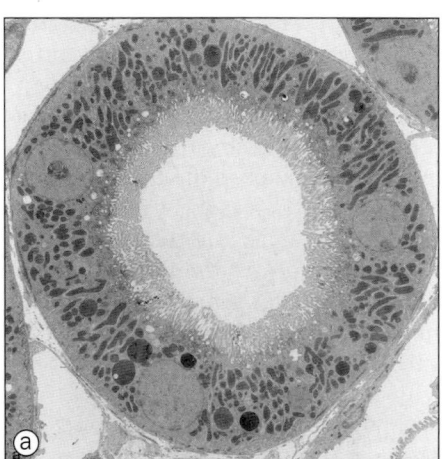
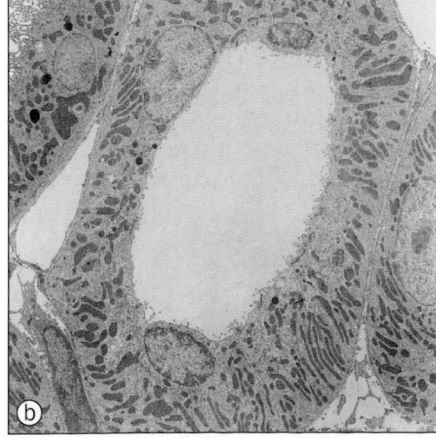

Figure 1.10 Tubules of the renal cortex.
(a) Proximal convoluted tubule is equipped with a brush border and a prominent vacuolar apparatus in the apical cytoplasm. The rest of the cytoplasm is occupied by a 'basal labyrinth' consisting of large mitochondria associated with basolateral cell membranes. (Transmission electron microscopy ×1530.) (b) Distal convoluted tubule also has interdigitated basolateral cell membranes intimately associated with large mitochondria; in contrast to the proximal tubule the apical surface is amplified only by some stubby microvilli. (Transmission electron microscopy ×1830.)

adaptations to this role. The proximal tubule has a prominent brush border (increasing the luminal cell surface area), and extensive interdigitation by basolateral cell processes (increasing the basolateral cell surface area). This lateral cell interdigitation extends up to the 'leaky' tight junction, thus increasing the tight junctional belt in length and providing a greatly increased passage for the passive transport of ions. Proximal tubules have large prominent mitochondria intimately associated with the basolateral cell membranes where the Na^+/K^+ ATPase is located; this machinery dominates the transcellular transport. The luminal transporter for Na^+ entry specific for the proximal tubule is the Na^+/H^+ exchanger. The high hydraulic permeability for water is rooted in abundant occurrence of the water channel protein aquaporin-1. A prominent lysosomal system is known as the apical vacuolar endocytotic apparatus and is responsible for the reabsorption of macromolecules (polypeptides and proteins such as albumin) that have passed through the glomerular filter. The proximal tubule is generally subdivided into three segments (known as S_1, S_2, S_3, or P_1, P_2, P_3) that differ considerably in cellular organization and, consequently, also in function[15].

The loop of Henle

The loop of Henle consists of the straight portion of the proximal tubule, thin descending and (in long loops) thin ascending limbs, and the thick ascending limb (see Figs 1.2 and 1.11). The thin descending limb, like the proximal tubule, is highly permeable for water (the channels are of aquaporin-1) whereas, beginning exactly at the turning point, the thin ascending limb is impermeable for water. The specific transport functions of the thin limbs contributing to the generation of the osmotic medullary gradient are under debate.

The thick ascending limb is often called the diluting segment. It is water impermeable but reabsorbs considerable amounts of salt, resulting in the separation of salt from water. The salt is trapped in the medulla, whereas the water is carried away into the cortex where it may return into the systemic circulation. The specific transporter for Na^+ entry in this segment is the luminal $Na^+/K^+/2Cl^-$ cotransporter, which is the target of diuretics such as furosemide (frusemide). The tight junctions of the thick ascending limb have a comparatively low permeability. The cells heavily interdigitate by basolateral cell processes, associated with large mitochondria supplying the energy for the transepithelial transport. The cells synthesize a specific protein, the Tamm–Horsefall protein, and release it into the tubular lumen. This protein is thought to be important later for preventing the formation of kidney stones. In contrast to the proximal tubule, the luminal membrane is only sparsely amplified by microvilli. Just before the transition to the distal convoluted tubule, the thick ascending limb contains the macula densa, which adheres to the parent glomerulus (see juxtaglomerular apparatus).

The distal convoluted tubule

The epithelium is fairly highly differentiated, exhibiting the most extensive basolateral interdigitation of the cells and the greatest density of mitochondria in all nephron portions (see Fig. 1.10). Apically, the cells are equipped with numerous microvilli. The specific Na^+ transporter of the distal convoluted

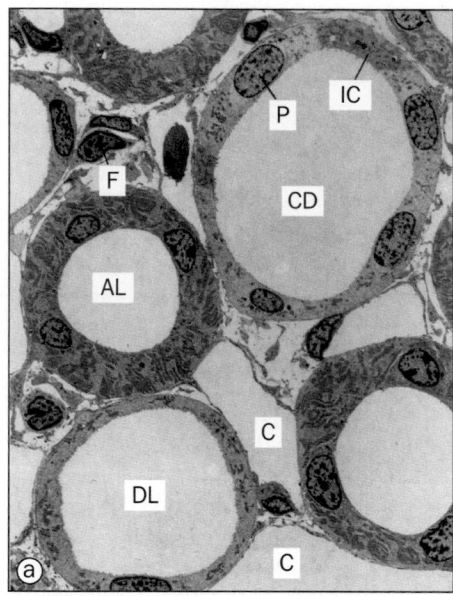

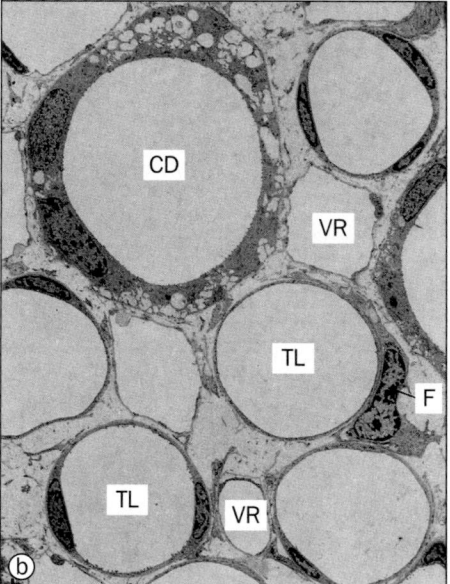

Figure 1.11 Tubules in the medulla. (a) Cross-section through the inner stripe of the outer medulla. A descending thin limb of a long loop (DL), medullary thick ascending limbs (AL), and a collecting duct (CD) with principal cells (P) and intercalated cells (IC) are shown. C, peritubular capillaries; F, fibroblast. (b) In the inner medulla cross-section, thin descending and ascending limbs (TL), a collecting duct (CD), and vasa recta (VR) are seen. (Transmission electron microscopy: (a) ×990; (b) ×1120.)

tubule is the luminal Na^+/Cl^- cotransporter, which is the target of thiazide diuretics.

THE COLLECTING DUCT SYSTEM

The collecting duct system (see Fig. 1.2) includes the connecting tubule (CNT) and the cortical and medullary collecting ducts. Two nephrons may join at the level of the connecting tubule, forming an arcade that, cytologically, is a connecting tubule. Two types of cell line the CNT: the connecting tubule cell (CNT cell), which is specific to the connecting tubules, and the intercalated cell, which also occurs later in the collecting duct. The CNT cells are similar in cellular organization to the collecting duct cells (CD cells). Both cell types share sensitivity to vasopressin (antidiuretic hormone, ADH) (see below); the CNT cell, however, lacks sensitivity to mineralocorticoids.

The collecting ducts

Collecting ducts (see Fig. 1.11) may be subdivided into cortical and medullary ducts, the latter into outer and inner medullary ducts; the transitions are gradual. Like the connecting tubule, the collecting ducts are lined by two types of cell: CD cells (principal cells) and intercalated cells (IC cells). The latter decrease in number as the collecting duct descends into the medulla and are absent from the papillary collecting ducts.

The CD cells (Fig. 1.12a) are simple, polygonal cells increasing in size towards the tip of the papilla. The basal surface of these cells is characterized by invaginations of the basal cell membrane (basal infoldings). The tight junctions have a large apico-basal depth and the apical cell surface has a prominent glycocalyx. Along the entire collecting duct these cells contain a luminal shuttle system for aquaporin-2 under the control of vasopressin, providing the potential to switch the water permeability of the collecting ducts from zero (or at least from low) to permeable[16]. A luminal amiloride-sensitive Na^+ channel is involved in the responsiveness of cortical collecting ducts to aldosterone.

The second cell type, the IC cell (Fig. 1.12b), is present in both the connecting tubule and the collecting duct. There are at least two types of IC, designated A and B cells, distinguished on the basis of structural, immunocytochemical, and functional characteristics. Type A cells have been defined as expressing H^+ ATPase at their luminal membrane; they secrete protons. Type B cells express the H^+ ATPase at their basolateral membrane; they secrete bicarbonate ions and reabsorb protons[17].

With these different cell types, the collecting ducts are the final regulators of fluid and electrolyte balance, playing important roles in the handling of Na^+, Cl^-, and K^+ as well as acid and base. The responsiveness of the collecting ducts to vasopressin enables an organism to live in arid conditions, allowing it to produce a concentrated urine, and, if necessary, a dilute urine.

THE JUXTAGLOMERULAR APPARATUS

The juxtaglomerular apparatus (JGA) (see Fig. 1.4) comprises the macula densa, the extraglomerular mesangium, the terminal portion of the afferent arteriole with its renin-producing granular cells (nowadays also often termed 'juxtaglomerular cells'), and the beginning portions of the efferent arteriole.

The macula densa (see Figs 1.5 and 1.13a) is a plaque of specialized cells in the wall of the thick ascending limb at the site where the limb attaches to the extraglomerular mesangium of the parent glomerulus. The most obvious structural feature is the narrowly packed cells with large nuclei, which accounts for the name 'macula densa'. The cells are anchored to a basement membrane, which blends with the matrix of the extraglomerular mesangium[4]. The cells are joined by tight junctions with very low permeability and have prominent lateral intercellular spaces. The width of these spaces varies under different functional conditions[1]. The most conspicuous immunocytochemical difference between macula densa cells and any other epithelial cell of the nephron is the high content of neuronal nitric oxide synthase-1[18].

The basal aspect of the macula densa is firmly attached to the extraglomerular mesangium, which represents a solid

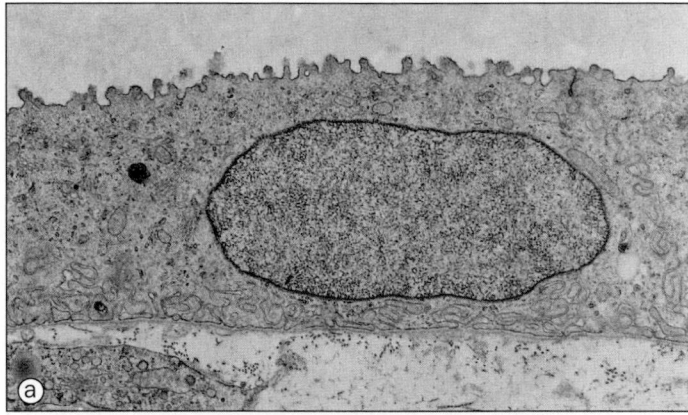

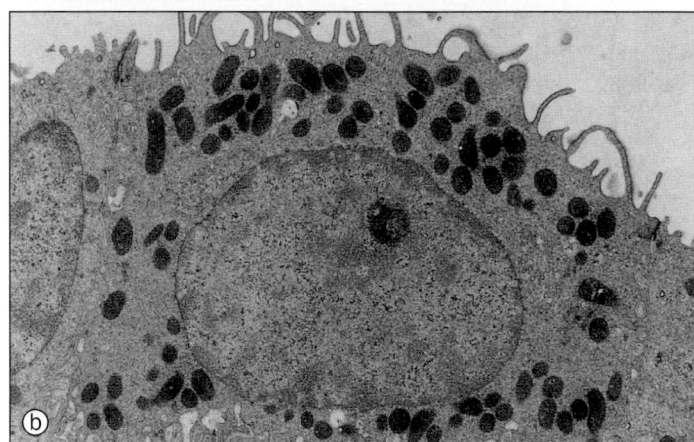

Figure 1.12 Collecting duct cells. (a) Principal cell (CD cell) of a medullary collecting duct. The apical cell membrane bears some stubby microvilli covered by a prominent glycocalyx; the basal cell membrane forms invaginations. Note the deep tight junction. (b) Intercalated cells, type A. Note the dark cytoplasm (dark cells) with many mitochondria and apical microfolds; the basal membrane forms invaginations. (Transmission electron microscopy: (a) ×8720; (b) ×6970.)

complex of cells and matrix that is penetrated neither by blood vessels nor lymphatic capillaries (see Figs 1.4 and 1.13a). Like the mesangial cells proper, extraglomerular mesangial cells are heavily branched. Their processes, interconnected among each other by gap junctions, contain prominent bundles of microfilaments and are connected to the basement membrane of Bowman's capsule as well as to the walls of both glomerular arterioles. As a whole, the extraglomerular mesangium interconnects all structures of the glomerular entrance[6].

The granular cells are assembled in clusters within the terminal portion of the afferent arteriole (Fig. 1.13b), replacing ordinary smooth muscle cells. Their name refers to the specific cytoplasmic granules in which renin, the major secretion product of these cells, is stored. They are the main site of the body where renin is secreted. Renin release occurs by exocytosis into the surrounding interstitium. Granular cells are connected to the extraglomerular mesangial cells, to adjacent smooth muscle cells, and to endothelial cells by gap junctions. They are densely innervated by sympathetic nerve terminals. Granular cells are modified smooth muscle cells; under conditions requiring enhanced renin synthesis (e.g., volume depletion or

Essential Renal Anatomy and Physiology

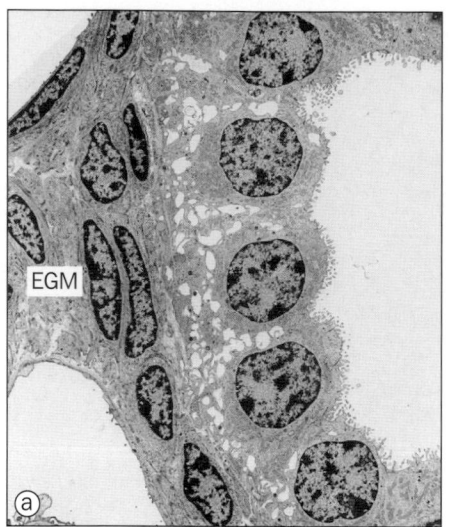

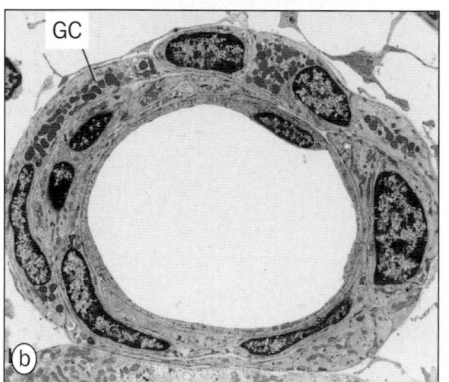

**Figure 1.13
Juxtaglomerular
apparatus.** (a) Macula
densa of a thick
ascending limb. The
cells have prominent
nuclei and lateral
intercellular spaces.
Basally they attach to
the extraglomerular
mesangium (EGM). (b)
Afferent arteriole near
the vascular pole.
Several smooth muscle
cells are replaced by
granular cells (GC)
containing
accumulations of renin
granules. (Transmission
electron microscopy:
(a) ×1730; (b) ×1310)

stenosis of the renal artery), additional smooth muscle cells located upstream in the wall of the afferent arteriole may transform into granular cells.

The structural organization of the JGA suggests a regulatory function. There is agreement that some component of the distal urine (probably Cl⁻) is sensed by the macula densa and this information is used first, to adjust the tone of the glomerular arterioles, thereby producing a change in glomerular blood flow and filtration rate. Even if many details of this mechanism are still subject to debate, the essence of this system has been verified by many studies and it is known as the tubular glomerular feedback mechanism[19]. Second, this system determines the amount of renin that is released – via the interstitium – into the circulation, thereby acquiring great systemic relevance.

THE RENAL INTERSTITIUM

The interstitium of the kidney is comparatively sparse. Its fractional volume in the cortex ranges from 5 to 7% (with a tendency to increase with age). It increases across the medulla from cortex to papilla: in the outer stripe it is 3–4% (the lowest value of all kidney zones; this is interpreted as forming a barrier to prevent loss of solutes from a hyperosmolar medulla into the cortex), in the inner stripe 10%, and in the inner medulla up to ~30%. The cellular constituents of the interstitium are resident fibroblasts, which establish the scaffold frame for renal corpuscles, tubules, and blood vessels.

In addition, there are varying numbers of migrating cells of the immune system, including macrophages and dendritic cells. The space between the cells is filled with extracellular matrix, i.e., ground substance (proteoglycans, glycoproteins), fibrils, and interstitial fluid[20].

From a morphologic point of view fibroblasts are the central cells in the renal interstitium. They are interconnected by specialized contacts, and they adhere by specific attachments to the basement membranes surrounding the tubules, the renal corpuscles, and the capillaries. They are in close touch with lymphatics, nerve terminals, and with all types of migrating interstitial cell.

Renal fibroblasts are difficult to distinguish from interstitial dendritic cells on a morphologic basis because both may show a stellate cellular shape and both display substantial amounts of mitochondria and endoplasmic reticulum. They may, however, easily be distinguished by immunocytochemical techniques. Dendritic cells constitutively express the major histocompatibility complex class II antigen whereas fibroblasts in the renal cortex (not in the medulla) contain the enzyme ecto-5'-nucleotidase (5'-NT)[21]. A subset of 5'-NT-positive fibroblasts of the renal cortex synthesize epoetin[21]. Under normal conditions, these fibroblasts are exclusively found within the juxtamedullary portions of the cortical labyrinth. When there is an increasing demand for epoetin, the synthesizing cells extend to more superficial portions of the cortical labyrinth and, to a lower degree, to the medullary rays[22].

Fibroblasts within the medulla, especially within the inner medulla, have a particular phenotype known as 'lipid-laden interstitial cells'. The cells are oriented strictly perpendicularly towards the longitudinal axis of the tubules and vessels (running all in parallel) and they contain conspicuous lipid droplets. These fibroblasts of the inner medulla produce large amounts of glycosaminoglycans and, possibly related to the lipid droplets, they produce vasoactive lipids, in particular prostaglandin E_2[20].

The intrarenal arteries are accompanied by a prominent sheath of loose interstitial tissue (Fig. 1.14); the renal veins are

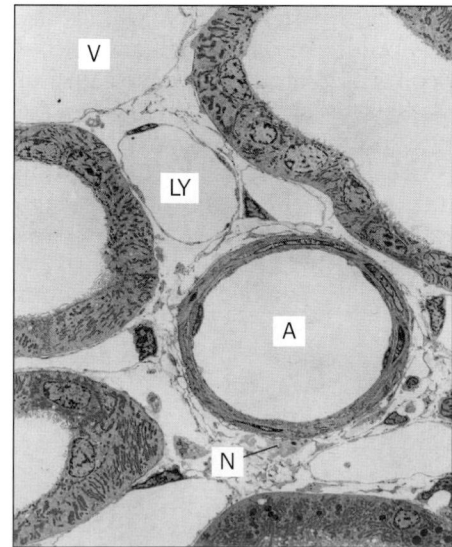

**Figure 1.14
Intrarenal arteries in
a periarterial
connective tissue
sheath.** Cross-section
through a cortical radial
artery surrounded by
the sheath containing
the renal nerves (N)
and lymphatics (LY).
A vein lies outside the
sheath. (Transmission
electron microscopy:
×830)

in apposition to this sheath but not included in it. Intrarenal nerve fibers and lymphatics run within this periarterial tissue. Lymphatics start in the vicinity of the afferent arteriole and leave the kidney running within the periarterial tissue sheath toward the hilum. Together with the lymphatics, the periarterial tissue constitutes a pathway for interstitial fluid drainage of the renal cortex; the renal medulla has no lymphatic drainage.

REFERENCES

1. Kriz W, Kaissling B. Structural organization of the mammalian kidney. In: Seldin DW, Giebisch G, eds. The kidney: physiology and pathophysiology. New York: Raven Press; 1992:707–77.
2. Kriz W, Bankir L. A standard nomenclature for structure of the kidney. The Renal Commission of the International Union of Physiological Sciences (IUPS). Pfluegers Arch. 1988;411:113–20.
3. Rollhäuser H, Kriz W, Heinke W. Das Gefässsystem der Rattenniere. Z Zellforsch. 1964;64:381–403.
4. Barajas L. Innervation of the renal cortex. Fed Proc. 1978;37:1192–201.
5. DiBona GF, Kopp UC. Neural control of renal function. Physiol Rev. 1997;77:75–197.
6. Elger M, Sakai T, Kriz W. The vascular pole of the renal glomerulus of rat. Adv Anat Embryol Cell Biol. 1998;139:1–98.
7. Inoue S. Ultrastructural architecture of basement membranes. Contrib Nephrol. 1994;107:21–8.
8. Miner JH. Renal basement membrane components. Kidney Int. 1999;56(6):2016–24.
9. Kriz W, Elger M, Mundel P, Lemley KV. Structure-stabilizing forces in the glomerular tuft. J Am Soc Nephrol. 1995;5:1731–9.
10. Rostgaard J, Qvortrup K. Electron microscopie demonstrations of filamentous molecular sieve plugs in capillary fenestrae. Microvascular Research 1997;53,1-13, Article No. MR961987.
11. Endlich K, Kriz W, Witzgall R. Update in podocyte biology. Curr Opin Nephrol Hypertens. 2001;10:331–40.
12. Kriz W, Kobayashi N, Elger M. New aspects of podocyte structure, function, and pathology. Clin Exp Nephrol. 1998;2:85–93.
13. Mundel P, Kriz W. Structure and function of podocytes: an update. Anat Embryol. 1995;192:385–97.
14. Drumond MC, Deen WM. Structural determinants of glomerular hydraulic permeability. Am J Physiol. 1994;266:F1–12.
15. Maunsbach AB. Functional ultrastructure of the proximal tubule. In: Windhager EE, ed. Handbook of physiology: renal physiology. New York: Oxford University Press; 1992:41–108.
16. Sabolic I, Brown D. Water channels in renal and nonrenal tissues. News Physiol Sci. 1995;10:12–17.
17. Madsen KM, Verlander JW, Kim JK, Tisher CC. Morphological adaptation of the collecting duct to acid–base disturbances. Kidney Int. 1991;40(Suppl 33):S57–63.
18. Mundel P, Bachmann S, Bader M, et al. Expression of nitric oxide synthase in kidney macula densa cells. Kidney Int. 1992;42:1017–19.
19. Schnermann JB, Briggs JP. The role of adenosine in cell-to-cell signaling in the juxtaglomerular apparatus. Semin Nephrol. 1993;13:236–45.
20. Lemley KV, Kriz W. Anatomy of the renal interstitium. Kidney Int. 1991;39:370–81.
21. Bachmann S, Le Hir M, Eckardt K-U. Co-localization of erythropoietin mRNA and ecto-5′-nucleotidase immunoreactivity in peritubular cells of rat renal cortex indicates that fibroblasts produce erythropoietin. J Histochem Cytochem. 1993;41:335–41.
22. Kaissling B, Spiess S, Rinne B, Le Hir M. Effects of anemia on the morphology of the renal cortex of rats. Am J Physiol. 1993;264:F608–17.

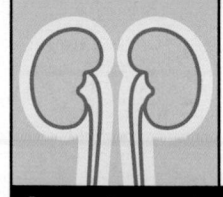

Section 1 Essential Renal Anatomy and Physiology

Chapter 2

Renal Physiology

David G Shirley, Giovambattista Capasso, and Robert J Unwin

The prime function of the kidney is to maintain a stable *milieu interieur* by the selective retention and elimination of water, electrolytes and other solutes. This is achieved by three processes: (i) filtration of circulating blood from the glomerulus to form an ultrafiltrate of plasma in Bowman's space; (ii) selective reabsorption (from tubular fluid to blood) across the cells lining the renal tubule; and (iii) selective secretion (from peritubular capillary blood to tubular fluid).

GLOMERULAR STRUCTURE AND ULTRASTRUCTURE

The process of urine formation begins by the production of an ultrafiltrate of plasma. Chapter 1 provides a detailed description of glomerular anatomy and ultrastructure, and only brief essentials to an understanding of how the ultrafiltrate is formed will be given here. The glomerulus is a tuft of capillaries supplied and drained by afferent and efferent arterioles, respectively. The pathway for ultrafiltration of plasma from the glomerulus to Bowman's space consists of the capillary endothelium, the capillary basement membrane and the visceral epithelial cell layer (podocytes) of Bowman's capsule; the podocytes have large cell bodies that float in Bowman's space and make contact with the basement membrane only by foot processes. Mesangial cells, which fill the spaces between capillaries, have contractile properties and are capable of altering the capillary surface area available for filtration.

What is filtered is determined principally by size and to a much lesser extent by charge. The size cut-off is not absolute; resistance to filtration begins at an effective molecular radius of slightly less than 2 nm, while substances with an effective radius exceeding ~4 nm are not filtered at all. The capillary endothelial cells have relatively large gaps (50–100 nm diameter) between them and the podocytes' foot processes have slit-like pores (30–40 nm diameter) between them, but the latter are partially occluded by zipper-like structures, so the real gap is much smaller. It is believed that these slit-like pores constitute the main filtration barrier, although both the endothelium (by preventing the passage of blood cells) and the basement membrane contribute. The glomerular membranes carry fixed negative charges from glycoproteins on their surface that further restrict the filtration of large negatively charged ions, mainly proteins (Fig. 2.1). This explains why albumin, despite an effective radius (3.6 nm) that would allow significant filtration on the basis of size alone, is normally virtually

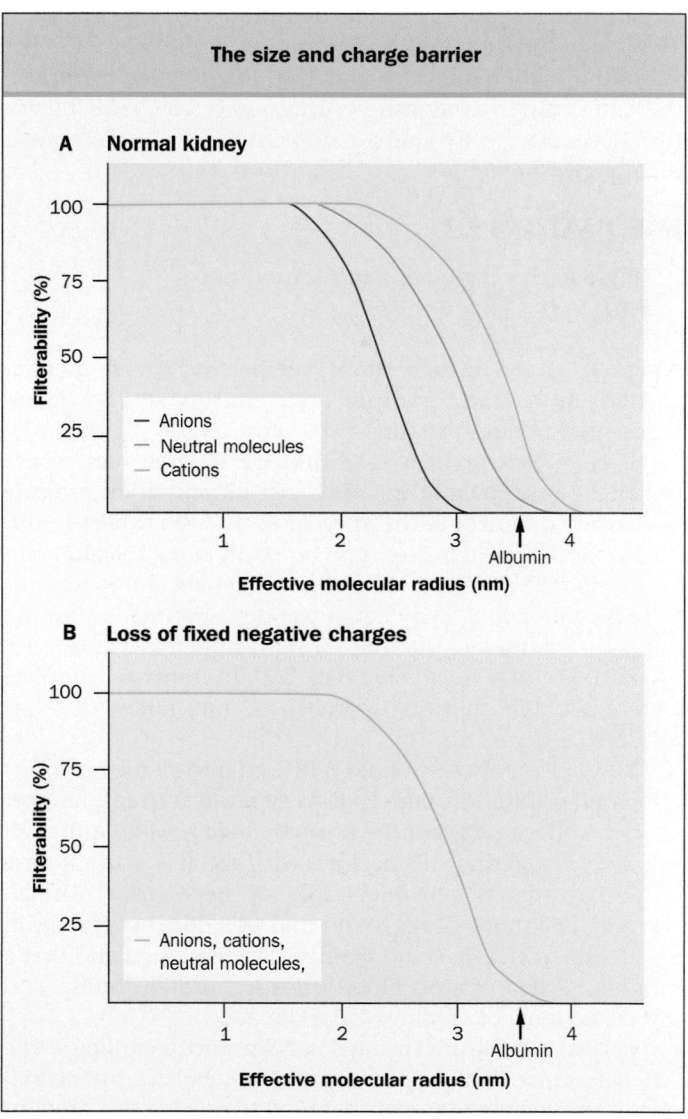

Figure 2.1 Effects of size and electrical charge on filterability. One hundred percent filterability indicates that the substance is freely filtered, i.e., its concentration in Bowman's space equals that in glomerular capillary plasma. For molecules and small ions (e.g., Na+, Cl-), charge has no effect on filterability, but for ions whose effective molecular radius exceeds ~1.6 nm, anions are filtered less easily than neutral molecules or cations. Thus, insignificant amounts of albumin (anion) are normally filtered. If the fixed negative charges of the glomerular basement membranes are lost, as in early minimal change nephropathy, charge no longer influences filterability; consequently, significant albumin filtration occurs.

excluded. If these fixed negative charges are lost, as in some forms of early or mild glomerular disease (e.g., minimal change nephropathy), albumin filterability increases and proteinuria results.

GLOMERULAR FILTRATION RATE AND RENAL BLOOD FLOW

At the level of the single glomerulus, the driving force for glomerular filtration (the *net ultrafiltration pressure*) is determined by the net hydrostatic and oncotic (colloid osmotic) pressure gradients between glomerular plasma and the filtrate in Bowman's space. The rate of filtration (single-nephron glomerular filtration rate) is determined by the product of the net ultrafiltration pressure and the *ultrafiltration coefficient*, the latter being a composite of the surface area available for filtration and the hydraulic conductivity of the glomerular membranes. Therefore:

■ EQUATION 2.1

Single-nephron glomerular filtration rate =
$$K_f((P_{gc} - P_{bs}) - (\pi_{gc} - \pi_{bs}))$$

where K_f is the ultrafiltration coefficient; P_{gc}, glomerular capillary hydrostatic pressure (~45 mmHg); P_{bs}, Bowman's space hydrostatic pressure (~10 mmHg); π_{gc}, glomerular capillary oncotic pressure (~25 mmHg); π_{bs}, Bowman's space oncotic pressure (0 mmHg). Thus, net ultrafiltration pressure is around 10 mmHg at the afferent end of the capillary tuft. As filtration of protein-free fluid proceeds along the glomerular capillaries, π_{gc} increases, and, at a certain point towards the efferent end, π_{gc} may equal the net hydrostatic pressure gradient; i.e., the net ultrafiltration pressure may fall to zero: so-called *filtration equilibrium* (Fig. 2.2). In humans, complete filtration equilibrium is approached, but rarely (if ever) achieved.

The total rate at which fluid is filtered into all the nephrons (glomerular filtration rate; GFR) is typically 120 mL/min per 1.73 m² surface area, but the normal range is wide. Although it is often stated that GFR declines with age, it is worth noting here that this is not inevitable or necessarily normal. Longitudinal studies have found that GFR does not change in up to 30% of elderly subjects (mean age 60 years) and that a fall in GFR depends on blood pressure, protein intake and associated renal or cardiovascular disease[1].

GFR can be measured using renal clearance techniques. The renal clearance of any substance not metabolized by the kidneys is the volume of plasma required to provide that amount of the substance excreted in the urine per unit time; this virtual volume can be expressed mathematically as follows:

■ EQUATION 2.2

$$C_y = U_y \times V/P_y$$

where C_y is the renal clearance of y, U_y is the urine concentration of y, V is the urine flow rate and P_y is the plasma concentration of y. If a substance is freely filtered by the glomerulus and is not reabsorbed or secreted by the tubule, then its renal clearance equals GFR; i.e., it measures the volume of plasma

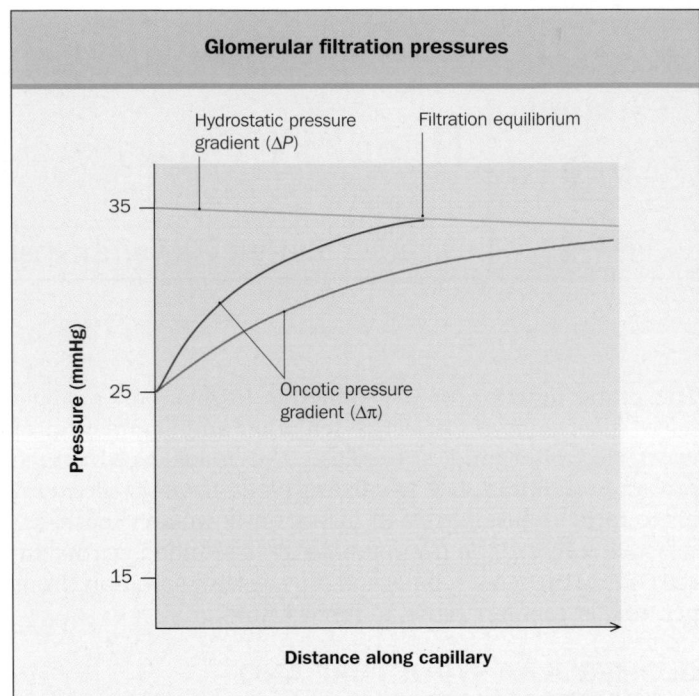

Figure 2.2 Filtration pressures along a glomerular capillary. The hydrostatic pressure gradient ($\Delta P = P_{gc} - P_{bc}$) is relatively constant along the length of a capillary, whereas the opposing oncotic pressure gradient ($\Delta\pi = \pi_{gc}$) increases as protein-free fluid is filtered, thereby reducing net ultrafiltration pressure. Two curves are shown, one where filtration equilibrium is reached and one where it is merely approached.

filtered through the glomeruli per unit time. Measurement of GFR and its pitfalls are described in detail in Chapter 3 and will be considered only briefly here. The substance that best fits the criteria for a marker of GFR is the polysaccharide inulin. However, partly because it has to be infused intravenously, measurement of inulin clearance is cumbersome and inappropriate for routine clinical investigation. In contrast, the clearance of endogenous creatinine is convenient and easy to measure, and provides a reasonable approximation of GFR in normal subjects; although because it is secreted into proximal tubules and because this secretion increases in renal failure, creatinine clearance will overestimate true GFR in this situation. Cimetidine administration inhibits the tubular secretion of creatinine and can therefore be used to improve creatinine clearance as an estimate of GFR in renal failure. As an alternative to creatinine clearance, the plasma disappearance of a glomerular marker radiolabelled with a gamma emitter (e.g., ⁵¹Cr EDTA, ⁹⁹ᵐTc DTPA), following a single intravenous injection, is often used.

Historically, the first estimate of GFR was obtained using urea clearance. However, in addition to the fundamental problem that approximately half the filtered urea is reabsorbed, urea clearance is affected by several factors unrelated to GFR. In severe congestive heart failure, dehydration, shock and cirrhosis with ascites, there is enhanced fractional reabsorption of urea, causing a reduction in urea clearance that is disproportionate to any change in GFR. The concentration of urea in blood, referred to as BUN (blood urea nitrogen), generally varies inversely with GFR, and consequently BUN is sometimes used clinically as an index of renal function. It should be noted, however, that BUN is also altered by many other factors including dietary protein, high catabolic rate associated with burn injuries or high fever, gastrointestinal hemorrhage, infections and a number of drugs, including corticosteroids and tetracycline antibiotics. For these reasons the finding of an elevated BUN does not necessarily mean a reduced GFR, and it is more usefully considered in relation to plasma creatinine, when it may indicate relative extracellular fluid volume depletion. A BUN of 3–14 mg/dL (1–5 mmol/L) almost certainly indicates a normal GFR, as long as protein intake is not restricted.

Plasma creatinine concentration, which also generally varies inversely with GFR, is less influenced by extrarenal factors than is BUN. Nevertheless, plasma creatinine is an insensitive index of renal function. It is affected by muscle mass, which may in turn reflect nutritional status; consequently, the range of normal values for plasma creatinine is wide.

MEASUREMENT OF RENAL PLASMA FLOW

Use of the clearance technique and the availability of substances that undergo both glomerular filtration and tubular secretion have made it possible to measure renal plasma flow (RPF). Para-amino hippurate (PAH) is an organic acid that is filtered by the glomerulus and actively secreted by the proximal tubule. The amount that is found in the final urine is the sum of the PAH filtered plus the component that is secreted. When the plasma concentration of PAH is lower than 10 mg/dL, most of the PAH reaching the peritubular capillaries is cleared by tubular secretion and little PAH appears in renal venous plasma. Mathematically, the amount of PAH transferred from the blood to the tubular lumen via filtration and secretion is equal to the amount found in the final urine:

■ EQUATION 2.3

$$RPF \times P_{PAH} = U_{PAH} \times V$$

or

■ EQUATION 2.4

$$RPF = (U_{PAH} \times V)/P_{PAH} = \text{PAH clearance}$$

where U_{PAH} and P_{PAH} are the concentrations of PAH in the urine and plasma, respectively, and V is the urine flow rate. Renal blood flow (RBF) can be calculated as follows:

■ EQUATION 2.5

$$RBF = (RPF/(100 - \text{hematocrit})) \times 100$$

The most important limitation of this method is the renal extraction of PAH. The latter is always less than 100%. At high plasma concentrations (> 10–15 mg/dL), fractional tubular secretion of PAH declines and significant amounts appear in the renal veins; under these circumstances, PAH clearance seriously underestimates RPF. There are also diseases that can either produce toxins or weak organic acids

(e.g., liver and renal failure) which interfere with PAH secretion or cause tubular damage, leading to inhibition of PAH transport. Finally, certain drugs, like probenecid, are organic acids and therefore compete with PAH for tubular secretion and reduce PAH clearance.

FACTORS AFFECTING RENAL BLOOD FLOW AND GLOMERULAR FILTRATION RATE

Although acute variations in arterial blood pressure inevitably cause corresponding changes in RBF and GFR, these are short-lived and, provided the blood pressure remains within the normal range, compensatory mechanisms come into play after a few seconds to return both RBF and GFR to near-normal[2]. This is the phenomenon of *autoregulation* (Fig. 2.3). Autoregulation is brought about predominantly by changes in the caliber of the afferent arterioles and is believed to result from a combination of two mechanisms:
1. A *myogenic reflex*, whereby the afferent arteriolar smooth muscle wall constricts automatically when renal perfusion pressure rises.
2. *Tubuloglomerular feedback* (*TGF*), whereby an increased delivery of NaCl to the *macula densa* region of the nephron (situated at the end of the loop of Henle), resulting from increases in blood pressure, RBF and GFR, causes vasoconstriction of the afferent arteriole supplying that nephron's glomerulus.

Because these mechanisms restore both RBF and P_{gc} towards normal, the initial change in GFR is also reversed. The TGF

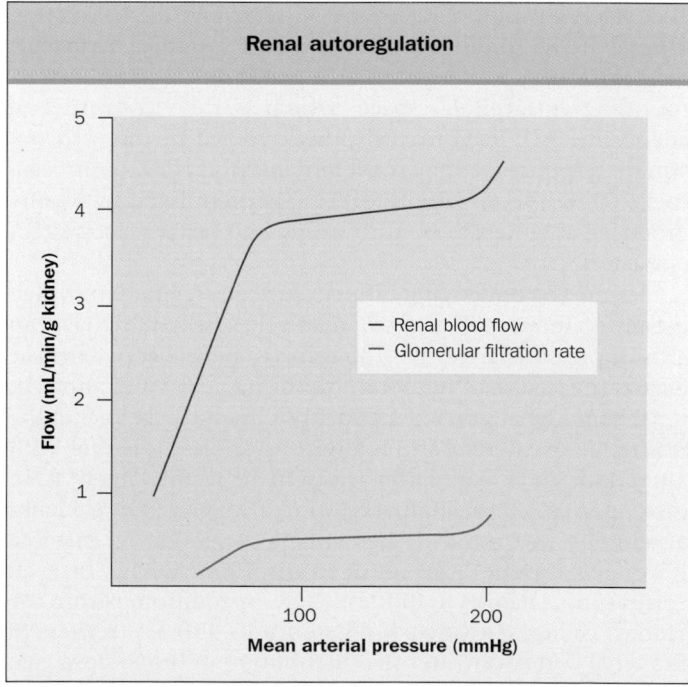

Figure 2.3 Autoregulation of renal blood flow and glomerular filtration rate. In the mean arterial blood pressure range ~80–180 mmHg, fluctuations in blood pressure have only marginal effects on renal blood flow and glomerular filtration rate. This is an intrinsic mechanism and can be modulated or overridden by extrinsic factors.

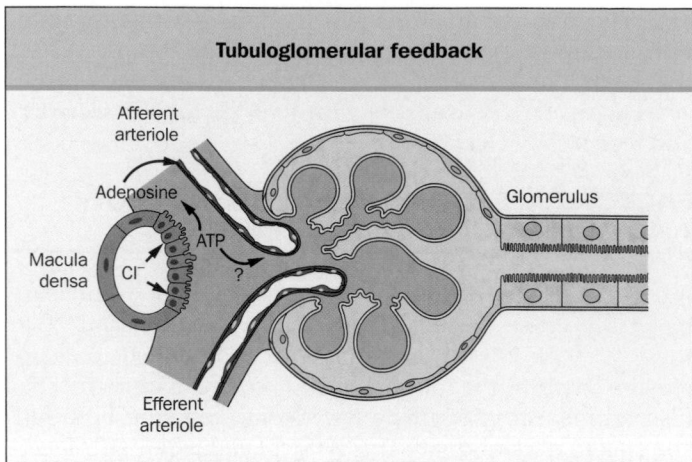

Tubuloglomerular feedback

Figure 2.4 Tubuloglomerular feedback. Changes in the delivery of Cl⁻ to the macula densa region of the thick ascending limb of the loop of Henle cause changes in afferent arteriolar caliber. The response is mediated by adenosine and/or ATP and modulated by other locally produced agents such as angiotensin II and nitric oxide. Increased macula densa Cl⁻ delivery results in afferent arteriolar constriction, thereby reducing GFR.

negative-feedback system is possible because of the anatomical arrangement in the kidney such that the macula densa region of each nephron is in close contact with its own glomerulus and afferent and efferent arterioles (Fig. 2.4). This structural complex is known as the *juxtaglomerular apparatus*.

There is good evidence that the major mediator of TGF is adenosine, acting on adenosine A₁ receptors in the afferent arteriole[3]. The stimulus is increased by Cl⁻ uptake by macula densa cells; this is thought to lead to ATP release into the surrounding extracellular space, which is then converted to adenosine. ATP itself may also be involved in the vasoconstrictor response (acting on afferent arteriolar P2X purinoceptors), while the sensitivity of TGF is modulated by locally produced angiotensin II, nitric oxide and certain eicosanoids (see later).

Despite the underlying influence of autoregulation, which usually maintains RBF and GFR relatively constant in the mean arterial pressure range ~80–180 mmHg, a number of extrinsic factors (nervous and humoral) can bring about alterations in renal hemodynamics. Independent or unequal changes in the resistance of afferent and efferent arterioles, together with alterations in K_f (the latter thought to result largely from mesangial cell contraction/relaxation, though recent evidence also implicates contractile elements in the podocytes that line Bowman's capsule), can result in disproportionate, or even contrasting, changes in RBF and GFR. In addition, within the kidney, changes in vascular resistance in different regions of the renal cortex can alter the distribution of blood flow, e.g., diversion of blood from outer to inner cortex in hemorrhagic shock[4]. Figure 2.5 indicates how, in principle, changes in afferent and efferent arteriolar resistance will affect net ultrafiltration. Some of the better known substances that influence renal hemodynamics are listed in Table 2.1; they will receive further attention in the final section of the chapter.

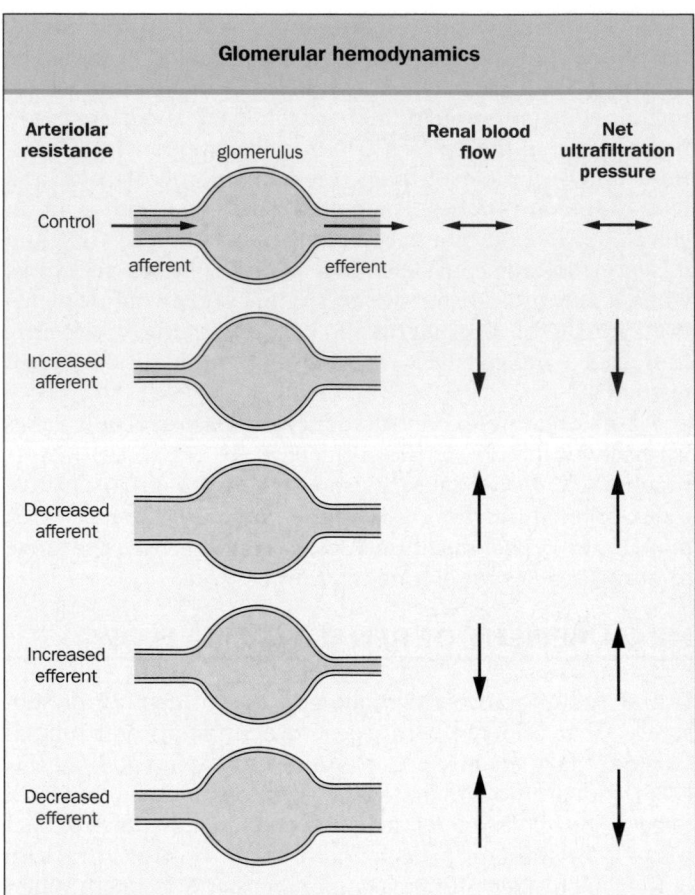

Glomerular hemodynamics

| Arteriolar resistance | glomerulus | Renal blood flow | Net ultrafiltration pressure |

Control
afferent   efferent

Increased afferent

Decreased afferent

Increased efferent

Decreased efferent

Figure 2.5 Glomerular hemodynamics. Changes in afferent or efferent arteriolar resistance will alter renal blood flow and (usually) net ultrafiltration pressure. However, the effect on ultrafiltration pressure depends on the *relative* changes in afferent /efferent arteriolar resistance. The overall effect on glomerular filtration rate will depend not only on renal blood flow and net ultrafiltration pressure but also on the ultrafiltration coefficient (K_f) (see Table 2.1).

TUBULAR TRANSPORT MECHANISMS: BASIC PRINCIPLES

Clearly, net movement of substances from tubular fluid to blood (reabsorption) and vice versa (secretion) requires vectorial transport, and the tubular cells are therefore polarized. This means that the membrane facing the tubular fluid (luminal or apical) has different properties from the membrane facing the blood (peritubular or basolateral). In non-polarized cells (e.g., red and white blood cells), transport proteins are distributed uniformly in the cell membrane, whereas in polarized cells (e.g., renal tubular cells and other epithelia) certain transport proteins are located in one membrane (apical or basolateral), while others are located in the other. The result is the movement of solutes through and across – in and then out – the cell (transcellular route). The tight junction, which is a contact point found close to the apical side of adjacent cells, limits water and solute movement between cells (paracellular route) and also helps to maintain polarity by preventing membrane proteins from moving from one side to the other (apical to basolateral or vice versa)[5].

Physiological and pharmacological factors with well-defined effects on glomerular hemodynamics						
	Afferent arteriolar resistance	Efferent arteriolar resistance	Renal blood flow	Net ultrafiltration pressure	K_f	GFR
Renal sympathetic nerves	↑↑	↑	↓	↓	↓	↓
Epinephrine	↑	↑	↓	→	?	↓
Adenosine	↑	→	↓	↓	?	↓
Cyclosporine	↑	→	↓	↓	?	↓
NSAIDs	↑↑	↑	↓	↓	?	↓
Angiotensin II	↑	↑↑	↓	↑	↓	↓→
Endothelin-1	↑	↑↑	↓	↑	↓	↓
High protein diet	↓	→	↑	↑	→	↑
Glucagon	↓	→	↑	↑	→	↑
Nitric oxide	↓	↓	↑	?	↑	↑(?)
Atrial natriuretic peptide (high dose)	↓	→	↑	↑	↑	↑
Prostaglandins E_2/I_2	↓	↓	↑	↑	?	↑
Calcium antagonists	↓	→	↑	↑	?	↑
ACE inhibitors/ angiotensin receptor antagonists	↓	↓↓	↑	↓	↑	↑→

The overall effect on glomerular filtration rate (GFR) will depend on renal blood flow, net ultrafiltration pressure and the ultrafiltration coefficient (K_f), the latter being controlled by mesangial cell contraction/relaxation. The effects shown are those seen when the agents are applied (or inhibited) in isolation; the actual changes that occur are dose-dependent and are modulated by other agents.

Table 2.1 Physiological and pharmacological factors with well-defined effects on glomerular hemodynamics.

There are several mechanisms of solute transport across cell membranes, which are either passive or active.

1. *Passive diffusion* always occurs down an electrochemical gradient, which is a composite of the concentration gradient and the electrical gradient. In the case of an undissociated molecule, only the concentration gradient is relevant, whereas in the case of a charged ion, the electrical gradient must also be considered. Passive diffusion does not require an energy source, although an active transport process (see below) is usually necessary to establish the initial concentration and/or electrical gradients.

2. *Facilitated diffusion* (or carrier-mediated diffusion) is also passive, but is more selective and depends on an interaction of the molecule or ion with a specific membrane carrier protein that eases, or facilitates, its passage across the cell membrane's lipid bilayer. It has the kinetic properties of an enzyme-substrate interaction.

3. *Diffusion through a membrane channel* (or pore) formed by specific integral membrane proteins is also a form of facilitated diffusion because it enables charged and lipophobic molecules to pass through the membrane at a high rate. However, channels are generally less discriminating than carrier-mediated transport. Channels are involved in the rapid and bulk transport of molecules or ions, whereas carriers are responsible for the highly selective transport of substances like sugars and amino acids[6].

4. The transport mechanisms described so far are dependent on the 'passive' electrochemical gradient across the cell membrane, which provides the driving force for entry or exit from the cell. In contrast, when a molecule is moved *against* an electrochemical gradient ('uphill'), a source of energy is required and this is known as *active* transport. In cells, this energy is derived from metabolism: adenosine triphosphate (ATP) production and its hydrolysis. The most important active cell transport mechanism is the 'sodium pump', which extrudes Na^+ from inside the cell in exchange for K^+ from outside the cell[7]; in the kidney it is located only in the basolateral membrane. It derives energy from the enzymatic hydrolysis of ATP; hence its more precise description as Na^+,K^+-ATPase. It exchanges $3Na^+$ ions for $2K^+$ ions, which makes it electrogenic, since it extrudes a net positive charge from the cell (inside negative – membrane hyperpolarization), and it is an example of a *primary* active transport mechanism. Other well-defined primary active transport mechanisms in the kidney are the proton-secreting H^+-ATPase, important in H^+ secretion in the distal nephron[8], and Ca^{2+}-ATPase, partly responsible for calcium reabsorption.

Activity of the basolateral Na^+,K^+-ATPase is key to the operation of all the passive transport processes outlined earlier. It ensures that the intracellular Na^+ concentration is kept low (10–20 mmol/L) and the K^+ concentration high

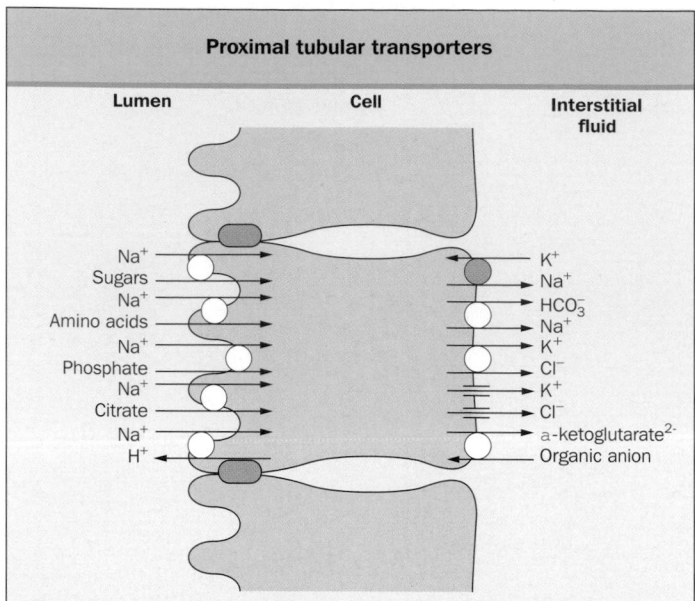

Figure 2.6 Major transport proteins in the apical and basolateral membranes of proximal tubular cells. Stoichiometry is not indicated; it is not 1 : 1 in all cases. Solid symbol represents primary active transport; open symbols, secondary active transport.

(~140 mmol/L), compared with their extracellular concentrations (~140 and ~4 mmol/L, respectively). Sodium entry into tubular cells down the electrochemical gradient maintained by the sodium pump is either through Na^+ channels (in the distal nephron) or linked (coupled) via specific membrane carrier proteins to the influx (*symport* or *cotransport*) or efflux (*antiport* or *counter-transport*) of other molecules or ions: in various parts of the nephron, glucose, phosphate, amino acids, K^+ and Cl^- can all be cotransported with Na^+ entry (symport), while H^+ and Ca^{2+} can be counter-transported against Na^+ entry (antiport). Figure 2.6 shows those mechanisms operating in the proximal tubule. In each case, the non-sodium molecule or ion is transported against its electrochemical gradient, using energy derived from the 'downhill' movement of sodium. Their dependence on the *primary* active sodium pump makes them *secondary* active transport mechanisms.

TRANSPORT IN SPECIFIC NEPHRON SEGMENTS

Given a typical GFR, approximately 180 L of (largely protein-free) plasma are filtered each day, necessitating massive reabsorption by the nephron as a whole. As indicated in Chapter 1, the first part of the nephron, the proximal tubule, is well adapted for bulk reabsorption. The epithelial cells have microvilli (brush border) on their apical surface, providing a large absorptive area, while the basolateral membrane is thrown into folds that similarly enhance surface area. The cells are rich in mitochondria (concentrated near the basolateral membrane) and lysosomal vacuoles; and the tight junctions between adjacent cells are in fact relatively leaky. The *proximal convoluted tubule* (PCT; pars convoluta) makes up the first two-thirds of the proximal tubule; the final third is the *proximal straight tubule* (pars recta).

On the basis of subtle structural and functional differences, the proximal tubule epithelium is subdivided into three types: S1 makes up the initial short segment of the PCT; S2, the remainder of the PCT and the cortical segment of the pars recta; and S3, the medullary segment of the pars recta. The proximal tubule as a whole is responsible for the bulk of Na^+, K^+, Cl^- and HCO_3^- reabsorption, and the near-complete reabsorption of glucose, amino acids and low-molecular-weight proteins (e.g., retinal binding protein, α- and β-microglobulins) that have evaded the filtration barrier. Most other filtered solutes are also reabsorbed to some extent in the proximal tubule (e.g., ~60% of calcium, ~80% of phosphate, ~50% of urea). The wall of the proximal tubule is highly permeable to water, so no quantitatively significant osmotic gradient can be established; thus, most filtered water (~65%) is also reabsorbed at this site. In the final section of the proximal tubule (late S2 and S3), there is some *secretion* of weak organic acids and bases, including most diuretics and *p*-aminohippurate.

The loop of Henle is defined anatomically as comprising the pars recta of the proximal tubule ('thick descending limb'), the thin descending and ascending limbs, the thick ascending limb (TAL) and the macula densa. In addition to its role in the continuing reabsorption of solutes (Na^+, Cl^-, K^+, Ca^{2+}, Mg^{2+}), this part of the nephron is responsible for the kidney's ability to generate a concentrated or dilute urine and will be discussed in more detail later.

Next is the distal tubule, which is made up of three segments: the *distal convoluted tubule* (DCT), where thiazide-sensitive NaCl reabsorption (via an apical cotransporter) occurs; the *connecting tubule*, whose function is essentially intermediate between that of the DCT and that of the next segment; and the *initial collecting tubule*, which is of the same epithelial type as the cortical collecting duct. Two cell types make up the late distal tubule and cortical collecting duct. The predominant type, the *principal cell* (Fig. 2.7), is responsible for Na^+ reabsorption and

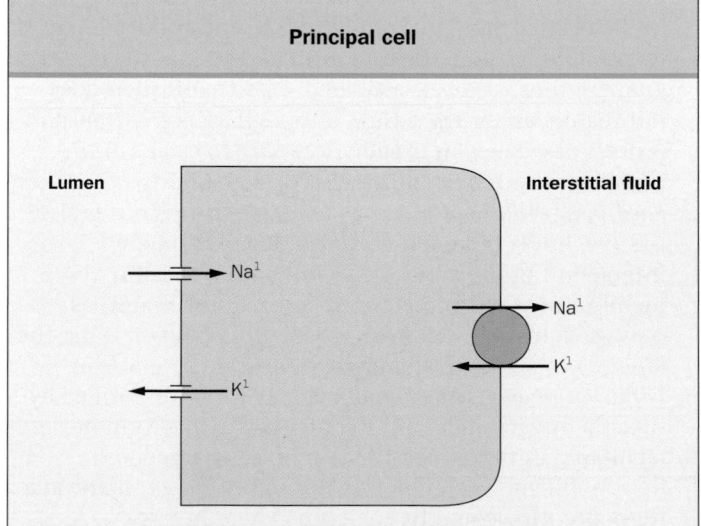

Figure 2.7 Sodium and potassium transport by principal cells of the late distal tubule and cortical collecting duct. Sodium enters from the lumen via apical Na^+ channels and potassium exits into the lumen via apical K^+ channels. Ultimately, both processes are driven by the basolateral Na^+/K^+ ATPase.

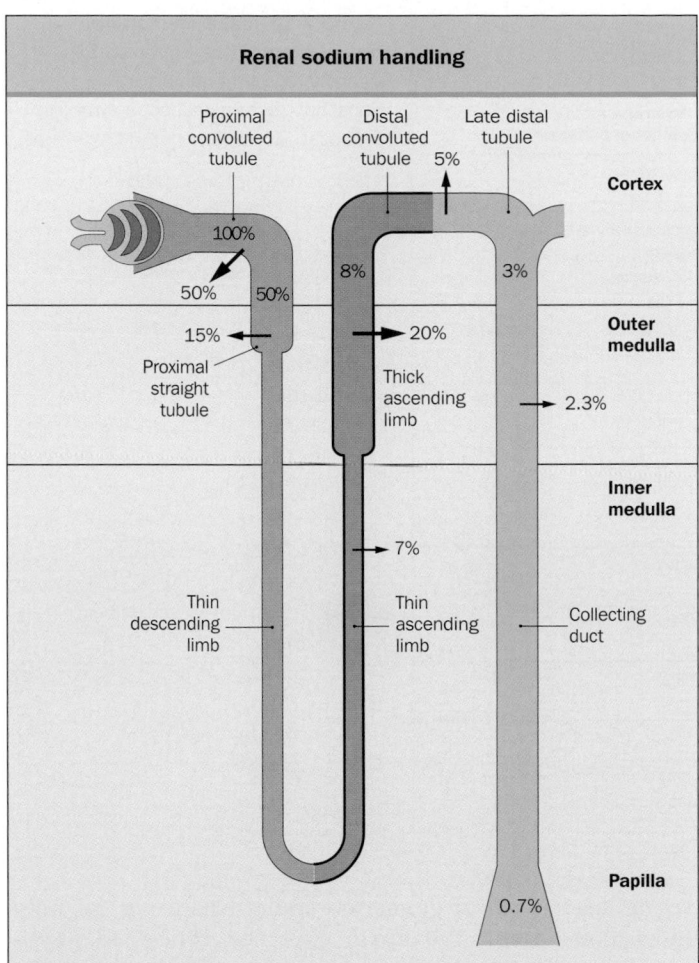

Figure 2.8 Sodium handling along the nephron. Figures outside the nephron represent the approximate percentage of the filtered load reabsorbed in each region. Figures within the nephron represent the percentages remaining. Most filtered sodium is reabsorbed in the proximal tubule and loop of Henle; normal day-to-day control of sodium excretion is exerted in the distal nephron.

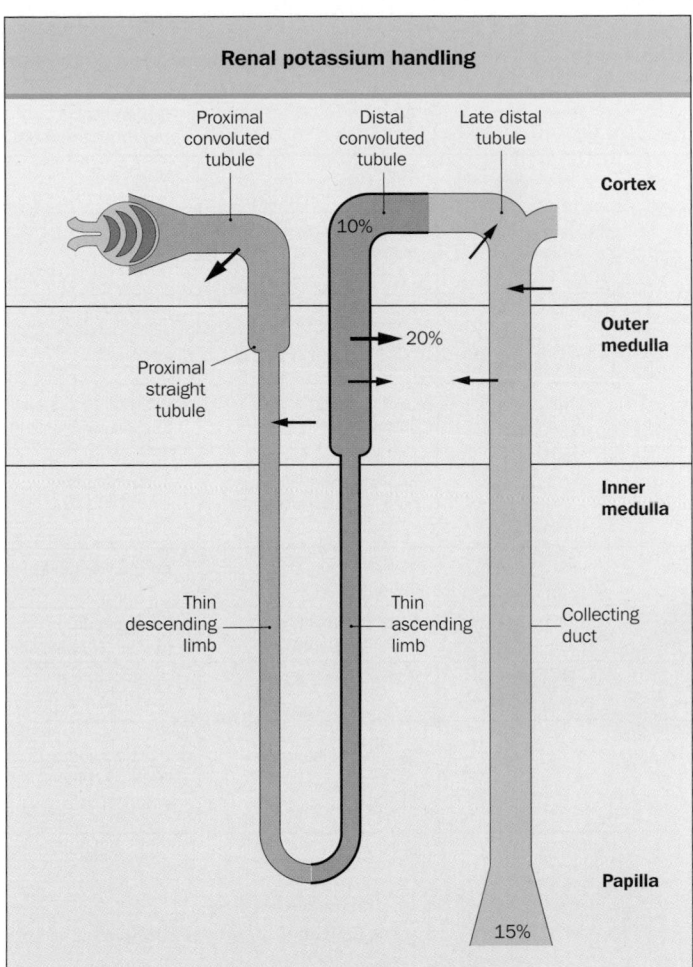

Figure 2.9 Potassium handling along the nephron. Figures are not given for percentages reabsorbed or remaining in each region because quantitative information is incomplete, but most filtered potassium is reabsorbed in the proximal convoluted tubule and thick ascending limb of Henle; approximately 10% of the filtered load reaches the early distal tubule. Secretion by principal cells in the late distal tubule/cortical collecting duct is variable and is the major determinant of potassium excretion.

K⁺ secretion, while the other type, the *intercalated cell*, is responsible for secretion of H^+ (by α-intercalated cells) or HCO_3^- (by β-intercalated cells) into the final urine. The medullary collecting duct consists largely of modified principal cells that reabsorb Na^+, but do not secrete K^+.

Figures 2.8 and 2.9 show schematically the sites of Na^+ and K^+ reabsorption/secretion along the nephron. Figure 2.10 lists the major transport mechanisms in the nephron, while Table 2.2 shows the pathophysiological consequences of known genetic defects in some of these transporters.

GLOMERULOTUBULAR BALANCE

Because the proportion of filtered sodium that is excreted in the urine is so small (normally <1%), it follows that, in the absence of any compensatory changes in reabsorption, even small changes in the filtered load would cause major changes in the amount excreted. For example, if GFR were to increase by 10% and the rate of reabsorption were to remain unchanged, sodium excretion would increase more than 10-fold. However, an intrinsic feature of tubular function is that the extent of sodium reabsorption in a given nephron segment is roughly proportional to the sodium delivery to that segment. This is the phenomenon of *glomerulotubular balance*. Perfect glomerulotubular balance would mean that both sodium reabsorption and sodium excretion changed in exactly the same proportion as the change in GFR, but in fact glomerulotubular balance is usually somewhat less than perfect. Thus, if GFR *were* to increase by 10%, reabsorption in the proximal tubule would increase, not by 10%, but by slightly less. Succeeding nephron segments exhibit the same property, so if the load to the loop of Henle and/or to the distal tubule is increased, some of the excess is mopped up. This is the reason why diuretics acting on the proximal tubule are relatively ineffective compared with those acting further downstream: with the latter there is less scope for buffering the effects. It is also the reason why combining two diuretics that act on different nephron segments is a particularly effective strategy.

Major membrane transporters in the nephron			
Transporter	Type	Segmental (nephron) location	Membrane location (apical/basolateral)
Na$^+$ / K$^+$ (solid)	Sodium pump	Ubiquitous	Basolateral
Na$^+$ / H$^+$ (open)	Sodium/hydrogen antiporter	Ubiquitous	Apical (NHE2 and 4) Basolateral (NHE1; 'housekeeping')
Na$^+$ / Glucose, amino acids phosphate, citrate (open)	Sodium-dependent cotransporter	Proximal tubule	Apical
Na$^+$ / HCO$_3^-$ (open)	Sodium/bicarbonate cotransporter	Proximal tubule and thick ascending limb	Basolateral
Na$^+$ / 2Cl$^-$ / K$^+$ (NH$_4^+$) (open)	Sodium/chloride/ potassium cotransporter	Thick ascending limb (NKCC2)	Apical (NKCC2)
Na$^+$ / Cl$^-$ (open)	Sodium/chloride cotransporter	Early distal tubule	Apical
K$^+$ / H$^+$ (solid)	Potassium/hydrogen exchange pump	Distal nephron (α intercalated cells)	Apical
Na$^+$ (channel)	Sodium channels	Distal nephron (principal cells)	Apical
K$^+$ (channel)	Potassium channels	Thick ascending limb Distal nephron Ubiquitous	Apical Apical Basolateral

Figure 2.10 Major membrane transporters in the nephron. Solid symbols represent primary active transport mechanisms; open symbols, secondary active transport mechanisms.

Defects in transport proteins resulting in renal disease	
Transporter	Consequence of mutation
Proximal tubule	
Apical Na$^+$/cystine cotransporter	Cystinuria
Apical Na$^+$/glucose cotransporter (SGLT2)	Renal glycosuria
Basolateral Na$^+$/HCO$_3^-$ cotransporter	Proximal renal tubular acidosis
Intracellular Cl$^-$ channel (ClC5)	Dent's disease
Thick ascending limb	
Apical Na$^+$/K$^+$/2Cl$^-$ cotransporter	Bartter syndrome type 1
Apical K$^+$ channel	Bartter syndrome type 2
Basolateral Cl$^-$ channel	Bartter syndrome type 3
Basolateral Cl$^-$ channel accessory protein	Bartter syndrome type 4
Distal convoluted tubule	
Apical Na$^+$–Cl$^-$ cotransporter	Gitelman's syndrome
Collecting duct	
Apical Na$^+$ channel (principal cells)	*Overexpression*: Liddle's disease
	Underexpression: Pseudohypoaldosteronism type 1a
Basolateral Cl$^-$/HCO$_3^-$ exchanger (intercalated cells)	Distal renal tubular acidosis
Apical H$^+$-ATPase (intercalated cells)	Distal renal tubular acidosis (with or without deafness)

Table 2.2 Defects in transport proteins resulting in renal disease.

The mechanism of glomerulotubular balance is not fully understood. As far as the proximal tubule is concerned, physical factors operating across peritubular capillary walls may be involved. Glomerular filtration of (essentially protein-free) fluid means that the plasma leaving the glomeruli in efferent arterioles and supplying the peritubular capillaries has a relatively high oncotic pressure, which favors uptake of fluid reabsorbed from the proximal tubules. Similarly, passage of blood through two sets of resistance vessels (afferent and efferent arterioles) means that the hydrostatic pressure in peritubular capillaries is particularly low, again favoring fluid uptake. If GFR were reduced in the absence of a change in RPF, peritubular capillary oncotic pressure would also be reduced, and the tendency to take up fluid reabsorbed from the proximal tubule would be diminished. It is thought that some of this fluid might leak back through the (leaky) tight junctions, thereby reducing net reabsorption (Fig. 2.11). This mechanism could only work if GFR changed in the absence of a corresponding change in RPF: if the two change in parallel (i.e., unchanged *filtration fraction*), there will be no change in oncotic pressure.

A second contributory factor to glomerulotubular balance in the proximal tubule might be the filtered loads of glucose and amino acids. If these increase (due to increased GFR), the rates of sodium-coupled glucose and amino acid reabsorption in the proximal tubule will also increase. This putative mechanism may be particularly relevant in tubular adaptation to the hyperfiltration seen in patients with diabetes mellitus.

Although the renal sympathetic nerves and certain hormones can influence reabsorption in the proximal tubule (e.g., angiotensin II) and loop of Henle (e.g., vasopressin), under normal circumstances the combined effects of autoregulation (see above) and glomerulotubular balance ensure that a relatively constant load of glomerular filtrate is delivered to the late distal tubule. It is in the final segments of the nephron that normal day-to-day control of sodium excretion is exerted: the hormone *aldosterone,* secreted from the adrenal cortex, stimulates the basolateral sodium pump in principal cells and increases the number of apical sodium channels (see Fig. 2.7). This not only stimulates sodium reabsorption but also facilitates potassium secretion in the late distal tubule/cortical collecting duct. The actions of aldosterone are mediated by mineralocorticoid receptors within principal cells. These receptors have equal affinity *in vitro* for aldosterone and adrenal *glucocorticoids.* Circulating concentrations of the latter vastly exceed those of aldosterone, but *in vivo* the mineralocorticoid receptors show specificity for aldosterone, due to the presence along the distal nephron of the enzyme *11β-hydroxysteroid dehydrogenase 2*, which inactivates glucocorticoids in the vicinity of the receptor[9].

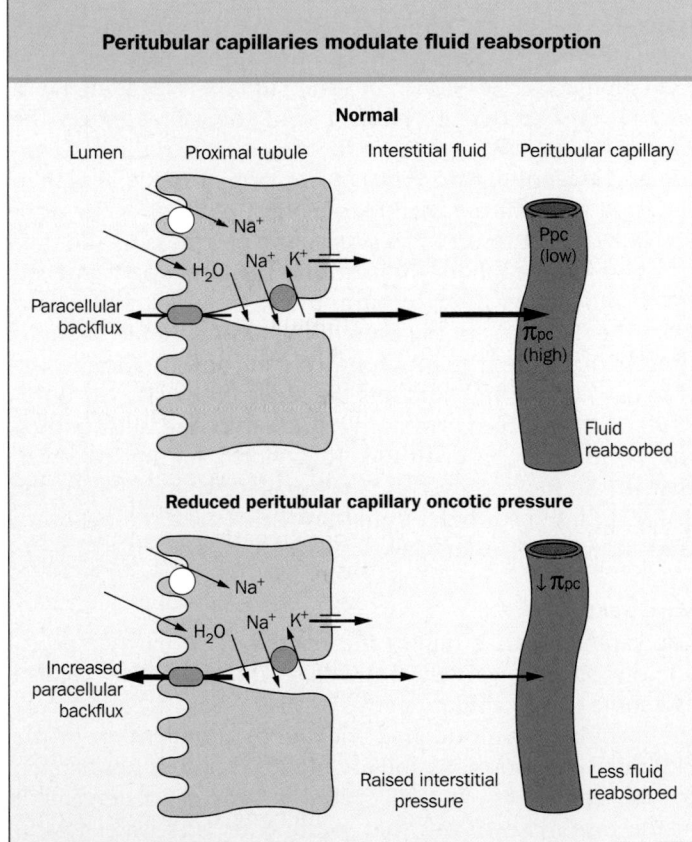

Figure 2.11 Influence of peritubular capillary oncotic pressure on net reabsorption in proximal tubules. Uptake of reabsorbate into peritubular capillaries is determined by the balance of hydrostatic and oncotic pressures across the capillary wall. Compared with those in systemic capillaries, the peritubular capillary hydrostatic (P_{pc}) and oncotic (π_{pc}) pressures are low and high, respectively, so that uptake of proximal tubular reabsorbate into the capillaries is favored. If peritubular capillary oncotic pressure falls (and/or hydrostatic pressure increases), less fluid is taken up, interstitial pressure rises, and more fluid leaks back into the lumen paracellularly; net reabsorption in proximal tubules is therefore reduced.

THE COUNTERCURRENT SYSTEM

A major function of the loop of Henle is the generation and maintenance of the interstitial osmotic gradient that increases from the renal cortex (~290 mOsm/kg) to the tip of the medulla (~1200 mOsm/kg). The anatomical loop of Henle reabsorbs approximately 40% of filtered Na[+], mostly in the TAL, and approximately 25% of filtered water, in the pars recta and thin descending limb. The thin descending limb is permeable to water, but relatively impermeable to Na[+], whereas both the thin ascending limb and TAL are essentially impermeable to water; in the thin ascending limb, Na[+] is reabsorbed passively, but in the TAL it is reabsorbed actively. Active Na[+] reabsorption is again energized by the basolateral sodium pump, which maintains a low intracellular Na[+] concentration, allowing Na[+] entry from the lumen via the Na[+]–2Cl[-]–K[+] cotransporter and, to a much lesser extent, the Na[+]–H[+] exchanger (Fig. 2.12). The apical Na[+]–2Cl[-]–K[+] cotransporter is unique to this nephron segment and is the site of action of loop diuretics like furosemide and bumetanide. Na[+] exits the cell via the sodium pump, and Cl[-] and K[+] exit via basolateral ion channels and a KCl cotransporter. K[+] also re-enters the lumen (recycles) through apical membrane potassium channels. Re-entry of K[+] into the tubular lumen is necessary for normal operation of the Na[+]–2Cl[-]–K[+] cotransporter, presumably because the availability of K[+] is a limiting factor for the transporter (the K[+] concentration in tubular fluid being much lower than those of Na[+] and Cl[-]). K[+] entry is also partly responsible for generating the lumen-positive potential difference (p.d.) found in this segment. This p.d. drives additional Na[+] reabsorption through the paracellular pathway: for each Na[+] reabsorbed transcellularly, there is one reabsorbed paracellularly (Fig. 2.12)[10]. Other cations (K[+], Ca[2+],

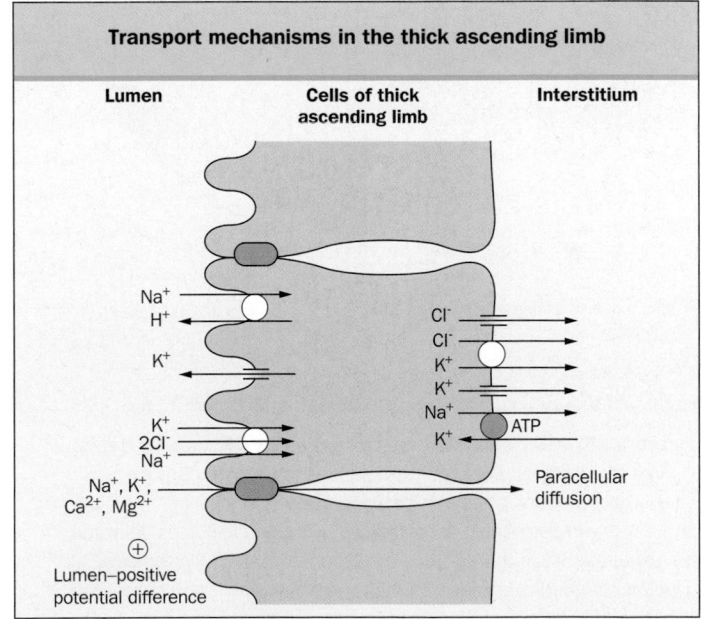

Figure 2.12 Transport mechanisms in the thick ascending limb of Henle. The major cellular entry mechanism is the Na[+]–K[+]–2Cl[-] cotransporter. The transepithelial potential difference drives paracellular transport of Na[+], K[+], Ca[2+] and Mg[2+].

Mg^{2+}) are also reabsorbed by this route. The reabsorption of Na^+ along the TAL in the absence of significant water reabsorption means that the tubular fluid leaving this segment is *hypotonic*, hence its other name of the *diluting segment*.

The U-shaped, countercurrent arrangement of the loop of Henle, the differences in permeability of the descending and ascending limbs to Na^+ and water, and active Na^+ reabsorption in the TAL, are the basis of *countercurrent multiplication* and generation of the medullary osmotic gradient (Fig. 2.13). Fluid entering the thin descending limb from the proximal tubule is isotonic (~290 mOsm/kg). However, the raised medullary osmolarity resulting from NaCl reabsorption in the water-impermeable ascending limb induces water reabsorption from the thin descending limb, thereby raising the osmolarity and NaCl concentration of the fluid delivered to the ascending

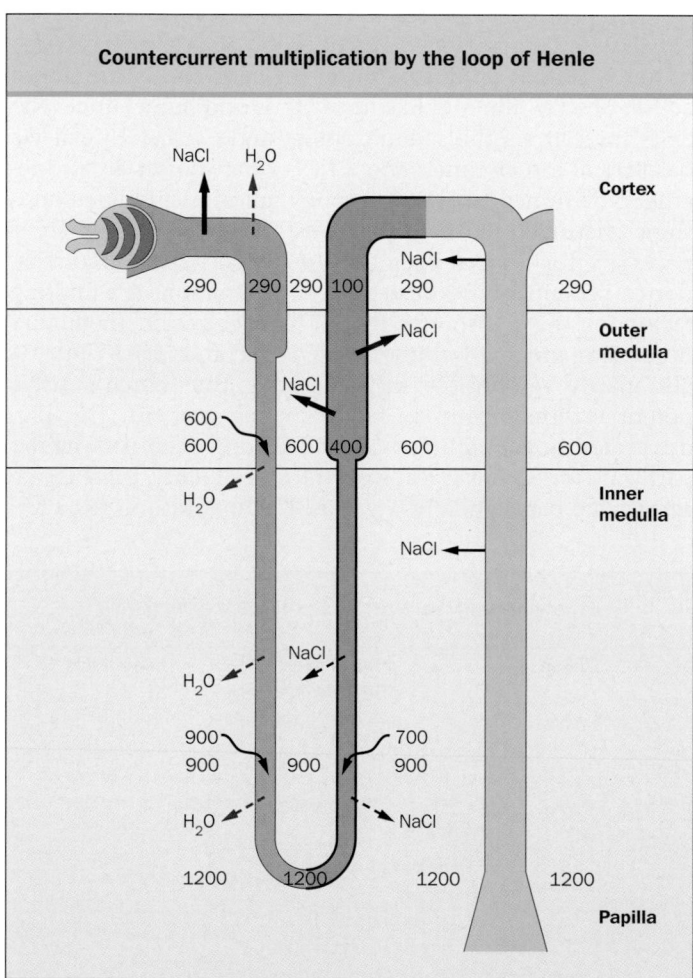

Figure 2.13 Countercurrent multiplication by the loop of Henle. Figures represent approximate osmolarities (mOsm/L). Osmotic equilibration occurs in the thin descending limb, while NaCl is reabsorbed in the water-impermeable ascending limb; hypotonic fluid is delivered to the distal tubule. In the absence of vasopressin, this fluid remains hypotonic during its passage through the distal tubule and collecting duct, despite the large osmotic gradient favoring water reabsorption. A large volume of dilute urine is formed. During maximal vasopressin secretion, water is reabsorbed down the osmotic gradient, so that tubular fluid becomes isotonic in the cortical collecting duct and hypertonic in the medullary collecting duct. A small volume of concentrated urine is formed.

limb. Further NaCl reabsorption in the ascending limb reinforces the effect, resulting in a progressive increase in medullary osmolarity from corticomedullary junction to papillary tip. A similar osmotic gradient exists in the thin descending limb, while at any level in the ascending limb the osmolarity is less than in the surrounding tissue. Thus, hypotonic (~100 mOsm/kg) fluid is delivered to the distal tubule. Ultimately, the energy source for countercurrent multiplication is active Na^+ reabsorption in the TAL. Na^+ reabsorption in the thin ascending limb is passive, and is made possible by a mechanism involving urea.

The role of urea

The thin limbs of the loop of Henle are relatively permeable to urea (ascending more than descending), but more distal nephron segments (TAL and beyond) are urea impermeable up to the final part of the inner medullary collecting duct. By this stage, vasopressin-dependent water reabsorption in the collecting ducts (see below) has led to a high urea concentration within the lumen, which in turn leads to reabsorption of urea into the interstitium by a vasopressin-sensitive urea transporter along the terminal portion of the inner medullary collecting duct[11]. The interstitial urea exchanges with *vasa recta* capillaries (see below), in which uptake is facilitated by a specific urea carrier mechanism, and some urea enters the urea-permeable S3 segment of the pars recta and the descending and ascending thin limbs of the loop of Henle; it is then returned to the inner medullary collecting ducts to be reabsorbed. The net result of this recycling process is to add urea to the inner medullary interstitium, thereby raising interstitial osmolality, which in turn increases water abstraction from the thin descending limb of the loop of Henle. It is this process that raises the intraluminal Na^+ concentration in the thin descending limb and sets the scene for passive Na^+ diffusion from the thin ascending limb into the surrounding inner medullary interstitium. It is worth noting, however, that in the final analysis it is *active* Na^+ reabsorption in the TAL, diluting the tubular fluid that enters the distal nephron, that allows the system to work.

Vasa recta

The capillaries that supply the medulla also have a special anatomical arrangement. If they passed through the medulla as a more usual capillary network, they would soon dissipate the medullary osmotic gradient due to equilibration of the latter with the isotonic capillary blood. This does not happen to any appreciable extent because the U-shaped arrangement of the *vasa recta* ensures that solute entry and water loss in the *descending* vasa recta are offset by solute loss and water entry in the *ascending* vasa recta. This is the process of *countercurrent exchange* and is entirely passive (Fig. 2.14).

VASOPRESSIN (ANTIDIURETIC HORMONE) AND WATER REABSORPTION

Vasopressin, or antidiuretic hormone, is a nonapeptide synthesized in specialized neurons of the supraoptic and paraventricular nuclei. It is transported from these nuclei to the posterior pituitary and is released in response to increases in

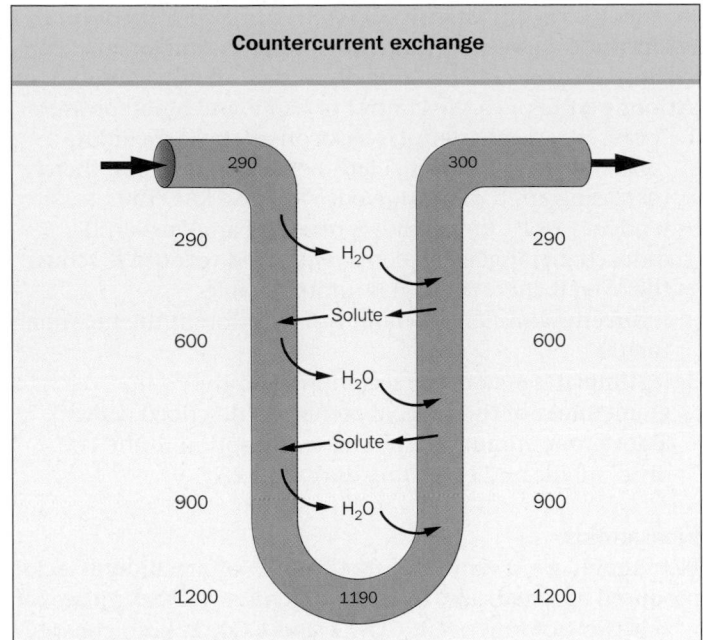

Figure 2.14 Countercurrent exchange by the vasa recta. Figures represent approximate osmolarities (mOsm/L). The vasa recta capillary walls are highly permeable, but the U-shaped arrangement of the vessels minimizes the dissipation of the medullary osmotic gradient. Nevertheless, because equilibration across the capillary walls is not instantaneous, a certain amount of solute is removed from the interstitium.

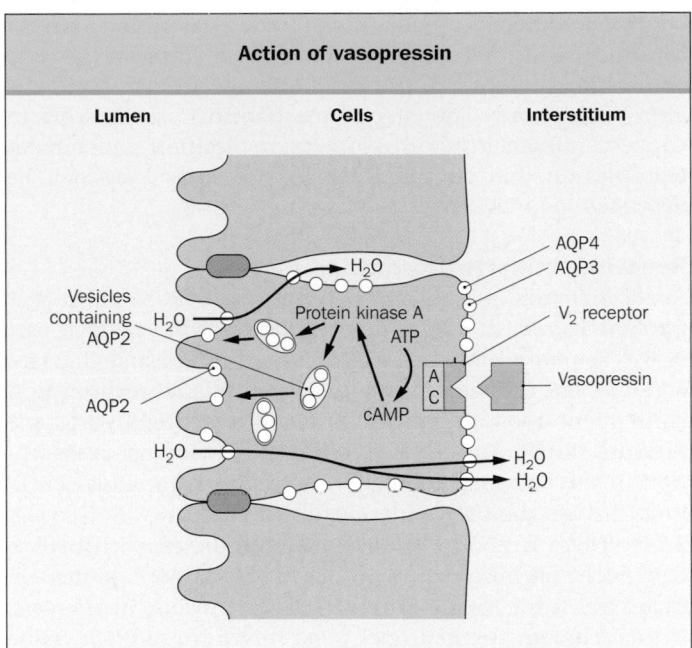

Figure 2.15 Mechanism of action of vasopressin (antidiuretic hormone). The hormone binds to V_2 receptors on the basolateral membrane of collecting duct principal cells and increases intracellular cAMP production, causing, via intermediate reactions involving protein kinase A, insertion of preformed water channels (aquaporin 2) into the luminal membrane. The water permeability of the basolateral membrane, which contains aquaporins 3 and 4, is permanently high, allowing transcellular movement of water from lumen to interstitium. AC, adenylate cyclase.

plasma osmolality and falls in blood pressure. Osmoreceptors are found in the hypothalamus and there is also input to this region from arterial baroreceptors and atrial stretch receptors. The actions of vasopressin are mediated by three receptor subtypes: V_{1a}, V_{1b} and V_2 receptors. V_{1a} receptors are found in vascular smooth muscle and are coupled to the phosphoinositol pathway; they cause an increase in intracellular Ca^{2+} resulting in contraction. (V_{1a} receptors have also been identified in the apical membrane of several nephron segments, though their role is not yet clear.) V_{1b} receptors are found in the anterior pituitary, where vasopressin modulates ACTH release. V_2 receptors are found in the basolateral membrane of principal cells in the late distal tubule and the whole length of the collecting duct; they are coupled to a G_s protein and thereby to cAMP generation, which leads to the insertion of water channels (aquaporins) into the apical membrane of this otherwise water-impermeable segment (Fig. 2.15). The V_2 receptor is defective in the X-linked form of nephrogenic diabetes insipidus[12].

Several aquaporins have been identified in the kidney[13]. Aquaporin 1 is found in the proximal tubule and thin descending limb of Henle, and is responsible for the permanently high water permeability of these segments. Aquaporins 3 and 4 are constitutively expressed in the basolateral membrane of principal cells in collecting duct epithelium. It is aquaporin 2 that is responsible for the variable water permeability of the collecting duct. Acute vasopressin release causes shuttling of aquaporin 2 from intracellular vesicles to the apical membrane, while chronically raised vasopressin levels increase aquaporin 2 expression. The apical insertion of aquaporin 2

allows reabsorption of water, driven by the high interstitial osmolality achieved and maintained by the countercurrent system[14]. Vasopressin also contributes to the effectiveness of this system by increasing Na^+ reabsorption in the TAL and urea reabsorption in the inner medullary collecting duct. In both the recessive and (even rarer) dominant forms of nephrogenic diabetes insipidus, aquaporin 2 is abnormal or fails to translocate to the apical membrane[13].

INTEGRATED CONTROL OF RENAL FUNCTION

Most regulatory mechanisms in the kidney are directed towards the control of 'effective circulating volume', a poorly defined and unmeasurable volume that reflects the degree of 'fullness' of the vasculature. Effective circulating volume normally varies in direct proportion to the extracellular fluid volume (ECFV). (However, this relationship breaks down in heart failure, cirrhosis and nephrotic syndrome, when effective circulating volume is reduced even though ECFV is not, triggering inappropriate renal fluid retention and contributing to the edema characteristic of these conditions.) Renal control of effective circulating volume is achieved by regulating the *sodium* content of the body. Osmoreceptor-mediated control of vasopressin secretion and thirst ensures that extracellular fluid osmolarity, and therefore sodium concentration, is closely regulated. Thus, by controlling the extracellular sodium *content*, extracellular *volume* is also

Essential Renal Anatomy and Physiology

controlled. Effective circulating volume is monitored largely by intravascular receptors located in the aorta and carotid sinuses (baroreceptors), the renal afferent arterioles and the atria of the heart. The effector mechanisms usually work in concert, influencing both glomerular filtration and tubular reabsorption, but in the interests of clarity they will be described individually.

Renal interstitial hydrostatic pressure

Acute increases in arterial blood pressure lead to natriuresis (*pressure natriuresis*). Since autoregulation is not perfect, part of this response is mediated by increases in RBF and GFR (see Fig. 2.3), but the main cause is reduced tubular reabsorption consequent upon an increase in renal interstitial hydrostatic pressure (RIHP). An elevated RIHP will reduce net reabsorption in the proximal tubule by increasing paracellular back-flux through the tight junctions in the tubular wall (see Fig. 2.11). There is good evidence that the increase in RIHP is dependent on intrarenally produced *nitric oxide*[15]. Moreover, increased nitric oxide production in macula densa cells (which contain the neuronal [type I] isoform of nitric oxide synthase) blunts the sensitivity of TGF (see below), thereby allowing increased NaCl delivery to the distal nephron without incurring a TGF-mediated fall in GFR[16]. A further renal action of nitric oxide results from the presence of inducible (type II) nitric oxide synthase in glomerular mesangial cells. Local production of nitric oxide counteracts the mesangial contractile response to agonists such as angiotensin II and endothelin (see below).

Renal sympathetic nerves

Reductions in arterial pressure and/or central venous pressure result in reduced afferent signaling from arterial baroreceptors and/or atrial volume receptors, which elicits a reflex increase in renal sympathetic nervous discharge. This reduces urinary sodium excretion in at least three ways:

- constriction of afferent and efferent arterioles (predominantly afferent), thereby directly reducing RBF and GFR and indirectly reducing RIHP;
- direct stimulation of sodium reabsorption in the proximal tubule and the TAL of Henle's loop;
- stimulation of *renin* secretion by afferent arteriolar cells (see below).

Renin–angiotensin–aldosterone system

The renin–angiotensin–aldosterone system is central to the control of ECFV and blood pressure. The enzyme renin is synthesized and stored in specialized afferent arteriolar cells that form part of the juxtaglomerular apparatus (see Fig. 2.4), and is released into the circulation in response to:

- increased renal sympathetic nervous discharge;
- reduced stretch of the afferent arteriole following a reduction in renal perfusion pressure (reduced arterial pressure);
- reduced delivery of NaCl to the macula densa region of the nephron. (This latter effect is in addition to the initiation of TGF described earlier.)

Renin catalyses the production of the decapeptide angiotensin I from circulating angiotensinogen (synthesized in the liver); angiotensin I is in turn converted to the octapeptide *angiotensin II* by the ubiquitous angiotensin converting enzyme (ACE). Angiotensin II has a number of actions pertinent to the control of ECFV and blood pressure:

1. It causes general arteriolar vasoconstriction, including renal afferent and (particularly) efferent arterioles, thereby increasing arterial pressure but reducing RBF. The tendency of P_{gc} to increase is offset by angiotensin II-induced mesangial cell contraction and reduced K_f; thus, the overall effect on GFR is unpredictable.
2. It directly stimulates sodium reabsorption in the proximal tubule.
3. It stimulates *aldosterone* secretion from the zona glomerulosa of the adrenal cortex. As described earlier, aldosterone stimulates sodium reabsorption in the late distal tubule and collecting duct (Fig. 2.7).

Eicosanoids

Eicosanoids are a family of metabolites of arachidonic acid, produced enzymatically by three systems: cyclo-oxygenase (of which two isoforms exist: COX 1 and COX 2, both constitutively expressed in the kidney), cytochrome P-450 and lipoxygenase. The major renal eicosanoids produced by the COX system are *prostaglandin E_2* and *prostaglandin I_2*, both of which are renal vasodilators and act to buffer the effects of renal vasoconstrictor agents such as angiotensin II and norepinephrine; and *thromboxane A_2*, a vasoconstrictor. Prostaglandin E_2 is also believed to have tubular effects, inhibiting sodium reabsorption in the TAL of Henle's loop and in the collecting duct.

The metabolism of arachidonic acid by renal cytochrome P-450 enzymes yields *epoxyeicosatrienoic acids* (EETs), *20-hydroxyeicosatetraenoic acid* (20-HETE) and *dihydroxyeicosatrienoic acids* (DHETs). These compounds appear to have a multiplicity of autocrine/paracrine/second messenger effects on the renal vasculature and tubules that are only now beginning to be unravelled[17]. Like prostaglandins, EETs appear to be vasodilator agents, whereas 20-HETE is a potent renal arteriolar constrictor and may be involved in the TGF mechanism. Recent work suggests that locally produced 20-HETE can also inhibit sodium reabsorption in the proximal tubule and TAL.

The third enzyme system that metabolizes arachidonic acid, the lipoxygenase system, is activated (in leucocytes, mast cells and macrophages) only during inflammation and injury, and will not be considered here.

Attention has been directed in recent years to the involvement of COX 2 in both renin release and TGF. COX 2 is present in macula densa cells and there is good evidence that it occupies a critical role in the stimulation of renin release in response to reduced NaCl delivery to the macula densa[18]. A low-sodium diet increases COX 2 mRNA and protein in the macula densa and simultaneously increases renin secretion, while selective inhibition of COX 2 blocks this renin response. More directly, it has been shown that in the rabbit isolated juxtaglomerular apparatus (JGA), COX 2 inhibition virtually abolishes renin release in response to reduced luminal NaCl at the macula densa. It seems likely, therefore, that the hyporeninemia observed during administration of nonsteroidal anti-inflammatory drugs is largely a consequence of COX 2 inhibition. The COX 2 product responsible for enhancing renin secretion is thought to be prostaglandin E_2, and it is notable that prostaglandin E_2 receptors in the JGA are upregulated during sodium depletion.

As already indicated, neuronal (type I) nitric oxide synthase (nNOS) is also present in macula densa cells, and nitric oxide produced at this site appears to be involved in modulating both renin release and TGF, possibly through an interaction with COX 2. Thus, the increase in macula densa COX 2 expression induced by a low-sodium diet is attenuated during administration of selective nNOS inhibitors, and this has led to speculation that nitric oxide is responsible for the increase in COX 2 expression and consequent increase in juxtaglomerular renin secretion[19]. Furthermore, in the rabbit isolated perfused JGA, inhibition of nNOS augmented the afferent arteriolar constrictor response to increased luminal NaCl in the macula densa, indicating that locally produced nitric oxide buffers the TGF response. These putative interactions between COX 2 and nNOS are shown diagrammatically in Figure 2.16.

Atrial natriuretic peptide

If blood volume increases significantly, the resulting atrial stretch stimulates the release of *atrial natriuretic peptide* (*ANP*) from atrial myocytes. This hormone increases sodium excretion, partly through suppression of renin and aldosterone

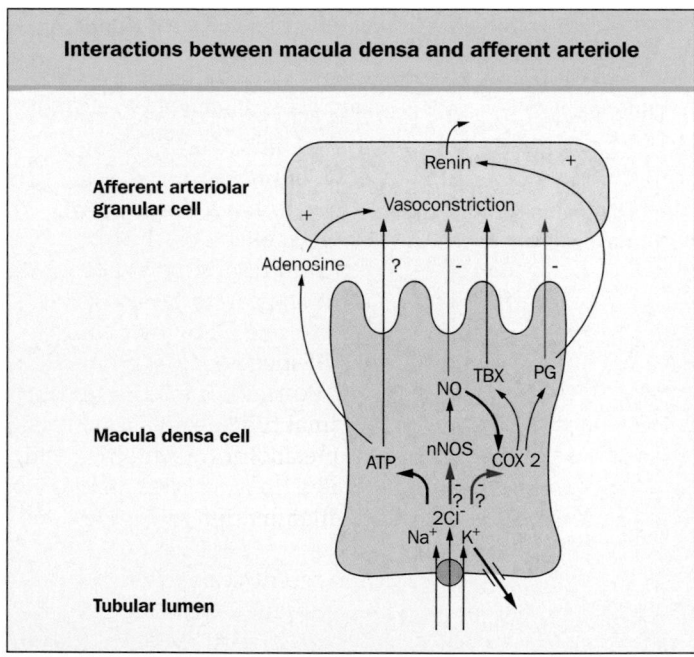

Figure 2.16 Proposed interactions between cyclo-oxygenase 2 (COX 2) and neuronal nitric oxide synthase (nNOS) in the control of renin secretion and tubuloglomerular feedback. Both enzyme systems are present in macula densa cells. Increased NaCl delivery to the macula densa stimulates NaCl entry into the cells via the $Na^+–K^+–2Cl^-$ cotransporter, which in turn causes afferent arteriolar constriction, through adenosine and/or ATP production, and inhibits COX 2 expression, possibly through inhibition of (nNOS-mediated) nitric oxide production. Generation of eicosanoids by COX 2 modulates the vasoconstriction (as does nitric oxide), while prostaglandin(s) (most likely E_2) stimulate(s) renin release. The latter effect is relatively well established, but many of the other interactions remain speculative.

release and partly through a direct inhibitory effect on sodium reabsorption in the medullary collecting duct. An additional action of ANP may be to increase GFR, since high doses cause glomerular arteriolar vasodilatation and mesangial cell relaxation (thus increasing K_f).

Endothelins

Endothelins 1–3 are a family of peptides with potent vasoconstrictor action, to which the renal vasculature is exquisitely sensitive[20]. Like nitric oxide, endothelins function primarily as autocrine or paracrine agents. The kidney is a rich source of endothelins, the predominant isoform being endothelin 1 (ET 1). ET 1 is generated throughout the renal vasculature, including afferent and efferent arterioles (where it causes vasoconstriction) and mesangial cells (where it causes contraction; i.e., decreases K_f). Consequently, renal ET 1 causes profound reductions in RBF and GFR. The effects, if any, of endothelins on tubular function are not yet clear; tubular endothelin receptors are found mainly in the collecting duct, and their activation inhibits sodium and water reabsorption. Although evidence is accumulating that ET 1 may be involved in disturbed renal function in pathological conditions such as congestive heart failure and radiocontrast-induced acute renal failure, its role in normal renal physiology remains to be clarified.

Purines

It is likely that an increasing number of autocrine or paracrine mechanisms will be added to the list of controlling factors. Evidence is accumulating that in addition to those humoral agents that can alter renal function by acting from the basolateral side of the tubule, several can act from within the tubular lumen. Prime candidates for such a role are the purines (ATP and adenosine). Purinoceptors are subdivided into P1 and P2 receptors. The former are responsive to adenosine, and are more usually known as adenosine receptors (A_1, A_{2a}, A_{2b} and A_3), while the latter, responsive to ATP, are further subdivided into P2X (ligand-gated ion channels) and P2Y (metabotropic) receptors. As indicated earlier, A_1 and P2X receptors are found in afferent arterioles and mediate vasoconstriction[21]. All three categories of purinoceptor are found along the nephron, sometimes on the basolateral membrane, sometimes on the luminal membrane, and sometimes both. Locally produced adenosine can enhance proximal tubular reabsorption, while either basolateral or luminal ATP can inhibit sodium reabsorption in the collecting duct[22]. The role of purines in normal tubular physiology, however, remains to be established.

CONCLUSION

The balance between glomerular filtration and tubular reabsorption allows precise control of overall sodium excretion and consequently of ECFV, the key to long-term blood pressure regulation. It is notable that, with the exception of aldosterone – the factor largely responsible for day-to-day fluctuations in sodium excretion, those agents prominent in the control of sodium excretion also have direct vascular effects, both within the kidney and systemically. Thus, there are elements in place for an integrated regulatory system that not only controls blood *volume* but contributes also to the circulatory *capacity*. It might not be too fanciful to hope that this concept could provide the opportunity for future antihypertensive therapeutic strategies capable of targeting both these variables.

REFERENCES

1. Fliser D, Ritz E, Franek E. Renal reserve in the elderly. Semin Nephrol. 1995;15:463–7.
2. Persson PB. Renal blood flow autoregulation in blood pressure control. Curr Opin Nephrol Hypertens. 2002;11:67–72.
3. Thomson SC. Adenosine and purinergic mediators of tubuloglomerular feedback. Curr Opin Nephrol Hypertens. 2002;11:81–6.
4. Shirley DG, Walter SJ. A micropuncture study of the renal response to haemorrhage in rats: assessment of the role of vasopressin. Exp Physiol. 1995;80:619–30.
5. Molitoris BA, Nelson WJ. Alterations in the establishment and maintenance of epithelial cell polarity as a basis for disease processes. J Clin Invest. 1990;85:3–9.
6. Stein WD. Channels, carriers, and pumps. An introduction to membrane transport. San Diego: Academic Press; 1990.
7. Skou JC. The influence of some cations on an adenosine triphosphatase from peripheral nerves. Biochim Biophys Acta. 1957;23:394–401.
8. Gluck S, Kelly S, Al-Awqati Q. The proton translocating ATPase responsible for urinary acidification. J Biol Chem. 1982;257: 9230–3.
9. Bailey MA, Unwin RJ, Shirley DG. In vivo inhibition of renal 11β-hydroxysteroid dehydrogenase in the rat stimulates collecting duct sodium reabsorption. Clin Sci. 2001;101:195–8.
10. Greger R. Ion transport mechanisms in thick ascending limb of Henle's loop of mammalian nephron. Physiol Rev. 1985;65: 760–95.
11. Sands JM, Timmer RT, Gunn RB. Urea transporters in kidney and erythrocytes. Am J Physiol. 1997;273:F321–F39.
12. Rosenthal W, Seibold A, Antaramian A, et al. Molecular identification of the gene responsible for congenital nephrogenic diabetes insipidus. Nature. 1992;359:233–5.
13. King LS, Agre P. Pathophysiology of the aquaporin water channels. Annu Rev Physiol. 1996;58:619–48.
14. Knepper MA. Molecular physiology of urinary concentrating mechanism: regulation of aquaporin water channels by vasopressin. Am J Physiol. 1997;272:F3–F12.
15. Nakamura T, Alberola AM, Salazar FJ, et al. Effects of renal perfusion pressure on renal interstitial hydrostatic pressure and Na^+ excretion: role of endothelium-derived nitric oxide. Nephron. 1998;78:104–11.
16. Thorup C, Persson AEG. Macula densa derived nitric oxide in regulation of glomerular capillary pressure. Kidney Int. 1996;49: 430–6.
17. Maier KG, Roman RJ. Cytochrome P450 metabolites of arachidonic acid in the control of renal function. Curr Opin Nephrol Hypertens. 2001;10:81–7.
18. Breyer MD, Harris RC. Cyclooxygenase 2 and the kidney. Curr Opin Nephrol Hypertens. 2001;10:89–98.
19. Welch WJ, Wilcox CS. What is brain nitric oxide doing in the kidney? Curr Opin Nephrol Hypertens. 2002;11:109–15.
20. Kohan DE. Endothelins in the normal and diseased kidney. Am J Kid Dis. 1997;29:2–26.
21. Chan CM, Unwin RJ, Bardini M, et al. Localization of the $P2X_1$ purinoceptors by autoradiography and immunohistochemistry in the rat kidney. Am J Physiol. 1998;274:F799–F804.
22. Leipziger J, Bailey MA, Unwin RJ. P2 receptors in the kidney. In: Schwiebert EM ed. Extracellular nucleotides and nucleosides (Current topics in membranes 54). San Diego: Academic Press; 2003.

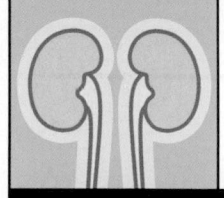

Section 2 Investigation of Renal Disease

Chapter 3

Assessment of Renal Function

Masaru Horio, Yoshimasa Orita, and Megumu Fukunaga

INTRODUCTION

The kidney has many functions including glomerular filtration, reabsorption and secretion in the tubules, concentration and dilution of urine, acidification of urine and production and metabolism of hormones. The most important parameter in assessing kidney function and the progression of renal disease is glomerular filtration rate (GFR), the renal excretory capacity. The correct assessment of GFR is the main focus of this chapter.

GLOMERULAR FILTRATION RATE AND THE CONCEPT OF RENAL CLEARANCE

GFR is the measurement of how much filtrate is made by the glomeruli. It is an excellent measure of the excretory function of the kidney. For each individual nephron the filtration is determined by the plasma flow, the net pressure gradient, the capillary surface area and the capillary permeability (see Chapter 2). The GFR of the whole organism corresponds to the sum of GFR for all nephrons (approximately 1 million per kidney).

GFR is described in terms of renal clearance, a concept originally developed by Homer Smith. The clearance of a substance is the volume of plasma from which all the substance is removed and excreted into the urine per unit time, and is a 'virtual' volume. In clinical practice, endogenous creatinine is usually the substance chosen for clearance measurements. More accurate estimation of GFR requires the administration of an exogenous substance by continuous infusion or single injection, for example inulin, iohexol, or ^{51}Cr-EDTA.

The renal clearance of a filtration marker, C, is defined as:

$$C = UV/P$$

where P is the plasma concentration of the marker, U is the urine concentration, and V is the urine flow rate. In actual clearance studies, the time over which urine is collected is required. Therefore this formula is written as:

$$C = U_{ex}/AUC$$

where U_{ex} is the amount of urine excretion of the marker and AUC is the area under the plasma concentration curve during the collection of urine (Fig. 3.1). This formula can be rewritten as:

$$C = U_{ex}/(P't)$$

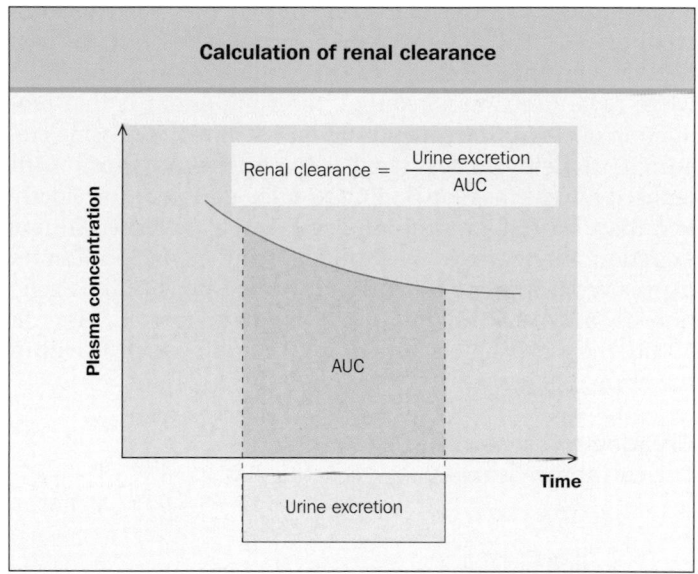

Figure 3.1 Calculation of renal clearance. Renal clearance of a substance is calculated by dividing the amount of the substance excreted in the urine by the area under the plasma concentration curve (AUC).

where P' is the mean plasma concentration of the marker during the urine collection and t is the period of urine collection.

The clearance of any chosen marker substance only equals GFR if a number of criteria for the measured substance are met. The substance must be freely filterable at the glomerulus, and neither secreted nor reabsorbed by the tubules. It must be in steady state concentrations in the blood, with no extrarenal route of excretion. It must also be easily and accurately measured.

MEASUREMENT OF GFR IN CLINICAL PRACTICE

Creatinine clearance is the usual method in clinical practice for estimation of GFR. Even simpler are the measurement of plasma urea and creatinine; these however have significant limitations.

Plasma urea

An elevated plasma urea suggests impaired renal function. However, urea is the main end product of protein catabolism, and individuals with a high protein intake may have elevated plasma urea without any renal dysfunction. Plasma urea also rises disproportionately to creatinine in the context of extra-cellular volume depletion, because tubular reabsorption of urea is increased.

Plasma creatinine

Creatinine is an endogenous substance mainly produced in muscle cells from creatine and phosphocreatine. The production rate is almost constant. Hence, the steady state concentration of plasma creatinine depends on its excretion, which mainly reflects GFR. However, large changes in GFR correspond to only small changes in plasma creatinine when patients have near normal renal function, making plasma creatinine a less sensitive marker of GFR in the early stages of renal disease (Fig. 3.2). Moreover, creatinine is not an ideal GFR marker since tubular secretion of creatinine is enhanced when renal function is reduced. Most important is that production of creatinine depends on muscle mass, so plasma creatinine underestimates renal impairment in those with reduced muscle mass, including women, children, the elderly and those with malnutrition[1]. For example, when creatinine excretion is 1 mg/min (1440 mg/day) and C_{cr} is 50 mL/min, plasma creatinine is 2.0 mg/dL. However, if creatinine excretion is only 0.5 mg/min (720 mg/day) and C_{cr} is still 50 mL/min, plasma creatinine is 1.0 mg/dL which is within the normal range.

Creatinine clearance

The creatinine clearance (C_{cr}) is defined as:

$$C_{cr} = U_{cr}V/P_{cr}$$

where P_{cr} is the plasma concentration of creatinine, U_{cr} is the urine concentration, and V is the urine flow rate. C_{cr} is a steady state estimation and therefore cannot be interpreted when renal function is rapidly changing, for example during the course of acute renal failure. Although superior to plasma creatinine as a measurement of GFR, C_{cr} has other significant limitations.

Timed urine collection

Measurement of C_{cr} requires a timed collection of urine with a single blood sample, ideally drawn during the collection. In practice a 24-h urine collection is undertaken and a blood sample drawn shortly after completion of the collection when the patient brings the urine to the office, surgery or hospital. Incomplete urine collection is a major source of inaccuracy in C_{cr} measurement in clinical practice. The patient should be instructed to pass urine into the toilet on rising, and then collect all urine subsequently passed over the next 24 h *including* the urine passed on rising the following day. Major inaccuracies are suggested by a low urine volume, but completeness of the urine collection is better assessed by comparing urinary creatinine with normal daily creatinine production: men 20–25 mg/kg/day (0.18–0.22 mmol/kg/day); women 15–20 mg/kg/day (0.13–0.18 mmol/kg/day).

Tubular secretion

Creatinine is secreted by the tubules as well as filtered by the glomerulus, therefore, C_{cr} consistently exceeds true GFR (Fig. 3.3). Cimetidine, trimethoprim, and probenecid inhibit

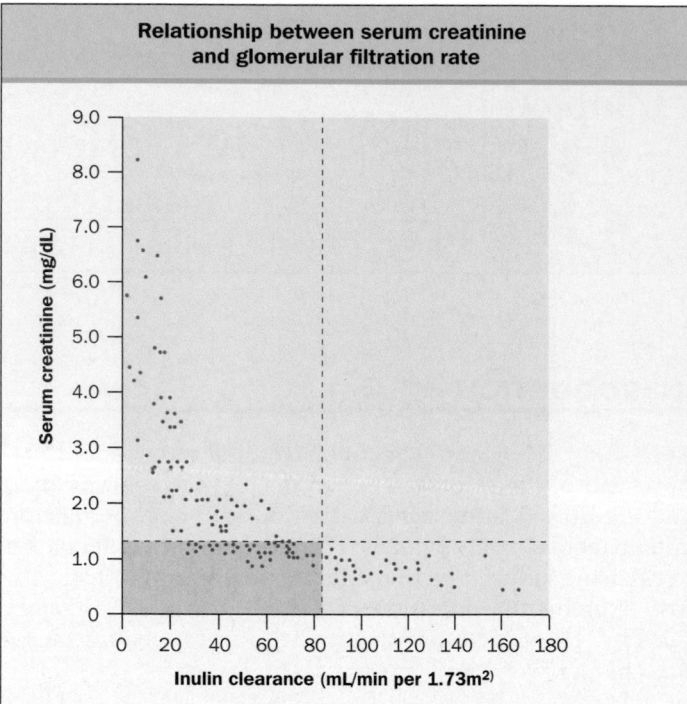

Relationship between serum creatinine and glomerular filtration rate

Figure 3.2 Relationship between serum creatinine and glomerular filtration rate. Simultaneous measurement of serum creatinine (Jaffé assay) and inulin clearance. The vertical dotted line represents the lower normal limit for inulin clearance (82 mL/min per 1.73 m²). The horizontal dotted line corresponds to the upper normal limit for serum creatinine concentration (1.4 mg/dL or 120 μmol/L). The shaded area includes values for patients in whom inulin clearance is reduced but serum creatinine concentration remains normal. (Adapted with permission from Levey et al.[10] and Shemesh et al.[2].)

proximal secretion of creatinine, elevate plasma creatinine and diminish creatinine clearance. Oral administration of cimetidine 600 mg before C_{cr} measurement has been recommended to inhibit creatinine secretion, thus producing values of C_{cr} closer to those of GFR, although this is not widely used in clinical practice[3].

Creatinine generation

Calculation of C_{cr} depends on the assumption that the concentration of plasma creatinine is constant. However, plasma creatinine level and urinary excretion of creatinine are both higher during the day than at night, mainly due to the absorption of exogenous creatinine contained in the diet. A transient increase in plasma creatinine and urinary creatinine excretion are observed after eating cooked meat, which contains a considerable amount of creatinine[4]. For this reason C_{cr} calculated from short-term daytime urine collections is about 20% higher than that calculated from a 24-h urine collection.

Assay methods for creatinine

There are two routine methods for assaying creatinine: a method using the Jaffé reaction and an enzymatic method. The Jaffé reaction in which creatinine reacts with an alkaline solution of picrate is still widely used but is not specific for

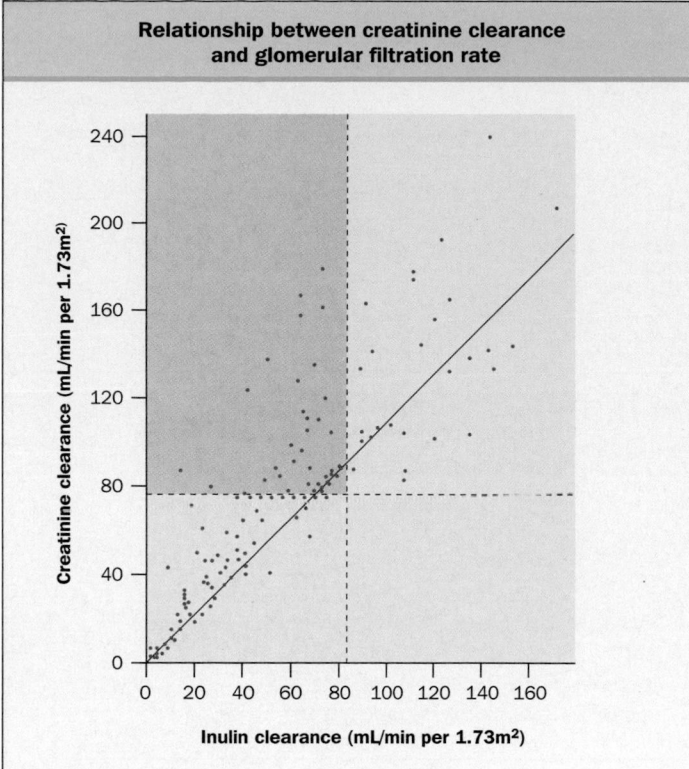

Figure 3.3 Relationship between creatinine clearance and glomerular filtration rate. Simultaneous measurements of creatinine clearance and inulin clearance. The vertical dotted line represents the lower normal limit for inulin clearance (82 mL/min per 1.73 m²). The horizontal dotted line represents the lower normal limit for creatinine clearance (77 mL/min per 1.73 m²). The shaded area includes values for patients in whom inulin clearance is reduced but whose creatinine clearance remains normal. (Adapted with permission from Levey et al.[10] and Shemesh et al.[2].)

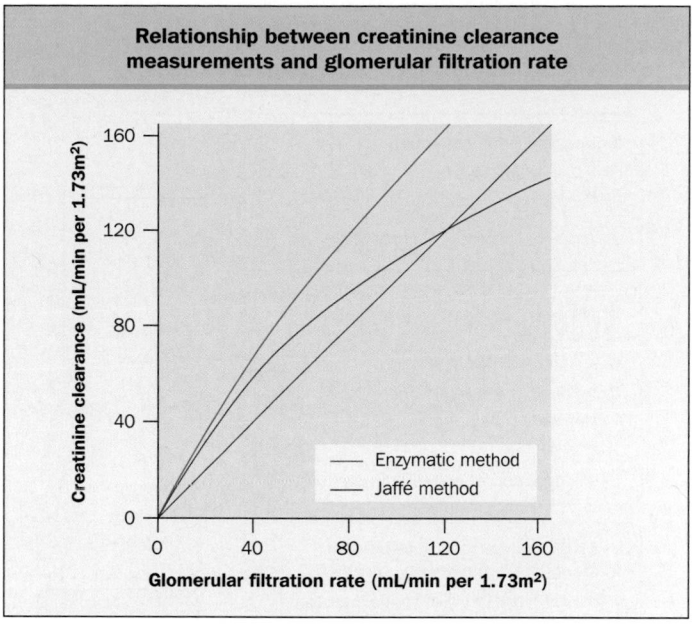

Figure 3.4 Relationship between creatinine clearance measurements and glomerular filtration rate. It has been assumed that creatinine excretion is constant (1500 mg/day), and that the positive bias of plasma creatinine value by Jaffé assay is 0.2 mg/dL at any creatinine level. Enzymatic assay represents true creatinine values. The ratio of tubular secreted creatinine to filtered creatinine gradually increases to 20% when GFR is 160 mL/min per 1.73 m² and to 100% when GFR is 10 mL/min per 1.73 m².

creatinine. Noncreatinine chromogens such as glucose, acetoacetate, ascorbic acid, and some cephalosporins, particularly cefoxitin, react positively and cause the Jaffé reaction to overestimate plasma creatinine. The Jaffé reaction overestimates plasma creatinine by about 0.2 mg/dL for normal plasma creatinine values, and by up to 0.4 mg/dL when plasma creatinine is 10 mg/dL. Overestimation of plasma creatinine is offset by tubular secretion of creatinine, with the net effect that C_{cr} by the Jaffé assay is close to GFR in normal individuals. The effect of the positive bias by the Jaffé assay becomes negligible as plasma creatinine increases, but creatinine secretion is greater with reduced GFR; hence the difference between C_{cr} and GFR expands in patients at lower GFR (Fig. 3.4).

The enzymatic method, now widely available in clinical use, is much more accurate and is recommended for creatinine measurement. The dissociation between C_{cr} by the enzymatic method and GFR is seen regardless of renal function (Fig. 3.4). Enzymatic assays are also prone to interference by drugs. For example, ethamsylate causes negative interference and reduces creatinine values in the peroxidase coupled reaction, and flucytosine causes positive interference in the creatinine deiminase coupled reaction. C_{cr} measurements must be

interpreted critically if they are to provide useful information about renal function (Fig. 3.5).

Predicted creatinine clearance – the Cockcroft–Gault formula

Rapid estimation of creatinine clearance from plasma creatinine values, without recourse to urine measurement, is clinically useful. Creatinine generation decreases linearly with advancing age, as muscle mass falls, and a number of formulae for the estimation of creatinine excretion have been derived to account for this. The most widely used formula is that of Cockcroft and Gault[5] (Fig. 3.6a). The formula overestimates the true C_{cr} values in obese patients, and also in those on a low protein diet. Equations which take body fat into account predict C_{cr} better than the Cockcroft–Gault formula, but are more complicated and not widely used[6].

Predicted GFR – a new equation from the MDRD study

An equation that predicts GFR from plasma creatinine concentration was developed from data obtained in the Modification of Diet in Renal Disease (MDRD) Study (Fig.3.6b)[7]. This equation proved more accurate than measured C_{cr} in both the MDRD study, and the African-American Study of Hypertension and Kidney Disease[7,8]. The equation has not yet been validated in children, the elderly or pregnant women, nor where there are extreme values for serum albumin concentration.

This equation is less quick than the Cockcroft–Gault formula to use in everyday clinical practice, and a nomogram to speed the estimation is shown in Figure 3.7.

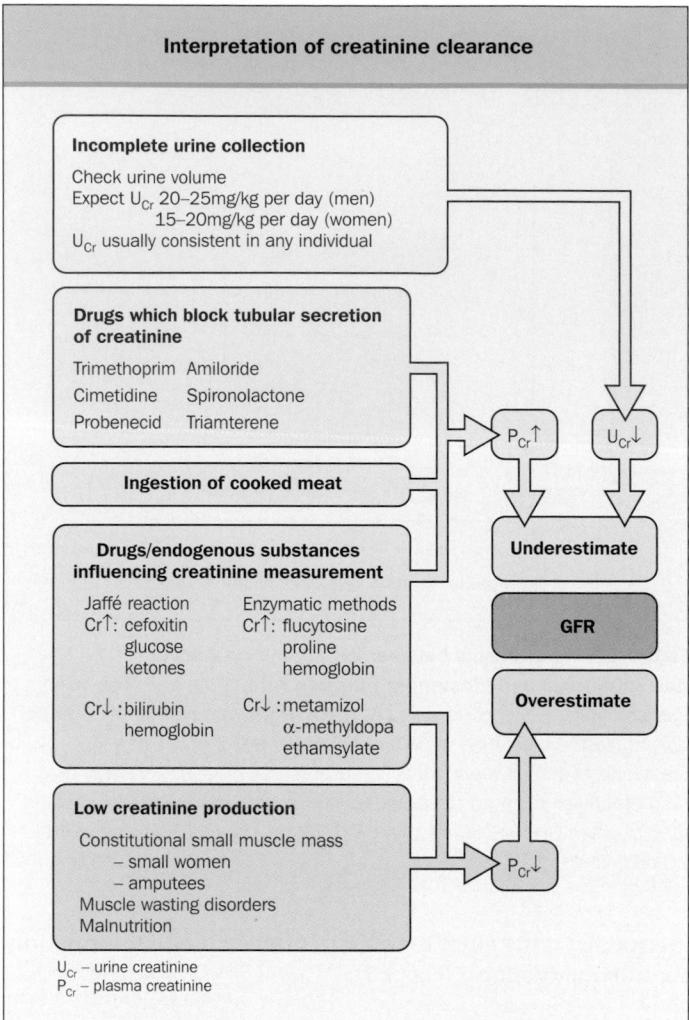

Figure 3.5 Interpretation of creatinine clearance.

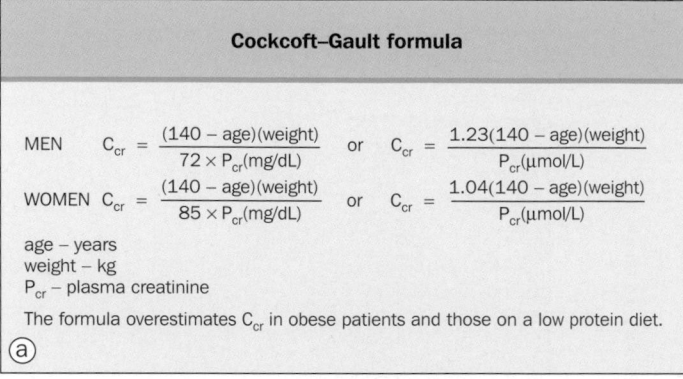

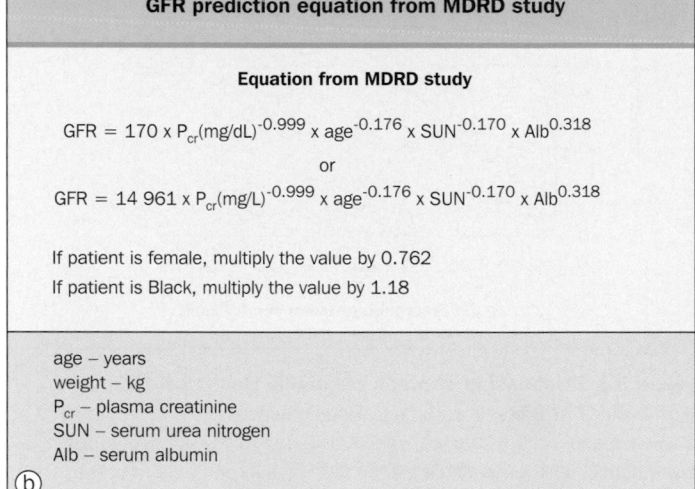

Figure 3.6 Formulae for estimation of GFR. (a) Cockcroft–Gault formula. Estimated creatinine clearance (C_{cr}) with respect to age, gender, serum creatinine, and body weight. (b) Prediction equation from MDRD study. Estimated GFR with respect to age, gender, ethnicity, serum creatinine, serum urea nitrogen, and serum albumin.

OTHER MEASUREMENTS OF GFR

Methods of measuring renal clearance more accurate than C_{cr} and its calculated estimates are required in some clinical settings and are also a valuable research tool. To avoid the inaccuracies of urine collection, the total plasma clearance is measured of an exogenous filtration marker which has little or no extrarenal excretion.

Plasma clearance with continuous injection – inulin clearance

Plasma clearance of a filtration marker, C, is defined as:

$$C = T_{ex}/AUC$$

where T_{ex} is the total amount excreted from plasma and AUC is the area under the plasma concentration curve (Fig. 3.1).

When a filtration marker is infused intravenously or subcutaneously at a constant rate, the plasma concentration reaches a steady state. At this point, the urinary excretion of the marker will be identical to the rate of infusion. Therefore, GFR can be calculated from plasma concentration and infusion rate of the marker. When the plasma concentration does not

reach a steady state, GFR will be overestimated; therefore this method requires a relatively long study period (3–24 h). Although cumbersome, this is the most accurate method and inulin clearance with continuous infusion is the 'gold standard' for measurement of GFR. Inulin, a 5200-Da uncharged polymer of fructose, satisfies the criteria for an ideal clearance substance since it is freely filtered at the glomerulus and is not reabsorbed, secreted, synthesized or metabolized by the tubules. But, as well as the practical disadvantages of a continuous infusion technique, the anthrone method, often used to assay inulin, is complicated and high glucose concentrations can give false-positive reactions. The alternative enzymatic assay of inulin is not widely available.

Plasma clearance with single injection

After a bolus intravenous injection, the disappearance curve of the plasma concentration represents two components: a rapid phase reflecting the distribution of the marker from intravascular space to extravascular space and a slow phase reflecting the renal excretion of the marker. A two-compartment model is required to describe the entire plasma disappearance curve,

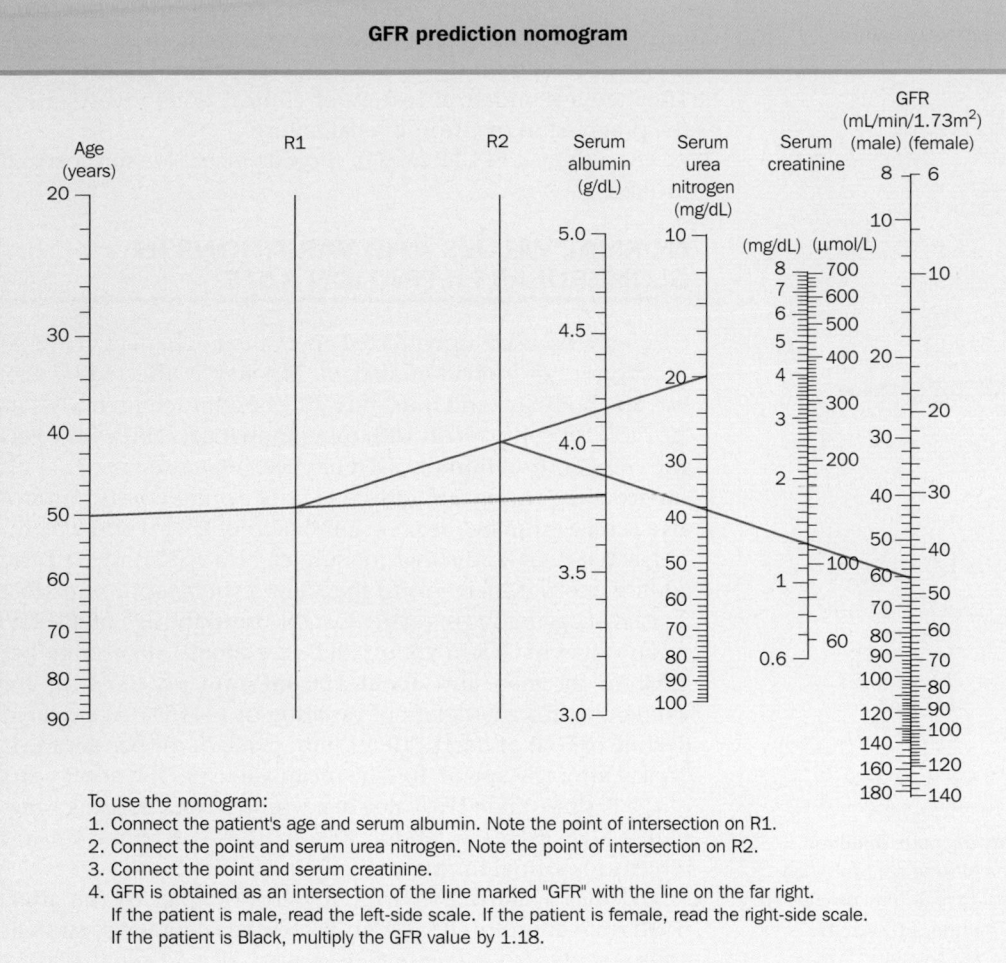

Figure 3.7 GFR prediction nomogram. The nomogram is mathematically identical to the equation developed from MDRD study (Fig.3.6b). The purple line shows a case (age: 50 years old, serum albumin: 3.8 mg/dL, serum urea nitrogen: 20 mg/dL, serum creatinine: 1.3 mg/dL). If the patient is a white male, the predicted GFR will be 60 mL/min per 1.73 m².

To use the nomogram:
1. Connect the patient's age and serum albumin. Note the point of intersection on R1.
2. Connect the point and serum urea nitrogen. Note the point of intersection on R2.
3. Connect the point and serum creatinine.
4. GFR is obtained as an intersection of the line marked "GFR" with the line on the far right.
   If the patient is male, read the left-side scale. If the patient is female, read the right-side scale.
   If the patient is Black, multiply the GFR value by 1.18.

but requires frequent blood sampling, which is impractical. Therefore, a one-compartment model is widely used which matches only the slow phase of the plasma disappearance curve.

This model is expressed as:

$$C(t) = Ae^{-Bt}$$

$$\ln C(t) = -Bt + A$$

where $C(t)$ is the plasma concentration of the marker at a given time (t), A is the zero-time intercept, and $-B$ is the rate constant, the falling slope of the marker in the semilogarithmic plot (see Fig. 3.8).

The line can usually be determined by two blood samples during the slow phase (e.g., at 90 and 120 min after injection), although a relatively long time (3–24 h) may be required to obtain the accurate falling slope of the marker in patients with impaired renal function. Plasma clearance is slightly overestimated in this simple one-compartment model, since it does not account for that part of the AUC resulting from the rapid phase[9]. Bröchener-Mortensen introduced the following equation to correct the clearance values:

Corrected plasma clearance = $0.990778C - 0.001218C^2$

Where C is the original clearance from the one-compartment model[9].

To enhance the convenience of these techniques, a single-sample method has been developed, using a sample taken 3–5 h after the bolus injection. Zero time intercept is calculated by dividing the injected dose by a distribution space of the marker estimated from body weight. However, the estimation of the distribution space is difficult in patients with severe edema or ascites.

Alternative filtration markers

[125]I-Iothalamate, ^{51}Cr-EDTA, ^{99m}Tc-diethylenetriaminepentaacetic acid (^{99m}Tc-DTPA; an analog of EDTA), and nonradioactive iothalamate and iohexol are also used as filtration markers. All can be used for measurement of GFR, most commonly in the single injection plasma clearance technique. The choice depends on local availability of methods to measure each marker. Iothalamate (Conray), a 614-Da ionic radiocontrast agent, is freely filtered by the glomerulus. It appears to have 1–8% protein-binding and proximal tubular secretion which accounts for about 10% of total urinary excretion. Nevertheless renal clearance of ^{125}I-iothalamate correlates reasonably with inulin clearance[10]. ^{125}I-iothalamate is administered as either a subcutaneous or intravenous single injection; subcutaneous injection has the advantage that slow absorption of the marker allows relatively stable plasma concentration and reduces the dose required. Preadministration of oral

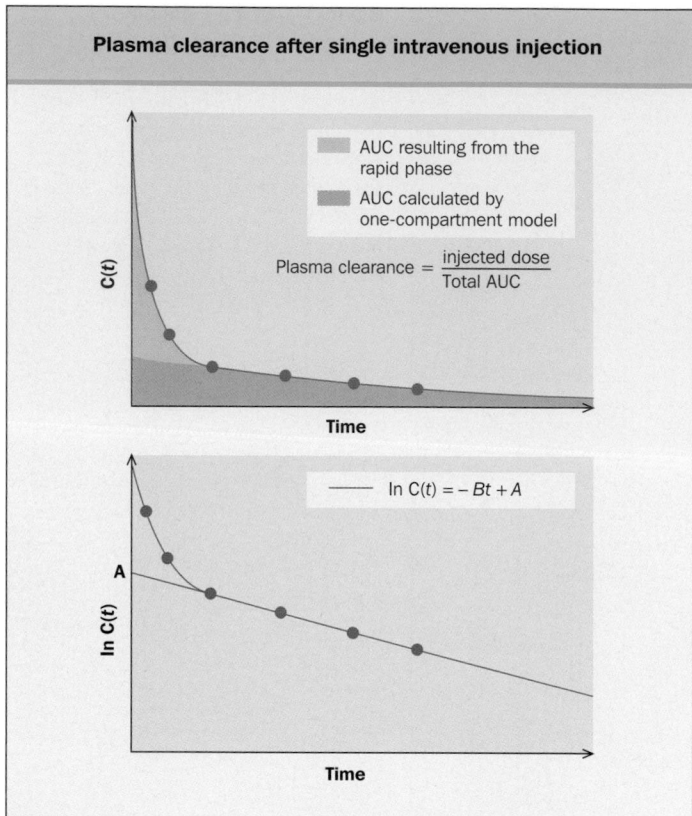

Plasma clearance after single intravenous injection

AUC resulting from the rapid phase

AUC calculated by one-compartment model

$$\text{Plasma clearance} = \frac{\text{injected dose}}{\text{Total AUC}}$$

$\ln C(t) = -Bt + A$

Figure 3.8 Plasma clearance after single intravenous injection.
Linear and semilogarithmic plots are shown. The plasma concentration during the slow phase is expressed as $\ln C(t) = -Bt + A$. The injected amount of the marker is assumed to be totally excreted. Therefore, plasma clearance is calculated by injected dose and total AUC. When a one-compartment model is assumed, the shaded area below the slope of the line is used as AUC for calculating clearance. This method needs a correction due to the part of AUC resulting from the rapid phase (see text).

iodine is required to prevent uptake and concentration of the isotope by the thyroid.

[51]Cr-EDTA is widely used as a filtration marker in Europe. The renal clearance of ^{51}Cr-EDTA is about 10% lower than simultaneously measured inulin clearance, which is probably due to plasma-protein binding, tubular reabsorption, or *in-vivo* dissociation of the chelate.

The renal clearance of ^{99m}Tc-DTPA is slightly lower than simultaneously measured inulin clearance probably as a result of plasma-protein binding. Plasma clearance of ^{99m}Tc-DTPA with the single injection method correlates well with inulin and ^{51}Cr-EDTA clearance. The advantage of ^{99m}Tc-DTPA is that its half-life is only 6 hours and so radiation exposure is minimized.

Nonradioactive materials have also been introduced as filtration markers. Levels of nonradioactive iothalamate and iohexol can be measured by X-ray fluorescence assay or high performance liquid chromatography. Iohexol has less protein-binding activity and tubular secretion compared with iothalamate. Its renal and plasma clearances correlate well with clearances of ^{125}I-iothalamate and inulin. Extrarenal clearance of iohexol is 2–3 mL/min per 1.73 m².

Although relatively cumbersome, these single injection filtration marker techniques for measurement of GFR are more accurate than those based on creatinine measurements. They are a mandatory feature of clinical trials investigating the progression of chronic renal failure.

The estimates of GFR used in clinical practice are summarized in Table 3.1.

NORMAL VALUES AND VARIATIONS IN GLOMERULAR FILTRATION RATE

GFR may be used uncorrected to evaluate changes in renal function in an individual patient. But GFR is affected by age, sex, and body size and must therefore be adjusted for body surface area for comparison with other individuals and with reference ranges. Traditionally, GFR has been expressed per 1.73 m² surface area, the mean surface area of young adults. Surface area can be estimated from a nomogram of height and weight.

Neonatal GFR adjusted for surface area is almost half the adult value[11]. It increases to the adult level by approximately 2 years of age[11] and thereafter is stable until the age of 40. The mean values of GFR in young adults are about 130 mL/min per 1.73 m² for men and about 120 mL/min per 1.73 m² for women, with a coefficient of variation of 14–18%. Age-related decline of GFR of nearly 10 mL/min per 1.73 m² per decade is typical after the age of 40. The mean value of GFR at 80 years of age is almost half the value of a young adult[12]. During pregnancy GFR increases about 50% in the first trimester and returns to normal immediately after delivery.

GFR has a diurnal rhythm; it is 10% higher in the afternoon than at midnight. A high-protein meal or an infusion of amino acids also increase GFR. Both GFR and renal plasma flow rise within an hour following a meal which includes meat. A transient reduction of GFR occurs during exercise.

MEASUREMENT OF RENAL PLASMA FLOW

p-Aminohippurate (PAH) is almost completely removed from the plasma during the first pass through the kidney. Therefore, renal clearance of PAH has been commonly used as an estimate of renal plasma flow (RPF). Renal blood flow (RBF) is obtained by dividing RPF by (1 – hematocrit). The RPF determined by the PAH clearance is termed the effective RPF (ERPF) because part of the renal blood flow perfuses a region which does not contribute to PAH secretion. The PAH clearance is approximately 10% lower than true RPF. The mean values of ERPF in young adults are about 650 mL/min per 1.73 m² for men and about 600 mL/min per 1.73 m² for women with a coefficient of variation of 25%. Conventional measurement of PAH clearance requires continuous infusion. PAH is secreted in the proximal tubule by carrier-mediated mechanisms. Excessive PAH administration results in underestimation of RPF since tubular secretion of PAH is saturated at high plasma concentrations. There is a larger variation in values for ERPF obtained by single injection with timed urine collection, probably because of the difference in arterial and peripheral venous PAH values. Plasma clearance with single injection of radioactive materials such as ^{131}I-hippuran or ^{99m}Tc-mercaptoacetyltriglycine (MAG3) are alternative methods for measurement of RPF.

Measurement of glomerular filtration rate in clinical practice		
Test	Method	Comments
Plasma creatinine	Random blood sample	Simple Inaccurate especially with mild renal impairment Reduced with low muscle mass Raised following cooked meat meal Affected by some drugs – altered tubule secretion (Fig. 3.5) Drug influences on assays (Fig. 3.5)
Creatinine clearance	24-h urine collection and blood sample	Urine collections unreliable Overestimates glomerular filtration rate (tubular secretion of creatinine) Drug influences creatinine assays (Fig. 3.5)
Estimated creatinine clearance (Cockcroft–Gault formula) (Fig. 3.6a)	Random blood sample	Avoids urine collection More accurate than plasma creatinine especially with mild renal impairment Underestimates in obesity Overestimates on low protein diet
Estimated glomerular filtration rate (equation from MDRD study) (Fig. 3.6b, Fig. 3.7)	Random blood sample	Avoid urine collection Better estimation of glomerular filtration rate than creatinine clearance or estimate by Cockcroft–Gault formula Not tested in persons with extreme low serum albumin concentration
Plasma clearance *isotopic*: ^{125}I-iothalamate ^{51}Cr-EDTA ^{99m}Tc-DTPA *non-isotopic*: iodothalamate iohexol	Single i.v. injection and at least two, timed blood samples	Best approximation to true glomerular filtration rate Invasive May use radioisotopes Not often needed in routine clinical care Mandatory in clinical trials investigating progressive renal failure

Table 3.1 Measurement of glomerular filtration rate in clinical practice.

MARKERS OF TUBULAR DAMAGE

Low molecular weight proteins

Low molecular weight proteins in plasma are readily filtered by the glomerulus, and are subsequently reabsorbed by the proximal tubule in normal subjects, with the result that only small amounts of the filtered proteins appear in the urine. The urinary excretion of these proteins rises when proximal tubular reabsorption is impaired. Since there is no distal tubular reabsorption, measurement of urinary low molecular weight proteins has been widely accepted as a marker of proximal tubular damage. β_2-Microglobulin (β_2-M; 11 800 Da), the light chain of the class I major histocompatibility antigens and α_1-Macroglobulin (α, M; 33 000 Da), a glycosylated protein synthesized in the liver, are measured in clinical practice. β_2-M is unstable in acidic urine (pH < 6.0), leading to underestimation; α_1-M is stable and not readily affected by urine pH.

N-acetyl-β-glucosaminidase

N-acetyl-β-glucosaminidase (NAG) is a hydrolytic enzyme distributed throughout the nephron, but its activity is two to four times higher in the proximal tubule than in other nephron segments. The molecular weight of 130 000–140 000 Da is too large for filtration by the glomerulus, so most urinary NAG originates from tubular cells. Urinary NAG excretion rises in tubular cell injury from a variety of insults including drug nephrotoxicity, renal transplant rejection, and tubulointerstitial nephritis. In renal diseases with glomerular proteinuria, a part of urinary NAG may have originated from the plasma and been filtered; since sustained glomerular proteinuria will damage the proximal tubule, this may cause a further rise in urinary NAG. Urinary NAG is therefore useful for the early diagnosis of tubular damage in the absence of glomerular injury. It has been used in the early diagnosis of renal transplant rejection with some success but its main value in clinical practice now lies in the early detection of drug nephrotoxicity. For example, an increase in urinary NAG excretion appears early in the course of aminoglycoside toxicity prior to any increase in plasma creatinine level or the appearance of β_2-M in urine[13].

MEASUREMENT OF TUBULAR FUNCTION

Techniques for assessing proximal and distal tubular function are discussed in the following chapters:
Sodium handling (see Chapter 7).
Concentrating and diluting capacity (see Chapter 8).
Potassium handling (see Chapter 9).
Urinary acidification (see Chapter 11).

REFERENCES

1. Levey AS, Perrone RD, Madias NE. Serum creatinine and renal function. Annu Rev Med. 1988;39:465–90.

2. Shemesh O, Bolbetz H, Kriss JP, Myers BD. Limitations of creatinine as a filtration marker in glomerulopathic patients. Kidney Int. 1985;28:830–8.

3. Hilbrands LB, Artz MA, Wetzels JFM, Koene RAP. Cimetidine improves the reliability of creatinine as a marker of glomerular filtration. Kidney Int. 1991;40:1171–6.

4. Jacobsen FK, Christensen CK, Mogensen CE, Heilskov NSC. Evaluation of kidney function after meals. Lancet. 1980;I:319.

5. Cockcroft DW, Gault MH. Prediction of creatinine clearance from serum creatinine. Nephron. 1976;16:31–4.

6. Horio M, Orita Y, Manabe S, et al. Formula and nomogram for predicting creatinine clearance from serum creatinine concentration. Clin Exp Nephrol. 1997;1:110–14.

7. Levey AS, Bosch JP, Breyer-Lewis J, et al. A more accurate method to estimate glomerular filtration rate from serum creatinine: A new prediction equation. Ann Intern Med. 1999;130:461–70.

8. Lewis J, Agodoa L, Cheek D, et al. Comparison of cross-sectional renal function measurements in African Americans with hypertensive nephrosclerosis and of primary formulas to estimate glomerular filtration rate. Am J Kidney Dis. 2001;38:744–53.

9. Bröchener-Mortensen I. A simple method for the determination of glomerular filtration rate. Scand J Clin Lab Invest. 1972;30:271–4.

10. Levey AS, Greene T, Schluchter MD, et al. Glomerular filtration rate measurements in clinical trials. J Am Soc Nephrol. 1993;14:1159–71.

11. Piepsz A, Pintelon H, Ham HR. Estimation of normal chromium-51 ethylenediamine tetraacetic acid clearance in children. Eur J Nucl Med. 1994;21:12–16.

12. Davies DF, Shock NW. Age changes in glomerular filtration rate, effective renal plasma flow and tubular excretory capacity in adult males. J Clin Invest. 1950;29:496–507.

13. Gibey R, Dupond JL, Alber D, Leconte des Floris R, Henry JC. Predictive value of urinary N-acetyl-β-D-glucosaminidase (NAG), alanine-aminopeptidase (AAP) and β-2-microglobulin (M) in evaluating nephrotoxicity of gentamicin. Clin Chim Acta. 1981;116:25–34.

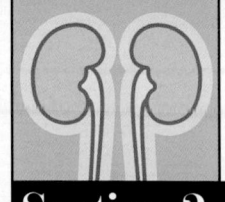
Chapter 4	**Urinalysis**
	Giovanni B Fogazzi

INTRODUCTION

Urinalysis is one of the basic tests to evaluate the presence and severity of kidney and urinary tract disease. This chapter describes the physico-chemical features of the urine as well as urine microscopy. Evaluation of urine chemistry, enzymuria and urine culture are covered elsewhere.

COLLECTION OF SPECIMENS

The way urine is collected and handled in the laboratory is of the highest importance since this can greatly influence the results. Recent European urinalysis guidelines[1] suggest that written instructions are given to the patient about urine collection. Strenuous physical exercise (e.g., running or a soccer match) must be avoided in the 72 h preceding the collection, to avoid exercise-induced proteinuria and/or hematuria or cylindruria[2]. In females, urinalysis should also be avoided during menstruation, since blood contamination can easily occur.

After the washing of hands, females should spread the labia, and males withdraw the foreskin of the glans. The external genitalia are then washed and wiped dry with a paper towel, and the urine is collected after discarding the first portion[1]. The same procedures can also be used for children, while for small infants bags for urine are often used, even though these carry a high probability of contamination. A suprapubic bladder puncture may occasionally be necessary. Urine can also be collected through a bladder catheter. However, this may cause hematuria in itself[3], while permanent indwelling catheters are almost invariably associated with bacteriuria, leucocyturia, hematuria, and candiduria.

The container for urine should be provided by the laboratory or bought in a pharmacy. It should be clean, and have a capacity of at least 50–100 mL, with a diameter opening of at least 5 cm to allow easy collection of urine by both female and male. It should also have a wide base to avoid accidental spillage and should be capped[1].

Several elements (but especially leukocytes) can lyse rapidly after collection, and the best means to preserve the specimens to minimize this is uncertain. Refrigeration of specimens at +2°C to +8°C assists preservation, but may allow precipitation of phosphates or urates, which can hamper examination of the sample. Formaldehyde, glutaraldehyde[4], and 'cellFIX', a formaldehyde-based fixative[5], have been found to be good particle preservatives for the formed elements of urine.

PHYSICAL PARAMETERS

Color

In normal conditions the color of urine ranges from pale to dark yellow and amber, depending on the concentration of the urochrome. Abnormal changes in color can be due to pathologic conditions, drugs, or foods.

The main *pathologic conditions* which can cause color changes of the urine are: gross hematuria, hemoglobinuria, myoglobinuria (pink, red, brown, or black urine); jaundice (dark yellow to brown urine); chyluria (white milky urine); massive uric acid crystalluria (pink urine); porphyrinuria and alkaptonuria (urine red to black upon standing).

The main *drugs* which can be responsible for abnormal urine color are: rifampin (rifampicin) (yellow-orange to red urine); phenytoin (red urine); chloroquine and nitrofurantoin (brown urine); triamterene and blue dyes of enteral feeds (green urine); methylene blue (blue urine); metronidazole, methyldopa, and imipenem-cilastatin (darkening upon standing).

Among *foods* it is worth remembering: beetroot (red urine), senna and rhubarb (yellow to brown or red urine), carotene (brown urine).

Turbidity

Normal urine is usually transparent. Urine can be turbid due to an increased concentration of any urine particle. The most frequent causes of turbidity are heavy hematuria, urinary tract infections, and contamination from genital secretions. The absence of turbidity is not a reliable criterion to judge a urine sample, since pathological samples can be perfectly clear.

Odor

Some rare pathologic conditions confer a characteristic odor to the urine. These are maple-syrup urine disease (maple syrup odor), phenylketonuria (musty or mousy odor), isovaleric acidemia (sweety feet odor) and hypermethioninemia (rancid butter or fishy odor). Ketones may confer a sweet or fruity odor to urine, while bacterial urinary tract infection is often associated with a pungent odor, which is due to the production of ammonia.

Relative density

Relative density can be measured by a number of methods:

Specific gravity is a function of the number and weight of the dissolved particles. It is usually measured by a urinometer, which is a weighted float marked with a scale from 1.000 to

1.060. The urinometer is simple and quick to use, but it needs at least 25 mL of urine. In addition, specific gravity is influenced by urine temperature, proteins, glucose, and radiocontrast media.

Refractometry is based on measurement of the refractive index, which depends on the weight of solutes per unit volume. Refractometers are simple to use and have the major advantage of requiring only one drop of urine. However, the factors which can interfere with specific gravity can also interfere with refractometry.

Osmolality depends on the number of particles present. It is not influenced by urine temperature and protein concentrations. However, high glucose concentrations significantly increases osmolality (10 g/L of glucose = 55.5 mOsmol/L).

Dry chemistry has been incorporated into dipsticks. In the presence of cations, protons are released by a complexing agent and produce a color change in the indicator bromthymol blue from blue via blue-green to yellow. This method is widely used, but does not strictly correlate with the results obtained by refractometry[6].

CHEMICAL PARAMETERS

pH

pH is generally evaluated by a dipstick in which a mixed pH indicator covers the pH range 5 to 8.5–9. Since significant deviations from true pH are observed for values less than 5.5 and greater than 7.5, a pH meter with a glass electrode is preferable for accurate measurements.

Hemoglobin

Hemoglobin is usually detected by a dipstick based on the pseudoperoxidase activity of the heme moiety of hemoglobin which catalyzes the reaction of a peroxide and a chromogen to produce a coloured product. The presence of hemoglobin is shown as green spots, which are due to intact erythrocytes, or as a homogenous diffuse green pattern. The latter is common with marked hematuria, due to the high number of erythrocytes which cover the whole pad surface. It may also be observed if lysis of erythrocytes has occurred on standing, or as a consequence of alkaline urine pH and/or a low relative density (especially below 1.010). A homogeneous pattern may also be found in the absence of hematuria due to free hemoglobinuria deriving from intravascular hemolysis or myoglobinuria secondary to rhabdomyolysis.

Glucose

Glucose is also commonly detected by dipstick. Glucose, with glucose oxidase as catalyst, is first oxidized to gluconic acid and hydrogen peroxide. Then, through the catalysing activity of a peroxidase, hydrogen peroxide reacts with a reduced colorless chromogen to form a colored product. This test is sensitive to concentration of 0.5 to 20 g/L. When more precise quantification of urine glucose is needed, enzymatic methods such as hexokinase are used.

Protein

Physiological proteinuria does not exceed 150 mg/24 h for adults and 140 mg/m² for children. In pathological conditions, the following types of proteinuria can be distinguished[7]:

- *Glomerular proteinuria.* This occurs in glomerular diseases and is due to abnormal glomerular permeability to proteins (example: albumin, globulins).
- *Tubular proteinuria.* This occurs in tubular and interstitial renal diseases and is caused by a reduced reabsorption of low molecular weight proteins which are normally ultrafiltered at glomerular level (example: α_1-microglobulin, β_2-microglobulin, retinol-binding protein).
- *Overload proteinuria.* This is due to the increased production or release of low molecular weight proteins which, after passing the glomerular barrier, exceed the reabsorption capacity of the tubules (example: light chain immunoglobulins (Bence-Jones proteinuria), lysozyme, myoglobin)
- *Benign proteinuria*, this includes idiopathic transient proteinuria, the proteinuria associated with physical exercise or fever, and orthostatic proteinuria.

Proteinuria is usually detected by dipstick. The test is based on the principle of the protein error of a pH indicator which reveals the presence of proteins through a sequential colour change from pale green to green and blue. This method is highly sensitive to albumin (detection limit 0.20 g/L), which has 16 binding sites for the chromogen contained in the pad, while it has little sensitivity to other proteins such as light chains immunoglobulins, which have only 1.5 to 2.0 binding sites for the chromogen. Thus, for Bence-Jones proteinuria, other detection methods should be used such as precipitation techniques, which are based on the turbidity occurring after proteins are precipitated by sulphosalicylic acid, trichloracetic acid or by heat and acetic acid–sodium acetate buffer.

Dipsticks allow only a rough quantification of urine proteins, which is expressed on a scale from 0 to +++ or ++++ according to the manufacturer. For reliable quantification of proteins other methods are necessary, such as turbidimetric, dye-binding, or biuret techniques. Biuret methods are among the most used and recommended. They are based on the interaction between copper ions and the carbamide group of proteins, and have the same sensitivity for all proteins, and minimal interference from drugs, radiographic contrast media, and colored metabolites.

Protein quantification is expressed as g/L or g/24 h. However, the 24-h urine collection is time consuming, subject to error, and scarcely practicable for a number of patients. A practical alternative to the 24-hour urine collection is the measurement of protein:creatinine ratio, which can be calculated in random urine samples[7]. The measurement obtained with this method correlates well with those obtained with the 24-h urine collection. Proteinuria > 3.5 g/24 h corresponds to a ratio > 3.5 (g protein : g creatinine) in single voided specimens, and proteinuria < 0.2 g/24 h corresponds to a ratio < 0.2[7]. The correlation between the two methods has been confirmed in several studies. However, since protein excretion follows a circadian rhythm (highest during the day and lowest overnight) while creatinine excretion is fairly constant over the 24 h, the time of collection may influence the results of protein : creatinine ratio. Therefore the spot sample for protein : creatinine ratio should always be collected at the same time of the day[8].

The qualitative analysis of proteinuria is currently performed by electrophoresis on cellulose acetate or agarose after protein concentration or using very sensitive stains such as silver or gold. Sodium dodecyl sulfate–polyacrylamide gel electrophoresis (SDS–PAGE) can be used to identify the different urine proteins on the basis of molecular weight[9]. Alternatively measurements can be made of the concentration of low molecular weight proteins, such as β_2-microglobulin[10], or a combination of glomerular and tubular proteins such as IgG and α_1-microglobulin[11]. These last techniques have all been used to demonstrate the presence of low-molecular-weight proteins in the urine of patients with glomerulonephritis and their value as predictors of a poor prognosis[9–11].

For the definition of a monoclonal component, immunofixation is the method of choice.

Selectivity of proteinuria in nephrotic syndrome is assessed by the ratio of the clearance of IgG, (molecular weight 160 000) to the clearance of transferrin (molecular weight 88 000)[12]. Highly selective proteinuria, ratio < 0.1, in nephrotic children, suggests the diagnosis of minimal change disease and predicts steroid responsiveness. A recent study suggests that the selectivity of proteinuria combined with SDS–PAGE and the excretion of α_1-microglobulin predicts the outcome and response to therapy in conditions such as minimal change disease, focal segmental glomerulosclerosis, and membranous nephropathy[13].

Leukocyte esterase

This dipstick evaluates the presence of leukocytes on the basis of an indoxyl esterase activity released from *lysed* neutrophil granulocytes and macrophages. This feature explains why, especially in urine with an alkaline pH and/or a low relative density, there frequently is a positive dipstick with negative microscopy.

Nitrites

This dipstick test reveals the presence of bacteria which have the capability of reducing nitrates to nitrites due to nitrate reductase activity, which is present in most Gram-negative uropathogenic bacteria, but low or absent in others such as *Pseudomonas* spp, *Staphylococcus albus*, and *Enterococcus* spp. Test positivity also requires a diet rich in nitrates (vegetables), which form the substrate for nitrite production, and sufficient bladder incubation time. Thus, it is not surprising that the sensitivity of this test is low (20–80%), while specificity is > 90%.

Ketones

This dipstick reveals the presence of acetoacetate and acetone, which are excreted into urine during diabetic acidosis, or during fasting, vomiting, or strenuous exercise. It is based on the reaction of the ketones with nitroprusside.

Table 4.1 shows the false-negative and false-positive results which can occur with the dipsticks described above. Better dipsticks, with fewer interferences, are expected for the future[14].

URINE MICROSCOPY

Urine microscopy is an integral part of urinalysis, and adds valuable information to the physicochemical investigation. However, reliable results can be achieved only with standardized methodology[1]. The urine sediment can contain cells, lipids, casts, crystals, and organisms.

Methods

The first or second urine of the morning should be collected, following the procedures described above (see

Table 4.1 Urine dipstick testing.
False-negative and false-positive results of urine dipsticks.

Urine dipstick testing		
Measurand	False-negative results	False-positive results
Specific gravity	Reduced values in the presence of glucose, urea, alkaline urine	Increased values in the presence of protein > 1 g/L, ketoacids
pH	Reduced values in the presence of formaldehyde	–
Hemoglobin	Ascorbic acid, high nitrite concentration, delayed examination, high density of urine, formaldehyde (0.5 g/L),	Myoglobin, microbial peroxidases, oxidizing detergents, hydrochloric acid
Glucose	Ascorbic acid, urinary tract infection	Oxidizing detergents, hydrochloric acid
Albumin	Immunoglobulin light chains, hydrochloric acid, tubular proteins, globulins, colored urine	Alkaline urine (pH 9), quaternary ammonium detergents, chlorhexidine, polyvinylpyrrolidone
Leukocyte esterase	Isotonic urine, vitamin C (intake g/day), protein > 5 g/L, glucose > 20 g/L, mucous specimen, cephalosporins, nitrofurantoin; mercuric salts, trypsin inhibitor oxalate, 1% boric acid	Oxidizing detergents, formaldehyde (0.4 g/L), sodium azide, colored urine due to beet ingestion, or bilirubin
Nitrites	No vegetables in diet, short bladder incubation time, vitamin C, Gram-positive bacteria	Colored urine
Ketones	Improper storage	Free sulfhydryl groups (e.g., captopril) L-dopa, colored urine

Procedures for preparation and examination of the urine sediment

- Written instructions to the patients for urine collection
- Collection in disposable containers of the second urine of the morning after discarding the first few mL of urine
- Sample handling and analysis within 2 h from collection
- Centrifugation of a 10 mL aliquot of urine at 400 **g** for 10 min
- Removal by suction of 9.5 mL of supernatant urine
- Gentle but thorough resuspension with a pipette of the sediment in the remaining 0.5 mL of urine
- Transfer by a pipette of 50 µL of resuspended urine to a slide
- Covering of sample with a 24 × 32 mm coverslip
- Examination of the urine sediment by a phase contrast microscope at ×160 and ×400
- Use of polarized light to identify doubtful lipids and crystals
- Match the microscopic findings with dipstick for pH, density, hemoglobin and leukocyte esterase
- Cells expressed as lowest–highest number seen/high power field, casts as number/low power field, all the other elements on a scale from 0 to ++++

Table 4.2 Procedures for preparation and examination of the urine sediment.

'Urine collection'). Then, as soon as possible to avoid the lysis of elements, an aliquot of urine is centrifuged and concentrated, after which a standardized volume of resuspended urine should be transferred to the slide and covered with a coverslip of defined size. Alternatively, a counting chamber can be used. A binocular phase contrast microscope equipped with adequate magnifications and polarizing light is requested (Table 4.2).

An adequate number of microscopic fields, in different areas of the sample, should be examined at both low and high magnification, with the use of polarizing light when necessary (e.g., for the identification of fatty particles containing cholesterol or to identify some types of crystals). For a correct examination, both pH and relative density of the sample should be known. Both alkaline pH and low relative density (especially < 1.010) favor the lysis of erythrocytes and leukocytes, which can cause discrepancies between dipstick readings and the microscopic examination (see above: 'Hemoglobin' and 'Leukocyte esterase'). In addition, alkaline pH prevents the formation of casts and favors the precipitation of phosphates.

When slides and coverslips are used, the elements observed are quantified as number/microscopic field, while when counting chambers are used the elements are quantified as number/mL.

Cells

The cells of the urine sediment derive from the circulation (i.e., erythrocytes and leukocytes) and from the epithelia lining the urinary tract (i.e., renal tubular cells, uroepithelial cells, and squamous cells).

Erythrocytes

There are two types of urinary erythrocytes: isomorphic, with regular shapes and contours, and dysmorphic, with irregular shapes and contours (Fig. 4.1a,b). The former derive from the

urinary excretory system, while dysmorphic erythrocytes are of glomerular origin[15]. When isomorphic erythrocytes predominate (≥ 80% of total erythrocytes) the hematuria is defined as nonglomerular, while when dysmorphic erythrocytes prevail (≥ 80% of total erythrocytes) the hematuria is defined as glomerular[16]. According to some investigators, a diagnosis of glomerular hematuria can also be made when the two types of cells are in the same proportion (so-called mixed hematuria)[17], or when at least 5% of erythrocytes examined are represented by acanthocytes[18]. These are a subtype of dysmorphic erythrocytes with a characteristic appearance which is due to the presence of one or more blebs protruding from a ring-shaped body (Fig. 4.1b). Erythrocyte dysmorphism is thought to be the result of a dual injury: deformation of the erythrocyte while passing through gaps of the glomerular basement membrane followed by physicochemical insults occurring while the erythrocyte passes through the tubular system[19].

This approach is of particular importance for the management of patients with isolated microscopic hematuria, allowing an early separation of patients with glomerular disease from those with a urological cause of the hematuria[20]. However, the evaluation of erythrocyte morphology is subjective and requires experience, which has limited its widespread introduction into clinical practice.

Leukocytes

Neutrophils are the leukocytes most frequently found in the urine. They are easily identified, due to their granular cytoplasm and lobulated nucleus (Fig. 4.1c).

Neutrophils are a marker of lower and upper urinary tract infections. However, especially in young women, they are frequently found due to urine contamination from genital secretions. They can also be found in glomerulonephritis, especially the proliferative forms, and interstitial nephritis.

Eosinophils, once considered a marker of acute allergic interstitial nephritis are now regarded as nonspecific elements, found in various types of glomerulonephritis, prostatitis, chronic pyelonephritis, urinary schistosomiasis, etc.[21,22].

Lymphocytes are an early marker of acute cellular rejection in renal allograft recipients, but their identification requires staining, and this technique is not used in clinical practice.

Renal tubular cells

These cells derive from the exfoliation of the tubular epithelium. Tubular cells in the urine differ in size and shape (from roundish to rectangular or columnar) (Figs 4.1d).

Tubular cells are found in acute tubular necrosis, acute interstitial nephritis, and acute cellular rejection of a renal allograft. In smaller numbers they are also found in glomerulonephritis. In the nephrotic syndrome they may contain variable amounts of lipids.

Uroepithelial cells

These cells derive from the exfoliation of the uroepithelium, which lines the urinary tract from calyces to the bladder in women, and to the proximal urethra in men. It is a multilayered epithelium, with small cells in the deep layers, and much larger cells in the superficial layers.

The cells of the deep layers (Fig. 4.1e), when in large amounts, are a marker of urological diseases, such as obstructing lithiasis or neoplasia, or uroepithelial damage caused by bladder or urethral catheters[23].

The cells of the superficial layers (Fig. 4.1f) are a common finding, especially in urinary tract infections.

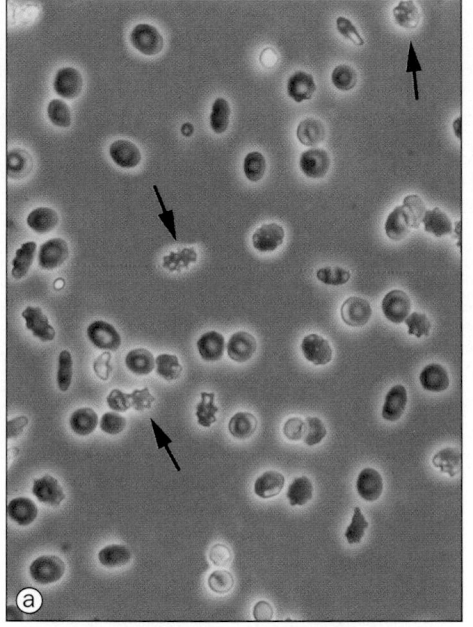

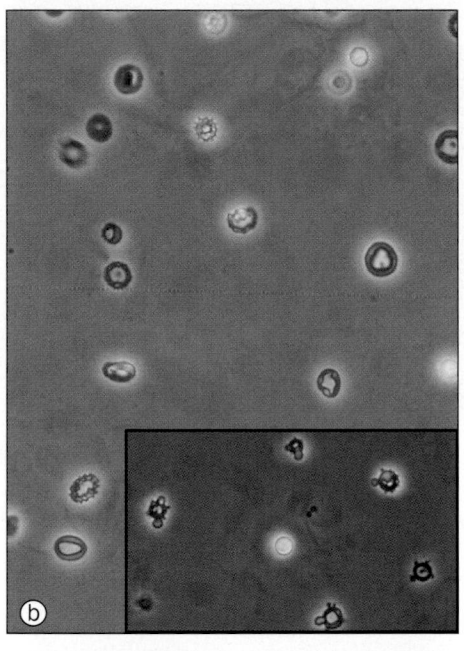

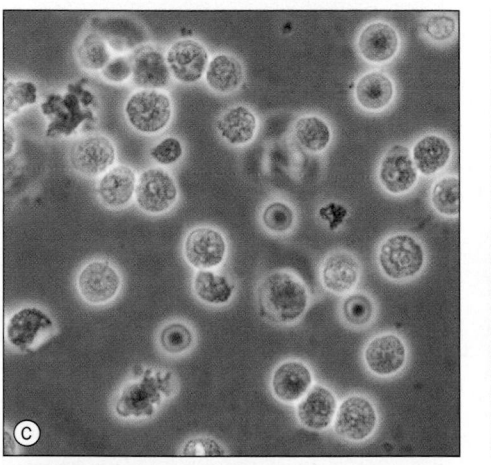

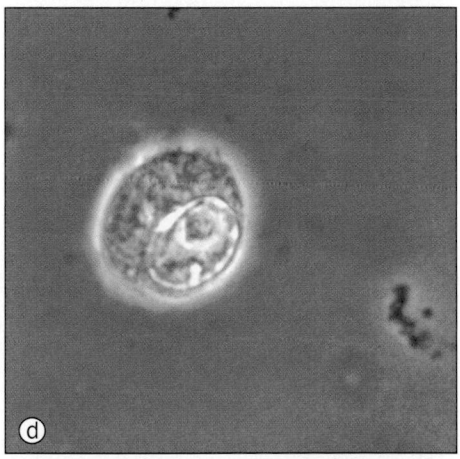

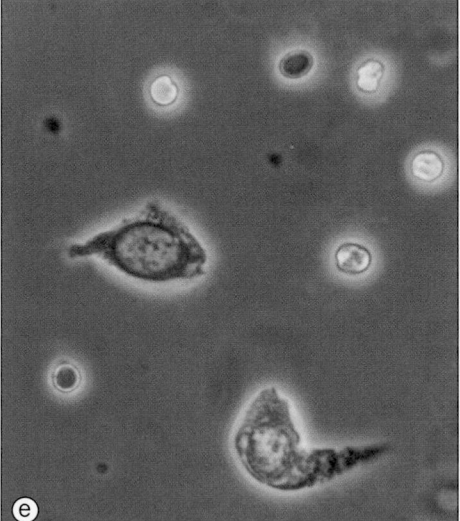

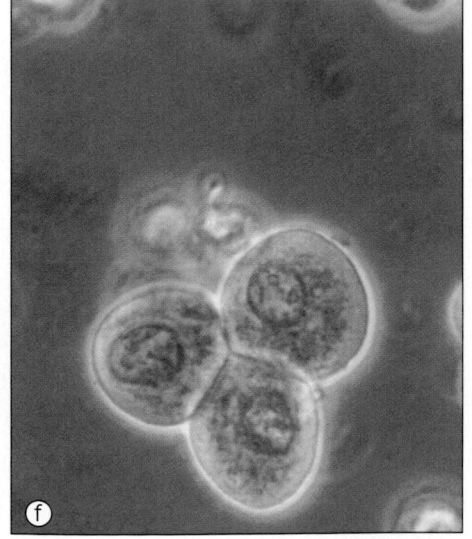

Figure 4.1 Urinary sediment cells.
(a) Isomorphic non-glomerular erythrocytes. The arrows indicate the so-called crenated erythrocytes, which are a frequent finding in non-glomerular hematuria. (b) Dysmorphic glomerular erythrocytes. The dysmorphism is mainly due to irregularities of the cell membrane (phase contrast microscopy, original magnification ×400). Inset: Acanthocytes. A ring-formed cell body with one or more blebs of different size and shape. These cells are the most reliable marker of a glomerular bleeding (phase contrast microscopy, original magnification ×400). (c) Neutrophils. Note their typical lobulated nucleus and granular cytoplasm (phase contrast microscopy, original magnification ×400). (d) An ovoid renal tubular cell. The nucleus is large and the cytoplasm is granular. (e) Two cells from the deep layers of the uroepithelium. (f) Three cells from the superficial layers of the uroepithelium. Note the difference in shape and nucleus/cytoplasm ratio existing between the two types of uroepithelial cells (phase contrast microscopy, original magnification ×400).

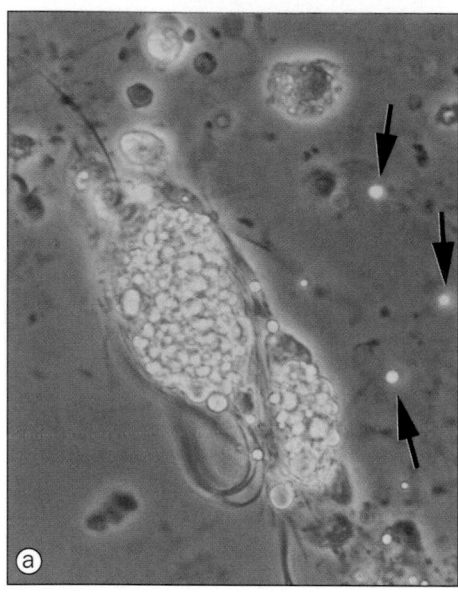
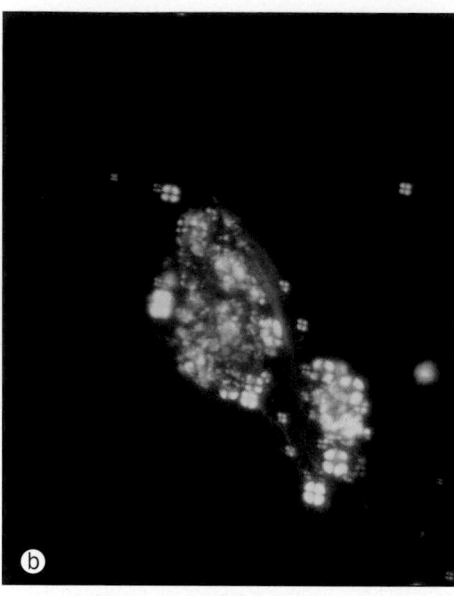

Squamous cells

These cells derive from the urethra or from the external genitalia. When in large amounts they indicate urine contamination from genital secretions.

Lipids

Lipids in the urine have the appearance of spherical, translucent and yellow drops of different size. They can be free in the urine (isolated or in clusters) or fill the cytoplasm of tubular epithelial cells or macrophages[24]. The latter are known as oval fat bodies. When entrapped within casts, lipids form fatty casts. Finally, they can also appear as cholesterol crystals (see Crystals).

Lipid drops contain mainly cholesterol esters and free cholesterol, and under polarized light appear as 'Maltese crosses' (Fig. 4.2).

Lipids in the urine are typical of glomerular diseases associated with marked proteinuria, usually but not invariably in the nephrotic range. They can also be found in sphyngolipidoses such as Fabry's disease. In this condition they appear as irregular large fat droplets, which form Maltese crosses under polarized light and show typical myelin bodies with electron microscopy.

Casts

Casts are elements with a cylindrical shape which form in the lumen of distal renal tubules and collecting ducts. Their matrix is Tamm–Horsfall glycoprotein, which is physiologically secreted by the cells of the thick ascending limb of the loop of Henle. Various factors such as increased concentration of urine electrolytes, hydrogen ions, ultrafiltered serum proteins, etc. stimulate the secretion and the polymerization of Tamm–Horsfall glycoprotein within the tubular lumen and hence increase the formation of casts.

Trapping of particles within the cast matrix, results in casts with different appearances and clinical significance (Table 4.3).

Hyaline casts are colorless elements, with a low refractive index (Fig. 4.3a). Therefore, they are easily seen with phase

Clinical significance of urinary casts	
Cast	**Main clinical Associations**
Hyaline	Normal subject Renal disease
Granular	Renal disease
Waxy	Renal insufficiency Rapidly progressive Glomerulonephritis
Fatty	Marked proteinuria Nephrotic syndrome
Erythrocyte	Glomerular bleeding Proliferative/necrotizing glomerulonephritis
Hemoglobin	Glomerular bleeding Proliferative/necrotizing glomerulonephritis Hemoglobinuria
Leukocyte	Acute pyelonephritis Acute interstitial nephritis Proliferative glomerulonephritis
Epithelial	Acute tubular necrosis Acute interstitial nephritis Glomerulonephritis
Myoglobin	Rhabdomyolysis

Table 4.3 Clinical significance of urinary casts.

contrast microscopy, but can be overlooked when bright field microscopy is used. Hyaline casts can be present in normal conditions. They are also seen in patients with a renal disease, when they are associated with other types of casts.

Granular casts contain fine granules (Fig. 4.3a), due to lysosomes containing ultrafiltered serum proteins, or coarse granules, due to degenerated cells entrapped in the matrix of the cast. Granular casts are typical of patients with a renal disease.

Waxy casts derive their name from their appearance, which is similar to that of melted wax (Fig. 4.3b). They are large with hard edges, which are often also indented. Waxy casts are typical of patients with renal failure. In the author's experience

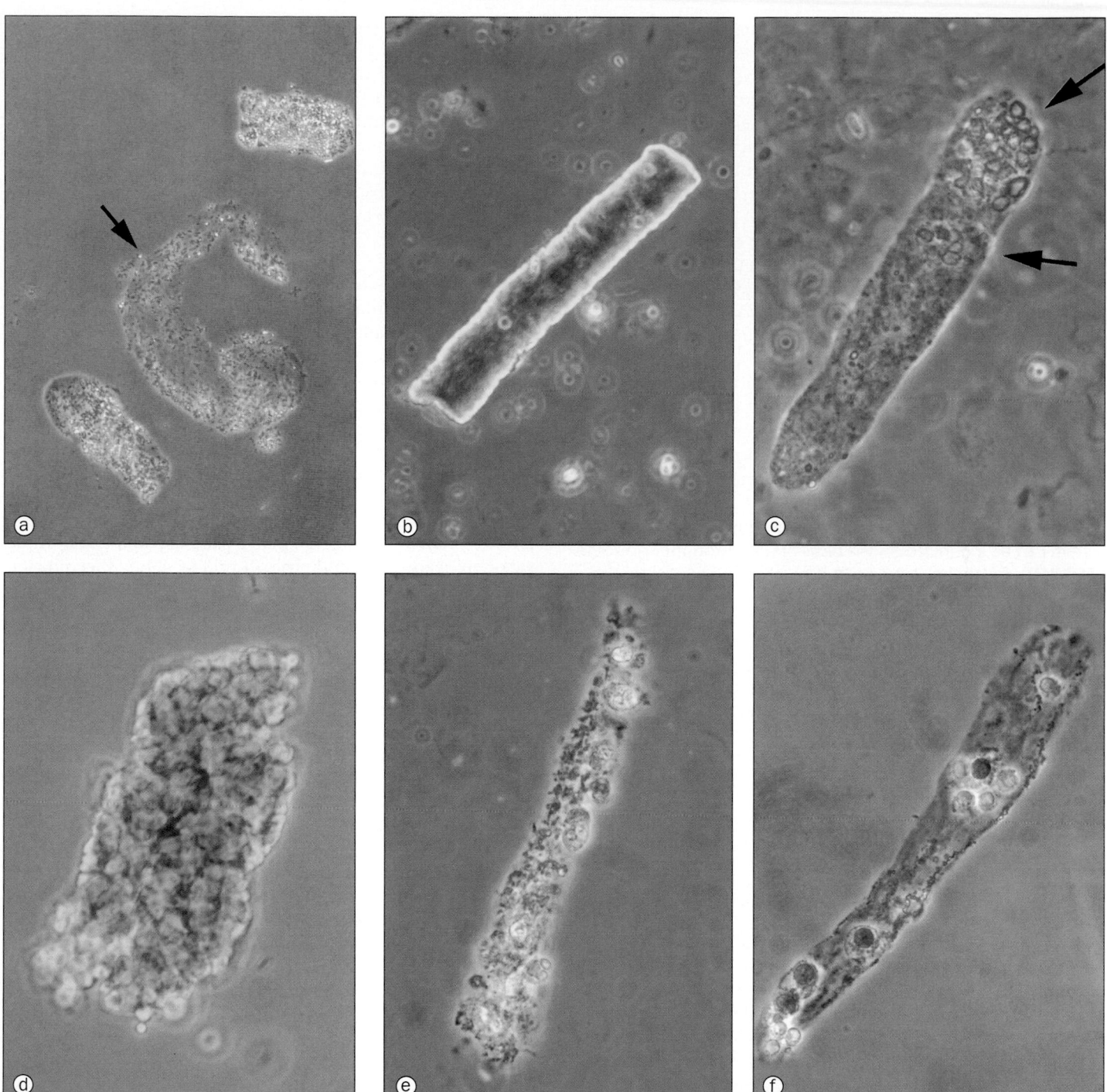

Figure 4.3 Casts. (a,b) **Finely granular cast** (arrow). The two other elements shown are hyaline granular casts, which are also frequent in patients with a glomerular disease (phase contrast microscopy, original magnification ×160). (b) **Waxy cast.** Note the typical appearance of melted wax and the hard edges (phase contrast microscopy, original magnification ×400). (c) **Erythrocyte cast.** The arrows indicate the erythrocytes embedded in the matrix of the cast. (d) **Hemoglobin cast.** It is identifiable by its typical brownish hue (phase contrast microscopy, original magnification ×400). (e) **Leukocyte cast.** The polymorphonuclear leukocytes are easily identifiable due to their lobulated nucleus (phase contrast microscopy, original magnification ×400). (f) **Epithelial cast.** It contains both large ovoid cells deriving from the proximal tubular segments (bottom) and smaller cells deriving from the distal tubular segments (top) (phase contrast microscopy, original magnification ×400).

they are also a frequent finding in the urine of patients with rapidly progressive glomerulonephritis.

Fatty casts contain variable amounts of lipid droplets, either isolated, in clumps, or packed. They are typical of glomerular diseases associated with marked proteinuria or the nephrotic syndrome.

Erythrocyte casts may contain a few erythrocytes, or so many that the matrix of the cast cannot be identified (Fig. 4.3c).

These casts are found in patients with hematuria, indicating that it is of glomerular origin. Therefore, erythrocyte casts are of particular importance in patients with isolated microscopic hematuria, since they orientate the diagnosis towards a renal disease. When looked for carefully they can be found in up to 85% of patients with a hematuric glomerulonephritis[25]. Erythrocyte casts also are a hallmark of proliferative glomerulonephritis, especially when this is associated with extracapillary/necrotizing lesions.

Hemoglobin casts have a brownish hue and, often, a granular appearance deriving from the degradation of erythrocytes entrapped within the casts (Fig. 4.3d). Therefore, hemoglobin casts have the same clinical meaning as erythrocyte casts. However, they may also derive from free hemoglobinuria in patients with intravascular hemolysis.

Leukocyte casts contain variable amounts of polymorphonuclear leukocytes (Fig. 4.3e). They are found in acute pyelonephritis and acute interstitial nephritis. However, they can also be found in proliferative glomerulonephritis, and especially in acute post-infectious glomerulonephritis and diffuse proliferative lupus nephritis.

Epithelial casts contain variable numbers of tubular cells, which can be identified on the basis of their prominent nucleus (Fig. 4.3f). Epithelial casts are a typical finding in acute tubular necrosis and acute interstitial nephritis of whatever cause. However, they are also frequent in glomerular disorders and in the nephrotic syndrome.

Myoglobin casts contain myoglobin and may be identical to hemoglobin casts (Fig. 4.3d), from which they can be distinguished through the knowledge of the clinical findings. They are found in the urine of patients with acute renal failure associated with rhabdomyolysis.

Crystals

There are several types of urine crystals, for whose identification the knowledge of morphology, urine pH, and appearance under polarizing light is mandatory[26,27]. The following are the main crystals of the urine:

Uric acid crystals and amorphous urates

Uric acid crystals have a typical amber color, and a wide spectrum of appearances, which range from rhomboids to barrels, to less defined shapes (Fig. 4.4a). These crystals are found only in acid urine (pH ≤ 5.8), and under polarizing light show a beautiful polychromatic appearance.

Amorphous urates are tiny granules of irregular shape, which also precipitate in acid urine. They are identical to amorphous phosphates, which however precipitate in alkaline pH. In addition, while urates polarize light, phosphates do not.

Calcium oxalate crystals

There are two types of calcium oxalate crystals. Bihydrated (or Wedellite) crystals most often a bipyramidal appearance (Fig. 4.4b), while monohydrated (or Whewellite) crystals are ovoid, dumb-bells, or biconcave disks (Fig. 4.4c). Both types of calcium oxalate crystals precipitate at pH 5.4 to 6.7. Bihydrated crystals do not polarize light while monohydrated crystals do.

Calcium phosphate crystals and amorphous phosphates

Calcium phosphate crystals are among the most pleiomorphic crystals, appearing as prisms, star-like particles, needles of various size and shape (Fig. 4.4d). They can also appear as plates with a granular surface. These crystals precipitate in alkaline urine (pH ≥ 7.0) and, with the exception of plates, they polarize light intensely.

Amorphous phosphates are tiny particles identical to amorphous urates. However, they precipitate at pH of ≥ 7.0 and do not polarize light.

Triple phosphate crystals

These crystals contain magnesium ammonium phosphate, and in most instances have the appearance of 'coffin lids' (Fig. 4.4e). They are found only in alkaline urine (pH ≥ 7.0) using polarized light.

Cholesterol crystals

They are transparent and thin plates, often clumped together, with sharp edges (Fig. 4.4f).

Cystine crystals

These crystals are hexagonal plates with irregular sides, which are often heaped one upon the other (Fig. 4.4g). They precipitate only in acid urine, especially after the addition of acetic acid and after overnight storage at 4°C.

2,8 Dihydroxyadenine crystals

They are spherical, brownish crystals with radial striations from the center, which polarize light strongly[28].

Crystals due to drugs

Many drugs can cause transient crystalluria. These may be crystals of the drug itself – including the sulphonamide sulfadiazine (Fig. 4.4h), the antiviral agents acyclovir (birefringent needles) and indinavir (Fig 4.4i), the diuretic triamterene, the coronary dilator piridoxylate, and the barbiturate primidone. Or the drug may promote monohydrated calcium oxalate crystals, as with naftidrofuryl oxalate or vitamin C[26,27] (Fig. 4.4i).

Clinical significance of crystals

The finding in the urine of a few uric acid, calcium oxalate, or calcium phosphate crystals is not uncommon. In most instances, it is a finding without clinical importance, since it reflects a transient supersaturation of the urine due to ingestion of some foods (e.g., meat for uric acid, spinach or chocolate for calcium oxalate, milk or cheese for calcium phosphate), or mild dehydration. However, such crystals may also be associated with pathological conditions. For instance, the persistence of a calcium oxalate, or uric acid crystalluria in repeated samples may reflect hypercalciuria, hyperoxaluria or hyperuricosuria. Large amounts of uric acid crystals may be associated with acute renal failure due to acute uric acid nephropathy, while large amounts of monohydrated calcium oxalate crystals may be associated with acute renal failure from ethylene glycol intoxication.

Some crystals are always pathologic. This is the case with: cholesterol, which is found in patients with marked proteinuria;

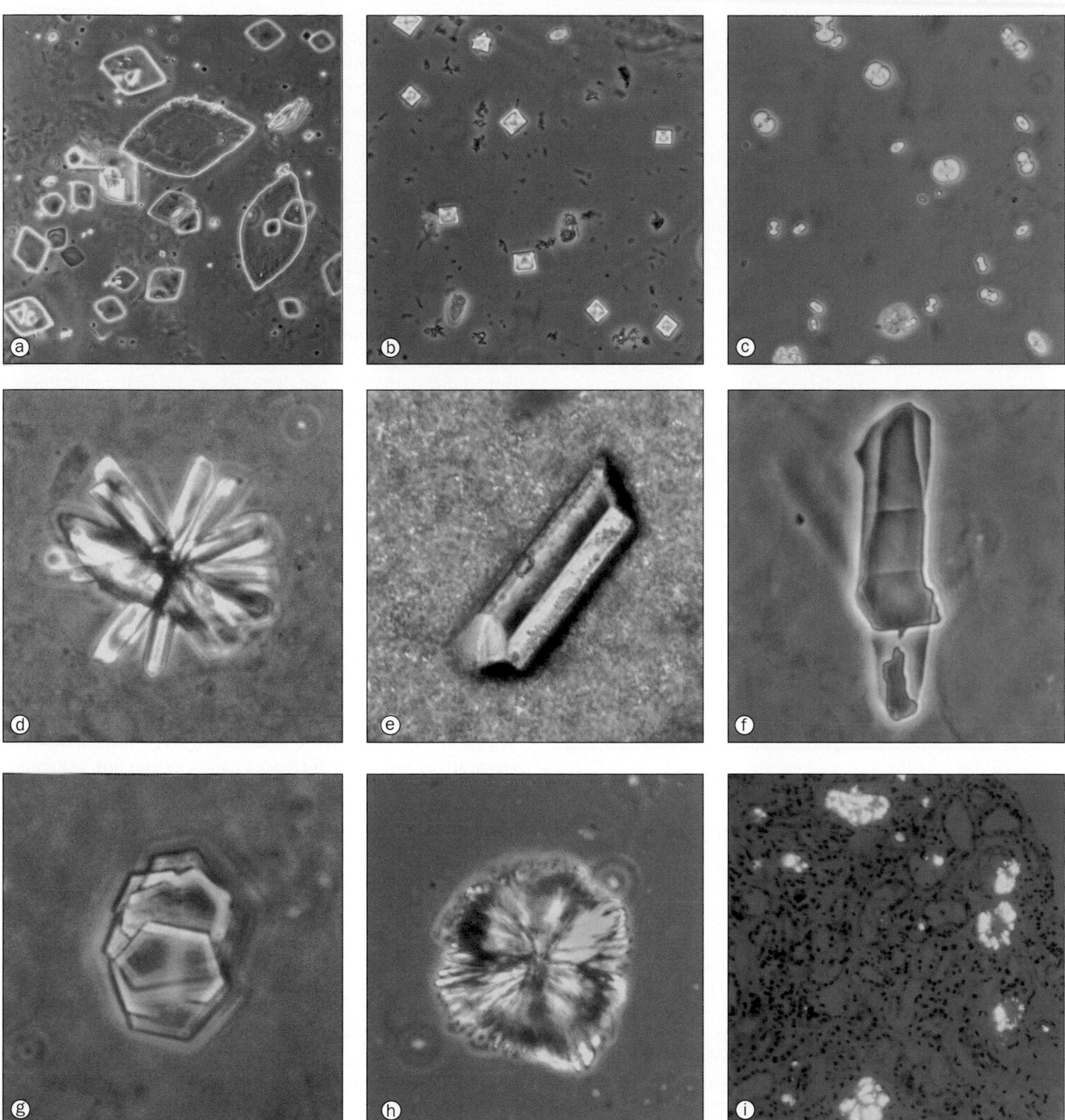

Figure 4.4 Crystals. (a) Uric acid crystals. This rhomboid shape is the most frequent (phase contrast microscopy, original magnification ×400). (b) Bihydrated calcium oxalate crystals. They have the typical appearance of 'letter envelope'. (c) Different types of monohydrated calcium oxalate crystals (phase contrast microscopy, original magnification ×400). (d) A star-like calcium phosphate crystal. (e) Triple phosphate crystal. On the background of a massive amount of amorphous phosphates particles (phase contrast microscopy, original magnification ×400). (f) Cholesterol crystal. (g) Cystine crystals (phase contrast microscopy, original magnification ×400). (h) Sulfadiazine crystal. This has a typical amber color and radial striations (phase contrast microscopy, original magnification ×400). (i) Intratubular precipitation of monohydrated calcium oxalate crystals seen on renal histology. This phenomenon can be caused by drugs such as naftidrofuryl oxalate or vitamin C (polarized light, original magnification ×250).

cystine, which is a marker of cystinuria; 2,8-dihydroxyade-nine, which is a marker of homozygotic deficiency of the enzyme adenine phosphoribosyltransferase, a condition which causes urinary stone formation and/or intra renal precipitation of crystals[28].

Crystalluria may be the only abnormality found, or may be associated with obstructive uropathy caused by stones due to the aggregation of drug crystals, as described for instance, with indinavir[29]), or may even be associated with acute tubular necrosis due to intratubular precipitation of crystals (Fig. 4.4i). This may happen with sulfadiazine, indinavir, naftidrofuryl oxalate, or vitamin C. Acute renal failure occurs especially when large doses of the drug are administered intravenously (for instance, grams of vitamin C are needed to produce oxalate crystalluria) or in the presence of dehydration or hypoalbu-minemia, which increase the blood concentration of the drug.

Organisms

Bacteria are a frequent finding, since urine is usually collected and handled under nonsterile conditions and examination is often delayed. Urine infection can be suspected only if bacteria are found in noncontaminated freshly voided midstream urine, especially if numerous leukocytes are also present[30]. *Candida*, *Trichomonas vaginalis*, and *Enterobius vermicularis* are mostly common contaminants deriving from genital secretions. *Schistosoma hematobium* is a parasite whose eggs are found in the urine, usually in association with hematuria and leukocyturia, as a consequence of infection of the bladder and/or the ureter (see Chapter 56).

INTERPRETATION OF THE MAIN URINE SEDIMENT FINDINGS

Examination of the urine sediment allows the identification of some urinary profiles which, integrated with other urine and blood findings, contribute to the diagnosis of diseases of the urinary tract. These are the main urine sediment profiles:

The nephrotic sediment

The typical nephrotic sediment contains casts, lipids, and tubular cells. Hyaline, hyaline-granular, granular, and fatty casts are seen, while erythrocyte/hemoglobin casts, leukocyte casts, and waxy casts are absent. Lipiduria has been reported in 63% of nephrotics, being more marked in membranous nephropathy and milder and less frequent in minimal change disease[31]. Erythrocytes may be totally absent, especially in minimal change disease, or may be in moderate numbers, which happens in membranous nephropathy and focal segmental glomerulosclerosis. Leukocytes are usually not found.

The nephritic sediment

Hematuria is the hallmark of the nephritic sediment. Moderate-to-marked hematuria is present in virtually all cases. More than 100 erythrocytes/high power field is not uncommon, especially in cases with extracapillary and/or necrotizing glomerular lesions. Leukocyturia is also frequent, about 65% of cases in the author's experience. However, it is usually mild, not exceeding 10 leukocytes/high power field. Erythrocyte/hemoglobin casts are frequent (about 80% of cases). Leukocyte and waxy casts can also be observed.

Under the effect of treatment the nephritic sediment may clear, while its reappearance indicates a relapse of the disease. Therefore, the study of the urine sediment is of special value in recurring proliferative glomerular diseases such as lupus nephritis[32] or systemic vasculitis[33]. However, in rare cases, there may be an active proliferative glomerular disease without the nephritic sediment.

The sediment of acute tubular necrosis

In acute tubular necrosis (ATN), the urine sediment contains marked granular and epithelial casts, and variable numbers of necrotic tubular cells. Epithelial cell casts may predominate at first if there is massive tubular cell injury, but as ATN progresses, the tubular cells become degraded during transit and granular casts are more characteristic, the so-called muddy brown casts of ATN. In addition, depending on the cause of the tubular damage, other elements can be seen. For instance, in rhabdomyolysis myoglobin pigmented casts can also be found, while in ATN due to intratubular precipitation of crystals (e.g., acute uric acid nephropathy, ethylene glycol poisoning, drugs) there may be massive crystalluria.

The sediment of urinary tract infection

Bacteriuria and leukocyturia are the hallmarks of this condition. The correlation between the urine sediment findings and the urine culture is usually good. However, false positive results may occur as a consequence of urine contamination from genital secretions or bacterial overgrowth upon standing. False negative results may be due to misinterpretation of bacteria (especially with cocci) or the lysis of leukocytes.

Minor urinary abnormalities

Besides the urine patterns described above, urine sediments can contain less defined changes, such as variable casts with or without mild erythrocyturia or leukocyturia, mild crystalluria, small number of superficial transitional cells, etc. In such cases the correct interpretation of the urinary findings requires adequate clinical information and the results of other diagnostic tests.

AUTOMATED ANALYSIS OF THE URINE SEDIMENT

Flow cytometry has recently been applied to the analysis of urine sediments. This technique has been incorporated into an instrument in which uncentrifuged samples are first stained with dyes for nucleic acid and cell membranes and then irradiated with laser light. The results appear on a screen as both 'scattergrams' and numeric data[34,35].

Flow cytometry allows the identification and quantification of most particles of urine sediments, including glomerular and nonglomerular erythrocytes based on their different size[36]. However, it does not recognize lipids and some types of crystals, casts, and epithelial cells (uroepithelial cells and renal tubular cells being all classified as 'small round cells')[34,35]. The instrument is programmed to point out the samples of particular complexity for which a microscopic analysis is preferable.

Today flow cytometry is used especially in large laboratories to screen large numbers of samples in short time. This approach greatly reduces the number of samples to be analyzed by microscopy.

REFERENCES

1. Kouri T, Fogazzi G, Gant V, et al. European urinalysis guidelines. Scand J Clin Lab Med. 2000;60(Suppl 231).
2. Fasset RG, Owen JE, Fairley J, et al. Urinary red-cell morphology during exercise. Br Med J. 1982;285:1455–57.
3. Hockberger RS, Schwartz B, Connor J. Hematuria induced by urethral catheterisation. Ann Emerg Med. 1987;16:500–2.
4. Anpalahan M, Birch DF, Becker GJ. Chemical preservation of urine sediment for phase contrast microscopic examination. Nephron. 1994;68:180–3.
5. Van der Snoek BE, Koene RAP. Fixation of urinary sediment. Lancet. 1997;350:933–4.
6. Dorizzi RM, Caputo M. Measurement of urine relative density using refractometer and reagent strips. Clin Chem Lab Med. 1998;36:925–8.
7. Ginsberg JM, Chang BS, Matarese RA, Garella S. Use of single voided urine samples to estimate quantitative proteinuria. N Engl J Med. 1983;309:1543–6.
8. Koopman MG, Krediet RT, Koomen GCM, et al. Circadian rhythm of proteinuria: consequences of the use of urinary protein:creatinine ratios. Nephrol Dial Transplant. 1989;4:9–14.
9. Bazzi C, Petrini C, Rizza V, et al. Characterization of proteinuria in primary glomerulonephritides. SDS–PAGE patterns: clinical significance and prognostic value of low molecular weight ('tubular') proteins. Am J Kidney Dis. 1997;29:27–35.
10. Reichert LJM, Koene RAP, Wetzels FM. Urinary excretion of β_2-microglobulin predicts renal outcome in patients with idiopathic membranous nephropathy. J Am Soc Nephrol. 1995;6: 1666–9.
11. Bazzi C, Petrini C, Rizza V, et al. Urinary excretion of IgG and α_1-microglobulin predicts clinical course better than extent of proteinuria in membranous nephropathy. Am J Kidney Dis. 2001;38:240–8.
12. Cameron JS, Blandford G. The simple assessment of selectivity in heavy proteinuria. Lancet. 1966;ii:242–7.
13. Bazzi C, Petrini C, Rizza V, et al. A modern approach to selectivity of proteinuria and tubulointerstitial damage in nephrotic syndrome. Kidney Int. 2001;58:1732–41.
14. Kutter D. The urine test strip of the future. Clin Chim Acta. 2000;297:297–304.
15. Fairley K, Birch DF. Hematuria: a simple method for identifying glomerular bleeding. Kidney Int. 1982;21:105–8.
16. Fasset RG, Horgan BA, Mathew TH. Detection of glomerular bleeding by phase contrast microscopy. Lancet. 1982;I:1432–4.
17. Rizzoni G, Braggion F, Zacchello G. Evaluation of glomerular and nonglomerular hematuria by phase-contrast microscopy. J Pediatr. 1983;103:370–4.
18. Dinda AK, Saxena S, Guleria S, et al. Diagnosis of glomerular hematuria: role of dysmorphic red cells, G1 cells and bright field microscopy. Scand J Clin Lab Invest. 1997;57:203–8.
19. Rath B, Turner C, Hartley B, Chantler C. What makes red cells dysmorphic in glomerular hematuria? Paediatr Nephrol. 1992;6: 424–7.
20. Schramek P, Gergopoulos M, Schuster FX, et al. Value of urinary erythrocytes morphology in assessment of symptomless microhematuria. Lancet. 1989;ii:1316–19.
21. Nolan CR III, Anger MS, Kelleher SP. Eosinophiluria – a new method of detection and definition of the clinical spectrum. N Engl J Med. 1986;315:1516–18.
22. Nolan CR, Kelleher SP. Eosinophiluria. Clin Lab Med. 1988;8: 555–65.
23. Fogazzi GB. Carboni N, Pruneri G. The cells of the deep layers of the urothelium in the urine sediment: an overlooked marker of severe diseases of the excretory urinary system. Nephrol Dial Transplant. 1995;10:1918–19.
24. Hotta O, Yusa N, Kitamura H, Taguma Y. Urinary macrophages as activity markers of renal injury. Clin Chim Acta. 2000;297: 123–33.
25. Koene RAP. Unexplained hematuria. Nephrol Dial Transplant. 1999;14:2025–7.
26. Fogazzi GB. Crystalluria: a neglected aspect of urinary sediment analysis. Nephrol Dial Transplant. 1996;11:379–87.
27. Fogazzi GB, Ponticelli C, Ritz E. The urinary sediment. An integrated view, 2nd edition. Oxford: Oxford University Press; 1999:91–114.
28. Arnadottir M, Laxdal T, Hardarson S, Asmundsson P. Acute renal failure in a middle-aged woman with 2,8 dihydroxyadeninuria. Nephrol Dial Transplant. 1997;12:1985–7.
29. Kopp JB, Miller KD, Mican JAM, et al. Crystalluria and urinary tract abnormalities associated with indinavir. Ann Intern Med. 1997;127:119–25.
20. Vickers D, Ahmad T, Coulthard MG. Diagnosis of urinary tract infection in children: fresh urine microscopy or culture? Lancet. 1991;338 767–70.
31. Ravigneaux M-H, Pellet H, Colon S, et al. Signification d'une cytolipidurie dans le cadre d'un syndrome néphrotique. Néphrologie. 1991;12:12–16.
32. Hebert LA, Dillon JJ, Middendorf DF, et al. Relationship between appearance of urinary red blood cell/white blood cell casts and the onset of renal relapse in systemic lupus erythemathosus. Am J Kidney Dis. 1995;26:432–8.
33. Fujita T, Ohi H, Endo M, et al. Levels of red blood cells in the urinary sediment reflect the degree of renal activity in Wegener's granulomatosis. Clin Nephrol. 1998;50:284–8.
34. Delanghe JR, Kouri TT, Huber AR, et al. The role of automated urine particles flow cytometry in clinical practice. Clin Chim Acta. 2000;301:1–18.
35. Regeniter A, Haenni V, Risch L, et al. Urine analysis performed by flow cytometry: reference range determination and comparison to morphological findings, dipsticks chemistry and bacterial culture results – A multicenter study. Clin Nephrol. 2001;55: 384–92.
36. Apeland T, Mestad O, Hetland Ø. Assessment of hematuria: automated urine flowmetry vs microscopy. Nephrol Dial Transplant. 2001;16:1615–19.

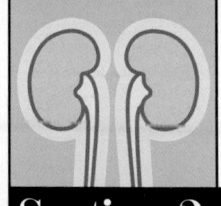

Section 2 | Investigation of Renal Disease

Chapter 5 | Imaging

Rosaleen B Parsons and William L Simpson, Jr

IMAGING STRATEGY

This chapter discusses the range of available imaging methods and their role in the diagnosis and management of renal disease. The correct choice of imaging will minimize the time and cost of effective evaluation. The first choice imaging techniques in common clinical situations are shown in Table 5.1.

RADIOLOGIC CONTRAST AGENTS

A triiodinated benzene ring forms the chemical basis for all intravascular contrast agents. Conventional contrast agents have high osmolality, approximately five times greater than plasma osmolality. This feature makes them excellent for renal opacification but also contributes to their toxicity. Modifications and additions to the benzene ring have led to the development of several additional categories of contrast agents. These newer compounds are low osmolar and both ionic and nonionic. Most contrast studies are now performed with low osmolar nonionic agents.

Intravascular contrast material rapidly passes through the capillary pores into the interstitial, extracellular space and into the renal tubules via glomerular filtration[1]. In patients with normal renal function, the kidneys eliminate almost all of the contrast agent. Extrarenal routes of excretion include the liver and bowel wall and account for less than 1% of elimination but can increase when renal function is compromised. The half-time for elimination in patients with normal renal function is 1–2 h compared with 2–4 h in dialysis patients[2,3].

The overall incidence of contrast reactions for all agents is 3.1–4.7%[4,5]. The most significant factor for development of a contrast reaction is a history of prior contrast reaction. It is estimated that 20% of patients will experience a reaction upon re-exposure that may be similar or worse than the prior reaction. Contrast reactions can be divided into two categories: anaphylactoid or chemotoxic reactions. The former mimic an allergic response while the latter are believed to be mediated by direct toxic effects of the contrast. The exact mechanism of contrast reaction is not known but is likely multifactorial. Formation of antigen–antibody complexes, complement activation, protein binding, and histamine release have all been cited as mechanisms responsible for mediating contrast reactions.

Reactions may be minor, intermediate, or severe. Minor reactions include heat sensation, nausea, and mild urticaria. Intermediate reactions include vasovagal reaction, bronchospasm,

First choice imaging techniques in renal disease	
Renal failure, unknown cause	Ultrasound (US)
Hematuria	Intravenous urography (IVU) or US + plain radiograph of kidneys, ureter and bladder (KUB)
Proteinuria/nephrotic syndrome	US
Hypertension	
with normal renal function	CT angiography including imaging of the adrenal glands
with impaired renal function	MRA
Renal artery stenosis	
with normal renal function	MRA
with impaired renal function	MRA
Renal infection	CT
Hydronephrosis detected by US	IVU (if renal function is preserved) or ^{99}Tc-DTPA renography
Retroperitoneal fibrosis	CT
Papillary necrosis	IVU
Cortical necrosis	Contrast enhanced CT
Renal vein thrombosis	Contrast enhanced CT
Renal infarction	Contrast enhanced CT
Nephrocalcinosis	Noncontrast CT
MRA, magnetic resonance angiography; CT, computerized tomography.	

Table 5.1 Imaging strategy: first choice imaging techniques in common clinical situations.

and generalized urticaria. Severe reactions include profound hypotension, pulmonary edema, and cardiac arrest. The use of nonionic contrast has been shown to reduce the incidence of minor and intermediate contrast reactions. The incidence of death related to ionic contrast is reported to be 1 in 40 000. Immediate treatment of reactions should be directed toward the symptoms.

Contrast nephrotoxicity

Renal failure associated with contrast administration has been reported as the third most common cause of in-hospital renal failure after hypotension and surgery[6]. Patients with normal renal function rarely develop contrast-induced renal failure. In patients with serum creatinine levels > 1.5 mg/dL (135 μmol/L), iodinated contrast should be used with caution

Risk factors for contrast nephrotoxicity
Pre-existing renal impairment (serum creatinine >1.5 mg/dL)*
Diabetes*
Age >75 years
Fluid depletion
Myeloma
Concurrent nephrotoxic drugs
Uricosuria
Ionic contrast media
* The greatest risk is presented by the coincidence of diabetes and pre-existing renal impairment.

Table 5.2 Risk factors for contrast nephrotoxicity.

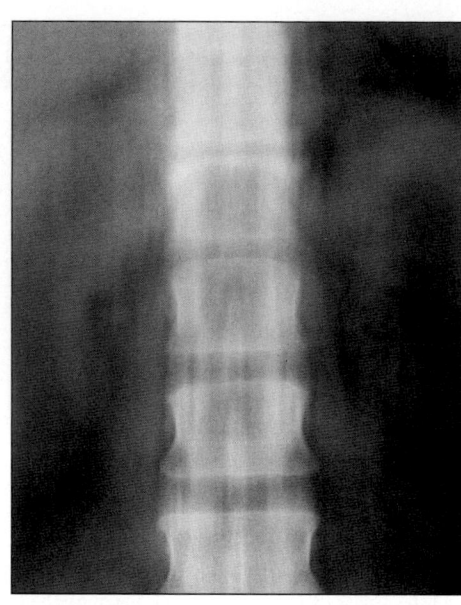

Figure 5.1 'Scout' tomogram of normal kidneys.

as the risk of contrast-induced renal failure is increased. Nephrotoxicity ranges in severity from nonoliguric transient renal dysfunction to severe renal failure requiring dialysis. The major risk factor for developing acute renal failure is the combination of pre-existing renal insufficiency and diabetes. Relative risk factors for development of contrast-induced renal failure include pre-existing renal insufficiency alone, diabetes, dehydration, cardiovascular disease and the use of diuretics, advanced age (> 75 years), multiple myeloma in dehydrated patients, hypertension, and uricosuria (see Table 5.2)[7]. Both ionic and nonionic contrast media can induce nephrotoxicity, although nonionic contrast is significantly less nephrotoxic. In end-stage renal disease (ESRD) fluid overload may follow the use of contrast because of thirst provoked by the osmotic load.

Contrast-induced renal failure is probably multifactorial. A vascular component manifested as vasoconstriction coupled with direct tubular injury is suspected. In the vast majority of patients the renal failure is transient and the patients recover without incident. The mainstay of prevention of contrast-induced renal failure is to endure adequate hydration using intravenous saline: for example 0.45% saline 1 mL/kg/h for 12 h before and after the examination, provided there is no contraindication to fluid loading. There is no evidence that dopamine or diuretics have a preventative role. Recent studies have shown that–acetylcysteine (600 mg b.i.d. before and after with saline)[8] and possibly the dopamine agonist fenoldopam[9] can reduce or prevent the nephrotoxic effects of low osmolality contrast agents. Contrast-induced renal failure is discussed further in Chapter 15.

PLAIN FILMS AND INTRAVENOUS UROGRAPHY

Intravenous urography (IVU) was the first radiographic examination with which the kidney, ureters and bladder could be identified. In many situations, it has now been replaced with computerized tomography (CT) and ultrasound. IVU still has particular utility for evaluation of genitourinary infections and occasionally for work up of painless hematuria. There is no standard filming sequence for an intravenous urogram; it varies depending on the clinical concerns and the interpreting physician's preferences.

Plain film
The typical urogram consists of a large plain film of the abdomen to include the region of the bladder (KUB: 'kidneys, ureter, bladder') and one smaller film, a tomogram through the renal regions prior to contrast administration (Fig. 5.1). The plain films are used to assess for soft tissue masses, the bowel gas pattern, calcifications, and renal location.

Renal calcification
The majority of renal calculi are radiodense and visible on plain films of the abdomen. Calculi that are radiolucent on plain films are usually detected as filling defects on the urogram. CT demonstrates nonopaque stones, which include uric acid, xanthine, struvite, and matrix stones. However, both CT and plain films do not detect calculi associated with protease inhibitor therapy[10]. Oblique films are sometimes obtained when a suspicious upper quadrant calcification is detected. Rotating the patient can aid in determining if such a calcification is renal in origin.

Nephrocalcinosis may be medullary (Fig. 5.2a,b) or cortical (Fig. 5.2c) and is localized or diffuse. The common causes of nephrocalcinosis are shown in Table 5.3 (and see Chapter 57).

Contrast films
Prior to administering contrast, an abdominal compression device may be placed. Its purpose is to maintain the excreted contrast in the upper tract and to distend the renal pelvis and calyces. A series of films are obtained following the contrast injection and their timing is somewhat variable. The first film is usually performed at 30 s; it is at this time that the renal parenchyma is at peak enhancement. Subtle renal masses are often only detected on these early films. Additional supine and oblique films of the entire abdomen are obtained when renal excretion of contrast is present, typically at 5 min. It is on these films that the ureters are best evaluated. Supine films are occasionally inadequate for visualization of the distal ureters because of their anterior location as they cross the pelvic brim, and prone films may be required. A filled bladder film is obtained and may also be supplemented with oblique

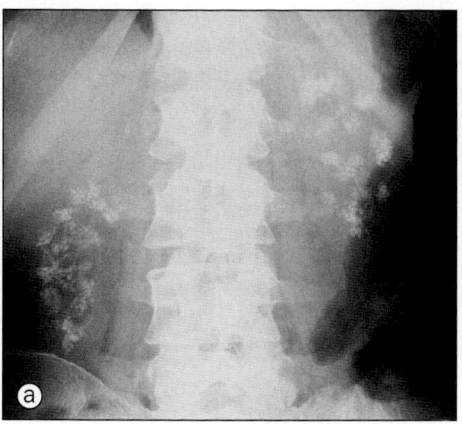
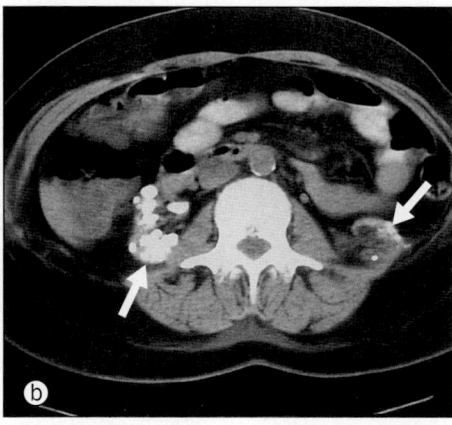
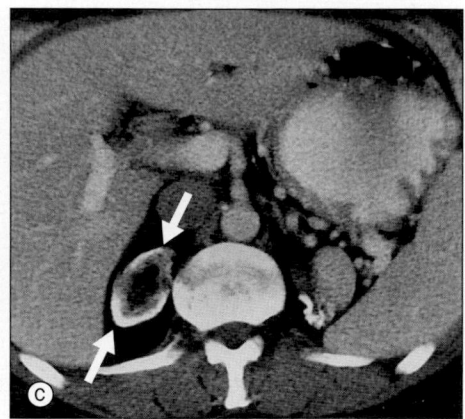

Figure 5.2 Nephrocalcinosis. (a) Plain film showing bilateral medullary nephrocalcinosis in a patient with distal renal tubular acidosis. (b) Noncontrast CT in a patient with hereditary oxalosis and dense bilateral renal calcification. The left kidney is atrophic. (c) CT showing cortical nephrocalcinosis in the right kidney following cortical necrosis.

or upright views. The last one is quite helpful for identification of bladder prolapse. A postvoid film of the bladder assesses bladder emptying and is useful for evaluation of the distal ureters, which may be obscured by a distended contrast-filled bladder[11].

Kidneys
Evaluation of the kidneys on IVU (and also on CT or magnetic resonance imaging (MRI)) should include their number, location, axis, size, contour, and degree of enhancement. In the normal patient, the kidneys are located in the superior portion of the retroperitoneum with the upper poles directed medially and the lower poles directed laterally. Ectopic kidneys can be identified lying as inferiorly as the bony pelvis and, rarely, within the chest. Renal size is variable but a normal kidney should be approximately three to four lumbar vertebral bodies in length. The renal outline should be smooth and sharply demarcated from the retroperitoneal fat. Benign cortical variations include a 'dromedary hump' and fetal lobulations. The dromedary hump is a contour deformity in the lateral upper kidney secondary to the spleen (Fig. 5.3). Fetal lobulation results from incomplete fusion of the fetal lobules and produces cortical indentations without associated parenchymal loss or calyceal irregularity.

Renal enhancement begins approximately 30 s after contrast administration and should be symmetric. Enhancement progresses centrally from the cortex, with excretion evident in the ureters by 5 min. Asymmetry of renal enhancement can be indicative of renal arterial disease.

Patterns and causes of nephrocalcinosis	
Area affected	**Causes**
Medullary	
Disturbed calcium metabolism	Hyperparathyroidism
	Sarcoidosis
	Idiopathic hypercalciuria
	Milk-alkali syndrome
	Hypervitaminosis D
Other systemic metabolic disease	Oxalosis
Other tubular disease	Distal renal tubular acidosis (RTA)
	Dent's disease
	Hyperoxaluria
	Bartter's syndrome
	Medullary sponge kidney
Other	Papillary necrosis
Cortical	Cortical necrosis
	Chronic glomerulonephritis
	Trauma

Table 5.3 Nephrocalcinosis. Patterns and common causes of nephrocalcinosis.

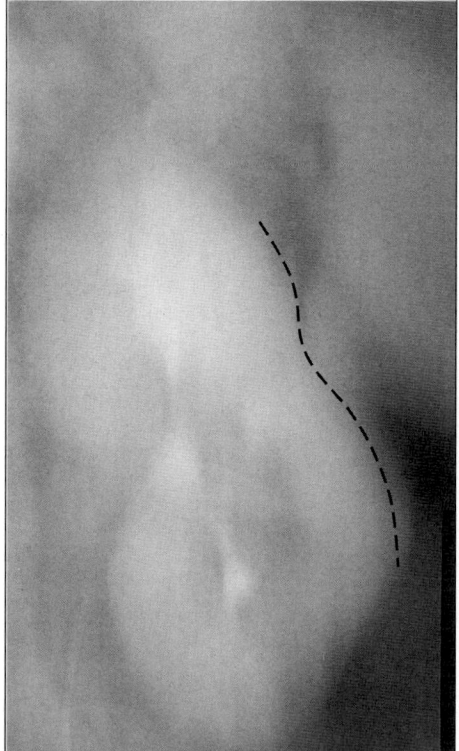

Figure 5.3 Intravenous urography showing 'dromedary hump'. This is a smooth contour depression (line) on the mid pole of the left kidney from the spleen.

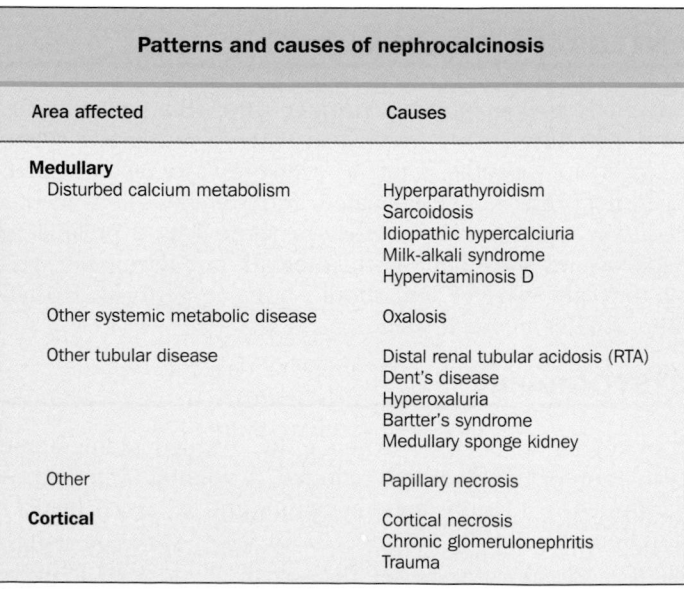

Investigation of Renal Disease

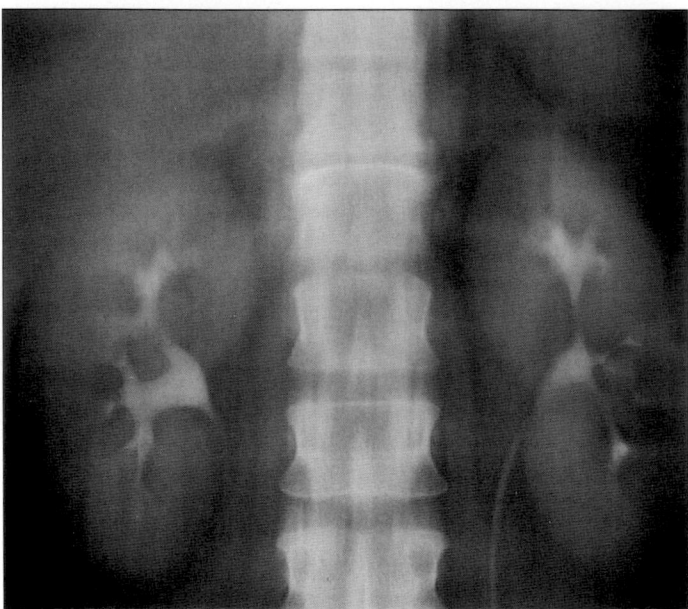

Figure 5.4 Normal parenchymal enhancement and normal renal excretion. Early postcontrast tomogram in IVU.

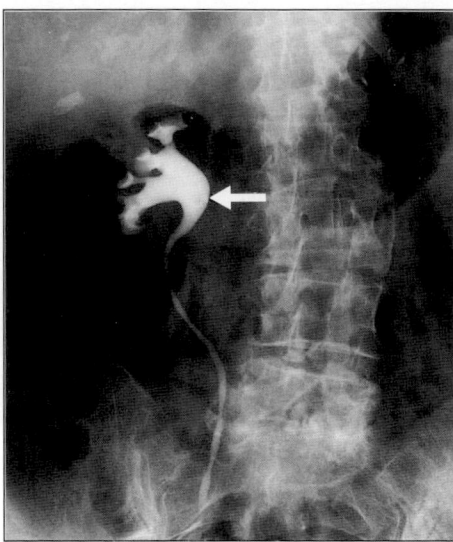

Figure 5.5 Retrograde pyelogram. The arrow indicates a small filling defect, which is a calculus in the renal pelvis. The remainder of the study is normal.

Pelvicalyceal system

The pelvicalyceal system is best evaluated on the early abdominal films. Normally there are about 10–12 calyces per kidney. The calyces drain into the infundibula, which in turn empty into the renal pelvis (Fig. 5.4). When more than one calyx drains into an infundibulum it is considered a compound calyx; this anatomic variation is frequently seen in the polar regions. The normal calyx is gently cupped. Calyceal distortion occurs with papillary necrosis and reflux nephropathy. The infundibulum and renal pelvis should have smooth contours without filling defects. Crossing vessels can mimic filling defects within the collecting system and should not be confused with significant pathology. Benign peripelvic and renal sinus fat can produce bowing of the infundibula.

Ureters

The ureters should be seen segmentally on the abdomen films after 5 min. Active peristalsis can lead to incomplete visualization of portions of the normal ureters and additional radiographs may be required for complete identification. The ureters should be free of filling defects and smooth. In the abdomen, the ureters lie in the retroperitoneum, passing anterior to the transverse processes of the vertebral bodies. In the pelvis, the ureters course laterally and posteriorly, eventually draining into the posteriorly located ureterovesicular junction.

At the vesico-ureteral junction, the ureters gently taper. Medial bowing or displacement of the ureter is often abnormal and should be further evaluated. Occasionally the active peristalsis creates a jet of urine into the bladder, which is seen as the more opaque contrast, containing urine, empties into the less opaque urine-filled bladder.

Bladder

The midline urinary bladder lies posterior to the symphysis pubis. Its cephalad extent varies in relation to bladder distension. The bladder should be rounded in configuration and smooth walled. Benign indentations on the bladder include the uterus, prostate gland, and bowel.

RETROGRADE PYELOGRAPHY

Retrograde pyelography is performed when the ureters are poorly visualized on other imaging studies or when samples of urine need to be obtained from the kidney for cytology or culture. Patients who have severe contrast allergies can be evaluated with retrograde pyelography. The examination is performed by placing a catheter through the ureteral orifice under cystoscopic guidance and advancing it into the renal pelvis. Using fluoroscopy, the catheter is slowly withdrawn while radiographic contrast material is injected (Fig. 5.5). This technique provides excellent visualization of the renal pelvis and ureter and can be used for cytologic sampling from suspect areas.

ANTEGRADE PYELOGRAPHY

Antegrade pyelography is performed through a percutaneous renal puncture and is resorted to when a retrograde pyelogram is not possible. Ureteral pressures can be measured, hydronephrosis can be evaluated, and ureteral lesions identified. The examination is often performed as a prelude to nephrostomy placement. Both antegrade and retrograde pyelography are invasive and should only be performed when other studies are inadequate.

CYSTOGRAPHY

A cystogram is obtained when more detailed radiographic evaluation of the bladder is required. A voiding cystogram is performed to identify ureteral reflux, and to assess bladder function and urethral anatomy. In the trauma setting, cystography is essential for evaluation of suspected bladder perforations, which can be missed on IVU or CT. A Foley catheter is placed into the bladder and the urine drained. Contrast is then placed through the catheter and the bladder filled under fluoroscopic guidance. Early supine frontal and oblique films are obtained while the bladder is filling. Ureteroceles are best identified on early films. When the bladder is full, multiple films are obtained with varying degrees of obliquity. Reflux may be seen on these films. To obtain a voiding cystogram, the catheter is removed and the patient voids. The contrast is followed into the urethra and spot films are obtained. Occasionally bladder diverticuli are only seen on the voiding films. When the patient has completely voided, a final film of the bladder is obtained which can be used to assess the amount of residual urine as well as the mucosal pattern.

ILEAL CONDUITS

Following cystectomy there are numerous types of urinary diversion that can be surgically created. There are continent or incontinent diversions; they are placed percutaneously or surgically by single or multistaged procedures. One of the most common diversions is the ileal conduit: an ileal loop is isolated from the small bowel and the ureters are reimplanted into the loop. This end of the loop is closed while the other end exits through the anterior abdominal wall. This type of conduit can be evaluated by an excretory study or a retrograde study. The excretory or antegrade study is performed and monitored in the same way as is an intravenous urogram. A retrograde examination, also referred to as a loop-o-gram, is obtained when the ureters and conduit are suboptimally evaluated on the excretory study. A Foley catheter is placed into the stoma and intravascular contrast is then slowly instilled. The ureters should fill via reflux since the ureteral anastamoses are not of the antireflux variety (Fig. 5.6). A postvoid film can be obtained to evaluate the emptying capacity of the system.

ULTRASOUND

Ultrasound examination of the kidneys is relatively inexpensive and provides a rapid way to assess renal location, contour, and size. Portable ultrasound is available and is essential in the pediatric or emergency setting. Clarification of renal masses as cystic or solid is quickly achieved and in cases of suspected obstruction the progression or regression of hydronephrosis is easily evaluated. Color Doppler imaging permits assessment of renal vascularity and perfusion. Unlike the other imaging modalities, ultrasound is highly dependent on the operator's skills.

Kidney size
The kidney is imaged in transverse and sagittal planes and is normally 9–12 cm in length in the adult. Abnormal renal size is the most common sign identified on renal imaging. Differences in renal size can be detected by ultrasound and also by contrast urography, CT, or MRI. The common causes of enlarged or shrunken kidneys are shown in Figure 5.7.

Renal echo pattern
The normal cortex is hypoechoic compared with the fat-containing echogenic renal sinus (see Fig. 5.8). The cortical echotexture may be isoechoic or hypoechoic compared with the liver or spleen[7]. In children, the renal pyramids are hypoechoic and the cortex is characteristically hyperechoic compared with the liver and the spleen[11]. In adults an increase in cortical echogenicity is a sensitive marker for parenchymal renal disease but is nonspecific (see Fig. 5.9). Decreased cortical echogenicity can be found in acute pyelonephritis and acute renal vein thrombosis.

The normal renal contour is smooth and the cortical mantle should be uniform and slightly thicker toward the poles. Two benign masses that can be seen with ultrasound include the dromedary hump (also see Fig. 5.3) and the column of Bertin. The column of Bertin results from bulging of cortical tissue into the medullary portion of the kidney. On ultrasound, it is seen as a mass with similar echotexture to the cortex but found within the central renal sinus (Fig. 5.10). The renal pelvis and proximal ureter are anechoic. An extrarenal pelvis refers to the renal pelvis location outside the renal hilum. The ureter is not identified beyond the pelvis in nonobstructed patients.

Obstruction can be identified by the presence of hydronephrosis (Fig. 5.11). The upper ureter will also be dilated if obstruction is distal to the pelviureteral junction. False-negative ultrasound examination with no hydronephrosis occasionally occurs in early obstruction.

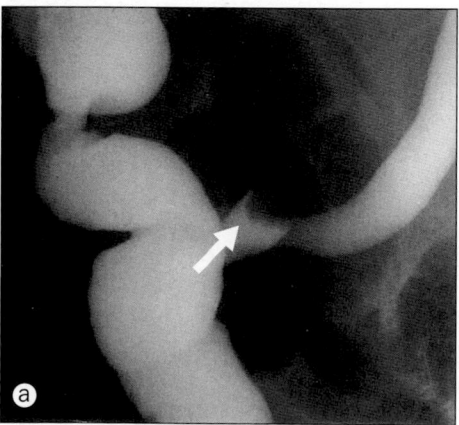

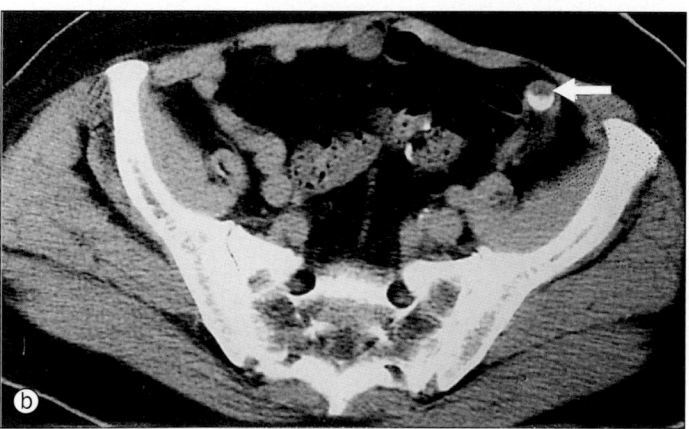

Figure 5.6 Ileal conduit. (a) 'Loop-o-gram'. A recurrent transitional carcinoma is present in the reimplanted left ureter (arrow). (b) CT scan clearly showing the tumor as a filling defect in the anterior aspect of the opacified ureter (arrow).

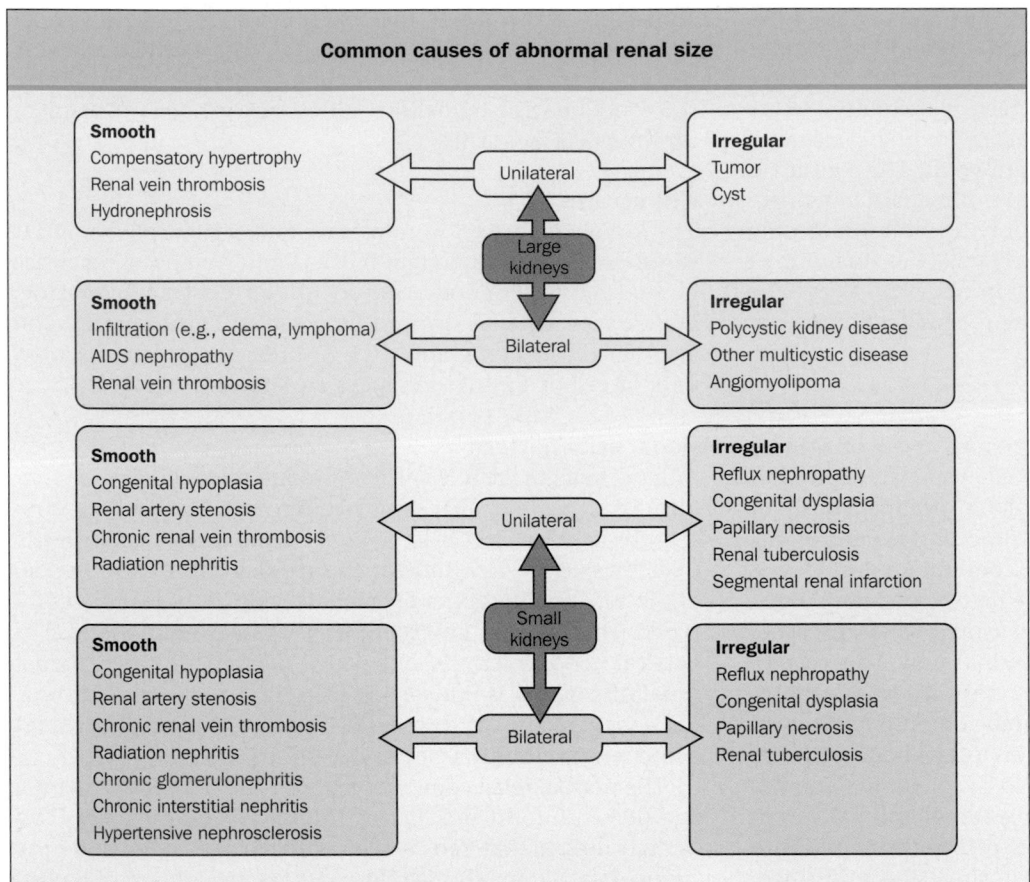

Figure 5.7 Common causes of abnormal renal size.

Common causes of abnormal renal size

Large kidneys

Unilateral

Smooth
Compensatory hypertrophy
Renal vein thrombosis
Hydronephrosis

Irregular
Tumor
Cyst

Bilateral

Smooth
Infiltration (e.g., edema, lymphoma)
AIDS nephropathy
Renal vein thrombosis

Irregular
Polycystic kidney disease
Other multicystic disease
Angiomyolipoma

Small kidneys

Unilateral

Smooth
Congenital hypoplasia
Renal artery stenosis
Chronic renal vein thrombosis
Radiation nephritis

Irregular
Reflux nephropathy
Congenital dysplasia
Papillary necrosis
Renal tuberculosis
Segmental renal infarction

Bilateral

Smooth
Congenital hypoplasia
Renal artery stenosis
Chronic renal vein thrombosis
Radiation nephritis
Chronic glomerulonephritis
Chronic interstitial nephritis
Hypertensive nephrosclerosis

Irregular
Reflux nephropathy
Congenital dysplasia
Papillary necrosis
Renal tuberculosis

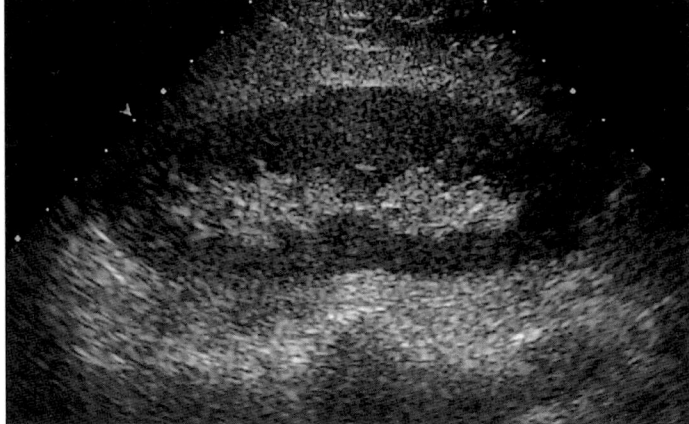

Figure 5.8 Normal sagittal renal ultrasound. The cortex is hypoechoic compared with the echogenic fat containing the renal sinus.

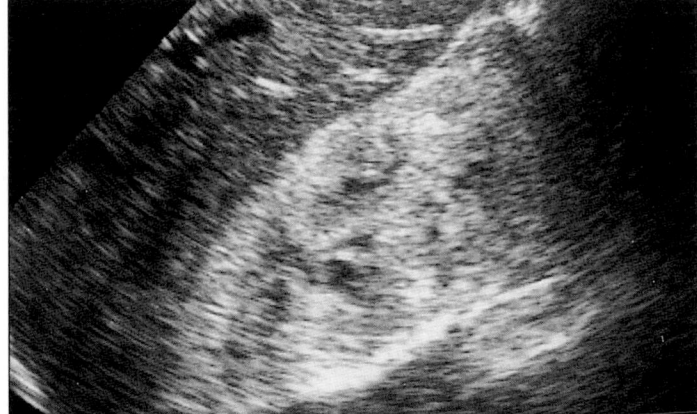

Figure 5.9 HIV nephropathy. Enlarged echogenic kidney with lack of corticomedullary distinction. Bipolar length of kidney = 14.2 cm.

Renal cysts

Cysts can be identified as anechoic lesions and are a frequent coincidental finding during renal imaging. Their differentiation into simple and complex cysts (Fig. 5.12) is required to plan intervention. The classification developed by Bosniak is widely used (Table 5.4)[12].

Simple cysts

A simple cyst on ultrasound is anechoic, has a thin or imperceptible wall, and demonstrates through transmission because of the relatively rapid progression of the sound wave through fluid compared with adjacent soft tissue.

Complex cysts

Complex cysts contain calcifications, septations, and mural nodules. Instead of being anechoic, they may contain internal echoes representing hemorrhage, pus, or protein. Complex cysts may be benign or malignant, the latter strongly suggested by cyst vascularity. Complex cysts identified by ultrasound require further evaluation by contrast CT (or MRI) to assess vascularity.

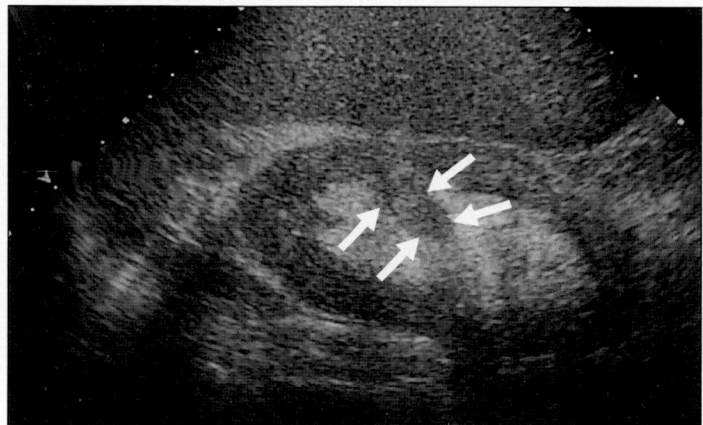

Figure 15.10 Sagittal renal ultrasound. Column of Bertin is present (arrows) and is easily identified because of the similar echo texture to the cortex.

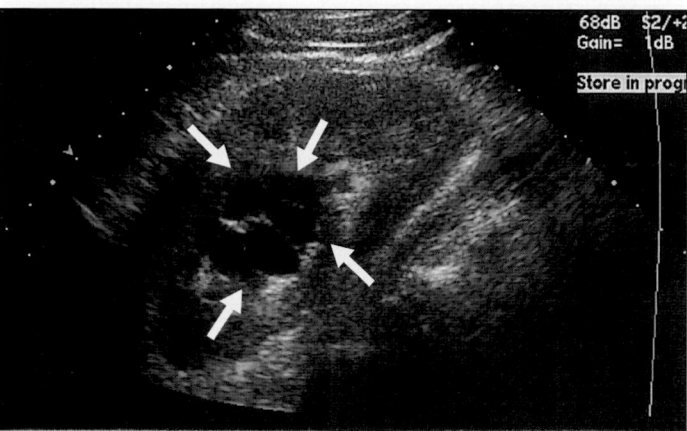

Figure 5.12 Sagittal renal ultrasound showing a complex cyst.

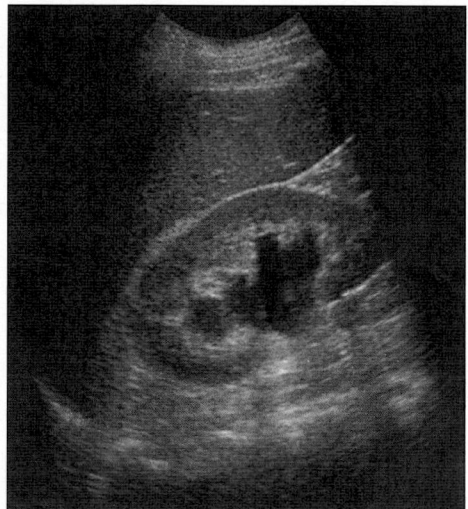

Figure 5.11 Sagittal renal ultrasound demonstrating hydronephrosis.

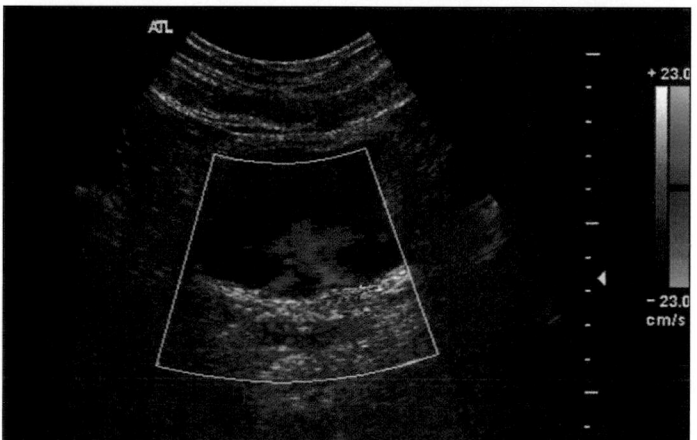

Figure 5.13 Bilateral ureteral jets detected with color Doppler ultrasound. This is a normal appearance

Bladder

Color flow Doppler evaluation of the bladder in well-hydrated patients can be used to identify a ureteral jet. The jet is produced when peristalsis propels urine into the bladder, the incoming urine having a specific gravity higher relative to the urine already in the bladder (Fig. 5.13). Absence of the ureteral jet can indicate total ureteral obstruction.

Renal vasculature

Color Doppler investigation of the kidneys provides a detailed evaluation of the renal vascular anatomy. The main renal arteries can be identified in most patients (Fig. 5.14). Power Doppler is a more sensitive indicator of flow than is color Doppler. Unlike color Doppler, it does not provide any information about flow direction and it can not be used to assess vascular waveforms. It is, however, exquisitely sensitive for detection of renal parenchymal flow and has been used to identify cortical infarction.

Renal artery duplex scanning

Renal artery stenosis is an uncommon cause of hypertension, but is potentially curable with angioplasty or surgery. The

Classification and evaluation of renal cysts		
Classification	Ultrasound characteristics	Intervention
Type I: simple cyst	Anechoic – thin walled	None
Type II: minimally complicated	Calcification, septation, mural nodules	Contrast CT to assess vascularity: if enhancement >12 HU use surgical intervention
Type III: complicated	Calcification, septation, mural nodules	Contrast CT to assess vascularity: if enhancement >12 HU use surgical intervention
Type IV: cystic malignancy	Calcification, septation, mural nodules, vascularization	Surgery

Table 5.4 Identification of simple and complex renal cysts[12].

role of gray scale and color Doppler sonography in screening for renal artery stenosis is controversial. The principle is that

Investigation of Renal Disease

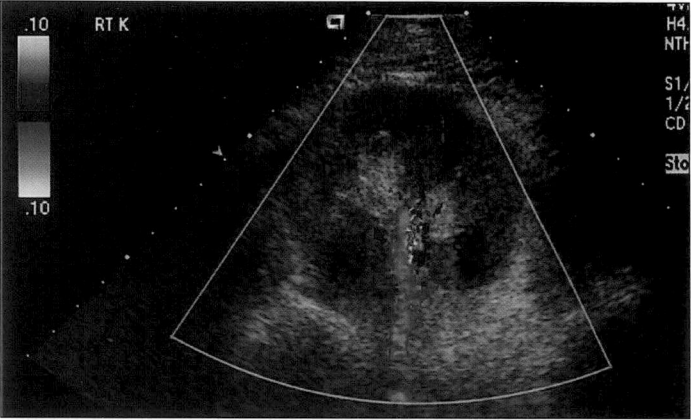

Figure 5.14 Transverse color Doppler ultrasound of the kidney. The artery is red and the vein is blue.

a narrowing in the artery will cause a velocity change commensurate with the degree of stenosis as well as a change in the normal renal arterial waveform downstream from the lesion. Longstanding renal artery stenosis often results in a decrease in renal size.

The entire length of the renal artery should be examined looking for the highest velocity signal. Usually the patient is positioned supine. The left renal vein is used as a landmark for the region of the aorta where the renal arteries originate. The origins of the renal arteries are important to identify since this is a common area affected by atherosclerosis. The mid and distal renal arteries as well as the branching artery in the hilum should be interrogated. Within the kidney medullary branches and cortical branches in the upper, mid and lower thirds should be included in the Doppler examination in order to attempt to detect stenosis in accessory renal arteries.

There are many limitations in renal artery duplex scanning. One of the major limitations is the inability to identify the entire course of the renal artery due to the patient body habitus or bowel gas. Scanning the patient after an overnight fast may reduce the amount of bowel gas[13]. In addition, the kidneys move with respiration. Patients must hold their breath to stop respiratory motion in order to obtain a good, reliable Doppler spectral tracing. There is a limit to the time patients can hold their breath for a Doppler study of the artery especially in the elderly. The Doppler angle should be kept at 60 degrees or less; the tortuosity of some renal arteries often makes this difficult.

Finally, 10–20% of patients have accessory renal arteries which are small and often missed on Doppler studies[14].

The criteria for diagnosing renal artery stenosis greater than 60% can be divided into proximal and distal categories. The proximal criteria detect changes in the Doppler signal at the site of stenosis. These include high systolic velocity and turbulence. The distal criteria detect a change in the arterial waveform downstream from a stenosis.

There are four proximal criteria:
- Peak systolic velocity of 200 cm/s or greater
- Ratio of peak systolic velocity in the renal artery to the aorta of greater than 3.5
- Turbulent flow in the poststenotic region
- Lack of detectable Doppler signal in a visualized renal artery denotes occlusion of the artery.

Using these criteria sensitivities and specificities ranged from 0–98% and 37–98% respectively have been reported[14,15]. The low sensitivity and specificity are attributable to a large number of technical failures in the study (42%).

The distal criteria are related to detection of a tardus parvus waveform distal to a stenosis. The normal renal arterial waveform demonstrates a rapid systolic upstroke and an early systolic peak (Fig 5.15a). The waveform becomes dampened downstream from a stenosis. This consists of a slow systolic acceleration (tardus) and a decreased and rounded systolic peak (parvus) (Fig. 5.15b).

There are four distal criteria:
- loss of the early systolic peak
- slope of the systolic upstroke (acceleration) reduced to less than 300 cm/s
- acceleration time of greater than 0.07 s
- resistive index change of greater than 5% between the left and right kidneys.

Using these distal criteria sensitivities and specificities of 66–100% and 67–94% respectively have been reported[16,17].

Combining the proximal and distal criteria improve the detection of stenoses. Sensitivity of 96.7% and specificity of 98% can be achieved when both the extrarenal and intrarenal arteries are examined[18]. However, it should be noted that reliable results require a skilled and experienced sonographer, long examination time and adequate prescreening of patients. These factors add to the controversy over duplex scanning as a screening tool and have led to the advocacy of contrast enhanced MRA as a faster and more reliable screening tool.

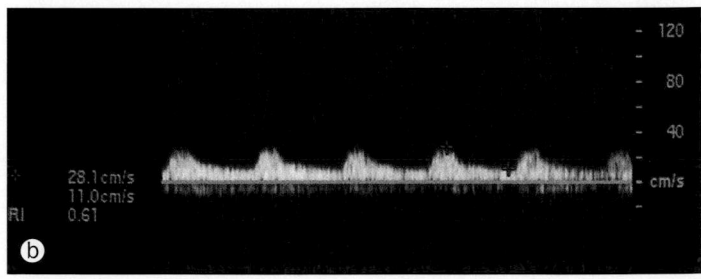

Figure 5.15 Renal artery color Doppler and spectral tracing. (a) Normal renal arterial tracing showing the rapid systolic upstroke and early systolic peak velocity (~100 cm/s). (b) Tardus parvus waveform demonstrating the slow systolic upstroke (acceleration) and decreased peak systolic velocity (~20 cm/s) associated with renal artery stenosis. Note different scales on vertical axis.

Contrast ultrasound

The contrast for ultrasound is a bubble-based perfluorooctyl bromide gas that is injected intravenously. The agent is expired after several minutes. Contrast agents are still under investigation and are not currently commercially available for clinical use.

COMPUTERIZED TOMOGRAPHY

CT examination of the kidneys is performed to evaluate suspect renal masses, to locate ectopic kidneys (Figs 5.16 and 5.17), to investigate calculi, to assess retroperitoneal masses, and for evaluating the extent of parenchymal involvement in patients with pyelonephritis (Figs 5.16 and 5.17). The major improvement in CT technology in the early 1990s was the introduction of helical scanners. With helical scans, a large volume of the body can be scanned in a fraction of the time required with the earlier machines. The abdomen and pelvis can be scanned at 3-mm intervals with one to two breath-held acquisitions. This eliminates motion artifact, which was previously a significant problem. In the late 1990s multidetector row CT was introduced. This results in up to four slices of information being acquired simultaneously. Therefore, the entire abdomen and pelvis can be covered in one breathhold using 1 mm intervals.

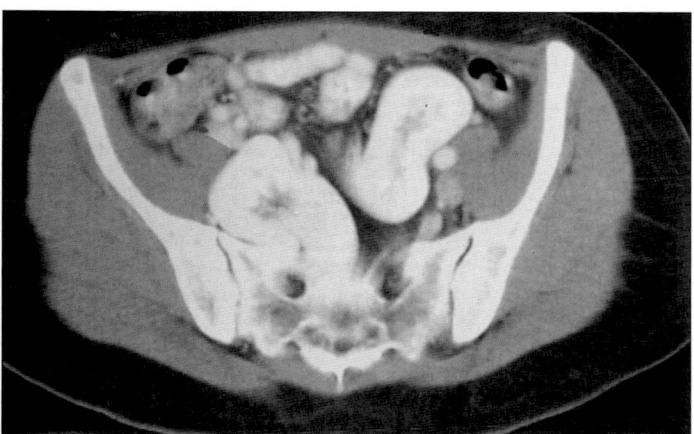

Figure 5.16 CT scan showing bilateral pelvic kidneys.

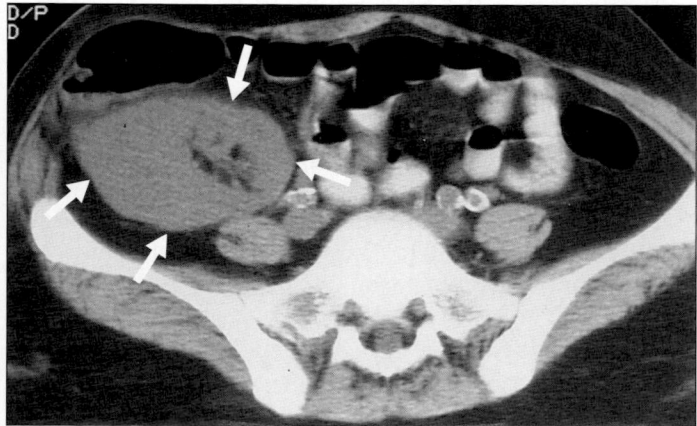

Figure 5.17 CT scan showing normal renal transplant.

The kidneys lie in the retroperitoneum. This space can be seen with MRI but is better detected with CT. It consists of three compartments: the anterior pararenal space, the perinephric space, and the posterior pararenal space. The anatomy of the spaces influences the spread of infectious and inflammatory processes (Figs 5.18 and 5.19). The perinephric space is open anteriorly across the midline and encompasses the aorta and inferior vena cava. Thus the right and left perinephric spaces are in potential communication across the midline. The perinephric space is bordered by the anterior and posterior perirenal fascia, also known as Gerota's fascia. The posterior pararenal space contains only fat and is not typically involved with inflammatory processes. The anterior pararenal space is open across the midline and contains the duodenum, pancreas, and ascending and descending colon (Fig. 5.18).

Tissue density

The Hounsfield unit (HU) is a measurement of relative tissue densities determined with CT. Simple benign renal cysts have densities ranging from –20 to +20 HU. Soft tissue measurements range between 30 and 80 HU. Bone density is high (400–1000 HU), while air is –1000 HU. Fat is –80 to –100 HU. The values vary somewhat among different machines and can vary depending on the imaging parameters selected. Fat, water, and some soft tissue densities can look identical to the eye, so such measurement is essential.

Contrast and noncontrast CT

CT examination of the kidneys can be performed with or without intravenous contrast. Noncontrast imaging allows the kidneys to be evaluated for the presence of calcium deposition and hemorrhage, which are obscured following contrast administration (see Fig. 5.2b). Noncontrast CT is the examination of choice in patients with renal colic and suspected nephrolithiasis[19,20].

Noncontrast CT followed by contrast-enhanced CT can be helpful in renal infection not only for identification of a

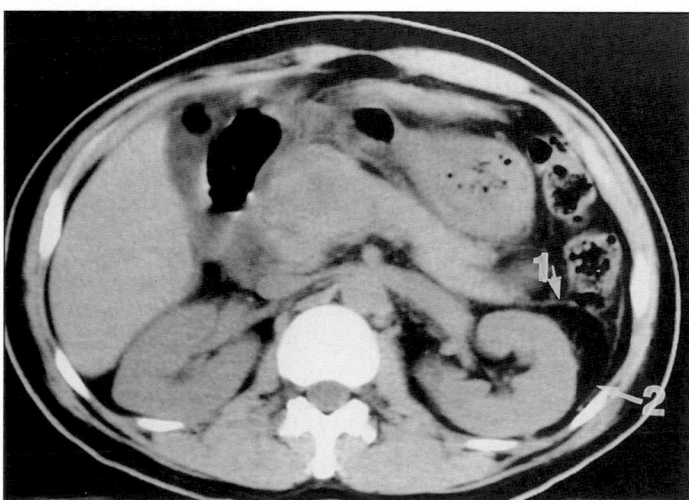

Figure 5.18 Noncontrast CT through the mid abdomen showing the retroperitoneal spaces. The kidney is situated in the perirenal space. The fascia surrounding the kidney is known as Gerota's fascia and comprises anterior (1) and posterior (2) fascial planes.

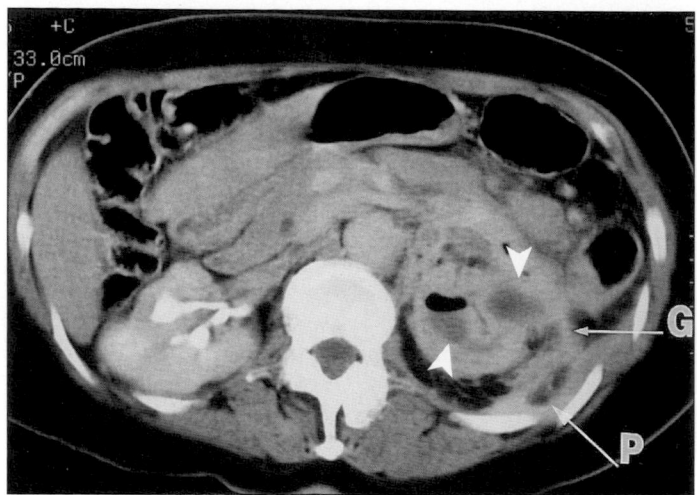

Figure 5.19 Emphysematous pyelonephritis. Contrast-enhanced CT showing gas within an enlarged left kidney and marked enhancement of Gerota's fascia (G) and the posterior perirenal space (P) indicative of inflammatory involvement.

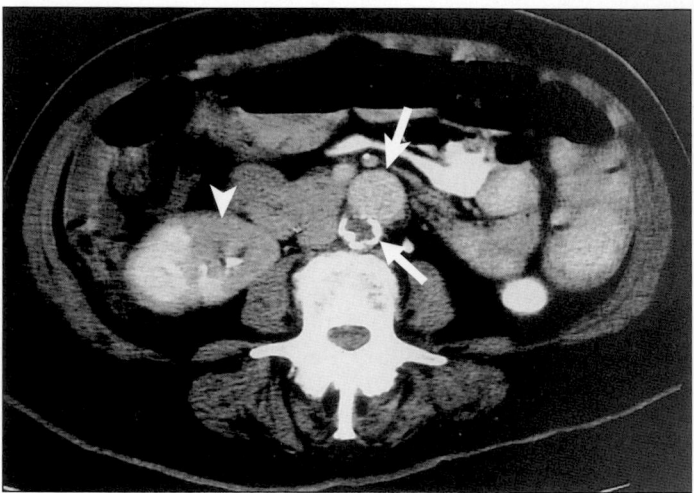

Figure 5.21 Renal infarction involving the medial half of the right kidney following aortic bypass surgery. CT scan shows densely calcified wall of the native aorta (arrow). The aortic graft is anterior to the native aorta (arrow).

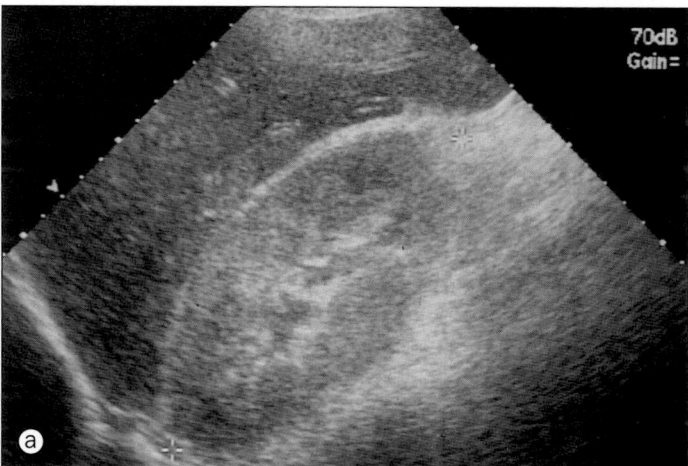

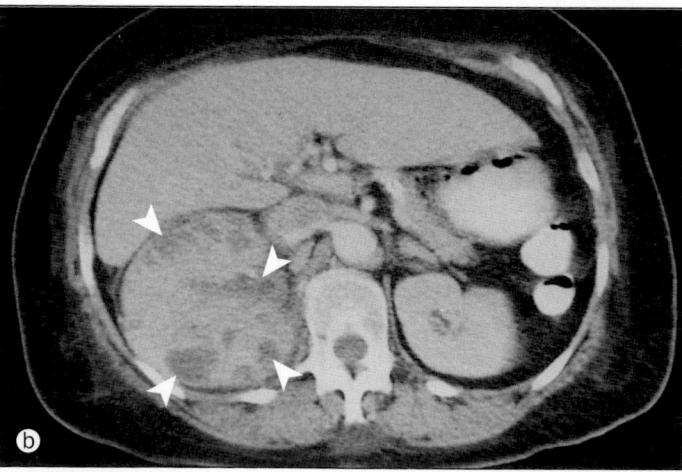

Figure 5.20 Acute pyelonephritis. (a) Ultrasound demonstrates an enlarged echogenic kidney. Bipolar length of kidney = 12.9 cm. (b) CT scan obtained 24 h later demonstrates multiple nonenhancing abscesses (arrowheads).

possible obstructing calculus but also for identification of the extent of parenchymal and perinephric involvement (Fig. 5.19).

Typically, the kidneys are imaged after contrast administration. With helical scans, the kidneys can be imaged initially during the cortical medullary phase and then later during the excretory phase. The kidneys should be similar in size and show equivalent enhancement and excretion. During the cortical medullary phase, there is brisk enhancement of the cortex. The cortical mantle should be intact. Any disruption of the cortical enhancement requires further evaluation: it may be caused by acute pyelonephritis (Fig. 5.20) or infarction (Fig. 5.21). During the excretory phase the entire kidney and renal pelvis enhance. Delayed excretion can be a finding in obstruction (Fig. 5.22) but also in renal parenchymal disease such as acute tubular necrosis.

CT angiography

One major advantage of helical scanning is the ability to perform CT angiography, which can produce images that are similar to conventional angiography and are less invasive. To perform CT angiography, a timed bolus of contrast is administered and the images are obtained at 0.5–3.0-mm consecutive intervals. The images are then reconstructed at a workstation. The aorta and branch vessels are well demonstrated. This technique has been used with success for assessment of the renal vascular supply in patients undergoing renal donor transplant evaluation. It can be used to screen for renal artery stenosis as well with sensitivity of 96% and specificity of 99% for the detection of hemodynamically significant stenosis when compared to digital subtraction angiography[21]. Advantages of CT angiography include the depiction of accessory renal arteries as well as non-renal causes of hypertension such as adrenal masses.

Limitations of CT

There are some limitations to CT. The cradle that the patient lies on has a weight limit, which varies by manufacturer:

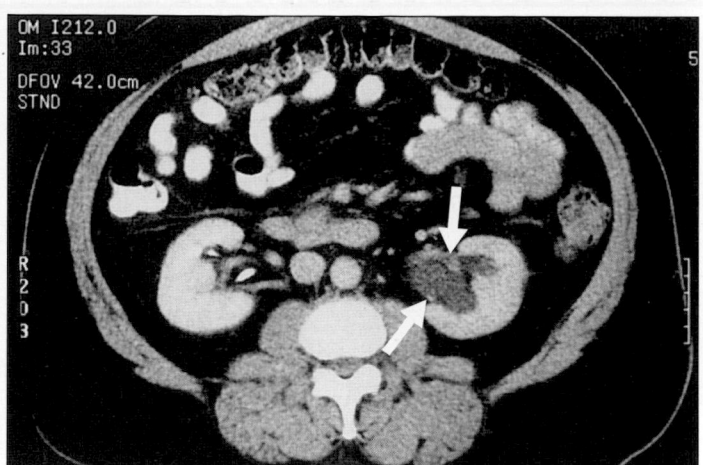

Figure 5.22 Delayed excretion in the left kidney secondary to a distal calculus. Contrast CT showing dilated left renal pelvis (arrows).

135 kg (300 lb) limits are typical. Large patients often have suboptimal scans because of poor intravenous access and extensive artifact caused by the excess weight. This can a particular problem in the abdomen and retroperitoneum. Ultrasound can be an alternative to CT in some situations. Finally, CT is very sensitive to metal. Retroperitoneal clips and intramedullary rods will cause extensive streak artifact, which severely degrades the images. In this situation, other imaging modalities should be considered.

MAGNETIC RESONANCE IMAGING

MRI should only rarely be the first examination used to evaluate the kidneys, but typically it is an adjunct to another imaging technique. The major advantage of MRI over the other imaging modalities is the capability of direct multiplanar imaging. CT is limited to slice acquisition in the axial plane of the abdomen. Coronal and sagittal planes are acquired by reconstruction of the axial data, which can lead to loss of information. MRI images can be directly acquired in other planes.

Tissues contain an abundance of hydrogen, the nuclei of which are positively charged particles called protons. These protons spin on their axis producing a magnetic field (magnetic moment). When a patient is placed in a strong magnetic field in an MRI scanner the protons align along the direction

of, or in the opposite direction to, the field. When the radio-frequency pulse is applied some of the protons aligned with the field will absorb energy and reverse their direction. This absorbed energy is given off as a radiofrequency pulse as the protons relax (return to their original alignment), producing a voltage in the receiver coil. The coil is the hardware that covers the region of interest. For renal imaging, a body coil or torso coil is used. Relaxation is a three-dimensional event giving rise to two parameters: T_1 relaxation results in the recovery of magnetization in the longitudinal (spin–lattice) plane while T_2 results from the loss of transverse (spin–spin) magnetization. A rapid sequence variant of T_2 in common use is fast spin echo (FSE). Hydrogen ions move at slightly different rates in the different tissues. This difference is used to select imaging parameters that can suppress or aid in the detection of fat and water. Fluid, such as urine, is dark or low in signal on T_1-weighted sequences and bright or high in signal on FSE sequences. Fat is bright on T_1 and not as bright on FSE sequences (Fig. 5.23). When MRI is performed, the sequences and imaging planes selected must be tailored to the individual case.

The standard imaging sequences usually include T_1 and FSE sequences. The imaging plane varies depending on the clinical concerns. Usually one sequence is performed in the axial plane. Sagittal images cover the entire length of the kidney and can make some subtle renal parenchymal abnormalities more conspicuous (Fig. 5.24).

On T_1-weighted sequences, the renal cortex is higher in signal than the medulla, producing a distinct corticomedullary differentiation. An indistinct corticomedullary junction is a feature of parenchymal renal disease. It is analogous to the echogenic kidney seen on ultrasound. On FSE sequences, the corticomedullary distinction is not as sharp but should still be present.

Contrast MRI

As with CT, intravenous contrast can be administered to allow further characterization of the lesions. Gadolinium is a paramagnetic contrast agent that is much less nephrotoxic than iodinated contrast and can be used in patients with depressed renal function[22-24]. Paramagnetic contrast agents are currently being investigated for use in evaluation of glomerular function.

Following injection of gadolinium, the vessels appears high in signal, or white, on T_1-weighted sequences. For renal

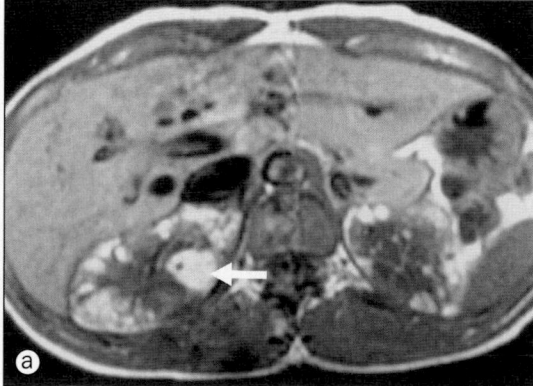

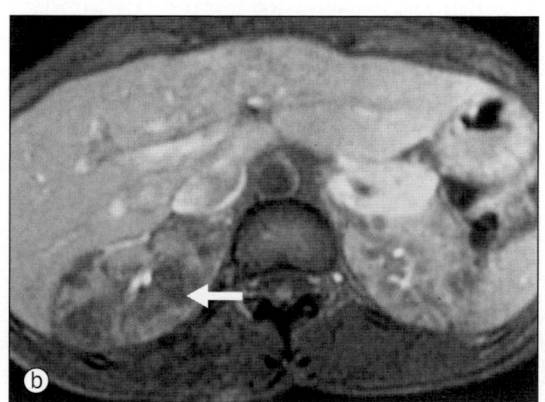

Figure 5.23 MRI in tuberous sclerosis. There are multiple renal angiomyolipomas. (a) T_1-weighted image. The tumors are high in signal on T_1 because of their fat – the largest is arrowed. (b) T_1-weighted image with fat suppression. The fat within the tumors is now low in signal.

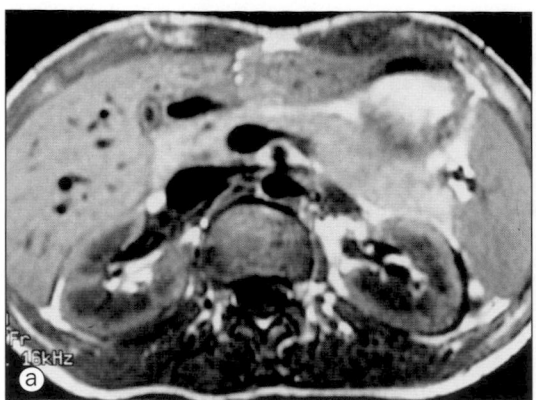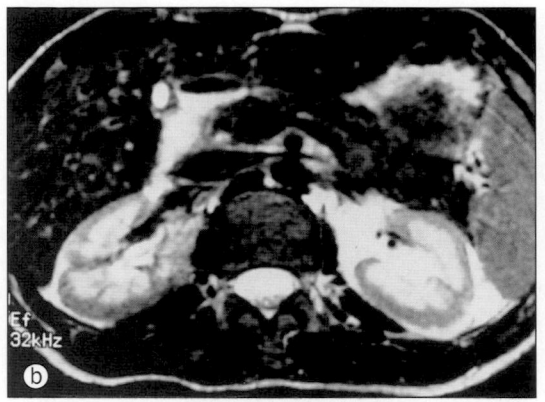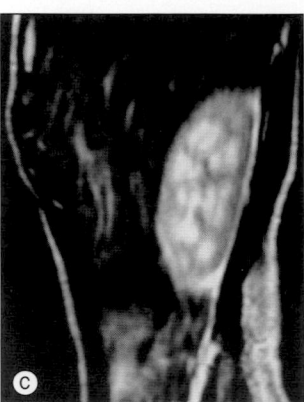

Figure 5.24 Normal MRI images through the kidneys. (a) T_1-weighted image. Note the distinct corticomedullary differentiation. (b) FSE image. The urine within the collecting tubules causes the high signal within the renal pelvis on this sequence. (c) FSE for normal sagittal image of the right kidney.

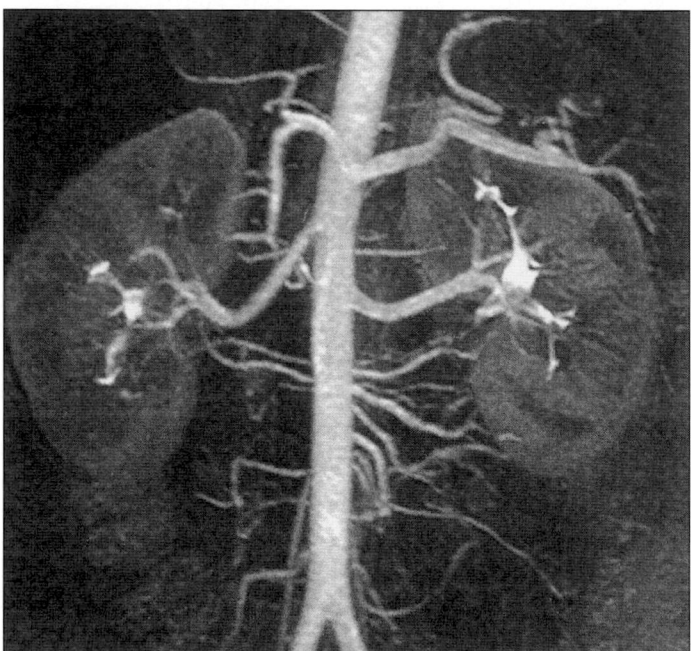

Figure 5.25 MR angiography. Coronal three-dimensional image following contrast administration showing normal renal arteries.

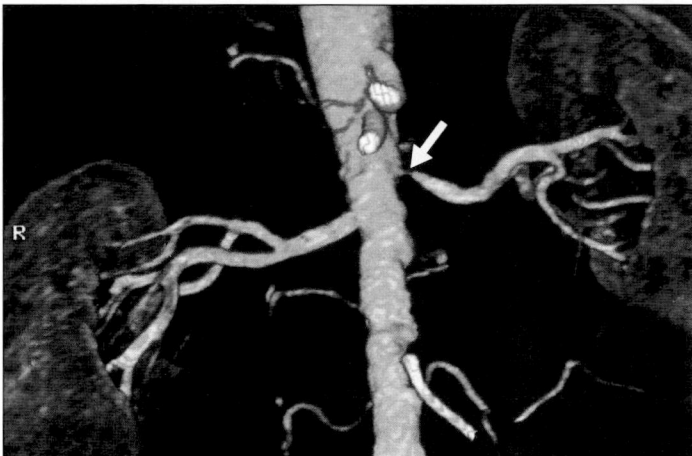

Figure 5.26 MR angiography. Coronal three-dimensional image showing left renal artery stenosis (arrow).

imaging, a bolus administration of gadolinium is administered followed by a rapid type of T_1 sequence called gradient echo imaging. Multiple images can be obtained in a single breath-held acquisition. This technique is useful for lesion characterization in patients who cannot obtain iodinated contrast. As with contrast-enhanced CT, the kidneys will initially demonstrate symmetric cortical enhancement, which eventually progresses to excretion. A delay in enhancement can be seen with renal artery stenosis.

MR angiography

MR angiography can be performed with or without intravenous contrast administration, although contrast is preferred. The aorta and branch vessels are beautifully demonstrated (Fig. 5.25). This technique is performed to evaluate the renal arteries for stenosis and is less invasive than angiography (Fig. 5.26). New technical advances in magnetic

resonance technology including faster sequences have greatly improved the current state of MR angiography. MRA has a sensitivity of 96% and a specificity of 93% when compared to digital subtraction angiography for the detection of renal artery stenosis[25]. It is becoming the primary screening modality in patients with hypertension, declining renal function and iodinated contrast allergy[26].

Disadvantages of MRI

MRI, like CT, has some disadvantages. The table and gantry are confining, so claustrophobic patients may be uncooperative for the study. Patients with some types of internal metallic hardware such as pacemakers cannot undergo MRI.

ANGIOGRAPHY

In the past, angiography was frequently performed for diagnosis, a role that has gradually been replaced by cross-sectional imaging. Angiography is now most often performed for therapeutic intervention such as embolotherapy or angioplasty. Diagnostic angiography is currently most frequently used for evaluation of the renal arteries to assess possible stenosis (Fig. 5.27) and, in many situations, correct it with angioplasty (Fig. 5.28). Although CT and MR angiography techniques are improving, they remain inferior to conventional angiography for detection of accessory renal arteries, which are often small and bilateral and a not infrequent cause of renal artery hypertension. There is also a role for diagnostic angiography in the evaluation of medium and large vessel vasculitis and detection of renal infarction.

The conventional arteriogram is performed through arterial puncture followed by catheter placement in the aorta. An abdominal aortogram is obtained to identify the renal arteries. Selective renal artery catheterization can be performed as necessary. The images can be obtained with conventional film or digital subtraction angiography. Conventional angiography is superior to digital angiography but requires higher doses of contrast material. Digital subtraction angiography uses computer reconstruction and manipulation to generate the images.

Renal venography

Venography is not routinely performed. Previously it was obtained for evaluation of renal vein thrombosis and gonadal vein thrombosis but it has largely been replaced with contrast-enhanced CT.

RADIONUCLIDE EVALUATION OF THE KIDNEYS

Unlike the other imaging modalities, scintigraphy provides a noninvasive means to obtain both qualitative and quantitative information about the kidneys. The gamma ray camera captures the photons from a radiotracer within the patient and generates an image. Images can be obtained over the entire body or portions of the body. Single-photon emission-computed tomography (SPECT) is a specialized type of imaging; the emitted photons are measured at multiple angles. There are three categories of radiotracers used in renal imaging, which differ in their mode of renal clearance: glomerular filtration, tubular secretion, and tubular retention agents (see Table 5.5).

Glomerular filtration agents

Glomerular filtration agents are cleared by the glomerulus and can be used to measure the glomerular filtration rate (GFR). [99]Technetium-labeled diethylenetriamine pentaacetic acid (DTPA), is the most common glomerular agent used for imaging. In patients with poor renal function, mercaptoacetyl triglycine (^{99}Tc-labeled MAG3) and o-iodohippurate, [^{131}I]OIH, are superior to DTPA (Fig. 5.29)[27,28].

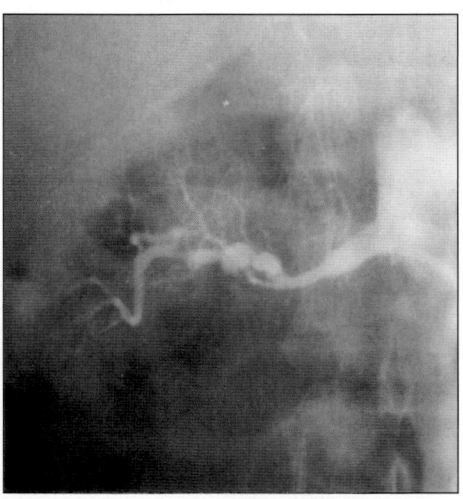

Figure 5.27 Fibromuscular dysplasia. Selective right renal arteriogram demonstrating typical beaded appearance. (Courtesy of Dr Harold Mitty.)

Choice of radionuclide in renal imaging	
Glomerular filtration rate	^{99}Tc-DTPA
Glomerular filtration rate with renal impairment	^{99}Tc-MAG3, ^{131}I-OIH
Effective renal plasma flow	^{99}Tc-MAG3, ^{131}I-OIH
Renal scarring	^{99}Tc-DMSA, ^{99}Tc-GH
Renal pseudotumor	DMSA
Upper renal tract obstruction	^{99}Tc-DTPA
Upper renal tract obstruction with renal impairment	^{99}Tc-MAG3

Table 5.5 Choice of radionuclide in renal imaging

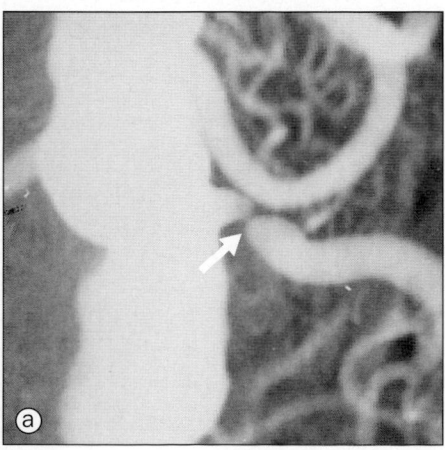
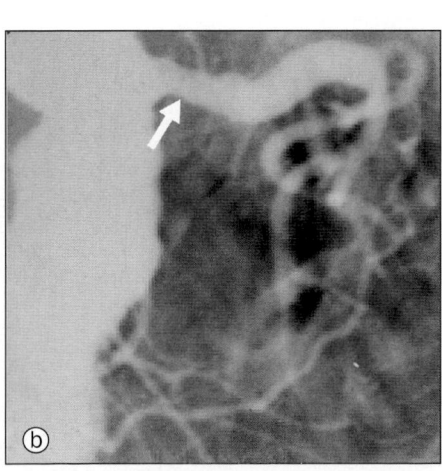

Figure 5.28 Left renal artery stenosis and angioplasty. (a) Aortogram demonstrating a tight left renal artery stenosis (arrow). (b) Postangioplasty image with marked improvement of the stenosis (arrow). (Courtesy of Dr Harold Mitty.)

Investigation of Renal Disease

Tubular secretion agents

Agents handled primarily by tubular secretion are used to estimate effective renal plasma flow because of their higher renal extraction and clearance. Both [131I]OIH and 99Tc-labeled MAG3 are secreted from the proximal tubule. The clearance rate for [131I]OIH in normal patients is 500–600 mL/min and for 99Tc-labeled MAG3 is 340 mL/min[29].

Tubular retention agents

Tubular retention agents include 99Tc-labeled dimercaptosuccinate (DMSA) and 99Tc-labeled glucoheptonate (GH). These agents provide excellent cortical imaging and can be used in suspected renal scarring and for clarification of renal pseudotumors.

The renogram

A renogram is generated by scintigraphy and provides information about blood flow, renal uptake, and excretion. Time–activity generated graphs are produced that plot flow of the radiotracer into each kidney relative to the aorta. Peak enhancement and clearance of the tracer are also plotted. DTPA, MAG3, and OIH can be used to generate the renogram. The relative radiotracer uptake can be measured and can provide split or differential information about renal function (Fig. 5.30).

The blood pool or flow images are obtained following injection of the radiotracers. Images are obtained with the gamma ray camera every several seconds for the first minute. The second component of the renogram evaluates renal function by measuring radiotracer uptake and excretion by the kidney. In normal patients, the peak concentration occurs between 3 and 5 min after injection tracer. Delayed transit of the isotope will alter the curve of the renogram.

In cases of suspected obstructive uropathy, a diuretic renogram can be obtained. A loop diuretic is injected intravenously when radiotracer activity is present in the renal pelvis; a computer-generated washout curve is obtained. In patients with true obstruction activity, it will remain in the renal pelvis, whereas it will quickly decrease in patients without an obstruction (Fig. 5.31).

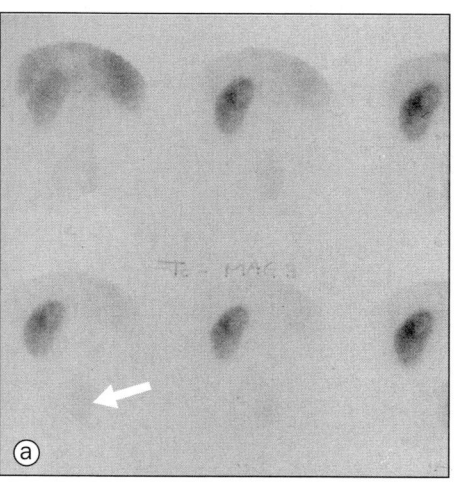

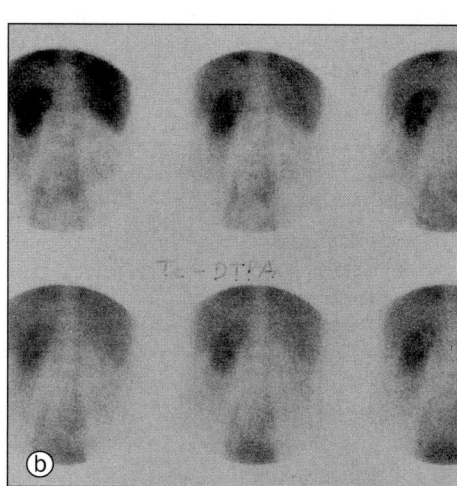

Figure 5.29 Advantage of 99Tc-labeled MAG3 in acute renal impairment. (a) Examination with 99Tc-labeled MAG3; note faint identification of the right pelvic kidney. (b) 99Tc-labeled DTPA examination obtained when renal function was markedly improved; however, the pelvic kidney is not identified. (Courtesy of Dr Chun Kim.)

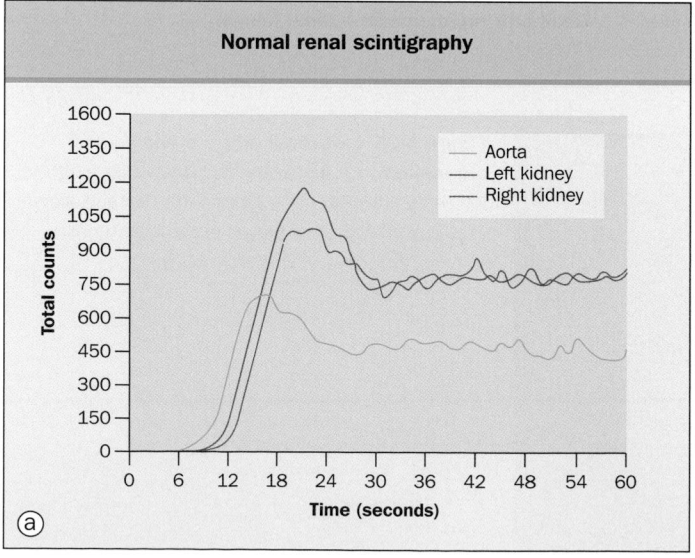

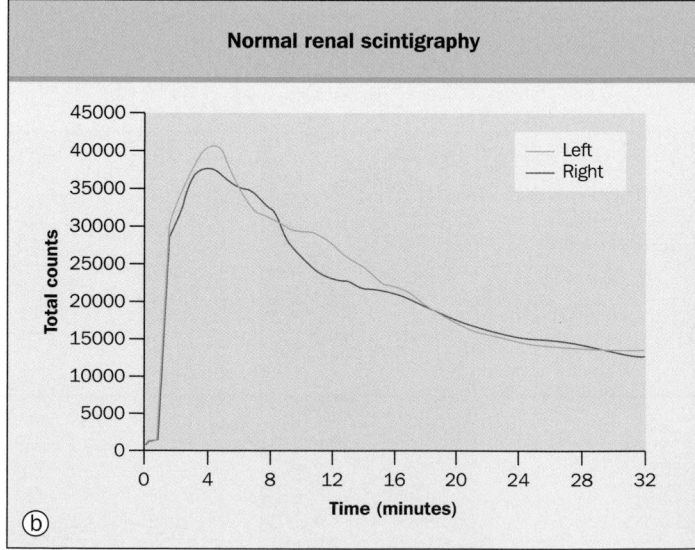

Figure 5.30 Normal 99Tc-labeled DTPA study – time activity curves. (a) Early (0–1 min), showing renal blood flow. (b) Later (0–30 min) showing renal uptake and excretion of tracer. (Courtesy of Dr Chun Kim.)

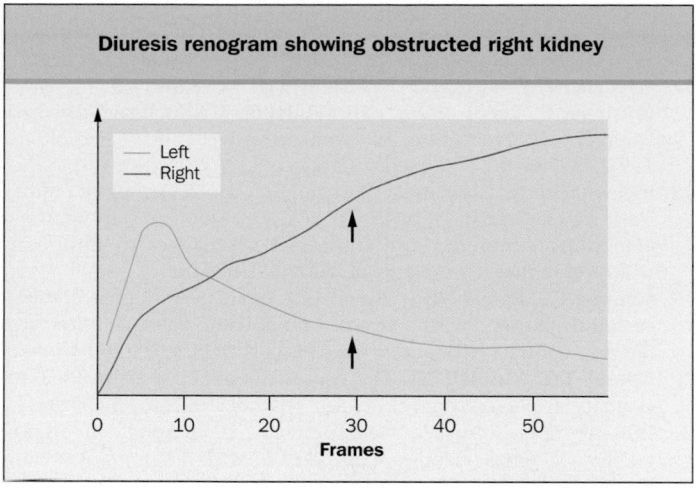

Diuresis renogram showing obstructed right kidney

Figure 5.31 Diuresis renogram showing obstructed right kidney. Isotope continues to accumulate in the right kidney despite intravenous furosemide (given at ↑). Isotope excretion in left kidney is normal.

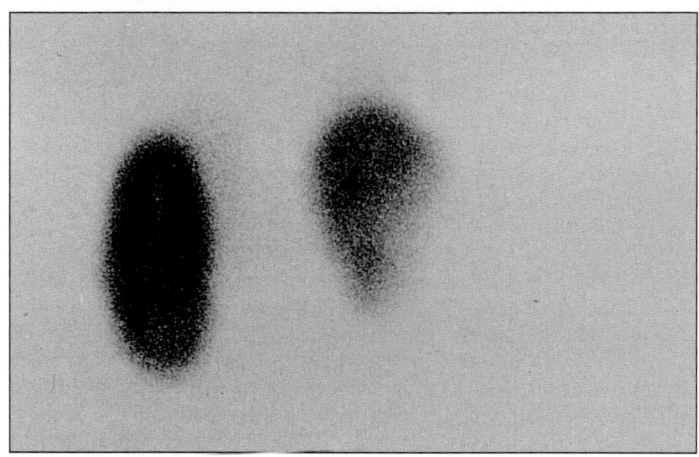

Figure 5.32 Renal infarct. DMSA scan in a newborn with a right lower pole infarct secondary to an embolus from an umbilical catheter. (Courtesy of Dr Chun Kim.)

Captopril renogram

An activated renin–angiotensin pathway occurs in the presence of renal artery stenosis. Angiotensin-converting enzyme (ACE) inhibitors prevent the conversion of angiotensin I to angiotensin II, thus reducing vasoconstriction of the efferent glomerular arterioles, with a subsequent decrease in the glomerular hydrostatic pressure. A decrease in glomerular filtration occurs in the affected kidney, which can be detected with the time–activity curve. Patients with suspected renal artery hypertension are examined initially with a standard renogram. Diuretics and ACE inhibitors are withheld several days prior to the study. A baseline renogram is performed using ^{99}Tc-labeled DTPA or ^{99}Tc-labeled MAG3. Flow and renogram curves are generated. The examination is then repeated following the administration of an ACE inhibitor, usually captopril. Findings indicative of renal artery stenosis include a delayed time to maximum radioactivity, cortical retention of the isotope, and a decrease in the GFR of the ipsilateral kidney. The sensitivity of captopril renography is decreased in the setting of renal insufficiency. It does not have a role in the evaluation small, nonfunctioning kidneys found in end-stage renal disease. However, if the small, nonfunctional kidney is unilateral, captopril renography can still be used to evaluate the contralateral kidney.

Cortical imaging

Renal cortical imaging is performed with ^{99}Tc-labeled GH or ^{99}Tc-labeled DMSA. Information about renal size, location, and contour can be obtained (Fig. 5.32). The study is most commonly used for evaluation of renal scarring, particularly in the pediatric age group, and for clarification of renal pseudotumors such as a suspected column of Bertin in which an apparent mass on ultrasound is found to produce no abnormality on radionuclide scanning. Split renal function can also be determined from cortical imaging. Pinhole imaging (using a pinhole collimator which magnifies the kidney so that you get more anatomic detail than with planar imaging) and, more recently, SPECT imaging have been found to be useful for detection of cortical defects caused by inflammation or scarring. Cortical imaging may be better than ultrasound in the evaluation of the young patient with urinary tract infection[30].

Vesicoureteral reflux

In children with suspected reflux causing pyelonephritis, a standard cystogram is obtained. The child is subsequently followed up with a radioisotope cystogram. The radioisotope cystogram exposes the child to a lower radiation dose and can be used to quantitate the bladder capacity when reflux occurs. The study is performed following placement of technetium pertechnetate into the bladder. Images are obtained during voiding.

Renal transplants

Renal transplants are easily evaluated with scintigraphy. As with the normal kidneys information about blood flow and function can be determined. Postoperative complications are also well delineated[31].

REFERENCES

1. Morris TW, Fischer HW. The pharmacology of intravascular radio-contrast media. Annu Rev Pharmacol Toxicol. 1986;26:143–60.
2. Norby A, Tvedt KE, Halgunset J, Haugen OA. Intracellular penetration and accumulation of radiographic contrast media in the rat kidney. Scanning Microsc. 1990;4:651–66.
3. Bahlmann J, Kruskemper HL. Elimination of iodine containing contrast media by hemodialysis. Nephron. 1973;19:25–55.
4. Shehadi WH. Adverse reactions to intravascularly administered contrast media. Am J Radiol. 1975;124:145–52.
5. Katayama H, Yamaguchi K, Kozuka T, et al. Adverse reactions to ionic and nonionic contrast media: a report from the Japanese committee on the safety of contrast media. Radiology. 1990;175:616–18.
6. Cohan RH, Dunnick NR. Intravascular contrast media: adverse reactions. Am J Radiol. 1987;149:665–70.
7. Katzberg RW. Urography into the 21st century: new contrast media, renal handling, imaging characteristics and nephrotoxicity. Radiology. 1997;204:297–312.
8. Tepel M, Van der Giet M, Schwartzfeld C, et al. Prevention of radiographic-contrast induced reductions in renal function by acetylcysteine. N Engl J Med. 2000;343:180–4.
9. Murphy, MB, Murray, C, Shorten, GD. Fenoldopam – a selective peripheral dopamine receptor agonist for the treatment of severe hypertension. N Engl J Med. 2001;345:1548–57.
10. Blake SP, McNicholas MM, Raptopoulos V. Nonopaque crystal deposition causing ureteric obstruction in patients with HIV undergoing Indinavir therapy. Am J Radiol. 1998;171:717–20.
11. Diagnostic and interventional techniques. In: Dunnick NR, Sandler CM, Amis ES, Newhouse JH, eds. Textbook of uroradiology, 2nd edn. Baltimore: Williams and Wilkins; 1997:44–87.
12. Bosniak MA. The current radiologic approach to renal cysts. Radiology. 1986;158:1–10.
13. Kohler TR, Zierler RE, Martin RL, et al. Noninvasive diagnosis of renal artery stenosis by ultrasonic duplex scanning. J Vasc Surg. 1986;4:450–6.
14. Berland LL, Koslin DB, Routh WD, Keller FS. Renal artery stenosis: Prospective evaluation of diagnosis with color duplex US compared with angiography. Radiology. 1990;174:421–3.
15. Olin JW, Piedmonte MR, Young JR, et al. The utility of ultrasound duplex scanning of the renal arteries for diagnosing significant renal artery stenosis. Ann Intern Med. 1995;122:833–8.
16. Kliewer MA, Tupler RH, Carroll BA, et al. Renal artery stenosis: analysis of doppler waveform parameters and tardus-parvus pattern. Radiology. 1993;189:779–87.
17. Schwerk WB, Restrepo IK, Stellwaag M, Klose KJ, Schade-Brittinger C. Renal artery stenosis: grading with image-directed Doppler US evaluation of renal resistive index. Radiology. 1994;190:785–90.
18. Radermacher J, Chavan A, Schaffer J, et al. Detection of significant renal artery stenosis with color Doppler sonography: combining extrarenal and intrarenal approaches to minimize technical failure. Clin Nephrol. 2000;53:333–43.
19. Sommer FG, Jeffrey RB Jr, Rubin GD, et al. Detection of ureteral calculi in patients with suspected renal colic. Value of reformatted non-contrast helical CT. Am J Radiol. 1995;165:509–13.
20. Lanoue MZ, Mindell HJ. The use of unenhanced helical CT to evaluate suspected renal colic. Am J Radiol. 1997;169:1579–84.
21. Wittenberg G, Kenn W, Tschammler A, et al. Spiral CT angiography of renal arteries: comparison with angiography. Eur Radiol. 1999;9:546–51.
22. Prince MR, Arnoldus C, Frisoli JK. Nephrotoxicity of high dose gadolinium compared with iodinated contrast. J Magn Reson Imaging. 1996;6:162–6.
23. Tombach B, Bremer C, Reimer P, et al. Renal tolerance of a neutral gadolinium chelate (gabobutrol) in patients with chronic renal failure: results of a randomized study. Radiology. 2001;218:651–7.
24. Townsend RR, Cohen DL, Katholi R, et al. Safety of intravenous gadolinium (Gd-BOPTA) infusion in patients with renal insufficiency. Am J Kidney Dis. 2000;36:1207–12.
25. Mittal TK, Evans C, Perkins T, Wood AM. Renal arteriography using gadolinium enhanced 3D MR angiography – clinical experience with the technique, its limitations and pitfalls. Br J Radiol. 2001;74:495–502.
26. Marcos HB, Choyke PL. Magnetic resonance angiography of the kidney. Semin Nephrol. 2000;20:450–55.
27. Taylor A, Nally JV. Clinical applications of renal scintigraphy. Am J Radiol. 1995;64:31–41.
28. Taylor A Jr, Ziffer JA, Echima D. Comparison of Tc-99m MAG3 and Tc-99m DTPA in renal transplant patients with impaired renal function. Clin Nucl Med. 1990;15:371–8.
29. Taylor A, Eshima D, Christian PE, et al. A technetium-99m MAG3 kit formulation: preliminary results in normal volunteers and patients with renal failure. J Nucl Med. 1988;29:616–62.
30. Mastin ST, Drane WE, Iravani A. Tc 99m DMSA SPECT imaging in patients with acute symptoms or history of UTI; comparison with ultrasonography. Clin Nucl Med.1995;20:407–12.
31. Genitourinary imaging. In: Thrall JH, Zeissman HA, eds. Nuclear medicine, the requisites. St Louis: Mosby; 1995:283–320.

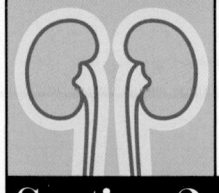

Chapter 6

Renal Biopsy

Michael Boulton-Jones

INTRODUCTION

The introduction of renal biopsy transformed the study of renal disease, particularly glomerular disease, by providing the pathologic information that formed the basis for a classification of disease still in current use and offering many insights into pathogenesis. Indeed the development of renal biopsy as a safe and informative technique was a key step in the evolution of nephrology as a specialty. Renal biopsy now plays a central role in the investigational approach of the nephrologist.

Iversen and Brun, in Copenhagen, adapted the liver biopsy technique (used since the 1930s) to attempt renal biopsies and published their first experiences in 1951[1]. They used intravenous urography to target the right kidney and the biopsy was obtained by suction with the patient in the sitting position. In Chicago, Kark and Muehrcke improved on the Danes' technique by using a modified Vim Silverman needle and lying the patient flat[2]. Their technique, reported in 1954, laid the foundation for the method used by nephrologists for the next 30 years. There have been two major modifications to the technique in recent years. First, the use of realtime ultrasound to localize the kidney[3] and observe the route of the biopsy needle. Second, improvements in the design of the needle used for biopsy with the introduction of the Trucut needle and subsequently the gun-mounted semiautomatic biopsy needle.

INDICATIONS FOR RENAL BIOPSY

Four groups of patients benefit most from the findings of renal biopsy: those with nephrotic syndrome, those with renal disease in the setting of a systemic disorder, those with acute renal failure and those with a renal transplant. Some patients with non-nephrotic proteinuria, hematuria, and chronic renal failure may also benefit.

Nephrotic syndrome

There are few exceptions to the general rule that renal biopsy is required in nephrotic syndrome (proteinuria > 3.5 g/day) to establish a diagnosis and plan therapy. The exceptions include:
- children from one year of age to puberty, who may be assumed to have minimal change nephrotic syndrome unless there is a reason to suspect otherwise, such as a low C3 concentration, hematuria, or renal impairment; these children should receive a trial of corticosteroids and biopsy is performed only if there is no response. Minimal change nephrotic syndrome is quite rare in infants less than 1 year old and a biopsy is necessary to identify other causes including congenital nephrotic syndrome of Finnish type or diffuse mesangial sclerosis.
- diabetics, who can be assumed to have diabetic nephropathy if they have a long history of diabetes with evidence of other diabetic microangiopathy including retinopathy, an inactive urine sediment and normal kidneys on ultrasound.

Systemic disease associated with proteinuria or renal failure

Many systemic diseases such as amyloid, drug reactions, myeloma and sarcoidosis may be diagnosed on renal biopsy. In other diseases, of which systemic lupus erythematosus is the best example, the biopsy may also indicate disease activity and be used to assess past treatment and plan future management.

Acute renal failure

The diagnosis of patients presenting with acute renal failure is often straightforward on clinical grounds as when acute tubular necrosis develops in the context of renal hypoperfusion. But in any patient with acute renal failure in whom the diagnosis is not clear, biopsy should be undertaken as soon as possible to make a diagnosis and start appropriate treatment with minimal delay.

The presence of hematuria and proteinuria with red cell casts is a useful pointer to a glomerular disease, as is a history characteristic of systemic vasculitis. Urgent biopsy is valuable in vasculitis to confirm the diagnosis and establish the severity of the acute inflammatory reaction and extent of fibrosis. However, if antineutrophil cytoplasmic antibodies (ANCA) are present and treatment is required for extrarenal manifestations of vasculitis, it can be argued that there is little reason for biopsy. It must be remembered, however, that a positive ANCA may occur in other settings such as endocarditis, and renal biopsy findings may help to clarify the diagnosis. Renal biopsy may also have a valuable role some time after initial treatment to assess severity and reversibility and, thus, to judge the value of continuing immunosuppressive therapy.

Non-nephrotic proteinuria

The value of renal biopsy in isolated non-nephrotic proteinuria (< 3.5 g/24 h) is less clear than in nephrotic syndrome. The REIN study showed a progressive acceleration in rate of loss of renal function with increasing proteinuria. Proteinuria

< 1.5 g/day was associated with a fall in GFR of 0.12 mL/min/month, with no significant benefit of ACE inhibitor treatment. The progressive fall in GFR was increased to 0.4 mL/min/month in those with proteinuria 1.5–3 g/day, and in this group ACE inhibitor treatment did slow this deterioration[4]. Therefore, it is worth establishing a diagnosis in patients with proteinuria > 1.5 g/day even if the immediate therapeutic implications are few. An additional indication is required to perform a biopsy with isolated proteinuria (< 1.5 g/24 h), for example, in patients with rheumatoid arthritis in whom the renal histology may influence management. Thus if AA amyloid is demonstrated, treatment should be intensified aiming to reduce the serum amyloid A (or C-reactive protein; CRP) level to normal but if membranous nephropathy is found, gold or penicillamine should be stopped and both avoided thereafter.

Mild proteinuria associated with hematuria

IgA nephropathy often presents with proteinuria of less than 1.5 g/24 h associated with microscopic hematuria. Making the diagnosis is important in that it identifies patients who require long-term follow-up. On the other hand, patients with postinfectious glomerulonephritis may have similar urinary findings but a better prognosis. Therefore, it is reasonable to delay 6 months and to biopsy only if the urinary abnormalities persist, provided renal function is normal.

When these urine abnormalities are associated with systemic disease such as vasculitis or lupus, renal biopsy has greater value in identifying the extent of glomerular injury and planning therapy.

Isolated hematuria

The investigation of patients with hematuria is controversial. Before biopsy is considered, other causes of hematuria should be excluded (see Chapters 57 and 59). However, the diagnoses most likely to be made by biopsy (such as thin membrane nephropathy and IgA nephropathy) are almost invariably benign unless proteinuria subsequently develops. Therefore, many nephrologists elect not to biopsy such patients but rather to follow them up for some years.

Unexplained chronic renal failure

Biopsy is valuable in unexplained renal impairment in patients with no more than minor proteinuria whose ultrasound image of the kidneys shows normal sized kidneys. If the kidneys are shrunken (< 9.5 cm in length in an average adult) the material recovered by biopsy is likely to show extensive glomerulosclerosis and interstitial fibrosis. Not only is it more difficult to arrive at a diagnosis in this sort of biopsy, but it is also unlikely to make a difference to treatment. Ultrasound evidence of increased echogenicity with loss of corticomedullary differentation is also a useful sign of advanced parenchymal disease, although less reliable than renal size.

Renal transplant dysfunction

Biopsy is particularly helpful in the period immediately following transplant in distinguishing between rejection and acute tubular necrosis. Later it can be used to differentiate acute rejection from chronic rejection, which does not require specific treatment, or from nephrotoxicity due to cyclosporine or tacrolimus. The relative ease of taking a biopsy from a transplanted kidney allows biopsy to be used repeatedly when necessary.

PREPARATION FOR RENAL BIOPSY

Workup for renal biopsy (Fig. 6.1) is required to exclude problems that may jeopardize the safety of the procedure and to identify contraindications to biopsy (Table 6.1). In particular the workup should establish that the patient has two kidneys of normal size and shape, that blood pressure is controlled, urine is sterile, and coagulation is normal. If any of these conditions cannot be fulfilled, the biopsy should be delayed until the abnormality has been corrected. Nearly all contraindications are relative rather than absolute and are influenced by the urgency of the clinical situation. For example, a patient with a solitary kidney and rapidly progressive renal failure may merit a biopsy in order to make a diagnosis so that treatment can be given to try to preserve some function in that kidney. While there are occasions when some of these clinical principles may need to be overruled, a biopsy should never be performed in the face of deranged coagulation. The tests of coagulation include platelet count, prothrombin time and activated partial thromboplastin time. Bleeding time has a traditional place because many biopsies complicated by hemorrhage are associated with an abnormal bleeding time. However, it has a very poor positive predictive value of about 5%[5]. Therefore, it should be used only in those with high risk which does not include uncomplicated renal failure[5].

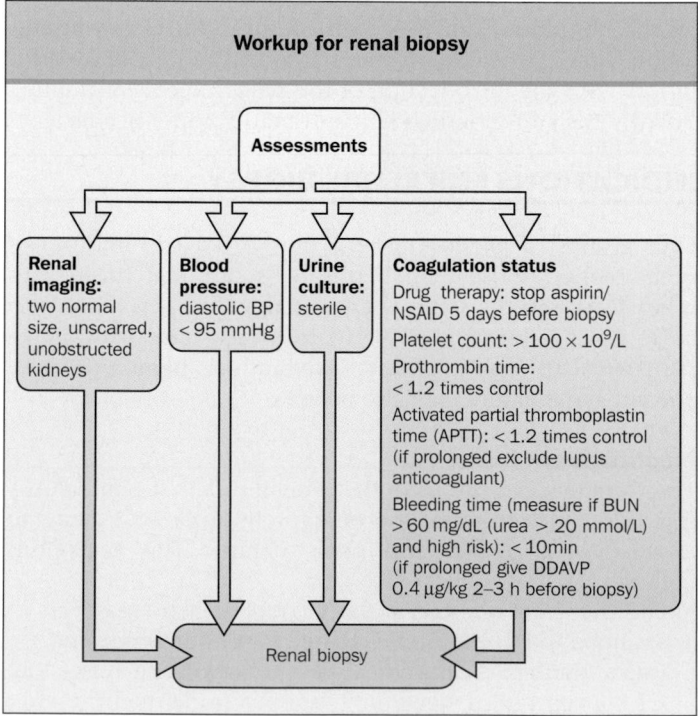

Figure 6.1 Workup for renal biopsy.

Contraindications to renal biopsy	
Kidney status	**Patient status**
Multiple cysts	Uncontrolled blood pressure
Solitary kidney	Uncontrolled bleeding diathesis
Acute pyelonephritis/perinephric abscess	Uremia
Renal neoplasm	Obesity
	Uncooperative patient
Most contraindications to renal biopsy are relative rather than absolute; when clinical circumstances necessitate urgent biopsy they may be overridden, apart from uncontrolled bleeding diathesis.	

Table 6.1 Contraindications to renal biopsy.

THE PROCEDURE

It is our practice to perform the biopsy under ultrasound control using a needle biopsy gun[6]. The biopsy should be performed where proper ultrasound facilities are available to identify the exact location of the kidney, preferably with a radiologist attending. There is no need to sedate the patient except in unusual circumstances. The patient should lie face down and some clinicians prefer a support under the upper abdomen to splint the kidney. Most prefer to biopsy the left kidney. The ultrasonographer (who may be a nephrologist with adequate experience) locates the lower pole of the kidney, and the skin over the target is marked. The chances of obtaining cortical tissue in the biopsy are increased if the needle is advanced at an angle of about 70° rather than vertically, so the skin entry site should be about 3 cm below the target area. The skin is then washed in antiseptic such as betadine or chlorhexidine. Local anesthetic is infiltrated down to

the capsule of the kidney but not into the kidney itself (see Fig. 6.2). A small stab incision is made through the skin. The biopsy needle is then mounted on a biopsy gun (see Fig. 6.3a) and the gun cocked (Fig. 6.3b). The needle is advanced under ultrasound control (the ultrasound probe should be placed in a sterile sleeve (Fig. 6.4)) to just short of the renal capsule. The patient should breathe normally during this phase. Following this, the movement of the kidney relative to the probe should be watched during some deep respiratory cycles and the patient told to hold their breath so that the kidney is in the correct position to biopsy the lower pole (Fig. 6.5). The gun is then fired and the needle withdrawn. The specimen of renal tissue is recovered (Fig. 6.6) and handed to the attendant pathologist or technician, who can examine it, preferably under an operating microscope, for glomerular content. The procedure should be repeated until two cores containing glomeruli are recovered, or the patient experiences discomfort.

One core of the biopsy should be fixed in formalin for light microscopy. The other should be divided so that both portions contain glomeruli. The larger part should be snap frozen in liquid nitrogen and processed for immunofluorescent techniques and the other fixed in gluteraldehyde for examination by electron microscopy. The division into three reduces the chances of all containing glomeruli. Attempts to develop a common way of processing the biopsy suitable for the three different modes of examination have been made but they are not widely applied[7,8].

The patient is then returned to the ward and asked to lie quietly in bed maintaining a high oral fluid intake for 24 h, during which time pulse, blood pressure, and urine output should be monitored. He or she can be discharged next day and asked to avoid strenuous exercise or violent movement for a week. If there is gross hematuria after the biopsy, discharge is delayed and bed rest maintained until the urine clears.

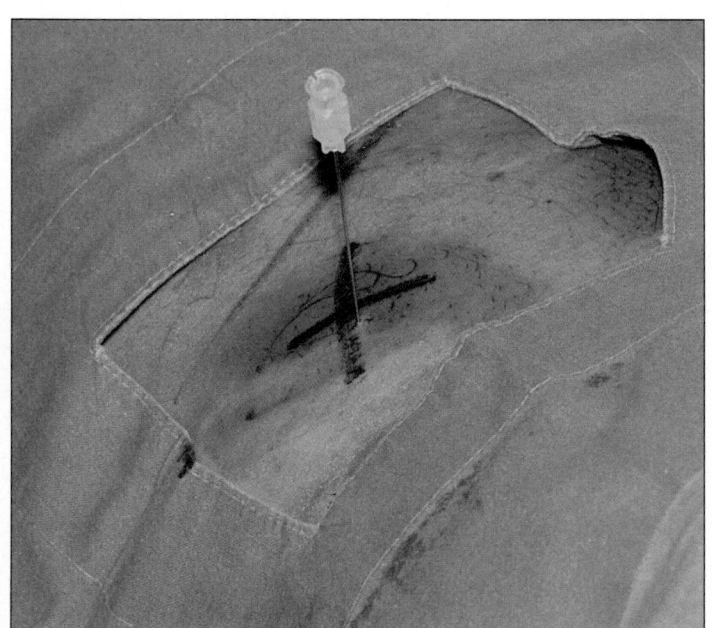

Figure 6.2 Renal biopsy. The skin has been cleaned with betadine, the lower pole of the left kidney identified, and the skin marked appropriately. A fine needle has been inserted for local anesthetic infiltration.

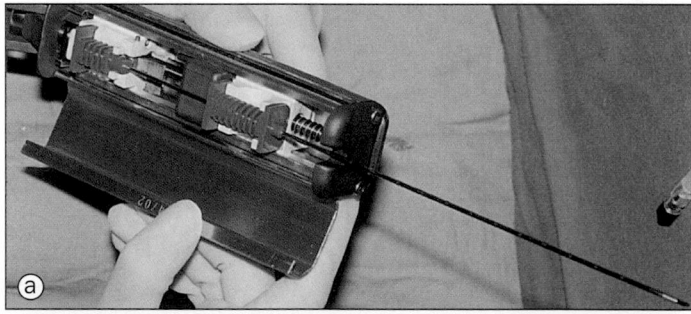

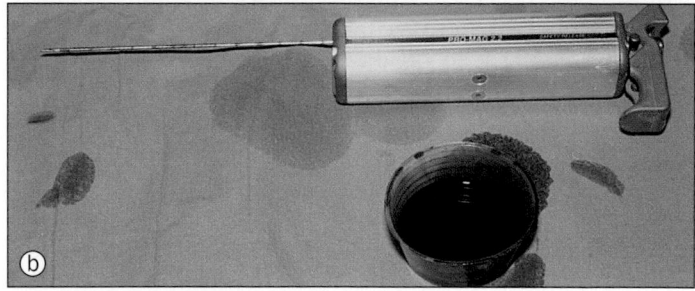

Figure 6.3 Renal biopsy gun. (a) A 16G needle is loaded in the gun. (b) The loaded gun is cocked. The trigger mechanism is on the right.

Investigation of Renal Disease

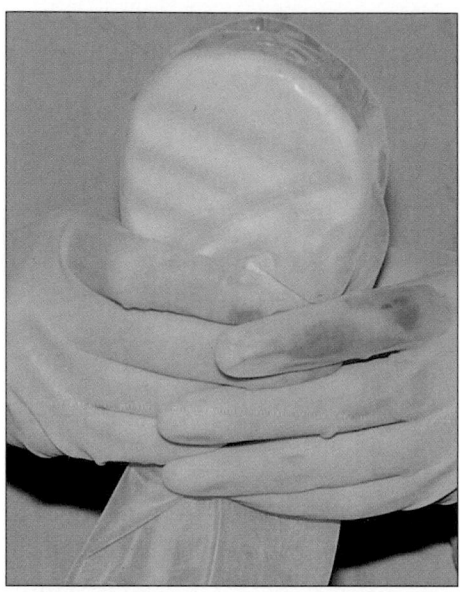

Figure 6.4 The ultrasound probe for renal biopsy. The probe is mounted in a sterile stocking for use during the biopsy.

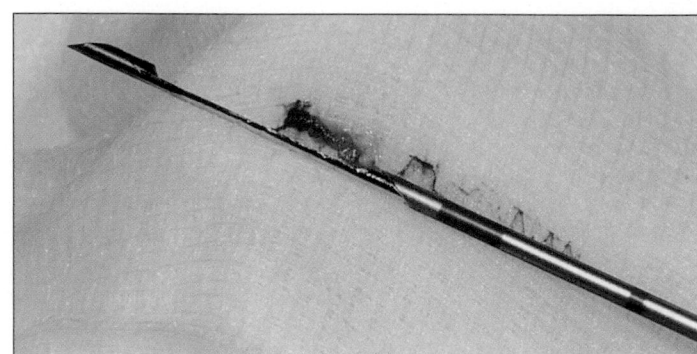

Figure 6.6 Renal biopsy specimen. Tip of biopsy needle and core of tissue obtained at biopsy: this core is only half the length of the needle.

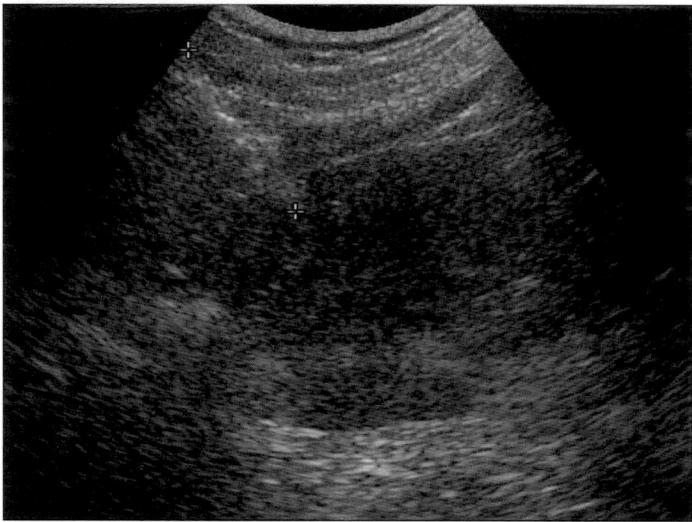

Figure 6.5 Renal biopsy. Ultrasound appearance of the lower pole of the left kidney with biopsy needle entering.

MODIFICATIONS OF THE BIOPSY PROCEDURE

Operator
Nephrologists perform most renal biopsies. However, the growth of interventional radiology has led to radiologists acquiring the necessary skills and it may be administratively easier for them to undertake the biopsy as it reduces the number of personnel who have to be present, especially if the biopsy needle is mounted on the ultrasound probe. However, a radiologist may not be available after hours for clinically urgent biopsies and nephrologists should still be trained and competent in renal biopsy.

Outpatient biopsy
The convention of a 24-h stay in hospital after renal biopsy is sometimes replaced by outpatient biopsy. The biopsy is performed in the morning and the patient lies supine for 8 h following the biopsy before being discharged home the same evening. About 80% of complications are detected within 8 h and 100% in 12 h[9]. Therefore, the outpatient approach carries a slight increase in risk which is probably acceptable in low-risk patients: those with asymptomatic urine abnormalities, normal blood pressure, and preserved renal function[10]. As well as patient convenience, the move toward outpatient biopsy is also influenced in some healthcare systems by the unwillingness of health insurers to reimburse for overnight stay.

Choice of needle and biopsy gun
If a biopsy gun is not available, a Trucut needle or even a modified Vim Silverman needle can be used. The needle should be advanced as before and inserted into the kidney just beyond the capsule. The operator should then take his or her hands off the needle and watch for movement with respiration and for transmitted pulsation, both signs that the needle tip is in the kidney. The biopsy should then be taken while the patient holds their breath.

The use of a biopsy gun has been compared directly with the hand-held Trucut needle. In one study, the success rate of a gun-mounted 18G needle was 93% compared with only 79% obtained with a 15G Trucut needle, and the complication rate was less, although not significantly so[11]. When needles of the same size were compared in another, larger study, no difference in diagnostic adequacy or complications between use of a 14G gun-mounted and a 14G hand-held needle[12] were noted.

The smaller the needle, the fewer the complications but the fewer glomeruli recovered. We find a gun-mounted 16G needle offers the best balance of success and risk.

Imaging
Ultrasound is now universally accepted as superior to intravenous urography for localization of the kidney. An alternative is the use of fluoroscopic screening following contrast injection to localize the needle in the kidney which is very effective in those with preserved renal function but involves the additional risks of contrast and radiation exposure. Ultrasound is used continuously in the procedure described above to observe the needle entering the kidney when using a gun-mounted needle. Alternatively, it is used in many centers to localize the kidney and set the co-ordinates of direction and depth. The actual procedure is then performed without

ultrasound checks. Since both of these techniques have shown a similar diagnostic adequacy (> 95%) and complication rate[13], the choice of techniques should rest with local experience and physician preference. Biopsy under CT localization has been recommended by some for biopsy in difficult or high-risk situations[14].

Position

Some patients cannot lie flat because of breathlessness or pain usually from arthritis. It is quite easy to modify the procedure with the patient sitting forward on the edge of the bed leaning forward onto a support set at a comfortable height.

Open biopsy

Open biopsy is reserved for higher risk patients, for example with a single kidney or with a hemorrhagic tendency or for those in whom the standard technique has failed. It ensures adequacy of specimen and secure hemostasis[15]. The additional cost and discomfort as well as the risk of general anesthesia must be weighed against these advantages. It is rarely used now.

The patient with a single kidney, especially if complicated by other relative contraindications, has, in the past, been regarded as requiring an open biopsy. However, in practice, ultrasound-guided needle biopsy is effective and safe in this setting; although postbiopsy observation should be vigilant and early radiologic intervention should be undertaken if substantial bleeding occurs[5].

The difficult/high-risk patient

In some circumstances the need for biopsy outweighs the potential contraindications. Additional more complex and time-consuming techniques that should be considered include biopsy guided by computed tomography or laparoscopy or biopsy using a transvenous approach. These techniques have not been compared directly in high-risk patients and the choice will depend on local expertise. They have been reviewed recently[5].

Biopsy of transplanted kidneys

Biopsy of transplanted kidneys is simplified by the accessibility of the transplant kidney just below the abdominal wall and its lack of movement on respiration. The biopsy is performed by biopsy gun or hand-held Trucut under ultrasound guidance. It can be a routine outpatient procedure. Repeated biopsy carries a low risk and many centers now perform protocol biopsies at fixed times after transplant as well as during workup for transplant dysfunction.

COMPLICATIONS

Complications compiled from large series of renal biopsies are shown in Table 6.2. The complications of hemorrhage have persisted in recent series despite the more sophisticated techniques in use, but there has been a reduction in severe life-threatening complications. However, recent series[9,10,12,16] have contained rather few patients with severe renal impairment, in whom there is known to be a higher incidence of complications[17].

Complications of renal biopsy		
	1952–77 (%)	1990s (%)
Number	14 492	2157
Hematoma	1	2 (33% on ultrasound)
Gross hematuria	3	1.5
Arteriovenous fistula	0.1	0.2 (10% by color Doppler)
Surgery	0.3	None
Death	0.12	None

The data for 1952–77 are taken from 20 series including 14 492 patients[15]. The 1990s data are from three series including 2157 patients[7,8,10,14]. In the latter group, there were no reports of deaths, infections, or nephrectomies for hemorrhage.

Table 6.2 Complications of renal biopsy.

Pain

A dull ache as the local anesthetic wears off is very common and may not require any treatment. However, sometimes the pain can be severe enough to require opiates, particularly if a large perinephric hematoma develops. The most severe pain results from clot colic.

Hemorrhage

Some hemorrhage with perirenal hematoma probably occurs after every renal biopsy. There is a mean fall of hemoglobin of 1 g/dL after renal biopsy[12]. Frank hematuria occurs in 1.5% of cases and painful perirenal hematoma develops in 2% of cases. Around 1% of patients may require transfusion. Occasionally, heavy hematuria may cause clot colic and/or clot retention. The patient should be rested until bleeding has stopped. If hemorrhage is severe and prolonged, angiography should be used to identify the feeding artery, which can be embolized. This procedure has rendered nephrectomy for post-biopsy bleeding virtually obsolete.

Arteriovenous fistula

This is a radiologic finding rather than a clinical problem. It occurs in about 10% of patients prospectively examined by arteriography or color Doppler; most cases resolve spontaneously. Rarely arteriovenous fistula formation is associated with persistent hematuria and the development of hypertension and renal impairment, in which case embolization may be necessary.

Other complications

A wide variety of other complications have been described. These include calyceal-peritoneal fistula, hemothorax and colonic perforation, as well as the more common hepatic or splenic biopsy. Even the pancreas has been biopsied which may lead to a short attack of pancreatitis. 'Page kidney' is a rare complication in which a subcapsular hematoma compresses the kidney provoking ischemia and high renin hypertension; surgical decompression may be necessary[17].

Death

A mortality of 0.12% is reported in series going back to the 1970s[18]. The great majority of fatalities result from hemorrhage in high-risk patients, particularly those with acute renal failure. No deaths are described in four large series from the 1990s[9,10,12,16].

RENAL BIOPSY FINDINGS: THE DIAGNOSTIC RANGE

The renal unit of the Glasgow Royal Infirmary, UK, carried out 890 biopsies between 1975 and mid-1996; the range of diagnoses is indicated in Table 6.3. This is typical of a northern European unit serving a population of about 1 million people. The biggest subgroup is primary glomerulopathies (55%), of which the most common is IgA nephropathy (29%). Steroid-sensitive nephropathy (23%) includes patients with minimal change and mesangial proliferative glomerulonephritis associated with negative immunofluorescence studies. Biopsy is no longer used in this unit in patients with isolated hematuria, so thin membrane nephropathy is under-represented.

Patients with systemic diseases accounted for 25% of biopsies. The most common class of disease was the vasculitides (including Henoch–Schönlein purpura), accounting for 35% of this group, followed by amyloid. Lupus is comparatively rare since this unit serves few Black or Asian patients. Diabetes is also under-represented because of the restrictive biopsy criteria used: 10% of biopsies show diabetic nephropathy whereas 20% of patients starting dialysis in our unit are diabetic.

THE VALUE OF RENAL BIOPSY

Biopsy adequacy

Most series describe effectiveness of renal biopsy in terms of diagnostic adequacy. This usually requires a minimum of 10–15 glomeruli with adequate material for immunofluorescence and electron microscopy as well as light microscopy. Thus enough tissue containing glomeruli should be available for each method of examination and the pathologist or technician attending the biopsy should be sufficiently experienced to decide when this is so. Further biopsy passes should be made until adequate material has been obtained unless there is a clinical contraindication to continuing. It should be remembered, however, that sometimes a single glomerulus will provide a diagnosis, for example in a nephrotic patient in whom the glomerulus shows amyloid.

Biopsy interpretation

The histopathologic classification of glomerular disease was established within 10 years of the introduction of renal biopsy and was based on light microscopic appearances; it has stood the test of time. The subsequent introduction of immunofluorescence identified IgA nephropathy and helped in the classification of crescentic nephritis. Electron microscopy led to the discovery of some new patterns, such as the various forms of fibrillary glomerulonephritis. While these histologic patterns do not necessarily define separate diseases (see Chapter 18), they have been extensively used in clinical practice and as the basis for treatment trials.

Diagnoses established by renal biopsy	
Biopsy result	**Number (%)**
Primary glomerulopathy	**490 (55)**
IgA nephropathy	142 (29)
Membranous nephropathy	95 (19)
Minimal change disease	68 (14)
Mesangial proliferative glomerulonephritis	43 (9)
Membranoproliferative glomerulonephritis	42 (9)
Thin membrane nephropathy	32 (6)
Focal glomerulosclerosis	38 (8)
Acute exudative glomerulonephritis	20 (4)
IgM nephropathy	10 (2)
Interstitial nephritis	**72 (8)**
Systemic disease	**222 (25)**
Vasculitis	45 (20)
Henoch–Schönlein purpura	30 (15)
Systemic lupus	21 (9)
Amyloid	40 (18)
Diabetes	23 (10)
Goodpasture's syndrome	15 (7)
Hypertension	13 (6)
Accelerated hypertension	10 (4)
Myeloma	9 (4)
Scleroderma	6 (3)
Infective endocarditis	5 (2.5)
Hemolytic uremic syndrome/thrombotic thrombocytopenic purpura	5 (2.5)
No clear diagnosis	**79 (9)**
Other diagnosis	**27 (3)**

Findings from 890 renal biopsies performed at Glasgow Royal Infirmary 1975–96.

Table 6.3 Diagnoses established by renal biopsy.

Immunofluorescence and electron microscopy are more useful in the diagnosis of an individual glomerular disease, and light microscopy is more useful in determining prognosis. The reasons for this observation are that the most common glomerular disease, IgA nephropathy, cannot be diagnosed by light microscopy alone and that others such as membranous nephropathy are more easily recognized by their electron microscopy or immunofluorescence appearance than by light microscopy. Immunofluorescence studies can often be used to determine which nephrotic patients with mesangial or focal proliferation merit a trial of corticosteroids: those with negative findings should be treated and those with positive findings should not.

Conversely, the prognosis for an individual patient cannot be accurately predicted by glomerular changes alone (apart from widespread glomerulosclerosis), and a sufficient quantity of tissue is required to evaluate the extent of the tubulointerstitial changes, which is best achieved by light microscopy. The tubulointerstitial changes correlate with renal function and prognosis better than do the glomerular changes.

Is renal biopsy really necessary?

At various times, the role of renal biopsy has been debated[13,19]; in particular, it was asserted that biopsy only infrequently altered treatment and an empirical trial of steroids in all adults with nephrotic syndrome without renal biopsy was advocated. This approach may treat patients with minimal change disease and focal glomerulosclerosis but would give unnecessary treatment to those with membranoproliferative glomerulonephritis and would under-treat some patients with membranous nephropathy. Furthermore, corticosteroids are not the only therapeutic approach to glomerular disease, and renal biopsy has an important role in providing precise diagnostic information before other therapies such as cytotoxic drugs or interferon are instituted for specific indications.

Prospective studies show that in 50–60% of patients, biopsy produces a diagnosis different from that predicted in advance by the clinician. This reclassification leads to a change in 20–50% of cases and is more common in symptomatic renal diseases such as nephrotic syndrome or acute renal failure[13]. This interpretation accepts that the diagnoses made by biopsy represent distinct diseases requiring distinct treatment regimens. However, these only differ subtly one from another. It is possible that the mechanism leading to proteinuria only has a few final pathways and that treatment with immunosuppressive agents affects the most common one. Nevertheless, the value of renal biopsy in guiding treatment is supported by a retrospective study which showed that renal biopsy altered management in 42% of all cases, but in 86% of those with nephrotic syndrome[20].

The role of biopsy in determining the quantity of treatment is also widely but not universally accepted. This is particularly true of lupus nephritis. Most nephrologists feel that the identification of patients with WHO class IV lupus nephritis is valuable since these patients have a worse prognosis and require more intensive treatment. Others argue that biopsy provides useful information about the degrees of activity and of scarring which help to decide treatment. There have been studies that support these claims but recent series have not found that prognosis correlated independently with any biopsy characteristic. However, these minority views have not shaken nephrologists' opinion that renal biopsy is an essential tool in the investigation of many forms of renal disease.

REFERENCES

1. Iversen P, Brun C. Aspiration biopsy of the kidney. Am J Med. 1951;11:324–30.
2. Kark RM, Muehrcke RC. Biopsy of the kidney in prone position. Lancet. 1954;1:1047–9.
3. Wiseman DA, Hawkins R, Numerow LM, Taub KJ. Percutaneous renal biopsy utilising real time, ultrasonic guidance and a semi-automated biopsy device. Kidney Int. 1990;38:347–9.
4. Ruggenenti P, Perna A, Gherardi, et al. Renoprotective properties of ACE-inhibition in non-diabetic nephropathies with non-nephrotic proteinuria. Lancet. 1999:354:359–364.
5. Stiles KP, Yuan CM, Ghurg EM, et al. Renal biopsy in high risk patients with medical diseases of the kidney. Am J Kidney Dis. 2000;36:419–33.
6. Bondestam S, Kontkanen T, Taavitsainen M, Tiula E. Technique of renal biopsy by ultrasound guided percutaneous puncture with a spring loaded 'gun'. Scand J Urol Nephrol. 1992;26:265–7.
7. Jackson R, Holme E, Phimister GM, et al. Immunoalkaline phosphatase technique applied to paraffin wax embedded tissues in diagnostic renal pathology. J Clin Pathol. 1990;43:665–70.
8. Pasquariello A, Innocenti M, Batini V, et al. Routine immunofluorescence and light microscopy processing with a single renal biopsy specimen: 18 years experience in a single center. J Nephrol. 2000;13:116–19.
9. Marwah, DS, Korbet SM. Timing of complications in percutaneous renal biopsy: what is the optimal period of observation? Am J Kidney Dis. 1996;28:47–52.
10. Fraser IR, Fairley K. Renal biopsy as an outpatient procedure. Am J Kidney Dis. 1995;25:876–8.
11. Cozens NJA, Murchison JT, Allan PL, Whinney RJ. Conventional 15G needle technique for renal biopsy compared with ultrasound guided spring loaded 18G needle biopsy. Br J Radiol. 1992;65:594–7.
12. Burstein DM, Korbet SM, Schwartz MM. The use of the automatic core biopsy system in percutaneous renal biopsies: a comparative study. Am J Kidney Dis. 1993;22:545–52.
13. Madaio MP. Renal biopsy. Kidney Int. 1990,38,529–43.
14. Lee SMK, King J, Spargo BH. Efficacy of percutaneous renal biopsy in obese patients under computerised tomographic control. Clin Nephrol. 1991;35:123–9.
15. Chodak GW, Gill WB, Wald V, Spargo B. Diagnosis of renal parenchymal diseases by a modified open kidney biopsy technique. Kidney Int. 1983;24:804–6.
16. Hergesell O, Felten H, Andrassy K, et al. Safety of ultrasound-guided percutaneous renal biopsy – retrospective analysis of 1090 consecutive cases. Nephrol Dial Transplant. 1998;13: 975–7.
17. McCune TR, Stone WJ, Breyer JA. Page kidney: case report and review of the literature. Am J Kidney Dis. 1991; 18: 593–9.
18. Parrish AE. Complications of percutaneous renal biopsy: a review of 37 years' experience. Clin Nephrol. 1992;38:135–41.
19. Adu D. The nephrotic syndrome: does renal biopsy affect management? Nephrol Dial Transplant. 1996;11:12–14.
20. Richards NT, Darby S, Howie AJ, et al. Knowledge of renal histology alters patient management in over 40% of cases. Nephrol Dial Transplant 1994; 9: 1255–9.

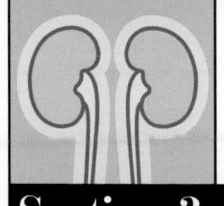

Chapter 7 Disorders of Extracellular Volume

Dinesh K Chatoth and Thomas E Andreoli

THE EXTRACELLULAR FLUID COMPARTMENT

In healthy adults, body water constitutes approximately 60% of the total body weight. It exists in two compartments: the intracellular fluid (ICF) compartment containing two-thirds of total body water and the extracellular fluid (ECF) compartment containing the remaining one-third. The capillary endothelial membrane further divides the ECF into two compartments. The intravascular or plasma fluid compartment makes up one-fourth of the ECF and the extravascular compartment makes up the remaining three-fourths of the ECF volume[1]. The extravascular compartment is comprised of two fractions: interstitial volume and transcellular water (25% and 4% of total body water respectively). Transcellular fluid includes cerebrospinal fluid, gastrointestinal fluids and the fluids in the eye and serous surfaces (Fig. 7.1).

The composition of the ECF is quite similar, with some difference as a result of disparity in the protein concentration between the plasma and interstitial space. The difference in the electrolyte concentration between these two compartments is determined by the effect of the Donnan equilibrium and

therefore, the concentration of diffusible cations are about 4% greater in plasma water and the concentration of diffusible anions are lower by the same percentage[2] (Table 7.1).

The ICF and ECF compartments are in osmotic equilibrium because virtually all cell membranes in the body are freely permeable to water. The ECF volume is determined primarily by the total amount of osmotically active solutes in the compartment. Sodium salts, by virtue of being the most abundant solutes in the ECF, are the most important determinants of ECF volume. The amount of sodium in the ECF is, therefore, regulated tightly. ECF sodium deficiency results in renal sodium retention and excess ECF sodium promotes increased urinary excretion of sodium.

The most fundamental characteristic of fluid and electrolyte homeostasis is the maintenance of ECF volume and circulatory stability. In normal humans, despite significant day-to-day variations in the intake of salt and water, the ECF volume is maintained within a normal range, varying by only 1–2%[3]. Maintaining the appropriate ECF volume is critical because it determines the mean arterial pressure and left ventricular filling volume. Furthermore, ECF bathes all cells and is therefore responsible for the delivery of oxygen and nutrients and the removal of metabolic products.

Effective arterial blood volume
The blood volume that is detected by volume sensors (see below) is sometimes referred to as the effective arterial blood

---

Distribution of total body water

Blood volume (3–5 L)

- Red blood cell volume
- Intravascular volume
- Transcellular volume (1–5 L)
- Interstitial volume (9 L)

Intracellular volume (28 L)

Extracellular volume (10–14 L)

Figure 7.1 Distribution of total body water into different compartments. The volumes are for an average 70-kg adult.

Concentrations of ions in plasma, plasma water, and interstitial fluid			
	Plasma (mmol/L)	Plasma water (mmol/L)	Interstitial fluid (mmol/L)
Sodium	140	151	148
Potassium	4.5	5.0	5.0
Calcium	2.5	2.8	2.0
Magnesium	0.85	0.9	0.75
Chloride	104	112	115
Bicarbonate	24	26	27
Phosphate	1.0	1.05	1.15

Table 7.1 Concentrations of ions in plasma, plasma water, and interstitial fluid.

The relationship of effective arterial blood volume and total extracellular fluid volume in various disease states					
Compartment	Volume depletion	Nephrosis	Congestive heart failure	Arteriovenous fistula with congestive state	Renal artery stenosis
Total extracellular fluid volume	↓	↑	↑	↑	↑
Total blood volume	↓	variable	↑	↑	↑
Arterial blood volume	↓	variable	↓	↑	↑
Effective arterial blood volume	↓	variable	↓	↓	↑
Renal blood flow	↓	variable	↓	↓	↓

Table 7.2 The relationship of effective arterial blood volume and total extracellular fluid volume in various disease states.

volume (EABV)[4]. In other words, EABV is the amount of arterial blood volume required to adequately 'fill' the capacity of the arterial circulation. ECF volume and EABV can be independent of each other (Table 7.2).

THE INTEGRATED HOMEOSTATIC RESPONSE

The characteristic feature of the body fluid homeostatic mechanism is that the composition of the body fluid compartments remains remarkably constant despite wide daily variations in solute and water intake[5]. The homeostatic mechanism also invariably protects the ECF volume in circumstances when multiple physiologic variables are threatened simultaneously; this can sometimes occur at the expense of aggravating another electrolyte disorder[6,7]. For example, a patient with volume depletion who is replenished with water, and not sodium, will retain water and become hyponatremic, thereby preventing circulatory collapse. Here, fluid balance is maintained at the expense of electrolyte imbalance, specifically, hypotonicity of body fluids.

The integrated homeostatic response involves two key components (Fig. 7.2): an afferent limb that contains sensors that detect changes in effective circulating volume and an efferent limb that regulates the rate of sodium excretion by the kidney[8,9].

The afferent limb: volume sensors

Volume detectors reside at several sites in the vasculature (Table 7.3) and serve as sensors that monitor changes in circulatory function within that compartment[10]. They can be broadly classified as:
- low-pressure baroreceptors
- high-pressure baroreceptors
- intrarenal sensors
- hepatic and central nervous system (CNS) sensors.

Low-pressure baroreceptors

Low-pressure baroreceptors are located on the venous side of the central circulation and assess the filling of the central venous circulation. They monitor changes in the intrathoracic volume and are designed to defend against ECF volume expansion and its deleterious pulmonary consequences. The low-pressure baroreceptors include the cardiac atria and the cardiopulmonary receptors.

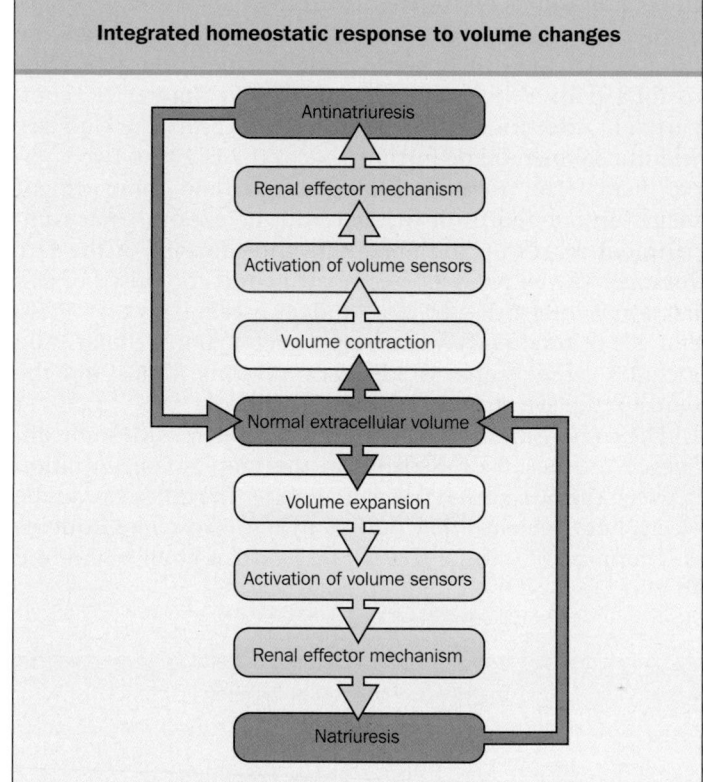

Figure 7.2 A general overview of the integrated homeostatic response system regulating extracellular fluid volume during volume contraction and expansion.

Cardiac atrial receptors

Receptors in the cardiac atria transduce atrial wall stretch. Increased venous return increases the discharge rate of these receptors, and stretch and tension impulses travel along cranial nerves IX and X to the hypothalamic and medullary centers in the brain. This, in turn, decreases the renal sympathetic nerve activity, leading to natriuresis. The resultant hemodynamic changes counteract the original stimuli from volume expansion.

Humoral alterations that assist in counteracting the increase in central blood volume also occur as a response to atrial stretch. The hypothalamus responds to an increase in atrial stretch by inhibiting the release of arginine-vasopressin (vasopressin, or

Afferent limb sensors of extracellular volume
Cardiopulmonary (venous circulation)
Atria
Ventricular and pulmonary
Arterial
Extrarenal: aortic arch, carotid sinus,
Intrarenal: juxtaglomerular apparatus
Others
Central nervous system
Hepatic

Table 7.3 The afferent limb (volume sensors) of the integrated homeostatic response system for extracellular volume.

antidiuretic hormone, abbreviated as ADH) and adrenocorticotropic hormone (ACTH). Vasopressin induces free water retention and ACTH stimulates mineralocorticoid release from the adrenal gland. The inhibition of these hormones in response to atrial stretch leads to salt and water diuresis. Furthermore, decreased renal sympathetic activity, specifically β-adrenergic activity, lowers renal renin production, which in turn decreases levels of angiotensin II[10]. This facilitates natriuresis and contributes to the lowering of blood pressure. Distention of the cardiac atria also results in release of atrial natriuretic peptide (ANP) from the myocytes. ANP induces renal excretion of sodium and water and may also increase the capacitance of the central circulatory bed, thus lowering central venous pressure (CVP). ANP does not seem to play an important role in daily salt and water balance and its most important role is in pathophysiologic states that affect ECF volume homeostasis. Volume contraction leads to a decrease in CVP, which in turn decreases the discharge rate of these atrial receptors, leading to renal salt and water conservation.

Cardiopulmonary sensors

The central circulation contains low-pressure receptors in the left ventricle and the pulmonary vascular bed. When CVP decreases, the rate of discharge from these cardiopulmonary receptors is low, which leads to a decrease in the inhibition of the vasomotor center in the brain and subsequent increase in sympathetic outflow. The net result is an increase in heart rate, peripheral vascular resistance, antinatriuresis and antidiuresis, all of which leads to increases in blood pressure and cardiac output and to volume conservation. Conversely, an increase in CVP increases the rate of discharge from these receptors, which eventually leads to natriuresis and sympathetic withdrawal.

High-pressure baroreceptors

High-pressure baroreceptors, located at the bifurcation of the carotid artery (carotid sinus body) and the aortic arch (aortic body), work independently from the low-pressure sensors. They assess the pressure of the arterial circulation and are designed to maintain mean arterial pressure at a constant level and protect the brain from wide fluctuations in perfusion pressure.

Underfilling of the arterial tree leads to activation of these receptors. Signals from these receptors travel to the vasomotor center in the brain, which in turn signals the kidney to retain sodium and water. The latter is accompanied by increased sympathetic nerve activity and increased plasma norepinephrine (noradrenaline) vasopressin, and endothelin levels[9,10]. The catecholamine response raises blood pressure by increasing the heart rate and arteriolar resistance. The increase in arteriolar resistance promotes transfer of fluid from the interstitium to the vascular compartment.

Overfilling of the arterial tree elicits the opposite response. It decreases the discharge rate from these baroreceptors, which finally results in natriuresis and decreased catecholamine response.

Intrarenal baroreceptor system: juxtaglomerular apparatus

The kidney plays an important role in the afferent limb of volume homeostasis. The intrarenal sensors are formed by the renal juxtaglomerular apparatus (JGA). Renin, an acid protease, is released from the JGA into the plasma when intrarenal sensors detect volume contraction. Renin catalyzes the release of angiotensin I from angiotensinogen. This is the rate-limiting step in the formation of angiotensin II. Subsequently, angiotensin converting enzyme (ACE) catalyzes the cleavage of angiotensin I to angiotensin II, which is the cardinal stimulus to aldosterone production and, by itself, is a potent vasoconstrictor.

Renin production is regulated by three major mechanisms[7]:

- *Change in renal perfusion pressure.* A decrease in perfusion pressure activates neuronal nitric oxide synthase (NOS-1) and cyclo-oxygenase-2 (COX-2) in the macula densa which then signals both renin secretion by granular cells in the afferent arteriole and juxtaglomerular apparatus.
- *Solute delivery to the macula densa cells.* A decrease in the concentration of sodium chloride in the vicinity of the macula densa cells also activates NOS-1, COX-2 and renin by a similar mechanism.
- *Influence of renal sympathetic nerves.* Activation of the β-adrenoceptors in the juxtaglomerular cells directly stimulates renin release from the macula densa cells.

In addition, it has been proposed that mild levels of hyperuricemia can activate renin production by juxtaglomerular cells[11].

Activation of NOS-1 and COX-2 by the macula densa cells in response to reductions in renal perfusion pressure or solute delivery to macula densa cells also results in afferent arteriolar dilation, mediated in part by prostacyclin (PGI$_2$) and also by nitric oxide (NO).

Other volume sensors

Several other volume sensors contribute to the afferent limb of the volume homeostasis loop. They are located in various organs in the body, for example the CNS and the portohepatic circulation. The physiologic significance and the exact mechanism of action of these sensors remain to be defined.

Efferent limb: effector elements

The stimulation of the afferent volume-sensing system leads to activation of the efferent limb, where the kidney is the

Major renal efferent mechanisms regulating extracellular fluid volume
Glomerular filtration rate
Physical factors
At the level of the proximal tubule
Beyond the proximal tubule
Humoral effector mechanisms
Renin–angiotensin–aldosterone system
Vasopressin
Catecholamines
Prostaglandins
Kinin–kallikrein system
Atrial natriuretic peptide
Endothelium-derived factors
Renal sympathetic nerves

Table 7.4 Major renal efferent mechanisms regulating excretion of sodium and controlling extracellular fluid volume.

major effector organ in the body fluid volume homeostasis loop. The ECF volume is mainly regulated by alteration in renal sodium excretion[12]. Several factors that influence renal sodium handling are listed in Table 7.4.

GLOMERULAR FILTRATION

The amount of sodium excreted by the kidney is dependent on the filtered load of sodium. The determinants of the filtered load of sodium include the glomerular filtration rate (GFR) and the serum sodium concentration. In the human kidney, more than 1000 mmol (23 g) of sodium are filtered each hour. Of this, about 990 mmol (22.8 g) are reabsorbed from the renal tubules. Consequently, any fluctuation in GFR can, in principle, affect the renal handling of sodium.

The transfer of fluid across a capillary wall is governed by the hydrostatic pressure gradients and plasma oncotic pressure gradients, expressed by the Starling equation[13].

$$J_v = K_f (\Delta P - \Delta \pi)$$

where J_v is the rate of fluid transfer between the capillary and interstitial compartments, K_f is the water permeability of the capillary bed (also termed the glomerular capillary ultrafiltration coefficient), ΔP is the hydrostatic pressure difference between capillary and interstitial fluids, and $\Delta \pi$ is the oncotic pressure difference between capillary and interstitial fluids.

Determinants of glomerular filtration
There are four major determinants of glomerular filtration[9]:
- The balance of Starling forces acting across the capillary wall; the glomerular capillary hydraulic pressure and the oncotic pressure of the Bowman's space favor filtration, whereas the Bowman space hydraulic pressure and glomerular oncotic pressure tend to retard it.
- The ultrafiltration coefficient K_f, which reflects the glomerular permeability and the total filtration area of the glomerular capillaries.

- Changes in plasma protein composition which affects the rate of filtrate formation.

The rate at which plasma flows through the glomeruli.

Renal autoregulation
Renal autoregulation is a phenomenon by which GFR is maintained fairly constant in the presence of perturbations that otherwise would result in its variation. For example, constricting the renal artery can lead to modest alteration in renal perfusion pressure without altering either GFR or renal blood flow (RBF).

The afferent arteriolar resistance is an important determinant of the net glomerular filtration pressure. The RBF and GFR are maintained under tight control by two intrarenal mechanisms that contribute to adjustments in arteriolar resistance during changes in arterial pressure. The first, known as the myogenic mechanism, is a pressure-sensitive mechanism that is an inherent property of smooth muscle cells. A rise in renal arterial pressure causes stretching of the afferent arteriolar smooth muscle cells. This in turn triggers afferent arteriolar constriction, preventing transmission of the high arterial pressure to the glomerular capillaries. A fall in renal arterial pressure results in the opposite effect.

The second mechanism, tubuloglomerular feedback (TGF), is a phenomenon whereby increased sodium delivery to the macula densa controls afferent arteriolar tone[14]. Here, a rise in intravascular pressure leads to an increase in GFR and increased delivery of sodium chloride to the macula densa. This causes an increase in afferent arteriolar resistance and subsequently decreases GFR back to normal[15]. These changes in afferent arteriolar tone are mediated principally by the interplay between vasodilatory factors – principally the prostaglandins, atrial natriuretic peptide and nitric oxide – and vasoconstrictive agents, primarily vasopressin, angiotensin II, and the adrenergic effectors epinephrine (adrenaline) and norepinephrine (noradrenaline). Finally, both the myogenic mechanism and TGF are impaired in circumstances which result in consistent renal hypoperfusion, such as renal artery stenosis.

Glomerulotubular balance
Glomerulotubular balance is a fundamental property of the kidney whereby changes in GFR automatically induce a proportional change in the rate of proximal tubular sodium reabsorption. Thus, the fractional excretion of sodium is maintained constant in the setting of increases or decreases in GFR.

Segmental tubular sodium reabsorption
The control of tubular sodium reabsorption is more important than GFR in the regulation of urinary sodium excretion. The net urinary sodium excretion is the balance between the filtered load of sodium and the amount of sodium reabsorbed from the nephron. As mentioned above, about 99% of the total filtered sodium is reclaimed from the renal tubules. This occurs via four major salt transporters located along the length of the nephron, as illustrated in Figure 7.3. The proximal nephron reclaims about 70% and Henle's loop accounts for about 20% of the glomerular filtrate. In the distal nephron, about 5% of the filtered sodium is reabsorbed in

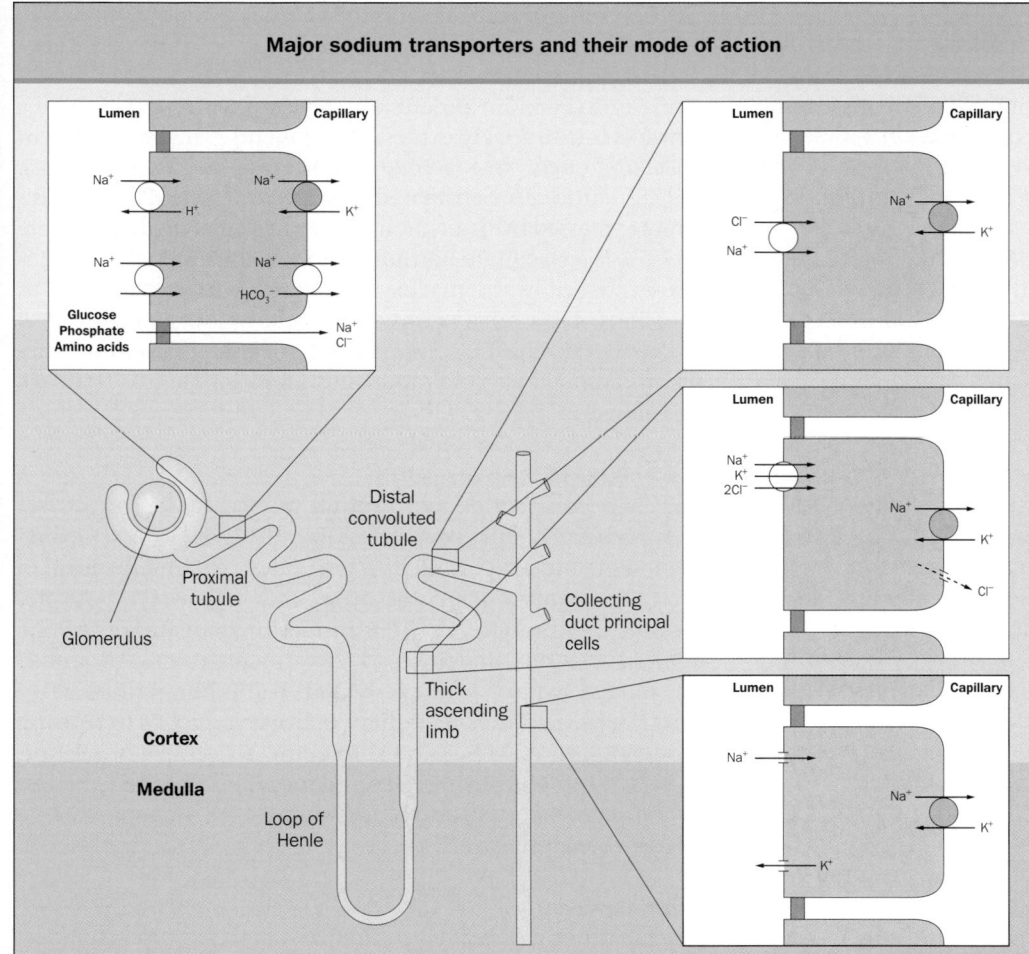

Figure 7.3 Structure of the nephron showing the four major sodium transporters and their mechanism of action.

the distal convoluted tubule and the final 2–4% is reabsorbed in the collecting duct.

Physical factors

Physical factors act through peritubular capillary Starling forces to influence the renal handling of sodium at the level of the proximal tubule as well as beyond this nephron segment. This effect is independent of GFR, hormones, and renal sympathetic nerves.

In the proximal nephron, the peritubular capillary network is closely linked to the glomerular capillary bed through the efferent arteriole. Consequently, changes in the physical determinants of GFR influence the hydrostatic and oncotic pressures in the peritubular capillaries[9]. The hydrostatic pressure is significantly lower in the peritubular capillaries than in the glomerular capillaries. Also, because the peritubular capillaries receive blood from the glomerulus, the plasma oncotic pressure is high at the outset as a result of prior filtration of protein-free fluid. The renal interstitial hydrostatic pressure and the peritubular oncotic pressure are important regulators of the absolute rate of reabsorption of proximal tubule absorbate[16].

Beyond the proximal tubule, there is substantial evidence that the natriuresis induced by volume expansion is also determined in part by physical factors. Increased distal delivery of fluid from the proximal tubule is associated with an increase in fractional sodium reabsorption along the loop of Henle. Furthermore, the loop of Henle has the capacity to increase fractional sodium reabsorption in response to changes in the delivered load of sodium from the proximal tubule. However, there also occurs, with an absolute increase in distal sodium delivery, an absolute increase in net sodium excretion.

Humoral mechanisms

Renin–angiotensin–aldosterone system

Volume contraction of the ECF leads to renal hypoperfusion, which enhances renin release by the JGA. Renal renin release into the plasma accelerates the formation of angiotensin II, the direct actions of which on the kidneys tend to be antinatriuretic[17]. These effects occur at relatively low concentrations of angiotensin II. The first effect of angiotensin II is a direct vasoconstrictor action predominantly on the efferent arteriole, with a subsequent increase in intraglomerular pressure and modulation of peritubular Starling forces; this results in enhanced proximal sodium and water reabsorption. Angiotensin II also directly stimulates the proximal tubular reabsorption of sodium independently of changes in renal or systemic hemodynamics. It stimulates catecholamine release from the renal nerves and enhances production of vasodilatory prostaglandins. Furthermore, it stimulates the adrenal gland to produce aldosterone, which increases the reabsorption of sodium in the distal parts of the nephron.

Vasopressin

The osmotic control for vasopressin release has been well characterized. Vasopressin is also released in response to a fall in EABV (non-osmotic volume stimulus). This hormone, when bound by the vasopressin V_2 receptors on basolateral membranes of medullary thick ascending limbs and collecting ducts, enhances water permeability and absorption from the collecting duct and also stimulates sodium chloride reabsorption from the thick ascending limb of the loop of Henle and from the cortical collecting duct. The systemic vasoconstrictor action of vasopressin, mediated by vasopressin binding to V_1 receptors in vascular smooth muscle, also helps in the defense against perceived ECF volume contraction.

Catecholamines

Epinephrine (adrenaline) and norepinephrine (noradrenaline) induce sodium retention by directly stimulating sodium reabsorption at the proximal tubule and the loop of Henle. They also activate the renin–angiotensin–aldosterone system and induce a preferential vasoconstriction at the level of the efferent arteriole to maintain the intraglomerular pressure in response to volume contraction. Dopamine, when administered in low concentrations, causes renal vasodilation and enhances glomerular filtration; dopamine may also have a direct role in augmenting renal sodium excretion by decreasing tubular sodium absorption.

Prostaglandins

Prostaglandins are autacoids derived from the metabolism of arachidonic acid. The important renal prostaglandins include prostaglandin E_2 (PGE_2), prostaglandin I_2, and thromboxane. Prostaglandins E_2 and I_2 have natriuretic properties and influence renal sodium handling in the collecting ducts and the loop of Henle. They also play an active role in regulating renal hemodynamics. PGE_2 also antagonizes the action of ADH on sodium reabsorption in the thick ascending limb and on water reabsorption in collecting ducts.

Two cyclo-oxygenase (COX) enzymes are involved in modulating prostaglandin production. Cyclo-oxygenase 1 (COX-1), which is constitutively expressed, augments PGE_2 production in collecting ducts, and facilitates natriuresis and water diuresis. COX-2, although considered inducible, is actually constitutively expressed by interstitial cells in the renal medulla (where it also acts to facilitate natriuresis and water diuresis). COX-2 is also expressed in the macula densa (and is further induced in situations of low renal perfusion pressure or low sodium intake) where it generates PGI_2 that stimulates afferent dilation, augments renin release, and modulates tubuloglomerular feedback (see above).

Atrial natriuretic peptide (ANP)

ANP is a polypeptide synthesized by the cardiac myocytes that has natriuretic properties. In the kidney, ANP exerts hemodynamic and tubular actions that eventually lead to increased urinary excretion of sodium and water[18]. At the level of the glomerulus, ANP induces vasodilatation of the afferent arteriole, thereby leading to increases in GFR and in the filtered load of sodium. ANP also inhibits sodium reabsorption in the inner medullary collecting duct by activating production of cGMP. ANP inhibits the action of several hormones; it inhibits renin release, reduces aldosterone secretion by the adrenal cortex, and blocks some of the vasoconstrictive effects of angiotensin II.

Other hormones

Several other hormones influence renal sodium excretion (Table 7.5). Whereas the renal sodium-regulating properties of some of these hormones have been elucidated, the exact roles of others in volume homeostasis have yet to be determined.

Hormones regulating renal sodium excretion			
Mediators	Site of production	Site of action	Tubular actions
Vasoconstrictors			
Angiotensin II	Circulating/local generation	Glomerular arterioles, proximal tubule	Na^+ retention
Aldosterone	Adrenal glands	Distal tubule	Na^+ retention
Vasopressin	Hypothalamus	Thick ascending limb of loop of Henle (TAL), distal tubule	Water retention, Na^+ retention
Catecholamines	Adrenal glands	Glomerular arterioles, proximal tubule	Na^+ retention
Renal sympathetics	Kidneys	Glomerular arterioles, proximal tubule	Na^+ retention
Endothelin I	Endothelium	Glomerular arterioles, IMCD	Natriuresis
Na^+/K^+ ATPase inhibitors	Adrenal glands	Tubular Na^+/K^+ ATPase	Natriuresis
Vasodilators			
Atrial natriuretic peptide	Cardiac atria	CCD/IMCD	Natriuresis
Brain natriuretic peptide	Brain	CCD/IMCD	Natriuresis
C-type natriuretic peptide	Endothelium	CCD/IMCD	Natriuresis
Urodilatin	Renal tubules	CCD/IMCD	Natriuresis
Nitric oxide	Endothelium	Glomerular arterioles, distal nephron	Natriuresis
Prostaglandins E_2 and I_2	Kidneys	Glomerular arterioles, TAL, IMCD, CCD	Natriuresis
Bradykinin-kallikrein	Distal nephron	Glomerular arterioles, IMCD	Natriuresis
Dopamine	Proximal tubular cells	Afferent arterioles, proximal nephron	Natriuresis
CCD, cortical collecting duct; IMCD, inner medullary collecting duct.			

Table 7.5 Characteristics of hormones regulating renal sodium excretion.

Renal nerves

The sympathetic nervous system is present in all segments of the renal vasculature and tubules. It innervates the afferent and efferent arterioles of the glomerulus and regulates urinary sodium and water excretion by changing hemodynamics[19]. It also exerts a direct effect on innervated tubules to regulate the renal reabsorption of sodium from the proximal nephron. ECF volume contraction increases the activity of the renal sympathetic nerves.

Sympathetic nerves, specifically β-adrenergic fibers, enhance the release of renin from the JGA, thereby increasing the level of angiotensin II and aldosterone. They also interact with other hormonal systems including vasopressin and ANP.

EXTRACELLULAR FLUID VOLUME CONTRACTION

Volume contraction has occurred when the functional ECF volume is less than 20% of the total body weight or less than 15 L in a 70 kg adult. The reduction in ECF volume usually occurs simultaneously from both the interstitial and intravascular compartments and is determined by whether the volume loss is primarily solute-free water or a combination of salt and water[20]. Since only 5% of the total body water resides in the vascular space, the loss of solute-free water has a lesser effect on intravascular volume[21]. However, most of the sodium is confined to the ECF space and a combined loss of sodium and water results in significant intravascular volume depletion.

Etiology and pathogenesis

Volume contraction is a result of increased salt and water loss from renal and extrarenal sources that exceeds total intake. Renal losses of salt and water (Table 7.6) can be secondary to either a loss of effector mechanisms for salt and water conservation or intrinsic renal diseases that cause alterations in the output mechanism[7]. Extrarenal fluid losses (Table 7.7), when inadequately replaced, can also lead to volume depletion.

Renal losses of salt and water
Chronic diuretic abuse

Chronic diuretic abuse is a frequent cause of ECF volume contraction seen in clinical practice and usually leads to renal salt wasting, volume contraction, and metabolic acid–base abnormalities. Acetazolamide and other proximal tubule diuretics inhibit proximal renal absorption of sodium bicarbonate, resulting in volume contraction and hyperchloremic, hypokalemic metabolic acidosis. Loop diuretics such as furosemide (frusemide) inhibit sodium chloride absorption in the thick ascending limb of the loop of Henle, thus causing renal salt and water loss and hypokalemic metabolic alkalosis. Competitive inhibitors of aldosterone, such as spironolactone, or nonaldosterone inhibitors of collecting duct sodium absorption, such as triamterene, can cause renal salt wasting, volume depletion, and hyperkalemic, hyperchloremic metabolic acidosis.

Osmotic and other diureses

Osmotic diuresis results in obligatory renal loss of salt and water. This can occur in uncontrolled diabetes secondary to the failure to reabsorb glucose from the tubular fluid; in mannitol diuresis; and in urea diuresis, which can occur in burn patients with abnormally high rates of urea production. Other common conditions associated with diuresis include postobstructive diuresis after relief of complete or partial urinary tract obstruction and the diuretic phase of acute tubular necrosis, where loss of sodium and water usually accompanies recovery from acute tubular necrosis.

Aldosterone deficiency

Aldosterone deficiency frequently leads to renal sodium wasting. It can occur from destruction of the adrenal gland, as seen in Addison's disease, or secondary to hyporeninemic hypoaldosteronism, which may occur in disease states like diabetes and other chronic renal interstitial disease.

Other causes

Less common conditions associated with excessive renal salt and water losses include renal tubular acidosis, Bartter's syndrome, and chronic tubular and interstitial renal diseases.

Renal water loss

Diabetes insipidus, either pituitary (impaired secretion of vasopressin) or nephrogenic (impaired renal response to vasopressin), can result in profound volume depletion from

Conditions associated with renal loss of salt and water
Salt and water
Diuretic abuse
Osmotic diuresis
Postobstructive diuresis
Salt-losing tubular nephropathies: medullary cystic disease, Bartter syndrome, chronic interstitial renal diseases
Aldosterone insufficiency: Addison's disease, hyporeninemic hypoaldosteronism
Water
Diabetes insipidus: pituitary, nephrogenic

Table 7.6 Conditions associated with renal loss of salt and water.

Conditions associated with extrarenal loss of salt and water
Dermal losses
Sweat
Burns
Insensible loss
Hemorrhage
Gastrointestinal losses
Upper: vomiting, nasogastric suction
Lower: diarrheal disorder, tube drainage, fistula
'Sequestrational' losses: intestinal obstruction, pancreatitis, muscle injury and rhabdomyolysis

Table 7.7 Conditions associated with extrarenal loss of salt and water.

obligatory loss of free water; which can sometimes exceed 10–15 L daily. This scenario is particularly manifest in patients with diabetes insipidus who are denied free access to water.

Extrarenal losses

Dermal fluid losses

Dermal fluid losses can result from excessive sweating caused by prolonged exercise or by high ambient temperature or fever. This is especially important when losses are not replaced by appropriate salt and water intake. Burns can lead to large amounts of fluid losses through the affected areas, with resultant profound ECF volume contraction.

'Sequestrational' losses

'Sequestrational' losses occur when ECF fluid is lost into body compartments. In intestinal obstruction, the fluid collects within the bowel lumen; in pancreatitis, the fluid is sequestered in the retroperitoneal space; and in cirrhosis, within the peritoneal cavity as ascites. Severe trauma and muscle injuries can cause significant sequestration of fluid, sufficient to cause volume depletion.

Hemorrhage

Hemorrhage, both internal and external, can lead to significant loss of intravascular volume and cause volume contraction.

Gastrointestinal losses

Gastrointestinal losses are commonly associated with volume contraction as a result of loss of significant amounts of digestive secretions. Upper gastrointestinal losses can occur from vomiting and from nasogastric suctioning; these are usually accompanied by metabolic alkalosis. Lower gastrointestinal alkaline fluid losses from diarrhea and fistula lead to metabolic acidosis.

Clinical manifestations

The clinical findings in states of volume contraction result from the underfilling of the arterial tree and the renal and hemodynamic responses to this underfilling. Signs and symptoms of volume depletion depend on the interplay of four major factors: the magnitude of fluid loss, the rate of volume loss, the nature of the losses, and, finally, the responsiveness of the vasculature to volume reduction.

An accurate history and a careful physical examination are extremely important in the clinical assessment of ECF volume contraction. A rapid reduction in body weight is a reliable indicator of ECF volume loss. The symptoms of ECF volume contraction are nonspecific and can range from minimal symptoms to severe circulatory collapse. In mild or partially compensated volume contraction, particularly when it is gradual, the patient may exhibit symptoms of mild postural dizziness, thirst, and weakness. In more advanced stages of volume depletion, particularly those occurring more acutely, the symptoms include recumbent hypotension, tachycardia, and a reduced urinary output. Finally, with severe volume contraction, the combination of profound fluid loss and sympathetic hyperactivity results in circulatory collapse characterized by confusion, oliguria, very low blood pressure (detectable by Doppler studies only), cold clammy extremities, and recumbent tachycardia.

The lack of physical findings does not exclude the presence of mild-to-moderate volume contraction. In postoperative patients, blood volume losses of 7–10% are frequently associated with normal blood pressure and only minimally reduced CVPs. Orthostatic hypotension may be one of the early manifestations of moderate volume depletion if accompanied by an increase in pulse rate. A low jugular venous pressure noted with the patient lying at 45° or less is also useful, particularly in patients with thin necks. Skin turgor and the moistness of the mucous membranes are valuable indicators of volume depletion in infants but are unreliable in adults. In young adults, reduction of skin turgor is usually associated with profound volume contraction; the normal loss of skin elasticity makes skin turgor difficult to assess in older patients. Furthermore, dry mucous membranes are a common occurrence in mouth breathers independent of external volume status and, therefore, may be unreliable.

Diagnosis

The blood pressure, pulse, loss of body weight, and clinical features provide an initial assessment of circulatory dynamics. Nevertheless, evaluation of hemodynamic parameters, serum, and urinary indices are helpful in characterizing the cause and severity of volume contraction[22].

Hemodynamic monitoring

Clinical findings may be unreliable or inconclusive in moderate degrees of volume contraction, and invasive hemodynamic monitoring may be required in critically ill patients who are hemodynamically unstable. The hemodynamic parameters frequently measured include CVP, pulmonary capillary wedge pressure (PCWP), cardiac output, arterial pressures, and systemic vascular resistance. However, most of these parameters may be within normal limits when blood volume has been reduced by 5–10%. Consequently, a fluid challenge may be necessary in the evaluation of patients in whom volume deficit is thought to be a contributing factor to a reduced cardiac output.

The exact volume of such a 'fluid challenge' is determined by the clinical circumstance. In individuals with no underlying cardiovascular disease, 500 mL of normal saline administered over 90 min is reasonable. In elderly patients, those with documented cardiovascular disease or starved individuals, it is prudent to reduce the volume administered to 300 mL of normal saline over a 3-h interval and then evaluate the patients' hemodynamic status before proceeding with more aggressive hydration.

Serum indices of volume contraction

Measurement of serum blood urea nitrogen (BUN) and creatinine concentration may assist in the diagnosis of volume contraction. Volume contraction causes increased tubular reabsorption of urea, leading to an increased serum BUN : creatinine ratio. This prerenal azotemia is characterized by a serum BUN : creatinine ratio (mg/dL : mg/dL) of greater than 20. Plasma volume contraction may also result in hemoconcentration (increased hematocrit) and a relative increase in serum albumin.

Urinary indices

The initial renal response to a decrease in EABV is a fall in urine volume and a reduction in sodium excretion. The urinary sodium concentration and fraction excretion of sodium are indices of renal sodium avidity. In a volume-contracted state, the urinary sodium concentration is generally less than 10–15 mmol/L and the fractional excretion of sodium is usually less than 1%.

The urinary sodium indices are not reliable determinants of volume contraction in some situations. The urinary sodium may be elevated in states of upper gastrointestinal fluid losses associated with vomiting and gastric drainage. Here, the metabolic alkalosis causes obligatory renal sodium wasting as a consequence of bicarbonaturia, which requires cations for electroneutrality. Therefore, in this situation, the urinary chloride concentration is a more reliable index of renal salt avidity. Volume-contracted states associated with obligatory renal sodium wasting, such as with diuretic use, will also make the urinary sodium indices unreliable. Finally, patients with pre-existing renal impairment and elderly patients may have higher than expected urinary sodium concentrations and fractional sodium excretion for the degree of volume contraction.

Other important urine parameters in volume-contracted states include urine osmolality and specific gravity. A urine : plasma creatinine ratio of greater than 40 : 1 also may be suggestive of a prerenal state.

Treatment

The most important goal in the treatment of volume contraction is the expansion of the ECF volume by replacing the fluid deficits. In general, the composition of the replacement fluid should resemble the lost fluid and the rate, amount, and route of administration will vary with the particular circumstance. Whereas increasing oral intake of salt and water may be sufficient with mild volume contraction, immediate administration of intravenous fluids is required in more severe states of ECF volume contraction. The amount of replacement fluid should be adjusted not only to correct the established volume contraction, but also to replace the ongoing fluid losses. However, in elderly patients and patients with congestive heart failure, one must be very careful to avoid volume overload and pulmonary congestion.

Solutions containing sodium as the principal solute preferentially expand the ECF volume. Infusion of 1 L normal saline can result in an increase in plasma volume by about 200 mL; the remaining portion is distributed in the interstitial compartment. Isotonic saline remains the fluid of choice in patients with hypernatremia and volume contraction because restoration of volume status takes preference over the correction of hypernatremia and hyperosmolality. Colloid-containing solutions such as albumin and plasma preferentially expand the intravascular compartment and should be limited to situations where patients are hemodynamically unstable and rapid correction of intravascular volume is critical. This is because the half-life of albumin is usually short, and the cost of albumin administration is very high. A recent meta-analysis also found an association between albumin infusion and mortality risk in critically ill patients[23]; however, it remains controversial as to whether this represents cause and effect or whether it simply reflects the fact that the more seriously ill patients were given greater amounts of colloid.

A physical examination should be performed frequently and laboratory parameters followed closely during the process of volume repletion. Monitoring of CVP and PCWP may be beneficial in patients who are critically ill with severe volume depletion. Hemodynamic monitoring may also be beneficial in patients with poor tolerance to volume expansion. It is important to remember that because volume contraction is accompanied by vasoconstriction, transient changes in PCWP may not accurately reflect the volume status of the patient. The initial elevation in wedge pressure is usually the result of fluid infusion onto a vasoconstricted, low-capacity vascular bed. This should not be misinterpreted to indicate adequacy of volume repletion.

EXTRACELLULAR FLUID VOLUME EXPANSION

ECF volume-expansion states are characterized by an increase in total body water, usually accompanied by an increase in total body sodium. They are associated with edema formation, which refers to the accumulation of excessive amount of salt and water in the interstitial space.

Etiology and pathogenesis

Volume expansion develops when the intake of salt and water exceeds the total renal and extrarenal volume losses. These disorders are usually associated with avid renal sodium and water retention that persists despite the ECF volume expansion. Three general kinds of physiologic derangement account for most edematous states (Table 7.8).

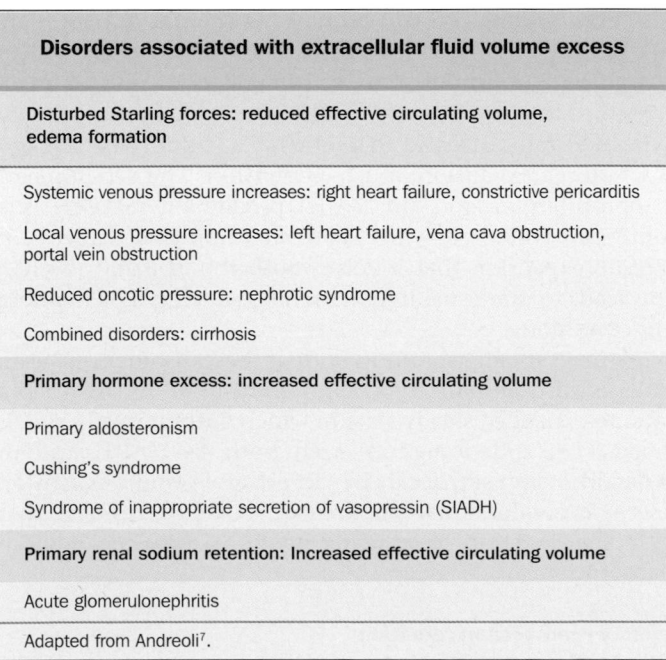

Disorders associated with extracellular fluid volume excess
Disturbed Starling forces: reduced effective circulating volume, edema formation
Systemic venous pressure increases: right heart failure, constrictive pericarditis
Local venous pressure increases: left heart failure, vena cava obstruction, portal vein obstruction
Reduced oncotic pressure: nephrotic syndrome
Combined disorders: cirrhosis
Primary hormone excess: increased effective circulating volume
Primary aldosteronism
Cushing's syndrome
Syndrome of inappropriate secretion of vasopressin (SIADH)
Primary renal sodium retention: Increased effective circulating volume
Acute glomerulonephritis
Adapted from Andreoli[7].

Table 7.8 Classification of disorders associated with extracellular fluid volume excess based on the type of physiologic derangement.

Disturbance in Starling forces

Derangement in the Starling forces leads to expansion of the interstitial compartment at the expense of the ECF volume. Volume-excess disorders are associated with a decrease in capillary oncotic pressure and/or an increase in capillary hydrostatic pressure. In other words, edema is a result of either an increase in movement of fluid to the interstitial space or a decrease in uptake of interstitial fluid into the intravascular compartment. Lastly, inadequacy in lymphatic drainage of the interstitial compartment can contribute to edema formation.

Cardiac disorders such as right heart failure or constrictive pericarditis are frequently associated with high systemic venous pressure[24]. Local elevations in pulmonary or venous pressures may also occur in conditions such as left heart failure, portal vein obstruction, or venacaval obstruction. In nephrotic syndrome, the reduction in plasma oncotic pressure may lead to a decrease in removal of interstitial fluid and a tendency for fluid to transude from the capillaries to the interstitium. In hepatic cirrhosis, there is a combination of increased venous pressures (portal hypertension) and decreased plasma oncotic pressure (hypoalbuminemia) that contributes to the development of ascites and edema[24,25].

Alterations in Starling forces across the capillary bed are responsible for the initiation of edema formation. However, the maintenance of edema occurs because the baroreceptors perceive a reduced effective circulating volume and this stimulates renal sodium and water retention[24]. This arterial 'underfilling' is, therefore, a result of the disease process limiting the ability of the heart to transfer blood from the venous to the arterial circuit. The combination of renal sodium and water retention coupled with continued salt and water intake leads to worsening of the edematous state.

Primary hormonal excesses

Disorders giving rise to primary hormonal excesses are characterized by increased circulating volume as a result of unregulated overproduction of mineralocorticoids or vasopressin. Mineralocorticoid excess states such as primary hyperaldosteronism lead to avid renal sodium retention and ECF volume expansion and hypertension. The syndrome of inappropriate vasopressin (ADH) production (SIADH) is a condition associated with water retention and subsequent volume expansion that involves both the ECF and the ICF. This leads to dilutional hyponatremia, which is a hallmark of this condition.

Edema is usually absent in both of these disorders. Instead, patients with primary hyperaldosteronism or SIADH reach a volume-expanded steady state in which output usually equals intake. This phenomenon, seen both in SIADH and in hyperaldosteronism, occurs in part because volume expansion resets glomerulotubular balance (see above) downwards, that is, in the direction of reducing fractional proximal sodium reabsorption.

Primary renal sodium retention

Abnormal renal sodium retention may sometimes occur when the effective circulating volume is normal. An example of such abnormal sodium retention is acute glomerulonephritis, where unidentified renal mechanisms are primarily responsible for salt retention and edema formation. This occurs without alteration in GFR or EABV, indicating that this disease clearly represents 'overfilling'.

Pathophysiology of renal salt retention

Congestive heart failure

Congestive heart failure (CHF) is associated with a reduction in the EABV along with increased filling pressures in the atrium and venous circuit 'behind' the failed ventricle. The 'backward' theory[12] suggests that the elevation of central venous pressures secondary to cardiac pump failure leads to increased peripheral venous pressure and subsequent alteration of the Starling forces at the capillary level, resulting in edema. The 'backward failure' theory certainly is adequate to explain the symptoms of congestive heart failure. However, the 'backward failure' theory does not account for fluid retention. Thus the most pure example of 'backward failure' is the sudden pulmonary edema, so-called 'flash' pulmonary edema, that occurs in patients with diastolic dysfunction.

The 'forward failure' theory argues that reduced filling of the arterial tree and, consequently, inadequate renal perfusion, results in sodium retention. In turn, if cardiac pump failure is present, much of this fluid will be accumulated on the venous side of the circulation. To summarize, 'backward failure' explains the accumulation of fluid on the venous side of the circulation, but 'forward failure' accounts for sodium retention by inadequate renal perfusion. In modern terms, the

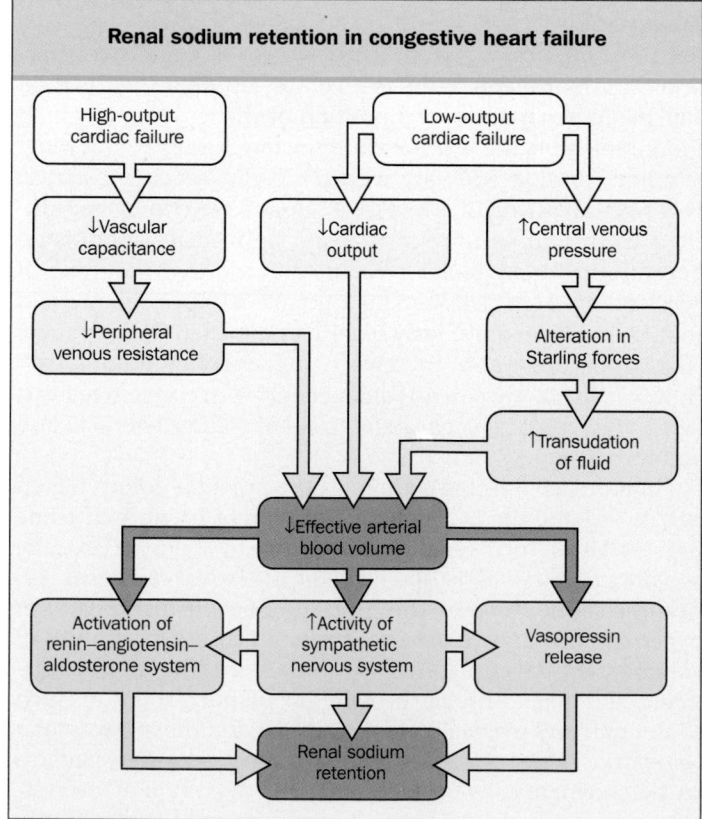

Figure 7.4 Pathophysiology of renal sodium retention in congestive heart failure.

purest form of 'backward failure' is, as noted above, the sudden pulmonary edema of diastolic dysfunction, while 'forward failure' is accounted for best by systolic pump failure and the attendant accumulation of fluid in the venous side of the circulation (Fig. 7.4).

In other words, an inability to transfer fluid either from the interstitium to veins, or from the veins to arteries, results in what has picturesquely been referred to as 'inadequate filling of the arterial tree'. The latter, whether in CHF, cirrhosis or the nephrotic syndrome, is perceived by the kidneys as a volume-contracted state[24,25]. Moreover, as a perceived reduction in effective blood volume becomes increasingly severe, there occurs not only sodium retention but water retention due to nonosmotic vasopressin release. As a consequence, hyponatremia in edematous states, particularly cirrhosis and congestive heart failure, is a particularly ominous condition. For example, several studies have indicated that, in cirrhosis, serum sodium concentrations less than 125 mmol/L are commonly associated with survival of less than 1 year.

There are significant alterations in the afferent limb of volume homeostasis in CHF[24,25,26]. There is blunting of the afferent signaling mechanisms emanating from the venous sensing sites. The reduction in cardiac output diminishes the blood flow to the critical sensors in the arterial circuit that detect an underperfused state. Abnormalities in the effector mechanisms are a consequence of primary disturbance in the afferent sensing mechanism. Alterations in glomerular hemodynamics in CHF include reduced GFR and a disproportionate increase in efferent arteriolar constriction, resulting in increased filtration fraction. As a direct consequence of the glomerular hemodynamics, there is an increase in proximal tubular reabsorption of filtered sodium load. Elevated angiotensin II, catecholamines, and vasopressin levels along with resistance to the action of ANP also contribute to the sodium retention in patients with CHF.

Cirrhosis

Cirrhosis results in disarray of hepatic architecture, with regenerating nodules compressing sinusoids and thus increasing intrasinusoidal hydrostatic pressure, with excessive loss of fluid from the hepatic surface into the peritoneal cavity causing ascites. Furthermore, portal hypertension, portosystemic shunting, splanchnic pooling and hypoalbuminemia characterize cirrhosis. The 'underfill' theory suggests that all these factors, along with peripheral vasodilation, leads to decreased EABV (see Fig. 7.5). Some investigators[27] have found evidence

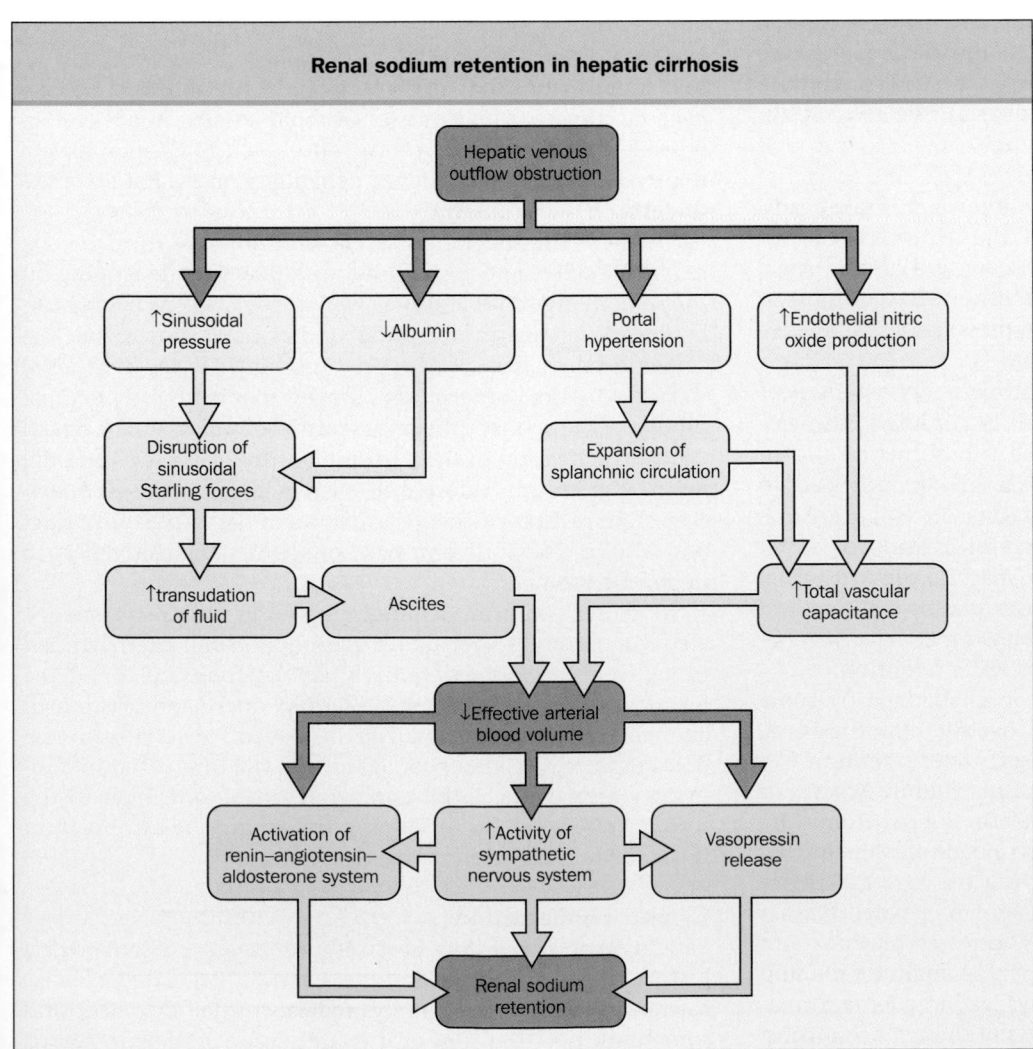

Figure 7.5 Pathophysiology of renal sodium retention on hepatic cirrhosis.

for increased total plasma volume in cirrhotic patients and therefore proposed the 'overfill' theory. However, it is quite likely that what has been termed 'overfilling' is the consequence of splanchnic vasodilatation[25]. The latter results, obviously, in a reduction in the volume/capacitance ratio in the systemic venous bed, a fall in systemic venous return and an attendant 'underfilling' of the arterial tree.

As in CHF, the abnormalities in the effector mechanism are multifactorial. Sodium retention occurs independently of a decrease in GFR and peritubular physical factors may enhance proximal tubular sodium reabsorption. Furthermore, there is activation of the renin–angiotensin–aldosterone axis, ANP resistance and sympathetic overactivity, all of which lead to renal tubular sodium retention.

The issue of ANP resistance warrants particular mention[24]. The inner medullary collecting duct is responsible for the net absorption of about 5% of the glomerular filtration rate, or approximately 1200–1500 mmol/day. ANP facilitates Na^+ excretion by binding specific receptors (ANP_A and ANP_B) and activating cGMP leading to an inhibition of the activity of the sodium channels, thus blocking apical entry of sodium[28,29].

There is now a considerable body of evidence indicating that ANP resistance is, in a sense, the last locus of action for producing renal retention of sodium. In experimental CHF, ANP resistance seems to be the result of a decrease in the density of ANP_A receptors; while in experimental cirrhosis and experimental nephrotic syndrome, ANP resistance is the consequence of an increase in cGMP-phosphodiesterase activity[30]. The resistance to ANP likely has a critical role for sodium retention in these edematous conditions.

Nephrotic syndrome

Nephrotic syndrome differs from CHF and cirrhosis because it is characterized by intrinsic renal disease and altered renal function in most patients. Consequently, this syndrome is associated with elevated mean arterial pressures and a relative impairment of renal sodium excretion.

The pathogenesis of edema in nephrotic syndrome involves two different mechanisms (see Fig. 7.6). According to the classic 'underfill' hypothesis, nephrotic syndrome results in increased urinary loss of albumin, which subsequently leads to hypoalbuminemia and decreased plasma oncotic pressure. Consequently, the alteration in Starling forces leads to the net efflux of fluid from the intravascular space to the interstitial compartment, which in turn decreases plasma volume and EABV. The reduction in EABV activates the effector mechanism that culminates in renal salt and water retention.

The 'underfill' hypothesis has been challenged by some investigators who have proposed the 'overfill' hypothesis[31,32]. According to this theory, renal salt and water retention is a primary phenomenon that leads to plasma volume expansion and subsequent exudation of fluid to the interstitium. The hypoalbuminemia and reduced plasma oncotic pressure further worsen the edema. Evidence supporting the 'overfill' hypothesis comes from studies that have shown elevated plasma volumes and blood pressure as well as decreased plasma renin and aldosterone levels. Furthermore, hypoalbuminemia and familial analbuminemia do not always lead to edema formation[31]. In evaluating the relative merits of these mechanisms,

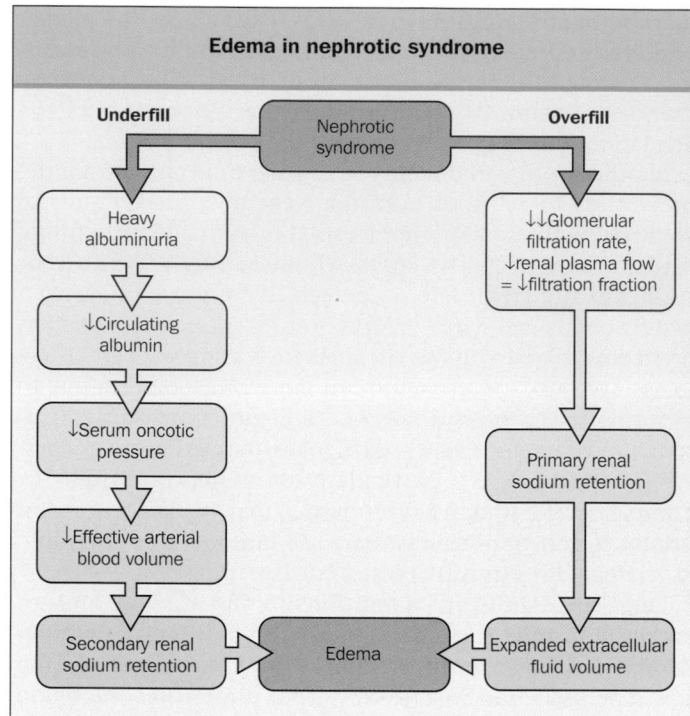

Figure 7.6 Pathophysiology of edema in nephrotic syndrome.

one should note that the nephrotic syndrome is a heterogeneous disease from a variety of renal lesions. It is therefore possible that both 'underfilling' and 'overfilling' may have a role in the formation of edema, depending on the nature of the underlying nephropathy.

The effector mechanisms for sodium retention in the nephrotic syndrome are complex and may vary depending on the underlying renal lesion as well as the stage of edema formation. Whereas some animal studies have shown that the collecting duct may be the predominant site for avid renal sodium retention, other studies suggest that increased proximal tubular sodium absorption may also be important. A fall in GFR and activation of the peritubular physical factors and the renin–angiotensin–aldosterone system also seem to be operative. ANP resistance in the inner medullary collecting duct may also be a final determinant of sodium acquisitiveness in nephrotic edema.

In general, minimal change disease in children is associated with minimal interstitial inflammation and arterial underfilling seems to be the dominant factor responsible for edema formation. However, in patients with glomerular diseases such as membranous nephropathy the overfill mechanism predominates. It has been postulated that the interstitial inflammatory cells in the latter conditions may contribute to the sodium retention by producing oxidants that inhibit local nitric oxide and by releasing angiotensin II[33].

Clinical manifestations

Patients with congestive heart failure usually present with a history of dyspnea on exertion, weakness, decreased exercise tolerance, orthopnea, paroxysmal nocturnal dyspnea, and sometimes nocturia. Physical examination reveals increased weight gain, distention of the jugular veins, pulmonary crackles, tachycardia, a third heart sound, and peripheral edema. Edema in cardiac disease is usually dependent and presents symmetrically in both lower extremities. Pretibial and ankle edema is frequently seen in the evening in ambulatory patients, and presacral edema is a feature of individuals on bed rest.

The edema of nephrotic syndrome is usually diffuse and manifests itself as anasarca. Periorbital edema is a characteristic feature of nephrotic syndrome. Some patients may present with pleural effusions or ascites.

Hepatic cirrhosis presents clinically as ascites and lower-extremity edema as a result of portal hypertension and hypoalbuminemia. Other signs of liver disease include jaundice, spider angiomas, palmar erythema, and gynecomastia.

Diagnosis and treatment

The management of ECF volume-expanded states is dependent on the accurate diagnosis and treatment of the underlying disorder. The cornerstone of therapy in these patients is sodium restriction and diuretics. For patients with mild volume expansion, a 3 g/day (130 mmol/day) sodium diet may be appropriate. For moderate-to-severe ECF volume expansion, a 2 g/day (86 mmol/day) sodium diet should be advocated. Restriction of daily fluid intake should occur only when patients are hyponatremic.

The management of volume-expanded states should aim to correct the underlying primary disorder. Drugs that predispose to sodium retention or alter the effect of diuretics need to be discontinued. For example, nonsteroidal anti-inflammatory agents promote renal sodium retention and interfere with the efficacy of some diuretics.

ACE inhibitors or angiotensin receptor antagonists (ATRA) are important in the treatment of nephrotic syndrome and heart failure. In the nephrotic syndrome, both ACE inhibitors and ATRA drugs minimize proteinuria. In heart failure, these agents reduce cardiac remodeling, and hence protect against diastolic dysfunction, and reduce afterload.

However, because blockade of the renin–angiotensin–aldosterone axis produces primarily efferent arteriolar relaxation, these agents should be used with caution in patients whose serum creatinine levels exceed 2.5–3.0 mg/dL (220–260 µmol/L)and not at all in cirrhotic patients, where efferent arteriolar dilatation can produce a sharp decline in GFR.

Diuretics

Diuretics are the mainstay of therapy in volume-expanded states and should be used only if symptomatic edema persists despite sodium restriction. The characteristics of commonly used diuretics are provided in Table 7.9. It should be recognized that diuretics such as acetazolamide, furosemide (frusemide), bumetanide and torsemide, as well as thiazide diuretics, are all derived from a common parent, sulfanilamide. Thus allergy to sulfa drugs must always be evaluated prior to instituting therapy with these agents.

A second factor relating to diuretics is the coadministration of agents intended to increase colloid osmotic pressure. For example, albumin infusions have been used in the hope of improving the efficacy of diuretics for many years[34]. However, there is no benefit in diuresis efficacy using an albumin/furosemide combination with respect to furosemide alone[35]. Finally, in chronic renal failure, the excretion of the diuretic agent is impaired and therefore, using the intravenous route and/or increasing the dose of the diuretic may be necessary.

Characteristics of the commonly used diuretics based on predominant site of action

Type of diuretic	Site of action	Potency	Primary effect	Secondary effect	Dosage (mg/day)	Complication
Carbonic anhydrase inhibitor	Proximal tubule		↓Na$^+$/H$^+$ exchange	↑K$^+$ loss, ↑HCO$_3^-$ loss		Hypokalemic hyperchloremic acidosis
Acetazolamide		+			250–500	
Loop	Loop of Henle		↓Na$^+$/K$^+$/2Cl$^-$ absorption	↑K$^+$ loss, ↑H$^+$ secretion		Hypokalemic alkalosis
Furosemide (frusemide)		+++			40–600	
Etacrynic acid (ethacrynic acid)		+++			50–400	
Thiazide	Distal tubule		↓Na$^+$ absorption	↑K$^+$ loss, ↑H$^+$ secretion		Hypokalemic alkalosis
Chlorothiazide		++			500–1000	
Hydrochlorothiazide		++			50–100	
Metolazone		++			2.5–10	
Potassium sparing	Collecting duct		↓Na$^+$ absorption	↓K$^+$ loss, ↓H$^+$ secretion		Hyperkalemic acidosis
Triamterene		+			100–300	
Amiloride		+			5–10	
Spironolactone		+			100–400	

Table 7.9 Characteristics of the commonly used diuretics based on predominant site of action.

Diuretics acting at the proximal tubule

Acetazolamide is the prototype of a proximal tubular diuretic. It is a carbonic anhydrase inhibitor and acts by blocking the proximal tubular reabsorption of sodium bicarbonate[34,35]. The proximal diuretics are relatively mild in their potency because the distal parts of the nephron compensate for the decrease in proximal sodium reabsorption. Prolonged use of acetazolamide can lead to increased urinary excretion of sodium, potassium, and bicarbonate and subsequent hyperchloremic metabolic acidosis. This modest alkaline diuresis may be beneficial in some patients with metabolic alkalosis and ECF volume expansion, where isotonic saline cannot be administered. These weak diuretics are used rarely in clinical practice as primary diuretic therapy. Acetazolamide is commonly used to treat open-angle glaucoma and to prevent acute mountain sickness.

Metolazone belongs to the thiazide class of diuretics and acts by a different mechanism from the carbonic anhydrase inhibitors. It blocks sodium chloride reabsorption in the proximal tubule and distal convoluted tubule by unknown mechanisms. Since the major tubular site for phosphate absorption is the proximal tubule, the phosphaturia accompanying metolazone administration exceeds that with other thiazide diuretics. Metolazone is more commonly used in conjunction with other classes of diuretic in instances where the latter are ineffective when used alone.

Diuretics acting at the loop of Henle

Furosemide, bumetanide, and torsemide are 'loop diuretics' that act by inhibiting the coupled entry of sodium, potassium, and chloride across apical plasma membranes in the thick ascending limb of the loop of Henle[34–36]. Approximately 25% of the filtered load of sodium chloride is reabsorbed along the loop of Henle. These diuretics are anions that are bound to protein; as a result, very little of the diuretic reaches the tubules via glomerular filtration. Loop diuretics are secreted into the lumen of the proximal tubule by the organic anion transport system and act on the luminal side of the thick ascending limb of Henle.

Loop diuretics are commonly referred to as 'high-ceiling' diuretics mainly because of their potency, and because the natriuretic dose–response characteristics of these diuretics are considered more linear than those of all other currently used diuretics. They inhibit potassium reabsorption along the thick ascending limb of the loop of Henle and increase potassium secretion along the distal nephron, which results in significant hypokalemia and metabolic alkalosis. These diuretics impair tubular reabsorption and increase the urinary excretion of calcium and magnesium.

Finally, with respect to the loop diuretics, some workers have proposed the use of continuous infusions of loop diuretics rather than oral pulses or intravenous boluses as a potential means of enhancing diuretic efficiency. Thus far, there are no controlled, paired clinical trials to support this contention.

Moreover, it should be recalled that the dose response curve for loop diuretics is nearly linear. Thus increasing the dosage of a single pulse of a loop diuretic – up to the equivalent of 200 mg furosemide (frusemide) intravenously, to avoid risk of ototoxicity – remains the most rational approach to diuresis in difficult patients, together with the simultaneous use of other diuretics, notably metolazone and spironolactone.

Diuretics acting at the distal convoluted tubule

Thiazides are the prototype for this class of diuretic. The distal convoluted tubule reabsorbs about 5–10% of the filtered sodium and chloride ions. These diuretics act on the distal convoluted tubule and interfere primarily with sodium and chloride reabsorption. They block sodium entry from the tubular fluid across apical plasma membranes into distal tubular cells[34,36]. Consequently, they limit the diluting ability of the distal nephron but have no effect on the concentration gradient generated by the loop of Henle. Distal convoluted tubule diuretics are anions, similar to the loop diuretics, and are secreted into the proximal nephron by the organic acid anion transport system. The effectiveness of this class of diuretic decreases when GFR drops below 40 mL/min.

Distal convoluted tubule diuretics, like loop diuretics, lead to hypokalemic metabolic alkalosis. Thiazides promote urinary magnesium losses; however, in contrast to the loop diuretics, they increase luminal calcium absorption and decrease urinary calcium losses. Accordingly, these drugs are useful in the treatment of hypercalciuric states, especially calcium nephrolithiasis. Hyponatremia occurs frequently and results from impaired distal tubular diluting mechanisms.

Diuretics acting at the collecting duct

Triamterene and amiloride are sodium channel blockers that predominantly inhibit sodium reabsorption from the luminal side of the collecting duct. Consequently, there is a fall in the transepithelial voltage in this segment with secondary inhibition of potassium and hydrogen ion secretion. This effect accounts for their potassium-sparing action. They are secreted in to the tubular fluid by the organic cation pathway.

Spironolactone is a competitive antagonist of aldosterone and causes mild natriuresis and potassium retention[34,3637]. It is a weak diuretic and its use is limited to conditions of aldosterone excess. Spironolactone is beneficial in treating disorders characterized by secondary hyperaldosteronism, such as cirrhosis with ascites.

These diuretics are relatively modest in their potency because they act on only a small part (about 3%) of the filtered sodium load. The most common use of collecting duct diuretics is in combination with other classes of diuretic to prevent potassium wasting. The predominant side effect of these agents is hyperkalemia. Spironolactone can cause painful gynecomastia in men and amenorrhea in women. Triamterene can sometimes crystallize in urine.

REFERENCES

1. Share L, Claybaugh JR. Regulation of body fluids. Annu Rev Physiol. 1972;34:235–60.
2. Oh MS, Carroll HJ. Regulation of intracellular and extracellular volume. In: Arieff AI, DeFronzo RA, eds. Fluid, Electrolyte, and Acid–Base Disorders, 2nd edn. New York, NY: Churchill Livingstone; 1995:1–28.
3. Simpson FO. Sodium intake, body sodium, and sodium excretion. Lancet. 1988;2:25–9.
4. Bichet DG, Schrier RW. Cardiac failure, liver disease, and nephrotic syndrome. In: Schrier RW, Gottschalk CW, eds. Diseases of the Kidney, 5th edn. Boston, MA: Little, Brown; 1993:2453–91.
5. Gauer OH, Henry JP, Behn C. The regulation of extracellular fluid volume. Annu Rev Physiol. 1970;32:547–95.
6. Briggs JP, Singh I, Sawaya BE, Schnermann J. Disorders of salt balance. In: Kokko JP, Tannen RL, eds. Fluid and Electrolytes, 3rd edition. Philadelphia, PA: WB Saunders Company; 1996:3–62.
7. Andreoli TE. Disorders of fluid volume, electrolytes and acid–base balance. In: Wyngaarden JB, Smith LH Jr, Bennett JC, eds. Cecil Textbook of Medicine, 18th edn. Philadelphia, PA: Saunders; 1992:499–527.
8. Schrier RW. Body fluid volume regulation in health and disease: a unifying hypothesis. Ann Intern Med. 1990;113:155–9.
9. Miller JA, Tobe SW, Skorecki KL. Control of extracellular fluid volume and the pathophysiology of edema formation. In: Brenner BW, ed. The Kidney, 5th edn. Philadelphia, PA: Saunders; 1996:817–62.
10. Gonzalez-Campoy JM, Knox FG. Integrated responses of the kidney to alterations in extracellular fluid volume. In: Seldin DW, Giebisch G, eds. The Kidney: Physiology and Pathophysiology, 2nd edn. New York: Raven Press; 1992:2041–97.
11. Mazzali M, Hughes J, Kim Y-G, et al. Elevated uric acid increases blood pressure in the rat by a novel crystal-independent mechanism. Hypertension. 2001;38:1101–6.
12. deWardener HE. The control of sodium excretion. Am J Physiol. 1978;235:F163–73.
13. Starling EH. On the absorption of fluid from the connective tissue spaces. J. Physiol (London). 1896;19:312–26.
14. Briggs JP, Schnermann J. The tubuloglomerular feedback mechanism. Functional and biochemical aspects. Annu Rev Physiol. 1989;49:251–73.
15. Thompson SC, Blantz RC. Homeostatic efficiency of tubuloglomerular feedback in hydropenia, euvolemia, and acute volume expansion. Am J Physiol. 1993;264:F930–6.
16. Brenner BM, Falchuh KH, Keinmowitz RI, Berliner RW. The relationship between peritubular capillary protein concentration and fluid reabsorption by the renal proximal tubule. J Clin Invest. 1969;48:1519–31.
17. Hall JE. Control of sodium excretion by angiotensin II: intrarenal mechanisms and blood pressure regulation. Am J Physiol. 1986;250:R960–72.
18. Ziedel ML, Brenner BM. Actions of atrial natriuretic peptides on the kidney. Semin Nephrol. 1987;7:91–7.
19. DiBona GF. Neural control of renal tubular sodium reabsorption and renin secretion: integrative aspects. Clin Exp Theor Pract. 1987;A9 (Suppl. 1):151–65.
20. Rose BD. Hypovolemic states. In: Rose BD, ed. Clinical Physiology of Acid-Base and Electrolyte Disorders, 2nd edn. New York: McGraw-Hill; 1989:279–309.
21. DuBose TD Jr. Salt wastage and salt depletion. In: Seldin DW, Giebisch G, eds. The Regulation of Sodium and Chloride Balance. New York: Raven Press;1990:419–32.
22. Gougoux A, Bichet DG. Extracellular fluid volume contraction. In: Jacobson HR, Striker GE, Klahr S, eds. The Principles and Practice of Nephrology, 2nd edn. St Louis, MO: Mosby; 1995:876–9.
23. Cochrane Injuries Group Albumin Reviewers. Human albumin administration in critically ill patients: systematic review of randomised controlled trials. Br Med J. 1998;317:235–40.
24. Andreoli TE. Edematous states: an overview. Kidney Int. 1997;51(Suppl. 59):S2–10.
25. Schrier RW, Ecder T. Unifying hypothesis of body fluid volume regulation: implications for cardiac failure and cirrhosis. Mt Sinai J Med. 2001;68:350–61.
26. Palmer BF, Alpern RJ, Seldin DW. Pathophysiology of edema formation. In: Seldin DW, Giebisch G, eds. The Kidney: Physiology and Pathophysiology, 2nd edn. New York: Raven Press; 1992: 2099–141.
27. Lieberman FL, Denison EK, Reynolds TF. The relationship of plasma volume, portal hypertension, ascites and renal sodium retention in cirrhosis: the overflow theory of ascites formation. Ann NY Acad Sci. 1970;170:202–10.
28. Zeidel ML, Silva P, Brenner BM, Seifter JL. cGMP mediates effects of atrial peptides on medullary collecting duct cells. Am J Physiol. 1987;252:F551–9.
29. Yechieli H, Kahana L, Haramati A, et al. Regulation of renal glomerular and papillary ANP receptors in rats with experimental heart failure. Am J Physiol. 1993;265: F119–5.
30. Lee EYW, Humphreys MH. Phosphodiesterase activity as a mediator of renal resistance to ANP in pathological salt retention. Am J Physiol. 1996;271:F3–6.
31. Seldin DW. Sodium balance and fluid volume in normal and edematous states. In: Seldin DW, Giebisch G, eds. The Regulation of Sodium and Chloride Balance. New York: Raven Press; 1990:261–92.
32. Koomans HA, Geers AB, Meiracker AH, et al. Effects of plasma volume expansion on renal salt handling in patients with nephrotic syndrome. Am J Nephrol. 1984;4:227.
33. Rodriguez-Iturbe B, Herrera-Acosta J, Johnson RJ. Interstitial inflammation, sodium retention, and the pathogenesis of nephrotic edema. Kidney Int. 2002;62:1379–84.
34. Dillingham MA, Schrier RW, Gregor R. Mechanism of diuretic action. In: Schrier RW, Gottschalk CW, eds. Diseases of the Kidney, 5th edn. Boston, MA: Little, Brown; 1993:2435–52.
35. Ghalasani N, Gorski JC, Horlander JC Sr, et al. Effects of albumin/furosemide mixtures on responses to furosemide in hypoalbuminemic patients. J Am Soc Nephrol. 2001;12:1010–16.
36. Brater DC. Drug-induced electrolyte disorders and use of diuretics. In: Kokko JP, Tannen RL, eds. Fluid and Electrolytes, 3rd edn. Philadelphia, PA: WB Saunders Company; 1996:693–728.
37. Brater C. The use of diuretics in congestive heart failure. Semin Nephrol. 1994; 14:479–84.

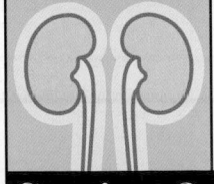

Chapter 8

Disorders of Water Metabolism

Chirag Parikh, Sumit Kumar, and Tomas Berl

PHYSIOLOGY OF WATER BALANCE

The maintenance of the tonicity of body fluids within a very narrow physiologic range is made possible by homeostatic mechanisms that control the intake of water and its excretion. Critical to this process are the osmoreceptors located in the hypothalamus, which control the secretion of vasopressin (antidiuretic hormone, ADH) in response to changes in tonicity. In turn, vasopressin governs the excretion of water by its end-organ effect on the renal collecting system.

Water balance and the control of renal water excretion

In steady-state situations, water intake matches water losses through all sources. Water intake, determined by thirst as well as by cultural and social behavior patterns, is finely balanced by the individual's need to maintain a physiologic serum osmolality of 285–290 mOsm/kg. Optimal water balance is achieved by a complex array of mechanisms that have evolved over millions of years; adaptation to a terrestrial life has evolved into the unique ability to excrete urine that can be either hypotonic or hypertonic in relation to plasma. Despite major fluctuations of solute and water intake, the total solute concentration (i.e., the tonicity) of body fluids is maintained virtually constant. The ability both to dilute and to concentrate the urine allows for a wide flexibility in urine flow. In conditions of water loading, the diluting mechanisms permit excretion of 20–25 L of urine per day. By comparison, in states of water deprivation, the urine volume may decrease to as little as 0.5 L per day[1].

The unique anatomic arrangement in the kidneys of tubular structures as well as vascular beds allows for the above described extremes of concentration and dilution possible (see Chapter 1). The nephron is organized into various components including the descending thin limb of the loop of Henle, which is in close proximity to the ascending thin limb of the loop of Henle, the thick ascending limb of the loop of Henle (TALH), and the collecting ducts. Interposed among these is the vascular component, the vasa recta, which has a descending and an ascending limb. There are two distinct populations of nephron in mammalian kidneys, those with short loops of Henle and those with long loops of Henle. The short loops originate in the superficial and midcortical glomeruli. They do not have a thin ascending limb: the thin descending limb turns directly into the TALH. The long loops form part of glomeruli that originate in the deep cortex and juxtamedullary region. The loops penetrate deep into the inner medulla. The transition between the thin and thick ascending limbs of the loops of Henle marks the transition between the anatomically distinct inner and outer medullary areas. This anatomic arrangement allows for countercurrent flow in the loop of Henle and vasa recta and the countercurrent mechanism for urinary concentration, discussed in more detail in Chapter 2.

Water reabsorption in the proximal tubule and the descending limb of the loop of Henle

At its origin, the glomerular filtrate is iso-osmotic to plasma. The proximal tubule and the descending limb of the loop of Henle are highly water permeable. About 70% of the filtrate, including solutes (bicarbonate, glucose, and amino acids) and water is iso-osmotically reabsorbed in the proximal tubule, with active Na^+ transport as the major driving force. Another 10% of the filtrate is absorbed in the descending limb of the loop of Henle with slight increase in osmolality. The volume of the fluid entering the bend of the loop sets the upper limit of the urine flow that can be excreted if no further water reabsorption were to occur in distal parts of the nephron. This is the mechanism whereby a reduction in the volume of filtrate delivered to the distal nephron can limit water excretion.

Water reabsorption in the ascending loop of Henle and the distal convoluted tubule

Short- and long-loop nephrons participate in the countercurrent exchange. In humans, 70–80% of the nephrons have short loops. It is generally accepted that in the descending and the ascending thin limbs, only passive solute transport occurs. In the TALH, separation of solute from water occurs. Sodium reabsorption occurs here via the $Na^+/K^+/2Cl^-$ cotransporter in the apical membrane, the only active step in the countercurrent multiplier system. Because of the low water permeability of the TALH, the osmolality of tubular fluid decreases along the length of this segment without any change in the volume. The tubular fluid that emerges from the loop is hypotonic and is further diluted in the early distal tubule. The efficiency of the countercurrent multiplier varies directly with the length of the TALH. This process predominantly occurs in the nephrons with long loops.

The electroneutral $Na^+/K^+/2Cl^-$ cotransporter belongs to a family of cotransporters that have been expressed in various tissues, most notably the kidney where they are found in the TALH, distal convoluted tubule, and the distal end of the collecting tubule. This major pathway for cellular uptake of Cl^- is critical for cell volume regulation and is the major target site for the action of loop diuretics. These agents interfere with both the diluting and concentrating mechanisms of the kidney. In contrast, thiazide-type diuretics act only in the cortical diluting segment and do not significantly impair the kidney's ability to generate interstitial tonicity, thus leaving the concentrating capacity intact. However, they do limit the urinary diluting capacity by inhibiting the Na^+/Cl^- cotransporter. In humans, the distal convoluted tubule is inert to the action of vasopressin and is impermeable to water regardless of the occurrence of vasopressin.

Water reabsorption in the collecting duct
Several distal tubules converge to form the collecting tubules in the cortex and these again merge as they descend through the outer medulla, with each terminal collecting duct drawing from as many as 7800 nephrons. At baseline, the water permeability of the collecting duct is extremely low, but it is increased markedly in the presence of vasopressin. It is here that the final volume and concentration of the urine is determined. In the presence of vasopressin, equilibration with the hypertonic interstitium results in excretion of a low volume of concentrated urine, whereas, in the absence of vasopressin, the collecting duct remains water impermeable and the dilute tubular fluid delivered from the distal tubule is excreted as urine. The presence or absence of vasopressin is, therefore, central to water homeostasis.

VASOPRESSIN

Physiology
Vasopressin (also known as arginine vasopressin or ADH) plays a critical role in determining the concentration of urine. It is a cyclic octapeptide (1099 Da) with a tail of three amino acid residues. It is synthesized and secreted by the specialized supraoptic and paraventricular magnocellular nuclei in the hypothalamus. Vasopressin has a short half-life of about 15 to 20 min and is rapidly metabolized in the liver and the kidney.

Osmotic stimuli for vasopressin release
Vasopressin is secreted in response to osmotic and nonosmotic stimuli. The 'osmoreceptor' cells are located in the anterior hypothalamus close to the supraoptic nuclei. Substances that are restricted to the extracellular fluid (ECF) such as hypertonic saline or mannitol decrease cell volume by acting as effective osmoles and enhancing osmotic water movement from the cell. This stimulates vasopressin release. Urea and glucose cross cell membranes freely and do not cause any change in cell volume. The osmoreceptors are sensitive to changes in plasma osmolality as small as 1%. In humans, the osmotic threshold for vasopressin release is 280–290 mOsm/kg (Fig. 8.1). This system is so efficient that the plasma osmolality usually does not vary by more than 1–2% despite wide fluctuations in water intake.

Nonosmotic stimuli for vasopressin release
There are several other nonosmotic stimuli for vasopressin secretion. In settings with decreased effective circulating volume (e.g., heart failure, cirrhosis, or vomiting), discharge from parasympathetic afferent nerves in the carotid sinus baroreceptors increases vasopressin secretion. Other nonosmotic stimuli include nausea, which can lead to a marked rise

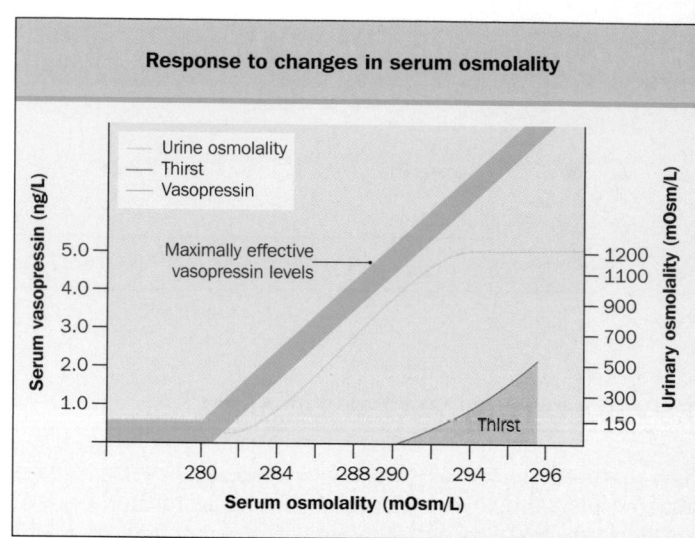

Figure 8.1 Mechanisms maintaining plasma osmolality. The response of thirst, vasopressin levels, and urinary osmolality to changes in serum osmolality. (Adapted with permission from Narins and Krishna[2].

in circulating vasopressin levels, postoperative pain, and pregnancy. Much higher vasopressin levels can be achieved with hypovolemia than with hyperosmolality, although a large (7%) fall in blood volume is required before this response is initiated. The complex interplay of these homeostatic mechanisms is in part effected by the thirst mechanism, which under normal conditions changes water intake in an effort to restore serum osmolality to normal.

Cellular mechanism of vasopressin action
The multiple actions of vasopressin are mediated by its interaction with at least three types of receptor coupled to G proteins: the V_{1a} (vascular and hepatic), V_{1b} (anterior pituitary), and V_2 receptors. The V_2 receptor is primarily localized in the kidney and leads to an increase in water permeability of the collecting duct. The cellular signaling pathway involved in vasopressin action is depicted in Figure 8.2 The final step in the process involves aquaporin 2 (AQP-2). This is a member of a growing family of cellular water transporters (Table 8.1)[3,4]. The first member of this family to be described and cloned AQP-1, is abundantly localized in the apical and basolateral region of the proximal tubule epithelial cells and the descending limb of Henle. This water channel accounts for the high water permeability of these nephron segments. Because AQP-1 is constitutively expressed in the proximal tubule, it is not subject to regulation by vasopressin. The water channel responsible for the high water permeability of the collecting duct luminal membrane in response to vasopressin has been designated AQP-2. This water channel is found exclusively in apical plasma membrane and in intracellular vesicles in the collecting duct principal cells. Vasopressin appears to be involved in both the short- and long-term regulation of AQP-2. The short-term regulation, also described as the 'shuttle hypothesis,' explains the rapid and reversible increase (within minutes) in collecting duct water permeability that is associated with vasopressin administration. This involves the insertion of water channels from

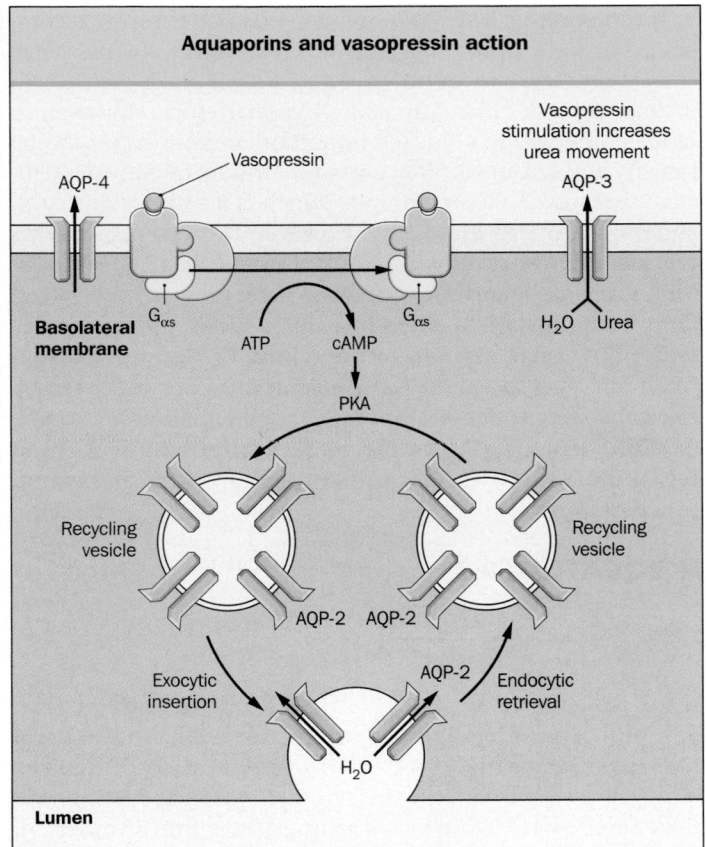

Figure 8.2 Cellular mechanism of vasopressin action. Vasopressin binds to V_2 receptors on the basolateral membrane and activates G proteins that initiate a cascade resulting in aquaporin-2 insertion in the luminal membrane. This then allows water uptake into the cell. (Adapted with permission from Bichet[3].)

subapical vesicles into the luminal membrane. Long-term regulation involves vasopressin-mediated increased transcription of genes involved in AQP-2 production and occurs if circulating vasopressin levels are elevated for 24 h or more. The maximal water permeability of the collecting duct epithelium is increased as a consequence of an increase in the total number of AQP-2 channels per cell. This process is not readily reversible[4].

The other members of the aquaporin family, AQP-3 and AQP-4, are located on the basolateral membranes (see Fig. 8.2 and Table 8.1) and are probably involved in water exit from the cell. AQP-3 is also urea permeable and under the stimulus of vasopressin increases the permeability of the collecting duct to urea, resulting in its movement into the interstitium. AQP-4 has also been identified in the hypothalamus and is a candidate osmoreceptor for the control of vasopressin release. A few more aquaporin molecules have been discovered in the kidney including AQP-6, AQP-7 and AQP-8 (see Table 8.1). AQP-5 and AQP-9 have been identified and are present elsewhere in the body but not in the kidney. Analysis of the molecular biology of these channels and the receptors responsible for vasopressin action have contributed to an understanding of the syndromes of genetically transmitted as well as acquired forms of vasopressin resistance.

The role of thirst in water balance

In humans and other terrestrial animals, the thirst mechanism plays an important role in water balance. Hypertonicity is the most potent stimulus for thirst, with a change of only 2–3% in plasma osmolality producing a strong desire to drink water. This absolute level of osmolality at which the sensation of thirst arises in healthy individuals is called the osmotic threshold for thirst. It usually occurs at approximately 290 to

Characteristics of aquaporins (AQPs)							
Characteristics	AQP-1	AQP-2	AQP-3	AQP-4	AQP-6	AQP-7	AQP-8
Size (amino acid residues)	269	271	285	301	282	269	263
Permeability to small solutes	No	No	Urea, glycerol	No	No	Glycerol, urea	Urea
Regulation by vasopressin	No	Yes	No	No	No	No	No
Site	Proximal tubules, descending thin limb	Collecting duct principal cells	Medullary collecting duct, colon	Hypothalamic, supraoptic and paraventricular nuclei; ependymal, granular, and Purkinje cells	Proximal tubules, collecting duct Intercalated cells	Testis, kidney	Kidney, pancreas, heart, liver, colon, brain
Cellular localization	Apical and basolateral membrane	Apical membrane and intracellular vesicles	Basolateral membrane	Basolateral membrane of the principal cells	Intracellular membrane vesicles	unknown	Intracellular membrane vesicles
Mutant phenotype	Concentrating defect (mice and humans)	Nephrogenic diabetes insipidus	Concentrating defect (mice)	Concentrating defect (mice)	unknown	unknown	unknown

Table 8.1 Characteristics of aquaporins (AQPs).

Fluid and Electrolyte Disorders

295 mOsm/kg H_2O and is above the threshold for vasopressin release (see Fig. 8.1). It closely approximates the level at which maximal concentration of urine is achieved. Hypovolemia, hypotension and angiotensin II are also stimuli for thirst. Between the limits imposed by the osmotic thresholds for thirst and vasopressin release, plasma osmolality may be regulated more precisely by small, osmoregulated adjustments in urine flow and water intake. The exact level at which balance occurs depends upon various factors, for example insensible losses through skin and lungs, the gains incurred from drinking water and eating, and water generated from metabolism. In general, overall intake and output come into balance at a plasma osmolality of 288 mOsm/kg, roughly half way between the thresholds for vasopressin release and thirst.

QUANTITATION OF RENAL WATER EXCRETION

Urine volume can be considered as having two components. The osmolar clearance (C_{osm}) is the volume needed to excrete solutes at the concentration of solutes in plasma. The free water clearance (C_{water}) is the volume of solute-free water that has been added to (positive C_{water}) or subtracted (negative C_{water}) from the isotonic portion of the urine (C_{osm}) to create either hypotonic or hypertonic urine.

Urine volume flow (V) comprises an isotonic portion (C_{osm}) and the free water clearance (C_{water}).

■ EQUATION 8.1

$$V = C_{osm} + C_{water}$$

$$C_{water} = V - C_{osm}$$

The term C_{osm} relates urine osmolality to plasma osmolality P_{osm} by

$$C_{osm} = \left(\frac{U_{osm} \times V}{P_{osm}} \right)$$

Therefore,

■ EQUATION 8.2

$$C_{water} = V - \left(\frac{U_{osm} \times V}{P_{osm}} \right)$$

$$= V \left(1 - \frac{U_{osm}}{P_{osm}} \right)$$

This relationship describes three key points:
- hypotonic urine: $U_{osm} < P_{osm}$ and C_{water} is positive;
- isotonic urine: $U_{osm} = P_{osm}$ and there is no C_{water};
- hypertonic urine: $U_{osm} > P_{osm}$ and C_{water} is negative (water retained).

A positive value for C_{water} represents the volume of water that must be removed from hypotonic urine and a negative value is the water that must be added to hypertonic urine to make it isotonic with plasma.

If excretion of free water in a polyuric patient is unaccompanied by water intake, the patient will become hypernatremic; conversely, the failure to excrete free water in settings of increased water intake can cause hyponatremia. However, in terms of predicting clinically important alterations in plasma tonicity and serum Na^+ concentration, this formulation is deficient, because it factors in urea, which is an important component of urinary osmolality. However, because urea crosses cell membranes readily, it does not establish a transcellular osmotic gradient and does not cause water movement between fluid compartments. Therefore, urea does not influence serum Na^+ concentration, or the release of vasopressin. As a result, changes in serum Na^+ concentration are predicted by electrolyte free water clearance ($C_{water}(e)$). Equation 8.2 can be modified, replacing P_{osm} by plasma Na^+ concentration (P_{Na}) and the urine osmolality by urinary sodium and potassium concentrations ($U_{Na} + U_K$):

■ EQUATION 8.3

$$C_{water}(e) = V \left(1 - \frac{U_{Na} + U_K}{P_{Na}} \right)$$

If the patient's value for $U_{Na} + U_K$ is less than the P_{Na}, then ($C_{water}(e)$) is positive and the serum Na^+ concentration will rise. However, if the $U_{Na} + U_K$ is greater than P_{Na}, then the ($C_{water}(e)$) is negative and the serum Na^+ concentration will tend to decrease. In clinical setting involving disorders of serum Na^+ concentration it is more appropriate to use Equation 8.3 since Equation 8.2 reflects water clearance with respect to total body osmolality. Clinical settings such as those associated with high urea excretion would predict negative water excretion and decrease in serum Na^+ concentration if Equation 8.2 were used; yet the serum Na^+ concentration rises – a fact that would be accurately predicted if Equation 8.3 were employed.

CONTROL OF SERUM SODIUM

The countercurrent mechanism of the kidneys, which allows for urinary concentration and dilution, acts in concert with the hypothalamic osmoreceptors via vasopressin secretion to maintain a finely tuned balance of water and to keep serum Na^+ and serum tonicity within a very narrow range (Fig. 8.3). A defect in the urine-diluting capacity when coupled with excess water intake leads to hyponatremia. Hypernatremia occurs when defects in urinary concentrating ability are not accompanied by adequate water intake.

Serum Na^+, along with its accompanying anions, accounts for nearly all of the osmotic activity of the plasma. Calculated serum osmolality is given by:

■ EQUATION 8.4

$$2[Na^+] + BUN\ (mg/dL)/2.8 + glucose\ (mg/dL)/18$$

where BUN is blood urea nitrogen. The addition of other solutes to ECF results in an increase in measured osmolality (Table 8.2). The nature of the solute plays an important role in determining whether there is an increase in measured

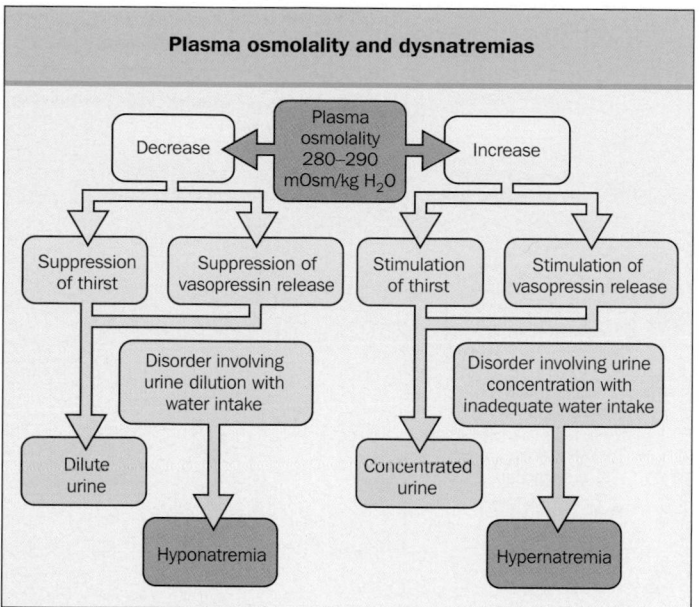

Figure 8.3 Maintenance of plasma osmolality and pathogenesis of dysnatremias. (Adapted with permission from Halterman and Berl[5].)

The effects of osmotically active substances on serum sodium levels	
Substances that increase osmolality without changing serum Na+	Substances that increase osmolality and decrease serum Na+ (translocational hyponatremia)
Urea	Glucose
Ethanol	Mannitol
Ethylene glycol	Glycine
Isopropyl alcohol	Maltose
Methanol	

Table 8.2 The effects of osmotically active substances on serum sodium levels.

osmolality or there is an actual increase in effective tonicity. Solutes that are permeable across cell membranes such as urea, methanol, ethanol, and ethylene glycol do not cause water movement and cause hypertonicity without causing cellular dehydration. Examples of increases in these solutes are a uremic patient with a high BUN and an ethanol-intoxicated individual. By comparison, a patient with diabetic ketoacidosis has an increase in plasma glucose, which cannot move freely across cell membranes in the absence of insulin. The presence of this glucose in ECF causes water to move from the cells to the ECF, thereby leading to cellular dehydration and concomitantly lowering serum Na+ concentration. This can be viewed as 'translocational' at the cellular level, as the serum Na+ concentration does not reflect change in total body water but rather reflects a movement of water from intracellular to extracellular space. Hyperglycemia accounts for 15% of hyponatremia in hospitalized patients. A decrease in serum Na+ of 1.6 mmol/L occurs for every 100 mg/dL (5.6 mmol/L) increase in plasma glucose. However, a recent study suggests that the calculation may underestimate the

impact of glucose to decreased concentration of serum sodium[6]. Other substances known to cause translocational hyponatremia are mannitol, maltose, and glycine[7]. Glycine is used as an irrigant solution during transurethral resection of the prostate and in endometrial surgery.

Pseudohyponatremia occurs when the solid phase of plasma (usually 6–8%) is greatly increased by large increments in either lipids or proteins (e.g., in hypertriglyceridemia and paraproteinemias). This false result occurs because the flame photometry method that measures the concentration of Na+ uses whole plasma and not just the liquid phase. The alternative method involves ion selective potentiometry – direct and indirect. However, only the direct (undiluted) potentiometry measurements, to which most laboratories are now moving, will give the true aqueous sodium activity. A rise in plasma lipids of 4.6 g/L leads to a decrease in serum Na+ concentration of 1 mmol/L; an increase in plasma protein greater than 10 g/dL has a similar effect.

Estimation of total body water

In the normal individual, total body water is approximately 60% of body weight (50% in women and in obese individuals). In patients with hyponatremia or hypernatremia, the change in total body water can be calculated from the serum Na+ concentration, using the following formulae:

■ EQUATION 8.5

$$\text{Water excess} = 0.6W \times \left(1 - \frac{(\text{Na}^+)_{obs}}{140}\right)$$

■ EQUATION 8.6

$$\text{Water deficit} = 0.6W \times \left(1 - \frac{(\text{Na}^+)_{obs}}{140}\right)$$

where $[\text{Na}^+]_{obs}$ is observed sodium concentration in mmol/L and W is body weight in kg. In general, a change in 10 mmol/L in the serum Na+ concentration in a 70-kg individual is equivalent to a change of 3 L in free water.

HYPONATREMIC DISORDERS

Disorders of urinary dilution underlie the development of hyponatremia. The components of normal urinary dilution are depicted in Figure 8.4. The disturbances of urinary dilution are reflected in perturbations of these components and include:

- intrarenal factors such as a diminished glomerular filtration rate (GFR), or an increase in proximal tubular fluid and Na+ reabsorption, or both, which decrease distal delivery to the diluting segments of the nephron;
- a defect in the Na+/Cl- transport out of the water-impermeable segments of the nephrons, i.e., in the TALH or distal convoluted tubule;
- and, most commonly the continued secretion of vasopressin despite the presence of serum hypo-osmolality, stimulated by nonosmotic mechanisms.

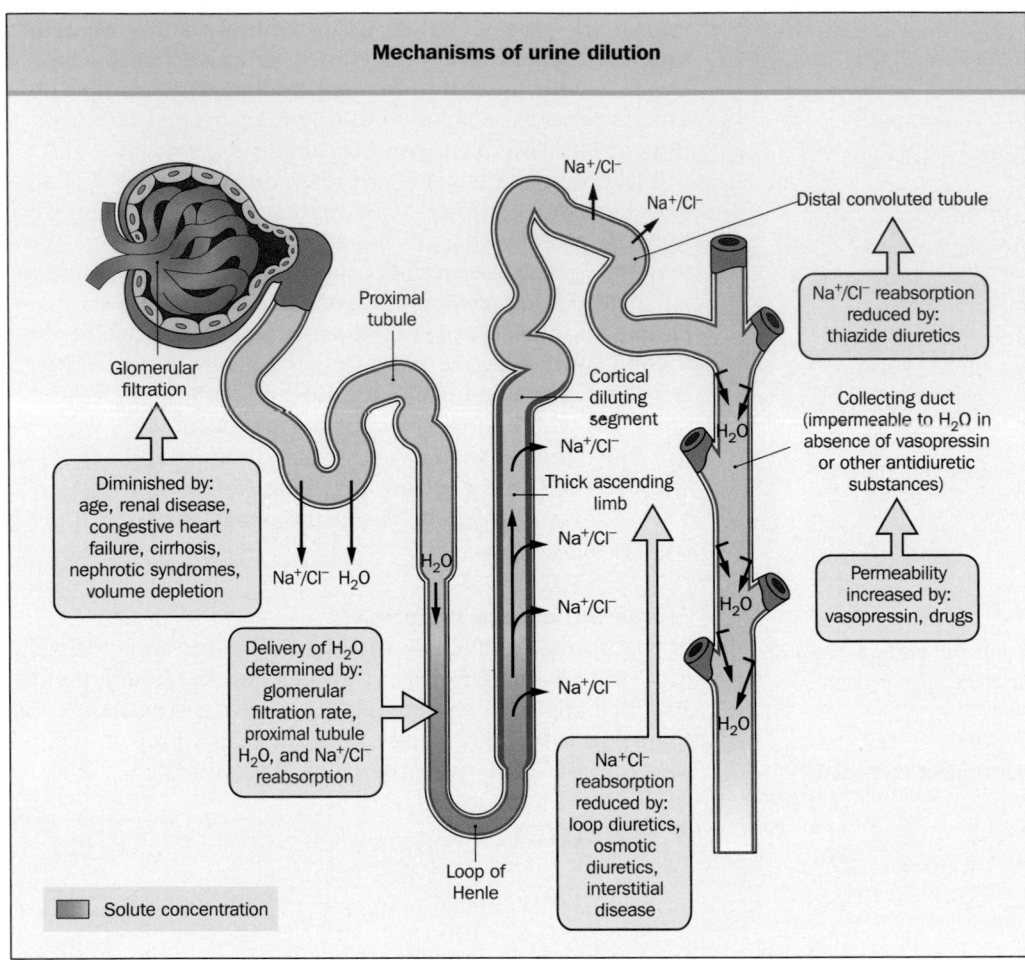

Mechanisms of urine dilution

Glomerular filtration

Diminished by: age, renal disease, congestive heart failure, cirrhosis, nephrotic syndromes, volume depletion

Proximal tubule

Delivery of H_2O determined by: glomerular filtration rate, proximal tubule H_2O, and Na^+/Cl^- reabsorption

Na^+/Cl^- H_2O

H_2O

Loop of Henle

Solute concentration

Na^+/Cl^-

Na^+/Cl^-

Cortical diluting segment

Na^+/Cl^-

Thick ascending limb

Na^+/Cl^-

Na^+/Cl^-

Na^+/Cl^-

Na^+Cl^- reabsorption reduced by: loop diuretics, osmotic diuretics, interstitial disease

Distal convoluted tubule

Na^+/Cl^- reabsorption reduced by: thiazide diuretics

Collecting duct (impermeable to H_2O in absence of vasopressin or other antidiuretic substances)

H_2O

H_2O

H_2O

Permeability increased by: vasopressin, drugs

Figure 8.4 Urinary dilution mechanisms. Normal determinants of urinary dilution and disorders causing hyponatremia. (Adapted with permission from Cogan[8].)

Approach to the hyponatremic patient

Once pseudohyponatremia and translocational hyponatremia are ruled out and the patient is established as truly hypo-osmolar, the next step is to classify the patient as hypovolemic, euvolemic, or hypervolemic (see Fig. 8.5)[5].

Hypovolemia: hyponatremia associated with decreased total body sodium

A patient with hypovolemic hyponatremia has both a total body Na^+ and a water deficit, with the Na^+ deficit exceeding the water deficit. This occurs in patients with high gastrointestinal and renal losses of water and solute accompanied by free water or hypotonic fluid intake. The underlying mechanism is the nonosmotic release of vasopressin stimulated by volume contraction, which maintains the secretion of the hormone despite the hypotonic state. Baroreceptors in the aortic arch and carotid sinus and vagal receptors located in the left atrium contribute to the release of vasopressin in response to volume contraction. Measurement of urinary Na^+ concentration is a useful tool in helping to diagnose these conditions (see Fig. 8.5).

Gastrointestinal and third-space sequestered losses

Patients with hyponatremia in the presence of gastrointestinal losses through either diarrhea or vomiting are extremely Na^+ avid, and the urinary Na^+ concentration tends to be very low

because the kidney responds to this state of volume contraction by conserving Na^+ and Cl^-. Third spacing of fluids occurs in the peritoneal cavity in peritonitis and pancreatitis or in the small bowel lumen with ileus and burns. In these situations, the urinary Na^+ concentration is usually < 10 mmol/L and the urine is hyperosmolar. In patients with vomiting and metabolic alkalosis, bicarbonaturia occurs; HCO_3^- is a nonreabsorbable anion and its excretion requires that cations are excreted as well. The urinary Na^+ in these situations may be > 20 mmol/L, despite severe volume depletion. The urinary Cl^-, however, is < 10 mmol/L. If renal function is severely impaired in the setting of chronic renal failure, renal salt conservation is impaired and maximal conservation does not occur.

Diuretics

Diuretic use is one of the most common causes of hypovolemic hyponatremia associated with a high urine Na^+ concentration. Hyponatremia occurs almost exclusively with the use of thiazide diuretics. The variation in the hyponatremic risk associated with loop or thiazide diuretics relates to their site of action. Loop diuretics inhibit the Na^+/Cl^- reabsorption in the TALH. This interferes with the generation of a hypertonic medullary interstitium. Therefore, even though volume contraction leads to increased vasopressin secretion, responsiveness to vasopressin is diminished because of the

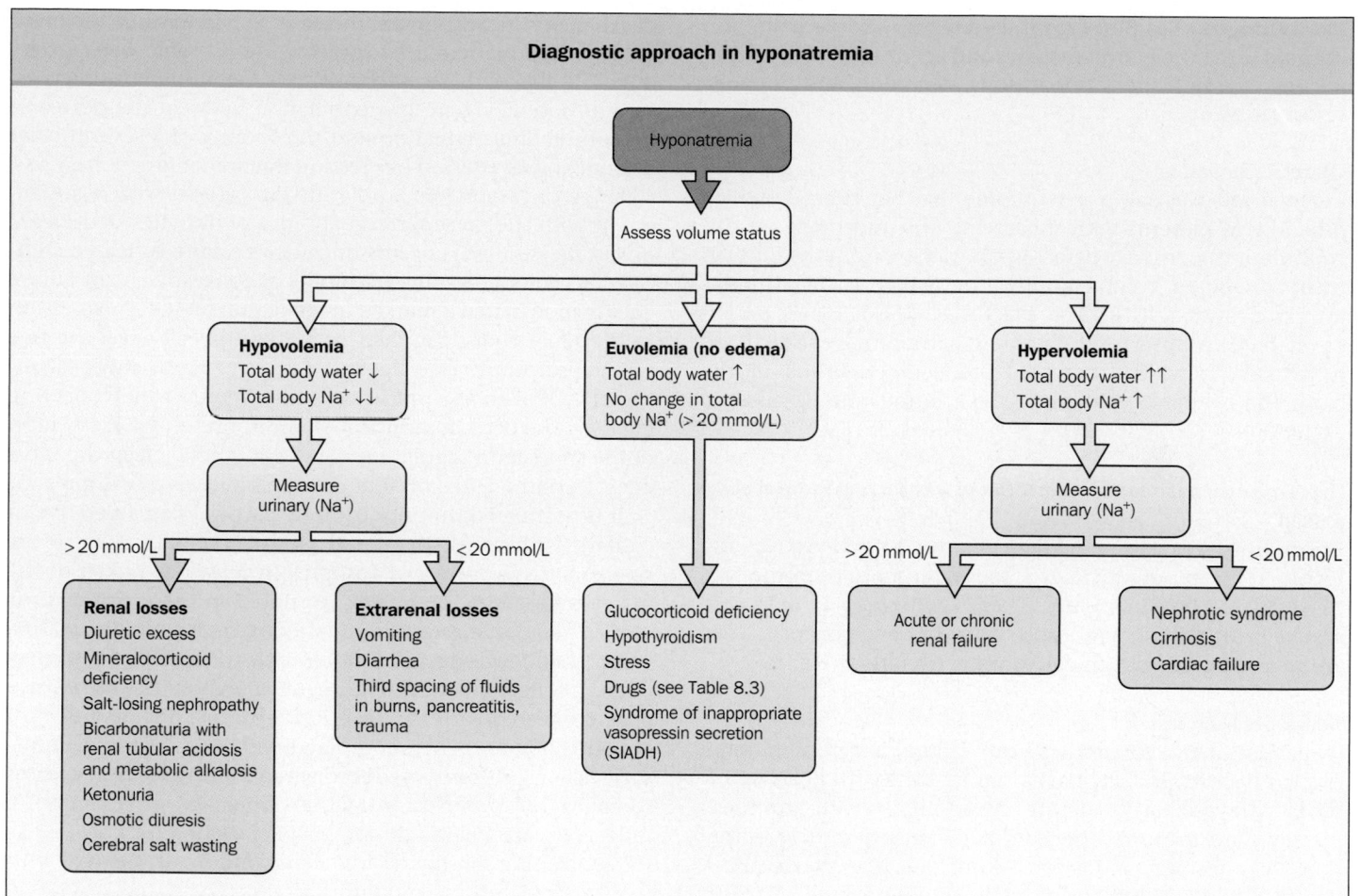

Figure 8.5 **Diagnostic approach for the patient with hyponatremia.** (Adapted with permission from Halterman and Berl[5].)

impairment in medullary hypertonicity. Thiazide diuretics, however, act in the distal tubule by interfering with urinary dilution rather than urinary concentration. Underweight women and elderly patients appear to be more prone to hyponatremia with thiazide diuretic use, which usually occurs within 14 days of initiation of therapy, although one-third present within 5 days of commencing therapy. Several mechanisms for diuretic-induced hyponatremia have been postulated:

- hypovolemia-stimulated vasopressin release and decreased fluid delivery to the diluting segment;
- impaired water excretion through interference with maximal urinary dilution in the cortical diluting segment;
- depletion, directly stimulating water intake by alterations in osmoreceptor sensitivity and increasing thirst.

It is interesting to note that water retention can mask the physical findings of hypovolemia, thereby making the patients with diuretic-induced hyponatremia appear euvolemic.

Salt-losing nephropathy
A salt-losing state sometimes occurs in patients with advanced chronic renal insufficiency (GFR < 15 mL/min) and is characterized by hyponatremia and hypovolemia. Such a state may occur in patients with medullary cystic disease, polycystic kidney disease, analgesic nephropathy, chronic pyelonephritis, and obstructive uropathy. Patients with proximal type II renal tubular acidosis exhibit renal Na^+ and K^+ wastage despite only moderate renal insufficiency. In these patients, bicarbonaturia obligates urine Na^+ excretion.

Mineralocorticoid deficiency
Hyponatremia with ECF volume contraction, urine Na^+ higher than 20 mmol/L, and high serum K^+, urea, and creatinine are indicative of mineralocorticoid deficiency. The decreased ECF volume, rather than the deficiency of the hormone *per se*, provides the nonosmotic stimulus for vasopressin release.

Osmotic diuresis
An osmotically active, nonreabsorbable solute obligates the renal excretion of Na^+ and results in volume depletion. With continuing water intake, the diabetic patient with severe glycosuria, the patient with a urea diuresis after relief of urinary tract obstruction, and the patient with mannitol diuresis all undergo urinary losses of Na^+ and water leading to hypovolemia and hyponatremia. The urinary Na^+ concentration is typically > 20 mmol/L. In diabetics, the Na^+ wasting is accentuated by ketonuria, which also causes obligatory Na^+ loss.

Fluid and Electrolyte Disorders

The ketone bodies β-hydroxybutyrate and acetoacetate also obligate urinary electrolyte losses and aggravate the renal Na+ wasting seen in diabetic ketoacidosis, starvation, and alcoholic ketoacidosis.

Cerebral salt wasting

Cerebral salt wasting is a syndrome that has been described primarily in patients with subarachnoid hemorrhage. In this condition, the primary defect is salt wasting from the kidneys with subsequent volume contraction, which is the stimulus for vasopressin release. The exact mechanism is not understood, but it is postulated that brain natriuretic peptide (BNP) is released from the hormone-producing neurons of the brain and is related to the increase in urine volume and Na+ excretion[9].

Hypervolemia: hyponatremia associated with increased total body sodium

In conditions causing hypervolemia, the total body Na+ and total body water are increased, the water more than the Na+, thus causing hyponatremia. These syndromes include congestive heart failure, nephrotic syndrome, and cirrhosis. They are all associated with impaired water excretion (Fig. 8.5).

Congestive heart failure

In patients with congestive heart failure, a defect in water excretion exists. In fact, edematous patients with heart failure have intravascularly volume contraction owing to lower systemic mean arterial pressure and the low cardiac output state. As a result, a reduction in the 'effective arterial blood volume', with a decrease in arterial filling sensed by aortic and carotid baroreceptors, causes stimulation of vasopressin release. In addition, the relative 'hypovolemic' state stimulates the renin–angiotensin axis and increases norepinephrine (noradrenaline) production, which in turn decreases GFR. The fall in GFR leads to a decrease in water delivery to the distal tubule and an increase in proximal tubular reabsorption. It is also interesting that both low cardiac output and higher angiotensin II levels are potent stimuli of thirst. The neurohumoral mediated decrease in delivery of tubular fluid to the distal nephron and/or an increase in vasopressin secretion mediate hyponatremia by limiting Na+/Cl− and water excretion. The goal of these mechanisms is to return perfusion pressure to normal. There is a correlation between the degree of neurohormonal activation and the severity of left ventricular dysfunction as assessed by ejection fraction or functional class.

Levels of vasopressin are elevated in patients with heart failure in both the presence and absence of diuretics. A decrease in vasopressin levels occurs once heart failure is treated clinically. Recent studies in a rat model of congestive heart failure have demonstrated a marked upregulation of AQP-2 expression in the renal collecting duct cells, resulting in excessive free water absorption[10] (see Fig. 8.6). Excessive intracellular targeting of AQP-2 to the apical cell membrane of the collecting duct has also been demonstrated, indicating a hyperactivation of the short-term regulation of AQP-2. These effects are most likely a consequence of high circulating levels of vasopressin.

It is postulated that nonosmotic pathways are operative in patients with congestive heart failure. The activation of the nonosmotic pathways of vasopressin release is linked to the increase in sympathetic activity noted in these patients. As cardiac function improves with afterload reduction, the plasma vasopressin levels decrease along with concomitant improvement in water excretion. The degree of hyponatremia has also been correlated with the severity of cardiac disease and with patient survival. When compared with eunatremic patients, survival is significantly reduced when the serum Na+ decreases to below 137 mmol/L. In fact, a serum Na+ of 125 mmol/L reflects severe heart failure. These patients are also at risk for worsening of heart and renal failure if treated with nonsteroidal anti-inflammatory agents (NSAIDs).

Hepatic failure

Patients with cirrhosis and hepatic insufficiency share some pathophysiologic mechanisms with patients with heart failure. They have increased extracellular volume (i.e., ascites and edema) and because of marked splanchnic venous dilatation have an increased plasma volume. Unlike patients with congestive heart failure, cirrhotic patients have an increased cardiac output because of multiple arteriovenous fistulae in

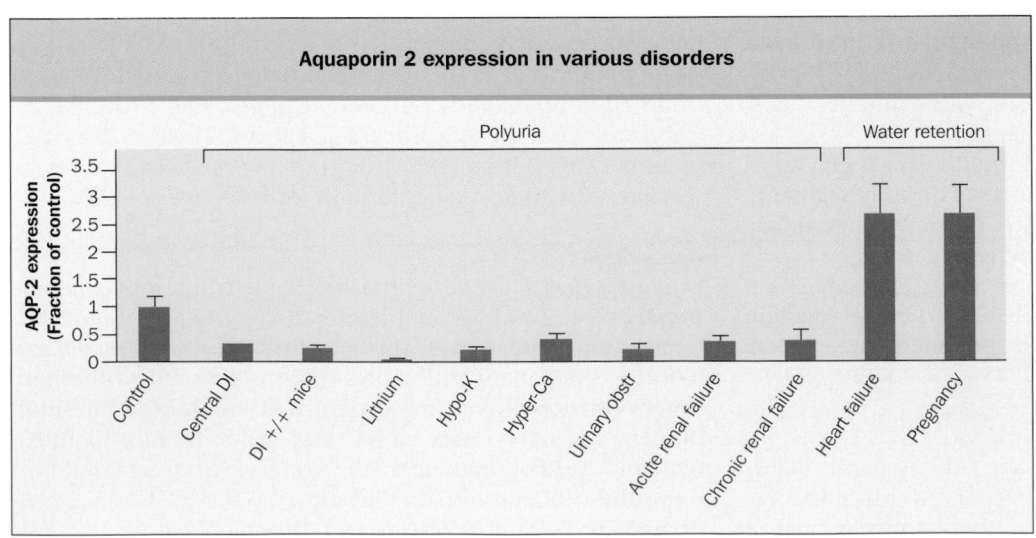

Figure 8.6 Changes in AQP-2 expression seen in association with different water balance disorders. Levels are expressed as a percentage of control levels (leftmost bar). AQP-2 expression is reduced, sometimes dramatically, in a wide range of hereditary and acquired forms of diabetes insipidus characterized by different degrees of polyuria. Conversely, congestive heart failure and pregnancy are conditions associated with increased expression of AQP-2 levels and excessive water retention. (With permission from Neilsen S, Schrier R, eds. Diseases of the kidney and urinary tract, 7th edn, Vol. 3. Philadelphia, PA: Lippincott Williams & Wilkins; 2001.)

their alimentary tract and skin. In patients with advanced chronic liver disease, arterial vasodilatation is prominent. Nitric oxide (NO), a vasodilator, plays a pivotal role in this process. Inhibition of NO synthesis corrects the arterial hyporesponsiveness to vasoconstrictors[11].

Splanchnic arterial vasodilatation and arteriovenous fistulae result in decreased mean arterial blood pressure and effective cardiac output. This fall in the effective arterial blood volume reduces the stimulation of the carotid and renal baroreceptors, causing increased vasopressin secretion, activation of the renin–angiotensin–aldosterone axis, and secretion of norepinephrine. The net effect is a hyperdynamic circulation and avid Na^+ and water retention. In patients with cirrhosis of increasing severity (ranging from patients with no ascites, through ascites, to patients with ascites and hepatorenal syndrome), a progressive increase in plasma renin, norepinephrine, vasopressin, and endothelin is noted. There is also an associated progressive decline in mean arterial pressure and in serum Na^+ levels.

The nonosmotic secretion of vasopressin is central to the water excretory defect and has been found to relate to increased hypothalamic vasopressin mRNA content in cirrhotic rats. In fact cirrhotic Brattelboro rats that lack vasopressin do not develop hyponatremia. Gene expression of vasopressin-regulated AQP-2 has also been shown to be increased in cirrhotic rats[12]. However, unlike in the heart failure model, an increase in intracellular trafficking of AQP-2 has not so far been demonstrated. Despite the disturbed hormonal milieu, the renal blood flow and GFR is maintained by endogenous vasodilatory prostaglandins: PGI_2 and PGE_2. This fine balance can be easily disturbed by the administration of NSAIDs and these should be avoided in patients with chronic liver disease. Other factors implicated in hyponatremia associated with cirrhosis include diuretic therapy, which can lead to intravascular volume contraction followed by nonosmotic release of vasopressin and water retention. Heavy beer drinkers usually consume hypotonic beer and worsen their hyponatremia ('beer drinkers' hyponatremia').

Nephrotic syndrome

Some patients with nephrotic syndrome, especially children with minimal change disease, have intravascular volume contraction through alteration in Starling's forces resulting from hypoalbuminemia and lowered plasma oncotic pressure. Most patients with nephrotic syndrome appear to have a renal defect in sodium excretion resulting in increased effective circulatory volume. In contrast to the water-retaining disorders discussed above, in which increased AQP-2 expression has been found, in rat models of nephrotic syndrome (i.e., treated with aminonucleoside or adriamycin (doxorubicin)), expression of AQP-2 and AQP-3 in the renal collecting ducts is downregulated. Downregulation of AQP-2 and AQP-3, together with a decrease in the urinary concentrating ability, is a response that may be appropriate to the extracellular volume expansion in these models[13].

Advanced chronic renal insufficiency

Patients with advanced renal insufficiency, either acute or chronic, have a profound increase in fractional excretion of Na^+ to maintain normal salt balance given the overall decreased number of functioning nephrons. Edema usually develops in patients when the Na^+ ingested exceeds the kidneys' capacity to excrete this load. The narrow range of water handling by the diseased kidney is probably also in large part the result of the smaller volumes of fluid that are filtered daily by the diseased kidney. At a GFR of 5 mL/min, only 7.2 L filtrate is formed daily, and perhaps 30%, or 2.2 L, of this filtered fluid will reach the diluting segment of the nephron. Therefore, even with total suppression of vasopressin, a maximum of 2.2 L of solute-free water can be excreted daily. If the water intake exceeds this threshold, then a positive water balance ensues and hyponatremia results.

Euvolemia: hyponatremia associated with normal total body sodium

Euvolemic hyponatremia is the most commonly encountered dysnatremia in hospitalized patients[14]. In these patients, no physical signs of increased total body Na^+ are detected. They may have slight excess of volume but are not edematous.

Glucocorticoid deficiency

Glucocorticoid deficiency causes the impaired water excretion seen in patients with primary and secondary adrenal insufficiency. Elevation of vasopressin levels accompanies the water-excretory defect resulting from anterior pituitary deficiency and adrenocorticotropic hormone (ACTH) deficiency. This can be corrected by physiologic doses of glucocorticoids. In addition vasopressin-independent factors, such as impaired renal hemodynamics and decreased distal fluid delivery to the diluting segments of the nephron, are also implicated in the defective water handling in glucocorticoid deficiency.

Hypothyroidism

Hyponatremia occurs in patients with hypothyroidism and myxedema. The cardiac output and GFR in severe hypothyroidism is often reduced. The decrease in cardiac output leads to nonosmotic release of vasopressin and a reduction in the GFR, which leads to diminished free water excretion through decreased delivery to the distal fluid. The exact mechanism, however, is less clear. In support of a vasopressin-independent mechanism, investigators have found normal suppression of vasopressin after water loading in patients with untreated myxedema[15]. However, elevated levels of vasopressin in the basal state and after a water load have been demonstrated in patients with advanced hypothyroidism. Though both vasopressin-dependent and vasopressin-independent factors may be operating, hyponatremia is readily reversed by treatment with levothyroxine (thyroxine).

Psychosis

Patients with acute psychosis have a propensity to develop hyponatremia. Although psychogenic drugs are commonly associated with hyponatremia, psychosis can cause hyponatremia independently. The pathophysiology involves increased thirst perception, a mild defect in osmoregulation that causes vasopressin to be secreted at lower osmolality, and an enhanced renal response to vasopressin.

Fluid and Electrolyte Disorders

Postoperative hyponatremia

Most hospitalized hyponatremic patients are asymptomatic, euvolemic, and have measurable vasopressin levels[16]. Postoperative hyponatremia occurs mainly in the setting of infusion of excessive amounts of electrolyte-free water (hypotonic saline or 5% dextrose in water) and the presence of vasopressin, which prevents the excretion of this electrolyte-free water. Hyponatremia can also occur in the postoperative setting despite near-isotonic saline infusion within 24 h of induction of anesthesia. This occurs mostly through the generation of electrolyte-free water by the kidneys in the presence of vasopressin[17]. In a small subgroup of young females, hyponatremia is accompanied by cerebral edema, leading to seizures and hypoxia with catastrophic neurologic events, particularly after gynecologic surgery.

Drugs causing hyponatremia

Drug-induced hyponatremia is mediated by vasopressin analogs such as desmopressin (DDAVP: deamino-D-arginine-vasopressin), drugs that enhance vasopressin release, or by agents potentiating the action of vasopressin. In other instances, the mechanism is unknown (Table 8.3).

Syndrome of inappropriate vasopressin secretion

Despite being the most common cause of hyponatremia in hospitalized patients, the syndrome of inappropriate vasopressin (ADH) secretion (SIADH) is a diagnosis of exclusion. It is characterized by a defect in osmoregulation of vasopressin. For the degree of hypotonicity, the plasma vasopressin levels

Drugs associated with hyponatremia*	
Vasopressin analogs	**Drugs that potentiate renal action of vasopressin**
Desmopressin (DDAVP) Oxytocin	Chlorpropamide Cyclophosphamide Nonsteroidal anti-inflammatory agents Acetaminophen (paracetamol)
Drugs that enhance vasopressin release	**Drugs that cause hyponatremia by unknown mechanisms**
Chlorpropamide Clofibrate *Carbamazepine–oxycarbazepine* Vincristine Nicotine Narcotics *Antipsychotics/antidepressants* Ifosfamide	*Haloperidol* *Fluphenazine* Amitriptyline Thioradazine Fluoxetine *Metamphetamine (MDMA or Ecstacy)* Sertraline
*Not including diuretics Modified with permission from Veis and Berl[19] Italics: The common causes	

Table 8.3 Drugs associated with hyponatremia.

are inappropriately stimulated, leading to urinary concentration. The more common causes of this syndrome are listed in Table 8.4.

Causes of the syndrome of inappropriate vasopressin release (SIADH)			
Carcinomas	**Pulmonary disorders**	**Nervous system disorders**	**Other**
Bronchogenic carcinoma	*Viral pneumonia*	*Encephalitis (viral or bacterial)*	*AIDS–HIV*
Carcinoma of the duodenum	Bacterial pneumonia	*Meningitis (viral, bacterial, tuberculous, and fungal)*	*Idiopathic (elderly)*
Carcinoma of the pancreas	Pulmonary abscess	Head trauma	Prolonged exercise
Thymoma	*Tuberculosis*	*Brain abscess*	
Carcinoma of the stomach	Aspergillosis	*Brain tumors*	
Lymphoma	Positive pressure breathing	Guillain–Barré syndrome	
Ewing's sarcoma	Asthma	Acute intermittent porphyria	
Carcinoma of the bladder	Pneumothorax	Subarachnoid hemorrhage or subdural hematoma	
Prostatic carcinoma	Mesothelioma	Cerebellar and cerebral atrophy	
Oropharyngeal tumor	Cystic fibrosis	Cavernous sinus thrombosis	
Carcinoma of the ureter		Neonatal hypoxia	
		Hydrocephalus	
		Shy–Drager syndrome	
		Rocky Mountain spotted fever	
		Delirium tremens	
		Cerebrovascular accident (cerebral thrombosis or hemorrhage)	
		Acute psychosis	
		Peripheral neuropathy	
		Multiple sclerosis	
With permission from Berl and Schrier[20] Italics: the common causes.			

Table 8.4 Causes of the syndrome of inappropriate vasopressin release (SIADH).

A few of the causes deserve special mention. Central nervous system (CNS) disturbances such as hemorrhage, tumors, infections, and trauma cause SIADH by releasing excess vasopressin. Small cell lung cancers, cancer of the duodenum, and pancreas and olfactory neuroblastoma cause ectopic production of vasopressin. The cells of these tissues are capable of increasing vasopressin secretion in response to osmotic stimulation *in vitro*. Human immunodeficiency virus (HIV) infection forms a category of patients with SIADH, with as many as 35% of hospitalized patients affected. In these patients, *Pneumocystis carinii* pneumonia (PCP), CNS infections, and malignancies play a role in the development of SIADH. Idiopathic cases of SIADH are unusual with the exception of elderly where in as many as 10% of the patients no cause was found for abnormal vasopressin secretion[18].

Several patterns of abnormal vasopressin release emerge from the careful studies of patients with clinical SIADH[1]. In a third of patients, vasopressin release varied appropriately with the serum Na^+ concentration but began at a lower threshold of serum osmolality, implying a 'resetting of the osmostat'. Consequently, any ingestion of free water above this threshold leads to its excretion, thus maintaining the serum Na^+ concentration at the new low level, usually 125–130 mmol/L. The remaining patients did not demonstrate any specific pattern of vasopressin release and revealed no correlation with the serum Na^+ concentration. These patients are unable to excrete a solute-free urine and, therefore, ingested water is retained, giving rise to moderate nonedematous volume expansion and dilutional hyponatremia. However, the degree of volume expansion and hyponatremia is limited by the phenomenon of 'vasopressin escape'. In classical animal experiments, it has been demonstrated that despite simultaneous water and vasopressin infusion, the animals increased their urine flow and decreased their urine osmolality. Recently, it was shown that escape from antidiuresis is caused by a marked and selective decrease in the expression of AQP-2, without a concomitant fall in the expression of the basolateral AQP-3 and AQP-4. However, in this model, the intracellular trafficking of AQP-2 to the apical membrane was intact[21]. The downregulation appears to be dependent upon the maintenance of volume expansion and independent of changes in plasma or interstitial osmolality.

The diagnostic criteria for SIADH are summarized in Table 8.5. When measured, plasma vasopressin levels may be in the 'normal' range (up to 10 ng/L). These levels are always abnormal given the hypo-osmolar state.

Symptoms of hyponatremia

The symptoms associated with hyponatremia and the rapidity of onset of hyponatremia are critical in determining the management strategy. Most patients with serum Na^+ concentration above 125 mmol/L are asymptomatic. Neuropsychiatric symptoms dominate the picture once the serum Na^+ concentration decreases below 125 mmol/L, mostly because of cerebral edema occurring through hypotonicity. These include headache, lethargy, reversible ataxia, psychosis, seizures, and coma. Uncommonly, the hypotonicity leads to severe cerebral edema manifested by increased intracerebral pressure, tentorial herniation, respiratory depression, and death. Hyponatremia-induced cerebral edema occurs primarily

Diagnostic criteria for the syndrome of inappropriate vasopressin release (SIADH)
Essential diagnostic criteria
Decreased extracellular fluid effective osmolality (<270 mOsm/kg H_2O)
Inappropriate urinary concentration (>100 mOsm/kg H_2O)
Clinical euvolemia
Elevated urinary Na^+ concentration under conditions of a normal salt and water intake
Absence of adrenal, thyroid, pituitary, or renal insufficiency or diuretic use
Supplemental criteria
Abnormal water-load test (inability to excrete at least 90% of a 20 mL/kg water load in 4 h and/or failure to dilute urine osmolality to <100 mOsm/kg)
Plasma vasopressin level inappropriately elevated relative to the plasma osmolality
No significant correction of plasma Na^+ level with volume expansion, but improvement after fluid restriction
With permission from Verbalis[22]

Table 8.5 Diagnostic criteria for the syndrome of inappropriate vasopressin release (SIADH).

with rapid development of hyponatremia, typically in hospitalized patients managed with hypotonic fluids in the postoperative setting and in those receiving diuretics. The mortality can be as high as 48% in patients with severe hyponatremia if left untreated. Neurologic symptoms in a hyponatremic patient call for prompt and immediate attention and treatment.

Factors affecting treatment strategy

The symptomatology of the patients and the rapidity of onset of hyponatremia guide the treatment strategy in a hyponatremic patient. Acutely hyponatremic patients (hyponatremia developing within 48 h) are at great risk for developing permanent neurologic sequelae from cerebral edema if the hyponatremia remains uncorrected; however, patients with chronic hyponatremia are at risk for osmotic demyelination if the hyponatremia is corrected too rapidly.

Cerebral adaptation to hypotonicity

Decreases in extracellular osmolality causes movement of water into the cells, increasing intracellular volume and causing tissue edema[23]. This cellular edema within the fixed confines of the cranium causes an increase in intracranial pressure, leading to the neurologic syndromes described above. In the vast majority of patients with hyponatremia, mechanisms geared towards volume regulation come into operation to prevent cerebral edema from developing.

Early in the course of hyponatremia, (within 1–3 h), a decrease in cerebral extracellular volume occurs by movement of fluid into the cerebrospinal fluid (CSF), which is then shunted back into the systemic circulation. This happens very promptly and is evident by the loss of extracellular solutes (Na^+ and Cl^-) as early as 30 min after the onset of hyponatremia (Fig. 8.7). If hyponatremia persists for longer than 3 h, the brain adapts by losing cellular electrolytes and organic solutes, which tends to lower the osmolality of the brain without substantial gain of water. This slower defense mechanism is indicated by a decrease in brain K^+ content 1–3 h after a hyponatremic insult. Thereafter, if hyponatremia persists, other organic osmolytes such as phosphocreatine, myoinositol, and amino acids (e.g., glutamine and taurine) are lost. The loss of these solutes markedly decreases cerebral swelling. In patients who have had a slower onset of hyponatremia (over 72–96 h or longer), the risk for osmotic demyelination rises, if hyponatremia is corrected too rapidly.

Acute cerebral edema in the hyponatremic patient
Certain patients are at risk for developing acute cerebral edema in the course of hyponatremia (Table 8.6). Hospitalized menstruant females with hyponatremia are more symptomatic

and more likely to develop complications of therapy than either postmenopausal females or men. This increased risk is independent of the rate of development or the magnitude of hyponatremia. The best approach to management of these patients is to prevent the problem. The administration of hypotonic fluids should not be used in the postoperative setting. Hyponatremia may occur in the postoperative state even if isotonic fluid is being used if the concentration of Na^+ plus K^+ in the urine exceeds that in the serum. However, the hyponatremia is mild and has not been reported to be associated with cerebral dysfunction[17]. Patients taking diuretics are also at risk for developing acute cerebral edema with the development of hyponatremia. Children are particularly vulnerable to the development of acute cerebral edema. This may be related to physical factors, such as the relatively high ratio of brain volume to skull volume. Psychiatric patients who have compulsive water-drinking disorders and high vasopressin levels may develop hyponatremia as well. It has also been observed that hypoxia increases brain edema and mortality.

Osmotic demyelination in the hyponatremic patient
Osmotic demyelination has been described worldwide in all age groups and can follow correction of hyponatremia of any cause. It appears to be common after orthotopic liver transplant, with a reported incidence of 13–29% at autopsy[25]. Table 8.6 lists the patients at risk for osmotic demyelination. The risk for development of central pontine myelinolysis (CPM) is related to the severity and chronicity of the hyponatremia. It rarely occurs if the serum Na^+ levels are more than 120 mmol/L and if the hyponatremia is acute in onset (< 48 h). The symptom complex follows a biphasic course. Initially, a generalized encephalopathy, associated with a rapid rise in serum Na^+, occurs. This is followed by the classic symptoms 2–3 days after correction of hyponatremia; these consist of behavioral changes, cranial nerve palsies, and progressive weakness culminating in quadriplegia with a 'locked-in' syndrome. On T_2-weighted magnetic resonance imaging (MRI), the lesions appear hyperintense (see Fig. 8.8). These lesions do not enhance with gadolinium and may not appear for 2 weeks after development. Therefore, a diagnosis of myelinolysis should not be excluded during the first 2 weeks of illness if the imaging is negative[25]. The pathogenesis of this

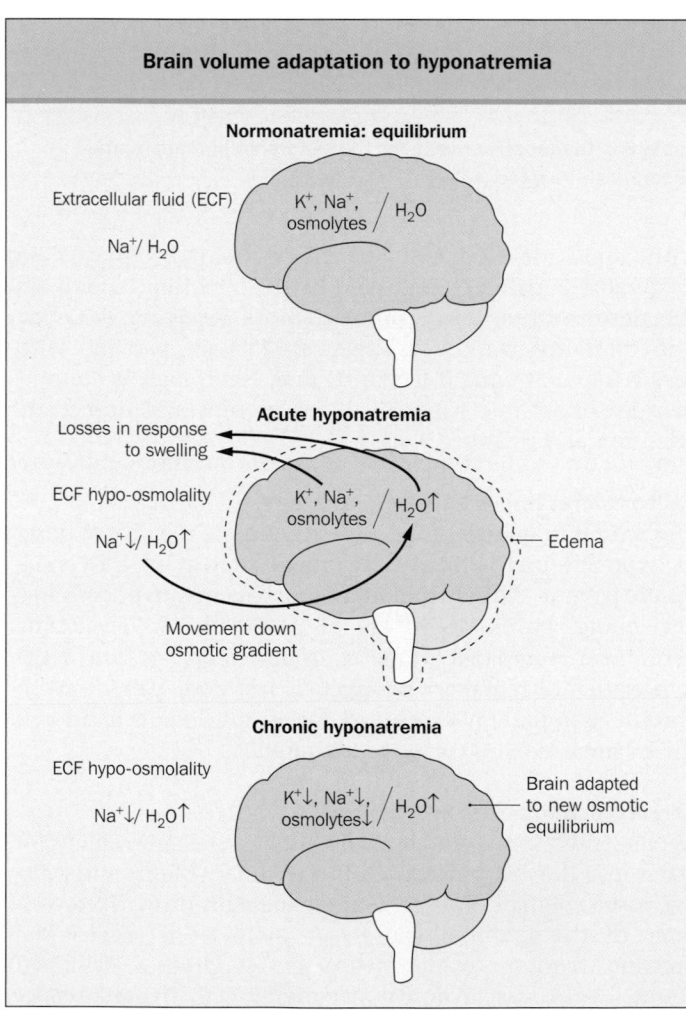

Figure 8.7 Brain volume adaptation to hyponatremia. Under normal conditions, brain osmolality and extracellular fluid (ECF) osmolality are in equilibrium. Following the induction of ECF hypo-osmolality, water moves into the brain down osmotic gradients, producing brain edema. In response, the brain loses both extracellular and intracellular solutes (see text for details). As water losses accompany the losses of brain solute, the expanded brain volume then decreases back to normal. In chronic hyponatremia, the brain volume eventually normalizes completely, and the brain becomes fully adapted to the ECF hyponatremia. (Adapted with permission from Verbalis[22].)

Hyponatremic patients at risk for neurologic complications	
Acute cerebral edema	**Osmotic demyelination syndrome**
Postoperative menstruant females	Alcoholics
Elderly women taking thiazides	Malnourished patients
Children	Hypokalemic patients
Psychiatric polydipsic patients	Burn victims
Hypoxemic patients	Elderly women on thiazide diuretics
	Hypoxemia
With permission from Lauriat and Berl[24]	

Table 8.6 Hyponatremic patients at risk for neurologic complications.

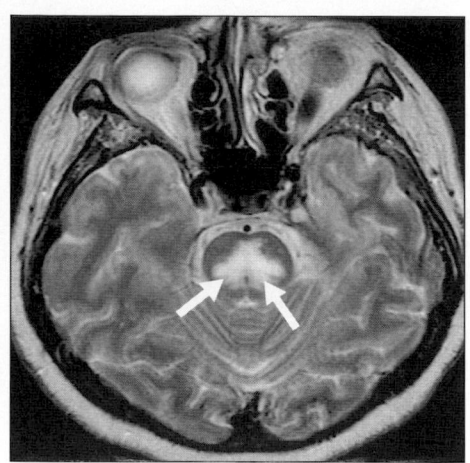

Figure 8.8 Central pontine myelinolysis. Magnetic resonance imaging T_2-weighted image. Arrows depict area of pontine demyelination. (With permission from Laureno and Karp[25].)

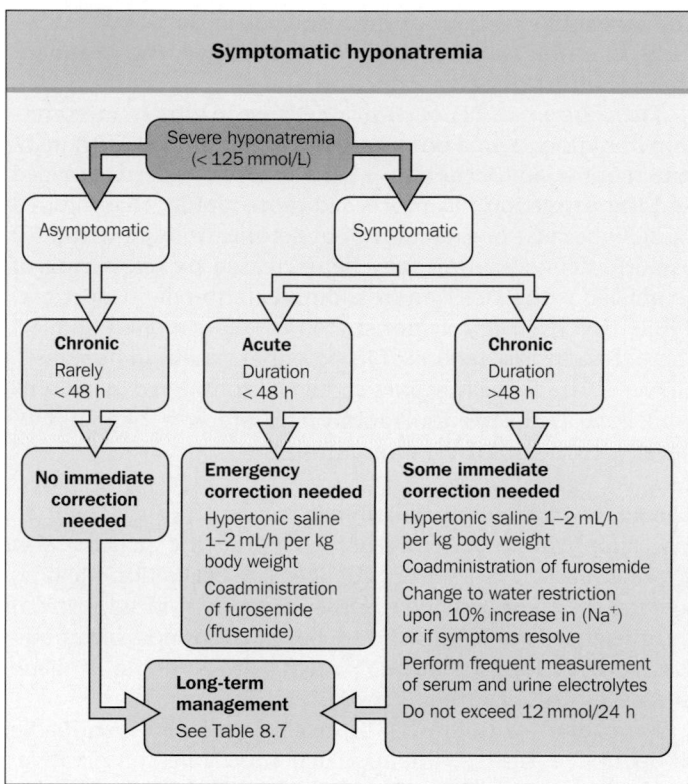

Figure 8.9 Treatment of the patient with symptomatic hyponatremia. (Adapted with permission from Halterman and Berl[5].)

syndrome continues to be investigated. As discussed above, the brain undergoes a several-step adaptation to hyponatremia. Once this adaptation occurs, the brain has no protection from the osmotic stress that accompanies the correction of hyponatremia. Though serum Na^+ and K^+ concentrations return to normal in a few hours, it takes several days for the osmotically active solutes in the brain to reach normal levels. This temporary imbalance causes cerebral dehydration and can lead to a potential breakdown of the blood–brain barrier.

Treatment of the hyponatremic patient

Acute, symptomatic hyponatremia

Acute symptomatic hyponatremia, especially associated with seizures or other neurologic manifestations, and developing in less than 48 h, almost always develops in hospitalized patients receiving hypotonic fluids (Fig. 8.9). In these patients, the treatment should be prompt as the risk for acute cerebral edema far exceeds the risk of osmotic demyelination. Attempts should be made to correct the serum Na^+ concentration by 2 mmol/L per hour until symptoms resolve, since the risk of severe hyponatremia is greater than the possible danger of overcorrection. It is not necessary to correct the serum Na^+ completely, though it does not appear to be unsafe to do so. Correction may be achieved by administration of hypertonic saline (3% Na/Cl) at the rate of 1–2 mL/h per kg body weight. The administration of a loop diuretic, like furosemide (frusemide), enhances free water excretion and hastens the process of normalization of serum Na^+ concentration. It should be noted that if the patient presents with severe neurologic symptoms, such as seizures, obtundation, or coma, 3% Na/Cl may be infused at higher rates (4–6 mL/h per kg body weight). A higher concentration of NaCl (50 mL of 29.2%) has also been used safely[26]. During treatment with hypertonic saline, the patient should be monitored carefully and serum electrolytes should be frequently checked.

Various formulae have been suggested to estimate the rise in serum Na^+ concentration after administration of intravenous fluids[27]. These formulae operate well in static conditions but fail to account for ongoing water and solute losses. A comprehensive formula incorporating the solute and water balance has been recently suggested by Barsoum et al.[28]. Although the formula is precise, it cannot be used routinely in clinical practice due to its complexity. Frequent monitoring of water and electrolyte intake and output is necessary in such acutely ill patients[5].

Chronic, symptomatic hyponatremia

If it is known that hyponatremia has taken more than 48 h to evolve or if the duration is not known, then therapy for correction of hyponatremia should be prescribed with caution (Fig. 8.9). Controversy exists as to whether it is the rate of correction or the magnitude of correction of hyponatremia that predisposes to neurologic complications. In clinical practice, it is difficult to dissociate these two variables since a rapid correction rate is usually accompanied by a greater absolute magnitude of correction over a given period of time. Therefore, each of these variables should be considered when designing a treatment regimen for the symptomatic hyponatremic patient. The following guidelines are fundamental to successful therapy[24]:

- Because cerebral water is increased only by approximately 10% in severe chronic hyponatremia, promptly increase the serum Na^+ level by 10%, or by approximately 10 mmol/L.
- After the initial correction, do not exceed a correction rate of 1.0–1.5 mmol/L per hour.
- Do not increase the serum Na^+ by more than 12 mmol/L per 24 h.

It is important to take into account the rate of infusion and the electrolyte content of infused fluids and the rate of production and electrolyte content of the urine. Once the desired increment in serum Na$^+$ concentration is obtained, the treatment should consist of water restriction.

There are a number of clinical settings in which the correction of hyponatremia can occur at a very rapid rate with institution of therapy. If the above parameters have been exceeded and the correction has proceeded more rapidly than desired (usually because of excretion of hypotonic urine), the risk for osmotic demyelination may be decreased by relowering of serum Na$^+$ with dDAVP and/or administration of 5% dextrose. While this has been demonstrated in experimental animals there are only case reports of its potential benefit in humans[29]. However, the above therapies should be considered in patients who have corrected too rapidly and are at a high risk of developing neurological symptoms.

Chronic, asymptomatic hyponatremia

The approach to the chronic, asymptomatic patient with hyponatremia is different. Initial bedside evaluation includes looking for an underlying disorder. Hypothyroidism, adrenal insufficiency, and SIADH should be sought as possible etiologies. A careful analysis of the patient's drugs should be made and necessary adjustments made.

For patients with SIADH, if the etiology is not identifiable or cannot be treated, the approach should be conservative, since rapid changes in serum tonicity lead to a greater degree of cerebral water loss and possible demyelination. Treatment options are summarized in Table 8.7.

Fluid restriction

Fluid restriction is the first-line therapy in patients with chronic asymptomatic hyponatremia. This approach is easy and usually successful if patients are compliant. It involves a calculation of the fluid restriction that will maintain a specific serum Na$^+$ concentration. The daily osmolar load (OL) and the minimal urinary osmolality $(U_{osm})_{min}$ determine a patient's maximal urine volume (V_{max}).

■ EQUATION 8.7

$$V_{max} = \frac{OL}{(U_{osm})_{min}}$$

The value of $(U_{osm})_{min}$ is a function of the severity of the diluting disorder. On a normal North American diet, the daily OL is approximately 10 mOsm/kg (700 mOsm for a 70-kg person). In a healthy person, $(U_{osm})_{min}$ (given no circulating vasopressin) it can be as low as 50 mOsm/kg. Therefore, the urine volume it can be as high as 14 L per day. Assuming a patient with SIADH whose U_{osm} cannot be lowered below 500 mOsm/kg, the same osmolar load of 700 mOsm per day allows for only 1.4 L of urine to be excreted per day. Therefore, if the patient drinks more than 1.4 L per day, the serum Na$^+$ concentration will fall. Measurement of urine Na and urine K can guide to the degree of water restriction that will be required in a given patient[30]. If the diluting defect is so severe that fluid restriction to less than 1 L is necessary, or if the patient's serum Na$^+$ remains low (< 130 mmol/L), an alternative approach to treatment such as increasing solute excretion or pharmacologic inhibition of vasopressin should be considered.

Maneuvers that increase solute excretion

If the patient remains unresponsive to fluid restriction, solute intake can be increased to facilitate an obligatory increase in excretion of solute and free water. This can be achieved by increasing oral salt and protein intake in the diet in order to increase the C_{osm} of the urine. The goal here is to increase the osmolality of the fluid or diet administered to exceed that of the urine. Loop diuretics combined with high Na$^+$ intake (2–3 g of additional salt) is effective in the management of hyponatremia. A single diuretic dose (furosemide, 40 mg) is usually sufficient in these patients. Diuretic doses should be doubled if the diuresis induced in the first 8 h is less than 60% of the total daily urine output. Likewise, the administration of

Treatment of chronic asymptomatic hyponatremia				
Treatment	Mechanism of action	Dose	Advantages	Limitations
Fluid restriction	Decreases availability of free water	Variable	Effective and inexpensive Not complicated	Non-compliance
Pharmacologic inhibition of vasopressin action				
Lithium	Inhibits the kidney's response to vasopressin	900–1200 mg daily	Unrestricted water intake	Polyuria, narrow therapeutic range, neurotoxicity
Demeclocycline	Inhibits the kidney's response to vasopressin	300–600 mg twice daily	Effective; unrestricted water intake	Neurotoxicity, polyuria, photosensitivity, nephrotoxicity
V$_2$ receptor antagonist	Antagonizes vasopressin action	–	Ongoing trials	–
Increased solute (salt) intake				
with furosemide (frusemide)	Increases free water clearance	Titrate to optimal dose; coadministration of 2–3 g NaCl	Effective	Ototoxicity, K$^+$ depletion
with urea	Osmotic diuresis	30–60 g daily	Effective; unrestricted water intake	Polyria, unpalatable, gastrointestinal symptoms

Table 8.7 Treatment of patients with chronic asymptomatic hyponatremia.

urea, by increasing the solute load, increases urine flow by causing an osmotic diuresis. This permits a more liberal water intake without worsening the hyponatremia and without altering urinary concentration. The dose for urea is usually 30–60 g daily. The major limitation is gastrointestinal distress and unpalatability. Quantitation of electrolyte C_{water} both before and after urea permits demonstration of the effect of the increased solute load. For an analysis of the manner in which urea increases C_{water}, the reader is referred to a recent review[24].

Pharmacologic inhibition of vasopressin

In patients who cannot comply with water restriction, pharmacologic agents can be used. Lithium was the first pharmacologic agent used to antagonize vasopressin action and to be used in the treatment of SIADH. However, because lithium has neurotoxicity and unpredictable reliability, demeclocycline is now the agent of choice. The drug inhibits the formation and action of cAMP in the renal collecting duct. The onset of action is usually 3 to 6 days after beginning treatment. Its action can be monitored by a decline in urine osmolality. The dose needs to be decreased to the lowest level that keeps the serum Na^+ concentration within the desired range with unrestricted water intake (usually a dose of 600–1200 mg daily). The drug is indicated in patients where water restriction is ineffective either because of high urine/plasma electrolyte ratio or due to poor compliance. The drug should be given 1 to 2 h after meals and calcium-, aluminum-, and magnesium-containing antacids should be avoided. Noncompliance remains a problem on account of the polyuria. Skin photosensitivity may occur and in the pediatric population tooth or bone abnormalities may result. Nephrotoxicity also limits its use. This commonly occurs in patients with underlying liver disease, in whom the hepatic metabolism of the drug may be impaired.

The novel V_2 receptor antagonists which block vasopressin binding to the collecting duct tubular epithelial cells are currently in clinical trials, may have the ability to precisely treat cases of hyponatremia due to SIADH and hypervolemic hyponatremia. However, one should remember that these drugs should not be used for treatment of hyponatremia due to hypovolemia (where saline is the treatment of choice) or for hyponatremia associated with advanced renal insufficiency (in which the hyponatremia is not mediated by vasopressin). There is a potential risk of rapid correction of hyponatremia, with these agents, if the ADH effect is completely eliminated. The V_2 receptor antagonists, or 'aquaretics' hold great promise, but are not yet available for clinical use.

Hypovolemic hyponatremia

Neurologic syndromes directly related to the hyponatremia are unusual in hypovolemic hyponatremia as both Na^+ and water loss limits any osmotic shifts in the brain. Restoration of ECF volume with crystalloids or colloids interrupts the nonosmotic release of vasopressin.

Hypervolemic hyponatremia

The treatment of hyponatremia in hypervolemic states is more difficult as it requires attention to the underlying disorder, be it heart failure or chronic liver disease, in order to reverse the pathophysiologic process responsible for hyponatremia. In patients with congestive heart failure, in addition to Na^+ restriction, water restriction is critical. Refractory patients may be treated with a combination of angiotensin-converting enzyme (ACE) inhibitors and diuretics. The increase in cardiac output that follows decreases the neurohumoral mediated processes that limit water excretion. Loop diuretics diminish the action of vasopressin on the collecting tubules, thereby decreasing water reabsorption. Demeclocycline also finds use in patients with chronic congestive heart failure and hyponatremia. It acts by enhancing C_{water}. However, nephrotoxicity limits its use in these patients. Thiazides should be avoided as they impair urinary dilution and may worsen hyponatremia. In patients with cirrhosis, water and sodium restriction is the mainstay of therapy. Loop diuretics increase C_{water} once a negative Na^+ balance has been achieved. In both of these disorders, the V_2 receptor antagonists, which are currently under active investigation, may be useful.

HYPERNATREMIC DISORDERS

The renal concentrating mechanism represents the first defense mechanism against water depletion and hyperosmolarity. The components of the normal concentrating mechanism are depicted in Figure 8.10. Disorders of urinary concentration reflect perturbations of these determinants:

- Decreased delivery of solute as GFR is decreased.
- Failure to generate interstitial hypertonicity as a consequence of decreased Na^+/Cl^- reabsorption in the ascending limb of the loop (loop diuretics), or decreased medullary urea accumulation (poor dietary intake), or alteration in medullary blood flow.
- Failure to release or respond to vasopressin.

Thirst is the first and most important defense mechanism in preventing water depletion.

Approach to the hypernatremic patient

As was the case with hyponatremic patients, patients with hypernatremia fall in to three broad categories based upon the volume status. A diagnostic algorithm is helpful in the evaluation of these patients (Fig. 8.11).

Hypovolemia: hypernatremia associated with low total body sodium

Patients with hypovolemic hyponatremia sustain losses of both Na^+ and water, but with a relatively greater loss of water. On physical examination, they manifest signs of hypovolemia such as orthostatic hypotension, tachycardia, flat neck veins, poor skin turgor, and sometimes altered mental status. Most patients with hypernatremia primarily have hypotonic water losses from the kidneys and/or the gastrointestinal tract. In the latter, the urinary Na^+ concentration will be low.

Hypervolemia: hypernatremia associated with increased total body sodium

Hypernatremia with increased total body Na^+ is the least common form of hypernatremia. It results from the administration

Fluid and Electrolyte Disorders

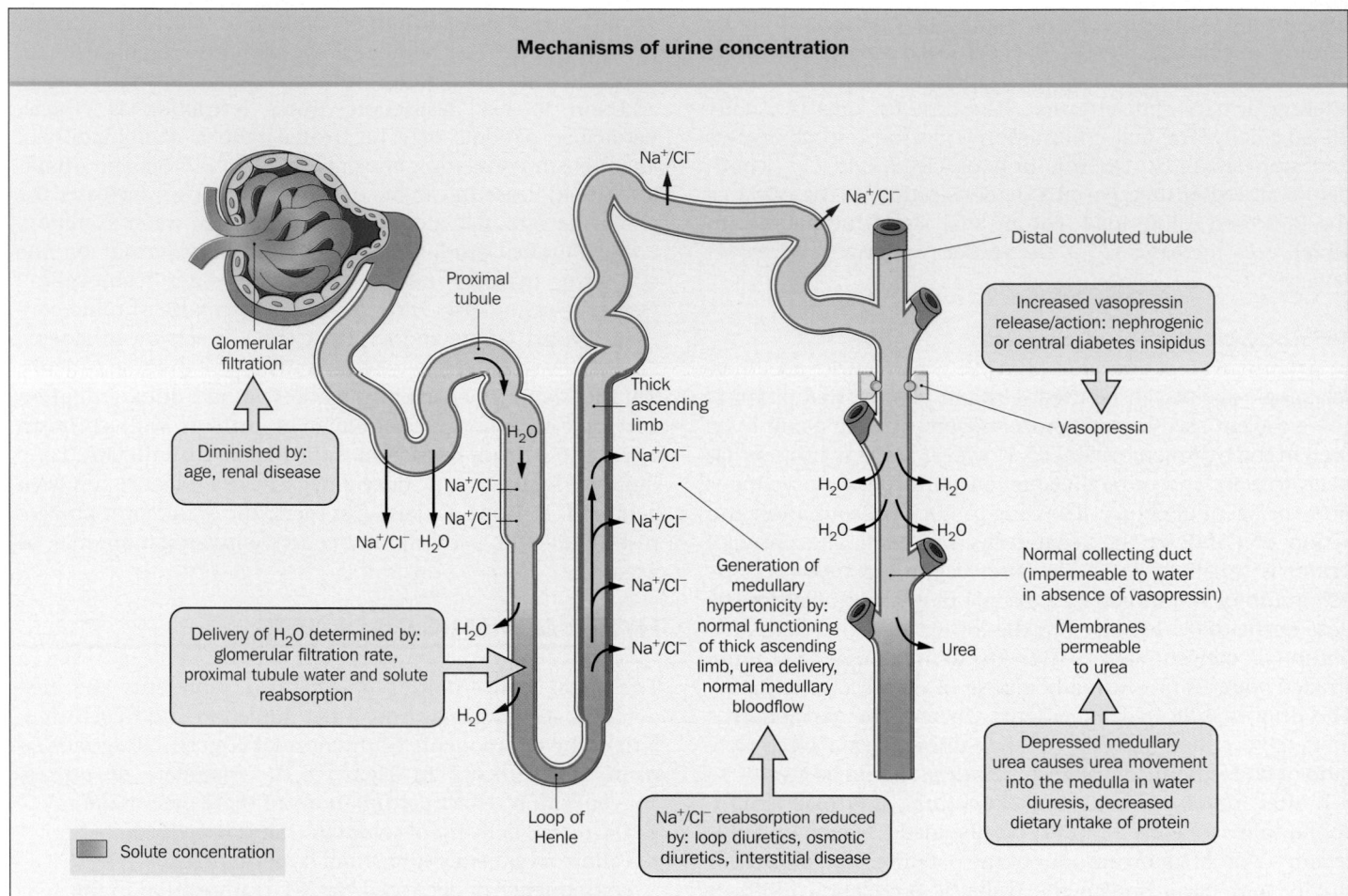

Figure 8.10 Urinary concentrating mechanisms. Determinants of normal urinary concentrating mechanism and disorders causing hypernatremia. (Adapted with permission from Cogan[8].)

of hypertonic solutions such as 3% Na/Cl, given as intra-amniotic instillation for therapeutic abortion, and the administration of $NaHCO_3$ for treatment of metabolic acidosis, hyperkalemia, and cardiorespiratory arrest. It may also result from inadvertent dialysis against a dialysate with a high Na^+ concentration or from consumption of salt tablets. Hypernatremia is increasingly recognized in hypoalbuminemic azotemic hospitalized patients who are edematous and unable to concentrate their urine[32].

Euvolemia: hypernatremia associated with normal body sodium

Most patients with hypernatremia secondary to water loss appear euvolemic with normal total body Na^+, since loss of water without Na^+ does not lead to overt volume contraction. Water loss *per se* need not result in hypernatremia unless it is unaccompanied by water intake. Since such hypodipsia is uncommon, hypernatremia usually supervenes in those who have no access to water and the very young and old, in whom there may be an altered perception of thirst. Extrarenal water loss occurs from the skin and respiratory tract in febrile or other hypermetabolic states. Urine osmolality is very high, reflecting an intact osmoreceptor–vasopressin–renal response.

Therefore, the defense against the development of hyperosmolality requires the appropriate stimulation of thirst and the ability to respond by drinking water. The urine Na^+ concentration varies with the intake. The renal losses of water that lead to euvolemic hypernatremia are a consequence of either a defect in vasopressin production and/or release (central diabetes insipidus) or a failure of the collecting duct to respond to the hormone (nephrogenic diabetes insipidus). Polyuric disorders can result from either an increase C_{osm} or an increase in C_{water} (see Equation 8.1). An increase in C_{osm} occurs in several settings, notably diuretic use, renal salt wasting, excess salt ingestion, vomiting (bicarbonaturia), and alkali administration, and with the administration of mannitol as a diuretic, for bladder lavage, and for the treatment of cerebral edema. An increase in C_{water} occurs either with an excess of ingested water (psychogenic polydipsia) or in abnormalities of the renal-concentrating mechanism (diabetes insipidus (DI)).

Diabetes insipidus

Diabetes insipidus is a disease characterized by polyuria and polydipsia and caused by defects in vasopressin action.

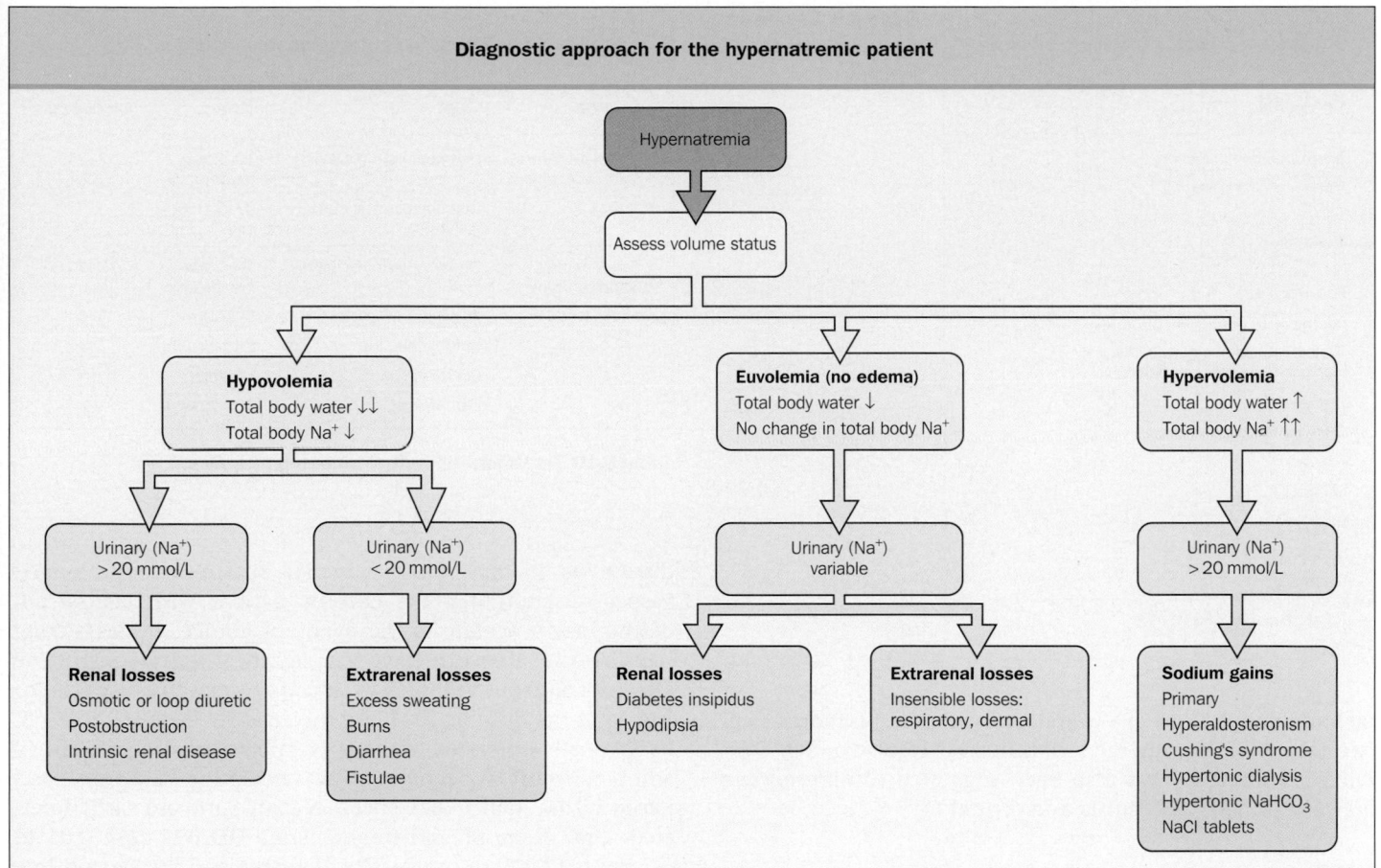

Figure 8.11 Diagnostic approach for the hypernatremic patient. (Adapted with permission from Halterman and Berl[5].)

Central diabetes insipidus

Clinical features

Patients with central and nephrogenic DI and primary polydipsia present with polyuria and polydipsia. The differentiation between these entities can be accomplished by
measurements of vasopressin levels and the response to a
water deprivation test followed by vasopressin administration
(Table 8.8). Other clinical features can distinguish compulsive
water drinkers from patients with central DI. The latter usually have an abrupt onset, whereas the compulsive water
drinker may give a vague history of the onset. Unlike patients
with compulsive water drinking, patients with central DI
have a constant need for water intake. Large variations in
water intake and urine output occur in compulsive water
drinkers. Nocturia is common in patients with central DI and
unusual in compulsive water drinkers. Finally, patients with
central DI have a predilection for cold water. A plasma osmolality of above 295 mOsm/kg suggests central DI and below
270 mOsm/kg suggests compulsive water drinking.

Measurements of circulating vasopressin by radioimmunoassay can be used as an alternative to the tedious water
deprivation test. Under basal conditions, the measurements
of vasopressin levels have not been of practical value since
there is a significant overlap among the polyuric disorders. Its

	Water deprivation test		
Condition	Urinary osmolality with water deprivation (mOsm/kg H_2O)	Plasma vasopressin after dehydration (ng/L)	Increase in urinary osmolality with exogenous vasopressin
Normal	>800	>2	Little or no increase
Complete central diabetes insipidus	<300	Undetectable	Substantially increased
Partial central diabetes insipidus	300–800	<1.5	Increase of greater than 10% of urinary osmolality after water deprivation
Nephrogenic diabetes insipidus	<300–500	>5	Little or no increase
Primary polydipsia	>500	<5	Little or no increase

With permission from Lanese and Teitelbaum[33]
Test Procedure: Water intake is restricted until the patient loses 3–5% of
his/her body weight or until three consecutive hourly determinations of urinary
osmolality are within 10% of each other. (Caution must be exercised to
ensure that the patient does not become excessively dehydrated.) Aqeous
vasopressin (5 U subcutaneously) is given and urinary osmolality is measured
after 60 min. The expected responses are given in the table.

Table 8.8 The water deprivation test.

Causes of central diabetes insipidus
Congenital
Autosomal dominant
Autosomal recessive
Acquired
Post-traumatic
Iatrogenic (postsurgical)
Tumors (metastatic from breast, craniopharyngioma, pinealoma)
Histiocytosis
Granuloma (tuberculosis, sarcoid)
Aneurysm
Meningitis
Encephalitis
Guillain–Barré syndrome
Idiopathic
Italics: The common causes.

Table 8.9 Causes of central diabetes insipidus.

Treatment of central diabetes insipidus			
Disease	**Drug**	**Dose**	**Interval (h)**
Complete central diabetes insipidus	Desmopressin (DDAVP)	10–20μg intranasally	12–24 12
	Desmopressin Acetate (DDAVP)	0.05–0.2mg oral	
Partial central diabetes insipidus	Desmopressin (DDAVP)	10–20μg intranasally	12–24
	Aqueous vasopressin	5–10U s.c.	4–6
	Chlorpropamide	250–500mg	24
	Clofibrate	500mg	6 or 8
	Carbamazepine	400–600mg	24

Table 8.10 Treatment of central diabetes insipidus.

measurement following a water deprivation test is more useful (see Table 8.9). Measurement of urinary excretion of AQP-2 by radioimmunoassay has also been suggested to differentiate between primary polydipsia and central DI[34].

Causes

The causes of central DI are listed in Table 8.9. In approximately 50% of patients, no cause is identified (idiopathic) and the other 50% are caused by infection, tumors, granuloma, and trauma affecting the CNS. In a survey of 79 children and young adults, the disease was idiopathic in 52%, with a significant number having tumors and Langerhans' cell histiocytosis. The latter group had an 80% chance of developing anterior pituitary hormone deficiency compared to 50% in patients with idiopathic disease[35]. An inherited autosomal dominant form of the disease has been described[36] that is caused by various point mutations in a precursor gene for vasopressin. Patients usually present with a mild polyuria and polydipsia in the first year of life. These children have normal physical and mental development. Rarely, an autosomal recessive central DI associated with diabetes mellitus, optic atrophy, and deafness (DIDMOAD or Wolfram syndrome) occurs. This has been linked to a defect in chromosome 4 and involves abnormalities in mitochondrial DNA. In patients with the Wolfram syndrome, the DI is usually partial and is gradual in onset.

Treatment

Central DI may be treated with hormone replacement or pharmacologic agents (Table 8.10). In acute settings, where renal water losses are extensive, aqueous vasopressin (Pitressin) is useful. It has a short duration of action, allows for careful monitoring, and avoids complications such as water intoxication. This drug should be used with caution in patients with underlying coronary artery disease and peripheral vascular disease as it may cause vascular spasm and prolonged vasoconstriction. For the chronic patient with central DI, desmopressin acetate is the agent of choice. It has a long half-life and does not have the significant vasoconstrictive effects of aqueous vasopressin. It can be conveniently administered at the dose of 10–20 μg intranasally every 12 to 24 h. It is usually tolerated well. It is safe to use in pregnancy and is resistant to degradation by circulating vasopressinase. Recently, oral tablets have been available and are easily tolerated. Oral desmopressin (brand name DDAVP, dose 0.05 to 0.5 mg q 12 h) are universally available and are second line of therapy. In patients with partial DI, in addition to desmopressin itself, agents that potentiate the release of vasopressin may be used. These agents include chlorpropamide, clofibrate, and carbamazepine.

Congenital nephrogenic diabetes insipidus

One form of congenital nephrogenic DI expresses itself in the complete clinical form only in males and is seen in a subclinical form in females, suggesting an X-linked dominant inheritance with variable penetrance in the female. The affected males have an inability to concentrate urine in response to vasopressin administration. Linkage analysis has located the defect to the X chromosome, where the V_2 receptor is encoded. Since the recognition of this mode of inheritance in certain families, 155 putative disease-causing mutations in the V_2 receptor gene in 239 presumably unrelated families with X-linked nephrogenic DI have been reported[37]. The autosomal recessive form of nephrogenic DI is caused by mutations in the gene for AQP-2. So far 26 mutations have been described in 25 families[38]. This form of nephrogenic DI is rare compared with the X-linked form of the disease. The disease may have variable penetrance and occurs with increased frequency in consanguineous marriages. Finally, it appears that mutations at the carboxy terminal of AQP-2 can cause an autosomal dominant form of nephrogenic DI which has been recently reported in three Japanese families[39].

Defects in water concentrating ability have also been described with other aquaporins like AQP-1[40] in mice and man, and AQP-3 and AQP-4 in mice only.

Acquired nephrogenic diabetes insipidus: causes and mechanisms				
Disease state	Defect in generation of medullary interstitial tonicity	Defect in cAMP generation	Downregulation of aquaporin 2	Other
Chronic renal failure	Yes	Yes	Yes	Downregulation of V$_2$ receptor message
Hypokalemia	Yes	Yes	Yes	–
Hypercalcemia	Yes	Yes	–	–
Sickle cell disease	Yes	–	–	–
Protein malnutrition	Yes	–	Yes	–
Demeclocycline therapy	–	Yes	–	–
Lithium therapy	–	Yes	Yes	–
Pregnancy	–	–	–	Placental secretion of vasopressinase

Table 8.11 Acquired nephrogenic diabetes insipidus: causes and mechanisms.

Clinical features

The diagnosis of congenital nephrogenic DI is usually made when an infant presents with hypo-osmolar urine together with severe dehydration, hypernatremia, vomiting, and fever. In the X-linked variety, unlike some of the females, with variable penetrance of the disease, male patients do not concentrate their urine despite severe dehydration and vasopressin administration. Affected patients suffer from repeated episodes of dehydration, hypernatremia, and hyperthermia early in infancy and may suffer from impaired growth and mental retardation. Hydronephrosis is not unusual in these patients as a consequence of the large urine output and some voluntary retention.

Treatment

Neither pharmacologic nor hormonal maneuvers are effective in patients with congenital nephrogenic DI: an intact thirst mechanism is indispensable to life. Since the excretion of solute requires further water losses, rehydration therapy should include hypotonic (2.5%) rather than isotonic (5%) glucose solutions. Solute intake should be kept low (low Na$^+$ and protein diet). The use of thiazide diuretics has met with some success. They decrease urine output by causing ECF volume contraction and thereby enhancing proximal tubular Na$^+$ and water reabsorption. The addition of amiloride to hydrochlorothiazide has also been found to be useful. NSAIDs such as tolmetin, especially in children, have been well tolerated. It should be realized that a change in urine osmolality from 50 to 200 mOsm/kg H$_2$O is very important, as it translates into substantial reduction in urine output from 10–12 L per day to 3–4 L per day.

Acquired nephrogenic diabetes insipidus

The acquired form of nephrogenic DI is more commonly encountered in practice. It is rarely as severe as congenital nephrogenic DI. In most affected patients, the ability to elaborate a maximal concentration of urine is impaired, but urinary concentrating mechanisms are partially preserved. For this reason, urinary volumes are < 3–4 L per day, which contrasts with the higher values seen in patients with congenital or central DI or compulsive water drinking. The causes and mechanisms of acquired nephrogenic DI are listed in Table 8.11.

Chronic renal failure

Most patients with advancing chronic renal failure develop a defect in the urinary concentrating ability. Advanced chronic renal insufficiency of any cause can lead to resistance to vasopressin associated with hypotonic urine. This may occur at any stage in the evolution of chronic renal failure. Disruption of inner medullary structures in tubulointerstitial diseases and diminished medullary concentration are thought to play a role. In rat models of chronic renal failure the vasopressin resistance may result from selective downregulation of the V$_2$ receptor in the inner medullary tubular membranes. Also AQP-2 decreases in obstruction and acute tubular necrosis (see Fig. 8.6). In caring for patients with chronic renal failure, it is important to recognize that a certain amount of fluid intake is necessary in most patients who still make urine, in order to effect daily osmolar clearance.

Electrolyte disorders

Hypokalemia causes a readily reversible abnormality in urinary concentrating ability. It does so by its effect on stimulating water intake and by a reduction in interstitial tonicity, which relates to the decreased Na$^+$/Cl$^-$ reabsorption in the TALH. Hypokalemia also affects intracellular cAMP accumulation and causes a reduction in the vasopressin-sensitive AQP-2 activity (Fig. 8.6). Hypokalemia resulting from diarrhea, chronic diuretic use, and primary aldosteronism may be associated with this defect in urinary concentration. Hypercalcemia also results in an abnormality in urinary concentrating ability. It occurs as a result of the mild polydipsia and an intrarenal defect along with decreased AQP-2 (Fig. 8.6). The pathophysiology is multifactorial. There is a reduction in medullary interstitial tonicity caused by decreased vasopressin-stimulated adenylate cyclase in the TALH, which leads to diminished solute reabsorption in this segment. In addition, a similar defect in adenylate cyclase activity caused by hypercalcemia in the collecting duct affects water reabsorption.

Pharmacologic agents

Several drugs cause a defect in urinary concentrating ability. In patients taking amphotericin and foscarnet, the concentrating defect may be related to their renal toxicity. Demeclocycline causes a dose-dependent reduction in human

Fluid and Electrolyte Disorders

renal medullary adenylate cyclase activity, decreasing the vasopressin effect on the collecting system and thereby elaborating a dilute urine. Lithium is commonly used in patients with manic–depressive psychosis. As many as 50% of patients taking lithium develop nephrogenic DI. It appears to affect vasopressin-mediated water transport in the collecting duct by causing downregulation of AQP-2 in this segment of the nephron (Fig. 8.6). The concentrating defect may persist in patients even when the drug is discontinued.

Sickle cell anemia
Patients with sickle cell disease and trait often have a urinary concentrating defect. In a hypertonic environment in the medullary interstitium, the 'sickled' red cells cause occlusion of the vasa recta and papillary damage. The resultant medullary ischemia may impair Na^+/Cl^- transport in the ascending limb and thus diminish medullary tonicity. Though initially reversible with normal blood, medullary infarcts occur with long-standing sickle cell disease and the concentrating defects become irreversible.

Dietary abnormalities
Extensive water intake leads to impairment of maximal urinary concentrating ability through a reduction in medullary interstitial tonicity. A marked decrease in salt and protein intake also causes a defect in urinary concentration, since Na^+ and urea (product of protein metabolism) are responsible for most of the interstitial tonicity. In experimental models of low-protein diets a decrease in vasopressin-stimulated osmotic water permeability associated with a decrease in AQP-2 has been demonstrated. There is also a downregulation of AQP-2 in the setting of excessive water intake.

Gestational diabetes insipidus
Gestational DI is typically vasopressin unresponsive. This occurs because of an increase in circulating vasopressinase, which is produced by the placenta. Desmopressin is usually effective in decreasing urine flow, as it does not undergo degradation by this enzyme.

Signs and symptoms of hypernatremia
There are certain groups of patients that are at increased risk for developing hypernatremia (Table 8.12). Hypernatremia always reflects a hyperosmolar state. The signs and symptoms mostly relate to the CNS and include altered mental status, lethargy, irritability, restlessness, seizures (usually in children), muscle twitching, hyper-reflexia, and spasticity. Fever, nausea or vomiting, labored breathing, and intense thirst can also occur. The morbidity and mortality of patients with acute hypernatremia is very high. In children, the mortality of acute hypernatremia ranges between 10 and 70%. As many as two-thirds of the survivors have neurologic sequelae. In contrast, mortality in chronic hypernatremia is 10%. In adults, serum Na^+ concentrations above 160 mmol/L are associated with a 75% mortality. Hypernatremia, in adults, occurs in the setting of serious disease and the mortality figures may reflect the mortality of the underlying diseases rather than hypernatremia *per se*.

Patient groups at risk for development of severe hypernatremia
Elderly patients or infants
Hospitalized patients receiving hypertonic infusions, tube feedings, osmotic diuretics, lactulose, mechanical ventilation
Altered mental status
Uncontrolled diabetes mellitus
Underlying polyuric disorders
With permission from Halterman and Berl[5].

Table 8.12 Patient groups at risk for development of severe hypernatremia.

Treatment of hypernatremic patients
Hypernatremia occurs in predictable clinical settings and thus preventing its development may be the best therapy. Elderly patients and hospitalized patients are at a very high risk due to impaired thirst mechanism or their inability to free water access. Certain clinical situations like recovery from acute renal failure, catabolic states, therapy with hypertonic solutions, uncontrolled diabetes, burns should prompt close attention to serum sodium and increased administration of free water.

The primary goal in the treatment of patients with hypernatremia is the restoration of serum tonicity. The treatment regimen depends upon the volume status. Specific management options are outlined in Figure 8.12. The following guidelines are helpful in the therapeutic approach to the hypernatremic patient.

- Hypovolemic hypernatremia with low total body Na^+ and orthostatic hypotension. These patients should be managed with isotonic saline until systemic hemodynamics are stabilized. Thereafter, fluid management generally involves 0.45% Na/Cl or 5% dextrose solution.
- Hypervolemic hypernatremia. The goal in therapy for these patients is to remove the excess Na^+, which is achieved with diuretics plus 5% dextrose. In patients who have renal impairment, dialysis may be needed.
- Euvolemic hypernatremia. In this group of patients, water losses far exceed solute losses and the mainstay of therapy is 5% dextrose. In order to correct the hypernatremia appropriately, an estimate of the total body water deficit must be made. This is calculated on the basis of the serum Na^+ concentration and on the assumption that 60% of the body weight is water.

The rapidity with which the hypernatremia should be corrected is a matter of some controversy. However, some animal studies and case series in pediatric patients suggest that a correction rate of > 0.5 mmol/L/h can cause seizures, probably due to the cerebral adjustments in hypernatremia. Cerebral edema can be caused by rapid correction of hypernatremia due to the net movement of water into the brain. Most of the clinicians feel that even in adults the correction should be achieved in more than 48 h and at a rate not greater than 2 mmol/h.

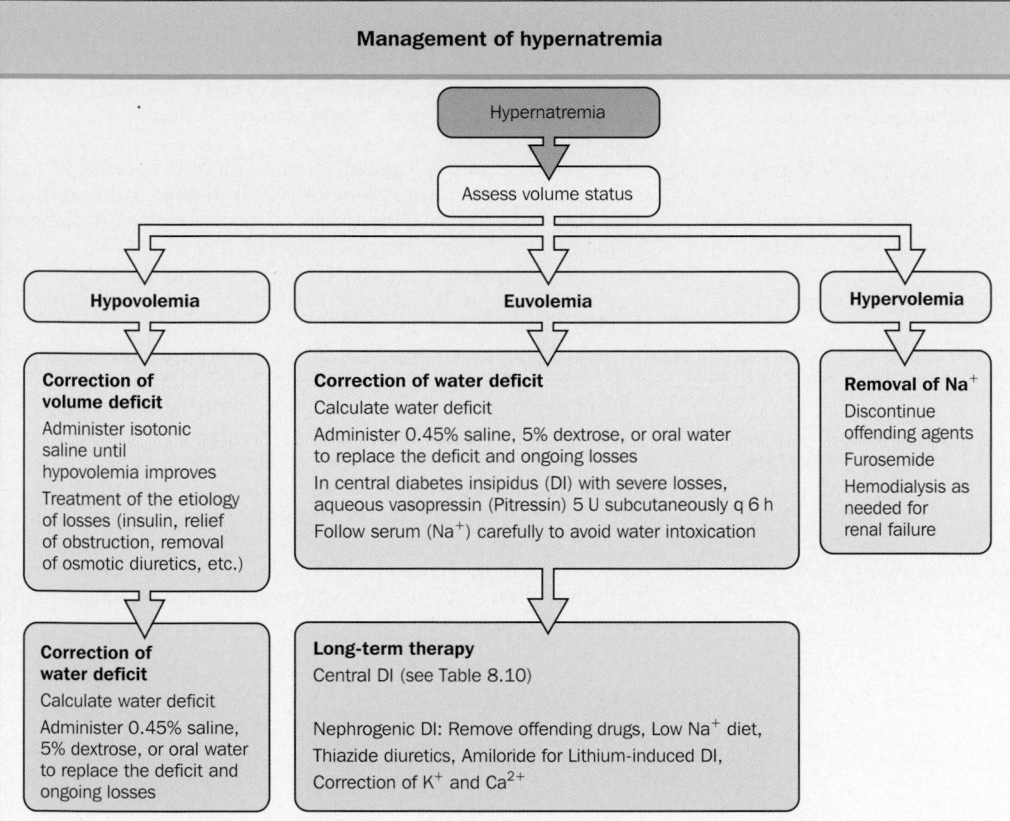

Figure 8.12 Management options for patients with hypernatremia. (With permission from Halterman and Berl[5].)

REFERENCES

1. Berl T, Robertson GL. Pathophysiology of water metabolism. In: Brenner BM, ed. The kidney, 6th edn. Philadelphia, PA: Saunders; 2000:866–924.

2. Narins RG, Krishna GC. Disorders of water balance. In: Stein JH, ed. Internal medicine. Boston: Little Brown; 1987:794.

3. Bichet D. Nephrogenic and central diabetes insipidus. In: Schrier R, ed. Diseases of the kidney and urinary tract, 7th edn, Vol. 3. Philadelphia ,PA: Lippincott Williams & Wilkins; 2001:2549–76.

4. Knepper MA. Molecular physiology of urinary concentrating mechanism: regulation of aquaporin water channels by vasopressin. Am J Physiol. 1997;272:F3–12.

5. Halterman R, Berl T. Therapy of dysnatremic disorders. In: Brady H, Wilcox C, eds. Therapy in nephrology and hypertension. Philadelphia, PA: Saunders; 1999:257–69.

6. Hiller TA, Abott RD, Barrett EJ. Hyponatremia: evaluating the correction factor for hypoglycemia. Am J Med 1999; 106:399–403.

7. Ayus JC, Arieff AI. Glycine-induced hypo-osmolar hyponatremia. Arch Intern Med. 1997;157:223–6.

8. Cogan M. Normal water homeostasis. In: Cogan M, ed. Fluid and electrolytes. Norwalk, CT: Lange; 1991:98–106.

9. Palmer BF. Hyponatremia in a neurosurgical patient: syndrome of inappropriate antidiuretic hormone secretion verses cerebral salt wasting. Nephrol Dial Transplant. 2000: 262–8.

10. Xu DL, Martin PY, Ohara M, et al. Upregulation of aquaporin-2 water channel expression in chronic heart failure rat. J Clin Invest. 1997;99:1500–5.

11. Martin PY, Gines P, Schrier RW. Nitric oxide as mediator hemodynamic abnormalities and sodium and water retention in cirrhosis. N Engl J Med. 1998;339:533–41.

12. Fujita N, Ishikawa SE, Sasaki S, et al. Role of water channel AQP-CD in water retention in SIADH and cirrhotic rats. Am J Physiol. 1995;269:F926–31.

13. Berl T. Aquaporin in health and disease. Kidney Int. 1998;53:1417–18.

14. Anderson RJ, Chung HM, Kluge R, Schrier RW. Hyponatremia: a prospective analysis of its epidemiology and the pathogenetic role of vasopressin. Ann Intern Med. 1985;102:164–8.

15. Iwasaki Y, Oiso Y, Yamauchi K, et al. Osmoregulation of plasma vasopressin in myxedema. J Clin Endocrinol Metab. 1990;70:534–9.

16. Anderson RJ. Hospital-associated hyponatremia (clinical conference). Kidney Int. 1986;29:1237–47.

17. Steele A, Gowrishankar M, Abrahamson S, et al. Postoperative hyponatremia despite near-isotonic saline infusion: a phenomenon of desalination. Ann Intern Med. 1997;126:20–5.

18. Miller M. Hyponatremia: age related risk factors and therapy decisions. Geriatrics. 1998;53:32–3, 37–8, 41–2.

19. Veis JH, Berl T. Hypernatremia. In: Jacobson HR, Striker GE, Klahr S, eds. The principles and practice of nephrology. St Louis, MO: Mosby; 1995: 888–93.

20. Berl T, Schrier R. Disorders of water metabolism. In: Schrier R, ed. Renal and electrolyte disorders, 6th edn. Philadelphia, PA: Lippincott-Raven; 2002.

21. Ecelbarger CA, Nielsen S, Olson BR, et al. Role of renal aquaporins in escape from vasopressin-induced antidiuresis in rat. J Clin Invest. 1997;99:1852–63.

22. Verbalis J. The syndrome of inappropriate antidiuretic hormone secretion and other hypoosmolar disorders. In: Schrier R, eds. Diseases of the kidney and urinary tract, Vol. 3. Philadelphia, PA: LLW; 2001: 2518.

23. Gross P. Treatment of severe hyponatremia. Kidney Int. 2001: 2417–27.

24. Lauriat S, Berl T. The hyponatremic patient: practical focus on therapy. J Am Soc Nephrol. 1997:1599–1607.

25. Laureno R, Karp BI. Myelinolysis after correction of hyponatremia. Ann Intern Med. 1997;126:57–62.
26. Soupart A, Decaux G. Therapeutic recommendations for management of severe hyponatremia: current concepts on pathogenesis and prevention of neurologic complications. Clin Nephrol. 1996;46:149–69.
27. Adrogue HJ, Madias NE. Hyponatremia. N Engl J Med. 2000;342:1581–9.
28. Barsoum N, Levine B. Current prescriptions for corrections of hypo- and hypernatremia: Are they too simple? Nephrol Dial Transplant. 2002;17:1176–80.
29. Goldszmidt MA, Iliescu EA. DDAVP to prevent rapid correction in hyponatremia. Clin Nephrol. 2000;53:226–9.
30. Furst H, Hallows KR, Post J, et al. The urine/plasma electrolyte ratio: a predictive guide to water restriction. Am J Med Sci. 2000;319:240–4.
31. Gross P, Reimann D, Henschkowski J, et al. Treatment of severe hyponatremia: conventional and novel aspects. J Am Soc Nephrol. 2001:suppl 17; S10–14.
32. Kahn T. Hypernatremia with edema. Arch Intern Med. 1999;159:93–8.
33. Lanese D, Teitelbaum I. Hypernatremia. In: Jacobson HR, Striker GE, Klahr S, eds. The principles and practice of nephrology, 2nd edn. St Louis, MO: Mosby 1995:893–8.
34. Saito T, Ishikawa S, Ito T, et al. Urinary excretion of aquaporin-2 water channel differentiates psychogenic polydipsia from central diabetes insipidus. J Clin Endocrinol Metab. 1999;84:2235–7.
35. Maghnie M, Cosi G, Genovese E, et al. Central diabetes insipidus in children and young adults. N Engl J Med. 2000;343:998–1007.
36. Rittig S, Robertson GL, Siggaard C, et al. Identification of 13 new mutations in the vasopressin-neurophysin II gene in 17 kindreds with familial autosomal dominant neurohypophyseal diabetes insipidus. Am J Hum Genet. 1996;58:107–17.
37. Bichet DG, Fujisawa I. Scriver SR (ed.) The metabolic and the molecular base of the disease. 8th edn. New York: McGraw Hill;2001:4181.
38. Canfield MC, Tamarappoo BK, Moses AM, et al. Identification and characterization of aquaporin-2 water channel mutations causing nephrogenic diabetes insipidus with partial vasopressin response. Hum Mol Genet. 1997;6:1865–71.
39. Kuwahara M, Iwai K, Ooeda T, et al. Three families with autosomal dominant nephrogenic diabetes insipidus caused by aquaporin-2 mutation in the C-terminus. Am J Hum Genet. 2001;69:738–48.
40. King LS, Choi M, Fernandez PC, et al. Defective urinary concentrating ability due to a complete deficiency of aquaporin-1. N Engl J Med. 2001;345:175–9.

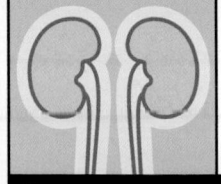

Chapter 9

Disorders of Potassium Metabolism

I David Weiner, Stuart L Linas, and Charles S Wingo

INTRODUCTION

Potassium disorders are some of the most commonly encountered fluid and electrolyte abnormalities in clinical medicine. They can be asymptomatic or associated with symptoms ranging from mild weakness to sudden death. When the serum potassium is verified as abnormal, correction is essential, but inappropriate treatment can worsen symptoms and even lead to death.

NORMAL PHYSIOLOGY OF POTASSIUM METABOLISM

Potassium intake

Potassium is essential for many cellular functions, is present in most foods, and is excreted primarily by the kidney. The typical Western diet contains approximately 70–150 mmol potassium/d. The gastrointestinal tract, particularly the jejunum and ileum, but also the colon, efficiently absorb potassium. Dietary potassium intake varies greatly with the composition of the diet. Table 9.1 summarizes the potassium content of several foods high in potassium content.

Potassium content of selected foods		
Food	**Portion size**	**mmol K+**
Artichoke, boiled	1, medium	27
Avocado	1, medium	38
Sirloin steak	8 oz	23
Hamburger, lean	8 oz	18
Cantaloupe, cut up	1 cup	13
Grapefruit juice	8 oz	10
Milk	8 oz	10
Orange juice	8 oz	12
Potato, baked	7 oz	22
Prunes	10	16
Raisins	2/3 cup	19
Squash	1 cup	15–20
Tomato paste	1/2 cup	31
Tomato juice	6 oz	10
Banana	medium size	12

Data adapted from Na-K-Phos Counter, published by the American Association of Kidney Patients, Inc, 1999.

Table 9.1 Potassium content of selected high potassium foods.

Potassium distribution

After absorption from the gastrointestinal tract, potassium distributes into the extracellular and intracellular fluid compartments. Potassium is the major intracellular cation, with values from ~100–120 mmol/L in the cytosol, and is primarily distributed intracellularly. Total intracellular potassium content is 3000–3500 mmol in healthy adults, which is primarily distributed in muscle (70%), with smaller amounts present in bone, red blood cells, liver, and skin (Table 9.2). Only 1–2% of total body potassium is present in the extracellular fluids. The electrogenic Na-pump, Na^+-K^+ ATPase, effects this asymmetrical potassium distribution by active uptake, which occurs in virtually all cells. Na^+-K^+-ATPase transports two potassium ions into cells in exchange for extrusion of three sodium ions, which results in high intracellular potassium, and low intracellular sodium activity. The ratio of intracellular to extracellular potassium concentration is a major determinant of cell membrane potential and intracellular electronegativity due to the action of potassium-selective ion channels. Normal maintenance of this ratio and membrane potential is critical for normal nerve conduction and muscular contraction.

With potassium addition to the extracellular fluid compartment, there is a concomitant shift of potassium from the extracellular to the intracellular fluid compartment. Conversely, potassium depletion results in cellular potassium release into the extracellular fluid, particularly from skeletal muscle. This serves to minimize changes in transcellular potassium ratio and membrane potential. Accordingly, small changes in extracellular potassium frequently are associated with substantial changes in total body potassium.

Distribution of total body potassium in organs and body compartments			
Organs and compartments		**Body compartment concentrations**	
Muscle	2650 mmol	Intracellular concentration	150 mmol/L
Liver	250 mmol	Extracellular concentration	4 mmol/L
Interstitial fluid	35 mmol		
Red blood cells	35 mmol		
Plasma	15 mmol		

Table 9.2 Distribution of total body potassium in organs and body compartments.

Fluid and Electrolyte Disorders

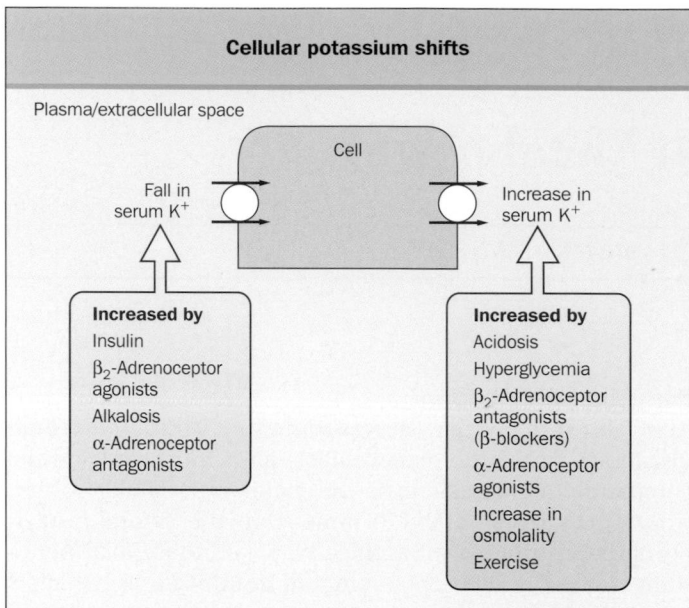

Figure 9.1 Regulation of extracellular/intracellular potassium shifts.

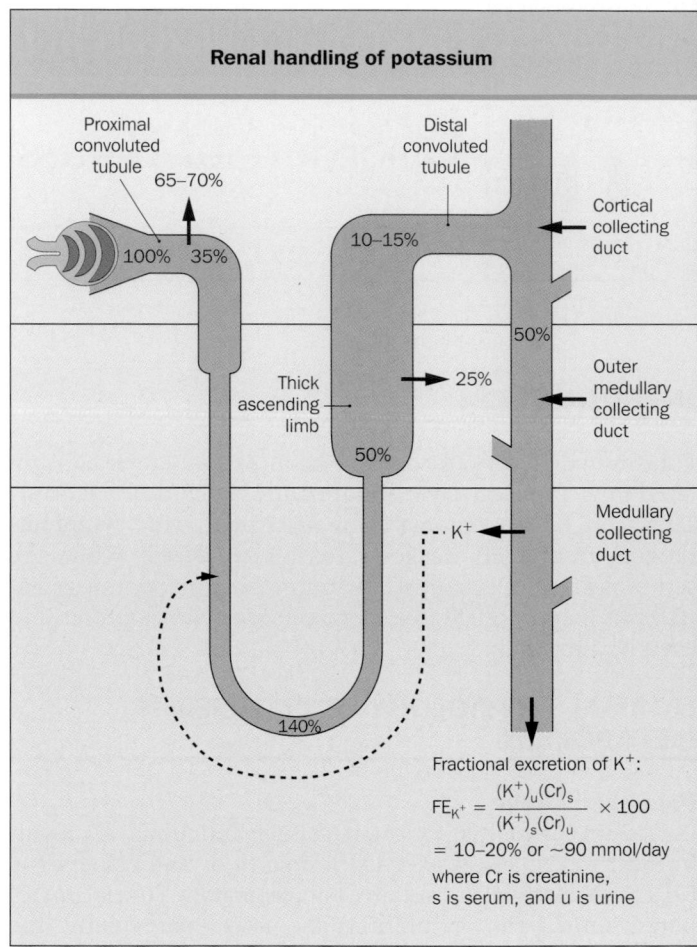

Figure 9.2 Renal handling of potassium.

There are several major factors that shift potassium from the extracellular to the intracellular pool or, conversely, block the shift and result in increases in the extracellular potassium concentration (Fig. 9.1). Acidosis associated with inorganic anions, such as NH_4Cl or HCl, is associated with hyperkalemia, but the mechanism is not fully understood. In contrast, with organic acidosis (such as lactic acidosis) there is minimal cellular shift of potassium.

Insulin and β_2-adrenergic receptor activation induce cellular potassium uptake by stimulating Na^+-K^+-ATPase. Insulin directly stimulates the Na^+-K^+-ATPase pump, resulting in cellular potassium uptake; this effect is independent of its stimulation of glucose entry. β_2-adrenergic receptor activation increases intracellular cAMP production, which stimulates Na^+-K^+-ATPase-mediated potassium uptake. α-Adrenergic activation opposes the effect of β_2-adrenergic receptor stimulation. The effects of insulin and β_2-adrenergic receptor activation are synergistic, as expected given the differing cellular mechanisms.

Aldosterone lowers serum potassium by two major mechanisms. Aldosterone stimulates potassium movement into cells, and aldosterone also increases potassium excretion in the kidney and to a lesser extent in the gut.

Changes in plasma osmolality can cause cellular potassium shifts. Hyperosmolality results in water movement out of the cells together with a mass movement of potassium; this results in hyperkalemia. In patients with diabetes mellitus, increased plasma glucose levels can increase plasma potassium due to the glucose-induced increase in extracellular osmolality.

Exercise may result in hyperkalemia due to α-adrenergic receptor activation that shifts potassium out of the skeletal muscle cells. The increased serum potassium induces arterial dilation, which increases skeletal muscle blood flow and acts as adaptive mechanism during exercise. Simultaneous β_2-adrenergic receptor activation stimulates skeletal muscle cellular potassium uptake and minimizes the severity of exercise-induced hyperkalemia, but this can lead to hypokalemia after the cessation of exercise[1]. In patients with pre-existent potassium depletion, postexercise hypokalemia may be severe and rhabdomyolysis may occur[2].

Renal potassium handling with normal renal function

Long-term potassium homeostasis is accomplished primarily via urinary potassium excretion that is regulated largely by active transport in the collecting duct. Potassium is almost completely ionized and not bound to plasma proteins, and is nearly completely filtered by the glomerulus (Fig. 9.2). The majority of filtered potassium is reabsorbed in the proximal tubule and the loop of Henle. Quantitatively, the majority (~65–70%) of filtered potassium is reabsorbed in the proximal tubule, but this segment exhibits little regulation in response to changes in dietary potassium intake. Potassium is secreted into the luminal fluid of the descending loop of Henle, at least in deep nephrons, and is reabsorbed from the ascending loop of Henle by the action of the Na^+-K^+-$2Cl^-$ cotransporter (Fig. 9.3a). Thus, modest net reabsorption of filtered potassium normally occurs in the loop of Henle. This absorption can be reversed to secretion, however, by administration of a loop diuretic or large levels of potassium loading. Nevertheless, the majority of potassium excretion is normally regulated by alterations in the rates of active secretion and absorption that occur in the distal convolution and collecting duct.

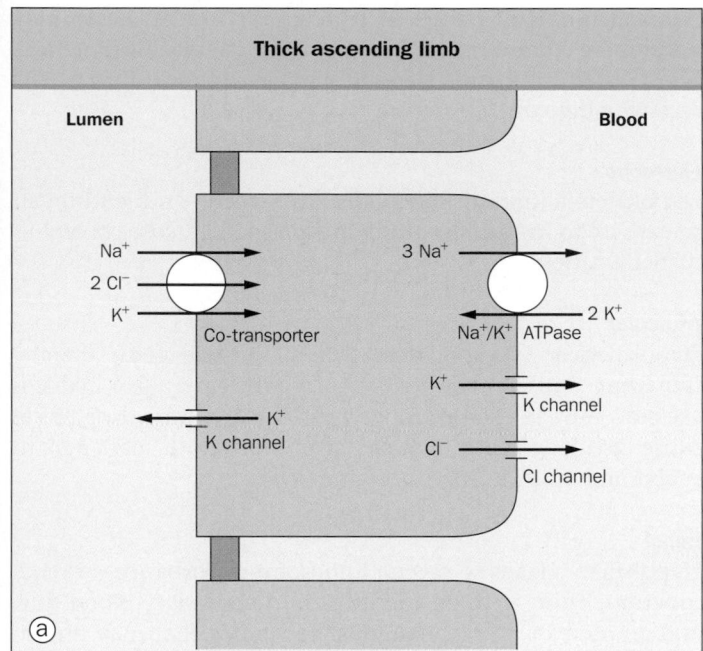

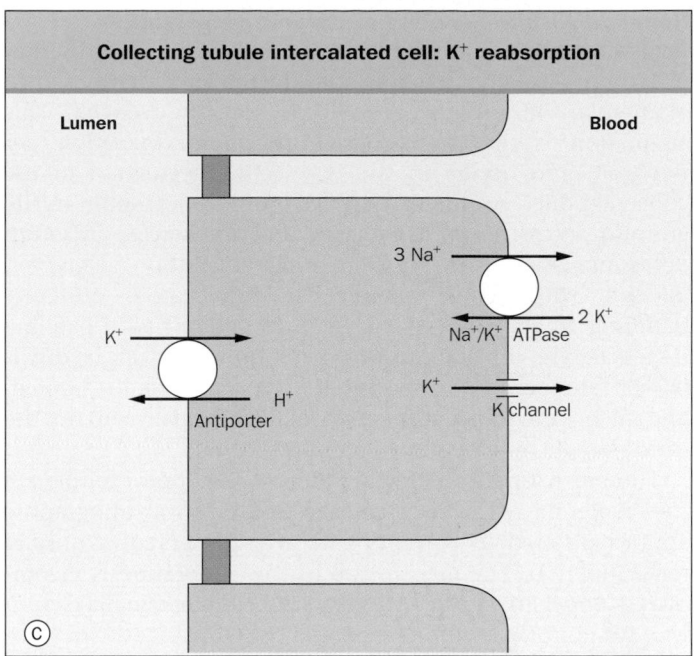

Figure 9.3 **Mechanisms of potassium reabsorption and secretion in the thick ascending limb and the collecting tubule principal and intercalated cells.**

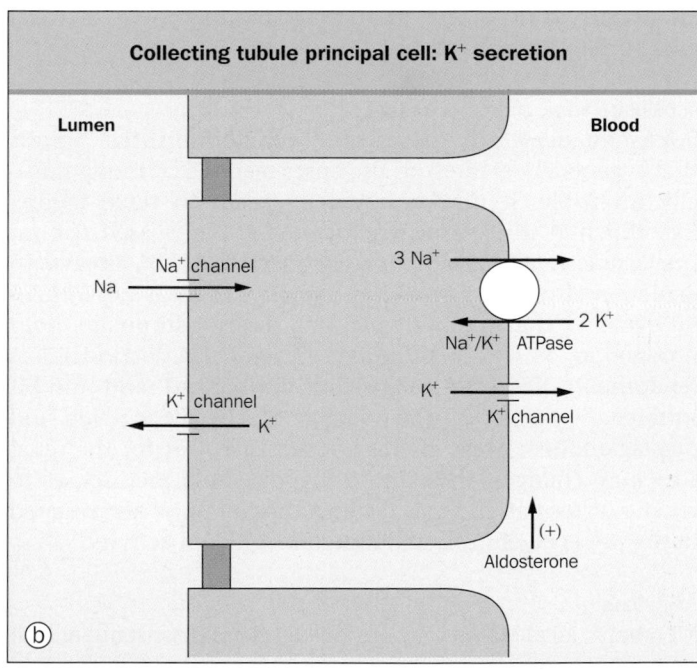

Net potassium transport in the collecting duct occurs through distinct cell types that allow fine control of renal potassium excretion. Potassium secretion is highly dependent on luminal flow rate within the normal physiological range. The principal cell of the cortical collecting duct is responsible for potassium secretion and Figure 9.3b illustrates the mechanism of potassium secretion by the principal cell. Sodium reabsorption through an apical sodium channel stimulates basolateral Na$^+$-K$^+$-ATPase, and the active turnover of this pump maintains high intracellular potassium concentrations. Subsequent to active basolateral potassium uptake, potassium is secreted into the luminal fluid by apical potassium channels and a KCl-cotransporter.

Several factors regulate potassium secretion by principal cells. In relative order of importance these are: luminal flow rate and distal sodium delivery, aldosterone, extracellular potassium and extracellular pH. An increase in luminal flow rate reduces luminal potassium concentration, thereby increasing the concentration gradient across the apical membrane, which stimulates potassium secretion. In addition, flow rate directly influences cellular potassium secretion, possibly by modulating the activity of potassium channels. Conversely, reduced luminal flow, such as occurs in pre-renal azotemia and obstruction, may result in hyperkalemia. Decreasing apical sodium reabsorption, whether from reduced luminal sodium delivery or by sodium channel inhibitors decreases potassium secretion by affecting the chemical and electrochemical driving forces for potassium secretion. The 'potassium-sparing diuretics' either directly or indirectly reduce these driving forces and inhibit potassium secretion. Conversely, aldosterone increases Na$^+$-K$^+$-ATPase expression and stimulates insertion of apical sodium channels and the apical potassium gradient, thereby stimulating potassium secretion. Increasing extracellular potassium directly stimulates Na$^+$-K$^+$-ATPase activity, leading to increased potassium secretion. Metabolic acidosis decreases potassium secretion, both through direct effects on potassium channels and through changes in interstitial ammonia concentration which then decreases potassium secretion[3].

The collecting duct also actively reabsorbs potassium (Fig. 9.3c) through the action of intercalated cells. Intercalated cells reabsorb potassium via an apical H$^+$-K$^+$-ATPase[4] that actively secretes H$^+$ into the luminal fluid in exchange for potassium reabsorption. In severe potassium deficiency, active potassium reabsorption by H$^+$-K$^+$-ATPase enables urinary potassium excretion to decrease to 15 mmol/d or less.

Renal potassium handling in chronic renal failure

Potassium homeostasis is relatively well-preserved and serum potassium usually remains in the normal range until glomerular filtration rate (GFR) is severely reduced. This adaptation is due to increased potassium excretion per nephron, and occurs in the connecting segment and the collecting duct. An increase in excretion of potassium in the gut also occurs. Both aldosterone and an increase in serum potassium may contribute to this adaptation. However, patients with renal insufficiency have more difficulty handling an acute potassium load. In patients with baseline hyperkalemia, the amount of potassium which can be distributed into cells in response to hyperkalemia is limited, and such individuals also often exhibit impairment in the maximal rate of potassium excretion.

Patients with chronic renal failure (CRF) appear to tolerate hyperkalemia with fewer cardiac and electrocardiographic abnormalities than patients with well-preserved or normal renal function. The mechanism of this adaptation is incompletely understood. Nevertheless, severe hyperkalemia (serum $K^+ > 6.0$ mmol/L or the presence of ECG changes) can have lethal effects and should be aggressively treated.

HYPOKALEMIA

Epidemiology

The incidence of potassium disorders is strongly dependent on the patient population. Less than 1% of normal adults not receiving medicines will develop hypokalemia or hyperkalemia; however, diets with large sodium and small potassium content may lead to potassium depletion. Thus, hypokalemia or hyperkalemia in a healthy adult not taking medicines should suggest the possibility of an underlying disease. In contrast, hypokalemia frequently occurs in the setting of specific disease states and with the use of medicines that affect renal potassium handling. For example, hypokalemia may be present in 50% of patients on diuretics[5], and is typical in subjects with primary or secondary hyperaldosteronism.

Clinical manifestations

Potassium deficiency alters the function of several organs, most prominently, the heart and blood vessels, nerves, muscles, and kidneys. Overall, children and young adults tolerate hypokalemia better than the elderly. Prompt correction is warranted in the presence of ischemic heart disease or in patients receiving digitalis.

Cardiovascular

Epidemiologic studies link a low potassium diet with an increased prevalence of hypertension. Experimentally hypokalemia has been shown to increase blood pressure (5–10 mmHg), and similarly, potassium supplementation can lower blood pressure[6]. Potassium deficiency probably increases blood pressure by stimulating sodium retention with expansion of intravascular volume and by sensitizing the vasculature to endogenous vasoconstrictors[6].

Hypokalemia increases the risk of a variety of ventricular arrhythmias, including ventricular fibrillation[7]. Diuretic-induced hypokalemia is of particular concern, as sudden death may occur more commonly in those treated with thiazide diuretics[7]. Ventricular arrhythmias are also more common in patients receiving digoxin.

Hormonal

Hypokalemia impairs both insulin release and end-organ sensitivity to insulin, resulting in worsened glucose control in diabetic patients[8].

Muscular

Hypokalemia hyperpolarizes skeletal muscle cells, thereby impairing muscle contraction. Hypokalemia also reduces skeletal muscle blood flow, possibly by impairing local nitric oxide release, which can predispose patients to rhabdomyolysis during vigorous exercise[9].

Renal

Hypokalemia leads to several important disturbances of renal function. These include a reduction in medullary blood flow and an increase in renal vascular resistance that may predispose to hypertension, tubulointerstitial and cystic changes, alterations in acid–base balance, and impairment of renal concentrating mechanisms.

Tubulointerstitial and cystic changes

Potassium depletion causes mild tubulointerstitial fibrosis that is generally greatest in the outer medulla. Although usually reversible, it may occasionally result in renal failure. Experimental studies suggest that there is increased risk for irreversible renal injury in the neonatal period[10]. Potassium depletion also causes renal hypertrophy. There is experimental evidence that hypokalemia may directly stimulate renin production, as well as stimulate intrarenal vasoconstrictors (endothelin, local angiotensin II formation) and inhibit intrarenal vasodilators (including kallikrein, nitric oxide, and prostaglandins); these alterations may account for the renal structural changes. In addition, hypokalemia predisposes to renal cyst formation. This finding appears to be accentuated in the presence of increased mineralocorticoid activity.

Acid–base

Metabolic alkalosis is a common acid–base consequence of potassium depletion and is due to increased renal net acid excretion[11]. Conversely, metabolic alkalosis may increase renal potassium excretion resulting in potassium depletion. Severe hypokalemia can lead to respiratory muscle weakness and the development of respiratory acidosis.

Polyuria

Severe hypokalemia also impairs concentrating ability and causes mild polyuria, averaging 2–3 L/d. Both increased thirst and mild nephrogenic diabetes insipidus contributes to the polyuria[12].

Hepatic encephalopathy

Hypokalemia increases renal ammonia production, approximately half of which returns to the systemic circulation via the renal veins and may worsen hepatic encephalopathy[13].

Etiology

Hypokalemia may be grouped into four etiologies: pseudohypokalemia, redistribution, extra-renal potassium loss and renal potassium loss.

Pseudohypokalemia

Large numbers of abnormal white blood cells, especially with acute myelogenous leukemia, can take up extracellular potassium when stored for prolonged periods at room temperature, resulting in a reduced plasma potassium concentration, 'pseudohypokalemia'. Rapid separation of the plasma or storing the sample at 4°C confirms the diagnosis, avoids this artifact, and prevents inappropriate treatment.

Redistribution

More than 98% total body potassium is present in the intracellular fluid; movement of relatively small amounts of potassium from the extracellular to the intracellular fluid compartment can alter the extracellular concentration markedly. As discussed above, many hormones, particularly insulin, aldosterone and β_2-adrenergic agonists, stimulate transcellular potassium uptake.

Rarely, hypokalemia is due to hypokalemic periodic paralysis[14]. Attacks frequently occur during the night or the early morning or after a carbohydrate-rich meal. They are characterized by flaccid paralysis that typically persists for 6–24 h. A genetic defect in a dihydropyridine-sensitive calcium channel has been identified in some cases[15].

Non-renal potassium loss

Both the skin and the gastrointestinal tract excrete potassium. Under normal conditions, fluid loss from these organs is small, limiting net potassium loss. Occasionally, excessive sweating or chronic diarrhea cause substantial potassium loss[16]. Vomiting or nasogastric suction may also result in loss of potassium, usually about 5–8 mmol/L of gastric contents. However, in these conditions a major mechanism for the development of hypokalemia is urinary potassium loss that results from the development of metabolic alkalosis and also from intravascular volume depletion with secondary hyperaldosteronism[16].

Renal potassium loss

The most common cause of hypokalemia is renal potassium loss. This can occur either from medications, endogenous hormone production or, in rare conditions, intrinsic renal defects.

Drugs

Both thiazide and loop diuretics increase urinary potassium excretion, and the incidence of diuretic-induced hypokalemia is both dose- and treatment duration-related. When adjusted for their natriuretic effect, thiazide diuretics cause more urinary potassium loss than loop diuretics. Certain antibiotics increase urinary potassium excretion. Some penicillin analogues, such as carbenicillin, increase distal tubular delivery of a non-reabsorbable anion which obligates the presence of a cation such as potassium, thereby increasing urinary potassium excretion[17]. The antifungal agent amphotericin B directly increases collecting duct potassium secretion, resulting in potassium wasting[18]. Aminoglycosides may cause hypokalemia either with or without simultaneous nephrotoxicity. The mechanism is incompletely understood, but may relate to magnesium depletion (see below). Cisplatin is a commonly used medication that can induce hypokalemia. Toluene exposure, from sniffing certain glues, can also cause renal tubular acidosis with renal potassium wasting leading to hypokalemia[19].

Endogenous hormones

Endogenous hormones are important and common causes of hypokalemia. Aldosterone is the most important hormone regulating total body potassium homeostasis, and causes hypokalemia both by stimulating potassium uptake into cells and by stimulating renal potassium excretion.

Other

Rarely, genetic defects lead to excessive aldosterone production (see Chapter 49). In glucocorticoid-remediable aldosteronism (GRA), an ACTH-regulated gene is linked to the gene for aldosterone synthase, the rate-limiting enzyme in aldosterone synthesis[20]. As a result, aldosterone synthesis expression is regulated by ACTH and hyperaldosteronism ensues. In congenital adrenal hyperplasia there is persistent adrenal synthesis of 11-deoxycorticosterone, a potent mineralocorticoid[21]. This condition can be recognized by the associated effects on sex steroid production.

Another rare condition is when glucocorticoid hormones activate the mineralocorticoid receptor. Under normal conditions, the enzyme 11β-hydroxysteroid dehydrogenase (11β-HSDH) rapidly metabolizes cortisol to cortisone, and thereby preventing inappropriate activation of mineralocorticoid receptors[22]. If this does not occur, glucocorticoid hormones are able to activate mineralocorticoid receptors. Some compounds, such as glycyrrhetinic acid, found in some chewing tobacco and licorice preparations, inhibit 11β-HSDH, allowing cortisol to exert mineralocorticoid-like effects[23]. In severe Cushing's syndrome circulating cortisol exceeds the metabolic capacity of 11β-HSDH and can cause hypokalemia[24]. Genetic deficiency of 11β-HSDH (type II) is rare, but leads to severe hypertension and hypokalemia.

Magnesium depletion

Magnesium deficiency inhibits the kidney's ability to retain potassium[25]. This is particularly true with diuretic-induced hypokalemia and in certain cases of aminoglycoside- and cisplatin-induced potassium wasting. This condition should be suspected in the individual in whom potassium replacement does not correct the hypokalemia.

Intrinsic renal defect

Intrinsic renal potassium transport defects leading to hypokalemia are rare, but have led to important advances in our understanding of renal solute transport. Patients with Bartter's syndrome have a reduced or normal blood pressure, hypokalemia, hypomagnesemia, hyperreninemia, metabolic alkalosis and hypercalciuria. They typically present at a young age with severe volume depletion. Gitelman's syndrome is similar to Bartter's syndrome, except patients have

Fluid and Electrolyte Disorders

hypocalciuria, milder clinical manifestations and usually are diagnosed later in life.

Liddle's syndrome is characterized by severe hypertension and suppressed renin and aldosterone levels. This condition appears to be due to defects in the collecting duct apical sodium channel, leading to excessive sodium reabsorption, potassium excretion, volume expansion, and hypertension[26].

Bicarbonaturia

Bicarbonaturia can result from either metabolic alkalosis, distal renal tubular acidosis or treatment of proximal renal tubular acidosis. In each case, the increased distal tubular bicarbonate delivery increases potassium secretion.

Diagnosis

The evaluation of hypokalemia is summarized in Figure 9.4. One should first rule out pseudohypokalemia or redistribution of potassium from the extra- to the intracellular space. Insulin, aldosterone or its synthetic analogue, fludrocortisone, and sympathomimetic agents, such as theophylline or β_2-adrenergic receptor agonists, are common causes of potassium redistribution.

If neither of these possibilities are present, then the hypokalemia probably represents total body potassium depletion due to renal, GI or skin losses. Renal potassium loss is most frequently due to diuretics. Secondary hyperaldosteronism is a common contributing cause. Hypomagnesemia-induced hypokalemia causes renal potassium wasting, and is frequently a complication of diuretic usage. Rarer causes of renal potassium loss include renal tubular acidosis (RTA), diabetic ketoacidosis and ureterosigmoidostomy. Primary aldosteronism, surreptitious diuretic use or vomiting, concomitant magnesium depletion and Bartter's or Gitelman's syndrome should be considered when the cause of the hypokalemia is not

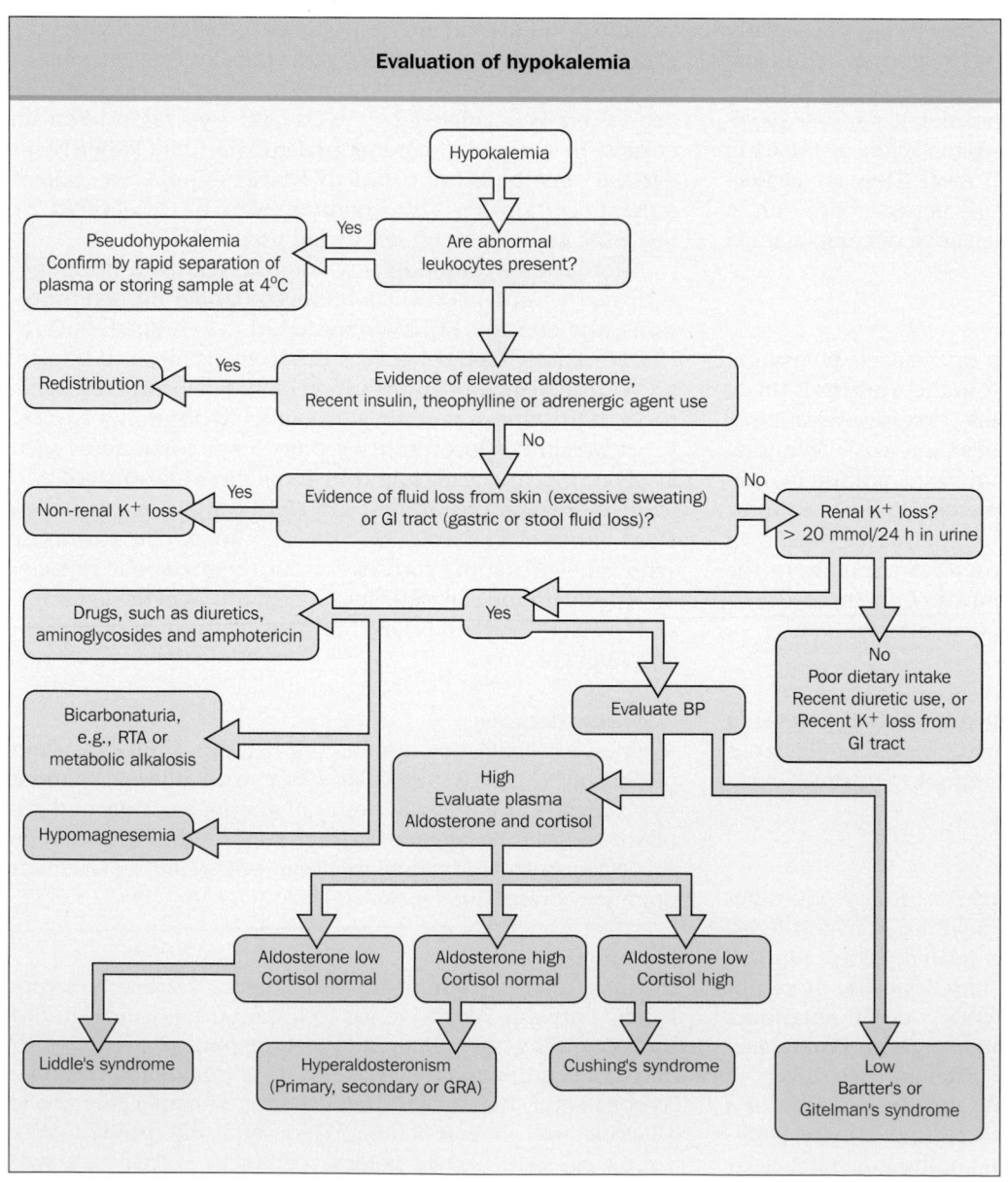

Figure 9.4 Diagnostic evaluation of hypokalemia. RTA, renal tubular acidosis; GRA, glucose remediable aldosteronism.

obvious. Finally, excessive potassium loss may result via the skin (excessive sweating) or from diarrhea, vomiting, NG suction, or a GI fistula. Occasionally, patients are reluctant to admit to self-induced diarrhea, and the diagnosis may need to be confirmed by sigmoidoscopy or direct testing of the stool for cathartic agents.

Treatment

The risks associated with hypokalemia must be balanced against the risks of therapy. Usually, the primary short-term risks are cardiovascular and neuromuscular. In contrast, the primary risk of over-aggressive replacement is acute hyperkalemia, with resultant ventricular asystole.

Conditions requiring urgent therapy are rare. The clearest indications are hypokalemic periodic paralysis, severe hypokalemia in a patient requiring emergency surgery, and the patient with an acute myocardial infarction and significant ventricular ectopy. In such cases, administration of 5–10 mmol of KCl intravenously over 15–20 min may be used, and can be repeated as needed. Close, continuous monitoring of the serum potassium concentration and the electrocardiogram (ECG) are necessary to reduce the risk of hyperkalemia.

The body responds to chronic hypokalemia due to potassium losses by shifting potassium from the intracellular to the extracellular space. This minimizes the apparent magnitude of the hypokalemia, and results in the amount of potassium needed to replace the deficit being much greater than predicted by the change in extracellular potassium concentration and the extracellular fluid volume. Figure 9.5 summarizes the expected total body potassium depletion that occurs in chronic hypokalemia, and illustrates that the total amount of potassium needed to correct hypokalemia may be quite large.

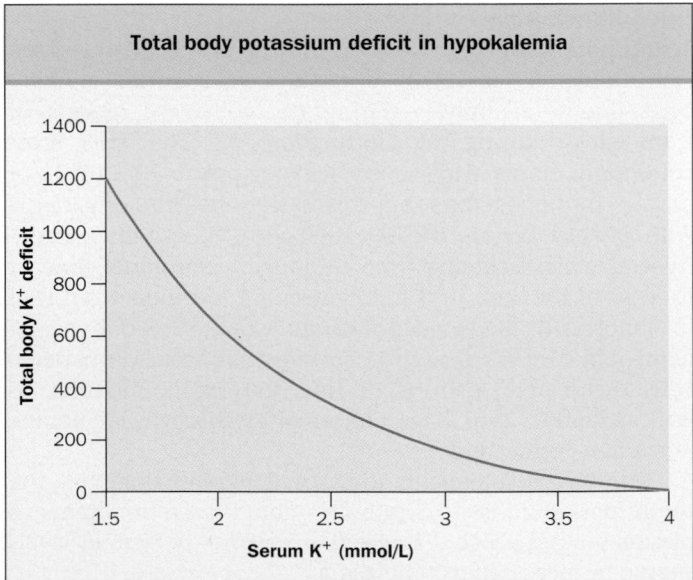

Figure 9.5 Total body potassium deficit in hypokalemia. Because of shift of potassium from the intracellular to the extracellular fluid compartment during chronic potassium depletion, the magnitude of deficiency can be masked, and is generally much larger than would be calculated solely from the change in plasma potassium and the extracellular fluid volume.

In most conditions, the choice of parenteral versus oral therapy depends on the ability of the patient to take oral medication and the ability of the gastrointestinal tract to function normally. If the patient is unable to take oral potassium safely or if gastrointestinal tract absorption is impaired, then intravenous KCl should be administered. When given via the intravenous route, replacement can be given safely at a rate of 10 mmol KCl/h. Although significant variations can occur between patients, administration of intravenous 20 mmol KCl typically increases the serum potassium by ~0.25 mmol/L[27]. If more rapid replacement is necessary, then 40 mmol/h can be administered through a central venous catheter, but simultaneous continuous ECG monitoring should be used under these circumstances.

The parenteral fluids used for potassium administration can affect the response. In patients without diabetes mellitus, dextrose administration increases serum insulin levels, which can cause redistribution of potassium from the extra- to the intracellular space. As a result, if KCl is administered in 5% dextrose in water, the dextrose load may stimulate cellular potassium uptake that exceeds the KCl replacement rate and may, paradoxically, decrease serum potassium levels[28]. Consequently, parenteral KCl should be administered in dextrose-free solutions.

The risk of hyperkalemia due to potassium replacement is less when potassium is given via the oral route. This probably reflects several factors, most prominently hepatic potassium uptake that minimizes changes in serum potassium levels.

The underlying condition should be treated whenever possible. Patients with diuretic-induced hypokalemia should be re-evaluated to reconsider the need for diuretics. If their use is required, concomitant use of potassium-sparing diuretics may be considered. When oral replacement therapy is required, KCl is the preferred drug in all patients, except those with metabolic acidosis. In the latter condition, either potassium bicarbonate or potassium citrate should be used. If indicated for other reasons, β-blockers or angiotensin converting enzyme inhibitors can assist in maintaining potassium levels.

Finally, hypomagnesemia can lead to refractoriness to potassium replacement[25]. Correction of the hypokalemia may not occur until the hypomagnesemia is corrected. Patients with unexplained hypokalemia or with diuretic-induced hypokalemia should have a serum magnesium checked and magnesium replacement therapy (such as 1 g intramuscularly daily for 3 d) begun, if indicated.

HYPERKALEMIA

Epidemiology

Less than 1% normal healthy adults develop hyperkalemia. This low frequency is a testament to the potent mechanisms for renal potassium excretion. Accordingly, hyperkalemia should suggest an underlying impairment of renal potassium excretion. Rarely, pseudohyperkalemia or conditions that shift potassium from the intracellular space to the extracellular space are present.

Clinical manifestations

Hyperkalemia may be asymptomatic or life-threatening. The most prominent effect of hyperkalemia is on the cardiac

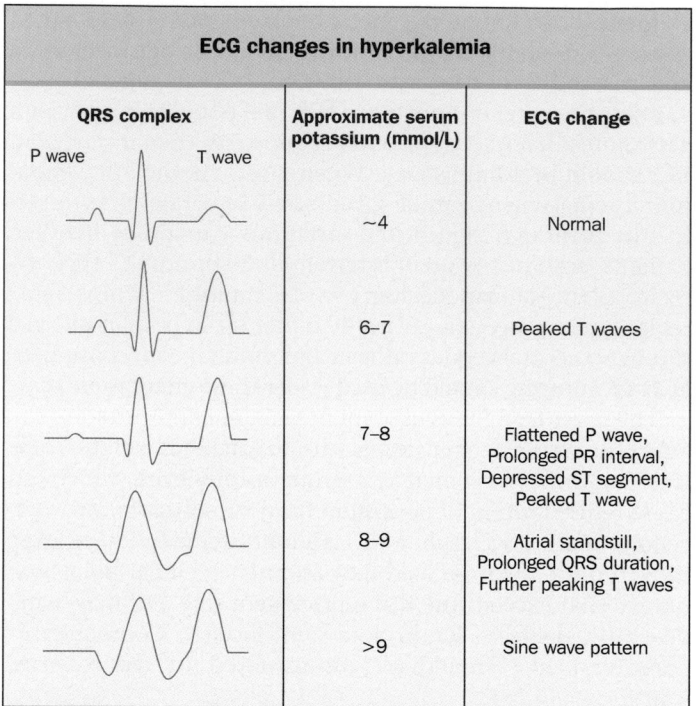

Figure 9.6 Electrocardiographic changes in hyperkalemia.
Progressive hyperkalemia results in identifiable changes in the electrocardiogram (ECG). These include peaking of the T wave, flattening of the P wave, prolongation of the PR interval, ST segment depression, prolongation of the QRS complex and, eventually, progression to a sine wave pattern. Ventricular fibrillation may occur at any time during this progression.

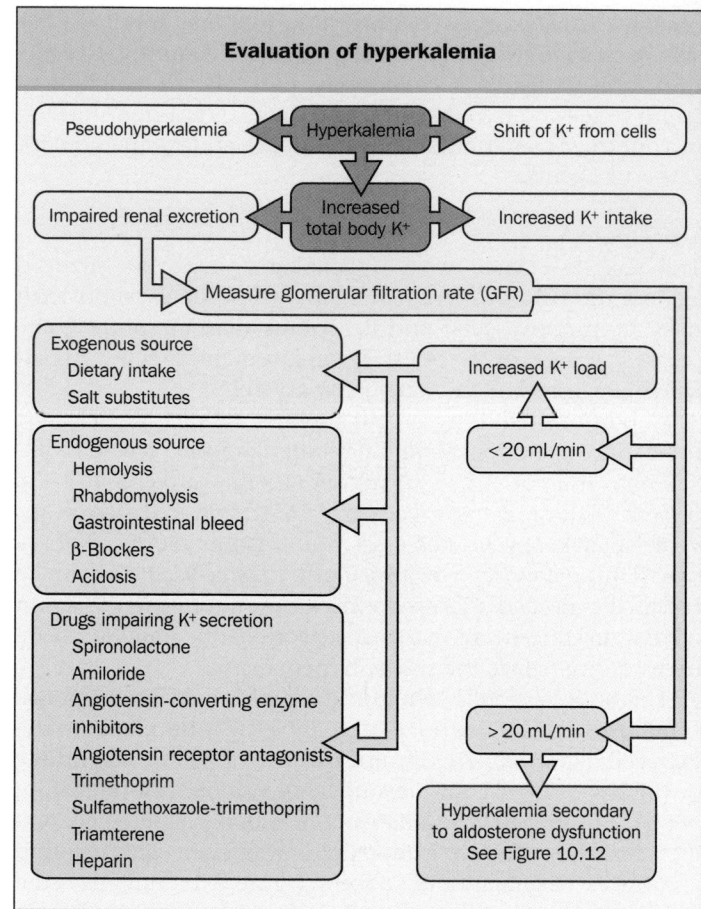

Figure 9.7 Workup of hyperkalemia.

conduction system. This is demonstrable in the electrocardiogram (ECG) (Fig. 9.6). The initial effect of hyperkalemia is a generalized increase in the height of the T waves, most evident in the precordial leads, known as 'tenting.' More severe hyperkalemia is associated with delayed electrical conduction, resulting in an increased PR interval and QRS interval. This is followed by progressive flattening and eventual absence of the P waves. Under extreme conditions, the QRS complex widens sufficiently that it merges with the T wave, resulting in a sine-wave pattern. Finally, ventricular asystole or fibrillation develops. Although a general correlation between the ECG findings and the degree of hyperkalemia is often observed, progression from mild to severe hyperkalemia may be unpredictable.

Hyperkalemia also affects cellular muscular contraction. Skeletal muscle cells are particularly sensitive to hyperkalemia, accordingly, hyperkalemia may cause weakness ('rubbery' or 'spaghetti' legs). With severe hyperkalemia respiratory failure may occur from paralysis of the diaphragm.

Etiology

Hyperkalemia can be due to either pseudohyperkalemia, redistribution of potassium from the intracellular to the extracellular space or imbalances between potassium intake and renal potassium excretion. A diagnostic approach is shown in Figure 9.7.

Pseudohyperkalemia

Serum potassium concentration may be artificially increased ('pseudohyperkalemia') by potassium release from erythrocytes due to hemolysis during the collection process or from release during the clotting process. The latter most commonly occurs with severe leukocytosis, $> 70 \times 10^9$/L, or marked thrombocytosis. Approximately one-third of patients with platelet counts of $500–1000 \times 10^9$/L exhibit pseudohyperkalemia. Ischemia from prolonged tourniquet time or exercise of the limb in the presence of a tourniquet can lead to abnormally increased potassium values. Pseudohyperkalemia may also occur with hemolysis that occurs in patients with rheumatoid arthritis or infectious mononucleosis, as well as families that have abnormal erythrocyte membrane potassium permeability.

Pseudohyperkalemia is diagnosed by showing that the serum potassium is > 0.3 mmol/L more than a simultaneous plasma sample. Once diagnosed, all further potassium levels should be measured using plasma.

Redistribution

Hyperkalemia may be observed in cases of severe hyperglycemia (due to effects of osmolarity), in association with severe acidosis due to nonorganic acids, and more rarely with β-blockers.

Potassium content of common enteral products				
	Calories/cc	Potassium (mmol/L)	Sodium (mmol/L)	Osmolality (mOsm/kg)
Ensure	1.06	40	37	470
Ensure Plus	1.50	54	49	690
Glucerna	1.00	40	40	375
Osmolite	1.06	26	27	300
Pulmocare	1.50	49	57	490
Suplena	2.00	29	34	615
Ultracal	1.06	41	41	310
Vivonex TEN	1.00	20	20	630

Table 9.3 Potassium content of common enteral products.

Excess intake

Excessive potassium ingestion is an infrequent cause of hyperkalemia in the absence of other contributing factors. Under normal conditions, the kidney can excrete hundreds of millimoles of potassium daily[29]. However, if renal potassium excretion is impaired, whether through drugs, renal insufficiency, or other causes, excessive potassium intake can produce hyperkalemia.

Common causes of excess potassium intake are potassium supplements, salt substitutes, enteral nutrition products and common foods. As many as 4% of patients receiving potassium supplements develop hyperkalemia. Typical salt substitutes contain 10–13 mmol potassium/g, or 283 mmol/tablespoon[30]. Many enteral nutrition products contain 40 mmol/L KCl or more; administration of 100 mL/h of such products can result in a potassium intake of ~100 mmol/d. Table 9.3 summarizes the potassium content of many common enteral products. Finally, many food products are particularly high in potassium content (Table 9.1), and many pharmacies routinely label diuretic medicine bottles with suggestions for the patient to increase potassium intake from dietary sources, such as bananas and fresh fruits. Table 9.1 summarizes the potassium content of many common foods with high potassium contents.

Impaired renal potassium secretion

The normal kidney possesses a remarkable ability to excrete potassium, so chronic hyperkalemia is difficult to produce unless renal potassium secretion is impaired. Factors that affect renal potassium excretion can be classified into those due to reduced nephron number and those due to intrinsic impairment of renal potassium handling.

Because the kidney is the primary organ regulating potassium excretion, impaired renal function decreases the maximal amount of potassium that can be excreted. In the absence of defects by other regulatory factors, renal potassium excretion is moderately well-preserved until glomerular filtration rate is markedly reduced. However, renal insufficiency, whether acute or chronic, impairs potassium excretion. This factor may be particularly important to consider in the elderly, because the decreased muscle mass may cause the serum creatinine level to be normal or only slightly elevated despite advanced renal insufficiency, and may therefore mask the degree of renal insufficiency.

Obstructive uropathy leads frequently to hyperkalemia through mechanisms that remain incompletely understood[31]. The hyperkalemia may occur either in association with metabolic acidosis or independent of acid–base changes. Mineralocorticoid resistance is present; whether this is a receptor deficiency, or is related to the interstitial nephritis that occurs, is unclear. In many cases, the hyperkalemia may persist for weeks following relief of the obstruction.

Specific drugs

The renin–angiotensin–aldosterone axis is the primary hormonal system regulating renal potassium excretion. Accordingly, medicines that either interfere with this system or that inhibit the cellular mechanisms of renal potassium excretion are frequent causes of hyperkalemia. Classes of medications that inhibit the renin–angiotensin–aldosterone axis are summarized in Table 9.4.

Prostaglandins increase renal potassium secretion by stimulating renin as well as by direct effects on the tubules. Nonsteroidal anti-inflammatory drugs (NSAIDs) as well as cyclo-oxygenase-2 (COX-2) inhibitors block prostaglandin formation and may be able to induce hyperkalemia.

Potassium-sparing diuretics, such as amiloride and triamterene, lead to hyperkalemia by decreasing urinary potassium excretion. The antibiotics trimethoprim and pentamidine have renal effects similar to amiloride and also cause hyperkalemia[32,33].

Digoxin inhibits the principal cell basolateral Na^+-K^+-ATPase, thereby inhibiting cellular potassium uptake. Hyperkalemia may occur in predisposed patients, such as those with renal failure, even in the absence of toxic levels[34].

The immunosuppressive medicines cyclosporine and tacrolimus can cause hyperkalemia by inhibiting distal nephron potassium secretion[35].

Certain agents that can depolarize skeletal muscle, such as succinylcholine, or that activate K-dependent amino acid exchangers, such as lysine or arginine, also can lead to hyperkalemia.

Distinguishing renal and non-renal mechanisms of hyperkalemia

In most circumstances, a 24-h urine potassium excretion rate will distinguish renal ($K^+ < 20$ mmol/L) from extrarenal ($K^+ > 40$ mmol/L) causes of hyperkalemia. Furthermore, in patients with a low urinary K^+ level, the administration of fludrocortisone may be used to distinguish aldosterone deficiency (urine K^+ increases to > 40 mmol/L) from aldosterone resistance (K^+ remains < 20 mmol/L). However, urinary K^+ measurements may be difficult to interpret, since potassium excretion is dependent on multiple factors, the most important being GFR, tubule lumen flow, and water reabsorption in the distal tubule. Fractional excretion of potassium has been postulated to help in differentiating renal from nonrenal causes of hyperkalemia, since it normalizes potassium excretion relative to GFR. However, when a result is particularly difficult to interpret (such as a urine K^+ of 30 mmol/L), the transtubular potassium gradient (TTKG) is used (Table 9.5).

Fluid and Electrolyte Disorders

Medications associated with hyperkalemia		
Class	Mechanism	Example*
Potassium-containing medicines	Increased potassium intake	KCl, PCN G, PolyCitra, PolyCitra K
β-adrenergic receptor blockers	Inhibit renin release	Propranolol, metoprolol, atenolol
ACE inhibitor	Inhibit conversion of Angiotensin I to Angiotensin II	Captopril, lisinopril
Angiotensin receptor blocker (ATRA)	Inhibit activation of AT1 receptor by Angiotensin II	Losartan, valsartan, irbesartan
Heparin	Inhibit aldosterone synthase, rate limiting enzyme for aldosterone synthesis	Heparin sodium
Aldosterone receptor antagonist	Block aldosterone receptor activation	Spironolactone
Potassium-sparing diuretic	Block collecting duct apical sodium channel, decreasing gradient for potassium secretion	Amiloride, triamterene, trimethoprim, pentamidine
NSAID and COX-2 inhibitors	Inhibit prostaglandin stimulation of collecting duct potassium secretion, inhibits renin release	Ibuprofen, rofecoxib
Digitalis glycosides	Inhibit Na^+-K^+-ATPase necessary for collecting duct potassium secretion	Digoxin
Calcineurin inhibitors	Inhibit Na^+-K^+-ATPase necessary for collecting duct potassium secretion	Cyclosporine, tacrolimus

Table 9.4 Medications associated with hyperkalemia.

Transtubular potassium gradient	
TTKG is a measurement of net K^+ secretion by the distal nephron after correcting for changes in urinary osmolality and is often used to determine if hyperkalemia is caused by aldosterone deficiency/resistance or if the hyperkalemia is secondary to nonrenal causes $$TTKG = (K_u/K_s) \times (S_{osm}/U_{osm})$$ where K_u and K_s are the concentration of K^+ in urine and serum, respectively and U_{osm} and S_{osm} are the osmolalities of urine and serum, respectively.	
TTKG value	Indication
6–12	Normal
> 10	Suggests normal aldosterone action and an extrarenal cause of hyperkalemia
< 5–7	Suggests aldosterone deficiency or resistance
After 0.05 mg 9α-fludrocortisone	
> 10	Hypoaldosteronism is likely
No change	Suggests a renal tubule defect from either K^+-sparing diuretics (amiloride, triamterene, spironolactone), aldosterone resistance (interstitial renal disease, sickle cell disease, urinary tract obstruction, pseudohypoaldosteronism type I), or increased distal K^+ reabsorption (pseudohypoaldosteronism type II, urinary tract obstruction)

Table 9.5 Transtubular potassium gradient.

The TTKG corrects the urinary potassium for changes in osmolality that occur with water reabsorption in the collecting duct. It provides an indirect measurement of the net K^+ secretion of the distal nephron. A value below 5–7 in the setting of hyperkalemia implies impaired distal tubular secretion of potassium owing to either aldosterone deficiency or resistance, whereas a value of >10 favors increased K+ intake and normal distal nephron handling of potassium.

Treatment

Therapies for hyperkalemia can be divided into those that minimize the cardiac effects of hyperkalemia, those that induce potassium uptake by cells resulting in a decrease in plasma potassium, and those that remove potassium from the body. Table 9.6 summarizes the available treatments, their mechanism of action, time of onset of action and duration of action.

Treatment of hyperkalemia should not include $NaHCO_3$ therapy unless the patient is frankly acidotic (pH < 7.2) or unless substantial endogenous renal function is present. Administration of hypertonic $NaHCO_3$ runs the risk of additional volume overload, a frequent issue in the patient with acute renal failure and no urine output, and it is well documented to have little benefit in patients without endogenous renal function[36].

Blocking cardiac effects

Intravenous calcium administration specifically antagonizes the effects of hyperkalemia on the myocardial conduction system and on myocardial repolarization. Calcium is the most rapid way to treat hyperkalemia, and should be given via the intravenous route if unambiguous ECG changes of hyperkalemia are present. All patients with prolonged PR intervals, widened QRS complexes, or absence of P waves should receive intravenous calcium without delay. Effects can be documented within 1–3 min, and last for 30–60 min. The dose may be repeated within 5–10 min if ECG changes persist. If a delay in the institution of dialysis is anticipated, a calcium infusion should be considered since the effect of a calcium bolus is transient.

Treatment of hyperkalemia				
Mechanism	Therapy	Dose	Onset	Duration
Antagonize membrane effects	Calcium	Calcium gluconate, 10% solution, 10 mL i.v. over 10 min	1–3 min	30–60 min
Cellular potassium uptake	Insulin	Regular insulin, 10 U i.v., with dextrose, 50%, 50 mL if plasma glucose < 250 mg/dL (14 mmol/L)	30 min	4–6 h
	β_2-adrenergic agonist	Nebulized albuterol, 10 mg	30 min	2–4 h
Potassium removal	Sodium polystyrene sulfonate	Kayexalate, 60 g p.o., in 20% sorbitol, or Kayexalate, 60 g in 250 mL water, per retention enema	1–2 h	4–6 h
	Hemodialysis	–	Immediate	Until dialysis completed

Table 9.6 Treatment of hyperkalemia.

There are several precautions to observe with intravenous calcium. First, it should not be administered in solutions containing $NaHCO_3$, because $CaCO_3$ precipitation can occur. Second, hypercalcemia, which occurs during rapid calcium infusion, can potentiate the myocardial toxicity of digoxin. Hyperkalemic patients taking digoxin should be given calcium as a slow infusion over 20–30 min.

Cellular potassium uptake

The second most rapid way to treat hyperkalemia is to stimulate cellular potassium uptake, with either insulin or β_2-adrenergic agonist administration. Insulin rapidly stimulates cellular potassium uptake, and should be administered intravenously to ensure predictable bioavailability. Effects on serum potassium concentration are generally seen within 10–20 min and will last for 4–6 h[37]. Glucose is generally coadministered to avoid hypoglycemia but may not be needed if hyperglycemia coexists. Extracellular glucose in patients with diabetes mellitus can function as an 'ineffective osmole' and can increase serum potassium. Therefore, further glucose administration should be avoided in patients with simultaneous hyperkalemia and hyperglycemia. If a delay in the institution of dialysis is anticipated, it may be wise to administer a continuous infusion of insulin 4–10 U/h with 10% dextrose in water with frequent measurements of serum glucose and potassium.

β_2-adrenergic receptor agonists directly stimulate cellular potassium uptake. Intravenous albuterol, 0.5 mg, rapidly increases potassium uptake, and can decrease serum potassium by ~1 mmol/L[38], but is not approved for intravenous use in the USA. Nebulized albuterol, at a dose of 10 or 20 mg, decreases serum potassium by ~0.6 or ~1.0 mmol/L, respectively, with a rapid onset of action and maximal effect at 90–120 min[39]. However, intravenous β_2-agonist therapy is limited frequently by tachycardia, and as many as 25% of patients do not respond when it is given by nebulizer[39]. A frequent mistake when administering nebulized albuterol is underdosage; the dose required is 2–8 times that usually given by nebulizer for bronchodilation, and is 50–100 times greater than the dose administered by metered dose inhalers. In severe hyperkalemia, combined therapy with insulin and albuterol may be more effective than either alone[40].

Potassium removal

Most cases of severe hyperkalemia are associated with increased extracellular fluid potassium content. Definitive treatment of these patients requires removing potassium from the extracellular fluid.

In selected cases, increasing renal potassium elimination may be adequate. With chronic or mild hyperkalemia, loop or thiazide diuretics increase renal potassium excretion and may be sufficient for therapy. In particular, loop diuretics may be the therapy of choice for patients with hyperkalemic renal tubular acidosis[41]. While synthetic mineralocorticoids, such as fludrocortisone, stimulate renal potassium excretion, the accompanying renal sodium retention and intravascular volume expansion is a relative contraindication to their use. Acute hyperkalemia generally should not be treated with diuretics, because the rate of renal potassium excretion usually will not be adequate. Also, most patients with hyperkalemia have underlying renal insufficiency as a contributing factor[42], which limits the effectiveness of diuretic therapy. If a rapidly reversible cause of renal failure is identified, such as obstructive uropathy, or prerenal azotemia, then treatment of the underlying condition with close observation of potassium values in association with continuous EKG observation may be adequate.

A second mode of potassium elimination is with sodium polystyrene sulfonate. This resin exchanges sodium for potassium in the gastrointestinal tract, thereby allowing potassium elimination. In general, 1 g of sodium polystyrene sulfonate removes ~0.5–1.0 mmol of potassium in exchange for 2–3 mmol of sodium. It can be administered either orally or per rectum as a retention enema. The rate of potassium removal is relatively slow, requiring ~4 h for full effect, although administering it as a retention enema results in more rapid onset of action. When given orally, sodium polystyrene sulfonate is generally administered with 20% sorbitol to avoid constipation. If given as an enema, sorbitol should be avoided, because rectal administration of sodium polystyrene sulfonate with 20% sorbitol may lead to colonic perforation[43].

Fluid and Electrolyte Disorders

Acute hemodialysis is the primary method of potassium removal when renal function is absent and hyperkalemia is persistent or severe. Serum potassium can decrease as much as 1.2–1.5 mmol/h with a potassium-free dialysate and may precipitate arrhythmias. It is generally proposed that the more severe the hyperkalemia, the more rapid should be the reduction in plasma potassium[44]. However, care should be exercised in the rapid reduction of serum potassium in patients with ischemic heart disease and those predisposed to arrhythmias. In general, the use of 0 or 1 mmol/L potassium dialysate fluids provides little additional benefit and runs the risk of precipitating serious hypokalemia. If a very low potassium dialysate is used, then the serum potassium should be rechecked after 2 h and in most cases the dialysate should contain 2 mmol/L potassium. Continuous dialysis modalities, such as peritoneal dialysis and chronic venovenous hemodialysis do not remove potassium sufficiently quickly to be recommended for use in life-threatening hyperkalemia.

Whereas dialysis is the most rapid method to treat most cases of hyperkalemia, other modes of treatment should not be delayed while waiting to institute dialysis. If dialysis is required at times other than a dialysis unit's regular hours or when hemodialysis vascular access is not already present then there is frequently a delay in beginning hemodialysis. In these conditions, other therapies should be instituted and continued until hemodialysis can be started.

Specific therapies may be quite valuable in certain causes of hyperkalemia. For example, digoxin-specific Fab fragments are beneficial in cases of severe digitalis toxicity[45]. Patients with acute urinary tract obstruction and subsequent hyperkalemia may be effectively treated with relief of the urinary tract obstruction. Since the rate of potassium excretion in the latter condition may be variable, frequent measurement of plasma potassium is necessary.

REFERENCES

1. Williams ME, Gervino EV, Rosa RM, et al. Catecholamine modulation of rapid potassium shifts during exercise. N Engl J Med. 1985;312:823.
2. Aizawa H, Morita K, Minami H, et al. Exertional rhabdomyolysis as a result of strenuous military training. J Neurol Sci. 1995; 132:239.
3. Hamm LL, Gillespie C, Klahr S. NH_4Cl inhibition of transport in the rabbit cortical collecting tubule. Am J Physiol. 1985; 248:F631.
4. Milton AE, Weiner ID. Intracellular pH regulation in the rabbit cortical collecting duct A-type intercalated cell. Am J Physiol. 1997;273:F340.
5. Bloomfield RL, Wilson DJ, Buckalew VM Jr. The incidence of diuretic-induced hypokalemia in two distinct clinic settings. J Clin Hypertens. 1986;2:331.
6. Barri YM, Wingo CS. The effects of potassium depletion and supplementation on blood pressure: a clinical review. Am J Med Sci. 1997;314:37.
7. Siscovick DS, Raghunathan TE, Psaty BM, et al. Diuretic therapy for hypertension and the risk of primary cardiac arrest. N Engl J Med. 1994; 330:1852.
8. Knochel JP. Diuretic-induced hypokalemia. Am J Med. 1984;77:18.
9. Singhal PC, Abramovici M, Venkatesan J, Mattana J. Hypokalemia and rhabdomyolysis. Miner Electrolyte Metab. 1991;17:335.
10. Ray PE, Suga S, Liu XH, Huang X, Johnson RJ. Chronic potassium depletion induces renal injury, salt sensitivity, and hypertension in young rats. Kidney Int. 2001;59:1850–8.
11. Tizianello A, Garibotto G, Robaudo C, et al. Renal ammoniagenesis in humans with chronic potassium depletion. Kidney Int. 1991;40:772.
12. Berl T, Linas SL, Alisenbrye GA, Anderson RJ. On the mechanism of polyuria in potassium depletion. The role of polydipsia. J Clin Invest. 1977;60:620–5.
13. Gabuzda GJ, Hall PW III. Relation of potassium depletion to renal ammonium metabolism and hepatic coma. Medicine. 1966;45: 481.
14. Ahlawat SK, Sachdev A. Hypokalaemic paralysis. Postgrad Med J. 1999;75:193.
15. Antes LM, Kujubu DA, Fernandez PC. Hypokalemia and the pathology of ion transport molecules. Semin Nephrol. 1998;18:31.
16. Knochel JP, Dotin LN, Hamburger RJ. Pathophysiology of intense physical conditioning in a hot climate. I. Mechanisms of potassium depletion. J Clin Invest 1972;51:242.
17. Gill MA, DuBe JE, Young WW. Hypokalemic, metabolic alkalosis induced by high-dose ampicillin sodium. Am J Hosp Pharm. 1977;34:528.
18. O'Regan S, Carson S, Chesney RW, Drummond KN. Electrolyte and acid–base disturbances in the management of leukemia. Blood. 1977;49:345.
19. Taher SM, Anderson RJ, McCartney R, et al. Renal tubular acidosis associated with toluene 'sniffing'. N Engl J Med. 1974;290:765.
20. Lifton RP, Dluhy RG, Powers M, et al. A chimaeric 11 beta-hydroxylase/aldosterone synthase gene causes glucocorticoid-remediable aldosteronism and human hypertension. Nature. 1992;355:262.
21. White PC, New MI, Dupont B. Congenital adrenal hyperplasia II. N Engl J Med. 1987;316:1580.
22. Funder JW, Pearce PT, Smith R, Smith AI. Mineralocorticoid action: target tissue specificity is enzyme, not receptor, mediated. Science. 1988;242:583.
23. Farese RV Jr, Biglieri EG, Shackleton CH, et al. Licorice-induced hypermineralocorticoidism. N Engl J Med. 1991;325:1223.
24. Ulick S, Wang JZ, Blumenfeld JD, Pickering TG. Cortisol inactivation overload: a mechanism of mineralocorticoid hypertension in the ectopic adrenocorticotropin syndrome. J Clin Endo Metab. 1992;74:963.
25. Whang R. Magnesium deficiency: pathogenesis, prevalence, and clinical implications. Am J Med. 1987;82:24.
26. Schild L, Canessa CM, Shimkets RA, et al. A mutation in the epithelial sodium channel causing Liddle disease increases channel activity in the Xenopus laevis oocyte expression system. Proc Natl Acad Sci USA. 1995;92:5699.
27. Kruse JA, Carlson RW. Rapid correction of hypokalemia using concentrated intravenous potassium chloride infusions. Arch Int Med. 1990;150:613.
28. Kunin AS, Surawicz B, Sims EAH. Decrease in serum potassium concentration and appearance of cardiac arrhythmias during infusion of potassium with glucose in potassium depleted patients. N Engl J Med. 1962;266:288.
29. Rabelink TJ, Koomans HA, Hene RJ, Dorhout ME. Early and late adjustment to potassium loading in humans. Kidney Int. 1990;38:942.

30. Sopko JA, Freeman RM. Salt substitutes as a source of potassium. J Am Med Assoc. 1977;238:608.

31. Batlle DC, Arruda JA, Kurtzman NA. Hyperkalemic distal renal tubule acidosis associated with obstructed uropathy. N Engl J Med. 1981;304:373.

32. Velazquez H, Perazella MA, Wright FS, Ellison DH. Renal mechanism of trimethoprim-induced hyperkalemia. Ann Intern Med. 1993;119:296.

33. Kleyman TR, Roberts C, Ling BN. A mechanism for pentamidine-induced hyperkalemia: Inhibition of distal nephron sodium transport. Ann Intern Med. 1995;122:103.

34. Papadakis MA, Wexman MP, Fraser C, Sedlacek SM. Hyperkalemia complicating digoxin toxicity in a patient with renal failure. Am J Kidney Dis. 1985;5:64.

35. Tumlin JA, Sands JM. Nephron segment-specific inhibition of Na+/K(+)-ATPase activity by cyclosporin A. Kidney Int. 1993;43:246.

36. Allon M. Hyperkalemia in end-stage renal disease: mechanisms and management. J Am Soc Nephrol. 1995;6(4):1134–42.

37. Clausen T, Hansen O. Active Na-K transport and the rate of ouabain binding. The effect of insulin and other stimuli on skeletal muscle and adipocytes. J Physiol (Lond). 1977;270:415.

38. Montoliu J, Lens XM, Revert L. Potassium-lowering effect of albuterol for hyperkalemia in renal failure. Arch Intern Med. 1987;147:713.

39. Allon M, Dunlay R, Copkney C. Nebulized albuterol for acute hyperkalemia in patients on hemodialysis. Ann Intern Med. 1989;110:426.

40. Allon M, Copkney C. Albuterol and insulin for treatment of hyperkalemia in hemodialysis patients. Kidney Int. 1990;38:869.

41. Sebastian A, Schambelan M, Sutton JM. Amelioration of hyperchloremic acidosis with furosemide therapy in patients with chronic renal insufficiency and type 4 renal tubular acidosis. Am J Nephrol. 1984;4:287.

42. Acker CG, Johnson JP, Palevsky PM, Greenberg A. Hyperkalemia in hospitalized patients: causes, adequacy of treatment, and results of an attempt to improve physician compliance with published therapy guidelines. Arch Intern Med. 1998;158:917.

43. Gerstman BB, Kirkman R, Platt R. Intestinal necrosis associated with postoperative orally administered sodium polystyrene sulfonate in sorbitol. Am J Kidney Dis. 1992;20:159.

44. Feig PU, Shook A, Stearns RH. Effect of potassium removal during hemodialysis on the plasma potassium concentration. Nephron. 1981;27:25.

45. Smith TW, Butler VPJ, Haber E, et al. Treatment of life-threatening digitalis intoxication with digoxin-specific Fab antibody fragments: experience in 26 cases. N Engl J Med. 1982;307:1357.

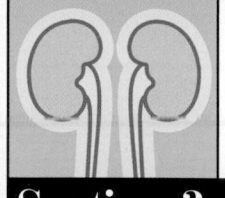

Chapter
10
Disorders of Calcium, Phosphate, and Magnesium Metabolism

Tilman B Drüeke and Bernard Lacour

HOMEOSTASIS OF CALCIUM AND DISORDERS OF CALCIUM METABOLISM

Distribution of calcium in the organism and calcium homeostasis

Calcium in the living organism is in either the bound or the free state. Most Ca is bound and associated with bony structures (99%). Most free Ca, either in diffusible (ultrafilterable) non ionized form or in ionized form (Ca^{2+}), is found in the intra- and extracellular fluid space. There is a steep concentration gradient between Ca^{2+} in the intra- and extracellular milieu. Figure 10.1 shows the distribution of Ca in the extracellular and intracellular fluid compartments.

Ca plays a crucial role in many biological processes and has an important mechanical function in the skeleton. The plasma concentration of Ca^{2+} is tightly regulated. The principal hormones implicated in this regulation are parathyroid hormone (PTH) and calcitriol (1,25-dihydroxycholecalciferol). The role of other Ca-regulatory hormones such as calcitonin, estrogens, and prolactin is less clear. Figure 10.2 shows the physiologic defense mechanisms used by the organism to counter changes of serum Ca^{2+} levels. Levels of Ca^{2+} are also altered by the acid–base status, with alkalosis causing a fall in ionized Ca^{2+} and acidosis having the opposite effect.

Long-term maintenance of Ca homeostasis depends on the adaptation of intestinal Ca^{2+} absorption to the needs of the organism, on the balance between bone accretion and resorption, and on the urinary excretion of Ca (see Fig. 10.3).

Intestinal, skeletal, and renal handling of calcium

Transport of Ca^{2+} across the intestinal wall occurs in two directions: absorption and secretion. Absorption can be subdivided into transcellular and paracellular flow (see Fig. 10.4)[1]. Many factors play a role in intestinal Ca^{2+} transport. Schematically, those that stimulate absorption can be distinguished from those that reduce absorption. Among the former, the daily amount of Ca ingested plays a major role (see Fig. 10.5), and its bioavailability is modified by a number of factors. Vitamin D synthesized in the skin from 7-dehydrocholesterol under the influence of sunlight or absorbed from the intestinal tract is first hydroxylated in the liver to 25(OH)vitamin D and then further hydroxylated to calcitriol in the kidney. Calcitriol is the most important hormonal regulatory factor[2]. After binding to its receptor (VDR) it increases active transport by inducing the synthesis of calbindin-D_{9k}, and probably also the synthesis or activity of Ca^{2+}-ATPase (see Fig. 10.4). Other hormones, including estrogens, prolactin,

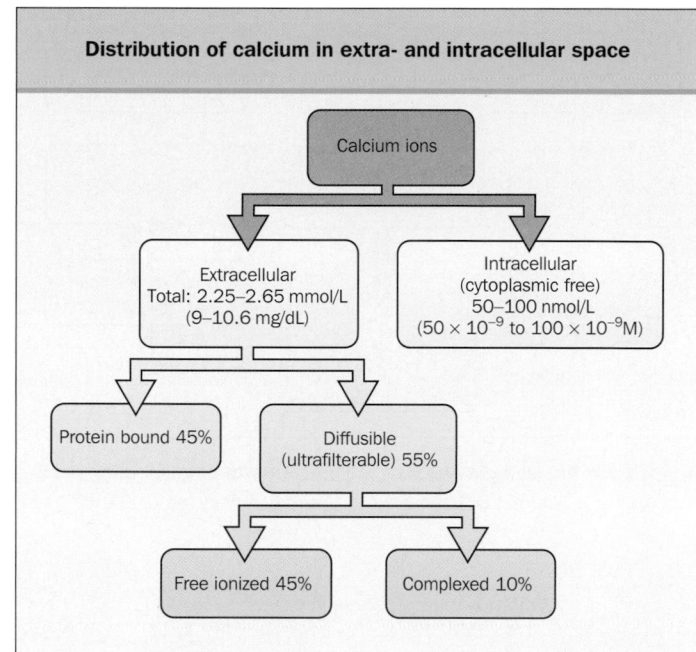

Figure 10.1 Distribution of calcium in extra- and intracellular space.

growth hormone, and PTH, can stimulate Ca^{2+} absorption, either directly or indirectly.

Increased Ca absorption is required in some physiological states, such as puberty, pregnancy, and lactation. In all these states, calcitriol synthesis is increased. Intestinal Ca^{2+} absorption is increased in at least two other pathological conditions: vitamin D excess and acromegaly. Other conditions are associated with a decrease in intestinal Ca^{2+} transport, including a low Ca^{2+}:phosphate ratio, a high vegetable fiber and fat content of the diet, glucocorticoid treatment, estrogen deficiency, advanced age, gastrectomy, intestinal malabsorption syndromes, diabetes mellitus, and renal failure. The decrease of Ca^{2+} absorption in the elderly probably results, in great part, from factors other than lowered serum calcitriol and intestinal VDR levels[3].

The skeleton constantly exchanges Ca with the surrounding milieu. The net balance between Ca^{2+} entry and exit is positive during skeletal growth in children, zero in young adults, and negative in the elderly. Exchangeable skeletal Ca^{2+} contributes to maintaining extracellular Ca^{2+} homeostasis. Several growth factors, hormones, and genetic factors participate in the differentiation from the mesenchymal precursor cell to the

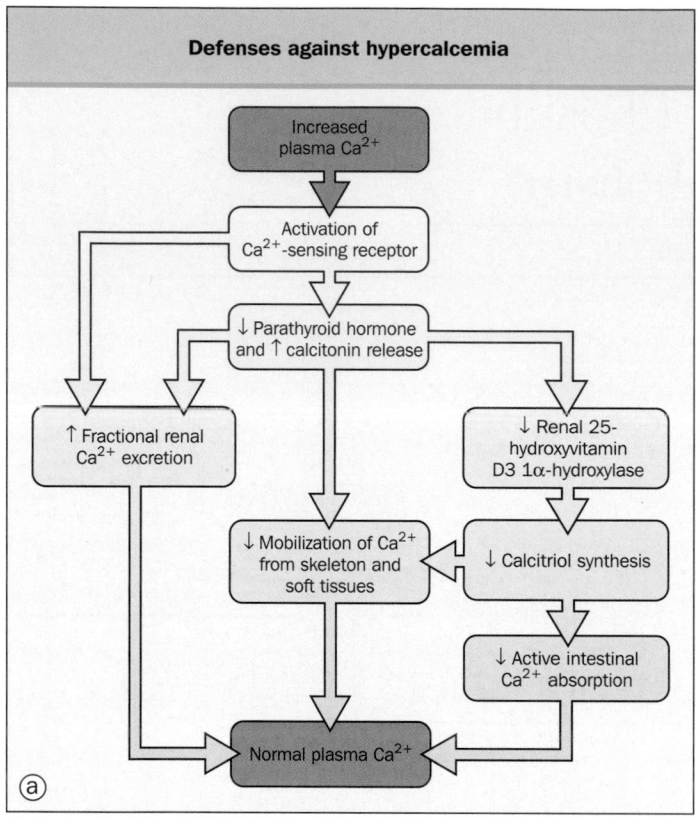

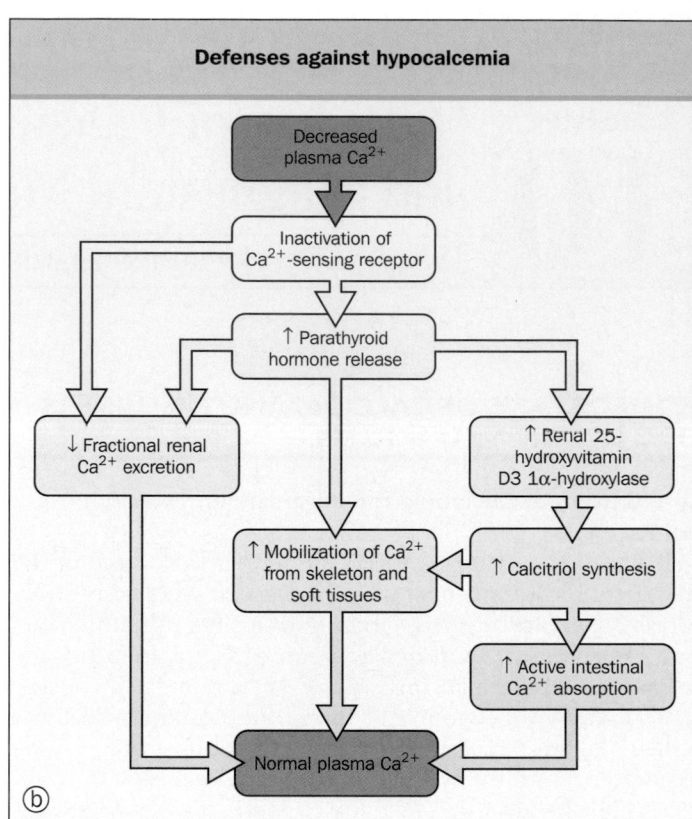

Figure 10.2 Physiologic defense mechanisms to counter changes in serum calcium. (a) Hypercalcemia. (b) Hypocalcemia. (Adapted with permission from Kumar R. Vitamin D and calcium transport. Kidney Int. 1991;40:1177–89.)

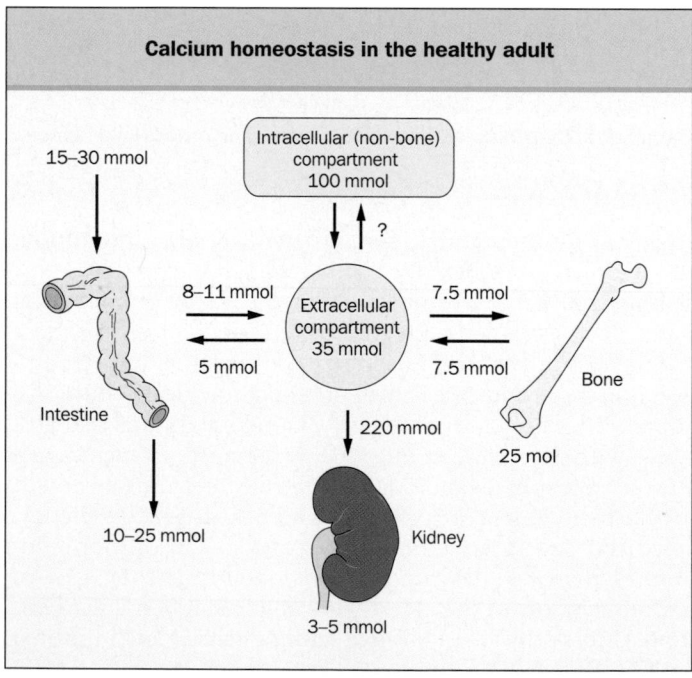

Figure 10.3 Calcium homeostasis in the healthy adult. Net zero Ca^{2+} balance is the result of net intestinal absorption (absorption minus secretion) and urinary excretion, which, by definition are the same. After its passage into the extracellular fluid, Ca^{2+} enters the extracellular space, is deposited in bone, or is eliminated via the kidneys. Entry and exit fluxes between the extra- and intracellular space (skeletal and nonskeletal compartments) are also of identical magnitude under steady-state conditions.

osteoblast (see Fig. 10.6). The regulation of bone formation and resorption also involves a large number of hormones, cytokines, and growth factors (see Fig. 10.7)[4,5].

The kidneys play a major role in the short-term, minute by minute regulation (see Fig. 10.8), while the intestine and the skeleton assure homeostasis in the mid and long term. The adjustment of blood Ca^{2+} is mainly achieved by modulation of tubular Ca^{2+} reabsorption in response to the body's needs, perfectly compensating minor increases or decreases in the filtered load of Ca at the glomerular level, which is normally about 220 mmol (8800 mg) in 24 h (see Fig. 10.3). In the proximal tubule, most of the Ca^{2+} is reabsorbed by convective flow (as for Na^+ and water) whereas in the distal segments of the tubule, the transport mechanisms are more complex. In the thick ascending loop, the transport of Ca^{2+} is primarily passive via the paracellular route, depending on the electrical gradient with the tubular lumen being positive, and also on the presence of claudin-16 in the tight junction. At this step, Ca^{2+} transport is regulated by the extracellular Ca^{2+} concentration, involving the Ca^{2+}-sensing receptor (CaR_G). In the distal tubule, Ca^{2+} transport is primarily active via the transcellular route, through a recently identified Ca channel (EcaC1) located in the apical membrane and coupled with a specific basolateral Ca-ATPase (PMCa1b) and a Na^+/Ca^{2+} exchanger. This step is regulated by PTH and calcitriol.

The factors that regulate the glomerular filtration and tubular reabsorption of Ca^{2+} are numerous[6,7]. Elevated renal blood flow and glomerular filtration pressure (during extracellular fluid volume expansion) lead to an increase in filtered load, as

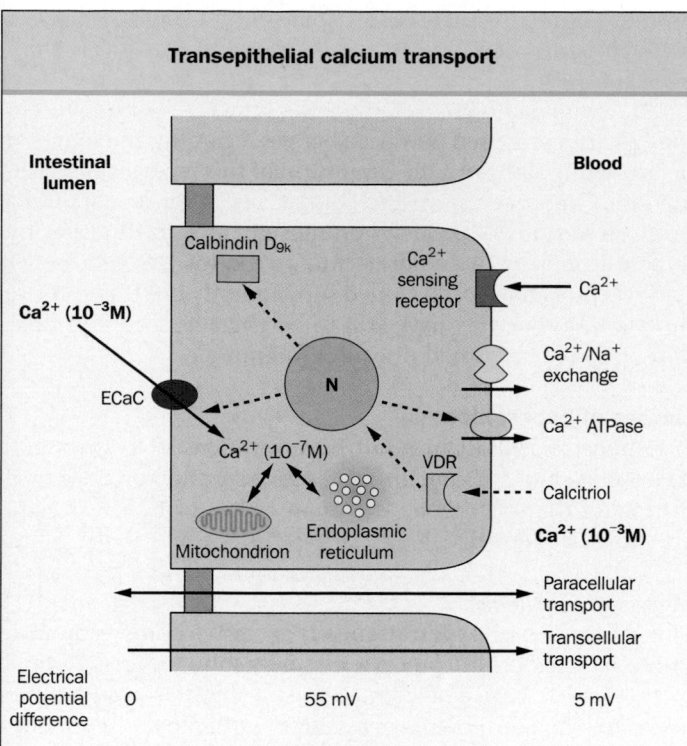

Figure 10.4 Transepithelial calcium transport in the small intestine. Calcium penetrates into the enterocyte via a recently discovered calcium channel (ECaC) via the brush border membrane along a favorable electrochemical gradient. Under physiologic conditions the cation is pumped out of the cell at the basolateral side against a steep electrochemical gradient by the ATP-consuming pump, Ca^{2+} ATPase. When there is a major elevation of intracytoplasmic Ca^{2+} the cation leaves the cell using the Ca^{2+}/Na^+ exchanger. Passive Ca^{2+} influx as well as efflux are sensitive to calcitriol.

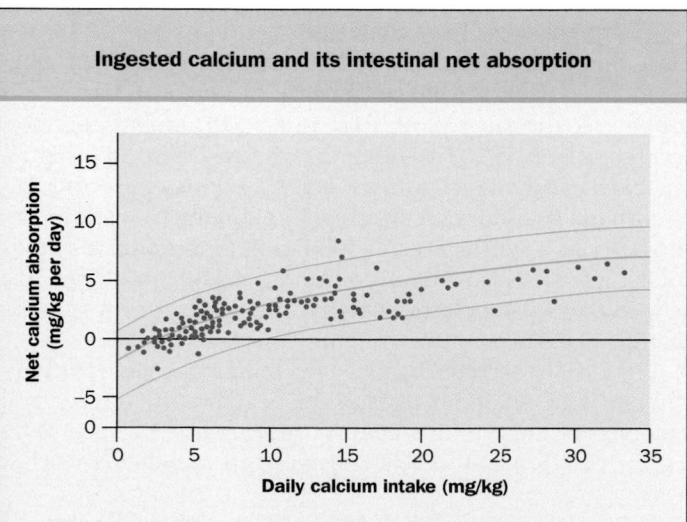

Figure 10.5 Relationship between ingested calcium and its absorption in the intestinal tract (net) in healthy young adults. (With permission from Wilkinson R. Absorption of calcium, phosphorus, and magnesium. In: Nordin BEC, ed. Calcium and magnesium metabolism. Edinburgh: Churchill Livingstone; 1976;36–112.)

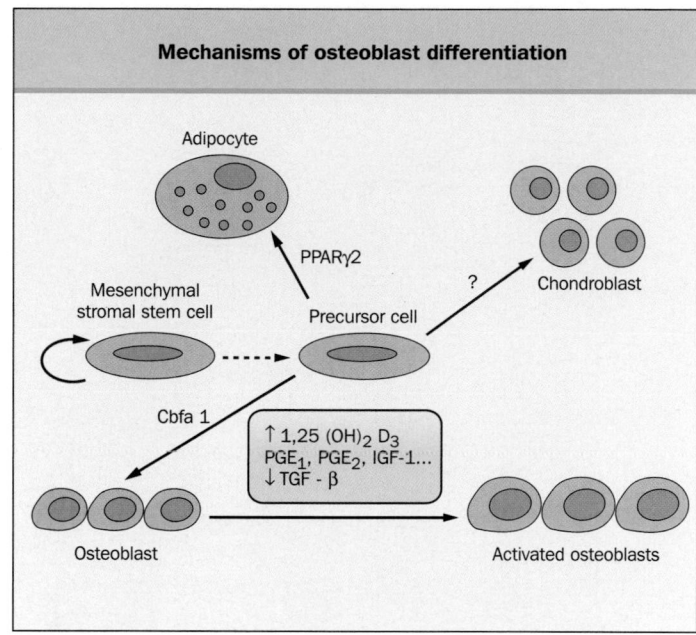

Figure 10.6 The major growth factors, and hormones controlling in the differentiation from the mesenchymal precursor cell to the osteoblast.

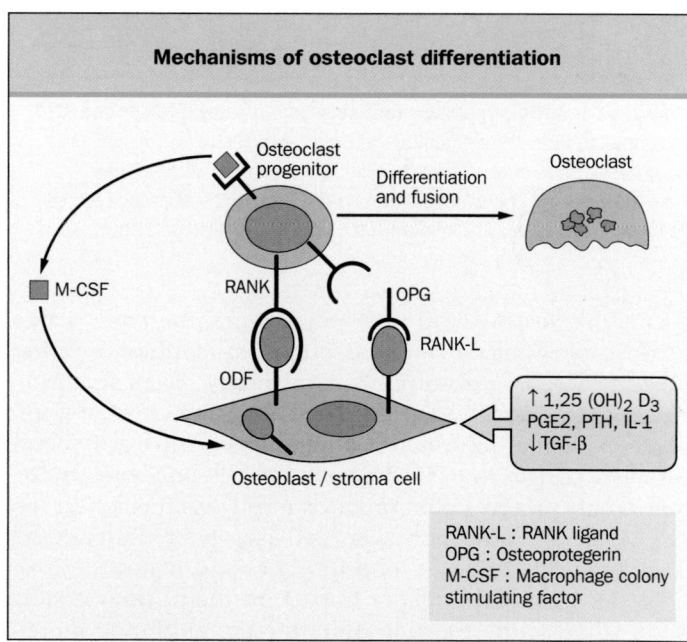

Figure 10.7 The major growth factors, cytokines and hormones controlling osteoblast and osteoclast activity.

do changes in the ultrafiltration coefficient K_f and an increase in glomerular surface. True hypercalcemia also increases ultra-filterable Ca whereas true hypocalcemia decreases it. PTH decreases glomerular K_f and thus reduces the ultrafiltered Ca load; it also increases Ca^{2+} reabsorption in the distal nephron. However, PTH and PTHrp (PTH-related peptide) also induce hypercalcemia and, because of the increase in serum Ca, the excretion of filtered Ca is elevated overall. Metabolic and

Fluid and Electrolyte Disorders

Calcium reabsorption in the kidney

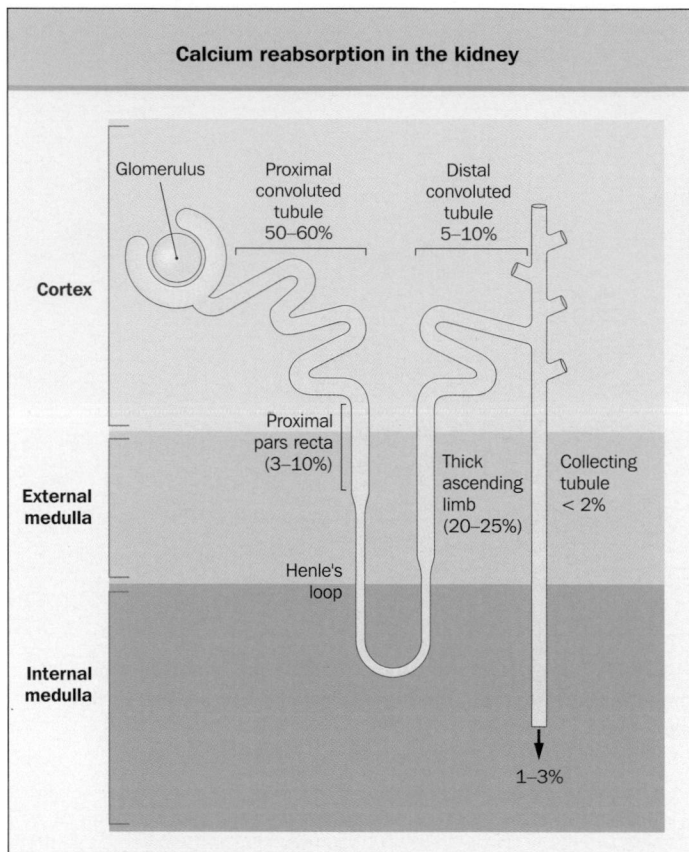

Figure 10.8 Sites of calcium reabsorption in various segments of the renal tubule. The percentage of Ca2+ absorbed in various sections following glomerular ultrafiltration is shown. (With permission from Puschett JB. Renal handling of calcium. In: Massry SG, Glassock RJ, eds. Textbook of nephrology. Baltimore, MD: Williams & Wilkins; 1989:293–9.)

respiratory acidosis lead to hypercalciuria, the latter via an increase in plasma Ca^{2+} and the former via an inhibitory effect on tubular Ca^{2+} reabsorption. Conversely, alkali ingestion reduces renal excretion of Ca. The enhancing effect of phosphate depletion on urinary Ca elimination can partly occur through changes in PTH and calcitriol secretion. Dietary factors modify urinary excretion of Ca mostly via their effects on intestinal Ca^{2+} absorption. Several classes of diuretics act directly on the tubules: loop diuretics and mannitol favor hypercalciuria, with a major impact on the thick ascending limb, whereas the thiazide diuretics and amiloride induce hypocalciuria.

HYPERCALCEMIA

Increased plasma total Ca concentration can result from an increase in plasma proteins ('false hypercalcemia') or from an increase in plasma ionized Ca^{2+} ('true hypercalcemia'). Only the latter leads to clinically relevant hypercalcemia. When only the value for the total plasma Ca is available rather than the free level ions, as is generally the case in clinical practice, plasma Ca^{2+} can be estimated by taking into account plasma albumin. This will give an estimate of how much Ca is

protein bound: an increase of albumin of 1.0 g/dL reflects a concomitant increase of 0.20–0.25 mmol/L (0.8–1.0 mg/dL) plasma Ca.

The cloning and characterization of the Ca^{2+}-sensing receptor CaR_G has provided new perspectives regarding the function of circulating Ca^{2+}, and the expression of this receptor has been identified in numerous tissues[8]. Mutations of the gene for CaR_G result in various clinical syndromes characterized either by hypercalcemia or by hypocalcemia (see below). Several other Ca^{2+} receptors have been cloned subsequently but their precise functional properties have still to be characterized and their potential role in human disease is unknown.

Causes of hypercalcemia

True hypercalcemia can result from an increase in intestinal Ca^{2+} absorption, a stimulation of bone resorption or a decrease in urinary Ca^{2+} excretion. The main causes of hypercalcemia are shown in Fig. 10.9.

Malignant neoplasias

The main cause of hypercalcemia is excessive bone resorption induced by neoplastic processes, usually solid tumors. Tumors of the breast, lung and kidney are the most common, followed by hematopoietic neoplasias, particularly myeloma; other types of lymphoma and leukemia cause hypercalcemia more rarely.

Most hypercalcemic tumors act on the skeleton either by direct invasion (metastases) or by producing factors that stimulate osteoclastic activity. The most important osteoclastic factor is PTHrp[9], others include osteoclastic activity factor (OAF), transforming growth factors (TGFs), prostaglandin E, rarely calcitriol and tumor necrosis factor-α (TNF-α) and very rarely PTH. Parathyroid cancer is an extremely infrequent cause of hypercalcemia. Its precise diagnosis is now possible, as a result of the discovery that it is associated with allelic loss in the retinoblastoma (RB) tumor-suppressor gene[10].

PTHrp has been fully characterized[9]. Only 8 of its 13 first amino acids are identical with those of the N-terminal fragment of PTH, but the effects of both hormones on target cells are mostly the same. Both PTH and PTHrp bind a common receptor (the PTH/PTHrp receptor) whereas a second receptor, the PTH_2 receptor, recognizes solely PTH, with similar or identical signal transduction systems. In pathological conditions, most PTHrp is synthesized by solid tumors, although its physiologic synthesis is widespread. Among its numerous actions, it stimulates osteoclastic activity and thus liberates excess quantities of Ca from the skeleton.

The OAF are secreted by myeloma plasmocytes and the lymphoblasts of malignant lymphomas. They include several members of the cytokine family, interleukins (ILs) such as IL-1α, IL-1β, IL-6, and also TNF, which can all stimulate osteoclast activity.

Prostaglandins of the E series (PGE_1 and PGE_2) can be secreted in large amounts by some tumors. They are also capable of stimulating osteoclastic resorption.

Some lymphoid tumors synthesize excess quantities of calcitriol. This capacity has been described in Hodgkin's disease, T-cell lymphoma and leiomyoblastoma.

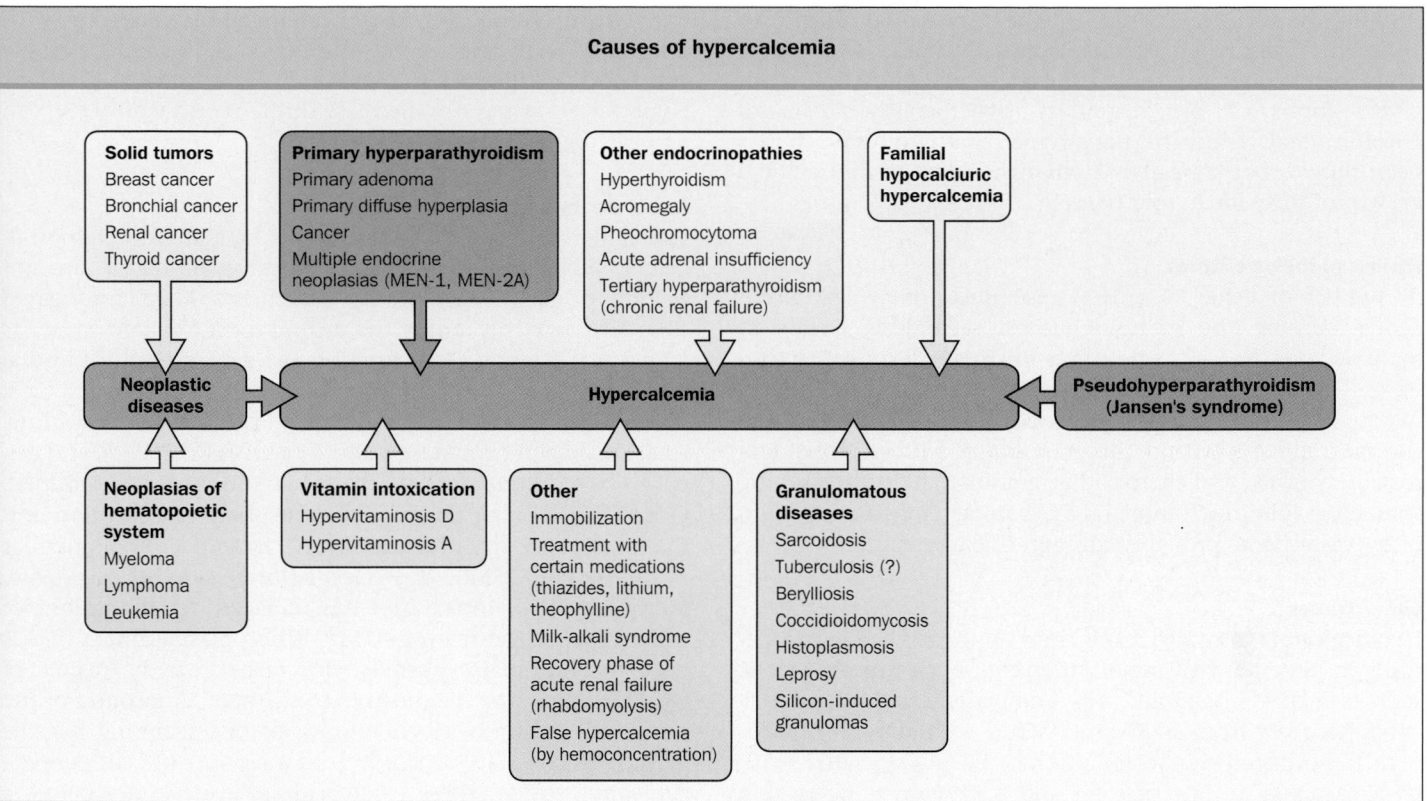

Figure 10.9 Causes of hypercalcemia. (With permission from Puschett JB. Renal handling of calcium. In: Massry SG, Glassock RJ, eds. Textbook of nephrology. Baltimore, MD: Williams & Wilkins; 1989:293–9.)

Primary hyperparathyroidism

The second most common cause of hypercalcemia is primary hyperparathyroidism. Early diagnosis is now achieved through the widespread use of routine plasma Ca determination. In over 80% of cases, the disease is caused by adenoma of a single parathyroid gland; in 10–15% there is diffuse hyperplasia of four or more glands, and in less than 5% a parathyroid cancer. Primary hyperparathyroidism can be inherited either as diffuse hyperplasia of the parathyroid glands alone or as a component in multiple glandular hereditary endocrine disorders. Patients with multiple endocrine neoplasia type 1 (MEN1) have various combinations of parathyroid, anterior pituitary, enteropancreatic, and other endocrine tumors, resulting in hypersecretion of prolactin and gastrin, in addition to PTH. This disease is caused by inactivating germ-line mutations of a tumor-suppressor gene (the *MEN1* gene) that is inherited as an autosomal dominant inherited trait. In the multiple endocrine neoplasia type 2 (MEN2A), the thyroid medulla and the adrenal medulla are involved with the parathyroid, resulting in hypersecretion of calcitonin and catecholamines. This disease is caused by activating mutations of the *RET* proto-oncogene. It is also inherited as an autosomal dominant inherited trait. Not all patients with mildly elevated plasma PTH levels develop hypercalcemia. The development of the latter may depend on a concomitant elevation of plasma calcitriol.

Jansen's syndrome

Jansen's syndrome is a rare hereditary form of short-limbed dwarfism, characterized by severe hypercalcemia, hypophosphatemia, and metaphyseal chondrodysplasia[11]. It is the result of activating mutations of the gene for the PTH/PTHrp receptor, a particular form of pseudohyperparathyroidism.

Familial hypocalciuric hypercalcemia

Familial hypocalciuric hypercalcemia is a hereditary disease with autosomal dominant transmission. It is characterized by moderate chronic hypercalcemia associated with hypophosphatemia, hyperchloremia and hypermagnesemia. Plasma PTH concentration is normal or moderately elevated. The fractional excretion of Ca is lower than observed in hyperparathyroidism, and the urine calcium : creatinine ratio (mg : mg) is usually less than 0.01. In patients suffering from this syndrome, hypercalcemia never leads to severe clinical signs (except during the neonatal period, in which malignant hypercalcemia can be observed in the context of severe hyperparathyroidism). This hereditary disease is due to inactivating mutations in the gene for CaR_G[12].

Other endocrine causes

Other endocrine disorders can be associated with moderate hypercalcemia, such as hyperthyroidism, acromegaly and pheochromocytoma. In addition, acute adrenal insufficiency should also be considered in the differential diagnosis, although here hypercalcemia is usually 'false' and results from hemoconcentration. Hypercalcemia also occurs in severe forms of the secondary hyperparathyroidism of chronic renal failure (tertiary hyperparathyroidism). It has been shown that the latter is often the result of monoclonal growth of the parathyroid tissue[13].

Various pathologic states

A number of other disorders sometimes involve hypercalcemia. Among the granulomatoses, sarcoidosis results in increased plasma Ca^{2+} particularly in patients exposed to sunlight. The cause is uncontrolled production of calcitriol by macrophages (owing to the presence of the 1α-hydroxylase in the macrophages within the granulomas). Tuberculosis, leprosy, berylliosis, and many other granulomatous diseases are sometimes (but much more rarely than sarcoidosis), the origin of hypercalcemia, probably through the same mechanism.

Other causes

Hypercalcemia may also result from prolonged bed rest (especially in patients with pre-existing high bone turnover rates, such as in children, adolescents, and patients with Paget's disease). Recovery from acute renal failure secondary to rhabdomyolysis-induced renal failure has been associated with hypercalcemia in 25% of cases and is thought to occur as a consequence of mobilization of soft tissue calcium deposits and through increases in PTH and calcitriol levels. Other causes include intoxication by vitamin D or one of its derivatives, vitamin A overload, and treatment by thiazide diuretics. Large doses of Ca (5–10 g/day), especially when ingested with alkali (antacids), can also lead to hypercalcemia and nephrocalcinosis (milk-alkali syndrome).

Clinical manifestations

The severity of clinical symptoms and signs caused by hypercalcemia depends not only on its degree but also on the velocity of its development. Rather severe hypercalcemia can be accompanied by few manifestations in some patients because of its slow, progressive development, whereas much less severe hypercalcemia can lead to major disorders if it develops rapidly.

Generally, the first symptoms are increasing fatigue, muscle weakness, nervousness, and other general manifestations. Subsequently, gastrointestinal signs may occur, such as constipation, nausea, and vomiting, and, rarely, peptic ulcer disease or pancreatitis. Renal-related signs include polyuria (secondary to nephrogenic diabetes insipidus), urinary tract stones and their complications, and occasionally tubulointerstitial disease with medullary and to a lesser extent cortical deposition of Ca (nephrocalcinosis). Neuropsychiatric manifestations include headache, loss of memory, somnolence, and stupor, and, rarely, coma. Ocular symptoms include conjunctivitis from crystal deposition and, rarely, band keratopathy. Osteoarticular pain in primary hyperparathyroidism has become rare in Western countries because of the generally early diagnosis of hypercalcemia. High blood pressure can be induced by hypercalcemia, but it is more frequently a chance association. Soft tissue calcifications can occur with long-standing hypercalcemia. The electrocardiogram may show shortening of the Q-T interval and 'coving' of the ST wave. Hypercalcemia may also increase cardiac contractility and can amplify digitalis toxicity.

Laboratory and causal diagnosis

The underlying cause should always be sought in hypercalcemia. When the history and clinical examination are not helpful, primary hyperparathyroidism should be investigated first. Although this is only the second most frequent cause, its laboratory diagnosis is at present easier than that of tumoral involvement. In addition to total plasma Ca and ionized Ca^{2+}, plasma albumin (or total protein), phosphate, creatinine, total alkaline phosphatases, and intact PTH (PTH_{1-84}), and urinary Ca, phosphate, and creatinine should be determined. From these results, the tubular phosphate reabsorption and the maximum amount reabsorbed factored for glomerular filtration rate (GFR), T_mP (see below), can be calculated. Measurement of intact PTH has replaced determinations of urinary nephrogenic cyclic AMP. When plasma intact PTH is high or abnormally normal with respect to the degree of hypercalcemia, the diagnosis is confirmed. Ultrasound of the neck and sesta-mibi (technetium) isotope scanning may be performed to locate a parathyroid adenoma but, in general, surgeons consider these examinations unnecessary before a first neck exploration. However, they are indispensable in case of recurrent hyperparathyroidism. If the plasma PTH level is low-normal or low, the possibility of a neoplastic disorder should be seriously considered. A low serum anion gap may be a clue to multiple myeloma (because occasionally the monoclonal IgG is positively charged). In addition to the usual examinations such as serum protein electrophoresis (SPEP), measurement of plasma PTHrp level can now be done in specialized laboratories. Exogenous vitamin D overload is associated with increased serum 25-hydroxyvitamin D levels, and granulomatous diseases such as sarcoidosis are associated with elevated calcitriol levels and with increased serum angiotensin-converting enzyme (ACE) activity.

Treatment

Treatment is aimed at the underlying cause. However, severe and symptomatic hypercalcemia requires rapid, effective treatment, whatever the cause. Initially, the patient must be rapidly rehydrated with isotonic saline to correct the often marked dehydration. Then loop diuretics can be used, for example intravenous furosemide (frusemide) at 100 to 200 mg every other hour, in order to facilitate urinary excretion of Ca. Oral intake and intravenous administration of fluids and electrolytes should be carefully monitored, and urinary, fecal, and gastric excretions measured if excessive, especially those of K, Mg and phosphate. Acid–base balance should also be carefully monitored. Severe cardiac failure or renal insufficiency are contraindications to massive extracellular fluid volume expansion in conjunction with diuretics.

Bisphosphonates have progressively become the treatment of first choice, especially in hypercalcemia associated with cancer[14]. They inhibit bone resorption as well as calcitriol synthesis. They can be administered orally in less severe disease or intravenously in severe hypercalcemia. The most frequently used bisphosphonates are clodronate (1600–3200 mg/day orally or 300 mg/day intravenously), pamidronate (15–90 mg/day intravenously), and alendronate (10 mg/day intravenously). For intravenous administration, doses should be infused in 500 mL isotonic saline or dextrose over at least 2 h and up to 24 h.

Calcitonin is theoretically an ideal drug for the treatment of hypercalcemia. Its effect is rapid (within hours), in particular after intravenous administration. Human, porcine, or salmon calcitonin can be given. Doses vary depending on the type of calcitonin used, for instance subcutaneous or intramuscular porcine calcitonin 4 IU/kg daily in two to four injections, or intravenous salmon calcitonin 4–8 IU/kg/day in 500 mL isotonic saline over 6 h. In clinical practice, however, calcitonin often has no effect or only a short-term effect because of the rapid development of tachyphylaxis.

Mitomycin (mitomycin C) is a cytostatic drug having a remarkable power to inhibit bone resorption. Administration of a single intravenous dose is generally followed by a rapid decline in plasma calcium within a few hours, and this effect lasts several days. However, its use is reserved for malignant hypercalcemia, and its cytotoxic effect and side effects (thrombocytopenia and liver function abnormalities) preclude prolonged administration. The maximal daily dose is 25 µg/kg.

Steroids (0.5–1.0 mg/kg prednisone daily) are mainly indicated in hypervitaminosis D of endogenous origin, such as sarcoidosis and tuberculosis, and of exogenous origin, such as vitamin D intoxication. The use of ketoconazole, an antifungal agent that can inhibit renal and extrarenal calcitriol synthesis and thus lower plasma calcitriol levels, has also been proposed in hypervitaminosis D.

Steroids can also be tried in treatment of hypercalcemia associated with some hematopoietic tumors such as myeloma and lymphoma, and even for some solid tumors such as breast cancer. Of course, prolonged treatment with corticosteroids exposes patients to the classic risks of such therapy.

In rare cases of malignant hypercalcemia, treatment with prostaglandin antagonists, for example indomethacin or aspirin, can be successful. Hyperkalemia and renal insufficiency my occur with indomethacin.

In moderate and nonsymptomatic hypercalcemia secondary to primary hyperparathyroidism, treatment with estrogens can also be tried, at least in females. Hypercalcemia caused by thyrotoxicosis can rapidly resolve with intravenous administration of propranolol, or less rapidly with oral administration.

A new, promising class of CaR agonists ('calcimimetics') is presently under clinical evaluation for the medical treatment of hyperparathyroidism. Short-term studies have shown that the calcimimetic drug R-568 can acutely reduce serum PTH and Ca^{2+} concentrations in hyperparathyroid postmenopausal women[15]. In uremic patients with secondary hyperparathyroidism, short-term experience from phase II studies with the calcimimetic drug R-568[16] have reported a reduction in plasma PTH of at least 30% and with a reduction in the Ca x phosphate product.

HYPOCALCEMIA

As with hypercalcemia, hypocalcemia can be secondary either to a change (reduction in this case) in plasma albumin ('false hypocalcemia') or to a change in ionized Ca^{2+} ('true hypocalcemia'). False hypocalcemia can be excluded by directly measuring ionized Ca^{2+}, by determining plasma total protein or albumin levels, by the clinical context, or by other laboratory results. Acute hypocalcemia is often observed during acute hyperventilation and the respiratory alkalosis that follows, regardless of the cause of hyperventilation. Hyperventilation can occur secondary to cardiopulmonary or cerebral diseases.

Causes of chronic hypocalcemia

After excluding false hypocalcemia linked to hypoalbuminemia, hypocalcemia can be divided into that associated with elevated or low plasma phosphate. The former is caused by hypoparathyroid states that are idiopathic or acquired (following surgery or radiotherapy, or secondary to AA amyloidosis). Sporadic cases of hypoparathyroidism can occasionally be seen in patients with pernicious anemia or adrenal insufficiency. Pseudohypoparathyroidism (Albright's hereditary osteodystrophy) is characterized by a particular phenotype (short neck, round face, and short metacarpals) with end-organ resistance to PTH. Chronic renal insufficiency, acute renal failure in its oligoanuric phase (such as secondary to rhabdomyolysis), and massive phosphate administration can also lead to hypocalcemia with hyperphosphatemia. At least one form of inherited, familial hypocalcemia is linked to activating mutations of CaR_G[12]. Hypocalcemia associated with low plasma phosphate may occur from vitamin D-deficient states. These can themselves be secondary to insufficient sunlight exposure, dietary deficiency of vitamin D, decreased absorption following gastrointestinal surgery, intestinal malabsorption syndromes (steatorrhea), or hepatobiliary disease (primary biliary cirrhosis). Magnesium deficiency may also result in hypocalcemia, often in conjunction with hypokalemia. The low serum Ca^{2+} appears to result from decreased PTH release and end-organ resistance. Acute renal failure in the polyuric phase may also be associated with hypocalcemia and hypophosphatemia. The main causes of hypocalcemia are shown in Figure 10.10.

Clinical manifestations

As with hypercalcemia, the symptoms of hypocalcemia depend as much on the rate of its occurrence as on the degree of reduction of plasma Ca^{2+}. The most common manifestations, in addition to fatigue and muscular weakness, are increased irritability, loss of memory, a state of confusion, hallucination, paranoia, and depression. The best known clinical signs are Chvostek's and Trousseau's signs. In acute hypocalcemia, there may be paresthesias of the lips and the extremities, muscle cramps, and sometimes frank tetany, laryngeal stridor, or convulsions. Chronic hypocalcemia can be associated with cataracts, brittle nails with transverse grooves, dry skin, and decreased, or even absent, axillary and pubic hair, especially in idiopathic hypoparathyroidism, which is often of autoimmune origin.

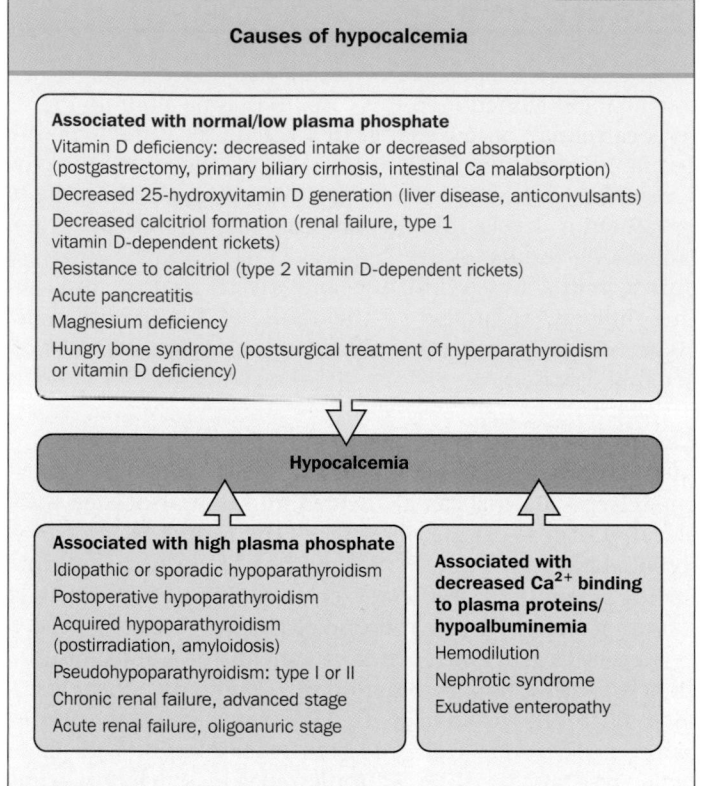

Causes of hypocalcemia

Associated with normal/low plasma phosphate
Vitamin D deficiency: decreased intake or decreased absorption (postgastrectomy, primary biliary cirrhosis, intestinal Ca malabsorption)
Decreased 25-hydroxyvitamin D generation (liver disease, anticonvulsants)
Decreased calcitriol formation (renal failure, type 1 vitamin D-dependent rickets)
Resistance to calcitriol (type 2 vitamin D-dependent rickets)
Acute pancreatitis
Magnesium deficiency
Hungry bone syndrome (postsurgical treatment of hyperparathyroidism or vitamin D deficiency)

Hypocalcemia

Associated with high plasma phosphate
Idiopathic or sporadic hypoparathyroidism
Postoperative hypoparathyroidism
Acquired hypoparathyroidism (postirradiation, amyloidosis)
Pseudohypoparathyroidism: type I or II
Chronic renal failure, advanced stage
Acute renal failure, oligoanuric stage

Associated with decreased Ca^{2+} binding to plasma proteins/hypoalbuminemia
Hemodilution
Nephrotic syndrome
Exudative enteropathy

Figure 10.10 Causes of hypocalcemia.

Laboratory and radiologic signs

Alterations in plasma and urinary electrolytes as well as in plasma intact PTH depend on the underlying cause. Plasma phosphate is elevated in hypoparathyroidism, pseudohypoparathyroidism, and advanced renal failure, whereas it is decreased in steatorrhea, vitamin D deficiency, acute pancreatitis, and the polyuric phase during recovery from acute renal failure. Plasma PTH is reduced in hypoparathyroidism and also during chronic magnesium deficiency, whereas it is normal or increased in pseudo-hypoparathyroidism and in chronic renal failure. Urinary Ca excretion is increased only in the treatment of hypoparathyroidism with calcium supplements and vitamin D derivatives ; it is low in all other cases of hypocalcemia. Fractional urinary Ca excretion is, however, high in hypoparathyroidism, in the polyuric phase during recovery from acute renal failure, and in severe chronic renal failure; it is low in all other cases of hypocalcemia. Urinary phosphate excretion is low in hypoparathyroidism, pseudohypoparathyroidism, and magnesium deficiency; it is high in vitamin D deficiency, steatorrhea, chronic renal failure, and during phosphate administration. Determination of serum 25-hydroxyvitamin D and calcitriol levels may also be useful.

Intracranial calcifications, notably of the basal ganglia, are observed radiologically in 20% of patients with idiopathic hypoparathyroidism, but much less frequently in patients with postsurgical hypoparathyroidism or pseudohypoparathyroidism.

On ECG, the corrected Q-T interval is frequently prolonged, and there are sometimes arrythmias. Electroencephalography shows nonspecific signs such as an increase in slow, high-voltage waves.

Treatment

As for hypercalcemia, the basic treatment is that of the underlying cause. Severe and symptomatic (tetany) hypocalcemia requires rapid and appropriate treatment. Acute respiratory alkalosis, if present, should be corrected if possible. When the cause is functional, the simple retention of carbon dioxide, for example by breathing into a paper bag, may suffice. In other cases and to obtain a prolonged effect, intravenous infusion of Ca salts is most often required. In the setting of seizures or tetany, calcium gluconate should be administered as a bolus (for instance 10 mL of a 10% solution which contains 90 mg Ca ions or 4.4 mmol) followed by 12–24 g over 24 h in 5% dextrose or isotonic saline. Calcium gluconate is preferred to calcium chloride because of its better clinical tolerance. Intravenously administered calcium chloride can lead to extensive skin necrosis in accidental extravasation.

Treatment of chronic hypocalcemia includes oral administration of varying doses of calcium salts, thiazide diuretics, or vitamin D. Several oral forms of Ca are available, each with their advantages and disadvantages. It should be remembered that the amount of elemental Ca of the various salts differs greatly. For example, the Ca content is 40% in carbonate, 36% in chloride, 12% in lactate, and only 8% in gluconate salts. The daily amount prescribed can be 2–4 g elemental Ca. Concurrent Mg deficiency (serum $Mg^{2+} < 0.75$ mmol/L) should be treated either with oral magnesium oxide (250–500 mg q6d) or with magnesium sulfate: intramuscular (4–8 mmol/day) or intravenous (for instance 12 mL 50% magnesium sulfate in 1000 mL 5% dextrose over 3–4 h).

Treatment of hypocalcemia secondary to hypoparathyroidism is difficult as urinary Ca excretion increases markedly with Ca supplementation and can lead to nephrocalcinosis and loss of renal function. To reduce renal Ca wasting, treatment often consists of adding thiazide diuretics in association with restricted sodium chloride intake.

Lastly, treatment with vitamin D, or rather its most active metabolite, calcitriol or its analog, 1α-hydroxycholecalciferol 0.25–1.0 µg/day, is the treatment of choice at present for idiopathic or acquired hypoparathyroidism, because these compounds are more easily taken by the patients than massive doses of Ca salts. Administration of vitamin D derivatives generally leads to hypercalciuria and, rarely, to nephrocalcinosis. It requires regular monitoring in order to avoid induction of hypercalcemia and renal disease.

HOMEOSTASIS OF PHOSPHATE

Distribution of phosphate in the organism and phosphate homeostasis

Phosphorus and Ca are the most abundant components of the skeleton. However, phosphate is also one of the main components of soft tissues and forms an integral part of the various cell structures. It is present in intra- and extracellular fluids and participates, directly or indirectly, in most metabolic processes. Phosphorus is found in the organism both as mineral phosphate and organic phosphate (phosphoric esters). The phosphate contained in laboratory samples (food, plasma, urine, feces, tissues) is generally expressed in terms of

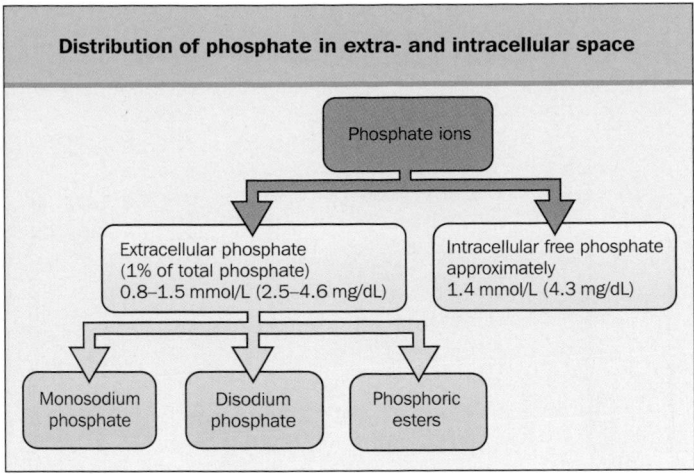

Distribution of phosphate in extra- and intracellular space

Figure 10.11 Distribution of phosphate in extra- and intracellular space.

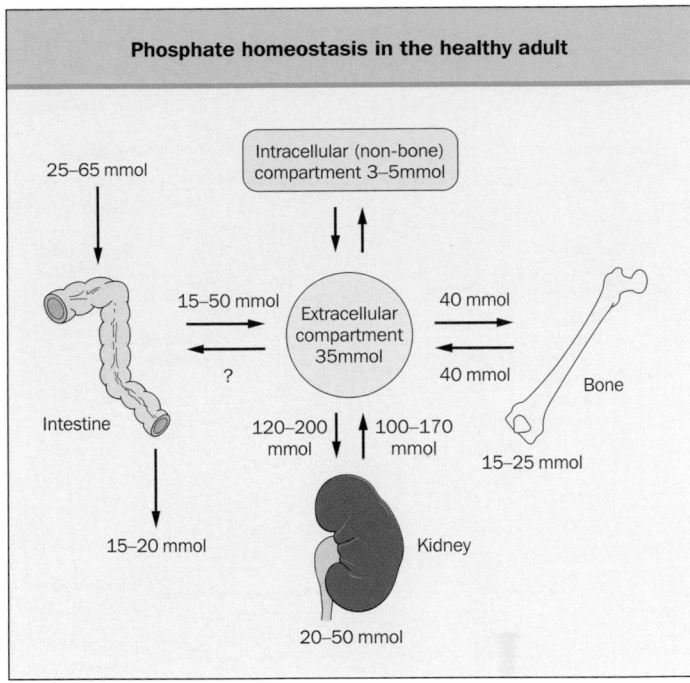

Phosphate homeostasis in the healthy adult

Figure 10.12 Phosphate homeostasis in healthy young adults. At net zero balance. Identical net intestinal uptake (absorption minus secretion) and urinary loss occurs. After its passage into the extracellular fluid, phosphate enters the intracellular space, is deposited in bone or soft tissue, or is eliminated via the kidneys. Entry and exit fluxes between the extra- and intracellular space (skeletal and nonskeletal compartments) are also the same under steady-state conditions.

elemental phosphorus. Phosphorus is, however, transported across cell membranes in the form of phosphate (31 mg/L elemental phosphorus = 1 mmol/L phosphorus in the form of phosphate). Figure 10.11 shows the distribution of phosphate in the extra- and intracellular fluid compartments.

Short-term variations in plasma phosphate are controlled by calciotropic hormones such as PTH and calcitriol. The existence of a specific hormone modulating phosphate has long been suspected and given the preliminary designation 'phosphatonin'. Recently, evidence has been provided that fibroblast growth factor-23 (FGF23) is the elusive phosphate regulatory hormone[17].

There are wide daily variations in blood phosphate levels, depending especially on food intake but also on dietary carbohydrates (negatively) and blood pH. Long-term maintenance of phosphate homeostasis depends mainly on the adaptability of renal tubular reabsorption of phosphate to the needs of the organism. Chronic deficiency in phosphate intake first leads to hypophosphatemia, then to intracellular depletion of phosphate. By comparison, hyperphosphatemia occurs in advanced renal failure even when dietary intake remains within normal limits.

Figure 10.12 shows the balance of ingestion, body distribution, and excretion of phosphate in a healthy human. A young adult requires around 0.5 mmol/kg phosphate daily. These needs are much higher in the child during growth. Phosphates are widely found in milk products, meat, eggs, and cereals.

Phosphate entrance into transport epithelia involves a secondary active Na+/phosphate cotransport. Three different Na+/phosphate cotransporters have been identified[18]. Type I cotransporter is present in the renal tubule and may also show anion channel function. Type II cotransporters serve rather specific epithelial functions, type IIa in the brush border of the proximal tubule and type IIb in the brush border of the small intestine, determining Na+-dependent phosphate reabsorption. Type III cotransporters are ubiquitous and could serve housekeeping functions. Type II cotransporters are regulated by altered phosphate intake, PTH, calcitriol, and pH. The exit of phosphate at the basolateral side probably occurs by both passive diffusion and anionic exchange.

The transcellular transport of phosphate is in addition controlled by several other metabolic, hormonal, and autocrine/paracrine factors, including growth hormone, insulin-like growth factor (IGF-1), insulin, and thyroid hormone[19].

Intestinal, skeletal and renal handling of phosphate

Phosphate transport across the intestinal wall occurs by both the transepithelial and the paracellular route (Fig. 10.13), most of it via Na+/phosphate cotransport. Absorption is a linear, non saturable function of phosphate intake (Fig. 10.14) and amounts to 60–75% of intake (15–50 mmol/day). Many factors affect phosphate uptake. Calcitriol stimulates Na+/phosphate cotransport whereas high Ca2+ concentrations decrease phosphate absorption.

Bone permanently exchanges phosphate with the surrounding milieu. Entry and exit of phosphate amount to about 100 mmol/day (slowly exchangeable phosphate), for a total skeleton content of about 19 000 mmol. The net balance is positive during growth, zero in the young adult, and negative in the elderly.

The kidneys play a major role in controlling extracellular phosphate homeostasis[18,19]. Normally, the daily amount of phosphate eliminated in urine equals that absorbed in the intestine. It usually comprises 5–20% of ultrafiltered phosphate. The amount of phosphate reabsorbed can be expressed in relation to the amount filtered as TRP which is calculated as $(1 - (C_p/GFR)) \times 100$, where C_p is phosphate clearance. TRP also equals $1 - (U_p S_{cr}/S_p U_{cr})$ where U_p S_p U_{cr} and S_{cr} are urinary

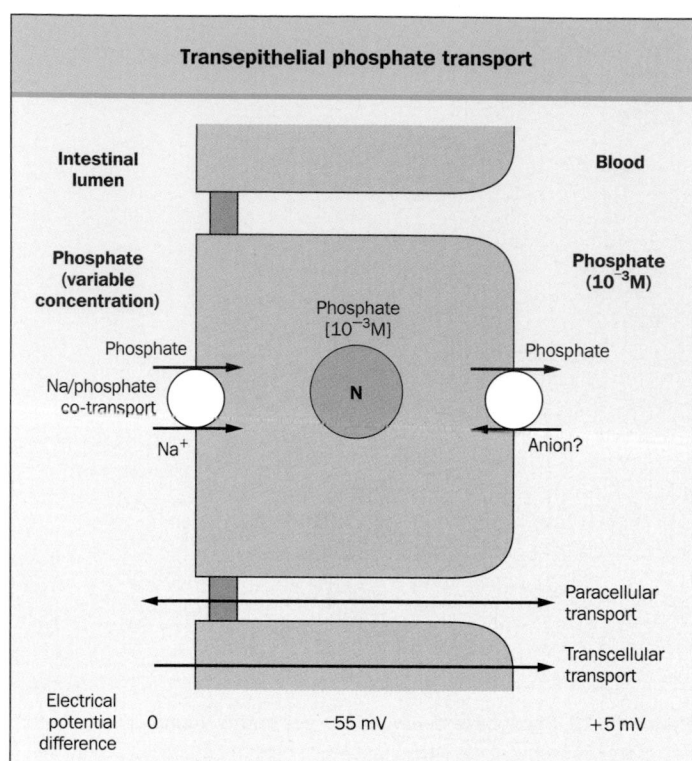

Figure 10.13 Transepithelial phosphate transport in the small intestine. Phosphate enters the enterocyte (influx) via the brush border membrane using the Na^+/phosphate cotransport system, with a stoichiometry of 2 : 1, operating against an electrochemical gradient. Phosphate exit at the basolateral side possibly occurs by passive diffusion or (more probably) by anion exchange.

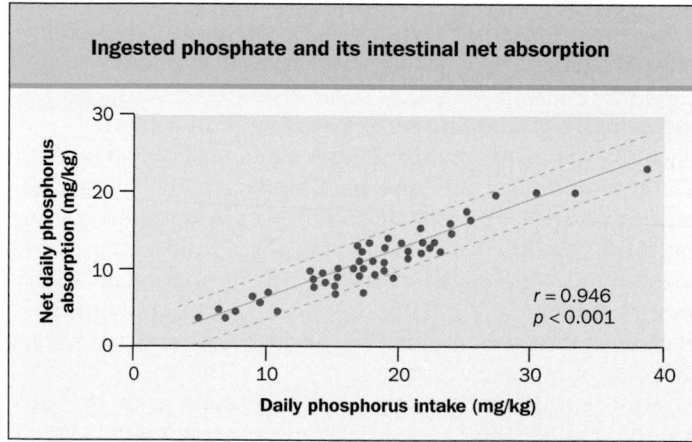

Figure 10.14 Relation between phophate ingested and that absorbed in the digestive tract (net absorption) in healthy young adults. (With permission from Wilkinson R. Absorption of calcium, phosphorus, and magnesium. In: Nordin BEC, ed. Calcium and magnesium metabolism. Edinburgh: Churchill Livingstone; 1976;36–112.)

and serum phosphate and creatinine concentrations, respectively. The maximal TRP factored for GFR (T_mP/GFR: 'Bijvoet index') represents the concentration above which most phosphate is excreted and below which most is reabsorbed. This can be calculated from the plasma phosphate and TRP (Fig. 10.15).

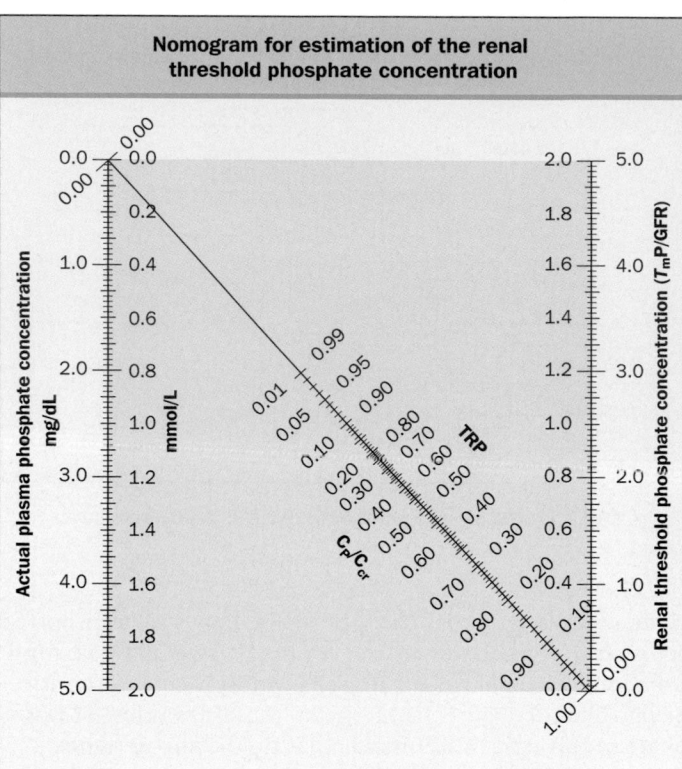

Figure 10.15 Nomogram for the estimation of renal threshold phosphate concentration (T_mP/GFR) without any calculation. A straight line through the appropriate values of phosphate concentration and TRP (amount of phosphate reabsorbed or C_P/C_{cr} where C is clearance for phosphate (P) or creatinine (cr)) passes through the corresponding value of T_mP/GFR. (With permission of Bijvoet OL. Relation of plasma phosphate concentration to renal tubular reabsorption of phosphate. Clin Sci. 1969;37:23–36.)

After its passage through the glomerular filter, part of the ultrafiltered phosphate is recovered by the tubule depending on the body's needs. The major part of phosphate is reabsorbed in the proximal convoluted tubule. A large number of endocrine and metabolic factors modulate urinary excretion of phosphate[19]. Factors increasing renal excretion of phosphate include PTH, FGF23, PHEX (phosphate-regulating gene, see below), dietary phosphate, and extracellular volume expansion, whereas calcitriol increases phosphate reabsorption. Adaptation of tubular reabsorption to dietary intake can occur independently of PTH and vitamin D.

Hyperphosphatemia

Causes of hyperphosphatemia

Increased levels of plasma phosphate can be observed in many clinical situations. The most common cause is reduced urinary excretion in renal failure[20]. Although hyperphosphatemia is seen particularly in conditions in which urinary phosphate excretion is perturbed, it can also be caused by increased exogenous or endogenous phosphate supply (see Fig. 10.16).

Renal failure

In advanced renal failure, hyperphosphatemia is a practically constant finding owing to phosphate retention[20]. This leads

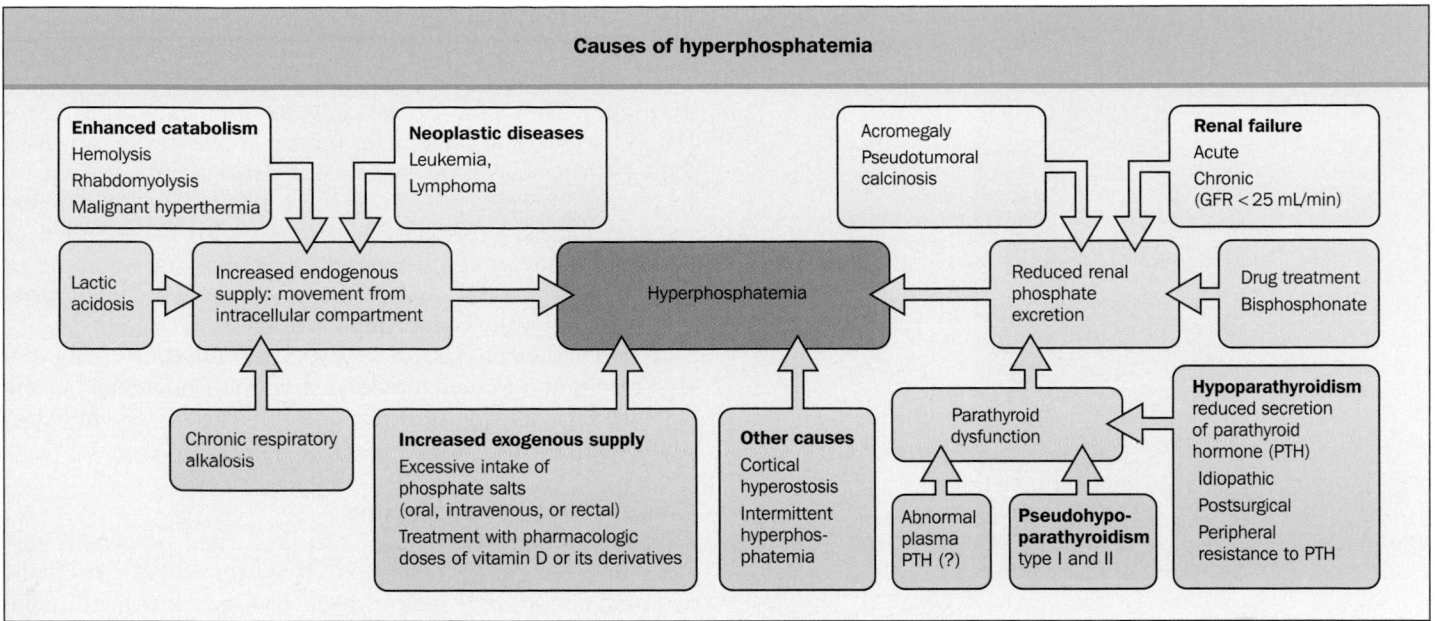

Figure 10.16 Causes of hyperphosphatemia.

to an increase in ultrafiltered phosphate by the remaining nephrons. At the same time, tubular reabsorption of phosphates progressively decreases under the influence of PTH. Thus fractional urinary excretion of phosphates can reach values as high as 60–90%. This progressive adaptation of tubular reabsorption maintains plasma phosphate within normal limits until GFR falls to < 25 mL/min. In patients with anuric end-stage renal disease, the increase in plasma phosphate results not only from decreased excretion but also from increased PTH, which may further increase plasma phosphate through its action to release Ca^{2+} and phosphate from bone. During acute renal failure, plasma phosphate is also high, sometimes even higher than in chronic renal failure, especially in association with infection or rhabdomyolysis.

Hypoparathyroidism
In states of reduced PTH secretion (idiopathic or postsurgical hypoparathyroidism) or resistance to its peripheral action (pseudohypoparathyroidism), tubular reabsorption of phosphate is increased and consequently urinary excretion is diminished. The resulting increase in plasma phosphate leads to an increase in the ultrafiltered load. This results in the regulation of plasma phosphate at a new level.

Chronic hypocalcemia
Hyperphosphatemia is sometimes observed in association with chronic hypocalcemia. As the plasma PTH levels are usually normal or high, in the absence of characteristic abnormalities of pseudohypoparathyroidism the existence of an abnormal form of plasma PTH has been suggested. The latter could result from an abnormal conversion of the prohormone to its secreted form.

Acromegaly and pseudotumoral calcinosis
The hyperphosphatemia of acromegaly results from an increase in tubular reabsorption of phosphate stimulated by

growth hormone. Pseudotumoral calcinosis is a condition seen primarily in African Americans, with hyperphosphatemia, an increased Ca x phosphate product (> 65 mg/dL × mg/dL), and metastatic soft tissue calcifications. The increase in plasma phosphate observed in pseudotumoral calcinosis is also associated with an exaggerated tubular phosphate reabsorption, either idiopathic or through excessive calcitriol levels. Circulating PTH is not decreased in these patients.

Treatment by bisphosphonates, in particular by etidronate in Paget's disease, can lead to hyperphosphatemia, possibly through an increased liberation of tissue phosphate and/or an increase in renal tubular reabsorption.

Hypercatabolism
Exaggerated phosphate loss by soft tissues can be observed in some states of increased cell lysis, as during the crush syndrome, or in some malignancies and their treatment (especially lymphomas and leukemias). Severe hypercatabolic states from infection or diabetic ketoacidosis can also cause hyperphosphatemia by increased cellular release of phosphate.

Phosphate salts and vitamin D
Massive supply of phosphate, as may occur by laxative or enema use, can sometimes lead to hyperphosphatemia. Similarly, administration of pharmacologic doses of vitamin D can lead to hyperphosphatemia. In this case, there is generally hypercalcemia as well.

Respiratory alkalosis by prolonged hyperventilation
Respiratory alkalosis resulting from prolonged hyperventilation is characterized by resistance to the renal action of PTH, hyperphosphatemia and hypocalcemia[21]. Functional pseudohypoparathyroidism may be present as well since renal phosphate clearance is diminished while plasma PTH is normal, despite hypocalcemia. There is no decrease in urinary Ca excretion.

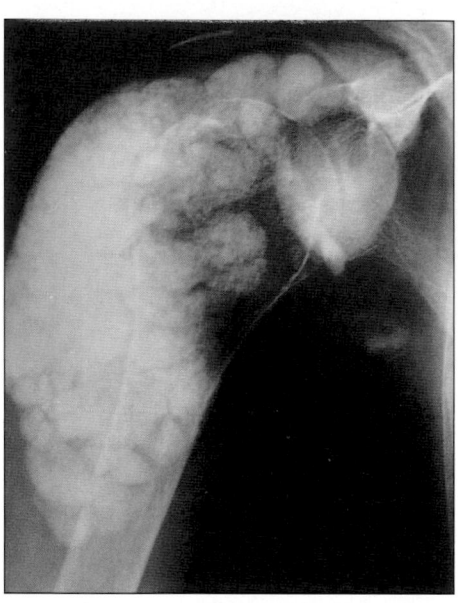

Figure 10.17 Tumor-like extraskeletal calcification.

Clinical manifestations

Severe hyperphosphatemia can induce hypocalcemia, which stimulates PTH secretion. In addition, it can inhibit renal synthesis of calcitriol, which tends to aggravate hypocalcemia further. The occurrence of severe hypocalcemia with tetany and ectopic calcifications is the most severe manifestation of hyperphosphatemia. Calcification may occur in joints and soft tissues, as well as in the lung, the kidney, and the conjunctiva. This syndrome is observed in several clinical situations, such as renal failure, hypoparathyroidism, pseudohypoparathyroidism and pseudotumoral calcinosis. Tumor-like extraskeletal calcifications, however, are more frequently observed in hyperphosphatemia associated with normal or increased plasma Ca^{2+} levels, either as a familial syndrome (very rare) or in uremic patients (rare). Figure 10.17 shows the radiographic aspect of a tumor-like, massive periarticular calcium phosphate deposit in a uremic patient with an extremely high serum Ca x phosphate product.

The stimulation of PTH secretion by high phosphate levels is both indirect, secondary to a decrease of plasma Ca^{2+} and calcitriol synthesis, and direct, secondary to a stimulatory effect on the parathyroid gland.

Treatment

Treatment of the underlying cause of hyperphosphatemia should be attempted whenever possible. In addition, oral phosphate binders can be given, such as aluminum salts or gels (up to 3 g/day), calcium salts (up to 6 g/day) and magnesium salts (2–3 g/day). These treatments have to be given very cautiously in uremic patients, especially aluminum-containing phosphate binders, because of the potential for aluminum accumulation and toxicity (see Chapter 68). A new, unabsorbable, aluminum- and calcium-free phosphate binding resin, sevelamer, has been marketed recently which has similar binding capacities and avoids calcium and aluminum overload. Another approach is dietary protein restriction, which results in reduced phosphate intake by the gut.

HYPOPHOSPHATEMIA

Decreased plasma phosphate levels may reflect phosphate deficiency. They can, theoretically, be observed during a prolonged decrease in phosphate intake. However, as shown in Figure 10.18, several defense mechanisms counter a decrease in plasma phosphate resulting from low intake. Moderately reduced plasma phosphate levels may also be observed in conditions not linked to overall deficiency, for example in maldistribution between the intra- and extracellular compartments during acute respiratory alkalosis.

When plasma phosphate is 0.8–0.3 mmol/L (2.5–1.0 mg/dL), the condition is termed 'moderate hypophosphatemia'. Below 0.3 mmol/L (1.0 mg/dL) it is considered to be 'severe hypophosphatemia'.

Causes of hypophosphatemia

Moderate hypophosphatemia can be caused by genetic diseases or by acquired conditions (see Fig. 10.19). The main acquired condition is malnutrition owing to low food intake or anorexia during severe disease or alcoholism ; its incidence varies greatly among countries. Another cause is a shift of phosphate into cells, which can occur through various mechanisms but especially with the administration of insulin. Although there are a large number of genetic diseases and syndromes, overall, these are rare. Severe forms of hypophosphatemia are all acquired.

Inherited forms of hypophosphatemia

Many inherited diseases are associated with chronic hypophosphatemia. These are generally diagnosed in childhood. Permanent low plasma phosphate usually leads to rickets or

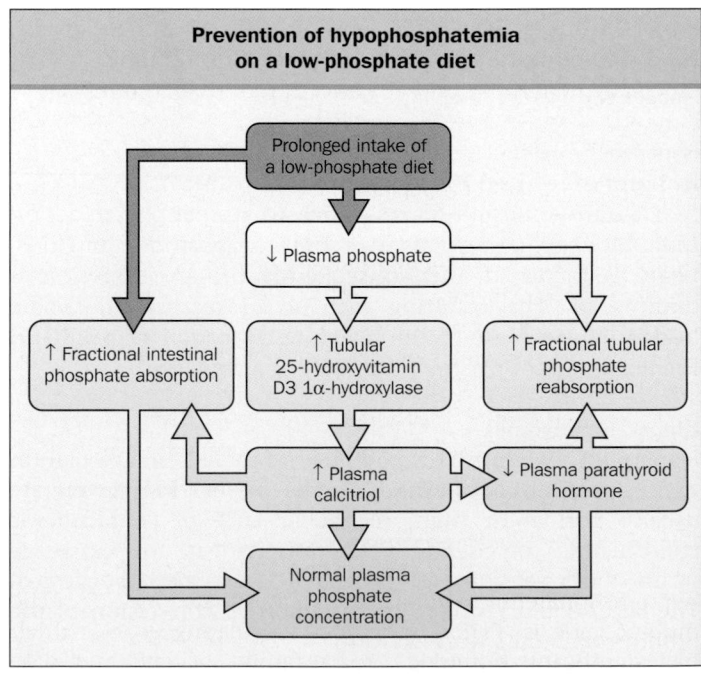

Figure 10.18 Compensatory mechanisms to prevent hypophosphatemia during a prolonged intake of a phosphate-poor diet.

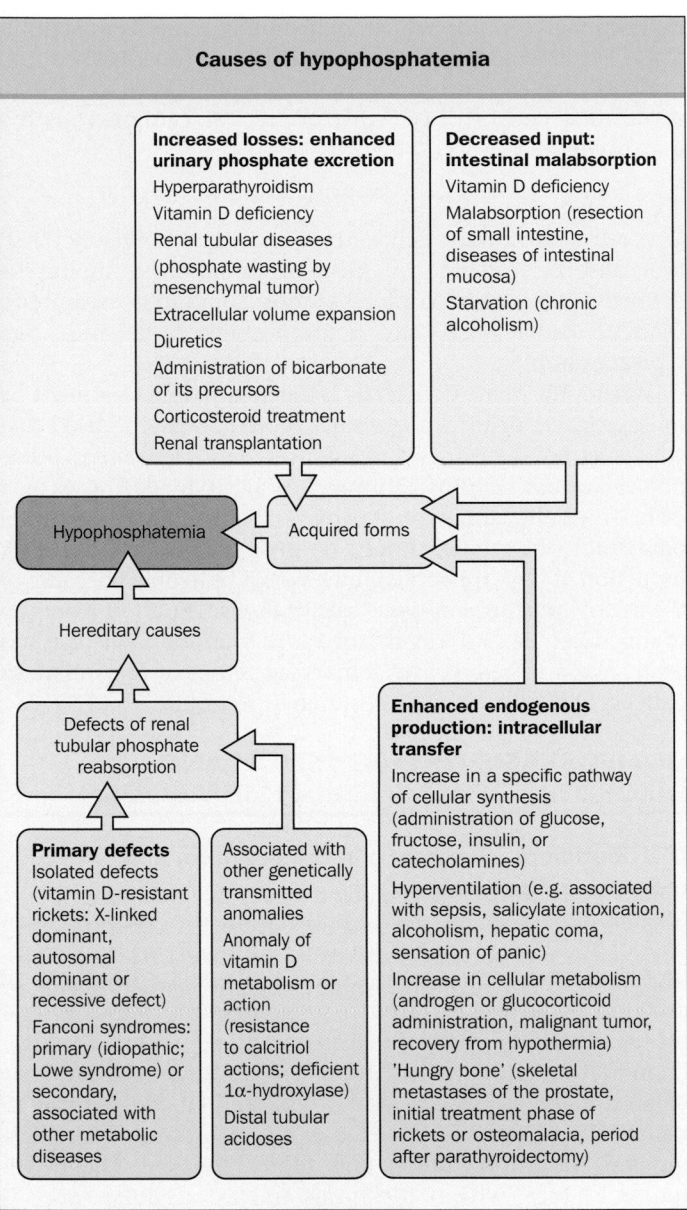

Figure 10.19 Causes of hypophosphatemia.

osteomalacia. The molecular genetic defect has not yet been identified in most cases.

Inherited hypophosphatemia can be subdivided into two groups: primary defects, which are either isolated or associated with tubular disorders (Fanconi syndrome), and defects that are secondary to another genetically transmitted disease, mainly metabolic disorders or disturbances in the action of vitamin D.

X chromosome-linked hypophosphatemia (XLH)

XLH is a rare dominantly transmitted disease characterized by hypophosphatemia and isolated phosphate wasting. The mutant gene is 'PHEX' (phosphate-regulating gene), which has significant homology to a family of endopeptidase genes[22]. The gene is mainly expressed in bone. The urinary leak of phosphate is secondary to a decrease in proximal tubular Na+/phosphate cotransport. Clinical signs are rickets in the

child and sometimes osteomalacia or bone deformation in the adult. Hypophosphatemia is associated with normal plasma Ca^{2+}, calcitriol, and PTH and with elevated serum alkaline phosphatases. The TRP is greatly lowered. Isolated inherited hypophosphatemia may also occur rarely in an autosomal dominant (see below) or autosomal recessive pattern.

Autosomal-dominant hypophosphatemic rickets (ADHR)

ADHR is a phosphate wasting disorder characterized by short stature, bone pain, fractures, and lower extremity deformity. It is caused by mutations of the *FGF23* gene[17]. The precise function of this recently cloned gene is not yet known. It may be the long-sought phosphate regulating hormone, or at least one of them, with a native phosphaturic action. Moreover, FGF23 may be a substrate for PHEX but further work is needed to prove this assertion.

The Fanconi syndrome

The Fanconi syndrome is characterized by a complex transport defect of the proximal tubule that results in decreased reabsorption of glucose, amino acids, and bicarbonate in addition to phosphate. The Fanconi syndrome is either primary (idiopathic, Lowe syndrome, Dent's disease) or associated with other metabolic diseases (cystinosis, Wilson's disease, and others). In Dent's disease and Lowe syndrome a defective recycling of megalin to the apical cell surface of the proximal tubule has been found, implicating a role in abnormal tubular endocytic function[23].

In addition to a tubular defect causing phosphate wasting, the activity of renal 1α-hydroxylase may be insufficient, resulting in decreased circulating calcitriol levels and bone disease such as rickets or osteomalacia. Functional disorders associated with the syndrome, such as polyuria and extracellular volume contraction, lead to hyperaldosteronism with hypokalemia and eventually to renal failure.

Hypophosphatemia linked to other inherited diseases

Several rare inherited diseases can be associated with hypophosphatemia, including vitamin D-dependent rickets type 1, caused by a defect of renal 1α-hydroxylase, and type 2 owing to peripheral resistance to the action of calcitriol. Clinical signs are similar to those of vitamin D deficient rickets, with alopecia occurring in 50% of cases. In type 1, calcitriol levels are low whereas in type 2 there is normal circulating 25-hydroxyvitamin D and high calcitriol. Treatment with low doses of calcitriol is sufficient to treat type 1, whereas extremely high doses of calcitriol or 1α-dihydroxy-vitamin D are required for type 2.

Distal renal tubular acidosis type I

Distal tubular acidosis type 1 is characterized above all by hypercalciuria and sometimes nephrocalcinosis. Hypophosphatemia is inconstant. It is possible that it is only secondary to concomitant vitamin D deficiency.

Acquired forms of hypophosphatemia

The number of acquired diseases that can be associated with hypophosphatemia is even greater than the inherited diseases and includes hyperparathyroidism and vitamin D deficiency

(Fig. 10.19). True phosphate deficiency associated with total body depletion must be distinguished from enhanced influx of phosphate from the extracellular to the intracellular space or increased skeletal mineralization.

Alcoholism

Alcoholism is the most common cause of severe hypophosphatemia in Western countries. The causes are multiple, including insufficient food intake, the use of phosphate binders for intestinal disorders, and excessive phosphate loss in urine secondary to hypomagnesemia, as well as phosphate transfer from the extra- to the intracellular compartment secondary to hyperventilation or glucose infusion in subjects with postalcoholic cirrhosis or in acute abstinence.

Acute respiratory alkalosis

In intense and short-term hyperventilation, plasma phosphate can sometimes fall considerably, to values as low as 0.1 mmol/L (0.3 mg/dL). Such a fall is never observed in acute metabolic alkalosis. Hypophosphatemia following acute and intense hyperventilation is probably the result of muscle sequestration of extracellular phosphate. However, it must be remembered that prolonged chronic hyperventilation leads to hyperphosphatemia (see above).

Diabetic ketoacidosis

During decompensated diabetes associated with acidosis provoked by accumulation of ketone bodies, glycosuria, and polyuria, plasma phosphate can be normal or high, even in the presence of hyperphosphaturia. Correction of this complication by insulin and refilling of the extracellular compartment leads to massive transfer of phosphate into the intracellular compartment, hypophosphatemia, and subsequently less urinary loss of phosphate. Generally, plasma phosphate does not fall below 0.3 mmol/L (0.9 mg/dL), except when there is pre-existing phosphate deficiency.

Oncogenic hypophosphatemic osteomalacia

Hypophosphatemia and osteomalacia resulting from renal phosphate wasting can occur in patients with mesenchymal tumors (hemangiopericytomas, fibromas, angiosarcomas). This condition can be healed by tumor resection. The humoral factor secreted by these tumors is *FGF23*[24].

Total parenteral nutrition

Hyperalimentation can also be associated with severe hypophosphatemia through the insulin mediated shift of phosphate into the cell, particularly if phosphate is omitted from the parenteral nutrition solution. Severe hypophosphatemia can also occur with acute feeding of starved patients (such as occurred in World War II).

Clinical manifestations

Clinical manifestations depend on the severity of the hypophosphatemia and the degree of phosphate deficiency. In practice they are rare. Nevertheless, some clinical symptoms and signs diagnostic of chronic hypophosphatemia should be known. They include metabolic encephalopathy, red blood cell dysfunction (by depletion of ATP and 2,3-diphosphoglycerate), which may induce hemolysis, anomalies of leukocyte function, and thrombocytopenia. Reduced muscle strength (and rarely rhabdomyolysis) and decreased myocardial contractility (with occasional cardiomyopathy) may occur.

Treatment

Generally, phosphate deficiency is not an emergency. First, the cause or at least the mechanism involved should be defined in order to determine the most appropriate treatment. Diabetic ketoacidosis and acute respiratory alkalosis are typical examples.

When phosphate deficiency is diagnosed, oral treatment by milk products or phosphate salts should always be tried first whenever possible. In severe, symptomatic deficiency, phosphates can also be infused intravenously, in divided doses over 24 h. In patients undergoing parenteral nutrition, 10–25 mmol potassium phosphate should be given for each 1000 kcal. Induction of hyperphosphatemia should be avoided because of the risk of inducing soft tissue calcifications. The administration of dipyridamole (300 mg divided into four doses per day) has been shown to reduce the urinary excretion of phosphate in patients with a low renal phosphate threshold[25].

HOMEOSTASIS OF MAGNESIUM AND DISORDERS OF MAGNESIUM METABOLISM

Distribution of magnesium in the organism and magnesium homeostasis

Magnesium (Mg) is, after potassium, the second most abundant cation in the intracellular fluid in living organisms. Mg^{2+} is involved in the majority of metabolic processes. In addition, it also plays a part in deoxyribonucleic acid and protein synthesis. It is involved in the regulation of mitochondrial function, in inflammatory processes and immune defense, allergy, growth, and stress, and in the control of neuronal activity, cardiac excitability, neuromuscular transmission, vasomotor tone, and blood pressure. The distribution of Mg^{2+} within the intra- and extracellular space is shown in Figure 10.20.

Figure 10.21 shows the balance of ingestion, body distribution and excretion of Mg^{2+} in healthy humans. Mg^{2+} influx into and efflux out of cells is linked to carbohydrate-dependent active transport systems. The stimulation of β-adrenoceptors favors Mg^{2+} outflux, while insulin, calcitriol, and vitamin B_6 favor Mg^{2+} entry into cells.

Intestinal and renal handling of magnesium

The intestinal absorption of dietary Mg^{2+} occurs by both a saturable and a passive transport process, the major part being absorbed in the small intestine. Absorption can vary by as much as 25–60%, with a mean absorption of approximately 30%. There appears to be no adaptation of intestinal Mg^{2+} transport in response to chronic changes of dietary Mg content.

Various factors modify intestinal Mg^{2+} absorption. High dietary phosphate intake is inhibitory, as is high phytate consumption. The effect of dietary calcium is complex, and vitamin D probably has an enhancing effect. Growth hormone

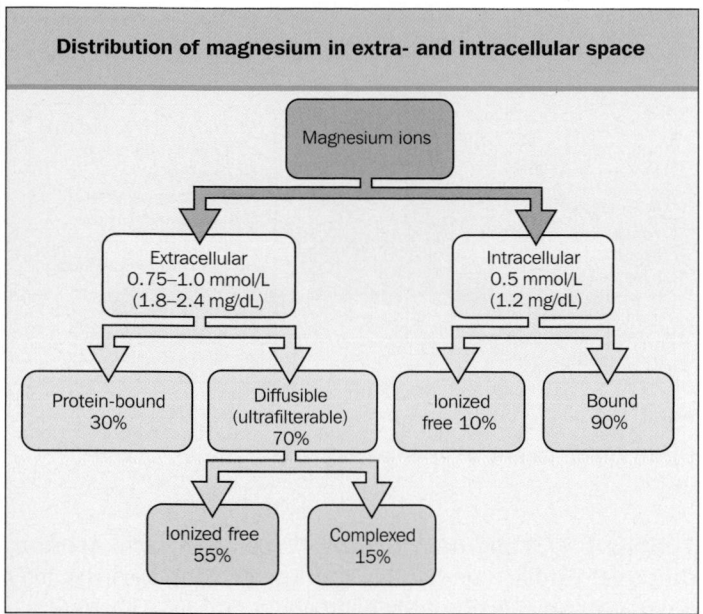

Figure 10.20 Distribution of magnesium in extra- and intracellular space.

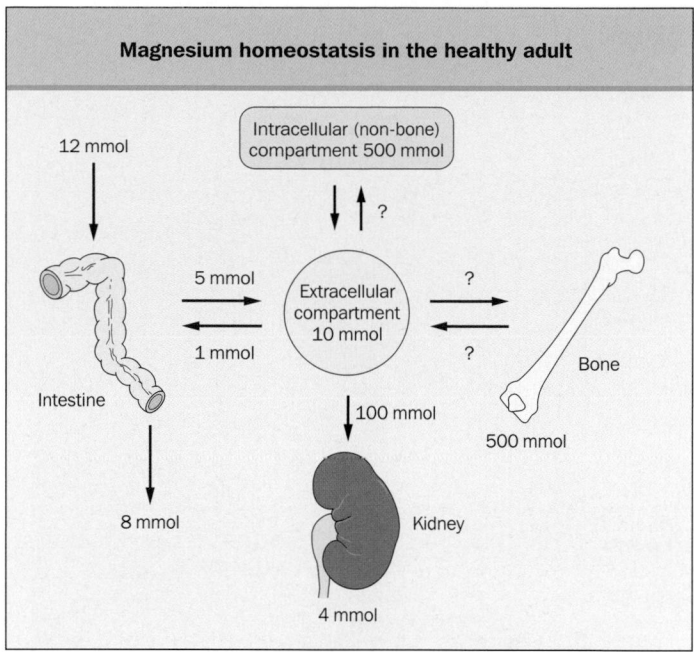

Figure 10.21 Magnesium homeostasis in the healthy young adult. Net zero balance results from net intestinal uptake (absorption minus secretion) equaling urinary loss. After its passage into the extracellular fluid Mg^{2+} enters the intracellular space, is deposited in bone or soft tissue, or is eliminated via the kidneys. Entry and exit fluxes between the extra- and intracellular space (skeletal and nonskeletal compartments) are also of identical magnitude; however, precise values of exchange are still debated.

slightly increases Mg^{2+} absorption whereas aldosterone and calcitonin appear to reduce it. Vitamin B_6 has been reported to enhance it.

Several conditions are associated with anomalies of intestinal Mg^{2+} absorption. A prolonged and severe reduction of dietary Mg may lead to hypomagnesemia, for example in chronic alcoholism. The fractional absorption of Mg^{2+} may be reduced in several malabsorption syndromes, intestinal bypass surgery or fistulae. Malabsorption also occurs with steatorrhea of various causes and in many diarrheal disorders. Severe diarrhea can cause magnesium deficiency quite rapidly. In alcoholism, diarrhea may contribute to reducing intestinal Mg^{2+} absorption.

An inborn error of intestinal absorption of Mg^{2+} has been reported. It is associated with profound hypomagnesemia and hypocalcemia. Reduction of intestinal Mg^{2+} absorption has also been observed in patients with hypercalciuria and nephrolithiasis.

Intake of large amounts of Mg-containing laxatives or antacids can cause a marked increase in Mg^{2+} absorption. However, clinical problems with hypermagnesemia caused by increased Mg intake arise only when the capacity to excrete Mg^{2+} is reduced.

Mg^{2+} is eliminated by the kidney. Losses via intestinal secretion and sweat are negligible under normal conditions. With an ultrafilterable plasma Mg concentration of 0.5–0.7 mmol/L, the filtered load of Mg amounts to approximately 104 mmol (or 2500 mg) per day. As the normal urinary Mg excretion rate is approximately 4 to 5 mmol (or 100 mg) per day, the urinary output represents about 5% of the filtered load. The major portion of filtered Mg is reabsorbed by the renal tubules (25% in proximal tubule, 65% in the thick ascending loop of Henle, and 5% in the distal convoluted tubule). Figure 10.22 shows a schematic view of the tubular reabsorption of Mg^{2+}.

Mg^{2+} transport in the thick ascending limb is primarily passive via the paracellular route. However, two conditions are necessary for normal Mg^{2+} reabsorption : firstly the generation of an electrical, lumen-positive gradient induced by NaCl reabsorption which creates the driving force required for the reabsorption of divalent cations, and secondly the expression of claudin-16 in the tight junction, which is responsible for the selectivity of the reabsorption of divalent cations. Different anomalies associated with either NaCl reabsorption or with claudin-16 (formerly called 'paracellin') expression result in hypermagnesuria[26] (see also below).

In the distal nephron, i.e., the distal convoluted tubule and the connecting tubule, Mg^{2+} is reabsorbed via the transcellular route, against an uphill electrochemical gradient. The precise nature and molecular identity of the proteins mediating this transport step remain elusive at present.

Tubular Mg^{2+} transport is modulated by serum Mg^{2+} and Ca^{2+} and extracellular fluid volume. An increase of plasma Mg^{2+} or Ca^{2+} concentration results in a depression of Mg transport. Extracellular volume expansion produces a decrease in proximal tubular Mg^{2+} reabsorption, in parallel with that of Na^+ and Ca^{2+}. Dietary phosphate restriction results in marked hypercalciuria and hypermagnesuria and can thereby lead to overt hypomagnesemia. PTH, vasopressin, calcitonin and glucagon increase tubular Mg^{2+} reabsorption, whereas acetylcholine, bradykinin and atrial natriuretic peptide (ANP) stimulate urinary Mg^{2+} excretion.

Finally, a number of drugs have been shown to increase renal Mg^{2+} excretion, including the loop diuretics such as

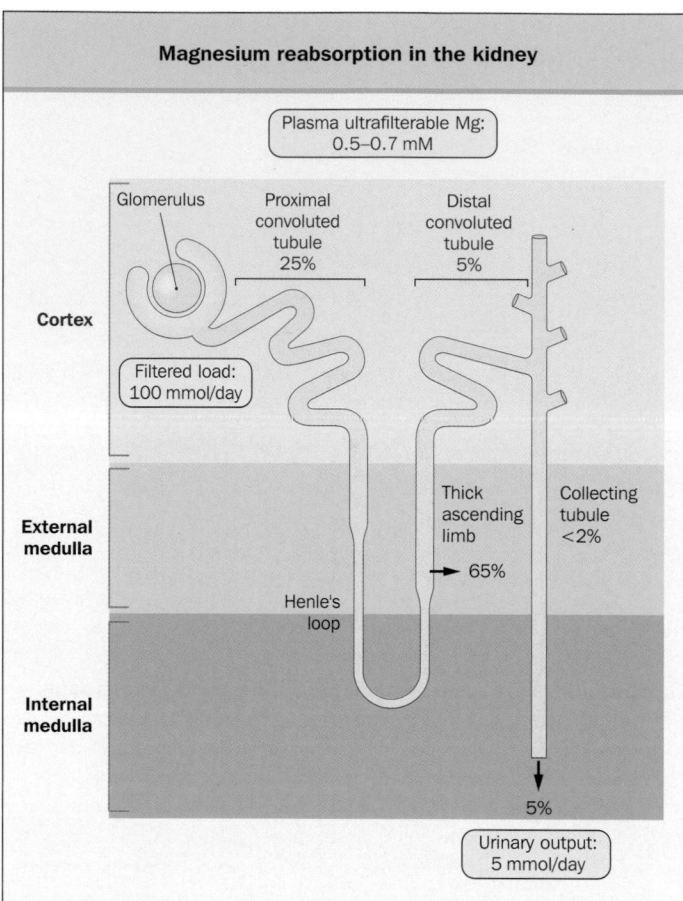

Magnesium reabsorption in the kidney

Plasma ultrafilterable Mg: 0.5–0.7 mM

Glomerulus

Proximal convoluted tubule 25%

Distal convoluted tubule 5%

Cortex

Filtered load: 100 mmol/day

External medulla

Thick ascending limb

Collecting tubule <2%

→ 65%

Henle's loop

Internal medulla

5%

Urinary output: 5 mmol/day

Figure 10.22 Sites of magnesium reabsorption in various segments of the renal tubule. The percentage absorbed various segments from the glomerular ultrafiltrate is shown. (With permission from Quamme GA. Control of magnesium transport in the thick ascending limb. Am J Physiol. 1989;256:F197–F210.)

furosemide, ethacrynic acid, distal diuretics such as thiazides, and osmotic diuretics such as mannitol and urea. Furthermore, renal Mg^{2+}-wasting syndromes have been observed in patients treated with antibiotics such as gentamicin, and antineoplastic agents such as cisplatin and cyclosporin. The precise mechanisms of action(s) of these agents are not all well understood.

HYPERMAGNESEMIA

Elevated plasma Mg^{2+} is seen in patients with acute or chronic renal failure, during the administration of pharmacological doses of Mg, in some infants born to mothers who received Mg for eclampsia, and with the use of oral laxatives or rectal enemas containing Mg^{27} (Fig. 10.23). Mild hypermagnesemia may also be present in patients with adrenal insufficiency, acromegaly, or familial hypocalciuric hypercalcemia.

Clinical manifestations
Symptoms and signs are the result of the pharmacological effects of increased Mg^{2+} concentrations on the nervous and cardiovascular system. At Mg^{2+} concentrations up to 1.5 mmol/L (3.6 mg/dL), hypermagnesemia is asymptomatic. Deep tendon reflexes are usually lost when plasma Mg is above

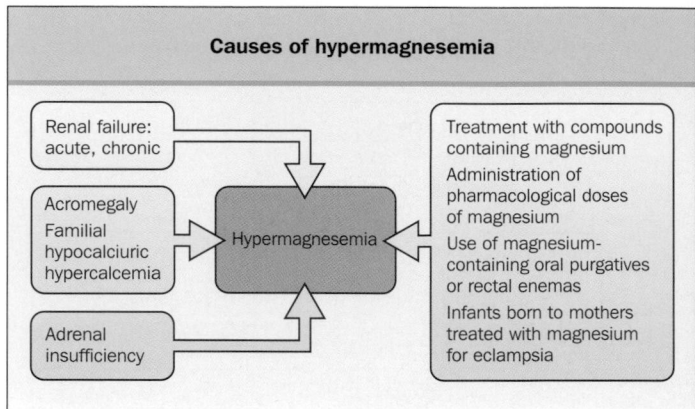

Causes of hypermagnesemia

Renal failure: acute, chronic

Acromegaly

Familial hypocalciuric hypercalcemia

Adrenal insufficiency

Hypermagnesemia

Treatment with compounds containing magnesium

Administration of pharmacological doses of magnesium

Use of magnesium-containing oral purgatives or rectal enemas

Infants born to mothers treated with magnesium for eclampsia

Figure 10.23 Causes of hypermagnesemia.

3 mmol/L (7.2 mg/dL). Respiratory paralysis, hypotension, abnormal cardiac conduction and loss of consciousness may occur as plasma levels of Mg approach 5 mmol/L (12 mg/dL).

Treatment
Treatment consists in cessation of Mg administration and reversal of the neural effects of hypermagnesemia with the intravenous infusion of Ca salts (1 ampul calcium gluconate, approximately 90 mg elemental Ca in 10 mL over 5–10 min intravenously) as initial steps for the management of symptomatic hypermagnesemia.

HYPOMAGNESEMIA AND MAGNESIUM DEFICIENCY

Magnesium deficiency is defined as a decrease in total body Mg content[27]. Poor dietary intake of Mg is usually not associated with a marked Mg deficiency because of the remarkable ability of the normal kidney to conserve Mg^{2+}. However, prolonged and severe dietary Mg restriction below 0.5 mmol/day can produce symptomatic Mg deficiency in humans. Severe hypomagnesemia is usually associated with Mg deficiency. Approximately 10% of patients admitted to a large city hospital in the USA were hypomagnesemic. The incidence may be as high as 65% in medical intensive-care units.

Underlying causes are usually diseases of the gastrointestinal tract, in particular malabsorption syndromes including nontropical sprue, and massive resection of the small intestine. Hypomagnesemia can also be induced by prolonged tube feeding without Mg supplements and by the excessive use of laxatives (Fig. 10.24).

Hypomagnesemia is encountered in about 25–35% of patients with acute pancreatitis, it is frequently observed in patients with chronic alcoholism and it can also be present in patients with poorly controlled diabetes mellitus.

Excessive urinary loss of Mg occurs in a variety of clinical conditions, leading to hypomagnesemia and Mg deficiency, even in the face of normal dietary intake. It may result from the overzealous use of diuretics and, therefore, it is important to monitor plasma Mg^{2+} levels in patients with congestive heart failure who are treated with digitalis derivatives and diuretic agents. The administration of other drugs, for example

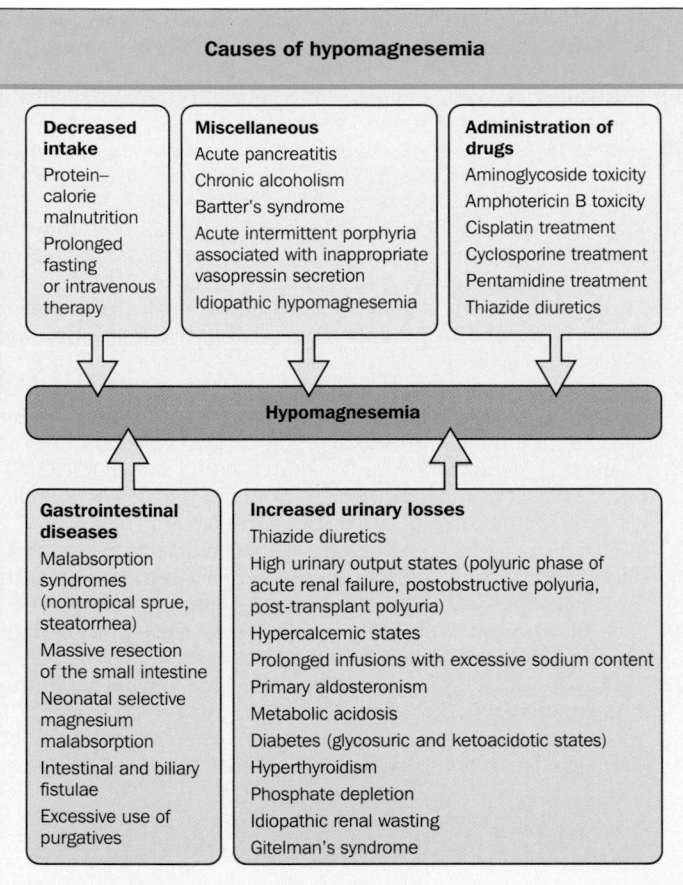

Causes of hypomagnesemia

Decreased intake
Protein–calorie malnutrition

Prolonged fasting or intravenous therapy

Miscellaneous
Acute pancreatitis

Chronic alcoholism

Bartter's syndrome

Acute intermittent porphyria associated with inappropriate vasopressin secretion

Idiopathic hypomagnesemia

Administration of drugs
Aminoglycoside toxicity

Amphotericin B toxicity

Cisplatin treatment

Cyclosporine treatment

Pentamidine treatment

Thiazide diuretics

Hypomagnesemia

Gastrointestinal diseases
Malabsorption syndromes (nontropical sprue, steatorrhea)

Massive resection of the small intestine

Neonatal selective magnesium malabsorption

Intestinal and biliary fistulae

Excessive use of purgatives

Increased urinary losses
Thiazide diuretics

High urinary output states (polyuric phase of acute renal failure, postobstructive polyuria, post-transplant polyuria)

Hypercalcemic states

Prolonged infusions with excessive sodium content

Primary aldosteronism

Metabolic acidosis

Diabetes (glycosuric and ketoacidotic states)

Hyperthyroidism

Phosphate depletion

Idiopathic renal wasting

Gitelman's syndrome

Figure 10.24 Causes of hypomagnesemia.

gentamicin, cis-platinum, and cyclosporine, can be responsible for hypomagnesemia as well.

Hypomagnesemia can also be observed in patients with hypercalcemic disorders and in primary aldosteronism. Hypermagnesuria, not always together with hypomagnesemia, can be associated with inactivating mutations of genes whose abnormal products are responsible for disturbed Mg^{2+} reabsorption in the thick ascending limb of Henle or in the distal nephron[26,28]. Inactivating mutations of the genes of the $Na^+/K^+/2Cl^-$ cotransporter, the rectifying K^+ channel (ROM-K), or the basolateral Cl^- channel in Bartter syndrome are responsible for the abolition of the driving force for Mg^{2+} reabsorption. This results in hypermagnesuria, which however is not always

associated with hypomagnesemia. Inactivating mutations of the CaR_G gene, whose protein product is a key regulator of NaCl reabsorption in the thick ascending limb via extracellular Ca^{2+} concentration, lead to hypermagnesuria and hypomagnesemia. Finally, a mutation of the *claudin-16* gene (3q27) has been also reported to induce a recessive disease characterized by hypomagnesemia, hypermagnesuria, hypercalciuria and nephrocalcinosis.

In the distal convoluted tubule, inactivating mutations of the thiazide-sensitive, electroneutral *NaCl cotransporter* gene in Gitelman disease are also responsible for selective renal Mg wasting and hypomagnesemia.

Recently, hypomagnesemia associated with inappropriate magnesuria has been reported in an autosomal-dominant, isolated familial hypomagnesemia syndrome, mapped to chromosome 11q23.

Clinical manifestations

The main clinical manifestations of moderate to severe Mg depletion include general weakness and neuromuscular hyperexcitability with hyperreflexia, carpopedal spasm, tremor, and rarely tetany. Cardiac findings include a prolonged Q-T interval and ST depression. There is a predisposition to ventricular arrhythmias and potentiation of digitalis toxicity. Mg deficiency can also be associated with hypocalcemia (decreased PTH release and end-organ responsiveness) and hypokalemia (urinary loss). In addition, intracellular K^+ is frequently decreased. Mg deficit constitutes a cardiovascular risk factor and also a risk factor in pregnancy for the mother as well as for the fetus.

The diagnosis of moderate degrees of Mg deficiency is not easy since clinical manifestations may be absent and blood Mg^{2+} levels may not reflect the state of body Mg. In contrast, a severe Mg deficit generally goes along with a decrease in blood Mg^{2+} level.

Treatment

Mg deficiency is managed with the administration of Mg salts. Magnesium sulfate is generally used for parenteral therapy (1500–3000 mg magnesium sulfate (150–300 mg elemental Mg) per day). A variety of Mg salts are available for oral administration, including sulfate, lactate, chloride, carbonate, oxide, and pidolate. Oral Mg salts may cause diarrhea and hence are poorly tolerated, although Mg oxide (400 mg) is often tolerated better than the other Mg salts.

REFERENCES

1. Wasserman RH, Chandler JS, Meyer SA, et al. Intestinal calcium transport and calcium extrusion process at the basolateral membrane. J Nutr (USA). 1992;122:662–71.
2. Wasserman RH, Fullmer CS. Vitamin D and intestinal calcium transport: facts, speculations and hypotheses. J Nutr (USA). 1995;125:1971S–9S.
3. Kinyamu HK, Gallagher C, Prahl JM, et al. Association between intestinal vitamin D receptor, calcium absorption, and serum 1,25 dihydroxyvitamin D in normal young and elderly women. J Bone Min Res. 1997;12:922–8.
4. Mundy GR, Chen D, Zhao M, et al. Growth regulatory factors and bone. Rev Endocr Metab Disord. 2001;2:105–15.
5. Wagner EF, Karsenty G. Genetic control of skeletal development. Curr Opin Genet Dev. 2001;11:527–32.
6. Bindels RJ. Molecular pathophysiology of renal calcium handling. Kidney Blood Press Res. 2000;23:183–4.
7. Hoenderop JG, Nilius B, Bindels RJ. Molecular mechanism of active Ca^{2+} reabsorption in the distal nephron. Annu Rev Physiol. 2002;64:529–49.

8. Brown EM, MacLeod RJ. Extracellular calcium sensing and extracellular calcium signaling. Physiol Rev. 2001;81:239–97.

9. Nissenson RA. Parathyroid hormone-related protein. Rev Endocr Metab Disord. 2000;1:343–52.

10. Cryns VL, Thor A, Xu HJ, et al. Loss of retinoblastoma tumor-suppressor gene in parathyroid carcinoma. N Engl J Med. 1994;330:757–61.

11. Schipani E, Langman CB, Parfitt AM, et al. Constitutively activated receptors for parathyroid hormone and parathyroid hormone-related peptide in Jansen's metaphyseal chondrodysplasia. N Engl J Med. 1996;335:708–14.

12. Pollak MP, Seidman CE, Brown EM. Three inherited disorders in calcium sensing. Medicine. 1996;75:115–23.

13. Arnold A, Brown MF, Ureña P, et al. Monoclonality of parathyroid tumors in chronic renal failure and in primary parathyroid hyperplasia. J Clin Invest. 1995;95:2047–54.

14. Delmas PD, Fontana A. Bone loss induced by cancer treatment and its management. Eur J Cancer. 1998;34:260–2.

15. Silverberg S, Bone HG, Marriott TB, et al. Short-term inhibition of parathyroid hormone secretion by a calcium-receptor agonist in patients with primary hyperparathyroidism. N Engl J Med. 1997;337:1506–10.

16. Drueke TB, Cunningham J, Goodman WG, et al. Short-term treatment of secondary hyperparathyroidism (SHPT) with the calcimimetic agent AMG 073 (Abstract A3992). J Am Soc Nephrol. 2001;12:764A.

17. White KE, Carn G, Lorenz-Depiereux B, et al. Autosomal-dominant hypophosphatemic rickets (ADHR) mutations stabilize FGF-23. Kidney Int. 2001;60:2079–86.

18. Murer H, Hernando N, Forster L, Biber J. Molecular mechanisms in proximal tubular and small intestinal phosphate reabsorption (plenary lecture). Mol Membr Biol. 2001;18:3–11.

19. Friedlander G. Autocrine/paracrine control of renal phosphate transport. Kidney Int Suppl. 1998;65:S18–23.

20. Delmez JA, Slatopolsky E. Hyperphosphatemia: its consequences and treatment in patients with chronic renal disease. Am J Kidney Dis. 1992;19:303–17.

21. Krapf R, Jaeger P, Hulter HN. Chronic respiratory alcalosis induces renal PTH-resistance, hyperphosphatemia and hypocalcemia in humans. Kidney Int. 1992;42:727–34.

22. TheHypConsortium. A gene (PEX) with homologies to endopeptidases is mutated in patients with X-linked hypophosphatemic rickets. Nat Genet. 1995;11:130–6.

23. Norden AG, Lapsley M, Igarashi T, et al. Urinary megalin deficiency implicates abnormal tubular endocytic function in Fanconi syndrome. J Am Soc Nephrol. 2002;13:125–33.

24. Shimada T, Mizutani S, Muto T, et al. Cloning and characterization of FGF23 as a causative factor of tumor-induced osteomalacia. Proc Natl Acad Sci USA. 2001;98:6500–5.

25. Prié D, Blanchet FB, Essig M, et al. Dipyridamole decreases renal phosphate leak and augments serum phosphorus in patients with low renal phosphate threshold. J Am Soc Nephrol. 1998;9:1264–9.

26. Cole DE, Quamme GA. Inherited disorders of renal magnesium handling. J Am Soc Nephrol. 2000;11:1937–47.

27. Nadler JL, Rude RK. Disorders of magnesium metabolism. Endocrinol Metab Clin North Am. 1995;24:623–41.

28. Yu AS. Evolving concepts in epithelial magnesium transport. Curr Opin Nephrol Hypertens. 2001;10:649–53.

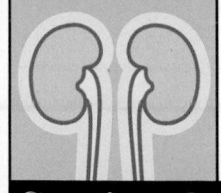

Section 3 Fluid and Electrolyte Disorders

Chapter 11 Normal Acid–Base Balance and Metabolic Acidosis

Biff F Palmer and Robert J Alpern

INTRODUCTION

The acid–base status of the body is carefully regulated to maintain the arterial pH between 7.35 and 7.45 and the intracellular pH between 7.0 and 7.3. This regulation occurs in the setting of continuous production of acidic metabolites and is accomplished by intracellular and extracellular buffering processes in conjunction with respiratory and renal regulatory mechanisms. The first part of this chapter provides a brief overview of normal acid–base homeostasis. The remainder of the chapter is devoted to the clinical entities that give rise to metabolic acidosis.

NET ACID PRODUCTION

Both acid and alkali are generated from the diet. Amino acids such as lysine and arginine yield acid upon metabolism, while the amino acids glutamate and aspartate, and organic anions such as acetate and citrate, yield alkali upon metabolism. Sulfur-containing amino acids (methionine and cysteine) are metabolized to sulfuric acid (H_2SO_4), and organophosphates are metabolized to phosphoric acid (H_3PO_4), both strong acids. In general, animal foods are high in proteins and organophosphates, which provide a net acid diet, while plant foods are higher in organic anions, which provide an alkaline load. In addition to acid/alkali produced from metabolism of the diet, there is a small daily production of organic acids such as acetic acid, lactic acid, and pyruvic acid. Lastly, a small amount of acid is generated by the excretion of alkali into the stool. Under normal circumstances, daily net acid production is approximately 1 mmol hydrogen ions (H^+) per kilogram body weight.

BUFFER SYSTEMS IN REGULATION OF pH

The immediate defense against addition of acid or alkali to the body is intracellular and extracellular buffers. Buffer systems minimize the change in pH during the addition of acid or base equivalents but do not remove acid/alkali from the body. The most important buffer system is that of the bicarbonate ion and carbon dioxide (HCO_3^-/CO_2). In this system, the CO_2 concentration is maintained at a constant level set by respiratory control. Addition of acid (HA) leads to conversion of HCO_3^- to CO_2 according to the reaction shown below.

■ EQUATION 11.1

$$HA + NaHCO_3 \rightleftharpoons NaA + H_2O + CO_2$$

HCO_3^- is consumed, but CO_2 concentration does not change because this is maintained by respiration. The net result is that the proton generated is no longer free and pH changes are minimal.

While the HCO_3^-/CO_2 buffer system is the most important of the buffers in extracellular fluid (ECF), other buffers such as plasma proteins and phosphate ions also participate in the maintenance of a stable pH. During metabolic acidosis, the skeleton becomes a major buffer source as acid-induced dissolution of bone apatite releases alkaline Ca^+ salts and HCO_3^- into the ECF. Within the intracellular compartment, pH is maintained by intracellular buffers such as hemoglobin, cellular proteins, organophosphate complexes, and HCO_3^-, as well as by the H^+/HCO_3^- transport mechanisms that serve to transport acid and alkali in and out of the cell.

RESPIRATORY SYSTEM IN REGULATION OF pH

While buffers minimize the changes in pH upon acid/alkali addition, they do not remove acid or alkali from the body. This is accomplished by the lungs and kidneys. The lungs regulate the CO_2 tension, while the kidneys regulate the HCO_3^- concentration. While the HCO_3^-/CO_2 buffer system is not the only buffer system, all buffer systems in the extracellular system are in equilibrium at a common pH. Because the concentration of HCO_3^- is far greater than that of other buffers, changes in the HCO_3^-/CO_2 buffer pair can easily titrate other buffer systems and, thus, set pH. To understand how the lungs and kidneys function in concert, it is useful to look at the Henderson–Hasselbalch equation.

■ EQUATION 11.2

$$pH = 6.1 + \log((HCO_3^-)/0.03 \times P_{CO_2})$$

As can be seen, pH is determined by the ratio of HCO_3^- to CO_2. Any condition associated with similar fractional changes in the concentrations of these components will not alter pH. Thus, if HCO_3^- and CO_2 concentrations are both halved, blood pH will not change.

The lungs defend pH by altering alveolar ventilation, which controls the P_{CO_2} of body fluids. An increase in nonvolatile acid production lowers blood pH and HCO_3^- concentration, which stimulates the respiratory center to lower the P_{CO_2}. As a result, the fall in blood pH will be less than that which would have occurred in the absence of respiratory compensation. If the fractional change in CO_2 tension were similar to that in HCO_3^- concentration, blood pH would not change. However, respiratory compensations generally do not return blood pH to normal, and, thus, the fractional change in CO_2 tension will be less than that in HCO_3^- concentration. The normal response of the respiratory system in metabolic acidosis is approximately a 1.2 mmHg decrease in P_{CO_2} for every 1 mmol/L fall in HCO_3^- concentration, while the response to metabolic alkalosis is a 0.6 mmHg increase in P_{CO_2} for every 1 mmol/L rise in HCO_3^- concentration.

RENAL REGULATION OF pH

While buffer systems and respiratory excretion of CO_2 provide partial defense of H^+ activity, the kidneys provide the ultimate defense against addition of nonvolatile acids to the body's fluids. The titration of the body's buffer systems would lead to their eventual depletion if no means were available for excretion of the nonvolatile acids generated by net acid production.

The kidney's role in the regulation of nonvolatile acid–base balance includes two components: (i) reclamation of filtered HCO_3^-, and (ii) regeneration of HCO_3^- consumed by net acid production. The kidney filters approximately 4000 mmol HCO_3^- a day, excretion of which would rapidly lead to metabolic acidosis. Thus, the kidney must reclaim this filtered HCO_3^-. Reclamation of HCO_3^- involves secretion of H^+ into the luminal fluid, leading to the net removal of luminal HCO_3^- and its addition to the plasma. Following reclamation, the kidney must then secrete an additional 1 mmol/kg of H^+ daily into the urine. This regenerates the HCO_3^- used to buffer the net acid production (Equation 11.2). The H^+ secreted for HCO_3^- regeneration is buffered in the tubular lumen by titratable buffers, and by ammonia (NH_3).

The net result of these processes is that to maintain acid–base balance the kidney must excrete net acid at a rate equal to the rate of extrarenal net acid production (~1.0 mmol/kg daily). The rate of net acid excretion (NAE) is given by the following equation.

■ EQUATION 11.3

$$NAE = U_{AM}V + U_{TA}V - U_{BC}V$$

where $U_{AM}V$ is the rate of NH_4^+ excretion, $U_{TA}V$ is the rate of titratable acid excretion, and $U_{BC}V$ is the rate of HCO_3^- excretion.

As shown above, the processes of HCO_3^- reclamation and HCO_3^- regeneration are both accomplished by the same general mechanism, acidification of the tubule fluid. This function is mainly accomplished along the nephron. The proximal tubule lowers luminal pH from 7.3 to approximately 6.7 and, thus, reclaims the major portion of filtered HCO_3^-. The thick ascending limb and distal nephron contribute to reclaiming any HCO_3^- that escapes the proximal tubule. Regeneration of HCO_3^- begins in the proximal tubule with titration of filtered buffers, but the key activities occur in the collecting duct where the final urinary acidification leads to titration of NH_4^+, PO_4^+, and other titratable buffers. Changes in glomerular filtration rate (GFR) can significantly affect renal acidification by altering the filtered load of HCO_3^-.

Mechanisms of proximal acidification

The proximal tubule is the site of reabsorption of most of the filtered HCO_3^-. This is accomplished through H^+ secretion into the luminal fluid[1]. Two-thirds of H^+ secretion across the apical (luminal) membrane is mediated by an Na^+/H^+ antiporter that exchanges one Na^+ for one H^+ while the remaining one-third is mediated by a vacuolar H^+ pump (Fig. 11.1). The driving force for H^+ secretion by the Na^+/H^+ antiporter is provided by the low cell Na^+ concentration, which is generated by the basolateral membrane Na^+/K^+ ATPase. The secretion of H^+ by the vacuolar H^+ pump is coupled directly to ATP metabolism. The H^+ secreted into the luminal fluid reacts with filtered HCO_3^- to form H_2CO_3. Intraluminal carbonic anhydrase then catalyzes the conversion of H_2CO_3 to CO_2 and H_2O. The CO_2 diffuses from the lumen into the cell, where in the presence of intracellular carbonic anhydrase it reacts with OH^- to form HCO_3^-. The HCO_3^- then exits the basolateral membrane by way of an $Na^+/HCO_3^-/CO_3^{2-}$ cotransporter. The thick ascending limb also reabsorbs a small amount of luminal HCO_3^- by a mechanism similar to that in the proximal tubule, except that there is no vacuolar H^+ pump.

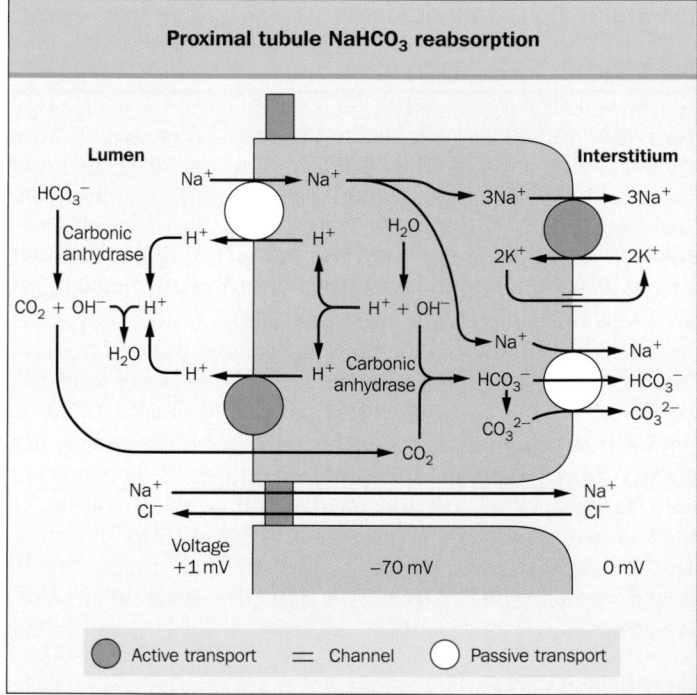

Figure 11.1 Cell model of proximal tubule NaHCO₃ reabsorption. The secretion of H^+ into the proximal tubule lumen involves an Na^+/H^+ antiporter and an H^+ ATPase. Apical membrane H^+ secretion generates OH^-, which reacts with CO_2 to form HCO_3^- and CO_3^{2-} and these exit with an Na^+ on the basolateral membrane $Na^+/HCO_3^-/CO_3^{2-}$ cotransporter. The Na^+ absorbed by the Na^+/H^+ antiporter exits the cell on the basolateral membrane Na^+/K^+ ATPase and the $Na^+/HCO_3^-/CO_3^{2-}$ cotransporter. The K^+ that enters the cell on the Na^+/K^+ ATPase exits on a basolateral membrane K^+ channel. Carbonic anhydrase catalyzes the conversion of HCO_3^- to CO_2 and OH^- in the lumen, and the reverse reaction in the cell. Electrogenic H^+ secretion generates a small lumen-positive voltage that generates a current flow across the paracellular pathway.

Mechanisms of distal acidification

Approximately 90% of the filtered HCO_3^- is reabsorbed in the proximal tubule, with most of the remainder absorbed in the thick ascending limb. One of the functions of the distal nephron is to reabsorb the remainder of the filtered HCO_3^-. In addition, the distal nephron must secrete a quantity of H^+ equal to that generated systemically by metabolism in order to maintain acid–base balance. While this quantity of H^+, approximately 50–80 mmol/day, is relatively small, H^+ secretion in the absence of adequate buffer would lead to a steep drop in intraluminal pH and create an unfavorable gradient, impairing further H^+ secretion. To prevent the development of a limiting pH gradient and ensure that the rate of H^+ secretion matches daily acid production, H^+ secreted in the distal tubule is buffered by NH_3, PO_4^{2-}, creatinine, and other miscellaneous buffers. Thus, the distal nephron reabsorbs a small fraction of filtered HCO_3^- and secretes 50–80 mmol/day of acid in the form of NH_4^+ and titratable acid.

The distal nephron is subdivided into several distinct portions that differ in their anatomy and acid secretory properties[2]. Most of these segments transport H^+ and HCO_3^- into the luminal fluid, but the main segments appear to be in the collecting duct. The segments of the collecting duct include the cortical collecting duct, the outer medullary collecting duct, and the inner medullary collecting duct. There are two distinct cell types in the cortical collecting duct, which can be distinguished histologically: the principal cell and the mitochondria-rich intercalated cell. Of these, most H^+/HCO_3^- transport can be attributed to the intercalated cell, while the principal cells reabsorb Na^+ and secrete K^+.

Absorption of HCO_3^- in the distal nephron is mediated by apical membrane secretion of H^+ (Fig. 11.2). While the greater part of H^+ secretion in the proximal nephron is mediated by an Na^+/H^+ antiporter, this is not true in the collecting duct. An Na^+/H^+ antiporter requires luminal Na^+ and can only create an H^+ gradient equal and opposite to the lumen-to-cell Na^+ gradient (approximately 10-fold). Because the luminal pH in the collecting duct may decrease to values as low as 4.5, a Na^+-independent mechanism is required. The secretion of H^+ in the collecting duct is Na^+ independent and is mediated by one of two pumps: a vacuolar H^+ ATPase or an H^+/K^+ ATPase (Fig. 11.2)[3]. The vacuolar H^+ ATPase is an electrogenic pump and resembles the H^+ pump present within many intracellular compartments, such as lysosomes, Golgi apparatus, and endosomes. The H^+/K^+ ATPase is similar to that present in the stomach and colon. This latter pump uses the energy derived from ATP hydrolysis to secrete H^+ into the lumen and reabsorb K^+ in an electroneutral fashion. The activity of the H^+/K^+ ATPase increases in K^+ depletion and thus provides a mechanism by which K^+ depletion enhances both collecting duct H^+ secretion and K^+ absorption.

Active H^+ secretion by the apical membrane generates base in the cell that must exit the basolateral membrane. Numerous studies suggest that a basolateral Cl^-/HCO_3^- exchanger is the mechanism by which this base exit occurs. The Cl^- that enters the cell in exchange for HCO_3^- exits the cell through a basolateral membrane Cl^- conductance channel (see Fig. 11.2).

In addition to the intercalated cell, the other cell type in the cortical collecting tubule is the principal cell. The principal

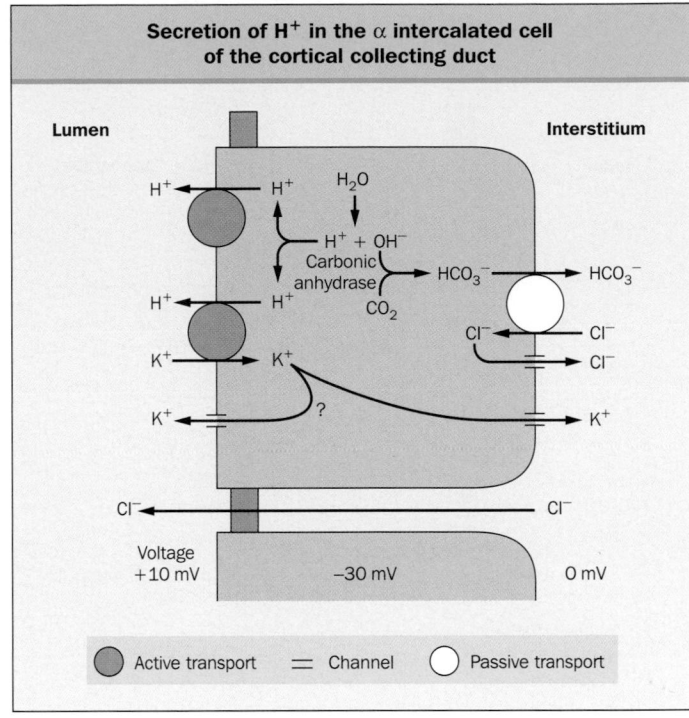

Secretion of H^+ in the α intercalated cell of the cortical collecting duct

Figure 11.2 Secretion of H^+ in the α intercalated cell. Secretion of H^+ into the lumen by an H^+ ATPase and an H^+/K^+ ATPase. Apical membrane H^+ secretion generates OH^-, which reacts with CO_2 to form HCO_3^-; this exits across the basolateral membrane on a Cl^-/HCO_3^- exchanger. The Cl^- that enters the cell on the exchanger recycles across a basolateral membrane Cl channel. The fate of K^+ that enters the cell on the H^+/K^+ ATPase is not clear. Carbonic anhydrase catalyzes the conversion of CO_2 and OH^- to HCO_3^- in the cell. Electrogenic H^+ secretion generates a lumen-positive voltage, which generates a current flow across the paracellular pathway.

cell contains an apical membrane amiloride-sensitive Na^+ channel. Sodium ions move from the lumen across the apical membrane through these Na^+ channels into the cell down its electrochemical potential gradient. It is extruded from the cell by the Na^+/K^+ ATPase located on the basolateral surface of the cell (Fig. 11.3). The process of Na^+ absorption generates a lumen-negative transepithelial potential. Although H^+ secretion is mediated by a separate cellular process, transport of Na^+ and H^+ are linked electrically. Factors that stimulate Na^+ reabsorption increase the luminal electronegativity, thereby reducing the electrochemical gradient against which H^+ secretion occurs. As a result, the rate of H^+ secretion is increased. Conversely, inhibition of Na^+ reabsorption leads to an increase in the electrochemical gradient and thus slows the rate of H^+ secretion. The principal cell of the cortical collecting duct also secretes K^+ into the luminal fluid. The basolateral membrane Na^+/K^+ ATPase transports K^+ from the interstitium into the cell, and cell K^+ enters the lumen through a K^+ channel.

Mineralocorticoid hormones play an important role in distal acidification through their effects on Na^+, K^+, and H^+ transport. Aldosterone directly stimulates Na^+ absorption, enhancing luminal electronegativity and, secondarily, stimulating K^+ and H^+ secretion. Aldosterone can also directly stimulate H^+ secretion in the intercalated cell both in the cortical and

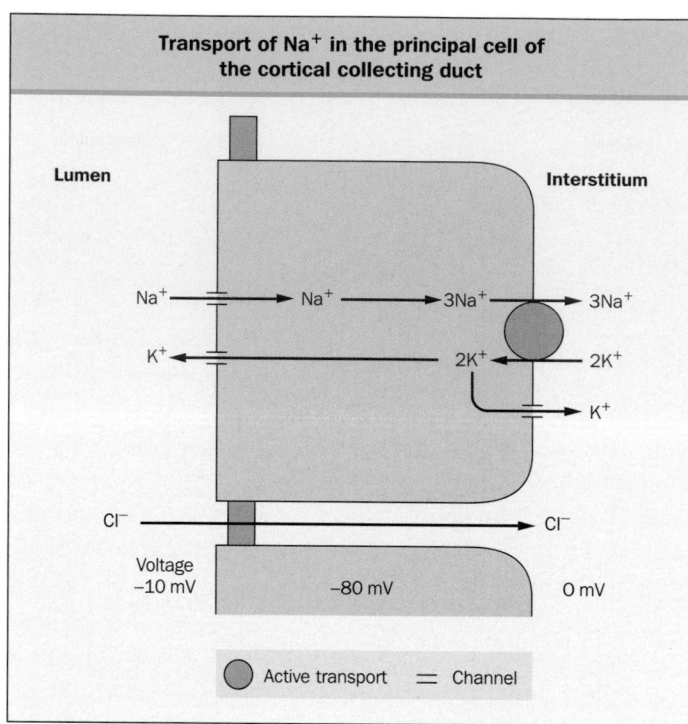

Figure 11.3 The transport of Na⁺ in the principal cell of the cortical collecting duct. Electrogenic Na⁺ absorption is mediated by a Na⁺ channel. The Na⁺ enters the cell across the apical membrane channel and exits the cell on the basolateral membrane Na⁺/K⁺ ATPase. The K⁺ that enters the cell on the Na⁺/K⁺ ATPase exits on a basolateral membrane K⁺ channel. Electrogenic Na⁺ absorption establishes a lumen negative voltage that drives a paracellular current.

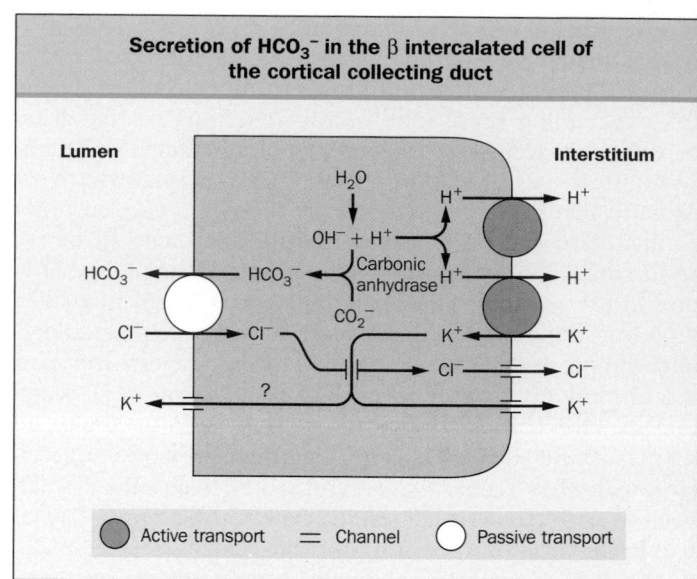

Figure 11.4 The secretion of HCO_3^- in the β intercalated cell. Here H^+ is secreted into the interstitium by an H^+ ATPase and an H^+/K^+ ATPase. The OH^- generated by basolateral membrane H^+ secretion reacts with CO_2 to form HCO_3^-, which exits across the apical membrane on a Cl^-/HCO_3^- exchanger. The Cl^- that enters the cell on the exchanger exits across a basolateral membrane Cl^- channel. The fate of K^+ that enters the cell on the H^+/K^+ ATPase is not clear. Carbonic anhydrase catalyzes the conversion of CO_2 and OH^- to HCO_3^- in the cell.

medullary collecting duct. Under conditions of aldosterone deficiency, distal H^+ secretion is markedly decreased through loss of this direct and indirect stimulatory effect. The development of hyperkalemia will further limit distal acidification by decreasing NH_3 availability to act as a urinary buffer.

Role of buffer in distal nephron acidification

In order for the distal nephron to secrete an adequate amount of H^+, buffer must be available to prevent extreme luminal acidity. Several weak acids such as creatinine, uric acid, and phosphate are filtered at the glomerulus and may act as titratable buffers. Of these, phosphate is the most important because of its favorable pK_a of 6.80 and its relatively high rate of urinary excretion. However, the buffer capacity of phosphate becomes exhausted as the urine pH falls below 5.5. Quantitatively, the most important urinary buffer is the NH_3/NH_4^+ system. Unlike other buffers, the rate of NH_3 production and excretion can be varied according to physiologic needs. Under normal circumstances, excretion of NH_4^+ accounts for more than half of the net acid excreted per day.

The majority of NH_4^+ excreted in the urine is derived from the metabolism of glutamine in the proximal tubule[4]. Synthesis of NH_3 is stimulated by a low pH and a low serum K^+ concentration, while synthesis is inhibited by an alkaline pH and hyperkalemia. Once synthesized, NH_3 is secreted selectively into the lumen of the proximal tubule by trapping of the NH_3 that diffuses across the apical membrane and by transport of

NH_4^+ on the apical membrane Na^+/H^+ antiporter. The NH_3 is then reabsorbed in the thick ascending limb of Henle such that only a small fraction reaches the distal nephron. Absorption of NH_4^+ in the thick limb occurs by pericellular and transcellular mechanisms. Pericellular diffusion is driven by the lumen-positive potential in this segment. Transcellular transport is mediated by the ability of NH_4^+ to substitute for K^+ on the apical membrane $Na^+/K^+/2Cl^-$ cotransporter and K^+ channel. The NH_3 then diffuses into the medullary interstitium where it can be trapped in the lumen of the collecting duct by an acidic pH (nonionic diffusion).

Distal nephron alkali secretion

The cortical collecting duct also possesses the capacity for HCO_3^- secretion[3]. In addition to the intercalated cells described above that secrete H^+ into the luminal fluid (α intercalated cells), there are intercalated cells that secrete HCO_3^- into the luminal fluid (β intercalated cells) (Fig. 11.4). In response to an alkaline diet or metabolic alkalosis, the activity of the β intercalated cells increases and the activity of the α intercalated cell decreases. The β intercalated cell is similar to an α intercalated cell but is somewhat reversed: H^+ is actively extruded across the basolateral membrane by H^+ pumps (either vacuolar or H^+/K^+) and HCO_3^- exits across the apical membrane on a Cl^-/HCO_3^- exchanger.

METABOLIC ACIDOSIS

Metabolic acidosis may result from renal or extrarenal processes. Extrarenal processes include increased endogenous acid production and accelerated extrarenal loss of HCO_3^-. The development of acidosis in this manner can actually be considered an extension of the normal physiologic process of acid–base balance but quantitatively greater.

Metabolic acidosis may also occur from a primary defect in renal acidification with no increase in extrarenal H^+ production. Metabolic acidosis occurs because either the renal input of new HCO_3^- is insufficient to regenerate the HCO_3^- lost in buffering endogenous acid as in distal renal tubular acidosis (RTA), or the filtered HCO_3^- is lost by renal HCO_3^- wasting as occurs in proximal RTA. In either condition, because of loss of either $NaHCO_3$ (proximal RTA) or NaA (distal RTA), effective extracellular volume is reduced and, as a result, the avidity for renal Cl^- reabsorption derived from the diet is increased and results in a hyperchloremic metabolic acidosis.

Metabolic acidosis is diagnosed by a low pH, a reduced HCO_3^- concentration, and respiratory compensation resulting in a decrease in the Pco_2. A low HCO_3^- concentration alone is not diagnostic of metabolic acidosis since it also results from the renal compensation to chronic respiratory alkalosis. Measurement of the arterial pH differentiates between these two possibilities. The pH is low in hyperchloremic metabolic acidosis and high in chronic respiratory alkalosis. The clinical approach to a patient with a low serum HCO_3^- concentration is given in Figure 11.5.

After confirming the presence of metabolic acidosis, calculation of the serum anion gap is a useful step in determining the differential diagnosis of the disorder. The anion gap is equal to the difference between the plasma concentrations of the major cation (Na^+) and the major measured anions ($Cl^- + HCO_3^-$).

■ EQUATION 11.4

$$Anion\ gap = (Na^+) - (Cl^-) - (HCO_3^-)$$

The normal value of the anion gap is approximately 12 ± 2. Most of the unmeasured anions consists of albumin, and, therefore, the normal anion gap changes in the setting of hypoalbuminemia (normal anion gap is approximately three times the serum albumin in g/dL). Because the total number of cations must equal the total number of anions, a fall in the serum HCO_3^- concentration must be offset by a rise in the concentration of other anions. If the anion accompanying excess H^+ is Cl^- then the fall in the serum HCO_3^- concentration is matched by an equal rise in the serum Cl^- concentration. The acidosis is classified as a normal gap or hyperchloremic metabolic acidosis. By contrast, if excess H^+ is accompanied by an anion other than Cl^- then the fall in HCO_3^- is balanced by a rise in the concentration of the unmeasured anion. The Cl^- concentration remains the same. In this setting, the acidosis is said to be a high anion gap metabolic acidosis. Figure 11.6 lists the causes of metabolic acidosis according to the anion gap.

A useful method to distinguish extrarenal and renal causes of metabolic acidosis is to measure urinary NH_4^+ excretion[5]. Extrarenal causes of metabolic acidosis are associated with an appropriate increase in net acid excretion primarily reflected by high levels of urinary NH_4^+ excretion. By contrast, net acid excretion and urinary NH_4^+ levels are low in metabolic acidosis of renal origin. Unfortunately, measurement of urinary NH_4^+ is not a test that is commonly available in clinical medicine. However, one can indirectly assess the amount of urinary NH_4^+ by calculating the urinary anion gap (UAG).

■ EQUATION 11.5

$$UAG = (U_{Na} + U_K) - U_{Cl}$$

Under normal circumstances, the UAG is positive, with values ranging from 30 to 50. A negative value for the UAG suggests

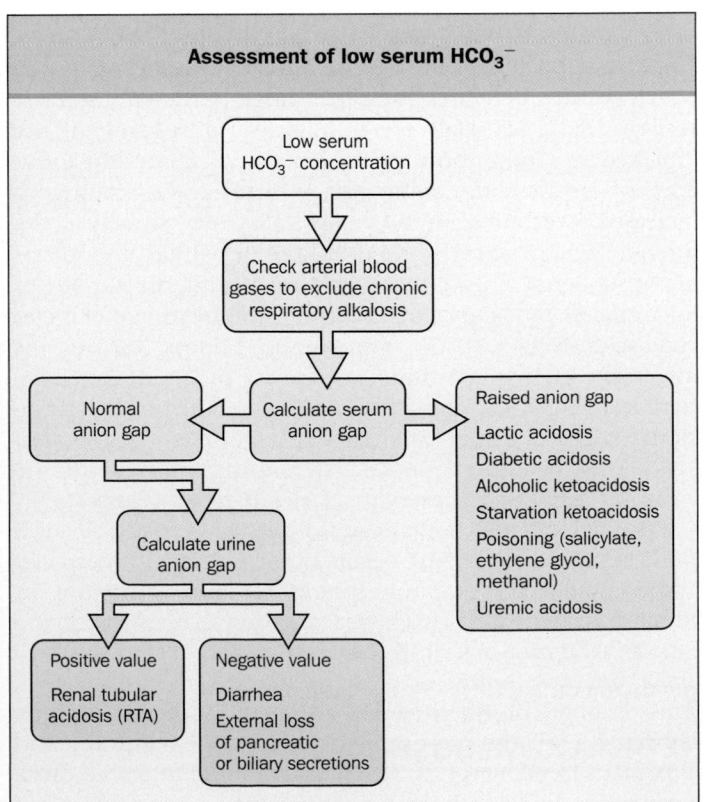

Figure 11.5 Approach to the patient with a low HCO_3^- concentration.

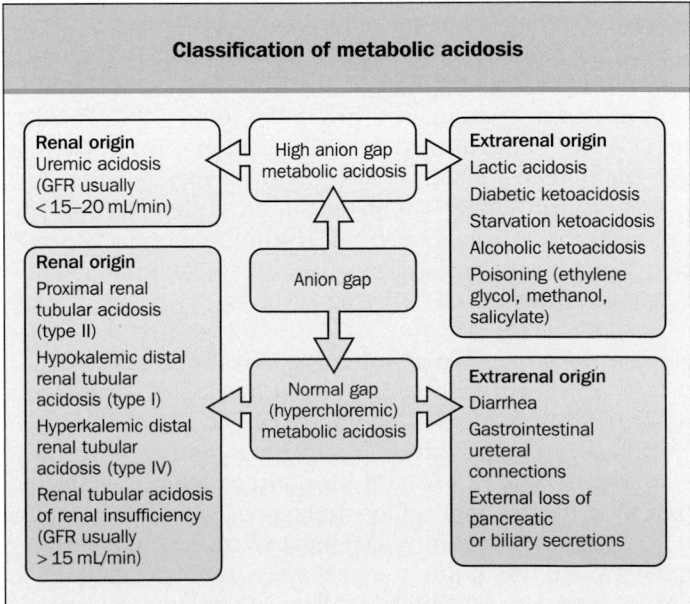

Figure 11.6 Classification of metabolic acidosis.

Fluid and Electrolyte Disorders

Urine anion gap (UAG) in evaluation of metabolic acidosis

Positive UAG

Decreased renal ammonia production
Proximal renal tubular acidosis (type II)
Hypokalemic distal renal tubular acidosis (type I)
Hyperkalemic distal renal tubular acidosis (type IV)
Renal tubular acidosis of renal insufficiency

Increased renal ammonia production and increased urinary excretion of sodium salts of acid
Sodium ketoacid salts (diabetic and alcoholic ketoacidosis)
Sodium hippurate and sodium benzoate (toluene poisoning)

Negative UAG

Increased ammonia production
Extrarenal acidosis

Table 11.1 Use of the urine anion gap (UAG) in evaluation of metabolic acidosis.

the presence of increased renal excretion of an unmeasured cation (i.e., a cation other than Na^+ or K^+). One such cation is NH_4^+. Metabolic acidosis of extrarenal origin is associated with a marked increase in urinary NH_4^+ excretion and, therefore, a large negative value will be obtained for the UAG. If the acidosis is of renal origin, urinary NH_4^+ excretion will be minimal and the UAG will usually be positive. One setting in which the UAG may not be useful is when there is increased excretion of Na^+ coupled to an anion other than Cl^-. For example, in diabetic and alcoholic ketoacidosis the UAG may remain positive despite an appropriate increase in urinary NH_3 excretion because of the increased urinary excretion of sodium keto acid salts. As discussed below a similar situation can occur in certain patients with toluene exposure due to increased urinary excretion of sodium salts of hippuric acid and benzoic acid. Table 11.1 describes the use of the UAG in the work up of metabolic acidosis.

In contrast to urinary NH_4^+ excretion, urine pH cannot reliably differentiate acidosis of renal origin from that of extrarenal origin. For example, an acid urine pH does not necessarily indicate an appropriate increase in net acid excretion. With a significant reduction in the availability of NH_4^+ to serve as a buffer, only a small amount of distal H^+ secretion will lead to a maximal reduction in urine pH. In this setting, the pH of the urine is acid but the quantity of H^+ secretion is insufficient to meet daily acid production. By contrast, an alkaline urine does not necessarily imply a renal acidification defect. In conditions where availability of NH_4^+ is not limiting, distal H^+ secretion can be massive and yet the urine remains relatively alkaline because of the buffering effects of NH_4^+.

Hyperchloremic normal anion gap metabolic acidosis

A hyperchloremic normal anion gap metabolic acidosis can be of renal or extrarenal origin. Metabolic acidosis of renal origin is the result of several types of abnormality in tubular H^+ transport. The RTA of early renal insufficiency is characterized by a normal gap acidosis; however, with severe reductions in the GFR an anion gap metabolic acidosis eventually develops. At this point the acidosis is often referred to as uremic acidosis. Metabolic acidosis of extrarenal origin is most commonly caused by gastrointestinal losses of HCO_3^-.

Other causes include the external loss of biliary and pancreatic secretions and ureteral diversion procedures.

Renal origin
Proximal renal tubular acidosis (type II)

Under normal circumstances, approximately 90% of the filtered load of HCO_3^- is reabsorbed in the proximal tubule. Normally the serum HCO_3^- concentration is maintained slightly below the threshold at which bicarbonaturia develops. In this manner, when the serum concentration of HCO_3^- exceeds 26–28 mmol/L, the excess HCO_3^- is excreted in the urine. In proximal RTA, the threshold for HCO_3^- reabsorption is reduced and results in a self-limited bicarbonaturia. This defect causes a portion of the filtered HCO_3^- to escape reabsorption in the proximal tubule and to be delivered into the distal nephron. The distal nephron has a low capacity for HCO_3^- reabsorption and, thus, HCO_3^- appears in the urine. The net effect is that the serum concentration and filtered load of HCO_3^- begin to fall. Despite the development of systemic acidemia, the urine pH is alkaline because of the presence of HCO_3^- in the urine. Eventually a steady state is reached at which point all the filtered HCO_3^- is reabsorbed. Now the delivery of HCO_3^- to the distal nephron may be abnormally increased, but it is of a magnitude that can be reabsorbed by the distal nephron. The urine is acidified to a pH of < 5.5, and net acid excretion is equal to endogenous acid production but at a lower serum HCO_3^- concentration. In the steady state, the serum HCO_3^- concentration is usually in the range 16–18 mmol/L.

One of the characteristic findings in proximal RTA is the presence of hypokalemia. The development of hypokalemia is the result of renal K^+ wasting caused by the coupling of increased aldosterone levels and increased distal Na^+ delivery. The loss of $NaHCO_3$ in the urine leads to volume depletion, which in turn activates the renin–angiotensin–aldosterone system. Distal Na^+ delivery is increased as a result of the impaired proximal reabsorption of $NaHCO_3$. Under the influence of aldosterone, some Na^+ is reabsorbed, leading to increased K^+ secretion. In the steady state when virtually all the filtered HCO_3^- is reabsorbed in the proximal and distal nephron, renal K^+ wasting is minimal and the degree of hypokalemia tends to be mild. By contrast, treatment of metabolic acidosis with HCO_3^- improves the acidosis but worsens the degree of hypokalemia. An increase in the filtered concentration of HCO_3^- above the reabsorptive threshold of the kidney will result in an increase in excretion of $NaHCO_3$ and $KHCO_3$. The persistent hyperaldosteronism combines with the increased distal Na^+ delivery to accelerate renal K^+ losses.

Proximal RTA may occur as an isolated defect in acidification alone but more commonly occurs in the setting of widespread dysfunction of the proximal tubule (Fanconi syndrome). In addition to decreased HCO_3^- reabsorption, patients with the Fanconi syndrome have impaired reabsorption of glucose, phosphate, uric acid, amino acids, and low-molecular-weight proteins. A variety of inherited and acquired disorders have been associated with the development of Fanconi syndrome and proximal RTA (Table 11.2). The most common inherited cause is cystinosis. Adults with the Fanconi syndrome most commonly have a dysproteinemic condition such as multiple myeloma.

Causes of proximal (type II) renal tubular acidosis	
Association	**Type**
Not associated with Fanconi syndrome	Sporadic
	Familial
	Disorder of carbonic anhydrase caused by drugs (e.g., acetazolamide; sulfanilamide)
	Carbonic anhydrase II deficiency
Associated with Fanconi syndrome	
Selective (no systemic disease present)	Sporadic
	Familial
Generalized (systemic disorder present)	Genetic disorders: cystinosis; Wilson's disease; hereditary fructose intolerance; Lowe's syndrome; metachromatic leukodystrophy
	Dysproteinemic states: myeloma kidney; light chain deposition disease
	Primary and secondary hyperparathyroidism
	Drugs: outdated tetracycline; ifosfamide; gentamicin; streptozocin
	Toxins: lead; cadmium; mercury
	Tubulointerstitial disease: post-transplant rejection Balkan nephropathy; medullary cystic disease
	Others: bone fibroma; osteopetrosis; paroxysmal nocturnal hemoglobinuria

Table 11.2 Causes of proximal (type II) renal tubular acidosis.

Unlike distal RTA, proximal RTA is not associated with nephrolithiasis or nephrocalcinosis. However, skeletal abnormalities are commonly present in these patients. Osteomalacia develops as a result of chronic hypophosphatemia owing to renal phosphate wasting. These patients may also have a deficiency in the active form of vitamin D because of an inability to convert 25-hydroxyvitamin D_3 to 1,25-dihydroxyvitamin D in the proximal tubule. In adults, osteopenia may be present as a result of acidosis-induced demineralization of bone.

The diagnosis of proximal RTA is suspected in a patient with a normal anion gap acidosis, hypokalemia, and an intact ability to acidify the urine to < 5.5 while in a steady state. Other findings of proximal tubular dysfunction such as glycosuria in the setting of a normal serum glucose concentration, hypophosphatemia, hypouricemia, and mild proteinuria help to support this diagnosis. The urine anion gap is normal. If the diagnosis is still in doubt, a $NaHCO_3$ infusion test can be performed (administration of $NaHCO_3$ at a rate of 0.5 to 1.0 mmol/h per kilogram body weight with measurement of urinary HCO_3^-). Raising the serum HCO_3^- concentration above the reabsorptive threshold will cause the pH of the urine to increase rapidly to > 7.5. In addition, the fractional excretion of $NaHCO_3$, which is normally < 5%, will increase to values > 15–20% as the plasma HCO_3^- concentration approaches normal.

The treatment of patients with proximal RTA is difficult. Correction of the acidosis is often not possible even with large amounts of HCO_3^- (3–5 mmol/kg daily) since exogenous alkali is rapidly excreted in the urine. In addition, such therapy leads to accelerated renal K^+ losses. Use of a thiazide diuretic to induce sufficient volume depletion to lower the GFR and, thus, decrease the filtered load of HCO_3^- may increase the effectiveness of alkali therapy. Potassium-sparing diuretics may limit the degree of renal K^+ wasting. Once therapy is initiated, close monitoring is required in order to guard against severe electrolyte derangements.

Hypokalemic distal renal tubular acidosis (type I)

In contrast to proximal RTA, patients with distal RTA do not acidify their urine despite severe metabolic acidosis. This disorder results from a reduction in net H^+ secretion in the distal nephron, which gives rise to an impairment in HCO_3^- regeneration. As a result, these patients are in a state of persistent positive acid balance, requiring bone buffers to prevent severe systemic acidemia. The pathophysiologic basis for this defect could be either impaired H^+ secretion (secretory defect) or an abnormally permeable distal tubule, resulting in increased backleak of normally secreted H^+ (gradient defect). One maneuver that has been utilized to differentiate these two possibilities has been to measure the urine to blood (U–B) P_{CO_2} gradient under conditions of an HCO_3^- infusion. In normal subjects given an HCO_3^- infusion to produce a high HCO_3^- excretion rate, distal H^+ secretion leads to the generation of a high P_{CO_2} in the urine (which is measured by collecting the urine under oil). Since the tubular fluid in the distal nephron is not in contact with carbonic anhydrase, H_2CO_3 formed by distal H^+ secretion disassociates at the uncatalyzed rate. As a result, most of the CO_2 is formed in the medulla and urinary pelvis, where the countercurrent system and surface–volume relationships are unfavorable for CO_2 diffusion. The magnitude of the U–B P_{CO_2} gradient has been used as an index of distal H^+ secretion. In most patients with distal RTA the U–B P_{CO_2} gradient is abnormally low (< 10 mmHg compared with > 30 mmHg in normals), suggesting that H^+ secretion is impaired. It should be noted that this is being measured in a setting where luminal pH is high and, thus, there is no gradient for back diffusion. This favors a secretory defect. The exceptions are those patients with amphotericin B-induced distal RTA. In these patients the U–B P_{CO_2} gradient is normal, suggesting an intact H^+ secretory mechanism. Rather, this disorder appears to be the result of a permeability defect such that secreted H^+ diffuses back into the cell.

For patients with a secretory defect, the inability to acidify the urine below pH 5.5 results from an abnormality in one or both of the H^+ secretory mechanisms. Some patients may have an isolated defect in the H^+/K^+ ATPase that impairs H^+ secretion and K^+ reabsorption. A defect confined to the vacuolar H^+ ATPase could also lead to renal K^+ wasting but would do so in a more indirect fashion. The development of systemic acidosis tends to diminish net proximal fluid reabsorption with an increase in distal delivery, volume contraction and activation of the renin–aldosterone system. Increased distal Na^+ delivery coupled to increased circulating levels of aldosterone would then lead to increased renal K^+ secretion. Patients with distal RTA exhibit low rates of NH_4^+ secretion given the degree of systemic acidemia. In part, the decreased secretion is caused by the failure to trap NH_4^+ in the tubular lumen of the collecting duct as a result of the inability to lower the pH of the fluid. In addition there is likely an impairment in the medullary transfer of NH_4^+ because of interstitial disease. Interstitial disease is frequently present in such patients through an associated underlying disease or as a result of nephrocalcinosis or hypokalemia-induced interstitial fibrosis.

Unlike proximal RTA, patients frequently manifest nephrolithiasis and nephrocalcinosis. This predisposition to renal calcification results from a number of factors. Urinary Ca^{2+} excretion is high secondary to acidosis-induced bone mineral dissolution. This increase in urinary Ca^{2+} excretion is made worse by the low intraluminal concentration of HCO_3^- in the distal nephron. Normally HCO_3^- acts to increase distal Ca^{2+} absorption. Systemic acidemia lowers the luminal concentration of HCO_3^- in the distal nephron; with the result that Ca^{2+} absorption is decreased and urinary Ca^{2+} excretion is further augmented. The increased Ca^{2+} excretion is more likely to result in supersaturation of the urine in the presence of an alkaline pH. The high urine pH decreases the solubility of calcium phosphate complexes. Stone formation is further enhanced as a result of low urinary citrate excretion. Citrate is metabolized to HCO_3^-, and thus its reabsorption contributes to correction of metabolic acidosis. Unfortunately, urinary citrate serves as the major Ca^{2+} chelator in the urine, and, therefore, its enhanced reabsorption in acidosis predisposes to nephrolithiasis and nephrocalcinosis.

Distal RTA may be a primary disorder, either idiopathic or inherited, but most commonly occurs in association with a systemic disease, of which one of the most common causes is Sjögren's syndrome (Table 11.3). There is a particularly striking association with hypergammaglobulinemic states. Several drugs and toxins have also been linked with the development of this disorder.

A common cause of acquired distal RTA is glue sniffing. Inhalation of toluene fumes found in model glue as well as spray paint and paint thinners can give rise to hypokalemic normal gap acidosis. First, toluene causes a secretory defect in distal hydrogen ion secretion as evidenced by the inability to normally increase urinary P_{CO_2} in the setting of a highly alkaline urine. This defect will be associated with low urinary ammonia excretion and a positive UAG. A second mechanism comes from the observation that some patients with this disorder have increased urinary ammonia excretion suggesting intact distal hydrogen ion secretion. The development of hypokalemic acidosis in these patients results from the metabolism of toluene to hippuric and benzoic acid, which are buffered by endogenous bicarbonate to form sodium hippurate and sodium benzoate. The excretion of these sodium salts by the kidney is equivalent to the loss of sodium bicarbonate from the body. The loss of these bicarbonate equivalents combined with ongoing sodium chloride reabsorption results in the development of a normal gap acidosis. During periods of active inhalation or in the setting of volume contraction production of these sodium salts may exceed renal excretion and the serum anion gap may be increased. Increased distal delivery of these sodium salts in the setting of high circulating levels of aldosterone will lead to renal potassium wasting and account for the development of hypokalemia. It is likely that both a secretory defect as well as increased urinary excretion of potential bicarbonate play a role in the electrolyte disturbances of patients with toluene toxicity. With prolonged and repetitive exposure to toluene the defect in distal acidification becomes more pronounced resulting in irreversible electrolyte abnormalities.

The diagnosis of distal RTA should be considered in a patient with hyperchloremic normal gap acidosis, hypokalemia, and an inability to lower the urine pH maximally[6]. A urine pH > 5.5 in the setting of systemic acidosis is consistent with a distal RTA, as is a positive urinary anion gap. The systemic acidosis tends to be more severe than in patients with a proximal RTA. The serum HCO_3^- concentration can reach values as low as 10 mmol/L. Hypokalemia can also be severe and present with musculoskeletal weakness and symptoms of nephrogenic diabetes insipidus. An abdominal radiograph may reveal nephrocalcinosis.

Correction of the metabolic acidosis in distal RTA can be achieved by administration of alkali in an amount equal to daily acid production (usually 1–2 mmol/kg per day). In patients with severe K^+ deficits, correction of the acidosis with HCO_3^- can transiently cause further lowering of the extracellular K^+ concentration and result in symptomatic hypokalemia. In this setting, the K^+ deficit should be corrected prior to correcting the acidosis. In addition to decreasing renal K^+ losses, correction of the acidosis will decrease urinary Ca^{2+} excretion and increase urinary citrate levels. Potassium citrate is the preferred form of alkali for those patients with persistent hypokalemia or with calcium stone disease.

Hyperkalemic distal renal tubular acidosis (type IV)

Type IV RTA is a disorder that is characterized by a disturbance in distal nephron function, resulting in impaired renal excretion of both H^+ and K^+ and giving a hyperchloremic normal gap acidosis and hyperkalemia[7]. The syndrome occurs most often in association with mild-to-moderate renal insufficiency; however, the magnitude of hyperkalemia and acidosis are disproportionately severe for the observed degree of renal insufficiency. While hypokalemic distal (type I) RTA is also a disorder of distal nephron acidification, this disorder

Type	Causes
Causes of hypokalemic distal (type I) renal tubular acidosis	
Primary	Idiopathic
	Familial
Secondary	Autoimmune disorders: hypergammaglobulinemia; Sjögren's syndrome; primary biliary cirrhosis; systemic lupus erythematosus
	Genetic diseases: Ehlers–Danlos syndrome; Marfan syndrome; hereditary elliptocytosis
	Drugs: amphotericin B
	Toxins: toluene
	Disorders with nephrocalcinosis: hyperparathyroidism; vitamin D intoxication; idiopathic hypercalciuria
	Tubulointerstitial disease: obstructive uropathy; renal transplantation

Table 11.3 Causes of hypokalemic distal (type I) renal tubular acidosis.

can be distinguished from type IV RTA on the basis of several important characteristics. First and foremost, patients with type IV RTA are distinguished from patients with type I RTA on the basis of plasma K^+ concentration, which is abnormally high in the former and abnormally low in the latter. Second, in type IV RTA, mild-to-moderate chronic renal failure is almost always present whereas in type I RTA renal function is normal or only mildly impaired. Third, in most cases of type IV RTA, the urine pH measured during spontaneous acidosis is appropriately low (< 5.5), whereas urine pH during spontaneous or induced acidosis in type I RTA fails to decrease appropriately (> 5.5). Fourth, metabolic acidosis in type IV RTA is mild, with plasma HCO_3^- concentration rarely below 15 mmol/L, but in type I RTA acidosis is often severe with plasma HCO_3^- concentrations less than 15 mmol/L. It should be remembered that type IV RTA is a much more common form of RTA and is, therefore, more likely to be encountered, particularly in adult patients.

The pathophysiologic basis for this disorder can either be a deficiency in circulating aldosterone or a disease of the cortical collecting duct. In either case, a defect in distal H^+ secretion develops. Impaired Na^+ reabsorption in the principal cell leads to a decrease in the luminal electronegativity of the cortical collecting duct, which impairs distal acidification as a result of the decrease in driving force for H^+ secretion into the tubular lumen. The H^+ secretion is further impaired in this segment as well as in the medullary collecting duct, as a result either of the loss of the direct stimulatory effect of aldosterone on H^+ secretion or of an abnormality in the H^+-secreting cell.

Another consequence of the decrease in luminal electronegativity in the cortical collecting duct is an impairment in renal K^+ excretion. In addition, an abnormality in the cortical collecting duct would also impair K^+ secretion. The development of hyperkalemia adds to the defect in distal acidification by decreasing the amount of ammonia available to act as a urinary buffer[8]. Hyperkalemia limits the availability of NH_3 by decreasing NH_3 production in the proximal tubule. NH_4^+ transport in the thick ascending limb is also inhibited because the large increase in luminal K^+ concentration effectively competes with NH_4^+ for transport on the $Na^+/K^+/2Cl^-$ cotransporter and apical K^+ channel. Net acid excretion decreases as a result of limited buffer availability for titration of secreted H^+.

The differential diagnosis of type IV RTA can be divided into those conditions associated with decreased circulating levels of aldosterone and conditions associated with impaired function of the cortical collecting duct (Table 11.4). Perhaps the most common disease associated with type IV RTA in adults is diabetes mellitus (Type 1 diabetes). In these patients, primary NaCl retention leads to volume expansion and suppression and atrophy of the renin-secreting juxtaglomerular apparatus. Several commonly used drugs such as nonsteroidal anti-inflammatory agents (NSAIDs), angiotensin-converting enzyme (ACE) inhibitors, and heparin can lead to decreased mineralocorticoid activity. Impaired function of the cortical collecting duct can be a feature of structural damage to the kidney, as in interstitial renal diseases such as in sickle cell nephropathy, urinary tract obstruction, or lupus; or it may also result from use of certain drugs.

Causes of hyperkalemic distal (type IV) renal tubular acidosis	
Defect	**Causes**
Mineralocorticoid deficiency	
Low renin, low aldosterone	Diabetes mellitus
	Drugs: nonsteroidal anti-inflammatory agents; cyclosporine; β-blockers
High renin, low aldosterone	Adrenal destruction
	Congenital enzyme defects
	Drugs: angiotensin-converting enzyme inhibitors; angiotensin receptor antagonists; heparin; ketoconazole
Abnormal cortical collecting duct	Absent or defective mineralocorticoid receptor
	Drugs: spironolactone; triamterene; amiloride; trimethoprim; pentamidine
	Chronic tubulointerstitial disease: chronic urinary tract obstruction; sickle cell nephropathy; systemic lupus

Table 11.4 Causes of hyperkalemic distal (type IV) renal tubular acidosis.

A type IV RTA should be suspected in a patient with a hyperchloremic normal gap metabolic acidosis associated with hyperkalemia. The typical patient is in the fifth to seventh decade of life with a long-standing history of diabetes mellitus with a moderate reduction in the GFR. The plasma HCO_3^- concentration is usually in the range of 18–22 mmol/L and the serum K^+ is in the range of 5.5–6.5 mmol/L. Most patients are asymptomatic; however, occasionally the hyperkalemia may be severe enough to cause muscle weakness or cardiac arrhythmias. The urinary anion gap is slightly positive, indicating little to no NH_4^+ excretion in the urine. Patients in which the disorder is caused by a defect in mineralocorticoid activity typically have a urine pH of < 5.5, reflecting a more severe defect in NH_3 availability than in H^+ secretion (Fig. 11.7). In patients with structural damage to the collecting duct, the urine pH may be alkaline reflecting both impaired H^+ secretion and decreased urinary NH_4^+ excretion.

Most patients with type IV RTA do not require treatment unless they have an intercurrent illness that may exacerbate hyperkalemia and acidosis. If treatment is required, the primary goal of therapy is to correct the hyperkalemia. In many instances, lowering the serum K^+ will simultaneously correct the acidosis[9]. Correction of the hyperkalemia allows for renal NH_4^+ production to increase, thereby increasing the buffer supply for distal acidification. The first consideration in the treatment of patients is to discontinue any drug that is known to interfere in the synthesis or activity of aldosterone. In patients who are not hypertensive or fluid overloaded, administration of a synthetic mineralocorticoid such as fludrocortisone (0.1 mg/day) is effective in conditions of aldosterone deficiency. An alternative choice would be administration of a thiazide diuretic in hypertensive patients or a loop diuretic in patients with a serum creatinine concentration < 2 mgdL (180 μmol/L). These diuretics increase distal Na^+ delivery and, as a result, stimulate K^+ and H^+ secretion in the collecting duct. Alkali therapy ($NaHCO_3$) can also be used to treat the acidosis and

Fluid and Electrolyte Disorders

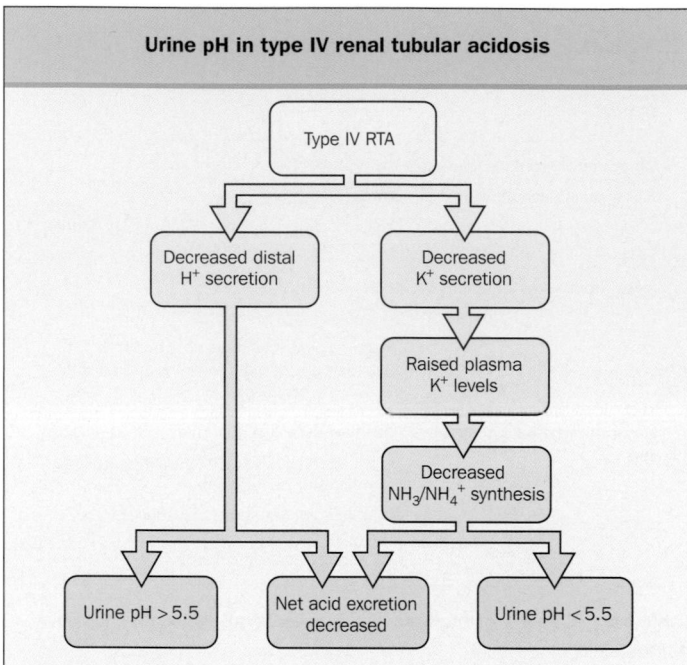

Urine pH in type IV renal tubular acidosis

Figure 11.7 Urine pH in type IV renal tubular acidosis. Net acid excretion is always decreased; however, the urine pH can be variable. In structural disease of the kidney, the predominant defect is usually decreased distal H+ secretion and the urine pH is > 5.5. In disorders associated with decreased mineralocorticoid activity, urine pH is usually < 5.5.

hyperkalemia, but one must closely monitor the volume status of the patient as administration of an alkaline salt can lead to volume overload.

Renal tubular acidosis of renal insufficiency

Metabolic acidosis occurs in chronic renal insufficiency caused by failure of the tubular acidification process to excrete the normal daily acid load. As functional renal mass is reduced by disease, there is an adaptive increase in NH_4^+ production and H+ secretion by the remaining nephrons. This adaptive increase eventually can no longer keep pace with daily acid production as the reduction in functioning renal mass continues. Net acid excretion becomes less than the quantity of acid produced endogenously and a hyperchloremic normal gap acidosis begins to develop. Patients with renal insufficiency initially develop a hyperchloremic normal gap metabolic acidosis associated with normokalemia as the GFR falls below 30 mL/min. With more advanced renal failure (GFR < 15 mL/min), the acidosis changes to predominately an anion gap metabolic acidosis.

The principal defect in net acid excretion is due to the inability to excrete adequate amounts of NH_4^+ in the urine. Despite increased production of NH_4^+ from each remaining nephron, overall production is decreased secondary to the decrease in total renal mass. In addition, there is less delivery of NH_4^+ to the medullary interstitium secondary to a disrupted medullary anatomy[10]. The ability to lower the urinary pH remains intact, reflecting the fact that the impairment in distal nephron H+ secretion is less than that in NH_3 secretion. Quantitatively, however, the total amount of H+ secretion is

small and the acidic urine pH is the consequence of very little buffer in the urine. The lack of NH_4^+ in the urine is reflected by a positive value for the urinary anion gap.

As renal insufficiency with a hyperchloremic metabolic acidosis progresses to a low GFR (< 10 mL/min), phosphate and other anions (sulfate and organic acids) accumulate, converting the acidosis to the anion gap form. The association between hypobicarbonatemia and an elevated anion gap in advanced renal insufficiency does not have the same pathogenic significance as it does with other forms of anion gap acidosis: in the overproduction form (lactic acidosis, diabetic ketoacidosis) or ingestion-associated form (methanol, ethylene glycol) the anions of the acids remain in the circulation in place of HCO_3^-. Therefore, in these types of organic acidosis, the decline in serum HCO_3^- usually bears a close quantitative relationship to the rise in unmeasured anions. In contrast, in uremic acidosis, the rise in unmeasured anions does not signify increased acid production or addition but merely reflects the associated renal insufficiency and consequent retention of anions normally excreted by filtration. As a result, plasma HCO_3^- in patients with renal insufficiency bears no predictable relationship to the rise in unmeasured anions.

Correction of the metabolic acidosis in patients with renal insufficiency is achieved by treatment with $NaHCO_3$ 0.5–1.5 mmol/kg/day beginning when the HCO_3^- level is < 18 mmol/L. Loop diuretics are often used in conjunction with alkali therapy to prevent volume overload. Eventually the acidosis becomes refractory to medical therapy, and dialysis needs to be initiated. Recent evidence suggests that metabolic acidosis in the setting of renal failure needs to be aggressively treated, as chronic acidosis is associated with metabolic bone disease and may lead to an accelerated catabolic state in patients with chronic renal failure[11]. An overall approach for workup of metabolic acidosis of renal origin is shown in Figure 11.8.

Extrarenal origin
Diarrhea
Intestinal secretions beyond the stomach including those of the pancreas and biliary tract are rich in HCO_3^-. Accelerated loss of this HCO_3^--rich solution from the body will lead to the development of metabolic acidosis. The resultant volume loss signals the kidney to increase the reabsorption of salt. Renal retention of NaCl combined with the intestinal loss of $NaHCO_3$ generates a hyperchloremic normal gap metabolic acidosis. The renal response to the systemic acidemia is to increase net acid excretion markedly. This is primarily accomplished by increasing the urinary excretion of NH_4^+. Hypokalemia, as a result of gastrointestinal losses, and the low serum pH both stimulate the synthesis of NH_3 in the proximal tubule. The increase in availability of NH_3 to act as a urinary buffer allows for a maximal increase in H+ secretion by the distal nephron.

Examination of the urine pH in diarrhea can be misleading when trying to determine whether the renal response to the systemic acidemia is appropriate. In fact, urine pH during chronic diarrheal states may be persistently > 6.0 despite the presence of systemic acidemia. In this regard, a patient who presents with hypokalemic hyperchloremic metabolic acidosis with a urine pH > 5.5 could either have a diarrheal state or a

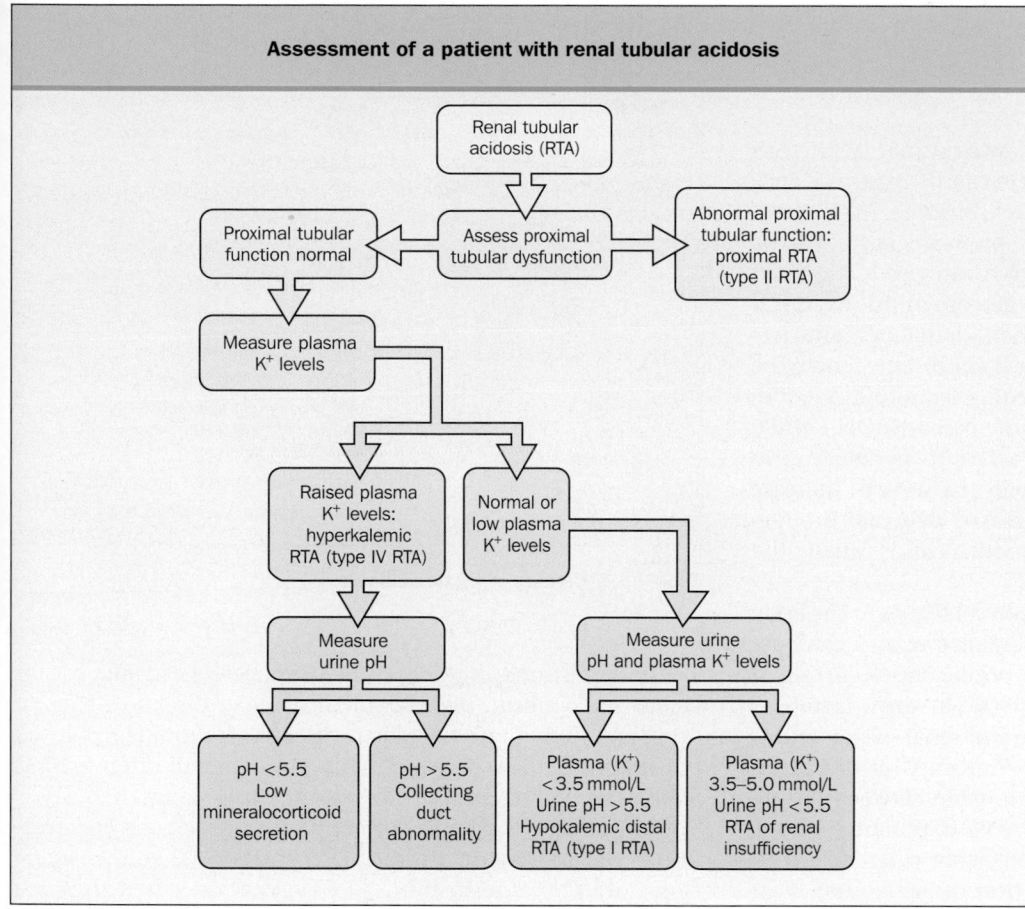

Assessment of a patient with renal tubular acidosis

Figure 11.8 Approach to the patient with renal tubular acidosis.

hypokalemic (type I) distal RTA. Although the clinical history would be the easiest way to distinguish between these two possibilities, in a patient with surreptitious laxative abuse this may not be helpful. Determination of the urinary anion gap is the best way to distinguish between them. In diarrhea, urine pH is high because of the large amount of NH_4^+ in the urine. This would be reflected by a negative urinary anion gap as most of the NH_4^+ is excreted in the urine as NH_4Cl. In hypokalemic distal RTA the urine pH is high because of the inability to secrete H^+ in the distal nephron. Urinary excretion of NH_3 is very low and the urinary anion gap is positive.

Ileal conduits

Surgical diversion of the ureter into an ileal pouch is a procedure often used in the treatment of patients with neurologic bladder abnormalities and urologic tumors. The procedure may rarely be associated with the development of a hyperchloremic normal gap metabolic acidosis. Acidosis may occur in part due to reabsorption of NH_4^+ and Cl^- from the urinary fluid by the intestine, which then metabolizes the NH_4^+ in the liver to NH_3 and H^+. Urinary Cl^- may also be reabsorbed in exchange for HCO_3^- through activation of the Cl^-/HCO_3^- exchanger on the intestinal lumen. In some patients, a renal defect in acidification can develop and exacerbate the degree of acidosis. Such a defect may result from tubular damage caused by pyelonephritis or high colonic pressures.

The main factors that influence the development and severity of acidosis are the length of time the urine is in contact with the bowel and the total surface area of bowel exposed to urine. In patients with a ureterosigmoid anastomosis, the acidosis tends to be more common and more severe than in those patients with an ileal conduit. The latter procedure was designed to minimize the time and area of contact between urine and intestinal surface. Patients undergoing this procedure who develop an acidosis should be examined for the possibility of an ileal loop obstruction, since this would lead to an increase in contact time between the urine and the intestinal surface.

Anion gap metabolic acidosis

Lactic acidosis

One of the most common causes of anion gap metabolic acidosis is lactic acidosis. Lactic acid is the end-product in the anaerobic metabolism of glucose, and is generated by the reversible reduction of pyruvic acid by lactic acid dehydrogenase and NADH.

■ EQUATION 11.6

$$\text{Pyruvate} + \text{NADH} + \text{H}^+ \rightleftharpoons \text{Lactate} + \text{NAD}$$

Under normal conditions, the reaction is shifted toward the right and the normal lactate to pyruvate ratio is approximately 10 : 1. The reactants in this pathway are interrelated as shown in the following equation.

■ EQUATION 11.7

$$(Lactate) = \frac{K(Pyruvate)(NADH)(H^+)}{(NAD^+)}$$

On the basis of this relationship, it is evident that lactate can increase, for three reasons. First, lactate can increase as a consequence of increased pyruvate production alone. In this situation the normal 10 : 1 lactate to pyruvate ratio will be maintained. An isolated increase in pyruvate production can be seen in the setting of intravenous glucose infusions, intravenous administration of epinephrine (adrenaline), and respiratory alkalosis. Lactate levels in these conditions tend to be only minimally elevated, rarely exceeding 5 mmol/L. Second, lactate can increase as a result of an increased NADH : NAD$^+$ ratio. Under these conditions, the lactate to pyruvate ratio can increase to very high values. Finally, lactate can increase when there is a combination of increased pyruvate production with an increased NADH : NAD$^+$ ratio. This is usually the case in severe lactic acidosis.

Under normal circumstances, virtually all tissues in the body metabolize glucose via the glycolytic pathway and generate lactate, with the greater part of lactate production occurring in brain, erythrocytes, and skeletal muscle. In turn, lactate is extracted predominately by the liver and renal cortex and is either reconverted to glucose or becomes fuel for oxidation for CO_2 and H_2O. This dynamic relationship between lactate and glucose is termed the Cori cycle. The importance of this cyclical relationship can best be appreciated when one considers that the normal daily production of lactate has been estimated to be 15–30 mmol/kg (equivalent to 15–30 mmol/kg H$^+$ per day). Since daily net acid excretion by the kidney is only 1 mmol/kg, the quantitative importance of this pathway in disposing of the H$^+$ produced during glycolysis becomes obvious. Furthermore, it is apparent that only a mild disruption in the equilibrium between lactate production and consumption in the Cori cycle can lead to the rapid development of devastating metabolic acidosis.

Lactic acidosis is generated whenever there arises an imbalance between the production and utilization of lactic acid[12]. The results of such an imbalance is an accumulation of serum lactate, most commonly accompanied by hypobicarbonatemia and systemic acidemia. The accumulation of a nonchloride anion accounts for the increase in anion gap. The pathogenesis of this imbalance can result from overproduction of lactic acid, underutilization, or both. Severe exercise and grand mal seizures are examples in which lactic acidosis can develop as a result of increased production. The short-lived nature of the acidosis in these conditions suggests that a concomitant defect in lactic acid utilization is present in most conditions of sustained and severe lactic acidosis.

A partial list of the disorders associated with the development of lactic acidosis is given in Table 11.5. Type A lactic acidosis is characterized by disorders in which there is underperfusion of tissue or acute hypoxia. Such disorders include patients with cardiopulmonary failure, severe anemia, hemorrhage, hypotension, sepsis, and carbon monoxide poisoning. Type B lactic acidosis occurs in patients with a variety of disorders that have in common the development of lactic acidosis in the absence of overt hypoperfusion or hypoxia.

Causes of lactic acidosis	
Types	**Causes**
Type A (tissue underperfusion and/or hypoxia)	Cardiogenic shock
	Septic shock
	Hemorrhagic shock
	Acute hypoxia
	Carbon monoxide poisoning
	Anemia
Type B (absence of hypotension and hypoxia)	Hereditary enzyme deficiency (glucose 6-phosphatase)
	Drugs: phenformin and metformin (especially in renal insufficiency); isoniazid; salicylate
	Toxins: cyanide; ethylene glycol; methanol
	Systemic disease: liver failure; malignancy

Table 11.5 Causes of lactic acidosis.

These conditions include congenital defects in glucose or lactate metabolism, diabetes mellitus, liver disease, effects of drugs and toxins, and neoplastic diseases. It should be pointed out that in clinical practice many patients will often exhibit features of type A and type B lactic acidosis simultaneously.

The primary goal in the therapy of lactic acidosis is correction of the underlying disorder. Every attempt should be made to restore tissue perfusion and oxygenation when they are compromised. The role of alkali in the treatment of lactic acidosis is controversial. The controversy has centered around experimental models and clinical observations that indicate administration of HCO$_3^-$ may depress cardiac function and exacerbate the acidemia. In addition, such therapy may be complicated by volume overload, hypernatremia, and rebound alkalosis after the acidosis has resolved. In general, HCO$_3^-$ should be given when the systemic pH falls below 7.1, as hemodynamic instability becomes much more likely with severe acidemia. However, attempts to normalize the pH or HCO$_3^-$ concentration should be avoided.

Diabetic ketoacidosis
Diabetic ketoacidosis is a metabolic condition characterized by the accumulation of acetoacetic acid and β-hydroxybutyric acid. The development of ketoacidosis is the result of insulin deficiency and a relative or absolute increase in glucagon concentration[13]. These hormonal changes lead to increased fatty acid mobilization from adipose tissue and, at the same time, alter the oxidative machinery of the liver such that delivered fatty acids are primarily metabolized into keto acids. In addition, peripheral glucose utilization is impaired and the gluconeogenic pathway in the liver is maximally stimulated. The resultant hyperglycemia results in an osmotic diuresis and volume depletion.

Ketoacidosis results when the rate of hepatic keto acid generation exceeds peripheral utilization and the blood keto acid concentration increases. The H$^+$ accumulation in the extracellular fluid disassociates HCO$_3^-$ while the keto acid anion concentration increases. The reduction in serum HCO$_3^-$

concentration approximates the increase in anion gap initially. The degree to which the anion gap is elevated will depend on the rapidity, severity, and duration of the ketoacidosis as well as the status of the extracellular fluid volume. While an anion gap acidosis is the dominant disturbance in diabetic ketoacidosis, a hyperchloremic normal gap acidosis is often present, depending upon the stage of the disease process. In the earliest stages of ketoacidosis when extracellular volume is near normal, keto acid anions that are produced are rapidly excreted by the kidney as Na^+ and K^+ salts. Excretion of these salts is equivalent to the loss of potential HCO_3^-. This loss of potential HCO_3^- in the urine at the same time as the kidney is retaining dietary NaCl results in a hyperchloremic normal gap acidosis. As the ketogenic process becomes more accelerated and as volume depletion becomes more severe, a larger proportion of the generated keto acid anions are retained within the body, thus increasing the anion gap. During treatment, the anion gap metabolic acidosis transforms once again into a hyperchloremic normal gap acidosis. Treatment leads to a termination in keto acid production. As the extracellular fluid volume is restored, there is increased renal excretion of the Na^+ salts of the keto acid anions. The loss of this potential HCO_3^- combined with the retention of administered NaCl accounts for the redevelopment of the hyperchloremic normal gap acidosis. In addition, K^+ and Na^+ administered in solutions containing NaCl and KCl enter into cells in exchange for H^+. The net effect is infusion of HCl into the extracellular fluid. The reversal of the hyperchloremic acidosis is accomplished over a period of several days as the HCO_3^- deficit is corrected by the kidney.

HCO_3^- levels may be as low as 10 mmol/L. Confirmation of the presence of keto acids can be achieved with use of nitroprusside tablets or reagent strips. However, this test can be misleading in assessing the severity of ketoacidosis as it only detects the presence of acetone and acetoacetate and does not permit reaction with β-hydroxybutyrate. Acetoacetic acid and β-hydroxybutyric acid are interconvertible, with the NADH : NAD^+ ratio being the primary determinant as to which moiety predominates. In the setting of a high ratio, formation of β-hydroxybutyric acid is favored and the nitroprusside test will become less positive or even negative despite significant ketoacidosis. This situation can occur when ketoacidosis is accompanied by lactic acidosis or in the setting of alcoholic ketoacidosis. During treatment, the NADH : NAD^+ ratio tends to decline, favoring the formation of acetoacetic acid. As a result, it is common for the nitroprusside test to register more strongly positive during the treatment of diabetic ketoacidosis.

Treatment of diabetic ketoacidosis involves the use of insulin and intravenous fluids to correct volume depletion. Deficiencies in K^+, Mg^{2+}, and phosphate are common and, therefore, these electrolytes are typically added to intravenous solutions. Alkali therapy is generally not required since administration of insulin leads to the metabolic conversion of keto acid anions into HCO_3^- and allows partial correction of the acidosis. However, HCO_3^- therapy may be indicated in those patients who present with severe acidemia (pH < 7.1).

D-Lactic acidosis

D-Lactic acidosis is a unique form of metabolic acidosis that can occur in the setting of small bowel resections or in patients with a jejunoileal bypass. Such short bowel syndromes create a situation in which carbohydrates that are normally extensively reabsorbed in the small intestine are delivered in large amounts to the colon. In the presence of colonic bacterial overgrowth, these substrates are metabolized into D-lactate and absorbed into the systemic circulation. Accumulation of D-lactate produces an anion gap metabolic acidosis in which the serum lactate is normal since the standard test for lactate is specific for L-lactate. These patients typically present after ingestion of a large carbohydrate meal with neurologic abnormalities consisting of confusion, slurred speech and ataxia. Ingestion of low carbohydrate meals and antimicrobial agents to decrease the degree of bacterial overgrowth are the principal treatments.

Starvation ketosis

Abstinence from food can lead to a mild anion gap metabolic acidosis secondary to increased production of keto acids. The pathogenesis of this disorder is similar to that of diabetic ketoacidosis in that starvation leads to relative insulin deficiency and glucagon excess. As a result, there is increased mobilization of fatty acids while the liver is set to oxidize fatty acids to keto acids. With prolonged starvation, the blood keto acid level can reach 5–6 mmol/L. The serum HCO_3^- concentration rarely falls to values below 18 mmol/L. More fulminant ketoacidosis is aborted by the fact that ketone bodies stimulate the pancreatic islets to release insulin and lipolysis is held in check. This break in the ketogenic process is notably absent in insulin-dependent diabetics. There is no specific therapy indicated in this disorder.

Alcoholic ketoacidosis

Ketoacidosis develops in patients with a history of chronic ethanol abuse, decreased food intake, and often a history of nausea and vomiting. As with starvation ketosis, a decrease in the insulin to glucagon ratio leads to accelerated fatty acid mobilization and alters the enzymatic machinery of the liver to favor keto acid production. However, there are features unique to this disorder that differentiate it from simple starvation ketosis. First, the presence of alcohol withdrawal combined with volume depletion and starvation markedly increases the levels of circulating catecholamines. As a result, the peripheral mobilization of fatty acids is much greater than that typically found with starvation alone. This sometimes massive mobilization of fatty acids can lead to marked keto acid production and severe metabolic acidosis. Second, the metabolism of alcohol leads to accumulation of NADH. The increase in the NADH : NAD^+ ratio is reflected by a higher β-hydroxybutyrate to acetoacetate ratio. As mentioned above, the nitroprusside reaction may be diminished by this redox shift despite the presence of severe ketoacidosis. Treatment of this disorder is centered on the administration of glucose. Glucose administration leads to the rapid resolution of the acidosis, since stimulation of insulin release leads to diminished fatty acid mobilization from adipose tissue as well as decreased hepatic output of keto acids.

Ethylene glycol and methanol poisoning

Ethylene glycol and methanol poisoning are characteristically associated with the development of a severe anion gap metabolic acidosis. Metabolism of ethylene glycol by alcohol

Fluid and Electrolyte Disorders

Table 11.6 Ethylene glycol and methanol poisoning
Time course of clinical symptoms and signs after ingestion
Ethylene glycol
0–12 h: inebriation progressing to coma
12–24 h: tachypnea, noncardiogenic pulmonary edema
24–36 h: flank pain, renal failure, urinary calcium oxalate crystals
Methanol
0–12 h: inebriation followed by asymptomatic period
24–36 h: pancreatitis, retinal edema progressing to blindness, seizures
>48 h: putamen and white matter hemorrhage leading to Parkinson-like state
Increased anion gap metabolic acidosis
Increased osmolar gap
Treatment
Supportive care
Fomepizole (4-methylpyrazole) is agent of choice (competitor of alcohol dehydrogenase)
15 mg/kg IV loading dose, then 10 mg/kg every 12 h for 48 h
After 48 h increase dose to 15 mg/kg every 12 h
Increase frequency of dosing to 4 h during hemodialysis
Intravenous ethanol if fomepizole unavailable (available as 5 or 10% solution)
Loading dose of 0.6 g/kg followed by hourly maintenance dose of 66 mg/kg
Increase maintenance dose with chronic alcohol use and during hemodialysis
Hemodialysis to accelerate removal of parent compound and metabolites
Bicarbonate therapy to treat acidosis

Table 11.6 Ethylene glycol and methanol poisoning.

dehydrogenase generates various acids, including glycolic, oxalic, and formic acids. Ethylene glycol is a component of antifreeze and solvents and is ingested by accident or as a suicide attempt. The initial effects of intoxication are neurologic and begin with drunkenness but can quickly progress to seizures and coma. If left untreated cardiopulmonary symptoms such as tachypnea, noncardiogenic pulmonary edema and cardiovascular collapse may appear. Twenty-four to 48 h after ingestion patients may develop flank pain and renal failure often accompanied by abundant calcium oxalate crystals in the urine (Table 11.6). A fatal dose is approximately 100 mL.

Methanol is also metabolized by alcohol dehydrogenase and forms formaldehyde, which is then converted to formic acid. Methanol is found in a variety of commercial preparations such as shellac, varnish, and de-icing solutions. As with ethylene glycol ingestion, methanol is ingested by accident or as a suicide attempt. Clinically, methanol ingestion is associated with an acute inebriation followed by an asymptomatic period lasting 24–36 h. At this point abdominal pain caused by pancreatitis, seizures, blindness, and coma may develop. The blindness is due to direct toxicity of formic acid on the retina. Methanol intoxication is also associated with hemorrhage in the white matter and putamen which can lead to the delayed onset of a Parkinson-like syndrome (Table 11.6). The lethal dose is between 60 and 250 mL. Lactic acidosis is also a feature of methanol and ethylene glycol poisoning and contributes to the elevated anion gap.

Together with the appearance of the anion gap, an osmolar gap also becomes manifest and is an important clue to the

diagnosis of ethylene glycol and methanol poisoning. The osmolar gap is the difference between the measured and calculated osmolality.

■ EQUATION 11.8

$$\text{Calculated osmolality} = \frac{2(\text{Na}^+)(\text{mmol/L}) + \text{BUN(mg/dL)}/2.8}{+ \text{Glucose(mg/dL)}/18}$$

where BUN is the blood urea nitrogen. The normal value for the osmolar gap is < 10 mOsm/kg. Each 100 mg/dL (161 mmol/L) ethylene glycol will increase the osmolar gap by 16 mOsm, while methanol contributes 32 mOsm/kg for each 100 mg/dL (312 mmol/L).

In addition to supportive measures, the therapy for ethylene glycol and methanol poisoning is centered on reducing the metabolism of the parent compound and accelerating the removal of the alcohol from the body (Table 11.6). Decreasing metabolism of the parent compound is important since the metabolites rather than the parent compound are primarily responsible for the toxic effects. Fomepizole (4-methylpyrazole) is now the agent of choice to inhibit the enzyme alcohol dehydrogenase and prevent formation of toxic metabolites[14].

If fomepizole is unavailable then intravenous ethanol can be utilized to prevent the formation of toxic metabolites. Ethanol has > 10-fold greater affinity for alcohol dehydrogenase than other alcohols. Ethanol has its greatest efficacy when levels of 100–200 mg/dL are obtained. With both fomepizole and ethanol therapy, hemodialysis therapy should be employed to remove both the parent compound and metabolites. One final aspect of management is correction of the acidosis. This can be accomplished with use of a HCO_3^--containing dialysate or by intravenous infusion of $NaHCO_3$.

Salicylate

Aspirin (acetylsalicylic acid) is one of the most widely available therapeutic agents and is associated with the largest number of accidental or intentional poisonings. At toxic concentrations, salicylate uncouples oxidative phosphorylation and, as a result, leads to increased lactic acid production. In children, keto acid production may also be increased. The accumulation of lactic, salicylic, keto, and other organic acids lead to the development of an anion gap metabolic acidosis. At the same time, salicylate has a direct stimulatory effect on the respiratory center. Increased ventilation lowers the $P\text{CO}_2$, contributing to the development of a respiratory alkalosis. Children primarily manifest an anion gap metabolic acidosis with toxic salicylate levels, while a respiratory alkalosis is most evident in adults.

In addition to conservative management, the initial goal of therapy is to correct systemic acidemia and to increase the urine pH. By increasing systemic pH, the ionized fraction of salicylic acid will increase and as a result there will be less accumulation of the drug in the central nervous system. Similarly, an alkaline urine pH will favor increased urinary excretion since the ionized fraction of the drug is poorly reabsorbed by the tubule. At serum concentrations of > 80 mg/dL or in the setting of severe clinical toxicity, hemodialysis can be used to accelerate the removal of the drug from the body.

REFERENCES

1. Alpern RJ. Cell mechanisms of proximal tubule acidification. Physiol Rev. 1990;70:79–114.

2. Alpern RJ, Giebisch G, Seldin DW. Renal electrolyte transport and its regulation. In: Seldin D, Giebisch G, eds. Diuretic agents: clinical physiology and pharmacology. San Diego, CA: Academic Press; 1997:31–72.

3. Alpern RJ, Rector FC. Renal acidification mechanisms. In: Brenner BM, ed. The kidney, 5th edn. Philadelphia, PA: Saunders; 1996:408–71.

4. Pitts RF. Control of renal production of ammonia. Kidney Int. 1972;1:297–305.

5. Halperin ML, Richardson RM, Bear R, et al. Urine ammonium: the key to the diagnosis of distal renal tubular acidosis. Nephron. 1988;50:1–4.

6. McSherry E, Sebastian A, Morris RC. Renal tubular acidosis in infants: the several kinds, including bicarbonate-wasting, classic renal tubular acidosis. J Clin Invest. 1972;51:499–514.

7. DuBose TD. Hyperkalemic hyperchloremic metabolic acidosis: pathophysiologic insights. Kidney Int. 1997;51:591–602.

8. Hulter HN, Ilnicki L, Harbottle J, Sebastian A. Impaired renal H^+ secretion and NH_3 production in mineralocorticoid-deficient glucocorticoid-replete dogs. Am J Physiol. 1977;232:F136–46.

9. Sebastian A, Schambelan M, Lindenfeld S, Morris RC. Amelioration of metabolic acidosis with fludrocortisone therapy in hyporeninemic hypoaldosteronism. N Engl J Med. 1977;297:576–83.

10. Buerkert J, Martin D, Trigg D, Simon E. Effect of reduced renal mass on ammonium handling and net acid formation by the superficial and juxtamedullary nephron of the rat. J Clin Invest. 1983;71:1661–75.

11. Alpern RJ, Sakhaee K. The clinical spectrum of chronic metabolic acidosis: homeostatic mechanisms produce significant morbidity. Am J Kidney Dis. 1997;29:291–302.

12. Madias N. Lactic acidosis. Kidney Int. 1986;29:752–74.

13. Foster DW, McGarry JD. The metabolic derangements and treatment of diabetic ketoacidosis. N Engl J Med. 1983;309:159–69.

14. Brent J, McMartin K, Phillips S, et al. Fomepizole for the treatment of ethylene glycol poisoning. Methylpyrazole for toxic alcohols study group. N Engl J Med. 1999; 340:832–8.

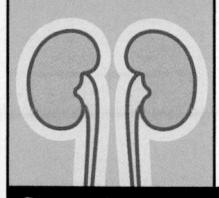

<table>
<tr><td>Chapter
12</td><td>

Metabolic Alkalosis

F John Gennari

</td></tr>
</table>

DEFINITION

Metabolic alkalosis is induced by the addition and retention of excess alkali, and is manifested by an increase in serum bicarbonate concentration, (HCO_3^-), to greater than 28 mmol/L (or serum (total CO_2) > 30 mmol/L). The rise in pH that results from retained HCO_3^- induces compensatory hypoventilation, producing an increase in arterial P_{CO_2}. Thus, the disorder is characterized by coexisting elevations in serum (HCO_3^-), arterial pH and P_{CO_2}. Because the kidney normally responds to an increase in (HCO_3^-) by rapidly excreting the excess alkali, sustained metabolic alkalosis only occurs when some additional factor disrupts the renal regulation of body alkali stores.

NORMAL PHYSIOLOGY OF RENAL REGULATION OF BICARBONATE

To maintain body alkali stores in the face of continuous metabolic acid production, the kidney normally reabsorbs all filtered HCO_3^-. Bicarbonate is removed from the tubular urine throughout the nephron by H^+ secretion. Secreted H^+ combines with filtered HCO_3^-, producing CO_2 and water, a process that removes HCO_3^- from the tubule and generates a new HCO_3^- in the peritubular vascular compartment[1,2]. Figure 12.1 illustrates the major epithelial H^+ secretory transporters and their linkages with the transport of Na^+, Cl^-, and K^+. In the proximal tubule H^+ is secreted via a Na^+-linked transporter (the Na^+/H^+ exchanger, NHE3), as well as by an H^+-ATPase (not shown in the figure). In the distal nephron, however, NHE3 is not present and H^+ secretion is accomplished primarily by the H^+-ATPase. The activity of this transporter in the distal tubule and collecting duct is regulated by aldosterone and by the rate of Na^+ delivery and reabsorption. In the presence of K^+ depletion, a second H^+ secretory transporter, the H^+/K^+-ATPase, is activated in the distal nephron, further promoting acid secretion and HCO_3^- reabsorption. When excess alkali is ingested and must be excreted, HCO_3^- can re-enter the tubular fluid in the distal nephron via an apical membrane Cl^-/HCO_3^- exchanger[3]. This transporter is activated by alkalemia and requires sufficient Cl^- delivery to the distal tubule for Cl^- to be reabsorbed in exchange for secreted HCO_3^-. Because continued H^+ secretion in the collecting duct results in further HCO_3^- reabsorption when this anion re-enters the tubular fluid, excretion of excess alkali requires both stimulation of the Cl^-/HCO_3^- exchanger and suppression

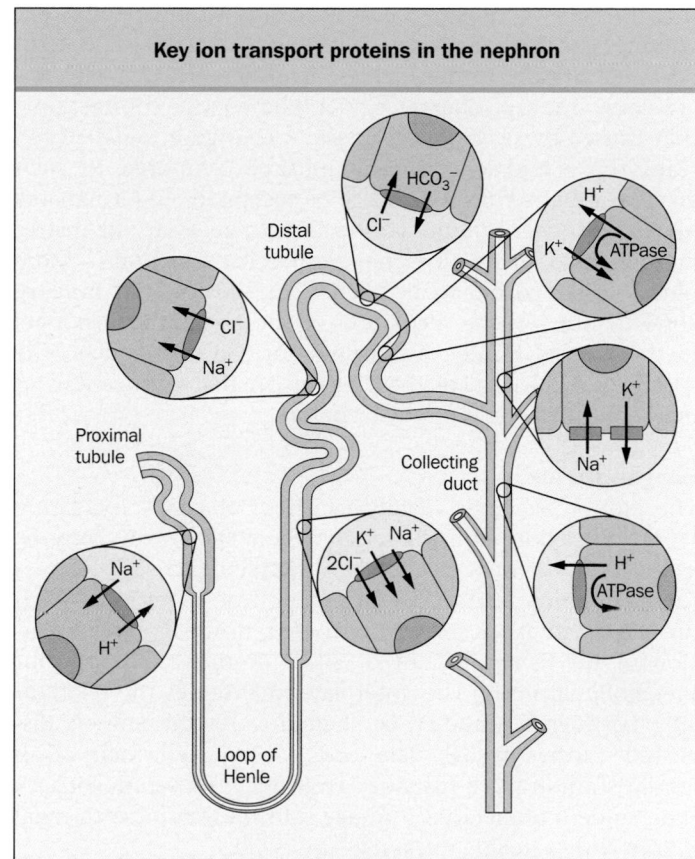

Figure 12.1 Key ion transport proteins and their linkages.
Bicarbonate reabsorption is accomplished by H^+ secretion throughout the nephron. This process is linked to Na^+ reabsorption directly in the proximal tubule (Na^+/H^+ exchanger) and indirectly in the collecting duct (Na^+ channel and parallel H^+-ATPase). Chloride-linked Na^+ reabsorption in the loop of Henle and early distal tubule is an important modulator of Na^+ delivery to the collecting duct. Bicarbonate secretion only occurs under conditions of alkalemia, via a Cl^--linked exchanger in the distal tubule and collecting duct. Potassium reabsorption in states of K^+ depletion is linked to H^+ secretion in the distal tubule and collecting duct. Reprinted with permission from Gennari[2].

of the normally active H^+-ATPase. Abnormal activation of any of these transporters, or changes in the activity of Na^+-linked Cl^- transporters in the loop of Henle and early distal tubule (see Fig. 12.1) can disrupt renal regulation of body alkali stores and produce metabolic alkalosis.

PATHOPHYSIOLOGY OF METABOLIC ALKALOSIS

Metabolic alkalosis can be produced experimentally by acutely administering HCO_3^- (or a HCO_3^- precursor), or by inducing K^+ or Cl^- depletion. Potassium and Cl^- depletion are closely linked events in causing sustained metabolic alkalosis and it is often difficult to assess which of these ions is the primary culprit. In clinical practice, the most common presentation of metabolic alkalosis is always associated with some degree of Cl^--depletion. Although the term 'contraction alkalosis' is often used as a synonym for Cl^--depletion alkalosis, this phrase is confusing because it implies incorrectly that volume contraction causes metabolic alkalosis. The term refers specifically to the increase in serum (HCO_3^-) that follows only one type of extracellular fluid volume contraction – that caused by selective Cl^- losses. A change in renal HCO_3^- reabsorption and acid excretion must occur in order for such an increase in serum (HCO_3^-) to be sustained, and it remains unclear whether volume contraction is necessary or instrumental in inducing this change in renal function[4,5]. More rarely, sustained metabolic alkalosis is the result of primary abnormalities in the regulation of specific ion transporters in the loop of Henle, distal tubule or collecting ducts. The specific role of each of these factors in the pathogenesis of metabolic alkalosis is discussed below.

Exogenous alkali

The kidney responds rapidly to excess alkali by increasing HCO_3^- excretion, and thus metabolic alkalosis can only be induced transiently. Even when supplemental $NaHCO_3$ is ingested daily, serum (HCO_3^-) does not increase[6]. When dietary Cl^- intake is severely restricted, however, daily ingestion of the same amount of alkali produces a significant metabolic alkalosis. This interplay underscores the relationship between Cl^- and HCO_3^- handling by the kidney, discussed further below. The one setting in which alkali administration has a sustained large effect on serum (HCO_3^-) independent of dietary Cl^- intake is in the patient with renal failure who is unable to excrete any alkali.

Potassium depletion

Induction of K^+ losses by severely restricting dietary K^+ intake produces a small but significant increase in serum (HCO_3^-) in normal human subjects[7]. When dietary Cl^- intake is concomitantly restricted, however, the resultant alkalosis is four times as great, illustrating the interplay between Cl^- and K^+ in regulating renal HCO_3^- reabsorption. Depletion of body K^+ stores is probably the most important factor in producing and sustaining the rarer Cl^--resistant forms of metabolic alkalosis (see later).

Chloride depletion

Selective Cl^- depletion, induced by nasogastric suction, produces a major increase in serum (HCO_3^-) (Fig. 12.2)[8]. The resultant metabolic alkalosis, moreover, is sustained until sufficient Cl^- is given to replenish losses. This form of metabolic alkalosis leads to concomitant K^+ depletion through renal K^+ losses, but Cl^- administration rapidly corrects the alkalosis

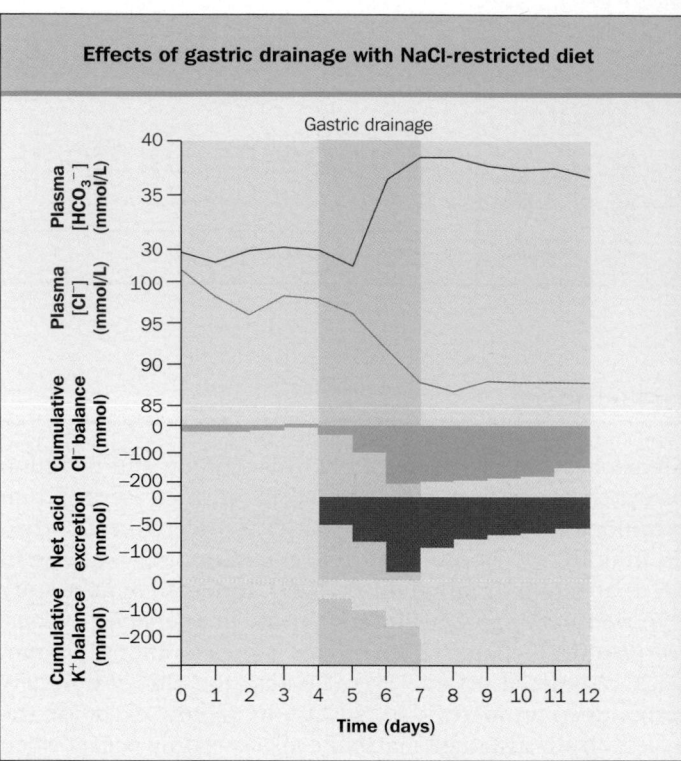

Figure 12.2 Effect of gastric drainage on plasma [HCO_3^-] and [Cl^-], on Cl^- and K^+ balance, and on net acid excretion in a normal individual ingesting a NaCl-restricted diet. In this subject, gastric drainage for 3 days increased plasma [HCO_3^-] by 9 mmol/L, a change that persisted despite replacement of gastric K^+ losses and ingestion of 73 mmol of K^+ each day. Potassium depletion occurs as a result of renal K^+ losses during the period of gastric drainage, and is not corrected in the postdrainage period. Net acid excretion decreases transiently during the period of gastric drainage, but then returns to control levels in the postdrainage period despite sustained metabolic alkalosis. Chloride depletion is maintained by the low dietary intake of this ion. Reprinted with permission from Excerpta Medica Inc from Kassirer and Schwartz[9].

even if the K^+ deficit is deliberately maintained[9]. The role of Cl^- depletion, as opposed to extracellular fluid (ECF) volume depletion, and the contribution of K^+ depletion in sustaining this form of metabolic alkalosis, remains controversial[4,5,7–9]. In the clinical setting, dissection of the contribution of each factor is of little importance, however, as most patients require both Cl^- and K^+ repletion to correct the volume depletion and hypokalemia that is almost always present.

Interplay of K^+, Cl^- and HCO_3^- transport by the kidney

When metabolic alkalosis is induced by Cl^- depletion and dietary Cl^- intake is restricted, a characteristic sequence of changes in renal electrolyte excretion occurs[8]. Sodium and HCO_3^- excretion increase transiently, then fall rapidly to low levels and K^+ excretion increases. The increase in K^+ excretion is also transient but nonetheless induces significant K^+ depletion (Fig. 12.2). In the new steady-state of alkalosis, urinary K^+ excretion matches intake despite persistent K^+ depletion. As a result, hypokalemia is a cardinal feature of metabolic alkalosis.

Chloride depletion promotes K+ secretion in the distal nephron through effects on several transport processes and may also impede K+ reabsorption in the ascending limb of the loop of Henle[10]. Potassium depletion stimulates both further H+ secretion (via the H+/K+-ATPase, Fig. 12.1) and renal NH4+ production by a direct effect, facilitating the acid excretion needed to sustain metabolic alkalosis (Fig. 12.3). Chloride depletion also impedes HCO3− secretion via the Cl−/HCO3− exchanger in the distal nephron[3,10]; continued secretion of aldosterone coupled with this impairment of distal HCO3− secretion promotes sustained acid excretion. Due to these interacting effects, acid excretion matches net acid production in the steady state despite systemic alkalemia. When K+ depletion is unusually severe, renal reabsorption of Cl− is also impaired, possibly due to a limitation in Cl− transport in the loop of Henle via the Na+/K+/2Cl− cotransporter (Fig. 12.1), resulting in persistent Cl− depletion despite intake or administration of this anion[10,11].

Primary abnormalities in renal ion transport

Metabolic alkalosis can be induced by acquired or inherited abnormalities in ion transport in the loop and distal tubule (Fig. 12.4). These Cl−-resistant forms of metabolic alkalosis probably account for less than 1% of all causes, and the most common of these is primary hyperaldosteronism[12,13]. In this disorder, persistently high and unregulated levels of aldosterone promote Na+ reabsorption and H+ and K+ secretion in the collecting duct by stimulating the activity of the epithelial Na+ channel (ENaC) as well as the H+-ATPase (Figs 12.1 and 12.4). The resultant K+ depletion promotes NH4+ production and stimulates the activity of the H+/K+-ATPase, facilitating acid excretion and producing metabolic alkalosis despite normal Cl− intake and serum concentration. Not surprisingly, the degree of alkalosis induced in primary hyperaldosteronism is modulated by both Cl− and K+ intake. Other forms of Cl-resistant alkalosis are caused by genetic mutations in the regulation and function of specific transporters in the loop of Henle and distal nephron (Fig. 12.4 and Chapter 49).

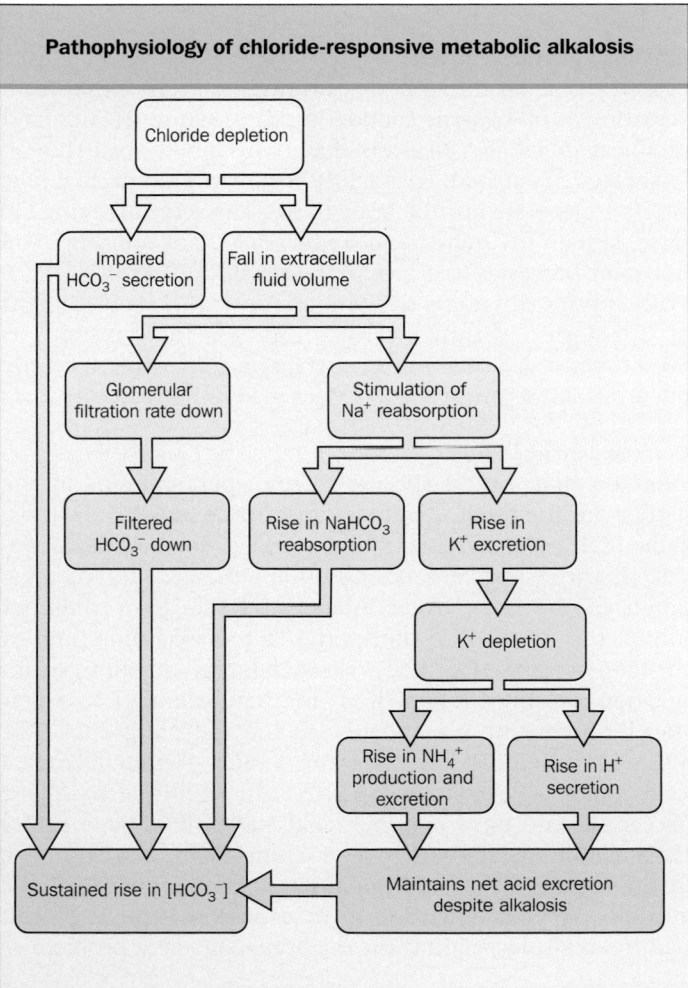

Figure 12.3 Pathophysiology of chloride-responsive metabolic alkalosis. Chloride depletion decreases extracellular (ECF) volume and glomerular filtration rate, increases HCO3− reabsorption by increasing the filtered load of this anion, increases K+ excretion, and impairs HCO3− secretion in the distal nephron. The resultant K+ depletion further stimulates H+ secretion and facilitates ammonium (NH4+) excretion. These events all contribute to a sustained increase in serum [HCO3−]. Reprinted with permission from Gennari[2].

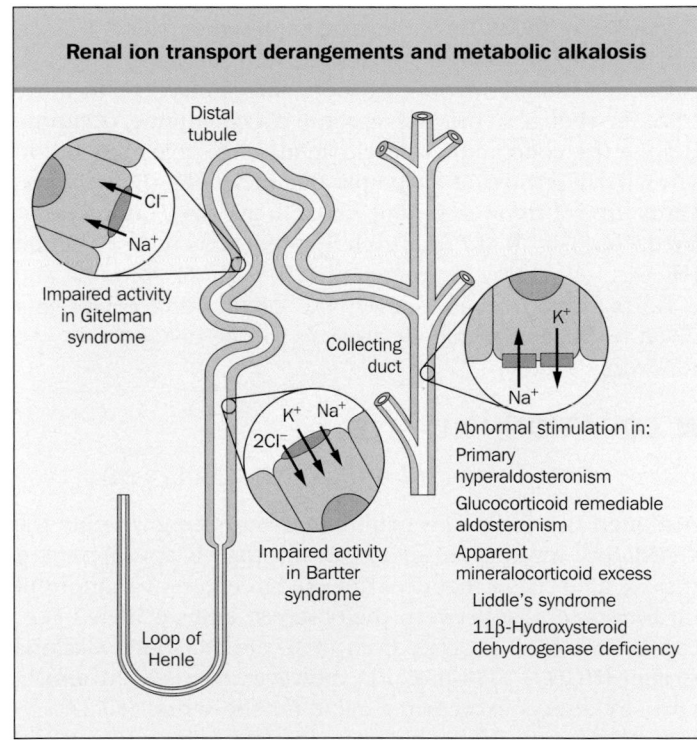

Figure 12.4 Primary derangements in renal ion transport that lead to sustained metabolic alkalosis. The epithelial Na+ channel in the collecting duct is stimulated abnormally in primary hyperaldosteronism and in three defined genetic abnormalities. One of these causes aldosterone secretion to respond to ACTH rather than angiotensin II (glucocorticoid-remediable aldosteronism); one blocks downregulation of the channel (Liddle's syndrome), and one allows cortisol to act as a mineralocorticoid (11β-hydroxysteroid dehydrogenase deficiency). Bartter and Gitelman syndrome are caused by genetic abnormalities that impede the activity of or inactivate Cl−-linked Na+ reabsorption in two separate transporters in the nephron.

Fluid and Electrolyte Disorders

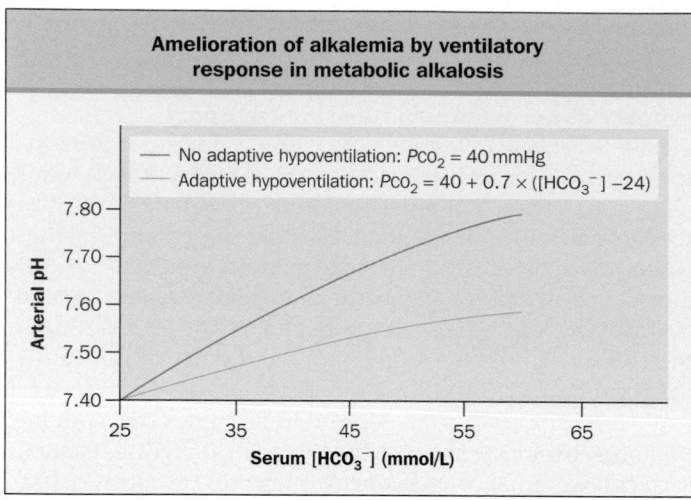

Figure 12.5 Amelioration of alkalemia by the normal ventilatory response to the increase in serum [HCO₃⁻] in metabolic alkalosis. The blue (upper) line in the graph illustrates the relationship between arterial pH and serum [HCO₃⁻] in the absence of adaptive hypoventilation (P_{CO_2} maintained at 40 mmHg) and the green (lower) line, the relationship when P_{CO_2} is increased by the expected level of hypoventilation.

Adaptive response to an increase in serum (HCO_3^-)

Regardless of the cause of the increase in serum (HCO_3^-), blood pH increases and elicits a characteristic ventilatory response. Alkalemia induces hypoventilation, increasing P_{CO_2} to minimize the change in pH. The response is a potent one, occurring despite the concomitant development of hypoxemia and, in virtually all settings of uncomplicated metabolic alkalosis, prevents the pH from exceeding 7.60. On average P_{CO_2} increases by 0.7 mmHg (0.1KP) for each 1 mmol/L increase in serum (HCO_3^-). Assuming a normal (HCO_3^-) of 24 mmol/L and a normal P_{CO_2} of 40 mmHg, the predicted P_{CO_2} for any given (HCO_3^-) in metabolic alkalosis can be calculated by the following formula:

■ EQUATION 12.1

$$P_{CO_2} \text{ (mmHg)} = 40 + 0.7 \times ((HCO_3^-) \text{ (mmol/L)} - 24)$$

Although this formula is helpful in determining whether the ventilatory response to metabolic alkalosis is appropriate, it implies a precision that does not exist in nature. Variations of up to 5–7 mmHg between the observed and calculated P_{CO_2} can be expected to occur. Even in severe metabolic alkalosis (serum (HCO_3^-) > 50 mmol/L), however, the P_{CO_2} in mmHg virtually always exceeds the value for the serum (HCO_3^-) in mmol/L. Figure 12.5 illustrates the ameliorating effect of increasing P_{CO_2} on pH in metabolic alkalosis. While it mitigates the alkalemia, the increase in P_{CO_2} also stimulates renal HCO_3^- reabsorption, increasing serum (HCO_3^-) further[14]. In the clinical setting, this latter effect is small and unimportant.

ETIOLOGIES

For ease of classification, the causes of metabolic alkalosis are subdivided into Cl⁻-responsive and Cl⁻-resistant forms. Metabolic alkalosis can also occur in certain settings as a result of alkali ingestion.

Table 12.1 Causes of chloride-responsive metabolic alkalosis.

Causes of chloride-responsive metabolic alkalosis
Acid loss from the stomach (common)
Vomiting
Nasogastric suction
Diuretic administration (common)
Thiazides
Metolazone
Loop diuretics: furosemide (frusemide), bumetanide, torasemide (torsemide), etacrynic acid (ethacrynic acid)
Recovery from chronic hypercapnia (rarer)
Chloride-depleting diarrhea (much rarer)
Congenital chloride diarrhea
Villous adenoma of the colon

Chloride-responsive metabolic alkalosis

Table 12.1 lists the main causes of Cl⁻-responsive metabolic alkalosis.

Acid loss from the stomach

Loss of HCl from the upper gastrointestinal tract either from vomiting or nasogastric suction increases serum (HCO_3^-) and produces metabolic alkalosis that is sustained until the Cl⁻ losses are replenished. For each H⁺ lost by the stomach, a new HCO_3^- is generated in the body fluids. The accompanying Cl⁻ losses sustain the increase in serum (HCO_3^-) by altering renal transport processes and promoting renal K⁺ losses (Fig. 12.2). With continued emesis or suction and with no replacement of Cl⁻ losses, serum (HCO_3^-) can rise to as high as 80–90 mmol/L. This form of metabolic alkalosis is the only one in which serum (HCO_3^-) values > 45 mmol/L occur.

Diuretic administration

Diuretics that inhibit specific Cl⁻ transport proteins in the kidney are the most common causes of metabolic alkalosis. Table 12.1 lists the diuretics that produce metabolic alkalosis. The thiazides and metolazone inhibit the Na⁺, Cl⁻ cotransporter in the early distal tubule, and the 'loop' diuretics inhibit the Na⁺/K⁺/2Cl⁻ transporter in the ascending limb of the loop of Henle (Fig. 12.1). These agents all impair Cl⁻ reabsorption, causing Cl⁻ depletion, and they stimulate K⁺ excretion by increasing Na⁺ delivery to the collecting duct. The alkalosis produced is typically mild (serum (HCO_3^-) < 36 mmol/L), except in patients who continue to ingest excess salt and have extreme renal Na⁺ avidity. Even under these conditions, it is rare to see a serum (HCO_3^-) > 40 mmol/L in the absence of an additional factor promoting metabolic alkalosis. Hypokalemia due to K⁺ depletion is more prominent than alkalosis and is the major management problem[15].

Recovery from chronic hypercapnia

The renal adaptive response to sustained hypercapnia results in an increase in HCO_3^- reabsorption and a decrease in Cl⁻ reabsorption. This response increases serum (HCO_3^-) but also causes Cl⁻ depletion. When P_{CO_2} is restored to normal, reduction in serum (HCO_3^-) to normal levels requires repletion of the Cl⁻ losses incurred during adaptation. If these losses are not replaced, recovery from hypercapnia can result in a persistent metabolic alkalosis.

Causes of chloride-resistant metabolic alkalosis	
	Examples
Mineralocorticoid excess	Primary hyperaldosteronism: adenoma, hyperplasia
	Cushing's syndrome
	ACTH-secreting tumor
	Renin-secreting tumor
	Glucocorticoid-remediable aldosteronism
	Adrenogenital syndromes
	Fluorocortisone treatment
Apparent mineralocorticoid excess	Licorice
	Carbenoxolone
	Liddle's syndrome
	11β-Hydroxysteroid dehydrogenase deficiency
Glucocorticoids (high dose)	
Impairment of Cl—linked Na$^+$ reabsorption	Bartter syndrome
	Gitelman syndrome
Severe K$^+$ deficiency	

Table 12.2 Causes of chloride-resistant metabolic alkalosis.

Chloride-losing diarrhea

In two rare forms of diarrhea, congenital chloride diarrhea and in the diarrhea caused by a Cl$^-$-secreting villous adenoma of the colon, Cl$^-$ losses in stool can produce metabolic alkalosis[5]. Although the alkalosis could, in theory, be corrected by Cl$^-$ administration, repletion of Cl$^-$ is difficult because of continued stool losses, and the alkalosis is often persistent despite adequate dietary intake.

Chloride-resistant metabolic alkalosis

Table 12.2 lists the causes of Cl$^-$-resistant metabolic alkalosis.

Mineralocorticoid excess

Aldosterone and other mineralocorticoids cause metabolic alkalosis by stimulating both the H$^+$-ATPase and epithelial Na$^+$ channel in the collecting duct (see Figs 12.1 and 12.4). The resultant Na$^+$ retention causes hypertension and also insures continued delivery of Na$^+$ to the distal nephron, facilitating continued H$^+$ and K$^+$ secretion. The metabolic alkalosis is typically mild (serum (HCO$_3^-$) 30–35 mmol/L), and is associated with more severe hypokalemia (K$^+$ often less than 3.0 mmol/L) than in most other causes of alkalosis[12,13]. Primary hyperaldosteronism is by far the most common cause of this form of Cl$^-$-resistant alkalosis (see Chapter 40), but it can also occur with rarer hereditary defects in cortisol synthesis or in the regulation of aldosterone secretion (Table 12.2). One of these, glucocorticoid-remediable aldosteronism, is caused by a mutation that results in aldosterone secretion being stimulated by ACTH rather than by angiotensin II[16]. Administration of the oral mineralocorticoid drug, fludrocortisone, can induce metabolic alkalosis if used inappropriately. Glucocorticoids, when administered in very high doses, increase renal K$^+$ excretion nonspecifically and produce a mild increase in serum (HCO$_3^-$).

Apparent mineralocorticoid excess syndromes

Several inherited abnormalities produce a Cl$^-$-resistant metabolic alkalosis that is clinically indistinguishable from hyperaldosteronism, but without measurable aldosterone. Liddle's syndrome results from a genetic mutation that prevents the removal of epithelial Na$^+$ channels from the urinary membrane of collecting duct epithelial cells (Fig. 12.4)[17]. As a result, Na$^+$ reabsorption cannot be downregulated, causing the same cascade of events seen in hyperaldosteronism. Because continuous stimulation of Na$^+$ reabsorption expands ECF volume, however, aldosterone levels are vanishingly low. In another rare familial disorder, termed 'the syndrome of apparent mineralocorticoid excess', a mutation inactivates 11-β-hydroxysteroid dehydrogenase, an enzyme adjacent to the mineralocorticoid receptor that rapidly converts cortisol to cortisone, preventing this normally abundant glucocorticoid from binding to the receptor and activating this signal pathway[18]. Because of this defect, cortisol binds to this receptor and behaves as a mineralocorticoid, stimulating Na$^+$ reabsorption and K$^+$ secretion and producing Cl$^-$-resistant metabolic alkalosis and hypertension with low aldosterone levels. Glycyrrhizic acid (a component of natural licorice), carbenoxolone and gossypol (an agent that inhibits spermatogenesis) all inhibit the activity of 11-β-hydroxysteroid dehydrogenase and can cause the same clinical picture.

Impairment of chloride-linked Na$^+$ transport

Bartter and Gitelman syndromes are two hereditary disorders manifested by Cl$^-$-resistant metabolic alkalosis and hypokalemia, but without hypertension (see Chapter 49). Gitelman syndrome becomes clinically apparent later in life than Bartter syndrome and differs from it in that hypomagnesemia and hypocalciuria are prominent features[19]. Gitelman syndrome is caused by genetic mutations that inactivate the thiazide-sensitive Na$^+$, Cl$^-$ cotransporter in the early distal tubule (Fig. 12.4), leading to hypokalemia and metabolic alkalosis similar to that caused by thiazide diuretics[20]. Bartter syndrome is caused by several mutations, all of which have the effect of impeding Cl$^-$-associated Na$^+$ reabsorption in the ascending limb of Henle's loop (via the Na$^+$/K$^+$/2Cl$^-$ cotransporter, see Fig. 12.4)[19,20]. Thus, patients with this syndrome show similarities to individuals abusing loop diuretics, most notably volume depletion. Although, in theory, Cl$^-$ repletion could correct these disorders, they are Cl$^-$-resistant because any administered Cl$^-$ is rapidly excreted due to the defective transporters.

Severe K$^+$ deficiency

In patients with severe K$^+$ depletion (serum (K$^+$) less than 2.0 mmol/L), metabolic alkalosis can be sustained despite Cl$^-$ administration[11]. Chloride resistance in this setting is due to impairment of renal Cl$^-$ reabsorption (see earlier discussion). Even partial repletion of K$^+$ stores rapidly reverses this problem, and makes the alkalosis Cl$^-$-responsive.

Alkali administration

Exogenous alkali can produce metabolic alkalosis in patients with normal renal function if they have deficient body K$^+$ or Cl$^-$ stores (Table 12.3, see earlier discussion)[6]. In patients with

Fluid and Electrolyte Disorders

Causes of metabolic alkalosis associated with alkali administration	
Renal status	Causes
Normal renal function (only in association with K+ depletion or low NaCl intake)	Alkali intake: NaHCO₃, citrate, lactate, acetate, amino acid anions
Renal failure	Milk alkali syndrome
	Alkali intake
	Aluminum hydroxide with K+ exchange resin

Table 12.3 Causes of metabolic alkalosis associated with alkali administration.

Potential sources of alkali	
Alkali/alkali precursor	Source
Bicarbonate	NaHCO₃: pills, intravenous solutions
	Proprietary brands, e.g. Alka Seltzer
	Baking soda
	KHCO₃: pills, oral solutions
Lactate	Ringer's solution, peritoneal dialysis solutions
Acetate Glutamate Propionate	Parenteral nutrition
Citrate	Blood products, plasma exchange, K+ supplements, alkalinizing agents
Calcium compounds (alkalinizing effect minimal when given by mouth) Acetate Citrate Carbonate	Calcium supplements, phosphate binders

Table 12.4 Potential sources of alkali.

acute or chronic renal failure, administration or ingestion of excess alkali produces a sustained metabolic alkalosis because the excess alkali cannot be excreted[21]. In such patients the alkalosis can usually be corrected by discontinuing the offending agent. Milk-alkali syndrome is characterized by the concomitant presence of metabolic alkalosis and renal insufficiency, brought on by the ingestion of $NaHCO_3$ in combination with excess calcium (either in milk or as $CaCO_3$)[22,23]. The renal insufficiency is caused by calcium deposition (facilitated by an alkaline urine) and damage to the kidney. The renal insufficiency in turn facilitates the development of metabolic alkalosis if alkali ingestion continues. Metabolic alkalosis is usually mild in these patients unless they develop concomitant vomiting. In hospitalized patients with renal failure, a wide variety of alkali sources or alkali precursors can cause metabolic alkalosis (Table 12.4). Although only rarely used now, administration of aluminum hydroxide in combination with sodium polystyrene sulfonate (kayexalate) can enhance gastrointestinal reabsorption of the HCO_3^- secreted by the pancreas, producing metabolic alkalosis in patients with renal failure[21].

Other causes

Refeeding after starvation causes an abrupt increase in serum (HCO_3^-) from the low levels characteristic of the fasting state. In some instances, serum (HCO_3^-) rises transiently above normal levels, causing a mild metabolic alkalosis. The causes are multiple, including new HCO_3^- generation from metabolism of accumulated organic anions, and K+ and Cl⁻ depletion. In experimental settings, sustained administration of either excess parathyroid hormone or vitamin D causes a small but significant increase in serum (HCO_3^-)[24,25]. Hyperparathyroidism in the clinic, however, is not associated with metabolic alkalosis. Hypercalcemia and vitamin D intoxication have been associated with metabolic alkalosis, but in most instances the alkalosis can be explained by the vomiting that characteristically accompanies these disorders. High aldosterone levels induced by hyperreninemia in renovascular or malignant hypertension are associated with hypokalemia and, occasionally, with very minor increases in serum (HCO_3^-)[21].

CLINICAL MANIFESTATIONS

Metabolic alkalosis is a well-tolerated disorder with few clinically important adverse effects. Patients with serum (HCO_3^-) levels as high as 40 mmol/L are usually asymptomatic. Perhaps the most concerning adverse effect of mild to moderate metabolic alkalosis is the associated hypokalemia. In patients with ischemic heart disease, the hypokalemia that occurs in metabolic alkalosis increases the likelihood of cardiac arrhythmias[26]. With more severe metabolic alkalosis, arterial hypoxemia (from hypoventilation) and a decrease in ionized calcium (due to alkalemia) become concerns. Arterial P_{O_2} can fall to less than 50 mmHg with severe alkalosis, and weakness and neurological symptoms can emerge. Patients with serum (HCO_3^-) > 50 mmol/L can present with seizures, tetany, delirium or stupor. These changes in mental status are probably multifactorial in origin, due to alkalemia, hypokalemia, hypocalcemia, and hypoxemia.

DIAGNOSIS

Diagnosis of metabolic alkalosis involves three basic steps (Fig. 12.6). The first step is detecting the presence of the disorder. The second step is to assure oneself that the disorder is not complicated by another acid–base abnormality that also requires attention. The third step is to uncover the specific cause. Detection of metabolic alkalosis is straightforward in most instances. The finding of a serum (HCO_3^-) (or (Total CO_2)) greater than 30 mmol/L in association with hypokalemia is virtually pathognomonic. The only other cause of an elevated serum (HCO_3^-) is chronic respiratory acidosis and hypokalemia is not a feature of this disorder (see Chapter 13). Because the diagnosis is usually evident and the disorder is almost always uncomplicated, one need not measure arterial pH and P_{CO_2} in most patients.

If the alkalosis is severe (serum (HCO_3^-) > 40 mmol/L), if the cause of the elevated (HCO_3^-) is unclear, or if a mixed acid–base disorder is suspected, however, one should always measure arterial pH and P_{CO_2} to fully characterize the disorder (Fig. 12.6). Measurement of pH and P_{CO_2} confirms the presence of alkalosis, and allows one to estimate whether the degree of

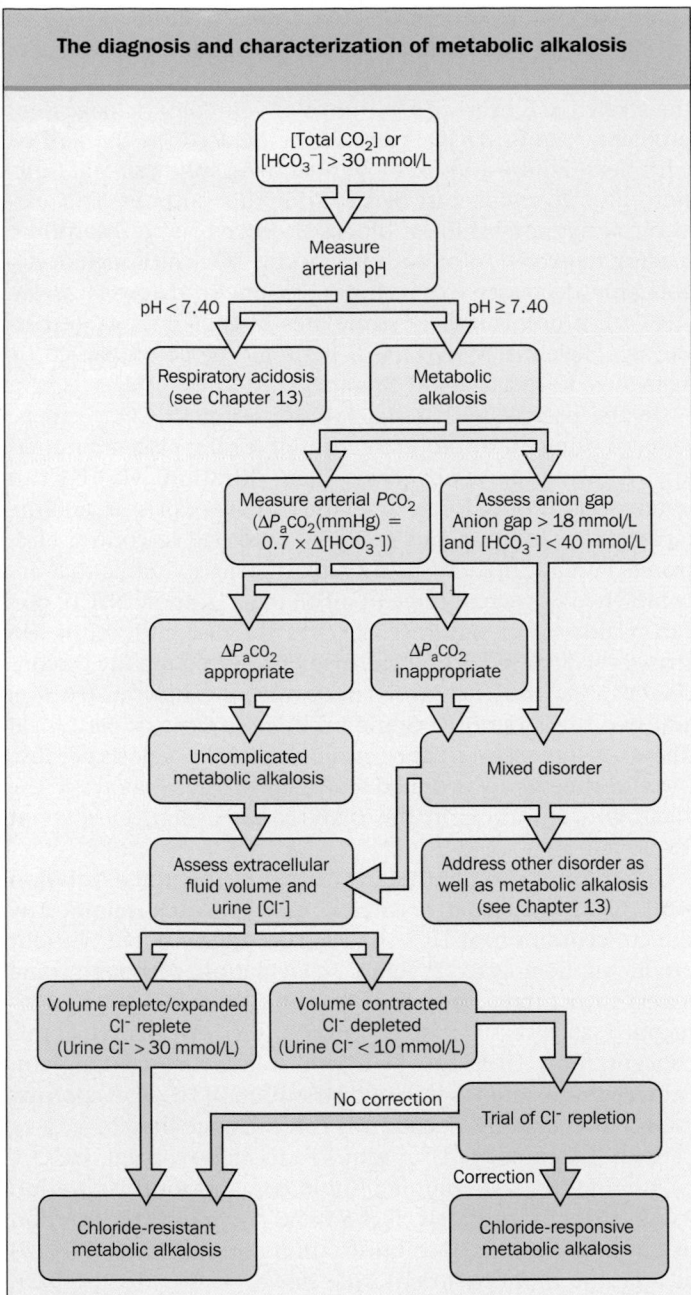

The diagnosis and characterization of metabolic alkalosis

Figure 12.6 Approach to diagnosis and characterization of metabolic alkalosis. To determine with certainty whether an increase in serum [HCO_3^-] signifies the presence of metabolic alkalosis, arterial pH and P_{CO_2} measurements are necessary. These measurements, along with a calculation of the anion gap, allow one to determine as well whether metabolic alkalosis is the only acid–base disturbance present. Once the acid–base disturbance has been characterized, one can assess extracellular fluid volume and/or measure urine Cl^- concentration to determine whether the disorder is Cl^- responsive or Cl^- resistant. Reprinted with permission from Gennari[2].

hypoventilation is appropriate for the degree of elevation in serum (HCO_3^-) (see earlier, Equation 1). A major deviation in P_{CO_2} from the expected value indicates the presence of a complicating respiratory acid–base disorder (either respiratory

acidosis or alkalosis, see Chapter 13). The anion gap, defined as $(Na^+) - ((Cl^-) + (HCO_3^-))$, is not increased in mild to moderate metabolic alkalosis, but can be increased by as much as 3–5 mmol/L when alkalosis is severe[21]. If the anion gap is greater than 20 mmol/L, the disorder is most likely complicated by a superimposed metabolic acidosis (Chapter 11).

In most instances, the third step, elucidating the cause, is also straightforward. Over 95% of metabolic alkalosis is caused either by diuretic usage or by Cl^- losses from the upper gastrointestinal tract. This historical information is usually easily obtainable, and attention can be directed towards the appropriate treatment. If the cause is unclear from the history, measurement of urinary Cl^- concentration can help. Unless the patient has recently taken a diuretic agent, urine (Cl^-) should be < 10 mmol/L. Surreptitious use of diuretics or self-induced vomiting (bulimia) can be a confounding problem. The former behavior presents the greater diagnostic dilemma, because continued diuretic-induced Cl^- excretion may lead one to undertake an extensive workup for rarer forms of metabolic alkalosis. Urinary screens for specific diuretic compounds may be necessary to establish the correct diagnosis. In bulimic patients, urinary Cl^- excretion should be low (spot urine (Cl^-) < 10 mmol/L). If the cause is not apparent from the above analysis, one should consider the Cl^--resistant forms of metabolic alkalosis. In these forms of metabolic alkalosis, urine (Cl^-) is typically greater than 30 mmol/L.

In the patient with hypertension and metabolic alkalosis who is not taking any diuretic agents, the most common cause of Cl^--resistant metabolic alkalosis is primary hyperaldosteronism. Measurement of serum renin and aldosterone levels can distinguish mineralocorticoid excess syndromes from the rarer syndromes of apparent mineralocorticoid excess (Table 12.2). The details of such a workup are presented in Chapter 49. In the normotensive or hypotensive patient with Cl^--resistant metabolic alkalosis, the diagnoses of either Bartter or Gitelman syndrome should be entertained. Aldosterone and/or renin levels are not helpful in making these diagnoses, because the levels can be low or high, depending on the patient's ECF volume at the time of measurement. Familial genetic studies can establish these diagnoses with high specificity.

TREATMENT

Chloride-responsive alkalosis

In the patient with metabolic alkalosis due to nasogastric drainage or vomiting, ECF volume depletion is always a concomitant feature and treatment is straightforward. Administration of intravenous NaCl will correct both the alkalosis and the volume depletion. Potassium losses should also be replaced by oral or intravenous KCl. Typically, the K^+ deficit is 200–400 mmol in patients with mild to moderate metabolic alkalosis induced by upper gastrointestinal Cl^- losses. When nasogastric drainage must be continued, HCl losses can be reduced by administration of drugs that inhibit gastric acid secretion, such as famotidine or omeprazole. In contrast to patients with upper gastrointestinal losses, NaCl administration is not usually required in patients with metabolic alkalosis caused by diuretics unless clinical signs of volume depletion are present. Potassium chloride supplements should be given to minimize K^+ depletion as well as the metabolic alkalosis. The addition of a K^+-sparing diuretic such as amiloride, triamterene or spironolactone, can assist in minimizing these abnormalities. Complete repair of diuretic-induced metabolic alkalosis is often difficult, because of continued Cl^- and K^+ losses. Fortunately, such a therapeutic goal is not necessary in most instances. As indicated above, mild metabolic alkalosis is well tolerated with no clinically significant adverse effects. One should always weigh the medical necessity of the diuretic agent. If the drug can be discontinued, the disorder will resolve so long as the diet contains adequate K^+ and Cl^-.

Chloride-resistant alkalosis

Management of Cl^--resistant alkalosis depends on the underlying cause. If the alkalosis is caused by an adrenal adenoma, the disorder is corrected by surgical removal of the tumor (see Chapter 40). In other forms of primary hyperaldosteronism, the alkalosis can be minimized by dietary NaCl restriction and by aggressive replacement of body K^+ stores, using supplemental KCl. Spironolactone, a competitive inhibitor of aldosterone, will also correct the disorder. In glucocorticoid-remediable aldosteronism, the disorder is corrected by dexamethasone administration, suppressing ACTH secretion and thereby reducing aldosterone secretion. In the hereditary forms of apparent mineralocorticoid excess (Liddle's syndrome and 11-β-hydroxysteroid dehydrogenase deficiency), amiloride is the most effective treatment. The metabolic alkalosis (and hypokalemia) seen in Bartter and Gitelman syndromes is the most difficult to correct. In additional to aggressively replacing K^+ (and magnesium, in Gitelman syndrome), nonsteroidal anti-inflammatory drugs have been used with moderate success. These drugs minimize renal Cl^- losses.

Alkali ingestion

Treatment here is directed at identifying and discontinuing the offending alkali (Table 12.4). One should be diligent in the intensive care unit to look for sources of exogenous alkali. A common offender is the use of acetate as a replacement for Cl^- in parenteral nutritional solutions.

SPECIAL PROBLEMS IN MANAGEMENT

Management of metabolic alkalosis is a more difficult undertaking in patients with severe congestive heart failure or renal failure. In most instances, one need not actively reduce serum (HCO_3^-) if the value is less than 42–45 mmol/L. If the alkalosis is more severe ((HCO_3^-) > 45 mmol/L or pH > 7.55), or if the alkalemia is causing symptoms or ventilator management problems, serum (HCO_3^-) should be reduced. In the patient with heart failure and fluid overload who still has renal function, acetazolamide can be used for this purpose. This carbonic anhydrase inhibitor blocks H^+-linked Na^+ reabsorption, leading to excretion of both Na^+ and HCO_3^-. Although acetazolamide decreases extracellular volume and lowers serum (HCO_3^-), it unfortunately stimulates K^+ excretion, exacerbating hypokalemia. When used, it should be accompanied by aggressive K^+ replacement therapy.

In the patient with renal failure, serum (HCO_3^-) can be reduced using the appropriate form of renal replacement therapy. Continuous venovenous hemofiltration (CVVH) can remove up to 20–30 L/day of an ultrafiltrate of plasma, and the replacement solution can easily be modified to control electrolyte composition. By using replacement solutions that are completely or partially free of alkali (e.g., isotonic NaCl), one can readily lower serum (HCO_3^-) to the desired level in less than 24 h. Serum (HCO_3^-) can also be lowered rapidly by continuous slow low-efficiency dialysis, with the dialysate (HCO_3^-) adjusted to 23 mmol/L. Standard hemodialysis or peritoneal dialysis is less useful in correcting metabolic alkalosis because these treatments are designed to add alkali to the blood and the alkali concentration in the dialysis bath solution is set at 35–40 mmol/L.

If renal replacement therapy cannot be instituted, titration with HCl is an alternative therapy. This approach is limited by the concentration of HCl that can be administered without producing hemolysis or venous coagulation. Although some investigators have used higher concentrations, the recommended safe level of H^+ is 100 mmol/L (0.1 N HCl). Even at this concentration, HCl must be administered via a central vein. Because the apparent space of distribution of HCO_3^- is approximately 50% of body weight, one can calculate that, in a 70-kg patient, 350 mmol of H^+ is required to reduce serum (HCO_3^-) by 10 mmol/L. The volume of fluid required for this titration using HCl, unfortunately, is 3.5 L. To provide H^+ for titration in a more concentrated solution, ammonium chloride (NH_4Cl) or arginine monohydrochloride has been used in the past. These solutions are no longer recommended because they both cause life-threatening problems[21]. The former can cause NH_3 intoxication and the latter, severe hyperkalemia.

REFERENCES

1. Gennari FJ, Maddox DM. Renal regulation of acid–base homeostasis. Integrated response. In: Seldin DW, Giebisch G, eds. The kidney. Physiology and pathophysiology, 3rd edn. Philadelphia: Lippincott Williams & Wilkins; 2000:2015–53.
2. Gennari FJ. Metabolic alkalosis. In: Jacobson HR, Striker, GE, Klahr S, eds. The principles and practice of nephrology, 2nd edn. St. Louis: Mosby; 1995:932–41.
3. Starr RA, Burg MB, Knepper MA. Bicarbonate secretion and chloride absorption in the rabbit cortical collecting ducts. Role of chloride/bicarbonate exchange. J Clin Invest. 1985;76:1123–30.
4. Jacobson HR, Seldin DW. On the generation, maintenance, and correction of metabolic alkalosis. Am J Physiol. 1983;245: F425–32.
5. Galla J. Metabolic alkalosis. J Am Soc Nephrol. 2000;11:369–75.
6. Cogan MG, Carneiro MW, Tatsumo J, et al. Normal diet NaCl variation can affect the set point for plasma pH – (HCO_3^-) maintenance. J Am Soc Nephrol. 1990;1:193–9.
7. Hernandez RE, Schambelan M, Cogan MG, et al. Dietary NaCl determines the severity of potassium depletion-induced metabolic alkalosis. Kidney Int. 1987;31:1356–67.

8. Kassirer JP, Schwartz WB. The response of normal man to selective depletion of hydrochloric acid. Am J Med. 1966;40:10–18.

9. Kassirer JP, Schwartz WB. Correction of metabolic alkalosis in man without repair of potassium deficiency. Am J Med. 1966;40:19–26.

10. Gennari FJ. Hypokalemia in metabolic alkalosis. A new look at an old controversy. In: Hatano M, ed. Nephrology. Tokyo: Springer Verlag; 1991:262–9.

11. Garella S, Chazan JA, Cohen JJ. Saline resistant metabolic alkalosis or 'chloride-wasting nephropathy'. Ann Intern Med. 1970; 73–81.

12. Bravo EL, Tarazi RC, Dustan HP, et al. The changing clinical spectrum of primary aldosteronism. Am J Med. 1983;74:641–51.

13. Holland OB. Primary hyperaldosteronism. Semin Nephrol. 1995;15:116–25.

14. Madias NE, Adrogue HJ, Cohen JJ. Maladaptive renal response to chronic metabolic alkalosis. Am J Physiol. 1980;238:F283–9.

15. Gennari FJ. Hypokalemia. N Engl J Med. 1998;339:451–8.

16. Lifton RP, Dluhy RG, Powers M, et al. A chimaeric 11β-hydroxylase/aldosterone synthase gene causes glucocorticoid-remediable aldosteronism and human hypertension. Nature. 1992;355:262–5.

17. Tamura H, Schild L, Enomoto N et al. Liddle disease caused by a missense mutation of β subunit of the epithelial sodium channel gene. J Clin Invest. 1996;97:1780–4.

18. Whorwood CB, Stewart PM. Human hypertension caused by mutations in the 11β-hydroxysteroid dehydrogenase gene: A molecular analysis of apparent mineralocorticoid excess. J Hypertension. 1996;14(Suppl 5):S19–S24.

19. Guay-Woodford LM. Bartter syndrome: Unraveling the pathophysiologic enigma. Am J Med. 1998;105:151–61.

20. Simon DB, Lifton RJ. The molecular basis of inherited hypokalemic alkalosis: Bartter and Gitelman syndromes. Am J Physiol. 1996;271:F961–6.

21. Rimmer JM, Gennari FJ. Metabolic alkalosis. J Intens Care Med. 1987;2:137–50.

22. Orwoll ES. The milk-alkali syndrome: Current concepts. Ann Intern Med. 1982;97:242–8.

23. Beall DP, Scofield RH. Milk-alkali syndrome associated with calcium carbonate consumption. Medicine. 1995;74:89–96.

24. Hulter HN, Sebastian A, Toto RD, et al. Renal and systemic effects of the chronic administration of hypercalcemia-producing agents: calcitriol, PTH and intravenous calcium. Kidney Int. 1982;21:445–58.

25. Hulter HN, Peterson JC. Acid–base homeostasis during chronic PTH excess in humans. Kidney Int. 1985;28:187–92.

26. Schulman M, Narins RG. Hypokalemia and cardiovascular disease. Am J Cardiol. 1990;65:4E–9E.

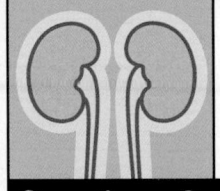

Chapter 13

Respiratory Acidosis, Respiratory Alkalosis, and Mixed Disorders

Horacio J Adrogué and Nicolaos E Madias

INTRODUCTION

Deviations of systemic acidity in either direction can have adverse consequences and, when severe, can be life threatening. Therefore, it is essential for the clinician to be able to recognize and properly diagnose acid–base disorders, understand their impact on organ function, and be familiar with their treatment and the potential complications of treatment[1,2]. Respiratory disorders, that is abnormalities of acid–base equilibrium initiated by a change in blood carbon dioxide tension (P_{CO_2}), as well as mixed acid–base disturbances, are frequently encountered in clinical practice, especially in critically ill patients. In the present chapter, we will focus on clinical diagnosis and management of respiratory acidosis, respiratory alkalosis, and mixed acid–base disorders.

RESPIRATORY ACIDOSIS (PRIMARY HYPERCAPNIA)

Definition

Respiratory acidosis is the acid–base disturbance initiated by an increase in CO_2 tension of body fluids. The secondary increment in plasma bicarbonate (HCO_3^-) observed in acute and chronic hypercapnia should be viewed as an integral part of the respiratory acidosis[3]. Whole-body CO_2 stores are increased and the level of arterial CO_2 tension (P_{aCO_2}) is > 45 mmHg (5.3 kP) in patients with simple respiratory acidosis (measured at rest and at sea level). An element of respiratory acidosis may still occur with lower levels of P_{aCO_2} in patients residing at high altitude (e.g., 4000 m or 13 000 feet) or with metabolic acidosis in whom a normal P_{aCO_2} is inappropriately high for this condition[4]. Another special case of respiratory acidosis is the presence of arterial eucapnia, or even hypocapnia, occurring together with severe venous hypercapnia, in patients having an acute, profound decrease in cardiac output but relative preservation of respiratory function[5,6]. This disorder is known as 'pseudorespiratory alkalosis' and is discussed under respiratory alkalosis.

Etiology and pathogenesis

The ventilatory system is responsible for maintaining P_{aCO_2} within normal limits by adjusting alveolar minute ventilation ($\dot{V}_A$) to match the rate of CO_2 production. The main elements of ventilation are the respiratory pump, which generates a pressure gradient responsible for air flow, and the loads that oppose such action. The inspiratory decrease in pleural pressure caused by the respiratory pump must be sufficient to counterbalance the opposing effect of the combined loads, including the airway flow resistance and the elastic recoil of the lungs and chest wall.

The determinants of CO_2 retention can be viewed as factors imposing an imbalance between the strength of the respiratory pump and the weight of the respiratory loads (Fig. 13.1). When the respiratory pump is unable to balance the opposing load, respiratory acidosis develops. Decreases in respiratory pump strength, increases in load, or a combination of the two can result in CO_2 retention. Respiratory pump failure can occur because of depressed central drive, abnormal neuromuscular transmission, or respiratory muscle dysfunction. Higher load can be caused by enhanced ventilatory demand, increased dead space ventilation, augmented airway flow resistance, and stiffness of the lungs or the pleural/chest wall. Respiratory acidosis is divided into acute and chronic forms, taking into consideration the usual mode of onset and duration of the various causes (see Tables 13.1 and 13.2). Life-threatening acidemia of respiratory origin can occur during severe, acute respiratory acidosis or during respiratory decompensation in patients with chronic hypercapnia.

Equation 13.1 presents the simplified form of the alveolar gas equation at sea level and when breathing room air (F_{iO_2}, 21%):

■ EQUATION 13.1

$$P_{AO_2} = 150 - 1.25\, P_{aCO_2}$$

where P_{AO_2} is alveolar O_2 tension in mmHg. Examination of this equation demonstrates that the major threat to life from CO_2 retention in patients breathing room air is the associated obligatory hypoxemia. In the absence of supplemental O_2, patients suffering respiratory arrest develop critical hypoxemia within a few minutes, long before severe hypercapnia occurs. The constraints of the alveolar gas equation establish that patients breathing room air cannot reach P_{aCO_2} levels much greater than 80 mmHg (10.6 kP) because the degree of hypoxemia that would occur at greater values is incompatible with life. Therefore, extreme hypercapnia occurs only during O_2 therapy, and severe CO_2 retention is often the result of uncontrolled O_2 administration.

Secondary physiologic response

Adaptation to acute hypercapnia elicits an immediate increment in plasma HCO_3^- concentration that is explained by titration of non-HCO_3^- body buffers; such buffers generate HCO_3^- by combining with H^+ derived from the dissociation of carbonic acid:

■ EQUATION 13.2 & 13.3

$$CO_2 + H_2O \rightleftharpoons H_2CO_3 \rightleftharpoons HCO_3^- + H^+$$
$$H^+ + B^- \rightleftharpoons HB$$

where B^- refers to the base component and HB refers to the acid component of non-HCO_3^- buffers. This adaptation is completed within 5 to 10 min from the rise in Pa_{CO_2}, and assuming a stable level of hypercapnia, no further change in

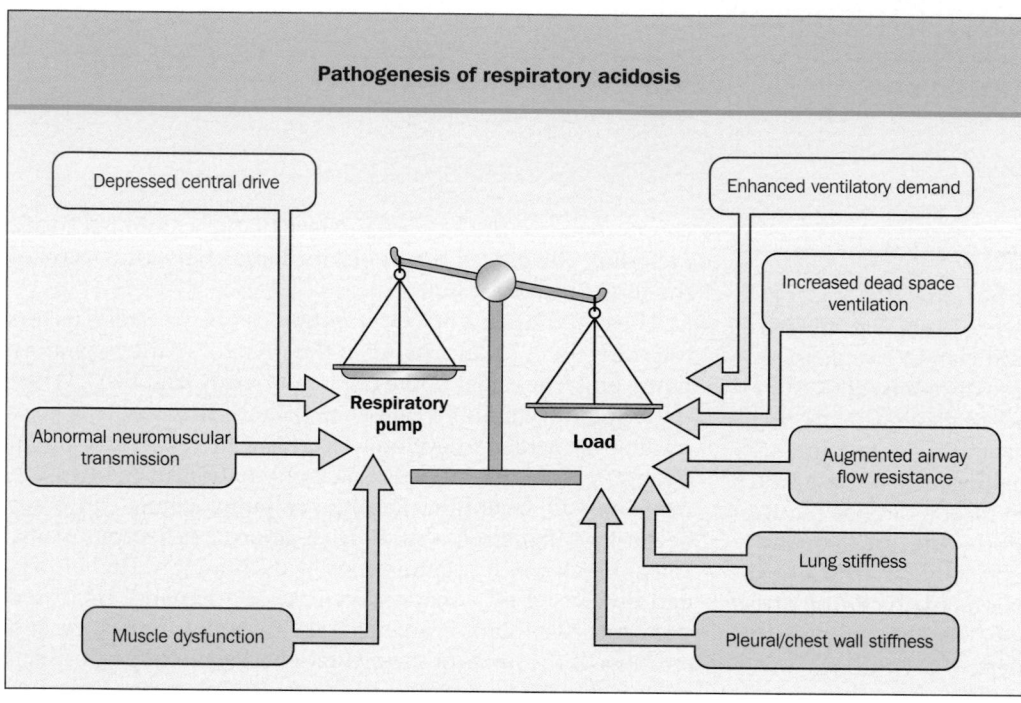

Pathogenesis of respiratory acidosis

Figure 13.1 Pathogenesis of respiratory acidosis.

Causes of acute respiratory acidosis

Table 13.1 Causes of acute respiratory acidosis.

Increased load	Depressed pump
Enhanced ventilatory demand	*Depressed central drive*
High carbohydrate diet	General anesthesia
High carbohydrate dialysate (peritoneal dialysis)	Sedative overdose
Sorbent-regenerative hemodialysis	Head trauma
	Cerebrovascular accident
Increased dead space ventilation	Obesity hypoventilation syndrome
Acute lung injury	Cerebral edema
Multi-lobar pneumonia	Brain tumor
Cardiogenic pulmonary edema	Encephalitis
Pulmonary embolism	Brain-stem lesion
Positive pressure ventilation	
Supplemental oxygen	*Abnormal neuromuscular transmission*
	High spinal cord injury
Augmented airway flow resistance	Guillain–Barré syndrome
Upper airway obstruction	Status epilepticus
Coma-induced hypopharyngeal obstruction	Botulism; tetanus
Aspiration of foreign body or vomitus	Crisis in myasthenia gravis
Laryngospasm	Familial periodic paralysis
Angioedema	Drugs or toxic agents (e.g., curare, succinylcholine,
Inadequate laryngeal intubation	aminoglycosides, organophosphate poisoning)
Laryngeal obstruction postintubation	
Lower airway obstruction	*Muscle dysfunction*
Status asthmaticus	Fatigue
Exacerbation of chronic obstructive pulmonary disease	Hyperkalemia
	Hypokalemia
Lung stiffness	
Atelectasis	
Pleural/chest wall stiffness	
Pneumothorax	
Hemothorax	
Flail chest	
Abdominal distension	
Peritoneal dialysis	

Causes of chronic respiratory acidosis

Increased load	Depressed pump
Increased dead space ventilation Emphysema Pulmonary fibrosis Pulmonary vascular disease	*Depressed central drive* Central sleep apnea Obesity hypoventilation syndrome Methadone/heroin addiction Brain tumor

Augmented airway flow resistance
Upper airway obstruction
  Tonsillar and peritonsillar hypertrophy
  Paralysis of vocal cords
  Tumor of the cords or larynx
  Airways stenosis postprolonged intubation
  Thymoma, aortic aneurysm
Lower airway obstruction
  Chronic obstructive pulmonary disease
	Bulbar poliomyelitis
	Hypothyroidism
	
	Abnormal neuromuscular transmission
	High spinal cord injury
	Poliomyelitis
	Multiple sclerosis
	Muscular dystrophy
	Amyotrophic lateral sclerosis
	Diaphragmatic paralysis

Lung stiffness Severe chronic interstitial lung disease	*Muscle dysfunction* Myopathic disease (e.g., polymyositis)
Pleural/chest wall stiffness Kyphoscoliosis Thoracic cage disease Thoracoplasty Obesity	

Table 13.2 Causes of chronic respiratory acidosis.

Secondary response to alterations in acid–base status

Condition	Initiating mechanism	Expected response: change in HCO_3^- ($\Delta[HCO_3^-]$) or in $PaCO_2$ ($\Delta PaCO_2$)	Maximal level of response

Respiratory acidosis
  Acute
  Chronic
	Rise in $PaCO_2$	
		Rise in (HCO_3^-) $\approx$ 0.1 $\Delta PaCO_2$
		Rise in (HCO_3^-) $\approx$ 0.3 $\Delta PaCO_2$
			
			30 mmol/L
			45 mmol/L

Respiratory alkalosis
  Acute
  Chronic
	Fall in $PaCO_2$	
		Fall in (HCO_3^-) $\approx$ 0.2 $\Delta PaCO_2$
		Fall in (HCO_3^-) $\approx$ 0.4 $\Delta PaCO_2$
			
			16–18 mmol/L
			12–15 mmol/L

Metabolic acidosis	Fall in $(HCO_3^-)_p$	Fall in $PaCO_2$ $\approx$ 1.2 $\Delta(HCO_3^-)$	10 mmHg (1.3 kP)
Metabolic alkalosis	Rise in $(HCO_3^-)_p$	Rise in $PaCO_2$ $\approx$ 0.7 $\Delta(HCO_3^-)$	65 mmHg (8.7 kP)

Table 13.3 Secondary response to alterations in acid–base status.

acid–base equilibrium is detectable for a few hours[7]. Empirical observations indicate that the overall limit of adaptation of plasma HCO_3^- is quite small. Moderate hypoxemia does not alter the adaptive response to acute respiratory acidosis. However, pre-existing hypobicarbonatemia (whether caused by metabolic acidosis or chronic respiratory alkalosis) enhances the magnitude of the HCO_3^- response to acute hypercapnia; this response is diminished in hyperbicarbonatemic states (whether caused by metabolic alkalosis or chronic respiratory acidosis)[8,9].

The adaptive increase in plasma HCO_3^- concentration observed in the acute phase of hypercapnia is amplified greatly during chronic hypercapnia as a result of HCO_3^- generation by the kidney. In addition, the renal response to chronic hypercapnia includes a reduction in the rate of Cl^- reabsorption, resulting in depletion of the body's Cl^- stores. Completion of the adaptation to chronic hypercapnia requires 3–5 days[7]. Quantitative aspects of the secondary physiologic responses to acute and chronic hypercapnia are depicted in Table 13.3. The renal response to chronic hypercapnia is not altered appreciably by dietary Na^+ or Cl^- restriction, moderate K^+ depletion, alkali loading, or moderate hypoxemia. However, recovery

from chronic hypercapnia is crippled by a diet deficient in Cl^-; in this circumstance, despite correction of the level of $PaCO_2$, plasma HCO_3^- concentration remains elevated so long as the state of Cl^- deprivation persists, thus creating the entity of 'posthypercapnic metabolic alkalosis.'

Clinical manifestations
Because clinical hypercapnia almost always occurs with some degree of hypoxemia, it is often difficult to determine whether a specific manifestation is the consequence of the elevated $PaCO_2$ or the reduced PaO_2. Nevertheless, one should bear in mind several characteristic manifestations of neurologic or cardiovascular dysfunction to diagnose the condition accurately and to treat it effectively[4,7].

Neurologic symptoms
Acute hypercapnia is often associated with marked anxiety, severe breathlessness, disorientation, confusion, incoherence, and combativeness. A narcotic-like effect is not uncommon in patients with chronic hypercapnia, and drowsiness, decreased alertness, inattention, forgetfulness, loss of memory, irritability, confusion, and somnolence can be observed.

Fluid and Electrolyte Disorders

Motor disturbances, including tremor, myoclonic jerks, and asterixis, are frequent accompaniments of both acute and chronic hypercapnia. Sustained myoclonus and seizure activity can also develop. Signs and symptoms of increased intracranial pressure (pseudotumor cerebri) are occasionally evident in patients with either acute or chronic hypercapnia, and they appear to be related to the vasodilating effects of CO_2 on cerebral blood vessels. Headache is a frequent complaint. Blurring of the optic discs and frank papilledema can be found when hypercapnia is severe. Hypercapnic coma characteristically occurs in patients with acute exacerbations of chronic respiratory insufficiency, who are treated injudiciously with 'high-flow' O_2.

Cardiovascular symptoms

Acute hypercapnia of mild-to-moderate degree is usually characterized by warm, flushed skin, a bounding pulse, sweating, increased cardiac output, and normal or increased blood pressure. By comparison, severe hypercapnia might be attended by decreases in both cardiac output and blood pressure. In the clinical setting, the cardiovascular manifestations of acute hypercapnia might well be altered significantly by the effects of concomitant hypoxemia, congestive heart failure, and vasoactive medications, including pharmacologic blockade of β-adrenoceptors. Cardiac arrhythmias occur frequently in patients with either acute or chronic hypercapnia, especially those receiving digitalis as therapy for cor pulmonale.

Renal symptoms

Retention of CO_2 affects the renal circulation and alters plasma levels of hormones that modify kidney function. Mild-to-moderate hypercapnia results in renal vasodilation, but acute increments in $PaCO_2$ to levels above 70 mmHg induce renal vasoconstriction and hypoperfusion. Salt and water retention commonly attends sustained hypercapnia, especially in the presence of cor pulmonale. In addition to the effects of heart failure on the kidney, multiple other factors might be at play, including the prevailing stimulation of the sympathetic nervous system and the renin–angiotensin–aldosterone axis, the increased renal vascular resistance, and the elevated levels of antidiuretic hormone and cortisol.

Diagnosis

In general, one should never rely on clinical examination alone to assess the adequacy of alveolar ventilation[10]. Whenever CO_2 retention is suspected, arterial blood gas determinations should be obtained. Indeed, accurate laboratory data are a prerequisite for establishing the diagnosis of respiratory acidosis.

If the patient's acid–base profile reveals hypercapnia in association with acidemia, at least an element of respiratory acidosis must be present. However, hypercapnia can be associated with a normal or even an alkaline pH if certain additional acid–base disorders are also present. Information from the patient's history, a physical examination, and ancillary laboratory data should be used to assess whether part or all of the rise in $PaCO_2$ reflects an adaptive response to metabolic alkalosis rather than being primary in origin. For moderate degrees of metabolic alkalosis (plasma $HCO_3^- < 40$ mmol/L),

secondary hypoventilation would be expected to raise $PaCO_2$ to levels no higher than about 50 mmHg.

Treatment

As previously noted, CO_2 retention, whether acute or chronic, is always associated with hypoxemia in patients breathing room air. In fact, hypoxemia, not hypercapnia or acidemia, is *the* critical factor that determines morbidity and mortality of patients with acute or chronic respiratory acidosis. Consequently, O_2 administration represents a critical element in the management of respiratory acidosis[1,11]. However, supplemental O_2 may lead to worsening hypercapnia especially in patients with chronic obstructive pulmonary disease. It was traditionally thought that this development was secondary to the removal of the hypoxic ventilatory drive. Although a depressed respiratory drive in CO_2 retention seems to play a role, other factors might largely account for the worsening hypercapnia in response to supplemental O_2 therapy. These include an increase in dead space ventilation and $\dot{V}/\dot{Q}$ mismatch due to the loss of hypoxic pulmonary vasoconstriction, and the Haldane effect (the decreased hemoglobin affinity for CO_2 in the presence of increased O_2 saturation) which mandates an increase in ventilation to eliminate the excess CO_2[12,13].

A synopsis of the management of acute respiratory acidosis and chronic respiratory acidosis is presented in Figures 13.2 and 13.3. Whenever possible, treatment must be directed at removing or ameliorating the underlying cause. Immediate therapeutic efforts should focus on securing a patent airway and restoring adequate oxygenation by delivering an O_2-rich inspired mixture. Mechanical ventilation must be initiated in the presence of apnea, severe hypoxemia unresponsive to conservative measures, or progressive respiratory acidosis ($PaCO_2 > 80$ mmHg (10.6 kP))[14]. Management of respiratory decompensation depends on the cause, severity, and rate of progression of CO_2 retention. Vigorous treatment of pulmonary infections, bronchodilator therapy, and removal of secretions can offer considerable benefit. Naloxone will reverse the suppressive effect of narcotic agents on ventilation. Avoidance of tranquilizers and sedatives, gradual reduction of supplemental oxygen (aiming at a PaO_2 of about 60 mmHg), and treatment of a superimposed element of metabolic alkalosis will optimize the ventilatory drive.

Whereas the early use of standard ventilator assistance is most appropriate for patients with acute respiratory acidosis, recent data indicate that patients with chronic obstructive pulmonary disease also have a high likelihood of being weaned from standard ventilators[4]. Noninvasive mechanical ventilation delivered through a nasal or full facial mask is being used with increasing frequency to avert possible complications of endotracheal intubation. This modality is effective in the management of acute asthma, the obesity hypoventilation syndrome and, especially, in patients with acute respiratory failure in the setting of chronic obstructive pulmonary disease[4]. However, if the patient is unstable or noninvasive ventilation fails, intubation should be carried out to allow invasive ventilatory support. Minute ventilation should be raised so that the $PaCO_2$ gradually returns to near its long-term baseline and excretion of excess HCO_3^- by the kidneys is accomplished (assuming that Cl^- is provided).

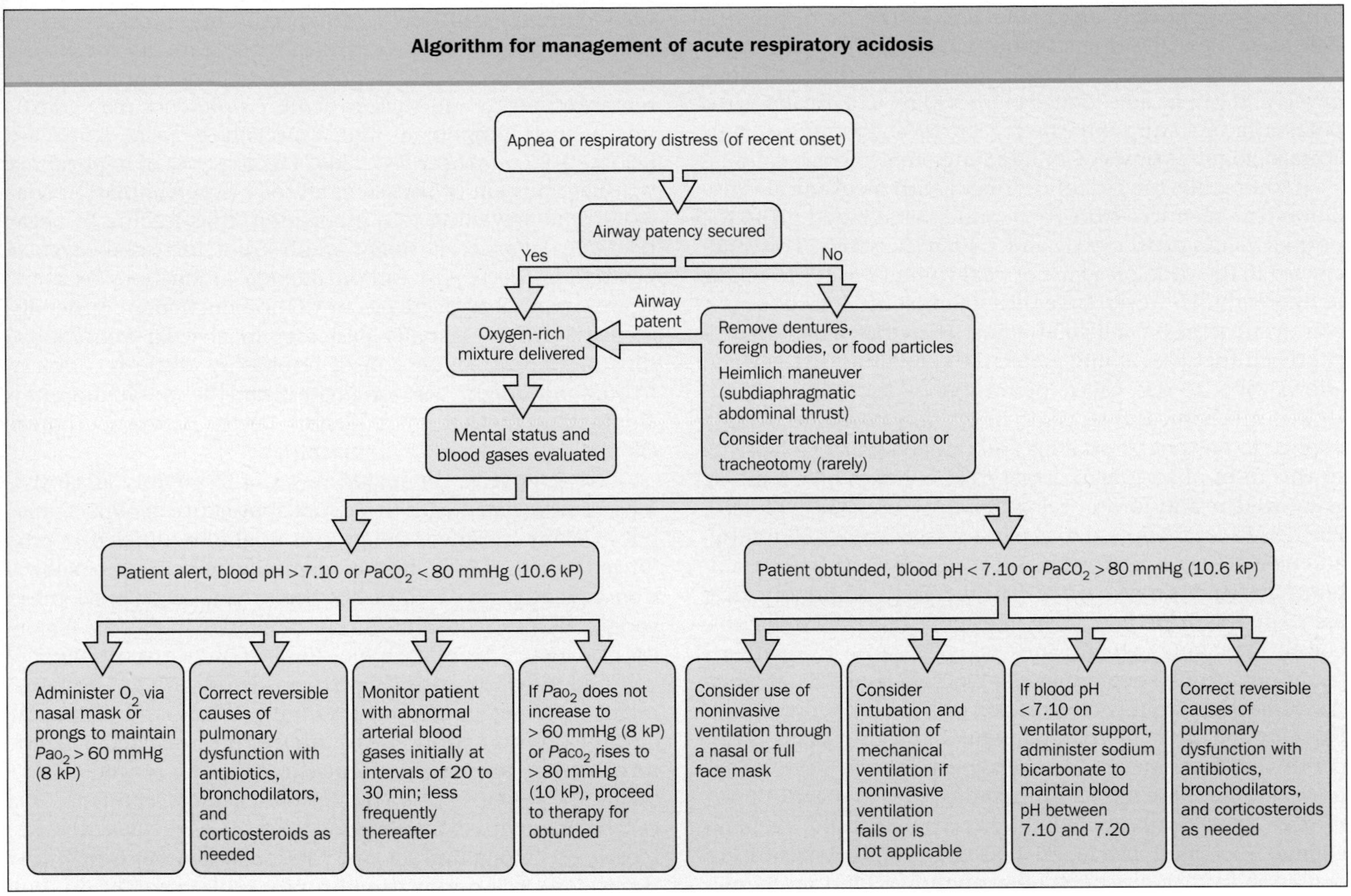

Algorithm for management of acute respiratory acidosis

Apnea or respiratory distress (of recent onset)

Airway patency secured

Yes — No

Airway patent

Oxygen-rich mixture delivered

Remove dentures, foreign bodies, or food particles

Heimlich maneuver (subdiaphragmatic abdominal thrust)

Consider tracheal intubation or tracheotomy (rarely)

Mental status and blood gases evaluated

Patient alert, blood pH > 7.10 or $PaCO_2$ < 80 mmHg (10.6 kP)

Patient obtunded, blood pH < 7.10 or $PaCO_2$ > 80 mmHg (10.6 kP)

Administer O_2 via nasal mask or prongs to maintain Pao_2 > 60 mmHg (8 kP)

Correct reversible causes of pulmonary dysfunction with antibiotics, bronchodilators, and corticosteroids as needed

Monitor patient with abnormal arterial blood gases initially at intervals of 20 to 30 min; less frequently thereafter

If Pao_2 does not increase to > 60 mmHg (8 kP) or $Paco_2$ rises to > 80 mmHg (10 kP), proceed to therapy for obtunded

Consider use of noninvasive ventilation through a nasal or full face mask

Consider intubation and initiation of mechanical ventilation if noninvasive ventilation fails or is not applicable

If blood pH < 7.10 on ventilator support, administer sodium bicarbonate to maintain blood pH between 7.10 and 7.20

Correct reversible causes of pulmonary dysfunction with antibiotics, bronchodilators, and corticosteroids as needed

Figure 13.2 Algorithm for management of acute respiratory acidosis.

Figure 13.3 Algorithm for management of chronic respiratory acidosis.

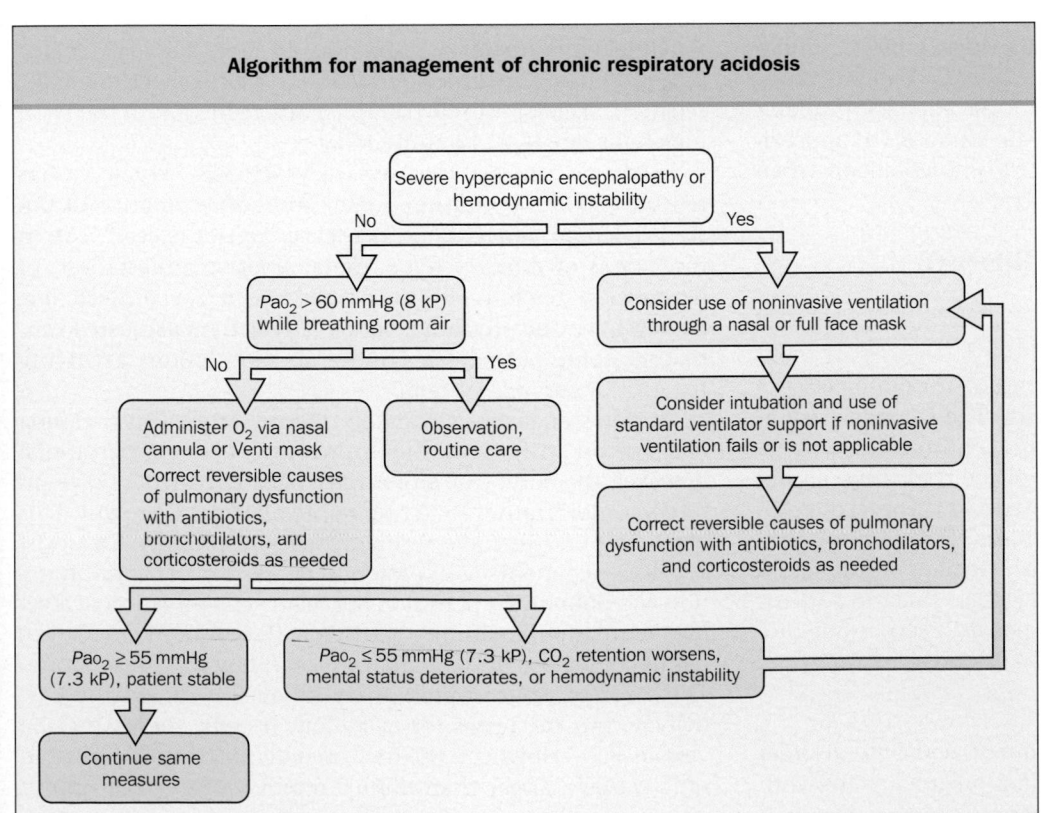

Algorithm for management of chronic respiratory acidosis

Severe hypercapnic encephalopathy or hemodynamic instability

No — Yes

Pao_2 > 60 mmHg (8 kP) while breathing room air

Consider use of noninvasive ventilation through a nasal or full face mask

No — Yes

Administer O_2 via nasal cannula or Venti mask

Correct reversible causes of pulmonary dysfunction with antibiotics, bronchodilators, and corticosteroids as needed

Observation, routine care

Consider intubation and use of standard ventilator support if noninvasive ventilation fails or is not applicable

Correct reversible causes of pulmonary dysfunction with antibiotics, bronchodilators, and corticosteroids as needed

Pao_2 ≥ 55 mmHg (7.3 kP), patient stable

Pao_2 ≤ 55 mmHg (7.3 kP), CO_2 retention worsens, mental status deteriorates, or hemodynamic instability

Continue same measures

Fluid and Electrolyte Disorders

By contrast, overly rapid reduction in the Pa_{CO_2} risks the development of posthypercapnic alkalosis, with potentially serious consequences. Should posthypercapnic alkalosis develop, it can be ameliorated by providing Cl^-, usually as the potassium salt, and administering the HCO_3^--wasting diuretic acetazolamide at doses of 250–375 mg once or twice daily.

Traditionally, the goal of treatment with mechanical ventilation had been to restore Pa_{CO_2} and arterial blood pH to the normal values of 40 mmHg and 7.40, respectively. This strategy led to the widespread use of tidal volumes of 10–15 mL/kg body weight. However, large tidal volumes often lead to alveolar overdistension and volutrauma. Therefore, an alternative approach that uses a lung-protective ventilatory strategy and allows Pa_{CO_2} to rise, called 'permissive hypercapnia' (or controlled mechanical hypoventilation), has been successfully applied to prevent barotrauma and cardiovascular collapse[4,15]. In this form of treatment, lower tidal volumes of < 6 mL/kg body weight and lower peak inspiratory pressures are used. Further, Pa_{CO_2} is allowed to rise but rarely exceeds 80 mmHg, and blood pH can decrease to as low as 7.00–7.10, while maintaining adequate oxygenation. The increased respiratory drive associated with permissive hypercapnia causes extreme discomfort, making sedation necessary. Because the patients commonly require neuromuscular blockade as well, accidental disconnection from the ventilator can cause sudden death. Furthermore, after the neuromuscular-blocking agent is discontinued, there may be weakness or paralysis for several days or weeks. There are several contraindications to the use of permissive hypercapnia, including cerebrovascular disease, brain edema, increased intracranial pressure, and convulsions; depressed cardiac function and arrhythmias; and severe pulmonary hypertension. Notably, most of these entities can develop as adverse effects of permissive hypercapnia itself, especially when hypercapnia is associated with substantial acidemia. In fact, some experimental evidence indicates that correction of acidemia attenuates the adverse hemodynamic effects of permissive hypercapnia[16]. It appears prudent, although still controversial, to keep the blood pH at approximately 7.30 by administering intravenous alkali when controlled hypoventilation is prescribed[1,17].

RESPIRATORY ALKALOSIS (PRIMARY HYPOCAPNIA)

Definition

Respiratory alkalosis is the acid–base disturbance initiated by a reduction in CO_2 tension of body fluids. The secondary fall in plasma HCO_3^- observed in acute and chronic hypocapnia should be viewed as an integral part of the respiratory alkalosis. Whole-body CO_2 stores are decreased and the level of Pa_{CO_2} is < 35 mmHg (4.7 kP) in patients with simple respiratory alkalosis who are at rest and at sea level. An element of respiratory alkalosis may still occur with higher levels of Pa_{CO_2} in patients with metabolic alkalosis, in whom a normal Pa_{CO_2} is inappropriately low for this primary metabolic disorder.

Etiology and pathogenesis

Respiratory alkalosis is the most frequent acid–base disorder encountered, since it occurs in normal pregnancy and with high-altitude residence[2,18]. It is also the most common acid–base abnormality in critically ill patients, occurring either as the simple disorder or as a component of mixed disturbances; indeed, in such patients, its presence may constitute a grave prognostic sign, especially if Pa_{CO_2} levels are below 20–25 mmHg (2.7–3.3 kP). The presence of hypocapnia signifies transient or persistent alveolar hyperventilation relative to the prevailing CO_2 production, thus leading to negative CO_2 balance; it might result from increased alveolar ventilation, decreased carbon dioxide production, or both. However, primary decreases in CO_2 production are generally accompanied by parallel decreases in alveolar ventilation, thus preventing expression of respiratory alkalosis. Primary hypocapnia might also originate from the extrapulmonary elimination of CO_2 by a dialysis device or extracorporeal circulation (e.g. heart–lung machine).

Table 13.4 gives the major causes of respiratory alkalosis[6]. Most are associated with the abrupt appearance of hypocapnia, but in many instances the process might be sufficiently prolonged to permit full, chronic adaptation to occur (see below). Consequently, no attempt has been made to separate these conditions into acute and chronic categories. In the vast majority of patients, primary hypocapnia reflects alveolar hyperventilation owing to increased ventilatory drive. The latter might represent signals arising from the lung, the peripheral chemoreceptors (carotid and aortic), or the brainstem chemoreceptors, or influences originating in other centers of the brain. The response of the brainstem chemoreceptors to CO_2 can be augmented by systemic diseases (e.g., liver disease, sepsis), pharmacologic agents, volition, and other influences. Hypoxemia is a major stimulus of alveolar ventilation, but Pa_{O_2} values lower than 60 mmHg (8 kP) are required to elicit this effect consistently. Not uncommonly, alveolar hyperventilation is the result of maladjusted mechanical ventilators. Potential mechanisms of respiratory alkalosis due to decreased CO_2 production include a reduction in physical activity (e.g., sedation, skeletal muscle paralysis) or a reduction in the basal metabolic rate (e.g., hypothermia).

In sharp contrast to respiratory acidosis, which always reflects a serious condition, some causes of respiratory alkalosis are benign. Since blood pH levels do not exceed 7.55 in most cases of primary hypocapnia, severe manifestations of decreased systemic acidity are usually absent. Severe alkalemia, however, may be produced, particularly with maladjusted ventilators, some psychiatric conditions, and lesions involving the central nervous system.

In states of severe circulatory failure, arterial hypocapnia may coexist with venous and, therefore, tissue hypercapnia; however, the body CO_2 stores have been enriched, and respiratory acidosis rather than respiratory alkalosis is present. This entity, which we have termed pseudorespiratory alkalosis, develops in patients with profound depression of cardiac function and pulmonary perfusion but relative preservation of alveolar ventilation, including patients with advanced circulatory failure and those undergoing cardiopulmonary resuscitation. The severely reduced pulmonary blood flow limits the CO_2 delivered to the lungs for excretion, thereby increasing the venous P_{CO_2}. However, the increased ventilation-to-perfusion ratio causes a larger than normal removal of CO_2 per unit of

Table 13.4 Causes of respiratory alkalosis.

Causes of respiratory alkalosis	

Hypoxemia or tissue hypoxia
  Decreased inspired O_2 tension
  High altitude
  Bacterial or viral pneumonia
  Aspiration of food, foreign body, or vomitus
  Laryngospasm
  Drowning
  Cyanotic heart disease
  Severe anemia
  Left shift deviation of HbO_2 curve
  Hypotension
  Severe circulatory failure
  Pulmonary edema
  Pseudorespiratory alkalosis
 	
Central nervous system stimulation
  Voluntary
  Pain
  Anxiety–hyperventilation syndrome
  Psychosis
  Fever
  Subarachnoid hemorrhage
  Cerebrovascular accident
  Meningoencephalitis
  Tumor
  Trauma
 	
Pulmonary diseases with stimulation of chest receptors
  Pneumonia
  Asthma
  Pneumothorax
  Hemothorax
  Flail chest
  Acute respiratory distress syndrome
  Cardiogenic and noncardiogenic pulmonary edema
  Pulmonary embolism
  Pulmonary fibrosis
	Drugs and hormones
	  Respiratory stimulants (doxapram, nikethamide,
	  ethamivan, progesterone, medroxyprogesterone)
	  Salicylates
	  Nicotine
	  Xanthines
	  Dinitrophenol
	  Pressor hormones (epinephrine, norepinephrine,
	  angiotensin II)
	
	Miscellaneous
	  Exercise
	  Pregnancy
	  Gram-positive septicemia
	  Gram-negative septicemia
	  Hepatic failure
	  Mechanical hyperventilation
	  Heat exposure
	  Recovery from metabolic acidosis
	  Hemodialysis with acetate dialysate

blood traversing the pulmonary circulation, thereby giving rise to arterial eucapnia or frank hypocapnia. A progressive widening of the arteriovenous difference in pH and $P\text{co}_2$ develops in these two settings of cardiac dysfunction, namely circulatory failure and cardiac arrest (Fig. 13.4). Severe O_2 deprivation prevails in the tissues in these two disorders, and it can be completely disguised by the reasonably preserved arterial O_2 values. Appropriate monitoring of acid–base composition and oxygenation in patients with advanced cardiac dysfunction requires mixed (or central) venous blood sampling in addition to the sampling of arterial blood.

Secondary physiologic response

Adaptation to acute hypocapnia is characterized by an immediate decrement in plasma HCO_3^- that results totally from nonrenal mechanisms and is explained principally by alkaline titration of the non-HCO_3^- body buffers (see Equation 13.2 and Table 13.3). This adaptation is completed within 5 to 10 min of the onset of hypocapnia, and, if one assumes no further changes in $P\text{aco}_2$, no additional, detectable changes in acid–base equilibrium occur for a period of several hours[7].

Adaptation to chronic hypocapnia entails an additional, larger fall in plasma HCO_3^- as a consequence of renal adjustments that reflect a dampening of H^+ secretion by the renal tubule[7]. Approximately 2–3 days are required for completion of the adaptation to chronic hypocapnia. Quantitative aspects of the secondary physiologic responses to acute and chronic hypocapnia are shown in Table 13.3.

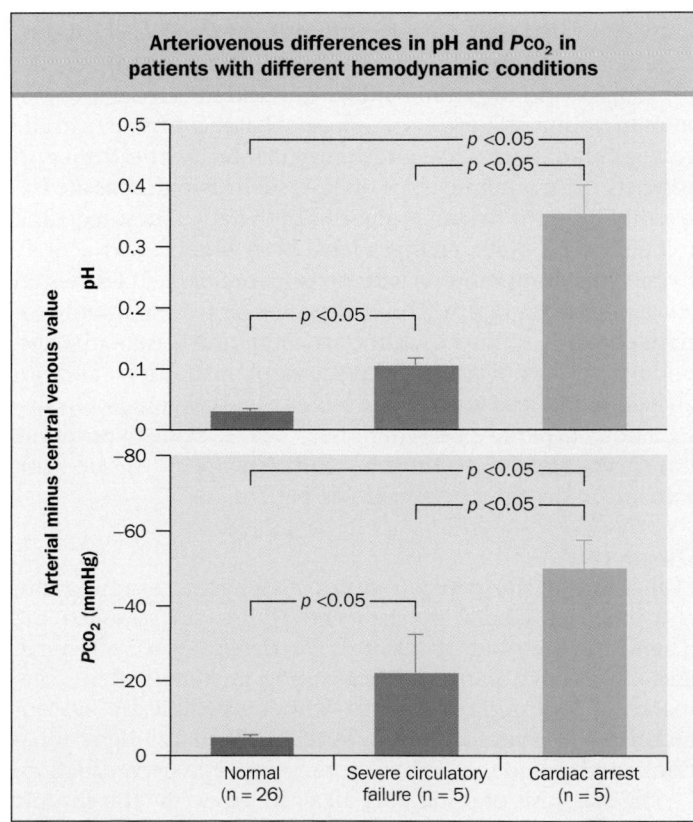

Figure 13.4 Arteriovenous differences in pH and $P\text{co}_2$ in patients with different hemodynamic conditions.

Clinical manifestations

A variety of neurologic and cardiovascular manifestations frequently occur in acute hypocapnia, but these are seldom evident in the chronic phase of the disorder. A rapid fall in Pa_{CO_2} to half normal values or lower is typically accompanied by numbness and paresthesias of the extremities, chest discomfort, circumoral numbness, lightheadedness, and mental confusion; muscle cramps, increased deep-tendon reflexes, carpopedal spasm, and generalized seizures occur infrequently. The neurologic manifestations of acute respiratory alkalosis have been attributed largely to the attendant cerebral hypoperfusion, although additional factors have been implicated[2,19], including alkalemia, the pH-induced shift to the left of the oxyhemoglobin dissociation curve (which lowers the O_2 extraction in the tissues), and the falls in the level of ionized Ca^{2+} and K^+. Cerebral vasoconstriction and reduced cerebral blood flow have been well documented during acute hypocapnia; in severe cases, cerebral blood flow might reach values lower than 50% of normal.

The cardiovascular manifestations of respiratory alkalosis differ in passive and active hyperventilation[7]. The induction of acute hypocapnia in anesthetized subjects (i.e., passive hyperventilation) results in a decrease in cardiac output, an increase in peripheral resistance, and a fall in the systemic blood pressure. By contrast, active hyperventilation does not change, or might even increase, cardiac output and leaves systemic blood pressure virtually unchanged. The discrepant response of cardiac output during hyperventilation probably reflects the fall in venous return caused by mechanical ventilation in passive hyperventilation and the reflex tachycardia consistently observed in active hyperventilation. Sustained hypocapnia induced by exposure to high altitude for several weeks results in a cardiac output equal to or higher than control values. Although acute hypocapnia does not lead to cardiac arrhythmias in normal volunteers, it appears that it contributes to the generation of both atrial and ventricular tachyarrhythmias in patients with ischemic heart disease; such arrhythmias are frequently resistant to standard forms of therapy. Chest pain and ischemic ST–T-wave changes have been observed in acutely hyperventilating subjects with no evidence of fixed lesions on coronary angiography. The pathogenesis of these manifestations remains unknown, although myocardial ischemia secondary to hypocapnia-induced vasoconstriction and an alkalemia-induced shift to the left of the oxyhemoglobin dissociation curve have been proposed. Indeed, acute hypocapnia has been shown to induce coronary-artery spasm and Prinzmetal's angina in susceptible patients.

Diagnosis

Evaluation of the patient's history, a physical examination, and ancillary laboratory data are required to establish the diagnosis of respiratory alkalosis[10,18]. Careful observation can detect abnormal patterns of breathing in some patients, yet marked hypocapnia can occur without a clinically evident increase in respiratory effort. Arterial blood gas determinations are required to confirm the presence of hyperventilation.

The diagnosis of respiratory alkalosis, especially the chronic form, is frequently missed; physicians often misinterpret the electrolyte pattern of hyperchloremic hypobicarbonatemia as indicative of normal anion gap metabolic acidosis. A differentiating clue is the fact that plasma K^+ concentration is typically within the normal range in chronic hypocapnia, whereas hypokalemia or hyperkalemia often accompanies the various types of hyperchloremic metabolic acidosis. If the patient's acid–base profile reveals hypocapnia in association with alkalemia, at least an element of respiratory alkalosis must be present. Yet hypocapnia might be associated with a normal or an acidic pH because of the concomitant presence of additional acid–base disorders. One should also note that mild degrees of chronic hypocapnia leave blood pH within the high-normal range. Careful examination of the patient's history, a physical examination, and ancillary laboratory data are required to assess whether part or all of a given fall in Pa_{CO_2} reflects an adaptive response to metabolic acidosis rather than being primary in nature. Once the diagnosis of respiratory alkalosis is made, a search for its cause should be carried out. The diagnosis of respiratory alkalosis can have important clinical implications; it often provides a clue to the presence of an unrecognized, serious disorder or signals the gravity of a known underlying disease.

Treatment

A synopsis of the management of respiratory alkalosis is presented in Figure 13.5. Whenever possible, treatment must be directed at removing or ameliorating the underlying cause. Because chronic respiratory alkalosis produces few or no symptoms, measures to treat the alkalemia itself are generally not required[2,7]. On the other hand, severe alkalemia requires corrective measures that depend on whether serious clinical manifestations are present. Such measures can be directed at reducing plasma HCO_3^- concentration, increasing Pa_{CO_2}, or both. Even if baseline plasma HCO_3^- is moderately decreased, reducing it further can be particularly rewarding in this setting, as this maneuver combines effectiveness with relatively little risk. For patients with the anxiety–hyperventilation syndrome, rebreathing into a closed system (e.g., a paper bag) might prove helpful, in addition to reassurance or sedation. Rebreathing in this way interrupts the vicious cycle that can result from the reinforcing effects of the symptoms of hypocapnia.

Respiratory alkalosis resulting from severe hypoxemia requires O_2 therapy. The oral administration of 250–500 mg acetazolamide can be beneficial in the management of signs and symptoms of high-altitude sickness, a syndrome characterized by hypoxemia and respiratory alkalosis[18]. Of course, patients undergoing mechanical ventilation lend themselves to an effective correction of hypocapnia (whether caused by maladjusted ventilator or other factors) by resetting the device.

MIXED ACID–BASE DISTURBANCES

Definition

Mixed acid–base disturbances are defined as the simultaneous presence of two or more acid–base disorders. Such association might include two or more simple acid–base disorders (e.g., metabolic acidosis and respiratory alkalosis), two or more forms of a simple disturbance having different time course or pathogenesis (e.g., acute and chronic respiratory acidosis, or

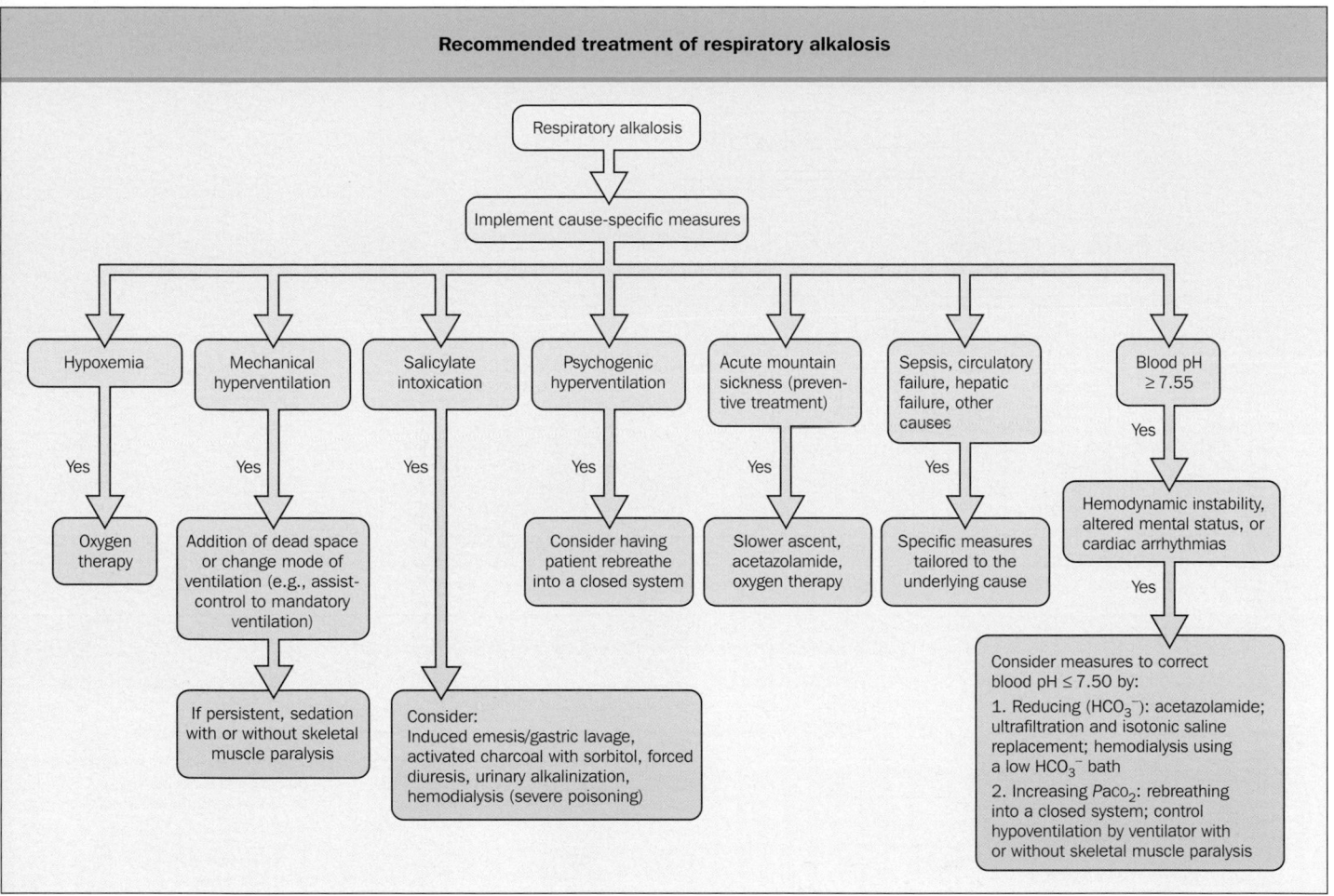

Figure 13.5 Recommended treatment of respiratory alkalosis.

high anion gap and hyperchloremic metabolic acidosis, respectively), or a combination of the previous two forms[20]. The secondary or adaptive response to a simple acid–base disorder cannot be taken as one of the components of a mixed disorder.

Etiology and pathogenesis

Mixed acid–base disturbances are commonly observed in hospitalized patients, especially those in critical care units[21]. Characterization of these disorders and proper identification of their pathogenesis can be challenging tasks and are a prerequisite for taking sound corrective action. Certain clinical settings are commonly associated with mixed acid–base disorders, including cardiorespiratory arrest, sepsis, drug intoxications, diabetes mellitus, and organ failure (especially renal, hepatic, and pulmonary failure). Patients with severe renal insufficiency or end-stage renal disease are prone to developing mixed acid–base disturbances of great complexity and severity[22]. Major relevant features of this state include presence of metabolic acidosis of the high anion gap type, which is frequently accompanied by a component of hyperchloremic acidosis; inability to mount an appropriate secondary response to chronic respiratory acidosis or alkalosis; inability to respond to a load of fixed acids (e.g., lactic acid) or a primary loss of alkali (e.g., diarrhea) with the expected increase in net acid

excretion; and inability to respond to an alkali load with bicarbonaturia despite the presence of an increased plasma HCO_3^- concentration. As a result, these patients are particularly vulnerable to the development of both extreme acidemia and extreme alkalemia.

A practical classification of mixed acid–base disorders recognizes three main groups of disturbances in accordance with the definition presented above (Fig. 13.6). Representative examples are depicted in Table 13.5, and some of these mixed disorders are reviewed below.

Metabolic acidosis and respiratory acidosis

Clinical examples of metabolic acidosis combined with respiratory acidosis include untreated cardiopulmonary arrest, circulatory failure in patients with chronic obstructive pulmonary disease (COPD), severe renal failure associated with hypercapnic respiratory failure, various intoxications, and hypokalemic (or less frequently hyperkalemic) paralysis of respiratory muscles in patients with diarrhea or renal tubular acidosis (see Table 13.5, example 4, and Fig. 13.7).

Metabolic alkalosis and respiratory alkalosis

Metabolic alkalosis combined with respiratory alkalosis might be encountered in patients with primary hypocapnia associated with chronic liver disease who develop metabolic

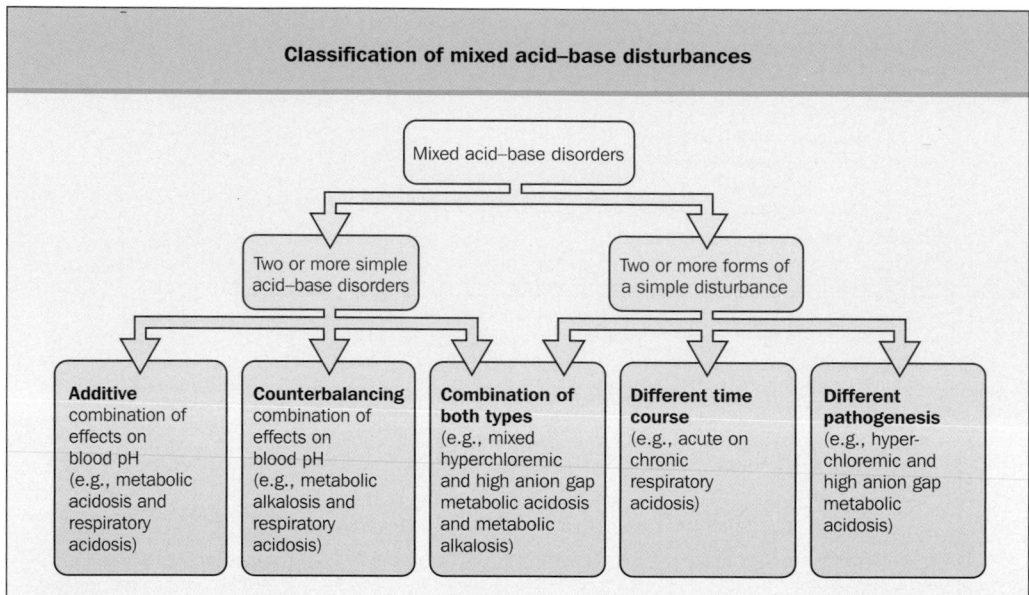

Figure 13.6 Classification of mixed acid–base disturbances.

Type of mixed disorder	Example No.	pH	$PaCO_2$ (mmHg)	HCO_3^-	Na^+	K^+	Cl^-	Anion gap	Clinical circumstances
				(← mmol/L →)					
Hyperchloremic and high anion gap metabolic acidosis	1	7.12	16	5	137	3.6	114	18	Diabetic ketoacidosis with adequate salt and water balance
Mixed high anion gap metabolic acidosis and metabolic alkalosis	2	7.36	31	17	132	4.0	89	26	Alcoholic liver disease, vomiting, and lactic acidosis
	3	7.40	40	24	143	5.5	95	24	Diabetic ketoacidosis and lactic acidosis after bicarbonate therapy
Mixed high anion gap metabolic acidosis and respiratory acidosis	4	7.18	44	16	133	5.7	100	17	Hepatic, renal, and pulmonary failure
Metabolic alkalosis and respiratory acidosis	5	7.44	55	36	135	3.8	84	15	Chronic obstructive pulmonary disease and diuretics
Metabolic alkalosis and respiratory alkalosis	6	7.60	40	38	131	3.6	77	16	Congestive heart failure and diuretics
Acute on chronic respiratory acidosis	7	7.22	80	32	141	4.3	99	10	Chronic obstructive pulmonary disease and therapy with O_2-rich mixtures

Anion gap is calculated as $(Na^+) - ((Cl^-) + (HCO_3^-))$

Table 13.5 Representative examples of mixed acid–base disorders

alkalosis owing to a variety of causes, including vomiting, nasogastric drainage, diuretics, profound hypokalemia, and alkali administration (e.g., absorption of antacids or infusion of Ringer's lactate solution, alimentation solutions, or citrated blood products), especially in the context of renal insufficiency. This entity also is observed in critically ill surgical patients, particularly those undergoing mechanical ventilation, and in patients with respiratory alkalosis caused by either pregnancy or heart failure who experience metabolic alkalosis attributable to diuretics or vomiting (see Table 13.5, example 6, and Table 13.4).

Metabolic alkalosis and respiratory acidosis
Metabolic alkalosis and respiratory acidosis represents one of the most frequently encountered mixed acid–base disorders. The usual clinical setting involves chronic lung disease caused by chronic bronchitis or emphysema in conjunction with diuretic therapy, but other causes of metabolic alkalosis (e.g., vomiting or administration of corticosteroids) might exist (see Table 13.5, example 5, and Fig. 13.10). Critically ill patients with respiratory failure caused by acute respiratory distress syndrome (ARDS) and, occasionally, those with profound hypokalemia also might develop this mixed disorder.

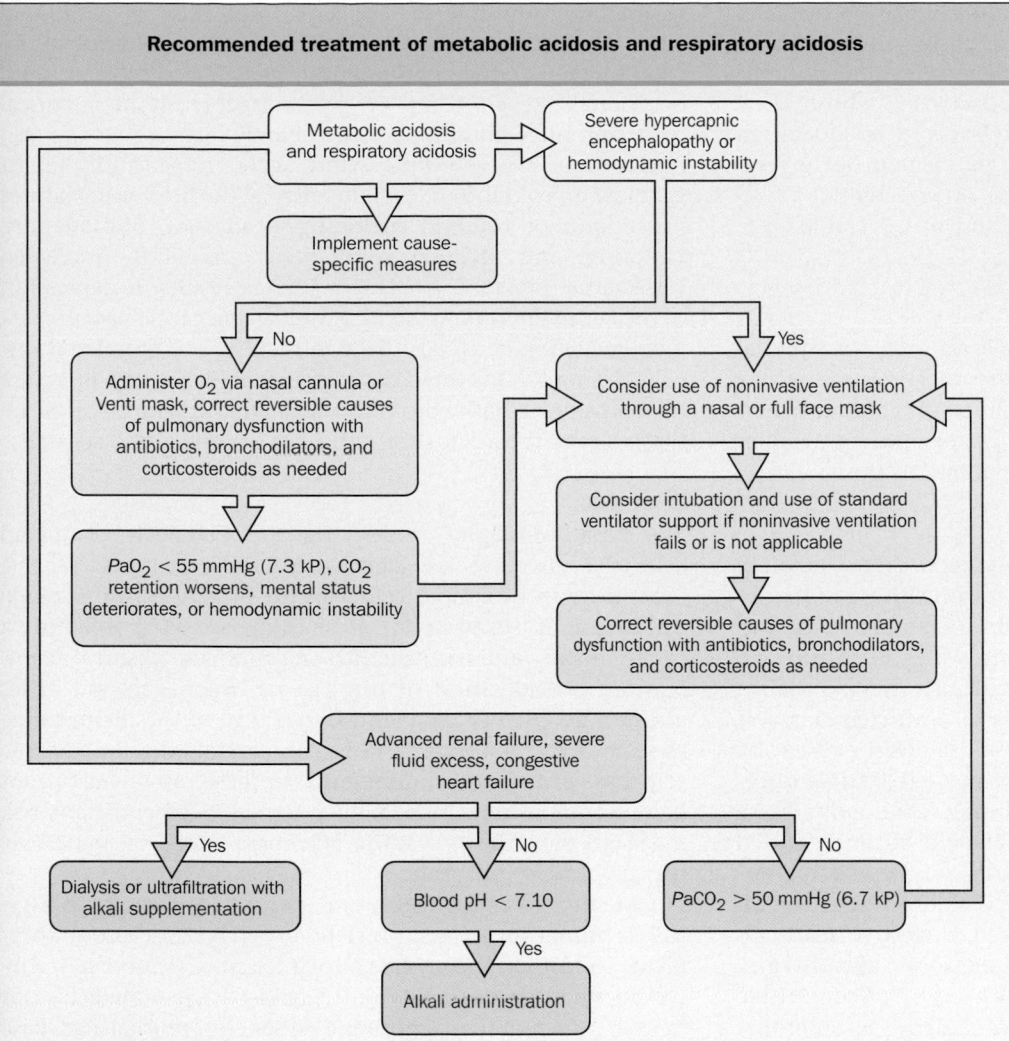

Figure 13.7 Recommended treatment of metabolic acidosis and respiratory acidosis.

Metabolic acidosis and respiratory alkalosis

The combination of metabolic acidosis and respiratory alkalosis, like respiratory acidosis and metabolic alkalosis, is characterized by normal or nearly normal blood pH; its two components exert offsetting effects on systemic acidity. This disorder is commonly observed in patients hospitalized in intensive care units and, as such, is generally associated with high mortality. Primary hypocapnia might result from a variety of causes, including fever, hypotension, Gram-negative septicemia, pulmonary edema, hypoxemia, or mechanical hyperventilation. The component of metabolic acidosis, in turn, might be attributable to lactic acidosis (e.g., complicating shock or hepatic failure) or renal acidosis. Salicylate intoxication represents another major cause of this mixed acid–base disorder. Stimulation of the ventilatory center in the brainstem accounts for the respiratory alkalosis, whereas the accelerated production of organic acids (including pyruvic, lactic, and keto acids) and, to a small extent, the accumulation of salicylic acid itself are responsible for the metabolic acidosis.

Metabolic acidosis and metabolic alkalosis

Metabolic acidosis and metabolic alkalosis is typically observed in patients with alcoholic liver disease who develop fasting ketoacidosis or lactic acidosis in conjunction with metabolic alkalosis caused by vomiting, diuretics, or other causes (see Table 13.5, examples 2 and 3). Protracted vomiting or nasogastric suction superimposed on uremic acidosis, diabetic ketoacidosis, or metabolic acidosis caused by diarrhea might also generate this offsetting metabolic combination. A similar picture might develop after administration of alkali during cardiopulmonary resuscitation or as therapy for diabetic ketoacidosis.

Mixed metabolic acidosis

Pathogenetically disparate entities of metabolic acidosis coexist in patients with mixed metabolic acidosis. Mixed high anion gap metabolic acidosis in patients with diabetic or alcoholic ketoacidosis may be combined with lactic acidosis consequent to circulatory failure. Uremic patients with associated lactic acidosis or ketoacidosis are another example of mixed high anion gap acidosis. Representative cases of mixed hyperchloremic metabolic acidosis are seen in patients with renal tubular acidosis or those being treated with carbonic anhydrase inhibitors who also suffer substantial fecal losses of HCO_3^- caused by severe diarrhea. Coexistence of hyperchloremic and high anion gap metabolic acidosis occurs

Fluid and Electrolyte Disorders

in patients with profuse diarrhea whose circulation becomes sufficiently compromised to generate, in turn, a high anion gap metabolic acidosis (as a result of renal failure or lactic acidosis). Patients with diabetic ketoacidosis, whose renal function is maintained at reasonable levels by adequate salt and water intake, might develop an element of hyperchloremic metabolic acidosis because of preferential excretion of ketone anions and conservation of Cl^- (Table 13.5, example 1)[23].

Mixed metabolic alkalosis

In a similar manner to mixed metabolic acidosis, the simultaneous presence of several processes that each contribute to a primary increment in plasma HCO_3^- (including diuretic therapy, vomiting, mineralocorticoid excess, or severe potassium depletion), will give rise to mixed metabolic alkalosis.

Triple disorders

The most frequent triple disorders comprise two cardinal metabolic disturbances in conjunction with either respiratory acidosis or respiratory alkalosis. A prime example of the former is illustrated by severely ill patients with COPD and CO_2 retention, who might develop simultaneously metabolic alkalosis (usually caused by diuretics and a Cl^--restricted diet) and metabolic acidosis (commonly lactic acidosis caused by hypoxemia, hypotension, or sepsis). This type of triple disorder also might be encountered during cardiopulmonary resuscitation, when an element of metabolic alkalosis caused by alkali administration is superimposed on pre-existing respiratory acidosis and metabolic (lactic) acidosis. Patients with respiratory alkalosis caused by advanced congestive heart failure also might have diuretic-induced metabolic alkalosis and lactic acidosis from tissue hypoperfusion. Such triple acid–base disorders can also be seen in patients with chronic alcoholism, who develop metabolic alkalosis from vomiting, lactic acidosis from volume depletion or ethanol intoxication, and respiratory alkalosis from hepatic encephalopathy or sepsis.

Less frequently, triple disorders encompassing two cardinal respiratory disturbances in combination with either metabolic acidosis or metabolic alkalosis are encountered. The typical presentation involves critically ill patients with chronic respiratory acidosis who experience an abrupt reduction in Pa_{CO_2} because of mechanical ventilation and superimposed metabolic acidosis (usually lactic acidosis, reflecting circulatory failure) or metabolic alkalosis (as a result of gastric fluid loss, diuretics, etc.). In the last circumstance, extreme alkalemia might ensue because of the concomitant presence of hypocapnia and hyperbicarbonatremia. Even more infrequently, this same clinical setting might give rise to a quadruple acid–base disorder in which all four cardinal acid–base disturbances coexist.

Clinical manifestations

As a general rule, the symptoms and signs of the underlying disease that gives rise to the observed mixed acid–base disorder dominate the clinical picture. Yet, the development of severe abnormalities in either Pa_{CO_2} (severe hypo- or hypercapnia) or systemic acidity (profound acidemia or alkalemia)

might be responsible for the superimposition of additional clinical manifestations. On the one hand, profound hypocapnia might induce obtundation, generalized seizures, and, occasionally, even coma or death as a result of a critical reduction in cerebral blood flow. Rarely angina pectoris also might occur. On the other hand, severe hypercapnia might generate a profound encephalopathy with the classic features ('pseudotumor cerebri') including headaches, obtundation, vomiting, and bilateral papilledema caused by increased intracranial pressure. Extreme acidemia results in depression of the central nervous system as well as the cardiovascular system. Reduction in myocardial contractility and peripheral vascular resistance triggered by acidemia might result in severe hypotension. Finally, profound alkalemia might elicit paresthesias, tetany, cardiac dysrhythmias, or generalized seizures.

Diagnosis

The basic principles underlying the diagnosis of mixed acid–base disorders are identical to those required for the identification of simple acid–base disturbances and include assessment of the accuracy of the acid–base data; obtaining a careful history and performance of a complete physical examination; consideration of the plasma anion gap and other ancillary laboratory data; and knowledge of the quantitative aspects of the adaptive response to each of the four simple acid–base disturbances. Adherence to these principles cannot be overemphasized. Indeed, even experienced clinicians risk misdiagnosing the prevailing acid–base status by bypassing this systematic approach.

Obtaining a careful history and performing a complete physical examination should precede any diagnostic pronouncement. The importance of this principle can be demonstrated by considering that normality of the acid–base parameters is not in itself sufficient to diagnose the presence of normal acid–base status; indeed, normal acid–base values might be the fortuitous end result of mixed acid–base disorders (e.g., high-anion-gap acidosis treated with alkali infusion, or diarrhea-induced metabolic acidosis in conjunction with vomiting-induced metabolic alkalosis). More broadly speaking, a given set of acid–base parameters is never diagnostic of a particular acid–base disorder, whether simple or mixed in nature, but rather is consistent with a range of acid–base abnormalities. What on the surface appears to be a clear-cut simple acid–base disorder might actually reflect the interplay of a number of coexisting acid–base disturbances. Information from the patient's history and findings from the physical examination frequently provide important insights into the prevailing acid–base status as well as useful clues to the differential diagnosis.

A critical component of the diagnostic process is the examination of the plasma anion gap (Table 13.6). This derived parameter provides important insights into the nature of the prevailing changes in plasma HCO_3^- concentration. Occasionally, an elevated plasma anion gap might offer the first readily available clue to the presence of disordered acid–base status despite the normalcy of the acid–base parameters themselves. In the presence of a plasma HCO_3^- deficit ($\Delta(HCO_3^-)_p$), a normal or subnormal value for the plasma anion gap denotes that the entire fall in HCO_3^- can be attributed to acidifying processes resulting in the loss of alkali (e.g., diarrhea,

Blood parameters in diagnosis of mixed metabolic acid–base disorders					
Blood composition	Normal	High anion gap acidosis	High anion gap and normal anion gap acidosis	Metabolic alkalosis	High anion gap acidosis and metabolic alkalosis
pH	7.40	7.29	7.10	7.50	7.38
$Paco_2$ (mmHg)	40	30	20	45	35
Bicarbonate (mmol/L)	24	14	6	34	20
Anion gap (mmol/L)	10	20	20	12	26
Δ Bicarbonate	0	–10	–18	+10	–4
Δ Anion gap	0	+10	+10	+2	+16

Table 13.6 Blood parameters in diagnosis of mixed metabolic acid–base disorders

renal tubular acidosis) or to respiratory alkalosis. By comparison, with a high anion gap metabolic acidosis, there is usually a close reciprocal stoichiometry between the fall in serum HCO_3^- and the rise in the anion gap, termed the Δ(anion gap). A reduction in serum HCO_3^- of 10 mmol/L is associated, therefore, with a Δ(anion gap) of 10 mmol/L. Addition of the value for the Δ(anion gap) to the prevailing level of serum HCO_3^- allows the derivation of the basal value of HCO_3^- existing prior to the development of the high anion gap metabolic acidosis. Appreciation of this reciprocal relation between the $\Delta(HCO_3^-)_p$ and the Δ(anion gap) is important in distinguishing between a pure high anion gap metabolic acidosis and a mixed high and normal anion gap metabolic acidosis, and in detecting a mixed

high anion gap metabolic acidosis and metabolic alkalosis. Additional diagnostic insights are often obtained by examination of other laboratory data, including the serum levels of K^+, glucose, urea nitrogen, and creatinine, semiquantitative measures for ketonemia or ketonuria, screening blood or urine for toxins, and estimation of the serum osmolar gap.

Mild acid–base disorders might pose particular diagnostic difficulty because of the considerable overlap of values for the simple disturbances near the range of normalcy. In such circumstances, any of several simple disorders or a variety of mixed disturbances might fully account for the acid–base data under evaluation. Again, careful correlation of all available clinical information should guide the diagnostic process.

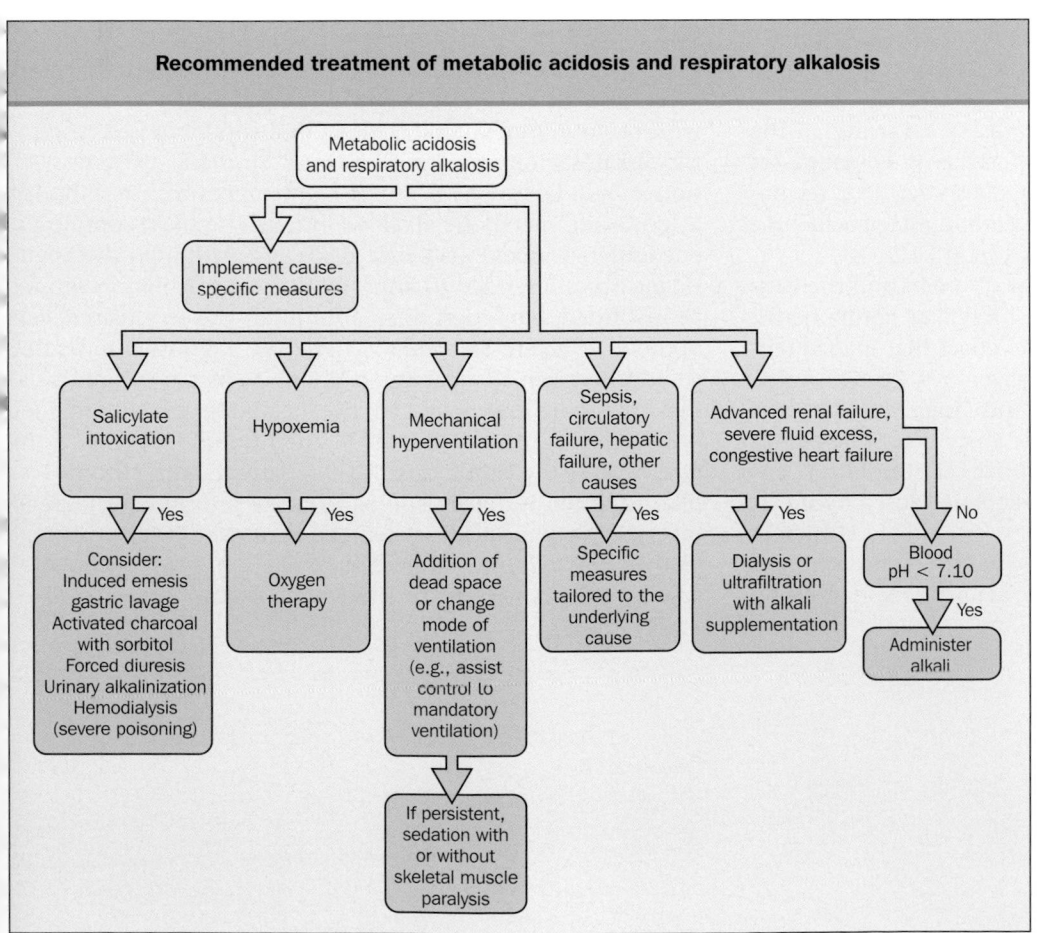

Figure 13.8 Recommended treatment of metabolic acidosis and respiratory alkalosis.

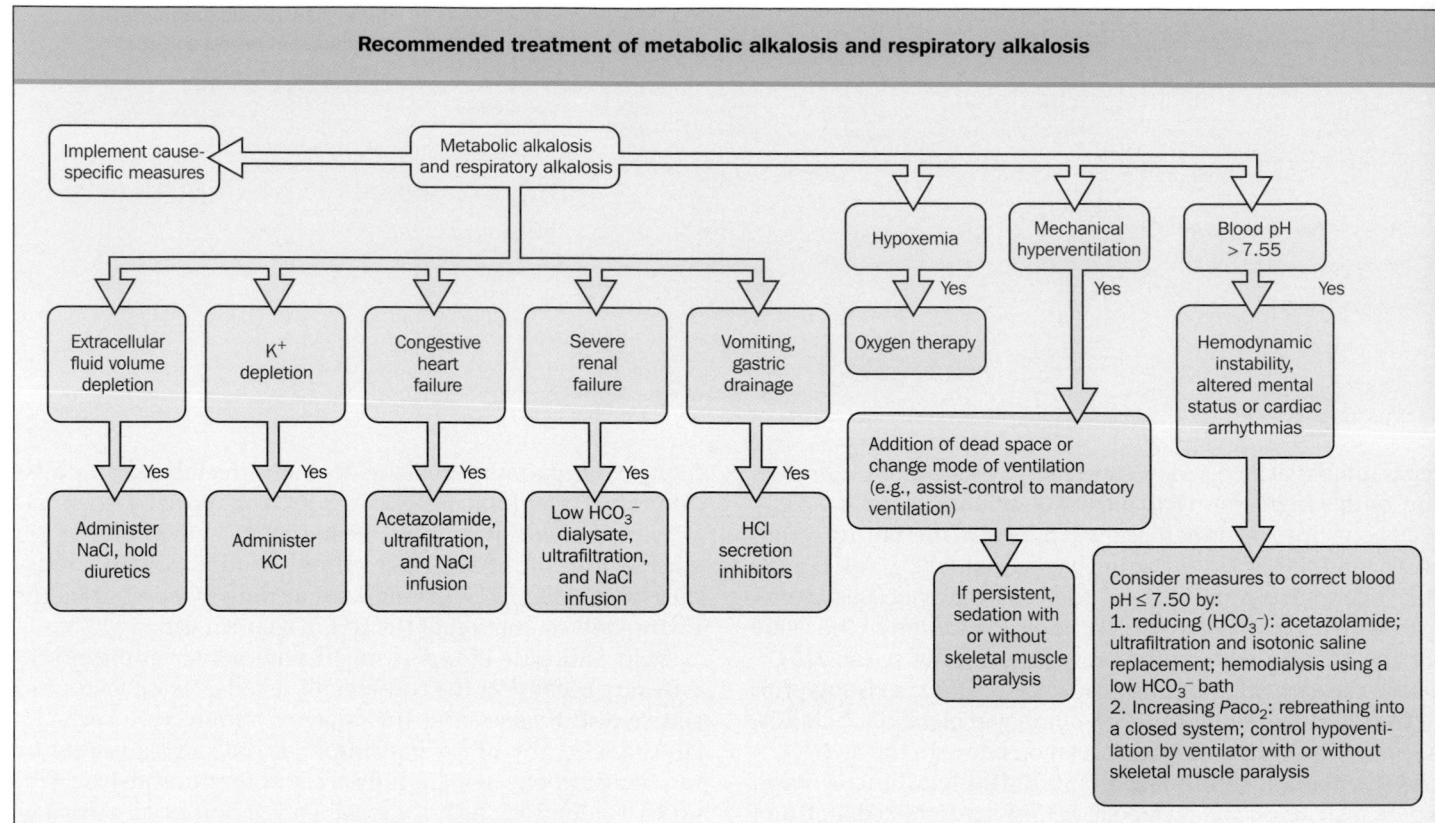

Figure 13.9 Recommended treatment of metabolic alkalosis and respiratory alkalosis.

Treatment

The management of mixed acid–base disturbances is aimed at restoring the altered acid–base status by reversing all the elemental components present[1,2,20,24]. Thus it encompasses the therapy of each simple acid–base disorder. Our recommendations for treatment of some common mixed acid–base disturbances are presented in Figures 13.7–13.10.

Given the nature of these different disorders and the variable response time to therapy of the individual components, it is crucial always to be aware of the effect that graded correction of a certain element might have on systemic acidity. The asynchronous reversal of the individual components might be used at times to therapeutic advantage, whereas on other occasions such practice might prove catastrophic. In this regard, patients featuring extreme acidemia caused by metabolic acidosis and respiratory acidosis, or extreme alkalemia caused by metabolic alkalosis and respiratory alkalosis, might derive prompt restitution of systemic acidity to safe levels by a rapid return of Pa_{CO_2} toward normal. By comparison, an asynchronous return of Pa_{CO_2} to normal values in a patient with profound metabolic acidosis and superimposed respiratory alkalosis might prove disastrous. Similarly, extreme caution should be exercised in treating patients with respiratory acidosis and metabolic alkalosis, one of the most commonly encountered mixed acid–base disorders. Although therapeutic measures intended to improve alveolar ventilation should be instituted, induction of an abrupt fall in Pa_{CO_2} risks development of severe alkalemia. Therefore, aggressive measures should be taken to treat the element of metabolic alkalosis, making certain that reversal of the metabolic component does not lag behind the treatment of the respiratory element. In fact, because the ventilatory drive in patients with chronic respiratory acidosis depends in part on the prevailing acidemia, reversal of a complicating element of metabolic alkalosis regularly results in improved alveolar ventilation, and consequently a fall in Pa_{CO_2} and a rise in Pa_{O_2} are realized.

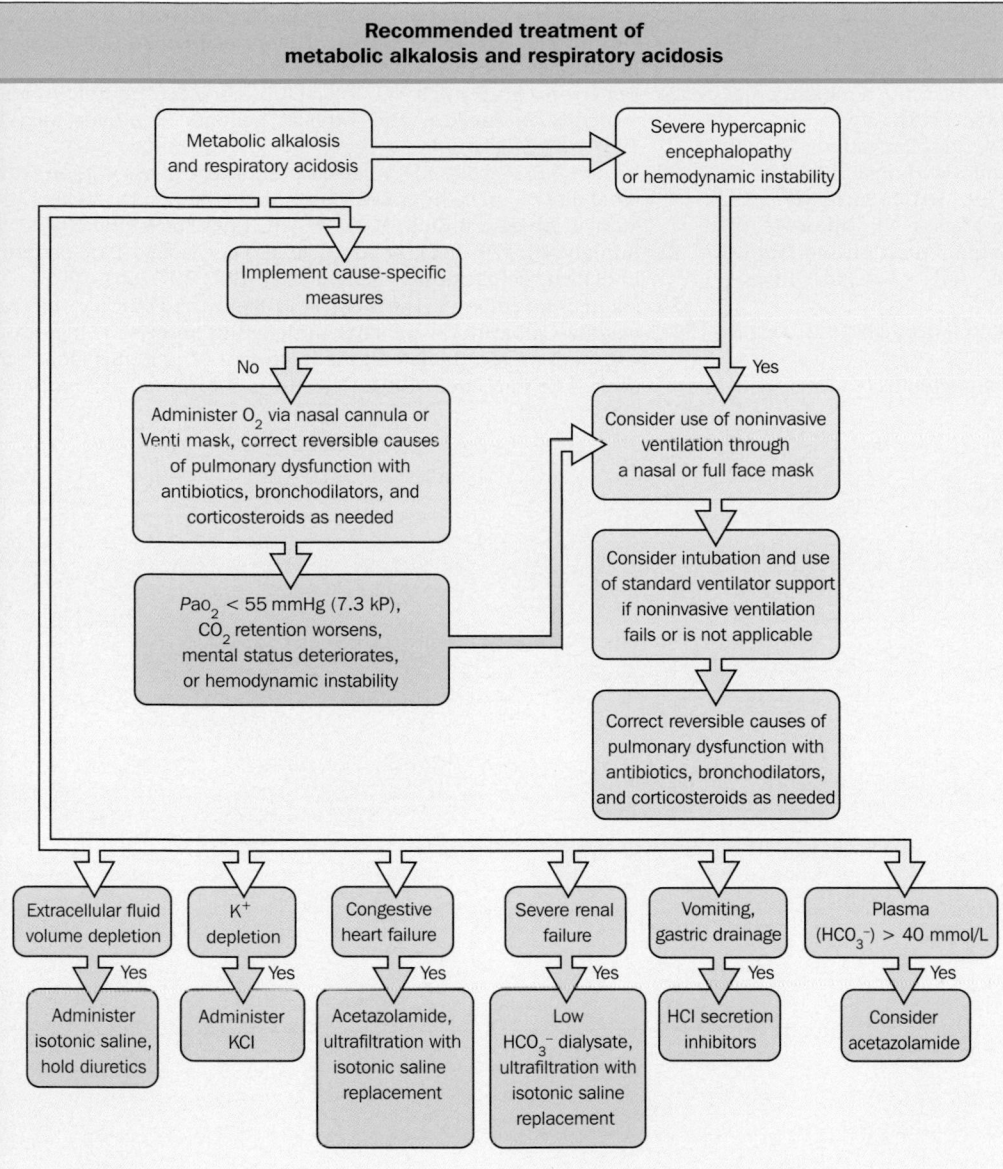

Figure 13.10 Recommended treatment of metabolic alkalosis and respiratory acidosis.

REFERENCES

1. Adrogué HJ, Madias NE. Management of life-threatening acid–base disorders (Part I). N Engl J Med. 1998;338:26–34.
2. Adrogué HJ, Madias NE. Management of life-threatening acid–base disorders (Part II). N Engl J Med. 1998;338:107–11.
3. Adrogué HJ, Wesson DE. Overview of acid–base disorders. In: Adrogué HJ, Wesson DE, eds. Blackwell's basics of medicine. Acid–base. Boston: Blackwell Science; 1994:49–133.
4. Epstein SK, Singh N. Respiratory acidosis. Respir Care. 2001;46:366–83.
5. Adrogué HJ, Rashad MN, Gorin AB, et al. Assessing acid–base status in circulatory failure. Differences between arterial and central venous blood. N Engl J Med. 1989;320:1312–16.
6. Adrogué HJ, Rashad MN, Gorin AB, et al. Arteriovenous acid–base disparity in circulatory failure: studies on mechanism. Am J Physiol. 1989;257:F1087–93.
7. Madias NE, Adrogué HJ. Acid–base disturbances in pulmonary medicine. In: Arieff AI, DeFronzo RA, eds. Fluid, electrolyte and acid–base disorders, 2nd edn. New York: Churchill Livingstone; 1995:223–53.

8. Madias NE, Adrogué HJ. Influence of chronic metabolic acid–base disorders on the acute CO_2 titration curve. J Appl Physiol. 1983;55:1187–95.
9. Adrogué HJ, Madias NE. Influence of chronic respiratory acid–base disorders on acute CO_2 titration curve. J Appl Physiol. 1985;58:1231–8.
10. Adrogué HJ, Madias NE. Arterial blood gas monitoring: acid–base assessment. In: Tobin MJ, ed. Principles and practice of intensive care monitoring. New York: McGraw-Hill; 1998:217–41.
11. Adrogué HJ, Tobin MJ. Management of respiratory failure. In: Adrogué HJ, Tobin MJ, eds. Blackwell's basics of medicine, Vol 6, Respiratory failure. Boston, MA: Blackwell Science; 1997:311–31.
12. Dick CR, Liu Z, Sassoon CS, Berry RB, Mahutte CK. O_2-induced change in ventilation and ventilatory drive of COPD. Am J Respir Crit Care Med. 1997;155:609–14.
13. Luft UC, Mostyn EM, Loeppky JA, Venters MD. Contribution of the Haldane effect on the rise of arterial P_{CO_2} in hypoxic patients breathing oxygen. Crit Care Med. 1981;9:32–7.

14. Tobin MJ. Mechanical ventilation. N Engl J Med. 1994;330: 1056–61.

15. Amato MBP, Barbas CSV, Medeiros DM, et al. Effect of a protective-ventilation strategy on mortality in the acute respiratory distress syndrome. N Engl J Med. 1998;338:347–54.

16. Cardenas VJ, Zwischenberger JB, Tao W, et al. Correction of blood pH attenuates changes in hemodynamics and organ blood flow during permissive hypercapnia. Crit Care Med. 1996;24:827–34.

17. Adrogué HJ, Brensilver J, Cohen JJ, Madias NE. Influence of steady-state alterations in acid–base equilibrium on the fate of administered bicarbonate in the dog. J Clin Invest. 1983;71:867–83.

18. Foster GT, Vaziri ND, Sassoon CSH. Respiratory alkalosis. Respir Care. 2001;46:384–91.

19. Hsia CCW. Respiratory function of hemoglobin. N J Engl Med. 1998;338:239–47.

20. Adrogué HJ, Madias NE. Mixed acid–base disorders. In: Jacobson HR, Striker GE, Klahr S, eds. The principles and practice of nephrology, 2nd edn. Philadephia: Decker; 1995:953–62.

21. Anderson LE, Henrich WL. Alkalemia-associated morbidity and mortality in medical and surgical patients. Southern Med J. 1987;80:729–33.

22. Madias NE, Perrone RD. Acid–base disorders in association with renal disease. In: Schrier SW, Gottschaid CW, eds. Diseases of the kidney, 5th edn. Boston: Little Brown; 1993:2669–99.

23. Adrogué HJ, Wilson H, Boyd AE, et al. Plasma acid–base patterns in diabetic ketoacidosis. N Engl J Med. 1982;307:1603–10.

24. Leung JM, Landow L, Franks M, et al. Safety and efficacy of intravenous Carbicarb in patients undergoing surgery: comparison with sodium bicarbonate in the treatment of mild metabolic acidosis. Crit Care Med. 1994;22:1540–9. [Erratum, Crit Care Med. 1995,23:420.]

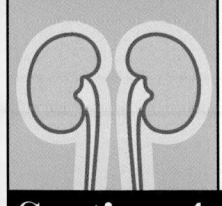

Chapter 14

Clinical Evaluation, Management, and Outcome of Acute Renal Failure

Niamh Kieran and Hugh R Brady

DEFINITIONS, INCIDENCE AND CLASSIFICATION

Acute renal failure (ARF) is a common clinical syndrome characterized by a rapid (over hours to weeks) decline in glomerular filtration rate (GFR), perturbation of extracellular fluid volume, electrolyte and acid–base homeostasis, and accumulation of nitrogenous waste products from protein catabolism, such as blood urea nitrogen (BUN) and creatinine[1–3].

ARF complicates approximately 5% of hospital admissions and up to 30% of admissions to intensive care units. ARF is usually asymptomatic and diagnosed when routine biochemical screening of hospitalized patients reveals a recent increase in BUN and serum creatinine levels. Oliguria (urine output < 400 mL/day) is a frequent (approximately 50%) but not invariable clinical feature. The kidney is remarkable among organs of the body in its ability to recover from almost complete loss of function, and most ARF is reversible. Nevertheless, ARF is associated with major in-hospital morbidity and mortality reflecting the serious and frequently lethal nature of the underlying illnesses and the high frequency of complications. It is important to appreciate that ARF can be prevented in many settings if predisposing conditions are recognized and promptly treated. A logical approach to the prevention, diagnosis and treatment of this important clinical syndrome is essential and requires an understanding of the causes and pathophysiologic mechanisms of ARF.

ARF may complicate a host of diseases that for purposes of diagnosis and management are conveniently divided into three categories: (1) prerenal ARF (also known as prerenal azotemia), a physiological response to renal hypoperfusion in which the integrity of renal parenchymal tissue is preserved; (2) intrinsic renal ARF (also known as renal azotemia) in which ARF is caused by diseases of renal parenchyma; and (3) postrenal ARF (also known as postrenal azotemia) due to acute obstruction of the urinary tract (see Chapter 15, Fig. 15.1). The percentage of cases attributed to prerenal and intrinsic renal ARF vary depending on the population studied and criteria (e.g., magnitude of increase in serum creatinine or BUN, oliguria) used to diagnose ARF. The majority of cases of ARF (> 85%) are due to either prerenal ARF or renal ARF secondary to acute tubular necrosis (ATN). More than 90% of intrinsic renal ARF in most series is caused by ischemia or nephrotoxins (often in combination) and is classically associated with ATN. Thus, the terms ischemic and nephrotoxic ATN are commonly used to denote ischemic or nephrotoxic ARF in clinical practice.

The diagnosis of ARF is usually based on serial analysis of BUN and serum creatinine. These are relatively insensitive indices of glomerular function, however, and several caveats must be entertained when extrapolating their levels to GFR. GFR may fall by approximately 50% before the serum creatinine levels rises outside the 'normal' range because the initial decline in creatinine filtration by glomeruli is matched by increased creatinine secretion by proximal tubule cells[1] (see Chapter 3, Fig. 3.2). Conversely, a relatively large increase in serum creatinine concentration may result from a relatively small decline in GFR in patients with pre-existing chronic renal insufficiency. GFR may fall without a marked elevation in creatinine or BUN level in patients with reduced muscle mass (such as the elderly) or reduced urea generation (e.g., malnutrition, liver disease), respectively. Furthermore, BUN or serum creatinine values may rise without an acute decline in GFR in patients with pre-existing chronic renal insufficiency and either enhanced urea or creatinine production, inhibition of proximal tubule creatinine secretion, or circulating substances that cross-react with creatinine in laboratory assays. Under the latter circumstances, BUN and serum creatinine values seldom rise above 30 mg/dL (serum urea 11 mmol/L) and 2.0 mg/dL (180 µmol/L) respectively, and simultaneous elevation of both parameters is rare. Despite these limitations, measurements of BUN and serum creatinine concentrations are likely to remain the principal method for diagnosis of ARF in the foreseeable future.

This chapter focuses on the clinical features, evaluation and management of prerenal ARF and ischemic ATN. The causes of intrinsic renal ARF and postrenal ARF are discussed further in Chapter 15 and other chapters in this book.

ETIOLOGY OF ACUTE RENAL FAILURE

Prerenal ARF

Prerenal ARF is the most common cause of ARF and represents an appropriate physiologic response to renal hypoperfusion of sufficient magnitude to impair glomerular filtration and the excretion of nitrogenous waste[1]. By definition, the integrity of renal parenchymal tissue is preserved and the reduction of GFR associated with prerenal failure is rapidly and completely reversed when the underlying cause of glomerular hypoperfusion is corrected. Renal blood flow, though reduced in prerenal failure, is sufficient to provide adequate oxygen and metabolic substrates to sustain the viability of renal tubular cells. However, if prerenal failure is not

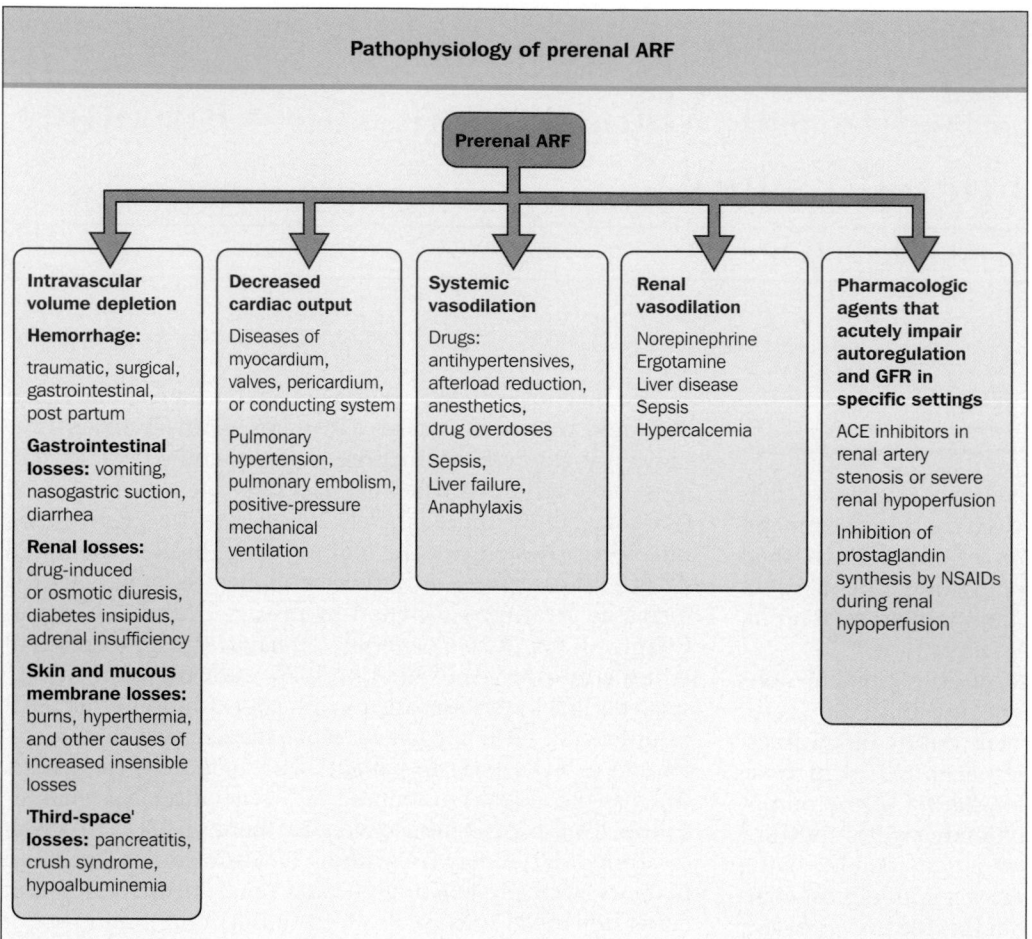

Figure 14.1 Major causes of prerenal ARF.

Pathophysiology of prerenal ARF

Prerenal ARF

Intravascular volume depletion

Hemorrhage:
traumatic, surgical, gastrointestinal, post partum

Gastrointestinal losses: vomiting, nasogastric suction, diarrhea

Renal losses: drug-induced or osmotic diuresis, diabetes insipidus, adrenal insufficiency

Skin and mucous membrane losses: burns, hyperthermia, and other causes of increased insensible losses

'Third-space' losses: pancreatitis, crush syndrome, hypoalbuminemia

Decreased cardiac output

Diseases of myocardium, valves, pericardium, or conducting system

Pulmonary hypertension, pulmonary embolism, positive-pressure mechanical ventilation

Systemic vasodilation

Drugs: antihypertensives, afterload reduction, anesthetics, drug overdoses

Sepsis, Liver failure, Anaphylaxis

Renal vasodilation

Norepinephrine
Ergotamine
Liver disease
Sepsis
Hypercalcemia

Pharmacologic agents that acutely impair autoregulation and GFR in specific settings

ACE inhibitors in renal artery stenosis or severe renal hypoperfusion

Inhibition of prostaglandin synthesis by NSAIDs during renal hypoperfusion

appropriately treated, it can lead to ischemic injury to renal tubular cells and to the development of ATN. Thus, prerenal ARF and ischemic ATN are part of a spectrum of manifestations of renal hypoperfusion. Indeed, clinical and biochemical features of prerenal ARF and ischemic ATN may coexist in some patients in a condition known sometimes as 'the intermediate syndrome'.

Prerenal ARF can complicate any disease characterized by hypovolemia, low cardiac output, systemic vasodilatation, or intrarenal vasoconstriction (Fig. 14.1). True hypovolemia and 'effective' circulatory volume depletion (e.g., in heart failure or septic shock) lead to a fall in mean systemic arterial pressure, which in turn activates arterial (e.g., carotid sinus) and cardiac baroreceptors and initiates a series of neural and humoral responses that include activation of the sympathetic nervous system and renin–angiotensin–aldosterone system and release of antidiuretic hormone (Fig. 14.2). Norepinephrine, angiotensin II and antidiuretic hormone act in concert in an attempt to maintain blood pressure and preserve cardiac and cerebral perfusion by stimulating vasoconstriction in relatively 'less important' vascular beds, such as the musculocutaneous and splanchnic circulations, by inhibiting salt loss through sweat glands, by stimulating thirst and salt appetite and by promoting renal salt and water retention. Glomerular perfusion, ultrafiltration pressure and filtration rate are preserved during mild hypoperfusion through several compensatory

mechanisms, including afferent arteriole vasodilatation triggered by a local myenteric reflex within the vessel wall, enhanced intrarenal biosynthesis of vasodilator prostaglandins (e.g., prostacyclin, prostaglandin E_2), kallikrein and kinins and possibly nitric oxide (NO) and preferential efferent arteriolar vasoconstriction induced by angiotensin II. As a result, intraglomerular pressure is preserved, the fraction of renal plasma that is filtered by glomeruli (filtration fraction) is increased, and GFR is maintained.

These compensatory renal responses are overwhelmed during states of moderate or severe hypoperfusion and ARF ensues. Autoregulatory dilatation of afferent arterioles is maximal at a mean systemic arterial blood pressure of approximately 80 mmHg and hypotension below this level causes a precipitous decline in glomerular ultrafiltration pressure and GFR. Lesser degrees of hypotension may provoke prerenal ARF in the elderly and in patients with diseases affecting the integrity of afferent arterioles (e.g., hypertensive nephrosclerosis, diabetic nephropathy). In addition, very high levels of angiotensin II, as found in patients with marked circulatory failure, stimulate constriction of both afferent and efferent arterioles, contrasting with the relatively selective effect of lower levels of this peptide on efferent arteriolar resistance.

Several classes of commonly prescribed drugs impair renal adaptive responses and can tip compensated renal

Figure 14.2 Pathophysiology of prerenal ARF.

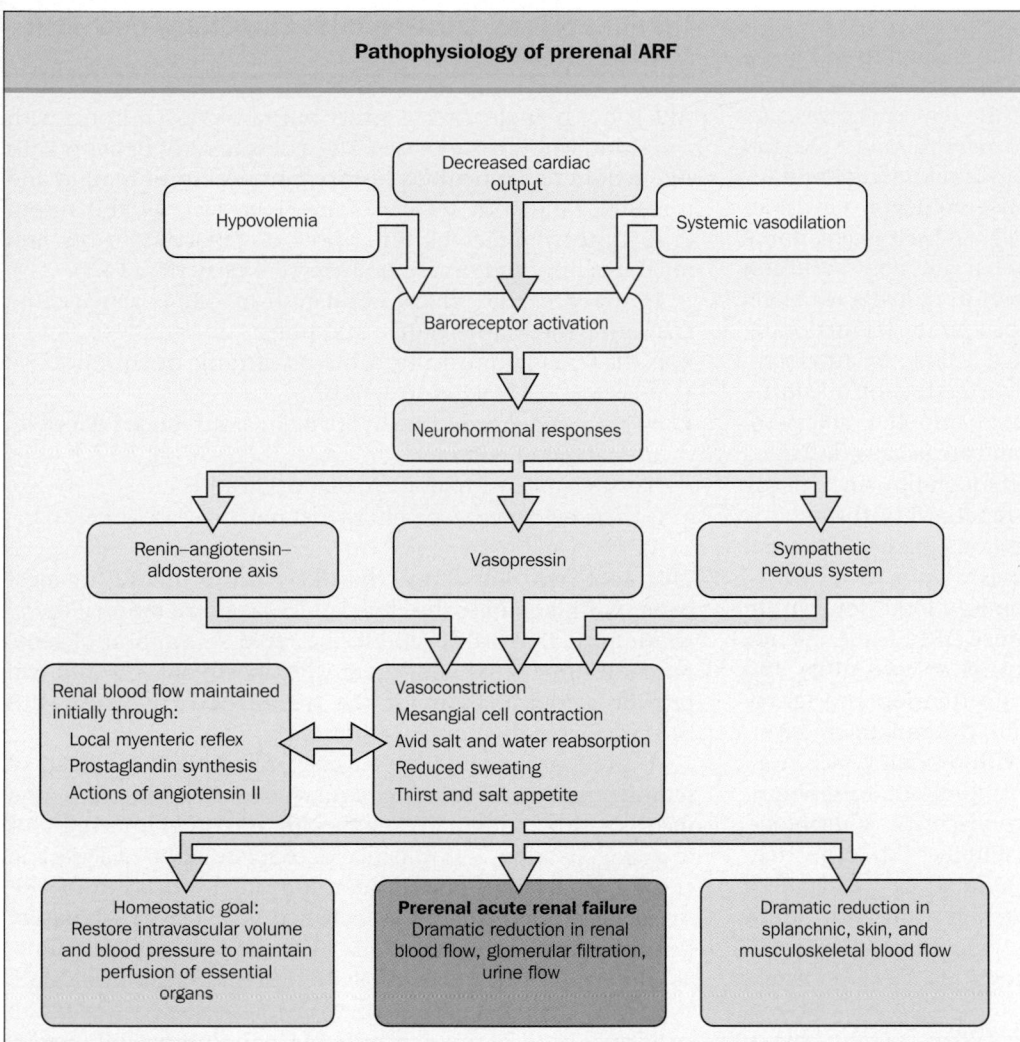

Pathophysiology of prerenal ARF

hypoperfusion into overt prerenal ARF, or indeed trigger progression of prerenal ARF to ischemic ATN. Nonsteroidal anti-inflammatory drugs (NSAIDs) inhibit renal prostaglandin biosynthesis. They do not compromise GFR in normal individuals but may precipitate prerenal ARF in subjects with true hypovolemia or decreased effective arterial blood volume, or in patients with chronic renal insufficiency in whom GFR is being maintained in part by prostaglandin-mediated hyperfiltration through a few remaining nephrons. Similarly, angiotensin converting enzyme (ACE) inhibitors and angiotensin II receptor antagonists (ATRA) may trigger prerenal ARF in individuals in whom intraglomerular pressure and GFR are dependent on angiotensin II. This complication is classically seen in patients with bilateral renal artery stenosis or with unilateral stenosis in a solitary functioning kidney. Here, angiotensin II preserves glomerular filtration pressure distal to renal arterial stenosis by increasing systemic arterial pressure and by triggering selective constriction of efferent arterioles. ACE inhibitors or ATRA blunt these compensatory responses and precipitate reversible ARF in approximately 30% of these patients, particularly in patients also taking diuretics. ACE inhibitors or ATRA, similar to NSAIDs, may also precipitate prerenal ARF in patients with compensated renal hypoperfusion of other etiologies and thus

serum creatinine should be closely monitored when these drugs are administered to high-risk individuals.

The classic urinary and biochemical sequelae of prerenal ARF can be predicted from the stimulatory actions of norepinephrine, angiotensin II and antidiuretic hormone on salt and water reabsorption and include concentrated urine (specific gravity > 1.018, osmolality > 500 mOsm/kg H_2O), low urinary Na^+ concentration (typically < 10 mmol/L) and 'benign' urine sediment containing transparent hyaline casts formed by precipitation of Tamm–Horsfall protein (normally secreted by the loop of Henle cells) in concentrated urine[1-3]. Some vasoactive mediators, drugs and diagnostic agents stimulate intense intrarenal vasoconstriction and induce glomerular hypoperfusion and ARF, with many of the functional, clinical and biochemical features of prerenal ARF. Examples include radiocontrast agents, cyclosporine, amphotericin B, hypercalcemia, endotoxin, epinephrine and norepinephrine (in therapeutic use or secreted by pheochromocytoma), ergotamine and high doses of dopamine. As many of these agents also induce injury to renal tubules, they are usually categorized as causes of acute intrinsic renal ARF and are discussed in subsequent sections. Definitive diagnosis of prerenal ARF hinges on rapid recovery of GFR after restoration of renal perfusion.

Intrinsic renal ARF

From a clinicopathologic viewpoint, it is helpful to categorize the causes of acute intrinsic renal ARF into (1) diseases involving large renal vessels; (2) diseases of the renal microvasculature and glomeruli; (3) ischemic and nephrotoxic ATN; and (4) other acute processes involving the tubulointerstitium.

Occlusion of large renal vessels, either arteries or veins, is an uncommon cause of ARF. To affect BUN and serum creatinine in patients with previously normal renal function, occlusion must be either bilateral or be unilateral in patients with pre-existing chronic renal insufficiency or a solitary functioning kidney. Renal arteries may be occluded acutely by atheroemboli, thromboemboli, thrombosis, dissection of an aortic aneurysm or, rarely, vasculitis. Atheroemboli (cholesterol emboli) are the most common cause and are usually dislodged from an atheromatous aorta during arteriography, angioplasty or aortic surgery. Thromboemboli, renal artery thrombosis complicating rupture of an atheromatous plaque and renal vein thrombosis are less frequent causes.

Virtually all diseases that compromise blood flow within the renal microvasculature may induce ARF. These include inflammatory (e.g., glomerulonephritis or vasculitis) and noninflammatory (e.g., malignant hypertension and scleroderma crisis) diseases of the vessel wall, thrombotic microangiopathies characterized by clotting within small vessels (e.g., hemolytic uremic syndrome (HUS), thrombotic thrombocytopenic purpura (TTP)) and hyperviscosity syndromes. Disorders of the tubulointerstitium that induce ARF, other than ischemia or tubule cell toxins, include allergic interstitial nephritis, severe infections, allograft rejection and, rarely, infiltrative disorders such as sarcoid, lymphoma or leukemia. A more comprehensive discussion of these diseases is presented in other chapters.

Ischemic ATN differs from prerenal ARF in that renal hypoperfusion has been severe enough to injure renal parenchymal cells, particularly tubule epithelium, and ARF does not resolve spontaneously upon restoration of renal blood flow. The pathogenesis of ATN is attributed to several inter-related pathologic processes that include enhanced vasomotor tone, with reduction in renal blood flow, renal tubular obstruction by ATN casts, backleak of glomerular filtrate through an ischemic epithelium and oxidant injury on reperfusion[1–4]. The causes and pathogenesis of ATN are described in Chapter 15.

Postrenal ARF

Urinary tract obstruction accounts for less than 5% of cases of ARF. Because one kidney has sufficient clearance capacity to excrete the nitrogenous waste products generated daily, ARF resulting from obstruction implies blockade of the urethra or bladder neck, bilateral ureteral obstruction, or unilateral ureteral obstruction in a patient with either one functioning kidney or pre-existing chronic renal insufficiency. It occurs in the absence of renal parenchymal disease and is potentially rapidly reversible when the cause of the urinary tract obstruction is treated. This syndrome is usually easily recognized by clinical assessment and ultrasonography of the urinary tract. If obstruction is allowed to persist untreated, irreversible renal parenchymal injury and chronic renal failure (CRF) can result. The pathophysiology and treatment of obstructive uropathy are discussed in Chapter 58.

DIFFERENTIAL DIAGNOSIS: ELUCIDATING THE CAUSE OF ARF

ARF is not a single disease entity but rather a syndrome with a multitude of diverse causes. The assessment of patients with ARF requires a meticulous history, physical examination and urinalysis, in-depth review of previous records and recent drug history, judicious utilization of laboratory tests and renal imaging, and occasionally renal biopsy (Fig. 14.3).

In practice, the clinical evaluation of ARF is achieved by answering the following five questions:
- Is the renal failure acute, acute-on-chronic or chronic?
- Is there renal tract obstruction?
- Is there evidence of true hypovolemia or reduced effective arterial blood volume?
- Has there been a major vascular occlusion?
- Is there evidence of parenchymal renal disease other than ATN?

This approach will reveal the likely cause of ARF in most patients. This enables the clinician to develop a rational therapeutic plan that will facilitate the rapid restoration of renal function in patients with prerenal or postrenal ARF and will provide a logical basis for the treatment of patients with intrinsic parenchymal renal disease[1–5].

A semilogarithmic plot, or even a simple flow sheet, of remote and recent serum creatinine values versus time and incorporating changes in drug therapy and other interventions (e.g., angiography) is invaluable for differentiation of acute and chronic renal failure and the identification of the cause of ARF. An acute process is easily established if review of laboratory records reveals a recent rise in BUN and serum creatinine. Spurious causes of increased BUN or serum creatinine values should be excluded. When previous measurements of serum creatinine or BUN are not available, the findings of anemia, hyperphosphatemia, hypocalcemia, neuropathy, band keratopathy on presentation, and radiologic evidence of renal osteodystrophy or small scarred kidneys are useful pointers to a chronic process. However, it should be noted that anemia, hyperphosphatemia, and hypocalcemia may also complicate ARF, if prolonged, and renal size can be normal or increased in a variety of chronic renal diseases (e.g., diabetic nephropathy, amyloid, polycystic kidney disease). A history of ingestion of a poison or nephrotoxic drug is also an essential component of a thorough history in a patient with ARF. In addition to nephrotoxic medications prescribed by the physician, the availability of nonprescription medications that are potentially nephrotoxic (such as NSAIDs and acetaminophen (paracetamol)) must also be considered.

Once a diagnosis of ARF is established, attention should focus on the differentiation between prerenal, intrinsic renal and postrenal ARF, and the identification of the specific causative disease.

Table 14.1 summarizes some clinical features, urinary findings and confirmatory tests that are useful for diagnosis of the most common causes of ARF.

Clinical evaluation
Prerenal ARF

Prerenal ARF should be suspected when serum creatinine rises after periods of volume depletion, including after hemorrhage;

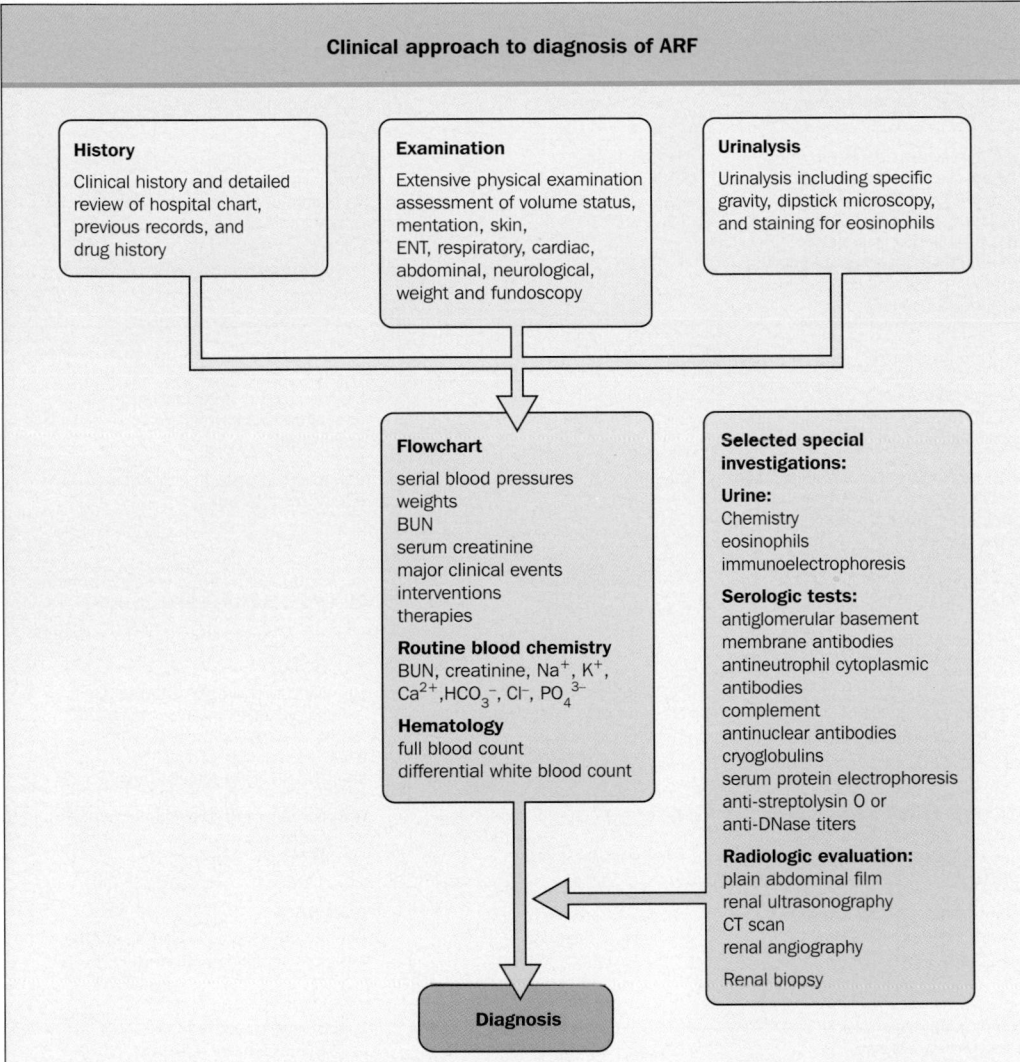

Figure 14.3 Clinical approach to the diagnosis of ARF. (Adapted with permission[1].)

excessive gastrointestinal, urinary, or insensible fluid losses; or extensive burns, particularly if access to fluids is restricted (e.g., comatose, sedated or obtunded patients). Supportive findings on clinical assessment include symptoms of thirst or postural dizziness and evidence of orthostatic hypotension (postural fall in diastolic pressure > 10 mmHg) and tachycardia (postural increase of more than 10 beats/min), reduced jugular venous pressure, decreased skin turgor and dry mucous membranes (Table 14.2). However, florid symptoms or signs of hypovolemia are usually not manifest until extracellular fluid volume has fallen by 10–20%. Nursing and pharmacy records should be reviewed for evidence of a progressive fall in urine output and body weight and for recent use of NSAIDs, ACE inhibitors or ATRA. Clinical examination may reveal stigmata of chronic liver disease and portal hypertension, cardiac failure or other causes of reduced effective arterial blood volume. Although clinical assessment provides a satisfactory index of cardiac output and tissue perfusion in most patients, invasive hemodynamic monitoring (central venous and/or Swan–Ganz catheterization) is often necessary in complicated cases. Definitive diagnosis of prerenal ARF rests on prompt resolution of ARF after restoration of renal perfusion.

Intrinsic renal ARF

There is a high likelihood of ischemic ATN if ARF follows a period of moderate or severe renal hypoperfusion and persists despite restoration of systemic blood pressure and tissue reperfusion. However, it should be noted that significant hypotension is recorded in the case notes of less than 50% of patients with postsurgical ATN. Diagnosis of nephrotoxic ATN requires examination of clinical, pharmacy, nursing and radiology records for a history of chronic renal failure (risk factor for ARF), recent periods of volume depletion, administration of nephrotoxic medications or radiocontrast agents.

Although most ARF is either prerenal, or due to ischemic and nephrotoxic ATN, patients should be assessed carefully for evidence of other renal parenchymal diseases because many of the latter are treatable and their diagnosis alters management and prognosis. Flank pain may be a prominent symptom of acute renal artery or vein occlusion, acute pyelonephritis and, occasionally, necrotizing glomerulonephritis. Skin examination may reveal the livido reticularis, subcutaneous nodules, digital ischemia and/or palpable purpura of atheroembolism or vasculitis, the butterfly rash of systemic lupus, impetigo in patients with postinfectious glomerulonephritis, a maculopapular rash suggestive of allergic interstitial nephritis, tell

Acute Renal Failure

Evaluation for the cause of ARF			
Cause of acute renal failure	Some suggestive clinical features	Typical urinalysis*	Some confirmatory tests
Prerenal ARF	Evidence of true volume depletion (thirst, postural or absolute hypotension and tachycardia, low jugular vein pressure, dry mucous membranes and axillae, weight loss, fluid output > input) or decreased effective circulatory volume (e.g., heart failure, liver failure), treatment with NSAIDs or ACE inhibitor	Hyaline casts FE_{Na} < 1% U_{Na} < 10 mmol/L SG > 1.018	Occasionally requires invasive hemodynamic monitoring; rapid resolution of ARF on restoration of renal perfusion
Intrinsic renal ARF *Diseases involving large renal vessels*			
Renal artery thrombosis	History of atrial fibrillation or recent myocardial infarct, nausea, vomiting, flank or abdominal pain	Mild proteinuria Occasionally red blood cells	Elevated lactate dehydrogenase with normal transaminases, renal arteriogram
Atheroembolism	Age usually > 50 years recent manipulation of aorta, retinal plaques, subcutaneous nodules, palpable purpura, livedo reticularis, vasculopathy, hypertension	Often normal, eosinophiluria, rarely casts	Eosinophilia, hypocomplementemia, skin biopsy, renal biopsy
Renal vein thrombosis	Evidence of nephrotic syndrome or pulmonary embolism, flank pain	Proteinuria, hematuria	Inferior venacavogram and selective renal venogram; Doppler flow studies; MRI
Diseases of small vessels and glomeruli			
Glomerulonephritis or vasculitis	Compatible clinical history (e.g., recent infection) sinusitis, lung hemorrhage, rash or skin ulcers, arthralgias, hypertension, edema	Red blood cell or granular casts, red blood cells, white blood cells, mild proteinuria	Low C3, antineutrophil cytoplasmic antibodies, antiglomerular basement membrane antibodies, antinuclear antibodies, antistreptolysin O, anti-DNase, cryoglobulins, renal biopsy
HUS or TTP	Compatible clinical history (e.g., recent gastrointestinal infection, cyclosporine, fever, pallor, ecchymoses, neurologic abnormalities	May be normal, red blood cells, mild proteinuria, rarely red blood cell or granular casts	Anemia, thrombocytopenia, schistocytes on blood smear, increased lactate dehydrogenase, renal biopsy
Malignant hypertension	Severe hypertension with headaches, cardiac failure, retinopathy, neurologic dysfunction, papilledema	Red blood cells, red blood cell casts, proteinuria	LVH by echocardiography or electrocardiography, resolution of ARF with control of blood pressure
ARF mediated by ischemia or toxins (ATN)			
Ischemia	Recent hemorrhage, hypotension (e.g., cardiac arrest), surgery	Muddy brown granular or tubule epithelial cell casts, FE_{Na} > 1%, U_{Na} > 20 mmol/L, SG = 1.010	Clinical assessment and urinalysis usually sufficient for diagnosis
Exogenous toxins	Recent radiocontrast study, nephrotoxic antibiotics or anticancer agents often coexistent with volume depletion, sepsis, or chronic renal insufficiency	Muddy brown granular or tubular epithelial cell casts, FE_{Na} > 1%, U_{Na} > 20 mmol/L, SG = 1.010	Clinical assessment and urinalysis usually sufficient for diagnosis
Endogenous toxins	History suggestive of rhabdomyolysis (seizures, coma, ethanol abuse, trauma)	Urine supernatant tests positive for heme	Hyperkalemia, hyperphosphatemia, hypocalcemia, increased circulating myoglobin, creatine kinase MM, uric acid
	History suggestive of hemolysis (blood transfusion)	Urine supernatant pink and positive for heme	Hyperkalemia, hyperphosphatemia, hypocalcemia, hyperuricemia, pink plasma positive for hemoglobin
	History suggestive of tumor lysis (recent chemotherapy), myeloma (bone pain), or ethylene glycol ingestion	Uric acid crystals, dipstick-negative proteinuria, oxalate crystals, respectively	Hyperuricemia, hyperkalemia, hyperphosphatemia (for tumor lysis); circulating or urinary monoclonal band (for myeloma); toxicology screen, acidosis, osmolal gap (for ethylene glycol)
Acute diseases of the tubulointerstitium			
Allergic interstitial nephritis	Recent ingestion of drug and fever, rash, or arthralgias	White blood cell casts, white blood cells (frequently eosinophiluria), red blood cells, rarely red blood cell casts, proteinuria (occasionally nephrotic)	Systemic eosinophilia, skin biopsy of rash area (leukocytoclastic vasculitis), renal biopsy
Acute bilateral pyelonephritis	Flank pain and tenderness, toxic state, febrile	Leukocytes, proteinuria, red blood cells, bacteria	Urine and blood cultures
Postrenal ARF	Abdominal or flank pain, palpable bladder	Frequently normal, hematuria if stones, hemorrhage, malignancy or prostatic hypertrophy	Plain film, renal ultrasonography, retrograde or anterograde pyelography, computed tomography

Clinical features, typical urinalysis and confirmatory tests for diagnosis of common causes of ARF. U_{NA}, Urine Na^+ concentration; SG, specific gravity. (Adapted with permission[1].)

Table 14.1 Evaluation for the cause of ARF.

Table 14.2 Clinical evaluation of volume status.

Clinical evaluation of volume status		
	Intravascular volume depletion	Volume overload/congestive heart failure
History and chart review	Thirst, dry mucosae, oliguria	Ankle swelling, weight gain
	Excessive fluid losses	Orthopnea, paroxysmal nocturnal dyspnea
	Fluid balance (intake/output, daily weights)	
Physical examination	Reduced skin turgor	Pitting edema
	Dry mucosae, absent axillary sweat	Jugular venous distension
	Reduced jugular venous pressure	Third heart sound
	Postural tachycardia or hypotension[a]	Pulmonary crackles
	Supine tachycardia or hypotension	Pleural effusion

[a]A rise in pulse rate of > 10 per min and/or a fall in systolic blood pressure of > 20 mmHg after standing for 1 min.

tale puncture marks of intravenous drug abuse, or the scarlatiniform eruption of staphylococcal toxic shock syndrome. The eyes should be assessed for hypertensive or diabetic retinopathy suggesting prior chronic renal failure; the bright orange retinal arteriolar stigmata of atheroembolism; the keratitis, scleritis, uveitis and iritis of autoimmune vasculitides; icterus; and the rare but nevertheless pathognomonic band keratopathy of hypercalcemia and flecked retina of hyperoxalemia. Examination of the ears, nose and throat may reveal conductive deafness and mucosal inflammation or ulceration suggestive of Wegener's granulomatosis or the neural deafness caused by aminoglycoside toxicity. Cardiovascular assessment may be notable for marked elevation in systemic blood pressure and suggest malignant hypertension or scleroderma, or it may reveal a new arrhythmia or murmur that is a potential source of thromboemboli or infective endocarditis (which may be associated with acute glomerulonephritis), respectively. Chest or abdominal pain and reduced pulses in the lower limbs should suggest aortic dissection or rarely Takayasu's arteritis, and widespread atheromatous disease increases the likelihood of atheroembolic disease. Pallor and recent bruising are important clues to the thrombotic microangiopathies, and the combination of bleeding and fever should raise the possibility of ARF in association with viral hemorrhagic fevers. A recent jejunoileal bypass may be a vital clue to acquired oxalosis a rare, but reversible cause of ARF in obese patients.

Postrenal ARF

Postrenal ARF may be asymptomatic if obstruction develops relatively slowly. More typically however, patients may present with suprapubic or flank pain if there is acute distention of the bladder or renal collecting system and capsule, respectively. Colicky flank pain radiating to the groin suggests acute ureteral obstruction. Prostatic disease should be suspected in patients with a history of nocturia, frequency and hesitancy and an enlarged or indurated prostate gland on rectal examination. Similarly, a rectal and/or pelvic examination may reveal obstructing tumors in female patients. Neurogenic bladder is a likely diagnosis in patients receiving anticholinergic medications (e.g., tricyclic antidepressants) or with physical evidence of neurologic disease and autonomic insufficiency (e.g., paralysis, abnormal rectal sphincter tone, postvoid urine volume more than 200–300 mL). Bladder distention may be evident on abdominal percussion and palpation in patients with bladder neck or urethral obstruction. Definitive diagnosis of postrenal ARF usually relies on judicious use of radiologic investigations, especially ultrasound, and rapid improvement in renal function after relief of obstruction.

Urinalysis
Urine volume
Urine volume is a relatively unhelpful parameter in differential diagnosis. Anuria suggests complete urinary tract obstruction but may be a complication of severe prerenal or intrinsic renal ARF (e.g., renal artery occlusion, severe proliferative glomerulonephritis or vasculitis, bilateral cortical necrosis due to severe ischemia). Wide fluctuations in urine output suggest intermittent obstruction. Patients with partial urinary tract obstruction may present with polyuria caused by secondary impairment of urine concentrating mechanisms.

Urine sediment
Analysis of the sediment and supernatant of a centrifuged urine specimen is valuable for distinguishing between prerenal, intrinsic renal and postrenal ARF and elucidating the precise etiology of intrinsic renal ARF (Table 14.3). Urine sediment should be inspected for the presence of cells, casts and crystals. The sediment is typically acellular in prerenal ARF and may only contain transparent hyaline casts (usually called a 'bland', 'benign', or 'inactive' urine sediment). Hyaline casts are formed in concentrated urine from normal constituents of urine, principally Tamm–Horsfall protein secreted by epithelial cells of the loop of Henle. Postrenal ARF may also present with a benign sediment, although hematuria and pyuria are common in patients with intraluminal obstruction (e.g., stones, sloughed papilla, blood clot) or prostatic disease. Pigmented 'muddy brown' granular casts and tubule epithelial cell casts are characteristic of ischemic or nephrotoxic ATN (Fig. 14.4). They are usually found in association with microscopic hematuria and mild 'tubular' proteinuria (< 1 g/day). Casts may be absent, however, in approximately 20–30% of patients with ischemic or nephrotoxic ATN. Red cell casts almost always indicate acute glomerular injury but may also be observed in acute interstitial nephritis. Dysmorphic red cells are a more common urinary finding in patients with glomerular injury but are a less specific finding than red cell casts. Urine sediment abnormalities vary in diseases involving preglomerular blood vessels, such as thrombotic

Urine sediment findings in ARF

Normal or few red blood cells or white blood cells

Prerenal acute renal failure

Arterial thrombosis or embolism

Preglomerular vasculitis

Hemolytic urea syndrome or thrombotic thrombocytopenic purpura

Scleroderma crisis

Postrenal acute renal failure

Granular casts

Acute tubular necrosis (muddy brown casts)

Glomerulonephritis or vasculitis

Interstitial nephritis

Red blood cell casts

Glomerulonephritis or vasculitis

Malignant hypertension

Rarely interstitial nephritis

White blood cell casts

Acute interstitial nephritis or glomerulonephritis (red cell casts much more common in the latter)

Severe pyelonephritis

Allograft rejection

Marked leukemic or lymphomatous infiltration

Eosinophiluria (>5%)

Allergic interstitial nephritis (antibiotics > NSAIDs)

Atheroembolic disease

Crystalluria

Acute uric acid nephropathy

Calcium oxalate (ethylene glycol toxicity)

Acyclovir

Examination of the urine sediment as a useful aid in the differential diagnosis of acute renal failure.

Table 14.3 Urine sediment findings in ARF.

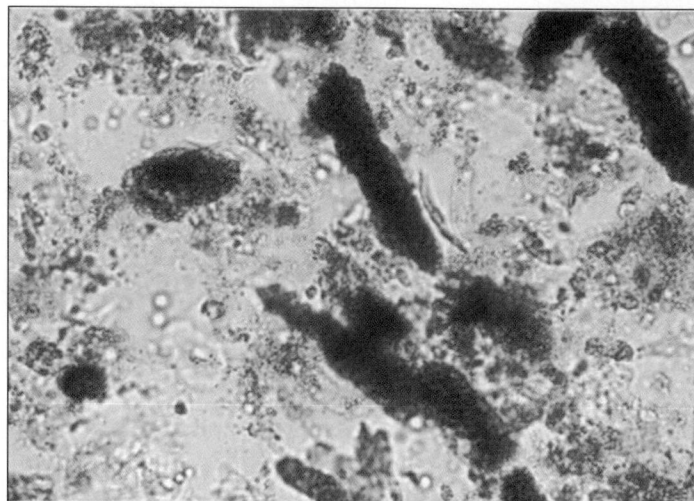

Figure 14.4 Muddy brown casts in acute tubular necrosis. Urine microscopy showing the typical muddy brown casts of ATN. (Courtesy of Dr Michael Ryan.)

microangiopathy, atheroembolic disease and vasculitis involving medium-sized or large vessels, and range from normal (benign) to frankly nephritic. White cell casts and nonpigmented granular casts suggest interstitial nephritis, and broad granular casts are characteristic of chronic renal disease and probably reflect interstitial fibrosis and dilatation of tubules (see Chapter 4, Fig. 4.3). Plasma cells are occasionally found in multiple myeloma. Eosinophiluria (between 1% and 50% of urine leukocytes) is a common finding (approximately 90%) in drug-induced allergic interstitial nephritis. Hansel's stain is significantly more sensitive than the traditional Wright's stain in this regard. However, eosinophiluria is only 85% specific for allergic interstitial nephritis, and eosinophiluria of 1–5% can occur in a variety of other diseases including atheroembolization, ischemic and nephrotoxic ARF, proliferative glomerulonephritis, pyelonephritis, cystitis, and prostatitis. Uric acid crystals (pleomorphic) may be seen in urine in prerenal ARF but should raise the possibility of acute uric acid nephropathy if seen in abundance. Oxalate (envelope shaped) and hippurate (needle shaped) crystals suggest a diagnosis of ethylene glycol toxicity (see Chapter 4, Fig. 4.4).

Proteinuria characteristically less than 1 g/day, is a common finding in ischemic or nephrotoxic ARF and reflects both failure of injured proximal tubule cells to reabsorb normally filtered protein and excretion of cellular debris (tubular proteinuria). Proteinuria greater than 1 g/day suggests injury to the glomerular ultrafiltration barrier (glomerular proteinuria) or excretion of myeloma light chains. The latter are not detected by conventional dipsticks (which detect albumin) and must be sought by other means (e.g., immunoelectrophoresis, or sulfosalicylic acid test). Heavy proteinuria is also a frequent finding (approximately 80%) in patients with allergic interstitial nephritis triggered by NSAIDs. These patients have a glomerular lesion that is almost identical to minimal change disease in addition to acute interstitial inflammation. A similar syndrome has been reported in patients receiving other agents such as ampicillin, rifampin and interferon-α. Hemoglobinuria or myoglobinuria should be suspected if urine is strongly positive for hemoglobin by dipstick but contains few red blood cells and if the supernatant of centrifuged urine is pink and also positive for free hemoglobin. Hemolysis and rhabdomyolysis can usually be differentiated by inspection of plasma. The latter is usually pink in hemolysis, but not in rhabdomyolysis, as free hemoglobin (65 000 Da) is a larger molecule than myoglobin (17 000 Da), which is heavily protein bound and filtered slowly by the kidney. Bilirubinuria may provide a clue to the presence of hepatorenal syndrome. The techniques of urine microscopy and the casts and crystals that can be seen in ARF are illustrated further in Chapter 4.

Urine chemistry in differential diagnosis of ARF		
Urine chemistry	Prerenal acute renal failure[a]	Ischemic Intrinsic acute renal failure[b]
Urine osmolality, U_{osm} (mOsm/kg H_2O)	>500	<250
Urine to plasma osmolality	>1.5	<1.1
Urine specific gravity	>1.018	<1.012
Plasma BUN : creatinine ratio	>20	<10–15
Urinary urea nitrogen : plasma urea nitrogen ratio	>8	<3
Urinary creatinine : plasma creatinine ratio	>40	<20
Urinary Na^+ concentration (mmol/L)	<10	>20
Fractional excretion of Na^+ (%)[c]*	<1	>2
Renal failure index[d]* $U_{Na}/U_{cr}/P_{cr}$	<1	>1
Urine sediment	Hyaline casts	Muddy brown granular casts

[a]Parameters suggesting prerenal failure are sometimes seen with nonoliguric acute tubular necrosis (ATN), acute glomerulonephritis and early obstruction.
[b]Parameters suggesting ATN may be misleading in prerenal failure in the elderly, in those with pre-exsisting renal impairment and following iuretic administration.
[c](Urine Na^+/plasma Na^+)/(urine creatinine/plasma creatinine) × 100.
[d]Urine Na^+/(urine creatinine/plasma creatinine) × 100.
[e]Most sensitive indices.

Table 14.4 Urine chemistry in differential diagnosis of ARF.

Urine chemistry

Analysis of urine and blood biochemistry is useful for discriminating between the major categories of ARF (Table 14.4). Urine chemistry has a role early in the evaluation of the oliguric patient, but only rarely will repeat estimations give further information. The fractional excretion of sodium (FE_{Na}) is the most sensitive index. FE_{Na} relates sodium (Na^+) clearance to creatinine clearance. Na^+ is reabsorbed avidly from glomerular filtrate in patients with prerenal ARF but inhibited in ATN as a result of tubule cell injury. Creatinine is reabsorbed to a much smaller extent than Na^+ in both conditions. The renal failure index (Table 14.4) provides comparable information, because clinical variations in serum Na^+ concentration are relatively small. Urinary Na^+ concentration is a less sensitive index for distinguishing prerenal ARF from ATN. Similarly, indices of urinary concentrating ability, such as urine specific gravity, urine osmolality, urine:plasma creatinine or urea ratios, and serum BUN:creatinine ratio, are of limited value in differential diagnosis. This is particularly true for elderly subjects, in whom urine concentrating mechanisms are frequently impaired while mechanisms for Na^+ reabsorption are preserved.

The urine in prerenal ARF will usually reflect the appropriate renal response to reduction in effective extracellular fluid volume, with avid sodium retention: urine sodium of approximately 10 mmol/L and fractional excretion of approximately 1%. The urine will also be markedly concentrated: urine osmolality of approximately 500 mosmol/kg and urine : plasma osmolality ratio 1.5 : 1. The finding of urine chemistry consistent with prerenal ARF is extremely useful and allows a further fluid challenge to be undertaken with a good chance of response. However, it must be appreciated that indices no different from those of prerenal ARF are also seen in early obstruction, in acute glomerulonephritis, in hepatorenal syndrome, following radiocontrast administration, occasionally in non-oliguric ATN and, rarely, early in rhabdomyolysis. Both FE_{Na} and the renal failure index have 90% specificity and sensitivity for the differentiation of ATN from prerenal ARF.

Typical indices of urine chemistry consistent with ATN must also be interpreted with caution. They may be found in prerenal ARF in the patient with pre-existing renal insufficiency and in many elderly patients, who will have impaired urine-concentrating ability. Furthermore, previous diuretic administration, acute or chronic, may promote a dilute urine with relatively high sodium content even if oliguria persists. Unfortunately, many patients with oliguria will already have been given a diuretic before the nephrologist has the opportunity to make an evaluation.

Approximately 15% of patients with nonoliguric ischemic or nephrotoxic ARF have $FE_{Na} < 1\%$, which probably reflects the 'intermediate' syndrome, a milder renal injury which has been described in ATN of a variety of causes, including ischemia, aminoglycosides, radiocontrast agents, rhabdomyolysis, hemolysis, burns, sepsis and hepatorenal syndrome. Under these circumstances, epithelial cell damage is probably localized to the corticomedullary junction and outer medulla with relative preservation of function in other Na^+ transporting segments. The apparent increase in incidence of the intermediate syndrome may reflect increasing attention by physicians to volume status and drug therapy in high-risk patients. FE_{Na} is usually less than 1% in ARF caused by urinary tract obstruction, glomerulonephritis and diseases of the renal vasculature, and other parameters must be employed to distinguish these conditions from prerenal ARF.

Serum creatinine

The pattern of change in serum creatinine often provides clues to the cause of ARF. Prerenal ARF is typified by rapid fluctuations in creatinine that parallel changes in hemodynamic function and renal perfusion. The serum creatinine level begins to rise within 24–48 h in patients with ARF after renal ischemia, radiocontrast and atheroembolization, three major diagnostic possibilities in patients undergoing emergency cardiac or aortic angiography and surgery. Serum creatinine usually peaks after 3–5 days in contrast nephropathy and returns to the normal range within 5–7 days. In contrast, creatinine levels typically peak later (7–10 days) in ischemic ATN and atheroembolic disease. ARF usually resolves in the next 7–14 days in ischemic ATN, whereas ARF is frequently irreversible in atheroembolic disease. These rapid changes are in marked contrast to the delayed elevation in serum creatinine levels (7–10 days) that is characteristic of many tubular epithelial cell toxins (e.g., aminoglycosides, cisplatin).

Other laboratory findings

Hyperkalemia, moderate hyperuricemia, hypocalcemia and hyperphosphatemia are all common in ARF of any cause. Only if urate is markedly elevated (> 15 mg/dL (900 μmol/L)) should acute uric acid nephropathy be considered. Hyperkalemia disproportionate to the severity of ARF (assuming that potassium-retaining medications have been withdrawn) is a feature of obstructive renal failure, is caused by type IV distal renal tubular acidosis, or it may indicate a hypercatabolic state. Hyperkalemia, hyperphosphatemia, hypocalcemia and elevated serum uric acid and creatine kinase (CK_3 isoenzyme) levels suggest a diagnosis of rhabdomyolysis. A similar biochemical profile occurs in ARF after cancer chemotherapy, but with higher levels of uric acid and normal or marginally elevated creatine kinase, and is typical of acute uric acid nephropathy and tumor lysis syndrome. Severe hypercalcemia of any cause can induce ARF. Widening of the serum anion gap ($Na^+ - (HCO_3^- + Cl^-)$) and osmolal gap (measured minus calculated serum osmolality) are clues to ethylene glycol toxicity.

Severe anemia in ARF in the absence of any source of blood loss raises the possibility of hemolysis, multiple myeloma or thrombotic microangiopathy. Other laboratory findings suggestive of thrombotic microangiopathy include thrombocytopenia, schistocytes and dysmorphic red blood cells on a peripheral blood smear, and elevated circulating levels of lactate dehydrogenase. The possibility of retroperitoneal hemorrhage (which can rarely cause urinary tract obstruction) should also be considered in severely anemic patients with ARF. This can be diagnosed by an abdominal ultrasound or computed tomography (CT) scan. The hematocrit is not a useful discriminant between ARF and CRF. A high white count may point to the presence of a systemic infection, lymphoma or leukemia, while the presence of eosinophilia suggests allergic interstitial nephritis, but may also be a prominent feature in other diseases such as atheroembolic disease, some types of vasculitis, particularly Churg–Strauss syndrome. Thrombocytopenia in patients with ARF should lead to a suspicion of thrombotic microangiopathy and may also occur in myeloma and in patients with sepsis and DIC.

Antibody titers (antinuclear, ANCA, anti-GBM and anti-streptozyme), complement levels and/or assays for cryoglobulins are indicated in patients with clinical manifestations that suggest the presence of a glomerular or vasculitic process. Blood

Value of renal ultrasound in differential diagnosis of ARF	
Observation	**Clue to diagnosis of:**
Shrunken kidneys	Chronic intrinsic renal disease
Normal size kidneys	
Echogenic	Acute glomerulonephritis, acute tubular necrosis
Normal echo pattern	Prerenal ARF, acute renal artery occlusion
Enlarged kidneys	Malignant infiltration, renal vein thrombosis, amyloid, HIV-associated nephropathy
Pelvicalyceal dilatation[a]	Obstructive nephropathy
[a]Pelvicalyceal dilatation is usual but not universal in the presence of obstruction.	

Table 14.5 Value of renal ultrasound in differential diagnosis of ARF.

cultures should be drawn if there is any possibility of infection in view of the strong association of sepsis with ARF.

Renal imaging
Ultrasound
Ultrasound is a key investigation for the diagnosis of obstruction or chronic renal disease (Table 14.5).

Obstruction of the urinary tract is recognized on renal ultrasound by the presence of dilatation of the calyces, pelvis, and ureters ('hydronephrosis') (see Chapter 5, Fig. 5.11). Ultrasound is a highly sensitive test for obstruction, positive in 98% of patients. It is less reliable in the first 24 h after the abrupt onset of obstruction. Furthermore, obstruction may rarely occur without hydronephrosis; for example, when dilatation of the collecting system is prevented by the process causing obstruction (e.g., retroperitoneal fibrosis and infiltration of the ureter by malignancy). Moreover, ultrasound is not a reliable method for identifying the anatomic site of obstruction.

Renal ultrasound is also useful in evaluating kidney size. Increased renal size without hydronephrosis may occur with acute glomerulonephritis, with infiltration by amyloid or malignancy, in diabetes, and in renal vein thrombosis. The finding of reduced renal size and increased echogenicity is the one piece of information that reliably points to a chronic element in the renal failure: the severity of the biochemical and hematologic abnormalities being an unreliable indication of chronicity. Even if the kidneys are reduced in size, the possibility of prerenal ARF or ATN superimposed on CRF must always be considered.

Other radiologic investigations
Since the advent of renal ultrasound, the intravenous urogram is rarely of diagnostic value in patients with ARF. Indeed, the systemic administration of radiocontrast agents should be avoided in view of the nephrotoxicity of these chemicals.

A plain radiograph of the abdomen (kidney, ureter and bladder; KUB) can demonstrate aortic and renal vascular calcification. More importantly, it identifies the presence of radio-opaque stones, will show small stones not found by ultrasound, and will show ureteral stones, which are poorly visualized by ultrasound. A KUB therefore is a mandatory investigation in any patient in whom an obstructive cause of ARF is suspected.

Clinical Evaluation, Management, and Outcome of Acute Renal Failure

The presence and site of obstruction is accurately diagnosed by pyelography. In retrograde pyelography, contrast is introduced into the distal end of the ureter via a cystoscope. In antegrade pyelography, contrast is injected into the renal pelvis by percutaneous puncture. If obstruction is present, a ureteral stent or percutaneous nephrostomy can be left in place to drain. Pyelography can therefore be therapeutic as well as diagnostic.

A CT scan performed without contrast is of comparable diagnostic value to the renal ultrasound for evaluation of ARF. Ultrasound is preferred because it is cheaper and more convenient. The one situation in which CT is superior is in the evaluation of ureteral obstruction, when CT can delineate the level of obstruction and define retroperitoneal inflammatory tissue (in retroperitoneal fibrosis) or a retroperitoneal malignant mass.

Renal angiography is only indicated in ARF in two settings. When renal artery occlusion (by embolization, thrombosis, or a dissecting aneurysm) is suspected on duplex scanning, angiography will be necessary to confirm the exact anatomy of the occlusion and to assess the potential for intervention by thrombolysis, angioplasty, or stenting. In this setting magnetic resonance angiography or spiral CT may soon be established as superior (see Chapter 5). Hepatic or renal angiography may also be extremely useful in diagnosing classical polyarteritis nodosa (see Chapter 26). Rarely, renal venography may be indicated to confirm the diagnosis of renal vein thrombosis.

Renal biopsy

Renal biopsy is reserved for patients in whom prerenal and postrenal failure have been excluded and the cause of intrinsic renal ARF is unclear. Renal biopsy is particularly useful when clinical assessment, urinalysis and laboratory investigation suggest diagnoses other than ischemic or nephrotoxic injury that may respond to specific therapy; for example, rapidly progressive glomerulonephritis (RPGN), thrombotic microangiopathy and allergic interstitial nephritis. In both acute interstitial nephritis and RPGN, it may sometimes be possible to establish the diagnosis with adequate confidence on the basis of clinical assessment, urine findings and serology. Nevertheless, renal histopathology still remains the gold

standard for establishing these diagnoses and is usually essential in RPGN to determine the cause as soon as possible so that the correct therapy can be started rapidly. As serologic tests that distinguish between these causes of RPGN become increasingly reliable and readily available, the need for renal biopsy in patients with RPGN may decrease. However, at present, the renal biopsy, if rapidly processed and interpreted by an experienced pathologist, remains the most reliable diagnostic tool. Renal biopsy should also be considered in ARF when there are symptoms or signs of a systemic illness, such as persistent fever or unexplained anemia. Unexpected causes of ARF, such as myeloma, interstitial nephritis, endocarditis or cryoglobulinemia, may be revealed by renal biopsy in these situations. In patients diagnosed with ATN who do not recover renal function after 4–6 weeks, a renal biopsy may be indicated to confirm the cause of ARF, exclude other treatable causes and determine the prognosis. Finally, renal biopsy is a routine diagnostic procedure in patients with ARF after transplantation when it is often essential for distinguishing between ischemic ATN, acute rejection and calcineurin inhibitor toxicity, and guiding further therapy.

MONITORING FOR COMPLICATIONS OF ACUTE RENAL FAILURE

The major complications of ARF are shown in Table 14.6.

Metabolic complications
Fluid balance
Intravascular volume overload is an almost inevitable consequence of diminished salt and water excretion in ARF and may present clinically as mild hypertension, increased jugular venous pressure, basal lung crackles, pleural effusions or ascites, peripheral edema, increased body weight and life-threatening pulmonary edema (Fig. 14.5). Hypervolemia may be particularly troublesome in patients receiving multiple intravenous medications, sodium bicarbonate for correction of acidosis, or enteral or parenteral nutrition. Moderate or severe hypertension is unusual in ATN and should suggest hypertensive nephrosclerosis, glomerulonephritis, renal artery stenosis and other diseases of the renal vasculature. Excessive

Complications of ARF					
Metabolic	Cardiovascular	Gastrointestinal	Neurologic	Hematologic	Infectious
Hyperkalemia	Pulmonary edema	Nausea	Neuromuscular	Anemia	Pneumonia
Metabolic acidosis	Arrhythmias	Vomiting	Irritability	Bleeding	Wound infections
Hyponatremia	Pericarditis	Malnutrition	Asterixis		Intravenous line infections
Hypocalcemia	Pericardial effusion	Gastritis	Seizures		Septicemia
Hyperphosphatemia	Hypertension	Gastrointestinal ulcers	Mental status changes		Urinary tract infection
Hypermagnesemia	Myocardial infarction	Gastrointestinal bleeding	Somnolence		
Hyperuricemia	Pulmonary embolism	Stomatitis or gingivitis	Coma		
	Pneumonitis	Parotitis or pancreatitis			

Table 14.6 Complications of ARF. (Adapted with permission of Brady et al.[1].)

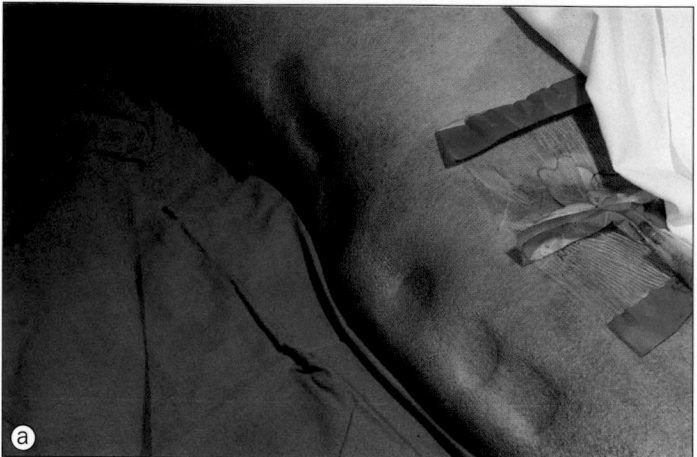

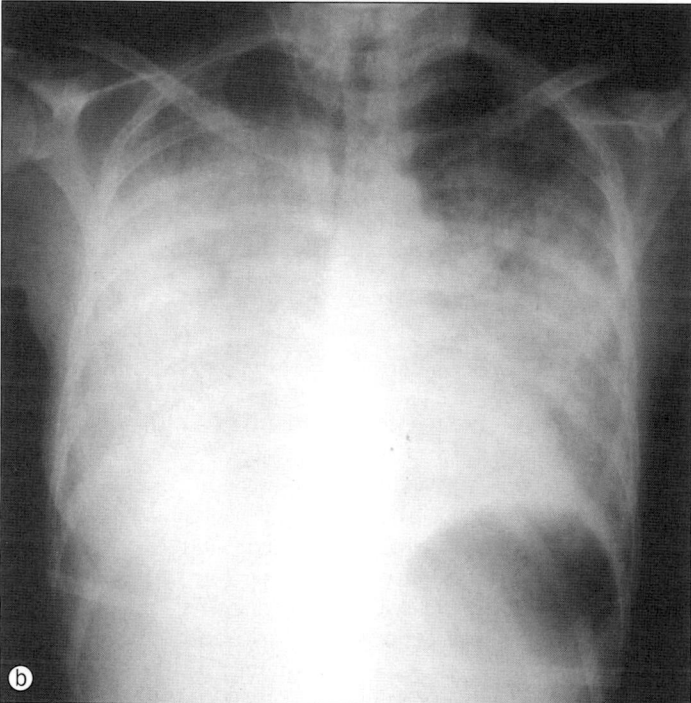

Figure 14.5 Fluid overload in ARF. (a) Gross pitting flank edema in a patient with ARF in whom femoral venous access has just been established to initiate hemodialysis. (b) Severe pulmonary edema.

water ingestion or administration of hypotonic saline or isotonic dextrose solutions can trigger hyponatremia, which, if severe, may cause cerebral edema, seizures and other neurologic abnormalities.

Potassium
Hyperkalemia is a common and potentially life-threatening complication of ARF. Serum K^+ typically rises by 0.5 mmol/L/day in oligoanuric patients and reflects impaired excretion of K^+ derived from diet, K^+-containing solutions, drugs administered as potassium salts (e.g., penicillin V) and K^+ released from injured tubular epithelium. Hyperkalemia may be compounded by coexistent metabolic acidosis that promotes K^+ efflux from cells. Severe hyperkalemia suggests massive tissue destruction such as rhabdomyolysis, hemolysis or tumor

lysis. Mild hyperkalemia (< 6.0 mmol/L) is usually asymptomatic. Higher levels are frequently associated with electrocardiographic abnormalities, typically peaked T waves, prolongation of the PR interval, flattening of P waves, widening of the QRS complex and left axis deviation (Fig. 14.6). These changes may antecede the onset of life-threatening cardiac arrhythmias such as bradycardia, heart block, ventricular tachycardia or fibrillation, and asystole. In addition, severe hyperkalemia may induce neuromuscular abnormalities such as paresthesias, hyporeflexia, weakness, ascending flaccid paralysis and respiratory failure. Hypokalemia is unusual in ARF but may complicate nonoliguric ATN caused by aminoglycosides, cisplatin or amphotericin B, presumably by causing epithelial cell injury in the thick ascending limb of the loop of Henle, the last major site of K^+ reabsorption.

Acid–base balance
Normal metabolism of dietary protein yields between 50 and 100 mmol/day of fixed nonvolatile acids (principally sulfuric and phosphoric acid), which must be excreted by the kidneys for preservation of acid–base homeostasis. Predictably, ARF is commonly complicated by metabolic acidosis, typically with a widening of the serum anion gap. Acidosis may be severe (daily fall in plasma $HCO_3^- > 2$ mmol/L) when the generation of H^+ is increased by additional mechanisms (e.g., diabetic or fasting ketoacidosis; lactic acidosis complicating generalized tissue hypoperfusion, liver disease or sepsis; metabolism of ethylene glycol). In contrast, metabolic alkalosis is an infrequent finding but may complicate overzealous correction of acidosis with HCO_3^- or loss of gastric acid by vomiting or nasogastric aspiration.

Uremia
Patients are unable to excrete nitrogenous waste products and may develop the uremic syndrome. In general, the severity of these complications mirrors the severity of renal injury and the catabolic state of the patient[1-3]. For example, the average daily increases in BUN and serum creatinine values in patients with nonoliguric, noncatabolic renal failure range from 10–20 mg/dL (serum urea 3.5–7 mmol/L) and 0.5–1.0 mg/dL (50–100 μmol/L), respectively. Comparable increments in oliguric, catabolic patients are BUN 20–100 mg/dL (serum urea 7–35 mmol/L) and creatinine 2–3 mg/dL (200–300 μmol/L). Clinical manifestations of the uremic syndrome include pericarditis, pericardial effusion and cardiac tamponade; gastrointestinal complications such as anorexia, nausea, vomiting and ileus; and neuropsychiatric disturbances including lethargy, confusion, stupor, coma, agitation, psychosis, asterixis, myoclonus, hyperreflexia, restless leg syndrome, focal neurologic deficit or seizures.

Uric acid
Uric acid is cleared from blood by glomerular filtration and secretion by proximal tubular cells, and asymptomatic hyperuricemia (12–15 mg/dL (715–900 μmol/L)) is typical in established ARF. Higher levels suggest increased production of uric acid and a possible diagnosis of acute uric acid nephropathy. In borderline cases, urinary uric acid/creatinine ratio, measured on a random specimen, may be helpful; the ratio is

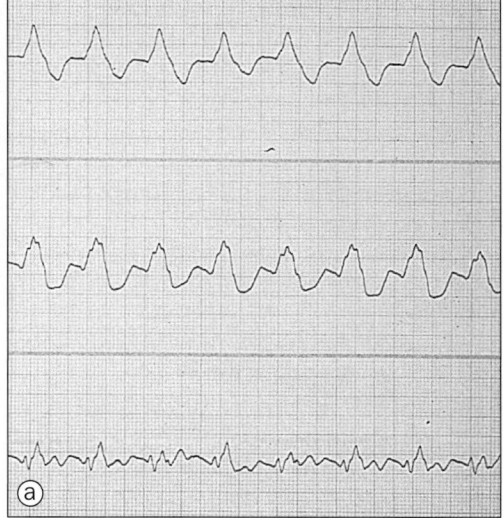
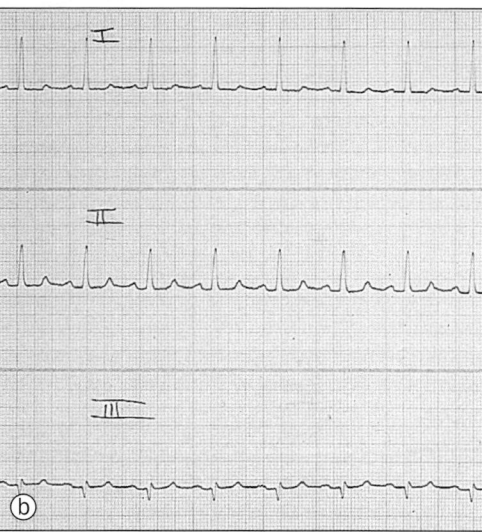

Figure 14.6 Electrocardiography (ECG) in hyperkalemia. (a) ECG recorded in a patient with ARF, serum potassium 6.8 mmol/L. Note the bizarre broad complex recording with no P waves, which is typical of hyperkalemia. (b) ECG in the same patient, 15 min later, following administration of 10 mL 10% calcium gluconate. Serum potassium is unchanged but the ECG has recovered.

typically > 1.0 when uric acid production is increased and < 0.75 in other patients with renal failure.

Calcium, phosphate and magnesium

Hyperphosphatemia (5–10 mg/dL (1.6–3.2 mmol/L)) is a common consequence of ARF and may be severe (10–20 mg/dL (3.2–6.4 mmol/L)) in highly catabolic patients or when ARF is associated with rapid cell death as in rhabdomyolysis, hemolysis, or tumor lysis. Metastatic deposition of calcium phosphate can lead to hypocalcemia, particularly when the product of serum calcium and phosphate exceeds 70 (mg × mg) or 5.5 (mmol × mmol). Other factors that may contribute to hypocalcemia include skeletal resistance to the actions of parathyroid hormone, reduced levels of 1,25-dihydroxy-vitamin D and Ca^{2+} sequestration in injured tissues.

Hypocalcemia is usually asymptomatic, possibly because of the counterbalancing effects of acidosis on neuromuscular excitability. However, symptomatic hypocalcemia can occur in rhabdomyolysis or acute pancreatitis, or after treatment of acidosis with sodium bicarbonate. Clinical manifestations of hypocalcemia include perioral paresthesias, muscle cramps, seizures, hallucinations and confusion, and prolongation of the QT interval and nonspecific T wave changes on an electrocardiogram. The Chvostek sign (contraction of facial muscles on tapping of the jaw over the facial nerve) and the Trousseau sign (carpopedal spasm after occlusion of arterial blood supply to the arm for 3 min with a blood pressure cuff) are useful indicators of latent tetany in high-risk patients.

Mild asymptomatic hypermagnesemia is usual in oliguric ARF and reflects impaired excretion of ingested magnesium (dietary magnesium, magnesium-containing laxatives, or antacids).

Hypomagnesemia occasionally complicates nonoliguric ATN associated with cisplatin or amphotericin B and, as with hypokalemia, probably reflects injury to the thick ascending limb of loop of Henle, the principal site for Mg^{2+} reabsorption. Hypomagnesemia is usually asymptomatic but may occasionally be manifest as neuromuscular instability, cramps, seizures, cardiac arrhythmias, or resistant hypokalemia or hypocalcemia.

Hematologic complications

Anemia develops rapidly in ARF and is usually mild. Contributing factors include inhibition of erythropoiesis, hemolysis, bleeding, hemodilution and reduced red blood cell survival time. Prolongation of the bleeding time and leukocytosis are also common. The former may result from mild thrombocytopenia, platelet dysfunction and/or clotting factor abnormalities (e.g., factor VIII dysfunction), and leukocytosis usually reflects sepsis, stress response, and/or other concurrent illness.

Infection

Infection is the most common and serious complication of ARF, occurring in 50–90% of cases and accounting for up to 75% of deaths. It is unclear whether this is due to defects in host immune responses or repeated breaches of muco-cutaneous barriers (e.g., intravenous cannulae, mechanical ventilation, bladder catheterization).

Other clinical features

Cardiac complications include arrhythmias, myocardial infarction and pulmonary embolism. Although these events may reflect primary cardiac disease, abnormalities in myocardial contractility and excitability may be triggered or compounded by hypervolemia, acidosis, hyperkalemia and other metabolic sequelae of acute ARF. The increased incidence of pulmonary embolism probably reflects protracted periods of immobilization. Mild gastrointestinal bleeding is common (10–30%) and is usually due to stress ulceration of gastric or small intestinal mucosa. Alterations in neurologic function may reflect the onset of the uremic syndrome, metabolic complications of ARF, impaired excretion of prescribed neuro-psychiatric medications, or primary neurologic disease.

Malnutrition

Malnutrition remains one of the most frustrating and troublesome complications of ARF. The majority of patients have net protein breakdown, which may exceed 200 g/day in catabolic subjects. Malnutrition is usually multifactorial in origin and may reflect (1) inability to eat or loss of appetite; (2) the catabolic nature of the underlying medical disorder (e.g., sepsis, rhabdomyolysis, trauma); (3) nutrient losses in drainage fluids or dialysate; (4) increased muscle catabolism and increased hepatic gluconeogenesis, probably through the actions of toxins, hormones (e.g., glucagon, parathyroid hormone), or other substances (e.g., proteases) which accumulate in ARF; and (5) inadequate nutritional support.

Recovery phase of ARF

A vigorous diuresis commonly occurs during the recovery phase of ARF. In most patients, this diuresis is appropriate and reflects excretion of salt and water retained during the oliguric phase. In a minority, however, this diuresis is inappropriate and may precipitate intravascular volume depletion and a delay in recovery of renal function. This diuretic response probably reflects the combined effects of an osmotic diuresis induced by retained urea and other waste products and delayed recovery of tubular function relative to glomerular filtration. Hypernatremia may also complicate this recovery phase if free water losses are not replenished or are inappropriately replaced by relatively hypertonic saline solutions. Hypokalemia, hypomagnesemia, hypophosphatemia and hypocalcemia are rarer metabolic complications during recovery from ARF. Mild transient hypercalcemia is relatively frequent during recovery and appears to be a consequence of hyperparathyroidism. In addition, hypercalcemia may complicate recovery from rhabdomyolysis because of mobilization of sequestered Ca^{2+} from injured muscle.

MANAGEMENT OF ACUTE RENAL FAILURE

Prerenal ARF

By definition, prerenal ARF is rapidly reversible on restoration of renal perfusion. Therapy is directed at the cause of hypoperfusion. The composition of replacement fluids for treatment of hypovolemia varies depending on the source of fluid loss. Hypovolemia due to severe hemorrhage is ideally corrected with packed red blood cells if the patient is hemodynamically unstable or if the hematocrit is dangerously low. In the absence of active bleeding or hemodynamic instability, isotonic saline may be used. The choice of replacement for non-hemorrhagic renal, extra-renal or third space losses is controversial. A recent critical review of randomized controlled trials comparing crystalloid with colloid replacement for the resuscitation in critically ill patients concluded that the routine use of colloids may be associated with an adverse outcome and is not justified[6]. Thus, isotonic saline is the appropriate replacement fluid for plasma losses (e.g., burns, pancreatitis). Urinary or gastrointestinal fluids vary greatly in composition but are usually hypotonic: initial replacement is best achieved with hypotonic solutions (e.g., 0.45% saline), and subsequent therapy should be based on measurements of the volume and ionic content of excreted or drained fluids (Table 14.7). Serum K^+ and acid–base status should be monitored in all subjects. K^+ supplementation of replacement fluids is rarely required unless sodium bicarbonate induces hypokalemia during treatment of metabolic acidosis.

Cardiac failure may require aggressive management with inotropes, antiarrhythmic drugs, preload- and afterload-reducing

Electrolyte composition of body fluids and intravenous replacement fluids							
	Electrolyte (mmol/L)[a]						
Fluids	Na$^+$	K$^+$	H$^+$	Cl$^-$	HCO$_3^-$	Ca^{2+}	Glucose (mmol/L (mg/dL))
Plasma, sweat, or gastrointestinal secretion							
Plasma	136–145	3.5–5.0	4×10^{-6} (40 mmol/L)	98–106	21–30	2.20–2.63	4.2–6.4 (75–115)
Sweat	30–50	5	–	45–55	–	–	–
Gastric secretions	40–65	10	90*	100–140	–	–	–
Pancreatic fistula	135–155	5	–	55–75	70–90	–	–
Biliary fistula	135–155	5	–	80–110	35–50	–	–
Ileostomy fluid	120–130	10	–	50–60	50–70	–	–
Diarrhea fluid	25–50	30–60	–	20–40	30–45	–	–
Common replacement fluids							
Isotonic saline (0.9%)	150	–	–	150	–	–	–
'Half normal' saline (0.45%)	75	–	–	75	–	–	–
Solution 18 (0.18%)	30	–	–	30	–	–	22.2 (400)
Ringers solution	147	4	–	156	–	2.2	–
Hartmans solution/ Ringer–Lactate solution	131	5	–	111	29	2	–
5% Dextrose	–	–	–	–	–	–	27.7 (500)

*Variable (e.g., lower in achlorhydria).

Table 14.7 Electrolyte composition of body fluids and intravenous replacement fluids.

agents, and mechanical aids such as an intra-aortic balloon pump. Invasive hemodynamic monitoring is invaluable for guiding therapy in complicated patients in whom clinical assessment of cardiovascular function and intravascular volume may be difficult and unreliable.

Fluid management may be particularly challenging in patients with ARF and cirrhosis. Although these subjects typically have intense intrarenal vasoconstriction and expanded total plasma volume because of pooling of blood in the splanchnic circulation, true hypovolemia or reduced effective systemic arterial blood volume may be an important contributory factor to ARF. Management may require fluid replacement with hemodynamic monitoring, abdominal paracentesis, porto-systemic shunting, and splanchnic vasoconstrictor therapy. Treatment of ARD in liver disease is discussed in more detail in Chapter 16.

Postrenal ARF

Management of postrenal ARF usually requires a multidisciplinary approach involving close collaboration among the nephrologist, urologist and radiologist. Prompt treatment is needed in order to relieve obstruction and avoid irreversible damage to the kidneys. Acute urinary tract obstruction at the level of the urethra or bladder neck is usually managed temporarily by insertion of a transurethral or suprapubic bladder catheter. Ureteral obstruction is usually treated initially by percutaneous placement of a nephrostomy tube into the dilated pelvis or ureter. Provided that the period of obstruction has not been of long duration, these measures usually restore urine flow, lower intratubular pressure and restore glomerular filtration. In addition, they provide a window of opportunity for identification of the obstructing lesion for treatment. Most patients experience an appropriate diuresis for several days after relief of obstruction; however, approximately 5% develop a transient salt-wasting syndrome, because of delayed recovery of tubule function relative to GFR, that may require intravenous fluid replacement to maintain blood pressure management. Urinary tract obstruction is discussed in greater detail in Chapters 58 and 59.

Intrinsic renal ARF: acute tubular necrosis (ATN)
Prevention
Hypovolemia
Prerenal ARF and ischemic ATN are part of the spectrum of manifestations of renal hypoperfusion[1-5]. Consequently, hypovolemia is a major risk factor for ATN during surgery, sepsis, or exposure to nephrotoxic drugs or radiocontrast. Meticulous monitoring of intravascular volume and correction of hypovolemia can dramatically reduce the incidence of ATN. Optimization of cardiovascular function and intravascular volume is the single most important maneuver in the management of ischemic ATN. There is compelling evidence that aggressive restoration of intravascular volume dramatically reduces the incidence of ATN after major surgery or trauma, burns and cholera.

Nephrotoxins
Volume depletion has been identified as a risk factor for ATN induced by a wide range of nephrotoxins. This has been demonstrated most convincingly with contrast nephropathy,

in which close attention to intravascular volume status ensures a low frequency of ARF[7] and prophylactic infusion of half-normal saline (1 mL/kg for 12 h pre and post procedure) is more effective in preventing ARF than mannitol or furosemide (frusemide)[8]. Oral administration of the antioxidant N-acetylcysteine has an additional effect in preventing contrast-induced ARF in patients with renal impairment (creatinine clearance < 50 mL/min)[9]. Diuretics, NSAIDs, ACE inhibitors and other vasodilators should be used with caution in patients with suspected true or effective hypovolemia or renovascular disease, as they may convert prerenal ARF to ischemic ATN and sensitize such patients to the actions of nephrotoxins. Careful monitoring of circulating drug levels appears to reduce the incidence of ARF associated with aminoglycoside antibiotics or cyclosporine, although as many as one-third of cases of aminoglycoside nephrotoxicity occur in patients with 'therapeutic' levels. Once-daily dosing with these agents affords equal antimicrobial activity and less nephrotoxicity than conventional regimens[10].

Other preventive agents
Several other agents are commonly employed to prevent ARF in specific clinical settings. Allopurinol is useful for limiting uric acid generation in patients at high risk for acute uric acid nephropathy; however, occasional patients receiving allopurinol still develop ARF, probably through the toxic actions of hypoxanthine crystals on tubular function. Forced diuresis and alkalinization of urine may attenuate renal injury caused by uric acid or methotrexate and after rhabdomyolysis. N-acetylcysteine limits acetaminophen-induced renal injury if given within 24 h of ingestion and dimercaprol, a chelating agent, may prevent heavy metal nephrotoxicity. Ethanol inhibits ethylene glycol metabolism to oxalic acid and other toxic metabolites, and fomepizole inhibits alcohol dehydrogenase; both are important adjuncts to hemodialysis in the emergency management of this intoxication.

Previously, there was a vogue for prophylactic use of mannitol and loop diuretics for prevention of nephrotoxic and ischemic ATN. It was hypothesized that loop diuretics would protect against ATN by increasing renal blood flow (through a weak vasodilatory action), by washing out intratubular casts, and by lowering renal ATP-dependent ion transport requirements and oxygen consumption. Similarly, mannitol was postulated to prevent ATN by increasing renal blood flow, washing out intratubular casts, decreasing cell swelling and scavenging free radicals. Unfortunately, these theoretic benefits were not borne out in subsequent controlled clinical trials, and there are insufficient data to support the use of these agents, except to treat hypervolemia[1-2].

Specific treatments in established ARF
The management of ATN still hinges on measures to prevent and treat uremic complications until patients recover renal function spontaneously. However, a variety of agents have been tested for their ability to attenuate injury or hasten recovery in ischemic and nephrotoxic ATN; unfortunately, none of these strategies has yet been proven to reduce the incidence of ATN or to reduce dialysis requirements or mortality in patients with established ATN when assessed in controlled clinical trials[1-5,11,12].

Diuretics

The administration of high dose intravenous diuretics to individuals with oliguric ARF is commonly practiced. While this strategy may minimize fluid overload, there is no evidence that it alters mortality or dialysis-free survival. Similarly, no adequate data exists to support the routine administration of mannitol to oliguric patients[5]; indeed, mannitol may trigger expansion of intravascular volume and pulmonary edema, and severe hyponatremia due to an osmotic shift of water from the intracellular to the intravascular space.

Dopamine

'Renal dose dopamine' (1–3 µg/kg/min) has been widely advocated for the management of oliguric ARF. In experimental animals and healthy human volunteers 'renal-dose dopamine' increases renal blood flow and, albeit to a lesser extent, GFR. Despite the attractive theoretic rationale, low-dose dopamine, in prospective controlled clinical trials does not prevent or alter the course of ischemic or nephrotoxic ATN, and is not recommended[13,14]. Furthermore, dopamine, even at low doses, is potentially toxic in critically ill patients, and can induce tachyarrythmias and myocardial ischemia, among other side effects. The rationale for using low-dose dopamine to achieve selective activation of dopamine receptors without activation of α- or β-adrenoceptors is derived from dopamine infusion into healthy subjects. In critically ill patients with pre-existing adrenergic activation and metabolic disturbances, low-dose dopamine is frequently associated with tachycardia and an increase in the cardiac index, suggesting adrenoceptor activation. Furthermore, low-dose dopamine may suppress central respiratory drive and induce arteriovenous shunting in the pulmonary circulation, both of which may exacerbate hypoxemia in compromised patients[13].

Other agents

A variety of newer strategies have been tested for their ability to prevent or reverse ATN (Fig. 14.7).

Endothelin-1, the most potent vasoconstrictor peptide found in humans, plays a pivotal role in persistent intrarenal vasoconstriction that is characteristic of ATN. Endothelin-1 receptor antagonists have given promising results in experimental ATN and are being assessed in clinical trials[12].

Atrial natriuretic peptide (ANP) is a 28 amino-acid polypeptide synthesized in cardiac atrial muscle. ANP augments GFR, renal blood flow and sodium and water excretion and confers protection against ischemic ATN in experimental models[1,12]. Although initial human studies were promising, a large multicenter trial of the ANP analogue anaritide, in critically ill patients with ARF failed to show any clinically significant improvement in dialysis free survival or overall mortality in ATN[15].

The epithelial cells of the proximal tubule and thick ascending limb of the loop of Henle are the major sites of injury in ATN. After ischemic or nephrotoxic injury, there is invariably loss of tubular epithelial continuity and sloughing of epithelial cells into the tubular lumen with attendant cast formation[3]. Clinically, recovery from ATN correlates with relief of intratubular obstruction and restoration of the continuity and function of the tubular epithelium. In animals, the administration of several growth factors accelerates tubular regeneration, recovery of GFR and anabolism[1-4]. In humans, insulin-like growth factor 1 administered postoperatively to patients who underwent renovascular surgery, improved creatinine clearance but not overall mortality or dialysis-free survival[16]. Disappointingly, no improvement in recovery of renal function was seen in a more representative study of patients with ATN in an intensive care setting with higher comorbidities[17].

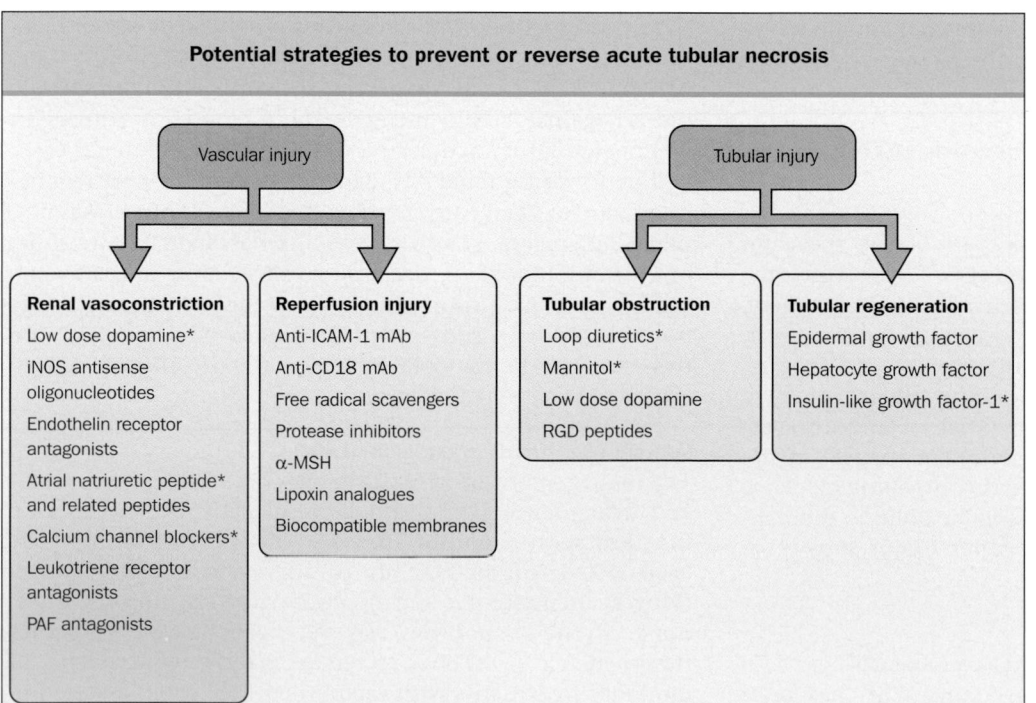

Potential strategies to prevent or reverse acute tubular necrosis

Vascular injury → Tubular injury

Renal vasoconstriction
Low dose dopamine*
iNOS antisense oligonucleotides
Endothelin receptor antagonists
Atrial natriuretic peptide* and related peptides
Calcium channel blockers*
Leukotriene receptor antagonists
PAF antagonists

Reperfusion injury
Anti-ICAM-1 mAb
Anti-CD18 mAb
Free radical scavengers
Protease inhibitors
α-MSH
Lipoxin analogues
Biocompatible membranes

Tubular obstruction
Loop diuretics*
Mannitol*
Low dose dopamine
RGD peptides

Tubular regeneration
Epidermal growth factor
Hepatocyte growth factor
Insulin-like growth factor-1*

Figure 14.7 Potential strategies to prevent or reverse acute tubular necrosis. iNOS, Inducible nitric oxide synthase; PAF, platelet activating factor; RGD peptide, peptides bearing the arginine-glycine-aspartic acid motif; mAb, monoclonal antibodies; ICAM-1, interstitial cell adhesion molecule-1; α-MSH, α-melanocyte stimulating hormone. *Tested in clinical trials with little or no benefit. (Adapted with permission[11].)

Table 14.8 Supportive management of ARF.

Supportive management of ARF	
Complication	Treatment
Intravascular volume overload	Restrict salt (1–2 g/day) and water (usually < 1 L/day) Diuretics (usually loop diuretics +/– thiazides) Ultrafiltration or dialysis
Hyponatremia	Restrict free water intake (< 1 L/day) Avoid hypotonic intravenous solutions (including dextrose solutions)
Hyperkalemia	Restrict dietary K^+ intake (usually < 40 mmol/day) Eliminate K^+ supplements and K^+ sparing diuretics Potassium-binding ion exchange resins Glucose (50 mL of 50% dextrose) and insulin (10 units) Sodium bicarbonate (usually 50–100 mmol) β_2 agonist inhaled (e.g., albuterol (salbutamol) 10–20 mg inhaled or 0.5–1 mg IV) Calcium gluconate (10 ml of 10% solution over 2–5 min)
Metabolic acidosis	Restrict dietary protein (usually 0.8–1.0 g/kg per day of high biologic value) Sodium bicarbonate (maintain serum bicarbonate > 15 mmol/L and arterial pH > 7.2)
Hyperphosphatemia	Restrict dietary phosphate intake (usually < 800 mg/day) Phosphate-binding agents (calcium acetate, calcium carbonate, aluminum hydroxide and sevelamer)
Hypocalcemia	Calcium carbonate (if symptomatic or if sodium bicarbonate to be administered) Calcium gluconate (10–20 mL of 10% solution)
Hypermagnesemia	Discontinue magnesium-containing antacids
Hyperuricemia	Treatment usually not necessary if uric acid < 15 mg/dL (< 900 µmol/L)
Nutrition	Restrict dietary protein (0.8–1.0 g/kg per day) if not catabolic Carbohydrate (100 g/day) Enteral or parenteral nutrition (if prolonged course or very catabolic)

Other strategies for the treatment of established ATN include maneuvers to relieve tubular obstruction (e.g., RGD peptides), reduce epithelial cell swelling (e.g., mannitol), replenish cell ATP levels (MgATP), scavenge oxygen free radicals (e.g., superoxide dismutase, catalase, mannitol), inhibit leukocyte-endothelial cell adhesion during reperfusion (e.g., anti-CD18, anti-ICAM-1, anti-P-selectin monoclonal antibodies and α-melanocyte stimulating hormone), and stimulate cellular regeneration (e.g., epidermal growth factor, amino acid infusions). Although many of these maneuvers afford some benefit in experimental models of ischemic or nephrotoxic ARF, their efficacy has yet to be proven in clinical trials[11,12].

Treatment for specific causes of ARF

Treatment of other intrarenal causes of ARF must be tailored to the causative disease. Systemic anticoagulation should be considered in patients with ARF caused by renal artery or vein thrombosis or in those suffering thromboembolization to the kidney. Patients with glomerulonephritis or vasculitis may respond to corticosteroids, alkylating agents and/or plasma exchange depending on the primary disease. Allergic interstitial nephritis typically resolves spontaneously when the inciting drug is stopped; however, corticosteroids appear to hasten recovery and may obviate the need for dialysis in some cases. Antiplatelet agents, plasma exchange and plasma infusion are useful in treatment of HUS and TTP. Aggressive control of systemic arterial pressure is of paramount importance in limiting renal injury in malignant hypertensive nephrosclerosis, toxemia of pregnancy, and other vascular diseases. Hypertension

and ARF associated with scleroderma may be exquisitely sensitive to treatment with ACE inhibitors. The specifics of treatment strategies for these disorders are discussed in other chapters.

Management of complications of established ARF

Management of the complications of ARF is summarized in Table 14.8. A careful clinical assessment is required daily or more often to identify such complications and initiate early treatment (Table 14.9).

Clinical assessment of ARF
• Search for reversible factors that may be exacerbating ARF, e.g., hypervolemia, ongoing administration of nephrotoxic medications
• Examine for clinical evidence of uremia (e.g., asterixis, confusion, hiccups, nausea, vomiting, pericarditis)
• Clinical assessment of intravascular volume
• Review most recent laboratory results for metabolic complications: hyperkalemia, acidosis, hyperphosphatemia
• Review drug prescription: discontinue all non-essential drugs and adjust dose or dose interval of drugs eliminated by kidney
• Review nutritional status: consider protein, salt, potassium and phosphate restriction: consider need for enteral nutrition or hyperalimentation

Table 14.9 Clinical assessment of ARF. Clinical assessment of patients with ARF. A 'bedside' checklist for daily assessment of patients with ARF.

Acute Renal Failure

Fluid balance

In patients with established ATN, hypovolemia can exacerbate renal injury and should be corrected with crystalloid solutions or blood, as outlined for prerenal ARF. Invasive hemodynamic monitoring (central venous and/or pulmonary capillary wedge pressure) is frequently necessary to guide volume replacement in patients with concomitant heart disease, who may be at risk of pulmonary edema, and in patients suffering massive shifts of fluid from the intravascular to the extravascular space (e.g., in sepsis, pancreatitis, burns, hypoalbuminemia or cirrhosis with ascites). Following correction of fluid deficits, preventive measures should be instituted to minimize hypervolemia. Salt and water intake should be adjusted to match losses (urinary, gastrointestinal, drainage sites, insensible losses), oral fluid intake can be reduced to 500–1000 mL/24 h and oral sodium intake restricted to 1–2 g/24 h. A more liberal approach can be adopted in nonoliguric ATN.

Despite these measures, expansion of the extracellular fluid volume is almost inevitable in sustained ARF. Hypertension if present is usually mild. If hypervolemia develops despite salt and water restriction, patients should receive a bolus injection of a loop diuretic such as furosemide (frusemide) 200 mg or bumetanide 5 mg. Patients who fail to diurese with bolus injection may respond if these agents are administered by continuous infusion (e.g., furosemide 10–40 mg/h), by intravenous bolus diluted in salt-poor albumin, or by intravenous bolus 30 min after a thiazide diuretic, such as hydrochlorthiazide or metolazone orally or chlorothiazide intravenously. The latter approach is intended to block sodium reabsorption at multiple sites along the nephron (loop diuretic: loop of Henle; thiazide: distal cortical nephron). In practice, combination regimens rarely provide a clinically significant augmentation in urine output by comparison with high-dose loop diuretic alone. Diuretic therapy should be discontinued in resistant patients as prolonged futile administration may induce ototoxicity. Mannitol should be avoided as it may precipitate pulmonary edema in patients with established ATN if mannitol-induced expansion of intravascular volume is not associated with diuresis. As in prevention of ATN, low-dose dopamine does not produce a clinically significant diuresis or accelerate recovery in patients with established ATN.

ATN impairs water excretion. Given that most patients have an obligatory water intake with meals, some dilutional hyponatremia and hypo-osmolality is almost inevitable in ATN. Hyponatremia can usually be controlled by restriction of free water intake to 500–1000 mL/24 h. It should be remembered that dextrose-containing solutions also constitute a hypotonic water load because dextrose is rapidly metabolized. Hypernatremia may complicate ATN in patients with large insensible or gastrointestinal losses who are denied access to water (e.g., if ventilated). If oral or nasogastric administration is not possible, hypotonic saline solutions or dextrose-containing solutions should be administered intravenously. The management of hyponatremia and hypernatremia is discussed further in Chapter 7.

Potassium

Hyperkalemia is almost inevitable in patients with oliguric ATN and is a potentially life-threatening complication that warrants urgent intervention. In the absence of clinical or electrocardiographic evidence of hyperkalemia, moderate hyperkalemia (5.5–6.5 mmol/L) can usually be controlled by restriction of dietary potassium or oral administration of potassium-binding ion-exchange resins, such as sodium polystyrene sulfonate (15–30 g in 50–100 mL 20% sorbitol every 3–4 h) or 'calcium resonium' (15–30 g three or four times daily). These resins can be administered as a retention enema when upper gastrointestinal function is impaired, but may cause constipation. Loop diuretics enhance potassium excretion in diuretic-responsive patients. Hyperkalemia is a medical emergency when levels exceed 6.5 mmol/L or when lower levels of hyperkalemia are accompanied by electrocardiographic abnormalities or clinical features of hyperkalemia (Fig. 14.6). In the presence of electrocardiographic abnormalities, calcium gluconate or calcium chloride (10 mL 10% solution intravenously over 5 min) is an interim measure to antagonize the cardiac and neuromuscular effects of hyperkalemia. Calcium gluconate does not lower serum potassium but protects against cardiac arrhythmias. Intravenous insulin (10 units soluble insulin) and glucose (50 mL 50% dextrose) shift potassium into cells within 30–60 min, and their administration is a useful temporizing measure while total body potassium is reduced by loop diuretics or dialysis. Frequent monitoring of blood glucose is advisable. Sodium bicarbonate (approximately 50 mmol over 5 min) also promotes rapid shift of potassium into cells (onset within 15 min, duration 1–2 h) and is often administered with insulin–dextrose, particularly in acidotic patients. Both sodium polystyrene sulfonate and sodium bicarbonate constitute a sodium load and must be used carefully in oliguric patients to avoid exacerbation of hypervolemia. Acute dialysis is mandatory if hyperkalemia is resistant to these conservative measures. From a practical viewpoint, dialysis is almost always required if hyperkalemia develops in oligoanuric diuretic-resistant patients.

Treatment with both sodium bicarbonate and insulin promotes flux of potassium into the intracellular compartment, as does treatment with β-agonists. If these are combined injudiciously with dialysis, postdialysis hypokalemia may result. In patients vulnerable to ventricular arrhythmia, for example after cardiac surgery, a high dialysate potassium concentration (e.g., 4 mmol/L) may be indicated to prevent hypokalemia.

Acid–base balance

Metabolic acidosis does not require treatment unless the serum bicarbonate and pH fall below 15 mmol/L and 7.2, respectively (some authorities recommend withholding therapy until serum bicarbonate and pH fall to approximately 12 mmol/L and 7.1, respectively). Acidosis is corrected by administration of sodium bicarbonate by mouth or intravenously. The initial rate of replacement should be based on estimates of bicarbonate deficit (bicarbonate deficit in mmol = 0.4 × lean body weight × (desired serum bicarbonate – measured serum bicarbonate)) and adjusted thereafter according to serum levels. In general, sodium bicarbonate is administered to maintain a serum concentration of 15–20 mmol/L. Initial therapy aims for partial correction of the plasma bicarbonate level, as excessive correction of severe metabolic acidosis (plasma bicarbonate less than 10 mmol/L) can have adverse consequences, including paradoxical acidification of the cerebrospinal fluid and an increase in the tissue production rate of lactic acid. Overzealous correction may result in metabolic alkalosis, hypocalcemia, hypokalemia, volume overload and pulmonary edema. Other disturbances of acid–base homeostasis are less frequent in patients with ATN and may reflect pulmonary comorbidity (e.g., respiratory acidosis or alkalosis in patients requiring mechanical ventilation) or gastrointestinal dysfunction (e.g., metabolic alkalosis caused by loss of gastric acid through vomiting or nasogastric aspiration).

Other biochemical changes

Mild hyperphosphatemia is common in ATN and can usually be controlled by restriction of dietary phosphate and oral administration of dietary phosphate binders (e.g., calcium carbonate 500 mg t.i.d.). Severe hyperphosphatemia may develop in highly catabolic patients and carries a risk of metastatic deposition of calcium phosphate when the serum calcium phosphate exceeds 70 (mg × mg) or 5.5 (mmol × mmol). Dialysis is advisable in this setting if serum phosphate cannot be lowered rapidly by dietary intervention and phosphate binders. Hypophosphatemia is a rarer complication of ARF, but may be seen in patients treated with total parenteral nutrition particularly in those with severe weight loss. Sustained hypophosphatemia may compromise respiratory muscle power and thereby hamper weaning of patients from ventilator support.

Mild hypocalcemia is relatively common in ATN and is typically asymptomatic. Treatment of hypocalcemia is not advisable in the absence of symptoms given the potential risk of calcium phosphate deposition. Hypermagnesemia is typically mild and does not require treatment unless clinically significant, as judged by hyporeflexia or respiratory depression (which are very rare). Hyperuricemia is also common in ATN, is usually mild (< 10 mg/dL (< 600 μmol/L)), and does not require treatment.

Malnutrition

Treatment of malnutrition requires a multidisciplinary approach involving physicians, nurses and dietitians. The objective of dietary modification during the maintenance phase of ARF is to provide sufficient calories to avoid protein catabolism and starvation ketoacidosis, while minimizing the generation of nitrogenous waste that may precipitate uremic syndrome. This is typically achieved by restricting intake prior to initiation of dialysis to protein of high biologic value (i.e., rich in essential amino acids) at approximately 0.8–1.0 g/kg body weight per day and providing most calories in the form of carbohydrate 3–5 g/kg body weight per day. Higher protein intake is advisable in catabolic patients or those with a prolonged maintenance phase[18], even if it precipitates the need for dialysis. Management of nutrition is easier in nonoliguric patients and after institution of dialysis. Vigorous parenteral hyperalimentation has been claimed to improve prognosis in ARF; however, a consistent benefit has yet to be demonstrated.

Hematologic complications

Anemia may require red cell transfusion in patients with symptoms or active bleeding. Erythropoetin is not useful in ARF because of its relatively delayed onset of action and the resistance of bone marrow in critically ill patients. The bleeding diathesis is typically mild and, if problematic, can be reversed temporarily by desmopressin, correction of anemia, estrogen therapy, or dialysis should hemorrhage develop or should patients require invasive procedures or surgery (see Chapter 70).

Gastrointestinal complications

Patients with ATN have an increased incidence of upper gastrointestinal hemorrhage caused by stress erosions and ulcers. Gastric stress ulcer prophylaxis, with histamine H_2 antagonists or proton pump inhibitors, is indicated if the patient is intubated or has a concurrent coagulopathy. Aluminum- and magnesium-based antacids should not be used for prolonged periods in patients with ATN as these cations may accumulate to toxic levels.

Infection

A high index of suspicion for infection is required, broad-spectrum antibiotics should be given while awaiting identification of specific organisms. Meticulous care of intravenous cannulae, bladder catheters and other invasive devices is mandatory. Prophylactic antibiotics have not been shown to reduce the incidence of infectious complications and may be harmful by promoting the emergence of resistant organisms.

INDICATIONS AND MODALITIES OF DIALYSIS

Dialysis does not hasten recovery from ARF, rather the goal of renal replacement therapy in ARF is to keep the patient alive while awaiting recovery in renal function. Initial studies suggesting that early dialysis therapy improved prognosis for patients with ARF have not been confirmed[19]. Similarly, it is unclear whether the choice of dialytic modality or the intensity of dialysis favorably affects outcome. Indeed, early and unnecessary hemodialysis may potentially exacerbate renal hypoperfusion, as transient hypotension is a common complication of this treatment modality, and leukocytes activated on exposure to dialysis membranes may potentially aggravate ischemic renal injury (see below). There is no firm consensus on the initiation of dialysis in ARF.

The absolute indications for the commencement of renal replacement therapy include symptoms or signs of uremia (asterixis, pericardial rub or effusion, encephalopathy) and acidosis, hyperkalemia or volume overload unresponsive to conservative management. Patients with ATN should be assessed daily, for these clinical features, which should prompt emergency dialysis (see Tables 14.9 and 14.10).

In practice, most nephrologists consider (and often initiate) dialysis in oliguric patients if blood urea and creatinine levels rise above 100 mg/dL (serum urea 35 mmol/L) and 8 mg/dL (800 μmol/L), respectively, in the absence of clinical (increased urine output) or biochemical evidence of renal recovery, on the basis that serious uremic complications are almost inevitable. The principal dialysis modalities are acute peritoneal dialysis (PD), acute intermittent hemodialysis (HD) and the various forms of slow continuous HD and

Indications for dialysis in ARF	
Indications	**Characteristics**
Uremia	• Obtundation, asterixis, seizures, nausea and vomiting, pericarditis
Hyperkalemia	• K⁺ >6.5 mmol/L • K⁻ > 5.5 mmol/L if ECG changes
Fluid overload	• Resistant to diuretics, especially pulmonary edema
Metabolic acidosis	• pH <7.2 despite sodium bicarbonate therapy • Sodium bicarbonate therapy not tolerated because of fluid overload

Table 14.10 Indications for dialysis in ARF.

hemofiltration (Table 14.11). The choice of dialysis modality is guided by the resources of the health care institution, the expertise of the nephrologists and intensivists, and the clinical status of the patient[20, 21]. In the context of the overall population of patients with ATN, each modality has the capacity to achieve adequate clearance of uremic toxins and to control uremic complications and hypervolemia.

Peritoneal dialysis

Peritoneal dialysis in ARF is effected through a temporary intraperitoneal catheter. Dialysis is typically achieved by either repeated 1-h exchanges, typically with a 10-min infusion time, a 30-min dwell and a 20-min drainage period or by slow continuous PD involving four dwells of dialysate in the peritoneal cavity for 6 h (continuous equilibrium PD). The continuous cycling technique has been greatly aided by the introduction of automated cyclers and offers better solute clearance than slow continuous therapy. Ultrafiltration rates can be varied by using dialysate of different osmotic strengths (i.e., different glucose concentrations). The use of peritoneal dialysis has declined in the acute setting, but it is still used in children and in regions where there is no access to acute or slow continuous hemodialysis[19,20].

Peritoneal dialysis has the advantage of being relatively 'low-tech' and portable, thus facilitating its use in remote or economically disadvantaged areas. Systemic hypotension is typically avoided as it provides gradual fluid removal, avoiding dramatic shifts in intravascular volume, and clearance toxins and ultrafiltration of excess intravascular volume is generally adequate. Other benefits include the avoidance of systemic anticoagulation, need for vascular access and exposure of blood to artificial membranes. Complications of PD include

Table 14.11 Dialytic modalities in ARF.

Dialytic modalities in ARF		
Modality	**Dialyzer**	**Physical principle**
Hemodialysis		
Conventional	Hemodialyzer	Intermittent diffusive clearance and ultrafiltration (UF) concurrently
Slow long extended daily dialysis (SLED)	Hemodialyzer	Intermittent diffusive clearance and ultrafiltration at low blood and dialysate flow rates
Sequential ultrafiltration and clearance	Hemodialyzer	Intermittent UF followed by diffusive clearance
Continuous arteriovenous hemodialysis (CAVHD)	Hemodialyzer	Slow diffusive clearance and UF concurrently without blood pump
Continuous venovenous hemodialysis (CVVHD)	Hemodialyzer	Slow diffusive clearance and UF concurrently with blood pump
Hemofiltration		
Continuous arteriovenous hemofiltration (CAVHF)	Hemofilter	Continuous convective clearance without a blood pump
Continuous venovenous hemofiltration (CVVHF)	Hemofilter	Continuous convective clearance with a blood pump
Hemodialysis plus hemofiltration		
Continuous arteriovenous hemodialysis plus hemofiltration (CAVHDF)	Hemofilter	Continuous convective plus diffusive clearance without a blood pump
Continuous venovenous hemodialysis plus hemofiltration (CVVHDF)	Hemofilter	Continuous convective plus diffusive clearance with a blood pump
Ultrafiltration		
Isolated ultrafiltration	Hemodialyzer	Intermittent UF alone without diffusive or convective clearance
Slow continuous ultrafiltration (SCUF)	Hemofilter	Continuous arteriovenous (no pump) or venovenous (pump) UF alone without diffusive or convective clearance
Peritoneal dialysis		
Continuous	Peritoneum	Continuous clearance and UF via exchanges performed at varying intervals
Intermittent	Peritoneum	Intermittent clearance and UF via exchanges performed for 10–12 h every 2–3 days

perforation of bowel or other organs at the time of peritoneal catheter insertion, peritonitis, and exacerbation of malnutrition as a result of loss of amino acids and proteins across the peritoneal membrane.

Acute intermittent hemodialysis

Acute intermittent hemodialysis has been the mainstay of renal replacement therapy in ARF over the past 30 years[19,20]. Typically, the patient undergoes dialysis for 3–4 h daily, or on alternate days, depending on their catabolic state. Clearance of uremic toxins, potassium and phosphate by diffusion is combined with fluid removal by ultrafiltration. The principles and practice of dialysis are discussed further in Chapters 78, 79 and 82.

Vascular access

Vascular access for short-term hemodialysis or hemofiltration is usually achieved using a double-lumen catheter inserted into the internal jugular vein. Subclavian vein cannulation for dialysis carries a higher complication rate than cannulation of the internal jugular vein, particularly for hemorrhage, pneumothorax and venous stenosis. Femoral vein catheterization is technically easy and relatively free of complications. It is useful in patients who cannot tolerate the Trendelenberg position or are likely to require only one or two dialysis treatments (e.g., poisoning). Jugular or subclavian lines are preferred for more prolonged treatment courses but, with careful nursing management, it is possible to maintain a femoral line *in situ* in the bedbound patient without incurring a significant infection risk[19].

Dialysis membranes

The choice of membrane used during dialysis may have an effect on outcome. Cellulose-based membranes cause activation of circulating complement and leukocytes, particularly neutrophils and monocytes. It is postulated that activated leukocytes, upon their return to the systemic circulation, traffic to the already injured kidney where they exacerbate nephrotoxic and ischemic renal injury. Synthetic noncellulosic membranes cause less complement and leukocyte activation, are more 'biocompatible'. Although some clinical trials have suggested an association between the use of biocompatible dialyzer membranes and clinical outcome in ARF[21–23], more recent studies have not confirmed these findings[24].

Anticoagulation

Anticoagulation with heparin is the standard method for preventing thrombosis of the extracorporeal circuit during acute intermittent dialysis[19]. Routine bedside measurement of the activated clotting time (ACT) allows heparin dosage adjustment as required to maintain a target ACT of baseline value plus 80%. Heparin-free dialysis can be performed in patients at high risk of hemorrhagic complications. This involves prerinsing the dialyzer with a heparinized solution (3000 U/L) and setting the blood flow rate at least 250–300 mL/min. A periodic saline rinse is then administered every 15–30 min to prevent the clotting in the extracorporeal circuit. Newer anticoagulation techniques include the administration of a single bolus of low-molecular weight heparin (LMWH) at the start of dialysis. Small-scale studies suggest that LMWH is a safe and effective anti-coagulant. LMWH does not alter the PT or APTT in the dosage range used, thus having the potential for fewer bleeding complications[19]. Alternative anticoagulant strategies include: (1) region heparinization with protamine infusion in the venous return line; (2) regional citrate anti-coagulation; (3) continuous prostacyclin infusion; (4) hirudin; and (5) serine protease inhibitors[19], but these agents have not been proven superior to low-dose heparin or heparin.

Initiation of dialysis

Several controlled studies have examined the effect of prophylactic dialysis on renal outcome (i.e., initiation of dialysis at a certain level of blood urea prior to development of absolute clinical or biochemical indications)[19]. However, there is no consistent evidence that earlier dialysis is associated with a superior renal outcome or reduced mortality.

Complications of dialysis

The major complications of acute intermittent hemodialysis relate to rapid shifts in plasma volume and solute composition, the vascular access procedure, the necessity for anticoagulation and dialysis membrane incompatibility (see Table 14.12)[19]. Intradialytic hypotension is common in patients undergoing acute intermittent hemodialysis; it impairs solute clearance and the efficiency of dialysis, and

Complications of dialysis in ARF	
Type	**Symptoms**
Related to vascular access	Pneumothorax
	Hemothorax
	Hemopericardium
	Air embolism
	Large vein thrombosis (particularly subclavian)
	False aneurysm following femoral artery catheterization
	Sepsis
Related to excessive ultrafiltration	Hypotension, cramps, exacerbation of ischemic acute tubular necrosis, exacerbation of myocardial ischemia
Related to clearance of solute	'First-use' syndrome, electrolyte disturbances
Related to dialysate contamination	Fever, chills (endotoxin), hemolysis (dilute dialysate
Related to dialysis membrane and circuitry	'First-use' syndrome
	Exacerbation of renal injury by leukocytes activated dialysis membrane
	Anaphylaxis and lesser hypersensitivity reactions (residual ethylene oxide in circuit)
	Air embolism resulting from air in the extracorporeal circuit
Miscellaneous	Systemic hemorrhage caused by anticoagulation therapy

Table 14.12 Complications of dialysis in ARF.

can further compromise renal perfusion and exacerbate tubular necrosis (see above). Intradialytic hypotension is typically triggered by excessive fluid removal during ultrafiltration. This, in turn, may occur if the degree of hypervolemia is overestimated, if the fluid removed is not matched by flux of fluid into the intravascular space from interstitial and cellular compartments, if the volume of fluid removed is excessive, or if the patient's compensatory responses are impaired as a result of microvascular disease or vasodilator medications (e.g., nitrates). Hypotension may be particularly problematic in critically ill patients with ATN and concurrent sepsis, hypoalbuminemia, malnutrition or large third space losses. Management of intradialytic hypotension requires careful assessment of intravascular volume, by invasive hemodynamic monitoring if necessary, prescription of realistic ultrafiltration targets and close observation for tachycardia or hypotension during dialysis.

The dialysis disequilibrium syndrome is a self-limiting condition characterized by nausea, vomiting, headache, altered consciousness and, rarely, seizures or coma[19]. It typically occurs after a first dialysis in very uremic patients. The syndrome is triggered by rapid movement of water into brain cells following the development of transient plasma hypo-osmolality as solutes are rapidly cleared from the bloodstream during dialysis. It can usually be avoided with the precise prescription of dialysis including such variables as membrane size, blood flow rate and sodium profile.

Slow continuous hemofiltration and hemodialysis

Many patient with ATN are critically ill, hypercatabolic and hemodynamically unstable. They frequently have large obligate fluid requirements, being on intravenous medication and parenteral alimentation. In this setting, ultrafiltration of large volumes of plasma over a relatively short period by acute intermittent hemodialysis may induce circulatory compromise. Even if tolerated hemodynamically, acute intermittent hemodialysis may not achieve adequate ultrafiltration or solute clearance to avoid life-threatening pulmonary or uremia. For these patients, a variety of slow-continuous dialytic therapies (Table 14.11) are now well established in the management of ARF[25,26]. Slow continuous techniques offer simplicity of operation, the ability to remove large volumes of fluid over a prolonged period with minimal hemodynamic compromise, and the capacity to control uremia, electrolyte and acid–base abnormalities with minimal perturbation of plasma osmolality.

Continuous venovenous hemodialysis (CVVHD) or continuous venovenous hemofiltration (CVVH) are the techniques favored by most centers. Clearance of low molecular weight solutes can be enhanced by an increase in the blood flow and dialysate rates, or by combining hemofiltration and hemodialysis (CVVHDF). Slow continuous ultrafiltration (SCUF) is a related technique in which the dialysis flow rate is set at zero and no replacement solution is administered. This technique yields 'pure' ultrafiltration and is typically used in the patient with marked volume overload as a result of obligate fluid intake and heart failure, or capillary leak syndrome in the absence of overt uremic or metabolic indications for renal replacement. Recently described sustained low efficiency dialysis is a promising technique for the treatment of critically ill patients with ARF. It uses conventional hemodialysis apparatus, performed daily at slow flow rates over an extended treatment time. It offers several advantages over CVVH, including less cumbersome technique, improved patient mobility between sessions and decreased requirement for anticoagulation, while providing similar hemodynamic stability and volume control. It is worth noting, however that CCVH requires no plumbing and can be set up easily in an intensive care setting, whereas slow extended HD requires pure water and plumbing, hemodialysis apparatus and trained dialysis nursing staff to initiate and supervise the procedure. The principles and practice of the various forms of continuous therapy are discussed in more detail in Chapter 82.

Choice of dialysis modality

Several retrospective studies have suggested an improved outcome in critically ill patients treated with continuous compared to intermittent forms of renal replacement[25-28] but, to date, there is limited prospective data on this issue. In most practices, continuous forms of renal replacement therapy are used in patients who are hemodynamically unstable or highly catabolic and intermittent HD is used in other patients.

Intensity of dialysis

Once renal replacement therapy has been initiated, the optimal intensity of dialysis has also been uncertain[19]. If intermittent HD is used in the intensive care setting, there is recent evidence that daily HD is associated with better control of symptoms of uremia and longer survival than conventional intermittent (typically alternate day) HD[29]. Using CVVH, there is now evidence in one large study that increasing ultrafiltration volume to at least 35 mL/h/kg may improve outcome[30].

OUTCOME

When ARF is severe enough to require renal replacement therapy, in-hospital mortality rates are extremely high, exceeding 50%[31-33]. The published intensive care and in-hospital mortality rates range from 40% to 80%[34]. Mortality rates have changed little over the past three decades, despite the introduction and refinement of dialytic techniques rates and major advances in intensive care procedures. This lack of improvement in outcome, despite significant advances in supportive care, may be more apparent than real and reflect the increasing proportion of patients who have ARF complicating multiple organ dysfunction in a critical care setting. Mortality in community-acquired ARF, which includes many patients with single organ renal failure, including reversible postrenal failure, is only 10–30%. Obstetric ARF now has a mortality of approximately 15%.

Before the development of dialysis and filtration techniques, the most common causes of death among patients with ARF were progressive uremia, hyperkalemia and complications of volume overload or bleeding diathesis. Currently, morbidity and mortality associated with dialysis dependent ARF are due to underlying disease and high frequency of superimposed complications rather than ARF *per se*[32–34]. Age, systemic inflammatory response syndrome, sepsis and multiple organ dysfunction all increase the mortality associated with ARF. Respiratory or central nervous system failure, hypotension, the need for vasoactive medications and persistent oliguria/anuria are all adverse prognostic signs in the intensive care unit[34]. Scoring systems which assess the severity of illness and likelihood of survival in critically ill patients, such as the acute physiology and chronic health evaluation II (APACHE II) score, when determined at the initiation of dialysis, predict patient survival[34]. Death is almost universal if ARF is associated with failure of more than three other organ systems. The costs of ARF in intensive care often exceed US $50 000 per quality-adjusted life year. In view of such high costs and poor outcome, the cost effectiveness and rationale for treating intensive care patients with ARF have been challenged. Dialysis in the acute setting should be seen as a bridge to recovery of renal function, rather than a proactive measure to accelerate recovery in the critically ill patient.

Patients who survive an episode of ATN generally recover sufficient renal function to live normal lives. However, 50% have subclinical functional defects in glomerular filtration, tubule solute transport, H^+ secretion and urinary concentrating mechanisms, and glomerular or tubulointerstitial scarring on renal biopsy[1]. ARF is irreversible in approximately 5% of patients, although, in the elderly, this is more common than was previously realized and may be as high as 16%[35]. Among other factors, this likely reflects the superimposition of ATN on underlying renovascular disease. An additional 5% of patients recover renal function but subsequently undergo progressive loss of renal function, probably as a consequence of compensatory glomerular hypertension and secondary focal and segmental glomerulosclerosis. These patients can usually be identified early by the failure of serum creatinine to return to the normal range and by persistent hypertension, although proteinuria will not necessarily be present from the time of ARF.

Because as many as 15% of patients with ARF may ultimately require dialysis at some stage during their lives, every effort should be made to protect the vessels in the nondominant arm of all patients with ARF as these will ultimately be required for the formation of an arteriovenous fistula. Venesection and arterial and venous cannulation should be avoided in that arm if at all possible.

REFERENCES

1. Brady HR, Brenner BM, Clarkson MR, Lieberthal W. Acute renal failure. In: Brenner BM, Rector FC, eds. The kidney, 6th edn. Philadelphia, PA: Saunders; 2000:1201–62.
2. Brady HR, Singer GG. Acute renal failure. Lancet. 1995;346:1533–40.
3. Thadhani R, Pascual M, Bonventre JV. Acute renal failure. N Engl J Med. 1996;334:1448–60.
4. Fisch BJ, Linas SL. Prerenal acute renal failure. In: Brady HR, Wilcox CS, eds. Therapy in nephrology and hypertension. Philadelphia, PA: Saunders; 1998:17–20.
5. Goligorsky MS, Allgren RL, Hammerman MR. Medical management of ischemic acute tubular necrosis. In: Brady HR, Wilcox CS, eds. Therapy in nephrology and hypertension. Philadelphia, PA: Saunders; 1998:21–8.
6. Schierhout G, Roberts I. Fluid resuscitation with colloid or crystalloid solutions in critically ill patients: a systemic review of randomised trials. Br Med J. 1998;316:961–4.
7. Barrett BJ, Parfrey PS. Contrast nephropathy. In: Brady HR, Wilcox CS, eds. Therapy in nephrology and hypertension. Philadelphia, PA: Saunders; 1998:41–4.
8. Solomon R, Werner C, Mann D, et al. Effects of saline, mannitol, and furosemide on acute decreases on renal function induced by radiocontrast agents. N Engl J Med. 1994;331:1416–20.
9. Tepel M, Van Der Giet M, Zidek W. Prevention of radiographic-contrast-agent-induced reductions in renal function by acetylcysteine. N Engl J Med. 2000;343:180–4.
10. Prins JM, Buller HR, Kuijper EJ, et al. Once versus thrice daily gentamicin in patients with serious infections. Lancet. 1993;341:335–9.
11. Kieran NE, Brady HR. Treatment of acute renal failure: promising experimental strategies and new therapeutic challenges. Semin Dialysis. 1999;12:275–7.
12. Rabb H, Bonventre J. Experimental strategies for acute renal failure – the future. In: Brady HR, Wilcox CS, eds. Therapy in nephrology and hypertension. Philadelphia, PA: Saunders; 1998:72–81.
13. Denton MD, Chertow G, Brady HR. 'Renal-dose' dopamine for the treatment of acute renal failure: scientific rationale, experimental studies and clinical trials. Kidney Int. 1996;49:4–14.
14. Bellomo R, Chapman M, Finfer S, et al. Low dose dopamine in patients with early renal dysfunction: a placebo-controlled randomized trial. Australian and New Zealand Intensive Care Society (ANZICS) Clinical Trials Group. Lancet 2000;356:2139–43.
15. Allgren RL, Marbury TC, Rahman SN, et al. Anaritide in acute tubular necrosis. N Engl J Med. 1997;336:828–34.
16. Franklin SC, Moulton M, Sicard GA, et al. Insulin-like growth factor 1 preserves renal function postoperatively. Am J Physiol. 1997;272:F257–9.
17. Hirschberg R, Kopple J, Capra W, et al. Multicenter clinical trial of recombinant human insulin-like growth factor 1 in patients with acute renal failure. Kidney Int. 1999;55:2423–32.
18. Druml W. Nutritional management of acute renal failure. Am J Kidney Dis. 2001;37:S89–94.
19. Daugirdas JT, Blake PG, Ing TS, eds. Handbook of dialysis. New York: Little, Brown; 2001.
20. Eustace J, Heffernan A, Watson A. Acute hemodialysis and acute peritoneal dialysis. In: Brady HR, Wilcox CS, eds. Therapy in nephrology and hypertension. Philadelphia, PA: Saunders; 1998:52–9.
21. Hakim RM, Wingard RL, Parker RA. Effect of the dialysis membrane in the treatment of patients with acute renal failure. N Engl J Med. 1994;331:1338–42.
22. Schiffl H, Lang SM, Konig A, et al. Biocompatible membranes in acute renal failure; prospective case-controlled study. Lancet. 1994;344:570–2.
23. Himmelfarb J, Tolkoff Rubin N, Chandran P, et al. A multicenter comparison of dialysis membranes in the treatment of acute renal failure requiring dialysis. J Am Soc Nephrol. 1998;9:257–66.
24. Jorres A, Gahl GM, Dobis C, et al. Hemodialysis-membrane biocompatibility and mortality of patients with dialysis-dependent acute renal failure: a prospective randomized multicentre trial. Lancet 1999;354:1337–41.
25. Manns M, Sigler MH, Teehan BP. Continuous renal replacement therapies: an update. Am J Kidney Dis. 1998;32:185–207.
26. Ronco C, Bellomo R, Ricci Z. Continuous renal replacement therapy in critically ill patients. Nephrol Dial Transplant. 2001;16(Suppl. 5):67–72.

27. Mehta RL, McDonald B, Kaplan RM, et al. A randomized clinical trial of continuous versus intermittent dialysis for acute renal failure. Kidney Int. 2001;60:1154–63.

28. Kumar VA, Craig M, Yeun JY, et al. Extended daily dialysis: a new approach to renal replacement for acute renal failure in the intensive care unit. Am J Kidney Dis. 2000;36:294–300.

29. Schiffl H, Lang SM, Fischer R. Daily hemodialysis and the outcome of acute renal failure. N Engl J Med. 2002;346:305–10.

30. Ronco C, Bellomo R, Homel P, et al. Effects of different doses of continuous veno-venous haemofiltration on outcomes of acute renal failure: a prospective randomized trial. Lancet. 2000;355:26–30.

31. Karsou SA, Jaber BL, Pereira BJ. Impact of intermittent hemodialysis variables on clinical outcomes in acute renal failure. Am J Kidney Dis. 2000;35:980–91.

32. Liano F, Junco E, Pascual J, et al. The spectrum of acute renal failure in the intensive care unit compared with that seen in other settings: The Madrid Acute Renal Failure Study Group. Kidney Int. 1998;53(Suppl. 66):S16–24.

33. Korkeila M, Ruokonen E, Takala J. Costs of care, long-term prognosis and quality of life in patients requiring renal replacement therapy during intensive care. Intens Care Med. 2000;26:1824–31.

34. Chen YC, Hsu HH, Kao KC, et al. Outcomes and APACHE II predictions for critically ill patients with acute renal failure requiring dialysis. Ren Fail. 2001;23:61–70.

35. Bhandari S, Turney JH. Survivors of acute renal failure who do not recover renal function. QJ Med.1996;89:415–21.

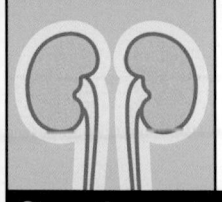

Chapter 15

Causes of Acute Renal Failure

Ashley Jefferson and Richard A Zager

INTRODUCTION

Acute renal failure (ARF) is a clinical syndrome characterized by an abrupt decline (days to a few weeks) in glomerular filtration rate (GFR) sufficient to decrease the elimination of nitrogenous waste products (urea and creatinine) and other uremic toxins. The urine volume in ARF is variable and is determined not only by GFR, but also by tubular reabsorption. Although ARF is defined by a reduced GFR, the cause of the renal impairment is usually due to tubular and vascular factors.

The incidence of ARF is difficult to determine from the literature due to wide variation in populations studied, and the varying diagnostic criteria which have been employed. However, it is generally accepted that in the hospital setting, ARF occurs in approximately 5% of all patients[1], and in 15–25% of intensive care/critically ill patients[2].

DIFFERENTIAL DIAGNOSIS

The differential diagnosis of ARF is broad and must be considered in a systematic fashion to avoid missing multiple factors which may be contributing to the condition. The traditional paradigm divides ARF into prerenal, renal and postrenal causes. Prerenal azotemia may be due to hypovolemia or a decreased effective arterial volume (see Chapter 14). Postrenal obstructive renal failure is usually diagnosed by urinary tract dilatation on renal ultrasound or CT scanning (see Chapter 58). Renal causes of ARF should be considered in five further categories according to the different anatomic components of the kidney (see Fig. 15.1). Major extra renal artery or venous occlusion must also be considered in the differential diagnosis (see Chapter 64).

In the hospital setting, prerenal uremia and acute tubular necrosis (ATN) account for the majority of ARF cases. One recent multicenter study from Spain detailed the incidence of hospital causes of ARF (Fig. 15.2)[3]. Patterns of ARF are changing with time as older patients undergo more complex surgery and often have substantial risk factors predisposing to ARF including underlying cardiovascular disease and diabetes, and are receiving multiple medications with nephrotoxic potential. In the community setting, the range of causes of ARF differs with a predominance of prerenal azotemia, ARF associated with pharmacological agents

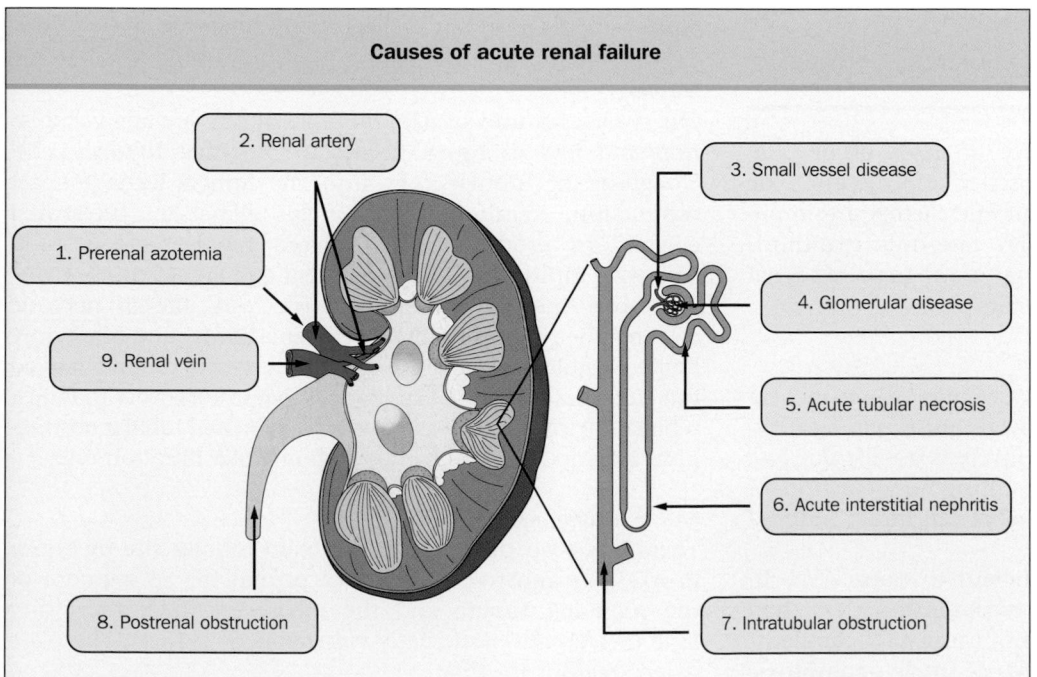

Figure 15.1 Causes of acute renal failure (ARF). ARF is divided into prerenal, renal and postrenal causes. Renal causes of ARF should be considered under the different anatomic components of the kidney (vascular, glomerular, tubular and interstitial disease).

Causes of acute renal failure

2. Renal artery
3. Small vessel disease
1. Prerenal azotemia
4. Glomerular disease
9. Renal vein
5. Acute tubular necrosis
6. Acute interstitial nephritis
8. Postrenal obstruction
7. Intratubular obstruction

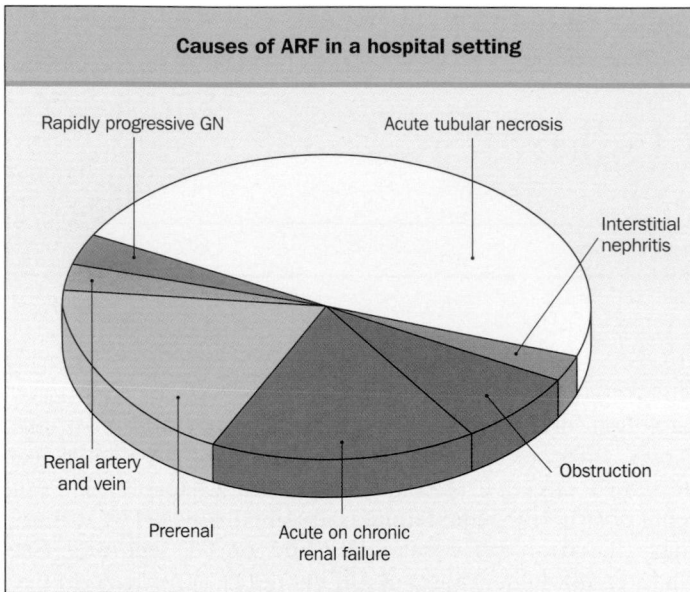

Causes of ARF in a hospital setting

Rapidly progressive GN

Acute tubular necrosis

Interstitial nephritis

Obstruction

Renal artery and vein

Prerenal

Acute on chronic renal failure

Figure 15.2 Causes of ARF in hospital setting[3].

(especially nonsteroidal anti-inflammatory drugs (NSAIDs) and angiotensin-converting enzyme (ACE) inhibitors), and obstructive nephropathy due to prostatic disease in older men.

There are also substantial geographical differences in the causes of ARF. In tropical countries, ATN is also the dominant cause, with hypovolemia caused by diarrheal disease being an important problem, particularly in children. Obstetric ARF remains more common in emerging countries. There are also different patterns of accidental and deliberate self-poisoning. In Africa herbal toxins are a common cause of ARF. Copper sulfate (widely used in the leather industry in India) has been a prominent cause. Severe hemolysis may also occur in malaria, with drugs in association with glucose 6-phosphate dehydrogenase deficiency, and following spider, snake and insect bites.

ACUTE TUBULAR NECROSIS

ATN is responsible for the majority of cases of hospital acquired ARF and is usually due to ischemic or nephrotoxic injury. In the majority of cases, multiple factors are implicated in the etiology. In the intensive care unit, two-thirds of cases of ARF are due to a combination of impaired renal perfusion, sepsis and nephrotoxic agents[2].

Clinical factors implicated in ATN

ATN commonly occurs in high risk settings which include post vascular and cardiac surgery, severe burns, pancreatitis, sepsis and chronic liver disease. The injury is usually due to a combination of ischemic injury resulting in depletion of cellular ATP and direct tubular epithelial cell injury induced by nephrotoxins.

Hypotension alone is rarely sufficient to cause ATN. In animal studies, severe, prolonged hypotension (less than 50 mmHg for 2–3 h in the rat) does not cause ATN. Similarly, animal models require very high doses of single nephrotoxic

agents to induce ARF. These features may reflect an inherent resistance to ATN in animal models, but also illustrate the fact that single insults alone are rarely sufficient to induce ATN.

Fever may exacerbate ATN by increasing renal tubular metabolic rate thereby increasing ATP consumption. In an experimental model (renal artery occlusion in the rat), renal ischemia for 40 min resulted in minimal renal injury at 32°C, but marked ARF at 39.4°C.

The management of ATN consists of optimizing renal hemodynamics, avoidance of nephrotoxins, management of the complications of ARF, judicious use of renal replacement therapy and general supportive care. These issues are discussed in Chapter 14.

Prognosis

The typical course of uncomplicated ATN is recovery over a 2–3-week period. However, superimposed renal insults may alter this pattern. For example, episodes of hypotension induced by dialysis in patients with established ARF can lead to additional ischemic lesions, potentially prolonging renal functional recovery.

Despite the increased ability to support critically ill patients, outcomes for hospital acquired ARF have changed little over the years with mortality in critically ill ARF patients ranging from 46 to 88%. This likely reflects the increasing age and severity of comorbid illnesses in those now treated for ARF. When disease severity and comorbidity are factored in, survival does appear to be improving, probably due to better supportive therapy and critical care.

Among those who survive an episode of ARF in an intensive care unit, approximately 90% of patients will recover independent renal function, albeit often with a degree of residual chronic renal impairment[4].

Pathophysiology of ATN

The pathophysiology of ATN is discussed in some detail as it is the most common cause of ARF and many of the underlying pathogenic features have relevance for other causes.

Histology

The typical features of ATN on renal biopsy include vacuolation and loss of brush border in proximal tubular cells. Sloughing of tubular cells into the lumen leads to cast obstruction, manifested by tubular dilatation. Interstitial edema can produce widely spaced tubules and a mild leukocyte infiltration is often present (see Fig. 15.3).

Despite the term acute tubular 'necrosis', frankly necrotic cells are not a common finding on renal biopsy and often only limited histological evidence of injury is present despite marked functional impairment. This implies that factors other than just tubular cell injury (such as vasoconstriction and tubular obstruction) are important in the loss of glomerular filtration rate.

Site of tubular injury in ATN

There has been debate over the main tubular site of injury in ATN, but most authorities accept that the S3 segment of the proximal tubule and the medullary thick ascending limb (mTAL) are particularly vulnerable (Fig. 15.4). There are several reasons for this:

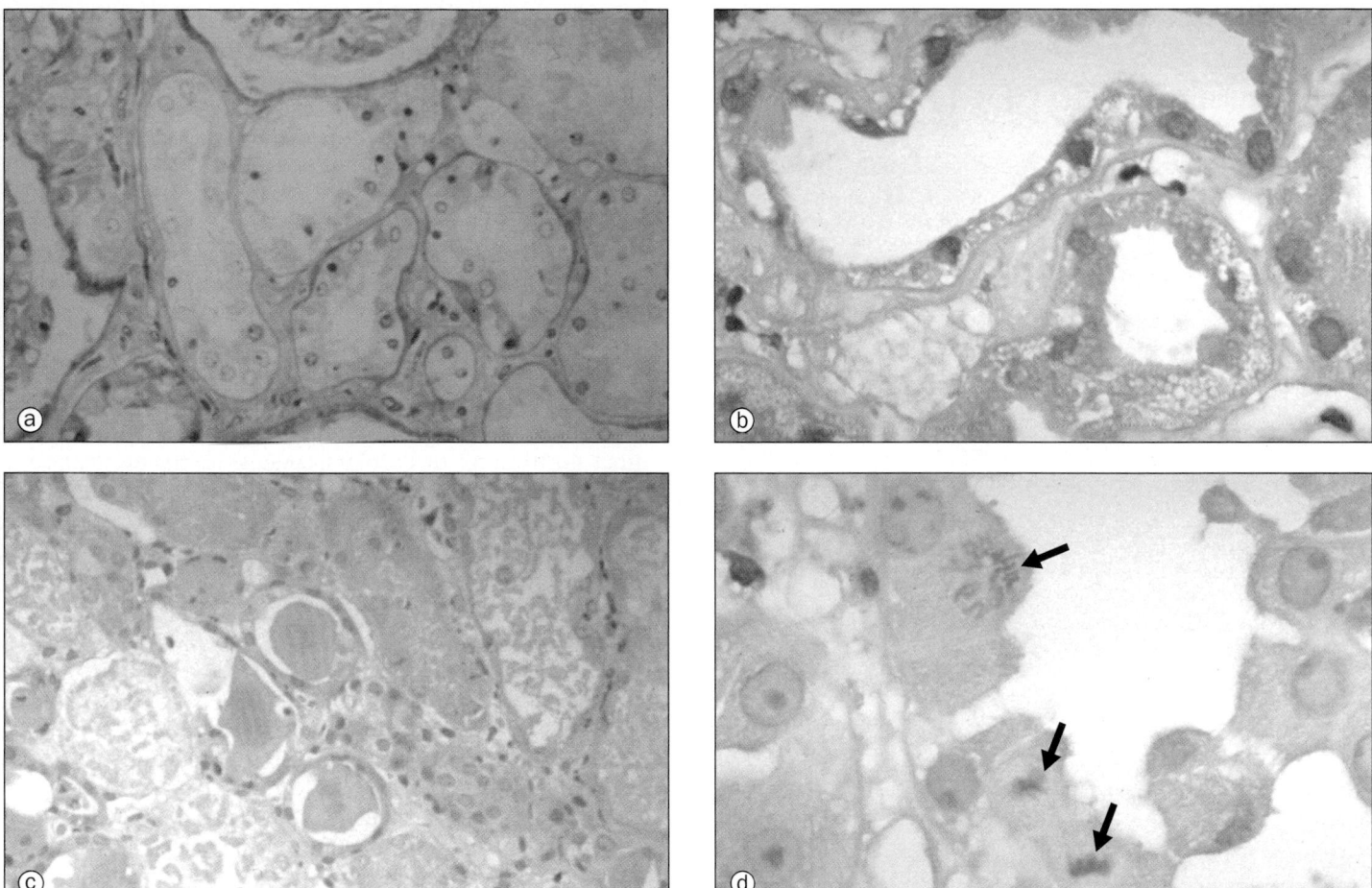

Figure 15.3 Renal pathology in acute tubular necrosis (ATN). (a) Normal cortical renal tubules. (b) ATN: note the flattened epithelium, bare basement membranes and (c) intraluminal cellular debris. (d) Recovering ATN: showing tubular epithelial cell mitotic figures (arrows).

Blood supply

The kidney receives about 25% of cardiac output. Thus, it seems paradoxical that this organ should be sensitive to ischemic or hypoxic injury. Furthermore, there is relatively low oxygen extraction across the kidney (high mixed venous Po_2 in renal veins) suggesting a more than adequate oxygen supply. However, the blood flow to the kidney is not uniform and the majority is directed to the renal cortex for glomerular filtration where the cortical tissue Po_2 is a luxuriant 50–100 mmHg (Fig. 15.4). By contrast, the outer medulla and medullary rays are watershed areas receiving their blood supply from vasa rectae. Countercurrent oxygen exchange occurs leading to a progressive fall in Po_2 from cortex to medulla. This results in medullary cells living on the 'brink of hypoxia' (medullary Po_2 as low as 10–15 mmHg). S3 segment proximal tubule cells and distal medullary thick ascending limbs are thus exposed to borderline chronic oxygen deprivation. Interestingly, chronic renal ischemia (e.g., cyclosporine nephrotoxicity) causes a striped pattern of fibrosis which corresponds to these vulnerable medullary rays.

High tubular energy requirements

The cells of the S3 region and mTAL have high metabolic activity, principally due to sodium reabsorption driven by basolateral membrane Na-K-ATPase. Indeed, blocking sodium reabsorption in the mTAL with loop diuretics raises the medullary tissue Po_2 from ~15 to 35 mmHg. The reduction of GFR in ARF may paradoxically protect the mTAL cells from injury by diminishing sodium filtration and hence sodium reabsorption which decreases ATP consumption.

Glycolytic capacity of tubular cells

Proximal tubular cells have minimal glycolytic machinery and rely almost solely on oxidative phosphorylation for the generation of ATP. In contrast, mTAL cells have a large glycolytic capacity (e.g., due to the presence of hexokinase, phosphofructokinase, pyruvate kinase) and are more resistant to hypoxic or ischemic insults.

Hemodynamic factors in the development of ATN

Intrarenal vasoconstriction

In established ATN, renal blood flow (RBF) is decreased by 30–50%. However, the decrease in GFR is generally > 90%, suggesting that other mechanisms are involved in the reduction in renal function. In addition to the absolute decrease in RBF, there is evidence of a selective reduction in blood supply to the outer medulla. A number of vasoconstrictors have been implicated in the response including angiotensin II,

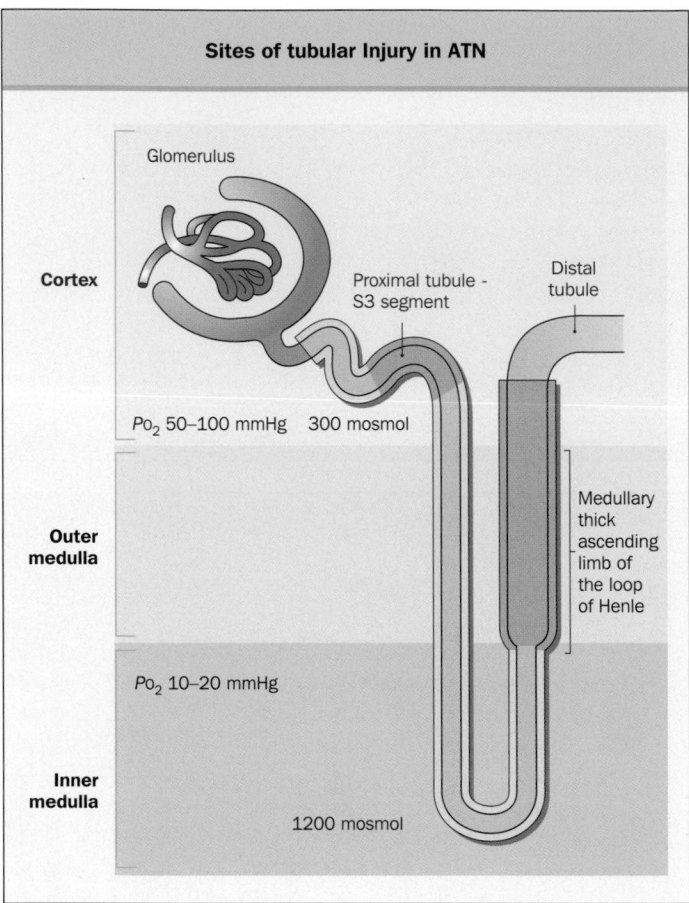

Sites of tubular Injury in ATN

Glomerulus

Cortex

Proximal tubule - S3 segment

Distal tubule

Po_2 50–100 mmHg   300 mosmol

Outer medulla

Medullary thick ascending limb of the loop of Henle

Po_2 10–20 mmHg

Inner medulla

1200 mosmol

Figure 15.4 Sites of tubular injury in ATN. The S3 segment of the proximal tubule and the medullary thick ascending limb are particularly vulnerable to ischemic injury due to the combination of borderline oxygen supply and high metabolic demands.

thromboxane A_2, prostaglandin H_2, leukotrienes C_4 and D_4, endothelin-1, adenosine and sympathetic nerve stimulation (reviewed in 5).

Impaired renal autoregulation

Normally RBF and GFR are maintained over a wide range of renal perfusion pressures, a phenomenon known as autoregulation. A number of factors contribute, including a myogenic response sensed by stretch receptors in the afferent arteriole, tubuloglomerular feedback, and a balance between renal vasodilator and vasoconstrictor influences. In settings of low renal perfusion (e.g., volume depletion, left ventricular failure, edematous states, renal artery stenosis), GFR may be dependent on autoregulation mediated by vasodilatory prostaglandins acting on the afferent arteriole, and angiotensin II mediated efferent arteriolar vasoconstriction to maintain glomerular pressure. Any interference with this mechanism (e.g., by NSAIDs or ACE inhibitors) may produce a precipitous fall in GFR.

Tubuloglomerular feedback (TGF)

This is essentially a protective mechanism to prevent volume depletion when sodium chloride reabsorption is impaired in the proximal nephron[6]. Raised luminal chloride levels are sensed by the macula densa (via the Na-K-2Cl cotransporter) which signals afferent arteriolar vasoconstriction and reduces the GFR. This reaction may be mediated by the local release of adenosine. Additional signals to the juxtaglomerular apparatus increase renin production which increases proximal sodium reabsorption and enhances TGF.

Tubular factors in the development of ATN

Factors which affect the integrity of the renal tubular epithelial cell lining of the nephron also contribute to the reduction in GFR (Fig. 15.5).

Loss of cell polarity

A characteristic feature of many injured cells is the disruption of the cellular actin cytoskeleton leading to alterations in the normal positioning of cellular proteins. In the tubular cell, this loss of polarity results in impaired reabsorption of filtrate in the proximal nephron and tubuloglomerular feedback. It also results in the weakening of cell–cell and cell–matrix adhesions.

Cast obstruction

Tubular cells are attached to the tubular basement membrane by specialized proteins called integrins. The movement of integrins from basolateral positions to the apical membrane results in impaired cell–matrix adhesion and cell detachment. Many of the detached cells are still viable and can be cultured from urine. Integrins recognize RGD (arginine–glycine–aspartate) sequences in matrix proteins. These sequences are present in Tamm–Horsfall protein promoting cast formation leading to intratubular obstruction. In models of ischemic ARF, the elevation in tubular pressure may be inhibited by synthetic RGD peptides which mitigate this obstructive process.

Backleak

The loss of adhesion molecules (E-cadherin) and tight junction proteins (ZO-1, occludin) weakens cells junctions, allowing filtrate to leak back into the renal interstitium. Cellular ATP depletion has recently been shown to disrupt tight junctions and adherens junctions by tyrosine phosphorylation of catenins. Although backleak does not alter the actual GFR, the net effect is a reduction in the measured GFR. In the renal allograft with ATN, backleak has been calculated to account for up to 50% of the reduction in GFR.

Inflammatory factors in the development of ATN

There is increasing evidence that the inflammatory response plays an important role in ATN. Leukocyte infiltration may be seen on renal biopsy and local tissue edema may compromise microvascular blood flow. The infiltrating leukocytes are most commonly neutrophils or macrophages.

Neutrophil activation with the release of proteases and reactive oxygen species can exacerbate injury in experimental ATN. By contrast, neutrophil depletion with antibody, or inhibiting neutrophil adhesion molecules (intracellular adhesion molecule-1; ICAM-1) with antibody or antisense oligonucleotides ameliorates injury in ischemic ATN. ICAM-1 'knockout' mice are similarly protected[7]. T lymphocytes have also been implicated, and CD4-/CD8- 'double knockout' mice are protected from ischemia reperfusion injury[8].

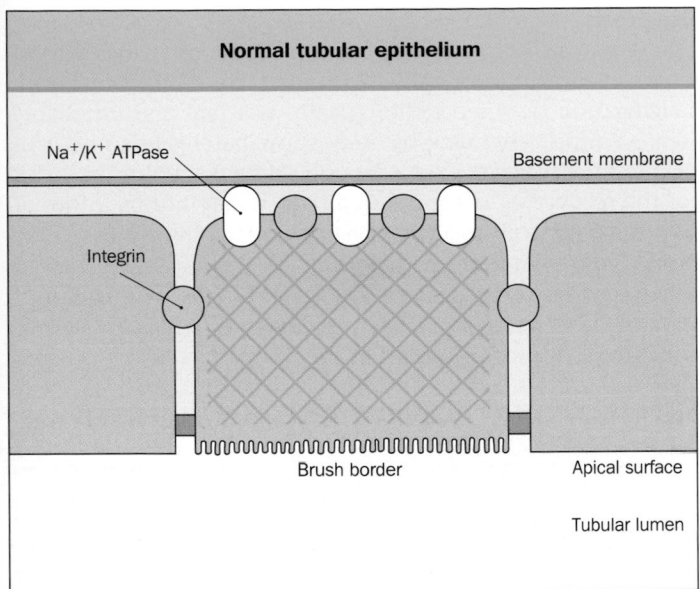

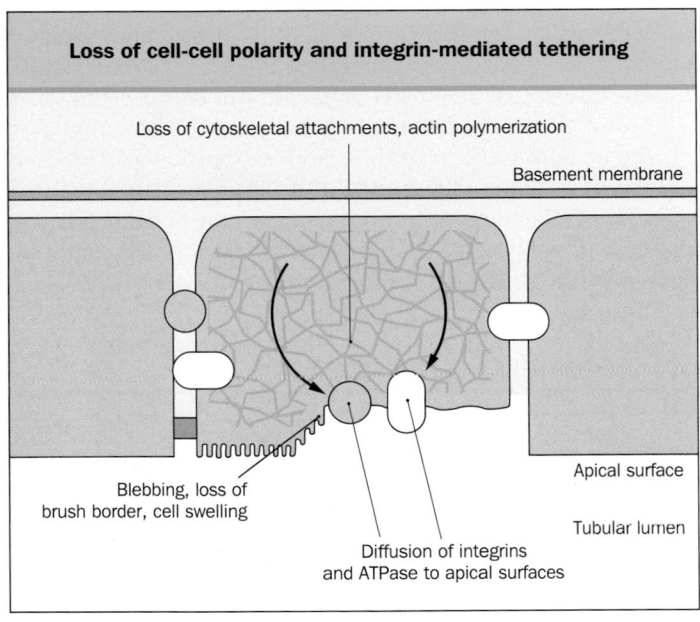

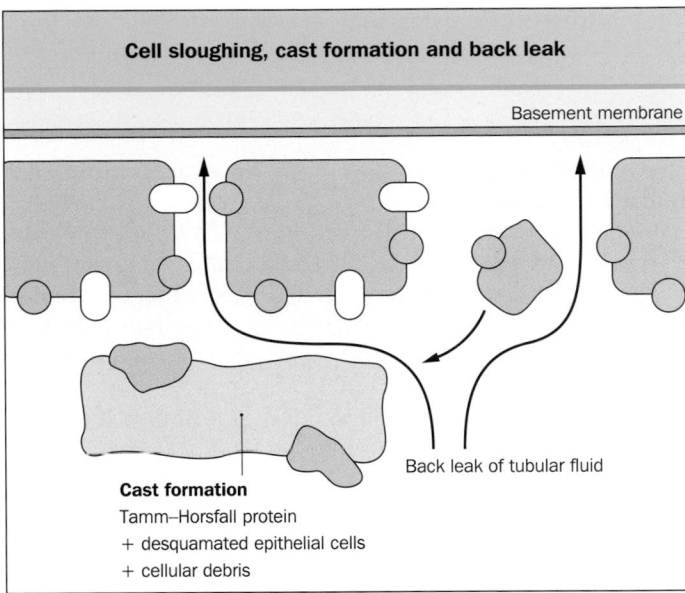

Figure 15.5 Tubular factors in the development of ATN. Loss of cell polarity results in weakening of cell–cell and cell–matrix adhesions resulting in cast obstruction and backleak of tubular fluid.

Calcium influx

Calcium influx is a common feature of cellular injury due to inhibition of Ca^{2+} ATPases in the plasma membrane. Calcium is also released from intracellular sequestration sites (e.g., mitochondria, endoplasmic reticulum). Several injurious processes may result including the calpain activation which degrades cytoskeletal proteins, activation of membrane phospholipases and inhibition of mitochondrial oxidative phosphorylation.

Phospholipase A_2

Activation of phospholipase A_2 leads to the breakdown of membrane phospholipids with diminished membrane integrity. The release of arachidonic acid may be directly toxic to mitochondria or may result in the generation of injurious eicosanoids.

Reactive oxygen species

A large body of evidence is accumulating to implicate reactive oxygen species (ROS) in the cellular injury of acute renal failure[10]. ROS may be derived from local sources (including xanthine oxidase, cyclo-oxygenases and secondary to mitochondrial injury) or from infiltrating leukocytes. In models of ischemic ATN, inhibition of ROS protects against renal injury. Interventions used include xanthine oxidase inhibitors (allopurinol), superoxide scavengers, hydroxyl radical scavengers (dimethlythiourea); thiol donors (N-acetylcysteine) and inhibitors of lipid peroxidation. Similarly, transgenic mice overproducing glutathione peroxidases are protected against ischemic injury.

Nitric oxide

This molecule has complex roles in ARF and may have beneficial properties including vasodilatation. However, hypoxia and cytokines stimulate inducible nitric oxide synthetase and

Mediators of tubular cell injury

At the level of the tubular cell, injury may be due to ischemia with resulting depletion of cellular energy stores (ATP) or direct cytotoxic injury. Following acute renal ischemia, much of the tubular cell injury may occur following the restoration of renal blood flow (reperfusion injury). Despite the term acute tubular 'necrosis', it is only a minority of cells that are lethally injured and many of these cells may die by apoptosis not necrosis[9]. Indeed, caspase inhibitors (which impair apoptosis) have been shown to protect against hypoxic injury in isolated proximal tubular cells.

There are several cellular factors mediating cell injury.

Cell swelling

ATP depletion inhibits Na-K-ATPase activity impairing cellular sodium export. The ensuing cell swelling may lead to cell membrane damage and tissue edema may inhibit local blood flow following relief of ischemia.

the resulting nitric oxide may combine with ROS to form the toxic peroxynitrite (OONO⁻). The value of inhibiting or augmenting NO in ATN has still to be clarified[11].

Complement

The complement system has been implicated in tubular epithelial cell injury possibly due to a direct toxic role of C5b–9. In keeping with this hypothesis, C3, C5, C6 (but not C4) deficient mice are protected against ischemic injury[12].

By contrast, there is experimental evidence that cells which have been sublethally injured may be more resistant to further injury. This 'acquired cytoresistance' may be to an enhanced protective mechanisms including the upregulation of heat shock proteins, antioxidant responses and proximal tubular cell membrane cholesterol accumulation.

Recovery phase

Tubular epithelial cells are normally highly differentiated and restoration of tubular cell number requires the dedifferentiation of surviving cells and cellular proliferation. A marked increase in proliferation occurs in human ATN and mitotic figures may be seen on histology (Fig. 15.3).

A number of growth factors have been implicated in the proliferative response[13], in particular insulin-like growth factor-1 (IGF-1). However, a therapeutic trial of subcutaneous recombinant IGF-1 in critically ill patients failed to show an acceleration in renal functional recovery[14].

Following tubular epithelial cell proliferation, the cells must migrate to areas of denuded tubular basement membrane, attach to the basement membrane and differentiate into mature polar tubular epithelial cells.

CORTICAL NECROSIS

A minority of patients who are subject to the same pathophysiologic processes do not develop ATN but instead develop acute cortical necrosis. If there is extensive cortical necrosis, renal failure is irreversible. More commonly, cortical necrosis is patchy and there may be partial recovery of renal function.

In cortical necrosis, there is microvascular thrombosis, including glomerular thrombosis, with extensive death of renal tissue. However, the process is distinct from that seen with infarction caused by arterial occlusion since some blood supply to the medulla is preserved. It appears it is not the severity of shock that predicts the risk of cortical necrosis but rather the type of shock. Cortical necrosis was formerly common in pregnancy, particularly following placental abruption. As these complications recede in importance, endotoxemia and disseminated intravascular coagulation become increasingly common predictors of the risk of cortical necrosis, although even in these settings, most patients will still develop ATN not cortical necrosis. Children are more susceptible to cortical necrosis than adults following severe volume depletion with gastroenteritis or in association with peritonitis or septicemia. Cortical necrosis may also follow thrombotic microangiopathy and snake bites where the venom may be directly toxic or produce its effects via hemorrhage or intravascular hemolysis.

Diagnosis

The diagnosis of cortical necrosis is most often considered when recovery from ARF attributed to ATN is delayed. Calcification detected radiologically is a late and unreliable sign. Contrast angiography may show patchy loss of perfusion but the contrast load is an unacceptable nephrotoxic risk for the recovering kidney. Renal biopsy may not be informative since cortical necrosis is patchy and a biopsy core may not be representative. In practice, it is usually necessary to continue renal replacement therapy and discover in hindsight whether there is sufficient recovery of renal function to conclude that most if not all of the injury was ATN.

NEPHROTOXIC AGENTS AND MECHANISMS OF NEPHROTOXICITY

The identification and avoidance of nephrotoxic agents in acute renal failure is critical in the management as ARF may be rapidly reversible with removal of the offending agent. Many nephrotoxins are tubular cell toxins and combine with ischemia to increase the risk of ATN. The range of other mechanisms of nephrotoxicity is very broad and include alterations in renal hemodynamics, allergic reactions resulting in interstitial nephritis and intratubular obstruction. Nephrotoxins may be both endogenous, for example myoglobin, hemoglobin and bilirubin, and exogenous, particularly radiocontrast and a wide range of drugs. The list of nephrotoxic agents is extensive but the more common are presented in Figure 15.6. The three commonest classes of drugs implicated in ARF are NSAIDs, ACE inhibitors and aminoglycoside antibiotics.

HEME PIGMENT NEPHROPATHY

Heme pigment nephropathy is a common cause of ARF and has been implicated in 10–15% of hospitalized patients with ARF in the USA[15]. The condition is usually secondary to the breakdown of muscle fibers (rhabdomyolysis) which release potentially nephrotoxic intracellular contents (particularly myoglobin) into the systemic circulation. Less commonly, heme pigment nephropathy may occur due to massive intravascular hemolysis.

Clinical features of heme pigment ARF

Heme pigment nephropathy typically presents with oliguric ARF following muscle injury, but it should be recognized that rhabdomyolysis may occur without ARF. Large amounts of fluid may be sequestered in injured muscle and volume depletion is prominent. Blood pressure may be preserved despite marked volume depletion due to the scavenging effect of myoglobin on nitric oxide. The injured muscle may not be clinically apparent on examination and muscle pain may be absent. In limb muscles confined to rigid compartments, cell swelling following injury may result in increased intracompartmental pressures impairing local microvascular circulation (Fig. 15.7).

Creatinine kinase is usually > 10 000 U/mL, although levels correspond poorly with the severity of renal failure. The release of other cellular constituents may produce hyperkalemia,

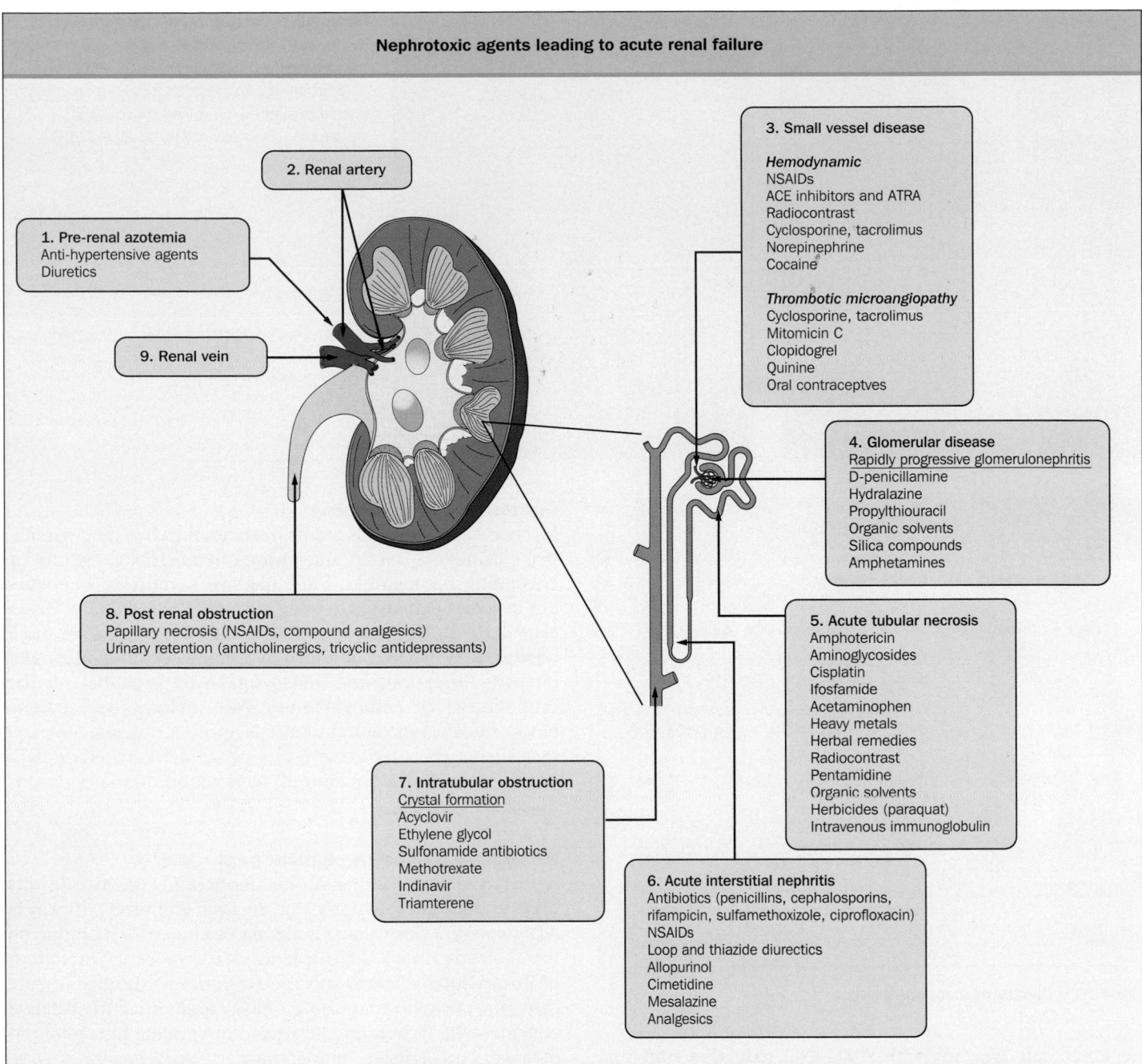

Nephrotoxic agents leading to acute renal failure

3. Small vessel disease

Hemodynamic
NSAIDs
ACE inhibitors and ATRA
Radiocontrast
Cyclosporine, tacrolimus
Norepinephrine
Cocaine

Thrombotic microangiopathy
Cyclosporine, tacrolimus
Mitomicin C
Clopidogrel
Quinine
Oral contraceptves

2. Renal artery

1. Pre-renal azotemia
Anti-hypertensive agents
Diuretics

9. Renal vein

4. Glomerular disease
Rapidly progressive glomerulonephritis
D-penicillamine
Hydralazine
Propylthiouracil
Organic solvents
Silica compounds
Amphetamines

8. Post renal obstruction
Papillary necrosis (NSAIDs, compound analgesics)
Urinary retention (anticholinergics, tricyclic antidepressants)

5. Acute tubular necrosis
Amphotericin
Aminoglycosides
Cisplatin
Ifosfamide
Acetaminophen
Heavy metals
Herbal remedies
Radiocontrast
Pentamidine
Organic solvents
Herbicides (paraquat)
Intravenous immunoglobulin

7. Intratubular obstruction
Crystal formation
Acyclovir
Ethylene glycol
Sulfonamide antibiotics
Methotrexate
Indinavir
Triamterene

6. Acute interstitial nephritis
Antibiotics (penicillins, cephalosporins,
rifampicin, sulfamethoxizole, ciprofloxacin)
NSAIDs
Loop and thiazide diurectics
Allopurinol
Cimetidine
Mesalazine
Analgesics

Figure 15.6 Common nephrotoxic agents leading to ARF.

hyperphosphatemia and hyperuricemia. Lactic acidosis may follow anerobic muscle metabolism. Hypocalcemia is typical in the acute stage due to calcium phosphate deposition in injured muscle, whilst hypercalcemia commonly occurs in the recovery phase as deposited calcium is mobilized from muscle.

Myoglobin is freely filtered and causes a red-brown discoloration of the urine and a positive dipstick urinalysis for heme. Urine microscopy reveals multiple pigmented casts. The absence of red cells with a positive urinalysis for heme implies myoglobinuria or hemoglobinuria. The finding of urine myoglobin is nonspecific as this test may be positive with only minor muscle injury. Fractional excretion of sodium is usually low due to volume depletion and renal vasoconstriction.

Causes of rhabdomyolysis

Muscle trauma is the commonest cause of rhabdomyolysis. The initial description was by Bywaters and Beall during the bombing of London in World War II[16]. Other common causes of muscle injury include seizures, pressure necrosis secondary to coma, alcohol abuse and limb ischemia (Table 15.1).

In the patient with alcohol abuse, rhabdomyolysis is often multifactorial due to pressure necrosis from coma ('found down'), direct myotoxicity from ethanol, electrolyte abnormalities (hypokalemia and hypophosphatemia) and seizures. With excessive exercise or seizures, ATP depletion from excessive metabolic activity may cause muscle injury. Muscle hyperthermia may potentiate injury by increasing the

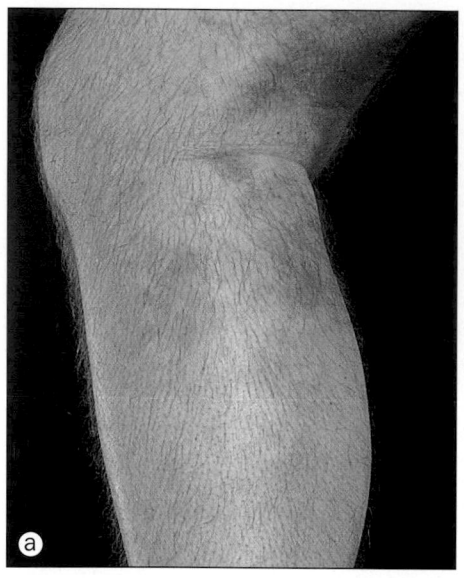

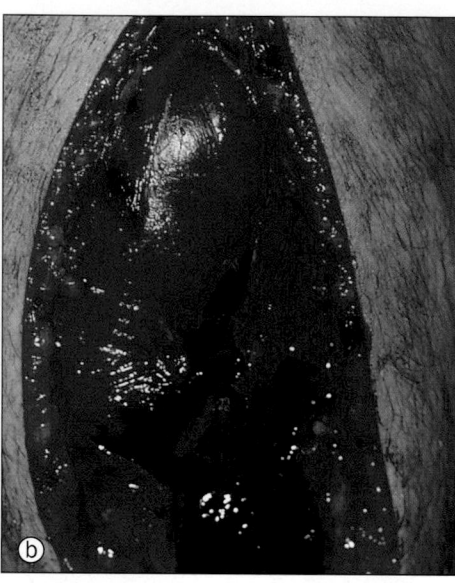

Figure 15.7 Compartment syndrome. (a) Severe calf swelling due to anterior and posterior compartment syndromes following ischemia-reperfusion. (b) Appearance following emergency fasciotomy: note edematous muscle and hematoma. (Courtesy of Mr. MJ Allen FRCS.)

Causes of rhabdomyolysis

Muscle injury/ischemia	Trauma; pressure necrosis; electric shock; burns; acute vascular disease
Myofiber exhaustion	Seizures; excessive exercise; heat exhaustion
Toxins	Alcohol; cocaine; heroin; amphetamines; Ecstasy; phencyclidine; snake bite
Drugs	Statins; fibrates; zidovudine; neuroleptic malignant syndrome; azathioprine; theophylline; lithium; diuretics
Electrolyte disorders	Hypophosphatemia; hypokalemia; excess water shifts (hyperosmolality)
Infections	Viral (influenza, HIV, Coxackie, Epstein–Barr virus); bacterial (*Legionella, Francisella, Strep. pneumoniae, Salmonella, Staph. aureus*)
Familial	McArdle's disease; carnitine palmitoyl transferase deficiency; malignant hyperthermia
Other	Hypothyroidism; polymyositis; dermatomyositis

Table 15.1 Causes of rhabdomyolysis.

metabolic rate. Therapy with HMG-CoA reductase inhibitors ('statins') may be associated with rhabdomyolysis. The risk is increased by concomitant therapy with fibrates, cyclosporine or erythromycin.

Electrolyte abnormalities may precipitate rhabdomyolysis. Hypophosphatemia may impair ATP production and hypokalemia may inhibit glycogen synthesis. Additionally, potassium is an important vasodilator in the muscle microcirculation. Hypokalemia may inhibit the hyperemia of exercising muscle and exacerbate ischemia. The release of potassium and phosphate from damaged cells may obscure these underlying causes of rhabdomyolysis. Familial myopathies are uncommon and usually due to inherited abnormalities of carbohydrate or lipid metabolism. They should be suspected in patients with a history of recurrent episodes of muscle pain, positive family history, onset in childhood and the absence of other identifiable causes[17].

Causes of hemoglobinuria

Intravascular hemolysis results in circulating free hemoglobin. If the hemolysis is mild, the released hemoglobin is bound by circulating haptoglobin. With massive hemolysis, haptoglobin becomes exhausted, hemoglobin (MW 69 000 kDa) dissociates into alpha–beta dimers (MW 34 kDa), which are small enough to be filtered, resulting in hemoglobinuria, hemoglobin cast formation, and heme uptake by proximal tubular cells. Causes of hemoglobinuric ARF include incompatible blood transfusion, autoimmune hemolytic anemia, malaria (Blackwater fever), glucose 6-phosphate dehydrogenase deficiency, paroxysmal nocturnal hemoglobinuria and toxins (dapsone, venoms).

Pathogenesis of heme pigment nephropathy

A variety of environmental, metabolic and infective insults may produce muscle injury, but the final common pathway is ATP depletion from tissue ischemia or altered ATP producing metabolic pathways. ATP depletion leads to the accumulation of intracellular calcium and the activation of proteases (e.g., calpain), phospholipases (e.g., PLA$_2$) and other degradative enzymes which cause myofibril and membrane phospholipid damage. Furthermore, mitochondrial injury generates large amounts of oxygen free radicals, culminating in oxidative tissue stress. During the period of tissue ischemia, cell viability may be maintained by limited calcium delivery, decreased production of oxidative radicals by mitochondria due to oxygen deprivation, and the protective effect of local acidosis. Reperfusion removes these protective mechanisms and much of the cellular damage occurs not during the ischemic period but following the restoration of blood flow (reperfusion injury). It is also during this time that myoglobin gains access to the systemic circulation and fluid sequestration in injured muscle occurs which can lead to intravascular volume contraction.

The renal injury is due to a combination of factors including volume depletion, renal vasoconstriction, direct heme-protein mediated cytotoxicity and intraluminal cast formation (Fig. 15.8). Volume depletion is often prominent due to sequestration

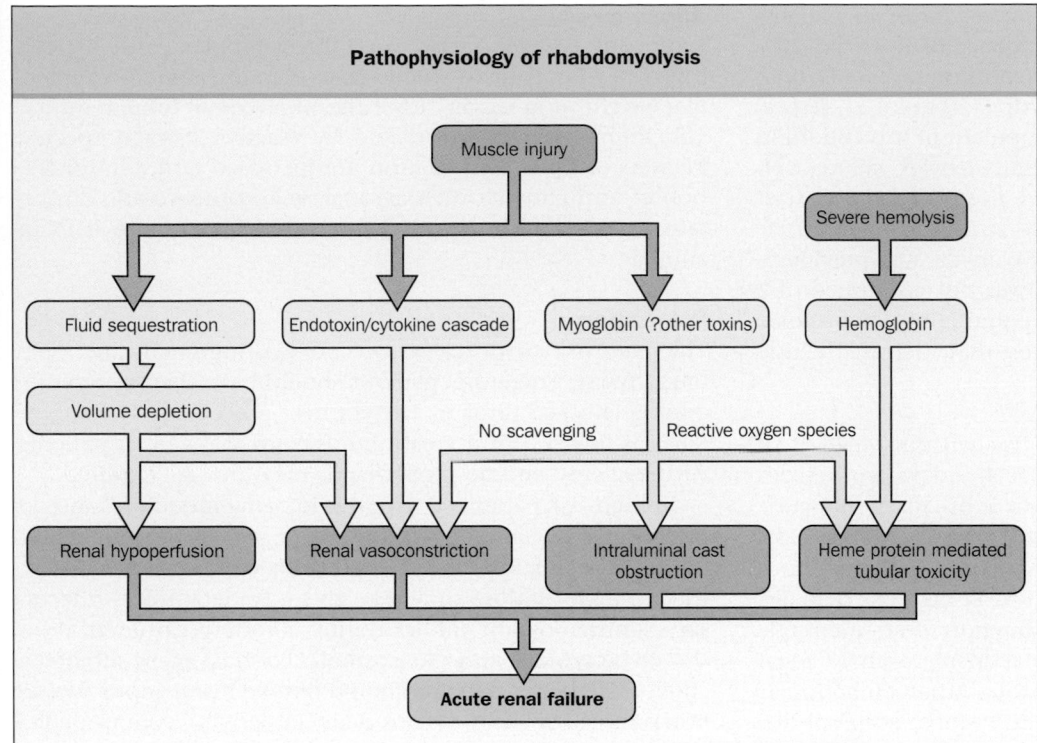

Pathophysiology of rhabdomyolysis

Figure 15.8 Pathophysiology of rhabdomyolysis. Renal impairment is due to multiple factors including volume depletion, renal vasoconstriction, direct tubular cell toxicity and intraluminal obstructing casts.

of large amounts of fluid (up to 15–20 L) in injured muscle. Volume depletion activates the sympathetic nervous system and renin–angiotensin system resulting in renal vasoconstriction, which may be exacerbated by the scavenging of nitric oxide by circulating heme proteins. Other vasoconstrictors such as endothelin and thromboxane A_2 may be involved. Activation of the endotoxin cytokine cascade has also been described due to intestinal ischemia.

Myoglobin (MW 17 kDa) is freely filtered at the glomerulus and is toxic to tubular epithelial cells. The heme center of myoglobin may directly induce lipid peroxidation and renal injury[18] and liberated free iron catalyzes the formation of hydroxyl radical by the Fenton reaction causing free radical induced injury. Mitochondria may be the principal site of heme protein free radical generation; free iron scavengers and various antioxidants are renoprotective in animal models.

Finally, the precipitation of myoglobin with Tamm–Horsfall protein and sloughed proximal tubular cells result in obstructing casts in the distal nephron. This is enhanced by increased concentrations of tubular heme protein due to volume depletion with low tubular fluid flow rates. The binding of heme protein to Tamm–Horsfall protein is enhanced in an acid urine.

Prevention and treatment

The key to the management of heme pigment nephropathy is early preventive therapy. Aggressive volume repletion should be begun as soon as possible. Large amounts of extracellular fluid may be sequestered in injured muscle and a typical regimen would be intravenous normal saline initially at 1–1.5 L/h, aiming for a urine output of 300 mL/h. Ten to 12 L may be required in the first 24 h with crush injuries[19]. Swelling of injured muscle may produce a compartment syndrome with impaired local tissue perfusion. Urgent fasciotomy may

be required when intracompartment pressures exceed 40 mmHg (Fig. 15.7).

In order to minimize heme protein toxicity an alkaline mannitol diuresis may be considered, but only when the urine output is sufficient to prevent bicarbonate and mannitol accumulation in serum. Alkalinization inhibits cast formation, and mannitol promotes an osmotic diuresis, increasing tubular fluid flow rates, thereby washing out obstructing casts. It has been hypothesized that mannitol can also scavenge hydroxyl radical, a presumed mediator of heme nephrotoxicity. Half normal saline containing 75 mmol/L $NaHCO_3$ may be used for intravenous fluid replacement aiming for a urine pH greater than 6.5 with a 15% mannitol infusion at 10 mL/h. Care must be taken to avoid a $NaHCO_3$-induced decrease in ionized calcium (due to metabolic alkalosis), which can trigger seizures and worsen existing muscle damage. An alkaline diuresis is ineffective if the patient already has established ARF and accumulation of mannitol in this setting may be deleterious, actually exacerbating renal injury.

Prolonged hemodialysis may be required to control the metabolic abnormalities of hyperkalemia and hyperphosphatemia. Serum potassium should be carefully monitored as rebound hyperkalemia may occur several hours after completion of a hemodialysis session. Hypocalcemia is often present during early stages, however, overtreatment of this may result in hypercalcemia in the recovery period due to the recycling of trapped calcium.

RADIOCONTRAST INDUCED NEPHROPATHY

Acute renal failure secondary to radiocontrast induced nephropathy (RCIN) is a well recognized complication of radiological procedures[20]. It typically occurs in patients with underlying renal impairment and is rarely seen in patients with normal renal function. The incidence of RCIN is ~20% and 50% in patients with a serum creatinine of greater than 2.0 mg/dL (180 µmol/L) and 5.0 mg/dL (450 µmol/L), respectively. Other risk factors for the development of this condition include diabetic nephropathy, congestive heart failure, volume depletion and high or repetitive doses of radiocontrast agent. High osmolar contrast agents are more nephrotoxic than low osmolar contrast agents. Myeloma was previously thought to be a risk factor but this was not confirmed in a recent study. Concurrent use of potentially nephrotoxic agents such as NSAIDs or ACE inhibitors may increase the risk.

Clinical features

Typically the creatinine begins to rise within 24–48 h of radiocontrast administration, peaks at 4–5 days and returns to baseline over 7–10 days. The patient is usually nonoliguric and examination of the urine sediment reveals granular casts and some tubular epithelial cells. Underlying atheromatous renovascular disease is common in those at high risk of RCIN. Failure to recover to baseline renal function after an episode of RCIN suggests an additional renal insult such as renal atheroembolism, sepsis or hypotension. Atheroembolism is suggested by the presence of embolic lesions, eosinophilia, and hypocomplementemia.

Pathogenesis

An alteration in renal hemodynamics leading to medullary hypoxia and direct tubular epithelial cell toxicity are the main factors in the pathogenesis of RCIN.

Altered renal hemodynamics

Typically a biphasic hemodynamic response is seen. An initial vasodilatation (lasting a few seconds to minutes) is followed by a more prolonged renal vasoconstriction. The consequent medullary hypoxia may be exacerbated by the osmotic diuresis leading to increased sodium delivery to the mTAL requiring greater O_2 consumption for reabsorption. The increased delivery of chloride to the macula densa activates tubuloglomerular feedback.

Alterations in the balance of renal vasoconstrictors and vasodilators mediates the renal hemodynamic changes. Vasoconstrictors include the renin angiotensin system, sympathetic nervous system, endothelin, and adenosine. Serum endothelin levels have been shown to increase within a few minutes of radiocontrast injection and persist for hours. In animal models, antagonism of the ET_A receptor prevented the decrease in renal blood flow and GFR, however, in a human study, a mixed ET_A and ET_B receptor antagonist was shown to exacerbate injury[21]. Adenosine acts as a vasoconstrictor in the renal circulation and is known to participate in tubuloglomerular feedback. Urinary levels of adenosine are increased by radiocontrast agents and adenosine antagonists have been shown to reduce nephrotoxicity in human studies[22]. Dipyridamole, an adenosine reuptake inhibitor, may exacerbate radiocontrast-mediated vasoconstriction. RCIN may also be exacerbated by impaired action of renal vasodilators: for example, nitric oxide inhibition and NSAIDs, which inhibit vasodilatory prostaglandins.

Tubular toxicity

Radiocontrast agents also cause direct tubular epithelial cell injury *in vitro*. Human studies have demonstrated low molecular weight proteinuria, suggestive of proximal tubular injury. The injury is partly mediated by reactive oxygen species. Markers of lipid peroxidation are increased and administration of antioxidants such as catalase and superoxide dismutase, or iron chelation with deferoxamine ameliorate RCIN in animals.

Prevention

The main risk factor for RCIN is pre-existing renal functional impairment. Therefore, patients should have their serum creatinine checked prior to any contrast procedure. The risk of RCIN is low if serum creatinine is normal (even in patients with diabetes) and no prophylactic measures are required.

In high-risk patients alternative imaging modalities should be considered. Gadolinium and other agents for magnetic resonance imaging appear non-nephrotoxic. If contrast must be used, the lowest dose should be given. For example, unnecessary ventriculogram studies during coronary catheterization should be avoided and a low osmolar contrast agent should be chosen. High-risk patients should receive intravenous hydration prior to the study to correct any underlying volume depletion and maintain urine flow rates (typically, half-normal saline at 100 mL/h for 12 h before and 12 h post procedure is recommended). Loop diuretics and mannitol have been shown to exacerbate RCIN[23].

Although vasodilators appear an attractive preventative therapy, they may cause systemic hypotension and exacerbate disease. Oral theophylline, an adenosine antagonist, can be considered to counteract the renal vasoconstriction. One study showed a benefit with oral theophylline (2.88 mg/kg q12h) for 48 h starting 1 h prior to procedure[22]. Protection has also been shown with *N*-acetylcysteine, a thiol containing antioxidant, given orally 600 mg q12h for 48 h commencing the day before the procedure, in addition to half-normal saline[24].

It should be noted that although a hemodialysis session can remove 80–90% of the radiocontrast dose, there appears to be no clinical benefit from immediate hemodialysis in preventing RCIN. However, patients with end-stage renal disease who are at risk of pulmonary edema from the large osmolal load may require urgent ultrafiltration.

NEPHROTOXIC DRUGS

Nonsteroidal anti-inflammatory drugs

NSAIDs are a common cause of ARF in the community due to the huge numbers of these drugs either prescribed or taken 'over the counter'. ARF may be due to a hemodynamically mediated reduction in GFR, acute tubular necrosis, an acute interstitial nephritis or rarely papillary necrosis[25]. The newer cyclo-oxygenase-2 (COX-2)-specific NSAIDs are not significantly less nephrotoxic[26].

Hemodynamically mediated ARF due to impaired renal autoregulation is discussed further in Chapter 14. This form of ARF is usually reversible in 2–7 days upon discontinuation of the drug. NSAIDs may also cause an acute interstitial nephritis, often with a subacute presentation, and typically with white cells and white cell casts in the urine. Approximately 85% of these patients will also have heavy proteinuria, due to coincident minimal change disease. Possibly due to the anti-inflammatory effects of these drugs, other typical features of acute interstitial nephritis, such as rash, fever and eosinophilia are often absent.

Other renal side effects of NSAIDs include sodium retention exacerbating hypertension and congestive heart failure, hyponatremia and hyperkalemia.

Angiotensin-converting enzyme inhibitors
ACE inhibitors may also cause a hemodynamically induced ARF in the setting of reduced renal perfusion due to impaired vasoconstriction of the efferent arteriole[27]. Angiotensin II receptor antagonists (ATRA) will cause ARF by the same mechanism. ACE inhibitors may also directly impair renal perfusion by their antihypertensive effects.

Aminoglycosides
Clinical features
Nonoliguric ARF usually occurs following 5–10 days of treatment. Involvement of distal tubular segments may produce polyuria and magnesium wasting. The risk of ARF correlates with the accumulation of aminoglycoside in proximal tubular cells, and is related to the daily dose, and duration of therapy. Prolonged accumulation in proximal tubular cells may allow development of ARF even after the drug has been discontinued. Renal biopsy may reveal ATN with coarse vacuolization in proximal tubular cells. Risk factors for aminoglycoside toxicity include increasing age, pre-existing renal disease, hypotension, concurrent liver disease, sepsis syndrome and concurrent nephrotoxins.

Pathogenesis
The nephrotoxicity of aminoglycosides has been best characterized for gentamicin, which is a polar drug with a small volume of distribution limited to the extracellular volume. It is excreted by glomerular filtration, cationic amino groups (NH_3^+) on the drug bind to anionic megalin on the brush border of proximal tubular epithelial cells and the drug is then internalized by endocytosis. The drug accumulates in proximal tubular cell lyzosomes and can reach 100–1000 times its serum concentration. The drug interferes with cellular energetics, impairs intracellular phospholipases, and induces oxidative stress, however, the exact pathways culminating in tubular necrosis remain unclear[28].

Prevention
Gentamicin serum levels should be monitored carefully to minimize nephrotoxicity. When possible, the drug may be administered in a single daily total dose, which leads to lower renal proximal tubular cell accumulation. Gentamicin, tobramycin and netilmicin appear to have similar nephrotoxic effects. However, amikacin which has fewer amino groups per molecule may be less nephrotoxic.

Amphotericin B
Clinical features
Early signs of nephrotoxicity include a loss of urine concentrating ability, followed by a decrease in GFR. Hypokalemia, hypomagnesemia and acidosis due to distal tubular toxicity are common. Nephrotoxicity relates to cumulative dosage, usually occurring after administration of 2–3 g.

Pathogenesis
Amphotericin B binds to sterols in the cell membranes of both fungal walls (ergosterol) and mammalian (cholesterol) cell membranes resulting in the formation of aqueous pores which increase membrane permeability. The increased sodium influx leads to increased Na-K-ATPase activity and depletion of cellular energy stores. Additionally, the standard amphotericin B formulation is suspended in the bile salt deoxycholate which has a detergent effect on cell membranes[29].

Prevention
Prevention of nephrotoxicity requires the maintenance of high urine flow rates by saline loading during amphotericin administration. Liposomal amphotericin preparations have less intrinsic nephrotoxicity. The binding of amphotericin B to ergosterol is more avid than to cholesterol and by delivering the drug as a cholesterol liposome, diminished binding to tubular epithelial cell membranes result without altering fungal binding. Additionally, liposomal preparations do not contain deoxycholate and studies have suggested this may account for much of the diminished toxicity of these agents. These compounds, however, are much more expensive than standard amphotericin B and at present are only recommended for those with a high risk of renal failure. Amphotericin B-induced ARF is usually reversible with discontinuing treatment, although distal injury manifest by magnesium wasting may persist.

Pentamidine
Pentamidine, used to treat *Pneumocystis carinii* infection in immunosuppressed patients, is associated with ATN in 25% of cases when used intravenously. Pentamidine also has an amiloride-like effect on the cortical collecting tubule and hyperkalemia is prominent. Magnesium wasting is also common. Risk of nephrotoxicity is enhanced by volume depletion and by the concomitant use of other nephrotoxic agents, such as aminoglycosides, amphotericin B and foscarnet, which may be necessary in AIDS patients with multiple opportunistic infections

Antiviral therapy
Acyclovir
Nephrotoxicity is typically seen following intravenous administration and may be due to the formation of intratubular acyclovir crystals, seen as birefringent needle shaped crystals on urine microscopy. However, crystals may also be seen without ARF patients and an acute interstitial nephritis may be the predominant mechanism of toxicity.

Oliguric ARF typically occurs within a few days of treatment and may be associated with abdominal or loin pain. High serum levels of acyclovir due to decreased renal clearance may also produce neurological toxicity. The ARF is usually mild and recovers on stopping the drug.

Foscarnet
This drug is a phosphate analog which inhibits proximal phosphate reabsorption. It is used in the treatment of severe

cytomegalovirus infection. ARF occurs in 10–20% of treated patients and may be due to an acute interstitial nephritis or intratubular crystal obstruction. The ARF is usually nonoliguric and associated with mild proteinuria (< 1 g) and a benign urine sediment. There may be hypocalcemia due to chelation of calcium. The renal failure is usually reversible although recovery may take several months.

Other antiviral agents

Most other antiviral agents are not nephrotoxic. In the treatment of hepatitis C, there have been rare reports of acute renal failure secondary to interferon-α. Although not nephrotoxic, doses of ribavirin must be reduced in patients with impaired renal function.

Acetaminophen (paracetamol)
Clinical features

Although isolated renal injury may occur, ARF secondary to acetaminophen toxicity is typically associated with acute hepatocellular injury. Renal and liver toxicity usually occur when > 15 g have been taken, but in alcoholics, normal doses may be toxic. Clinical manifestations usually present 3–4 days following ingestion. Renal impairment is due to acute tubular necrosis.

Pathogenesis

Acetaminophen is conjugated in the liver and undergoes renal excretion. Less than 5% undergoes metabolism by P-450 (CYP2E1) enzymes to form a toxic metabolite, N-acetylimidoquinone, which is inactivated by the thiol group of glutathione. With high levels of acetaminophen, glutathione becomes depleted and N-acetylimidoquinone can bind to thiol groups on intracellular proteins resulting in cell injury. Liver and renal injury only begin once glutathione levels are depleted.

Prevention

N-acetylcysteine administration can be protective, if administered early, as it provides a free thiol group, substituting for glutathione.

Immunosuppressive agents (see Chapter 85)
Calcineurin inhibitors

Both cyclosporine and tacrolimus may cause acute renal impairment due to afferent arteriolar vasoconstriction partly mediated by endothelin. This is usually reversible upon dose reduction. Persistent injury may lead to chronic interstitial fibrosis in a striped pattern along medullary rays reflecting the ischemic nature of the insult. Associated clinical features may include hypertension, hyperkalemia and wasting of phosphate and magnesium from tubular injury. Calcineurin inhibitors may also cause endothelial injury leading to thrombotic microangiopathy, which may be poorly reversible.

Other immunosuppressive agents

The monoclonal anti-CD3 antibody (OKT3) or polyclonal antilymphocyte preparations (ALG, ATG) may cause a first dose cytokine release syndrome and prerenal azotemia secondary to capillary leak. OKT3 has rarely been associated with thrombotic microangiopathy. Intravenous immunoglobulin can cause ARF which may be partly mediated by the high sucrose concentration in these products. The latter is thought to induce tubular cell swelling, resulting in luminal occlusion. Methotrexate is toxic to proximal tubular epithelial cells and rarely may cause intratubular crystal obstruction.

Chemotherapeutic agents
Cisplatin

Cisplatin is commonly associated with nonoliguric ARF. Nephrotoxic injury affects both the proximal and distal nephron and clinically may be associated with magnesium wasting. Chloride ions in the *cis* position on the molecule may be replaced by water, releasing toxic hydroxyl radicals. Prophylaxis against nephrotoxicity includes volume loading, possibly with hypertonic saline, and the use of the antioxidant amifostine as a thiol donor. The alternative agent carboplatin appears to be less nephrotoxic. Once renal impairment is present, recovery may be poor and magnesium wasting may persist.

Ifosfamide

Ifosfamide is a cyclophosphamide analog with a nephrotoxic metabolite, chloracetaldehyde. Cyclophosphamide itself has no significant nephrotoxicity since it does not generate chloracetaldehyde. ARF is usually mild, although proximal tubular dysfunction (Fanconi syndrome) and hypokalemia may be prominent.

Ethylene glycol

Ethylene glycol found in antifreeze remains a cause of both deliberate and accidental injury. It is rapidly metabolized by alcohol dehydrogenase to glycoaldehyde and glyoxylate which are toxic to tubular cells. Further metabolism generates oxalic acid which can precipitate in renal tubules leading to intratubular obstruction.

The diagnosis is suggested by the presence of a severe anion gap metabolic acidosis and the presence of a serum osmolal gap. Oxalate crystals are typically, but not always, seen on urine microscopy (Chapter 4, Fig. 4.4(c)). Management includes inhibition of alcohol dehydrogenase with intravenous ethanol (aiming for blood levels of 100–200 mg/dL) or the specific alcohol dehydrogenase inhibitor, fomepizole. Hemodialysis should be performed to remove the ethylene glycol and metabolites when the level is greater than 20 mg/dL and continued until less than 5 mg/dL. Methanol intoxication may present with similar metabolic abnormalities, but rarely causes acute renal failure.

Illicit drug use

Acute renal failure is a common condition in those who abuse drugs and may be due to nephrotoxicity of the drug, coexistent viral infection (HIV, Hepatitis C), sepsis, infective endocarditis, rhabdomyolysis, or alcohol abuse.

Cocaine

Cocaine induces intense vasoconstriction which may lead to severe hypertension and rhabdomyolysis[30]. Mechanisms for rhabdomyolysis include coma and pressure necrosis; vasospasm leading to ischemic muscle injury; adrenergic stimulation and hyperpyrexia leading to increased cellular metabolism. It typically occurs in those who inject cocaine and the patient often presents with fever, hypertension, tachycardia and impaired mental state.

Other illicit drugs associated with ARF include opiates (coma associated pressure induced rhabdomyolysis); phencyclidine (rhabdomyolysis secondary to hyperpyrexia and vasoconstriction); and amphetamines (ARF secondary to rhabdomyolysis, acute interstitial nephritis or acute necrotizing angiitis).

Occupational toxins
Heavy metals
Lead intoxication usually causes a chronic nephropathy with hyperuricemia, hypertension, proximal tubular disease and chronic interstitial nephritis. Rarely acute tubular injury occurs which may be associated with Fanconi syndrome. ATN may also occur in cadmium and mercury poisoning.

Organic solvents
These may cause acute tubular injury due to peroxidation of membrane lipids. A subacute renal failure due to antiglomerular basement membrane disease has also been reported with exposure to halogenated hydrocarbons.

Herbal remedies
Specific herbs used in traditional African medicine are common causes of ARF in parts of Africa. A subacute form of renal failure due to aristolochic acid found in certain herbs used in traditional Chinese medicine is also described (Chinese herb nephropathy, see chapter 64).

ATHEROEMBOLIC RENAL DISEASE

Atheroembolic renal disease is an important cause of ARF, predominantly in older patients with atherosclerotic renovascular disease and may be precipitated by arteriography, vascular surgery, thrombolysis and anticoagulation. Destabilization of atherosclerotic plaques primarily in the aorta results in showers of cholesterol that lodge in small arteries in the kidneys and typically the lower extremities. At times, significant embolization of extrarenal intra-abdominal vessels can occur inducing ischemic injury (e.g., gut and pancreas). Needle shaped clefts may be seen on renal or skin biopsy, denoting the pretissue fixation localization of cholesterol plaques. The cholesterol emboli produce a marked and progressive inflammatory reaction resulting in occlusion of the involved vasculature. Typically, a subacute renal failure occurs which is progressive and is usually associated with systemic embolic phenomena including digital infarcts, livedo reticularis and distal cyanosis ('purple toes'). Eosinophilia and hypocomplementemia may also be found, and the condition may mimic systemic vasculitis. The condition is an important differential diagnosis in older patients undergoing vascular interventions. There is currently no effective treatment for this condition. Atheroembolic renal disease is discussed further in Chapter 63.

ACUTE INTERSTITIAL NEPHRITIS

This is most commonly a drug-induced phenomenon and is an important differential diagnosis in ARF as removal of the offending agent can result in reversal of the condition. Classic cases present with nonoliguric ARF, eosinophilia, skin rash and fever. Urine microscopy may reveal granular casts, white cell casts and urinary eosinophilia, although these are inconstant. Acute interstitial nephritis may not be clinically detectable until several weeks after commencement of the relevant drug. AIN is discussed further in Chapter 60 .

ARF IN SPECIFIC CLINICAL SITUATIONS

Determining the etiology of acute renal failure is often aided by recognizing common patterns of presentation and determining the likely causes arising in each of these situations.

ARF in the patient with sepsis syndrome
Approximately 20% of patients with sepsis syndrome and 50% of those with septic shock develop ARF. The cause of the ARF in this setting is usually multifactorial and due to a combination of hypotension, impaired renal perfusion, sepsis and nephrotoxic agents[2]. A similar syndrome termed the systemic inflammatory response syndrome (SIRS) may occur secondary to noninfectious insults such as acute pancreatitis, major trauma or ischemia reperfusion.

Sepsis syndrome is characterized by an exaggerated inflammatory response with widespread endothelial injury leading to peripheral vasodilatation, increased vascular permeability and leukocyte infiltration[31,32]. A wide range of cellular and humoral mediator systems are activated, including the cytokine cascade (tumor necrosis factor (TNF)-α, interleukin (IL)-1β, IL-6)[33], the complement, coagulation and fibrinolytic systems, and the release of mediators such as eicosanoids, platelet activating factor and endothelin-1 and nitric oxide (Fig. 15.9).

Clinical features
Diagnostic criteria for sepsis/SIRS include tachypnea (> 20 breaths/min or $Paco_2$ < 32 mmHg), tachycardia (> 90 beats/ min), and fever (> 38°C or hypothermia < 36°C). Leukocytosis with a left shift or leukopenia may be present.

Systemic vasodilatation produces a hyperdynamic circulation with warm extremities. The blood pressure is initially maintained by a markedly increased cardiac output, but at later stages, sepsis has depressant effects on myocardial function and hypotension develops. Organ dysfunction is manifest by ARF, acute respiratory distress syndrome, liver dysfunction and hypoperfusion with lactic acidosis. This combination has been described as the multiple organ dysfunction syndrome. Renal dysfunction is an early feature of sepsis syndrome. Initially there is a prominent prerenal element from systemic hypotension and intrarenal vasoconstriction. In this setting the kidneys are highly susceptible to further insults leading to ATN.

Treatment of ARF in SIRS
Many of the aspects of management of ARF in SIRS are covered in Chapter 14. There is no specific therapy for ARF in this

219

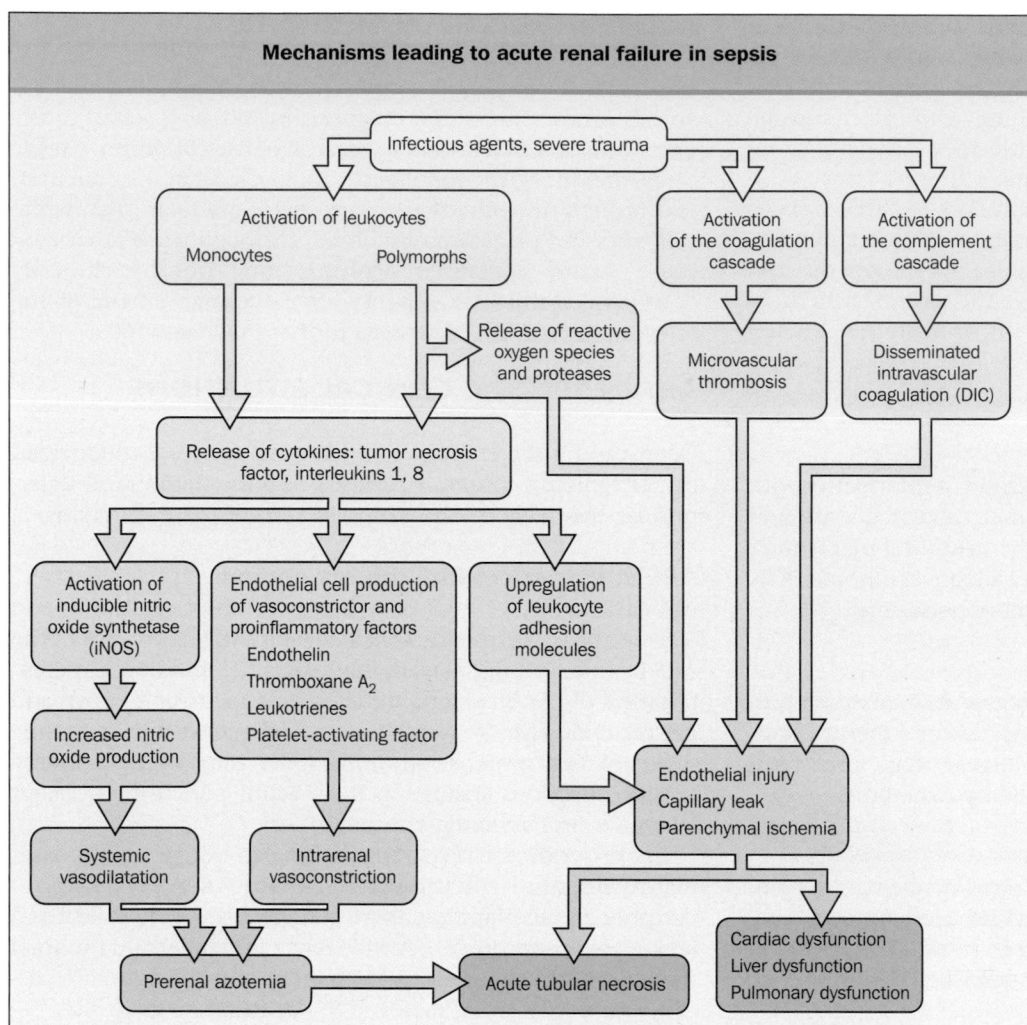

Mechanisms leading to acute renal failure in sepsis

Infectious agents, severe trauma

Activation of leukocytes
Monocytes · Polymorphs

Activation of the coagulation cascade

Activation of the complement cascade

Release of reactive oxygen species and proteases

Microvascular thrombosis

Disseminated intravascular coagulation (DIC)

Release of cytokines: tumor necrosis factor, interleukins 1, 8

Activation of inducible nitric oxide synthetase (iNOS)

Endothelial cell production of vasoconstrictor and proinflammatory factors
Endothelin
Thromboxane A$_2$
Leukotrienes
Platelet-activating factor

Upregulation of leukocyte adhesion molecules

Increased nitric oxide production

Endothelial injury
Capillary leak
Parenchymal ischemia

Systemic vasodilatation

Intrarenal vasoconstriction

Prerenal azotemia

Acute tubular necrosis

Cardiac dysfunction
Liver dysfunction
Pulmonary dysfunction

Figure 15.9 Mechanisms leading to acute renal failure in sepsis.

condition. The underlying cause of the SIRS should be identified and treated. Nephrotoxic agents should be avoided and the dose of drugs with renal elimination appropriately adjusted. Intravenous fluids should be administered to ensure adequate filling pressures and circulatory hemodynamics optimized to enhance renal perfusion. There appears to be no benefit in the use of colloids compared to crystalloids for volume replacement in the critically ill. Volume expansion is often limited by a capillary leak syndrome which may exacerbate the adult respiratory distress syndrome. Vasopressors (such as norepinephrine or dopamine) and inotopes are frequently required. Systemic hypoxia should be corrected and the role of supranormal oxygen delivery to treat tissue hypoxia may warrant consideration. General supportive measures, physiotherapy and good nutrition are vital.

Specific treatments for SIRS are often disappointing[34]. Attempts to inhibit the cytokine cascade with corticosteroids, anti-TNF-α antibodies, soluble TNF-α receptors and IL-1 receptor antagonists have been unsuccessful. Similarly, antiendotoxin therapy (monoclonal antibody HA-A1) has not shown benefit.

A recent study showed very promising results using recombinant activated protein C, which enhances the natural fibrinolytic system, suggesting that the procoagulant state induced by endothelial activation plays an important role in

the pathogenesis of SIRS. In a multicenter double-blind study of 1690 patients with severe sepsis, although changes in renal function were not described, overall mortality was reduced from 31 to 25%[35].

Other therapies currently being investigated include recombinant tissue factor pathway inhibitor, inhibition of nitric oxide (e.g., methylene blue) and antibodies to macrophage migration inhibitory factor.

ARF in the postoperative patient
ARF in the postoperative period is commonly due to problems with fluid balance or as a consequence of perioperative hemodynamic instability. Hypotension is generally insufficient to cause ARF, and an additional renal insult, such as a nephrotoxic agent, should be sought. The critically ill postoperative patient may develop SIRS. ARF is particularly common following vascular, cardiac and hepatobiliary surgery.

There is evidence that anesthetic agents may impair renal function. This may be partly due to their hypotensive effects, but the metabolism of fluorinated agents can lead to the production of potentially nephrotoxic fluoride ions. Modern inhaled agents, including isoflurane, halothane, and enflurane, all cause a transient decrease in GFR, and use of methoxyfluorane had to be discontinued due to nephrotoxicity.

Post vascular surgery

Patients with peripheral vascular disease have a very high incidence of atherosclerosis in other vessels and are at high risk for complications. Prior ischemic renal disease is often present and preoperative renal function is the strongest predictor of the risk for postoperative ARF. In aortic aneurysm surgery, ARF occurs in ~5% of elective cases and up to 50% of emergency cases[36]. The majority of aortic aneurysms are infrarenal; however, surgery that directly involves the renal arteries, or aortic cross clamping above the renal arteries can result in severe renal ischemia. Furthermore, aortic manipulation may dislodge atherosclerotic plaque resulting in renal atheroembolism. Peripheral limb surgery may be complicated by rhabdomyolysis and radiocontrast is frequently used for diagnostic purposes.

Post cardiac surgery

A transient rise in creatinine is found in up to 30% of patients undergoing coronary artery bypass grafting with approximately 2% of patients requiring dialysis[37]. Risk factors for postoperative ARF include duration of cardiac bypass, preoperative renal function, age, diabetes and poor cardiac function. The surgery is usually performed with the patient cooled to less than 30°C to protect cells against ischemic injury, however, systemic hypothermia may cause intravascular coagulation. Aortic instrumentation and clamping may lead to dislodgment of atherosclerotic plaques and renal atheroembolism. Cardiopulmonary bypass exposes blood to a nonendothelialized plastic surface in the extracorporeal circuit resulting in activation of neutrophils, platelets, complement and fibrinolytic systems. Significant hemolysis may also occur, potentially resulting in hemoglobinuria. Low cardiac output may impair renal perfusion postoperatively, although this is often transient and recovers within 24–48 h. Atrial fibrillation is a common complication and may be associated with peripheral embolization.

Post hepatobiliary surgery

Surgery to relieve obstructive jaundice is more commonly associated with ARF than other forms of abdominal surgery. This may be due to the absence of bile salts in the gut lumen which normally break down lipopolysaccharide endotoxin, preventing absorption. One study suggested a decreased incidence of postoperative endotoxemia when treated with oral bile salts. Other factors may include direct nephrotoxic effects of bilirubin or bile salts on renal tubular cells and an increased incidence of biliary sepsis.

Pulmonary–renal syndrome

Pulmonary–renal syndrome describes patients who present with a combination of renal and respiratory failure, and is usually restricted to a combination of pulmonary hemorrhage and ARF due to immune-mediated disease including antiglomerular basement membrane disease (Goodpasture's disease), systemic vasculitis and systemic lupus. Conditions which may masquerade as a pulmonary– renal syndrome include pulmonary edema secondary to volume overload in ARF, bacterial pneumonia complicated by acute tubular necrosis or post-infectious glomerulonephritis, and *Legionella* infection causing a severe atypical pneumonia with acute interstitial nephritis or rhabdomyolysis (see Chapter 25 Tables 25.4 and 25.5).

Thrombotic microangiopathy

Thrombotic microangiopathy should be considered when a patient presents with ARF and thrombocytopenia, although it may occur in the absence of a low platelet count. Endothelial activation is followed by the formation of platelet thrombi which occlude small vessels and lead to downstream ischemic injury. The microthrombi cause mechanical injury to erythrocytes and produce a hemolytic anemia which may be confirmed on blood film by the presence of fragmented red cells (schistocytes). The differential diagnosis and management are discussed in Chapter 31.

ARF and liver disease

The patient with liver cirrhosis is predisposed to the development of ARF and the differential diagnosis typically falls between prerenal uremia, hepatorenal syndrome and acute tubular necrosis (see Chapter 16). Alternatively, the same etiological agent may be responsible for both the liver and renal injury. This occurs with certain infections and nephrotoxic agents (Table 15.2).

Leptospirosis

This zoonosis is caused by the spirochete, *Leptospira interrogans*. The organism infects a wide range of mammals and the bacterium is shed in the urine. The rat is the commonest vector for human disease and the portal of entry usually breaks in the skin or mucous membranes. The disease course

Causes of ARF in patients with liver disease	
Prerenal uremia	Diuretic use
	Gastrointestinal loss
	Peritoneal aspiration
	Hypoalbuminemia
Hepatorenal syndrome (see Chapter 16)	
Acute tubular necrosis	Hyperbilirubinemia
	Sepsis
	Toxic shock syndrome
Drugs	Acetaminophen (paracetamol)
	NSAIDs
	Tetracycline
	Rifampin (rifampicin)
	Isoniazid
	Anesthetic agents
	Sulfonamides
	Allopurinol
	Methotrexate
Infections	Hepatitis C and cryoglobulinemia
	Hepatitis B and polyarteritis nodosa
	Epstein–Barr virus
	Leptospirosis
	Hantavirus
	Gram-negative sepsis
Other	Inhalation of chorinated hydrocarbons
	Mushroom poisoning (*Amanita phalloides*)

Table 15.2 Causes of ARF in patients with liver disease.

may be mild or follow a fulminant course (Weil's disease). The classical pattern is of a biphasic disease. Initial symptoms include the abrupt onset of fevers, myalgias, arthralgias, headache and conjunctival suffusion. In the second phase, jaundice with a mild transaminitis occurs, but liver failure is rare. Renal failure develops subsequently and may be due to either an acute interstitial nephritis, ATN or direct endothelial cell/vascular injury[38]. Rhabdomyolysis may also complicate the course of this disease and contribute to ARF.

The diagnosis can be made from blood cultures (in the first 10 days), urine cultures (up to day 30) or by serology for antibody titers. Antibiotic treatment with either intravenous penicillins or oral doxycycline form the cornerstone of therapy. A Jarisch–Herxheimer reaction due to the release of lipopolysaccharide from dying spirochetes may occur. Hypercatabolism is a feature of this condition and aggressive nutritional support with daily hemodialysis may be required. The renal failure typically recovers over 3–4 weeks, although there may be residual chronic renal damage.

Hantavirus

Hantavirus infection may cause hemorrhagic fever and renal syndrome (HFRS; also known as Korean hemorrhagic fever, Songo fever, epidemic hemorrhagic fever or nephropathica epidemica). The virus is widely distributed in Europe and Asia and infections with it must be differentiated from other forms of hemorrhagic fever such as Dengue fever. The severity of infection is dependent on the viral species, but the most severe varieties are mostly found in Asia with mortality rates as high as 10–25%. The infection is acquired by inhaling live virus which is excreted in the saliva, urine and feces of rodent vectors.

HFRS presents with a prodromal illness with an abrupt onset of fever, myalgias and headache with progression to a systemic inflammatory response syndrome. Loin pain may be prominent. Thrombocytopenia is often severe with petechial bruising and gastrointestinal bleeding. Abnormal liver function tests, particularly elevations of transaminases and bilirubin, may be present. Oliguric renal failure develops secondary to severe hypotension, a marked tubulointerstitial nephritis and renal vascular endothelial injury with cortical necrosis[39] (Fig. 15.10). Respiratory failure may develop secondary to noncardiogenic pulmonary edema. Hantavirus pulmonary syndrome is a separate entity due to Hantavirus infection which is rarely associated with renal failure.

The infection is diagnosed by high titers of anti-Hantavirus antibodies. Treatment is mainly supportive, although recent evidence suggests a benefit from antiviral therapy with ribavarin.

ARF in the patient with HIV infection

ARF in the patient with HIV infection may be related to the disease itself, the therapy, opportunistic infections, or coexistent intravenous drug abuse (Table 15.3). A wide range of causes are found and renal biopsy should be considered when ARF does not respond to supportive measures[40]. In the HIV-infected intravenous drug user, ARF may be due to concomitant hepatitis C infection-associated membranoproliferative

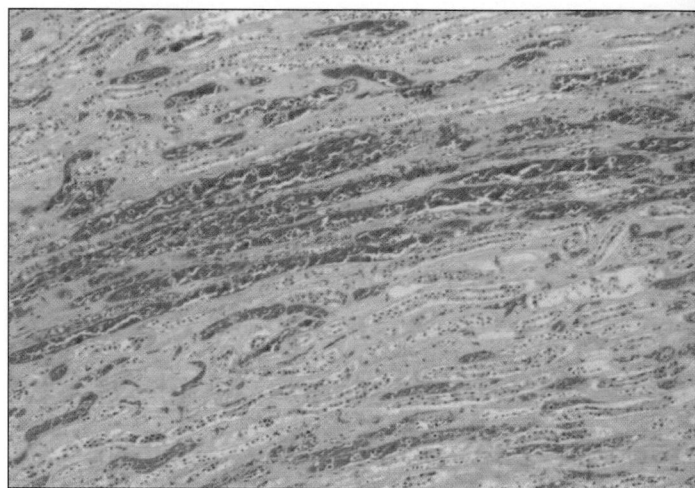

Figure 15.10 Renal histology in Hantavirus infection. Extensive tubular and interstitial injury with medullary hemorrhage.

Causes of ARF in patients with HIV infection	
HIV associated nephropathy (see Chapter 21)	
Thrombotic microangiopathy	HIV associated hemolytic–uremic syndrome
Acute tubular necrosis	Sepsis Nephrotoxins (aminoglycosides, amphotericin B, acyclovir, cidofovir, pentamidine) Rhabdomyolysis
Immune complex glomerulonephritis	Postinfectious glomerulonephritis HCV associated MPGN; cryoglobulinemia
Acute interstitial nephritis	Cotrimoxazole Rifampin (rifampicin) Foscarnet
Drug-induced intratubular obstruction	Sulfadiazine Indinavir Foscarnet Acyclovir
Associated with IV drug abuse	Sepsis Endocarditis Hepatitis C Heroin associated nephropathy (FSGS) Rhabdomyolysis

MPGN, membranoproliferative glomerulonephritis; FSGS, focal segmental glomerular sclerosis.

Table 15.3 Causes of ARF in patients with HIV infection.

glomerulonephritis or due to complications related to intravenous drug use (most notably endocarditis associated renal disease or rhabdomyolysis).

HIV nephropathy (HIVAN) is a collapsing glomerulopathy associated with severe cystic tubular changes (see Chapter 21). It has a subacute presentation with proteinuria and progressive renal failure. The disease most commonly affects African American patients and is typically associated with advanced HIV disease, but may also occur early. Thrombotic microangiopathy has also been described in HIV infection which may respond to plasma exchange.

Causes of ARF in patients with cancer	
Prerenal	Nausea and vomiting Hypercalcemia
Vascular	Thrombotic microangiopathy (adenocarcinoma of stomach, pancreas, prostate; radiation nephropathy) Renal vein thrombosis secondary to hypercoagulability Disseminated intravascular coagulation (acute promyelocytic leukemia)
Thrombotic microangiopathy	Mitomycin C; Bleomycin Cisplatin
Glomerular	Rapidly progressive glomerulonephritis
Acute tubular necrosis	Sepsis and antibiotic nephrotoxicity Hypercalcemia
Tubular toxicity	Cisplatin Ifosfamide Plicamycin (mithramycin) 5-fluorouracil Tioguanine (6-thioguanine) Cytarabine (cytosine arabinoside)
Malignant interstitial infiltration	Lymphoma, Acute lymphoblastic leukemia
Intraluminal obstruction	Tumor lysis syndrome Myeloma cast nephropathy Methotrexate
Postrenal obstruction	Transitional cell carcinoma ureters/bladder Extrinsic ureteric compression (tumor mass, nodes, retroperitoneal fibrosis)
Other mechanisms	Capillary leak syndrome (IL-2 therapy) Acute interstitial nephritis (interferon-α)

Table 15.4 Causes of ARF in patients with cancer.

Drug therapy

Protease inhibitors may cause ARF in patients with HIV infection. This occurs most commonly with indinavir which can cause intratubular crystal obstruction or obstructing renal calculi, but it has also been reported with ritonavir. Reverse transcriptase inhibitors may also produce ARF (e.g., adefovir). Although not nephrotoxic, zidovudine can produce a severe type B lactic acidosis due to mitochondrial dysfunction.

Treatment of opportunistic infections often requires the use of potentially nephrotoxic drugs such as aminoglycosides or amphotericin B. *Pneumocystis* infection may be treated with high dose cotrimoxazole, which may provoke acute interstitial nephritis or intratubular crystal obstruction. Alternatively, Pneumocystis may be treated with pentamidine and resistant cytomegalovirus infection may require foscarnet therapy, both of which are potentially nephrotoxic, and are further discussed above.

ARF in the cancer patient

The patient with cancer is prone to acute renal failure both as a consequence of the malignancy and of its treatment[41]. Some nephrotoxic chemotherapeutic agents are discussed above. There is also a high incidence of prerenal azotemia in cancer patients due to the high frequency of nausea, vomiting and diarrhea (Table 15.4).

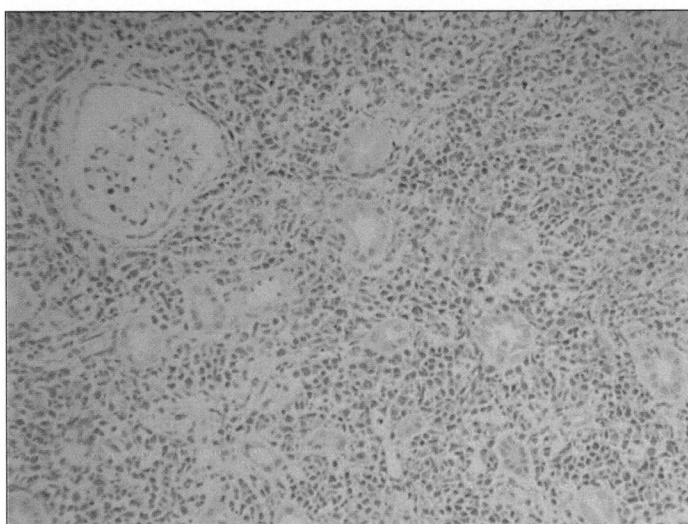

Figure 15.11 Lymphomatous infiltration of the kidney. Note the normal glomerular and tubular morphology and extensive infiltration of the interstitium by lymphoid cells.

Tumor lysis syndrome

Extensive necrosis of tumor cells, typically following chemotherapy, may release large amounts of nephrotoxic intracellular contents (uric acid, phosphate, xanthine) into the circulation[42]. This commonly occurs with lymphomas (particularly Burkitt's lymphoma) and leukemias, but may be seen with solid tumors. Rarely a spontaneous form of tumor lysis syndrome occurs in rapidly growing tumors that outstrip their blood supply.

In earlier days, hyperuricemia resulted in acute uric acid nephropathy due to intratubular crystal obstruction and interstitial nephritis. This condition is now uncommon due to the prophylactic use of allopurinol prior to chemotherapy. Other intracellular components are now more commonly involved, for example phosphate release leading to intratubular precipitation of calcium phosphate.

The ARF is typically oligoanuric and the condition should be suspected in patients with high lactate dehydrogenase levels suggestive of massive cell lysis. Markedly elevated phosphate and uric acid levels may also be found. Hyperkalemia may be prominent and life threatening.

Preventive measures include the use of high dose allopurinol (600–900 mg/day) started 2–3 days before chemotherapy, and either oral or intravenous fluid loading to ensure a urine output greater than 2.5 L/day. Urine alkalinization is not recommended as it may promote tubular calcium phosphate deposition. If the patient develops ARF and is markedly hyperuricemic or hyperphosphatemic, early dialysis should be considered to remove these potential causes of further renal damage. Frequent (12–24-hourly) or prolonged dialysis treatments should be considered to rapidly lower levels of waste and after nephotoxic components.

Hypercalcemia

Volume depletion secondary to hypercalcemia induced nausea and vomiting may cause ARF which may be exacerbated by hypercalcemia induced nephrogenic diabetes insipidus. Other hypercalcemia associated factors which may contribute

Acute Renal Failure

to ARF include direct intrarenal vasoconstriction, acute interstitial nephritis or intra-tubular obstruction.

Renal infiltration

Direct infiltration of the kidneys by tumor is not uncommon, however this rarely results in renal failure. ARF may be seen with slow growing lymphomas or leukemias, when the patient presents with nonoliguric ARF, a benign urine sediment and enlarged kidneys on ultrasound scan. Renal histology shows interstitial infiltration of tumor cells (Figure 15.11). Renal function may improve depending on the responsiveness of the tumor to treatment.

REFERENCES

1. Hou SH, Bushinsky DA, Wish JB, Cohen JJ, Harrington JT. Hospital-acquired renal insufficiency: a prospective study. Am J Med. 1983;74(2):243–8.
2. Brivet FG, Kleinknecht DJ, Loirat P, Landais PJ. Acute renal failure in intensive care units – causes, outcome, and prognostic factors of hospital mortality; a prospective, multicenter study. French Study Group on Acute Renal Failure. Crit Care Med. 1996;24(2):192–8.
3. Liano F, Pascual J. Epidemiology of acute renal failure: a prospective, multicenter, community-based study. Madrid Acute Renal Failure Study Group. Kidney Int. 1996;50(3):811–8.
4. Spurney RF, Fulkerson WJ, Schwab SJ. Acute renal failure in critically ill patients: prognosis for recovery of kidney function after prolonged dialysis support. Crit Care Med. 1991;19(1):8–11.
5. Conger J. Hemodynamic factors in acute renal failure. Adv Ren Replace Ther. 1997;4(2 Suppl 1):25–37.
6. Schnermann J, Traynor T, Yang T, et al. Tubuloglomerular feedback: new concepts and developments. Kidney Int Suppl. 1998;67:S40–5.
7. Kelly KJ, Williams WW, Jr., Colvin RB, et al. Intercellular adhesion molecule-1-deficient mice are protected against ischemic renal injury. J Clin Invest. 1996;97(4):1056–63.
8. Rabb H, Daniels F, O'Donnell M, et al. Pathophysiological role of T lymphocytes in renal ischemia-reperfusion injury in mice. Am J Physiol Renal Physiol. 2000;279(3):F525–31.
9. Rana A, Sathyanarayana P, Lieberthal W. Role of apoptosis of renal tubular cells in acute renal failure: therapeutic implications. Apoptosis. 2001;6(1–2):83–102.
10. Nath KA, Norby SM. Reactive oxygen species and acute renal failure. Am J Med. 2000;109(8):665–78.
11. Goligorsky MS, Noiri E. Duality of nitric oxide in acute renal injury. Semin Nephrol. 1999;19(3):263–71.
12. Zhou W, Farrar CA, Abe K, et al. Predominant role for C5b-9 in renal ischemia/reperfusion injury. J Clin Invest. 2000;105(10):1363–71.
13. Humes HD, Liu S. Cellular and molecular basis of renal repair in acute renal failure. J Lab Clin Med. 1994;124(6):749–54.
14. Hirschberg R, Kopple J, Lipsett P, et al. Multicenter clinical trial of recombinant human insulin-like growth factor I in patients with acute renal failure. Kidney Int. 1999;55(6):2423–32.
15. Zager RA. Rhabdomyolysis and myohemoglobinuric acute renal failure. Kidney Int. 1996;49(2):314–26.
16. Bywaters EGL, Beall D. Crush injuries with impairment of renal function. Br Med J. 1941;1:427–432.
17. Lofberg M, Jankala H, Paetau A, Harkonen M, Somer H. Metabolic causes of recurrent rhabdomyolysis. Acta Neurol Scand. 1998;98(4):268–75.
18. Holt S, Moore K. Pathogenesis of renal failure in rhabdomyolysis: the role of myoglobin. Exp Nephrol. 2000;8(2):72–6.
19. Better OS, Stein JH. Early management of shock and prophylaxis of acute renal failure in traumatic rhabdomyolysis. N Engl J Med. 1990;322(12):825–9.
20. Murphy SW, Barrett BJ, Parfrey PS. Contrast nephropathy. J Am Soc Nephrol. 2000;11(1):177–82.
21. Wang A, Holcslaw T, Bashore TM, et al. Exacerbation of radiocontrast nephrotoxicity by endothelin receptor antagonism. Kidney Int. 2000;57(4):1675–80.
22. Katholi RE, Taylor GJ, McCann WP, et al. Nephrotoxicity from contrast media: attenuation with theophylline. Radiology. 1995;195(1):17–22.
23. Solomon R, Werner C, Mann D, D'Elia J, Silva P. Effects of saline, mannitol, and furosemide to prevent acute decreases in renal function induced by radiocontrast agents. N Engl J Med. 1994;331(21):1416–20.
24. Safirstein R, Andrade L, Vieira JM. Acetylcysteine and nephrotoxic effects of radiographic contrast agents – a new use for an old drug. N Engl J Med. 2000;343(3):210–2.
25. Venturini CM, Isakson P, Needleman P. Non-steroidal anti-inflammatory drug-induced renal failure: a brief review of the role of cyclo-oxygenase isoforms. Curr Opin Nephrol Hypertens. 1998;7(1):79–82.
26. Harris RC, Jr. Cyclooxygenase-2 inhibition and renal physiology. Am J Cardiol. 2002;89(6A):10D-17D.
27. Textor SC. Renal failure related to angiotensin-converting enzyme inhibitors. Semin Nephrol. 1997;17(1):67–76.
28. Swan SK. Aminoglycoside nephrotoxicity. Semin Nephrol. 1997;17(1):27–33.
29. Fanos V, Cataldi L. Amphotericin B-induced nephrotoxicity: a review. J Chemother. 2000;12(6):463–70.
30. Nzerue CM, Hewan-Lowe K, Riley LJ, Jr. Cocaine and the kidney: a synthesis of pathophysiologic and clinical perspectives. Am J Kidney Dis. 2000;35(5):783–95.
31. Thijs A, Thijs LG. Pathogenesis of renal failure in sepsis. Kidney Int Suppl. 1998;66:S34–7.
32. Adrie C, Pinsky MR. The inflammatory balance in human sepsis. Intens Care Med. 2000;26(4):364–75.
33. Ulevitch RJ, Tobias PS. Receptor-dependent mechanisms of cell stimulation by bacterial endotoxin. Annu Rev Immunol. 1995;13:437–57.
34. Wheeler AP, Bernard GR. Treating patients with severe sepsis. N Engl J Med. 1999;340(3):207–14.
35. Bernard GR, Vincent JL, Laterre PF, et al. Efficacy and safety of recombinant human activated protein C for severe sepsis. N Engl J Med. 2001;344(10):699–709.
36. Kashyap VS, Cambria RP, Davison JK, L'Italien GJ. Renal failure after thoracoabdominal aortic surgery. J Vasc Surg. 1997;26(6):949–55; discussion 955–7.
37. Ostermann ME, Taube D, Morgan CJ, Evans TW. Acute renal failure following cardiopulmonary bypass: a changing picture. Intens Care Med. 2000;26(5):565–71.
38. Yang CW, Wu MS, Pan MJ. Leptospirosis renal disease. Nephrol Dial Transplant. 2001;16(Suppl 5):73–7.
39. Papadimitriou M. Hantavirus nephropathy. Kidney Int. 1995;48(3):887–902.
40. Rao TK. Acute renal failure syndromes in human immunodeficiency virus infection. Semin Nephrol. 1998;18(4):378–95.
41. Kapoor M, Chan GZ. Malignancy and renal disease. Crit Care Clin Med. 2001;17(3):571–98, viii.
42. Jeha S. Tumor lysis syndrome. Semin Hematol. 2001;38(4 Suppl 10):4–8.

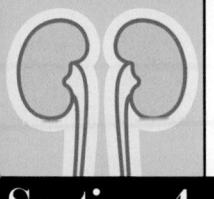

Chapter 16

Hepatorenal Syndrome

Ignatius KP Cheng

INTRODUCTION AND DEFINITION

Hepatorenal syndrome

Hepatorenal syndrome (HRS) can occur in patients with acute or chronic liver disease, advanced hepatic failure, and portal hypertension. It is characterized by impaired renal function and marked abnormalities in the arterial circulation and endogenous vasoactive systems. In the kidney, there is marked vasoconstriction resulting in low glomerular filtration rate (GFR). In the extrarenal circulation, there is a predominance of arteriolar dilatation, resulting in reduction of systemic vascular resistance and arterial hypotension[1].

Oliguric renal failure in advanced liver disease in the absence of significant histologic changes in the kidneys was first described by Austin Flint in 1863. However, the existence of HRS was not generally accepted until the detailed description by Hecker and Sherlock in the 1950s. The functional nature of the renal failure was subsequently established by studies which showed that kidneys from patients suffering from HRS function normally after being transplanted into patients with chronic renal failure and that renal failure is rapidly reversed after successful orthotopic liver transplantation (OLT). Studies since the 1970s have focused on the pathogenesis and treatment of HRS. With a better understanding of its pathogenesis, medical therapy (apart from OLT) for HRS has started to emerge in the last few years.

Pseudohepatorenal syndrome

Pseudohepatorenal syndrome was introduced by Conn in 1973 to describe concurrent hepatic and renal dysfunction secondary to a wide variety of infectious, systemic, circulatory, genetic, and other diseases and after the administration of drugs and toxins. These conditions must be excluded before the diagnosis of HRS can be established.

ETIOLOGY AND PATHOGENESIS

The renal and systemic hemodynamic changes that occur in HRS are the result of complex interactions among a multitude of neurohumoral disturbances. HRS most likely represents one end of the spectrum of homeostatic abnormalities that accompany liver failure and portal hypertension.

Renal and systemic hemodynamic changes

The renal and systemic hemodynamic changes observed in patients with HRS differ from those observed in patients with other causes of renal failure. In HRS, reduction in GFR occurs mainly as a result of renal cortical hypoperfusion consequent upon intense cortical renal vasoconstriction. The latter can be demonstrated angiographically as marked beading and tortuosity of the interlobular and proximal arcuate arteries and the absence of a distinct cortical nephrogram and vascular filling of the cortical vessels (Fig. 16.1)[2]. The ^{133}Xe washout

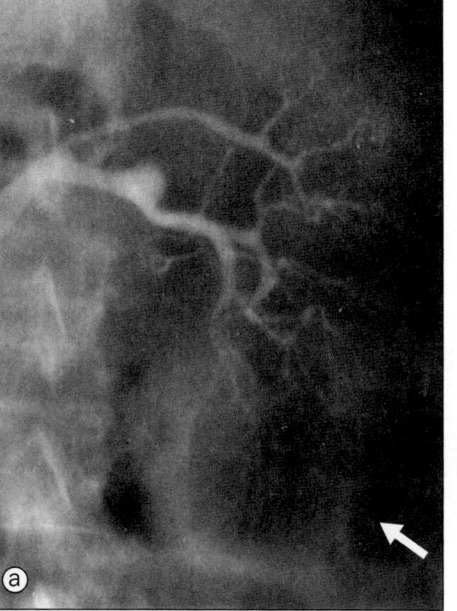
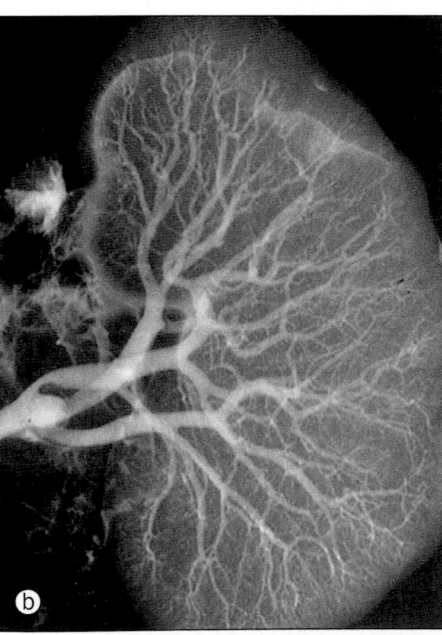

Figure 16.1 Hepatorenal syndrome (HRS).
(a) Renal angiogram (the arrow marks the edge of the kidney). (b) The angiogram carried out in the same kidney at autopsy. Note complete filling of the renal arterial system throughout the vascular bed to the periphery of the cortex. The vascular attenuation and tortuosity seen previously in (a) is no longer present. The vessels are also histologically normal. This indicates the functional nature of the vascular abnormality in HRS. (Reprinted with permission from Excerpta Medica Inc. From Epstein, et al.[2].)

Acute Renal Failure

technique shows that the vasomotor abnormality in HRS is variable with time. Intense renal vasoconstriction occurs in the presence of coexisting splanchnic and systemic vasodilatation. The latter gives rise to a low systemic mean arterial blood pressure (MAP), which together with a raised renal venous pressure caused by ascites further compromises renal perfusion. This occurs because intense renal vasoconstriction results in blunting of the autoregulation of renal blood flow and so renal perfusion becomes more pressure dependent. In HRS, filtration fraction is also reduced, reflecting a dominant increase in afferent arteriolar tone and a decrease in the ultrafiltration coefficient.

Neurohumoral abnormalities

A multitude of neurohumoral abnormalities have been detected in HRS[3–7]. The sympathetic nervous system (SNS) is activated in HRS and the sympathetic discharges via the renal nerves are markedly increased. Abnormalities in the plasma and urinary levels of a number of endogenous vasoactive substances are also observed (Tables 16.1 and 16.2). Most of the neurohumoral abnormalities found in HRS are also detected, albeit to a lesser extent, in decompensated cirrhosis (with ascites) with normal renal function and in compensated cirrhosis (without ascites). This observation supports the hypothesis that HRS represents one end of the spectrum of homeostatic abnormalities that occur in liver failure and portal hypertension.

The role of each of the neurohumoral abnormalities and their complex interactions in the pathogenesis of HRS is still being debated. They can be broadly divided into several groups according to their postulated pathogenetic roles in HRS.

Initiators of vasodilatation

Circulating and vascular vasodilators increase in concentration, which contributes to the initiating event of peripheral vasodilatation. The most important of these dilators is nitric oxide; its enhanced vascular release is reflected by increased circulating levels of plasma nitrite and nitrate. Increased shear stress in portal hypertension and endotoxemia associated with portosystemic shunting are thought to induce vascular nitric oxide release through the activation of the constitutive and inducible forms of nitric oxide synthetase[6]. Other endogenous vasodilators that may also be involved include glucagon and other gut hormones, prostacyclin, and possibly false neurotransmitters.

Adaptive responses to decreased effective arterial blood volume

Increases in the levels of some circulating vasoconstrictors may be viewed as an adaptive response to a decrease in effective arterial blood volume (EABV) and in MAP consequent to systemic and splanchnic vasodilatation and peritoneal and interstitial fluid sequestration. These vasoconstrictors include arginine-vasopressin, hormones of the renin–angiotensin–aldosterone system (RAAS), and norepinephrine (noradrenaline). Although increased levels of these vasoactive hormones may also contribute to active renal vasoconstriction, pharmacologic blockade of these hormones invariably leads to systemic hypotension (and in the case of angiotensin blockade, also a reduction in filtration fraction), thus negating any potential beneficial effect on GFR in patients with HRS.

Responses to endotoxemia or oxidant stress

Some increase in the levels of circulating and intrarenal vasoconstrictors occurs not as an adaptive response to hemodynamic changes but rather as a consequence of the endotoxemia or oxidant stress that accompanies portal hypertension, portosystemic shunting, and liver failure. These agents include endothelins, leukotrienes, thromboxanes, platelet-activating factors, and F_2-isoprostanes (noncyclo-oxygenase-derived prostanoids produced *in vivo* as products of free

Endogenous vasomotor substances in plasma in cirrhosis and hepatorenal syndrome			
Vasomotor substances	Compensated cirrhosis	Cirrhosis with ascites	HRS
Vasodilators			
Endotoxin	↔	↑	↑↑
Nitrite/nitrate	↑	↑↑	↑↑
Glucagon	↑	↑	↑↑
Vasoconstrictors			
Renin activity	↔↓	↑	↑↑
Norepinephrine	↔↓	↑	↑↑
Vasopressin	↔	↑	↑↑
Platelet-activating factor	↔	↑	↑
Endothelin	↔	↑	↑↑
Isoprostanes (F_2)	↔	↔	↑
Adapted with permission from Badalamenti et al.[3].			

Table 16.1 Endogenous vasomotor substances in plasma in cirrhosis and hepatorenal syndrome.

Endogenous vasomotor substances in the urine in cirrhosis and hepatorenal syndrome			
Vasomotor substances	Compensated cirrhosis	Cirrhosis with ascites	HRS
Vasodilators			
Kallikrein	↔	↑	↓
Prostaglandin E_2	↔	↑	↓
6-Keto-PGF$_{1\alpha}$, a stable metabolite of renal prostacyclin	↔	↑	↓
2, 3-Dinor-6-keto-PGF$_{1\alpha}$ (PG$_1$-M), a stable metabolite of systemic prostacyclin	↑	↑	↑
Vasoconstrictors			
Thromboxane β_2, a stable metabolite of thromboxane A_2	↔	↑	?
Leukotrienes	↔	↑	↑
Adapted with permission from Badalamenti et al.[3].			

Table 16.2 Endogenous vasomotor substances in the urine in cirrhosis and hepatorenal syndrome.

radical-catalyzed lipid peroxidation). This group of vasoactive hormones are putative renal vasoconstrictors in HRS and potential targets for pharmacotherapy. Since they do not appear to increase as an adaptive response to changes in EABV and MAP, their blockade would be less likely to affect systemic hemodynamics adversely.

Intrarenal changes
The renal effects of circulating and intrarenal vasoconstrictors are also modulated by intrarenal (urinary) vasodilators. Falls in the levels of these substances are thought to be an important precipitating factor for the development of HRS. They include prostaglandins, prostacylin (prostaglandin I_2), and kallikrein.

Summary of the pathogenetic events
Figure 16.2 is a simplified diagram of the pathogenetic events that lead to HRS, related to the changes in neurohumoral mediators described above. Liver failure and portal hypertension increase circulating and vascular levels of vasodilators. These, together with opening up of anatomic vascular shunts, lead to splanchnic and systemic vasodilatation, which is thought to be the initiating event in the homeostatic disturbances accompanying advanced liver disease. Peripheral vasodilatation decreases vascular filling and reduces the EABV. The subsequent stimulation of the central volume receptors leads to compensatory increases in arginine-vasopressin and

in RAAS and SNS activities, which help to restore EABV. This restoration is achieved in patients with compensated cirrhosis but not in patients with decompensated cirrhosis. In the latter group of patients, increasing severity of the homeostatic abnormalities, combined with a progressive fall in plasma oncotic pressure consequent to decreased albumin synthesis by the diseased liver, causes an imbalance of the Starling equilibrium, resulting in ascites and edema formation. The resultant sequestration of fluid in the peritoneal and interstitial space aggravates vascular underfilling, lowers systemic MAP, and leads to further nonosmotic release of arginine-vasopressin (hence the tendency for hyponatremia) and continuous stimulation of the RAAS and SNS. The SNS activity is further enhanced by stimulation of the hepatorenal neural reflex arc as portal hypertension progresses. Progressive liver failure and portal hypertension also lead to increased levels of potent circulating or locally produced renal vasoconstrictors. These, together with increasing renal SNS activity are thought to lead to the progressive renal vasoconstriction that characterizes HRS. Normally, the effect of renal vasoconstrictors is counterbalanced by the reactive production of intrarenal vasodilators. It is postulated that HRS develops when the balance of activities between the renal vasoconstrictors and intrarenal vasodilators finally breaks down. The likelihood that this will occur increases with progressive deterioration in liver function or increasing severity of portal hypertension and is precipitated by events that lead to further volume contraction and reduction of the EABV e.g., spontaneous bacterial peritonitis or by the administration of substances e.g., nonsteroidal anti-inflammatory drugs, (NSAIDs) that further suppress intrarenal generation of vasodilators (e.g., prostaglandins).

CLINICAL MANIFESTATIONS

There are two common clinical presentations of HRS[1]. An acute form (type 1) is characterized by rapid spontaneous deterioration in renal function defined as doubling of serum creatinine to a level > 2.5 mg/dL (> 220 μmol/L) or a 50% or more reduction of the baseline creatinine clearance in less than 2 weeks. This is most often observed in patients suffering from acute liver failure, acute alcoholic hepatitis, or acute decompensation on a background of cirrhosis. This group of patients tend to have severe jaundice and coagulopathy. Acute decompensation may be precipitated by bacterial infection (including spontaneous bacterial peritonitis), gastrointestinal bleeding, vigorous diuretic therapy, or abdominal paracentesis.

A chronic form (type 2) is characterized by insidious onset and slowly progressive deterioration in renal function. This is most often observed in patients with decompensated cirrhosis and portal hypertension. This group of patients tends to be less severely jaundiced and has refractory ascites.

PATHOLOGY

HRS is by definition a functional renal disorder and the presence of significant glomerular and tubular pathology excludes the diagnosis. Glomerular abnormalities, including mesangial

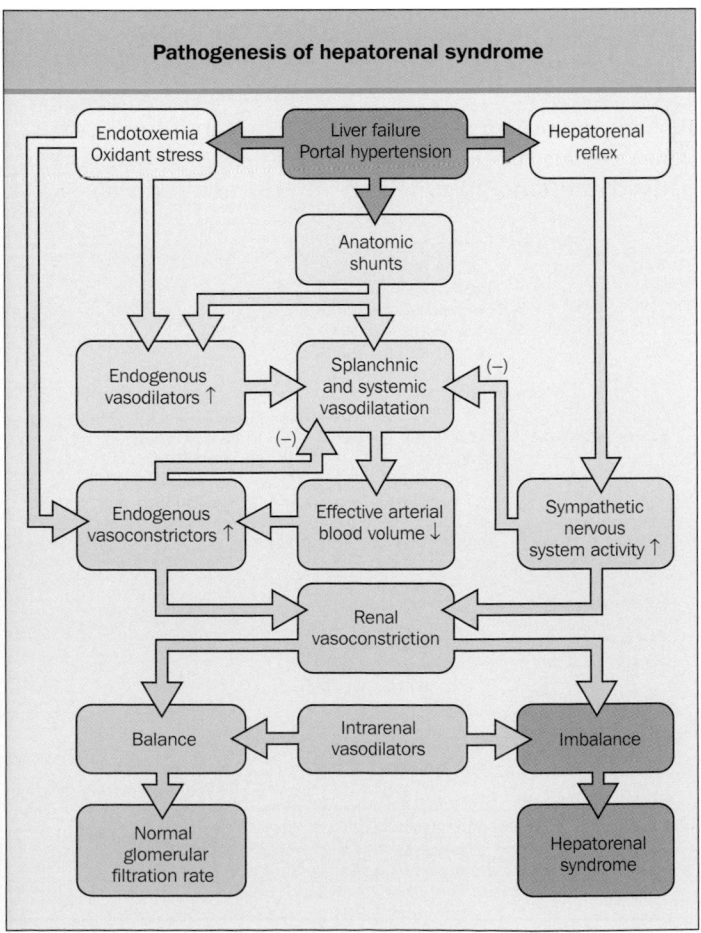

Figure 16.2 The pathogenesis of hepatorenal syndrome.

expansion, capillary wall thickening, mesangial and capillary wall electron-dense deposits, and immune deposits of C3 and the immunoglobins IgA, IgM, and IgG are frequently found in cirrhotic patients with normal renal function and minimal urinary abnormalities. The presence of such glomerular abnormalities in a cirrhotic patient, therefore, does not exclude the diagnosis of HRS. Reflux of the proximal tubular epithelium into the Bowman's space (glomerulotubular reflux) is described, but is not specific for HRS and is found in other conditions associated with profound renal ischemia and terminal hypotension. Although early autopsy studies have demonstrated normal tubular morphology in patients dying from HRS, recent detailed light and electron microscopic studies have documented proximal tubular lesions consistent with ischemic injury. Therefore, the demonstration of such lesions is consistent with the diagnosis of HRS.

DIAGNOSIS AND DIFFERENTIAL DIAGNOSIS

The diagnostic criteria of HRS have recently been updated by the International Ascites Club (Table 16.3)[1]. The diagnosis of HRS is mainly one of exclusion (see major criteria, Table 16.3) although measurement of urinary electrolytes and osmolarity and plasma sodium may provide supportive evidence for the diagnosis.

HRS should be suspected in any patient with acute or chronic liver disease with advanced liver failure and portal hypertension who develops progressive renal insufficiency. Significant renal insufficiency may be present despite a normal serum creatinine or blood urea nitrogen (BUN) because these patients are frequently malnourished, with reduced lean body mass, and often have a low urea generation rate because of liver failure and low protein intake. Severe hyperbilirubinemia, which is often present in patients with HRS, interferes with the measurement of serum creatinine, and in these patients alternative methods (e.g., $[^{125}I]$iothalamate, $[^{51}Cr]$-labeled EDTA, or inulin clearance) may be needed to measure GFR accurately.

Pseudohepatorenal syndrome (see Table 16.4)[8] is usually easy to exclude because the etiological agent is frequently known and both renal and liver functional abnormalities are often found at first clinical presentation, whereas evidence of advanced liver failure and portal hypertension is usually not initially present. This is in contrast to HRS, which invariably occurs after liver failure and portal hypertension are fully established and frequently develops when the patient is undergoing treatment for these conditions or their complications in hospital.

Diagnostic criteria for hepatorenal syndrome

Major criteria

Chronic or acute liver disease with advanced hepatic failure and portal hypertension

Low glomerular filtration rate, as indicated by serum creatinine >1.5 mg/dL (135 µmol/L) or 24-h creatinine clearance <40 mL/min

Absence of shock, ongoing bacterial infection, and current or recent treatment with nephrotoxic drugs

Absence of gastrointestinal fluid losses (repeated vomiting or intense diarrhea)

Absence of renal fluid losses (weight loss >500 g/day for several days in patients with ascites without peripheral edema or 1000 g/day in patients with peripheral edema)

No sustained improvement in renal function (decrease in serum creatinine to 1.5 mg/dL (135 µmol/L) or less or increase in creatinine clearance to 40 mL/min or more) following diuretic withdrawal and expansion of plasma volume with 1.5 L of isotonic saline

Proteinuria <500 mg/day and no ultrasonographic evidence of obstructive uropathy or parenchymal renal disease

Additional criteria

Urine volume < 500 mL/day

Urine sodium < 10 mmol/L

Urine osmolality greater than plasma osmolality

Urine red blood cells < 50 per high power field

Serum sodium concentration < 130 mmol/L

With permission from Arroyo et al.[1].

Table 16.3 Diagnostic criteria for hepatorenal syndrome.

Causes of pseudohepatorenal syndrome

Potential causes	Predominantly tubulointerstitial involvement	Predominantly glomerular involvement
Infections	Sepsis, leptospirosis, brucellosis, tuberculosis, Epstein–Barr virus, Hepatitis A virus	Hepatitis B, C virus. HIV virus, *Schistosoma mansoni*, liver abscess
Drugs	Tetracycline, rifampin (rifampicin), sulphonamide, phenytoin, allopurinol, methoxyflurane, fluroxene, methotrexate (high dose), acetaminophen (overdose)	
Toxins	Carbon tetrachloride, trichloroethylene, chloroform, elemental phosphorus, arsenic, copper, chromium, barium, amatoxins[a], raw carp bile toxins[b]	
Systemic disease	Sarcoidosis, Sjögren's syndrome	Systemic lupus, vasculitis, cryoglobulinemia, amyloidosis
Circulatory failure	Hypovolemic or cardiogenic shock	
Malignancy	Lymphoma, leukemia	
Congenital and genetic disorders	Polycystic liver and kidney disease, nephronophthisis and congenital hepatic fibrosis	
Miscellaneous	Fatty liver of pregnancy. Reye syndrome	Eclampsia, HELLP syndrome Cirrhotic glomerulopathy

[a] Accidental poisoning after ingestion of mushroom of the *Amanita* genus.
[b] Accidental poisoning after ingestion of the raw gall bladder or bile of the fresh water of grass carp (a common practice in rural East Asia).
Adapted with permission from Levenson et al.[8].

Table 16.4 Causes of pseudohepatorenal syndrome.

In patients with pre-existing liver failure and portal hypertension, nephrotoxic agents (e.g., NSAIDs or aminoglycosides) must be stopped and conditions leading to renal failure must be excluded by careful history, physical examination, urine examination, and ultrasonography before the diagnosis of HRS can be considered. Ultrasonography helps to exclude obstructive uropathy and parenchymal renal disease. The absence of shock, gastrointestinal bleeding, bacterial infection (especially spontaneous bacterial peritonitis), and excess gastrointestinal, peritoneal, or renal fluid loss must also be documented. Prerenal azotemia must be excluded by withdrawal of diuretics and fluid challenge (1.5 L isotonic saline or 100 g albumin in 500 mL saline). The presence of oliguria < 500 mL, urine sodium < 10 mmol/L, urine osmolarity greater than plasma osmolarity, urinary red blood cells < 50 per high-power field, and urinary protein < 500 mg/L help to exclude significant coexisting glomerular or tubulointerstitial disease leading to renal failure and provide supportive evidence for the diagnosis of HRS. However, the absence of these abnormalities does not exclude the diagnosis of HRS. A low plasma sodium is often present in patients with HRS and its presence provides additional evidence for the diagnosis. The absence of debris or casts in the urine sediment is not a diagnostic criterion since they may appear late in the course of HRS owing to ischemic tubular injury.

NATURAL HISTORY

The probability of developing HRS in cirrhotic patients is estimated at 18% at 1 year and 39% at 5 years[5]. Neither the etiology (alcoholic versus nonalcoholic) nor the Child–Pugh score have predictive value on the incidence of HRS. A multivariate analysis showed that there are only three independent predictors of HRS: low serum sodium concentration, high serum renin activity, and absence of hepatomegaly[8]. Abnormal renal duplex Doppler ultrasonography (resistive index > 0.7) has also been shown recently to be an independent predictor of the occurrence of HRS.

The prognosis of HRS is extremely poor. Without OLT, the mortality rate is between 80 and 95% depending on the etiology of the underlying liver disease. Recovery in renal function coincides with recovery of liver function and liver regeneration. Renal failure is infrequently an immediate cause of death, and most patients succumb to the other complications of liver failure and portal hypertension such as hepatic encephalopathy, gastrointestinal bleeding, and sepsis.

TREATMENT

General approach to treatment

If one accepts the hypothesis that HRS represents one end of the spectrum of the homeostatic abnormalities in liver failure and portal hypertension and is precipitated by such events as volume contraction, sepsis, or the administration of potential nephrotoxic agents, it follows that a major focus of treatment must be to avoid the occurrence of such events, to have high awareness of their existence, and to treat them promptly when they occur. In patients with decompensated liver disease, the common events that lead to volume contraction

include gastrointestinal bleeding, injudicious use of lactulose (for treatment of hepatic encephalopathy) resulting in profuse diarrhea, and over-rigorous diuretic therapy and/or paracentesis for the treatment of ascites. To avoid the last, a stepwise approach for the treatment of ascites is recommended and has recently been published[10]. The threshold for antibiotic therapy for suspected sepsis should be low. Spontaneous bacterial peritonitis must be excluded by regular examination of ascites fluid and treated not only with broad spectrum antibiotics but also with albumin infusion (1.5 g/kg initially and 1 g/kg 2 days later) as the latter has been shown to prevent the subsequent development of HRS[11]. The use of potential nephrotoxic agents including angiotensin-converting enzyme (ACE) inhibitors, NSAIDs, aminoglycosides, and radiologic contrast media should be avoided as far as possible. Therapeutic agents (e.g., β-blockers and somatostatin) that are employed for the treatment of bleeding esophageal and gastric varices may lead to a reduction of GFR, and their use must be monitored carefully.

Figure 16.3 is an algorithm for the management of HRS[3–5,7]. Currently, there is no established treatment for HRS except OLT. In view of the poor prognosis of HRS without liver transplantation and because the diagnosis of HRS is mainly one of exclusion, conditions that mimic HRS and that are more amenable to treatment or have a better prognosis must

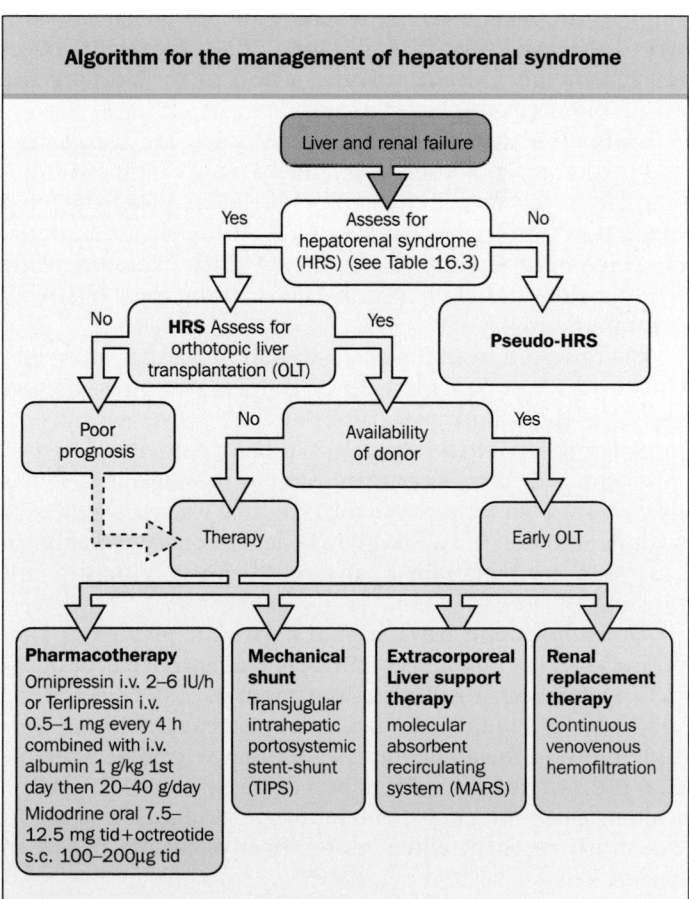

Figure 16.3 Algorithm for the management of hepatorenal syndrome.

be diligently excluded. Once the diagnosis of HRS is made, the patients should be assessed for their suitability for OLT. If they are suitable candidates they should be put onto the urgent waiting list for cadaveric liver transplantation. In places where cadaveric donor livers are scarce and where the surgical expertise is available, a search for a suitable living donor should also be explored. In patients who are potential transplant candidates, treatments that have been shown to be potentially useful for the treatment of HRS should be instituted as a bridge to OLT. These include pharmacotherapy, interventional procedures, extracorporeal liver support therapy and, in patients with advancing uremia, renal replacement therapy. In patients who are not transplant candidates, the use of these forms of therapy is more controversial but recent studies have shown that prolonged survival in terms of months may be achievable even in some of these patients.

Pharmacotherapy

From a pathogenetic viewpoint, the appropriate form of pharmacotherapy for HRS would be the administration of an agent, or a combination of agents, that induces simultaneous renal vasodilatation and splanchnic vasoconstriction. The former effect would theoretically alleviate renal cortical vasoconstriction, a functional hallmark of HRS, while the latter would reduce portal pressure and restore a previously depressed EABV resulting from peripheral vasodilatation back to normal. This in turn would reduce renal SNS activity and suppress the generation of circulating and intrarenal vasoconstrictors. These agent(s) may achieve their therapeutic effect either through a direct vascular action or by blocking the action of putative vasoactive substances.

Nonspecific vasodilators (e.g., acetylcholine and papaverine) and α-adrenergic blockers (e.g., phentolamine) infused intra-arterially at low dose to patients with HRS may increase renal blood flow but do not enhance GFR. At higher intra-arterial dose or as intravenous infusion, they invariably cause systemic hypotension and their use in HRS is, therefore, relatively contraindicated.

The observation that administration of NSAIDs often precipitates HRS in patients with decompensated cirrhosis suggests an important role of intrarenal prostaglandins in modulating renal hemodynamics in these patients. However, intravenous or intra-arterial infusion of prostaglandin E_1 has not been shown to improve the GFR, free water clearance, or sodium excretion in HRS, while a beneficial effect of oral misoprostol (a prostaglandin E_2 analog) in this condition is not proven.

Intravenous and intra-arterial dopamine given at a subpressor dose (1–3 μg/kg per min) acts as an intrarenal vasodilator and has been used in the treatment of HRS with limited success[12]. Although dopamine increased cortical blood flow and improved the angiographic appearance in these patients, GFR did not consistently improve. Despite this, dopamine remains a popular choice of pharmacological agents to use in HRS until recently when more effective agents began to emerge.

Vasopressin analogs have recently attracted the most attention as potential therapeutic agents in HRS. Vasopressin has a preferential vasoconstrictor action on the splanchnic versus

the renal vascular bed and its use could theoretically reverse splanchnic vasodilatation without compromising renal perfusion. Ornipressin (8-ornithine vasopressin) and terlipressin (triglycyl-lysine-vasopressin) are synthetic polypeptide analogs of arginine-vasopressin which have equipotent vasoconstrictor activity to the parent compound but have markedly reduced antidiuretic properties. Short term administration of these agents has been shown to increase MAP, reduce SNS and renin activities, and increase renal blood flow and GFR[13–14]. Prolonged intravenous administration of ornipressin for 15 days at 2 IU/h in combination with daily albumin infusion (1 g/kg on the first day followed by 20–40 g daily) reversed HRS (type unspecified) in four of eight patients[14] while administration of ornipressin (6 IU/h for up to 27 days) given with dopamine at a subpressor dose has been shown to reverse type 1 HRS in four of seven patients[15]. The longest patient survival following treatment without OLT was 8 months[15]. The main limitation of treatment was ischemic complications which was observed in 5 of these 15 patients and included intestinal ischemia, tongue necrosis and ventricular arrhythmia. In a recent pilot study, terlipressin (0.5–1 mg i.v. 4-hourly) in combination with daily albumin infusion for up to 15 days was shown to successfully reverse HRS (six with type 1 and three with type 2) in seven of nine patients with the longest survivor living up to 4 months without OLT and without any severe ischemic complication which necessitated early termination of treatment[16]. If this finding is confirmed by further studies, terlipressin may prove to be the most convenient and safest vasopressin analog which is currently available for use in the treatment of HRS.

Vasoconstrictors apart from vasopressin analogs have also been used in the treatment of HRS. Intravenous metaraminol (200–1000 μg/min), a synthetic sympathomimetic agent with both α- and β-agonist actions, given to raise mean arterial blood pressure by 30–40 mmHg increases peripheral vascular resistance and improves water and sodium excretion and GFR. However, the proarrhythmogenic effect of this agent greatly limits its use. Intravenous norepinephrine (0.45 μg/kg/min), raises the MAP by 10–20 mmHg but has no effect on renal blood flow and GFR and reduces water and sodium excretion. Similarly, short term administration of midodrine, an orally active α-mimetic drug, resulted in an increase in MAP and systemic vascular resistance and a reduction in plasma renin activity but no improvement in renal blood flow or GFR[17].

Specific inhibitors or antagonists of endogenous vasoactive substances thought to be important in the pathogenesis of HRS have also been studied for their therapeutic benefit. ACE inhibition and angiotensin blockade with saralasin led to profound hypotension and adversely affected renal function, and are therefore, relatively contraindicated in HRS. This underscores the important adaptative role of RAAS in maintaining systemic hemodynamics in this condition. Inhibition of thromboxane A_2 generation using dazoxiben, a specific thromboxane synthetase inhibitor, fails to improve renal function in patients with HRS. Since thromboxane inhibition leads to accumulation of the prostaglandin endoperoxides PGG_2 and PGH_2, which mimic the renal effect of thromboxane A_2 by interacting with the same receptor, this cannot be used as conclusive evidence against a therapeutic role of thromboxane blockade in HRS. A preliminary short-term study showed that a specific endothelin A receptor antagonist increased renal blood flow and GFR in three patients with HRS in the absence of any change of systemic vascular resistance and cardiac output but no long term survival data are available[18]. In another preliminary study, improvement of renal function and prolonged survival (58% at 3 months) was observed in 12 patients with HRS after intravenous infusion of N-acetylcysteine (150 mg/kg over 2 h followed by continuous infusion of 100 mg/kg daily for 5 days)[19]. This occurred without demonstrable improvement of liver function and systemic hemodynamics and presumably works by relieving the oxidant stress that accompany portal hypertension, portosystemic shunting and liver failure thereby reducing the level of circulating and intrarenal vasoconstrictors. Finally, octreotide, an inhibitor of glucagon release but unlike somatostatin with no adverse effect on renal hemodynamic and function, was recently shown in a preliminary study to improve renal function and urine output in four of five patients with HRS when given intravenously at 25 µg/h for 5 days with one patient surviving up to 5 months while being maintained on a subcutaneous tapering dose of 1500 to 500 µg/day[20].

In order to achieve simultaneous intrarenal vasodilatation and systemic and splanchnic vasoconstriction, combinations of intravenous prostacyclin and norepinephrine and low-dose dopamine and norepinephrine have been used for the treatment of HRS with limited success. Recently, a combination of oral midodrine (7.5–12.5 mg tid) and subcutaneous octreotide (100–200 µg tid) was successful in reverting type 1 HRS in all of five treated patients compared to only one of eight patients treated with subpressor dose dopamine. The longest survivor lived for 15.5 months without OLT. The dose was titrated to achieve an increase in MBP of 15 mmHg and treatment was maintained for up to 2 months (at home in three patients). Reversion of HRS coincided with an increase in MAP and a reduction in plasma serum renin activity, aldosterone, ADH, glucagon and nitrite and nitrate levels[21].

Interventional procedures

In patients with HRS and tense ascites, paracentesis of 2 L of ascitic fluid reduces intra-abdominal pressure. This is associated with a parallel decline in the pressure of the hepatic vein and inferior vena cava (and presumably the renal vein) and a transient increase in renal blood flow, GFR, and urine flow rate[22]. The lack of a sustained renal hemodynamic response to paracentesis is partly attributed to the reaccumulation of ascites fluid and partly to volume contraction owing to redistribution of fluid from the vascular to the peritoneal space. This may be overcome by the creation of a peritoneovenous shunt (PVS).

Leveen peritoneovenous shunt

In 1974, Leveen designed a one-way pressure-activated valve that could be implanted to create a permanent shunt between the peritoneal cavity and the superior vena cava for the treatment of ascites. Reversal of HRS was reported following the implantation of this shunt, but the diagnosis of HRS was not always well documented in these reports and some of these patients may have been suffering from prerenal azotemia rather than HRS[4]. Two recent randomized controlled studies comparing PVS and medical therapy in the treatment of HRS

showed that renal function appears to be better preserved in patients receiving a PVS but survival is only minimally or not affected[23,24]. PVS is not without side effects, which include fever, disseminated intravascular coagulation, shunt occlusion, infection, and ascites leak, and it has a reported operative mortality rate of 26% and a morbidity rate of over 65%. Its use in HRS is therefore not generally recommended[5].

Transjugular intrahepatic portosystemic stent-shunt

Portal hypertension plays a central role in the pathogenesis of the homeostatic abnormalities in cirrhosis and hepatic failure and in HRS. Early studies have shown that side-to-side portocaval shunt may improve renal function in patients with HRS but the high operative mortality precludes its use in this group of patients. Transjugular intrahepatic portosystemic stent-shunting (TIPS) is a recently described technique in which a metallic stent is used to reinforce a parenchymal track created by balloon dilatation between a branch of the hepatic vein and a branch of the portal vein (Fig. 16.4). In experienced hands, this technique is associated with an operative mortality rate of 1–2% and a morbidity rate of 10%. Procedure related complications include intra-abdominal bleeding, cardiac arrhythmia, fever, shunt migration and thrombosis, hemolytic anemia, fever, infection and reaction to radiocontrast media (including nephrotoxicity). The resultant diversion of portal blood flow from the liver to the systemic circulation may result in transient deterioration of liver function and development of encephalopathy. The successful application of TIPS to the treatment of HRS is supported by both short-term and long-term studies[25,26]. Reversal of HRS was associated with a decrease in SNS and RAAS activity, which indicates re-expansion of a previously depressed EABV[25]. In a recent phase II long-term study[26], improvement of renal function was observed in 31 nontransplantable cirrhotic patients with HRS but without severe liver failure (bilirubin < 15 mg/dL, Child–Pugh scores < 12 and absence of spontaneous severe encephalopathy) in whom limited portal decompression was achieved using 8–10-mm stents. For the whole group, the survival rates were 81%, 71%, 48% and 35% at 3, 6, 12 and 18 months and for 14 patients with type 1 HRS, they were 64%, 50% and 20% at 3, 6 and 12 months. There was one procedure-related death. Shunt stenosis and occlusion was seen in seven patients of whom patency was re-established in six patients by balloon dilatation or stent prolongation. Transient deterioration of liver function and development or worsening of hepatic encephalopathy was observed in 11 patients.

Extracorporeal liver support therapy

Extracorporeal liver support therapy has been used as a bridge to OLT and utilizes either biological or nonbiological methods. The biological method used hepatocytes or whole liver organ from human or animal source in an ex-vivo perfusion system while the non-biological methods have included hemodialysis, hemofiltration, plasma exchange and hemoperfusion through charcoal or other absorbents. Recently, in a prospective randomized controlled trial, molecular adsorbent recirculating system (MARS), a modified dialysis method using an albumin-containing dialysate that is recirculated

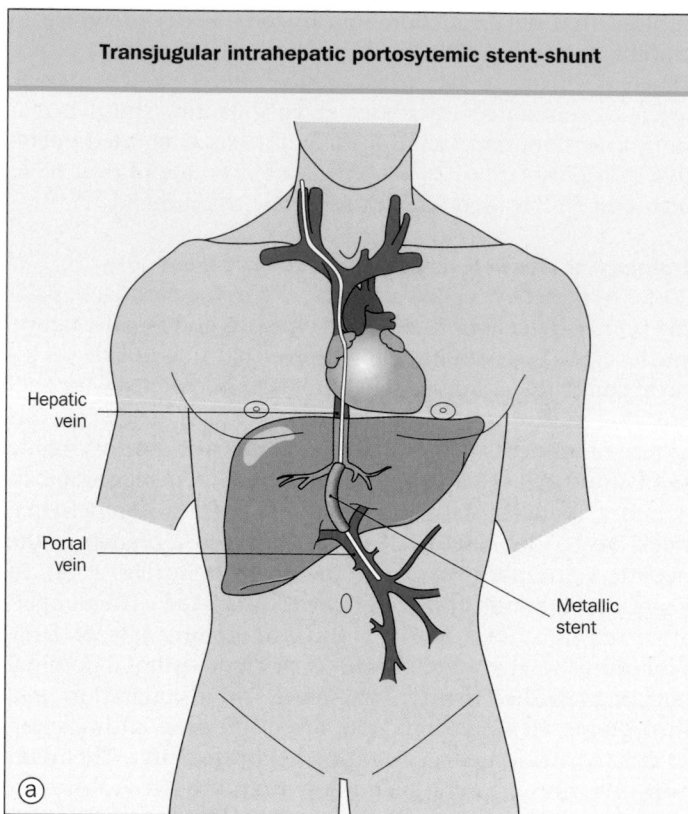

Transjugular intrahepatic portosytemic stent-shunt

Hepatic vein

Portal vein

Metallic stent

(a)

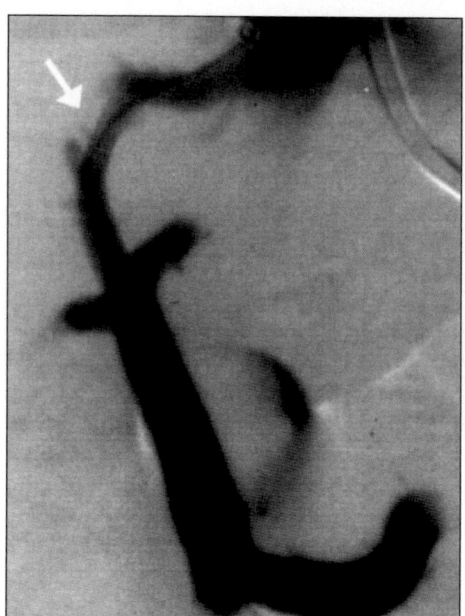

Figure 16.4 Transjugular intrahepatic portosystemic stent-shunt (TIPS). (a) An intrahepatic tract has been created between the right hepatic vein and the right portal vein. The tract is dilated and stented, creating a shunt as demonstrated on shuntogram (b). (Courtesy of Dr WK Tso.)

and perfused online through charcoal and anion-exchanger columns (Fig. 16.5), was shown to effectively remove strongly albumin bound toxic metabolites (i.e., bilirubin and bile acids) and to improve renal function and prolong survival in eight patients with type 1 HRS with severe liver failure (bilirubin > 15 mg/dL) compared to five untreated patients[27]. MARS treatment was associated with a reduction in plasma renin activity which was partly attributed to direct removal but mainly due to increase in EABV secondary to an increased systemic vascular resistance[28]. The latter was in turn hypothesized to be due to the removal of nitric oxide which is transported primarily bound to albumin as an *S*-nitrosothiol.

Renal replacement therapy

Hemodialysis and peritoneal dialysis have been used for the treatment of advancing uremia in patients suffering from HRS but both are fraught with difficulties. Systemic hypotension, which is invariably present, often means that conventional hemodialysis is not feasible or can only be carried out with difficulty. The presence of large amounts of ascites creates a huge 'dead space' that reduces the efficency of peritoneal dialysis. This may be overcome by complete drainage of the abdominal fluid between cycle exchange, but this would result in substantial derangement of body fluid distribution, with resultant hypotension. Continuous arteriovenous or venovenous hemofiltration (CAVH or CVVH) has been advocated for the treatment of advancing uremia in HRS[29]. The continuous nature of the procedure together with lack of osmotic shifts allows adequate removal of fluid and uremic toxins with minimal hemodynamic compromise. In addition, this allows the administration of nutritional support, which

is often vital to the survival of these patients and would optimize their condition before OLT. Furthermore, continuous hemofiltration is associated with a fall in intracranial pressure in patients with HRS, whereas an increase is observed with intermittent hemofiltration or hemodialysis. It is, therefore, also safer to use in patients who suffer from severe hepatic encephalopathy. While continuous hemofiltration is generally recommended for patients with HRS, anticoagulation should be minimized by giving the replacement fluid in the predilutional mode. Bicarbonate should be used instead of lactate as the buffer for the replacement solution, to minimize metabolic acidosis. In liver transplant candidates, the site of dialysis catheter placement should be carefully chosen so the right jugular and right femoral veins may be preserved for cannulation when going into bypass at the time of liver transplantation.

Orthotopic liver transplantation

OLT is the only definitive treatment for patients suffering from HRS. A recent study compared the clinical outcome of OLT in 56 patients with HRS with that of 513 patients without HRS under immunosuppression based on steroid and cyclosporine[30]. The patient and graft survival rates were slightly lower in the HRS group compared with the non-HRS group (60 versus 68% and 51 versus 61%, respectively, at 5 years). Although renal function improved after transplantation in HRS patients, it never reached a level of function demonstrable in non-HRS patients. The HRS group required a longer stay in an intensive-care unit, longer hospitalization, and more dialysis treatment after transplantation; however, pretransplant or post-transplant dialysis did not affect the clinical outcome. The incidence of end-stage renal disease in the HRS group was 7% compared with 2% in the non-HRS group. There was no significant difference in the retransplantation rate and no difference in the long-term liver function between the two groups. It would, therefore, appear that OLT is associated with an acceptable renal and liver outcome and is the treatment of choice for patients suffering from HRS.

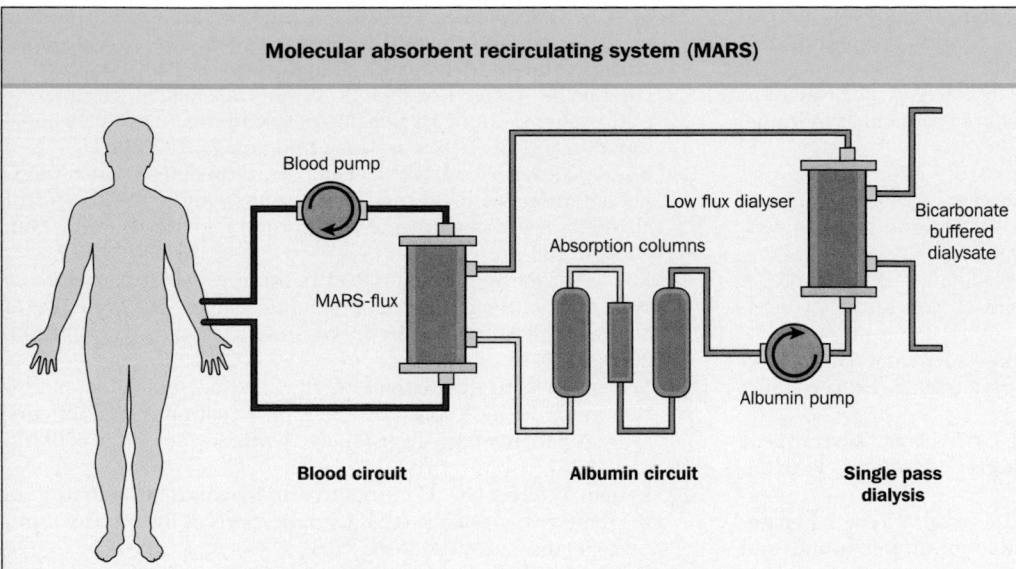

Figure 16.5 Molecular absorbent recirculating system (MARS). The system contains three circuits: the blood circuit, an albumin circuit, and an open-loop, single-pass dialysis circuit. Blood is passed through a non-albumin-permeable high flux dialysis membrane (MARS-flux). The albumin circuit, containing 20% albumin, is passed through the MARS-flux and subsequently regenerated by dialysis against a bicarbonate-buffered dialysate, followed by passage through two sequential columns; the first contains uncoated charcoal and the second contains an anion exchanger resin. (Adapted with permission from Mitzer et al.[28].)

THERAPEUTIC STRATEGY AND CHOICE OF TREATMENT MODALITIES

While OLT is undoubtedly the treatment of choice for patients suffering from HRS, other treatments described above may be used a bridge to OLT, and they may improve the renal outcome following successful OLT. In patients who are not transplant candidates, these treatments are their only chance for increased survival and in some cases, may improve their condition to an extent that may allow them to be reconsidered for transplantation. The choice of therapeutic modalites depends on the availability of resources and expertise on one hand and the severity of underlying renal and liver failure and the general condition of the patient on the other. In patients with relatively well preserved liver function (bilirubin < 15 mg/dL) with no or mild hepatic encephalopathy, pharmacotherapy or TIPS would the therapy of choice while in those with severe liver failure and hepatic encephalopathy, MARS should be considered as a therapeutic option. In patients with advancing renal failure, CVVH is the treatment of choice and may be combined with the therapeutic modalities previously mentioned. Among the numerous pharmacotherapies, the regimen of intravenous ornipressin or terlipressin combined with daily albumin infusion and that of oral midodrine combined with subcutaneous octreotide appear most promising. The latter regimen has the advantage of home treatment.

REFERENCES

1. Arroyo V, Gines P, Gerbes AL, et al. Definition and diagnostic criteria of refractory ascites and hepatorenal syndrome in cirrhosis. Hepatology. 1996;23:164–76.
2. Epstein M, Berk P, Hollenberg NK, et al. Renal failure in the patient with cirrhosis. The role of active vasoconstriction. Am J Med. 1970;49:175–85.
3. Badalamenti S, Graziani G, Salerno F, Ponticelli C. Hepatorenal syndrome. New perspectives in pathogenesis and treatment. Arch Intern Med. 1993;153:1957–67.
4. Epstein M. Hepatorenal syndrome: emerging perspectives of pathophysiology and therapy. J Am Soc Nephrol. 1994;4:1735–53.
5. Moore K. The hepatorenal syndrome. Clin Sci. 1997;92:433–43.
6. Epstein M, Goligorsky MS. Endothelin and nitric oxide in hepatorenal syndrome: a balance reset. J Nephrol. 1997;10:120–35.
7. Bataller R, Gines P, Arroyo V, et al. Hepatorenal syndrome. Clin Liver Dis. 2000;4:487–507.
8. Levenson D, Korecki KL, Narins RG. Acute renal failure associated with hepatobiliary disease. In: Brenner BM, Lazarus JM, eds. Acute renal failure. New York: Churchill Livingstone; 1988:535–80.
9. Gines A, Escorsell A, Gines P, et al. Incidence, predictive factors, and prognosis of the hepatorenal syndrome in cirrhosis with ascites. Gastroenterology. 1993;105:229–36.
10. Roberts LR, Kamath PS. Ascites and hepatorenal syndrome: pathophysiology and management. Mayo Clin Proc. 1996;71:874–81.
11. Sort P, Navasa M, Arroyo V, et al. Effect of intravenous albumin on renal impairment and mortality in patients with cirrhosis and spontaneous bacterial peritonitis. N Engl J Med. 1999;341:403–9.
12. Bennett W, Keefe E, Melnyk C, et al. Response to dopamine hydrochloride in the hepatorenal syndrome. Arch Intern Med. 1975;135:964–71.
13. Lenz K, Hortnagl H, Druml W, et al. Ornipressin in the treatment of functional renal failure in decompensated liver cirrhosis. Effects on renal haemodynamics and atrial natriuretic factor. Gastroenterology. 1991;101:1060–7.
14. Guevara M, Gines P, Fernandez-Esparrach G, et al. Reversibility of hepatorenal syndrome by prolonged administration of ornipressin and plasma volume expansion. Hepatology. 1998;27:35–41.

15. Gulberg V, Bizer M, Gerbes AL. Long term therapy and retreatment of hepatorenal syndrome type 1 with ornipressin and dopamine. Hepatology. 1999;30:870–5.

16. Uriz J, Gines P, Cardenas A, et al. Terlipressin plus albumin infusion: an effective and safe therapy of hepatorenal syndrome. J Hepatol. 2000;33:43–8.

17. Angelli P, Volpin R, Piovan D, et al. Acute effects of the oral administration of midodrine, an α-adrenergic agonist, on renal haemodynamics and renal function in cirrhotic patients with ascites. Hepatology. 1998;987:937–43.

18. Sopor CP, Latif AB, Bending MR. Amelioration of hepatorenal syndrome with selective endothelin-A antagonist. Lancet. 1996;347:1842–3.

19. Holt S, Goodier D, Marley R, et al. Improvement in renal function in hepatorenal syndrome with N-acetylcysteine. Lancet. 1999; 353:294–5.

20. Kaffy F, Borderie C, Chagneau C, et al. Octretide in the treatment of hepatorenal syndrome in cirrhotic patients. J Hepatol. 1999;:30:174.

21. Angeli P, Volpin R, Gerunda G, et al. Reversal of type 1 hepatorenal syndrome with the administration of midodrine and octretide. Hepatology. 1999;29:1690–7.

22. Cade R, Wagemaker H, Vogel S, et al. Hepatorenal syndrome. Studies of the effect of vascular volume and intraperitoneal pressure on renal and hepatic function. Am J Med. 1987;82:427–38.

23. Linas SL, Shaefer JW, Moore EE, et al. Peritoneovenous shunt in the management of the hepatorenal syndrome. Kidney Int. 1986;30:756–40.

24. Stanley MM, Ochi S, Lee KK, et al. Peritoneovenous shunting as compared with medical treatment in patients with alcoholic cirrhosis and massive ascites. N Engl J Med. 1989;321:1632–8.

25. Guevara M, Gines P, Bandi JB, et al. Transjugular intrahepatic portosystemic shunt in hepatorenal syndrome: effects on renal function and vasoactive systems. Hepatology. 1998;28:416–22.

26. Brensing KA, Textor J, Perz J, et al. Long term outcome after transjugular intrahepatic portosystemic stent-shunt in non-transplant cirrhotics with hepatorenal syndrome: a phase II study. Gut. 2000;47:288–95.

27. Mitzer SR, Stange J, Klammt S, et al. Improvement of hepatorenal syndrome with extracorporeal albumin dialysis MARS: results of a prospective, randomized, controlled trial. Liver Transpl. 2000;6:277–86.

28. Mitzer SR, Stange J, Klammit S, et al. Extracorporeal detoxification using the molecular adsorbent recirculating system for critically ill patients with liver failure. J Am Soc Nephrol. 2001;12: S75–S82.

29. Epstein M, Perez GO. Continuous arteriovenous ultrafiltration in the management of the renal complications of liver disease. Int J Artif Organs. 1985;9:215–16.

30. Gonwa TA, Klintmalm GB, Levy M, et al. Impact of pretransplant renal function on survival after liver transplantation. Transplantation. 1995;59:361–5.

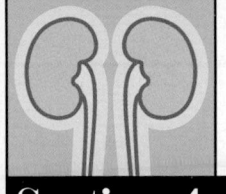

Chapter 17 Myeloma Kidney

Christopher G Winearls

INTRODUCTION

Patients with paraproteinemias present to nephrologists in a number of ways and circumstances but the most urgent and grave is with acute renal failure (Table 17.1). This chapter will describe acute renal failure in patients with multiple myeloma, a lymphoid malignancy. Among the various causes of acute renal failure in myeloma (Table 17.2), the specific characteristic cause is myeloma cast nephropathy (Fig. 17.1). The presentation and special problems of other paraproteinemic conditions, such as Waldenström's macroglobulinemia and AL amyloid (see Chapter 29), and acute cryoglobulinemic nephritis (see Chapter 23). are discussed elsewhere.

EPIDEMIOLOGY

Myeloma is a disease of the elderly: the median age of onset in males is 60–65 years and it is more common in African Caribbeans than in Caucasians. In the UK, the incidence of myeloma is 30–40 new cases per million population per year but only 2% of these are under 40 years of age at the time of diagnosis[1].

Renal impairment of some degree (plasma creatinine > 1.5 mg/dL (> 130 μmol/L)) is observed in 50% of patients who present with myeloma[2]. In most of these patients, the renal failure is reversible, but in about 10% the renal failure is severe enough to require dialysis. In three-quarters of these patients, the myeloma and renal failure are diagnosed within a month of each other[3].

ETIOLOGY/PATHOGENESIS

Myeloma: the nature of the disease

Myeloma is a lymphoid malignancy, the precursor cell of which is a memory B lymphocyte that evolves into the malignant plasma cell producing and usually secreting a monoclonal protein (the M protein)[4]. The M protein may be whole immunoglobulin, free light chain, both or neither (nonsecretory myeloma). The malignant cells are usually found throughout the bone marrow but may be isolated to one site as a plasmacytoma or may even spill into the blood stream as plasma cell leukemia. Their growth is sustained in the microenvironment of the bone marrow by interleukin-6 (IL-6). The clinical manifestations will reflect the load of tumor, its rate of accumulation, and the biologic properties of both the cells and the M protein. In about 50% of patients, the

paraprotein is whole IgG with or without free light chains, in a quarter it is IgA; in one-fifth, light chains alone are detected and in < 1% it is IgD or IgE (Fig. 17.2).

Table 17.1

Paraproteinemias and patterns of renal disease		
	Renal disease	Characteristics
Myeloma (IgG, IgA, IgD, and light chains)	Acute reversible renal failure	Hypercalcemia
		Hyperuricemia
		Dehydration
		Contrast nephrotoxicity
		Cast nephropathy
		Infiltration by plasma cells
	Chronic renal failure	AL amyloid
		Cast nephropathy
		Immunoglobulin deposition disease
	Proteinuria and the nephrotic syndrome	Immunoglobulin deposition disease
		AL amyloid
		Light chain deposition disease
		Heavy chain deposition disease
	Tubular dysfunction	Fanconi syndrome
Macroglobulinemia (IgM)	Waldenström's macroglobulinemia	Hyperviscosity
	Type I cryoglobulinemia	Obstruction of small vessels

Table 17.1 Paraproteinemias and patterns of renal disease.

Table 17.2

Renal pathology in myeloma
Acute tubular necrosis
Cast nephropathy
Interstitial nephritis without casts
AL amyloid
Light chain deposition disease
Plasma cell infiltration

Table 17.2 Renal pathology in myeloma. A spectrum of pathological changes are found in renal biopsies.

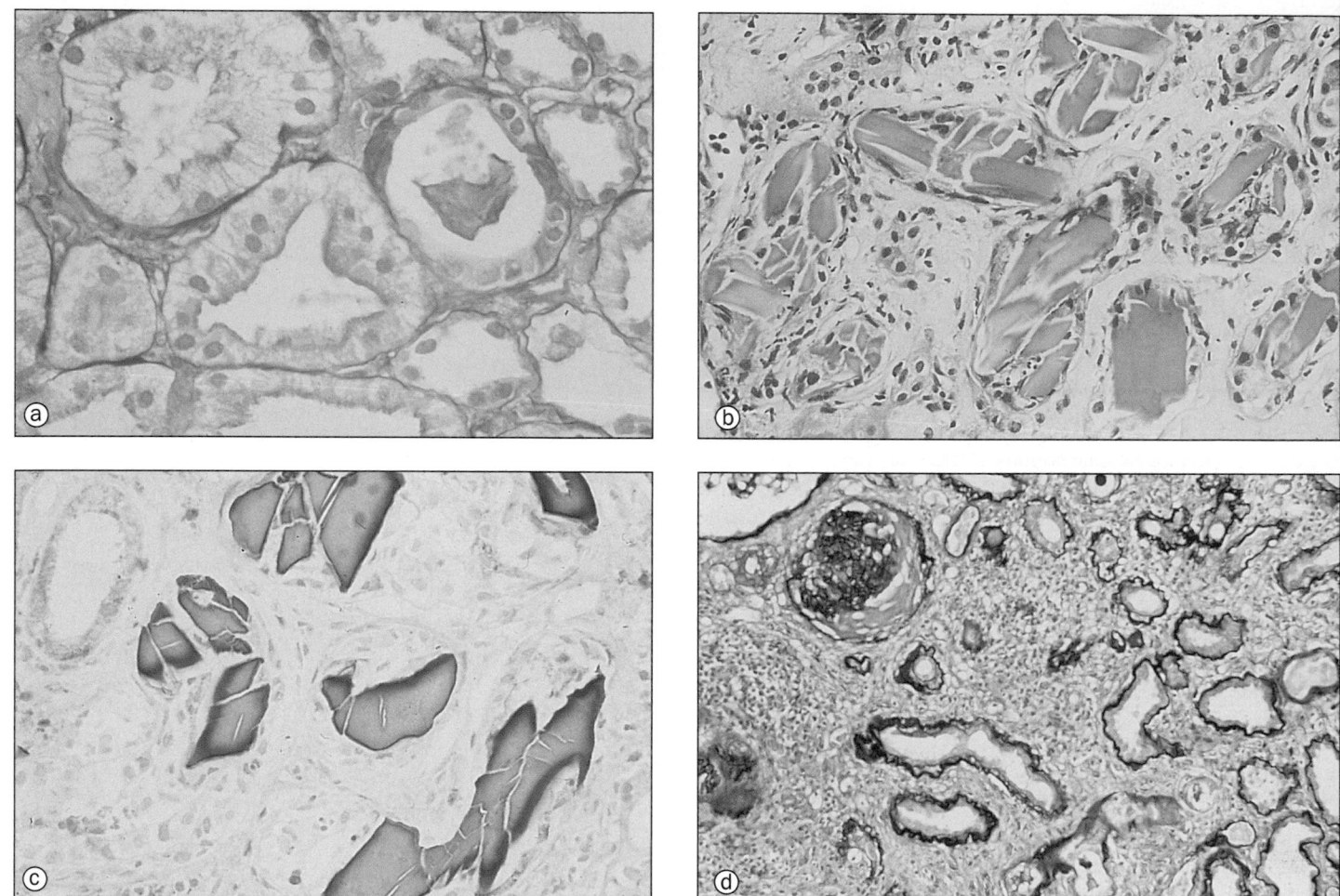

Figure 17.1 Renal histology in myeloma kidney. (a) A cast forming in the distal tubule. The proximal tubules can be distinguished by their brush borders. (b) Classic fractured casts in the distal tubules of a patient with acute renal failure and myeloma and (c) these casts stained by immunoperoxidase for kappa light chain. (d) Severe tubulointerstitial damage with tubular atrophy and interstitial fibrosis in a patient with myeloma kidney and irreversible renal failure.

Pathophysiology of cast nephropathy

Although over half of patients with myeloma have some degree of renal impairment at or after diagnosis, this can in most cases be simply attributed to a combination of dehydration, infection, hypercalcemia, and the effects of nephrotoxic drugs (Fig. 17.3). It is only a minority of patients who develop severe renal failure caused by cast nephropathy[5]. Development of cast nephropathy requires not only the presence of urinary light chains, but also that the light chains should have a predilection for cast formation and be delivered to the distal tubule at a critical concentration.

Cast nephropathy depends on the presence of free light chains so it is very rare to make this diagnosis without detecting light chains in the urine. The explanation for not finding them in a few cases is that they are present but below the limit of detection, for example in IgD myeloma, or that they have all precipitated within the kidney. Patients with pure light-chain myeloma are more likely to develop renal failure and such patients are over-represented in series of acute myeloma kidney (one third of patients with acute myeloma kidney have pure light-chain myeloma compared with 20% of myeloma as

a whole; see Fig. 17.2). There are several pieces of evidence that indicate that the development of cast nephropathy depends in part on the load of the disease. Renal impairment is seen in 40% of patients judged to have a high tumor load compared with 3% of those with a low tumor load. The risk of renal impairment increases with the amount of light chain being excreted: it is 7, 17, and 39% in patients with < 0.005, 0.005–2.0, and > 2 g per day, respectively.

There are several reasons to support the belief that the development of the renal lesion depends on the properties of the light chain. First, although the risk depends on tumor load, it is still only a minority of patients with advanced myeloma that have renal failure. Second, patients with myeloma kidney tend to present with the myeloma and renal failure simultaneously. Third, the specific renal lesion of a patient can be reproduced in laboratory animals injected with the light chain purified from the urine[6]. Patients are equally susceptible to cast nephropathy whether they have free kappa or free lambda light chains. Nor is it the charge (pI) of the light chain that is important but its ability to bind to a specific peptide portion of Tamm–Horsfall protein in the distal tubule, aggregate,

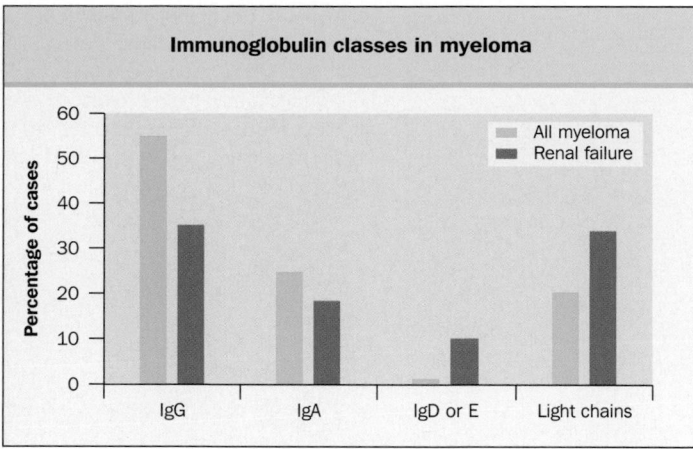

Figure 17.2 Immunoglobulin classes in myeloma. The distribution of monoclonal proteins in all myelomas compared with those in patients with acute renal failure. Note the excess of pure light chain myeloma among those with acute renal failure.

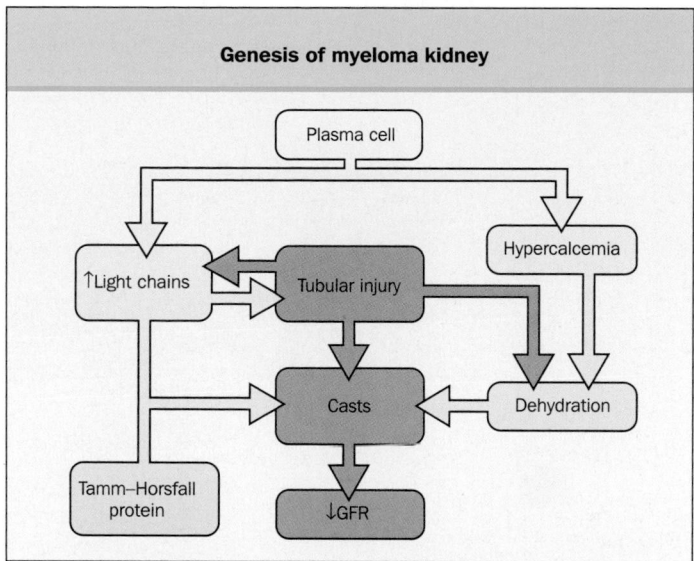

Figure 17.3 Genesis of myeloma kidney. Factors that provoke and aggravate the renal injury in myeloma.

and precipitate in that site. It is interesting that administration of colchicine to experimental animals (which alters the glycosylation of Tamm–Horsfall protein) can prevent the binding of light chains[7]. The results of a number of experiments including those using an isolated tubule perfusion model allow the following hypothesis to be proposed[8].

The kidney is itself responsible for disposal of light chains, which when monomeric are freely filtered, absorbed, and catabolized in the proximal tubular cells (Fig. 17.4). The light chains bind to the proximal tubule brush-border membrane via a single class of low-affinity high-capacity receptors called cubulins (gp280) that function as part of the endocytotic pathway. The concentration of light chains that leave the proximal portion of the nephron will depend, therefore, on the filtrate concentration and the capacity of the tubular cells to absorb and catabolize them. Therefore, any reduction in the glomerular filtration rate (GFR), for example caused by dehydration or damage to the proximal tubule, will reduce the amount of light chain cleared by the kidney and lead to an increase in the plasma and filtrate concentration of light chains. Certain light chains are themselves toxic to the proximal tubule. They can be identified in the endosomes and activated lysosomes of the tubules, and electron microscopy reveals cellular desquamation, cytoplasmic vacuolation, and focal loss of the microvillus border of the cell[9,10]. Damage to the proximal tubule and a reduction in GFR cause reduced tubular clearance of the light chains and lead to a higher concentration of light chains being presented to the distal tubule. It is here, when a critical concentration is reached, that they aggregate, co-precipitate with Tamm–Horsfall protein in the distal nephron and form casts. These casts obstruct tubular fluid flow, leading to disruption of the basement membrane and to leakage into the interstitium (Fig. 17.5). This explains why a patient without renal impairment can suddenly develop a catastrophic and irreversible renal injury and renal failure.

This process will be accelerated and aggravated by dehydration, diuretics, hypercalcemia, and the effects of prostaglandin synthetase inhibitors on glomerular filtration and sodium handling.

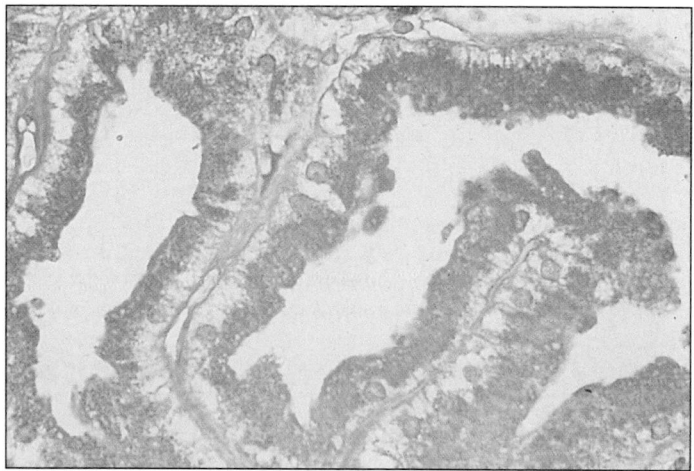

Figure 17.4 Uptake of light chains by proximal tubular cells. Renal biopsy from a patient excreting kappa light chains. Immunoperoxidase staining showing kappa chains along the brush border and in the cytoplasm of proximal tubular cells.

PATHOLOGY

There are a range of findings which are consistent with 'myeloma kidney' but these are not diagnostic (Table 17.2)[9]. In addition to the characteristics of cast nephropathy, there are other features that need to be defined by a biopsy:

- Tubular casts – the number, site, and characteristics of tubular casts should be noted. They are usually in the distal tubules, hyaline, fractured and contain the appropriate light chain on immunostaining (see Fig. 17.1a–c). They may be surrounded by multinucleate cells of macrophage origin.
- Glomerulus – the glomeruli are usually normal but there will rarely be coincident amyloid deposition.

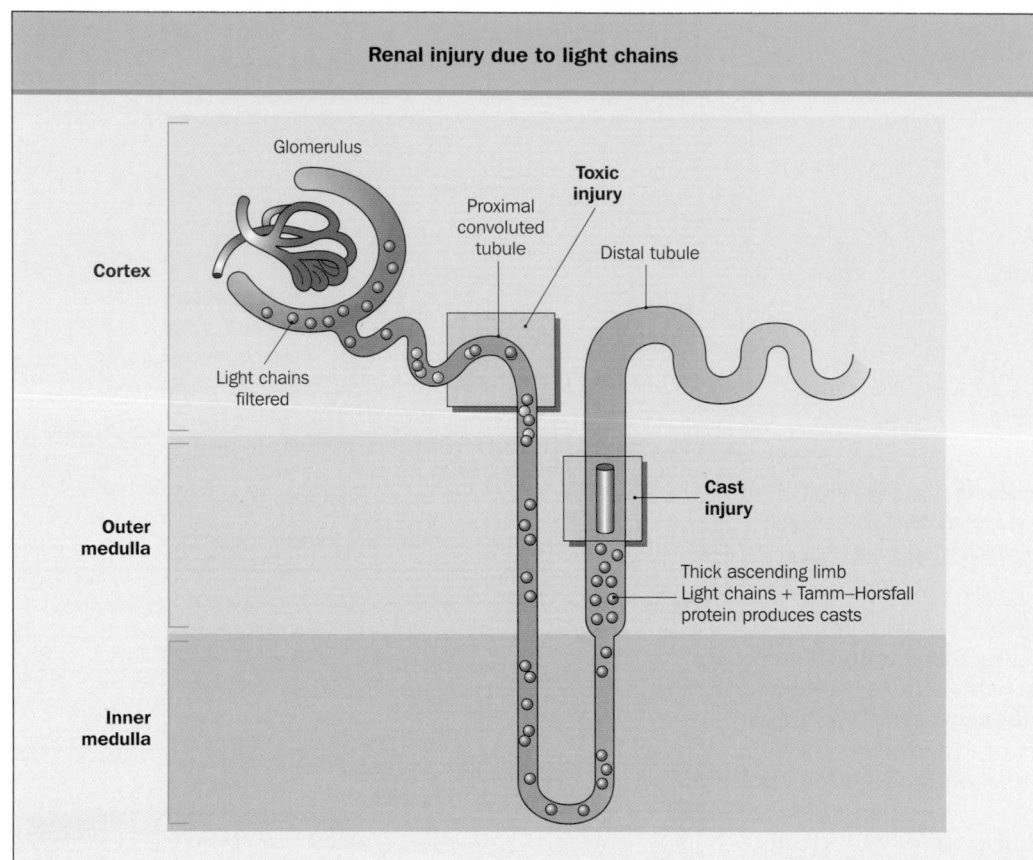

Renal injury due to light chains

Glomerulus

Proximal convoluted tubule

Toxic injury

Distal tubule

Cortex

Light chains filtered

Outer medulla

Cast injury

Thick ascending limb
Light chains + Tamm–Horsfall protein produces casts

Inner medulla

Figure 17.5 Renal injury caused by light chains. Sites (shaded boxes) where light chains injure the tubule. In the proximal tubule there is direct tubular cell toxicity. In the distal tubule there is cast injury.

- Tubulointerstitium– a marked interstitial infiltrate of chronic inflammatory cells with accompanying fibrosis and tubular atrophy predicts a small chance of improvement of renal function (see Fig. 17.1d).

CLINICAL MANIFESTATIONS AND DIAGNOSIS

The diagnosis of myeloma, which is often delayed because of the nonspecific symptoms of the patients, requires a minimum of two of the four criteria listed in Table 17.3. These criteria allow the important distinction to be made between myeloma and benign paraproteinemias, including benign monoclonal gammopathy, or MGUS (monoclonal gammopathy of uncertain significance).

The usual clinical problem facing the nephrologist is the combination of severe renal failure and untreated myeloma[3]. The possibility of myeloma should be considered in any patient with unexplained renal failure, normal sized kidneys, and a bland urine deposit. Urine dipstick testing may be negative since it identifies albumin but not light chains. The suspicion is heightened in the elderly, particularly if there is a history of nonspecific ill health for 3–6 months prior to presentation. Other renal and nonrenal features of myeloma are inconsistently present; these include Fanconi syndrome (proximal renal tubular acidosis), a low anion gap (caused by cationic paraprotein), hyperglobulinemia, and osteopenia.

The diagnosis may require, or even first be suggested by, a renal biopsy. But, even if there is characteristic cast nephropathy, it is essential to request urgent protein electrophoresis of

Diagnostic criteria for multiple myeloma

At least two of:

Bone marrow aspirate contains >20% plasma cells or if <20% the cells are a monoclonal population

Monoclonal serum protein detected in the serum (IgG >30 g/L; IgA >20 g/L)

Monoclonal light chain in the urine

Lytic lesions on skeletal survey

Table 17.3 Diagnostic criteria for multiple myeloma. Two or more of the four criteria are required to establish the diagnosis.

serum and spot urine (concentrated 100-fold) and total serum immunoglobulins. If these are abnormal, further assessment requires serum and urine immunoelectrophoresis. Acute myeloma kidney is very uncommon in patients without detectable monoclonal urinary light chains but it is worth emphasizing that the serum protein electrophoresis may not reveal a band in patients with pure light-chain myeloma. If these tests confirm the diagnosis, additional data are required to stage the disease and plan treatment. These include a radiologic skeletal survey, bone marrow aspiration and trephine biopsy, quantitation of the paraprotein, and assay of serum β_2-microglobulin and C-reactive protein concentrations.

The clinical assessment should also include a review of recent drug treatment especially with nonsteroidal anti-inflammatory drugs (NSAIDs), the volume status of the patient, the presence of hypercalcemia and infection, and evidence of marrow failure from the full blood count. This information will be used to make a judgment on the extent to which the renal failure is acute and, therefore, potentially reversible.

A renal biopsy is only useful in patients with confirmed myeloma in three circumstances:

- If it will guide treatment. Aggressive chemotherapy with or without plasma exchange to reduce the light chain concentration may be justified in the hope that some recovery of renal function will be achieved in those patients without severe tubulointerstitial injury.
- If there is doubt about the predominant cause of renal failure. Biopsy may reveal an explanation other than cast nephropathy, for example acute tubular necrosis, hyperuricemic injury, or amyloidosis.
- If prognostic information is essential. For example if there is doubt in a frail, elderly patient with substantial comorbidity whether any supportive therapy is appropriate.

The risks of renal biopsy will, however, be increased in these uremic, anemic and sometimes thrombocytopenic patients.

NATURAL HISTORY

Myeloma

Myeloma is staged in a number of ways. The Durie and Salmon system estimates the tumor cell mass as low (I), intermediate (II), or high (III) from the hemoglobin, calcium, and paraprotein concentrations and bone lesions. It subclassifies patients into those with relatively normal renal function (A) and those with abnormal renal function (B)[11]. Alternative staging methods rely on the concentration of β_2 microglobulin (which rises in proportion to the tumor burden and renal function); C-reactive protein (reflecting IL-6 secretion); or bone marrow plasma cell morphology and the degree of infiltration. The stage of the disease gives an indication of the likely survival. For patients with stage I, the median survival is 36 months and for stage III it is 14 months.

Renal function

Some improvement in renal function can be expected in about 50% of patients, but most of the series from which this figure is obtained include patients with varying degrees and duration of renal functional impairment. The Oxford experience of 47 dialysis-dependent patients was very disappointing in that only seven (15%) recovered sufficient function to be independent of renal replacement treatment[12]. The chances of improvement are greater in those with less severe renal dysfunction and with an obvious and reversible precipitant. Age, stage, infection, hypercalcemia, and the pI of the light chain are not useful predictors of recovery of renal function. The appearance of the renal biopsy gives useful information. Tubular atrophy and interstitial fibrosis were found more commonly in patients with only minor improvement in renal function or with totally irreversible renal failure[13].

Myeloma with renal failure

The presence of renal failure has long been recognized as a sinister sign and a herald of a poor prognosis in patients with myeloma. This is because patients with renal failure often have more advanced disease. This is supported by the data of Alexanian et al., who reported that 40% of patients with a high tumor mass had plasma creatinine concentrations > 2 mg/dL (> 180 μmol/L) compared with 11% with intermediate and only 3% with low tumor mass[14]. It is illustrated too by the finding in the large UK MRC trials that plasma creatinine (after rehydration) at the time of presentation predicts prognosis[2]. The effect is still apparent for even modest degrees of renal impairment. Some early reports however will have included patients who were not offered renal replacement therapy, even for acute support, and therefore die of renal failure not of myeloma. But the adverse impact of renal dysfunction is also seen in later studies where renal failure was actively managed. In our series of 42 patients with acute presentation of renal failure, the median survival was 8 months[3] and in the total of 40 patients who survived 30 days from presentation and started maintenance dialysis it was 8.5 months[12]. All the patients had stage II or III disease for which the overall predicted median survival is 14 months. This supports the view that having dialysis-dependent renal failure is an additional adverse factor for patients with advanced myeloma. Nevertheless, there is a sufficient, albeit small, number of patients who enjoy a good-quality prolongation of life to justify an energetic approach to treatment and dialysis support.

TREATMENT

Treatment of the renal lesion

The aim of urgent treatment is to correct easily reversible causes of acute renal failure including dehydration, hyperuricemia, and hypercalcemia. Rehydration by saline diuresis in those who are not already fluid overloaded or oliguric, may also prevent further cast precipitation. (The recommendation that this diuresis should be 'alkaline' is not of proven benefit; it is based on theoretical considerations of the relative insolubility of the light chains at acid pH.) Hypercalcemia should be reversed with intravenous biphosphonates (e.g., pamidronate 30–90 mg) if rehydration alone has not proved sufficient. NSAIDs should obviously be stopped. Hyperuricemia should be minimized with allopurinol.

An immediate effect on the plasma cells intended to reduce light chain production can be obtained by the administration of high-dose dexamethasone (40 mg daily). Antiproliferative agents such as melphalan and vincristine take longer to act. Plasma exchange has been recommended by many for the removal of light chains, and the literature is full of anecdotal reports of its efficacy. However evidence from controlled trials is less convincing. Zucchelli et al. compared hemodialysis and plasma exchange with peritoneal dialysis alone. Eleven of thirteen dialysis-dependent patients treated with plasma exchange were able to discontinue treatment compared with only two of eleven in the control group[15]; interpretation of this study is complicated by five early deaths in the control group. The report of Johnson et al. also favored plasma exchange but the benefical effect did not reach statistical significance[16]. The possible benefits should be viewed with caution since a 4 L plasma exchange can have only a small effect on the plasma concentration of light chains which are distributed throughout the extracellular fluid. On available evidence plasma exchange may increase the chance of renal recovery or prevent progression to dialysis dependence, but its application should be confined to those with acute renal injury.[17] A further randomized clinical trial is needed.

Renal replacement therapy

Dialysis should be started early, preferably hemodialysis because the patients are usually elderly, frail, hypercatabolic, and already hypoalbuminemic. There is no particular reason to use high-flux dialyzers as they are unlikely significantly to reduce the concentration of light chains. These patients have a major systemic illness and the synergistic effect of uremia can only increase the risk to life. Dialysis will improve the bleeding diathesis, provide 'space' for blood transfusions, help to control hypercalcemia and hyperuricemia, and minimize the inevitable increase in blood urea that will follow the administration of chemotherapeutic regimens containing high-dose corticosteroids. Because recovery from renal failure is delayed and infrequent, and the risks of infection are high, a permanent dialysis catheter should be placed as soon as possible. If renal failure does prove irreversible, continuous ambulatory peritoneal dialysis (CAPD) is an option and the decision to switch to this treatment will be based on the usual considerations. The risk of peritonitis is often quoted as a reason to prefer hemodialysis but this ignores the equal risk of bacteremia and septicemia from the vascular access[18]. A review of myeloma patients in the USRDS who started renal replacement therapy between 1992 and 1997 showed an all cause two year mortality of 58% compared to 31% in all other patients[19]. There are prejudices but no evidence that the choice of dialysis modality influences outcome[20]. It is said that the need for renal replacement therapy itself does not worsen the prognosis of patients with myeloma, which is dependent on the stage of the disease and the response to chemotherapy. Intuitively, this seems unlikely given the increased risk of death on renal replacement therapy of patients with other renal disease even in the absence of comorbid conditions. Younger patients in whom stable remission of the myeloma has been achieved may be candidates for renal transplantation[21].

Treatment for myeloma

The aim of treatment is usually to prolong survival and prevent or ameliorate complications rather than attempt cure. It is directed at reducing the bulk of the tumor but the emergence of therapy-resistant subclones leads eventually to an overwhelming tumor burden and death. In a minority of patients, attempts are made at cure by the administration of high-dose chemotherapy supported by autologous or allogeneic bone marrow transplantation, or stem cell support.

There are no specific trials to guide choice of therapy for myeloma complicated by renal failure. Oral melphalan and prednisolone given as 4-day pulses at intervals of 4–6 weeks will produce a response in about 50% of patients. The dose of melphalan is usually reduced by 50% in patients with GFR < 10 mL/min but this may not actually be necessary[22]. Weekly pulses of cyclophosphamide are an equivalent and convenient option for initial induction treatment.

In younger patients and those in whom a more rapid response is needed, combination regimens such as 'VAD' (vincristine, daunorubicin (adriamycin), and dexamethasone) are preferred and well tolerated.

Myeloablative treatment with high-dose melphalan and autologous stem-cell support has been applied in patients with renal failure including those on dialysis. The treatment related mortality is ~10% but overall survival > 50% at 3 years[23]. It is still being evaluated. Allogeneic bone marrow transplantation is an even higher-risk treatment but has a lower relapse rate. These more aggressive treatment schedules are not commonly used in patients with renal failure but there are anecdotal reports of their successful application in younger dialysis-dependent subjects[1].

Maintenance interferon-α may prolong the plateau phase by 6 to 12 months but does not prolong survival. Adverse effects on renal function in patients with renal involvement have been reported[24].

Patients require adequate analgesia for the bone lesions and this will often include opiates and local radiotherapy. NSAIDs should be used with caution and not at all if renal function is impaired or the patient dehydrated or infected. Monthly infusions of pamidronate provide significant protection against skeletal complications and may even modify disease progression in advanced myeloma. This benefit is not confined to patients with hypercalcemia[25].

In elderly patients with advanced disease, it is reasonable to withhold chemotherapy that will cause immediate side effects and is unlikely to prolong life or improve its quality. It is our practice to use dialysis for such patients and support them with blood transfusions, analgesics, antibiotics, and palliative radiotherapy to skeletal deposits.

Treatment summary

Although the treatment plan for each patient should be designed individually and modified according to response or complications, our approach can be summarized as follows:

- For elderly patients (age > 75 years) with advanced disease, we provide supportive treatment and commence dialysis if it is the patient's wish.
- If the prognosis for survival in the elderly patient is judged to be more than 3–6 months, immediate treatment with dexamethasone followed by a standard melphalan–prednisolone regimen is also recommended.
- Younger patients and those with less severe complications are treated with VAD and will be considered for myeloablative treatment with autologous stem-cell support.

REFERENCES

1. UK myeloma forum. British Committee for Standards in Haematology. Diagnosis and management of multiple myeloma. Br J Haematol. 2001;115:522–40
2. MacLennan IC, Cooper EH, Chapman CE, et al. Renal failure in myelomatosis. Eur J Haematol Suppl. 1989;51:60–5.
3. Winearls CG. Acute myeloma kidney. Kidney Int. 1995;48:1347–61.
4. Bataille R, Harousseau J. Medical progress. Multiple myeloma. N Engl J Med. 1997;336:1657–64.
5. Iggo N, Winearls CG, Davies DR. The development of cast nephropathy in multiple myeloma. Q J Med. 1997;90:653–6.
6. Solomon A, Weiss DT, Kattine AA. Nephrotoxic potential of Bence Jones proteins. N Engl J Med. 1991;324:1845–51.
7. Sanders PW. Potential role of colchicine in the prevention of cast nephropathy from Bence Jones proteins. Contrib Nephrol. 1993;101:104–8.
8. Sanders PW, Booker BB, Bishop JB, Cheung HC. Mechanisms of intranephronal proteinaceous cast formation by low molecular weight proteins. J Clin Invest. 1990;85:570–6.
9. Striker LJ, Olson JL, Striker GE. Renal diseases associated with lymphoplasmacytic disorders. Philadelphia, PA: Saunders; 1990:195–223.
10. Pirani CL, Silva F, D'Agati V, et al. Renal lesions in plasma cell dyscrasias: ultrastructural observations. Am J Kidney Dis. 1987;10:208–21.
11. Durie BGM, Salmon SE. A clinical staging system for multiple myeloma. Correlation of measured myeloma cell mass with presenting clinical features, response to treatment, and survival. Cancer. 1975;36:842–54.
12. Irish AB, Winearls CG, Littlewood T. Presentation and survival of patients with severe renal failure and myeloma. Q J Med. 1997;90:773–80.
13. Rota S, Mougenot B, Baudouin B, et al. Multiple myeloma and severe renal failure: a clinicopathologic study of outcome and prognosis in 34 patients. Med Baltimore. 1987;66:126–37.
14. Alexanian R, Barlogie B, Dixon D. Renal failure in multiple myeloma. Pathogenesis and prognostic implications. Arch Intern Med. 1990;150:1693–5.
15. Zucchelli P, Pasquali S, Cagnoli L, Ferrari G. Controlled plasma exchange trial in acute renal failure due to multiple myeloma. Kidney Int. 1988;33:1175–80.
16. Johnson WJ, Kyle RA, Pineda AA, et al. Treatment of renal failure associated with multiple myeloma. Plasmapheresis, hemodialysis, and chemotherapy. Arch Intern Med. 1990;150:863–9.
17. Moist L, Nesrallah G, Kortas C, Eet al. Plasma exchange in rapidly progressive renal failure due to multiple myeloma. A retrospective case series. Am J Nephrol. 1999;19:45–50.
18. Tapson JS, Mansy H, Wilkinson R. End-stage renal failure due to multiple myeloma – poor survival on peritoneal dialysis. Int J Artif Organs. 1988;11:39–42.
19. Abbott KC, Agodoa LY. Multiple myeloma and light chain-associated nephropathy at end-stage renal disease in the United States: patient characteristics and survival. Clin Nephrol. 2001;56:207–10.
20. Iggo N, Palmer AB, Severn A, et al. Chronic dialysis in patients with multiple myeloma and renal failure: a worthwhile treatment. Q J Med. 1989;73:903–10.
21. van Bommel EFH. Multiple myeloma treatment in dialysis-dependent patients: to transplant or not to transplant? Nephrol Dial Transplant. 1996;11:1486–7.
22. Tricot G, Alberts DS, Johnson C, et al. Safety of autotransplants with high-dose melphalan in renal failure: a pharmacokinetic and toxicity study. Clin Cancer Res. 1996;2:947–52.
23. Badros A, Barlogie B, Siegel E, et al. Results of autologous stem cell transplant in multiple myeloma patients with renal failure. Br J Haematol. 2001;114:822–9.
24. Fahal IH, Murry N, Chu P, Bell GM. Acute renal failure during interferon treatment. Br Med J Clin Res. 1993;306:973.
25. Berenson JR, Lichtenstein A, Porter L, et al. Efficacy of pamidronate in reducing skeletal events in patients with advanced multiple myeloma. Myeloma Aredia Study Group. N Engl J Med. 1996;334:488–93.

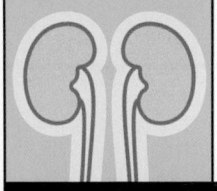

Chapter 18 | Introduction to Glomerular Disease: Pathogenesis and Classification

Richard J Johnson, Helmut Rennke, and John Feehally

INTRODUCTION

Numerous inflammatory and noninflammatory diseases affect the glomerulus and lead to alterations in glomerular permeability, structure, and function. Many glomerular diseases come under the generic title glomerulonephritis (GN), which implies that there is an immune pathogenesis. Not all glomerular disease is caused by GN and other causes need to be considered in its differential diagnosis. Particularly important are diabetic nephropathy and amyloidosis, as well as the hereditary nephropathies, most commonly Alport syndrome.

GN may be primary, restricted in clinical manifestations to the kidney, or it may be part of a multisystem disease, most frequently systemic lupus or vasculitis. While the likelihood of a patient having GN can be estimated with varying degrees of confidence from the clinical setting and laboratory tests, it cannot ultimately be diagnosed without histologic examination of cortical renal tissue.

CLASSIFICATION

GN is classified by the different patterns of histologic injury seen on a renal biopsy examined by light microscopy, immunofluorescence, and electron microscopy. This classification is not ideal since it cannot always be assumed that one histologic pattern has a single etiology or that it will have a single clinical presentation. Furthermore, one etiology may produce a variety of histologic patterns (for example the varied glomerular disease seen in association with hepatitis B infection or lupus).

It is more helpful to regard the renal biopsy appearance as a 'pattern' rather than a 'disease': a 'pattern' that may frequently have a number of clinical correlates, a number of putative etiologic agents, and which may eventually prove to have more than one immune mechanism. Nevertheless, the classification of GN remains largely based on renal pathology and the approach taken in this book chiefly subdivides GN on this basis.

HISTOPATHOLOGY

The full assessment of a renal biopsy requires light microscopy, electron microscopy, and examination for immune deposits stained by immunofluorescence or immunoperoxidase.

Light microscopy

In GN, the dominant, but not the only, histologic lesions are in glomeruli (see Fig. 18.1). GN is described as focal (only some glomeruli are involved) or diffuse. In any individual glomerulus, injury may be segmental (affecting only part of any glomerulus) or global. There is a potential for sampling error in a renal biopsy: the extent of a focal lesion may be misjudged in a small biopsy specimen and sections through glomeruli may miss segmental lesions. Lesions may also be hypercellular due to either an increase in endogenous endothelial or mesangial cells (termed 'proliferative') and/or to an infiltration of inflammatory leukocytes (termed 'exudative'). Severe acute inflammation may produce glomerular necrosis, which is often segmental. The walls of the glomerular capillaries can also be thickened by a number of processes, which include increase in glomerular basement membrane (GBM) material and immune deposits. Methenamine silver staining is helpful because the silver stains basement membranes and other matrix black. It may, for example, reveal a double contour to the GBM because of the interposition of cellular material, or it may show increased mesangial matrix not easily seen with other techniques. Segmental sclerosis and scarring may also occur, and is characterized by segmental capillary collapse with the accumulation of hyaline material and mesangial matrix, and often with attachment of the capillary wall with Bowman's capsule ('synechiae' or adhesion formation).

Crescents are inflammatory collections of cells in Bowman's space. Crescents develop when severe glomerular injury results in local rupture of the capillary wall or Bowman's capsule allowing plasma proteins and inflammatory material to enter into Bowman's space. Crescents consist of proliferating parietal epithelial cells, infiltrating fibroblasts, and lymphocytes and monocytes/macrophages, often with local fibrin deposition. They are called crescents because of their appearance when the glomerulus is cut in one plane for histology. They are destructive, rapidly increasing in size and squeezing the glomerular tuft until it is occluded (Fig. 18.1f). Even if the acute injury is stopped, the crescents heal by fibrosis, causing irretrievable loss of renal function. Crescents are most commonly observed with vasculitis, in Goodpasture's disease, and in severe, acute GN of any etiology.

Abnormalities are not confined to the glomeruli in GN. Tubulointerstitial inflammation is common, the more so with acute and severe GN. In advanced GN, as glomeruli fail their associated tubules will atrophy, leading to interstitial fibrosis in a pattern no different from other progressive chronic renal diseases (see Chapter 66).

Glomerular Disease

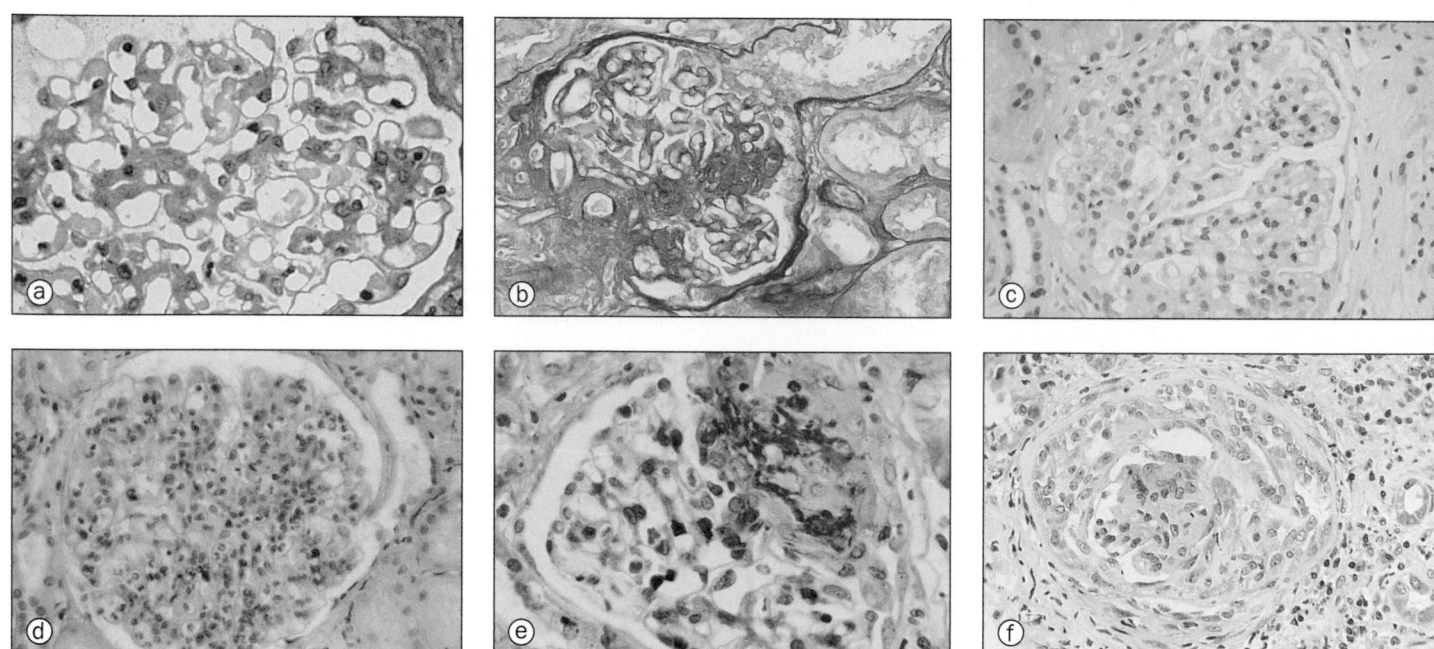

Figure 18.1 Pathology of glomerular disease. Light microscopy. Characteristic patterns of glomerular disease illustrating the range of histologic appearances and the descriptive terms used. (a) Normal glomerulus; minimal change disease. (b) Segmental sclerosis; focal segmental glomerulosclerosis. (c) Diffuse mesangial hypercellularity; IgA nephropathy. (d) Diffuse endocapillary hypercellularity; poststreptococcal glomerulonephritis. (e) Segmental necrosis; renal vasculitis. (f) Crescent formation; antiglomerular basement membrane disease.

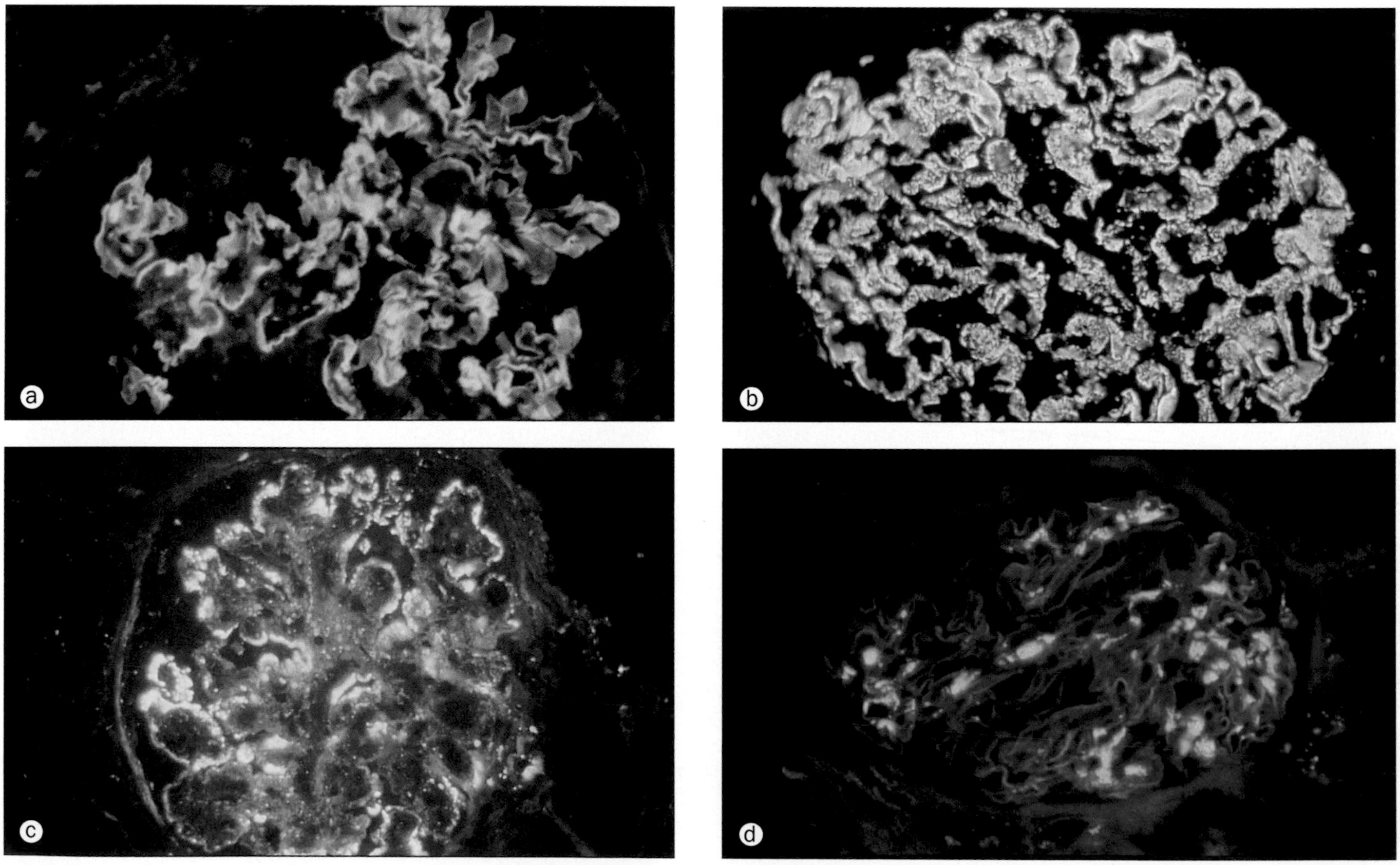

Figure 18.2 Pathology of glomerular disease. Immunofluorescence microscopy. Common patterns of glomerular staining found by immunofluorescence. (a) Linear capillary wall IgG; antiglomerular basement membrane disease. (b) Fine granular capillary wall IgG; membranous nephropathy. (c) Coarse granular capillary wall IgG; membranoproliferative GN type I. (d) Granular mesangial IgA; IgA nephropathy.

Immunofluorescence microscopy

Indirect immunofluorescence and immunoperoxidase staining are both used to identify immune reactants (Fig. 18.2). It is routine to look for the deposition of immunoglobulins IgG, IgA, and IgM, for components of both classic and alternative pathway (usually C3, C4, and C1q) and for the presence of fibrin, which is commonly observed in crescents and in capillaries in thrombotic disorders (such as hemolytic–uremic syndrome and the antiphospholipid syndrome). Immune deposits may occur along the capillary loops or in the mesangium. They may be continuous (linear) or discontinuous (granular) along the capillary wall or in the mesangium.

Granular deposits in glomeruli are sometimes called 'immune complexes'. This implies the deposition or local formation of an antigen–antibody complex in the glomerulus. However, in very few situations is the putative antigen known and only rarely is there definite evidence of antigen deposition along with antibody in human GN. The term 'immune complex' harks back to experimental models of GN where there is strong evidence of antigen–antibody complexes directly initiating glomerular injury. The more general term, immune deposit, is preferable.

Electron microscopy

Electron microscopy is valuable for defining the anatomy of the basement membranes (abnormal in some forms of hereditary nephropathy, e.g., Alport syndrome and thin basement membrane nephropathy (see Chapter 48)) and for localizing the site of immune deposits (which are usually homogeneous and electron dense; Fig. 18.3). Electron-dense deposits are seen in the mesangium or along the capillary wall on the subepithelial or subendothelial side of the GBM. Uncommonly the electron-dense material lies linearly within the GBM. The sites of immune deposits are helpful in the classification of the types of GN.

PATHOGENESIS OF GLOMERULAR INJURY

The type of glomerular injury depends not only on the initial immune response but also on the extent to which that response is perpetuated and provokes glomerular injury. It also depends on the extent to which the initial inflammation resolves without scarring or proceeds to glomerular destruction, either by rapid inflammation and necrosis or by slowly progressive glomerulosclerosis and tubulointerstitial fibrosis (see Fig. 18.4).

Immune glomerular injury

Events involved in the initiation of glomerular disease are still poorly understood. Most glomerular diseases develop as a result of immune dysregulation, either an inappropriate immune response to self-antigens occurring through a failure of tolerance ('autoimmunity') or an ineffectual response to a foreign antigen.

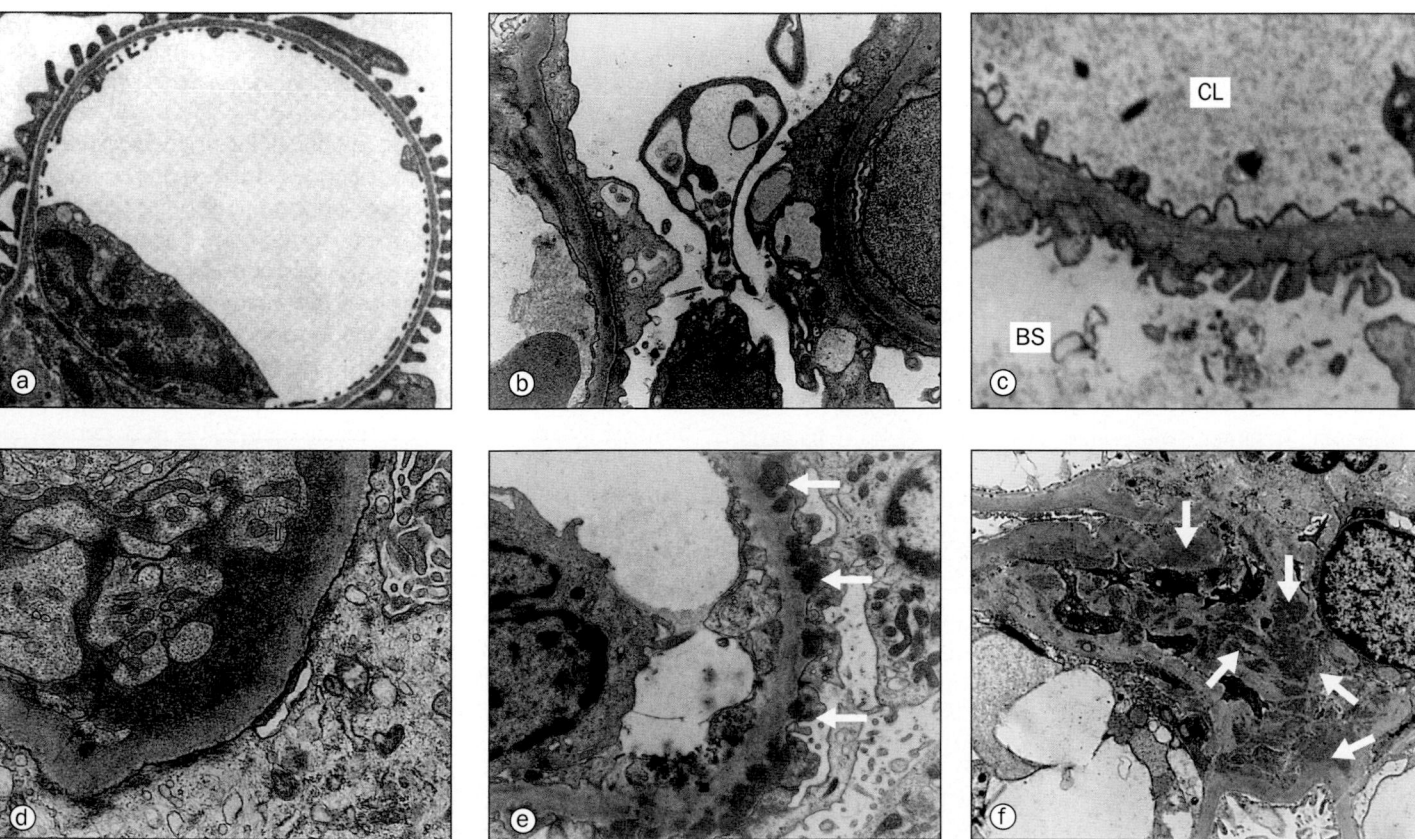

Figure 18.3 Ultrastructural pathology of glomerular disease. Some characteristic patterns of electron-dense deposits (EDD) and glomerular basement membrane (GBM) abnormalities seen in glomerular disease. (a) Normal. (b) Foot process effacement; minimal change disease. (c) GBM thickening and splitting; Alport syndrome. (d) Subendothelial EDD; membranoproliferative glomerulonephritis (MPGN) type I. (e) Subepithelial EDD (arrows); membranous nephropathy. (f) Mesangial EDD (arrows); IgA nephropathy.

Glomerular Disease

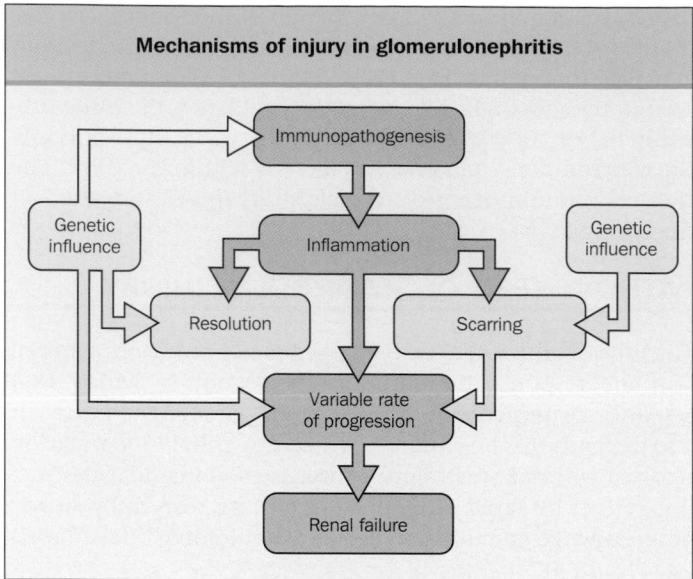

Mechanisms of injury in glomerulonephritis

Figure 18.4 Mechanisms of injury in glomerulonephritis.

Autoimmunity

In health, a tension exists between the normal immune response to foreign antigen and 'tolerance', which is the cellular process that prevents an immune response to self-antigen. Tolerance develops because self-reactive T and B cells are clonally deleted during fetal and neonatal life, although small numbers survive outside the thymus. Under certain conditions, these peripheral self-reactive T and B cells can be stimulated to generate a cellular and humoral response to a 'self-antigen'. Infection or toxins may play a role in initiating the response by releasing antigens from sequestered sites so they have access to T cells, by altering host proteins to make them more immunogenic, or by 'molecular mimicry' in which antibodies to an exogenous antigen (for example in an infecting organism) cross-react with a native protein. Recently it has been shown that oxidants, such as may occur with smoking or with aging, can alter GBM to expose the Goodpasture antigen from an otherwise cryptic site that may not only allow it to function as a neoantigen but also to be recognized by anti-glomerular basement membrane antibody[1]. Certain bacteria and viruses also express 'superantigens', which can activate T cells directly and may lead to polyclonal B cell expansion. Once there is an inflammatory response, the further release of antigens may result in the generation of additional auto-antibodies, a process known as 'determinant spreading'. Activation of T cells may be further enhanced by the release of cytokines and lymphokines, and the conversion of normally innocuous cells into antigen-presenting cells via the upregulated or *de novo* expression of HLA class II molecules.

Genetic background to glomerulonephritis

Variations in human leukocyte antigen (HLA) molecules and the T cell receptor are under strong genetic influence. For that reason, immunogenetic associations particularly between HLA expression and various patterns of GN have been studied in great detail, but none of the reported associations is absolutely specific[2]. Consequently, while HRA-DR2 identifies

a powerful relative risk for the development of Goodpasture's disease, it is still possible to develop the disease without HRA-DR2; and the vast majority of individuals with HRA-DR2 never develop this rare disease. Furthermore, the HLA associations often differ among racial groups with different distributions of HLA. This suggests that the associations so far identified are not the disease susceptibility genes themselves but are adjacent to them and associated by linkage disequilibrium, and that there may be other susceptibility genes not yet identified, perhaps on remote chromosomes. It also suggests that environmental events may have great importance, acting on genetic background, in inducing GN and that additional genes might influence disease severity rather than susceptibility. HLA associations have no practical diagnostic or therapeutic implications as yet, and HLA typing is not needed in the clinical management of GN.

Ineffectual response to a foreign antigen

Some glomerular diseases may occur as a consequence of an inability to eliminate a foreign antigen. A classic example is hepatitis B (HBV) infection, in which infection, particularly in fetal or early life, results in tolerance and a chronic carrier state. Despite a strong humoral response, viral infection persists because the cell-mediated response required for elimination of HBV from the liver is impaired. The consequence is a state of persistent antigenemia with circulating antigen–antibody complexes, which predisposes to glomerular injury.

Mechanisms of immunecomplex formation within the glomerulus

In most cases of GN, there is immunoglobulin deposition in glomeruli, often codeposited with components of the complement cascade, which is presumed to represent immunecomplex formation[3].

Circulating immune complexes (CIC) may localize to the glomerulus by passive deposition from the circulation. Normally, complexes of antibody and foreign antigen engage complement and are cleared from the circulation by binding of the complex to the C3b receptors on erythrocytes; the immune complexes are then removed and degraded during transit of the erythrocytes in the liver and spleen. If antigenemia persists or clearance of complexes is impaired (such as in chronic liver disease or due to defective immune-complex binding by erythrocytes), immune complexes may deposit in the glomerulus by binding to Fc receptors on mesangial cells or by passive deposition in the mesangium or subendothelial space. Physical characteristics of the complexes may also favor deposition, including avidity, charge, and size. Measurement of CIC in patients with GN has not, however, shown close correlation with glomerular events, nor has analysis of CIC led to identification of many pathogenetic antigens.

A second mechanism for immunecomplex localization involves local *in situ* formation. Antibody may bind directly to an intrinsic glomerular antigen. Alternatively, a nonglomerular antigen, such as a viral or food antigen, may first localize to a glomerular structure ('planted antigen') followed by antibody binding. This situation may be more likely when the antigen has characteristics favoring binding to glomeruli (such as cationic antigens that can bind the anionic basement membrane) or when the antibody has low avidity (thereby favoring dissociation of the immune complexes in the circulation).

Identification of antigens

Most of the specific antigens involved in human GN remain unknown. The best characterized antigen that is involved with autoimmunity is the α3 chain of type IV collagen, which is the target antigen in anti-GBM disease (Goodpasture's disease)[4]. Recently a form of congenital membranous nephropathy was identified in which the mother, who genetically lacked a glomerular epithelial antigen (neutral endopeptidase, NEP), generated antibodies to NEP from a previous miscarriage and passively transferred them to her infant during delivery[5]. The best example of a response to foreign antigen is poststreptococcal GN, where streptococcal antigens (glyceraldehyde 3-phosphate dehydrogenase (GAPDH)/nephritis-associated plasmin receptor and exotoxin B precursor/zymogen) can be found in the glomerular deposits[6]. Another example is HBV-associated GN.

The failure to identify the antigens within immune deposits in GN may be due to the fact that the relevant antigens may not have been considered, or because the initiating antigen may no longer be present, and the immune deposits are being perpetuated by a secondary anti-idiotype antibody response directed against the original antibody. In some cases an antigen may never have been present in the first place, the immunoglobulin being deposited not in response to antigen but for other reasons, possibly physicochemical.

Cell-mediated immune mechanisms

In contrast to the immune-complex mechanisms discussed above, certain glomerular diseases develop primarily through cell-mediated immunity. Studies in experimental models of crescentic nephritis have provided convincing evidence for a direct role for T cells in mediating proteinuria and crescent formation[7]. It is thought that T cells sensitized to endogenous or exogenous antigen present in the glomeruli recruit macrophages, which leads to a local delayed-type hypersensitivity reaction. In certain models, CD8+ T cells have also been shown to mediate crescent formation via perforins (enzymes that act similarly to the complement membrane attack complex). Cell-mediated immunity has also been incriminated in minimal change disease; here, it has been postulated to result from a T cell product that injures the glomerular epithelial cell and induces a permeability defect (see below).

Effector mechanisms

What really decides the severity of glomerular injury is the way in which this initial immune event recruits inflammatory mediators. In immune-complex disease, the amount of inflammation is dependent on the amount, mechanism of formation, and biologic properties of the complexes as well as their site of deposition.

Complement

The complement system is an amplifying cascade of proteins that produces cell injury and promotes inflammation (Fig. 18.5). The central event in the complement cascade is the cleavage of C3 which leads to the production of the membrane attack complex and to C3 fragments, which are active in inflammation. Complement can be activated by immune complexes via the classical pathway, initiated by the binding of C1q to the Fc portion of antibody. Classic pathway activation typically occurs in diffuse proliferative lupus nephritis, cryoglobulinemia, and membranoproliferative GN (MPGN) type I. In this setting both serum C3 and C4 are usually low. Complement can also be activated via the mannose-binding pathway initiated by a lectin (mannose-binding lectin; MBL), which has a similar structure to C1q. The role of the mannose-binding pathway in GN has not yet been clearly established.

Finally, the complement cascade can also be initiated via the alternative pathway, an amplification loop for C3 activation, which is independent of immune complexes but is triggered by polysaccharide antigens, aggregated IgA, injured cells, or endotoxins. This pathway appears to be activated in MPGN type II, and in some cases of poststreptococcal GN. Serum C3 is typically low, but C4 normal. Nephritic factors are autoantibodies that stabilize various convertases in the complement pathway, and modify their action; they play a key role in the pathogenesis of MPGN (see Chapter 23).

Activation of the complement pathway has several consequences. Leukocyte recruitment is facilitated by the chemotactic factor C5a, and C3b binding is important in the binding and opsonization of the immune complexes by the infiltrating leukocytes. The terminal membrane attack complex of the cascade, C5b–9, inserts into cell membranes where it can kill cells or activate them to secrete cytokines, oxidants, and extracellular matrix. C5b–9 is thought to be important in mediating injury to the glomerular epithelial cell in membranous nephropathy, a disease in which immune deposits and complement activation occur in the subepithelial space.

Inflammatory cells

The infiltration by inflammatory cells is largely determined by the site of immune deposits. Immune deposits with direct access to the circulation (i.e., those in mesangial, subendothelial and basement membrane locations) are usually associated with a pronounced leukocyte accumulation. In contrast, immune deposits in the subepithelial space (such as in membranous nephropathy) generally are not associated with inflammatory cells, as the release of chemotactic factors such as C5a are not sensed by leukocytes due to the intervening basement membrane and the filtration forces wash the C5a into the urine. Leukocyte infiltration tends to be more severe in acute forms of GN such as MPGN. Infiltrating cells are neutrophils (typically in postinfectious GN), T cells, or monocytes/macrophages.

Intrinsic glomerular cells (epithelial, mesangial, and endothelial) may also be activated by the injury to become inflammatory-like cells. Mesangial cells, for example, can be activated to produce oxidants, proteases, cytokines, vasoactive mediators and extracellular matrix; mesangial cell proliferation and matrix expansion are critical pathogenic features in IgA nephropathy.

Soluble factors

The biology of these soluble factors is very complex, but already known to be important are cytokines, vasoactive mediators, growth factors, reactive oxygen species, proteases, and proteins of the coagulation cascade. These factors variously promote the recruitment and activation of inflammatory cells,

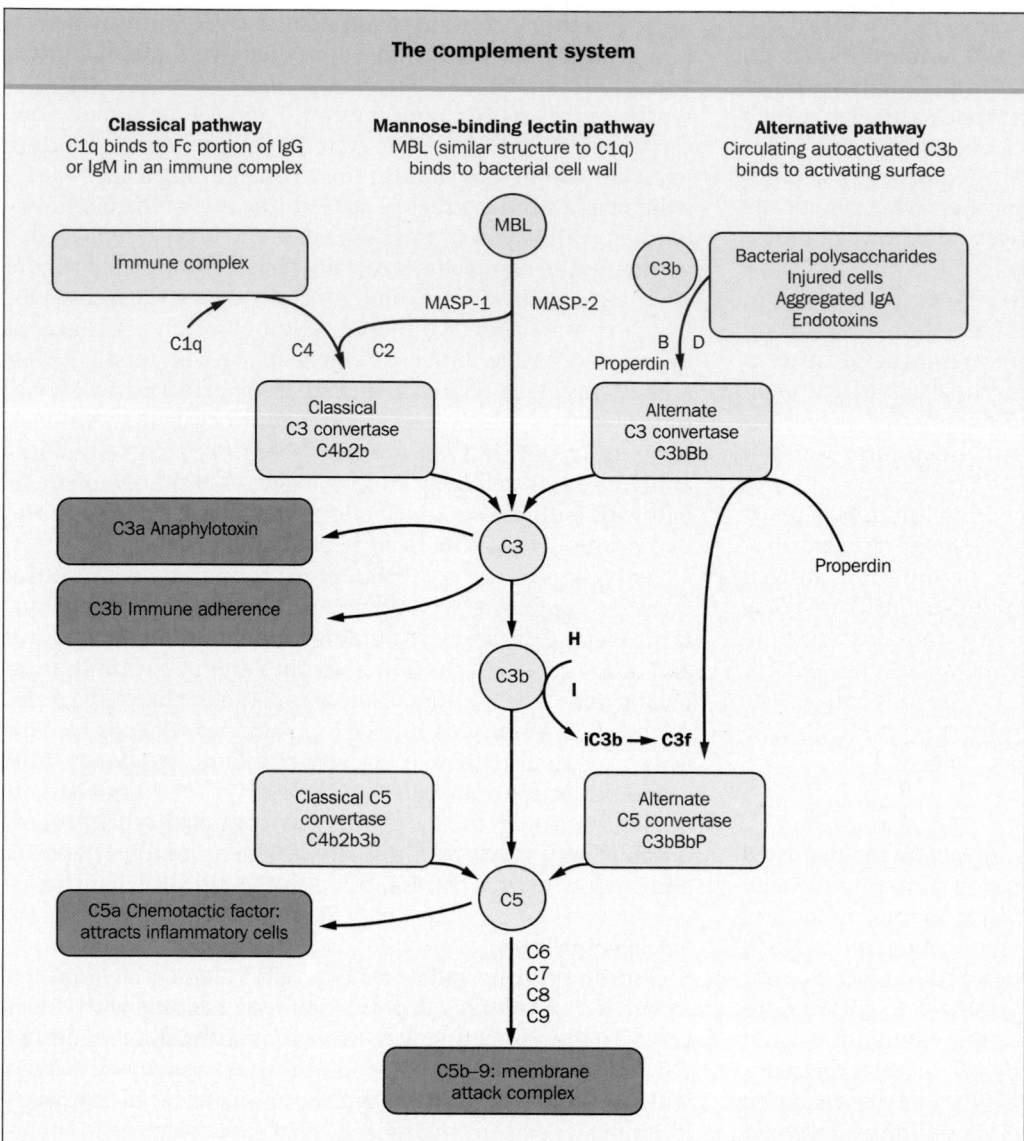

The complement system

Classical pathway
C1q binds to Fc portion of IgG
or IgM in an immune complex

Mannose-binding lectin pathway
MBL (similar structure to C1q)
binds to bacterial cell wall

Alternative pathway
Circulating autoactivated C3b
binds to activating surface

MBL

Immune complex

C3b

Bacterial polysaccharides
Injured cells
Aggregated IgA
Endotoxins

MASP-1 MASP-2

C1q C4 C2

B D
Properdin

Classical
C3 convertase
C4b2b

Alternate
C3 convertase
C3bBb

C3a Anaphylotoxin

C3

Properdin

C3b Immune adherence

H

C3b

I

iC3b → C3f

Classical C5
convertase
C4b2b3b

Alternate
C5 convertase
C3bBbP

C5a Chemotactic factor:
attracts inflammatory cells

C5

C6
C7
C8
C9

C5b–9: membrane
attack complex

Figure 18.5 The complement system. The complement system is a self-amplifying cascade of proteins that generates a membrane attack complex, which is cytolytic; the cascade promotes inflammation by the activity of the fragments it produces. The amplifying cascades occur because activated fragments of the components combine to make convertase enzymes that degrade C3 and C5. The complement cascade is controlled in part by the very short active life of many of its components. There are also inhibitory regulatory proteins, most notably factors H and I inhibiting C3b. Activated fragments of any component are designated b, e.g., C3b; anaphylatoxic fragments are designated a, e.g., C5a. Inflammatory functions of complement components are shown in orange.

activate resident glomerular cells, directly cause tissue injury, stimulate production of matrix proteins (which forms the basis of scarring), and may either block or promote inflammation.

Mechanisms of proteinuria

Proteinuria is the hallmark of glomerular disease. In the normal individual, minimal protein is filtered because of the charge and size selectivity of the glomerular capillary wall. Proteins, which are mainly negatively charged, are repelled by negative charges both within the GBM (mainly heparan sulfate proteoglycans) and on the surface of glomerular endothelial cells and epithelial cells (GEC) (primarily sialoproteins). In addition, the slit diaphragms between the podocyte foot processes act as the primary site for the size barrier to protein filtration (Fig. 18.6).

The slit diaphragm consists of several transmembrane proteins that extend from adjacent interdigitating foot processes to form a zipper-like scaffold on the outer side of the GBM. Recently it has been recognized that several genetic causes of nephrotic syndrome are associated with mutations in genes for proteins related to or associated with the slit diaphragm. Mutations in the *NHPS1* gene, which codes for nephrin, are responsible for the autosomal recessive congenital nephrotic syndrome of the Finnish type[8]. Mutations in *NHPS2*, which codes for podocin, is responsible for a different autosomal recessive steroid-resistant nephrotic syndrome[9] and also occasional cases of sporadic focal segmental glomerular sclerosis (FSGS). The cytoplasmic binding protein, CD2-associated protein (CD2AP), which interacts with nephrin and podocin, has also been shown to be critical for the glomerular permeability barrier, as gene knockout mice lacking CD2AP also develop nephrotic syndrome[10]. Mutations in *ACTN4*, which encodes the podocyte cytoplasmic protein α-actinin-4, have also been shown to be a cause of familial FSGS[11].

The key role for the GEC slit diaphragm in the permeability barrier to protein has renewed interest in the role of podocyte in diseases associated with massive proteinuria. It is now recognized that the foot process fusion that is commonly observed in most proteinuric states is not simply a 'secondary

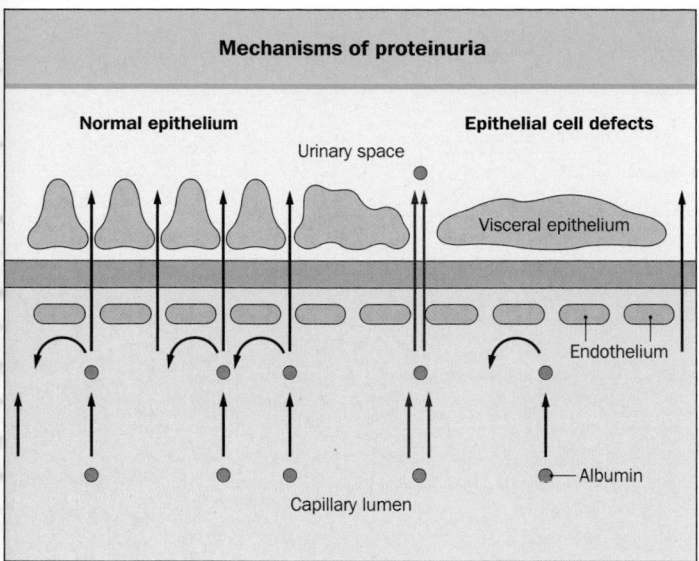

Mechanisms of proteinuria

Normal epithelium

Epithelial cell defects

Urinary space

Visceral epithelium

Endothelium

Albumin

Capillary lumen

Figure 18.6 Mechanisms of proteinuria. Normally negatively charged proteins, such as albumin, are retarded by the negatively charged proteins in the endothelium (sialoglycoproteins) and basement membrane (heparan sulfate proteoglycans), as well as by a size barrier in the GBM and at the slit diaphragm. In most proteinuric states the podocytes are injured, leading to foot process swelling and injury to the slit diaphragm; in these situations protein (albumin) can pass through the GBM and between gaps between the fused foot processes.

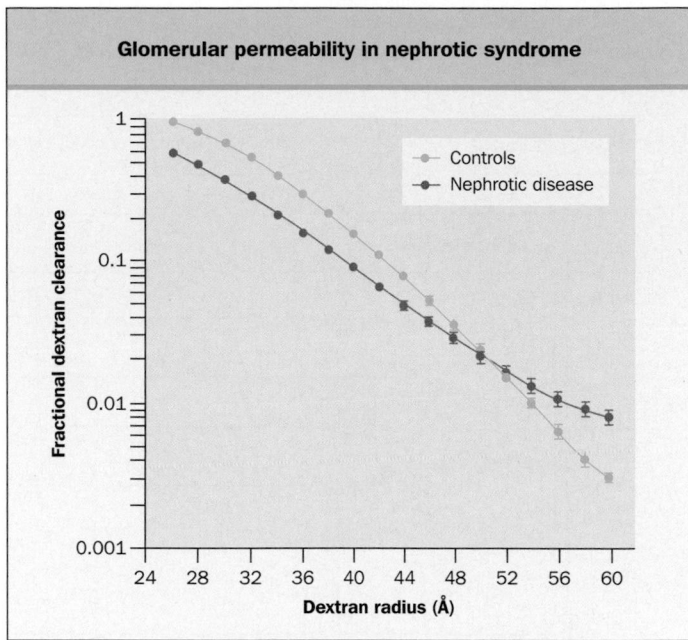

Glomerular permeability in nephrotic syndrome

Controls

Nephrotic disease

Fractional dextran clearance

Dextran radius (Å)

Figure 18.7 Glomerular permeability in nephrotic syndrome. A dextran sieving curve showing the relative glomerular permeability of different sized dextrans in normal subjects and nephrotic patients with membranous nephropathy and minimal change disease. Nephrotic subjects actually have a lower fractional dextran clearance for small dextrans (26–48 Å (2.6–4.8 nm)) but have an increased clearance for dextrans of larger molecular weight (52–60 Å (5.2–6.0 nm)). This is consistent with large 'pores' appearing in the GBM. (Adapted with permission from Myers and Guasch[12].)

consequence' of proteinuria but rather that it represents podocyte injury that is likely the cause of proteinuria. The injury may be mediated by immune deposits with complement activation, such as in membranous nephropathy, or due to injury by an as yet unidentified toxin or cytokine such as occurs in minimal change disease. Filtration is actually reduced at sites where the foot processes fuse (which may account for the reduction of the filtration coefficient, K_f, seen in nephrotic syndrome) but there are gaps where the GEC are detached from the GBM. It is at these sites that massive protein filtration occurs; structurally the capillary wall defects are likely to correspond to the large 'pores' noted in functional studies (Fig. 18.7)[12]. The principal mechanisms responsible for proteinuria in the different patterns of glomerular disease are described below and shown in Fig. 18.8.

Minimal change disease and focal segmental glomerulosclerosis
In minimal change disease and FSGS there are no deposits of immunoglobulin and the disease does not appear to be mediated by immune-complex deposition (see Chapter 20). There appears to be a circulating factor that directly alters glomerular permeability to protein[13]. It has long been proposed that this factor was T cell derived, and it has been shown that T cell hybridomas from patients with minimal change disease secrete a factor that provokes heavy proteinuria in rats[14]. Although it has not been shown that this factor is directly toxic to GEC, heavy proteinuria can be provoked by antibodies or toxins against the GEC.

In some patients, focal and segmental sclerotic changes develop, and consist of segmental collapse of the capillary tuft, often with hyalinosis and adhesions (synechiae) to Bowman's

capsule. The pathogenesis of segmental sclerosis is unclear, although it has been suggested that it results from increased protein trafficking across the GBM[15] or as a consequence of the increase in net ultrafiltration pressure that occurs secondary to the hypoalbuminemia and low oncotic pressure[16]. It is not known if focal segmental sclerosis represents part of the spectrum that includes minimal change disease or whether they are separate entities. However, both conditions are characterized by generalized foot process fusion and massive proteinuria.

Membranous nephropathy
In membranous nephropathy (see Chapter 22), immune deposits are localized to the subepithelial space. Although small complexes can cross the GBM and deposit at this site, experimental studies suggest that deposits are formed *in situ* by accretion of antibody to intrinsic or planted antigens on the GEC. In animal studies (passive Heyman nephritis), the intrinsic antigen (megalin) has been defined in detail, but there is as yet no evidence for a similar antigen in humans other than the rare congenital form of membranous nephropathy induced by antibodies to the podocyte antigen, neutral endopeptidase. GEC injury is then mediated by local complement activation with insertion of C5b–9 into the cell membrane of the GEC[3]. Although the chemotactic factor C5a is generated in the subepithelial space, the intervening GBM and filtration forces limit its access to the circulation and infiltration of leukocytes does not occur.

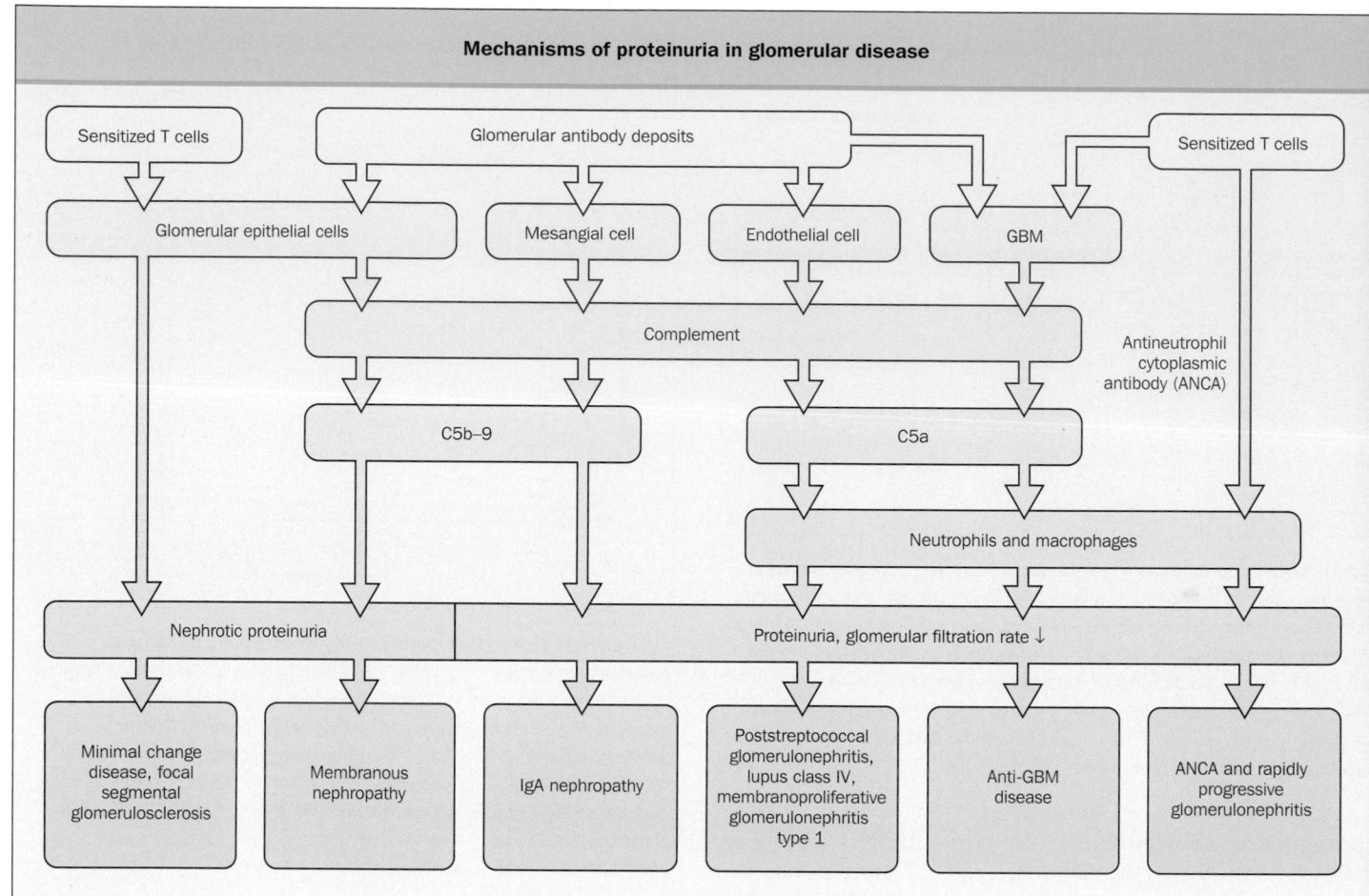

Figure 18.8 Mechanisms of proteinuria in glomerular disease. The main immune mechanisms involved in glomerular injury and the common glomerular diseases in which they occur. (With acknowledgment to Dr William G Couser.)

Mesangial proliferative glomerulonephritis

IgA nephropathy (see Chapter 24) is the most common etiology for mesangial proliferative GN. Here the immune complexes deposit in the mesangium, the glomerular capillary wall is relatively spared, and proteinuria is not commonly a major feature of the clinical presentation. Mesangial cell injury is probably mediated by binding of the immune complexes to Fcα and Fcγ receptors on the mesangial cell, resulting in the release of chemokines and growth factors that provokes leukocyte infiltration and mesangial cell proliferation (driven primarily by platelet-derived growth factor), and mesangial matrix production (mediated by transforming growth factor-β)[17]. While it had generally been thought that the mesangial cell was a specialized cell that was strictly resident within the glomerulus, recent experimental studies suggest that mesangial cell progenitors may be bone marrow-derived[18]. The role of these bone marrow-derived mesangial progenitors in mesangial diseases such as IgA nephropathy is not yet known.

Membranoproliferative glomerulonephritis

In MPGN the immune deposits localize both to the mesangium and the subendothelial space (see Chapter 23). A similar pattern is observed in cryoglobulinemic GN in which the immune complexes contain a monoclonal IgM (type II) or polyclonal IgM (type III) cyroglobulin that acts as a rheumatoid factor by binding to the IgG in the immune complex. In both cases the disease is thought to occur by passive deposition from the circulation. When this pattern is seen in lupus nephritis, it may be facilitated by the binding of nucleosomes to the complexes (nucleosomes are cationic nuclear proteins that can interact with the negatively charged proteins within the glomerulus).

Studies in experimental models suggest that the intraglomerular immune complexes cause local complement activation with the generation of chemotactic factors (including C5a, chemokines, leukotrienes, and platelet activating factor). Leukocyte adhesion molecules on endothelial cells are upregulated (intracellular adhesion molecule-1) or expressed *de novo* (E- and P-selectins)[19]. Proinflammatory cytokines (interleukin-1 and tumor necrosis factor-α) are generated locally and augment the inflammatory response. Neutrophils, platelets, and monocytes/macrophages then localize in the glomerulus and release oxidants (particularly hypohalous acids generated by neutrophil myeloperoxidase) and proteases (elastase, cathepsin G, and metalloproteinases) that cause local cellular injury and GBM degradation.

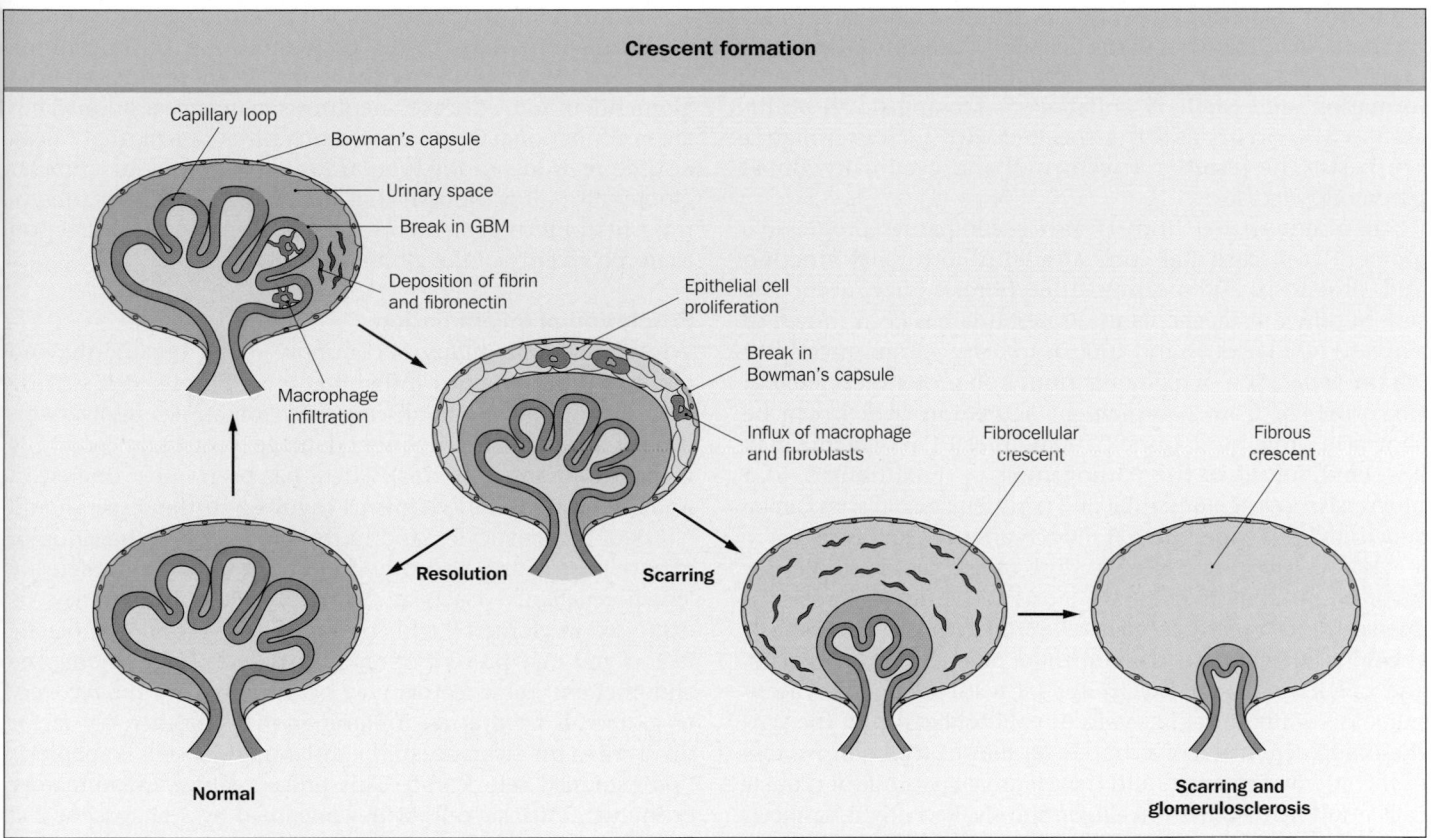

Crescent formation

Figure 18.9 Crescent formation. In early crescent formation, cytokines and growth factors cross the GBM to initiate proliferation of the parietal epithelial cells. Small breaks in the GBM occur secondary to injury from oxidants and proteases from neutrophil and macrophages, thus allowing macrophages to enter Bowman's space where they can proliferate. Breaks in Bowman's capsule secondary to the periglomerular inflammation also occur, allowing the entrance of more inflammatory cells as well as fibroblasts. The proliferation of parietal epithelial cells and macrophages is associated with fibrin deposition, slowly choking the glomerular tuft until filtration becomes impossible. In the late stages the crescent becomes fibrotic and the glomerulus end-stage.

Poststreptococcal GN

Poststreptococcal GN has long been considered to be an equivalent of acute serum sickness in rabbits. It is thought that 'nephritogenic' strains of group A streptococcus release specific antigens, especially nephritis associated plasmin receptor (recently identified as GAPDH) and zymogen into the circulation where they bind to antibody and localize to glomeruli[6]. The zymogen antigen is cationic and may preferably localize to the subepithelial space; the plasmin-binding receptor protein also activates the alternative pathway of complement and may augment the inflammatory response independent of antibody. Activation of complement in the proximity of the endothelium leads to a brisk inflammatory reaction with local endothelial and mesangial cell proliferation and manifestations of the nephritic syndrome.

Pathogenesis of crescent formation

Crescent formation can occur with any severe glomerular injury, most notably in vasculitis (see Chapter 26), anti-GBM disease (see Chapter 25) and in severe forms of immune complex GN (such as in IgA nephropathy or poststreptococcal GN). The crescent is a proliferation of extracapillary cells within Bowman's space. There is evidence that crescent formation is initiated by cytokine-driven proliferation of the parietal and possibly the visceral GEC. Local breaks in the GBM or Bowman's capsule, mediated by activated leukocytes, is followed by macrophage infiltration, myofibroblast accumulation, and local fibrin deposition (Fig. 18.9). Most evidence suggests that crescent formation is a manifestation of cell-mediated rather than humoral immune mechanisms[7].

Pathogenesis of progressive renal failure in glomerular disease

Two key processes characterize progressive renal failure: glomerulosclerosis and interstitial fibrosis. Although the original disease contributes to these processes, there is abundant evidence that progression is largely mediated by common nonimmunologic mechanisms[20]. These are discussed in more detail in Chapter 66.

Glomerulosclerosis may be a direct consequence of the original glomerular injury, but in addition a secondary form of FSGS may develop (see Chapter 21). It appears to be a consequence of reduced nephron number, which is followed by glomerular capillary hypertension (in response to afferent arteriolar vasodilatation) and hypertrophy (in response to cytokines and growth factors). Death of GEC results in capillary collapse and activation of the coagulation system. At the same time, progressive expansion of the capillary wall during glomerular hypertrophy results in denuded GBM since GEC proliferation is ineffectual; the denuded GBM abuts Bowman's capsule, initiating synechiae formation, subsequent hyalin formation, and capillary collapse[21,22]. Mesangial cell proliferation also occurs and is associated with increased matrix synthesis. The result is a segmental and eventually global glomerulosclerosis.

Tubulointerstitial fibrosis also accompanies progressive glomerular disease and correlates with both renal function and prognosis. Tubulointerstitial fibrosis may occur via several different mechanisms. Proteinuria has been shown to activate tubular cells and induce toxicity, either directly or via the generation of oxidants (from iron proteins excreted in the urine) or from complement activation (which can be shown in proteinuric urine). Tubulointerstitial ischemia may also be involved in the pathogenesis of renal fibrosis, as a progressive loss of glomerular and peritubular capillaries can be shown in both experimental models and human disease.

There is growing understanding of the cellular responses involved in tubulointerstitial fibrosis[23]. The fibrotic process is characterized by early tubular cell proliferation with release of chemotactic factors, the recruitment of monocyte/macrophages, and to a lesser extent, T cells, the local stimulation and accumulation of fibroblast-like cells (myofibroblasts) with the synthesis and deposition of extracellular matrix, a progressive loss of the microvasculature, and the eventual apoptosis of tubular cells resulting in a dense acellular fibrosis. Recently it has been recognized that the myofibroblast may derive from a resident population of fibroblasts, or by 'transdifferentiation' from injured tubular cells[24].

The mechanism by which tubulointerstitial fibrosis impairs renal function relates to the progressive loss of functioning nephrons. However, recently it has been recognized that glomeruli in some diseased nephrons may appear normal, but are nonfunctional due to tubulointerstitial fibrosis that causes a stricture or loss of the tubular lumen (resulting in 'atubular glomeruli')[25]. It is thought that this may explain why tubulointerstitial fibrosis often correlates better with renal function than the severity of the glomerular lesion.

Resolution of inflammation

While irreversible injury is common in GN because the end result of the glomerular inflammation is fibrosis, it is striking that acute forms of the disease may sometimes resolve with little or no apparent permanent damage (poststreptococcal GN is the best example of this). There has been much interest in understanding the mechanisms involved in the dispersal and efflux of the leukocytes, and in the proteolytic degradation of extracellular matrix. Recently it has been shown that there are 'chemorepellants' (such as Slit-1 and Robo) that may be expressed in glomeruli and counter the effects of chemotactic factors and may prevent or repel leukocytes from binding the endothelium; these factors may be important in the recovery of glomeruli from acute inflammation[26]. Another key factor involved in the clearance of the inflammatory cells is apoptosis ('programmed cell death'). This process allows inflammatory or injured, intrinsic cells to be consumed by a phagocytic cell rather than to necrose and liberate their injurious contents[27]. Research aimed at identifying these natural restorative mechanisms may provide insights into new approaches for therapy.

REFERENCES

1. Kalluri R, Cantley LG, Kerjasckhi D, Neilson EG. Reactive oxygen species expose cryptic epitopes assocated with autoimmune Goodpasture Syndrome. J Biol Chem. 2000;275:20027–32.
   Rees AJ. The immunogenetics of glomerulonephritis. Kidney Int. 1994;45(2):377–83.
3. Couser WG. Pathogenesis of glomerular damage in glomerulonephritis. Nephrol Dial Transplant. 1998;13(Suppl 1):10–15
4. Kalluri R, Wilson CB, Weber M, et al. Identification of the alpha 3 chain of type IV collagen as the common autoantigen in anti-basement membrane disease and Goodpasture syndrome. J Am Soc Nephrol. 1995;6(4):1178–85.
5. Debiec H, Guigonis V, Mougenot B, et al. Antenatal membranous glomerulonephritis due to anti-neutral endopeptidase (NEP) antibodies. N Engl J Med. 346:2053–60.
6. Yoshizawa N, Oshima S, Sagel I, et al. Role of a streptococcal antigen in the pathogenesis of acute poststreptococcal glomerulonephritis. J Immunol. 1992;148:3110–16.
7. Atkins RC, Nikolic-Patterson DJ, Song Q, et al. Modulators of crescentic glomerulonephritis. J Am Soc Nephrol. 1996; 7:2271–8.
8. Kestila M, Lenkkeri U, Manikko M, et al Positionally cloned gene for a novel glomerular protein-nephrin-is mutated in congenital nephrotic syndrome. Mol Cell. 1998;1:575–82.
9. Boute N, Gribouval O, Roselli S, et al. NHPS2, encoding the glomerular protein, podocin, is mutated in autosomal recessive steroid-resistant nephrotic syndrome. Nat Genet. 2000;24:349–54.
10. Shih N-Y, Li J, Karpitskii V, et al. Congenital nephrotic syndrome in mice lacking CD2-associated protein. Science. 1999; 286:312–15.
11. Kaplan JM, Kim SH, North KN, et al. Mutations in ACTN4, encoding alpha-actinin-4, cause familial focal segmental glomerulosclerosis. Nat. Genet. 2000; 24:251–6.
12. Myers BD, Guasch A. Mechanisms of proteinuria in nephrotic humans. Pediatr Nephrol. 1994;8:107–12.
13. Savin VJ, Sharma R, Sharma M, et al. Circulating factor associated with increased glomerular permeability to albumin in recurrent focal segmental glomerulosclerosis. N Engl J Med. 1996;334: 878–83.
14. Koyama A, Fukisaki M, Kobayashi M, et al. A glomerular permeability factor produced by human T cell hybridomas. Kidney Int. 1991;40:453–60.
15. Remuzzi G. A unifying hypothesis for renal scarring linking protein trafficking to the different mediators of injury. Nephrol Dial Transplant. 2000;15 (Suppl 6):58–60.
16. Johnson RJ. Have we ignored the role of oncotic pressure in the pathogenesis of glomerulosclerosis? Am J Kid Dis. 1997;29:147–52.
17. Peters H, Noble NA, Border WA. Transforming growth factor-beta in human glomerular injury. Curr Opin Nephrol Hypertens. 1997;6:389–93.
18. Cornacchia F, Fornoni A, Plati AR, et al. Glomerulosclerosis is transmitted by bone marrow-derived mesangial cell progenitors. J Clin Invest. 2001;108:1649–56.
19. Adler S, Brady HR. Cell adhesion molecules and the glomerulopathies. Am J Med. 1999;107(4):371–86.
20. Brenner BM, Mackenzie HS. Nephron mass as a risk factor for progression of renal disease. Kidney Int Suppl. 1997;63:S124–7.

21. Rennke HG. How does glomerular epithelial cell injury contribute to progressive glomerular damage? Kidney Int Suppl. 1994;45:S58–63.

22. Kriz WR. Progressive renal failure – inability of podocytes to replicate and the consequences for development of glomerulosclerosis. Nephrol Dial Transplant. 1996;11:1738–42.

23. Eddy A. Molecular insights into renal interstitial fibrosis. J Am Soc Nephrol. 1996;7:2495–508.

24. Jinde K, Nikolic-Paterson DJ, Huang XR, et al. Tubular phenotypic change in progressive tubulointerstitial fibrosis in human glomerulonephritis. Am J Kidney Dis. 2001;38:761–9.

25. Marcussen N. Tubulointerstitial damage leads to a tubular glomeruli: significance and possible role in progression. Nephrol Dial Transplant. 2000;15:S74–5.

26. Kanellis J, Li P, Garcia GE, et al. Modulation of inflammation by slit protein in vivo in experimental crescentic glomerulonephritis. J Am Soc Nephrol. in press.

27. Savill J, Apoptosis in resolution of inflammation. Kidney Blood Press Res. 2000;23(3–5):173–4.

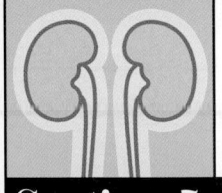

Chapter 19

Introduction to Glomerular Disease: Clinical Presentations

John Feehally and Richard J Johnson

INTRODUCTION

Glomerular disease has clinical presentations that vary from the asymptomatic individual who is found to have hematuria or proteinuria at a routine medical assessment to a patient with a fulminant illness with acute renal failure possibly associated with life-threatening extrarenal disease (Fig. 19.1). The most dramatic symptomatic presentations are uncommon. Asymptomatic urine abnormalities are much more common but less specific; they may also indicate a wide range of nonglomerular urinary tract disease.

CLINICAL EVALUATION OF GLOMERULAR DISEASE

History, physical examination, and investigation is aimed at excluding nonglomerular disease, finding evidence of associated multisystem disease, and establishing glomerular function.

History

A family history of renal disease (especially with hearing loss) should suggest Alport syndrome, although there are also uncommon familial forms of IgA nephropathy, focal segmental glomerulosclerosis (FSGS) and hemolytic–uremic syndrome (HUS). Certain drugs and toxins may cause glomerular disease, including minimal change disease (nonsteroidal anti-inflammatory agents (NSAIDs) and interferon), membranous nephropathy (gold, penicillamine, NSAIDs, mercury present in skin-lightening creams), FSGS (heroin), or HUS (cyclosporine, tacrolimus, mitomycin C, oral contraceptives). Recent or persistent infection may also be associated with a variety of glomerular diseases (especially streptococcal infection, infective endocarditis, and certain viral infections) (see Chapter 28).

Various malignancies are associated with glomerular disease including lung, breast, and gastrointestinal carcinoma (membranous nephropathy), Hodgkin's disease (minimal change disease), non-Hodgkin lymphoma (membranoproliferative glomerulonephritis (MPGN)) and renal carcinoma (amyloid) (see Chapter 30). Occasionally patients will present with the renal disease as the first manfestation of their tumor.

Multisystem diseases associated with glomerular disease include diabetes, amyloid, lupus, and vasculitis.

Physical examination

The presence of dependent pitting edema suggests the nephrotic syndrome, heart failure, or cirrhosis. In the nephrotic

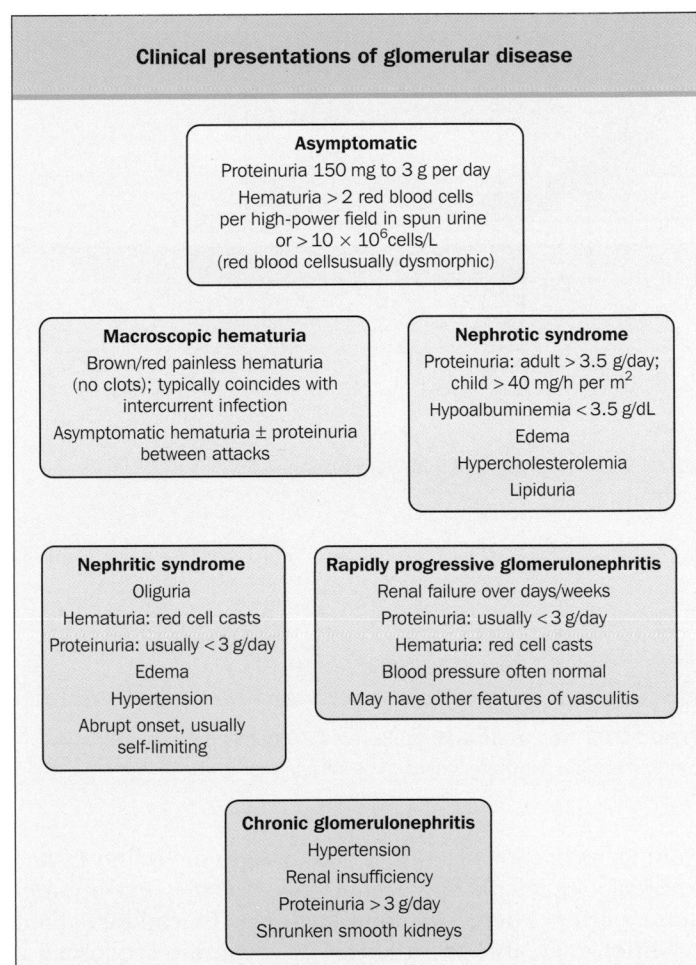

Figure 19.1 Clinical presentations of glomerular disease.

subject, edema is often periorbital in the morning (see Fig. 19.2) whereas the face is not affected overnight in edema associated with heart failure (because of orthopnea resulting from pulmonary congestion) or cirrhosis (because the patient cannot lie flat due to pressure on the diaphragm from ascites). As it progresses, edema of genitals and abdominal wall becomes apparent, and accumulation of fluid in body spaces leads to ascites and pleural effusions. Edema is unpleasant; it leads to feelings of tightness in the limbs and a bloated abdomen. There are practical problems of clothes and shoes no longer fitting. Yet surprisingly, edema may become massive in nephrotic syndrome before patients seek medical help;

Glomerular Disease

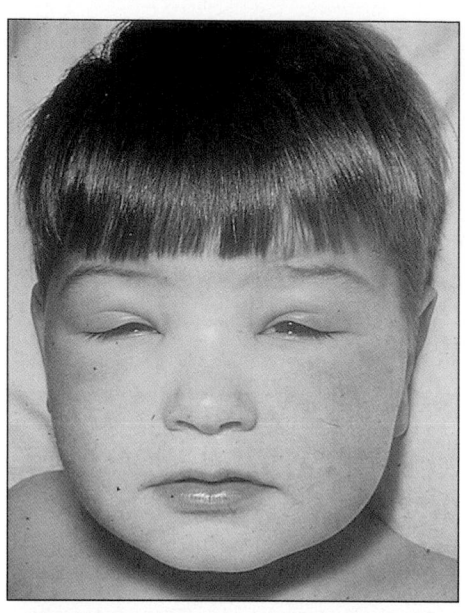

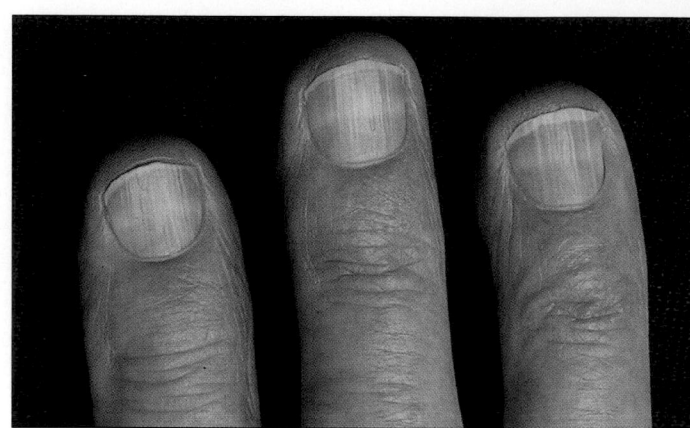

**Figure 19.2
Nephrotic edema.**
Periorbital edema in
the early morning in a
nephrotic child. The
edema resolves during
the day under the
influence of gravity.

Fig 19.4 Muehrcke's bands in nephrotic syndrome. The white band
grew during a transient period of hypoalbuminemia caused by the
nephrotic syndrome.

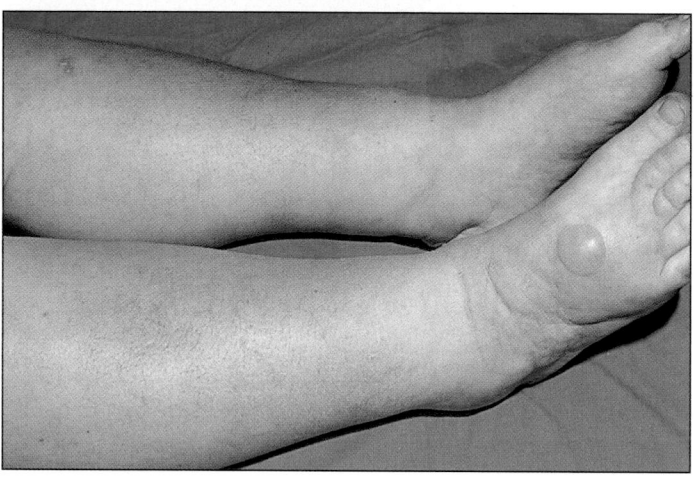

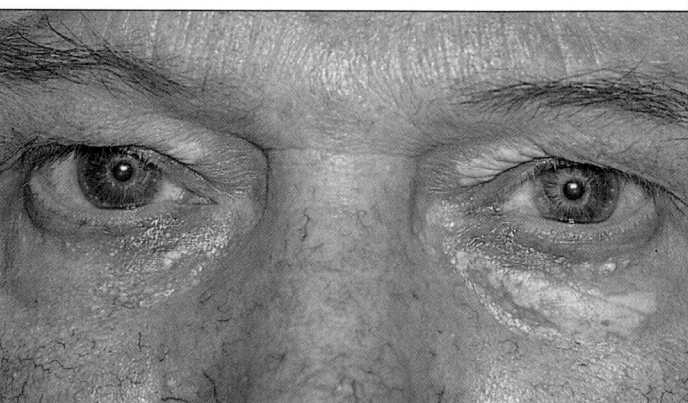

Figure 19.3 Nephrotic edema. Severe peripheral edema in nephrotic
syndrome; note the blisters caused by intradermal fluid.

Figure 19.5 Xanthelasma in nephrotic syndrome. These prominent
xanthelasma developed within a period of two months in a patient with
recent onset of severe nephrotic syndrome and serum cholesterol
550 mg/dL (14.2 mmol/L).

fluid gains of 20% of normal body weight are by no means
unusual (Fig. 19.3). The edema only becomes brawny and
stops pitting when very long standing. In children, fluid
retention may also be striking with nephritic syndrome: a
useful clinical sign to help to distinguish nephrotic from
nephritic syndrome is the paper-thin, floppy ears (Heyman's
sign) typical of nephrotic syndrome. Chronic hypoalbuminemia is also associated with loss of normal pink color under
the nails, resulting in white nails or white bands if the
nephrotic syndrome is transient (Muehrcke's bands, Fig 19.4).
Xanthelasma may also be present as a result of the hyperlipidemia associated with the nephrotic syndrome (Fig. 19.5).

The presence of pulmonary signs should suggest one of
the pulmonary–renal syndromes (see Table 25.4). Palpable
purpura may be seen in vasculitis, systemic lupus, cryoglobulinemia or endocarditis.

Laboratory studies

Assessing renal function and careful examination of the urine
(see Chapter 4) are critical. The quantity of urine protein and

the presence or absence of dysmorphic red cells and casts will
help to classify the clinical presentation (see Fig. 19.1).

Certain serologic tests are also helpful, including antistreptolysin O titer or streptozyme test (poststreptococcal glomerulonephritis (GN)); antinuclear and anti-DNA antibodies (lupus);
cryoglobulins and rheumatoid factor (both suggestive of cryoglobulinemia); antiglomerular basement membrane (anti-GBM)
antibodies (Goodpasture's syndrome); and antineutrophil
cytoplasmic antibodies (ANCA) (vasculitis). Serum and urine
electrophoresis will detect monoclonal light chains or heavy
chains (myeloma-associated amyloid or light-chain deposition
disease).

Testing for the presence of ongoing bacterial or viral infections is also useful and includes blood cultures and testing for
hepatitis B, hepatitis C, and human immunodeficiency virus
(HIV) infection.

Measurements of systemic complement pathway activation
by testing for serum C3, C4, and CH_{50} (50% hemolyzing
dose of complement) is particularly helpful in limiting the
differential diagnosis (Table 19.1).

Hypocomplementemia in glomerular disease			
Pathway affected	Complement changes	Glomerular diseases	Non-glomerular diseases
Classical pathway activation	C3 ↓, C4 ↓, CH$_{50}$ ↓	Lupus nephritis (especially class IV), mixed essential cryoglobulinemia,	
	+ C4 nephritic factor	Membranoproliferative GN type I	
Alternative pathway activation	C3 ↓, C4 normal, CH$_{50}$ ↓	Poststreptococcal GN	Atheroembolic renal disease
		GN associated with other infection[a] endocarditis shunt nephritis hepatitis B	
		Hemolytic–uremic syndrome	
	+ C3 nephritic factor	Membranoproliferative GN type II	
Reduced complement synthesis	Acquired		Hepatic disease
			Malnutrition
	Hereditary C2 deficiency Factor H deficiency	Lupus nephritis Familial hemolytic–uremic syndrome	

CH$_{50}$ - 50% hemolyzing dose of complement
[a]Glomerulonephritis (GN) associated with visceral abscesses is generally associated with normal or raised complement (elevations occur because complement components are acute phase reactants).

Table 19.1 Hypocomplementemia in glomerular disease.

Imaging

Ultrasonography is recommended in the workup to ensure the presence of two kidneys, to rule out obstruction or anatomic abnormalities, and to assess kidney size. Renal size is often normal in GN, although sometimes large kidneys (> 14 cm) are seen in nephrotic syndrome associated with diabetes, amyloid, or HIV infection. Large kidneys can also occasionally be seen with any acute severe GN. The occurrence of small kidneys (< 9 cm) suggests chronic renal disease and should limit enthusiasm for renal biopsy or aggressive, immunosuppressive therapies.

Renal biopsy

Renal biopsy is generally required to establish the type of glomerular disease and to guide treatment decisions. The principles and practice of renal biopsy are discussed in Chapter 6. There are some situations, however, where renal biopsy is not performed. If there are no unusual clinical features in nephrotic children the probability of minimal change disease is so high that corticosteroids can be initiated without biopsy (see Chapter 20). In acute nephritic syndrome, if all features point to poststreptococcal GN, especially in an epidemic, biopsy can be reserved for the minority who do not show early spontaneous improvement (see Chapter 28). In anti-GBM disease (see Chapter 25), the presence of lung hemorrhage and rapidly progressive renal failure with high titers of circulating anti-GBM antibody establishes the diagnosis without the need for a biopsy, although a biopsy may still provide prognostic information. In patients with systemic features of vasculitis, a positive ANCA, negative blood cultures, and a tissue biopsy from another site showing vasculitis are sufficient to secure a diagnosis of renal vasculitis. Biopsy is also not generally performed in long-standing diabetics with characteristic findings suggestive of diabetic nephropathy and other evidence of microvascular complications of diabetes. Biopsy may also not be indicated in many patients with mild glomerular disease presenting with asymptomatic urine abnormalities as the prognosis is excellent and histologic findings will not alter management.

ASYMPTOMATIC URINE ABNORMALITIES

Urine testing that detects proteinuria or microscopic hematuria is often the first evidence of glomerular disease. The random nature of urine testing in most communities inevitably means that much mild glomerular disease remains undetected. In some countries, symptomless individuals may only have a urine test if they require medical approval for some key life event: to obtain life insurance, to join the armed forces, or sometimes for employment purposes. In other countries, for example Japan, urinalysis is performed routinely in school or for employment. These different practices may partly account for the apparently variable incidence of certain diseases such as IgA nephropathy. Asymptomatic proteinuria and hematuria, and the combination of the two, increase in prevalence with age (see Fig. 19.6)[1]. Nevertheless there is no evidence to justify routine population-wide screening for asymptomatic urine abnormalities, as renal biopsy and/or therapeutic intervention is rarely required when renal function is preserved.

Asymptomatic microscopic hematuria

Microscopic hematuria is defined as the presence of more than two red blood cells per high power field in a spun urine sediment (3000 r.p.m. for 5 min) or red blood cells > 10 × 10^6/L.

Microscopic hematuria is common in many glomerular diseases, especially IgA nephropathy and thin membrane nephropathy, although there are many other causes of hematuria (discussed further in Chapter 59). A glomerular origin

Glomerular Disease

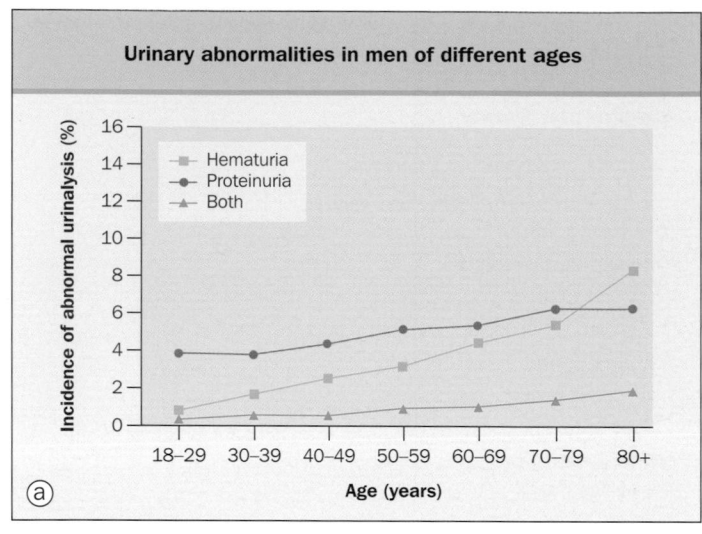

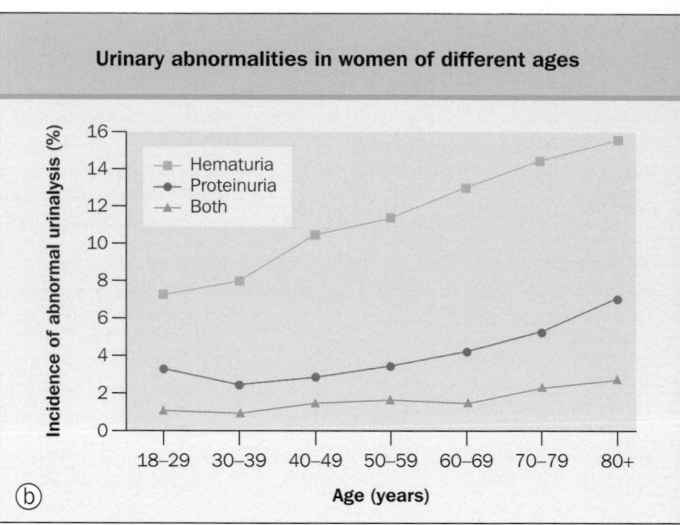

Figure 19.6 Prevalence of asymptomatic proteinuria and hematuria with age. Mass screening of a population of 107 192 adult men (a) and women (b) in Okinawa, Japan. Hematuria is more common in women. (Adapted with permission from Iseki et al.[1].)

should especially be considered if the red blood cells appear dysmorphic (see Chapter 4) or if the hematuria is accompanied by red cell casts or proteinuria.

Pathogenesis

Glomerular hematuria is thought to result from small breaks in the GBM that allow extravasation of RBCs into the urinary space. This may occur in the peripheral capillary wall but more commonly occurs in the paramesangial basement membrane, particularly in diseases where there is injury to the mesangium ('mesangiolysis').

Evaluation

The evaluation of microscopic hematuria begins with urine culture to exclude urinary or prostatic infection. If cultures are negative, renal imaging is performed to exclude anatomic lesions such as polycystic kidneys, stones, tumor, or arteriovenous malformations. Assessment of renal function and protein excretion will increase suspicion of an underlying glomerular disease if there is persistent proteinuria or reduced glomerular filtration rate (GFR). A sickle cell screen is required in appropriate populations and tuberculosis should also be excluded by tuberculin test and urine cultures in patients at high risk. Serum and urine calcium and uric acid should be measured because painless hematuria from calcium or uric acid crystals ('sand' or 'gravel') is well recognized, particularly in children.

In those over 40 years of age, cystoscopy is mandatory to exclude uroepithelial malignancy. Below 40 years, such malignancy is so rare that cystoscopy is not recommended. If all of the prior studies are negative, glomerular etiology is likely, of which IgA nephropathy and thin basement membrane disease are the most likely at any age[2]. The glomerular etiology can only be determined by renal biopsy but this is rarely done since the prognosis is excellent in the setting of normal renal function, normal blood pressure, and low-grade proteinuria (< 0.5 g/day). However, repeated evaluation is indicated every

12 months while hematuria persists, as in occasional patients progression to a more serious clinical presentation can occur.

Asymptomatic non-nephrotic proteinuria

The hallmark of glomerular disease is the excretion in urine of protein. Normal urine protein excretion is < 150 mg/24 h (consisting of 20–30 mg albumin, 10–20 mg of low-molecular-weight proteins that are freely filtered, and 40–60 mg secreted proteins such as Tamm–Horsfall protein and IgA). Proteinuria is identified and quantitated by dipstick testing or by assay in timed urine collections. The interpretation of these methods is discussed in Chapter 4.

Microalbuminuria is defined as the excretion of 30–300mg albumin/day (equivalent to a urine albumin : creatinine (g : g) ratio of 0.03–0.3) and is detected by quantitative immunoassay or by special urine dipsticks, as this is below the sensitivity of the normal dipstick. This measurement is primarily used to identify diabetic subjects at risk for developing nephropathy.

Non-nephrotic proteinuria is defined as a urine protein excretion of less than 3.5 g/24 h, or a urine protein : creatinine (g : g) ratio < 3. Although nephrotic-range proteinuria is absolutely characteristic of glomerular disease, asymptomatic proteinuria (< 3.5 g/24 h) is much less specific and may occur with a wide range of nonglomerular parenchymal disease as well as with nonparenchymal renal and urinary tract conditions that must be excluded by clinical evaluation and investigation.

Selectivity of proteinuria is measured by the ratio of IgG and albumin clearances. Highly selective proteinuria – IgG : albumin clearance ratio < 10% – (i.e., loss of the glomerular charge barrier with an intact glomerular size barrier) is characteristic of minimal change disease. In other nephrotic diseases, nonselective proteinuria (i.e., loss of both size and charge barriers) is more usual. Urine protein selectivity now rarely influences clinical decision making and need not be measured routinely.

Raised urine protein excretion may result from alterations in glomerular permeability or tubulointerstitial disease, although only in glomerular disease is it in the nephrotic range. It can also occur from increased filtration through normal glomeruli: 'overflow' proteinuria.

Overflow proteinuria

Overflow proteinuria is typical of urinary light-chain excretion. It is seen in myeloma but can occur in other settings (such as the release of lysozyme by leukemic cells) and should be suspected when the urine dipstick is negative for albumin despite detection of large amounts of proteinuria by other tests.

Tubular proteinuria

Tubulointerstitial disease can also be associated with low-grade (usually < 2 g/day) proteinuria. In addition to the loss of tubular proteins (such as β_2-microglobulin), there will also be some albuminuria owing to impaired tubular reabsorption of filtered albumin.

Glomerular proteinuria

Glomerular proteinuria is further classified into that which is transient or hemodynamic ('functional'), that which is present only during the day (orthostatic), and that which is persistent or 'fixed'.

Functional proteinuria

Functional proteinuria refers to the transient non-nephrotic proteinuria that can occur with fever, exercise, heart failure, and hyperadrenergic or hyper-reninemic states. Functional proteinuria is benign; it is usually assumed to be hemodynamic in origin and to be the consequence of increases in single nephron flow or pressure.

Orthostatic proteinuria

In children and young adults, low-grade glomerular proteinuria may be orthostatic, meaning that proteinuria is absent when urine is generated in the recumbent position. If there is no proteinuria in early morning urine, the diagnosis of orthostatic proteinuria can be made. The mechanism of orthostasis is not understood. Total urine protein in orthostatic proteinuria is usually less than 1 g/24 h; hematuria and hypertension are absent. Renal biopsy usually shows normal morphology or occasionally mild glomerular change. The prognosis is uniformly good and renal biopsy is not indicated[3].

Fixed non-nephrotic proteinuria

Fixed non-nephrotic proteinuria is usually caused by glomerular disease. If GFR is preserved, the benefits of renal biopsy are controversial. Biopsy is not indicated in this setting but prolonged follow-up is necessary so long as significant proteinuria persists to rule out the possibility of the disease progressing, although this is unusual. Previous studies indicate that the range of biopsy findings in these patients will be similar to those seen in nephrotic syndrome, although milder lesions are more common, particularly mesangial proliferative GN without immune deposits. The finding of no light microscopic change without immune deposits is also common, with varying degrees of foot process effacement. Although the histologic features are those of minimal change

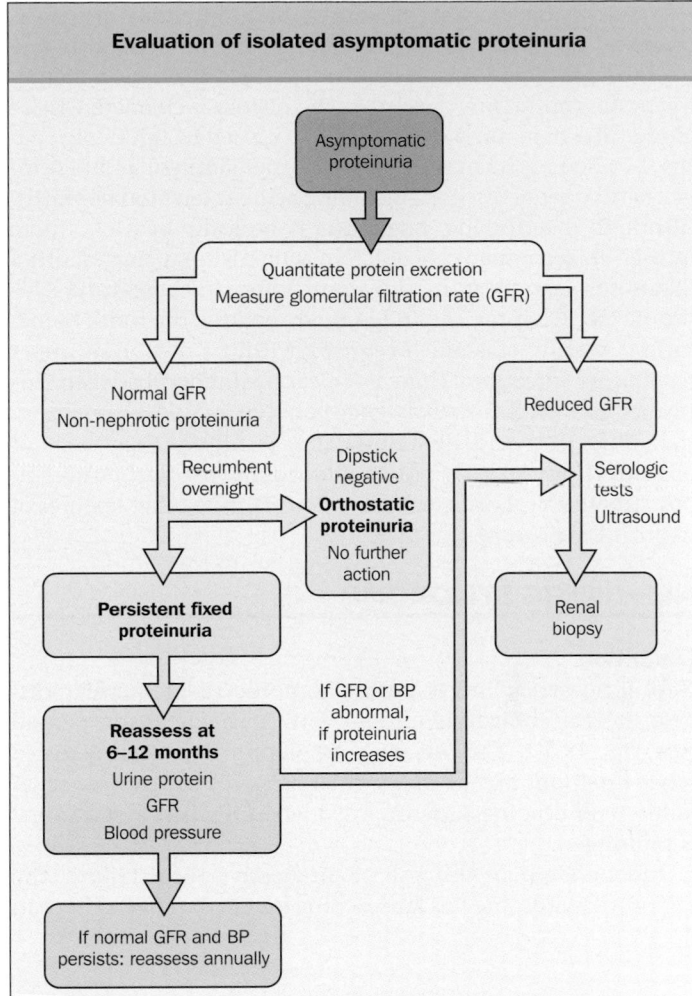

Figure 19.7 Evaluation of patients with isolated asymptomatic proteinuria.

disease, the proteinuria is not steroid responsive, as would be the case if there were a nephrotic presentation. Generally no treatment is necessary.

The evaluation of isolated asymptomatic proteinuria is summarized in Figure 19.7.

Asymptomatic proteinuria with hematuria

When asymptomatic hematuria and proteinuria coincide there is a much greater risk of significant glomerular injury, hypertension, and progressive renal dysfunction. Minor histologic changes are less common. Renal biopsy is indicated even if urine protein is only 0.5–1 g/24 h if there is also persistent microscopic hematuria with casts.

MACROSCOPIC HEMATURIA

Episodic painless macroscopic hematuria associated with glomerular disease is often brown or 'smoky' rather than red, and clots are unusual. It must be distinguished from other causes of red or brown urine, including hemoglobinuria, myoglobinuria, and consumption of food dyes, particularly beetroot.

Macroscopic hematuria caused by glomerular disease is observed primarily in children and young adults and is rare over the age of 40 years. It requires urologic evaluation including cystoscopy at any age unless the history is characteristic of glomerular hematuria. Most cases are caused by IgA nephropathy, but hematuria may occur with other glomerular and nonglomerular renal diseases, including acute interstitial nephritis. Although macroscopic hematuria is typically painless, there may be an accompanying dull loin ache that may suggest other diagnoses such as stone disease or loin-pain hematuria syndrome (see Chapter 57). In IgA nephropathy, the frank hematuria is usually episodic, occurring within a day of an upper respiratory infection. There is a clear distinction between this history and the 2–3 week latency between an upper respiratory tract infection and hematuria that is highly suggestive of postinfectious (usually poststreptococcal) GN; furthermore in poststreptococcal disease, there will usually be other features of nephritic syndrome.

NEPHROTIC SYNDROME

Definition

Nephrotic syndrome is pathognomonic of glomerular disease. It is a clinical syndrome with a characteristic pentad (see Fig. 19.1)[4]. Patients may be nephrotic with preserved renal function, but in many circumstances progressive renal failure will become superimposed when nephrotic syndrome is prolonged.

Independent of the risk of progressive renal failure, the nephrotic syndrome has far-reaching metabolic effects that can influence the general health of the patient. Fortunately, some episodes of nephrotic syndrome are self-limiting and a few respond completely to specific treatment (e.g., corticosteroids in minimal change disease). However, for most patients, it is a chronic condition. Not all patients with proteinuria over 3.5 g/24 h will have a full nephrotic syndrome; some have a normal serum albumin and no edema. This difference presumably reflects the varied response of protein metabolism: some patients sustain an increase in albumin synthesis in response to heavy proteinuria and some maintain a normal serum albumin.

Etiology

The major causes of nephrotic syndrome are shown in Table 19.2. Proteinuria in the nephrotic range in the absence of edema and hypoalbuminemia has similar etiologies. The relative frequency of the different glomerular diseases varies with age (Table 19.3). Although predominant in childhood, minimal change disease remains common at all ages[5]. There is an increased prevalence of FSGS in African Americans, and historical comparisons indicate that FSGS is becoming more common and MPGN less common in all adults[6].

Hypoalbuminemia

Hypoalbuminemia is a consequence of urinary losses. It may also be the result of increased reabsorption and catabolism of albumin by the proximal tubules, although this remains controversial[7]. The liver responds by increasing albumin synthesis, but this compensatory mechanism appears to be blunted in nephrotic syndrome. Furthermore, increasing protein intake does not improve albumin metabolism since

Table 19.2 Common glomerular diseases presenting as nephrotic syndrome in adults

Common glomerular diseases presenting as nephrotic syndrome in adults		
Disease	**Associations**	**Serologic tests helpful in diagnosis**
Minimal change disease	Allergy, atopy, NSAIDs, Hodgkin's disease	None
Focal segmental glomerulosclerosis	African Americans	–
	HIV infection	HIV antibody
	Heroin	–
Membranous nephropathy	Drugs: gold, penicillamine, NSAIDs	–
	Infections: hepatitis B, C; malaria	Hepatitis B surface antigen, anti-HCV antibody
	Lupus nephritis	Anti-DNA antibody
	Malignancy: breast, lung, gastrointestinal tract	–
Membranoproliferative glomerulonephritis (Type I)	C4 nephritic factor	C3 ↓, C4 ↓
Membranoproliferative glomerulonephritis (Type II)	C3 nephritic factor	C3 ↓, C4 normal
Cryoglobulinemic MPGN	Hepatitis C	Anti-HCV antibody, rheumatoid factor, C3 ↓, C4 ↓, CH$_{50}$ ↓
Amyloid	Myeloma	Serum protein electrophoresis, urine immunoelectrophoresis
	Rheumatoid arthritis, bronchiectasis, Crohn's disease (and other chronic inflammatory conditions), familial Mediterranean fever	–
Diabetic nephropathy	Other diabetic microangiopathy	None

Age-related variations in nephrotic syndrome					
		Prevalence (%)			
	Child	Young adult		Middle and old age	
	(<15 years)	Whites	Blacks	Whites	Blacks
Minimal change disease	78	23	15	21	16
Focal segmental glomerulosclerosis	8	19	55	13	35
Membranous nephropathy	2	24	26	37	24
Membranoproliferative glomerulonephritis (MPGN)	6	13	0	4	2
Other glomerulonephritis	6	14	2	12	12
Amyloid	0	5	2	13	11
Data adapted from Haas et al.[6] and Cameron[5].					

Table 19.3 Age-related variations in nephrotic syndrome

the hemodynamic response to an increased intake is a rise in glomerular pressure, producing enhanced urine protein losses. The end result is that serum albumin falls further. White bands in the nails (Muehrcke's bands) are a characteristic clinical sign of hypoalbuminemia (Fig. 19.4). The increase in protein synthesis in response to proteinuria is not discriminating; as a result, proteins that are not being lost in the urine may actually increase in concentration in plasma. This is chiefly determined by molecular weight; large molecules will not spill into the urine and will increase in the plasma; smaller proteins although synthesized to excess will enter the urine and be diminished in the plasma. These variations in plasma proteins are clinically important in two areas: hypercoagulability and hyperlipidemia (see below).

Edema

At least two major mechanisms are involved in the formation of nephrotic edema (Fig. 19.8)[8]. In the first mechanism, which is more common in children with minimal change disease, the edema appears to be the consequence of the low serum albumin producing a fall in plasma oncotic pressure, which allows increased transudation of fluid from capillary beds into the extracellular space according to the laws of Starling. The consequent fall in circulating blood volume ('underfill') produces a secondary stimulation of the renin–angiotensin system resulting in aldosterone-induced sodium retention in the distal tubule. This attempt to compensate for hypovolemia merely aggravates edema because the low oncotic pressure alters the balance of forces across the capillary wall in favor of hydrostatic pressure, forcing more fluid into the interstitial space rather than retaining it within the vascular compartment.

Figure 19.8 Mechanisms of nephrotic edema.

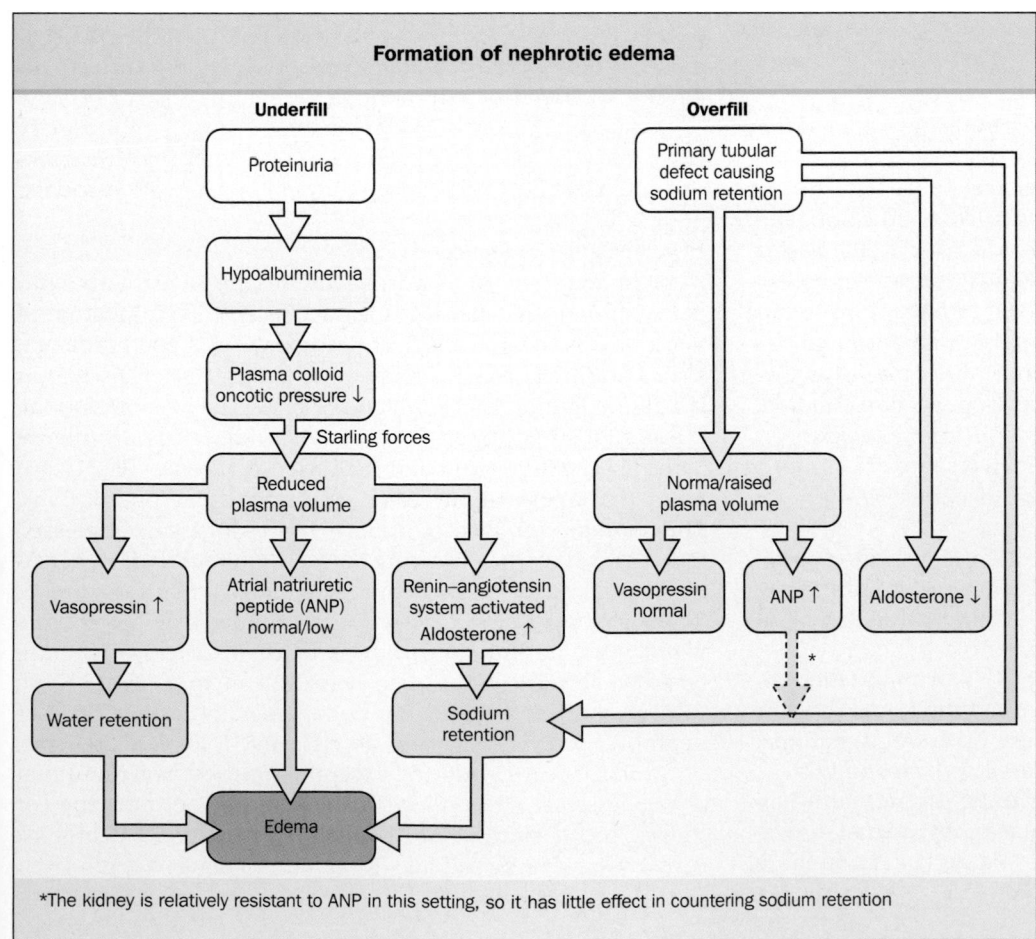

Formation of nephrotic edema

*The kidney is relatively resistant to ANP in this setting, so it has little effect in countering sodium retention

In many nephrotic patients, however, there appears to be a primary defect in the ability of the distal nephron to excrete sodium. As a result, there is an increased blood volume, suppression of renin–angiotensin and vasopressin, and a tendency to hypertension rather than hypotension; the kidney is also relatively resistant to the actions of atrial natriuretic peptide. An elevated blood volume results ('overfill'), which in association with the low plasma oncotic pressure provokes transudation of fluid into the extracellular space and edema. The mechanism for the defect in sodium excretion remains unknown, although it has been hypothesized that the presence of inflammatory leukocytes in the interstitium, found in many glomerular diseases, may impair sodium excretion due to their ability to produce angiotensin II and oxidants (the latter which inactivates local nitric oxide which is natriuretic)[9].

Metabolic consequences of nephrotic syndrome

Negative nitrogen balance

The heavy proteinuria leads to marked negative nitrogen balance, usually measured in clinical practice by serum albumin. Nephrotic syndrome is a wasting illness but the degree of muscle loss is masked by edema and not fully apparent until the patient is rendered edema free. Loss of up to 10–20% of lean body mass is not uncommon. Albumin turnover is increased in response to the tubular catabolism of filtered protein rather than merely to urinary protein loss. High protein intake will lead to increased albumin synthesis rate but also increases proteinuria. A low-protein diet will reduce proteinuria but also reduces albumin synthesis rate and, in the longer term, may increase the risk of worsening negative nitrogen balance.

Hypercoagulability

Multiple proteins of the coagulation cascade have altered levels in nephrotic syndrome; in addition, platelet aggregation is enhanced[10]. The net effect is a hypercoagulable state that is enhanced further by immobility, coincidental infection, and hemoconcentration if the patient has a contracted plasma volume (see Fig. 19.9). Not only is venous thromboembolism common at any site, but spontaneous arterial thrombosis may occur. In adults, arterial thrombosis may occur in the context of atheroma promoting coronary and cerebrovascular events in particular; but it also occurs in nephrotic children, where spontaneous thrombosis of major limb arteries is an uncommon but feared complication. Up to 10% of nephrotic adults and 2% of children will have a clinical episode of thromboembolism.

The elevated fibrinogen produces an increase in erythrocyte sedimentation rate (ESR). Values up to 100 mm/h are not unusual, so ESR loses its clinical value as a marker of an acute-phase response in nephrotic patients.

Renal vein thrombosis (see Chapter 64) is an important complication of nephrotic syndrome. At one time it was thought that renal vein thrombosis could cause nephrotic syndrome; this is no longer considered true. Renal vein thrombosis is reported clinically in up to 8% of nephrotic patients but when sought systematically (by ultrasonography or contrast venography) the frequency increases to 10–50%. It may be more common in membranous nephropathy than other disease

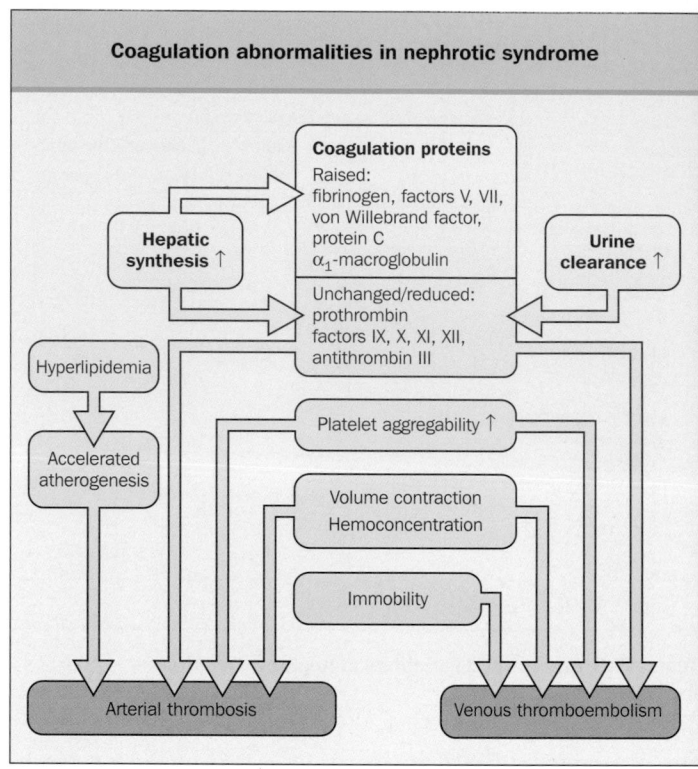

Figure 19.9 Coagulation abnormalities in nephrotic syndrome.

patterns, although there is no explanation for this observation. Symptoms when the thrombosis is acute may include flank pain and hematuria; rarely, acute renal failure (ARF) can occur if the thrombosis is bilateral. However, often the thrombosis develops insidiously with minimal symptoms or signs because of the development of collateral blood supply. Pulmonary embolism is an important complication. Renal vein thrombosis should not be screened for routinely in nephrotic patients.

Hyperlipidemia and lipiduria

Hyperlipidemia is such a frequent finding in patients with heavy proteinuria that it is regarded as an integral feature of nephrotic syndrome[11]. Clinical stigmata of hyperlipidemia, such as xanthelasma, may have a rapid onset (see Fig. 19.5). It is not uncommon for serum cholesterol to be over 500 mg/dL (13 mmol/L), although serum triglyceride levels are highly variable. The lipid profile in nephrotic syndrome (Fig. 19.10) is known to be highly atherogenic in other populations. The presumption that coronary heart disease is increased in nephrotic syndrome owing to the combination of hypercoagulation and hyperlipidemia has been difficult to prove. Many patients who are nephrotic for more than 5–10 years will develop additional cardiovascular risk factors, including hypertension and uremia, so it is difficult to separate these influences. However, it is now generally accepted that nephrotic patients do carry about a five-fold increased risk of coronary death, with the exception of those with minimal change disease. Presumably this is because the transience of the nephrotic state before remission with steroid treatment does not subject the patient with minimal change to prolonged hyperlipidemia.

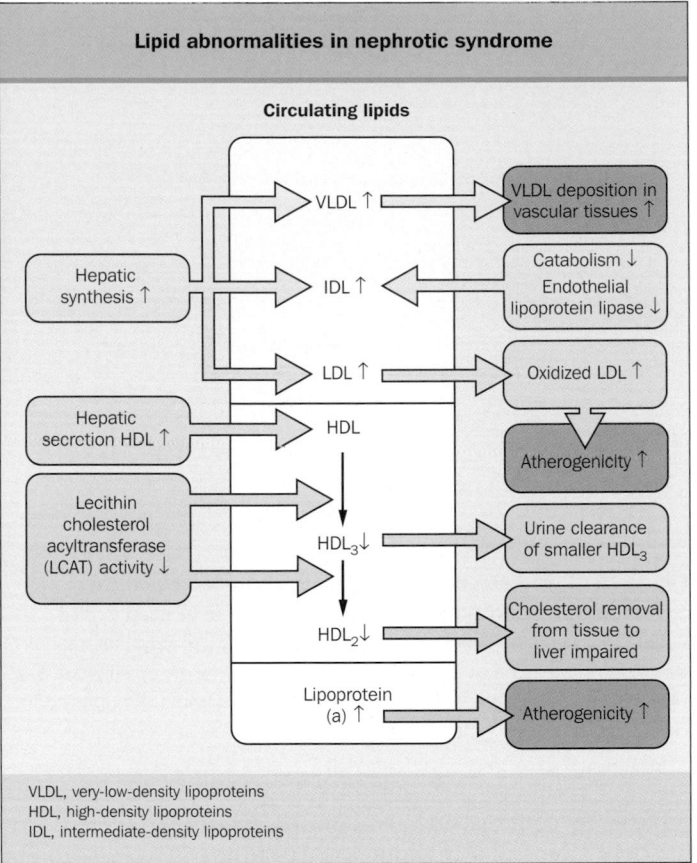

Figure 19.10 **Lipid abnormalities in nephrotic syndrome.** Changes in high-density lipoproteins (HDL) are more controversial than those in very-low-density lipoproteins (VLDL).

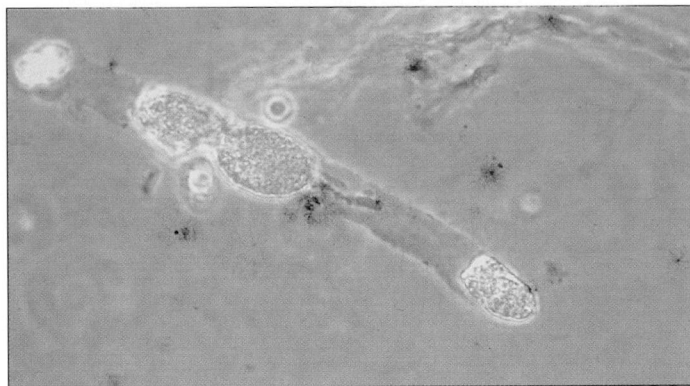

Figure 19.11 **Fat in the urine.** A hyaline cast containing oval fat bodies, which are tubular epithelial cells full of fat. Oval fat bodies often appear brown in color.

is usually normal and overt osteomalacia or uncontrolled hyperparathyroidism is very unusual in nephrotic syndrome in the absence of renal insufficiency. Thyroid-binding globulin is lost in the urine and total circulating thyroxine is reduced, but free thyroxine and thyroid-stimulating hormone are normal and there are no clinical alterations in thyroid status. Occasional cases of copper, iron, or zinc deficiency have been described as a consequence of the loss of binding proteins in the urine.

Drug binding may be altered by the decrease in serum albumin. Although most drugs do not require dose modifications, one important exception is clofibrate, which at normal dosage in nephrotic patients produces a severe myopathy. Altered protein binding may also change the dosage of warfarin (Coumadin) required to achieve adequate anticoagulation.

Infection

Nephrotic patients are prone to bacterial infection. Before steroids were shown to be effective in childhood nephrotic syndrome, sepsis was the commonest cause of death and it remains a major problem in the developing world. Primary peritonitis, especially caused by pneumococci, is particularly characteristic of nephrotic children. It is less common with increasing age: by the age of 20 years, most adults have antibodies against pneumococcal capsular antigens. Peritonitis caused by both β-hemolytic streptococci and Gram-negative organisms occur, but staphylococcal peritonitis is not reported. Cellulitis, especially in areas of severe edema, is also common, most frequently caused by β-hemolytic streptococci.

There are several explanations for the increased risk of infection. Large fluid collections are sites for bacteria to grow easily; nephrotic skin is fragile, creating sites of entry; and edema may dilute local humoral immune factors. Loss of IgG and complement factor B (of the alternative pathway) in the urine impairs host ability to eliminate encapsulated organisms such as pneumococci. Zinc and transferrin are lost in the urine and both are required for normal lymphocyte function. Polymorph phagocytic function is impaired in nephrotic syndrome and a number of *in vitro* T-cell dysfunctions are described, although their clinical significance is uncertain.

There is also experimental evidence that hyperlipidemia may contribute to progressive renal disease by lipid deposition in both glomeruli and interstitium, with protection afforded by lipid-lowering agents. However, although a meta-analysis suggests lipid-lowering may slow the rate of progression of chronic renal disease[12], there are not yet adequate prospective clinical studies to support the use of lipid lowering agents with this goal in mind.

Several mechanisms account for the lipid abnormalities in nephrotic syndrome, including increased hepatic synthesis of low-density and very-low-density lipoproteins (LDL and VLDL) and lipoprotein (a) secondary to the hypoalbuminemia, defective peripheral lipoprotein lipase activity resulting in increased VLDL, and urinary losses of high-density lipoproteins (HDL) (see Fig. 19.10).

Lipiduria, the fifth component of the nephrotic syndrome, is manifested by the presence of refractile accumulations of lipid in cellular debris and casts (oval fat bodies and fatty casts (see Fig. 19.11)). However, the lipiduria appears to be a consequence of the proteinuria and not of the plasma lipid abnormalities.

Other metabolic effects of nephrotic syndrome

Vitamin D-binding protein is lost in the urine, resulting in low plasma 25-hydroxyvitamin D levels, but free vitamin D

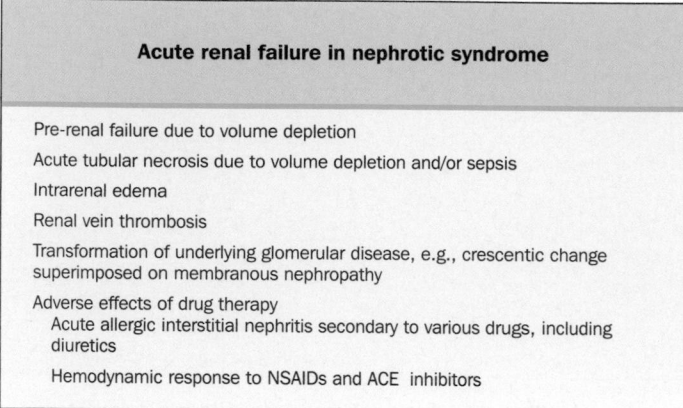

Acute renal failure in nephrotic syndrome

Pre-renal failure due to volume depletion

Acute tubular necrosis due to volume depletion and/or sepsis

Intrarenal edema

Renal vein thrombosis

Transformation of underlying glomerular disease, e.g., crescentic change superimposed on membranous nephropathy

Adverse effects of drug therapy
 Acute allergic interstitial nephritis secondary to various drugs, including diuretics

 Hemodynamic response to NSAIDs and ACE inhibitors

Table 19.4 Acute renal failure in nephrotic syndrome. Problems to consider when evaluating acute deterioration in renal function in nephritic syndrome.

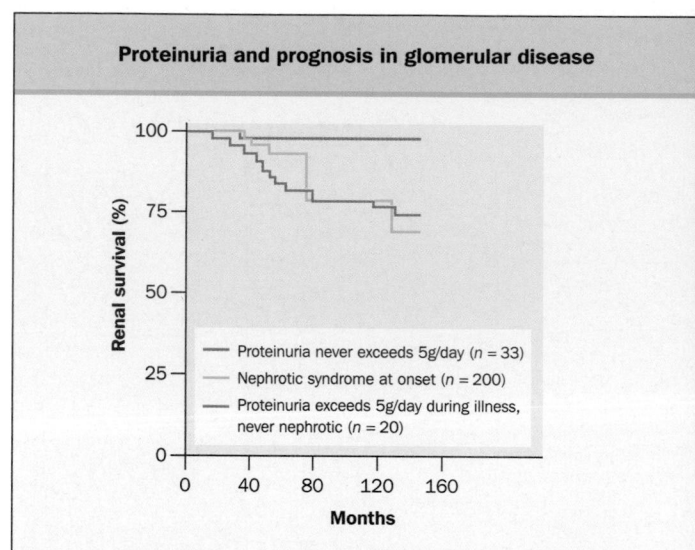

Figure 19.12 Proteinuria and prognosis in glomerular disease. The influence of heavy proteinuria on long-term renal function in 253 patients with primary glomerular disease at Manchester Royal Infirmary, UK. Heavy proteinuria at any time during long-term follow-up substantially worsens prognosis even without frank nephrotic syndrome. (Courtesy of Dr CD Short.)

Acute and chronic changes in renal function in nephrotic syndrome

Acute renal failure

Patients with nephrotic syndrome are also at risk for the development of ARF[13], which can occur by a variety of mechanisms which are summarized in Table 19.4). These include volume depletion and/or sepsis resulting in either prerenal azotemia or acute tubular necrosis[14]; transformation of the underlying disease (such as the development of crescentic nephritis in a patient with membranous nephropathy); the development of bilateral renal vein thrombosis; an increased disposition to azotemia from NSAIDs and angiotensin-converting enzyme (ACE) inhibitors; and an increased risk for allergic interstitial nephritis secondary to drugs, including diuretics. It has also been postulated that some patients develop ARF from intrarenal edema with compression of tubules[15]; these patients respond with diuresis to albumin infusions coupled with a loop diuretic.

Chronic renal insufficiency

With the exception of minimal change disease, most causes of nephrotic syndrome are associated with some risk for the development of progressive renal failure. In this regard, one of the greatest risk factors for progression is the degree of proteinuria (see Chapter 66). Progression is uncommon if proteinuria is less than 2 g/day and the risk increases in proportion to the severity of the proteinuria (Fig. 19.12), with marked risk for progression when protein excretion is more than 5 g/day. This may be because proteinuria identifies patients with severe glomerular injury, but there is also experimental and clinical evidence that proteinuria, *per se*, may be toxic, especially to the tubulointerstitium. In several experimental models, measures that reduce proteinuria, such as ACE inhibitors or low-protein diet, also prevent tubulointerstitial disease and progressive renal failure.

NEPHRITIC SYNDROME

In nephrotic syndrome, the glomerular injury manifests primarily as an increase in permeability of the capillary wall to protein. By contrast, in the nephritic syndrome, there is evidence of glomerular inflammation resulting in a reduction in GFR, non-nephrotic proteinuria, edema and hypertension (secondary to sodium retention), and hematuria with red-cell casts.

The classic nephritic syndrome presentation is that seen with acute poststreptococcal GN in children. These children usually present with the rapid onset of oliguria, weight gain, and generalized edema over a few days. The hematuria results in brown rather than red urine, and clots are not seen. The urine contains protein, red cells, and red-cell casts. Since proteinuria is rarely in the nephrotic range, serum albumin is usually normal. Circulating volume increases with hypertension, and pulmonary edema follows without evidence of primary cardiac disease.

The distinction between typical nephrotic syndrome and nephritic syndrome is usually straightforward on clinical and laboratory grounds (see Table 19.5) and the use of these clinical descriptions is particularly helpful in the approach to patients with suspected GN at first presentation, helping to narrow the differential diagnosis. However, the classification systems are imperfect and patients with certain glomerular disease patterns, for example MPGN, may present with either a nephrotic or nephritic picture.

Etiology

The primary glomerular diseases associated with the nephritic syndrome and the serologic tests helpful in diagnosis are shown in Table 19.6. The classification is even more challenging than for nephrotic syndrome as some diseases are identified by histology (IgA nephropathy), others by serology and histology (ANCA-associated vasculitis and lupus nephritis), and others by etiology (postinfectious GN).

Differentiation between nephrotic syndrome and nephritic syndrome		
Typical features	Nephrotic	Nephritic
Onset	Insidious	Abrupt
Edema	++++	++
Blood pressure	Normal	Raised
Jugular venous pressure	Normal/low	Raised
Proteinuria	++++	++
Hematuria	May/may not occur	+++
Red-cell casts	Absent	Present
Serum albumin	Low	Normal/slightly reduced

Table 19.5 Differentiation between nephrotic syndrome and nephritic syndrome.

RAPIDLY PROGRESSIVE GLOMERULONEPHRITIS

Rapidly progressive glomerulonephritis (RPGN) describes the clinical situation in which glomerular injury is so acute and severe that renal function deteriorates over days or weeks. The patient may present as a uremic emergency, with nephritic syndrome that is not self-limiting but moves on rapidly to renal failure, or with rapidly deteriorating renal function when being investigated for extrarenal disease (many of the patterns of GN associated with RPGN occur as part of a systemic immune illness).

The histologic counterpart of RPGN is crescentic GN: the proliferative cellular response outside the glomerular tuft but within Bowman's space that is known as a crescent because of its shape on histologic cross-section. Typically, the glomerular tuft also shows segmental necrosis – focal segmental necrotizing GN – and this is particularly characteristic of the vasculitis syndromes.

Common glomerular diseases presenting as nephritic syndrome		
Disease	Association	Serologic tests helpful in diagnosis
Poststreptococcal glomerulonephritis	Pharyngitis, impetigo	ASO titer, streptozyme antibody
Other postinfectious disease		
Endocarditis	Cardiac murmur	Blood cultures, C3 ↓
Abscess	–	Blood culture, C3, C4 normal or raised
'Shunt'	Treated hydrocephalus	Blood cultures, C3 ↓
IgA nephropathy	Upper respiratory or gastrointestinal infection	Serum IgA ↑
Systemic lupus	Other multisystem features of lupus	Antinuclear antibody, anti-double stranded DNA antibody, C3 ↓, C4 ↓

Table 19.6 Common glomerular diseases presenting as nephritic syndrome.

The term RPGN is, therefore, often used to describe acute deterioration in renal function in association with a crescentic nephritis. Unfortunately, not all patients with a nephritic urine sediment and ARF will fit this syndrome. For example, ARF may also occur in milder forms of glomerular disease if complicated by accelerated hypertension, renal vein thrombosis, or acute tubular necrosis. This emphasizes the need to obtain histologic confirmation of the clinical diagnosis.

Etiology

The primary glomerular diseases associated with RPGN and helpful serologic tests are shown in Table 19.7. As with nephritic syndrome, different assessment methods are useful for different diseases causing RPGN.

Common glomerular diseases presenting as rapidly progressive glomerulonephritis (RPGN)		
Disease	Association	Serologic tests helpful in diagnosis
Goodpasture's disease	Lung hemorrhage	Antiglomerular basement membrane (anti-GBM) antibody (occasionally antineutrophil cytoplasmic antibodies (ANCA) present)
Vasculitis		
Wegener's granulomatosis	Upper and lower respiratory involvement	cANCA (cytoplasmic)
Microscopic polyangiitis	Multisystem involvement	pANCA (perinuclear)
Pauci-immune crescentic glomerulonephritis	Renal involvement only	pANCA
'Immune complex'		
Systemic lupus	Other multisystem features of lupus	Antinuclear antibody, anti-double stranded DNA antibody, C3 ↓, C4 ↓
Poststreptococcal glomerulonephritis	Pharyngitis, impetigo	Asotiter, streptozyme antibody, C3 ↓, C4 normal
IgA nephropathy/Henoch–Schönlein purpura (HSP)	Characteristic rash ± abdominal pain in HSP	Serum IgA ↑ (30%), C3 and C4 normal
Endocarditis	Cardiac murmur; other systemic features of bacteremia	Blood cultures, ANCA (occasionally) C3 ↓, C4 normal

Note the overlap between the diseases in this figure and those in Table 19.5. A number of glomerular disease may present with either a nephritic syndrome or with RPGN.

Table 19.7 Common glomerular diseases presenting as rapidly progressive glomerulonephritis (RPGN).

CHRONIC RENAL FAILURE

The natural history of many types of GN is of slowly progressive renal impairment. If no clinical event early in the course of the disease brings them to medical attention, patients may present late with established hypertension, proteinuria, and renal impairment. In very long-standing GN, the kidneys shrink (but remain smooth and symmetrical). Renal biopsy at this stage is more hazardous and less likely to provide diagnostic material. Light microscopy often shows nonspecific features of 'end-stage kidney', consisting of focal or global glomerulosclerosis and dense tubulointerstitial fibrosis, and it may not be possible to define with confidence that a glomerular disease was the initiating renal injury, let alone define the pattern further. Immunofluorescence may be more helpful; in particular, mesangial IgA may be present in adequate amounts to allow a diagnosis of IgA nephropathy to be made. However, when renal imaging shows small kidneys, only rarely will biopsy be appropriate. For this reason 'chronic GN' has often been a presumptive diagnosis in patients presenting late with shrunken kidneys, proteinuria, and renal impairment. This is imprecise and in the past has led to an overestimate of the frequency of GN as a cause of end-stage renal disease in registry data. GN should only be diagnosed if there is confirmatory histologic evidence.

TREATMENT OF GLOMERULAR DISEASE

General principles

Treatment of glomerular disease consists of both general supportive treatment and disease-specific therapy. The former includes measures to reduce proteinuria, control edema, treat blood pressure, and address other metabolic consequences of nephrotic syndrome. The latter may involve immunosuppressive drugs and plasma exchange or may require elimination of persistent antigen by adequate treatment of infection.

Treatment of nephrotic edema

Before the era of effective diuretics, treatment of nephrotic edema was very unsatisfactory (Fig. 19.13). In contemporary practice, the mainstay of treatment is diuretics accompanied by moderate dietary sodium restriction (60–80 mmol/24 h). Significant hypovolemia is not often a clinical problem provided that fluid removal is controlled and gradual. Daily weight is the best measurement of progress. Nephrotic children are much more prone to hypovolemic shock than adults, and diuresis must be induced with caution. Nephrotic patients are diuretic resistant even if GFR is normal: loop diuretics must reach the renal tubule to be effective and transport from the peritubular capillary requires protein binding which is reduced in hypoalbuminemia; once drug reaches the renal tubule it will become 70% bound to protein present in the urine and, therefore, less effective. Oral diuretics are usually preferred as efficacy relates to 'area under the curve' (AUC), which is greater than with intravenous diuretic; twice-daily dosing also improves AUC for oral diuretics. However, in severe nephrosis, gastrointestinal absorption of the diuretic may be uncertain because of intestinal wall edema, and intravenous diuretic, by bolus injection or infusion, may be

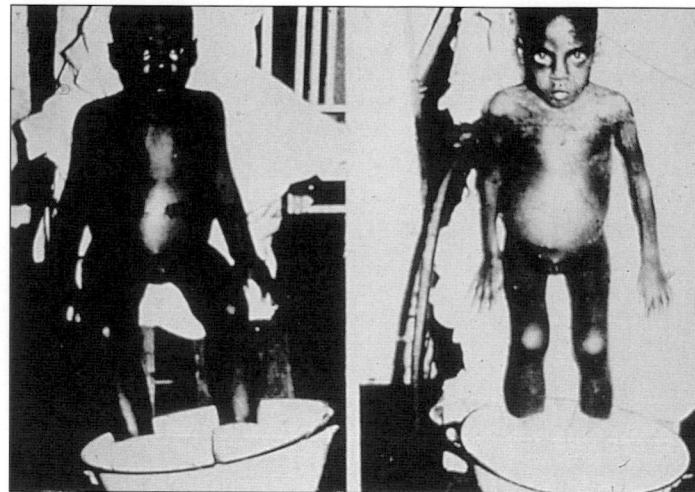

Figure 19.13 Treatment of nephrotic edema before the availability of diuretics. Edema in nephrotic syndrome was very difficult to treat: this child with anasarca, pictured in 1953, stands in a bowl while edema fluid drips out through small tubes placed through needles in the skin of the feet. This was nevertheless effective treatment: the two pictures of the same child were taken four days apart – during which time the child lost 4.5 kg (10 lb); 18% of body weight. (Courtesy of Dr Robert Vernier.)

necessary to provoke an effective diuresis. The characteristics of different diuretics are discussed in Chapter 7. A stepwise approach to diuretic use is required, aiming at fluid removal in adults of no more than 2 kg daily, moving on to the next drug level if this is not achieved (Fig. 19.14).

Treatment of proteinuria

Currently, much attention has focused on measures to reduce urinary protein excretion in patients with glomerular disease. There are several benefits from this approach. First, if proteinuria can be reduced to a non-nephrotic range, serum proteins may rise, with alleviation of many of the metabolic complications of nephrotic syndrome. Second, most studies suggest that the progressive loss of renal function observed in many glomerular diseases can largely be prevented if proteinuria can be reduced to the non-nephrotic range. This may be because many of the measures to reduce protein excretion, such as the use of ACE inhibitors, also reduce glomerular hypertension, which is frequently observed in progressive renal diseases. However, there is also increasing evidence that proteinuria or factors present in proteinuric urine may be toxic to the tubulointerstitium[16]. Finally, if proteinuria can be reduced with relatively nontoxic therapies, there may be less need for disease-specific therapies, which often include immunosuppressive agents that themselves have multiple side effects.

Most of the agents used to reduce urinary protein excretion do so hemodynamically, either reducing glomerular afferent arteriolar dilatation (NSAIDs, low-protein diet, or dipyridamole) or blocking efferent arteriolar constriction (ACE inhibitors or angiotensin receptor antagonists, ATRA). Some of the agents, such as ACE inhibitors, may also have direct effects on reducing the increased glomerular capillary wall

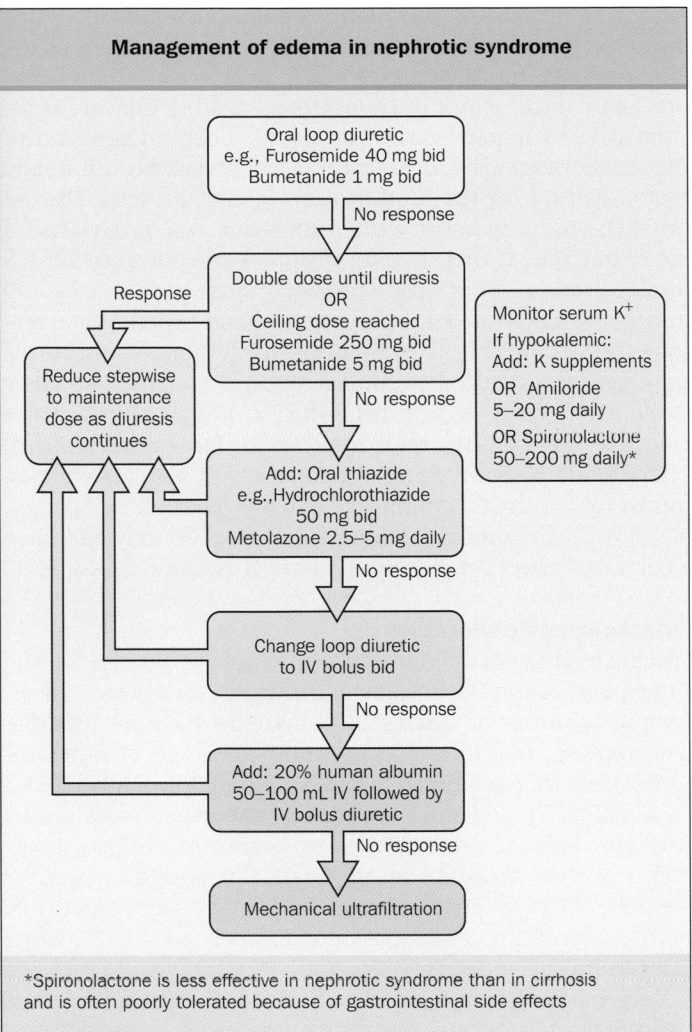

Management of edema in nephrotic syndrome

Oral loop diuretic
e.g., Furosemide 40 mg bid
Bumetanide 1 mg bid

No response

Double dose until diuresis
OR
Ceiling dose reached
Furosemide 250 mg bid
Bumetanide 5 mg bid

No response

Response

Reduce stepwise
to maintenance
dose as diuresis
continues

Monitor serum K+
If hypokalemic:
Add: K supplements
OR Amiloride
5–20 mg daily
OR Spironolactone
50–200 mg daily*

Add: Oral thiazide
e.g.,Hydrochlorothiazide
50 mg bid
Metolazone 2.5–5 mg daily

No response

Change loop diuretic
to IV bolus bid

No response

Add: 20% human albumin
50–100 mL IV followed by
IV bolus diuretic

No response

Mechanical ultrafiltration

*Spironolactone is less effective in nephrotic syndrome than in cirrhosis and is often poorly tolerated because of gastrointestinal side effects

Figure 19.14 Management of edema in nephrotic syndrome. Edema is often diuretic resistant, but the response is not predictable. Therefore, stepwise escalation of therapy is appropriate until diuresis occurs. Even when there is anasarca, diuresis should not proceed faster than 2 kg daily in adults, to minimize the risk of clinical significant hypovolemia. Mechanical ultrafiltration is rarely required for nephrotic edema, unless there is associated renal insufficiency.

permeability. A consequence of this type of therapy is a reduction in the GFR; however, in general, the decrease in GFR is of a lower magnitude than the decrease in protein excretion.

The most common agents used are ACE inhibitors, which reduce proteinuria by an average of 40–50%, particularly if the patient is on dietary salt restriction. Although less-studied, ATRA appear equally effective. While other classes of antihypertensive agent will reduce proteinuria coincident with a fall in systemic blood pressure (particularly the nondihydropyridine calcium channel blockers such as diltiazem), both ACE inhibitors and ATRA appear to reduce proteinuria independent of blood pressure. There is also evidence that ACE inhibitors and ATRA have an additive effect in reducing proteinuria[17].

Other therapies less commonly used include NSAIDs, which lessen proteinuria by reducing intrarenal prostaglandin production, and dipyridamole, which lowers proteinuria through adenosine-mediated afferent arteriolar vasoconstriction. All of these therapies must be used cautiously as the fall in GFR may be profound, particularly with ACE inhibitors or NSAIDs, and other complications may also manifest, such as hyperkalemia with ACE inhibitors and salt retention and diuretic resistance with NSAIDs.

A low-protein diet will lessen proteinuria, but must be advised with great care because of the risk of malnutrition. Adequate compensation must be made for urine protein losses[18] and the patient carefully monitored for evidence of malnutrition (see Chapter 74).

Finally, in the rare setting where proteinuria is so severe that the patient is dying from the complications of nephrotic syndrome, one may have to resort to nephrectomy to prevent continued protein losses. This may be done as a 'medical' nephrectomy: the deliberate use of NSAIDs and/or ACE inhibitors to lessen proteinuria by removal of residual GFR. If medical nephrectomy alone does not adequately reduce proteinuria, bilateral renal artery embolization should be considered. This is a surprisingly well-tolerated procedure, but is not always as successful as might be expected (perhaps because of collateral arterial supply to the kidneys, which is not blocked by the embolization). A final alternative is bilateral nephrectomy, which carries significant mortality in these severely ill hypoproteinemic patients and is rarely used in adults, although it is a conventional part of management of infants with congenital nephrotic syndrome.

Correction of hypoproteinemia

It is logical to attempt to increase serum proteins even if proteinuria cannot be lessened, but it is not easy. Although it has been shown in hospital inpatients that dietary protein intake can be increased in nephrotic patients to sustain positive nitrogen balance, this is rarely achieved in practice. This is because increased dietary protein may merely result in increased urinary protein loss, and in any case compliance is poor: nephrotic patients have anorexia and easy satiety, related to gut edema and ascites. There is also considerable experimental evidence that sustained high protein intake may be detrimental to renal function. Low protein diet lessens proteinuria and may, therefore, allow improvement in serum proteins, but great care must be taken to avoid malnutrition. In practice, adequate dietary protein should be ensured (0.8–1.0 mg/kg daily) with a high carbohydrate intake to maximize utilization of that protein which is eaten.

Treatment of hypercoagulability

The nephrotic patient is at increasing risk of thrombotic events as serum albumin falls and the risk becomes progressively more important from albumin values of 2.5 g/dL downwards. Immobility as a consequence of edema or intercurrent illness further aggravates the risk. Prophylactic anticoagulation is indicated at times of high risk such as relative immobilization in hospital (e.g., heparin 5000 units subcutaneously twice daily). Whether a nephrotic patient should also receive long-term anticoagulation, at least while albumin remains below 2.5 g/dL, remains controversial, although at least one decision analysis suggests it is beneficial[19].

Glomerular Disease

However, if a thrombosis or pulmonary embolism is documented, the patient should receive long-term anticoagulation while still nephrotic (or at least while albumin is still < 2.5 g/dL). Heparin is used for initial anticoagulation but increased dosage may be needed since part of the action of heparin depends on antithrombin III, which is often reduced in the plasma in nephrotic patients. Warfarin (Coumadin) (target international normalized ratio (INR) 2–3) is the long-term treatment of choice but should be manipulated with especial care because of altered protein binding, which may require dosage reductions. In the setting of an acute renal vein thrombosis, there are also anecdotal reports using thrombolytic therapy or surgical thrombectomy. While occasional successes are described, no convincing evidence has been provided that any treatment improves long-term renal function.

Treatment of hyperlipidemia

Although there is no absolute proof that the hyperlipidemia of nephrotic syndrome is associated with increased risk of cardiovascular disease, extrapolation of evidence in the general population strongly supports attempts to reduce lipid levels in nephrotic patients. Dietary restriction alone has only modest effects. Until the introduction of statins (hydroxymethylglutaryl (HMG) CoA reductase inhibitors) there was no acceptable drug treatment. Previously available lipid-lowering agents were either ineffective or not tolerated (e.g. myositis provoked by fibrates). Statins (such as simvastatin, lovastatin, pravistatin) have now been shown to reduce total and LDL cholesterol in nephrotic patients, with some increase in HDL and additional reduction in triglyceride. They are well tolerated. The addition of bile acid sequestrants (cholestyramine) may lower LDL further and increase HDL but is usually not tolerated because of gastrointestinal effects. Second-line treatments are probucol (which has a more modest effect on lipids but is well tolerated) and newer fibrates (gemfibrozil, bezafibrate), provided patients are monitored for drug-induced muscle injury. Conventional dosing is used.

Infection

A high order of clinical suspicion for infection is vital in nephrotic patients. Because spontaneous bacterial peritonitis is common, especially in nephrotic children, ascitic fluid should be examined microscopically and cultured if there is any suspicion of systemic infection. Bacteremia is common even if clinical signs are localized. ESR is elevated in nephrotic syndrome *per se* and so is unhelpful, but an elevated C-reactive protein may be more informative. Parenteral antibiotics should be started once cultures are taken and the regimen should include benzylpenicillin (to cover pneumococci). If repeated infections occur, serum immunoglobulins should be measured. If serum IgG is less than 600 mg/dL, there is evidence in an uncontrolled study that infection risk is reduced by monthly administration of intravenous immunoglobulin 10–15 g to keep the IgG levels above 600 mg/dL[20].

Hypertension

Hypertension is very common in GN and virtually universal as chronic GN progresses towards end-stage renal disease. Sodium and water overload is an important part of the pathogenetic process and high-dose diuretics with moderate dietary sodium restriction are usually an essential part of the treatment. As in other chronic renal disease, the aim of blood pressure control is not only to protect against the cardiovascular risks of hypertension but also to delay progression of the renal disease. The ideal target blood pressure is not finally established but in the Modification of Diet in Renal Disease (MDRD) study, patients with proteinuria (> 1 g/day) had a better outcome if their blood pressure was reduced to 125/75 mmHg rather than the previous standard of 140/90 mmHg[21,22]. There are strong theoretical and experimental reasons for ACE inhibitors to be first-choice therapy and this is now well documented in clinical studies[23–25]. ATRA are likely to be as effective as ACE inhibitors although clinical trials evidence to support their use is so far rather limited. They should be reserved for the minority of patients who are intolerant of ACE inhibitors, usually because of cough. Nondihydropyridine calcium channel blockers may also have a beneficial effect on proteinuria as well as blood pressure.

Disease-specific therapies

Specific treatments for glomerular diseases are discussed in the subsequent chapters; the general principles are discussed here. As most glomerular disease is thought to have an immune pathogenesis, treatment has generally consisted of immunosuppressive therapy aimed at blocking both the systemic and local effects. In the setting where glomerular disease results from an ineffectual elimination of a foreign antigen, treatment involves measures to eliminate this antigen whenever possible (such as antibiotics in endocarditis-associated GN or interferon-α for cryoglobulinemia associated with hepatitis C infection).

In general, the more severe and acute the presentation of GN, the more successful is immune treatment; there has been little success for immunosuppression in chronic GN. In situations where renal function is declining rapidly, there is 'little to lose' and the toxicity of intensive regimens becomes acceptable for a short period where it would be unacceptable if prolonged. Furthermore, the nonspecific nature of most immune treatments results in widespread interruption of immune and inflammatory events at multiple levels. In the acute situation, this broad-based attack is a virtue; in more indolent disease more specific treatment is needed but is unavailable. Despite great increases in the understanding of immune mechanisms in glomerular disease since the 1970s, immune therapies have not yet become more specific and precise. The mainstays of treatment remain agents that were available in the 1960s: corticosteroids, azathioprine, and cyclophosphamide. Cyclosporine, for example, despite 20 years use in clinical transplantation, does not yet have a fully defined role in the treatment of glomerular disease. Other newer immunosuppressive agents developed for use in transplantation including tacrolimus, mycophenolate and rapamycin, do not yet have established indications in glomerular disease.

The use of immunosuppressive therapies to treat GN carries certain drawbacks. In many diseases, treatment is based on small series, and good prospective controlled trials are lacking. Because of both the rarity and the variable natural history of GN, proof of efficacy for a particular therapy often requires a multicenter approach with prolonged follow-up, which is logistically difficult. It should also be recognized that if sufficient glomerular damage is present, proteinuria and progressive deterioration of renal function may occur by nonimmune pathways that may not be responsive to immunosuppressive therapies. Given the frequent uncertainty of the response to immunosuppressive therapy, it becomes mandatory to weigh the potential benefits against the risks of therapy.

Immunosuppression may be associated with reactivation of tuberculosis and hepatitis B infection and can also lead to a 'hyperinfection' syndrome in patients with *Strongyloides* sp. infection. Therefore, high-risk patents should be screened for these diseases prior to embarking on therapy.

Alkylating agents, such as cyclophosphamide and chlorambucil, have considerable toxicity. In the short term, leukopenia is common, as is alopecia, although hair will regrow within a few months of discontinuing therapy. These agents can cause infertility (observed in adults with cumulative doses of cyclophosphamide above 200 mg/kg and chlorambucil 10 mg/kg). There is also an increased incidence of leukemias (observed with total doses of cyclophosphamide above 80 g and chlorambucil 7 g). Cyclophosphamide is also a bladder irritant and treatment can result in hemorrhagic cystitis and bladder carcinoma, particularly after therapy lasting more than 6 months[26]. Irritation of the bladder is caused by a metabolite, acrolein. The effect can be minimized in patients receiving intravenous cyclophosphamide by enforcing a good diuresis and administering mesna, given by intravenous infusion at the same dose as the cyclophosphamide. Chlorambucil and cyclophosphamide also require dose reduction in the setting of renal insufficiency. Given all these concerns, oral treatment with these agents should ideally be limited to 12 weeks.

The modes of action and potential adverse effects of corticosteroids, azathioprine, and other immunosuppressives occasionally used in glomerular disease, are discussed further in Chapter 85.

REFERENCES

1. Iseki K, Iseki C, Ikemiya Y, Fukiyama K. Risk of developing end-stage renal disease in a cohort of mass screening. Kidney Int. 1996;49:800–5.
2. Topham PS, Harper SJ, Furness PN, et al. Glomerular disease as a cause of isolated microscopic haematuria. Q J Med. 1994;87:329–36.
3. Springberg PD, Garrett LE, Thompson AL, et al. Fixed and reproducible orthostatic proteinuria. Results of a 20 year follow up study. Ann Intern Med. 1982;97:516–19.
4. Orth SR, Ritz E. The nephrotic syndrome. N Engl J Med. 1998;338:1201–12.
5. Cameron JS. Nephrotic syndrome in the elderly. Semin Nephrol. 1996;16:319–29.
6. Haas M, Meehan SM, Karison TG, Spargo BH. Changing etiologies of unexplained adult nephrotic syndrome: a comparison of renal biopsy findings from 1976–1979 and 1995–1997. Am J Kidney Dis. 1997;30:621–31.
7. Kaysen G, Gambertoglio J, Felts J, Hutchison F. Albumin synthesis, albuminuria and hyperlipidemia in nephrotic syndrome. Kidney Int. 1987;31:1368–76.
8. Humphreys MH. Mechanisms and management of nephrotic edema. Kidney Int. 1994;45:266–81.
9. Rodriguez-Iturbe B, Herrera-Acosta J, Johnson RJ. Interstitial inflammation, sodium retention and the pathogenesis of nephrotic edema. Kidney Int. 2002;62:1379–84.
10. Rabelink TJ, Zwaginga JJ, Koomans HA, Sixma JJ. Thrombosis and hemostasis in renal disease. Kidney Int. 1994;46:287–96.
11. Wheeler DC, Bernard DB. Lipid abnormalities in nephrotic syndrome. Am J Kidney Dis. 1994;23:331–46.
12. Fried LF, Orchard TJ, Kasiske BL. Effect of lipid reduction on the progression of renal disease: a meta-analysis. Kidney Int. 2001;59:260–9.
13. Smith JD, Hayslett JP. Reversible renal failure in the nephrotic syndrome. Am J Kidney Dis. 1992;19:201–13.
14. Jennette JC, Falk RJ. Adult minimal change glomerulopathy with acute renal failure. Am J Kidney Dis. 1990;16:432–7.
15. Lowenstein J, Schacht RG, Baldwin DS. Renal failure in minimal change nephritic syndrome. Am J Med. 1981;70:227–33.
16. Burton C, Harris KPG. The role of proteinuria in the progression of chronic renal failure. Am J Kidney Dis. 1996;27:765–75.
17. Nakao N, Yoshimura A, Morita H, et al. Combination treatment of angiotensin-II receptor blocker and angiotensin-converting enzyme inhibitor in non-diabetic renal disease [COOPERATE]: a randomised controlled trial. Lancet. 2003;361:117–34.
18. Maroni BJ, Staffield C, Young VR, et al. Mechanisms permitting nephrotic patients to achieve nitrogen equilibrium with a protein restricted diet. J Clin Invest. 1997;99:2479–87.
19. Sarasin FP, Schifferli JA. Prophylactic oral anticoagulation in nephrotic patients with idiopathic membranous nephropathy. Kidney Int. 1994;45:578–85.
20. Ogi M, Yokoyama H, Tomosui N, et al. Risk factors for infection and immunoglobulin replacement therapy in adult nephrotic syndrome. Am J Kidney Dis. 1994;24:427–36.
21. Klahr S, Levey AS, Beck GJ, et al. The effects of dietary protein restriction and blood pressure control on the progression of chronic renal disease. N Engl J Med. 1994;330:877–84.
22. National Health and Nutritional Examination Survey. The Sixth Report of the Joint National Committee on Prevention, Detection, Evaluation and Treatment of High Blood Pressure. Arch Intern Med. 1997;157:2413–15.
23. Maschio G, Alberti D, Janin G, et al. Effect of the angiotensin-converting-enzyme inhibitor, benazepril, on the progression of chronic renal insufficiency. N Engl J Med. 1996;334:939–45.
24. The GISEN group. Randomised placebo-controlled trial of effect of ramipril on decline in glomerular filtration rate and risk of terminal renal failure in proteinuric, non-diabetic nephropathy. Lancet. 1997;349:1857–63.
25. Jafar TH, Schmid CH, Landa M, et al. Angiotensin-converting enzyme inhibitors and progression of non-diabetic renal disease. A meta-analysis of patient-level data. Ann Intern Med. 2001;135:73–87.
26. Talar-Williams C, Hijazi C, Walther M, et al. Cyclophosphamide-induced cystitis and bladder cancer in patients with Wegener's granulomatosis. Ann Intern Med. 1996;124:477–84.

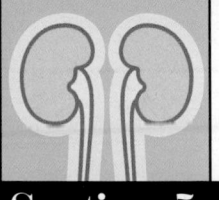

Section 5 Glomerular Disease

Chapter 20

Minimal Change Disease and Primary Focal Segmental Glomerulosclerosis

Phil D Mason

INTRODUCTION AND DEFINITIONS

Minimal change disease (MCD) and focal segmental glomerulosclerosis (FSGS) are the cause of the nephrotic syndrome in about 90% of children aged under 10 years, about 50–70% of older children, and 20–35% of adults. The relationship between the two conditions, in particular whether or not they share a common pathogenesis, is not yet defined. They are considered together since both are characterized by a diffuse capillary wall defect in the absence of immune deposits, they share many clinical features, and are treated in a similar way, at least initially.

MCD is defined by the absence of histologic glomerular abnormality, other than ultrastructural evidence of epithelial cell foot process fusion, in a patient presenting with nephrotic syndrome, who is typically steroid responsive.

FSGS is defined on histologic criteria by segmental capillary obliteration with increased mesangial matrix deposition, intracapillary hyaline deposits, and focal adhesions of the capillary tuft to Bowman's capsule. Primary FSGS occurs in a patient presenting with nephrotic syndrome in the absence of any of the known causes of secondary FSGS, which are discussed in Chapter 21.

Steroid-responsive or steroid-sensitive nephrotic syndrome are the terms used to describe the disease occurring in children with nephrotic syndrome who respond to steroids but have not had a renal biopsy to provide the histologic proof of MCD.

The conditions are defined by a combination of the pathologic features and the clinical presentation. This is an important point because similar histopathologic appearances may be seen with proteinuria in the absence of nephrotic syndrome. Such patients may have different conditions with different prognosis and, therefore, different requirements for management.

ETIOLOGY AND PATHOGENESIS

In a minority of patients with MCD, there is a clear association with a factor that appears to provoke the nephrotic syndrome (Table 20.1). FSGS occurs in association with a wide variety of infections, nonrenal conditions, and pre-existing renal diseases that appear to be causally related to the glomerular injury (see Table 21.1). These secondary forms of FSGS are more likely if the proteinuria is not in the nephrotic range. They are discussed in Chapter 21.

In normal glomeruli, the barrier to protein filtration is provided by a combination of size barriers and charge selectivity.

Factors associated with the onset of nephrotic syndrome in minimal change disease
Drugs
Nonsteroidal anti-inflammatory drugs
Interferon-α
Lithium: rare (usually causes chronic interstitial nephritis)
Gold: rare (usually causes membranous nephropathy)
Allergy
Pollens
House dust
Insect stings
Immunizations
Malignancy
Hodgkin's disease
Mycosis fungoides
Chronic lymphocytic leukemia: uncommon (usually associated with membranoproliferative glomerulonephritis)

Table 20.1 Factors associated with the onset of nephrotic syndrome in minimal change disease.

Neutral molecules larger than 4–4.5 nm are excluded; although albumin molecules are smaller than this, they are excluded because they are anionic and are repelled by the negative charge on the epithelial cells and glomerular basement membrane (GBM) (mainly owing to heparan sulfate). In MCD and FSGS (as well as in some other causes of the nephrotic syndrome) the clearance of small neutral molecules is actually less than normal, suggesting that the massive albumin filtration is primarily the result of loss of GBM surface charge.

Although the injury is manifest as a change in glomerular capillary permeability, it is probable that the underlying problem is toxic epithelial cell injury, which results in foot process fusion and epithelial cell detachment, and alters capillary wall function. There is increasing circumstantial evidence that a circulating factor is involved in the pathogenesis and that there may be an abnormality, of cell-mediated immunity. The close clinical relationship between MCD and FSGS has led some to suggest a shared pathogenesis, but the increasing evidence of differences makes this less likely.

Minimal change disease

Evidence for an immune abnormality is particularly found in MCD, which seems likely to be a systemic condition rather than an intrinsic disease of the kidney. In the precortico-steroid era it was observed that the nephrotic syndrome often remitted in children who contracted measles, which is known to have powerful depressive effects on cell-mediated immunity. MCD is also associated with lymphomas (especially Hodgkin's disease) and atopy (up to 30% of children in some series), and responds to immunosuppressive drugs. There are also many reports of abnormal humoral and cellular immunity in patients with MCD during relapse and sometimes in remission as well, but not in those with other causes of nephrotic syndrome. Finally, an association has been reported with HLA-DR7, at least in steroid-responsive individuals. There are many reports of MCD relapse following exposure to an allergen in sensitive individuals. As a result, patients with identified food allergies have been managed with exclusion diets with reported complete or partial remissions, and relapse following reintroduction of the offending food. However, even if the relationship is real, it is possible that the allergic events merely trigger relapse, as may infections.

The histopathology does not give any clues to pathogenesis although the absence of immune deposits implies that immune mechanisms are likely to be cellular rather than humoral. The characteristic podocyte foot process fusion is seen in other patients with heavy proteinuria (e.g., due to FSGS) and also in children with severe hypoalbuminemia, but no proteinuria, dying of kwashiorkor[1], but the mechanism may differ in these conditions, with reduced levels of dystroglycans (adhesion molecules believed to anchor podocytes to the glomerular basement membrane) in MCD but not in FSGS, with normalization following steroid treatment[2].

A circulating factor acting on podocytes has not yet been identified. Lymphocyte-derived cytokines have been proposed for many years but remain elusive, although studies in which the supernatant from T-cell hybridomas derived from these patients provokes proteinuria and foot process fusion when infused into rats are suggestive of such a mechanism[3]. Hemopexin, an acute phase reactant extracted from human plasma, is capable of inducing proteinuria in rats[4]. Evidence for a circulating factor in humans is also supported by the observation that proteinuria resolved within days following transplantation from a cadaveric donor with minimal change nephropathy[5].

Focal segmental glomerulosclerosis

In FSGS, evidence for a circulating factor is more substantial, mainly based on the high incidence of recurrence following transplantation, with heavy proteinuria developing sometimes within hours. Initially the histologic picture is MCD developing later into FSGS. Plasma exchange and elution with protein A or anti-IgG columns can lead to remission in transplant recurrence of FSGS, and eluates from the columns may induce proteinuria[6]. A soluble factor that causes proteinuria in rats and increased protein permeability in cultured human glomeruli has also been described[7]. This has not yet been characterized, but it may form the basis of a predictive test for deciding if and when a patient should have a further

transplant or to plan pre-emptive treatment of recurrence[8]. Upregulated expression of transforming growth factor-β (TGF-β), a profibrotic cytokine, has been described in patients with FSGS, but it is unclear whether this is a primary or secondary phenomenon.

There are also a number of well-described, but rare, familial cases of FSGS that probably have a different etiology. Mutations of the gene encoding an actin filament binding protein, α-actinin-4 (which may be involved in cytoskeletal function of glomerular podocytes) have been described in autosomal dominant FSGS[9]. Mutations of NPHS2, a gene encoding an integral membrane protein, podocin, expressed in podocytes have been reported in autosomal recessive and some sporadic FSGS[10].

A further conundrum to answer is the segmental nature of the sclerotic process in FSGS given that the capillary wall abnormalities that allow proteinuria to occur appear to be global, suggesting that epithelial cell injury may also be widespread. It has been suggested that segmental sclerosis is often hilar because the high net filtration pressures consequent upon heavy proteinuria are maximal at the beginning of the glomerular capillaries.

EPIDEMIOLOGY

Although more common in childhood (the most common age of onset being 2 to 7 years), MCD is also an important cause of the nephrotic syndrome in adults of all ages. However, the incidence varies geographically: as low as 1 per million in the UK and up to 27 per million in the USA. It is more common in South Asians and Native Americans but is rarer in Africans, who are much more likely to have FSGS and to have steroid-resistant nephrotic syndrome. Boys are twice as likely to be affected than girls, but the sex incidence is equal in adolescents and adults.

Primary FSGS is the cause of nephrotic syndrome in < 10% of children, the middle aged, and the elderly but is the diagnosis in up to 20% of nephrotic adolescents and young adults. It has an incidence of about two per million in a white European population[11]. It is more common in African Americans in the USA and the incidence appears to be rising[12]. Overall it is the cause of renal failure in about 2.5% of patients on renal replacement therapy, but represents a greater proportion of younger patients since the median age is 48 years at the start of renal replacement therapy[13].

Familial focal segmental glomerulosclerosis

Rare familial forms of FSGS have been described in both Caucasians and African Americans. Affected individuals usually present in the first to fourth decades with nephrotic syndrome, hypertension, and progressive renal insufficiency. They are usually steroid resistant, with the majority progressing to end-stage renal disease (ESRD) within 10 years. In a series describing 60 families in whom two or more (up to 37) individuals have developed FSGS, both dominant and recessive patterns of inheritance was suggested by the involvement of multiple and single generations respectively[14]. Twins were concordant in 3/4 monozygotic sets and dysmorphic features were evident in two families. Patients from single generation kindreds deteriorated more rapidly than those from kindreds in whom multiple generations were affected. The causes of familial FSGS may be different from sporadic cases, especially since recurrence after transplantation occurred in only 1/41 transplants suggesting that a defect in the native kidneys, rather than a circulating factor, is responsible. This is consistent with recent data reporting mutations in genes coding for podocyte structural proteins in these families (see above).

CLINICAL MANIFESTATIONS

Typically, patients present with edema that develops over a short period of time, with fluid retention exceeding 3% of the body weight and often very much more. Up to two-thirds of presentations and relapses follow an infection, most commonly in the upper respiratory tract, but whether or not these are of causative significance is uncertain.

The clinical signs and symptoms are the same as those for the nephrotic syndrome from any cause (see Chapter 19), although the nephrotic syndrome may be of very rapid onset, increasing the risk of hypovolemia, particularly in children. Pleural effusions and ascites are common, particularly in children, who may present with abdominal pain, a symptom that may suggest peritonitis or herald hypovolemia. Pericardial effusions may occur but pulmonary edema is uncommon except following treatment with albumin or with coexisting cardiac disease. Hepatomegaly is frequent in children and this may be painful. The distribution of the edema is gravitational but facial puffiness is common and genital swelling may be very uncomfortable, especially in men. Gross edema may predispose to ulceration and infection of dependent skin; striae often appear even without steroids, and lacerations or needlestick punctures weep fluid profusely. Edema of the bowel may cause diarrhea with significant albumin loss from the gut. Other clinical features include white nails, sometimes in bands (Muehrcke's bands) correlating with periods of clinical relapse (see Fig. 19.4). Occasionally, xanthomata are associated with gross hyperlipidemia.

Microscopic hematuria is rare in MCD but is more common in FSGS. Hypertension is not usually regarded as typical of MCD but was a feature at presentation in 30% of 89 adults reported from Guy's Hospital, UK[15]; hypertension has also been described in 14–21% of children, when making comparisons with appropriate age- and sex-matched blood pressure reference ranges. This usually resolves during remission, especially in children. Hypertension is sometimes associated with expansion of the intravascular volume but may paradoxically be related to hypovolemia and stimulation of the renin–angiotensin axis. Hypertension is more common in FSGS, especially with impaired function and irrespective of age.

Before the introduction of corticosteroids, the morbidity and mortality of patients with MCD were high because of complications of nephrotic syndrome, particularly infection. This continues to be a serious problem and 6 out of 389 children with MCD reported by the International Study of Kidney Disease in Children in 1984 died of sepsis[16]. Peritonitis is still a major cause of mortality in the Third World, mainly in children. *Streptococcus pneumoniae*, *Haemophilus* and other encapsulated bacteria are commonly implicated. Children with persistent nephrotic syndrome should be immunized against *S. pneumoniae* and *H. influenzae* and given prophylactic oral penicillin. Peritonitis is rare in adults, who usually have protective antibodies against these bacteria, and prophylactic antibiotics are not indicated.

The risk of thromboembolism increases in MCD and FSGS, as in all nephrotics. Venous thromboembolism may occur in the common sites and, in addition, nephrotic children occasionally have other catastrophic events such as intracerebral venous thombosis. Arterial thrombosis is also a rare and feared complication that seems to affect children almost exclusively and may result in loss of limb.

Acute renal failure is a complication particularly seen in adults. It may follow hypovolemia, which should be avoided especially during intensive diuretic treatment, but acute renal failure may also occur in patients who are volume replete. It may be more common than generally accepted and its etiology is discussed further in Chapter 19.

Non-nephrotic proteinuria

Identical histologic changes of MCD and FSGS may be found in adults and children investigated for asymptomatic proteinuria who never become nephrotic. The different management of these patients is discussed below.

PATHOLOGY

Minimal change disease

Classically, MCD is associated with a completely normal appearance in the glomeruli on light microscopy and immunohistology. Podocyte (epithelial cell) foot process effacement seen with electron microscopy (Fig. 20.1) is the only abnormality, but this is a nonspecific finding. However, mild mesangial hypercellularity is now accepted as an infrequent finding (3–5%), and small amounts of mesangial IgG, complement C3, and occasionally IgA are sometimes seen in patients whose clinical course is indistinguishable from classical MCD. The presence of mesangial IgM is considered by

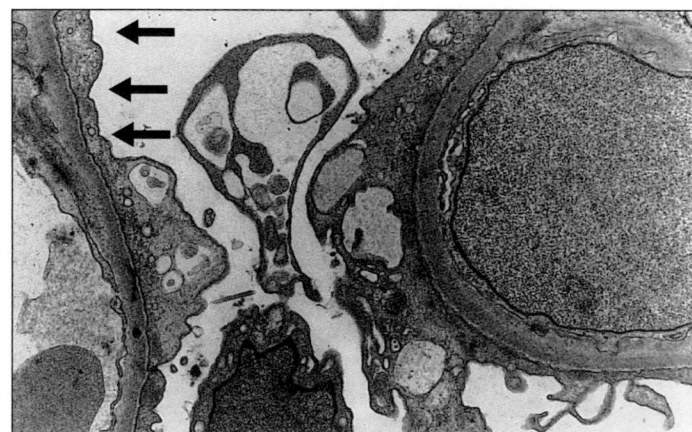

Figure 20.1 Podocyte foot process fusion in minimal change disease. The epithelial cells (arrows) are completely effaced along the glomerular basement membranes. (Electron micrograph × 6000.) The normal appearance of epithelial cell foot processes is shown in Figure 1.7.

some to define a separate entity (see below). Hyaline casts obstructing tubules, foam cells, and occasionally appearances consistent with acute tubular necrosis may be seen, especially if acute renal failure is present at the time of biopsy.

Focal segmental glomerulosclerosis

Light microscopy
As the name implies, FSGS is characterized histopathologically by segmental glomerular scarring (see Fig. 20.2). In the affected segments, the capillary is obliterated by accumulation of acellular matrix and hyaline deposits, associated with adhesions to Bowman's capsule. The juxtamedullary glomeruli are typically the first to be affected. It is, therefore, possible to miss the diagnosis, especially if there are only a few glomeruli in the biopsy sample. A glomerulus containing a sclerotic segment may also be missed on a single section; when careful serial sections are performed the incidence of lesions will increase. As the disease progresses, an increasing proportion of the glomeruli are affected, some with segmental sclerosis, some with global sclerosis. As more glomeruli become sclerotic, tubular atrophy and interstitial fibrosis develop. If a biopsy sample is small, and focal tubular atrophy and interstitial fibrosis are identified with normal looking glomeruli, this should suggest FSGS, especially in the context of the nephrotic syndrome. Serial sections may then reveal typical changes.

Immunofluorescence
Sclerotic segments are often positive for IgM and C3 complement, but this is almost certainly a nonspecific effect of the injury, caused by passive trapping of large molecules in the damaged capillary loops, rather than being a causal factor of the sclerosis.

Electron microscopy
Foot process fusion on electron microscopy, even of unaffected glomeruli, is often indistinguishable from that seen in MCD and in other causes of the nephrotic syndrome. However, diffuse foot process fusion predominates in the sclerotic segments, with partial effacement in surrounding apparently normal lobules. It may also be seen in patients with low-level proteinuria in the absence of the nephrotic syndrome. Glomerulosclerosis occurs spontaneously with age (although much less in humans than in some experimental animals, particularly the rat), which influences the interpretation of the histologic findings.

In FSGS, only the presence of interstitial fibrosis correlates with the eventual prognosis, which not surprisingly also correlates with serum creatinine levels at the time of biopsy[17].

Histologic variants of primary focal segmental glomerulosclerosis
There is considerable overlap in the descriptions of histologic variants of FSGS and continuing uncertainty whether they should be regarded as distinct entities.

Collapsing variant
Collapsing FSGS is now recognized as a distinct entity in which segmental sclerotic lesions are associated with collapse of the glomerular tuft. The clinical context is nephrotic syndrome complicated by rapid loss of renal function. It bears many similarities to the secondary form of FSGS that occurs in association with HIV infection and it is, therefore, discussed further in Chapter 21.

The glomerular 'tip' lesion
In primary FSGS, the segmental scars vary in position and have been described as 'hilar' when related to the vascular pole, 'peripheral' when opposite the tubular pole, or 'intermediate'. The 'tip' lesion describes peripheral segmental sclerosis adjacent to the tubular pole of Bowman's capsule, with protrusion into the tubular lumen (Fig. 20.3). The glomerular capillary loops adjacent to the proximal tubule are dilated, with accumulation of foamy cells, sometimes accompanied by hyalinosis but without significant increase in mesangial cells or matrix. These lesions frequently show adhesion to Bowman's capsule and at times prolapse into the proximal tubules. Visceral epithelial cells surrounding the lesion are prominent and contain large protein resorption droplets. Glomerular changes at the tubular origin are common in many disorders and appear to be a result of proteinuria. The 'tip' lesion is, therefore, seen in glomeruli that otherwise appear normal on light microscopy and, in its absence, would have been called MCD. This explains why it has been associated with a greater likelihood of steroid responsiveness and a better long-term prognosis. Contradictory data have since been reported, and most series do not support an association with a better prognosis, but this may reflect the more

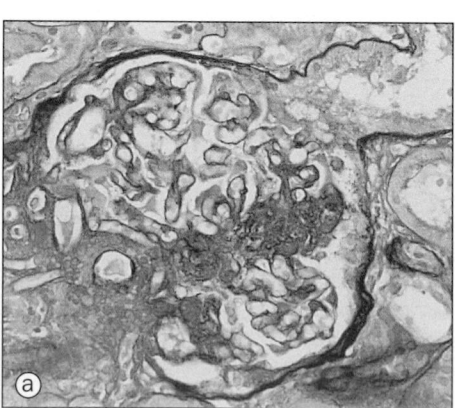
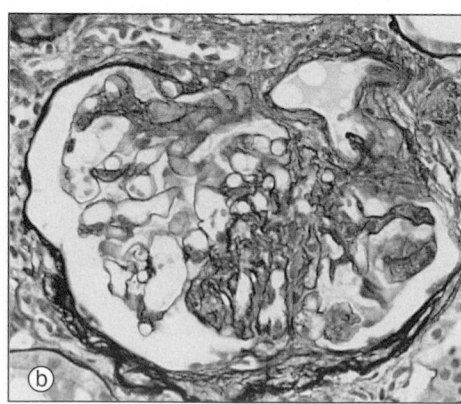

Figure 20.2 Light microscopic appearances in focal segmental glomerulosclerosis.
Segmental scars with capsular adhesions in otherwise normal glomeruli. ((a) Periodic acid–Schiff, ×300; (b) Methenamine silver stain ×300.) (Courtesy of Dr D Davies.)

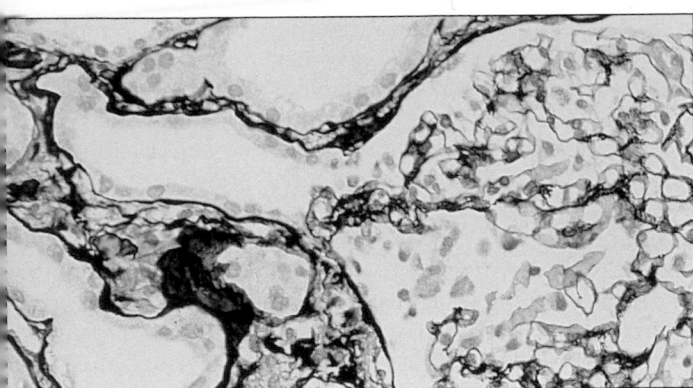

Figure 20.3 The glomerular 'tip' lesion. A glomerulus in a renal biopsy from an adult with steroid-responsive nephrotic syndrome. The glomerular tuft is normal away from the tubular origin, but at the tubular origin there is adhesion to Bowman's capsule with protrusion into the tubular lumen. (Methenamine silver stain ×300.) (Courtesy of Dr D Davies.)

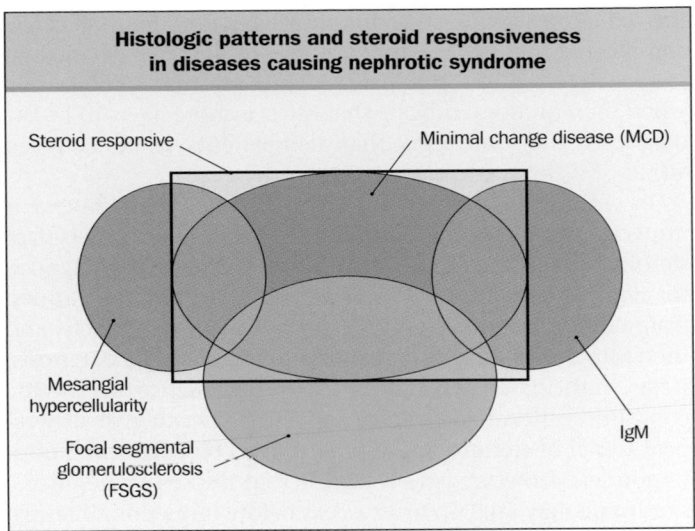

Figure 20.4 Histologic patterns and steroid responsiveness in nephrotic syndrome. The inter-relationships between steroid responsiveness and minimal change disease, focal segmental glomerulosclerosis, mesangial hypercellularity, and mesangial IgM deposition.

widespread use of the term 'tip' lesion when glomerular changes at the tubular origin occur in other glomerular disorders with proteinuria, including membranoproliferative glomerulonephritis, IgA nephropathy, and renal allografts. Perhaps the most important reason to recognize the lesion is to prevent a misdiagnosis of a proliferative glomerulonephritis.

Cellular variants

Visceral cell hyperplasia and proliferation may overlie segmental scars or an area of collapsed capillary loops. In areas of segmental sclerosis there may also be endocapillary hypercellularity, foam cells, leukocytes, and nuclear debris, mimicking proliferative glomerulonephritis. It is not clear that this variant has any useful clinicopathologic correlates.

More diffuse mesangial hypercellularity may also be seen in FSGS. While the presence of mesangial hypercellularity in MCD may be a better predictor of resistance to steroid therapy and a poor clinical prognosis, attempts to correlate its significance in FSGS have yielded conflicting results[18]. Some consider mesangial hypercellularity to be an intermediate step in the evolution (progression) of MCD to FSGS.

IgM nephropathy

Some patients presenting with nephrotic syndrome have mesangial deposits of IgM, often with a minor degree of mesangial hypercellularity. Patients are more likely to have microscopic (and occasionally macroscopic) hematuria and are said to be less likely to respond to steroids (50% compared with 90% for MCD[18]). Others challenge the existence of this condition, pointing out that IgM deposits, at least to some degree, are seen in MCD, FSGS, and mesangial proliferative glomerulonephritis in a similar proportion of patients.

The relationship between MCD, FSGS, and IgM nephropathy is poorly defined, but steroid responsiveness is a shared feature (Fig. 20.4). The lesions may form part of a continuum and some believe that FSGS develops in a proportion of patients with MCD, while others believe that they have different etiologies. Undoubtedly, some patients with FSGS behave as if they had MCD, and it is possible that the segmental lesions

may be coincidental, especially in adults over 40 years of age in whom sclerotic lesions become increasingly common. There have been some reports that increased expression of TGF-β may distinguish between prognostic groups[19], but more studies are needed to confirm these claims. Operationally a distinction is unnecessary, at least for the initial phase of management.

DIAGNOSIS AND DIFFERENTIAL DIAGNOSIS

The clinical diagnosis of nephrotic syndrome is straightforward, with edema in the presence of heavy proteinuria, usually without microscopic hematuria on urine dipstick testing. Urine microscopy reveals hyaline casts and sometimes lipid casts. There is hypoalbuminemia and nephrotic range proteinuria (> 3.5 g/24 h in adults or > 40 mg/h/m² in children) with hyperlipidemia. Hyponatremia and hemoconcentration may be seen, even before treatment. Elevated urea and creatinine concentrations occur more often in adults. Typically, IgG levels are low while IgM is raised. Serum complement levels are normal. In children, steroid-responsive MCD is usually associated with 'selective' proteinuria of smaller molecules including albumin and transferrin but not of larger molecules such as immunoglobulins and ferritin. A selectivity index is usually derived from the ratio of IgG clearance to albumin clearance:

■ EQUATION 20.I

$$\text{Selectivity index} = \frac{[\text{IgG}]_u \, [\text{Albumin}]_s}{[\text{IgG}]_s \, [\text{Albumin}]_u}$$

where subscript u is concentration in urine and s is that in serum. If the selectivity index is < 10%, the proteinuria is 'highly selective', if > 20% it is 'nonselective'. This is of limited clinical value since highly selective proteinuria is less common in adult MCD and does not influence a decision to treat with steroids. However, highly selective proteinuria, when present, does indicate that MCD is more likely to be the diagnosis, and some argue that such patients should be given a trial of steroids without a renal biopsy.

In children, aged between 1 and 12 years, renal biopsy is unnecessary unless the patient does not respond to corticosteroid treatment. In adults there is a wide differential diagnosis for nephrotic syndrome that can only partially be clarified from clinical criteria, steroid responsiveness is less likely, and therefore a renal biopsy is required to establish the diagnosis. It has, in the past, been argued that, in the absence of a specific contraindication to steroid therapy, it is safer to give a therapeutic trial of steroids and reserve a renal biopsy for the non-responders. However, adults with steroid-responsive nephrotic syndrome may take up to 12 weeks before induction of remission and so the morbidity from steroids does become significant and will outweigh the risks of a renal biopsy. Therefore, a renal biopsy is routinely recommended for the investigation of adults with nephrotic syndrome. In the context of the nephrotic syndrome and a typical biopsy appearance, it is always important to consider whether the patient may have a secondary cause of MCD or FSGS.

NATURAL HISTORY

There is a tendency for patients with MCD to run a relapsing–remitting course, and this is more frequent in children. Those presenting at an earlier age are more likely to have a longer disease course before long-term remission occurs (see Fig. 20.5). Relapse occurs in more than two-thirds of children and nearly 50% relapse more than four times, usually following steroid cessation or reduction. If relapse occurs during steroid reduction, the patient is described as steroid dependent. Long-term remission can be expected in 75% of initial responders who do not relapse within 6 months, while those

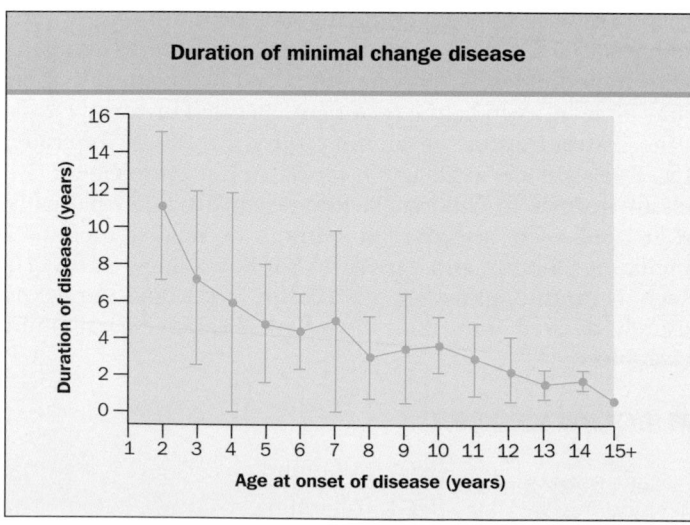

Figure 20.5 Long-term outcome in childhood-onset minimal change disease. The duration of disease is inversely related to the age of presentation. (Adapted with permission from Trompeter et al.[21].)

who do relapse become non-relapsing after an average of 3 years[20]. However, it is reassuring that < 5% of children with MCD enter adulthood still having relapses, although the younger the onset of the first attack, the longer the child is likely to continue having relapses[21]. In general, increasing time since last relapse reduces the risk of further relapse, but occasionally adults will have a relapse after an interval of 10 years or more.

MCD does not progress to renal failure, although a number of patients with this diagnosis are found to have FSGS on subsequent biopsies. It is still unclear whether the focal nature of the disease resulted in the correct diagnosis being missed on the initial biopsy or whether evolution from MCD to FSGS does occur. The incidence of progressive renal failure in primary FSGS is often quoted as around 50%, although there may be variation in the exact diagnostic criteria and prognosis is clearly related to the level of proteinuria and the response to treatment[22] (Fig. 20.6). Non-nephrotic patients with normal plasma albumin and proteinuria of > 3 g/day have a 10-year incidence of renal failure of just 10–15%. Many with non-nephrotic proteinuria will have secondary FSGS.

TRANSPLANTATION

Relapse of FSGS following transplantation is common; the overall risk of relapse of FSGS in a first transplant is said to be 20–30% (with graft loss in half of these). However, in some reports, a diagnosis of recurrent FSGS may be based on histopathologic findings alone, which can be misleading because FSGS is seen in the later stages of other disease (see Chapter 21). The risk of relapse for nephrotic patients with primary FSGS is not adequately defined but is probably higher than the quoted figure of 20–30%. Relapse risk is highest in children, especially when renal failure progressed rapidly in their native kidneys. The recurrence rate is 60% or more if a previously transplanted kidney has been lost through recurrent disease, and it rises to over 80% for the third transplant. Since recurrence is so common, many groups have been cautious about living related donor transplantation, especially for high-risk patients. Transplant recurrence of primary FSGS is discussed further in Chapter 91.

TREATMENT

Steroid treatment induces remission in almost all patients with MCD and in about 40% of those with FSGS. Before remission is achieved, and in nonresponders, it is important that the general management of the nephrotic syndrome is optimal through control of edema, consideration of prophylactic measures for the thrombotic tendency and infection, control of hypertension and, in the longer term, control of hyperlipidemia (see Chapter 19).

Although steroids form the core of treatment, at least initially, there is considerable variation in doses and duration recommended, and many individual regimens have not been compared in adequate controlled trials. The management guidelines described here are widely, but not universally, accepted. They are justified, where possible, by evidence from clinical trials.

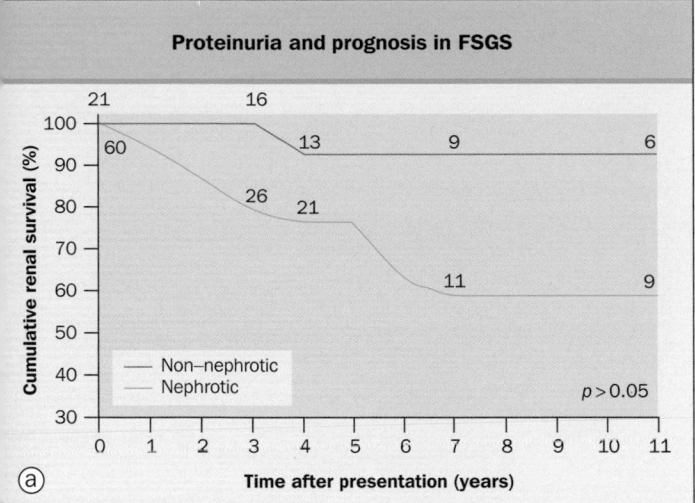

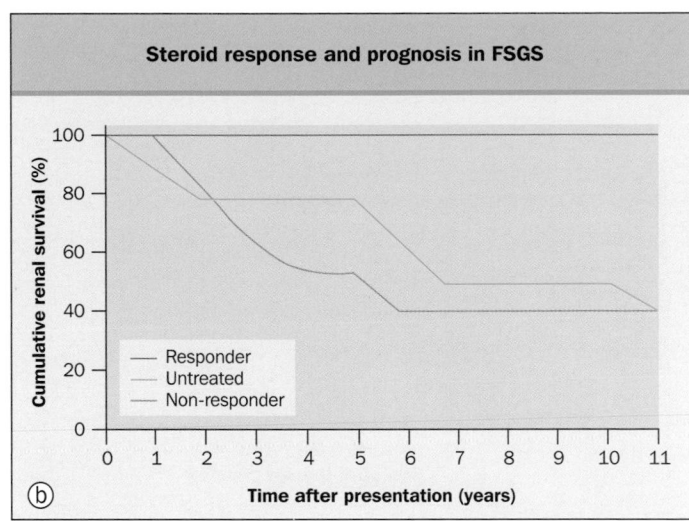

Figure 20.6 Prognosis in primary focal segmental glomerulosclerosis. (a) The risk of developing renal failure is related to the extent of proteinuria. Those with nephrotic-range proteinuria are much more likely to develop renal failure than those with low-grade proteinuria. The figures indicate the number of at-risk patients at different time points. (b) Steroid-responsive patients are significantly less likely to develop renal failure than nonresponders and untreated patients. (Adapted with permission from Rydel et al.[22].)

Childhood minimal change disease

Treatment of first episode

Children should be treated with oral prednisolone 60 mg/m² or 1 mg/kg daily or 2 mg/kg alternate days (all calculated on the basis of estimated 'dry' weight). About 75% respond within 2 weeks, 80–85% within 4 weeks, and over 90% within 8 weeks. Steroids should be continued at the initial dose for a further 4 weeks once the urine is protein free and then the dosage should be switched to alternate day dosing for 4–8 weeks (see below) followed by subsequent tapering (e.g., reducing every 2 weeks by 15 mg/m² on alternate days until steroid withdrawal is completed). The aim of this regimen is to keep patients on steroids for 3–4 months since this appears to be associated with a lower 1-year relapse rate compared with children receiving steroids for 2 months or less (19 and 64%, respectively)[23]. If proteinuria persists for more than 4 weeks on steroids, there is some anecdotal evidence that increasing the steroid dose or giving an intravenous pulse of methylprednisolone (1 g/1.73 m²) will improve the probability of inducing a remission. Other reasons for treatment failure include noncompliance and poor absorption from an edematous bowel, and especially in the presence of diarrhea it is logical to give intravenous steroids. Even in the absence of diarrhea, prescription of nonenteric-coated steroid formulations is recommended, since occasionally patients will absorb enteric-coated tablets inadequately. Increased appetite, hyperactivity, and mood swings may be particular problems in children on high-dose corticosteroids.

Diagnosis and treatment of relapses

The urine should be tested daily during and after treatment. The rationale is that relapses should be treated on the basis of proteinuria (usually requiring at least 3+ (dipstick measurement) proteinuria for 3 consecutive days to initiate a further course of steroids). The aim is to treat relapse early to avoid complications.

Management of relapsing children is intended to maintain the child in a non-nephrotic state with the lowest possible dose of steroids. The first relapse is generally treated with a second induction course of steroids, although a shorter course (about 2 weeks at full dose followed by 2 weeks of alternate day treatment) is probably adequate[24]. Subsequent relapses may be treated similarly or by tapering the prednisolone to 15 mg/m² on alternate days and continuing for 12–18 months (assuming this is above the 'steroid threshold' at which relapse occurs in that individual). Clearly the acceptability of this approach depends on the 'steroid threshold'.

Frequent relapsers

There is even more variation in the management of frequent relapsers, with a paucity of controlled data, but generally 'second-line' drugs are used to avoid steroid toxicity, most commonly alkylating agents (cyclophosphamide and chlorambucil), levamisole, and cyclosporine.

Alkylating agents were used first for many years, although increasingly other agents are now being tried first, mainly because of the potential side effects of alkylating agents (immediately infection and alopecia, and subsequently sterility[25], hemorrhagic cystitis, and longer-term risks of hematologic malignancy), which although probably minor, especially for a 3-month course, need to be balanced against the fact that MCD is usually self-limiting. In addition, the permanent remission rate is not very high. Cyclophosphamide (2–2.5 mg/kg daily) is often effective, and some studies suggest that a 12-week course gives a 2-year remission rate of 60% versus 30% for an 8-week course[26] (Fig. 20.7). Chlorambucil (0.2 mg/kg daily) for 2 months appears to have a similar effect to cyclophosphamide and, apart from not provoking hemorrhagic cystitis, has the same range of adverse effects. There are data suggesting that frequent relapsers are more likely to have a long-term remission following an 8-week course of cyclophosphamide or chlorambucil than steroid-dependent children (75 versus 35%). There

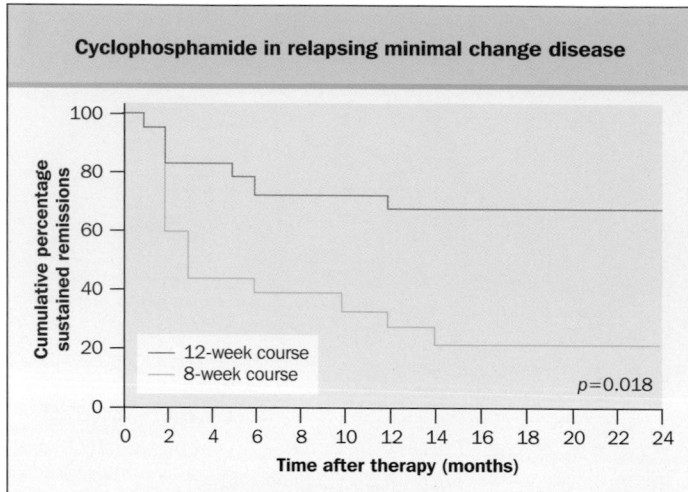

Figure 20.7 Cyclophosphamide therapy in relapsing minimal change disease. A 12-week course of cyclophosphamide ($n = 18$) was associated with a lower risk of subsequent relapse than an 8-week course ($n = 18$)[26].

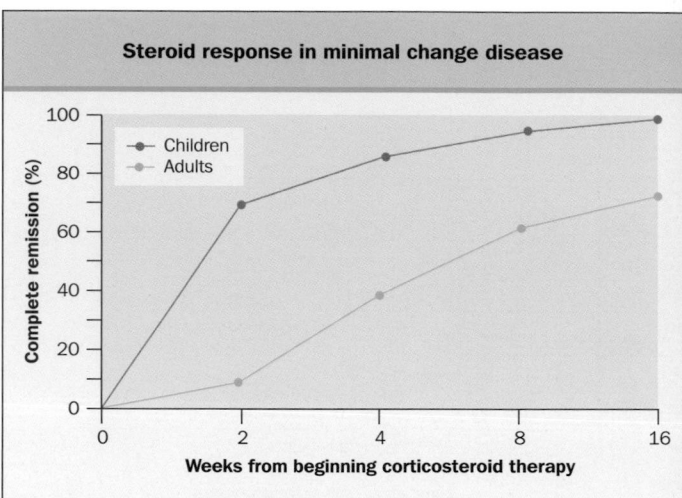

Figure 20.8 Steroid response in adults and children with minimal change disease. Adults with nephrotic syndrome and minimal change disease take longer to respond and are less likely to remit than children. (With permission from Nolasco et al.[15].)

are few data on second courses of alkylating agents, which are not recommended partly because the maximum acceptable cyclophosphamide cumulative dose of 150–250 mg/kg[25] is likely to be exceeded and because the response rates are lower than for the initial course. During treatment with cyclophosphamide or chlorambucil, blood counts should be checked weekly and dose reductions made to avoid cytopenias. Herpes zoster infection carries a particular risk for non-immune children, who should receive hyperimmune immunoglobulin if there is an unavoidable contact with active zoster.

Azathioprine has no proven role in the management of children with MCD and was ineffective in a randomized trial. It may perhaps have a place as a 'steroid-sparing' agent in steroid-dependent children resistant to second-line treatments who have to be maintained on long-term alternate day steroids.

Cyclosporine (up to 150 mg/m² or 4 mg/kg per day) is usually effective in children with both steroid-dependent and frequently relapsing nephrotic syndrome[27]. However, relapse is almost invariable within 3 months of stopping treatment and there is a risk of cyclosporine nephrotoxicity even with low-dose regimens and careful monitoring of blood levels, glomerular filtration rate, and blood pressure. The aim of therapy is that cyclosporine will maintain remission without steroids until the underlying disease remits. The optimum duration of therapy is not established but treatment for 1 year followed by its slow withdrawal is a well-used regimen.

Levamisole, an antihelminthic drug, has also been used successfully (2.5 mg/kg on alternate days for 3 months)[28] but most patients relapse within 3 months of stopping the drug. Nevertheless, as with cyclosporine, it may provide a relatively nontoxic alternative to steroids until spontaneous remission of the condition eventually occurs.

Newer agents
The role of newer immunosuppressive regimens, including tacrolimus and mycophenolate which are being used in some centers, is yet to be defined and advice on the use of these agents must await publication of trial data.

Adult minimal change disease
There are fewer good studies comparing different steroid regimens in adults with MCD, and conventional treatment recommendations are extrapolated from successful approaches in children, although using slightly lower doses of oral prednisolone (1 mg/kg daily, up to 80 mg/day). However, response is often delayed in comparison with children and 25% fail to remit after 3–4 months (Fig. 20.8)[15]. The reasons for this are unclear. It has been suggested that many adults are often given a smaller dose of steroids, maximum of 60 mg prednisolone daily rather than 1 mg/kg daily, or it may be that a greater proportion of adults have FSGS, missed on the original biopsy, which is more steroid resistant (see below). The prednisolone should be reduced to half-dose 1 week after remission (the absence of protein on urine dipstick) for 4–6 weeks, followed by tailing off over a further 4–6 weeks, aiming, as in children, for a total initial steroid course of at least 4 months (although this principle is not evidence-based).

Frequent relapsers
Adults relapse less often than children (30–50%). As with children, some adults develop transient non-nephrotic relapses; treatment, initially with a repeat course of steroids, should await firm evidence of relapse with more than 5 consecutive days of proteinuria > 2+ on urine dipstick and a significant weight gain and/or the development of edema. Frequently relapsing and steroid-dependent patients should be treated with cyclophosphamide, which induces a permanent remission more often than in children (75 and 66% at 2 and 5 years, respectively)[15]. Although there are no satisfactory studies comparing 8- and 12-week courses in adults, a 12-week course may be logical by extension of the pediatric experience, especially since adults may be less susceptible to gonadal damage, and men can be given the opportunity to bank sperm prior to treatment.

For patients who relapse after cyclophosphamide treatment, cyclosporine (4–6 mg/kg daily) is also effective, but relapse usually follows dose reduction or withdrawal. It is worth considering as a short- to medium-term management strategy, since there is evidence that remission eventually occurs in 50–75% of patients even without treatment[15]. However, careful monitoring is required since nephrotoxicity is common after more than 1 year's treatment[29]. Some nephrologists prefer to try this before cyclophosphamide, especially in younger adults. Several uncontrolled reports suggest that mycophenolate may also have a place in managing steroid- and cyclosporine-dependent patients[30,31].

'Minimal change' with non-nephrotic proteinuria

This should not be treated except for controlling hypertension if present (usually with an ACE-inhibitor or angiotensin II receptor antagonist, ATRA), with long-term monitoring to detect increasing proteinuria or renal impairment in which case a repeat biopsy is usually indicated.

Focal segmental glomerulosclerosis

Traditionally, FSGS has been thought to have a poor prognosis, with a low rate of response to treatment and about 50% of patients progressing to ESRD in 10 years[32] although only those who are nephrotic seem to be at particular risk (see Fig. 20.6). However, it is now clear that up to 40% of nephrotic patients (adults and children alike) respond to steroids with complete remission, and in those who respond, the 5-year actuarial renal survival exceeds 95%[22].

Unfortunately, there does not presently seem to be any way of identifying patients who will or will not respond. In a number of studies, the only retrospective factor seems to be the duration of steroid treatment. For example, one study showed that 87% of responders received 60 mg prednisolone for 1 month and 67% for 2 months and that the median response time was 3.7 ± 2 months[33]. My own practice is to treat nephrotic adults with FSGS with prednisolone 1 mg/kg daily for at least 3 months (2 months in children). Responders, in whom the proteinuria reduces or remits, are treated with reducing doses for about 6 months, while the steroids are tapered and stopped within 4 weeks in the nonresponders. Patients should be monitored for steroid side effects and decisions to abandon treatment need to be made on an individual basis.

Frequent relapsers and those who become steroid dependent may benefit from a 3-month course of cyclophosphamide[34], but steroid-unresponsive patients rarely, if ever, obtain a sustained remission[34,35] and the risks probably outweigh the benefits.

Cyclosporine is usually effective, in steroid-dependent and steroid-resistant patients[32,36], and in adults and children[36,37]. It is beneficial even though, as in MCD, relapse usually follows withdrawal of the drug (although there anecdotal reports that patients kept in remission for 12 months followed by cyclosporine withdrawal without relapse[38]). There are several small randomized controlled trials, although the reported response is variable (20–70%). Currently the largest randomized trial of cyclosporine includes only 49 adults. The patients were all steroid resistant (and 40% had also received cyclophosphamide). They received prednisolone (0.15 mg/kg/day) and

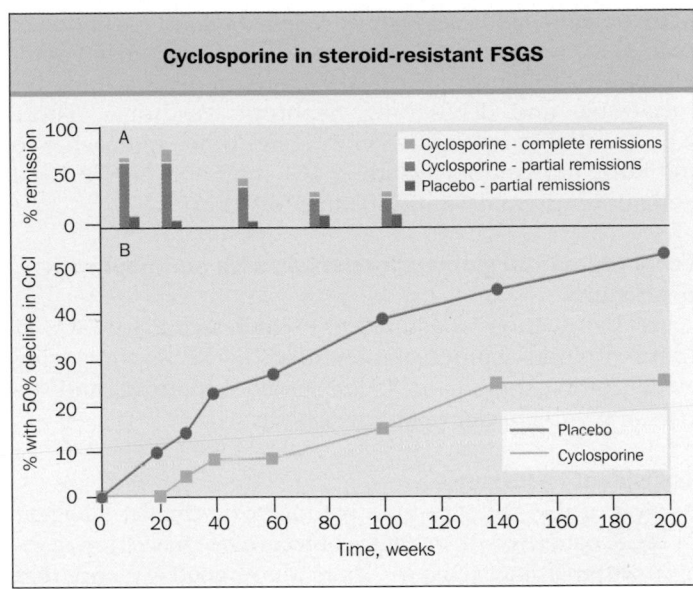

Figure 20.9 Cyclosporine in steroid-resistant FSGS; a randomized controlled trial of 6 months treatment with prednisolone and either cyclosporine or placebo. Upper panel (A) cyclosporine induces a partial or complete remission significantly more often than placebo. Lower panel (B) cyclosporine treatment results in a lower rate of decline in renal function than placebo even after 4 years. (Adapted with permission from Cattran et al.[34].)

either 6 months of cyclosporine (3.5 mg/kg/day adjusted to trough levels 125–225 ng/mL) or placebo. In the cyclosporine-treated patients complete or partial remission was induced in 12% and 58% respectively compared with 4% (combined) in the placebo treated controls (Fig. 20.9). Although the relapse rate was high (4 and 35% were still in remission at 1 and 4 years respectively) the treated cohort had a significantly lower rate of progression of renal failure (Fig. 20.9)[34]. In addition to the potential long-term benefit of cyclosporine, control of the nephrotic syndrome with even partial remission is advantageous to the patient, and the incidence of cyclosporine nephrotoxicity in the long term appears to be low[37]. Although not entirely evidence-based, I recommend treating steroid relapsers and non-responders with cyclosporine (aiming for trough levels of 125–175 ng/mL) for 6 months if remission is not achieved, but continuing for 1 year with tapering over about 3 months if remission does occur. If the patient subsequently relapses I consider restarting long-term cyclosporine, to control the nephrotic syndrome with careful monitoring of renal function.

More aggressive regimens such as prolonged courses of daily cyclophosphamide (up to 2 years), extended therapy with pulse steroids and intravenous cyclophosphamide, or cyclical treatments with corticosteroids and chlorambucil, similar to that introduced by Ponticelli for the treatment of membranous nephropathy have been tried. One study reported that tacrolimus induced a significant number of complete or partial 2-year remissions even in cyclosporine-resistant patients[40]. More recently mycophenolate has been reported by several groups to be effective[30,31,39]. Although impressive results have been reported, no controlled trials are available and the risks

Glomerular Disease

of treatment need to be carefully weighed against likelihood of success as well as the alternatives, even if these include progression to ESRD with medical or surgical nephrectomy for intractable and debilitating nephrotic syndrome. Those who are steroid resistant should receive other approaches to minimize proteinuria, including ACE inhibitors or ATRA and perhaps nonsteroidal anti-inflammatory drugs.

Focal segmental glomerulosclerosis with non-nephrotic proteinuria

Careful evaluation is required to exclude secondary FSGS in those with non-nephrotic proteinuria. There is no convincing evidence that these patients are steroid responsive, and the risks of treatment outweigh the benefits.

Transplant recurrence

In view of the evidence for a pathogenetic circulating agent in FSGS, patients with evidence of recurrence have been managed with plasma exchange. There is now good evidence that plasma exchange can reduce proteinuria, although the response is not absolutely reliable[41]. The best chance of a lasting response occurs when plasma exchange is initiated as soon as possible after the appearance of proteinuria and in those whose recurrence is in the first few weeks after transplantation. The effect can be dramatic and long lasting (Fig. 20.10) but unfortunately the nephrotic syndrome frequently recurs within a few months of discontinuing plasma exchange and there is much less evidence that a further course of plasma exchange also gives benefit. Treatment of recurrence of primary FSGS is discussed further in Chapter 91.

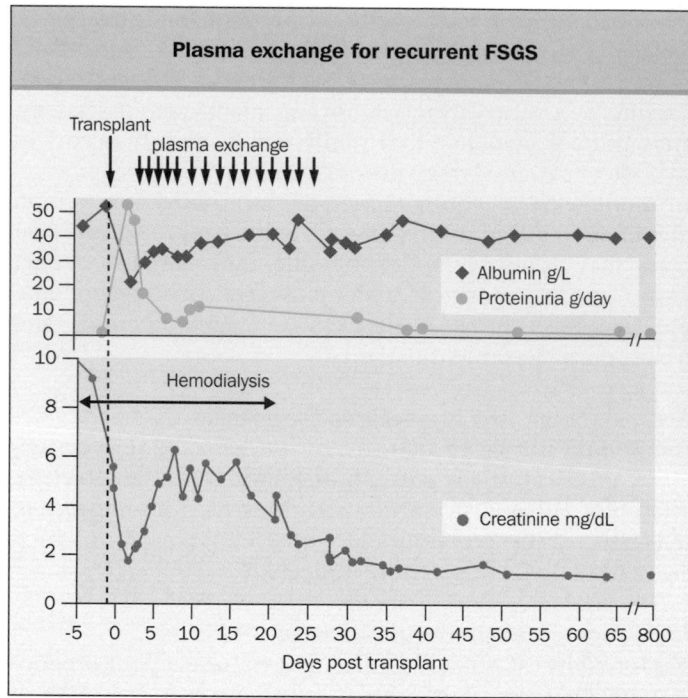

Figure 20.10 Response of recurrent FSGS in a renal transplant to plasma exchange. Following transplantation serum creatinine initially fell, but there was heavy proteinuria by day 3 and acute renal failure (with no evidence of rejection on biopsy) developed. The patient was plasma exchanged daily for 5 days from day 3 and then alternate days until day 26. Remission followed which has been sustained, currently for nearly 3 years.

REFERENCES

1. Golden MH, Brooks SE, Ramdath DD, Taylor E. Effacement of glomerular foot processes in kwashiorkor. Lancet. 1990;336: 1472–4.
2. Regele HM, Fillipovic E, Langer B, et al. Glomerular expression of dystroglycans is reduced in minimal change nephrosis but not in focal segmental glomerulosclerosis. J Am Soc Nephrol. 2000; 11:403–12.
3. Koyama A, Fujisaka M, Kobayashi M, et al. A glomerular permeability factor produced by human T cell hybridomas. Kidney Int. 1991;40:453–60.
4. Cheung PK, Klok PA, Baller JF, Bakker WW. Induction of experimental proteinuria in vivo following infusion of human plasma hemopexin. Kidney Int. 2000;57(4):1512–20.
5. Ali AA, Wilson E, Moorhead JF, et al. Minimal-change glomerular nephritis. Normal kidneys in an abnormal environment? Transplantation. 1994;58:849–52.
6. Dantal J, Godfrin Y, Koll R, et al. Antihuman immunoglobulin affinity immunoadsorption strongly decreases proteinuria in patients with relapsing nephrotic syndrome. J Am Soc Nephrol. 1998;9:1709–15.
7. Savin VJ, Artero M, Sharma R, et al. Circulating factor associated with increased glomerular permeability to albumin in recurrent focal segmental glomerulosclerosis. N Engl J Med. 1996;334: 878–83.
8. Dall'Amico R, Ghiggeri G, Carraro M, et al. Prediction and treatment of recurrent focal segmental glomerulosclerosis after renal transplantation in children. Am J Kidney Dis. 1999;34: 1048–55.
9. Kaplan JM, Kim SH, North KN, et al. Mutations in ACTN4, encoding alpha-actinin-4, cause familial focal segmental glomerulosclerosis. Nat Genet. 2000;24:251–6.
10. Karle SM, Uetz B, Ronner V, et al. Novel mutations in NPHS2 detected in both familial and sporadic steroid-resistant nephrotic syndrome. J Am Soc Nephrol. 2002;13:388–93.
11. Schena FP. Survey of the Italian Registry of Renal Biopsies. Frequency of the renal diseases for 7 consecutive years. The Italian Group of Renal Immunopathology. Nephrol Dial Transplant. 1997;12:418–26.
12. Haas M, Meehan SM, Karrison T, Spargo BH. Changing etiologies of unexplained adult nephrotic syndrome: a comparison of renal biopsy findings in 1976–1979 and 1995–1997. Am J Kidney Dis. 1997;30:621–31.
13. 2001 Atlas of ESRD in the US, USRDS Annual report Reference Table A9 pp286. http://www.usrds.org/atlas.htm
14. Conlon PJ, Lynn K, Winn MP, et al. Spectrum of disease in familial focal and segmental glomerulosclerosis. Kidney Int. 1999;56:1863–71.
15. Nolasco F, Cameron JS, Heywood EF, et al. Adult-onset minimal change nephrotic syndrome: a long term follow-up. Kidney Int. 1986;29:1215–23.
16. International Study of Kidney Disease in Children. Minimal change nephrotic syndrome in children: deaths during the first 5 to 15 years' observation. Report of the International Study of Kidney Disease in Children. Pediatrics. 1984;73:497–501.
17. Schwartz MM, Korbet SM, Rydell J, et al. Primary focal segmental glomerular sclerosis in adults: prognostic value of histologic variants. Am J Kidney Dis. 1995;25:845–52.

18. Border WA. Distinguishing minimal change disease from mesangial disorders. Kidney Int. 1988;34:419–34.
19. Strehlau J, Schachter AD, Pavlakis M, et al. Activated intrarenal transcription of CTL-effectors and TGF-beta1 in children with focal segmental glomerulosclerosis. Kidney Int. 2002;61:90–5.
20. Tarshish P, Tobin JN, Bernstein J, Edelmann CM, Jr. Prognostic significance of the early course of minimal change nephrotic syndrome: report of the International Study of Kidney Disease in Children. J Am Soc Nephrol. 1997;8:769–76.
21. Trompeter RS, Lloyd BW, Hicks J, et al. Long-term outcome for children with minimal change nephrotic syndrome. Lancet. 1985;i:368–70.
22. Rydel JJ, Korbet SM, Borok RZ, Schwartz MM. Focal segmental glomerular sclerosis in adults: presentation, course, and response to treatment. Am J Kidney Dis. 1995;25:534–42.
23. Hodson EM, Knight JF, Willis NS, Craig JC. Corticosteroid therapy for nephrotic syndrome in children (Cochrane Review). Cochrane Database Syst Rev. 2001;2:CD001533.
24. Mendoza SA, Tune BM. Treatment of childhood nephrotic syndrome. J Am Soc Nephrol. 1992;3:889–94.
25. Trompeter RS, Evans PR, Barratt TM. Gonadal function in boys with steroid-responsive nephrotic syndrome treated with cyclophosphamide for short periods. Lancet. 1981;i:1177–9.
26. Arbeitsgemeinschaft für Padiatrische Nephrologie. Cyclophosphamide treatment of steroid-dependent nephrotic syndrome: comparison of eight weeks with 12 weeks course. Arch Dis Child. 1987;62:1102–6.
27. Durkan AM, Hodson EM, Willis NS, Craig JC. Immunosuppressive agents in childhood nephrotic syndrome: a meta-analysis of randomized controlled trials. Kidney Int. 2001; 59:1919–27.
28. British Association for Paediatric Nephrology. Levamisole for corticosteroid-dependent nephrotic syndrome in childhood. Lancet. 1991;337:1555–7.
29. Melocoton TL, Vanni ES, Cohen AS, Fine RN. Long-term cyclosporin A treatment of steroid-resistant nephrotic and steroid-dependent nephrotic syndrome. Am J Kidney Dis. 1991:18:583–8.
30. Choi MJ, Eustace JA, Gimenez LF, et al. Mycophenolate mofetil treatment for primary glomerular diseases. Kidney Int. 2002; 61:1098–114.
31. Day CJ, Cockwell P, Lipkin GW, et al. Mycophenolate mofetil in the treatment of resistant idiopathic nephrotic syndrome. Nephrol Dial Transplant. 2002;17:2011–13.
32. Korbet, SM. Primary focal segmental glomerulosclerosis. J Am Soc Nephrol. 1998;9:1333–40.
33. Banfi G, Moriggi M, Sabadini E, et al. The impact of prolonged immunosuppression on the outcome of idiopathic focal-segmental glomerulosclerosis with nephrotic syndrome in adults. A collaborative retrospective study. Clin Nephrol. 1991;36:53–9.
34. Siegal NJ, Gaudio KM, Krassner LS, et al. Steroid-dependent nephrotic syndrome in children: histopathology and relapses after cyclophosphamide treatment. Kidney Int. 1981;19:454–9.
35. Tarshish P, Tobin JN, Bernstein J, Edelmann CM Jr. Cyclophosphamide does not benefit patients with focal segmental glomerulosclerosis. A report of the International Study of Kidney Disease in Children. Pediatr Nephrol. 1996;10:590–3.
36. Cattran DC, Appel GB, Hebert LA, et al. A randomized trial of cyclosporin in patients with steroid-resistant focal segmental glomerulosclerosis. North America Nephrotic Syndrome Study Group. Kidney Int. 1999;56:2220–6.
37. Niaudet P. Treatment of childhood steroid-resistant idiopathic nephrosis with a combination of cyclosporin and prednisone. French Society of Pediatric Nephrology. J Pediatr. 1994;125(6 Pt 1):981–6.
38. Lieberman KV, Tejani A. A randomized double-blind placebo-controlled trial of cyclosporin in steroid-resistant idiopathic focal segmental glomerulosclerosis in children. J Am Soc Nephrol. 1996;7:56–63.
39. Matalon A, Valeri A, Appel GB. Treatment of focal segmental glomerulosclerosis. Semin Nephrol. 2000;20:309–17.
40. Segarra A, Vila J, Pou L, et al. Combined therapy of tacrolimus and corticosteroids in cyclosporin-resistant or -dependent idiopathic focal glomerulosclerosis: a preliminary uncontrolled study with prospective follow-up. Nephrol Dial Transplant. 2002;17: 655–62.
41. Artero ML, Sharma R, Savin VJ, Vincenti F. Plasmapheresis reduces proteinuria and serum capacity to injure glomeruli in patients with recurrent focal segmental glomerulosclerosis. Am J Kidney Dis. 1994;23:574–81.

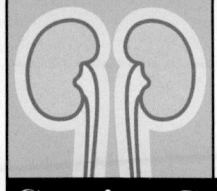
Chapter 21 Secondary Focal Segmental Glomerulosclerosis

TK Sreepada Rao and Praveen N Chander

INTRODUCTION

Focal segmental glomerulosclerosis (FSGS), first described in 1957, is now a common pathologic glomerular lesion identified in patients with both nephrotic- and non-nephrotic-range proteinuria, and accounts for 10% to 30% of all chronic glomerulonephritis. The prevalence of FSGS is increasing throughout the world. FSGS is a histologic lesion characterized by segmental glomerular capillary obliteration with increased mesangial matrix deposition, and is accompanied at times by intracapillary foam cells and/or hyaline deposits, and/or focal adhesions (synechiae) of the capillary tuft to the Bowman's capsule.

Primary FSGS (idiopathic), a common lesion observed in young patients with nephrotic syndrome, is discussed in Chapter 20. FSGS is also seen in a spectrum of diseases with diverse etiologies, such as viral infections, illicit drug use, vesicoureteric reflux, sickle cell disease and other disorders. Furthermore, in the remnant model of experimental renal disease and its clinical correlates in humans, such as unilateral renal agenesis, renal dysplasia and others, FSGS is the commonest lesion encountered. Despite the fact that, in many such instances, a causal or precise relationship cannot be established with certainty between morphologic renal manifestations and the underlying disturbance, they are referred to as secondary FSGS. A classification of FSGS is shown in Table 21.1.

COLLAPSING FOCAL SEGMENTAL GLOMERULOSCLEROSIS

Introduction and definition

Collapsing FSGS is a histologic variant of FSGS characterized by extensive focal or global glomerular capillary tuft collapse, podocytic hypertrophy and hyperplasia (Fig. 21.1), and varying degrees of tubulointerstitial injury. Collapsing FSGS has no known cause in a proportion of patients. However, it is increasingly clear that the same histologic pattern occurs with a variety of viral and drug-induced toxicities (Table 21.2). In particular, it shares many common features with one of the most important forms of secondary FSGS: HIV-associated nephropathy (HIVAN).

Idiopathic collapsing FSGS

The prevalence of idiopathic collapsing FSGS, an unrecognized lesion prior to 1979, is increasing. In a study of 240 patients with idiopathic FSGS, 18% showed features of collapsing FSGS, none were intravenous drug addicts (IVDA),

Classification of focal segmental glomerulosclerosis (FSGS)
Primary (Idiopathic)
Focal and segmental glomerulosclerosis with hyalinosis Progression from minimal change disease Progression from IgM nephropathy Progression from mesangial proliferative glomerulonephritis Superimposed on other primary glomerulonephritis (membranous nephropathy, IgA nephropathy)
Variants of primary FSGS
Collapsing form Cellular variant (endo and extra capillary hypercellularity) FSGS with mesangial hypercellularity FSGS with glomerular tip lesions
Secondary

Drugs	Intravenous heroin, pamidronate	
Viruses	Hepatitis B, human immunodeficiency virus, parovirus	
Hemodynamic		
Reduced renal mass	Solitary kidney, renal allograft, renal dysplasia, oligomeganephronia, segmental hypoplasia, vesicoureteral reflux, surgical ablation	
Without reduced renal mass	Obesity, sickle cell nephropathy, congenital cyanotic heart disease	
Malignancies	Lymphomas, other malignancies	
Miscellaneous	Hypertensive nephrosclerosis, Alport syndrome, sarcoidosis, radiation nephritis	
Scarring	Postinflammatory in postinfectious GN Postnecrotic in SLE, and other vasculitis	

Primary (idiopathic) FSGS is discussed in Chapter 20.

Table 21.1 Classification of focal segmental glomerulosclerosis (FSGS).

or had evidence of HIV infection[1]. Idiopathic FSGS is seven times more prevalent in African Americans than in Caucasians, and the association is even stronger in the collapsing variant. In FSGS associated with heroin addiction and HIV infection, African Americans outnumber Caucasians by a ratio of greater than 9 : 1. Whether the racial predilection is related to genetic or enviromental factors, altered cytokine production, such as transforming growth factor β (TGF-β), or poor control of hypertension, is unknown.

Glomerular Disease

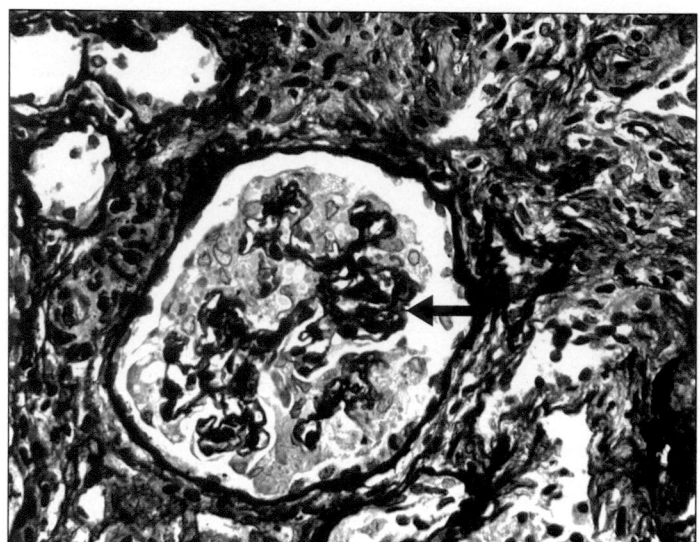

Figure 21.1 Collapsing variant of focal segmental glomerulosclerosis (FSGS). Glomerulus from an HIV-negative nephrotic patient showing moderate collapse of capillary tuft with segmental sclerosis (arrowed) and diffusely hypertrophic and markedly vacuolated visceral epithelium. (Jones methenamine silver ×300).

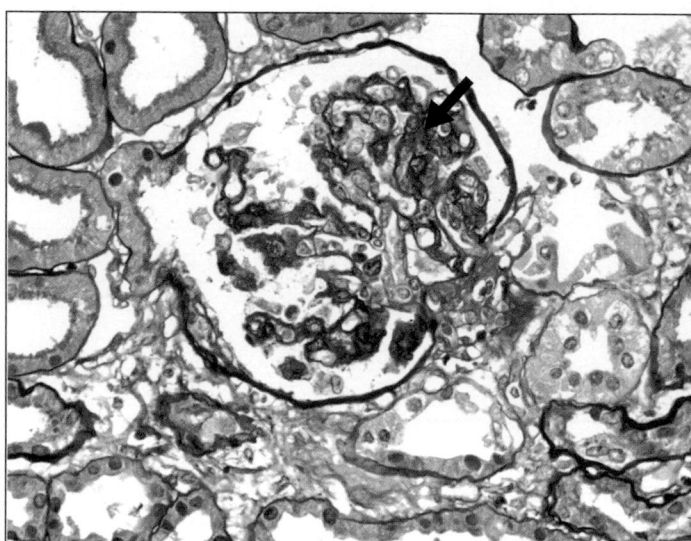

Figure 21.2 Pamidronate-associated collapsing FSGS. Glomerular capillary tuft shows moderate global collapse with wrinkled basement membrane and an area of segmental sclerosis (arrow). Podocytes are markedly hypertrophied, focally detached and contain foci of large vacuoles. Tubular epithelium shows degenerative changes and focal necrosis (Periodic acid–Schiff ×450).

Causes of collapsing FSGS
Etiologic factors associated with the collapsing form of FSGS
Idiopathic
Heroin
HIV
Parvovirus
Pamidronate

Table 21.2 Causes of collapsing FSGS.

Collapsing FSGS is characterized by severe nephrotic syndrome on presentation, steroid resistance, and rapid development of end-stage renal disease (ESRD) (median time of 13 months compared to 65 months in other primary forms of FSGS). The prognosis is similar in African Americans and Caucasians[1].

In the original reports, none were IVDA, and only one patient developed acquired AIDS later during follow-up. Even though many clinical and pathologic features noted in these patients with collapsing FSGS resembled those with HIVAN, the main distinguishing features were negative HIV serology and lack of endothelial tubuloreticular inclusions on electron microscopy (described below under HIVAN).

Parvovirus-associated collapsing FSGS
In sickle cell patients with aplastic crisis, a number of glomerular lesions have been associated with parvovirus infection, including FSGS, diffuse proliferative glomerulonephritis, and membranoproliferative glomerulonephritis (MPGN). *De novo* development of collapsing FSGS in the renal allograft of a recipient with red cell aplasia and persistent parvovirus B19

(PVB19) infection has also been described. In a recent report, PVB19 DNA was demonstrated in renal biopsy specimens in 78% of patients with collapsing FSGS, 16% with HIVAN, 22% with idiopathic FSGS and 14% of controls[2]. In the peripheral blood, PVB19 was detected in 87.5% of patients with collapsing FSGS, but only in 14% with HIV infection, and 3% of healthy volunteers. PVB19 was identified in glomerular parietal and epithelial cells and in tubular cells. These data suggest that, in susceptible individuals, renal epithelial cell infection with PVB19 may induce collapsing FSGS[2].

Pamidronate-associated collapsing FSGS
Pamidronate, a biphosphonate, is an effective agent in the management of hypercalcemia associated with malignancy and osteolytic metastasis. Seven patients (six with multiple myeloma and one with metastatic breast carcinoma) receiving chemotherapy or radiotherapy have been described who developed collapsing FSGS following pamidronate therapy[3]. All seven were Caucasians, age range 50–77 years, and HIV negative. Although pamidronate was administered initially at the monthly recommended dose, five patients subsequently received larger doses. They presented with nephrotic syndrome and renal insufficiency 15–48 months after starting pamidronate. Four patients developed ESRD, two of whom had continued to receive pamidronate. Among those who stopped pamidronate, renal function stabilized or improved. Renal histology showed collapsing FSGS characterized by retraction of glomerular basement membrane (GBM), hyperplasia of podocytes, and severe tubular degeneration (Fig. 21.2). On electron microscopy, there was marked podocyte injury, with extensive degenerative changes in proximal tubular cells. It has been proposed that the mechanism for the renal epithelial toxicity of pamidronate may be similar to its complex effects in osteoclasts.

HIV-ASSOCIATED FOCAL SEGMENTAL GLOMERULOSCLEROSIS

Introduction and definition

FSGS is one of a number of renal disorders that are frequent in patients with HIV infection (Table 21.3 and chapter 28). Here, we will only discuss HIVAN, a comprehensive name that replaces the old term AIDS-associated nephropathy. HIVAN refers to a syndrome of massive proteinuria, microhematuria and azotemia, usually with rapid progression to ESRD and occurring predominantly in Black patients with HIV infection[4]. Histologic characteristics are a collapsing form of FSGS with unusual light and electron microscopic features.

Pathogenesis

Although nephropathy may be an initial manifestation leading to the diagnosis of HIV disease, the number of circulating CD4 cells in patients with HIVAN is generally below 200×10^6 cells/L, suggesting that renal disease usually occurs late in the course of HIV infection. However, HIVAN often occurs before the onset of opportunistic infections and may be the first manifestation of HIV infection. HIVAN has also been reported in a HIV seronegative patient with $> 500 \times 10^6$ CD4 cells/L, and plasma viral load of $> 700\ 000$ copies per mL, suggesting that renal disease can occur during acute HIV infection[5]. Because glomerular immune deposits are scanty in HIVAN, and viral antigens have not been localized in glomeruli, it is unlikely that antigen–antibody-mediated mechanisms are involved. Viral genome has been demonstrated in various glomerular cells in renal biopsies from patients with HIVAN[6]. However, HIV genome is also found in renal tissue in HIV-infected patients without nephropathy suggesting that, in addition to viral infection, individual host responses or other triggering mechanisms may be necessary to produce HIVAN[6]. It is still unclear whether viral proteins in glomerular cells represents a causal role in the pathogenesis of HIVAN or are a secondary phenomenon. Early studies performed in vitro suggested that HIV can infect and survive in glomerular endothelial cells and, to a lesser extent, in mesangial cells, but epithelial cells were considered resistant to infection, making it difficult to explain the predominance of epithelial cell injury in HIVAN. However, recent studies have demonstrated active HIV infection of epithelial cells even in patients receiving highly active antiretroviral agents (HAART) and with undetectable plasma viral burden[7,8]. Host response to HIV infection may be the critical factor that determines who develops nephropathy. Genetic and environmental factors likely play a major role as the disease is very rare among Caucasians and common in African Americans. In experimental models, nephritogenicity varies with different HIV strains; for example, the macrophage-tropic strain is more implicated in inducing FSGS lesions than the lymphotropic strain.

Transgenic mice with a noninfectious HIV-1 construct (lacking certain structural proteins but preserving the envelope and regulatory genes) develop FSGS with gross nephrotic syndrome and progressive renal failure, which are all features resembling HIVAN in humans[9]. In these transgenic mice, envelope and regulatory viral genomes are expressed in the glomerular and tubular epithelium, and there is upregulation of basic

Renal disorders in patients with HIV infection
HIV associated (specific?) glomerular syndromes
• Focal and segmental glomerulosclerosis
• IgA nephropathy
• Immune complex glomerulonephritis
• Other forms of glomerulopathy
Unrelated renal diseases in HIV infected patients
• Heroin associated nephropathy
• Obstructive nephropathy
Acute renal failure
HIV infection in patients receiving renal replacement therapy
• Maintenance dialysis (peritoneal and hemodialysis) patients acquiring HIV infection from blood transfusions, intravenous drug abuse, and sexual contacts
• Renal transplant recipients developing HIV infection through renal allograft, blood transfusions, intravenous drug abuse, and sexual contacts

Table 21.3 Renal disorders in patients with HIV infection.

fibroblast growth factor and TGF-β. The whole virus may therefore not be necessary to evoke nephropathy; rather one or more viral proteins can trigger renal disease by acting either directly on renal cells or indirectly through the release of soluble mediators that affect the kidney. A direct viral pathogenetic effect is suggested by studies in which normal kidneys transplanted into HIV transgenic mice remain disease free, while HIVAN develops in transgenic kidneys transplanted into nontransgenic litter mates[10]. The levels of cytokines (TGF-β, interleukin-8) are increased in renal biopsies from patients with HIVAN, as well as there being overexpression of TGF-β in renal cells. HIV infection is associated with dysregulation of various host cytokines. Studies performed in vitro have shown multiple nephropathogenetic effects of HIV proteins. The HIV transactivator protein stimulates cell proliferation and production of TGF-β by macrophages; and the HIV glycoprotein, gp120, can modulate immune-cell functions, promote apoptosis and decrease extracellular matrix (ECM) degradation. Increased renal cellular expression of TGF-β, as a result of either direct viral infection or exposure to circulating HIV peptides, may be a key contributor to the glomerulosclerosis seen in HIVAN[11].

Thus, the pathogenesis of HIVAN is a complex process involving an interplay of direct viral infection, expression of viral genes in various renal cells, dysregulated cytokine system, persistence of virus in the kidney, and environmental and genetic factors.

Epidemiology

In approximately one-third of patients, nephropathy may be the initial manifestation prompting clinicians to investigate for the presence of HIV infection. HIVAN is seen in patients irrespective of the route of HIV infection: whether by sexual contact, via needle sharing in IVDA, contaminated blood products, or in children born to HIV-infected mothers. In IVDA, renal disease may be related either to drug abuse (heroin-associated nephropathy (HAN)), or secondary to HIV infection (HIVAN). HIV-infected drug addicts are three times

Glomerular Disease

more likely to develop renal disease than those addicts who are persistently HIV seronegative[12]. Most subjects with HIVAN are young African American men (mean age 33 years, male : female ratio 10 : 1), and approximately 50% are IVDA. HIVAN is now the third leading cause of renal failure in African Americans aged 20–64 years[13]. In Miami and Brooklyn, 30–40% of patients with HIVAN are Haitian immigrants, while the remainder are homosexual or bisexual men, heterosexual contacts of infected persons, or children with AIDS. The incidence of HIVAN in children has dramatically declined in the past decade and has practically disappeared at our institution (see below). In San Francisco, where the majority of patients with HIV disease are Caucasian homosexual men, nephropathy is distinctly rare, as is the case at other centers in the US and elsewhere.

Clinical manifestations

The usual presenting feature of HIVAN is nephrotic syndrome, often of rapid onset. Occasionally, mild proteinuria (< 2 g/day) may be discovered during the evaluation of an unrelated medical problem. Proteinuria is accompanied by either normal renal function or varying degrees of azotemia, with or without gross or microscopic hematuria. In children born with HIV infection, the mean age of onset of proteinuria or azotemia ranges from 2.5–4.9 years. In adults, it is difficult to determine the time course to development of nephropathy to the time of HIV infection.

Serum complement levels are normal, but there is hypergammaglobulinemia with increases in IgA, IgG and IgM. The absolute number of CD4+ lymphocytes is usually $< 200 \times 10^6$ cells/L, and the CD4 : CD8 cell ratio in the blood is reversed, along with HIV seropositivity and high plasma viral levels. Although HIVAN is seen in asymptomatic HIV-seropositive individuals, they usually have low CD4 cell counts and high plasma viral load. A patient has been reported who developed severe nephrotic syndrome with HIVAN during acute retroviral infection before seroconversion[5]. A recent prospective cohort study established a strong association between both increasing HIV RNA levels and decreasing CD4 lymphocyte count with the presence of proteinuria and occurrence of renal failure. This study also found an association between proteinuria and positive hepatitis C antibody[14].

Patients are usually normotensive, often with low serum cholesterol levels and, even in the presence of severe azotemia, hypertension is rare. On ultrasonography, or at autopsy, the kidneys are enlarged and highly echogenic, a nonspecific finding in the nephrotic stage of the illness. Amyloidosis with large kidneys and nephrotic syndrome can occur in patients with AIDS and should be considered in the differential diagnosis.

Pathology

The most common renal pathology in HIVAN is the collapsing variant of FSGS. If the mesangial lesions assumed to be an early precursor of glomerulosclerosis are also included, then FSGS accounts for approximately 95% of all renal histologic changes reported in HIVAN. Histologically, HIVAN is characterized by a classic constellation of glomerular and tubulo-interstitial pathology.

Light microscopy

Frequent findings are focal and segmental or global collapse of glomerular capillary tufts accompanied, in later stages, by global glomerulosclerosis. Dilated Bowman spaces are filled with abundant eosinophilic proteinaceous material. Sclerotic and collapsed capillary tufts in general are devoid of hyaline deposits, foam cells and excessive mesangial matrix. Globally collapsed glomeruli have shrunken tufts retracted towards the vascular pole, giving the appearance of a rapidly progressive event, which may explain the fulminant clinical deterioration. Focal mesangial hyperplasia and increased matrix may be seen in other areas of the same biopsy. Diffuse mesangial proliferation has also been described, usually in Caucasians, and may represent immune-complex glomerulonephritis associated with bacterial and other viral infections. Podocytes are markedly hypertrophied, focally hyperplastic and contain abundant protein resorption droplets (Fig. 21.4a). Some are multinucleated and occasional cells display mitosis. Tubulointerstitial disease often coexists. The proximal renal tubular cells contain numerous protein absorption droplets. However, the most striking feature is the presence of enormously dilated tubules, reaching microcystic proportions, filled with large hyaline casts and lined by flattened or swollen reactive epithelium (Fig. 21.3). Interstitial infiltrate varies from moderately dense in early lesions to scant as the disease approaches end stage. At this stage, the interstitium appears edematous and is replaced by homogeneous acidophilic material. The interstitial infiltrate consists mostly of CD8+ T lymphocytes mixed with few plasma cells, B lymphocytes, and monocytes. Chronic changes, such as severe interstitial fibrosis, arterial and arteriolosclerosis, are usually absent.

Immunofluorescence

Albumin, IgG and IgA are found in hypertrophic and hyperplastic podocytes overlying the collapsing glomerular capillary tufts (Fig. 21.4b). Segmental coarse granular deposits of

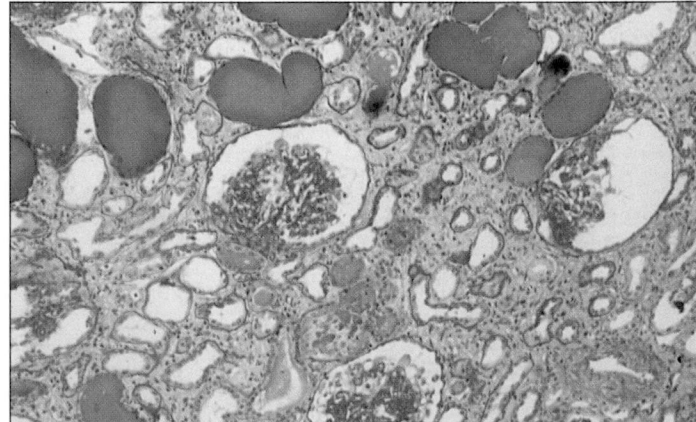

Figure 21.3 HIV-associated nephropathy. Glomerular tufts show variable degrees of collapse, with segmental to global sclerosis. Many tubules show microcystic dilatation, with eosinophilic proteinaceous casts. The remaining tubules are lined by simplified epithelium with features suggestive of degeneration and regeneration. Interstitium contains excessive fibrosis and sparse mononuclear infiltrate (Periodic acid–Schiff ×130).

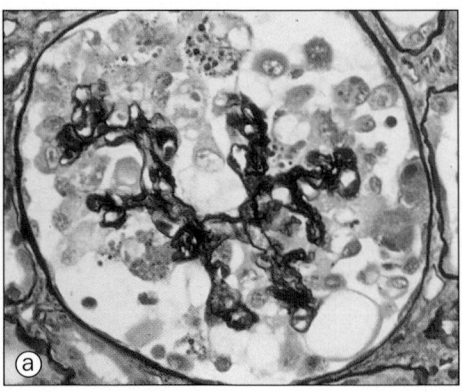 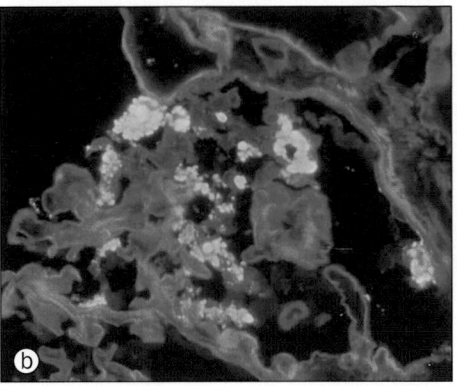 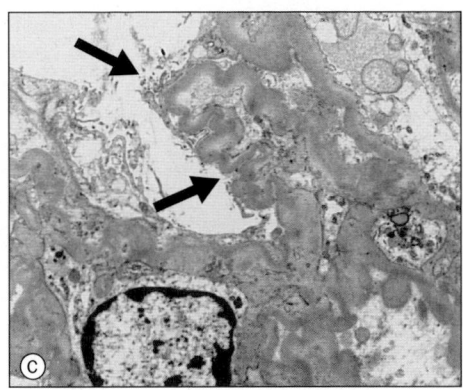

Figure 21.4 Glomerular changes in HIV-associated nephropathy. (a) Light microscopy showing a glomerular tuft undergoing global collapse. Markedly hypertrophic and focally proliferating visceral epithelial cells contain large vesicular nuclei, focally prominent protein resorption droplets, and vacuoles of variable size. (Jones methenamine silver ×530.) (b) Immunofluorescence photomicrograph stained with antialbumin shows enormous resorption droplets in visceral epithelium overlying segmentally collapsing capillary tuft (×330). (c) Low-power electron micrograph showing moderate segmental retraction of glomerular capillary tuft with consequent wrinkling of peripheral basement membranes. There is no significant increase in mesangial matrix. Visceral epithelial cells are detached and focally degenerated overlying the sclerosing lesion (arrows). The remaining foot processes are completely effaced (×5900).

IgM and C3 are also seen in the mesangium and sclerotic areas, findings similar to those in heroin-associated nephropathy and idiopathic FSGS. Additionally, in the adjacent unaffected glomeruli, variable scattering of C1q, IgG and IgA may be seen, mostly in the mesangium and rarely in the periphery. These immune deposits may represent deposited immune complexes or nonspecific trapping of immunoglobulins in the mesangium or sclerotic areas. In HIV-associated IgA nephropathy, the circulating immune complexes are composed of IgA idiotypic antibodies, and glomerular mesangial IgA deposits contain HIV antigens.

Electron microscopy
Ultrastructurally, wrinkling and collapse of GBM, with or without excessive accumulation of mesangial matrix, are seen in collapsed or sclerosed glomeruli (Fig. 21.4c). There is diffuse effacement and focal detachment of podocyte foot processes. Podocytes are markedly swollen, hypertrophic with

frequent villous transformation, and may contain protein resorption droplets. Scattered mesangial and rare subendothelial and subepithelial electron-dense deposits may be seen. However, the most striking feature is the abundant tubuloreticular inclusions (TRI), in the glomerular, and particularly in the peritubular capillary endothelial cells. In the glomeruli, multiple aggregates of TRI are present in different endothelial cells of a single capillary loop, as well as within a single endothelial cell (Fig. 21.5a). TRI are also present in the infiltrating leukocytes, interstitial fibroblasts (Fig. 21.5b) and, rarely, in mesangial cells and myocytes in the arteriolar media. The presence of abundant TRI in endothelial cells, particularly in conjunction with their presence in non-endothelial cells, is of high predictive value in suspecting HIV infection in otherwise asymptomatic individuals. A variety of unusual ultrastructural changes best described as viral footprints are also noted in HIVAN[15]. These include an increase in the number and complexity of nuclear bodies (Fig. 21.5b),

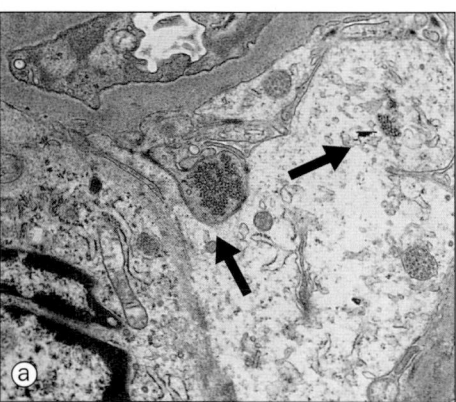 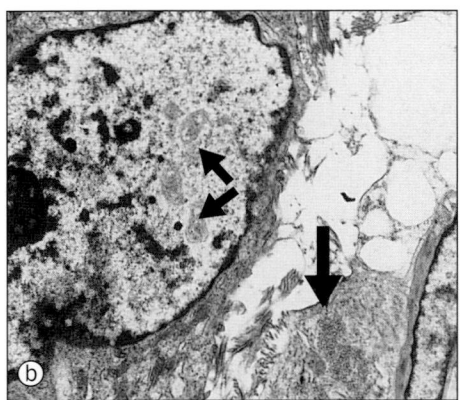 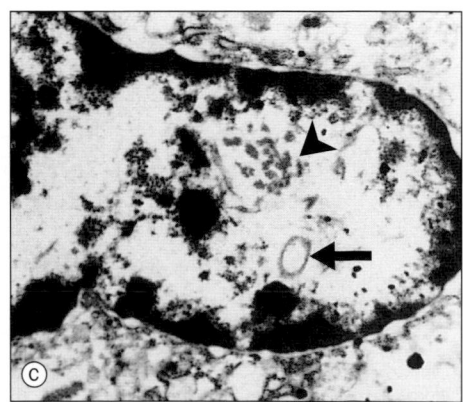

Figure 21.5 Electron micrographs of tubuloreticular inclusions (TRI) and nuclear bodies in HIV-associated nephropathy. (a) A glomerular capillary loop showing aggregates of TRI (arrows) in swollen endothelial cells and in a mesangial cell (on the left). Note multiple aggregates in an individual cell and within a single capillary loop (×13 500). (b) Renal interstitium displaying two fibroblasts, one with a large aggregate of TRI (large arrow) and another with multiple (up to seven) types I and II nuclear bodies (two labeled with small arrows) (×8000). (c) The nucleus of an interstitial cell showing fibrillary inclusions (arrowhead) and intranuclear cylindrical confronting cisternae (arrow) (previously termed 'test tube and ring-shaped forms') (×12 000).

and a peculiar granulofibrillary transformation of nuclear chromatin in the tubular and interstitial cells. In addition, intranuclear inclusions seen in the interstitial fibroblasts include filamentous crystalline and fibrillary inclusions, membranous lamellae, vacuoles, lipid and granular vesicles and, rarely, cylindrical confronting cisternae (Fig. 21.5c).

Natural history

Before the availability of antiretroviral drugs, the typical natural history consisted of a rapid deterioration in renal function from the onset of nephrotic range proteinuria, leading to ESRD in 3–4 months (median 11 weeks). In children, mean duration from the onset of proteinuria to development of ESRD was 8–9 months. In some patients, the use of azidothymidine (AZT, zidovudine) and/or corticosteroids delays the onset of ESRD. In the present era of highly active antiretroviral agents (HAART), the natural history of HIVAN is rapidly changing. Excellent responses to HAART are increasingly being described. A growing number of case reports show that patients with HIVAN and receiving HAART have improvement in proteinuria, and prolonged stabilization of glomerular filtration rate (GFR). However, in many urban facilities, including ours, noncompliant patients who refuse to take HAART still present with rapid onset of irreversible renal failure.

Earlier patients with HIVAN who developed ESRD had a dismal prognosis with median survival of only 2–3 months while receiving maintenance dialysis, reflecting the progress of HIV infection rather than of renal disease. Survival has improved significantly with newer therapies for HIV infection[16]. In many renal centers, it is now common to see HIV patients surviving beyond 5–6 years while receiving maintenance dialysis.

Transplantation

Renal transplantation has not generally been advocated for ESRD patients with HIV infection. The fear was an unacceptable increase in opportunistic infections and/or malignancies with the use of immunosuppressive drugs in an already immunocompromised host. However, in a small number of renal transplants performed without prior knowledge of HIV infection (before the introduction of serologic markers), there has not been any recurrence of HIVAN in the allograft. With the success of HAART in arresting HIV infection, many centers are now undertaking renal transplantation in stable patients with very low or undetectable plasma viral load with acceptable short-term results[17]. Because cyclosporine and mycophenolate mofetil have some antiretroviral effects, these are the preferred immunosuppressive agents along with corticosteroids. Despite immunosuppression, viral load remains undetectable, with stable CD4 cell counts. While there is no need to modify the dose of protease inhibitors or nucleoside reverse transcriptase inhibitors, the dose of immunosuppressive drugs should be reduced: cyclosporine to 25% of standard dose, sirolimus and tacrolimus to 1–2 mg per day. It will be important to see whether or not HAART can prevent the development of HIVAN in the allograft.

Differential diagnosis

FSGS is a very common disease in African American men aged between 18 and 45 years. Differentiation between the idiopathic form, HAN or HIVAN, is often difficult. The distinction between HAN and idiopathic FSGS may at times be impossible except for the history of IVDA. However, there are clear differences between HAN and HIVAN (Table 21.4). HIVAN shows a larger percentage of 'collapsed' glomeruli, conspicuous tubulointerstitial pathology, and the presence of microcystic

Comparison of HIV-associated and heroin-associated nephropathies		
Features	**HIV-associated nephropathy**	**Heroin-associated nephropathy**
Epidemiology		
HIV infection	**Positive**, all routes of infection	Not necessarily positive
Racial/genetic grouping	>95% African Americans	>90% African Americans
Intravenous drug addicts (%)	50	100
Male : female ratio	10 : 1	8 : 1
Clinical features		
Nephrotic	Yes	Yes
Hematuria	Yes	Yes
Hypertension	**Mostly normotensive**	**Hypertensive**
Time to reach end-stage renal diease (ESRD) (months)	3–4	7–48
Pathology		
Kidney size	Large echogenic kidneys	Large kidneys at first, shrink with ESRD
Focal segmental glomerulosclerosis	Collapsing form	Yes
Histology	**Tubuloreticular inclusions**	**Vascular changes with hypertension**
Interstitial fibrosis	**None**	**Yes**

Table 21.4 Differing clinical and pathologic features of HIV-associated (HIVAN) and heroin-associated (HAN) nephropathies. Main distinguishing features are shown in bold.

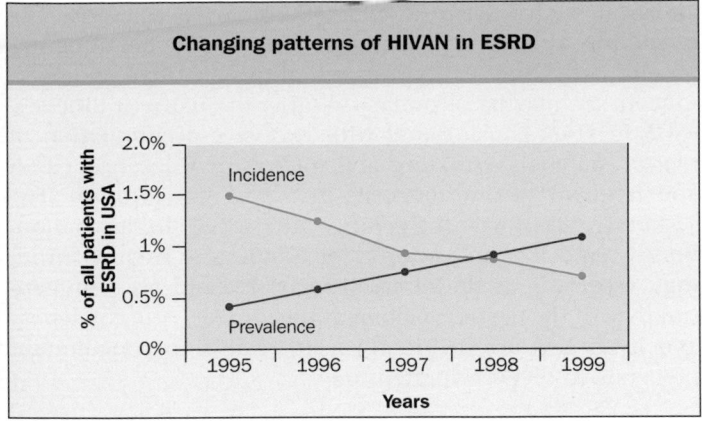

Figure 21.6 Changing incidence and prevalence of HIV-associated nephropathy in patients with end-stage renal disease (ESRD). The fall in incidence of HIV-associated nephropathy (HIVAN) among ESRD patients may indicate the efficacy of highly active antiretroviral agents (HAART) both in preventing HIVAN and delaying its progression. The increasing prevalence likely represents improved survival of those with ESRD.

dilatation of renal tubules. Ultrastructurally, there is an abundance of TRI in the glomerular endothelial cells in HIVAN, which are rare or absent in other forms of FSGS. There are several other major points of distinction between the two entities. A fulminant clinical course to ESRD in 3–4 months, large highly echogenic kidneys and persistent normotension seen in HIVAN contrasts with HAN, which comprises a disease marked by severe hypertension as renal function declines gradually. In HAN, as ESRD approaches, shrunken kidneys are a reflection of progression of FSGS to global glomerulosclerosis, along with severe tubular atrophy, interstitial fibrosis and scarring. It should be remembered that children and non-addicts constitute over 50% of patients with HIVAN.

HIVAN is very rare in Caucasians. Several recent reports of IgA nephropathy in Caucasians and Hispanics with HIV infection suggest a racial difference in glomerular immunologic response to HIV infection. Other uncommonly reported lesions in HIV-positive patients include minimal change disease, membranous nephropathy, MPGN and amyloidosis[4] (Table 21.3).

Treatment

In addition to symptomatic treatment of edema and hypoalbuminemia, specific treatment options for HIVAN are limited because of a lack of prospective controlled studies. Early experience suggested that prolonged AZT therapy (the only antiretroviral drug then available) might be efficacious if started early, but that abrupt discontinuation of AZT, either because of side effects or noncompliance, may lead to an accelerated deterioration in renal function[18]. Two studies have suggested that angiotensin converting enzyme (ACE) inhibitors may have a favorable role in HIVAN by reducing proteinuria and preserving renal function[19]. A recent retrospective cohort study of severe HIVAN concluded that a limited course of corticosteroids in selected patients was beneficial and safe[20]. However, concerns about life-threatening infections limit the use of corticosteroids in HIVAN. There are recent reports of the effectiveness of HAART in reducing proteinuria and prolonged preservation of renal function[21-25]. Improvement in renal function and reduction in proteinuria seem to correlate with reduction in plasma viral load. It is not yet clear whether antiretroviral therapy can prevent the development of nephropathy if administered before the clinical onset of renal disease. However this possibility is supported by the near disappearance of HIVAN in children, perhaps explained by diagnosis of HIV infection at birth, followed by early initiation of HAART. It is also supported by a recent decline in the incidence of HIVAN in the USA (Figs 21.6 and 21.7). Present speculation is that the widespread deployment of HAART has not only improved the overall morbidity and mortality in HIV-infected patients, but also slowed the epidemic of both acute renal failure and ESRD from HIVAN in urban areas.

HEROIN-ASSOCIATED FOCAL SEGMENTAL GLOMERULOSCLEROSIS

Introduction and definition

Heroin-associated nephropathy (HAN) refers to a syndrome of massive proteinuria seen after prolonged intravenous addiction to heroin, accompanied typically by FSGS. It is unresponsive to immunosuppressive therapy and progresses

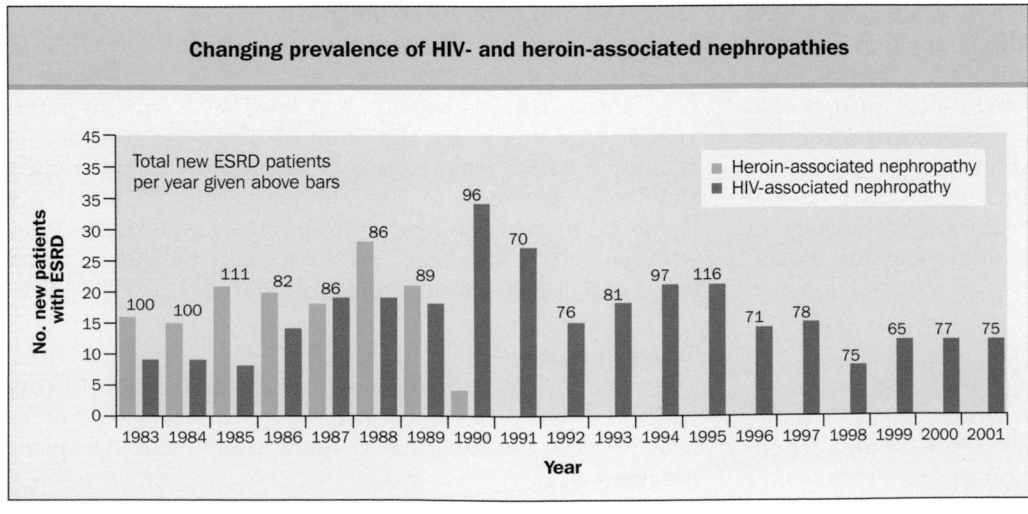

Figure 21.7 Changing prevalence of heroin- and HIV-associated nephropathies. Data from new patients with ESRD at King County Hospital, New York, USA 1983–1999.

to irreversible uremia in 7–48 months[26]. First described in the early 1970s, HAN is a disappearing entity.

Etiology and pathogenesis

The pathogenesis of HAN is not clear. Because of the many immunologic alterations observed in addicts (both serologic and clinical), immune-mediated damage to the kidney has been postulated, but no compelling evidence exists. Perhaps heroin, or more likely one of its diluents such as quinine, is toxic to the podocytes. There are undefined hemodynamic alterations which may be injurious to the glomerulus, and also responsible for progression of the disease even after cessation of heroin abuse. Glomerulosclerosis has been produced in rats by chronic intravenous administration of heroin and adulterants, but lactose is also capable of producing the lesion in the absence of heroin. Because more than 90% of reported patients are African American, there may be a strong genetic predisposition to HAN, perhaps aggravated by unknown environmental factors.

Epidemiology

In the Buffalo Metropolitan area in 1980, heroin addicts accounted for 26% of new cases of sclerosing glomerular disease and 13% of new-onset ESRD cases in patients between the ages of 18 and 45 years[27]. In the same age group, the estimated annual incidence of sclerosing glomerular disease in IVDA was 30 times higher than in the overall non-addict population. In other urban centers across the USA, the prevalence of HAN as a cause of ESRD was reported as 11.4%[27]. While HAN was a major cause of ESRD at our institutions in the 1970s and 1980s, the disease gradually disappeared in the 1990s (Fig. 21.7)[28]. HAN as a cause of ESRD has not been observed at our institution since 1991. The same observation has been made at other institutions in New York, Miami and elsewhere.

Clinical manifestations

The typical patient with HAN is a young African American male (age of onset 18–45 years, male : female ratio 8 : 1, African American : Caucasian ratio 45 : 1) who presents with severe nephrotic syndrome (proteinuria up to 40 g/24 h). Occasionally, microscopic or gross hematuria accompanied by proteinuria may be an early clinical feature. Creatinine clearance may still be normal at presentation but ESRD, when first seen, is also not uncommon. Proteinuria and/or azotemia may also be discovered incidentally while an addict seeks medical attention for an unrelated illness, such as viral hepatitis or pneumonia. Serum C3 complement levels are normal or increased, and concentrations of IgM and IgG in the blood are usually elevated. Ultrasound shows normal or slightly enlarged kidneys in the early nephrotic stage of the illness, but small and shrunken kidneys as the disease progresses to ESRD.

Pathology

Light microscopy

In drug addicts with the nephrotic syndrome, FSGS is the most frequent lesion (approximately 80% of all disease patterns). 'Minimal changes' are found in some patients, as are focal, global sclerosis and diffuse global sclerosis. The remaining glomerular lesions, such as membranous nephropathy and various forms of proliferative glomerulonephritis, may be secondary to other intercurrent illnesses. FSGS in HAN is associated with excessive accumulation of matrix material, wrinkling and folding of thickened GBM, and frequent hyaline deposits in a perihilar location (Fig. 21.8a). Pericapsular thickening, interstitial inflammation, fibrosis, and loss and atrophy of tubules are frequent findings, especially as the disease progresses, and are commensurate with the degree of glomerulosclerosis[26]. Arteriosclerosis and hyalinosis are frequently seen, related to concomitant moderate-to-severe hypertension.

Immunofluorescence

Immunofluorescence studies are either negative or show focal, segmental deposition of IgM and C3 in the sclerotic lesions, as seen in primary FSGS (see Chapter 20). These deposits represent a nonspecific trapping of serum proteins rather than being evidence of a causative immune mechanism. The C3 and IgM seem to accumulate in areas of wrinkled capillary loops and altered mesangium, contributing to the 'hyalinosis' seen in association with focal sclerosis (Fig. 21.8b).

Electron microscopy

Electron microscopy reveals severe focal damage to podocytes, cytoplasmic vacuolization and degeneration, and often separation of podocytes from basement membranes. Foot processes are diffusely effaced in sclerotic areas, and variably effaced elsewhere.

All the glomerular lesions of HAN described above are nonspecific and may not be distinguishable from those seen in idiopathic and other forms of FSGS. This contrasts with the characteristic ultrastructural features and tubular lesions in HIVAN (described above).

Natural history

HAN typically pursues a course of gradual deterioration in renal function complicated by the development of moderate-to-severe hypertension, terminating in ESRD in 7–48 months from the time of diagnosis.

Diagnosis and differential diagnosis

Since the histologic features do not distinguish HAN from other forms of FSGS, the diagnosis relies on the history of drug abuse. HAN is usually associated with current intravenous drug use. When the onset of nephrotic syndrome is associated with a remote history of drug use, the differential should be widened to include idiopathic FSGS, HIVAN (Table 21.4), membranous nephropathy or MPGN associated with hepatitis B infection, and MPGN and cryoglobulinemia associated with hepatitis C infection.

Transplantation

There is little experience in renal transplantation for patients with HAN. The poor compliance with medication and unreliable lifestyle usually exclude them from renal transplant programs.

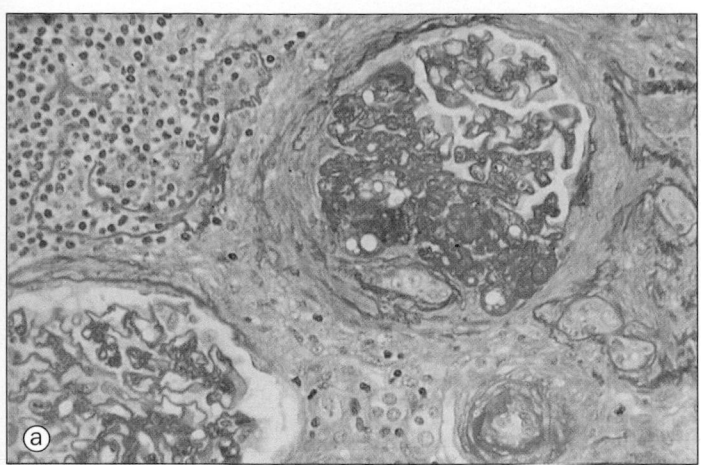
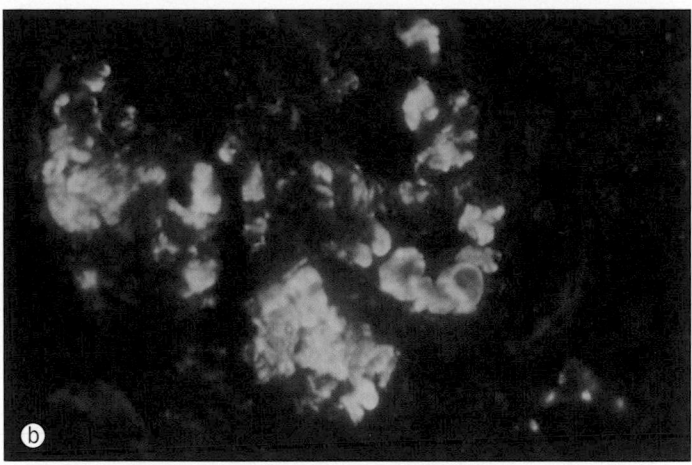

Figure 21.8 Heroin-associated nephropathy. (a) A glomerulus (on upper right) with large area of segmentally obliterated capillary tuft, adhesions to Bowman's capsule, prominent increase in mesangial matrix, and focal accumulations of hyaline deposits containing lipid droplets. Variable pericapsular thickening is noted in this and an adjacent relatively normal appearing glomerulus. Atrophying tubules are surrounded and invaded by moderately dense mononuclear infiltrate. Also, note a markedly thickened arteriole with sclerosis and hyalinosis. (Periodic acid–Schiff ×265.) (b) Immunofluorescence photomicrograph demonstrating coarsely granular deposits of complement C3 in a glomerular lesion with segmental sclerosis and hyalinosis extending from the vascular pole (×330).

Treatment

In one report of four patients, the cessation of narcotic drug abuse was associated with an improvement in renal function along with marked reduction in proteinuria[29]. However, such a favorable outcome is the exception in most drug addicts. The usual sequence of events is hypertension, edema and poor compliance by patients to any medical regimen, with many being lost to follow-up or progressing to ESRD. ACE inhibitors may have a role by reducing proteinuria and controlling hypertension but no studies have specifically addressed their use in HAN.

FOCAL SEGMENTAL GLOMERULOSCLEROSIS ASSOCIATED WITH GLOMERULAR HEMODYNAMIC CHANGES

The secondary forms of FSGS resulting from functional and structural adaptations mediated by hemodynamic and growth factors fall into two categories (Table 21.1). In some diseases, there is a reduction in nephron mass, with hemodynamic responses that are designed to cause compensatory increases in GFR in the remaining nephrons but which, ultimately, are maladaptive. FSGS may also be found in situations where, despite lack of renal functional loss, the normal nephron population is subjected to an excessive hemodynamic stress. The general features of these conditions are described, followed by specific features of some of them.

Etiology

Examples of conditions in which FSGS may develop in association with reduced nephron number or renal mass include patients with partial surgical ablation of a solitary kidney and renal allograft recipients, as well as patients with inherited abnormalities, including renal dysplasia, renal agenesis, oligomeganephronia and segmental hypoplasia. Patients with advanced primary renal diseases, particularly reflux nephropathy, are also in this category.

Conditions where FSGS occurs with no reduction of functioning renal mass, but where the normal nephron population is subjected to excessive hemodynamic stress, include morbid obesity with or without sleep apnea; sickle cell disease; and congenital cyanotic heart disease. Generally, these diseases are associated with cardiomegaly, increased cardiac output and, presumably, hemodynamic alterations in the glomeruli, leading to glomerular hyperfiltration and increased glomerular capillary pressure.

Pathogenesis

In experimental animals, surgical reduction of renal mass results in the development of segmental glomerulosclerosis in the remaining functioning nephrons. Within 2 to 3 weeks of subtotal nephrectomy in rats, there is functional hypertrophy of remnant nephrons, as demonstrated by an increase in both kidney weight and single nephron GFR. These functional adaptations consist of high glomerular plasma flow mediated by afferent arteriolar vasodilatation and increased glomerular capillary pressure secondary to efferent arteriolar vasoconstriction, leading to hyperfiltration[30]. These adaptive processes eventually become maladaptive, resulting in structural alterations. Morphologic changes that follow include expansion of matrix components, endothelial and mesangial cell proliferation, microthrombosis, microaneurysms, accumulation of hyaline material and podocyte effacement and detachment. Segmental and, ultimately, global glomerulosclerosis ensues. The process is self-perpetuating depending on the number of glomeruli lost, with an increasingly heavy hemodynamic load imposed on a dwindling number of glomeruli. In addition, a host of growth factors that promote glomerular cell growth and ECM deposition are involved in the genesis of glomerulosclerosis (see Chapter 66). In humans, the critical limit of

Glomerular Disease

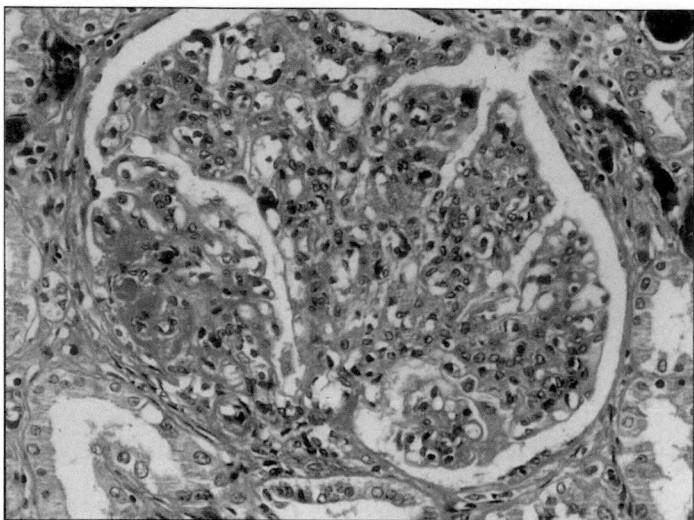

Figure 21.9 Focal segmental glomerulosclerosis associated with congenital cyanotic heart disease. Marked glomerulomegaly, mesangial hypercellularity and segmental sclerosis with focal hyalinosis (left side) seen in the autopsy of a child with moderate proteinuria, who died of complications of tetralogy of Fallot (Hematoxylin & eosin ×265).

nephron loss that leads to initiation of compensatory adaptive changes terminating in glomerulosclerosis is unclear. For example, the long-term study of healthy living related renal donors has failed to reveal an increased incidence of proteinuria or hypertension, even though the remaining kidney is enlarged and hypertrophied. In unilateral renal agenesis, the development of proteinuria, FSGS and renal failure is an indication that the solitary kidney is abnormal. Studies in patients with renal carcinoma undergoing partial nephrectomy of a single remaining kidney show that the highest risk of developing FSGS and ESRD is seen in those with > 75% reduction in renal mass.

Clinical manifestations
The common presentation is low-grade proteinuria (< 3 g/24 h), and frank nephrosis is less frequent. Hypertension is common despite nephrotic-range proteinuria in some, hypoalbuminemia, edema and hyperlipidemia are typically absent. Possible explanations are differences in the rate of hepatic albumin synthesis, and in the absorption/catabolism of proteins in the proximal tubules in these patients.

Pathology
In these secondary forms of FSGS, glomeruli are enlarged and hypertrophied (Fig. 21.9). In vesicoureteral reflux, there is a good correlation between glomerular size and azotemia[31]. The mean proportion of the glomerular surface area affected by foot process fusion in FSGS associated with obesity and vesicoureteral reflux is significantly less than that in those with primary FSGS[31,32].

Differential diagnosis
If diagnosis rests solely on the morphologic appearance of the kidney lesions, these secondary forms of FSGS are easily

misdiagnosed as primary FSGS. This confusion may result in inappropriate treatment of such patients with corticosteroids and/or cytotoxic agents, which are not only ineffective, but may also cause serious side effects. The differences in glomerular size and in the proportion of glomerular surface area covered by foot process fusion, although helpful at times, are not adequate to distinguish confidently between primary and secondary forms of FSGS. The distinction therefore relies on careful assessment of the clinical context for any likely cause of FSGS.

Treatment
There is no evidence that corticosteroids or other immunosuppressive agents are effective in these secondary forms of FSGS and they are not recommended.

FOCAL SEGMENTAL GLOMERULOSCLEROSIS ASSOCIATED WITH VESICOURETERAL REFLUX

Proteinuria in reflux nephropathy, which may not occur for several years after the scarring has occurred, is a bad prognostic marker, and its severity increases with worsening of renal function. There is a strong positive correlation between the extent of glomerular involvement and the magnitude of proteinuria and reduction in GFR[33]. Hypertension is a relatively late complication. Many of these patients with severe bilateral reflux, proteinuria and hypertension develop ESRD. The histologic hallmark in this group of patients is FSGS with hyalinosis involving unscarred areas of the kidney, or in the contralateral normal kidney in those with unilateral reflux nephropathy.

FSGS is the most common renal lesion described both in children and adults with reflux nephropathy who have developed chronic renal failure. Widespread glomerulomegaly has been reported. Deposits of IgM, complement and properdin in the sclerosed glomeruli, along with subendothelial electron-dense deposits, are observed. Some workers have also reported only interstitial changes and severe scarring with no evidence of FSGS in nephrectomized specimens.

FOCAL SEGMENTAL GLOMERULOSCLEROSIS ASSOCIATED WITH OBESITY

In a review of 1000 obese subjects, proteinuria was seen in 410, but nephrotic syndrome was seen in 12 patients only[34,35]. Among these 12, five had evidence of FSGS, one had membranous nephropathy, and no significant glomerular abnormality was seen in the other six. No patient had significant renal impairment and, in almost all patients, there was a remission of nephrotic syndrome with weight loss. If proteinuria does not cease with weight loss in obese patients, another disorder must be suspected. Even in those patients with obesity-associated FSGS and nephrotic range proteinuria, hypoalbuminemia and edema are either minimal or absent.

A U.S. study of obesity-related FSGS showed a progressive increase in the incidence from 0.2% of all renal biopsies in 1986–90 to 2% in 1996–2000[36]. Patients had a mean age of 43 years, were more often Caucasian, and had a lower incidence of nephrotic syndrome. Renal biopsy showed fewer lesions of segmental sclerosis, more glomerulomegaly, and less extensive foot process effacement.

Glomerular visceral cell hyperplasia is infrequently seen. Some have found abundant lipid deposits in the glomeruli, suggesting a pathogenetic role for altered lipid metabolism in obesity-associated FSGS. Although hypoxemia and polycythemia in conjunction with sleep apnea are common features in this disease, these are not universally present. The condition rarely leads to renal failure.

FOCAL SEGMENTAL GLOMERULOSCLEROSIS ASSOCIATED WITH SICKLE CELL DISEASE

The renal hemodynamic abnormalities that follow medullary ischemia in sickle cell disease and their functional consequences are discussed further in Chapter 51. The most common clinical manifestation is hematuria (microscopic and gross). Renal papillary necrosis and urinary tract infection are also seen, and defects in tubular function are common.

Proteinuria has also been reported in one-quarter of adults with sickle cell disease, although nephrotic range proteinuria is less common[37]. Although a variety of glomerular histology has been described in nephrotic patients, FSGS is the most commonly observed lesion (Fig. 21.10) along with marked glomerulomegaly. Glomerular area is twice that seen in normal controls[36]. The administration of ACE inhibitors resulted in a 57% (range 23–79%) decrease in proteinuria in ten patients reported by Falk et al[37]. FSGS is also found in children with sickle cell disease. In patients with sickle cell disease, functional studies showing an increase in renal hemodynamics, and clinical evidence for a reduction in proteinuria with ACE inhibitors, strongly support the contention that hyperfiltration makes them more prone to develop FSGS.

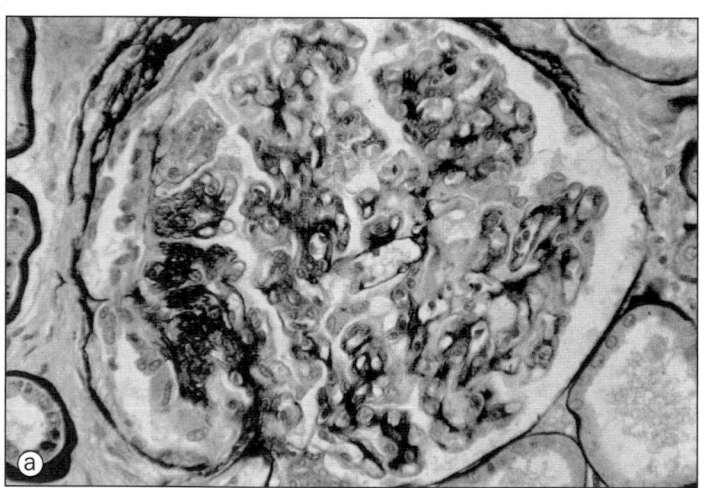 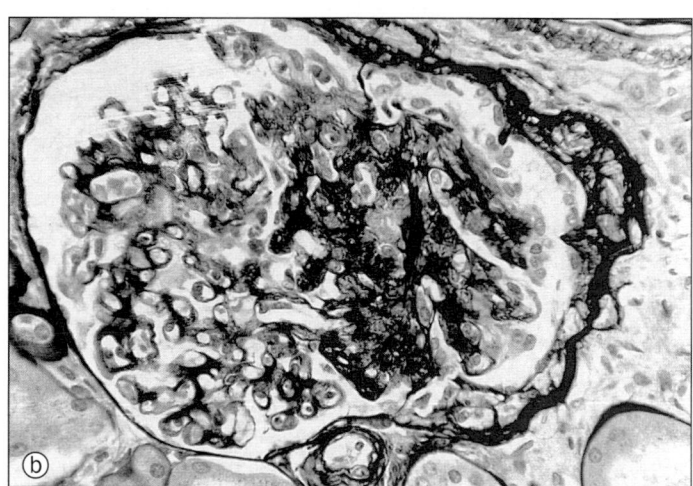

Figure 21.10 Glomerular pathology in sickle cell nephropathy. Mild (a) and moderate (b) perihaler focal segmental glomerulosclerosis. (Courtesy of Dr Charles Jennette.)

REFERENCES

1. Valeri A, Barsoni L, Appel GB, et al. Idiopathic collapsing focal segmental glomerulosclerosis: a clinicopathologic study. Kidney Int. 1996;50:1734–46.

2. Moudgil A, Nast CC, Bagga A, et al. Association of parvovirus B19 infection with idiopathic collapsing glomerulopathy. Kidney Int. 2001;59:2126–33.

3. Markowitz GS, Appel GB, Fine PL, et al. Collapsing focal segmental glomerulosclerosis following treatment with high dose Pamidronate. J Am Soc Nephrol. 2001;12:1164–72.

4. D'Agati V, Appel GB. HIV infection and the kidney. J Am Soc Nephrol. 1997;8:138–52.

5. Levin ML, Palella F, Shah S, et al. HIV-associated nephropathy occurring before HIV antibody seroconversion. Am J Kidney Dis 2001;37:39.

6. Cohen AH, Sun NCJ, Shapshak P, Imagawa DT. Demonstration of human immunodeficiency virus in renal epithelium in HIV-associated nephropathy. Mod Pathol. 1989;2:125–8.

7. Conaldi PG, Biancone L, Bottelli A, et al. HIV-1 kills renal tubular epithelial cells in vitro by triggering an apoptotic pathway involving caspase activation and Fas up-regulation. J Clin Invest. 1998;102:2041–9.

8. Bruggerman LA, Ross MD, Tanji N, et al. Renal epithelium is a previously unrecognized site of HIV-1 infection. J Am Soc Nephrol. 2000;11:2079–87.

9. Kopp JB, Ray PE, Adler SH, et al. Nephropathy in HIV-transgenic mice. Contrib Nephrol. 1994;107:194–204.

10. Bruggeman LA, Dickman S, Meng C, et al. Nephropathy in human immunodeficiency virus-1 transgenic mice is due to transgene expression. J Clin Invest. 1997;100:84–92.

11. Yamamoto T, Noble NA, Miller DE, et al. Increased levels of transforming growth factor beta in HIV-associated nephropathy. Kidney Int. 1999;55:579–92.

12. Coresh J, Caiaffa WT, Vlahov D, et al. HIV infection and the risk of renal disease among injection drug users: a prospective study in the alive cohort. J Am Soc Nephrol. 1997;8:135A.

13. Winston JA, Burns GC, Klotman PE. The human immunodeficiency virus (HIV) epidemic and HIV-associated nephropathy. Semin Nephrol. 1998;18:373–7.

14. Szczech LA, Gange SJ, Horst CV, et al. Predictors of proteinuria and renal failure among women with HIV infection. Kidney Int. 2002;61:195–202.

15. Chander P, Agarwal A, Soni A, et al. Renal cytomembranous inclusions in idiopathic renal disease as predictive markers for the acquired immunodeficiency syndrome. Hum Pathol. 1998; 19:1060–4.

16. Ahuja TS, Borucki M, Grady J. Highly-active antiretroviral therapy improves survival of HIV-infected hemodialysis patients. Am J Kidney Dis. 2000;36:574–80.

17. Stock P, Roland M, Carlson L, et al. Solid organ transplantation in HIV-positive patients. Trans Proc. 1999;33:3646–8.

18. Ifudu O, Rao TKS, Tan CC, et al. Zidovudine is beneficial in human immunodeficiency virus associated nephropathy. Am J Nephrol. 1995;15:217–21.

19. Burns GC, Paul SK, Toth IR, Sivak SL. Effect of angiotensin-converting enzyme inhibition in HIV-associated nephropathy. J Am Soc Nephrol. 1997;8:1140–6.

20. Eustace JA, Nuermberger E, Choi M, et al. Cohort study of severe HIV-associated nephropathy with corticosteroids. Kidney Int. 2000;58:1253–60.

21. Wali RK, Drachenberg CI, Papadimitriou JC, et al. HIV-1-associated nephropathy and response to highly-active antiretroviral therapy. Lancet. 1998;352:783–4.

22. Dellow E, Unwin R, Miller R, et al. Protease inhibitor therapy for HIV infection: the effect on HIV-associated nephrotic syndrome. Nephrol Dial Transplant. 1999;14:744–7.

23. Viani RM, Dankner WM, Muelenaer PA, Spector SA. Resolution of HIV-1-associated nephrotic syndrome with highly active antiretroviral therapy delivered by gastrostomy tube. Pediatrics. 1999;104:1394–6.

24. Navarette JE, Pastan SO. Effect of highly active antiretroviral treatment and prednisone in biopsy proven HIV associated nephropathy. J Am Soc Nephrol. 2000;11:93A.

25. Cosgrove CJ, Abu-Alfa AK, Perazella MA. Effects of highly active antiretroviral therapy on HIV patients with renal disease. J Am Soc Nephrol. 2001;12:198A.

26. Rao TKS, Nicastri AD, Friedman EA. The nephropathies of drug addiction and acquired immunodeficiency syndrome. In: Tisher CC, Brenner BM, eds. Renal pathology. New York: Lippincott; 1989:340–56.

27. Cunningham EE, Brentjens OR, Zielezny MA, et al. Heroin nephropathy a clinicopathologic and epidemiologic study. JAMA. 1980;68:47–53.

28. Friedman EA, Rao TKS. Disappearance of uremia due to heroin associated nephropathy. Am J Kidney Dis. 1995;25:689–93.

29. Llach F, Descoeudres C, Massry SG. Heroin associated nephropathy: clinical and histological studies in 19 patients. Clin Nephrol. 1979;11:7–12.

30. Meyer TW, Baboolal K, Brenner BM. Nephron adaptation to renal injury. In: Brenner BM, ed. The kidney. Philadelphia, PA: Saunders; 1996:2031–7.

31. El-Khatib MT, Becker GJ, Kincaid-Smith PS. Morphometric aspects of reflux nephropathy. Kidney Int. 1987;32:261–6.

32. Barisoni L, Szabolcs M, Ward L, D'Agati V. Visceral epithelial cell alterations in focal segmental glomerulosclerosis. Mod Pathol. 1994;7:157A.

33. Kincaid-Smith PS, Walker RG. Reflux nephropathy. Med J Aust. 1987;146:563–8.

34. Klahr S. Kidney in nutritional disorders. In: Massry SG, Glassock RJ, eds. Textbook of nephrology. Philadelphia, PA: William & Wilkins; 1995:1124–35.

35. Verani RR. Obesity associated focal segmental glomerulosclerosis: pathologic features of the lesion and relationship with cardiomegaly and hyperlipidemia. Am J Kidney Dis. 1992;10:629–34.

36. Kambham N, Markowitz GS, Valeri AM, et al. Obesity-related glomerulopathy: an emerging epidemic. Kidney Int. 2001;59:1498–1509.

37. Falk RJ, Scheinman J, Phillips G, et al. Prevalence and pathologic features of sickle cell nephropathy and response to inhibition by angiotensin converting enzyme inhibition. N Engl J Med. 1992; 326:910–15.

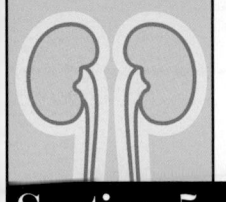

Chapter 22

Membranous Nephropathy

William G Couser and Stuart J Shankland

INTRODUCTION AND DEFINITION

Membranous nephropathy (MN) is a glomerular disease in which immune deposits of IgG and complement components develop predominantly or exclusively on the subepithelial surface of the glomerular capillary wall. Deposition is associated with a marked increase in glomerular permeability to protein, which is manifested clinically as nephrotic syndrome[1]. The disease occurs in association with a variety of other conditions, some of which are likely causal and some of which probably represent only associations (Table 22.1)[2]. However, most occurrences (two-thirds) are without obvious initiating events: idiopathic. MN is the most common cause of idiopathic nephrotic syndrome in older (age over 60 years) Causasian adults and is rare in children.

Although the term 'membranous', which refers to thickening or expansion of the glomerular capillary wall, has been in use in renal pathology for most of the 20th century, the entity now referred to as MN was clearly defined only following the advent of immunofluorescence and electron microscopy as routine tools in the study of renal biopsies in the 1950s and 1960s. These techniques first revealed the presence early in the development of the disease of the diffuse, finely granular immune deposits in the subepithelial space that are now regarded as pathognomonic of MN. Consequently, MN is a pathologic diagnosis made when glomeruli exhibit these deposits without associated hypercellularity or inflammatory change.

Considerable evidence supports the hypothesis that idiopathic MN is an autoimmune disease, although the nephritogenic autoantigens have not been identified in humans. Whether MN that occurs in association with various systemic disorders such as lupus, hepatitis, and malignancy represents a similar process or is consequent to other mechanisms is not known. The principal consequence of formation of subepithelial immune deposits is the development of increased glomerular permeability to protein, with increased protein excretion and nephrotic syndrome, and about half of all patients with MN progress eventually to renal failure over a period of several years[1].

ETIOLOGY AND PATHOGENESIS

Etiology

The pathogenesis of human MN is not known. However, the frequent occurrence of this lesion in autoimmune disorders such as lupus and diabetes, as well as its remarkable similarity to a lesion induced in rats with antibody to antigens

Conditions and agents associated with membranous nephropathy		
Groups	Common	Uncommon
Immune diseases	Systemic lupus erythematosus, diabetes mellitus	Rheumatoid arthritis, Hashimoto's disease, Graves' disease, mixed connective tissue disease, Sjögren's syndrome, primary biliary cirrhosis, bullous pemphigoid, small bowel enteropathy syndrome. dermatitis herpetiformis, ankylosing spondylitis, graft-versus-host disease, Guillain–Barré syndrome
Infectious or parasitic diseases	Hepatitis B	Hepatitis C, syphilis, filariasis, hydatid disease, schistosomiasis, malaria, leprosy
Drugs and toxins	Gold, penicillamine, nonsteroidal anti-inflammatory agents	Mercury, captopril, formaldehyde, hydrocarbons, bucillamine
Miscellaneous	Tumors, renal transplantation	Sarcoidosis, sickle cell disease. Kimura disease, angiofollicular lymph node hyperplasia

The list excludes conditions where only a single case has been reported or where the lesions were atypical of membranous nephropathy. With permission from Couser and Alpers[2].

Table 22.1 Conditions and agents associated with membranous nephropathy.

expressed on the surface of the glomerular epithelial cell (GEC), have fueled speculation that the disease is caused by deposits of autoantibody to fixed components of the GEC membrane[3]. A large number of agents appear to be capable of initiating this process in genetically susceptible individuals (Table 22.1), and include viruses such as hepatitis B (HBV) and hepatitis C (HCV), drugs including gold, penicillamine, and nonsteroidal anti-inflammatory agents (NSAIDs), and toxins such as hydrocarbons and formaldehyde, and a variety of chronic immune disorders such as lupus, thyroiditis, graft-versus-host disease, and renal allografts. In about two-thirds of patients no obvious etiologic agent or condition can be identified; doubtless this is a manifestation of the paucity of knowledge about the disease rather than the absence of such agents.

Recently there has been one well-documented case of congenital MN that was shown to be mediated by an antibody to an endogenous antigen (neutral endopeptidase, NEP) on the glomerular podocyte. In this situation, the mother, who had a

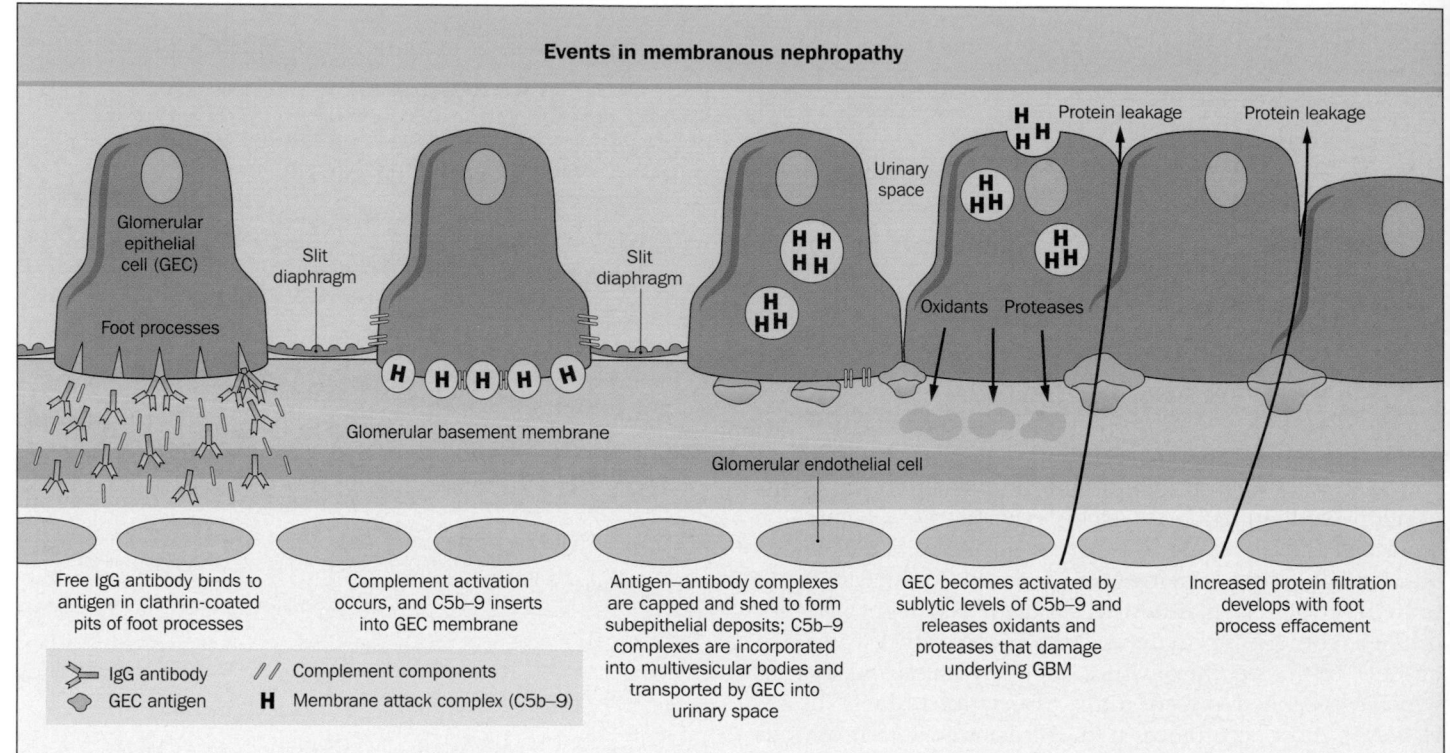

Figure 22.1 Events in a rat model of membranous nephropathy. Immune deposit formation, C5b–9 insertion, and GEC activation lead to proteinuria (see text).

hereditary deficiency in NEP, became sensitized during pregnancy and passively transferred anti-NEP IgG to her infant at birth, resulting in a lesion of MN[4].

Mechanisms of immune deposit formation

Regardless of the initiating event(s), the disease appears to be mediated primarily by the humoral immune response, which leads to deposition of IgG and complement on the outer surface of the glomerular capillary wall. Experimental evidence suggests that this is unlikely to be the consequence of passive glomerular trapping of preformed immune complexes directly from the circulation. However, such deposits can be produced by local or *in situ* immune-complex formation involving antigens that could be exogenous or endogenous and could act in three ways. First, exogenous antigens could localize on the subepithelial surface because of their cationic charge and small size or, second, they could form immune complexes on the inner surface of the capillary wall that dissociate, traverse the glomerular basement membrane (GBM) and reform in the subepithelial space. Finally, the antigens could be endogenous constituents of a subepithelial component of the capillary wall such as the GEC, or podocyte, membrane[3]. The total absence of deposits at subendothelial (and mesangial) sites in idiopathic MN, as well as the ability to duplicate the lesion with anti-GEC antibodies, strongly favors the third or autoimmune explanation for the unique localization of deposits in this disease. In rat models of MN, which closely simulate the human disease (Heymann nephritis), the antigens responsible are components of the Heymann

nephritis antigenic complex: a large (516 kDa) glycoprotein, called megalin, bound to a smaller receptor-associated protein (RAP) expressed in the clathrin-coated pits of the podocyte foot processes[5]. While antibodies to small antigenic determinants on both molecules can form subepithelial immune-complex deposits, an additional antigen–antibody system involving an unidentified glycolipid antigen that activates complement is required to induce proteinuria. Once formed, these complexes of antigen and antibody are capped and shed from the cell surface, where they bind to underlying GBM, resist degradation, and persist for weeks or months as immune deposits detectable by immunofluorescence and electron microscopy (Fig. 22.1)[3].

However, other than the rare case of congenital MN due to antibody to NEP, such autoantibodies have not been identified in human MN, and the two exogenous antigen mechanisms have not been excluded (although in the authors' judgment they are unlikely), particularly in disease induced by foreign agents such as viruses.

Mechanism of glomerular injury

Based entirely on studies in animal models, the mechanism by which damage to the glomerular filtration barrier occurs that is sufficient to cause proteinuria, appears to involve sublytic effects of complement C5b–9 (a multimer comprising several complement components and also known as the membrane attack complex, MAC) on the GEC (Fig. 22.2)[2,3]. Complement activation and cleavage of C5 generates the chemotactic factor C5a, which presumably is flushed by filtration forces into the

Glomerular injury in membranous nephropathy

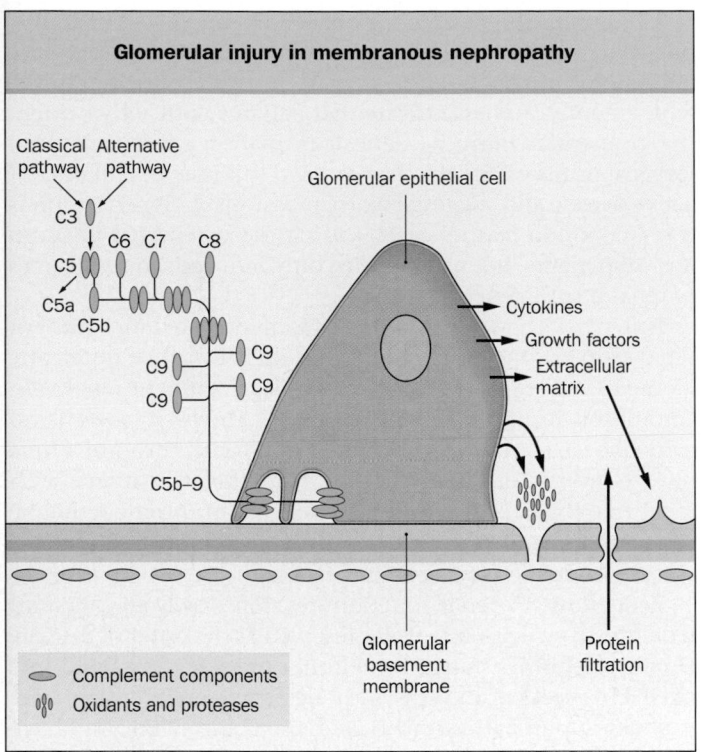

Figure 22.2 Postulated mechanism of glomerular injury in membranous nephropathy. Antibodies against the glomerular epithelial cells (GEC) induce complement activation via the classical or alternative pathway, leading to formation of C5b–9. Insertion of C5b–9 is insufficient to cause lysis but stimulates the GEC to release a host of inflammatory mediators that damage the underlying glomerular basement membrane, leading to increased protein filtration.

Diagnosis and management of patients with membranous nephropathy

Patient groups	Test
All patients	
General	Renal function (serum creatinine and creatinine clearance)
	Blood pressure
	Urine protein excretion (24-h urine or urine protein : creatinine ratio)
	Serum albumin
	Serum cholesterol
	Urinalysis
	Renal biopsy
Associated disease	Hepatitis B (HBs antigen)
	Hepatitis C (HCV antibody)
	Antinuclear antibody (ANA), anti-double-stranded DNA (the hallmark of systemic lupus erythematosus)
	Complement C3, C4 (usually normal in idiopathic membranous nephropathy)
Selected patients	
With suspected thromboembolic events, flank pain, hematuria, acute renal failure	Renal vein angiography
With sudden decrease in renal function, development of active urine sediment	Antiglomerular basement membrane antibody
Over 50 years of age	Cancer screening (see text)

Table 22.2 Diagnosis and management of patients with membranous nephropathy.

urinary space and does not move backwards across the GBM to attract circulating inflammatory cells. The other product of C5 cleavage, C5b, combines with C6 to form a lipophilic complex that inserts into the lipid bilayer of the GEC where C7, C8, and multiple C9 molecules are added to create a pore-forming complex, C5b–9 (see Figs 22.1 and 22.2). The GEC is resistant to lysis and endocytoses the C5b–9, transporting it intracellularly in multivesicular bodies and extruding it into the urinary space (see Fig. 22.1). However, the membrane insertion of C5b–9, although insufficient to cause cell lysis, does induce cell activation and signal transduction, with increased production of multiple potentially nephritogenic molecules, including oxidants, proteases, cytokines, growth factors, vasoactive molecules, and extracellular matrix (see Fig. 22.2)[3]. Current evidence is strongest for the role of GEC-derived oxidants in producing the GBM damage that leads to increased protein filtration in MN, but an equivalent role for unique GEC-derived proteases has not been excluded. During the period when antibody deposition, deposit formation, and complement activation are occurring, increased excretion of C5b–9 can be measured in the urine[3].

Consequences of injury induced by C5b–9

The glomerular injury mediated by C5b–9 induces a nonselective proteinuria through loss of both the size- and the charge-selective properties of the glomerular capillary wall.

The subsequent reduction in GFR that occurs in progressive MN has both glomerular and interstitial components. In the glomerulus, there is thickening of the GBM resulting from overproduction of several different extracellular matrix molecules, which are deposited between and around the immune deposits to form subepithelial 'spikes'. These are characteristic of this disease when a biopsy is studied with silver–methenamine staining, (see Fig. 22.3c). This appears to occur in part through upregulation of GEC production of transforming growth factors TGF-β_2 and TGF-β_3 as well as increased expression of TGF-β receptors in response to C5b–9. The GEC itself has limited ability to proliferate due to overexpression of cyclin kinase inhibitors and undergoes hypertrophy and detachment[6]. In the interstitium, there is an increased macrophage infiltrate and overproduction of matrix by interstitial fibroblasts, leading to interstitial fibrosis[7,8]. This response is likely common to all nonselective proteinuric disorders and results from toxic effects of normal serum proteins, lipid-derived chemotactic factors, iron, intratubular C5b–9 activation, and other glomerular-derived mediators on the tubular cells and the milieu in which they live[5,8]. When nephrotic-range proteinuria persists, the consequence is glomerular sclerosis as well as interstitial fibrosis and progression to renal failure, which are directly related to both the magnitude and the duration of increased protein filtration.

EPIDEMIOLOGY

The disease is uncommon in children, accounting for 2–12% (usually less than 5%) of pediatric patients undergoing biopsy for nephrotic syndrome. In adults, about 30% of all biopsies for idiopathic nephrotic syndrome reveal MN, and the disease accounts for about 50% of biopsied cases of idiopathic nephrotic syndrome in older adults, a population in which MN remains the leading cause of idiopathic nephrotic syndrome[1]. There is some variation in these figures among different countries, with slightly lower numbers in the UK and higher numbers in Greece and Macedonia. The US Renal Data System records 1392 patients with end-stage renal disease (ESRD) owing to established MN in 1991–1995, or about 0.5% of the total ESRD population[9]. However, if one includes patients with lupus MN and an estimated 5% of patients classified only as chronic GN, the total is probably twice that. Further, if only 50% of patients progress to renal failure, and another 20–30% are clinically silent, the real prevalence of this disease is probably around 2000 patients per year in the USA or about eight patients per million population per year.

There is a three-fold increased risk for MN in patients with HLA-DR3, and associations with HLA-B8 and HLA-B18 have also been reported[2]. HLA-DR5, in addition to HLA-DR3, appears to increase the risk of progression. In Japan, MN is associated with HLA-DR2, some Caucasian patients have a deletion of C4 with the HLA-B8-DR3 haplotype. Rare examples of familial MN have also been reported, usually presenting in brothers.

CLINICAL MANIFESTATIONS

Idiopathic disease

MN is a disorder of insidious onset in which the only clinical manifestations of early disease are an increase in urine protein excretion and the consequences thereof. Most patients present with a gradual development of peripheral edema without other signs or symptoms. The disease has been reported in children less than 1 year of age and in adults over 90 years, but it is uncommon in patients under 30. MN is more common in men than women by about a 2–3 : 1 ratio, and individual peaks occur between ages 30 and 40 and again between ages 50 and 60 years[1,2].

About 80% of patients have overt nephrotic syndrome at the time of presentation, with urine protein excretion exceeding 3.5 g/day, reduced serum albumin levels, and elevated serum lipids, as well as fluid retention and edema (see Chapter 19). However, the disease likely develops over a period of several weeks or months before proteinuria of this magnitude occurs, and about 20% of patients are detected with asymptomatic non-nephrotic proteinuria (< 3.5 g/day). Proteinuria is always nonselective and generally in the 5–15 g/day range. Urine protein excretion exceeding 15 g is more suggestive of minimal change disease, but this is not absolute. Day-to-day fluctuations in protein excretion are frequent in MN and likely reflect changes in protein intake, posture, exercise, and hemodynamic variables more than changes in the activity of the disease.

Microscopic hematuria may be seen in up to 50% of adults, but macroscopic hematuria and red blood cell casts are extremely unusual and suggest a different diagnosis. Experimental studies indicate that patients with active, ongoing glomerular immune deposit formation exhibit elevated levels of urinary C5b–9 excretion, and this may be a marker of active disease and suggest a worse prognosis[2,3]. Hypertension is not a common feature of MN. It has been reported in up to 30% of patients, but usually with only more advanced degrees of renal insufficiency[1].

Patients with MN appear to have an increased incidence of renal vein thrombosis, above that seen in other nephrotic glomerular diseases. Prospective studies document renal vein thrombosis in up to 40% of patients[1,2]. However, there is no evidence that the presence of renal vein thrombi alters disease severity or renal function. Nonetheless, patients with renal vein thrombosis are at increased risk of thromboembolic phenomena, and prophylactic anticoagulation treatment is recommended for such patients (see below).

Reductions in renal function develop slowly in MN, and renal function is usually well preserved at the onset of disease. Usually, nephrotic-range proteinuria precedes any fixed loss of GFR by weeks or months, although some prerenal azotemia may develop in patients who are hypoalbuminemic and have depleted extracellular fluid volume. Less than 20% of patients have a reduction in GFR at the time of initial diagnosis[1,2,10,11].

The diagnostic studies that should be performed in patients with known or suspected MN are listed in Table 22.2.

Common secondary causes

While the typical clinical features of MN are not unique or different from several other diseases that cause idiopathic nephrotic syndrome, about one-third of patients have MN as a manifestation of some other systemic disease process. Several of these associations are sufficiently common to warrant separate mention.

Membranous lupus nephritis

The class V, or membranous, form of lupus nephritis may be indistinguishable from idiopathic MN clinically and even serologically[12]. This lesion accounts for about 20% of patients with lupus nephritis and often presents as nephrotic syndrome in young women who do not have other clinical or serologic manifestations of systemic lupus, although they usually develop these later. In patients with lupus MN, anti-DNA antibody levels and antinuclear antibody titers (ANA) are often low, and the antibody is of very low avidity compared with that in patients with class IV lesions (diffuse proliferative lupus nephritis). Complement levels are also often normal. While the glomerular lesion of lupus MN closely mimics the idiopathic form of the disease, the presence of deposits of immunoglobulins other than IgG (i.e., IgA and IgM), particularly in the mesangium, as well as tubuloreticular structures seen by electron microscopy suggest lupus as an underlying etiology[1,2,12]. The natural history of lupus MN is similar to that of the idiopathic form of the disease, with about 85% renal survival at 10 years. Treatment generally is similar to that suggested for idiopathic MN.

Hepatitis B

Worldwide there is a strong association between MN and a chronic carrier state for HBV, particularly in young males between the ages of 2 and 12 years. However, the incidence of HBV in MN varies widely in different parts of the world, from about 30–40% of adult patients in Asia to less than 1% in the USA[13]. In children, the rate is much higher, ranging from 20–64% in the USA to over 80% in eastern Europe, Asia, and Africa. The presence of HBV antigens, particularly HBe antigen (HBeAg), in glomeruli, together with antibody to it, suggests that HBV antigens participate in *in situ* immune-complex formation, leading to disease development in patients who cannot clear antigens and remain in persistent antigen excess or exhibit low-avidity antibodies.

Clinically, HBV MN presents like idiopathic MN with nephrotic syndrome. It occurs in patients who often have a history of viral hepatitis, laboratory evidence of low-grade chronic hepatitis, and evidence of HBs antigen (HBsAg), and often HBeAg, in the circulation. Complement levels are more often reduced in HBV MN than in the idiopathic form of the disease (30–50% of patients), and hematuria and hypertension are also more common[13]. The course is more benign than in idiopathic MN, with most children undergoing spontaneous remission within 5 years and only 10–20% of adults progressing to chronic renal failure. Treatment is generally supportive, with diuretics and angiotensin-converting enzyme (ACE) inhibitors to reduce protein excretion. In symptomatic or progressive disease, a trial of antiviral therapy with interferon-α is probably indicated[13]. Many adults enter remission following antiviral therapy if renal function is well preserved. Steroids are without obvious benefit to the glomerular lesion and may induce viral replication and worsen liver disease. Similar problems beset the use of cytotoxic drug therapy, including the immuno-suppressive regimens required for transplantation.

MN has also been reported with HCV infection, sometimes in the absence of cryoglobulins or rheumatoid factor, although this association is less well established than that with HBV.

Cancer

An association between MN and solid tumors is well established, particularly in adults over 50 years, where the incidence of malignancy in MN in some reports has approached 20%[1,14]. The most common associated cancers are those of the lung, breast, and gastrointestinal tract, but cases of MN have been reported with most forms of cancer. In patients with cancer-associated MN, the nephrotic syndrome may precede clinical evidence of the tumor by 12–18 months[1,2,14]. A careful search for malignancy is, therefore, mandatory in older patients who present with MN. This should include a chest X-ray, colonoscopy, stool guaiac test for occult blood, mammography in women, and measurement of tumor markers such as CEA (carcinoembryonic antigen) and PSA (prostate-specific antigen). In patients with other signs to suggest cancer, such as unexplained weight loss or pain, an abdominal computed tomographic (CT) scan is indicated. The glomerular lesion and nephrotic syndrome have been reported to resolve following successful resection of early tumors, although this does not always occur. Prognosis is generally determined more by the tumor than by the MN,

and no form of immunosuppressive therapy has been shown to be useful in inducing remission or slowing progression in such patients.

Membranous nephropathy in renal allografts

MN may recur occasionally in allografts; this usually occurs in patients with severe disease who progress from onset of symptoms to renal failure in 3 years or less. Recurrent MN generally appears in the first 6–12 months following transplantation[15]. More commonly, MN develops *de novo* in the allograft, where it accounts for up to 30% of transplant recipients with nephrotic syndrome. It is second only to transplant glomerulopathy as a cause of nephrotic syndrome in transplant recipients and generally presents 2 or more years following transplantation[15]. In patients with renal allografts and *de novo* MN, 60% are nephrotic and 40% have non-nephrotic proteinuria. As in idiopathic MN, the pathogenesis of the lesion is unknown, although some cases are associated with HCV infection. The presence of *de novo* MN does not appear to be a significant risk factor for allograft survival, and most such grafts are lost from chronic rejection. There are no data to document a benefit of disease-specific therapy in reducing proteinuria or prolonging graft survival beyond the immunosuppressive regimen utilized for transplantation.

Membranous nephropathy and rapidly progressive glomerulonephritis

A rare but well-documented event in MN is the super-imposition of a crescentic glomerular lesion with sudden deterioration in renal function accompanied by an active urine sediment. Usually this results from the development of anti-GBM antibodies. In such patients, an anti-GBM antibody assay should be performed since linear staining of the GBM may be difficult to distinguish from the very finely granular deposits that characterize uncomplicated MN. When this does occur, for anti-GBM disease, usually including cyclo-phosphamide and plasma exchange (see Chapter 25), should be instituted.

PATHOLOGY

The pathologic features of MN evolve from the initial formation of subepithelial immune complexes of IgG and complement along the outer surface of the capillary wall. Changes occur first in the GEC, then in glomerular barrier function leading to proteinuria, then in the renal interstitium (probably as a consequence of the proteinuria), and finally in the GBM itself, which becomes thickened (membranous) through the accumulation of additional matrix material along the outer surface, often in an irregular, or spike-like pattern[2,10]. With time, the immune deposits become surrounded by GBM material. This sequence of events, observed primarily by electron microscopy, has led pathologists to classify the glomerular changes into 'stages' ranging from minimal change with only small deposits (stage I) through the evolution to thickened basement membrane with resolution of deposits (stage IV)[2]. The extent to which individual patients will exhibit these sequential changes depends on the duration of the underlying immunopathologic process and its severity. Doubtless, there

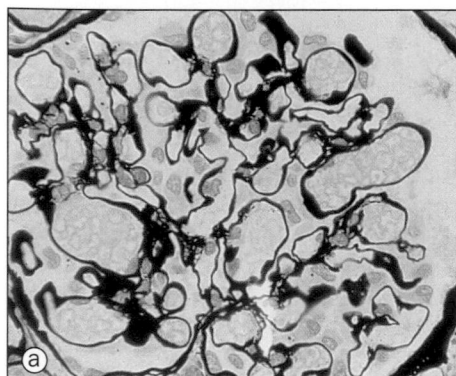 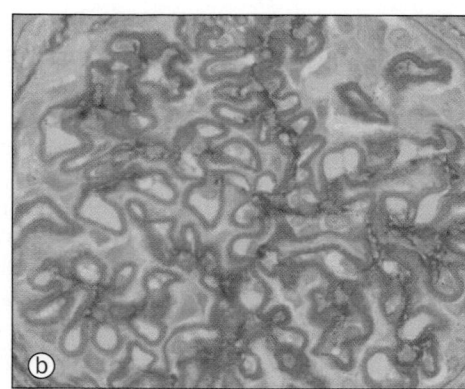 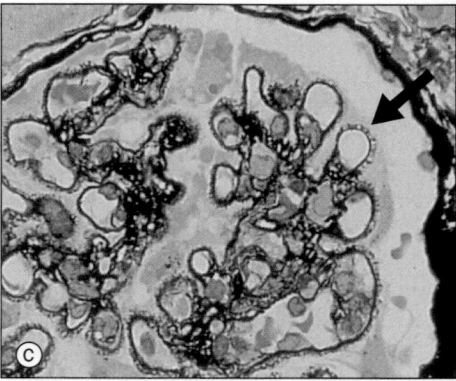

Figure 22.3 Light microscopy in membranous nephropathy (MN). (a) Early MN: a glomerulus from a patient with severe nephrotic syndrome and early MN, exhibiting normal architecture and peripheral capillary basement membranes of normal thickness (Silver–methenamine ×400). (b) morphologically advanced MN: uniform increase in the thickness of the glomerular capillary walls throughout the glomerulus without any increase in glomerular cellularity (×400). (periodic acid–Schiff.) (c) Morphologically more advanced MN (same patient as in (b)): discrete spikes of matrix emanating from the outer surface of the basement membrane (arrow) indicative of advanced MN are revealed by silver–methenamine stain (×400). (Courtesy of CE Alpers.)

are other factors that modulate the GEC response to injury and also contribute to progression or resolution of the disease. It has generally not been possible to draw meaningful clinical correlations between these different pathologic stages and disease severity, prognosis, or response to therapy.

Light microscopy
In the earliest stages of the disease, the glomeruli and interstitium may be essentially normal by light microscopy, and the diagnosis can be made only by application of immunofluorescence and electron microscopy (see Fig. 22.3a). However, the disease progresses early to a homogeneous thickening of the capillary wall, seen in light microscopy in sections stained with hematoxylin and eosin or with periodic acid–Schiff reagent (see Fig. 22.3b). By silver–methenamine staining, early projections of the GBM between deposits may be detected in a characteristic spike-like configuration (see Fig. 22.3c).

In contrast to diseases in which similar quantities of immune deposits are formed along the subendothelial surface of the capillary wall or in the mesangium, no glomerular leukocyte infiltration occurs in MN. This is presumably because chemotactic products of complement activation follow filtration forces into the urinary space rather than diffusing backward into the capillary lumen, and the intervening GBM prevents immune adherence mechanisms from being operative. Although similar deposits at other sites may induce proliferation of glomerular endothelial and, particularly, mesangial cells, GECs *in vivo* seem terminally differentiated and rarely proliferate[6]. As a result, the pathologic lesion of MN is characterized only by changes in GECs and basement membrane without any associated glomerular hypercellularity.

The GECs response to this form of injury does include effacement of foot processes, which is visible only by electron microscopy. A variety of molecules are upregulated in damaged or activated GEC in experimental MN including cysteine-rich acidic secreted protein (SPARC), desmin, platelet-derived growth factor, TGF-β, TGF-β receptors, and several other cytokines. There are no visible mesangial or endothelial cell

abnormalities. The presence of significant mesangial hypercellularity suggests immune deposit formation in the mesangium and is more consistent with a secondary MN such as class V lupus nephritis (see above). In some patients with heavy proteinuria and progressive disease, glomeruli exhibit areas of focal sclerosis similar to the appearance of idiopathic focal segmental glomerulosclerosis (see Chapter 20). These patients often have a more rapidly progressive course and a poor response to therapy. These sclerotic lesions may be a consequence of glomerular hypertrophy accompanied by an inability of the terminally differentiated GEC to proliferate[6], leading to areas of denuded GBM, attachment to Bowman's capsule, and subsequent capillary collapse (see Chapter 18).

As in all nephrotic glomerular diseases, interstitial changes predict renal function and outcome better than glomerular abnormalities do. The degree of interstitial change reflects the magnitude of proteinuria and its duration. Interstitial changes include a diffuse mononuclear cell infiltrate comprising T cells, monocytes, macrophages, and B cells. Tubular degeneration and atrophy and interstitial fibrosis (composed predominantly of type I collagen) evolve over time. In the experimental setting, a number of mediators are overexpressed in the interstitium, including osteopontin (a macrophage chemotactic and adhesive protein made by tubular cells), TGF-β (derived from tubular cells), macrophages, fibroblasts, and thrombospondin (an activator of TGF-β)[3]. It is likely that several cell types, including tubular epithelial cells, fibroblasts, and perhaps macrophages, contribute to the overproduction of extracellular matrix, which leads to interstitial scarring and ultimately to loss of renal function[3].

Immunofluorescence microscopy
The pattern of IgG staining in MN is characteristic and easily recognizable by immunofluorescence (Fig. 22.4). Positive staining for IgG marks the finely granular subepithelial deposits, which are present in all portions of all capillary loops[2]. The predominant IgG subclass in idiopathic MN is IgG4. Staining in MN is positive only for IgG. Positive staining

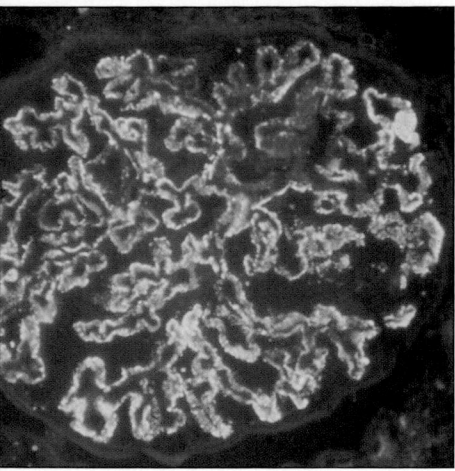

Figure 22.4 Immunofluorescence in membranous nephropathy. A glomerulus with diffuse, finely granular deposition of IgG along the outer surface of all capillary walls. The antibody is believed to represent autoantibody directed at some constituent of the glomerular epithelial cell membrane (original magnification ×400). (Courtesy of CE Alpers.)

for IgA or IgM, or significant staining in the glomerular mesangium, suggests lupus as an underlying mechanism. In idiopathic MN, immune deposit formation occurs only in a subepithelial distribution. Complement C3 is also present in about 50% of patients and usually reflects staining for C3c, a breakdown product of C3b that is rapidly cleared. Consequently, positive C3 staining likely reflects active, ongoing immune deposit formation and complement activation at the time of the biopsy, whereas the absence of C3 suggests that the process of forming deposits has ceased. When looked for, staining for C5b-9 is generally present as well, which is consistent with the proposed pathogenetic role of C5b-9 in this disease (see above)[2,3]. C1 and C4 are often absent, which is consistent with activation of complement through the alternative pathway as a consequence of

GEC damage or downregulation of complement regulatory proteins expressed on the GEC membrane.

Electron microscopy

The presence of subepithelial electron-dense deposits by electron microscopy parallels IgG staining. These deposits in early stages of the disease process are homogeneous and may even be confluent in some areas with overlying GEC foot process effacement and little change in the underlying GBM (stage I). As the disease persists, there is projection of basement membrane material up between the deposits to form subepithelial spikes that can be detected by light microscopy using a silver–methenamine stain and are easily visible by electron microscopy (stage II) (Fig. 22.5a). Later, the spikes extend and the deposits may become surrounded by new basement membrane-like material (stage III) (Fig. 22.5b). In stage IV disease, the basement membrane is overtly thickened, the deposits incorporated in it become more lucent, and the spikes are less apparent (Fig. 22.5c). Although these changes clearly reflect the severity and duration of disease, they do not correlate well with clinical manifestations or outcome.

DIFFERENTIAL DIAGNOSIS

The differential diagnosis of MN before biopsy is the differential diagnosis of idiopathic nephrotic syndrome (see Chapter 19) and includes minimal change/FSGS, membranoproliferative glomerulonephritis types I and II, and dysproteinemias such as amyloid and light chain deposition disease. The pathogenetic antibody is not known (and is likely to be present in the circulation only intermittently anyway), and so there are no laboratory tests that establish the diagnosis.

An outline of appropriate studies to perform in patients with known or suspected MN was presented in Table 22.2.

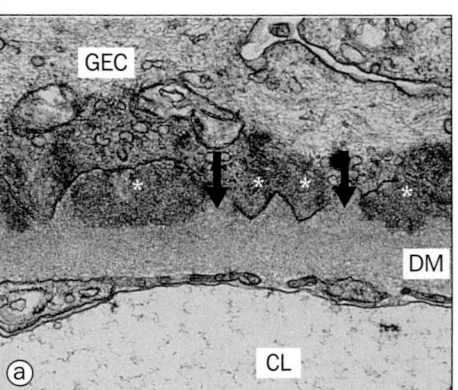
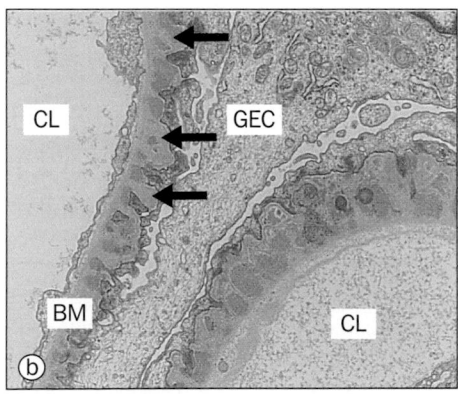
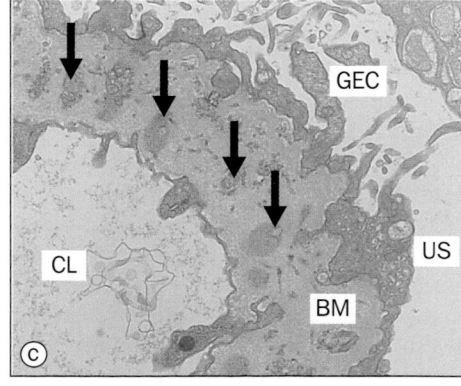

Figure 22.5 Electron microscopy in membranous nephropathy (MN). (a) Early (stage II) disease: glomerular capillary wall with discrete electron-dense deposits on the subepithelial surface of the basement membrane (BM) corresponding to granular deposits of IgG detected by immunofluorescence microscopy (corresponding to the light micrograph in Fig. 22.3b). There are diffuse, granular immune-complex deposits (asterisks) along the outer surface of the capillary wall with effacement of overlying glomerular epithelial cell (GEC) foot processes. Small extensions of BM between deposits (arrows) are also evident and represent the projections that are seen as spikes by light microscopy with silver–methenamine staining. (b) More advanced disease (stage III): two glomerular capillary loops showing involvement of the BM by the immune-complex deposition. There is prominent membrane synthesis surrounding and incorporating these deposits into the BM (corresponding to the spikes seen on silver-stained histologic preparations). Overlying cells continue to demonstrate widespread effacement of foot processes. (c) Morphologically advanced MN (stage IV): the capillary BM is diffusely thickened; scattered electron-dense immune deposits (arrows) are present throughout its thickness in addition to scattered subepithelial deposits. Overlying GECs continue to demonstrate effacement of foot processes. CL, capillary lumen; US, urinary space (original magnifications ×18 000). (Courtesy of CE Alpers.)

The presence of hypocomplementemia is more suggestive of MN associated with lupus or HBV. MN is rare in children as a cause of idiopathic nephrotic syndrome (< 5%) but is the most common cause in adults over 50 years, particularly in Caucasian patients. It is generally associated with lower levels of protein excretion than usually seen in minimal change disease, averaging about 10 g/day, and less hypertension than in focal glomerular sclerosis or membranoproliferative glomerulonephritis[1,2]. However, a definitive diagnosis can only be made with a diagnostic renal biopsy, which is indicated in all patients with idiopathic nephrotic syndrome.

Once the diagnosis has been established, it is mandatory to look for other causes of MN: particularly hepatitis B, systemic lupus, and malignancy (see Table 22.1). These disorders can usually be excluded by appropriate clinical and serologic evaluation.

NATURAL HISTORY AND PROGNOSIS

Before considering approaches to therapy, which remain controversial, it is imperative to understand the nature of untreated MN and its prognosis. Although not proven, it is likely that the onset of disease probably precedes development of overt nephrotic syndrome by weeks or months. In fact, it is probable that the period of ongoing antibody deposition that characterizes active disease has ceased in some patients by the time a diagnosis is made. This is made more likely by the observation that the fully developed lesion of MN requires weeks or months to resolve after the initiating pathogenetic process is abrogated. Therefore, the presence of severe nephrotic syndrome does not necessarily imply the presence of active immunologic disease, and the clinical course of MN in terms of proteinuria and renal function may be substantially dissociated from the initiating disease mechanism.

When MN is drug induced, the disease always resolves but can take years to do so. In idiopathic MN, spontaneous resolution occurs in over 50% of children within 5 years, and 10-year renal survival exceeds 90%. Most children and most women will experience spontaneous remissions, and disease-specific therapy is rarely indicated unless there is a documented loss of GFR[1,11]. In adult men, the prognosis is worse. Three outcomes are possible: spontaneous remission, persistent proteinuria without progression, and persistent proteinuria with progressive loss of GFR[16,17]. The approximate prevalence of each of these at various time points after diagnosis is illustrated in Figure 22.6. However, it should be emphasized that these figures were obtained before the availability of some more effective, nonspecific therapies for nephrotic patients, such as lipid-lowering agents, better blood pressure control, and treatments (e.g., ACE inhibitors) that significantly reduce protein excretion in most patients. About 25% of patients eventually have a spontaneous complete remission (normal protein excretion), usually within 3–5 years, and another 25% have partial remissions (< 2 g/day proteinuria) with persistent proteinuria but no loss of GFR. About 25% of patients who enter remission suffer a subsequent relapse of nephrotic syndrome. For patients who exhibit partial remissions or maintain normal GFR for over 3 years, the prognosis is excellent[17].

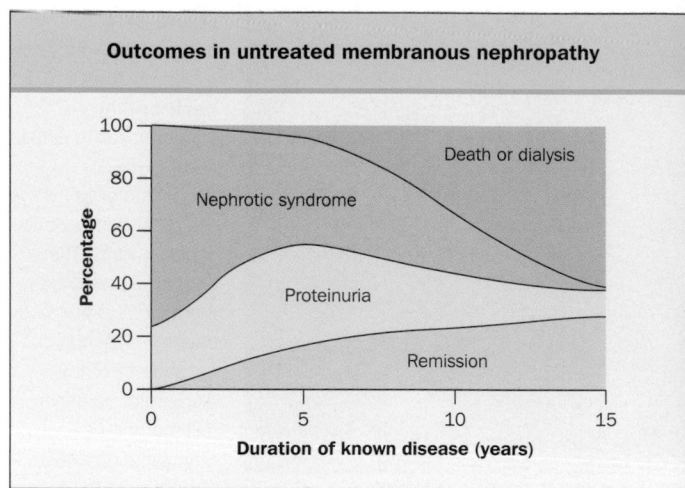

Figure 22.6 Possible outcomes in untreated membranous nephropathy. Approximate prevalence of outcomes in untreated patients with time after diagnosis. These results do not account for the likely benefits of newer nondisease-specific therapies for hypertension, elevated lipid levels, or proteinuria on the course of the disease (Adapted with permission from Cameron[16].)

However, about 50% of patients do have persistent proteinuria in the nephrotic range with a progressive course. About 15% of all patients are dead or on dialysis in about 5 years, about 35% by 10 years and over 40% at 15 years[11,17]. The mean time to doubling of serum creatinine in patients with progressive disease is about 30 months, but a subset of patients with a more rapidly progressive course can develop ESRD within 3 years or less. In this group of patients, there is an increased probability of recurrence of MN in the renal allograft. Since disease-specific therapy is generally associated with significant side effects, it is important to try to identify patients at substantial risk of progression to receive such treatment and to spare those patients who are likely to have a benign course independent of cytotoxic immunosuppressive therapy. Table 22.3 lists the factors that have been established or suggested to portend a poor prognosis in MN[18,19].

Reichert et al. have recently analyzed the literature on prognostic factors in MN and have provided estimates of the predictive value of these factors in identifying patients whose disease will subsequently progress (Table 22.3)[18]. Since the overall rate of progression in most studies is only 25–40%, it is apparent that many of these factors are not of high predictive value. Of most use is the presence of persistent proteinuria (> 8 g for over 6 months, > 6 g for over 9 months or > 4 g for over 1 year) and increased serum creatinine at the time of diagnosis or during follow-up, which documents that progression is already in progress[18]. Other variables, such as urinary excretion of IgG (an index of urine protein selectivity), β_2-microglobulin (an index of tubular function), and C5b-9 (an index of both glomerular disease and intratubular complement activation), are either too preliminary to be considered established or not readily available. Although electron microscopy staging had some predictive value in this study, most other reports have found this variable to be less useful.

Factors associated with progression of membranous nephropathy		
Factors	Predictor	Positive predictive value %
Clinical features		
Age	Older > younger	43
Sex	Male > female	30
HLA type	HLA/B18/DR 3/Bff1 present	71
Hypertension	Present	39
Serum albumin	< 1.5 g/dL	56
Serum creatinine	Above normal	61
Urine protein		
Nephrotic syndrome	Present	32
Proteinuria	> 8 g for >6 months	66
IgG excretion	> 250 mg/day	80
β_2-Microglobulin excretion	> 500 mg/min	79
C5b–9 excretion	> 7 µg/mg creatinine	67
Biopsy changes		
Focal sclerosis	Present	34
Tubulointerstitial disease	Present	48
Electron microscopy	Stages III, IV	67

Factors associated with increased likelihood of progression and their predictive value.
Positive predictive values adapted from Reichert et al.[18]

Table 22.3 Likelihood of progression of membranous nephropathy.

THERAPY

Despite the fact that MN is a relatively common glomerular disease and has been subjected to multiple controlled trials of various steroid and immunosuppressive regimens, the therapy of MN is still controversial[20–22]. Some experienced investigators advocate no disease-specific treatment because of the relatively benign course, while others treat all patients with aggressive cytotoxic drug protocols. Multiple factors complicate interpretation of such studies, including the limited number of patients or short duration of most studies, failure to measure or control for some variables that are likely to affect prognosis (Table 22.3), failure to understand other variables that are likely to be of significance such as etiologic and immunogenetic factors, and inability to incorporate the likely benefits for nephrotic patients of current nonspecific therapies such as those achieving good blood pressure control, modern lipid-lowering agents, and drugs or dietary manipulations that nonspecifically lower the level of urine protein excretion (such as protein restriction, ACE inhibitors, or angiotensin II receptor antagonists, ATRA). The therapeutic options for treating patients with MN are listed in Table 22.4.

Treatment that is not disease specific
Nondisease-specific variables have been shown to impact the prognosis of all glomerular diseases adversely, including MN. These variables include elevated blood pressure, elevated

Therapeutic options in membranous nephropathy
Nondisease-specific therapy: in all patients
Blood pressure control (125/75 mmHg): sodium restriction; drug therapy, angiotensin-converting enzyme (ACE) inhibitors or angiotensin II receptor antagonists (ATRA) preferred
Reduction in lipid levels
Reduction in urine protein excretion
Dietary protein restriction (0.8 g/kg daily): ACE inhibitors or ATRA, nonsteroidal anti-inflammatory agents (selected patients), anticoagulation (selected patients)
Disease-specific therapy: in selected patients
Low-dose steroids and cytotoxic drugs
Oral cyclophosphamide (1.5–2.0 mg/kg daily) for 6–12 months
Alternating monthly cycles of oral chlorambucil (0.1–0.2 mg/kg daily) and pulse steroids for 6 months
Possibly mycophenolate motil 1.0 g twice daily
Low-dose cyclosporine (2.5–5.0 mg/kg daily) for 12–24 months
Intravenous immunoglobulin
Therapies suitable for selected patients are discussed in the text.

Table 22.4 Therapeutic options in membranous nephropathy.

serum lipid levels, and urine protein excretion rates > 2–3 g/day (see Table 22.3).

The importance of good blood pressure control, to values of 125/75 mmHg or less, is stressed elsewhere in this book with suggested approaches to treatment (see Chapter 19). In nephrotic syndrome, sodium restriction and the use of agents that reduce intraglomerular as well as systemic blood pressure are of particular importance. Although hypertension is not a common initial sign in MN, patients who develop any degree of renal insufficiency, or patients subjected to therapy with drugs such as steroids or cyclosporine, may require careful attention to blood pressure control. Increased blood pressure increases the risk of progressive disease in MN two- or three-fold. Therefore, appropriate combinations of dietary sodium restriction, diuretics, and long-acting ACE inhibitors or ATRA are appropriate considerations for all patients[20–23].

Increased lipid levels, including total cholesterol > 220 mg/dL, low high-density-lipoprotein to low-density-lipoprotein (HDL:LDL) ratios, or LDL cholesterol above 190 mg/dL, contribute to an increased risk of coronary disease in nephrotic patients. Experimental data suggest that elevated lipids may also adversely impact renal function. Therefore, the judicious use of hydroxyglutaryl coenzyme A (CoA) reductase inhibitors (statins) is also appropriate in patients with prolonged elevations in urine protein excretion and secondary hyperlipidemia[22].

There is little question now that progression in all glomerular diseases is closely linked to the magnitude and duration of urine protein excretion, probably because of the adverse effects of proteinuria on the renal interstitium (see above)[3]. Therefore, any measures that can lower levels of proteinuria, even if independent of an effect on the underlying disease process, are likely to slow the rate of progression or perhaps even prevent progression entirely in patients with more moderate disease. Several studies have documented the benefit of moderate dietary protein restriction (usually 0.8 g/kg daily) in reducing proteinuria by 15–25% and slowing progression of renal disease, without significant side effects or adverse changes in serum protein levels, especially in patients with urinary protein excretion between 2 and 10 g/day[24]. Some clinicians advocate adding back to the diet the amount of protein excreted in the urine, but the necessity for this is not established. Similarly, it is not known at what level of hypoalbuminemia protein restriction becomes detrimental. An additional approach for reducing proteinuria in a nonspecific manner is through the effects of ACE inhibitors, or ATRA, which likely exhibit their effects primarily by altering glomerular hemodynamics. ACE inhibitors can lower protein excretion in early MN by an average of 35% without having adverse effects on blood pressure or GFR; this effect does appear to result in a clinically significant reduction in the rate of disease progression[25]. ATRA appear to achieve similar effects[23]. Some patients respond to the use of both an ACE inhibitor and an ATRA together with a further reduction in proteinuria. These agents are generally employed in long-acting form and titrated to the maximal dose that can be tolerated without adversely affecting systemic blood pressure, GFR, or serum potassium levels. They should be utilized cautiously in older patients with possible renal vascular disease or significant renal insufficiency. ACE inhibitors may require several weeks to achieve maximal effects on proteinuria, and these effects may persist for weeks or months after the drug is discontinued, suggesting an effect on nonhemodynamic variables that modulate glomerular permeability to protein.

A third approach for reducing urine protein excretion nonspecifically is by judicious use of a NSAID. Such agents should probably be employed only in patients who have not achieved a reduction in proteinuria by 40–50% with dietary protein restriction and ACE inhibitors or ATRA, and great caution should be utilized in older patients and in those with renal insufficiency, hypertension, or upper gastrointestinal symptoms, including patients receiving steroid therapy. It must be kept in mind that NSAIDs can occasionally cause renal failure and rarely cause MN (see Table 22.1). However, drugs such as indomethacin or meclofenamate can sometimes reduce protein excretion by 30–50% and have been shown to have additive effects with ACE inhibitors, sometimes achieving reductions in protein excretion of over 50%. Such a regimen is likely to be of benefit only at the expense of some reduction in GFR, although this is usually reversible upon discontinuation of the drug.

A fourth nonspecific therapy to consider is the use of oral anticoagulants in severely nephrotic patients with MN. The apparent increased risk of renal vein thrombosis and thromboembolic phenomena in these patients is discussed above. Studies now document a benefit of prophylactic anticoagulation in reducing fatal thromboembolic episodes in nephrotic patients without a concomitant excessive risk of bleeding[26]. In patients who are severely nephrotic (proteinuria of > 10 g/day and serum albumin of < 2.5 g/dL), subjected to intensive diuretic therapy, or placed at bedrest, prophylactic anticoagulant therapy should be employed if no contraindications are present.

The advent of better measures to reduce urinary protein excretion nonspecifically, as well as to control blood pressure and lipid levels, almost certainly means that the natural history of MN without disease-specific therapy is better than that discussed above or illustrated in Figure 22.6. However, there are a significant number of patients who have persistent nephrotic syndrome with progressive loss of renal function despite vigorous application of all of these nonspecific measures. These patients are candidates for treatment directed specifically at the underlying disease process.

Disease-specific therapy

As mentioned above, the selection of patients for more aggressive therapy, and the efficacy of such therapy, remain topics of significant controversy[20–22]. The authors' approach to therapy of MN is outlined in Figure 22.7 and is described at the end of this section. The following summarizes what we regard as the most salient current information in this area.

Based on several controlled studies, there is a consensus that utilization of high-dose oral steroids alone is not beneficial in MN[1,2]. A more promising approach has been the use of oral steroids combined with cytotoxic drugs. The best and most convincing studies of this approach have been those of

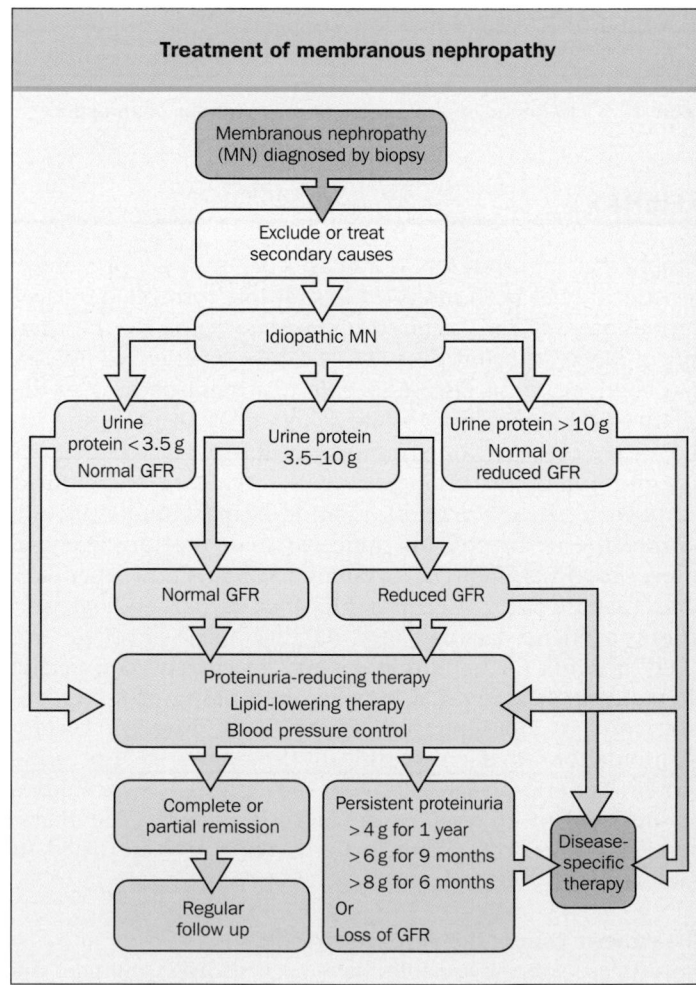

Figure 22.7 Algorithm for the treatment of membranous nephropathy. Details of possible therapies are discussed in the text.

Ponticelli and his Italian colleagues, who have employed a regimen of a 3-day course of methylprednisolone 1.0 g intravenously followed by high-dose (0.4–0.5 mg/kg daily) oral prednisone for 1 month alternating with 1 month of oral chlorambucil (0.2 mg/kg daily) for a total treatment period of 6 months[20]. After 5 years of follow-up, renal function had deteriorated in about 50% of the control group and 10% of the treated patients; progression to dialysis occurred in 4 of 39 in the control group and only 1 of 42 treated patients[27]. At 10 years, 88% of treated and only 47% of control patients had complete or partial remissions of nephrotic syndrome, and of the treated group only 8% were in renal failure compared with almost 40% of controls[21,27]. Decision analysis of these data using an average 40-year-old patient with MN suggests a reduction in quality-adjusted life expectancy of 4 years with this therapy compared with 11 years in untreated patients. The Italian group has treated all types of patients with MN, making the results even more impressive since many patients would likely have had a benign course without therapy.

Although the Ponticelli studies provide compelling evidence for the efficacy of combined steroid/cytotoxic drug therapy in MN, the protocol employed has not been widely utilized in the USA because of problems with bone marrow suppression and infection in chlorambucil-treated patients, particularly if any renal insufficiency is present. More popular has been oral cyclophosphamide, usually 1.5–2.0 mg/kg daily, in combination with low-dose prednisone (0.5 mg/kg daily), for periods of 3–6 months. This regimen has been less extensively studied than the one employed by Ponticelli, but the results have generally been favorable. Ponticelli et al. have compared chlorambucil and cyclophosphamide in their treatment regimen and found them to give comparable results[28]. In one small study of 10 treated patients with persistent nephrotic syndrome and documented loss of GFR, renal function improved in nine and daily urine protein excretion decreased from a mean of 11.9 g to 2.3 g[29]. Other small studies in high-risk patients have shown similar benefits[30,31]. Of interest, one controlled trial of intravenous cyclophosphamide in MN did not show any significant benefit. Meta-analysis of the existing literature covering the use of cytotoxic drugs in MN confirms a benefit in reducing proteinuria but not in preserving renal function, probably because of the relatively short-term nature of most such studies[32].

In the authors' judgment, the data cited above, and a host of other smaller studies, do establish a benefit of combined low-dose prednisone and cytotoxic drug therapy in preserving renal function in MN, although more and better data are clearly needed. The necessity for the steroids is unclear, although steroids alone do not appear beneficial and one study of oral cyclophosphamide without steroids also did not show a benefit. However, the benefits of current therapy are not dramatic, as they are, for example, in minimal change nephrotic syndrome, and the toxicity is significant. Therefore, it is imperative that only patients at high risk of progression should be treated and that the search continues for other more effective and less toxic alternatives.

The best-studied alternative to steroid/cytotoxic drug therapy for MN is cyclosporine, usually employed in relatively low doses of 3.5–5.0 mg/kg daily. Cyclosporine does reduce protein excretion in MN, usually by 30–50%, and some studies have reported a 60–70% rate of complete or partial remission[33,34]. The disease often relapses after short (4–6 months) courses of cyclosporine, but more prolonged courses (1–2 years) may produce more permanent remissions. In patients who do respond, a stabilization of renal function has also been reported. In the authors' judgment, cyclosporine is a second choice to cytotoxic drug therapy because of the lower incidence of complete remissions, the tendency to relapse when therapy is discontinued, the potential nephrotoxic effects of the drug itself, and the problems of hypertension and hyperkalemia encountered during treatment.

Among alternative therapies that have only preliminary data to support their use, mycophenolate mofetil (a significantly less-toxic immunosuppressive agent than cyclophosphamide or chlorambucil) may be beneficial in some patients with MN, especially patients intolerant of, or dependent on, cyclophosphamide or cyclosporine[35,36]. One study has reported benefit from azathioprine with steroids in progressive MN, but other studies are conflicting[37]. Another therapy with some promising results is intravenous immunoglobulin. In one study, eight of nine patients had a complete or partial remission following intravenous immunoglobulin therapy, including four of five with normal GFR and three of four with some renal impairment[38]. The treatment consisted of 0.4 g/day for 3 days with three additional 3-day courses at 3-week intervals, followed by 6–9 months of 1-day courses every 3 weeks[38]. Of interest, intravenous immunoglobulin has a complement inhibitory effect as well as an effect on the humoral immune response through idiotype/anti-idiotype interactions. However, problems with intravenous immunoglobulin therapy include cost, volume expansion, and occasional occurrences of acute renal failure. Preliminary data have also suggested that pentoxyfylline, a TNF-α suppressing agent, may also reduce proteinuria in MN[39].

With the above data in mind, the author's suggested approach to the treatment of idiopathic MN is illustrated in Figure 22.7 and outlined here. Patients with less than 1 g/day of proteinuria generally have an excellent prognosis and do not require therapy, although careful follow-up to ensure that the disease is not worsening is mandatory. In patients with proteinuria of 1.0–10 g daily, there is also no compelling need to initiate disease-specific therapy if renal function is well maintained. All patients should be treated aggressively using nondisease-specific therapy, as discussed above, to control blood pressure, lower lipid levels, and reduce proteinuria by at least 50% (dietary protein restriction, ACE inhibitors and/or ATRA, and, possibly, NSAIDs if GFR is normal), and they should be followed for 6 months if GFR is stable. If there is any evidence of loss of GFR, and/or if proteinuria in excess of 8 g/day persists for over 6 months (or 6 g for over 9 months, or 4 g for over 1 year), despite maximal therapy to reduce proteinuria, then disease-specific therapy should be instituted. If initial levels of protein excretion exceed 10 g/day, other risk factors should be examined. For example, in a woman with normal GFR and normal blood pressure, a trial of nonspecific therapy is probably a reasonable initial approach. However, if the patient is male, has any reduction in GFR, or has any predictive signs of progression on biopsy such as focal glomerular sclerosis or interstitial fibrosis, disease-specific therapy is indicated if the serum creatinine is < 3.5 mg/dL. There is little evidence that disease-specific therapy is efficacious in patients with serum creatinine levels > 3.5 mg/dL. Patients being treated with steroids and immunosuppressive agents for MN should also receive full treatment to control blood pressure and lipids, and to reduce urinary protein excretion by other mechanisms.

If a course of steroid/cytotoxic drug therapy is indicated, the authors generally start with prednisone, 0.5 mg/kg daily or 1 mg/kg on alternate days, together with cyclophosphamide 1.5mg/kg daily. The patient's white blood cell count should be monitored weekly, and good hydration maintained, particularly if there is a reduction in GFR. Treatment should continue until a complete or partial remission (< 2.0 g/day proteinuria) is achieved or for up to 6 months. In patients who do not achieve a complete or partial remission on this protocol, therapy can be changed to cyclosporine 3–6 mg/kg daily for 3 months. The Ponticelli protocol of alternate monthly cycles of high-dose steroids and chlorambucil can be considered if the patient seems resistant and GFR remains above 50 mL/min. Mycophenolate mofetil would be an alternative to steroids and cyclophosphamide or chlorambucil in patients who are intolerant or resistant to these drugs, but its long-term efficacy in MN is less well established. Trials of intravenous immunoglobulin or pentoxyfylline would only be warranted in resistant patients.

In treating patients with MN, the long lag-time between successful interruption of the immune response and a corresponding reduction in urine protein excretion must be kept in mind. Adjunct therapy to be considered in patients receiving steroids and immunosuppressive drugs include co-trimoxale (trimethoprim and sulfamethoxazole) sulfa for prophylaxis against *Pneumocystis carinii* pneumonia and bisphosphonates along with calcium and vitamin D to prevent steroid-induced osteopenia.

Finally, we must always remind ourselves as nephrologists that renal replacement therapy is effective and often safer than prolonged and repeated courses of very toxic immunosuppressive medication in patients with compromised renal function who are resistant to treatment. The issue of recurrence of MN or development of *de novo* MN in renal allografts is discussed in Chapter 91.

REFERENCES

1. Cattran DC. Idiopathic membranous glomerulonephritis. Kidney Int. 2001;59:1983–94.
2. Couser WG, Alpers CE. Membranous nephropathy. In: Neilson EG, Couser WG, eds. Immunologic renal diseases, Ch. 43. Philadelphia, PA: Lippincott Williams & Wilkins; 2001:1029–36.
3. Couser WG. Pathogenesis of glomerular damage in glomerulonephritis. Nephrol Dial Transplant. 1998;13(Suppl. 1):10–15.
4. Debiec H, Guignis V, Mougenot B, et al. Antenatal membranous glomerulonephritis due to anti-neutral endopeptidase (NEP) antibodies. N Engl J Med. 2002;346:2053–60.
5. Kerjaschki D. Pathogenetic concepts of membranous glomerulopathy (MGN). J Nephrol. 2000;13(Suppl. 3):S96–100.
6. Shankland SJ, Pippin JW, Couser WG. Complement (C5b-9) induces glomerular epithelial cell DNA synthesis but not proliferation *in vitro*. Kidney Int. 1999;56:536–48.
7. Papagianni AA, Alexopoulos E, Leontsini M, Papadimitriou M. C5b-9 and adhesion molecules in human idiopathic membranous nephropathy. Nephrol Dial Transplant. 2002;17:57–63.
8. Nangaku M, Pippin J, Couser WG. C6 inhibits chronic progressive renal disease in remnant kidney rats. J Am Soc Nephrol. 2002;13:928–36.
9. US Renal Data System. USRDS 2001 Annual Data Report. Atlas of End-Stage Renal Disease in the United States. National Institutes of Health, National Institute of Diabetes and Digestive and Kidney Diseases, Bethesda, MD, 2001.
10. Zucchelli IP, Cagnoli L, Pasquali C. Clinical and morphologic evolution of idiopathic membranous nephropathy. Clin Nephrol. 1986;25:282–8.
11. Hogan SL, Muller KE, Jennette JC, Falk RJ. A review of therapeutic studies of idiopathic membranous glomerulopathy. Am J Kidney Dis. 1995;25:862–8.
12. Appel GB, Silva FG, Pirani CL, et al. Renal involvement with systemic lupus erythematosus: a study of 56 patients emphasizing histologic classification. Med (Baltimore). 1978;57:371–92.
13. Johnson RJ, Couser WG. Hepatitis B infection and renal disease: clinical, immuno-pathogenetic and therapeutic considerations. Kidney Int. 1990;37:663–76.
14. Burstein DM, Korbet SM, Schwartz MM. Membranous glomerulonephritis and malignancy. Am J Kidney Dis. 1993;22:5–17.
15. Hariharan S, Peddi VR, Savin VJ, et al. Recurrent and de novo renal diseases after renal transplantation: a report from the Renal Allograft Registry. Am J Kidney Dis. 1998;31:928–31.
16. Cameron J. Pathogenesis and treatment of membranous nephropathy. Kidney Int. 1979;15:88–103.
17. Schieppati A, Mosconi L, Perna A, et al. Prognosis of untreated patients with idiopathic membranous nephropathy. N Engl J Med. 1993;329:85–9.
18. Reichert LJM, Koene RAP, Wetzels JFM. Prognostic factors in idiopathic membranous nephropathy [editorial review]. Am J Kidney Dis. 1998;31:1–11.
19. Wu Q, Jinde K, Nishina M, et al. Analysis of prognostic predictors in idiopathic membranous nephropathy. Am J Kidney Dis. 2001;37:380–7.
20. Kincaid-Smith P. Pharmacological management of membranous nephropathy. 2002;11:149–54.
21. Ponticelli C, Passerini P. Treatment of membranous nephropathy. Nephrol Dial Transplant. 2001;16(Suppl. 5):8–10.
22. Cattran DC. Management of membranous nephropathy. Minerva Urol Nefrol. 2002;54:19–27.
23. Miyauchi N, Nakamura Y. Antiproteinuric effect of an angiotensin II receptor antagonist in membranous nephropathy. Nephrology. 2001;88:183–4.
24. Klahr S, Levey A, Beck G, et al. The effects of dietary protein restriction and blood-pressure control on the progression of chronic renal disease. N Engl J Med. 1994;330:877–84.
25. Praga M, Hernandez E, Montoyo C, et al. Long-term beneficial effects of angiotensin-converting enzyme inhibition in patients with nephrotic proteinuria. Am J Kidney Dis. 1992;20:240–8.
26. Sarasin F, Schifferli J. Prophylactic oral anticoagulation in nephrotic patients with idiopathic membranous nephropathy. Kidney Int. 1994;45:578–85.
27. Ponticelli C, Zucchelli P, Passerini P, et al. A 10-year follow up of a randomized study with methylprednisolone and chlorambucil in membranous nephropathy. Kidney Int. 1995;48:1600–4.
28. Ponticelli C, Altieri P, Scolari F, et al. A randomized study comparing methylprednisolone plus chlorambucil versus methylprednisolone plus cyclophosphamide in idiopathic membranous nephropathy. J Am Soc Nephrol. 1998;9:444–50.

29. Bruns FJ, Adler S, Fraley DS, Segel DP. Sustained remission of membranous glomerulonephritis after cyclophosphamide and prednisone. Ann Intern Med. 1991;114:725–30.

30. Branten AJ, Wetzels JF. Short- and long-term efficacy of oral cyclophosphamide and steroids in patients with membranous nephropathy and renal insufficiency; Study Group. Clin Nephrol. 2001;56:1–9.

31. Torres A, Dominguez-Gil B, Carreno A, et al. Conservative versus immunosuppressive treatment of patients with idiopathic membranous nephropathy. Kidney Int. 2002; 61:219–27.

32. Imperiale TF, Goldfarb S, Berns JS. Are cytotoxic agents beneficial in idiopathic membranous nephropathy? A meta-analysis of the controlled trials. J Am Soc Nephrol. 1995;5:1553–8.

33. Cattran DC, Appel GB, Hebert LA, et al. North American Nephrotic Syndrome Study Group. Kidney Int. 2001;59:1484–90.

34. Yao X, Chen H, Wang Q, et al. Cyclosporin A treatment for idiopathic membranous nephropathy. Chin Med J (Engl). 2001;114: 1305–8.

35. Briggs WA, Choi MJ, Scheel PJ. Successful mycophenolate mofetil treatment of glomerular disease. Am J Kidney Dis. 1998;31:213–16.

36. Choi MJ, Eustace JA, Gimenez LF, et al. Mycophenolate mofetil treatment for primary glomerular disease. Kidney Int. 2002;61:1098–108.

37. Brown JH, Douglas AF, Murphy BG, et al. Treatment of renal failure in idiopathic membranous nephropathy with azathioprine and prednisolone. Nephrol Dial Transplant. 1998;13:443–9.

38. Palla R, Cirami C, Panichi V, et al. Intravenous immunoglobulin therapy of membranous nephropathy: efficacy and safety. Clin Nephrol. 1991;35:98–102.

39. Ducloux D, Bresson-Vautrin C, Chalopin J. Use of pentoxyfylline in membranous nephropathy. Lancet. 2001;357:1672–3.

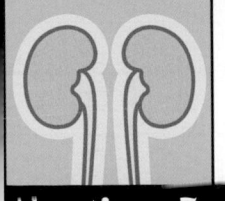

Section 5 Glomerular Disease

Chapter 23
Membranoproliferative Glomerulonephritis and Cryoglobulinemic Glomerulonephritis

F Paolo Schena, Richard J Johnson and Charles E Alpers

INTRODUCTION AND DEFINITION

Membranoproliferative glomerulonephritis (MPGN), or mesangiocapillary glomerulonephritis, is characterized by diffuse proliferative lesions and widening of the capillary loops, often with a double contoured appearance. MPGN may be primary (idiopathic) or secondary to chronic infections, cryoglobulinemia, or systemic autoimmune disorders that result in aberrant immune complex formation. Based on the histomorphological pattern, three types of MPGN can be described. Type I is defined by the presence of immune deposits in the subendothelial space (capillary wall thickening) and in the mesangium. Type II is characterized by the presence of 'dense deposits' within the mesangium and in the basement membranes of the glomeruli, tubules and Bowman's capsules. Type III, which is a variant of type I, is defined by the presence of immune deposits that are diffusely present in the subendothelium, within the glomerular basement membrane (GBM), and in the subepithelial space. This deposition process is accompanied by alterations and remodeling of the lamina densa of the basement membrane and newly elaborated lamina densa-like material.

ETIOLOGY AND PATHOGENESIS

A variety of diseases or conditions may be associated with MPGN (Table 23.1)[1]. Although frequently idiopathic, the histologic diagnosis of MPGN should provoke a search for secondary causes, including those associated with infections, cryoglobulinemia, complement abnormalities or deficiencies, malignancy, chronic liver disease, and collagen vascular diseases. In children and young adults (< 30 years) with MPGN, the disease is often associated with the presence of nephritic factors, which are IgG or IgM autoantibodies that bind to and stabilize the C3 convertase of the alternative (C3bBb), classical (C4b2b) or common pathway (Fig. 23.1), thus resulting in continued complement activation with a reduction in various complement components. In older adults (> 30 years), MPGN is frequently associated with cryoglobulinemia and hepatitis C virus (HCV) infection.

MPGN type I is most likely to occur in the setting of chronic immune-complex disease. One mechanism may be present in situations where the host defenses cannot eliminate a foreign antigen effectively despite a humoral response. This may account for the MPGN observed with chronic bloodborne viral (HCV, human immunodeficiency (HIV) and hepatitis B virus (HBV)), bacterial (endocarditis, infected ventriculoatrial shunt)

Etiology of membranoproliferative glomerulonephritis	
Type	**Secondary causes**
MPGN type I	
With mixed (type II or III) cryoglobulinemia	Hepatitis C virus (70–90% of patients) Other infections: bacterial endocarditis, chronic hepatitis B viral infection Collagen vascular disease: systemic lupus, Sjögren's syndrome Malignancy: chronic lymphocytic leukemia, nonHodgkin's lymphoma
Without cryoglobulinemia	Bacterial infections: endocarditis, abscess, infected ventriculoatrial shunt Viral infections: hepatitis B, C and G, HIV, hantavirus Malarial (*Plasmodium malariae*) Collagen vascular disease (systemic lupus, hypocomplementic urticarial vasculitis) Hereditary complement deficiency (C1q, C2, C4, or C3) Acquired complement deficiency (presence of C4 nephritic factor) Chronic liver disease (especially associated with hepatitis B or C infection, chronic schistosomal infection, with splenorenal shunt for liver fibrosis, and with α_1-antitrypsin deficiency) Sickle cell disease Malignancy: chronic lymphocytic leukemia, lymphoma, thymoma, renal cell carcinoma
MPGN type II	
Associated with C3 Nephritic factor (C3Nef)	With or without partial lipodystrophy and retinal abnormalities
Associated with factor H defect	Factor H deficiency Autoantibodies to factor H Hereditary defect
MPGN type III	
Associated with or without terminal complement nephritic factor (Nef$_t$)	Secondary causes similar to MPGN type I (hepatitis C or B, and others)

Table 23.1 Etiology of membranoproliferative glomerulonephritis.

and malarial infection (*Plasmodium malariae*). A histologic pattern resembling MPGN can also be observed in chronic immune-complex diseases associated with collagen vascular diseases (such as lupus) or with malignancy (especially chronic lymphocytic leukemia). Chronic immune-complex disease and MPGN are also more likely to occur if the host has a defect in clearing immune complexes, such as in complement deficiency or when the reticuloendothelial system is impaired, as occurs with liver or splenic disease. Hereditary deficiencies of the

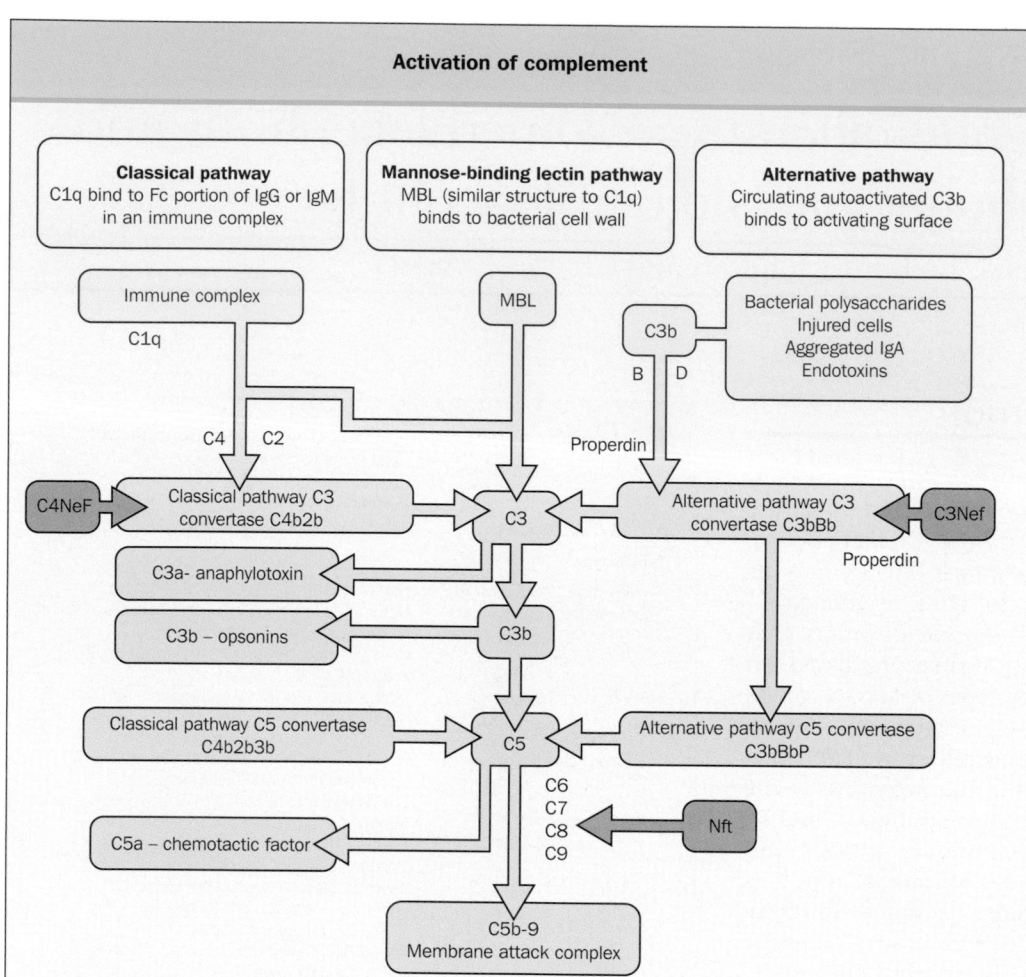

Figure 23.1 Mechanisms of activation of complement pathways including nephritic factors. See text for details.

classical pathway of complement (C1q, C2, C4) and of C3 are associated with the development of MPGN in addition to predisposing to lupus and bacterial infections. MPGN is also observed in patients with chronic liver disease, particularly associated with chronic HCV infection (HCV antigens), schistosomiasis (schistosomal antigens), α_1-antitrypsin deficiency (in which the circulating PI Z protein elicits an immune response), and with splenorenal shunts (in which there is increased exposure of enteric antigens to the circulation). Similarly, splenic dysfunction may account for decreased clearance of immune complexes and for the association of MPGN with conditions such as sickle cell disease.

The pathogenesis of MPGN type I is believed to result from the glomerular deposition of immune complexes from the circulation that preferentially localize in the mesangium and subendothelial space. Once localized, the immune complexes activate complement via the classical pathway, leading to the generation of chemotactic factors (C5a), opsonins (C3b) and the membrane attack complex (C5b–9). The hypocomplementemia is caused by activation of the classical pathway and is associated with low C3 and C4 levels. In some patients, complement is activated by the nephritic factor, C4NeF; in other cases, activation of complement may occur by the mannose-binding lectin (MBL) pathway (Fig. 23.1). MBL is a lectin that binds IgG and activates the complement pathway, and MBL has been localized to the immune deposits of some patients

with MPGN type I[2]. Complement activation results in the release of chemotactic factors that stimulates platelet and leukocyte accumulation (Fig. 23.1 and 23.2). Leukocytes release oxidants and proteases that mediate capillary wall damage and cause proteinuria and a fall in the glomerular filtration rate. Cytokines and growth factors released by both exogenous and endogenous glomerular cells lead to mesangial proliferation and matrix expansion.

The pathogenesis of MPGN type II ('dense deposit' disease) is intricately linked to continual overactivation of the alternative pathway of complement (Fig. 23.1). This can occur in humans through the dysfunction of a constitutive inhibitor (factor H) or through the presence of an IgG or IgM autoantibody (C3 nephritic factor, C3Nef) that binds the alternative pathway C3 convertase (C3bBb) and prevents its inactivation by factor H, thus resulting in continuing complement activation and consumption (Fig. 23.1). Although patients with MPGN and hereditary deficiency of factor H (from homozygous or heterozygous factor H deficiency) have been described, most patients with MPGN type II have C3Nef which has also been referred to as the nephritic factor of the amplification loop (NFa). This factor activates C3 rapidly when added to serum, does not activate terminal components, and does not require properdin. The consequence is a low C3 level in the setting of normal classical (C2 and C4) and terminal (C5–C9) components. C3c or C3d split products of C3 are present in

Pathogenesis of membranoproliferative glomerulonephritis type I

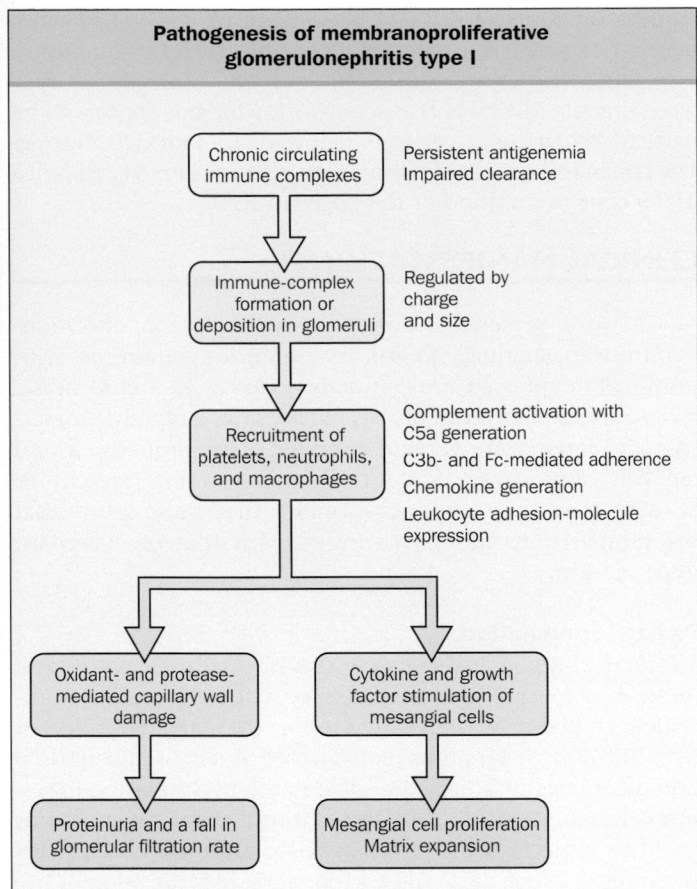

Figure 23.2 Pathogenesis of membranoproliferative glomerulonephritis type I.

Classification of cryoglobulins

Type	Composition	Associated disease
I	Monoclonal IgG, IgA, or IgM	Multiple myeloma (IgG, IgM)
		Chronic lymphocytic leukemia
		Waldenström's macroglobulinemia (IgM)
		Idiopathic monoclonal gammopathy
		Lymphoproliferative disorders
II	Polyclonal IgG and monoclonal IgM (with rheumatoid factor activity)	Hepatitis C virus
		Neoplasms: chronic lymphocytic leukemia, diffuse lymphoma, B lymphocytic neoplasia
		Essential
III	Polyclonal IgG and polyclonal IgM	Infections: viral (hepatitis B and C, Epstein–Barr virus, cytomegalovirus), bacterial (endocarditis, leprosy, poststreptococcal glomerulonephritis), parasitic (schistosomiasis, toxoplasmosis, malaria)
		Autoimmune disorders: systemic lupus erythematosus, rheumatoid arthritis, etc.
		Lymphoproliferative disorders
		Chronic liver disease
		Essential

Table 23.2 Classification of cryoglobulins.

the dense deposits. Interestingly, MPGN type II may also be associated with partial lipodystrophy which is characterized by a gradual loss of subcutaneous fat from the face and upper body, often acutely and sometimes following a viral infection such as measles. The lipodystrophy results from complement-dependent loss of the adipocyte, mediated by activation of complement on the adipocyte surface due to both the presence of C3Nef as well as to overproduction by the adipocyte of adipsin, a protein that is identical to factor D of the alternative pathway (Fig. 23.1)

The pathogenesis of MPGN type III appears to be similar to MPGN type I, except that certain characteristics of the immune complexes may also favor localization in the subepithelial space. The nephritic factor of the terminal pathway (NFt) may be present in this form. NFt activates C3 slowly, activates terminal components and requires properdin (Fig. 23.1). In addition to a depressed C3 level, there is a reduced level of properdin, depressed levels of C5, depressed levels of one or more of the other four terminal components and elevated levels of C5b-9. NFt seems to be solely responsible for hypocomplementemia in MPGN type III.

Cryoglobulinemia may also be associated with MPGN. Cryoglobulins are immunoglobulin-containing proteins that precipitate in the cold and can be categorized as type I if the immunoglobulin is monoclonal (such as in Waldenström's macroglobulinemia), type II if it consists of a monoclonal

(usually IgMk) and a polyclonal component (IgG), and type III if both antibodies are polyclonal (Table 23.2). The 'mixed' cryoglobulinemias (types II and III) are the types most commonly associated with MPGN; these have been strongly associated with chronic HCV infection in 90% and 70% of patients, respectively. The non-HCV cases have been associated with other infections (chronic HBV, bacterial endocarditis), collagen vascular diseases (systemic lupus) and other immunologic disorders (notably poststreptococcal glomerulonephritis). Chronic lymphocytic leukemia may also be associated with cryoglobulinemia or MPGN; interestingly, some of these patients are also infected with HCV and have a circulating monoclonal IgMk.

The mechanism by which chronic HCV infection causes cryoglobulinemia is not entirely known. Most patients with HCV infection and cryoglobulinemia will have an IgMk monoclonal antibody that has intrinsic rheumatoid factor activity, and this rheumatoid factor can be found with anti-HCV IgG and HCV RNA in the cryoprecipitates. It has been postulated that the IgM is produced as a consequence of dysregulation of the B cell, which can also be infected with HCV. Cryoglobulinemia does not develop until many years (> 10) after HCV infection, but by the time chronic active hepatitis or cirrhosis develop, as many as 30–40% of patients will have circulating cryoglobulins. Most of these patients will not develop renal disease, but in some patients, particularly those in which the cryoglobulins have an affinity for fibronectin, the cryoglobulins containing HCV antigens will deposit in glomeruli (Fig. 23.3)[3].

EPIDEMIOLOGY

MPGN is one of the major causes of nephrotic syndrome. In North America and Europe, MPGN characterizes 5% to 20% of all primary glomerulonephritides, although there are

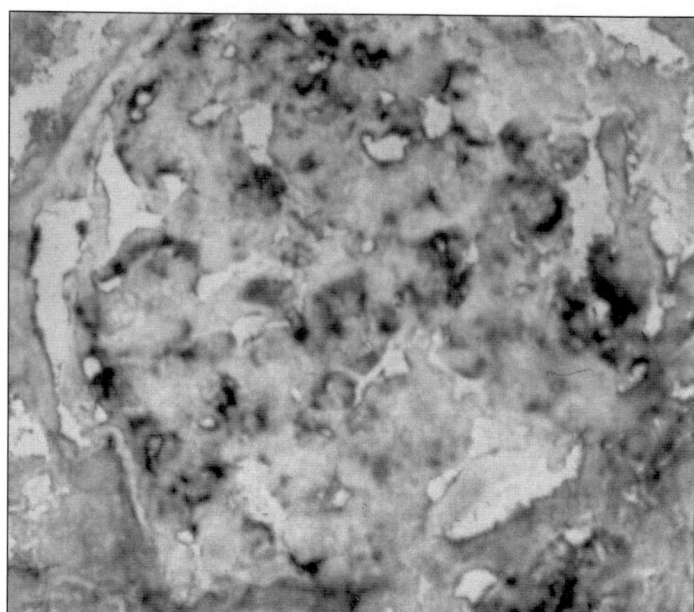

Figure 23.3 Hepatitis C-related antigen (c22–3) in the capillary wall of a glomerulus from a patient with cryoglobulinemic membranoproliferative glomerulonephritis (light microscopy × 100).

factors. By contrast, MPGN presenting in adults (typically over age 18 years) is usually type I or type III and is commonly associated with cryoglobulinemia and HCV infection. Cryoglobulinemic MPGN is also seen worldwide but appears to be particularly frequent (or well reported) in southern Europe. The Italian registry of renal biopsies reports an annual incidence of 0.9 cases per million of the population[4].

CLINICAL MANIFESTATIONS

MPGN may present as microscopic hematuria and non-nephrotic proteinuria (35%), as nephrotic syndrome with minimally depressed renal function (35%), as a chronically progressive glomerulonephritis (20%), or as a rapidly progressive and deteriorating renal function with proteinuria and red cell casts (10%). Systemic hypertension is present in 50–80% of patients and, occasionally, may be so severe that the presentation may be confused with that of malignant hypertension.

Pediatric population

MPGN in children and young adults is usually idiopathic and presents as a primary kidney disease without systemic manifestations. Recently, there was a report that Japanese children with MPGN type I who were diagnosed as a consequence of a urinalysis screening program at school had lower blood pressures, less proteinuria and less chronic renal disease compared to subjects who were diagnosed after presenting with symptoms[5]. These data suggest that early identification of the disease by urinary screening may allow for early treatment and improve the prognosis of the disease.

Twenty to 25% of patients with MPGN type II may also manifest partial lipodystrophy that preferentially involves the face and upper body (Fig. 23.4a) and, occasionally, patients with MPGN type II will have mild visual field and color defects and prolonged dark adaptation with mottled retinal pigmentation (drusen bodies) (Fig. 23.4b). Indocyanine green angiography of the retina may reveal dense deposits in the ciliary epithelial basement membrane (abnormal fluorescent dots) and choroidal neovascularization[6,7].

several reports that the incidence has decreased to 4% to 6% in the last two decades. In Asia (Saudi Arabia), South America (Peru) and Africa (Nigeria), MPGN remains one of the most common causes of nephrotic syndrome and may account for 30–40% of all cases because of the association of chronic infections with type I MPGN.

The disease may be familial in rare cases and different histological lesions may occur in family members (i.e., type I in one member and type III in another).

MPGN occurs equally in males and females and in the USA is relatively more common in Caucasians than in African Americans. Two distinct presentations of MPGN are particularly common. MPGN presenting in childhood (primarily between age 8 and 14 years) includes all three types of MPGN and is frequently idiopathic or associated with nephritic

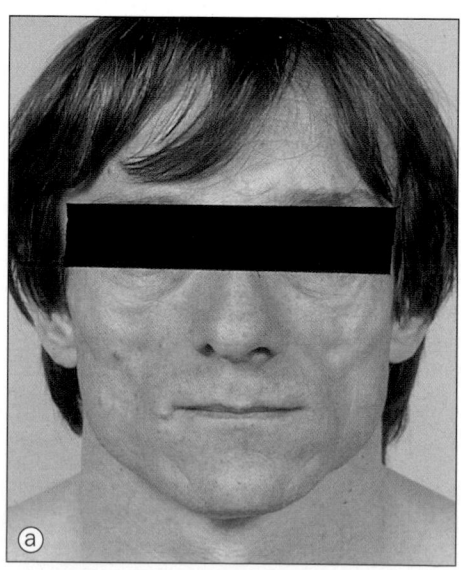

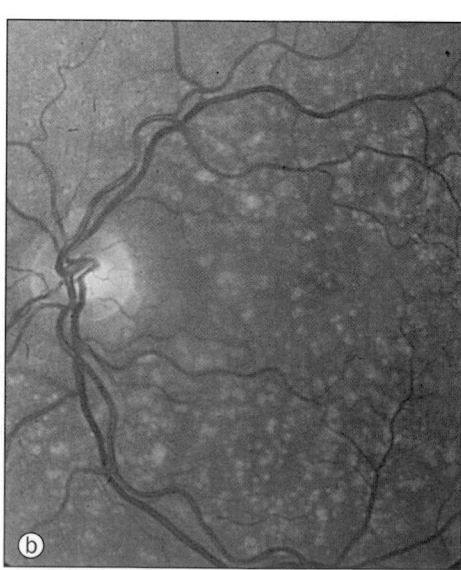

Figure 23.4 Membranoproliferative glomerulonephritis type II. (a) Partial lipodystrophy; note the absence of subcutaneous fat from the face. (b) Drusen bodies in the retina. (Courtesy of Dr C D Short.)

(a)

(b)

Adult population

MPGN in adults is also often limited to the kidney in its presentation but occasionally can be associated with systemic cryoglobulinemia. These patients, who usually have chronic HCV infection, may present with the triad of weakness, arthralgias and purpura. The arthralgias are only rarely accompanied by arthritis, are usually symmetric, and classically involve the knees, hips and shoulders. The purpura (Fig. 23.5) is usually painless, palpable, nonpruritic, occurs in 'crops' that last 4–10 days, and preferentially localizes to the extremities. Other manifestations may include ulcerative, vasculitic lesions that classically involve the lower extremities (Fig. 23.5) and buttocks (Fig. 23.6), Raynaud's phenomenon, digital necrosis (Fig. 23.7), peripheral neuropathy, hepatomegaly, and, rarely, signs of cirrhosis (clubbing, spider angiomata, ascites). Although most patients with cryoglobulinemia have a chronic waxing and waning course, occasionally patients may have a more fulminant presentation, with congestive heart failure (from an HCV-induced cardiomyopathy), nodular infiltrates in the lung from deposition of cryoglobulins (Fig. 23.8), pulmonary hypertension, severe systemic hypertension, or mesenteric ischemia[8].

In view of the conditions associated with MPGN (Table 23.1), signs of bacterial infection (endocarditis, dental and visceral abscess), viral infection (HCV, HBV and HIV), systemic lupus, malignancy (especially chronic lymphocytic leukemia) and chronic liver disease should be sought.

Laboratory findings

MPGN is associated with depressed complement levels (C3 and total hemolytic complement (CH_{50})), although complement levels may be normal. In type I MPGN, and in cryoglobulinemic MPGN, the classical pathway is preferentially activated (normal or low C3, low C4, and low CH_{50}); in

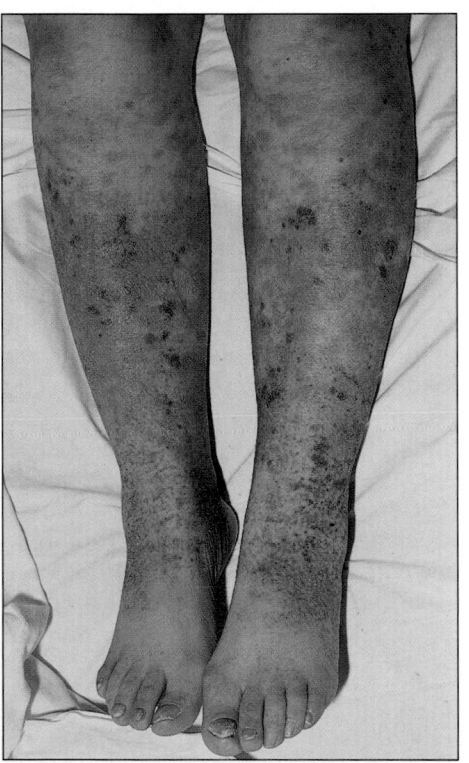

Figure 23.5 Purpura in a patient with hepatitis C-associated cryoglobulinemia. Raised purpuric lesions are present on the legs of this individual. The differential diagnosis of purpura and renal disease includes cryoglobulinemia, Henoch–Schönlein purpura, vasculitis and endocarditis.

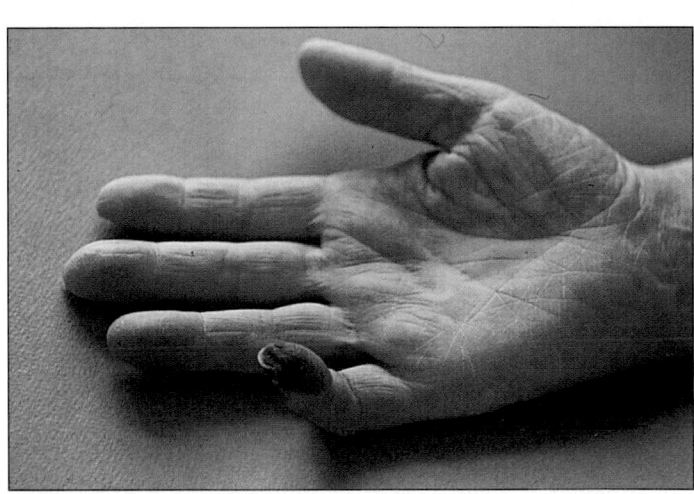

Figure 23.7 Necrosis of the distal portion of the little finger in a young woman with essential mixed cryoglobulinemia.

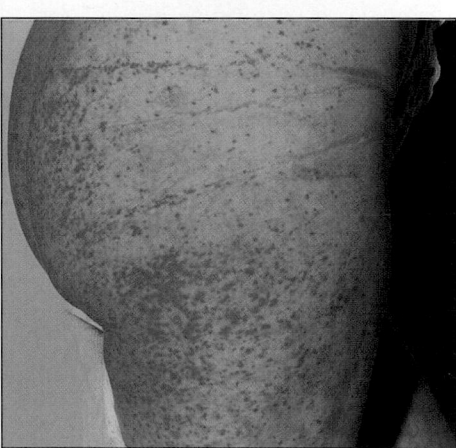

Figure 23.6 Purpura in a patient with hepatitis C-associated cryoglobulinemia. Purpuric lesions are present on the buttocks and thigh of the patient. Interestingly note the presence of purpuric lesions along the superior and inferior elastic border of the undergarment line.

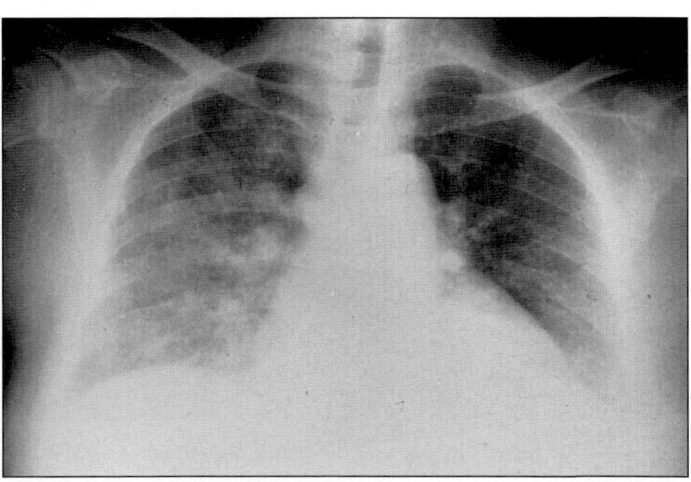

Figure 23.8 Chest radiograph showing nodular infiltrate in the lung secondary to cryoglobulinemic vasculitis in a patient with hepatitis C infection.

Glomerular Disease

MPGN type II the alternative pathway is activated (low C3, normal C4 and low CH_{50}); and in type III, C3 is generally low in association with a depression of terminal complement components (C5–C9)[9]. C3Nef activity is usually detected in plasma by the hemolytic test or the C3 NeF IgG solid phase assay[10]. The presence of rheumatoid factors or cryoglobulins should prompt testing for anti-HCV antibody (second- or third-generation enzyme immunoassay) and HCV RNA (by polymerase chain reaction (PCR) or branch chain DNA methodology). However, MPGN can be associated with HCV infection in the absence of cryoglobulinemia or rheumatoid factors[11]. Failure to detect the cryoglobulins may result from improper handling of specimens or occur because the cryo-globulinemia was transient; however, in some patients (especially in renal transplant recipients) tests for cryoglobulinemia may be persistently negative. Clinical or laboratory evidence of liver disease should prompt a search for causes of chronic liver disease, including HCV, HBV and, if appropriate, rare entities such as schistosomiasis or α_1-antitrypsin deficiency.

PATHOLOGY

MPGN is diagnosed by renal biopsy. By light microscopy, MPGN type I is classically described as hypercellular owing to both the influx of circulating leukocytes and intrinsic glomerular cell proliferation (typically mesangial cells), leading to a lobular appearance in some cases (Fig. 23.9a). Accumulation of extracellular material, predominantly matrix, contributes to the mesangial expansion that occurs in most cases of MPGN. The proportion of cells to matrix may change during the evolution of the disease process. This results in glomerular appearances that can range from markedly hypercellular to predominantly sclerotic, which, in the latter case in its most advanced form, can be manifest as nodules of accumulated mesangial matrix indistinguishable from the nodular mesangial sclerosis of severe diabetic nephropathy. Using the methenamine silver stain, which stains glyco-proteins within the GBM, a double contouring of the GBM can often be appreciated ('tram tracks') as a result of the inter-position of mesangial cells, leukocytes and/or endothelial

cells in the capillary wall with the synthesis of new basement membrane material (Fig. 23.10). Monocytes and macrophages are also commonly present in the glomerulus and the peri-glomerular areas[12]. Type II MPGN is characterized by dense deposits within the mesangium and the basement membranes of the glomeruli, tubules and Bowman's capsules, often visible with conventional eosin and periodic acid–Schiff (PAS) stains. The hallmark of type III MPGN is the inter-ruption of lamina densa associated with subendothelial and subepithelial deposits, often confluent, and interspersed with multilayers of new lamina densa. However, cases of type I and type III MPGN may form a morphologic continuum and thus not always be separable.

Immunofluorescence in type I and type III MPGN frequently shows the deposition of IgM, IgG and C3 in a granular capillary wall distribution (Fig. 23.9b), although the immunoglobulin deposits may be scant. Staining for C3 in a peripheral (lobular) pattern involving capillary walls and mesangial areas is the most constant and strongest, while staining for classical complement components (C1q, C4) may also be seen in MPGN type I. In contrast, in MPGN type II, the immunofluorescence pattern is positive for C3 but is negative for both classical complement components and for immunoglobulins. The absence of staining for immunoglobu-lin is a critical feature of type II MPGN that helps to distinguish it from other types of injury with an MPGN pattern. The C3 stain binds to the surface of the dense deposits and occasion-ally gives an appearance of 'tram tracks' or 'mesangial rings'.

By electron microscopy, discrete immune deposits can be observed in the subendothelial portions of the capillary walls and mesangial regions in type I MPGN, often in association with platelet and leukocyte infiltration (Fig. 23.9c). The deposits are often discrete, but may be confluent in their involvement of the capillary wall. They can be small and sparse, or large and numerous such that they are visible by light microscopy. In addition, a separation of the endothelium from the GBM can occasionally be observed, usually with some synthesis of new basement membrane material under the endothelial cells that have become detached from the original basement membrane. Between these layers (old and new) of

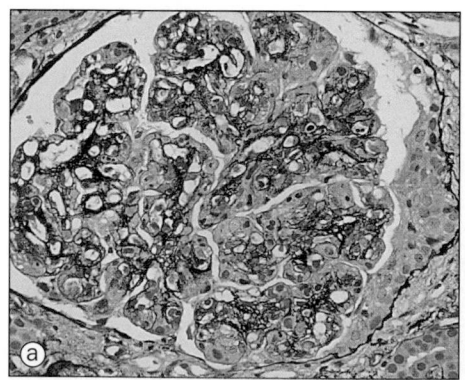
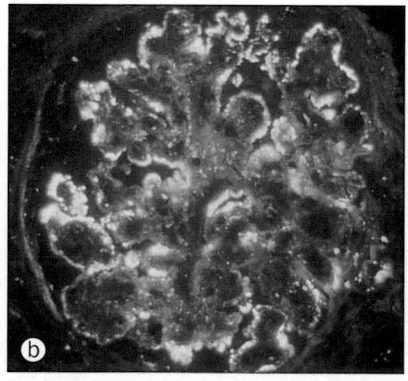
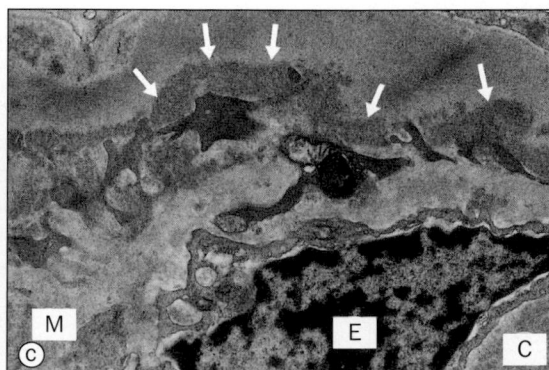

Figure 23.9 Pathology of membranoproliferative glomerulonephritis type I. (a) Light microscopy shows a hypercellular glomerulus with accentuated lobular architecture and a small cellular crescent (methenamine silver). (b) Immunofluorescence usually shows discrete, granular staining of the peripheral capillary wall for immunoglobulin (Ig)G (seen here) and C3, and occasionally for IgM and earlier complement components (C1q and C4). (c) By electron microscopy, numerous subendothelial deposits are observed (arrows) between the duplicated basement membrane; these deposits extend into the mesangium (M). (C, capillary lumen; E, endothelial cell nucleus).

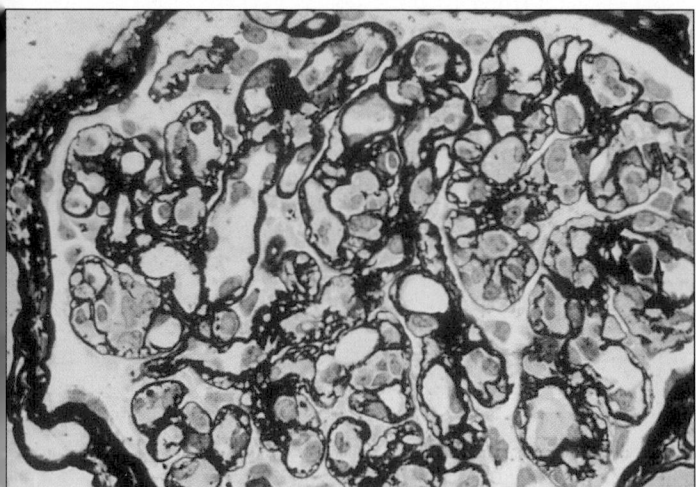

Figure 23.10 'Tram tracks' in membranoproliferative glomerulonephritis type I. By silver stain, a double contouring of the glomerular basement membrane can be observed in MPGN type I, resembling 'tram tracks'.

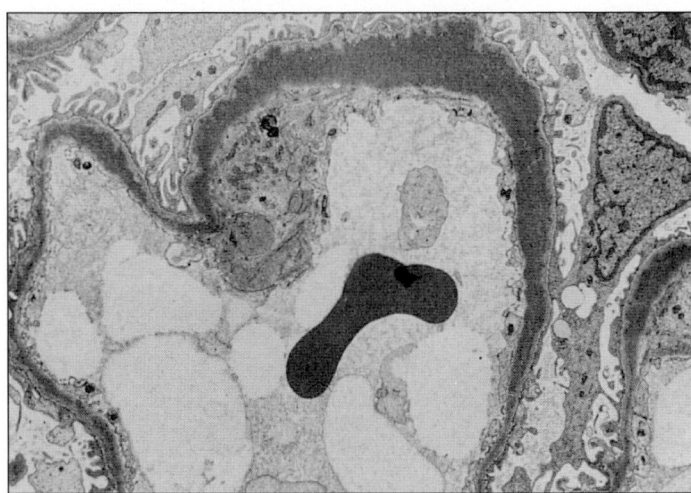

Figure 23.11 Electron microscopy of membranoproliferative glomerulonephritis type II. Dense material replaces sections of the glomerular basement membrane.

basement membranes interposed cells of mesangial, endothelial, or leukocyte origin may be found, as well as immune deposits and matrix. In contrast, in MPGN type II, electron microscopy shows replacement of large sections of the GBM with an extremely electron dense band of homogenous material (Fig. 23.11). Sometimes, the deposits are relatively small and irregularly distributed. Involvement of mesangial regions, Bowman's capsules, and tubular basement membranes by the deposits is common. Perhaps 15% of cases of MPGN demonstrate both subendothelial and subepithelial deposits that are associated with minute disruptions of the lamina densa and newly elaborated lamina densa-like material (type III MPGN). After a number of years of normocomplementemia, the type III lesions can also disappear but there is no evidence that this will inevitably occur[13].

Cryoglobulinemic MPGN may appear histologically identical to MPGN type I by light, immunofluorescence, and electron microscopy. However, the cryoprecipitates can occasionally be observed by light microscopy as intracapillary hyaline-like deposits, and there is often a more pronounced infiltration of macrophages within capillary lumina. Electron microscopy may also show the highly organized tubular or finely fibrillar structures consisting of the precipitated cryoglobulins (Fig. 23.12).

Certain histologic features carry prognostic relevance. For example, the presence of cellular crescents can be associated with a rapidly progressive course and worse prognosis. In addition, the degree of tubulointerstitial damage may be the best predictor of both the current renal function and the long-term prognosis.

DIAGNOSIS AND DIFFERENTIAL DIAGNOSIS

MPGN is diagnosed by renal biopsy in patients presenting with nephrotic or non-nephrotic proteinuria, especially when accompanied by microhematuria. The light microscopic finding of a hypercellular, lobulated glomerulus with an increase

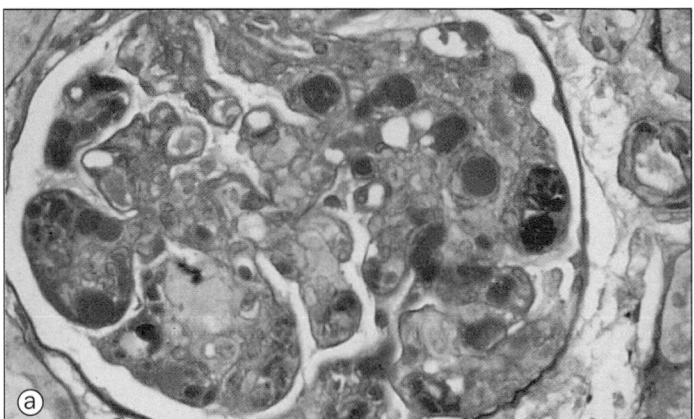

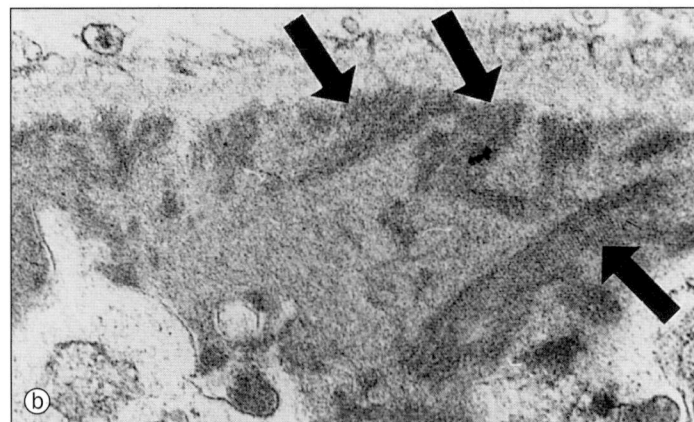

Figure 23.12 Pathology of cryoglobulinemic membranoproliferative glomerulonephritis. (a) Although cryoglobulinemic MPGN may histologically appear similar to MPGN type I (Fig. 23.9), occasionally discrete precipitates of cryoglobulins may be found occluding individual capillary loops. (Reproduced with permission[6].) (b) In addition, electron microscopy shows organized fibrillar or tubular structures consistent with cryoglobulins (arrows). (Reproduced with permission from the New England Journal of Medicine, Johnson et al., 1993;328:465–70. Massachusetts Medical Society, all rights reserved.)

Glomerular Disease

Diseases that histologically resemble membranoproliferative glomerulonephritis
Paraproteinemias: especially fibrillary glomerulonephritis, light chain nephropathy
Thrombotic microangiopathies: hemolytic uremic syndrome, scleroderma, radiation nephropathy, malignant hypertension
Hepatic glomerulosclerosis
Postinfectious glomerulonephritis
'Transplant' glomerulopathy
Rare diseases: collagen III glomerulopathy, C1q nephropathy, lipoprotein nephropathy

Table 23.3 Diseases that histologically resemble membranoproliferative glomerulonephritis.

in mesangial matrix should suggest a diagnosis of MPGN, but other entities may appear histologically similar, including poststreptococcal glomerulonephritis, the thrombotic micro-angiopathies, paraproteinemias, fibrillary glomerulonephritis, and several rare diseases (Table 23.3). Immunofluorescence and electron microscopy is critical for separating these diseases. The finding of IgG, C3 and C4 by immunofluorescence and subendothelial immune deposits by electron microscopy should limit the diagnosis to either MPGN type I or systemic lupus; the latter can be largely eliminated by serologic (antinuclear and anti-double-stranded DNA antibody) testing.

Other useful tests are serum C3, C4 and CH_{50} levels. Low complement levels can also be observed in atheroembolic renal disease (low C3 with eosinophilia), in thrombotic micro-angiopathy, in chronic liver disease (because of decreased synthesis) and in several glomerular diseases including lupus (low C3 and C4) and poststreptococcal glomerulonephritis (low C3). The detection of C3NeF activity in plasma suggests the presence of MPGN type II.

Once MPGN is diagnosed, careful evaluation for secondary causes should be conducted (see Chapter 28). Bacterial infection should be suspected in patients with fever or ventriculo-atrial shunts, and blood or other appropriate cultures should be obtained. Chronic infection from HCV, HBV and HIV should be ruled out by testing for anti-HCV antibody (enzyme immunoassay), HBsAg, and HIV antibody. Chronic malarial infection should be suspected in patients from West Africa where *P. malariae* (the Plasmodium species associated with MPGN) is endemic. The finding of an absent CH_{50} should suggest a hereditary deficiency in a complement component.

NATURAL HISTORY

Idiopathic MPGN in childhood has a relatively poor prognosis, with 40–50% of untreated patients progressing to renal failure over 10 years. Risk for progression is greater for those presenting with an elevated creatinine, nephrotic proteinuria, a renal biopsy showing > 50% crescents or marked interstitial fibrosis, or severe hypertension. Renal failure may also be more likely to develop in patients with type II MPGN[14].

Idiopathic MPGN in adults also carries an unfavorable prognosis because, 5 years after biopsy, 50% of patients either die

or need renal replacement therapy (dialysis or transplant). This proportion increases to 64% after 10 years[15]. The unfavorable outcome appears to be influenced by the severity of the tubulointerstitial lesions and interstitial fibrosis.

TRANSPLANTATION

MPGN recurs in renal transplant recipients with a frequency of 20–30% in type I and 80–90% in type II and type III. Although the disease is often milder, it is associated with a reduced graft survival and may warrant treatment (see Chapter 91). In patients in which MPGN recurs, there is a high frequency that it will recur with a second or third transplant. It is important to distinguish MPGN in the transplant patient from transplant glomerulopathy, which has identical features by light microscopy. MPGN is associated with immune deposits of IgG, IgM and C3 (MPGN types I and III) or C3 (type II) and with immune deposits or dense deposits, respectively, by electron microscopy. In contrast, transplant glomerulopathy is not associated with immune deposits, but rather by lifting of the endothelium with the accumulation of flocculent material in the subendothelial space[16]. Diagnosing MPGN is important, as the relative risk of graft failure is double in patients with recurrent or *de novo* MPGN. Furthermore, anecdotal reports suggest that the immunosuppressive medications should be modified to include cyclophosphamide while continuing calcineurin inhibitors and prednisone[17].

HCV-associated MPGN can also occur *de novo* or recur in renal transplant recipients and has also been observed in HCV-infected patients after liver transplantation. In these patients, marked proteinuria and reduced renal function appear, and interestingly, cryoglobulinemia is frequently absent and complement levels may be normal. Treatment with interferon (IFN)-α may reverse renal dysfunction and stabilize proteinuria but is not recommended because it may occasionally precipitate rejection.

TREATMENT

The initial treatment plan in MPGN is based on identifying the etiology, if possible, and on general supportive measures to reduce proteinuria and control blood pressure (see Chapters 18 and 19). Treatment plans for the various types of MPGN are discussed below (Table 23.4).

Idiopathic disease in childhood
Some studies that primarily used historical or nonrandomized controls have shown a beneficial role of alternate day steroids in childhood MPGN, particularly if administered within the first year of presentation[18]. While this data is not definitive, we recommend an initial treatment approach using alternate day steroids in this population. For children with MPGN with moderate proteinuria (< 3 g/day), and normal renal function, we administer prednisone (40 mg/m² on alternate days) for 3 months. In patients with nephrotic syndrome and/or impaired renal function, the high dose of steroids is administered for 2 years (40 mg/m² on alternate days). In case of benefit, prednisone is tapered to a maintenance dose of 20 mg on alternate days for 3–10 years[18].

Suggested management of membranoproliferative glomerulonephritis	
Type	**Treatment**
Idiopathic MPGN in children	Mild proteinuria, normal renal function: follow with 3-month visits
	Normal renal function and moderate proteinuria (<3 g/day): prednisone 40 mg/m² on alternate days for 3 months
	Nephrotic or impaired renal function: prednisone 40 mg/m² on alternate days (80 mg maximum) for 2 years, tapering to 20 mg on alternate days for 3–10 years
	In the presence of chronic renal failure: ACE inhibitors
Idiopathic MPGN in adults	Non-nephrotic, normal renal function: follow with 3-month visits
	Nephrotic or impaired renal function: 6-month course of corticosteroid with/without cytotoxic agents
	Rapidly progressive renal failure with diffuse crescents: treat as for idiopathic rapidly progressive glomerulonephritis (see Chapter 26)
	In the presence of chronic renal failure or nephrotic proteinuria: ACE inhibitors
MPGN associated with hepatitis C or cryoglobulinemia	Non-nephrotic, normal renal function: treat with interferon-α based on severity of liver disease (diagnosed by biopsy)
	Nephrotic syndrome, reduced renal function, or signs of cryoglobulinemia: interferon-α 3 mU three times a week and ribavirin (15 mg/kg/day) for 6 months, followed by a short-term course of corticosteroids at low dosage; if relapse occurs, consider high dose interferon-α (10 mU daily for 2 weeks, then every alternate day for 6 more weeks)
	Rapidly progressive renal failure or severe symptoms of vasculitis (heart failure, pulmonary disease): methylprednisolone 1 g intravenous daily for 3 days, followed by oral prednisone 60 mg daily with slow taper over 2–3 months
	Cyclophosphamide (2 mg/kg/day with adjustment for renal function) and cryofiltration may be added as adjunctive therapy. When the prednisone is reduced to 20 mg/day and the cyclophosphamide is discontinued, add interferon-α
	MPGN in the renal or liver transplant recipient: consider course of oral ribavirin (0.6–1.0 g/day)

Table 23.4 Suggested management of membranoproliferative glomerulonephritis.

Treatment may be associated with a reduction in hematuria (80%), proteinuria (remitting in 25–40%) and better preservation of renal function (80% at 10 years versus 50% in historical controls). The most important side effects are exacerbation of hypertension, growth retardation, weight gain, and obesity. If no benefit is seen after 1 year of treatment, conservative therapy may be undertaken with withdrawal of the steroids and with treatment solely aimed at controlling blood pressure and reducing proteinuria with angiotensin converting enzyme (ACE) inhibitors. A recent study suggests that the response to alternate day steroids is superior in children with type I MPGN, whereas children with type III MPGN are more likely to have a progressive reduction in renal function, slower reduction of serum C3, more persistent urinary abnormalities and more frequent relapses[19].

Idiopathic disease in adults

For patients with normal renal function and asymptomatic non-nephrotic range proteinuria, no specific therapy is necessary. Close follow-up every 3–4 months is recommended[18]. In patients with nephrotic syndrome and normal or impaired renal function, a 6-month course of corticosteroids (prednisone 1 mg/kg body weight per day) may be prescribed. If there is considerable reduction of proteinuria, corticosteroids may be continued at the minimal effective dose. If no response is observed within 4–6 months, corticosteroids should be stopped and conservative therapy is recommended. The administration of ACE inhibitors or angiotensin receptor antagonists (ATRAs) should also be used to reduce proteinuria. Antiplatelet agents have also been used to treat MPGN in adults[20]; however, a reanalysis of the original trial suggests that it may not provide real benefit[21].

HCV-associated disease and cryoglobulinemia

HCV-associated cryoglobulinemic MPGN has been treated with interferon-α (3 million U three times weekly for 6–12 months) and while clinical remission is achieved in approximately 60% of patients, relapse occurs in nearly 100% of subjects within 3–6 months[11]. Recently, several controlled trials have demonstrated that a combined therapy with interferon-α and ribavirin is superior in the treatment of chronic HCV hepatitis, especially in the presence of high levels of viremia, such as is frequent in patients with cryoglobulinemia[22]; there is also evidence that this combination may attenuate the clinical manifestations of mixed cryoglobulinemia and reduce cryoglobulin production. Therefore, in patients with chronic low-grade HCV associated MPGN or cryoglobulinemic MPGN, antiviral treatment with interferon-α (3 million U three times weekly) and ribavirin (15 mg/kg/day) for 6 months followed by a short-term course of corticosteroids at low dosage is recommended[23]. However, ribavirin may be associated with the development of hemolysis, and its toxicity is increased in the setting of renal insufficiency. Therefore, alternative regimens may also be considered. For example, a prolonged course of high dose interferon-α has been used in some patients with significant success. This may be particularly useful in patients with persistent hypocomplementemia, cryoglobulinemia and nephrotic syndrome, in which a course of high dose interferon-α (10 million U/day for 2 weeks) followed by 10 million U three times a week for an additional 6 weeks may result in negative HCV RNA and cryoglobulins, normal complement levels and remission of the nephrotic syndrome[24]. However, interferon-α at high dose may be associated with unacceptable side-effects, including severe influenza-like symptoms, depression or psychosis, the development of hypothyroidism and, rarely, the development of proteinuria (with a minimal change type of lesion).

Recently, cryofiltration has been introduced as a means to remove cryoglobulins. Cryofiltration utilizes double filtration plasmapheresis with a cooling unit, and is an online technique to remove cryoglobulins. The combination of cryofiltration and interferon-α with corticosteroids may be effective. For example, when the patient is elderly and infection is caused by HCV genotype Ib (which is more resistant to interferon-α), cryofiltration and low doses of oral corticosteroids may improve proteinuria and renal function without adverse effects. The addition of cryofiltration can remove cryoglobulins to an undetectable level. This combination therapy can reduce proteinuria and prevent the progressive deterioration of renal function, but the major adverse effects of this therapy are represented by bleeding and myelosuppression[24].

In patients with acute exacerbation and/or rapidly progressive MPGN, the initial treatment is represented by corticosteroids (methylprednisolone 1 g i.v. daily for 3 days followed by oral prednisone 60 mg daily with slow tapering over 2–3 months) and cytotoxic drugs (cyclophosphamide 2 mg/kg/day with adjustment for renal function) followed by the above antiviral therapy[14]. Acute oliguric renal failure may also be reversed by cryofiltration and oral administration of prednisolone. Finally, splenectomy may be considered when liver cirrhosis and pancytopenia secondary to splenomegaly are present.

Other types of MPGN

MPGN associated with infections other than HCV is discussed in Chapter 28. MPGN associated with α_1-antitrypsin deficiency has been reported to be cured by liver transplantation, which cures the genetic defect. MPGN associated with malignancy generally responds to effective treatment of the underlying cancer.

REFERENCES

1. Rennke HG. Secondary membranoproliferative glomerulonephritis (clinical conference). Kidney Int. 1995;47:643–56.
2. Lhotta K, Würzner R, König P. Glomerular deposition of mannose-binding lectin in human glomerulonephritis. Nephrol Dial Transplant. 1999;14:881–6.
3. Fornasieri A, Armelloni S, Bernasconi P, et al. High binding of immunoglobulin M kappa rheumatoid factor from type II cryoglobulins to cellular fibronectin: a mechanism for induction of in situ immune complex glomerulonephritis? Am J Kidney Dis. 1996;27:476–83.
4. Schena FP and the Italian Group of Renal Immunopathology. Survey of the Italian Registry of Renal Biopsies. Frequency of the renal diseases for 7 consecutive years. Nephrol Dial Transplant. 1997;12: 418–26.
5. Kawasaki Y, Suzuki J, Nozawa R, Suzuki H. Efficacy of school urinary screening for membranoproliferative glomerulonephritis type I. Arch Dis Child. 2002;86:21–5.
6. Kim RY, Faktorovich EG, Kuo CY, Olson JL. Retinal function abnormalities in membranoproliferative glomerulonephritis type II. Am J Opthalmol. 1997;123:619–28.
7. Parrat E, Arndt CF, Labalette P, et al. Retinochoroidal involvement of type II membranoproliferative glomerulonephritis. An angiographic study with indocyanine green. J Fr Ophtalmol. 1997;20: 430–8.
8. Johnson RJ, Alpers CE, Gretch D, et al. Renal diseases and the liver. In: Gitlin N, ed. Liver and systemic disease. Edinburgh: Churchill Livingstone; 1997:43–58.
9. Jelezarova E, Schlumberger M, Sadallah S, et al. A C3 convertase assay for nephritic factor functional activity. J Immunol Meth. 2001;251:45–52.
10. Schwertz R, Rother U, Anders D, et al. Complement analysis in children with idiopathic membranoproliferative glomerulonephritis: a long-term follow-up. Pediatr Allergy Immunol. 2001;12:166–72.
11. Johnson RJ, Gretch DR, Couser WG, et al. Hepatitis C virus-associated glomerulonephritis. Effect of alpha-interferon therapy. Kidney Int. 1994;46:1700–4.
12. Gesualdo L, Grandaliano G, Ranieri E, et al. Monocyte recruitment in cryoglobulinemic membranoproliferative glomerulonephritis: a pathogenetic role for monocyte chemotactic peptide-I. Kidney Int. 1997;51:155–63.
13. West CD, McAdams AJ. Membranoproliferative glomerulonephritis type III: association of glomerular deposits with circulating nephritic factor-stabilized convertase. Am J Kidney Dis. 1998;32: 56–63

14. Cameron JS, Turner DR, Heaton J, et al. Idiopathic mesangiocapillary glomerulonephritis: comparison of types I and II in children and adults and long-term prognosis. Am J Med. 1983;74:175–90.
15. Schmitt H, Bohle A, Reincke T, et al. Long-term prognosis of membranoproliferative glomerulonephritis type I. Significance of clinical and morphological parameters: an investigation of 220 cases. Nephron. 1990;55:242–50.
16. Andreosdottir MB, Assmann KJM, Koene RAP, Wetzels JFM. Immunohistological and ultrastructural differences between recurrent type I membranoproliferative glomerulonephritis and chronic transplant glomerulopathy. Am J Kidney Dis. 1998;32: 582–8.
17. Hariharan S, Adams MB, Brennan DC, et al. Recurrent and de novo glomerular disease after renal transplantation. Transplant. 1999;68:635–41.
18. Levin A. Management of membranoproliferative glomerulonephritis: evidence-based recommendations. Kidney Int. 1999;55: S41–6.
19. Braun MC, West CD, Strife CF. Differences between membranoproliferative glomerulonephritis types I and III in long-term response to an alternate-day prednisone regimen. Am J Kidney Dis. 1999;34:1022–32
20. Donadio JV, Anderson CF, Mitchell JC, et al. Membranoproliferative glomerulonephritis. A prospective clinical trial of platelet-inhibitor therapy. N Engl J Med. 1984;310: 1421–6.
21. Donadio JV, Offord KP. Reassessment of treatment results in membranoproliferative glomerulonephritis, with emphasis on life-table analysis. Am J Kidney Dis. 1989;14:445–51.
22. McHutchinson JG, Gordon SC, Schiff ER, et al. Interferon alfa-2b alone or in combination with ribavirin as initial treatment for chronic hepatitis C. Hepatitis Interventional Therapy Group. N Engl J Med. 1998;339:1485–92.
23. Daghestani L, Pomeroy C. Renal manifestations of hepatitis C infection. Am J Med. 1999;106:347–54.
24. Sarac E, Bastacky S, Johnson JP. Response to high-dose interferon-α after failure of standard therapy in MPGN associated with hepatitis C virus infection. Am J Kidney Dis. 1997;30:113–15.
25. Kiyomoto H, Hitomi H, Hosotani Y, et al. The effect of combination therapy with interferon and cryofiltration on mesangial proliferative glomerulonephritis originating from mixed cryoglobulinemia in chronic hepatitis C virus infection. Ther Apher. 1999;3:329–33.

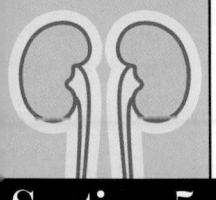

Section 5 Glomerular Disease

Chapter 24

IgA Nephropathy and Henoch–Schönlein Nephritis

John Feehally

INTRODUCTION AND DEFINITIONS

IgA nephropathy

IgA nephropathy (IgAN) is a mesangial proliferative glomerlonephritis characterized by diffuse mesangial deposition of IgA. IgAN was first recognized when immunofluorescence techniques were introduced for the study of renal biopsy. It was described in 1968 by a Parisian pathologist, Jean Berger (it has also been called 'Berger's disease'). Although its most common clinical presentation is visible hematuria provoked by mucosal infection, this is neither universal nor necessary for the diagnosis. IgAN is unique among glomerular diseases in being defined by the presence of an immune reactant rather than by any other morphologic feature found on renal biopsy, and the light microscopic changes are very variable. IgAN is the most prevalent pattern of glomerular disease seen in countries where renal biopsy is widely practiced. At one time the term 'benign recurrent hematuria' was also used for IgAN but it is now known to be an important cause of end-stage renal disease (ESRD).

Henoch–Schönlein purpura

Henoch–Schönlein purpura (HSP) is a small-vessel vasculitis affecting the skin, joints, gut, and kidney. It is defined by tissue deposition of IgA. Henoch–Schönlein purpura was described separately by Schönlein in 1837 and Henoch in 1874. Typically there is clinical involvement in the skin, gut, and kidneys. The nephritis associated with HSP is also characterized by mesangial IgA deposition; indeed, the renal histologic features of Henoch–Schönlein nephritis are indistinguishable from those of IgAN. Henoch–Schönlein nephritis is differentiated from IgAN by the extrarenal manifestations.

ETIOLOGY AND PATHOGENESIS

Although infective episodes precede HSP in up to 50% of cases, there is no evidence of a role for any specific antigen. The clinical association of visible hematuria with upper respiratory tract infection in IgAN indicates that the mucosa may be a site of entry for foreign antigens. An infectious source has long been suspected and there have been occasional reports of IgAN in association with microbial infection, both bacterial (including *Campylobacter*, *Yersinia*, *Mycoplasma*, and *Haemophilus*) and viral (including cytomegalovirus, adenovirus, coxsackie and Epstein–Barr virus). None, however, has been consistently implicated by finding microbial antigen in glomerular deposits. Food antigens have also been proposed (particularly gliadin) but their involvement is not proven. The mesangial IgA may represent a common immune response to a variety of foreign antigens, the original antigen having disappeared from the deposits by the time of the biopsy. Alternatively it may be an autoimmune disease directed against mesangial antigens, or it may develop through an antigen-independent mechanism such as altered IgA glycosylation[1].

The regular recurrence of IgAN and Henoch–Schönlein nephritis after renal transplantation strongly implies an abnormality in the host IgA immune system.

The IgA immune system

IgA is the most abundant immunoglobulin in the body and is chiefly concerned with mucosal defence. It has two subclasses, IgA1 and IgA2. Mucosal antigen challenge provokes polymeric IgA (pIgA) production by plasma cells of the mucosa-associated lymphoid tissue; the pIgA is transported across epithelium into mucosal fluids. The function of circulating IgA is less clear; it is bone-marrow derived and mostly monomeric IgA1 (mIgA1). Circulating IgA1 is cleared by the liver through hepatocyte asialoglycoprotein receptors and Kupffer cell Fcα receptors.

The mesangial IgA in IgAN is pIgA1. The clinical association with mucosal infection originally suggested that the mesangial pIgA1 comes from the mucosal immune system, as most pIgA is mucosally derived. In IgAN, however, pIgA1 production is downregulated in the mucosa and upregulated in the bone marrow. Moreover, the pIgA response to systemic immunization with common antigens is increased, whereas the response to mucosal immunization is impaired. Impaired mucosal IgA responses allowing enhanced antigen challenge to the marrow could be the primary abnormality in IgAN, although this remains unproven. Tonsillar pIgA1 production is also increased, although IgAN can occur after tonsillectomy and the tonsil is a very minor source of IgA production compared to the mucosa or marrow. Hepatic clearance of IgA is reduced in IgAN but there is no direct evidence that this is caused by liver cell receptor dysfunction.

Serum IgA levels are increased in one-third of patients with IgAN and HSP. There are elevations in both mIgA and pIgA. High serum IgA *per se* is not, however, sufficient to cause IgAN; high circulating levels of monoclonal IgA (in myeloma) or polyclonal IgA (in AIDS) only infrequently provoke mesangial IgA deposition.

Circulating macromolecular IgA is characteristic of IgAN. It is often described as IgA immune complexes, although the antigen is only rarely identified. There are circulating IgA rheumatoid factors (IgA against the constant domain of IgG) in 30% of those with IgAN and 55% of those with HSP. IgA-fibronectin complexes, at one time thought to be diagnostic for IgAN, are a function of the general increase in serum IgA. Studies *in vitro* indicate that IgA production by mononuclear cells is exaggerated in IgAN and that these cells show abnormal patterns of cytokine production. The direct relevance of these observations to events *in vivo* is uncertain, however.

IgA glycosylation

IgA1 carries distinctive O-linked sugars at its hinge region; IgA2 has no hinge and carries no such sugars. There is good evidence that circulating IgA1 in IgAN and HS nephritis has abnormal O-linked hinge-region sugars with reduced galactosylation and sialylation[2]. It has recently been shown that mesangial IgA1 in IgAN has the same abnormalities of O-glycosylation[3,4]. The altered glycosylation may promote mesangial IgA1 deposition by predisposing to the formation of circulating IgA1-immune complexes, or by directly modifying IgA1 interactions with matrix proteins and mesangial cell Fc receptors. It may also impair IgA1 clearance, by inhibiting IgA1 interactions with hepatic IgA receptors.

Glomerular injury following IgA deposition

Polymeric IgA deposition in the mesangium is typically followed by mesangial proliferative glomerulonephritis (GN). In animal models codeposition of IgG and complement is necessary for inflammation but this is not mandatory in human disease. Circulating anti-mesangial IgG has been associated with disease activity in IgAN; this remains unconfirmed, however. Complement deposits are usually C3 and properdin without C1q and C4, indicating alternative pathway activation. The extent to which IgA engages inflammatory cells in the circulation and especially in the kidney will also determine the intensity of inflammation. Fc receptors for IgA (Fcα receptors) on myeloid and mesangial cells may play a key role.

The mechanisms of mesangial proliferative GN have been studied in detail in animal models, particularly anti-Thy 1 nephritis in the rat. These studies[5] have shown the key role of cytokines and growth factors in mesangial cell proliferation (particularly platelet-derived growth factor[5] (PDGF) and basic fibroblast growth factor (bFGF)) and in the subsequent matrix production and sclerosis (particularly transforming growth factor-β (TGF-β)). Studies of renal biopsies in human IgAN also support a role for PDGF and TGF-β. These mechanisms are not unique to IgAN but are likely to be involved in all forms of mesangial proliferative GN, including those without IgA deposition. As yet these pathogenetic insights (Fig. 24.1) provide no specific approaches to treatment.

Animal models of IgA nephropathy

Animal IgA does not have the same characteristics as human IgA1, and some animals also have IgA clearance mechanisms distinct from those in humans. It follows that animal models, even if they provoke mesangial IgA deposits, are not

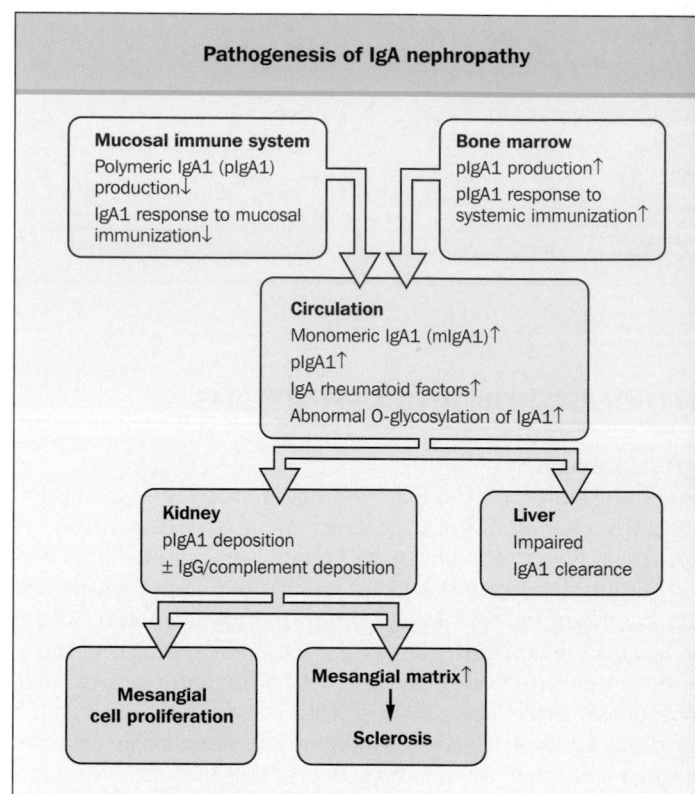

Figure 24.1 Pathogenesis of IgA nephropathy. Abnormalities in IgA immunity leading to mesangial IgA deposition and injury.

particularly informative about the mechanisms that underlie human mesangial pIgA1 deposition, although they have provided many insights into events after IgA deposits have developed. There is no animal model in existence for HSP.

Relationship between IgA nephropathy and Henoch–Schönlein purpura

Despite some differences in age of onset and natural history of IgAN and HS nephritis[6] there is much evidence to support a close pathogenetic link between the two conditions. Monozygotic twins who developed IgAN and HSP respectively at the same time have been reported. The evolution of IgAN into HSP in the same patient is described in both adults and children. Many of the abnormalities of IgA production and handling reported in IgAN are also detected in HSP.

IgA–anti-neutrophil cytoplasmic antibody (IgA–ANCA) has been proposed as a marker of the systemic features that differentiate HSP from IgAN. Circulating IgA–ANCA has been described in HSP, although findings are not consistent. IgA–ANCA is not found in IgAN.

EPIDEMIOLOGY

IgA nephropathy (IgAN) is the most prevalent pattern of glomerular disease in all countries where renal biopsy is widely used as an investigative tool. However, there is striking geographic variation (Fig. 24.2). Genetic variations may be important. For example, in North America IgAN is less common in African Americans than Caucasians of European

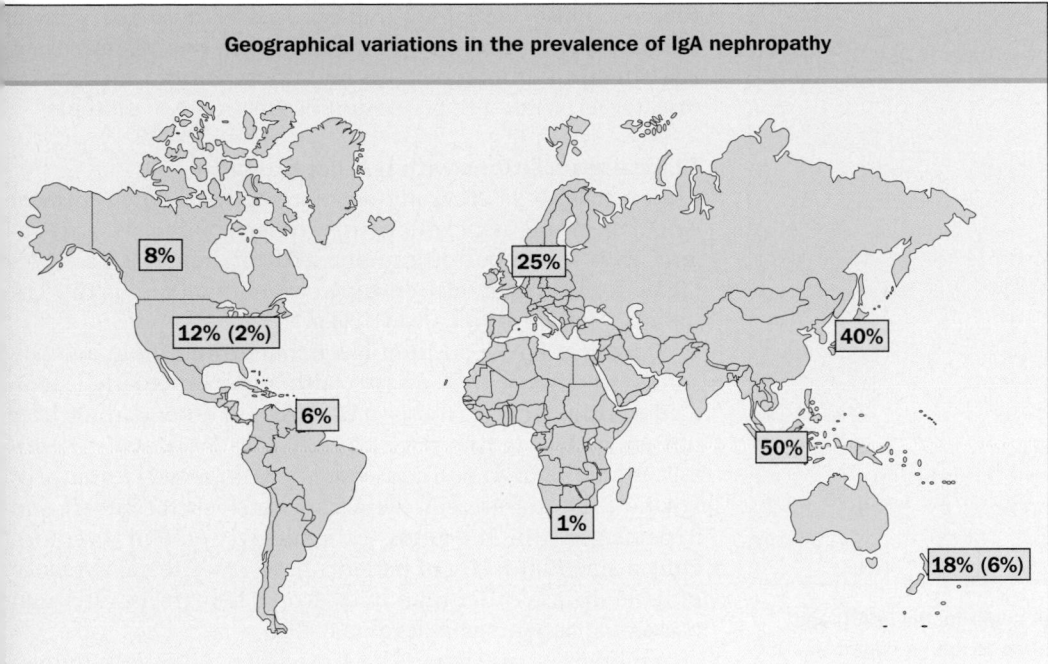

Geographical variations in the prevalence of IgA nephropathy

8%

25%

12% (2%)

40%

6%

50%

1%

18% (6%)

Figure 24.2 Geographical variations in the prevalence of IgA nephropathy (IgAN). Percentages of patients with glomerular disease who have IgAN. The figures in brackets are percentages of glomerular disease in minority racial groups: among African Americans in the USA and among Polynesians in New Zealand.

origin. It is also very uncommon among black South Africans. In New Zealand, IgAN is much less common among Polynesians than among Caucasians of European origin, even though Polynesians have an increased prevalence of many other renal diseases. Perceived prevalence of IgAN may also be influenced by attitudes to the investigation of microscopic hematuria. A country with an active program of routine urine testing will inevitably identify more individuals with microscopic hematuria, but IgAN will be identified only if renal biopsy is performed.

In children, HSP is usually diagnosed on clinical grounds without biopsy confirmation of tissue IgA deposition. Transient urine abnormalities are very common in the acute phase. However, only those with persistent urine abnormalities or with more overt renal disease will come to renal biopsy. Therefore the incidence of Henoch–Schönlein nephritis is almost certainly underestimated with many unidentified mild and transient cases. There is no information on geographic variations in HSP.

Genetic basis of IgA nephropathy

Urine abnormalities increase in frequency among the relatives of those with IgAN, although only in a few pedigrees is IgAN found in multiple generations. One very large pedigree has been described in Kentucky, USA, and other large families have been found in Italy. However, more than 90% of all cases of IgAN are sporadic.

Many studies have sought genes associated with disease susceptibility[7]. However, encouraging recent work has identified a region on chromosome 6 which shows much promise as a disease susceptibility gene and further characterization is awaited[8]. As yet, these studies have had no impact on clinical management.

A deletion allele (D) in the angiotensin-converting enzyme (ACE) gene increases serum and tissue ACE levels and has been associated with risk of progression of IgAN[8]. The findings are not confirmed in all studies, however. The link is unlikely to be specific for IgAN: an association between increased rate of progression of chronic renal failure and DD genotype has been found in patients with other causes of renal failure[8].

CLINICAL MANIFESTATIONS OF IgA NEPHROPATHY

The wide range of clinical presentations of IgAN vary in frequency with age (Fig. 24.3). No clinical pattern is pathognomonic of IgAN. It is more common in males than in females by a ratio of 3 : 1.

Macroscopic hematuria

In 40–50% of cases the clinical presentation is episodic macroscopic hematuria, most frequently in the second and third decades of life. The urine is usually brown rather than red and clots are unusual. There may be loin pain due to renal capsular swelling. Hematuria usually follows intercurrent mucosal infection, commonly in the upper respiratory tract (the term 'synpharyngitic' hematuria has been used) or occasionally in the gastrointestinal tract. Hematuria is usually visible within 24 h of the onset of the symptoms of infection, differentiating it from the 2–3-week delay between infection and subsequent hematuria in post-infectious (for example post-streptococcal) GN. Exercise alone will provoke hematuria in a few patients. The macroscopic hematuria resolves spontaneously in the course of a few days. There is persistent microscopic hematuria between attacks. Most patients have only a few episodes of frank hematuria. These become less frequent and resolve over a few years at most. Such episodes are only rarely associated with acute renal impairment.

Asymptomatic hematuria and proteinuria

Asymptomatic urine testing identifies 30–40% of patients with IgAN. Microscopic hematuria with or without proteinuria

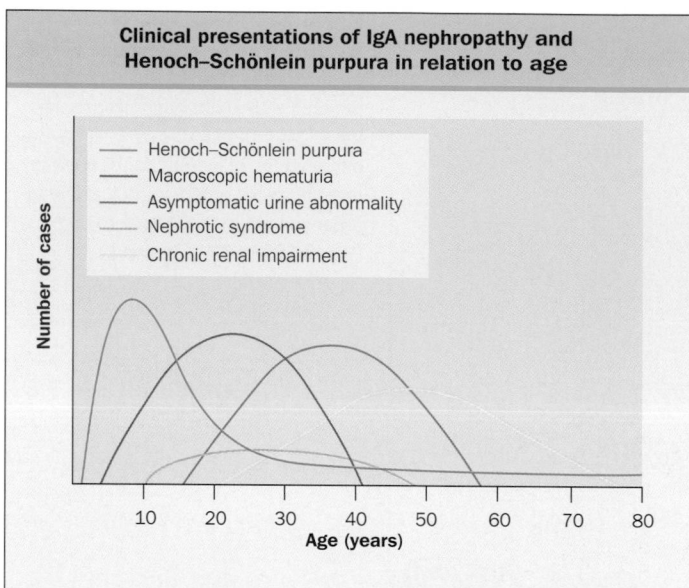

Figure 24.3 Clinical presentations of IgA nephropathy (IgAN) and Henoch–Schönlein purpura (HSP) in relation to age at diagnosis. HSP is most common in childhood but may occur at any age. Macroscopic hematuria is very uncommon over the age of 40 years. The importance of asymptomatic urine abnormality as the presentation of IgAN will depend on attitudes to routine urine testing and renal biopsy. It is uncertain whether those presenting late with chronic renal impairment have a disease distinct from that of those presenting younger with macroscopic hematuria.

(usually < 2 g/24 h) is noted. The number of patients identified in this way will depend on local attitudes to urine screening as well as the use of renal biopsy in patients with isolated microscopic hematuria.

Proteinuria and nephrotic syndrome

It is rare for proteinuria to occur without microscopic hematuria. Nephrotic syndrome is uncommon, occurring in only 5% of all patients with IgAN. Nephrotic syndrome may occur early in the course of the disease, with minimal glomerular change or with active mesangial proliferative GN. Alternatively, it may occur as a late manifestation of advanced chronic glomerular scarring.

Acute renal failure

Acute renal failure is very uncommon in IgAN (< 5% of all cases) and develops by two distinct mechanisms. There may be acute severe immune injury with necrotizing GN and crescent formation – 'crescentic IgA nephropathy'; this may be the first presentation of IgAN or may develop superimposed on established less aggressive disease. Alternatively acute renal failure can occur with mild glomerular injury when heavy glomerular hematuria leads to tubule occlusion by red cells (see Fig. 24.6). Rapid deterioration in IgAN may occur in pregnancy due to crescentic transformation.

Chronic renal failure

Some patients already have renal impairment and hypertension when first diagnosed. These patients tend to be older, and it is probable that they have long-standing disease

that previously remained undiagnosed because the patient neither had frank hematuria nor underwent routine urinalysis. Hypertension is common as in other chronic glomerular disease; accelerated hypertension occurs in 5% of patients.

Clinical associations with IgA nephropathy

Although IgAN is clinically restricted to the kidney in most cases, there are associations with other conditions, particularly with a number of immune and inflammatory diseases (Table 24.1). Their relationship to abnormalities of the IgA immune system is not always clear.

Mesangial IgA deposition is a frequent finding in autopsy studies in chronic liver disease. Although particularly associated with alcoholic cirrhosis, it can occur in other chronic liver disease, including that caused by hepatitis B and schistosomiasis. It is thought to be a consequence of impaired clearance of IgA by the Kupffer cells (which express Fcα receptors) and hepatocytes (which express the asialoglycoprotein receptor). Only a small minority of patients have any clinical evidence of renal disease other than microscopic hematuria, although occasional patients will develop ESRD.

A number of case reports have associated IgAN with human immunodeficiency virus/acquired immune deficiency syndrome (AIDS). The polyclonal increase in serum IgA, which is a feature of AIDS, has been cited as a predisposing factor. Autopsy studies indicate, however, that IgAN is not unduly common in large populations of AIDS patients[9].

CLINICAL MANIFESTATIONS OF HENOCH–SCHÖNLEIN PURPURA

HSP is most prevalent in the first decade of life but may occur at any age. A palpable purpuric rash, which may be recurrent, occurs on extensor surfaces (Fig. 24.4). There may be polyarthralgia (usually without joint swelling) and abdominal pain caused by gut vasculitis. This may be severe, with bloody diarrhea if intussusception develops. In practice, the diagnosis is made by clinical criteria in the great majority of children in whom HSP is a self-limiting illness. In adults clinical features are little different from those of other forms of small-vessel vasculitis, and tissue confirmation of IgA deposition is necessary to establish the diagnosis.

Much renal involvement in HSP is transient. Urine abnormalities are noted during the acute presentation, but disappear. Of those referred to a nephrologist, asymptomatic urine abnormality is still the most frequent clinical manifestation. Nephrotic syndrome occurs in 20% of patients. Acute renal failure may develop as a result of crescentic GN.

PATHOLOGY

The respective renal histopathologies in IgAN and HS nephritis may be indistinguishable from each other (Fig. 24.5).

Immune deposits

Diffuse mesangial IgA, shown in Figure 24.5(b), is the defining hallmark. C3 is codeposited in up to 90% of cases. IgG in 40% and IgM in 40% of cases may also be found in the same distribution. IgA also deposits sometimes along capillary loops

Diseases reported in association with IgA nephropathy			
Disease	Common	Reported	Rare
Rheumatic and autoimmune disease	Ankylosing spondylitis Rheumatoid arthritis Reiter's syndrome Uveitis	Behçet's syndrome* Takayasu's arteritis† Myasthenia gravis	Sicca syndrome
Gastrointestinal disease	Celiac disease	Ulcerative colitis	Crohn's disease Whipple's disease
Hepatic disease	Alcoholic liver disease Nonalcoholic cirrhosis Schistosomal liver disease		
Lung disease	Sarcoid		Pulmonary hemosiderosis
Skin disease	Dermatitis herpetiformis		
Malignancy		IgA monoclonal gammopathy	Bronchial carcinoma Renal carcinoma Laryngeal carcinoma Mycosis fungoides Sézary syndrome
Infection	Human immunodeficiency virus Hepatitis B (in endemic areas)	Brucellosis	Leprosy
Miscellaneous		Wiskott–Aldrich syndrome‡	

* Behçet's syndrome: a systemic vasculitis typified by orogenital ulceration and chronic uveitis
† Takayasu's arteritis: a systemic vasculitis involving the aorta and its major branches, most often found in young women
‡ Wiskott–Aldrich syndrome: an X-linked disorder in which raised serum IgA is associated with the triad of recurrent pyogenic infection, eczema and thrombocytopenia

Table 24.1 Diseases reported in association with IgA nephropathy (IgAN) – common, reported and rare. 'Rare' associations have been made in one or two reported cases only. In a disease as common as IgAN it is therefore uncertain if they are truly related.

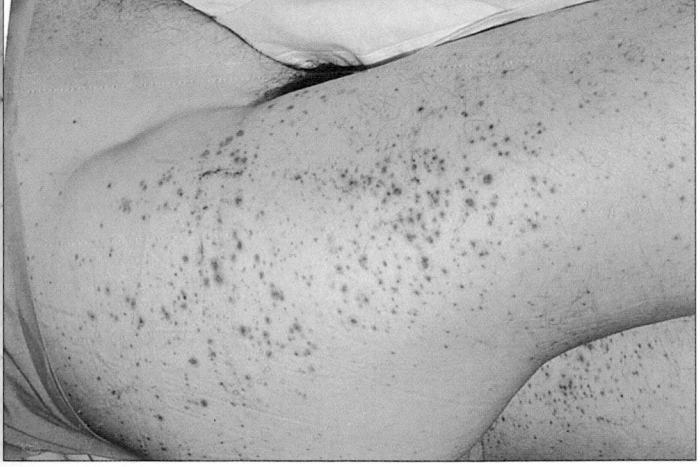

Figure 24.4 Henoch–Schönlein purpura. The rash is a palpable purpuric vasculitis on the lower limbs spreading on extensor surfaces to the buttocks and occasionally to the upper limbs. Histology shows leukocytoclastic vasculitis with IgA deposits in blood-vessel walls.

(a pattern more common in HS nephritis); in IgAN this pattern is associated with a worse prognosis. C5b-9 is found with properdin but not C4, indicating alternative complement pathway activation. Disappearance of IgA deposits after prolonged clinical remission has been documented in Japanese children but not yet in adults.

Light microscopy

Light microscopic changes are remarkably variable and do not correlate topographically with the IgA deposits.

The glomeruli may be virtually normal or there may be mesangial hypercellularity, either global (Fig. 24.5a) or segmental. In long-standing disease, there will be varying degrees of glomerular sclerosis in association with tubulointerstitial scarring. Classification of the morphology is of value in predicting prognosis, although there has not yet been universal agreement as to the ideal classification. The classifications of both Haas[10] and Lee[11] are most widely used, but each has some limitations as a prognostic indicator[12].

Two distinct patterns are seen in acute renal failure: necrotizing GN with crescent formation; or tubular occlusion by red cells without acute glomerular injury (see Fig. 24.6).

Electron microscopy

Electron-dense deposits correspond to the mesangial (or capillary loop) IgA, as shown in Figure 24.5c. Up to one-third of patients will have some focal thinning of the glomerular basement membrane (GBM). Occasionally there will be extensive GBM thinning suggesting a coincident diagnosis of thin membrane nephropathy (see Chapter 48).

DIFFERENTIAL DIAGNOSIS

The diagnosis of IgAN or HS nephritis requires identification of mesangial IgA in the glomeruli. It cannot be made, therefore,

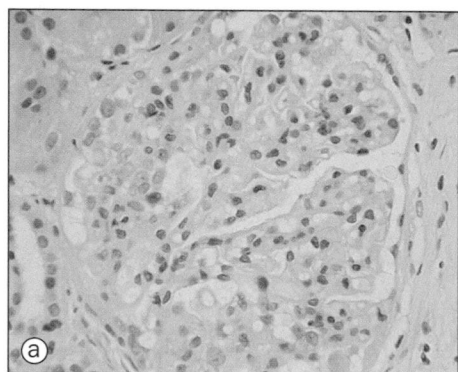
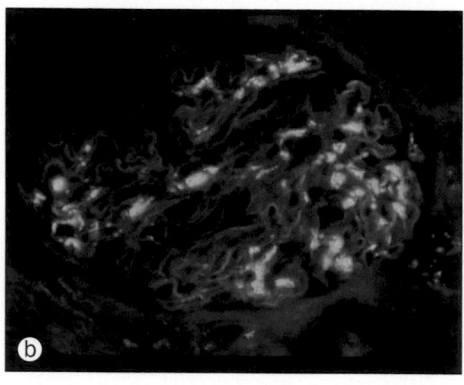
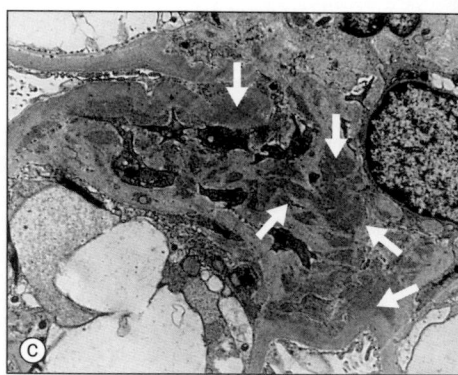

Figure 24.5 Renal pathology in IgA nephropathy (IgAN). (a) Light microscopy: diffuse mesangial hypercellularity, hematoxylin–eosin ×300. (Micrograph courtesy of Prof P Furness.) (b) Immunofluorescence microscopy: diffuse mesangial IgA. Indirect immunofluorescence with FITC–anti-IgA ×300. (Reproduced with permission of Chapman & Hall.) (c) Electron microscopy: mesangial electron-dense deposits. The deposits are shown by arrows . Electron micrograph ×16 000. (Micrograph courtesy of Prof P Furness.)

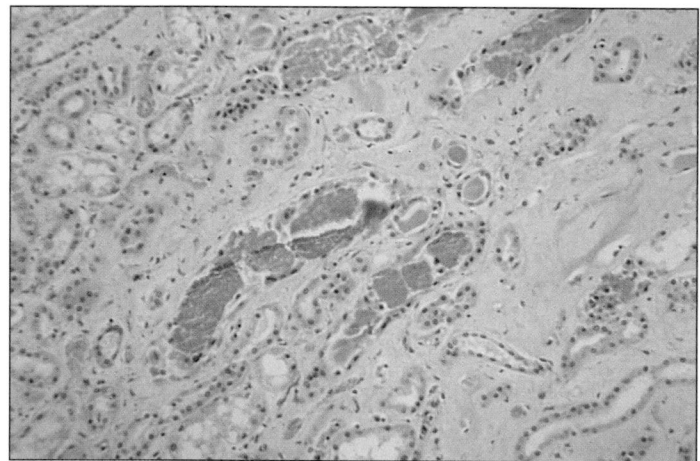

Figure 24.6 Acute renal failure in IgA nephropathy. Tubular occlusion by red cells, hematoxylin–eosin ×300. This appearance was usually associated with only minor glomerular changes. (Reproduced with permission of Chapman & Hall.)

Conditions associated with mesangial IgA deposition
IgA nephropathy
Henoch–Schönlein nephritis
Lupus nephritis
Alcoholic liver disease
IgA monoclonal gammopathy
Schistosomal nephropathy
Distinguishing lupus nephritis (especially WHO Classes II and III) may cause difficulty. The finding of C1q deposition is useful. It indicates classical pathway involvement found in lupus nephritis but not in IgAN.

Table 24.2 Differential diagnosis of IgA nephropathy (IgAN): conditions associated with mesangial IgA deposition.

without a renal biopsy, no matter how suggestive the clinical presentation may be. Serum IgA is often raised and there may be IgA in cutaneous blood vessels in IgAN, and in both affected and unaffected skin in HSP. Neither finding, however, is reliable enough to support the diagnosis without a renal biopsy. Serum complement components are normal unless the C4 null allele is carried.

Mesangial IgA occurs in other conditions (Table 24.2) which can usually be differentiated on clinical, serologic and histologic criteria. None of the light-microscopic features are of themselves diagnostic of IgAN.

Hematuria

Non-glomerular causes of hematuria, particularly stones and neoplasia, must be excluded by appropriate urologic investigation (see Chapter 59). In its most characteristic clinical setting (recurrent macroscopic hematuria coinciding with mucosal infection in a male in the second or third decade of life) the diagnosis can be strongly suspected. Such a diagnosis, however, cannot be made without a biopsy, since recurrent macroscopic hematuria also occurs in other glomerular diseases, particularly in children and young adults.

Nephrotic syndrome

Patients with IgAN occasionally develop nephrotic syndrome, which is indistinguishable from that in minimal change disease. There is a sudden onset of nephrosis, with biopsy evidence of glomerular epithelial cell foot process effacement and a prompt absolute remission of proteinuria in response to corticosteroids. Only hematuria and mesangial IgA deposits persist after treatment. This pattern occurs particularly in children. These patients are usually regarded as having two separate common glomerular diseases, IgAN and minimal change disease[13].

Other patients with IgAN may develop nephrotic syndrome with more structural glomerular damage and lack the response to corticosteroids. The clinical differential diagnosis includes common causes of nephrotic syndrome appropriate for the age of the patient (see Chapter 19).

Chronic renal disease: hypertension, proteinuria, renal impairment

In this context IgAN will be clinically indistinguishable from many forms of chronic renal disease. The renal biopsy may be diagnostic, by identifying mesangial IgA, even when structural damage is so advanced on light microscopy that it has the non-specific features of 'end-stage kidney'.

Acute renal failure

Urgent renal biopsy is mandatory to differentiate the tubular occlusion from acute tubular necrosis which occasionally follow heavy glomerular hematuria from crescentic IgAN, or other coincidental causes of acute renal failure (see Fig. 24.6).

Differential diagnosis of Henoch–Schönlein purpura

In children the diagnosis of HSP is usually made on the basis of clinical criteria. Confirmatory evidence of tissue IgA deposition will not be obtained unless persistence of renal disease results in a renal biopsy. In adults the differential diagnosis is much wider and includes other forms of systemic vasculitis requiring diagnosis by clinical, serologic and histologic characteristics (see Chapter 26).

NATURAL HISTORY

Natural history of IgA nephropathy

The overall prognosis of IgAN has now been defined in long-term natural history studies[14]. Although the evidence shows clinical remission (disappearance of hematuria and proteinuria) in up to one-third of patients with mild disease, large studies with prolonged follow-up indicate a slow attrition. By 20 years, one quarter of patients will have ESRD; a further 20% will have impaired renal function and hence will also eventually suffer progressive disease.

Although an active approach to the investigation of microscopic hematuria will increase the size of the cohort of patients found to have IgAN, it will include more with a good prognosis, thus altering the perceived risk of disease progression. Episodes of macroscopic hematuria do not confer a worse prognosis. This may indicate that such episodes only occur early in the natural history of the disease, and that patients doing less well from the point of diagnosis in fact were only identified at a later stage in their disease. This is also suggested by the adverse influence on outcome of advancing age at diagnosis.

The risk of renal failure is not uniform. As in any chronic glomerular disease, the presence of hypertension, proteinuria and renal impairment at presentation, as well as histologic evidence of glomerular and interstitial fibrosis, identify at the time of diagnosis those with a poor prognosis[14] (see Table 24.3). Hyperuricemia is also an independent risk factor for progression. However, during follow up, only hypertension and proteinuria are reliable predictors of risk of progression. Some evidence suggests geographical variation in risk of progression. A Canadian study indicates risk of progression is negligible when proteinuria remains < 0.2 g/24 h with normal blood pressure[15]. However, in contrast, a study from Hong Kong suggests that among those presenting with isolated microscopic hematuria, as many as 44% may subsequently develop proteinuria, hypertension or renal impairment over a 7-year follow up[16].

Natural history of Henoch–Schönlein nephritis

This is less well defined than IgAN. Observations are restricted to those referred for renal biopsy. This therefore

Prognostic markers at presentation in IgA nephropathy	
Clinical	**Histopathologic**
Poor prognosis	**Poor prognosis**
Increasing age	Glomerular sclerosis
Duration of preceding symptoms	Tubular atrophy
Severity of proteinuria	Interstitial fibrosis
Hyperuricemia	Vascular wall thickening
Hypertension	Capillary-loop IgA deposits
Renal impairment	
Good prognosis	
Recurrent macroscopic hematuria	
No impact on prognosis	**No impact on prognosis**
Gender	Intensity of IgA deposits
Serum IgA level	
None of the clinical or histopathologic adverse features, except capillary-loop IgA deposits, are specific to IgAN.	

Table 24.3 Prognostic markers at presentation in IgA nephropathy.

excludes the majority of patients with minor transient renal involvement, who have an excellent prognosis. Up to 40% will have chronic renal failure 5 years after biopsy.

TRANSPLANTATION

Recurrent IgA nephropathy

There is no evidence from transplant registry data that transplant outcome is inferior if IgAN is the primary renal disease. Nevertheless mesangial IgA deposits recur in the donor transplant kidney in up to 60% of patients with IgAN[17]. They may occur within days or weeks, but the risk increases with the duration of the transplant. The deposits seem benign in the short term and are not often associated initially with light-microscopic changes. Graft failure, associated with proteinuria and hypertension, has been reported to occur in up to one-half of those with recurrent IgA deposits. It seems likely that recurrent IgAN will increasingly emerge as an important long term cause of graft failure as prevention of rejection improves. One Chinese study suggests that the risk of recurrence is increased in living related transplants[18], but numerous other studies do not support this. There is no evidence that newer immunosuppressive agents have modified the frequency of recurrent IgA deposits. Recurrence of crescentic IgAN with rapid graft failure occurs uncommonly, and is generally resistant to treatment.

In a few unwitting experiments, cadaver kidneys with IgA deposits have been transplanted into recipients without IgAN. In all cases the IgA rapidly disappeared, supporting the concept that abnormalities in IgAN lie in the IgA immune system and not in the kidney.

Recurrent Henoch–Schönlein nephritis

Recurrence of IgA deposits is also common in HSP, occurring in about 50% of transplants, although a full recurrence of HSP with systemic involvement including a rash is rare. As in IgAN, transplant registry data show no worsening of outcome if HSP is the primary disease. Delaying transplantation once ESRD is reached does not reduce the risk of recurrence. Unconfirmed evidence from one series of studies in children suggests that the risk of recurrence is increased in live donor transplants.

TREATMENT

Although specific early treatment intervention might influence the IgA immune system abnormalities that underlie IgAN, the mechanisms of chronic disease progression are unlikely to be unique. It is probable, therefore, that studies of such IgAN patients will provide information applicable to many forms of chronic GN for which IgAN is the paradigm.

The balance of risk against benefit for immunosuppressive therapy is often unfavorable in IgAN, except in the unusual circumstance of crescentic IgAN.

The need for randomized controlled trials of adequate power to answer questions about the prevention of chronic renal failure in IgAN is pressing. It is disappointing, despite the prevalence of IgAN and consensus about its definition and natural history, that there are so few such studies[19]. They are shown in Table 24.4. Patients with HSP have been excluded from almost all treatment studies, so it is uncertain whether any strategies developed for IgAN are applicable to HS nephritis.

TREATMENT OF IgA NEPHROPATHY

Treatment recommendations are summarized in Table 24.5.

Reduction of IgA production

Tonsillectomy reduces the frequency of episodic hematuria when tonsillitis is the provoking infection. A long-term retrospective study from Japan suggests tonsillectomy may reduce the risk of renal failure[20] but this is not supported by a German study[21]. The lack of controlled trials is particularly important as the natural history is for macroscopic hematuria to become less frequent with time, independent of any specific treatment. There is no role for prophylactic antibiotics. Dietary gluten restriction, used to reduce mucosal antigen challenge, has not been shown to preserve renal function.

Prevention and removal of IgA deposits

The ideal treatment for IgAN would remove IgA from the glomerulus and prevent further IgA deposition. This remains a remote prospect while the pathogenesis remains incompletely understood.

Randomized controlled trials in IgA nephropathy			
Treatment	Country/Year	Study group	Outcome
Phenytoin	Australia 1980	Adults	No benefit
Corticosteroids	Hong Kong 1986	Adults: nephrotic	16 weeks treatment No benefit: response in subgroup with minimal change
	USA 1992	Children: low-grade proteinuria	12 weeks treatment No benefit
	Italy 2001	Adults: proteinuria	6 months treatment Proteinuria lessened, renal function preserved
Corticosteroids/azathioprine	Japan 1999	Children: low-grade proteinuria	2 years treatment Proteinuria lessened, renal function unchanged, less glomerulosclerosis
Cyclophosphamide	UK 2001	Adults: proteinuria, progressive	Renal failure delayed
Cyclophosphamide/dipyridamole/warfarin	Singapore 1991 Australia 1990	Adults: proteinuria, progressive Adults: proteinuria, progressive	Renal failure delayed Proteinuria lessened, no benefit on renal function
Dipyridamole/warfarin	Hong Kong 1987 Singapore 1989	Adults: proteinuria Adults: proteinuria, progressive	No benefit Renal function preserved
ACE inhibitors	Italy 1994 Australia 1995	Adults: proteinuria, normotensive Adults: proteinuria, hypertensive	Proteinuria reduced Proteinuria reduced: glomerular filtration rate no different at 1 year
	Hong Kong 1999	Adults: proteinuria, hypertensive	No benefit
Fish oil	Australia 1989 Hong Kong 1990 USA 1991 Sweden 1994	Adults: proteinuria, progressive Adults: advanced renal impairment Adults: proteinuria, progressive Adults: proteinuria, progressive	No benefit No benefit Renal failure delayed: proteinuria unchanged No benefit
These are reviewed in Feehally[19].			

Table 24.4 Randomized controlled trials in IgA nephropathy.

Treatment recommendations for IgA nephropathy		
Recurrent macroscopic hematuria (preserved renal function)		
no specific treatment (no role for antibiotics or tonsillectomy)		
Macroscopic hematuria with acute renal failure		
renal biopsy mandatory		
acute tubular necrosis – supportive measures only		
crescentic IgAN –	induction	prednisolone 0.5–1 mg/kg/day for up to 8 weeks
		cyclophosphamide 2 mg/kg/day for up to 8 weeks
	(no evidence favoring oral or intravenous route – follow local practice)	
	maintenance	prednisolone in reducing dosage
		azathioprine 2.5 mg/kg/day
Proteinuria < 1 g/24 h (± microscopic hematuria)		
no specific treatment		
Nephrotic syndrome – with minimal change on light microscopy		
prednisolone 0.5–1 mg/kg/day (children 60 mg/m²/day) for up to 8 weeks		
Proteinuria > 1 g/24 h (± microscopic hematuria)		
ACE inhibitor		
If proteinuria still > 1 g/24 h on maximal ACE inhibitor, serum creatinine < 1.5 mg/dL		
consider corticosteroids – 0.5 mg/kg per alt day for 6 months ± azathioprine		
If proteinuria still > 1 g/24 h on maximal ACE inhibitor, serum creatinine > 1.5 mg/dL		
consider fish oil – 12 g daily for 6 months		
Hypertension		
ACE inhibitors are agent of first choice		
target blood pressure	135/85 *if* proteinuria < 1 g/24 h	
	125/75 *if* proteinuria > 1 g/24 h	
Transplantation		
no special measures required		

Table 24.5 Treatment recommendations for IgA nephropathy.

Altering immune and inflammatory events that follow IgA deposition

Rapidly progressive renal failure associated with crescentic IgA nephropathy

In this uncommon situation the risk–benefit balance is most strongly placed in favor of intensive immunosuppressive therapy since, untreated, there will be rapid progression to ESRD. Treatment has usually combined plasma exchange with prednisolone and cyclophosphamide[22]. Early clinical response is favorable, as in other crescentic nephritis. Medium-term results, however, are disappointing: one-half of the reported patients have reached ESRD within 12 months[21]. A subset of patients with circulating IgG–ANCA may have a more favorable response to immunosuppressive therapy similar to that seen in other ANCA-positive crescentic nephritis[23]. There have been no controlled trials of treatment so it is not possible to be certain which elements of the regimen (corticosteroids, cyclophosphamide, or plasma exchange) are mandatory.

Early treatment with immunosuppressive or anti-inflammatory regimens

Corticosteroids

Corticosteroids have been given in two short-term randomized controlled trials: one in nephrotic adults, one in children with low-grade proteinuria. Neither trial showed benefit. Among the nephrotic adults, however[24], there was a small group with very minor histologic changes which responded rapidly to treatment. Nephrotic syndrome may occur in this setting when minimal change disease and IgAN coincide, in which case the nephrotic syndrome will be fully and promptly steroid-responsive. A trial of high-dose corticosteroid therapy is therefore justified in IgAN when there is nephrotic syndrome associated with minimal glomerular injury.

Despite the generally negative outcome of the two short-term studies, uncontrolled data have favored the use of prolonged administration of alternate-day steroids, and this approach is further supported by a randomized controlled trial suggesting that 6 months of alternate-day corticosteroids in adults with low-grade proteinuria may protect renal function[25].

Another small controlled trial of corticosteroids with antiplatelet agents in patients with non-nephrotic proteinuria, showed some reduction in protein excretion but was not powered to study protection of renal function[26]. Corticosteroids combined with azathioprine have also been used in a two year randomized trial in children with early disease[27], in whom proteinuria lessened and glomerulosclerosis was avoided, although there was no effect on renal function.

Cyclophosphamide

Cyclophosphamide has been used in combination with warfarin and dipyridamole in two randomized controlled trials, the results of which are not mutually consistent. Both showed modest reduction in proteinuria but only one, preserved renal function. Cyclophosphamide combined with prednisolone preserved renal function in a controlled trial in patients with a poor prognosis[28]. Cyclophosphamide has not been used alone in IgAN. Many physicians regard the toxicity of cyclophosphamide as unacceptable in young adults with IgAN.

Dipyridamole and warfarin

These have also been given in two controlled trials that showed mutually inconsistent results. There was no benefit in one and preserved renal function in the other.

Cyclosporine

Cyclosporine has been used in one controlled trial. There was a reversible fall in proteinuria. This went in parallel with a fall in creatinine clearance, suggesting that the changes were a hemodynamic effect of cyclosporine rather than an immune modulating effect.

Pooled human immunoglobulin

Pooled human immunoglobulin has given encouraging preliminary results in IgAN: proteinuria lessened, deterioration in GFR slowed and histologic activity lessened on repeat renal biopsies[29]. No controlled trial is yet available for this promising approach.

Treatment of slowly progressive IgAN

There is little evidence to indicate that the events of progressive glomerular injury are unique to IgAN. Treatments available are non-specific approaches for chronic glomerular disease, of which IgAN is the commonest and most easily defined.

Hypertension

There is compelling evidence for the benefit of lowering blood pressure (BP) in the treatment of chronic progressive glomerular disease such as IgAN. In IgAN there is also evidence that casual clinic BP readings underestimate BP load as judged by ambulatory BP monitoring and echocardiographic evidence of increased left ventricular mass[30]. Although there is no prospective controlled trial evidence to support the use of ACE inhibitors in IgAN, there is very powerful evidence from studies on other proteinuric renal disease that ACE inhibitors or angiotensin receptor antagonists (ATRA) should be the first choice hypotensive agent to minimize proteinuria as well as control blood pressure. Low target BP (< 135/85 if proteinuria < 1 g/24 h, 125/75 if proteinuria > 1 g/24 h) are recommended from a number of large studies of chronic progressive renal disease (see Chapter 66), although there is no specific evidence for this in IgAN. It is unfortunate that available randomized controlled trials of corticosteroids, immunosuppressive agents and fish oil in IgAN have not controlled BP rigorously to these low targets, and have not uniformly used ACE inhibitors; it is therefore not possible to be certain whether the apparent benefits in these trials would be sustained if tight BP control with ACE inhibition is maintained. ACE inhibitors have an equivalent effect to ATRA on proteinuria and BP in IgAN, and there is some evidence that the two classes of agents may have additive effects on proteinuria[31].

Fish oil

The favorable effects of supplementing the diet with ω-3 fatty acids in the form of fish oil include reductions in eicosanoid and cytokine production, changes in membrane fluidity and rheology, and reduced platelet aggregability. These features should significantly reduce the adverse influence of many mechanisms thought to impact on progression of chronic glomerular disease.

A randomized controlled trial provides convincing evidence of protection from 2 years' treatment with fish oil of patients with proteinuria and a rising serum creatinine[32]. It is, however, surprising that fish oil did not significantly reduce proteinuria, a major risk factor for progression. A further study showed no advantage for high over low dose fish oil[33]. However other smaller controlled trials have shown no benefit[34], although severity of renal impairment before treatment was not equivalent in all these studies. Fish oil treatment does not have the drawbacks associated with immunosuppressive treatment. It is safe apart from a decrease in blood coagulability, which is not usually a practical problem, and an unpleasant taste, with flatulence, which may make compliance difficult. A further confirmatory study of fish oil would be of great value.

Recommendation

The treatment of IgAN with proteinuria > 1 g/24 h remains controversial. Physicians are increasingly using corticosteroids when there is preserved renal function (serum creatinine < 1.5 mg/dL (140 μmol/L)) and fish oil when there is renal impairment (serum creatinine > 1.5 mg/dL). However in this author's opinion the case is not yet made for either of these therapies. Tight control of blood pressure with ACE inhibitors or ATRA should be the first line of treatment. Fish oil or corticosteroids should only be considered if proteinuria > 1 g/24 h persists on maximal ACE inhibitor therapy with BP < 125/75.

Transplant recurrence

The majority of recurrences do not worsen graft outcome and require no specific treatment. When crescentic IgAN recurs with rapidly deteriorating graft function, treatment as for primary crescentic IgAN has been used although evidence of its success is sparse.

TREATMENT OF HENOCH–SCHÖNLEIN NEPHRITIS

Many patients have transient nephritis during the early phase of HSP, which spontaneously remits and requires no treatment. There are no prospective randomized controlled trials to guide the treatment of HS nephritis. Most therapeutic studies of IgAN exclude those with HSP, so it is uncertain whether a number of potential treatments have a role in HS nephritis. Treatment recommendations are summarized in Table 24.6.

Rapidly progressive renal failure caused by crescentic nephritis

Crescentic nephritis is more common in HS nephritis than in IgAN, particularly early in the course of HSP. There is little specific information on treatment in adults or children, but regimens based on those for other forms of systemic vasculitis are widely used. These have included corticosteroids, and cyclophosphamide, with the addition of plasma exchange or pulse methylprednisolone in some cases. There have been no controlled trials and HS nephritis has usually been excluded from trials of severe nephritis in systemic vasculitis. It is not possible to define the best regimen on available evidence.

Active HS nephritis without renal failure

There is little information about less aggressive HS nephritis. Corticosteroids alone have never been shown to be beneficial. It has been proposed, but not confirmed, that early use of corticosteroids in HSP may prevent nephritis[35]. Promising findings with combination therapy of corticosteroids, cyclophosphamide and antiplatelet agents have only been reported in small nonrandomized studies[36]. A nonrandomized study reported that prednisolone/azathioprine preserved renal function and improved histological appearances, but relied on historical controls[37]. There are very few patients with HS nephritis included in the promising studies of immunoglobulin.

Slowly progressive renal failure

While the renal histology and clinical course of slowly progressive HS nephritis and IgAN may be indistinguishable, patients with HS nephritis have not been included in studies of fish oil. Tight blood pressure control with ACE inhibitors or ATRA is recommended for proteinuric HS nephritis as for IgAN.

Transplant recurrence

No treatment is known to reduce the risk of recurrence. There is some evidence that recurrence is more common and more

Treatment recommendations for Henoch–Schönlein nephritis

Crescentic nephritis
regimen as for crescentic IgA nephropathy (Table 24.5)

All other Henoch–Schönlein nephritis (including nephrotic syndrome)
no specific treatment – supportive measures only

Hypertension
ACE inhibitor – agent of first choice
target blood pressure   135/85 *if* proteinuria < 1 g/24 h
        125/75 *if* proteinuria > 1 g/24 h

Transplantation
cadaveric donor may be preferable to live related donor in children

Table 24.6 Treatment recommendations for Henoch–Schönlein nephritis.

likely to lead to graft loss in children receiving live donor kidneys than cadaver kidneys[38], although this is not confirmed in adults[39]. If crescentic HS nephritis recurs, intensive immunosuppression may be justified as for primary disease. This, however, has not been thoroughly evaluated.

REFERENCES

1. Smith AC, Feehally J. New insights into the pathogenesis of IgA nephropathy. Springer Semin Immunopathol. 2002 (in press).
2. Allen AC, Bailey EM, Barratt J, et al. Analysis of IgA1 O-glycans in IgA nephropathy by fluorophore assisted carbohydrate electrophoresis. J Amer Soc Nephrol. 1999;10:1763–71.
3. Allen AC, Bailey EM, Brenchley PEC, et al. Mesangial IgA1 in IgA nephropathy exhibits abberant O-glycosylation: observations in three patients. Kidney Int. 2001;60:969–73.
4. Hiki Y, Odani H, Takahashi M, et al. Mass spectrometry proves underglycosylation of glomerular IgA1 in IgA nephropathy. Kidney Int. 2001;59:1077.
5. Johnson RJ. The glomerular response to injury. Mechanisms of progression or resolution. Kidney Int. 1994;45:1769–82.
6. Davin JC, ten Berge IJ, Weening J. What is the difference between IgA nephropathy and Henoch-Schönlein purpura nephritis? Kidney Int. 2001;59:823–34.
7. Gharavi AG, Yan Y, Scolari F, et al. IgA nephropathy, the most common glomerulonephritis, is linked to 6q22–23. Nat Genet. 2000;26:354.
8. Hsu SI, Ramirez B, Winn MP, et al. Evidence for genetic factors in the development and progression of IgA nephropathy. Kidney Int. 2000;57:1818–35.
9. Cohen AH. Human immunodeficiency virus and IgA nephropathy. Nephrology. 1997;3:51–4.
10. Haas M. Histologic classification of IgA nephropathy: a clinicopathologic study of 244 cases. Am J Kidney Dis. 1997;29:829–42.
11. Lee SM, Rao VM, Franklin WA, et al. IgA nephropathy: morphological predictors of progressive renal disease. Hum Pathol. 1982;13:314–22.
12. Feehally J. Predicting prognosis in IgA nephropathy. Am J Kidney Dis. 2001;38:881–3.
13. Clive DM, Galvanek EG, Silva FG. Mesangial immunoglobulin-A deposits in minimal change nephrotic syndrome: a report of an older patient and a review of the literature. Am J Nephrol. 1990;10:31–6.
14. D'Amico G: Natural history of IgA nephropathy: role of clinical and histological prognostic factors. Am J Kidney Dis. 2000;36:227–37.
15. Bartosik L, Lajoie G, Sugar L, Cattran DC. Predicting progression in IgA nephropathy. Am J Kidney Dis. 2001;38:728–35.
16. Szeto CC, Lai FM, To KF, et al. Natural history of immunoglobulin A nephropathy presenting with hematuria and minimal proteinuria. Am J Med. 2001;110:434–7.
17. Floege J, Burg M, Kliem V. Recurrent IgA nephropathy after kidney transplantation: not a benign condition. Nephrol Dial Transplant. 1998;13:1933.
18. Mang AYM, Lai FM, Yu AW-Y, et al. Recurrent IgA nephropathy in renal transplant allografts. J Amer Soc Nephrol. 2001;38:588.
19. Feehally J. IgA nephropathy and Henoch-Schönlein purpura. In: Brady HR, Wilcox CS, eds. Therapy in Nephrology and Hypertension. Philadelphia, PA: WB Saunders; 2003 (in press).
20. Hotta OF, Miyazaka M, Furuta T, et al. Tonsillectomy and steroid pulse therapy significantly impact on clinical remission in patients with IgA nephropathy. Am J Kidney Dis. 2001;38: 736–43.
21. Rasche FM, Schwarz A, Keller F. Tonsillectomy does not prevent a progressive course in IgA nephropathy. Clin Nephrol. 1999; 51:147.
22. Roccatello D, Ferro G, Cesano D, et al. Steroid and cyclophosphamide in IgA nephropathy. Nephrol Dial Transplant. 2000;15:833–5.
23. Haas M, Jafri J, Bartosh SM, et al. ANCA-associated crescentic glomerulonephritis with mesangial IgA deposits. Am J Kidney Dis. 2000;36:709–18.
24. Lai KN, Lai FM, Ho CP, et al. Corticosteroid therapy in IgA nephropathy with nephrotic syndrome: a long-term controlled trial. Clin Nephrol. 1986;26:174–80.
25. Locatelli F, Pozzi C, Del Vecchio L, et al. Role of proteinuria reduction in the progression of IgA nephropathy. Renal Failure. 2001;23: 495–505.

26. Shoji T, Nakanashi I, Suzuki A, et al. Early treatment with corticosteroids ameliorates proteinuria, proliferative lesions, and mesangial phenotypic modulation in adult diffuse proliferative IgA nephropathy. Am J Kidney Dis. 2000;35:194–201.

27. Yoshikawa N, Ito H, Sakai T, et al. A controlled trial of combined therapy for newly diagnosed severe childhood IgA nephropathy. J Amer Soc Nephrol. 1999;10:101–9.

28. Ballardie FW, Roberts IDS. Controlled prospective trial of prednisolone and cytotoxics in progressive IgA nephropathy. J Amer Soc Nephrol. 2002;13:142–8.

29. Rostoker G, Desvaux-Belghiti D, Pilatte Y, et al. High-dose immunoglobulin therapy for severe IgA nephropathy and Henoch– Schönlein purpura. Ann Intern Med. 1994;120:476–84.

30. Stefanski A, Schmidt KG, Waldherr R, Ritz E. Early increase in blood pressure and diastolic left ventricular malfunction in patients with glomerulonephritis. Kidney Int. 1995;54:926–31.

31. Russo D, Minutolo R, Pisani R, et al. Additive antiproteinuric effect of converting enzyme inhibitor and losartan in normotensive patients with IgA nephropathy. Am J Kidney Dis. 2001;33:851–6.

32. Donadio JV, Grande JP, Bergstralh EJ, et al. The long-term outcome of patients with IgA nephropathy treated with fish oil in a controlled trial. J Amer Soc Nephrol. 1999;10:1772.

33. Donadio JV, Larson TS, Bergstralh EJ, Grande JP. A randomised trial of high-dose compared with low-dose omega-3 fatty acids in severe IgA nephropathy. J Am Soc Nephrol. 2001;12:791.

34. Dillon JJ. Fish oil therapy for IgA nephropathy: efficacy and inter-study variability. J Amer Soc Nephrol. 1997;8:1739–44.

35. Mollica F, LiVolti S, Garozzo R, et al. Effectiveness of early prednisone treatment in preventing the development of nephropathy in anaphylactoid purpura. Eur J Pediatr. 1992;151:140.

36. Oner A, Tinaztepe K, Erdogan O. The effect of triple therapy on rapidly progressive type of Henoch-Schönlein nephritis. Pediatr Nephrol. 1995;9:6.

37. Foster BJ, Bernard C, Drummond KN, Sharma AK. Effective therapy for Henoch–Schönlein purpura nephritis with prednisone and azathioprine: a clinical and histopathologic study. J Pediatr. 2000;136:370–5.

38. Hasegawa A. Fate of renal grafts with recurrent Henoch– Schönlein purpura nephritis in children. Transplant Proc. 1989;21:2130.

39. Meulders Q, Pirson Y, Cosyns J-P, et al. Course of Henoch– Schonlein nephritis after renal transplantation. Transplantation. 1994;48: 1179–86.

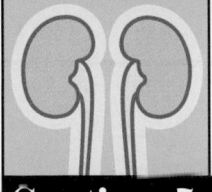

Chapter 25

Antiglomerular Basement Membrane Disease and Goodpasture's Syndrome

Richard G Phelps and A Neil Turner

INTRODUCTION

The syndrome of renal failure and lung hemorrhage was associated with the name of Ernest Goodpasture by Stanton and Tange in their description of nine cases in 1958[1,2]. All nine patients presented with pulmonary hemorrhage and acute renal failure, and died within hours or days, largely as a result of massive pulmonary hemorrhage. These features had been prominent in the case of a young man who died during the influenza pandemic of 1919, whose postmortem findings were memorably reported by Goodpasture:

The lungs gave the impression of having been injected with blood through the bronchi so that all the air spaces were filled (Fig. 25.1).

It is almost certain that the patients described by Goodpasture, Stanton, and Tange had different diseases but with similar dominant clinical features. Several diseases are now recognized as being associated with alveolar hemorrhage and rapidly progressive renal glomerulonephritis (RPGN). Nevertheless this remains a striking clinical entity with relatively few causes and few pathogenetic mechanisms.

Because the first recognized mechanism was antiglomerular basement membrane (anti-GBM) antibody formation and deposition, Goodpasture's name is firmly associated with anti-GBM (Goodpasture's) disease, even though this is responsible for only a proportion of patients with Goodpasture's syndrome of lung hemorrhage and RPGN. The terminology used in this chapter is defined in Table 25.1.

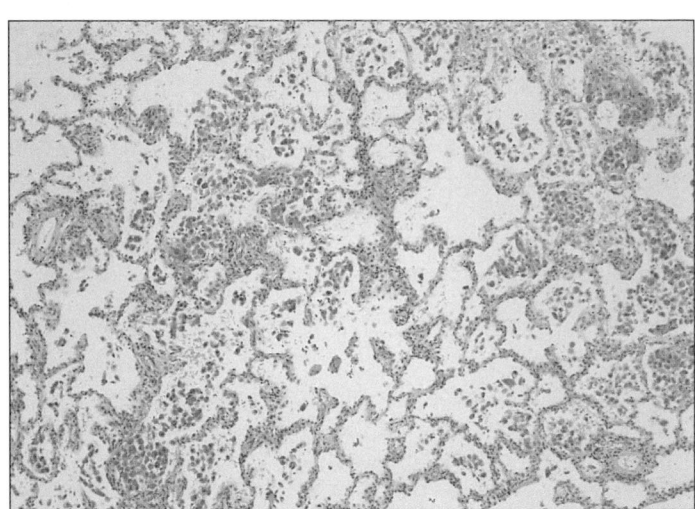

Figure 25.1 Alveolar hemorrhage in a patient with Goodpasture's disease. Open lung biopsy. (Courtesy of Dr E Mary Thompson.)

Table 25.1 Definition of terms.

Definition of terms		
Term	**Definition**	**Pathogenesis**
Pulmonary renal syndrome	Renal and respiratory failure	Many causes (see Table 25.4)
Goodpasture's syndrome	RPGN and alveolar hemorrhage	Several causes (see Fig. Table 25.5)
Anti-GBM disease	Disease associated with antibodies specific for (any) components of the GBM	Most important are Goodpasture's disease and Alport post-transplant anti-GBM disease
Goodpasture's disease	Disease associated with autoantibodies specific for α3(IV)NC1. May include RPGN, lung hemorrhage or both	Autoimmunity to α3(IV)NC1
Alport post-transplant anti-GBM disease	Glomerulonephritis associated with anti-GBM antibodies developing after renal transplantation in patients with Alport syndrome	Immunity to 'foreign' collagen IV chains not expressed in Alport patients (usually α3 or α5(IV)NC1)

ETIOLOGY AND PATHOGENESIS

Autoimmunity to a component of the glomerular basement membrane

Goodpasture's disease is caused by autoimmunity to a specific component of the GBM that has been identified as the carboxyl-terminal, noncollagenous (NC1) domain of a type IV collagen chain, α3(IV)NC1, also known as the Goodpasture antigen[3,4]. Type IV collagen is an essential constituent of all basement membranes. In most tissues it is composed of trimers comprising two α1 and one α2 chains, but there are also four tissue-specific chains, α3–6[5,6]. Three of these, α3–α5, are found in GBM as well as in the basement membranes of the alveolus, the cochlea, parts of the eye (including corneal basement membrane and Bruch's membrane), the choroid plexus of the brain, and some endocrine organs.

All patients with RPGN, lung hemorrhage, and anti-GBM antibodies have antibodies to α3(IV)NC1, usually binding predominantly to a single or a very restricted set of epitopes. Some patients also have antibodies to other basement membrane constituents, including other collagen IV chains, usually in low titer.

Predisposing factors

As is mostly the case in autoimmune disease, both environmental and genetic factors appear to be important in etiology. Genetic influences are apparent from reports of the disease occurrence in siblings and twins and from the strong association between Goodpasture's disease and human leukocyte antigen (HLA) class II alleles. One of the alleles contributing to the DR2 specificity, HLA-DRB1*1501, is carried by 64–91% of patients but only 20–31% of controls. There is a less pronounced but significant association with HLA-DR4 alleles and 90–97% of patients carry DRB1*1501 or DR4. Most other HLA class II alleles have a neutral influence on susceptibility to Goodpasture's disease (Fig. 25.2) but DR1 and DR7 confer strong and dominant protection. Possible mechanisms are discussed by Phelps and Rees[7].

Precipitating factors

Reports of the temporal and geographic clustering of cases suggest an environmental trigger[8]. No specific infectious agent has been consistently identified. Hydrocarbon exposure has been linked to disease onset in several striking case reports but in some cases such exposure may simply trigger pulmonary hemorrhage in patients who already have the disease. Furthermore, exposures of this kind are very common in the modern world. Similarly, cigarette smoking may precipitate pulmonary hemorrhage in patients who already have circulating autoantibodies, but whether it plays a role in causation is less clear.

Intriguingly, there are several instances where renal trauma or inflammation (Table 25.2) has preceded the development of the disease. These may alter α3(IV)NC1 turnover and metabolism qualitatively or quantitatively, providing an opportunity for self-tolerance to be broken. A possible qualitative change is the accessibility of relevant epitopes within the basement membrane which is increased, for example, by exposure to

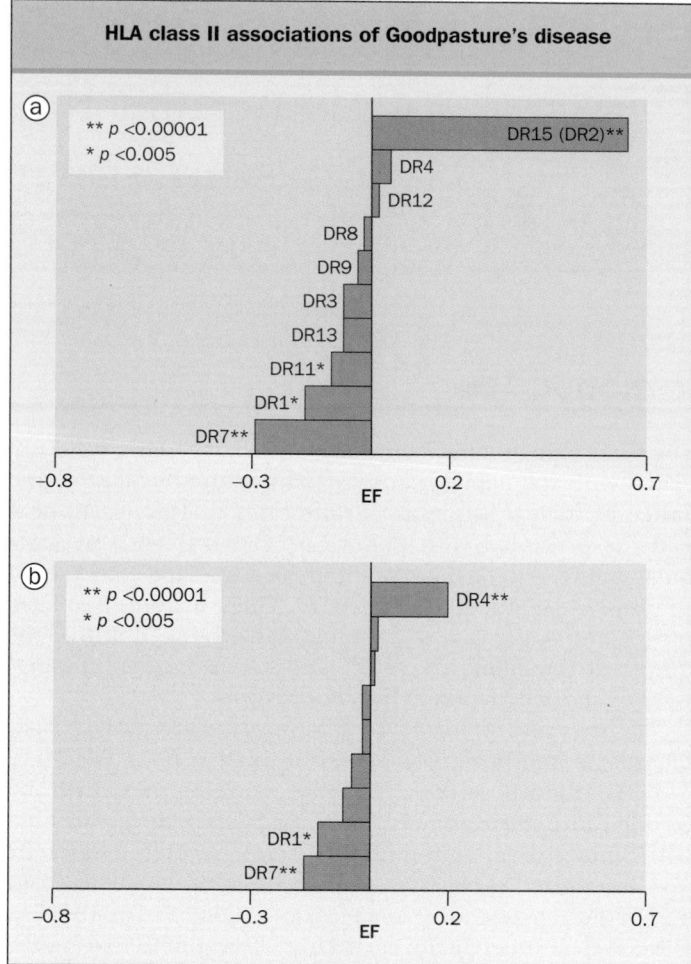

Figure 25.2 HLA class II associations of Goodpasture's disease. The association between HLA class II alleles and Goodpasture's disease is shown as the etiologic fraction (EF), calculated using allele frequency data for 139 Caucasian patients assembled from published studies[7]. The preponderance of DR15 (a DR2 allele) distorts the frequencies of other alleles (a), so these are also shown analyzed alone (b). This procedure, called relative predispositional analysis, shows the positive association with DR4 to be highly significant. The EF is calculated in the same way as population attributable risk and unlike the relative risk, indicates disease association irrespective of allele frequencies. The EF ranges between −1 and 1, representing complete negative and positive associations respectively. An EF of 0 indicates no association. EF is calculated thus: $EF = (f_p - f_c)/(1 - f_c)$, where f_p is frequency of allele in patients and f_c = frequency of allele in controls.

reactive oxygen species likely to be abundant in inflamed glomeruli. The quantity of α3(IV)NC1 presented to T cells may be greater where there has been damage to the basement membrane, as occurs in systemic small vessel vasculitis (see Chapter 26); the outcome of treatment and other features suggest that the anti-GBM response may be a secondary phenomenon in most of these patients[9,10]. The association with membranous nephropathy is interesting as the thickened GBM in that disease contains increased amounts of the tissue-specific type IV collagen chains, including the α3 chain, which bears the Goodpasture antigen.

Conditions and events associated with the presentation of Goodpasture's disease
Possibly induce autoimmune response and disease
Systemic small vessel vasculitis affecting glomeruli
Membranous nephropathy
Lithotripsy of renal stones
Urinary obstruction
Precipitate pulmonary hemorrhage
Cigarette smoke
Hydrocarbon exposure
Pulmonary infection
Fluid overload

Table 25.2 Conditions and events associated with the presentation of Goodpasture's disease.

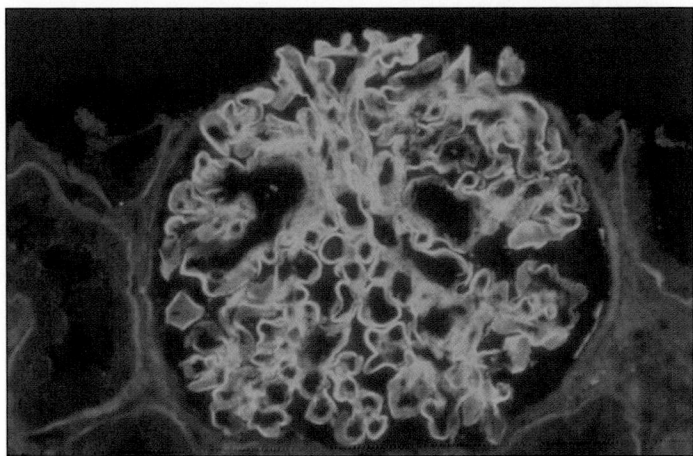

Figure 25.3 Autoantibodies to the Goodpasture antigen bound to a normal glomerulus. Shown by direct immunofluorescence in a patient with lung hemorrhage and hematuria. (Courtesy of Dr Richard Herriot.)

Mechanisms of renal injury

Several lines of evidence support a direct role for anti-$\alpha3(IV)NC1$ autoantibodies (Fig. 25.3) in the pathogenesis of Goodpasture's disease[11]. Over 30 years ago, Lerner, Glassock and Dixon[12] showed that antibodies eluted from the kidneys of patients who had died from Goodpasture's disease, rapidly bound to the GBM and caused glomerulonephritis when injected into squirrel monkeys. Furthermore, the deposited antibodies are predominantly IgG1 and are complement fixing. Experimental models have shown that contributions to renal injury mediated by such antibodies come from complement, and neutrophil and macrophage infiltration. However, it is very likely that T cells are essential for driving autoantibody production by T dependent B cells, and in experimental renal disease they are critical in producing glomerular crescents[13], which are a usual feature of Goodpasture's disease.

Agents that downregulate inflammation by inhibiting interleukin (IL)-1 or tumor necrosis factor-α (TNF-α), or that inhibit recruitment of inflammatory cells by blockade of adhesion molecules or chemoattractants, suppress injury in experimental models of anti-GBM disease. There is supportive evidence in humans and in experimental animals that the severity of renal injury may be increased by proinflammatory cytokines, or by stimuli likely to elicit them, such as bacteremia[14].

Crescent formation is seen in aggressive, inflammatory glomerulonephritis. The mechanism by which it is believed to occur is described in Chapter 18 (Figure 18.8).

Pulmonary hemorrhage

Lung hemorrhage in Goodpasture's disease (but not in small vessel vasculitis – the other major cause of Goodpasture's syndrome) only occurs if there is an additional insult to the lung, which is usually cigarette smoke. However, infection, fluid overload, toxicity from inhaled vapors or other irritants, and the effects of systemic administration of some cytokines are also possibilities. This is probably because the alveolar capillary endothelial cell provides more of a barrier between circulating immunoglobulin and the underlying basement membrane than the diaphragm-free fenestrations of the glomerular capillary endothelial cell.

In the glomerulus, antibodies have direct access to the GBM because of the fenestrations of glomerular endothelium. Other sites at which the Goodpasture antigen is found are not involved in Goodpasture's disease, except possibly the choroid plexus, where the endothelium is again fenestrated, and more rarely, the eye.

EPIDEMIOLOGY

Goodpasture's disease is rare, with an estimated incidence in Caucasian populations of between 0.5 and 0.9 cases/million per annum[15]. The incidence in Black and South Asian populations appears to be lower. The incidence in other racial groups is uncertain because of sparse reports, but is probably also very low. There is a slight male predominance. Most are young men in their second and third decades, with a smaller peak incidence in the sixth and seventh decades; but cases of either sex and all ages are reported.

Lung hemorrhage is more common in younger male patients, but it is unclear whether this reflects age-related susceptibility or demographic differences in smoking.

CLINICAL MANIFESTATIONS

The principal clinical manifestations of Goodpasture's disease arise from lung hemorrhage and/or rapidly progressive glomerulonephritis[15]. Between 50 and 75% of patients present with acute symptoms of lung hemorrhage and are found to be in a state of advanced renal failure. Usually symptoms are confined to the preceding few weeks or months, but very rapid progression (over days) or much slower progression (over many months) may occur. A lack of systemic symptoms, other than those related to anemia, is typical although it is common for an apparently minor infection to trigger the clinical presentation.

Pulmonary hemorrhage

Lung hemorrhage may occur with renal disease or in isolation. Presenting symptoms may include cough, hemoptysis, exertional dyspnea, and fatigue. Hemorrhage into alveolar spaces

Glomerular Disease

occurs and may result in marked iron-deficiency anemia and exertional dyspnea, even in the absence of hemoptysis. Depending on the degree and chronicity of lung hemorrhage, examination findings may include pallor, scattered dry inspiratory crackles, signs of consolidation, or respiratory distress. Recent pulmonary hemorrhage is usually apparent on a chest radiograph (Fig. 25.4), typically appearing as central shadowing that may traverse fissures and give rise to the appearance of an air bronchogram. However even pulmonary hemorrhage sufficient to reduce the hemoglobin concentration may cause only minor or transient radiographic changes, and these cannot be confidently distinguished from other causes of alveolar shadowing (notably edema, infection) by radiological appearances alone. The most sensitive indicator of recent pulmonary hemorrhage is an increased uptake of inhaled carbon monoxide ($D_L CO$). Patients with lung hemorrhage are usually current cigarette smokers.

In isolated lung disease, progressive alveolar or fibrotic disease or pulmonary hemosiderosis may be suspected, although at least hematuria is usually present. This may continue for months or in rare cases recurrently for years before significant renal disease occurs.

Glomerulonephritis

Patients with glomerulonephritis may notice dark or red urine but sometimes progression to oliguria is so rapid that this phase, if it occurs, is missed. In one-third to one-half of patients, glomerulonephritis occurs in the absence of lung hemorrhage. In this subgroup, because systemic symptoms are generally not prominent, progression is silent unless disease is signaled by hematuria, and presentation is often late with renal failure.

Whatever the early pattern of disease, once significant renal impairment has occurred further deterioration in renal function is usually rapid. Presentation at the time of, or very shortly after acceleration of the disease process, is common, and patients may demonstrate very rapid loss of renal function and life-threatening lung hemorrhage. Urinalysis always reveals hematuria (even in almost all patients with apparently isolated pulmonary disease), usually modest proteinuria, and on microscopy, dysmorphic red cells and red-cell casts. The kidneys are generally of normal size, but may be enlarged. Hematuria may be substantial or associated with loin pain in acute disease. In a few patients with a subacute presentation, proteinuria is in the nephrotic range, and the rate of progression of the disease is slow.

PATHOLOGY

Renal biopsy is essential as it provides diagnostic and prognostic information. Typical appearances are of diffuse proliferative glomerulonephritis with variable degrees of necrosis, crescent formation, glomerulosclerosis, and tubular loss (Fig. 25.5). The degree of crescent formation and tubular loss

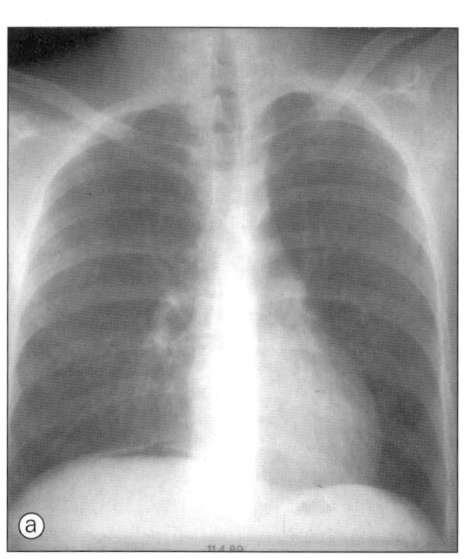
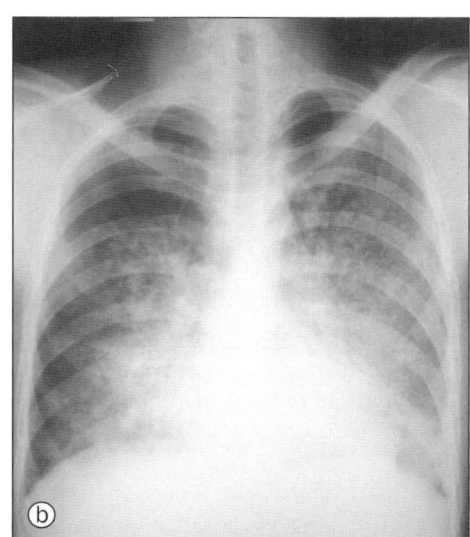

Figure 25.4 Chest radiographs of a patient with lung hemorrhage. Radiographs (a) and (b) taken 4 days later show the evolution of alveolar shadowing caused by lung hemorrhage.

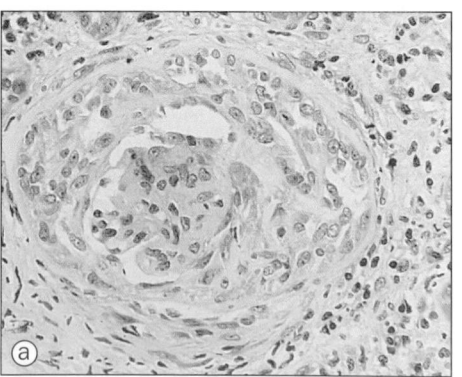
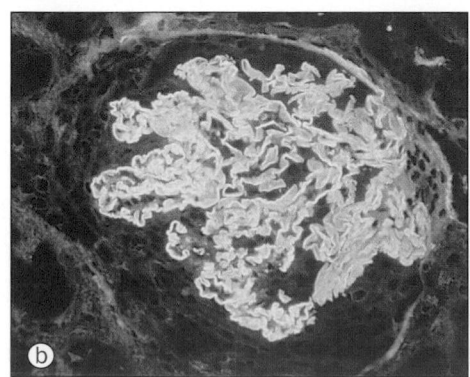

Figure 25.5 Renal biopsy in Goodpasture's disease. (a) Glomerulus from a patient with Goodpasture's disease, showing a recent, mostly cellular crescent. (b) Direct immunofluorescence study showing ribbon-like linear deposition of IgG along the glomerular basement membrane (GBM). The glomerular tuft is slightly compressed by cellular proliferation, forming a crescent (arrows). (Courtesy of Dr Richard Herriot.)

correlate with renal prognosis. Characteristically the crescents all appear to be of similar age and cellularity. When biopsied earlier in the disease, changes may be limited to focal and segmental mesangial expansion, with or without necrosis. This progresses to hypercellularity and then to more general changes including fractures of the GBM and Bowman's capsule, neutrophils in the glomeruli, and glomerular capillary thrombosis[16].

Immunohistology

In the presence of severe glomerular inflammation, linear deposition of immunoglobin along the GBM is pathognomonic. The immunoglobulin is usually IgG, sometimes (10–15%) with IgA or IgM, but very rarely IgA alone is detected. Linear deposition of C3 is detectable in about 75% of biopsies. Linear immunofluorescence with anti-immunoglobulin reagents is occasionally seen in other conditions (Table 25.3), usually without glomerular inflammation. In most instances the deposited immunoglobulin is less abundant than in Goodpasture's disease and is either nonspecifically deposited or bound to GBM components other than type IV collagen chains.

Circulating IgG anti-GBM antibodies are almost invariably present, even in the rare instances where only IgM or IgA has been reported to be bound to the GBM. They may be detected and quantified using immobilized Goodpasture antigen in an immunoassay. The titer of anti-GBM antibody at presentation correlates with the severity of nephritis. Treatment and relapse are often mirrored by changes in titer.

Pathology in other tissues

Pathologic changes in lung tissue (see Fig. 25.1) can be difficult to interpret because the changes in Goodpasture's disease, including immunoglobulin deposition, are often patchy and may be missed. Frequently, the only findings are mild, chronic inflammation and hemosiderin-laden macrophages, which is consistent with other more common pathologic diagnoses. This makes negative bronchoscopic or open lung biopsies unhelpful in excluding the diagnosis.

Other tissues in which α3(IV)NC1 is expressed are rarely available for pathologic analysis, but if antibody is deposited in other sites, then pathology is rarely associated with it. A number of case reports describe neurologic syndromes, particularly convulsions, which might be related to antibody deposition in the choroid plexus (Fig. 25.6) but may have other explanations in patients with acute renal failure. Other reports have described retinal detachment, in one instance with antibody deposition, but again this is rare.

DIFFERENTIAL DIAGNOSIS

Diagnosis of Goodpasture's disease in patients who present with Goodpasture's syndrome does not usually present difficulties once the possibility has been raised, although the urgency is often not appreciated. Direct immunofluorescence on renal tissue and assay for circulating anti-GBM antibodies are the most rapid techniques. Diagnosis is often delayed when patients present with subacute disease affecting lung or kidney in isolation. Patients with subacute lung hemorrhage may never report hemoptysis and present as cases of diffuse lung disease, of which there are many causes.

Detection of antiglomerular basement membrane antibodies

Detection of tissue-deposited, anti-GBM antibodies is usually achieved by direct immunofluorescence on frozen tissue sections using fluorochrome-conjugated antibodies that are specific for different classes of immunoglobulin. The technique is very sensitive for detecting anti-GBM antibody production, as the GBM selectively adsorbs and concentrates low levels of circulating antibody from the circulation. However, in some circumstances GBM may also adsorb antibody nonspecifically (see Table 25.3). Detection of anti-GBM antibodies in serum was previously by indirect immunofluorescence onto frozen sections of normal kidney, but this technique is too insensitive for routine use. Most assays are now solid-phase enzyme-linked immunosorbent assay (ELISA) or radioimmunoassay based on preparations of human or

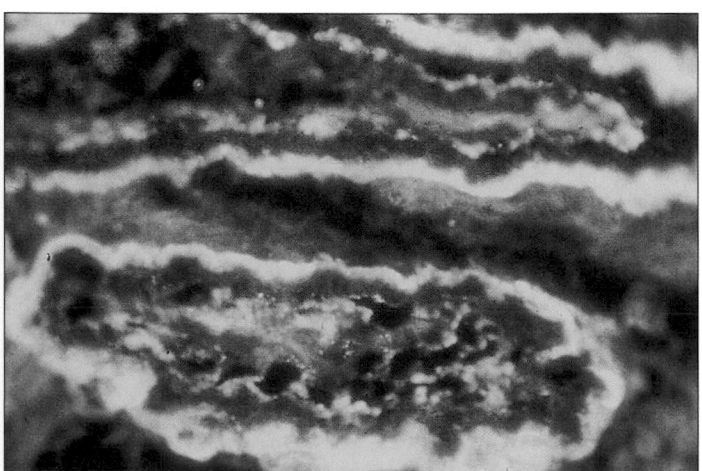

Figure 25.6 Direct immunofluorescence study showing binding of IgG to the choroid plexus of a patient who died from Goodpasture's disease. (Courtesy of Dr Stephen Cashman.)

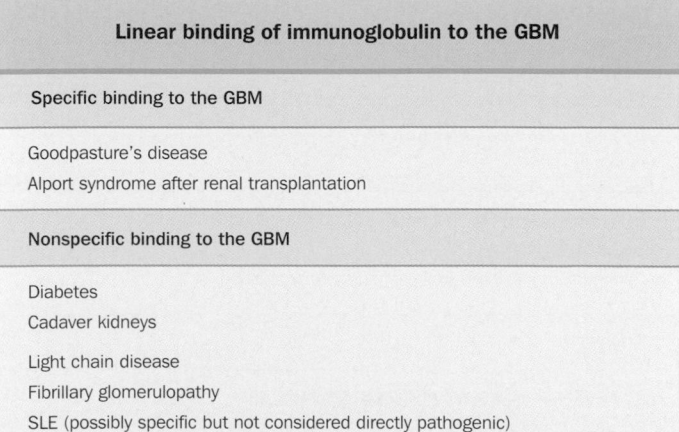

Linear binding of immunoglobulin to the GBM
Specific binding to the GBM
Goodpasture's disease Alport syndrome after renal transplantation
Nonspecific binding to the GBM
Diabetes Cadaver kidneys
Light chain disease Fibrillary glomerulopathy SLE (possibly specific but not considered directly pathogenic)

Table 25.3 Conditions associated with linear binding of immunoglobulin to the GBM.

animal GBM or recombinant antigen. The quality of these assays is variable. Confirmation of the specificity of anti-GBM antibodies may be obtained by Western blotting of serum onto solubilized human GBM or recombinant α3(IV)NC1, usually at a reference laboratory.

False-positive results may be encountered in various assays, particularly in sera from patients with inflammatory diseases that often exhibit increased nonspecific binding. This places greater emphasis on the purity of antigen used for anti-GBM assays. False-negative results are usually encountered in patients with low titers of antibodies in association with isolated lung disease or with very early or subacute renal disease. But low titers may occasionally be associated with anti-GBM disease that occurs after renal transplantation in patients with Alport syndrome (see below).

In very advanced disease, linear antibody deposition may not be seen because of extensive destruction of GBM structure. Otherwise deposited immunoglobulin remains detectable by direct fluorescence for some months after circulating immunoglobulin ceases to be detectable by ELISA.

Patients with antiglomerular basement membrane antibodies and other diseases

Antineutrophil cytoplasmic antibody and systemic small vessel vasculitis

Anti-GBM antibodies are sometimes detected in patients with sera that contain antineutrophil cytoplasmic antibody (ANCA), especially in those ANCA with specificity for myeloperoxidase (see Chapter 26). Such 'double-positive' patients may have a clinical course and response to treatment more typical of vasculitis than of Goodpasture's disease, and have possibly developed anti-GBM antibodies secondary to vasculitic glomerular damage[8-10]. Some patients have symptoms and signs in other organs, which suggest that they have systemic vasculitis. Anti-GBM titers tend to be lower in ANCA+/anti-GBM+ patients than in patients with anti-GBM antibodies alone.

Recovery of renal function may be more likely if ANCA are present, even if patients are dialysis-dependent when treatment is started, although some recent observations have failed to detect the differences described in early reports.

Membranous nephropathy

Anti-GBM antibodies are occasionally identified in patients with membranous nephropathy, usually coincident with an accelerated decline in renal function and the formation of glomerular crescents[5,17,18]. In approximately two-thirds of the two dozen or so published reports there was evidence of evolution from pre-existing nephrotic syndrome and in about half a previous kidney biopsy showed typical membranous nephropathy. Progression to end-stage renal disease (ESRD) has usually been rapid, but the diagnosis has rarely been made at an early enough stage to expect intensive treatment to be successful. Two patients with Goodpasture's disease later developed typical membranous nephropathy.

Differential diagnosis of Goodpasture's syndrome

A wide variety of conditions may cause simultaneous pulmonary and renal disease. The term 'pulmonary–renal syndrome' implies failure of both organs; the most common cause being fluid overload in a patient with renal failure of any cause. This may resemble Goodpasture's syndrome particularly if there is hematuria and pre-existing cardiac dysfunction. However, a number of diseases may mimic Goodpasture's syndrome (pulmonary hemorrhage with RPGN) to varying degrees by causing acute renal failure with acute lung disease (Table 25.4). Diseases associated with the syndrome fall into the two pathogenetic classes: those characterized by systemic vasculitis; and those associated with anti-GBM antibodies (Goodpasture's disease) (Table 25.5).

These diseases can sometimes be confidently differentiated clinically, but usually serology and renal biopsy are required. Renal biopsy also provides valuable prognostic information.

Causes of pulmonary renal syndrome
With pulmonary edema
Acute renal failure with hypervolemia Severe cardiac failure
Infective
Severe bacterial pneumonia (e.g., Legionella) with renal failure Hantavirus infection Opportunistic infections in the immunocompromised
Other
ARDS with renal failure in multiorgan failure Paraquat poisoning Renal vein/IVC thrombosis with pulmonary emboli

Table 25.4 Causes of pulmonary renal syndrome.

Causes of Goodpasture's syndrome (lung hemorrhage and rapidly progressive glomerulonephritis)
Diseases associated with antibodies to the GBM (20–40% of cases)
Goodpasture's disease (spontaneous anti-GBM disease)
Diseases associated with systemic vasculitis (60–80% of cases)
Wegener's granulomatosis ⎤ ⎬ Common Microscopic polyangiitis ⎦ Systemic lupus erythematosus Churg Strauss syndrome Henoch–Schönlein purpura Behçet's disease Essential mixed cryoglobulinemia Rheumatoid vasculitis Drugs: penicillamine, hydralazine, propylthiouracil

Table 25.5 Causes of Goodpasture's syndrome (lung hemorrhage and rapidly progressive renal glomerulonephritis).

NATURAL HISTORY

There is some variability in the pattern of early disease. Most patients present acutely with lung hemorrhage and/or advanced renal failure and report that the illness developed over only weeks or a few months. However, there are several reports of patients presenting with mild respiratory symptoms or incidental microscopic hematuria and with disease progressing much more slowly over months or years. It is unclear to what extent these reports indicate differences in clinical course or earlier detection, as patients with slowly progressive or static disease may abruptly develop the full acute syndrome.

Once RPGN has developed, renal function is rapidly and often irretrievably destroyed. Progression is often much more rapid than in RPGN occurring in other contexts such as microscopic polyangiitis, perhaps because more glomeruli are simultaneously affected. Consequently there is a much narrower window of opportunity for effective treatment.

Although a severe exacerbation of lung disease commonly coincides with deterioration of renal function, the natural history of isolated lung disease critically depends on continued exposure to irritants. For example, avoidance of smoking frequently results in symptomatic remission and ironically may convince the patient to delay medical assessment, while the renal disease progresses unnoticed. The same danger is inherent in treating patients with isolated lung disease with less intensive immunosuppressive regimens.

TREATMENT

Immunosuppressive regimens

Before the introduction of immunosuppressive treatment, most patients died shortly after the development of renal impairment or pulmonary hemorrhage[18]. Powerful immunosuppressive regimes have transformed the prognosis. Pulmonary hemorrhage can usually be arrested within 24–48 h. Renal function can be protected if impairment is mild, and in some circumstances even severe renal impairment can be reversed. But dialysis-dependent patients rarely recover kidney function despite immunosuppression, and should probably only be immunosuppressed if pulmonary hemorrhage occurs.

A chart recording treatment of a patient with Goodpasture's disease is shown in Figure 25.7. Recommended treatment for acute severe disease is shown in Table 25.6. The regimen was devised to reduce levels of circulating pathogenic antibodies as rapidly as possible, and to curtail their contribution to the rapid glomerular destruction that can occur during acute severe disease, and is very effective. Once the disease is controlled, immunosuppression can usually be tailed off over 3 months and subsequent relapse is uncommon. The immune response is also self-limiting if renal function is supported, with antibodies disappearing over 1–2 years.

Plasma exchange and immunosuppression

Only one element, plasma exchange, has been tested in a randomized controlled trial, but the regimen dramatically

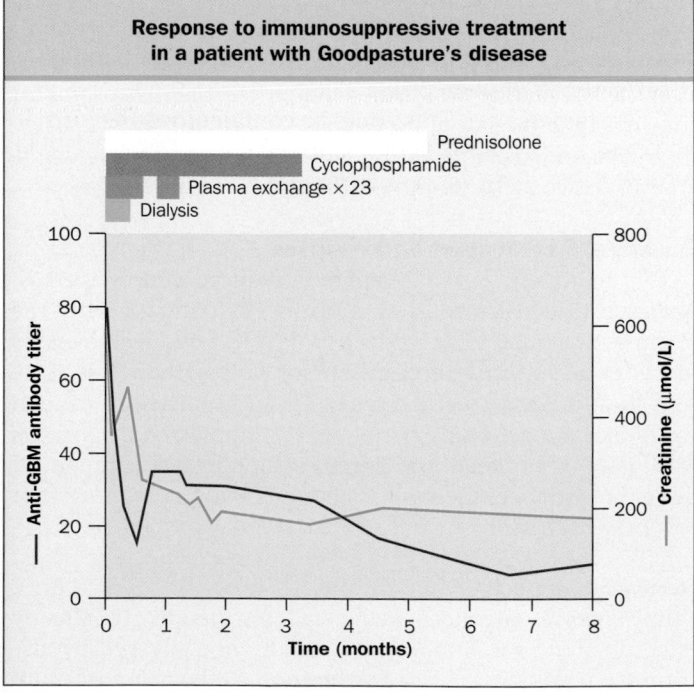

Figure 25.7 Response to immunosuppressive treatment in a patient with Goodpasture's disease. The patient required dialysis for renal disease but had no lung hemorrhage. The good response to treatment was unusual but not unique. The renal biopsy showed 85% of glomeruli contained recent (mostly cellular) crescents, suggesting very acute disease, which may be indicative of a more favorable response to treatment. (With permission from W.B. Saunders & Co. Turner and Rees[18].)

Treatment regimen for acute Goodpasture's disease	
Prednisolone	1 mg/kg/24 h orally. Reduce at weekly intervals to achieve one-sixth of this dose by 8 weeks. For a starting daily dose of 60 mg, use weekly reductions to 45 mg, 30 mg, 25 mg, 20 mg, 15 mg; then 2 weekly to 12.5 mg, 10 mg. Maintain this dose to 3 months; then stop by 4 months.
Cyclophosphamide	3 mg/kg/24 h orally, rounded down to the nearest 50 mg. Patients > 55 years receive a reduced dose of 2.5 mg/kg.
Plasma exchange	Daily exchange of 4 L of plasma for 5% human albumin for 14 days or until the circulating antibody is suppressed. In the presence of pulmonary hemorrhage, or within 48 h of an invasive procedure, 300–400 mL of fresh, frozen plasma is given at the end of each treatment.
Monitoring	Daily blood count during plasma exchange and while antibody titer remains elevated. At least twice weekly during first month, weekly thereafter. If white blood cell count falls below 3.5, stop cyclophosphamide until it recovers. Resume at lower dose if cessation has been necessary. Baseline D_LCO, with further measurements as indicated. Daily coagulation tests during plasma exchange to monitor for significant depletion of clotting factors. Initially, daily checks of renal and hepatic function, glucose
Prophylaxis against complications of treatment	Oral antifungal lozenges or rinse; H_2 antagonist. Cotrimoxazole prophylaxis against *Pneumocystis carinii*. Avoid nonessential lines, catheters

(With permission: W.B. Saunders & Co, Turner and Rees[18].)

Table 25.6 Treatment regimen for acute Goodpasture's disease.

improved the outlook for patients when it was introduced in the 1970s. The trial[19] suggested some additional benefit of plasma exchange, but the interpretation was complicated by the fact that the recipient group had less severe disease at presentation. It showed that milder disease can be effectively treated with corticosteroids and cyclophosphamide alone, although the overall outcomes for all patients were not as good as have been described with more intensive regimens[18].

Historical evidence suggests that treatment with corticosteroids alone, or corticosteroids with azathioprine, is less effective. Plasma exchange is only of value if accompanied by adjunctive immunosuppressive therapy. Immunoadsorption to protein-A also lowers anti-GBM antibodies rapidly; it does not deplete complement components or clotting factors and a few reports suggest that it is as effective as plasma exchange.

Lung hemorrhage occurring alone tends to be relapsing and remitting, so there have been many reports of treatments (including bilateral nephrectomy) which may help. Use of pulse methylprednisolone is particularly popular. High doses of corticosteroids fail to alter the underlying pathogenetic immune response and put the patient at increased risk of infective and other complications. Therefore, administration of these drugs alone is not recommended. Seriously ill patients should be treated with moderate doses of corticosteroids plus plasma exchange and cyclophosphamide.

Anecdotal experience in other acute severe diseases suggests that daily administration of cyclophosphamide may be more rapidly and consistently effective than pulse administration, and this remains our usual practice. Patients unable to take the drug orally can be given daily intravenous therapy at the usual oral dose. Dosage does not need to be reduced in severe renal failure but reductions for older patients are important (Table 25.6), and close monitoring of leukocyte counts is imperative in all patients.

Results from all series show that recovery of renal function is unlikely if at the time it is commenced the patient is oliguric, has a very high proportion of glomeruli with circumferential crescents, or has a creatinine serum level of over 5–6 mg/dL (500–600 µmol/L)[20]. This is a notably different experience from that encountered in systemic vasculitis or idiopathic RPGN (see Chapter 26), in which renal disease of apparently similar severity (judged by histology and creatinine level) can be salvaged by similar treatment protocols[21]. It has led to the suggestion that immunosuppressive treatment should be withheld from patients in whom the chance of recovery is slight, to protect them from the risks of the treatment itself. This is considered further below.

Supportive treatment
The most likely cause of death in the first few days is respiratory failure caused by lung hemorrhage. Lung hemorrhage may be precipitated or exacerbated by:
- fluid overload;
- smoking and other pulmonary irritants possibly including high fractional inspired oxygen concentrations;
- local or distant infection;
- anticoagulation used during dialysis or plasma exchange;
- the thrombocytopenia and defibrination that occur as a consequence of plasma exchange.

It is therefore sensible to ensure correct fluid balance, prohibit smoking, use the lowest fractional inspired oxygen concentration that gives adequate oxygenation, and minimize the use of heparin.

Plasma exchange should be monitored by daily blood counts and coagulation tests, and if pulmonary hemorrhage occurs, diminished clotting factor levels should be replenished by administering fresh frozen plasma or clotting factor preparations at the end of each plasma exchange session.

After the first few days the major cause of morbidity and mortality is infection. Infection carries the added risk of potentiating glomerular and lung inflammation and injury so precautions to reduce the risk of infection, such as minimizing the number of indwelling cannulae, are particularly important. The neutrophil count should be monitored and if neutropenia develops, cyclophosphamide should be discontinued and resumed at a lower dose when the neutrophil count recovers, if necessary with the assistance of granulocyte colony-stimulating factor (G-CSF).

Monitoring effect of treatment on disease activity
The effect of treatment on the renal disease may be monitored by following serum creatinine levels. Indicators of recent pulmonary hemorrhage include hemoptysis, falls in hemoglobin concentration, chest radiograph changes, and rises in the $D_L CO$, the latter being the most sensitive. Any worsening of symptoms during treatment may indicate inadequate immunosuppression but frequently it is a consequence of intercurrent infection exaggerating immunologic injury, or fluid overload or other factors precipitating pulmonary hemorrhage.

Monitoring anti-GBM titers during and particularly 24 h after the last planned plasma exchange treatment is useful for confirming effective suppression of autoantibodies. They should be undetectable within 8 weeks, but remain detectable for an average of 14 months without treatment.

Duration of treatment and relapses
Steroid treatment may be gradually reduced and cyclophosphamide discontinued at 3 months. In contrast with the treatment of small vessel vasculitis, it is not usually necessary to continue immunosuppression for longer than this. Late rises in anti-GBM level may auger clinical relapse, although antibodies are generally permanently suppressed in patients who have completed the immunosuppressive regimen. If there is recurrence, success has been achieved by treating as at first presentation.

Electing not to treat
Unfortunately advanced renal failure, frequently already established at presentation, is generally not salvaged by any current treatment[18,20,22]. Furthermore, the immunosuppressive regimen outlined above carries significant risks, the plasma exchange element is expensive, and assiduous monitoring is required. For these reasons it may be reasonable not to commence potentially dangerous immunosuppression in patients who present with advanced renal failure without pulmonary hemorrhage. The decision not to treat is strengthened if renal biopsy shows widespread glomerulosclerosis and

Factors influencing treatment decisions in Goodpasture's disease		
	Factors favoring aggressive treatment	Factors against aggressive treatment
Pulmonary hemorrhage	Present	Absent
Oliguria	Absent	Present
Creatinine	< 6.6 mg/dL (600 μmol/L)	>6.6 mg/dL (600 μmol/L) and ANCA negative Severe damage on biopsy No desire for early transplantation
Other factors	Creatinine >600 μmol/L BUT Rapid and recent progression ANCA positive Glomerular damage less severe than expected Crescents recent, nonfibrous Early renal transplantation desired	
Associated disease	Absent	Unusually high risk from immunosuppression

Table 25.7 Factors influencing decision to treat/not treat aggressively in Goodpasture's disease.

tubular loss and the patient is dialysis-dependent at presentation (Table 25.7). The risk of developing late pulmonary hemorrhage in these circumstances seems to be very low, but warrants particular care to avoid the major precipitating factors, smoking and pulmonary edema, in at least the first few months.

However, patients who are dialysis dependent should be treated if the renal biopsy changes are unexpectedly mild or very recent (highly cellular crescents, even if 100% of glomeruli are involved) as several reports describe good outcomes in these circumstances even after prolonged oliguria.

Treatment of 'double positive' patients

Patients with ANCA as well as anti-GBM antibodies ('double positive' patients) should usually be treated even when dialysis-dependent, as a useful renal response is more likely. Furthermore these patients may have other extrarenal disease requiring treatment (Table 25.7). 'Double positive' patients should receive an immunosuppressive regimen similar to that given for small vessel vasculitis with continuing immunosuppression with azathioprine after 3 months of cyclophosphamide.

In RPGN where there is no evidence of an infective etiology, immunosuppressive therapy should be started immediately, sometimes before the renal biopsy findings are available. If therapy is stopped after a few days the patient will have incurred very little risk (as long as pulsed high-dose corticosteroids are avoided), but sometimes has a great deal to gain from earlier treatment.

In contrast to advanced renal failure where treatment is unlikely to lead to recovery of renal function, even severe pulmonary hemorrhage is likely to respond to treatment with full or nearly full recovery of lung function.

TRANSPLANTATION

Renal transplantation in patients who have had Goodpasture's disease carries the additional risk of disease recurrence. Recurrence with consequent loss of the graft has been reported and appears more likely when circulating anti-GBM antibodies are still detectable at the time of transplantation. For this reason it is reasonable to delay transplantation until circulating anti-GBM antibodies have been undetectable for 6 months and monitor graft function, urinary sediment, and circulating anti-GBM antibody levels to detect recurrent disease. Biopsies of well-functioning grafts sometimes show linear deposition of immunoglobulin on the GBM without clinical or histologic disease, nor apparently an adverse prognosis.

ALPORT POST-TRANSPLANT ANTI-GBM DISEASE

Patients with Alport syndrome have mutations in a gene encoding one of the tissue-specific type IV collagen chains, usually α5. Because these chains assemble with each other during biosynthesis, the resulting phenotype in the case of most mutations has all the tissue-specific chains (α3–α5) missing from the basement membranes, where they are normally coexpressed. Altered expression may lead to absent or inadequate immunologic tolerance to these proteins and to the preservation of the capacity to mount a powerful (allo)immune response to the type IV collagen chains expressed in a normal donor kidney after renal transplantation. Most Alport patients accommodate renal transplants with conventional immunosuppression without developing anti-GBM glomerulonephritis. However, the development of low titers of anti-GBM antibodies is shown by the fact that many such patients have linear deposition of IgG on the GBM of the transplanted kidney (by direct immunofluorescence).

A minority of patients (up to about 5%) develop RPGN clinically indistinguishable from Goodpasture's disease but without pulmonary hemorrhage. This is more likely if they have a large gene deletion causing the disease, rather than a point mutation, with the inference that their immune system has never been exposed to the mature protein. Typically, graft function is lost despite treatment for presumed acute rejection. Disease is usually encountered some months or longer after a first renal transplant; after weeks in a second; and after days in a third. In the past the diagnosis has only rarely been appreciated before glomeruli have been largely destroyed.

Experience with regrafting patients who have lost kidneys to Alport post-transplant anti-GBM disease is limited and generally depressing. However, regrafting has been successful in two cases known to us and in two further cases in the literature. If the disease is recognized early, there are sound theoretical reasons for treating with the regimen recommended for Goodpasture's disease, but there are few data on its effectiveness.

Glomerular Disease

In contrast to spontaneous Goodpasture's disease, the specificity of anti-GBM antibodies in Alport post-transplant anti-GBM disease is not always to α3(IV)NC1. In many patients, possibly in most, the autoantibodies are specific for α5(IV)NC1, encoded by the gene usually implicated in causation of the disease[23]. This is important because immunoassays for anti-GBM antibodies have usually been optimized for detection of the anti-α3(IV)NC1 antibodies of spontaneous Goodpasture's disease, and they may have very low sensitivity for anti-α5(IV)NC1 antibodies. In the absence of widely available assays for these uncommon antibodies, renal biopsy with immunohistology is the only reliable method of diagnosis.

REFERENCES

1. Goodpasture EW. The significance of certain pulmonary lesions in relation to the etiology of influenza. Am J Med Sci. 1919;158:863–70.
2. Stanton MC, Tange JD. Goodpasture's syndrome (pulmonary haemorrhage associated with glomerulonephritis). Aust NZ J Med. 1958;7:132–44.
3. Saus J, Wieslander J, Langeveld J, et al. Identification of the Goodpasture antigen as the α3(IV) chain of collagen IV. J Biol Chem. 1988;263:13374–80.
4. Turner N, Mason PJ, Brown R, et al. Molecular cloning of the human Goodpasture antigen demonstrates it to be the a3 chain of type IV collagen. J Clin Invest. 1992;89:592–601.
5. Kashtan CE, Michael AF. Alport syndrome. Kidney Int. 1996;50:1445–63.
6. Aumailley M. Structure and supramolecular organization of basement membranes. Kidney Int.1995;49:54–7.
7. Phelps RG, Rees AJ. The HLA complex in Goodpasture's disease: A model for analyzing susceptibility to autoimmunity. Kidney Int. 1999;56(5):1638–54.
8. Bolton WK. Goodpasture's syndrome. Kidney Int. 1996;50:1753–66.
9. Bosch X, Mirapeix E, Font J, et al. Prognostic implications of anti-neutrophil cytoplasmic autoantibodies with myeloperoxidase specificity in antiglomerular basement membrane disease. Clin Nephrol. 1991;36:107–13.
10. Jayne DRW, Marshall PD, Jones SJ, Lockwood CM. Autoantibodies to glomerular basement membrane and neutrophil cytoplasm in rapidly progressive glomerulonephritis. Kidney Int. 1990;37:965–70.
11. Phelps RG, Turner AN. Goodpasture's syndrome: new insights into pathogenesis and clinical picture. J Nephrol. 1996;9:111–17.
12. Lerner RA, Glassock RJ, Dixon FJ. The role of antiglomerular basement membrane antibody in the pathogenesis of human glomerulonephritis. J Exp Med. 1967;126:989–1004.
13. Atkins RC, Nikolic-Paterson DJ, Song Q, Lan HY. Modulators of crescentic nephritis. J Am Soc Nephrol. 1996;7:2271–8.
14. Savill J, Rees AJ. Mechanisms of glomerular injury. In: Cameron JS, Davison AM, Grunfeld JP, et al. eds. Oxford Textbook of Nephrology. Oxford: OUP; 1997:403–39.
15. Turner AN, Rees AJ. Antiglomerular basement membrane disease. In: Cameron JS, Davison AM, Grunfeld JP. Oxford Textbook of Nephrology. Oxford: OUP; 1997:647–66.
16. Heptinstall RH. Schönlein–Henoch syndrome; lung hemorrhage and glomerulonephritis. In: Heptinstall RH, ed. Pathology of the Kidney. Boston: Little Brown; 1983:761–91.
17. Thitiarchakul S, Lal SM, Luger A, Ross G. Goodpasture's syndrome superimposed on membranous nephropathy. A case report. Int J Artif Org. 1995;18:763–5.
18. Turner AN, Rees AJ. Anti-glomerular basement membrane antibody disease. In: Brady HR, Wilcox N, eds. Therapy in Nephrology and Hypertension: a companion to Brenner and Rector's The Kidney. Philadelphia: W.B. Saunders; 1999:152–7.
19. Johnson JP, Moore JJ, Austin HA, et al. Therapy of anti-glomerular basement membrane antibody disease: analysis of prognostic significance of clinical, pathologic and treatment factors. Medicine (Baltimore). 1985;64:219–27.
20. Levy JB, Turner AN, Rees AJ, Pusey CD. Long-term outcome of anti-glomerular basement membrane antibody disease treated with plasma exchange and immunosuppression. Ann Intern Med. 2001;134:1033–42.
21. Hind CRK, Paraskevakou H, Lockwood CM, et al. Prognosis after immunosuppression of patients with crescentic nephritis requiring dialysis. Lancet. 1983;1:8319:263–5.
22. Flores JC, Taube D, Savage COS, et al. Clinical and immunological evolution of oliguric anti-GBM nephritis treated by haemodialysis. Lancet. 1986;1:8471:5–8.
23. Brainwood D, Kashtan C, Gubler MC, et al. Targets of alloantibodies in Alport anti-glomerular basement membrane disease after renal transplantation. Kidney Int. 1998;53:762–6.

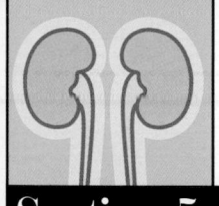

Chapter 26

Renal and Systemic Vasculitis

J Charles Jennette and Ronald J Falk

INTRODUCTION

The kidneys frequently are targets for a variety of systemic vasculitides, especially those that affect small vessels[1-4]. This is not surprising given the large number and variety of renal vessels. Vasculitis involving the kidneys can produce a wide variety of clinical manifestations depending in large measure upon the type of renal vessel affected. As demonstrated in Figures 26.1, 26.2 and Table 26.1, vasculitides can be categorized as large vessel vasculitis, medium-sized vessel vasculitis, and small vessel vasculitis. The categorization of systemic vasculitides is controversial. For the purposes of the discussion in this chapter, the Chapel Hill Consensus Conference definitions will be used (see Table 26.1).

A number of the vasculitides listed in Figure 26.2 are covered elsewhere in the book and will not be reviewed in detail here except in the context of differential diagnosis: for example, cryoglobulinemic vasculitis (see Chapter 23), Henoch–Schönlein purpura (see Chapter 24), and anti-glomerular basement membrane (GBM) disease (see Chapter 25). Nephrologists most often encounter patients with small vessel vasculitis, which will receive the most attention in this chapter.

Large vessel vasculitis

Large vessel vasculitis is chronic granulomatous arteritis that affects predominantly the aorta and its major branches. When there is renal involvement, the ostia of the renal arteries and the main renal arteries are most often affected. The most common clinical renal manifestation is renovascular hypertension.

Medium-sized vessel vasculitis

Medium-sized vessel vasculitis is necrotizing arteritis that affects predominantly major visceral arteries and may involve any renal arteries, including the main renal artery, interlobar arteries, arcuate arteries, and interlobular arteries. Inflammation and necrosis of arteries may result in thrombosis or rupture, which causes renal infarction and hemorrhage.

Small vessel vasculitis

Small vessel vasculitis is necrotizing polyangiitis that affects predominantly vessels smaller than arteries, including capillaries, venules, and arterioles; however, arteries also may be involved. The most common renal targets for small vessel vasculitides are the glomeruli and, therefore, the most common clinical renal manifestations are those of glomerulonephritis.

SMALL VESSEL PAUCI-IMMUNE VASCULITIS

Wegener's granulomatosis, Churg–Strauss syndrome, and microscopic polyangiitis share an indistinguishable form of necrotizing small vessel vasculitis that affects capillaries, venules, arterioles, and small arteries[3,4]. Some patients, however, have no evidence for involvement of arteries, but involvement of glomerular capillaries, causing glomerulonephritis; pulmonary alveolar capillaries, causing pulmonary hemorrhage; or dermal venules, causing purpura. These so-called pauci-immune small vessel vasculitides are distinguished from clinically and histologically similar forms of immune-complex small vessel vasculitis, such as cryoglobulinemic vasculitis and Henoch–Schönlein purpura, by the absence or paucity of immune-complex deposits in vessel walls. The diagnosis for the specific subtypes of pauci-immune small vessel vasculitides can be made on the basis of the accompanying syndrome.

- Wegener's granulomatosis occurs in association with necrotizing granulomatous inflammation, which most often affects the respiratory tract.
- Churg–Strauss syndrome is vasculitis occurring in association with asthma, eosinophilia, and necrotizing granulomatous inflammation.
- Microscopic polyangiitis is pauci-immune vasculitis occurring in the absence of evidence for Wegener's granulomatosis or Churg–Strauss syndrome, i.e., in the absence of asthma, eosinophilia, and evidence for necrotizing granulomatous inflammation.

Microscopic polyangiitis, Wegener's granulomatosis, and, less frequently, Churg–Strauss syndrome also share an indistinguishable pattern of glomerulonephritis that is the expression of the vasculitis in glomerular capillaries. The glomerulonephritis usually has necrosis and crescent formation and an absence or paucity of immunoglobulin deposition and is often designated pauci-immune crescentic glomerulonephritis. When pauci-immune crescentic glomerulonephritis occurs in the apparent absence of systemic vasculitis, it is sometimes referred to as 'renal vasculitis', 'renal-limited vasculitis', or 'idiopathic rapidly progressive glomerulonephritis' (RPGN).

Pathogenesis

Wegener's granulomatosis, microscopic polyangiitis, Churg–Strauss syndrome, and isolated pauci-immune crescentic glomerulonephritis are all associated with the presence in serum of autoantibodies against components of the cytoplasm

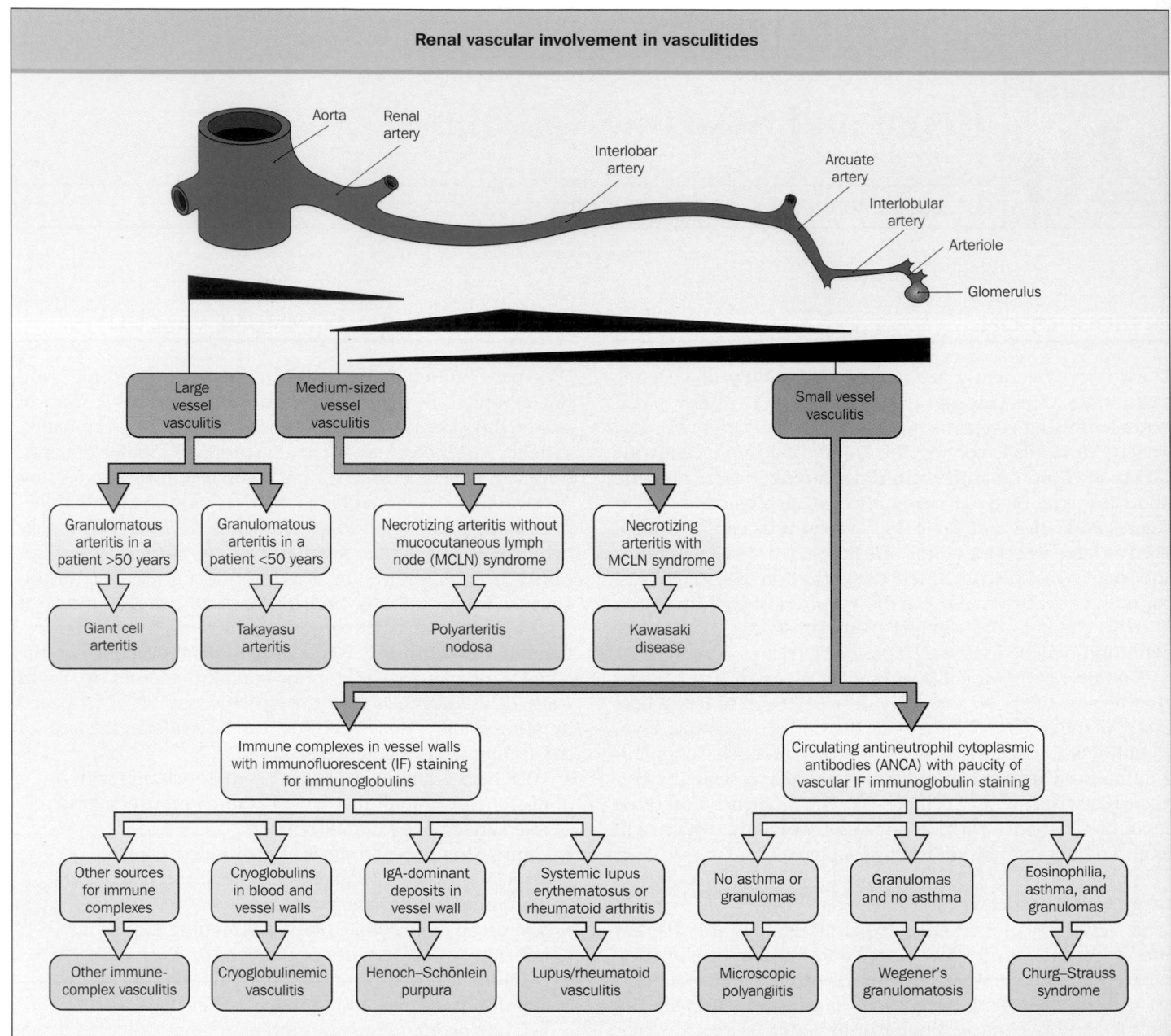

Figure 26.1 Renal vasculitis: the predominant distribution of renal vascular involvement by a variety of vasculitides. The heights of the trapezoids represent the relative frequency of involvement of different portions of the renal vasculature by the three major categories of vasculitis. (Adapted with permission from Jennette and Falk[3].)

of neutrophils: circulating antineutrophil cytoplasmic auto-antibodies (ANCA)[5–7]. The most common antigen specificities of ANCA in patients with vasculitis and glomerulonephritis are for proteinase 3 (PR3) and myeloperoxidase (MPO). This association with ANCA has led to the development of hypotheses that incriminate ANCA in the pathogenesis of these vasculitides[8].

A number of clinical observations, in addition to the association alone, raise the possibility that ANCA are involved in the pathogenesis of pauci-immune small vessel vasculitis. ANCA disease responds to immunosuppressive treatment. This is very nonspecific because many other potential pathogenetic mechanisms also would respond to immunosuppression. The observation that ANCA titers correlate with disease activity is more specific; however, this is not a very tight correlation. Most suggestive is the observation that administration of certain drugs, such as propylthiouracil, hydralazine, and penicillamine, can induce ANCA concurrent with the development of pauci-immune crescentic glomerulonephritis and small vessel vasculitis.

A number of *in vitro* observations suggest mechanisms by which ANCA could cause vascular injury. Priming of neutrophils by cytokines, as would occur with a viral infection, causes neutrophils to express antigens on their surfaces where

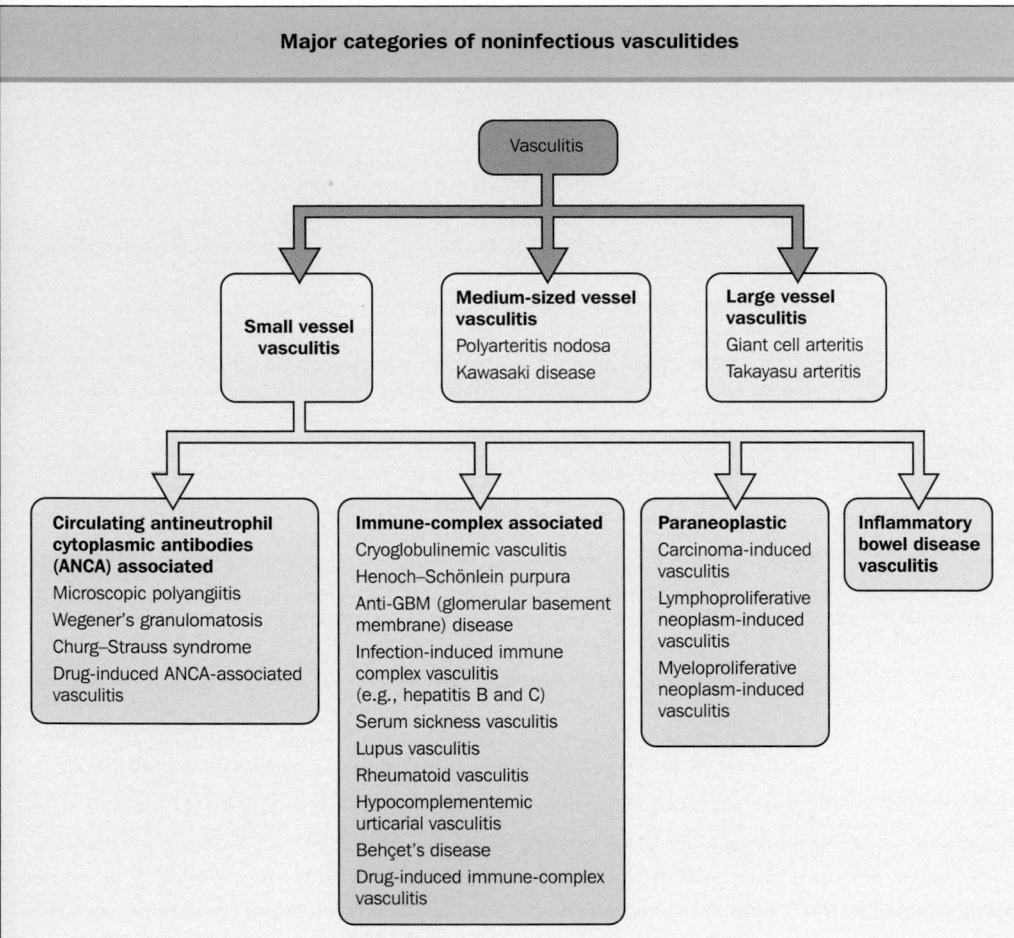

Major categories of noninfectious vasculitides

Figure 26.2 The major categories of noninfectious vasculitis. Not included are vasculitides that are known to be caused by direct invasion of vessel walls by infectious pathogens, such as rickettsial vasculitis and neisserial vasculitis.

they are accessible to interact with ANCA. Cytokine-primed neutrophils that are exposed to ANCA release IgG from granules, release toxic oxygen metabolites, and kill cultured endothelial cells. ANCA–antigen complexes adsorb onto endothelial cells where they could participate in *in situ* immune-complex formation. Endothelial cells may synthesize PR3, which could participate in *in situ* immune-complex formation, although the existence of this synthetic capability is controversial. ANCA activation of neutrophils is mediated by both F(ab)′$_2$ binding to neutrophils and Fc receptor engagement. If these events occurred *in vivo* they would lead to vasculitis as a result of neutrophils adhering to, penetrating, and destroying vessel walls (Fig. 26.3)[8].

A number of observations in experimental animal models support a pathogenetic role for ANCA. Rats immunized with human MPO develop anti-MPO that cross-reacts with rat MPO. Subsequent renal perfusion with MPO results in glomerulonephritis and vasculitis with only transient low-level immune-complex formation in glomeruli. In another model, rats injected with low doses of anti-GBM antibodies develop crescentic glomerulonephritis and vasculitis in the presence of circulating anti-MPO but not in the absence of the anti-MPO[9]. The low-level anti-GBM injury may serve as a priming event that synergizes with the anti-MPO (ANCA) to cause severe glomerulonephritis and vasculitis. Recent studies have used MPO knock out mice as sources for anti-MPO antibodies and

antibody producing lymphocytes. Adoptive transfer of anti-MPO antibody-producing lymphocytes or passive infusion of anti-MPO antibodies into immune deficient mice recipients causes severe necrotizing and crescentic glomerulonephritis and small vessel vasculitis[10]. This is the compelling evidence that ANCA cause glomerulonephritis and vasculitis.

Thus, the *in vitro* and the experimental animal data support the hypothesis that ANCA can activate neutrophils and cause vasculitis, especially if there is a concurrent synergistic proinflammatory stimulus. The requirement for a synergistic inflammatory process may be reflected in the very frequent association of the onset of ANCA small vessel vasculitis with a flu-like syndrome. A flu-like syndrome is a manifestation of high levels of circulating cytokines, for example as induced by a viral respiratory tract infection, which could serve as priming factors for neutrophils. In a normal person, circulating primed neutrophils would be more efficient at localizing at sites of appropriate inflammation; however, in a patient with ANCA, the interaction between primed neutrophils and ANCA could result in vasculitis and glomerulonephritis. At the current time, this scenario remains unproven.

Epidemiology

Wegener's granulomatosis, microscopic polyangiitis, and Churg–Strauss syndrome usually begin during the fifth, sixth, and seventh decades of life, although they may occur at any

Names and definitions of vasculitis adopted by the Chapel Hill Consensus Conference on the nomenclature of systemic vasculitis		
Category	Type	Definition
Large vessel vasculitis	Giant cell (temporal) arteritis	Granulomatous arteritis of the aorta and its major branches, with a predilection for the extracranial branches of the carotid artery. Often involves the temporal artery. Usually occurs in patients older than 50 and often is associated with polymyalgia rheumatica
	Takayasu arteritis	Granulomatous inflammation of the aorta and its major branches. Usually occurs in patients younger than 50
Medium-sized vessel vasculitis	Polyarteritis nodosa (classic polyarteritis nodosa)	Necrotizing inflammation of medium-sized or small arteries without glomerulonephritis or vasculitis in arterioles, capillaries, or venules
	Kawasaki disease	Arteritis involving large, medium-sized, and small arteries, and associated with mucocutaneous lymph node syndrome. Coronary arteries are often involved. Aorta and veins may be involved. Usually occurs in children
Small vessel vasculitis	Wegener's granulomatosis	Granulomatous inflammation involving the respiratory tract, and necrotizing vasculitis affecting small to medium-sized vessels, e.g., capillaries, venules, arterioles, and arteries. Necrotizing glomerulonephritis is common
	Churg–Strauss syndrome	Eosinophil-rich and granulomatous inflammation involving the respiratory tract, and necrotizing vasculitis affecting small to medium-sized vessels; associated with asthma and blood eosinophilia
	Microscopic polyangiitis (microscopic polyarteritis)	Necrotizing vasculitis with few or no immune deposits, affecting small vessels, i.e., capillaries, venules, or arterioles. Necrotizing arteritis involving small and medium-sized arteries may be present. Necrotizing glomerulonephritis is very common. Pulmonary capillaritis often occurs
	Henoch–Schönlein purpura	Vasculitis with IgA-dominant immune deposits affecting small vessels, i.e., capillaries, venules, or arterioles. Typically involves skin, gut and glomeruli and is associated with arthralgias or arthritis
	Essential cryoglobulinemic vasculitis	Vasculitis with cryoglobulin immune deposits, affecting small vessels, i.e., capillaries, venules, or arterioles; associated with cryoglobulins in serum. Skin and glomeruli are often involved
	Cutaneous leukocytoclastic angiitis	Isolated cutaneous leukocytoclastic angiitis without systemic vasculitis or glomerulonephritis

Note that all three categories affect arteries, but only small vessel vasculitis has a predilection for vessels smaller than arteries. (Modified with permission from Jennette et al[4].

Table 26.1 Names and definitions of vasculitis adopted by the Chapel Hill Consensus Conference on the nomenclature of systemic vasculitis.

age. There is a slight male predominance. Caucasians have a disproportionately greater incidence than African Americans. Crude estimates of the annual incidence of these diseases in North America and Europe are approximately 1 to 2 per 100 000 population. Although not documented with adequate data, there is a suspicion that Wegener's granulomatosis is more frequent in colder compared with warmer climates, whereas microscopic polyangiitis has the opposite trend.

Clinical manifestations

The clinical manifestations of Wegener's granulomatosis, microscopic polyangiitis, and Churg–Strauss syndrome are extremely varied because they are influenced by the sites of involvement, and the activity versus the chronicity of involvement. All three categories of vasculitis share features caused by the small vessel vasculitis, and patients with Wegener's granulomatosis and Churg–Strauss syndrome have the additional features that define each of these syndromes[2,4,11,12].

Renal involvement is very common in Wegener's granulomatosis and microscopic polyangiitis and less frequent in Churg–Strauss syndrome (Table 26.2). The most common renal manifestations are caused by glomerular involvement and include hematuria, proteinuria, and renal failure. The renal failure often has the characteristics of RPGN in patients with Wegener's granulomatosis and microscopic polyangiitis but usually is less severe in those with Churg–Strauss syndrome.

Wegener's granulomatosis and microscopic polyangiitis also can present as a subacute or chronic nephritis.

Generalized nonspecific manifestations of systemic inflammatory disease often are present, such as fever, malaise, anorexia, weight loss, myalgias, and arthralgias. Many patients trace the origin of their disease to a 'flu-like' illness.

Cutaneous involvement is frequent. Purpura caused by dermal venulitis is a common manifestation of Wegener's granulomatosis, microscopic polyangiitis, and Churg–Strauss syndrome (Fig. 26.4). The purpura is most common on the lower extremities and tends to occur as recurrent crops. The purpura may be accompanied by small areas of ulceration. Nodular cutaneous lesions occur with Wegener's granulomatosis and Churg–Strauss syndrome but are very rare with microscopic polyangiitis. Nodules can be caused by dermal or subcutaneous arteritis and by the necrotizing granulomatous inflammation of Wegener's granulomatosis and Churg–Strauss syndrome.

Upper and lower respiratory tract involvement is most common in Wegener's granulomatosis and Churg–Strauss syndrome but also occurs in those with microscopic polyangiitis. All three categories can have pulmonary hemorrhage caused by hemorrhagic capillaritis. Wegener's granulomatosis and Churg–Strauss syndrome also can have pulmonary injury caused by necrotizing granulomatous inflammation, which may be detected radiographically as nodular or cavitary lesions.

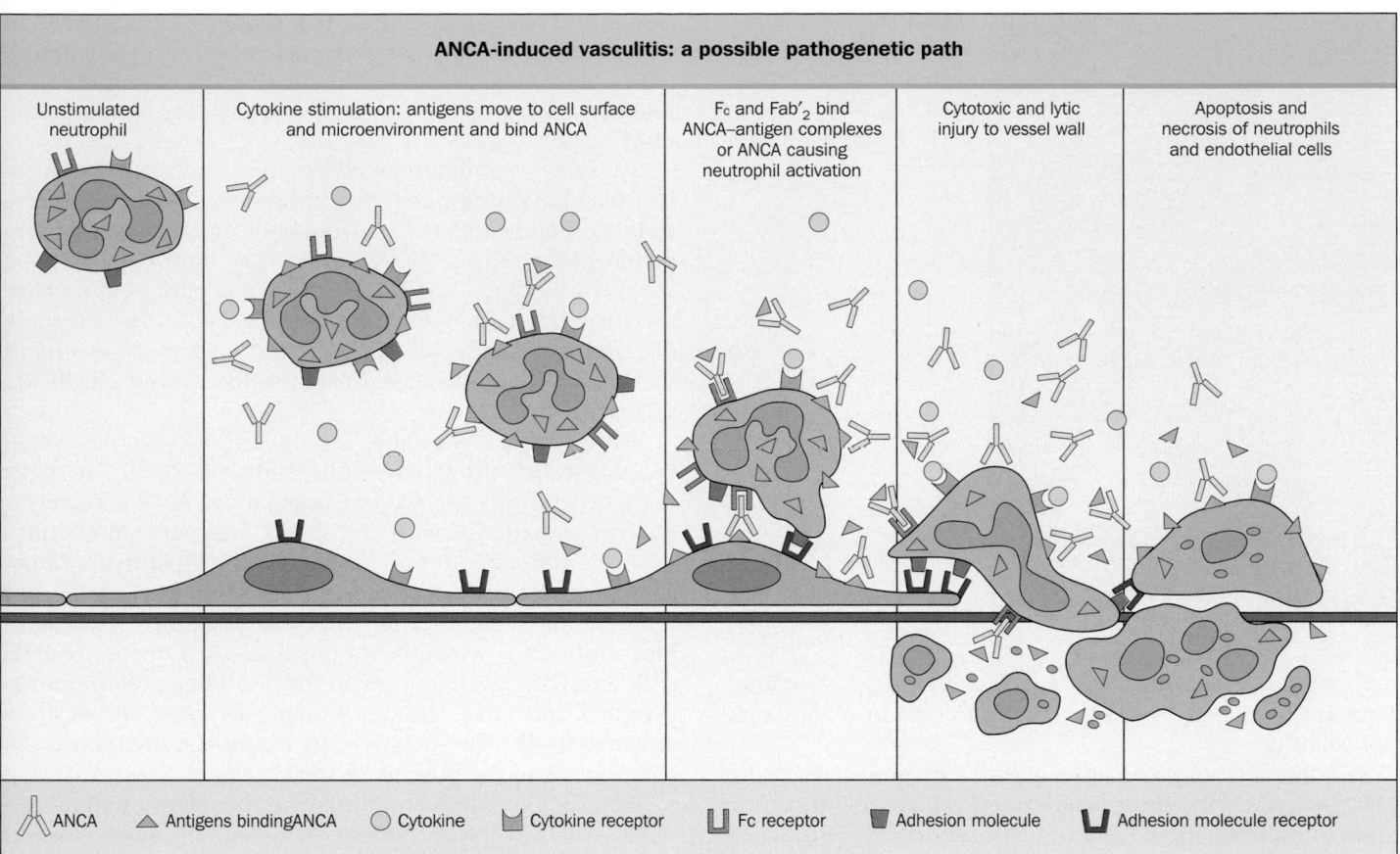

Figure 26.3 Vasculitis induced by antineutrophil cyloplasmic antibodies (ANCA): a hypothetical sequence of pathogenetic events. (Adapted with permission from Jennette and Falk[8].)

	Organ system involvement in small vessel vasculitis				
	Frequency of involvement (%)				
Organ system	Microscopic polyangiitis	Wegener's granulomatosis	Churg–Strauss syndrome	Henoch–Schönlein purpura	Cryoglobulinemic vasculitis
Kidney	90	80	45	50	55
Skin (cutaneous)	40	40	60	90	90
Lungs	50	90	70	<5	<5
Ear, nose, and throat	35	90	50	<5	<5
Musculoskeletal system	60	60	50	75	70
Neurologic system	30	50	70	10	40
Gastrointestinal system	50	50	50	60	30

Modified with permission from Jennette JC, Falk RJ. Small vessel vasculitis. N Engl J Med. 1997;337:1512–23.

Table 26.2 Organ system involvement in small vessel vasculitis.

By definition, patients with microscopic polyangiitis do not have granulomatous respiratory tract lesions.

Manifestations of upper respiratory tract disease include sinusitis, rhinitis, otitis media, and ocular inflammation. These features are most common in Wegener's granulomatosis but may occur in Churg–Strauss syndrome and microscopic polyangiitis. The upper respiratory tract inflammation in microscopic polyangiitis is caused by angiitis alone, without granulomatous inflammation. Destruction of bone, for example resulting in septal perforation and saddle nose

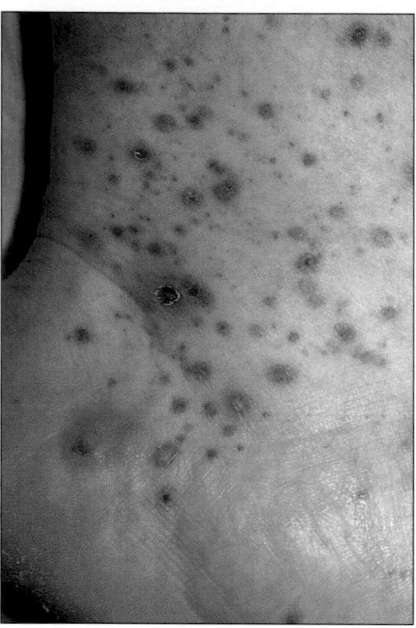

deformity, appears to require necrotizing granulomatous inflammation and, therefore, does not occur in microscopic polyangiitis.

Peripheral neuropathy, usually with a mononeuritis multiplex pattern, is the most common neurologic manifestation and is most frequent in Churg–Strauss syndrome. Central nervous system involvement is less common, and includes vasculitis within the meninges. Gastrointestinal involvement typically causes abdominal pain and blood in the stool, with mesenteric ischemia and, rarely, intestinal perforation. Vasculitis in the pancreas and liver can mimic pancreatitis and hepatitis symptomatically and with respect to elevated serum enzymes.

Antineutrophil cytoplasmic autoantibodies

Serologic testing for ANCA is a useful diagnostic procedure for pauci-immune small vessel vasculitis and pauci-immune crescentic glomerulonephritis but should be interpreted in the context of other patient characteristics[5–7,13–15]. Laboratory testing for ANCA should include both indirect immunofluorescence microscopy assay (IFA) and enzyme immunoassay (EIA)[13].

IFA using normal human neutrophils as substrate produces two major staining patterns, cytoplasmic (c-ANCA), where staining occurs diffusely throughout the cytoplasm, and peripheral (p-ANCA) (Fig. 26.5). By EIA, most c-ANCA have specificity for proteinase 3 (PR3-ANCA) and most p-ANCA have specificity for myeloperoxidase (MPO-ANCA). For adequate diagnostic accuracy, all serologic testing for ANCA should include an immunochemical analysis for antigen specificity, such as an EIA.

ANCA testing has good sensitivity for pauci-immune small vessel vasculitis and glomerulonephritis (80–90%). The specificity depends on the patient population. Approximately a quarter of patients with anti-GBM crescentic glomerulonephritis and a quarter of patients with idiopathic immune-complex crescentic glomerulonephritis are ANCA positive, but less than 5% of patients with all other categories of glomerulonephritis and vasculitis are positive. Most of the patients with anti-GBM glomerulonephritis and idiopathic immune-complex crescentic glomerulonephritis who are positive are analytically true positives in whom the ANCA may be contributing to the phenotype of the disease.

Table 26.3 provides an estimate of the relative frequencies of PR3-ANCA/c-ANCA and MPO-ANCA/p-ANCA in the different phenotypes of pauci-immune small vessel vasculitis and crescentic glomerulonephritis based on our own experience and a crude synthesis of current literature. PR3-ANCA/c-ANCA is most prevalent in Wegener's granulomatosis and MPO-ANCA/p-ANCA is most prevalent in renal-limited pauci-immune crescentic glomerulonephritis. Patients with microscopic polyangiitis have a more even distribution of PR3-ANCA/c-ANCA and MPO-ANCA/p-ANCA. These data make it clear that ANCA antigen specificity cannot be used to determine the clinicopathologic phenotype of pauci-immune small vessel vasculitis.

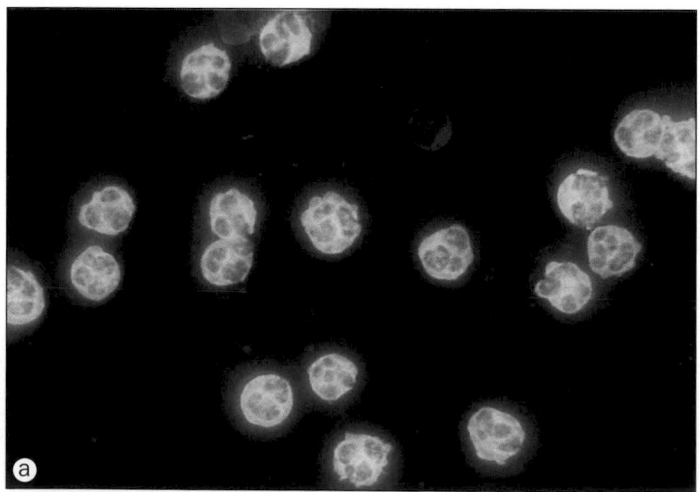

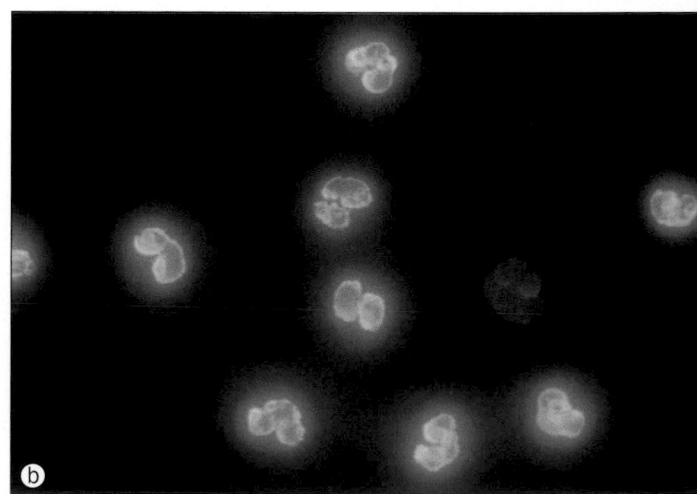

Figure 26.5 Indirect immunofluorescence for antineutrophil cytoplasmic antibodies (ANCA). Staining pattern of alcohol-fixed normal human neutrophils. (a) Cytoplasmic pattern (cANCA) caused by ANCA with specificity for proteinase 3 (PR3). (b) Perinuclear staining (pANCA pattern) caused by ANCA with specificity for myeloperoxidase (MPO). (Anti-IgG, original magnification ×250.)

Antineutrophil cyloplasmic antibodies (ANCA) in small vessel vasculitis			
	Frequencies (%)		
	Proteinase 3 (PR3/cANCA)	Myeloperoxidase (MPO/pANCA)	Negative
Wegener's granulomatosis	70	25	5
Microscopic polyangiitis	40	50	10
Churg–Strauss syndrome	10	60	30
Pauci-immune glomerulonephritis	20	70	10
Approximate frequencies of ANCA with specificity for proteinase 3 (PR3/pANCA) and for myeloperoxidase (MPO/pANCA) in patients with different categories of pauci-immune small vessel vasculitis and crescentic glomerulonephritis.			

Table 26.3 Antineutrophil cyloplasmic antibodies (ANCA) in small vessel vasculitis.

Changes in ANCA titers over time correlate to a degree with disease activity but are not infallible markers and thus must be interpreted with much caution[5,14,15]. Titers usually fall with treatment and rise with disease recurrence. A rise in ANCA titer should prompt careful evaluation of the patient for corroborating evidence of exacerbation, but most physicians do not modify treatment on the basis of a rise in titer without associated clinical or laboratory evidence for increased disease activity.

ANCA may sometimes be positive with other inflammatory conditions, which may need to be considered in the differential diagnosis, including inflammatory bowel disease, rheumatoid disease, chronic inflammatory liver disease, bacterial endocarditis, and cystic fibrosis. In this setting, specificity of the ANCA may not be against PR3 or MPO but against other neutrophil antigens including lactoferrin, cathepsin G, and antibactericidal/permeability-increasing protein.

Pathology

The basic shared acute vascular lesion of the pauci-immune small vessel vasculitides is segmental fibrinoid necrosis, often accompanied by leukocyte infiltration and leukocytoclasia (leukocyte fragmentation) (Figs 26.6 and 26.7)[1,2]. The earliest vasculitic lesions have infiltrating neutrophils, which are quickly replaced by predominantly mononuclear leukocytes. The acute necrotizing lesions evolve into sclerotic lesions and may be complicated by thrombosis.

These focal necrotizing lesions can affect many different vessels, thus causing many different signs and symptoms: for example, involvement of glomerular capillaries causing nephritis, alveolar capillaries causing pulmonary hemorrhage, dermal venules causing purpura, upper respiratory tract mucosal venules causing rhinitis and sinusitis, abdominal visceral arteries causing abdominal pain, and epineural arteries causing mononeuritis multiplex.

The histology of pauci-immune small vessel vasculitis cannot be accurately distinguished from that of immune-complex-mediated small vessel vasculitides, such as Henoch–Schönlein purpura and cryoglobulinemic vasculitis. Immunohistology can make this distinction by demonstrating immunoglobulin in the walls of vessels injured by immune-complex-mediated vasculitis.

The shared glomerular lesion of the pauci-immune small vessel vasculitides is a necrotizing glomerulonephritis, usually with resultant crescent formation (Figs 26.8 and 26.9). Early mild lesions have segmental fibrinoid necrosis with or without an adjacent small crescent (see Fig. 26.8). Severe acute lesions may have essentially global necrosis with large circumferential crescents (see Fig. 26.9). In our experience with over 200 specimens of ANCA-linked glomerulonephritis, on average 50% of glomeruli have necrosis and crescents at the time of initial biopsy, but the frequency ranges from < 5% to 100%. Non-necrotic segments within segmentally injured glomeruli (see Fig. 26.8) and glomeruli without necrosis typically have little or no histologic abnormalities. This differs from immune-complex-mediated crescentic glomerulonephritis, such as that caused by lupus nephritis, IgA nephropathy, or

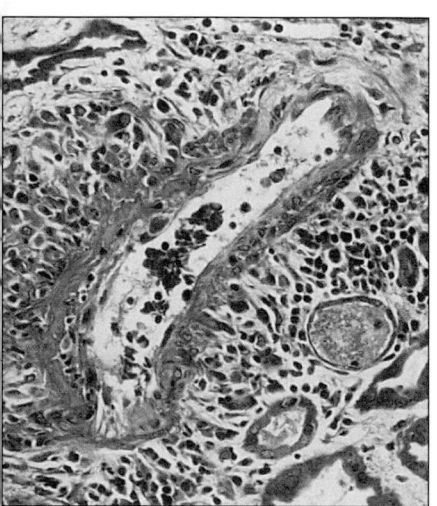

Figure 26.6 Necrotizing arteritis in an interlobular artery from a patient with ANCA-associated small vessel vasculitis. There is segmental fibrinoid necrosis with adjacent perivascular leukocyte infiltration. (Hematoxylin–eosin stain, original magnification ×50.)

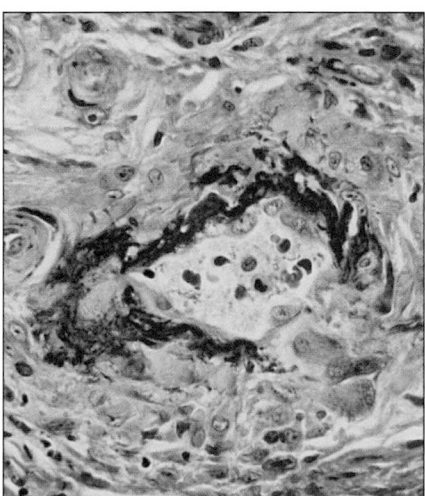

Figure 26.7 Necrotizing arteritis in an interlobular artery from a patient with ANCA-associated small vessel vasculitis. The fibrinoid necrosis is accentuated by the red staining of the trichrome stain. (Masson trichrome stain, original magnification ×100.)

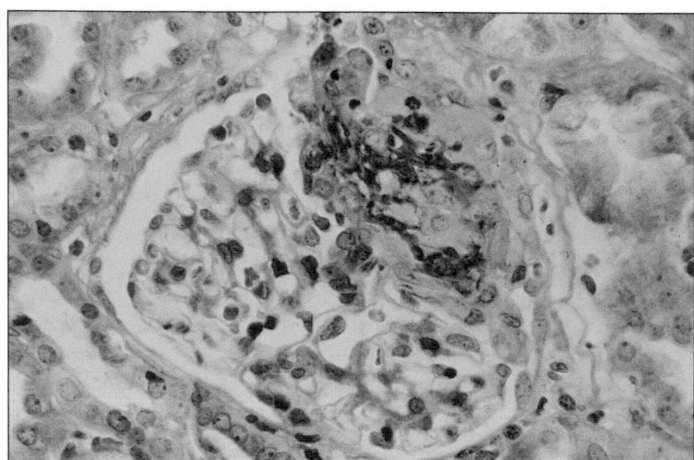

Figure 26.8 Segmental glomerular necrosis and crescent formation in a patient with ANCA-associated small vessel vasculitis. The fibrinoid material is red. The uninvolved segments appear normal. (Masson trichrome stain, original magnification ×150.)

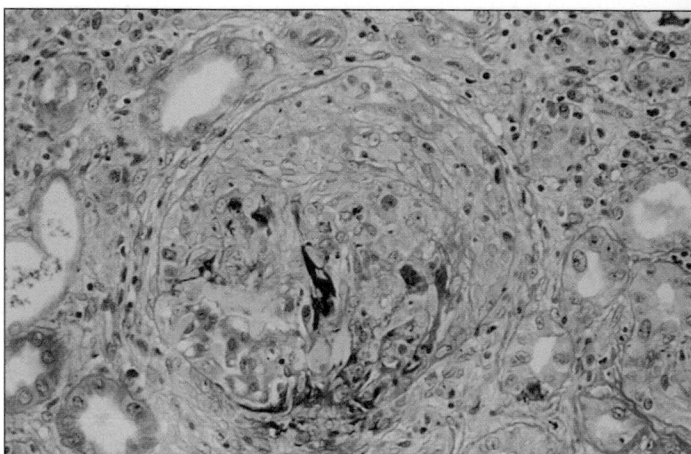

Figure 26.9 Global glomerular necrosis and circumferential crescent formation in a glomerulus from a patient with ANCA-associated small vessel vasculitis. (Masson trichrome stain, original magnification ×150.)

membranoproliferative glomerulonephritis, which typically have endocapillary hypercellularity and capillary wall thickening in non-necrotic segments. Anti-GBM glomerulonephritis causes glomerular necrosis and crescent formation without endocapillary hypercellularity that is indistinguishable from pauci-immune crescentic glomerulonephritis by light microscopy. Immunohistology readily demonstrates the linear GBM staining for IgG in anti-GBM glomerulonephritis, whereas the glomerulonephritis of the pauci-immune small vessel vasculitides has little or no staining for immunoglobulin. However, as mentioned above, approximately a quarter of patients with anti-GBM crescentic glomerulonephritis and a quarter of patients with immune-complex-mediated crescentic glomerulonephritis will be ANCA positive. By contrast, less than 5% of patients with immune-complex glomerulonephritis who do not have crescents will be ANCA positive. Therefore, even in patients with immune-complex glomerulonephritis, the presence of ANCA is associated with an increased incidence of crescents (and also inflammation in vessels other than glomerular capillaries).

In addition to glomerulonephritis, patients with pauci-immune small vessel vasculitis also may have renal arteritis, most often affecting interlobular arteries (see Figs 26.6 and 26.7), and medullary angiitis affecting the vasa recta (Fig. 26.10). The medullary angiitis may be severe enough to cause papillary necrosis, although this appears to be a rare complication. A mononuclear interstitial infiltrate is also seen when glomerular and arteritic lesions are severe; eosinophils are occasionally prominent in the infiltrate.

Patients with Wegener's granulomatosis and Churg–Strauss syndrome have pathologic lesions in addition to the necrotizing small vessel vasculitis that they have in common with microscopic polyangiitis patients[2-4]. The necrotizing granulomatous inflammation of Wegener's granulomatosis occurs most often in the respiratory tract and is characterized by zones of necrosis surrounded by mixed infiltrates of neutrophils, lymphocytes, monocytes, and macrophages, often including scattered multinucleated giant cells. Varying numbers of

eosinophils may be present in the lesions of Wegener's granulomatosis, but these are more conspicuous and may predominate in the necrotizing granulomatous inflammation of Churg–Strauss syndrome. Eosinophils also are typically conspicuous in the vasculitic lesions of Churg–Strauss syndrome, but this is not a pathognomonic observation because numerous eosinophils may be present in the vasculitic lesions of Wegener's granulomatosis, microscopic polyangiitis, polyarteritis nodosa, and other vasculitides.

Differential diagnosis

The ANCA-associated small vessel vasculitides must be differentiated from other forms of small vessel vasculitis that can produce the same signs and symptoms[2]. In addition, an attempt should be made to distinguish between microscopic polyangiitis, Wegener's granulomatosis, and Churg–Strauss syndrome, although sometimes this cannot be accomplished conclusively and is not required for initiation of therapy.

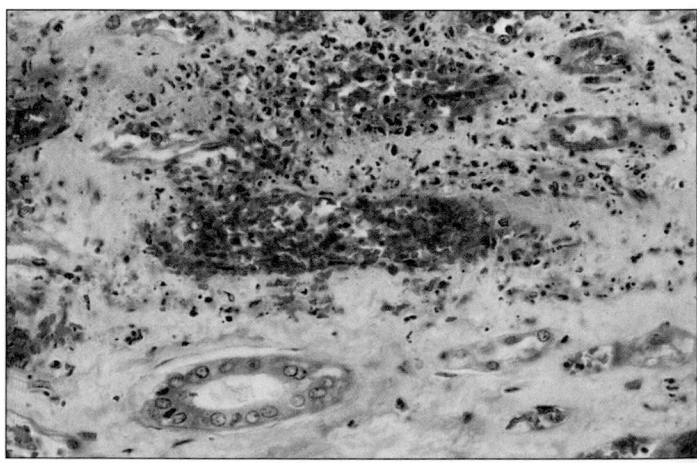

Figure 26.10 Medullary leukocytoclastic angiitis involving the vasa recta in a patient with Wegener's granulomatosis. (Hematoxylin–eosin stain, original magnification ×150.)

Differential diagnostic features of selected forms of small vessel vasculitis					
Features	Microscopic polyangiitis	Wegener's granulomatosis	Churg–Strauss syndrome	Henoch–Schönlein purpura	Cryoglobulinemic vasculitis
Vasculitic signs and symptoms[a]	+	+	+	+	+
IgA-dominant immune deposits	–	–	–	+	–
Cryoglobulins in blood and vessels	–	–	–	–	+
Antineutrophil cytoplasmic antibodies (ANCA) in blood	+	+	+	–	–
Necrotizing granulomas	–	+	+	–	–
Asthma and eosinophilia	–	–	+	–	–

Modified with permission from Jennette and Falk[4].
[a] All of these vessel vasculitides can manifest any or all of the shared features of small vessel vasculitides, such as nephritis, purpura, abdominal pain, peripheral neuropathy, myalgas, and arthralgias. Each is distinguished by the presence and just as importantly the absence of certain specific features.

Table 26.4 Differential diagnostic features of selected forms of small vessel vasculitis.

Table 26.4 indicates a number of features that discriminate among several important categories of small vessel vasculitis.

All forms of small vessel vasculitis listed in Figure 26.2 are capable of producing clinically indistinguishable overlapping features of disease, such as nephritis, purpura, peripheral neuropathy, myalgias, arthralgias, and abdominal pain. Accurate differentiation among them is very important for proper patient management because the natural histories and appropriate treatments vary greatly. For example, a patient presenting with nephritis, arthralgias, and abdominal pain could have Henoch–Schönlein purpura, microscopic polyangiitis, cryoglobulinemic vasculitis, or a number of other small vessel vasculitides. A number of serologic and pathologic observations are useful for reaching the correct diagnosis (see Table 26.4). A positive ANCA assay (confirmed by EIA to be MPO-ANCA or PR3-ANCA) supports a diagnosis of microscopic polyangiitis or one of the other pauci-immune small vessel vasculitides. A negative ANCA assay and positive cryoglobulin assay (especially if accompanied by hypocomplementemia and positive hepatitis C serology) support a diagnosis of cryoglobulinemic vasculitis. A negative ANCA assay, negative cryoglobulin assay, and normal complement levels support a diagnosis of Henoch–Schönlein purpura, especially in a patient younger than 21 years of age. The age of a patient influences the likelihood of a specific diagnosis. For example, approximately 80% of children younger than 10 years who have purpura, nephritis, and arthralgias will have Henoch–Schönlein purpura, whereas approximately 80% of adults over 60 years old with the same symptoms will have an ANCA-associated small vessel vasculitis. However, each disease can occur at any age. For example, we have been involved with the care of several children who were initially diagnosed clinically as having Henoch-Schönlein purpura and given a good prognosis and no specific therapy who returned after a week or two with advanced renal failure and were found to have ANCA-positive microscopic polyangiitis.

Exposure to drugs that may provoke vasculitis must be considered, including penicillamine, hydralazine, and propylthiouracil. Cholesterol embolization (see Chapter 63) can also mimic the clinical features of small vessel vasculitis but ANCA is negative. The differential diagnosis of lung hemorrhage and nephritis is discussed further in Chapter 25.

Natural history

Prior to the advent of immunosuppressive therapy, the survival of patients with Wegener's granulomatosis, microscopic polyangiitis, and Churg–Strauss syndrome was dismal, with most patients dying in less than a year. With adequate immunosuppressive therapy, 1-year renal survival and patient survival is 70–80%. The most life-threatening component of ANCA-associated small vessel vasculitis is massive pulmonary hemorrhage caused by alveolar capillaritis. The likelihood of success of long-term maintenance of renal function is inversely correlated with the serum creatinine when therapy begins, which indicates the importance of early diagnosis and prompt initiation of appropriate treatment.

When severe glomerulonephritis is present, the renal prognosis is similar for patients with Wegener's granulomatosis, microscopic polyangiitis, Churg–Strauss syndrome, and isolated pauci-immune crescentic glomerulonephritis. Renal involvement, however, is not usually present or is mild in patients with Churg–Strauss syndrome. Cardiac involvement is the most frequent cause of death in patients with Churg–Strauss syndrome. Wegener's granulomatosis has a broad spectrum of clinical manifestations, from very localized indolent disease to fulminant multisystem disease. For example, some patients have disease limited to the upper respiratory tract, or to the upper and lower respiratory tract. Such limited disease may have a more benign natural history than systemic disease with substantial renal involvement and may warrant less aggressive treatment. The goal should be not to overtreat mild disease and not to undertreat severe disease.

Treatment

This section will focus on patients with ANCA-associated small vessel vasculitis affecting the kidneys. Glomerulonephritis that is severe enough to cause renal impairment is an indication for immunosuppressive treatment in patients with Wegener's granulomatosis, microscopic polyangiitis, Churg–Strauss syndrome, and isolated pauci-immune crescentic glomerulonephritis. Treatment involves three phases: induction of remission, maintenance of remission, and treatment of relapse[16].

Induction therapy

The consensus is that corticosteroids alone are not as effective for induction therapy as corticosteroids combined with a cytotoxic agent such as cyclophosphamide[16–18]. Combined treatment with corticosteroid and cyclophosphamide induces improvement in over 90% of patients and essentially complete remission in 75%. The specifics of combined induction regimens vary with respect to agents, doses, route of administration, and duration. Our induction approach is to begin with 7 mg/kg intravenous methylprednisolone daily for 3 days followed by oral prednisone 60 mg daily tapering to 10 mg daily by 3 months[18]. This is combined with 2 mg/kg oral cyclophosphamide daily, or intravenous cyclophosphamide at 0.5 g/m^2 per month adjusted upward to 1 g/m^2 based on the leukocyte count. The role of plasma exchange in induction therapy is controversial, but it may be beneficial, especially with severe disease such as dialysis-dependent renal failure or life-threatening pulmonary hemorrhage[19]. Treatment with pooled intravenous gamma globulin has appeared to offer benefits in anecdotal reports, but the effectiveness of this treatment has not been adequately documented[20].

Maintenance therapy

The duration of induction therapy and the intensity of maintenance therapy should be reduced as much as possible to reduce toxic side effects. This is a difficult challenge because of the tendency of the pauci-immune small vessel vasculitides to recur. Corticosteroids may be discontinued after remission is achieved, which usually occurs within 6 months. Cyclophosphamide therapy may be continued for 6 to 12 months to sustain the remission. Treatment with azathioprine is an alternative strategy for maintenance of remission[21,22]. For example, cyclophosphamide can be terminated after 3 months and replaced by 2 mg/kg per day azathioprine to maintain remission. Methotrexate is another possible alternative for maintaining remission, but this agent cannot be used when the serum creatinine is > 2 mg/dL and its efficacy is not clearly established.

The role of antimicrobial agents, such as trimethoprim–sulfamethoxazole, in maintenance of remission is controversial. Some studies have suggested a benefit but others have not[23,24]. Trimethoprim–sulfamethoxazole alone is not sufficient maintenance treatment without immunosuppression.

Relapse therapy

Approximately a quarter to a half of patients with pauci-immune small vessel vasculitis and glomerulonephritis will experience a relapse within several years. The best treatment for relapses is unsettled. Reinstitution of treatment similar to an induction regimen is used most often[18], but less intensive therapy may be adequate if relapse is diagnosed early.

Transplantation

There are a few reports of recurrent disease in renal transplants given to patients with end-stage renal disease caused by pauci-immune crescentic glomerulonephritis but they are not numerous enough to be a contraindication to transplantation. Although the data are limited, the frequency of recurrence appears to be approximately 20%, but graft loss caused by recurrence may be less than 5%. A positive ANCA titer at the time of transplantation does not increase the risk of recurrent disease in the transplant[25,26].

POLYARTERITIS NODOSA

Polyarteritis nodosa is a systemic necrotizing arteritis that affects predominantly main visceral arteries and their intraparenchymal branches[11]. There is still much confusion over the relationship between polyarteritis nodosa and microscopic polyangiitis (which also has been referred to as microscopic polyarteritis). We adhere to the approach of the Chapel Hill Consensus Conference, which confines the diagnosis of polyarteritis nodosa to patients who have only arteritis[4]. The presence of vasculitis in vessels other than arteries, such as capillaries, venules, or arterioles, excludes a diagnosis of polyarteritis nodosa and indicates some form of small vessel vasculitis. By this approach, the presence of glomerulonephritis excludes a diagnosis of polyarteritis nodosa. When polyarteritis nodosa is distinguished from microscopic polyangiitis by this approach, the two categories of vasculitis have not only different pathologic characteristics but also different clinical features and natural histories, which justifies the nosologic distinction between polyarteritis nodosa and microscopic polyangiitis[11,27,28].

Pathogenesis

The etiology and pathogenesis of polyarteritis nodosa are unknown. When polyarteritis nodosa is separated from microscopic polyangiitis, the latter but not the former is associated with ANCA. An immune-complex trigger for polyarteritis nodosa has been proposed but has not been confirmed as the major pathogenetic process. A minority of patients have hepatitis B virus infection, especially in France, which has raised the possibility that the hepatitis B infection is producing immune complexes that are localizing in artery walls and inducing inflammation. However, the evidence that hepatitis B infection is causing vascular immune-complex deposition is stronger in certain forms of glomerulonephritis and small vessel vasculitis than in polyarteritis nodosa.

Epidemiology

Polyarteritis nodosa is a rare disease, occurring much less frequently than microscopic polyangiitis. Polyarteritis nodosa affects males and females equally and is found in all races. Onset is most frequent between the ages of 40 and 60 years.

Clinical manifestations

The usual clinical presentation of polyarteritis nodosa includes nonspecific constitutional symptoms, such as fever, malaise, arthralgias, myalgias, and weight loss, as well as manifestations of arteritis. Peripheral neuropathy, typically in the form of a mononeuritis multiplex, is a common manifestation. This is caused by inflammation of small epineural arteries and is clinically indistinguishable from the peripheral neuropathy caused by other forms of vasculitis that can affect epineural arteries, such as microscopic polyangiitis, Wegener's granulomatosis, and Churg–Strauss syndrome. Gastrointestinal involvement occurs in about half of patients, usually manifesting as abdominal pain and blood in the stool. Bowel infarction is uncommon and perforation is rare. Renal involvement produces infarction and hemorrhage, which are indicated by flank pain and hematuria. Rupture of an arterial aneurysm with retroperitoneal or peritoneal hemorrhage is an uncommon but potentially lethal renal complication. Approximately a third of patients develop hypertension, which rarely reaches malignant range. Red, tender inflammatory nodules are the most common cutaneous manifestation. Infarction, ulceration and livedo reticularis may be present.

Arterial aneurysms may be detected by angiography in patients with polyarteritis nodosa (Fig. 26.11). This is not a completely specific determination because any necrotizing arteritis that affects arteries large enough to be seen by angiography can produce this finding.

Pathology
Any artery in the kidney can be affected by polyarteritis nodosa, from the main renal artery to the interlobular arteries. Nodular inflammatory lesions and aneurysms (pseudoaneurysms) can be observed grossly when medium-sized arteries are involved. Inflammation in small arteries can only be observed by microscopy.

The characteristic acute lesion is segmental transmural fibrinoid necrosis of arteries, usually accompanied by infiltrating leukocytes with leukocytoclasia (Fig. 26.12)[3]. The earliest lesions have numerous neutrophils and later lesions have predominantly mononuclear leukocytes. Acute lesions may be complicated by thrombosis or hemorrhage. Older lesions develop fibrosis and endarterial remodeling. The aneurysms of necrotizing arteritis are not true aneurysms but rather are inflammatory pseudoaneurysms. That is, the walls of

the arteries are not dilated but rather have been eaten away by the necrotizing inflammation, which then erodes into the surrounding perivascular tissue to create an enlarged lumen at the site of inflammation. This explains the propensity for such lesions to induce thrombosis or to undergo rupture.

The necrotizing arteritis of polyarteritis nodosa cannot be distinguished by light microscopy from arteritis caused by other necrotizing vasculitides affecting arteries. For example, necrotizing arteritis in a skeletal muscle biopsy or a peripheral nerve biopsy is histologically identical whether it is caused by polyarteritis nodosa, microscopic polyangiitis, Wegener's granulomatosis, or Churg–Strauss syndrome. To distinguish these vasculitides requires additional clinical and serologic information.

Differential diagnosis
Polyarteritis nodosa must be distinguished from other forms of vasculitis, especially other forms of necrotizing vasculitis that can affect arteries, such as microscopic polyangiitis. Guillevin and his associates have identified clinical features that assist in the differential diagnosis (Table 26.5)[11,28].

A positive ANCA test supports the presence of one of the ANCA-associated small vessel vasculitides rather than polyarteritis nodosa. The presence of glomerulonephritis indicates some form of small vessel vasculitis rather than polyarteritis nodosa. Vasculitic pulmonary disease is rare in polyarteritis nodosa but is frequent in microscopic polyangiitis, Wegener's granulomatosis, and Churg–Strauss syndrome. Peripheral neuropathy or muscle tenderness with arteritis in epineural or skeletal muscle arteries are not useful differentiating features because they are frequent in polyarteritis nodosa as well as the ANCA-associated small vessel vasculitides. Kawasaki disease causes necrotizing arteritis but is distinguished from polyarteritis nodosa by the presence of the mucocutaneous lymph node syndrome.

Natural history
The natural history of polyarteritis nodosa is difficult to determine because most of the early studies of outcome grouped

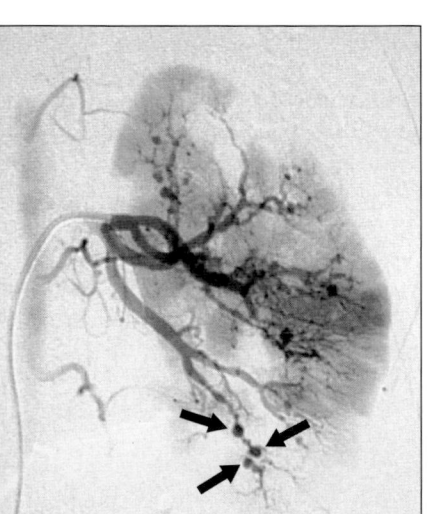

Figure 26.11 Renal angiogram in polyarteritis nodosa. Angiogram shows patchy renal perfusion defects and aneurysms (arrows).

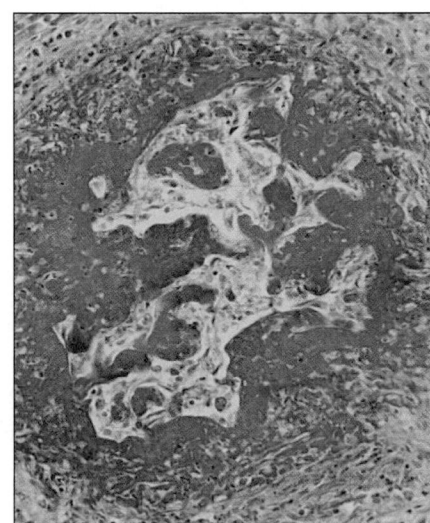

Figure 26.12 Necrotizing arteritis in an arcuate artery of a patient with polyarteritis nodosa. The lumen is partially occluded by thrombotic material that is continuous with the fibrinoid material which has replaced the entire wall of the artery. (Hematoxylin–eosin stain, original magnification ×50.)

polyarteritis nodosa together with microscopic polyangiitis. Polyarteritis nodosa with multisystem involvement has a very poor prognosis without therapy. With therapy, the 10-year patient survival is approximately 80%. The natural history of the disease appears to differ from that of microscopic polyangiitis in that it is less likely to recur once the initial episode resolves[28].

Treatment

Polyarteritis nodosa in patients with no evidence for hepatitis B infection is treated with corticosteroids and cytotoxic drugs, usually cyclophosphamide[11,28]. The regimens vary and include treatment approaches similar to those described earlier for microscopic polyangiitis and Wegener's granulomatosis. However, in patients with no risk factors for poor outcome (such as age over 50 years, cardiac involvement, gut involvement, or renal involvement), corticosteroids alone may be adequate and are less toxic therapy than corticosteroids combined with cytotoxic agents.

Aggressive immunosuppressive therapy is contraindicated in patients with hepatitis B-associated polyarteritis nodosa because of potential adverse effects on the outcome of the hepatitis B infection. Guillevin et al. advocate short-term steroid treatment combined with antiviral agents and plasma exchange for such patients[29]. Their regimen calls for 1 mg/kg prednisone daily for 1 week followed by tapering during the second week. If there is continued disease activity or relapse, additional daily courses of 1 mg/kg may be required. A 3-week course of antiviral agents, such as vidarabine or interferon-α, is added after 1 week. The Guillevin regimen used three plasma exchanges per week for the first 2 weeks, followed by four to five exchanges per week for the following 3 weeks, then three exchanges per week for 3 weeks, and two exchanges per week for 2 weeks.

KAWASAKI DISEASE

Definition

Kawasaki disease is an acute febrile illness that usually occurs in young children, often less than 1 year old[30,31]. The mucocutaneous lymph node syndrome is the characteristic clinical presentation of Kawasaki disease. This includes fever (usually 38–40°C), erythema of the oropharyngeal mucosa, polymorphous erythematous rash, erythema of the palms and soles, and indurative edema of the extremities, followed by desquamation, conjunctivitis, and nonsuppurative lymphadenopathy. Necrotizing arteritis is a complication of Kawasaki disease that is present in some but not all patients. Clinically significant renal involvement is very rare; therefore, Kawasaki disease is rarely encountered by nephrologists.

Pathogenesis

The occasional occurrence of Kawasaki disease as endemic and epidemic disease suggests that the cause may be an infectious agent or an environmental toxin. Both cell-mediated and antibody-mediated mechanisms have been incriminated, including a possible role for antiendothelial antibodies. At the current time, the etiology and pathogenesis of Kawasaki disease are unproven.

Clinical differences between polyarteritis nodosa and microscopic polyangiitis		
Clinical feature	Polyarteritis nodosa	Microscopic polyangiitis
Microaneurysms by angiography	Yes	No (?rare)
Rapidly progressive nephritis	No	Yes (very common)
Pulmonary hemorrhage	No	Yes
Renovascular hypertension	Yes (10–33%)	No
Peripheral neuropathy	Yes (50–80%)	Yes (10–20%)
Positive hepatitis B serology	Uncommon	No
Positive ANCA serology	Rare	Frequent
Relapses	Rare	Frequent

Modified with permission from Lhote F, Guillevin L. Polyarteritis nodosa, microscopic polyangiitis, and Churg–Strauss syndrome. Clinical aspects and treatment [review]. Rheum Dis Clin North Am. 1995;21:911–47.

Table 26.5 Clinical differences between polyarteritis nodosa and microscopic polyangiitis.

Epidemiology

Kawasaki disease usually occurs in children less than 5 years old and has a peak incidence in the first year of life. It was first described in Japan, but it occurs worldwide. The disease is more common in Asians and Polynesians than in Whites and Blacks. Kawasaki disease occasionally occurs in an endemic or epidemic pattern but usually is sporadic.

Clinical manifestations

The mucocutaneous syndrome is the characteristic clinical manifestation of Kawasaki disease[4]. This includes fever (usually 38–40 °C), mucosal inflammation, swollen red tongue ('strawberry tongue'), polymorphous erythematous rash, indurative edema of the extremities, erythema of palms and soles, desquamation from the tips of digits, conjunctival injection, and enlarged lymph nodes.

The frequency of active arteritic lesions peaks during the first week of the illness and is markedly reduced after 1 month. Arteritis most often manifests as cardiac disease. Thrombosis of inflamed coronary arteries in patients with Kawasaki disease is the most common cause for childhood myocardial infarction. Clinically significant renal disease is uncommon. This is somewhat surprising because autopsy reveals arteritis in renal vessels in up to three-quarters of patients[30].

Pathology

The arteritis of Kawasaki disease involves small and medium-sized arteries. The acute histologic lesion is necrotizing inflammation with less fibrinoid necrosis than is usually observed with polyarteritis nodosa (Fig. 26.13). Aneurysm (pseudoaneurysm) formation and thrombosis may occur.

The most frequent site of arteritis is the coronary arteries followed by the renal arteries[23]. Arteritis most often affect interlobar arteries, occasionally arcuate arteries, and only rarely interlobular arteries.

Differential diagnosis

Kawasaki disease has sometimes been misdiagnosed as childhood polyarteritis nodosa. The differentiation of Kawasaki disease from polyarteritis nodosa is very important because corticosteroid treatment may increase the risk of coronary artery aneurysms in Kawasaki disease. The histologic lesions and the aneurysms observed by angiography cannot be distinguished from the lesions of polyarteritis nodosa. The presence or absence of the mucocutaneous lymph node syndrome is the basis for distinguishing between Kawasaki disease and other forms of arteritis[4].

Natural history

Kawasaki disease usually is self limited with an uneventful recovery. Recurrence is rare. Only about 1% of patients develop severe arteritic complications, usually affecting the coronary arteries.

Treatment

Aspirin (30 mg/kg daily) and intravenous gammaglobulin are the standard therapy for Kawasaki disease[30]. Corticosteroid treatment may increase the risk of adverse coronary artery complications, although the data supporting this are limited.

TAKAYASU ARTERITIS AND GIANT CELL ARTERITIS

Takayasu arteritis and giant cell arteritis affect the aorta and its major branches[4]. Giant cell arteritis has a predilection for the extracranial branches of the carotid artery but can affect arteries in almost any organ. Takayasu arteritis has a predilection for major arteries supplying the extremities. Both diseases cause chronic vascular inflammation, often with a granulomatous appearance that may include multinucleated giant cells. Giant cell arteritis, but not Takayasu arteritis, is associated with polymyalgia rheumatica.

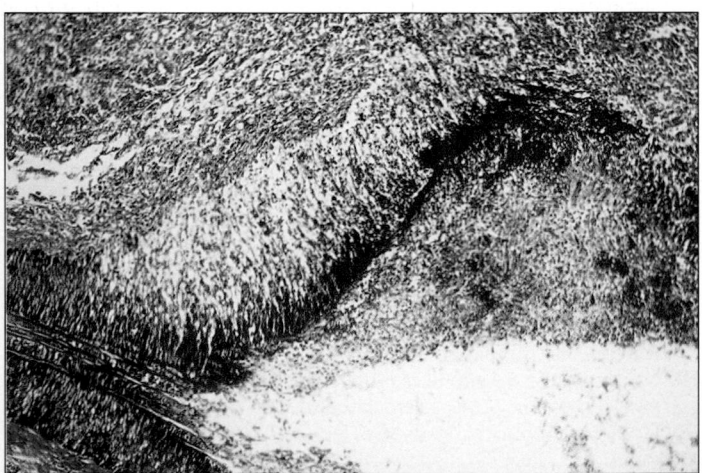

Figure 26.13 Kawasaki disease arteritis affecting a renal interlobar artery in a young child. The artery wall is intact on the far left. The remainder of the wall has extensive edema, infiltration by mononuclear leukocytes, and a band of fuchsinophilic (red) fibrinoid material roughly at the junction between the inflamed intima and muscularis. (Masson trichrome stain, original magnification ×25.)

Pathogenesis

The etiology and pathogenesis of giant cell arteritis and Takayasu arteritis are unknown. Because of the histologic changes and the nature of the infiltrating leukocytes, cell-mediated immune mechanisms are incriminated. The inciting antigen or autoantigen has not been identified.

Epidemiology

Takayasu arteritis is seen most frequently in Asia. Giant cell arteritis is most frequent in individuals of northern European ancestry. Takayasu arteritis has a female to male ratio of approximately 9 : 1, and giant cell arteritis has a female to male ratio of 2–5 : 1. Takayasu arteritis usually is diagnosed in those between the ages of 10 and 20 years and is very rare after 50 years of age. Giant cell arteritis is very rare before age 50 years.

Clinical manifestations

In addition to nonspecific constitutional symptoms such as fever, arthralgias, and weight loss, the major clinical manifestations of Takayasu arteritis and giant cell arteritis are caused by arterial narrowing and resultant ischemia.

The major clinical manifestations of Takayasu arteritis are reduced pulses (95% of patients), vascular bruits, claudication, and renovascular hypertension. Renovascular hypertension is a major cause for morbidity and mortality and results from renal ischemia caused by renal artery stenosis or aortic coarctation[32]. Reduced aortic elasticity and impairment of carotid artery baroreceptors also may play a role in some patients.

Headache is the most common presenting symptom in patients with giant cell arteritis. Temporal artery tenderness, nodularity, or decreased pulsation is present in about half of patients. Additional common symptoms include blindness, deafness, jaw claudication, tongue dysfunction, extremity claudication, and reduced pulses. More than half of patients with giant cell arteritis have polymyalgia rheumatica, which is characterized by stiffness and aching in the neck and the proximal muscles of the shoulders and hips. Clinically significant renal disease is much rarer in giant cell arteritis than in Takayasu arteritis. There are case reports of necrotizing and crescentic glomerulonephritis associated with giant cell arteritis, but these may represent examples of Wegener's granulomatosis or microscopic polyangiitis with temporal artery involvement.

Pathology

The aortitis and arteritis of Takayasu arteritis and giant cell arteritis cannot be confidently distinguished from each other by pathologic examination. Both are characterized in the active phase by inflammation with a predominance of mononuclear leukocytes, often with scattered multinucleated giant cells (Fig. 26.14). The chronic phase is characterized by progressive fibrosis that may cause severe narrowing of vessels, with resultant ischemia. Major renal arteries are often found to be involved at autopsy in both Takayasu arteritis and giant cell arteritis patients. However, clinically significant renal disease is relatively common in Takayasu arteritis but rare in giant cell arteritis. A glomerular lesion characterized by nodular mesangial matrix expansion and mesangiolysis may occasionally be a component of Takayasu arteritis[33].

Differential diagnosis

There is a great deal of overlap between the clinical manifestations and pathologic features of Takayasu arteritis and giant cell arteritis. The age of the patient and the presence or absence of polymyalgia rheumatica are the best features for discriminating between these two vasculitides.

Giant cell arteritis also has been called temporal arteritis. This is a misleading designation because all patients do not have temporal artery involvement and patients with other types of vasculitis, such as polyarteritis nodosa, Wegener's granulomatosis, and microscopic polyangiitis, can have involvement of the temporal arteries. Some of the reported examples of necrotizing glomerulonephritis associated with 'temporal arteritis' probably represent Wegener's granulomatosis or microscopic polyangiitis with temporal artery involvement.

Treatment

Corticosteroids are the usual treatment for giant cell arteritis and Takayasu arteritis, for example initial daily therapy with 0.5–1 mg/kg for 1 to 2 months followed by tapering over several months. More prolonged treatment may be dictated by persistent disease activity. Cytotoxic agents such as cyclophosphamide may be required in patients with recalcitrant disease.

Management of renal disease is not an issue with typical giant cell arteritis although rare patients have ischemic renal manifestations. Renovascular hypertension is the major renal problem caused by Takayasu arteritis. When bilateral renal

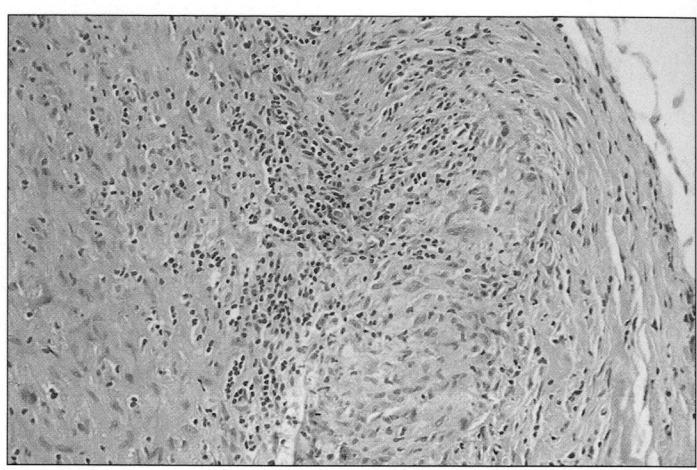

Figure 26.14 Severe giant cell arteritis affecting a main renal artery. This caused marked renal atrophy and renovascular hypertension. (Hematoxylin–eosin stain, original magnification ×50.)

artery involvement occurs, angiotensin-converting enzyme inhibitors may precipitate renal failure in patients with Takayasu arteritis[34]. When medical management fails, the renovascular hypertension in patients with Takayasu arteritis may be controlled by bypass surgery or angioplasty[32,35]. The management of renovascular hypertension is covered in Chapter 39.

REFERENCES

1. Jennette JC, Falk RJ. The pathology of vasculitis involving the kidney. Am J Kidney Dis. 1994;24:130–41.
2. Jennette JC, Falk RJ. Small vessel vasculitis. N Engl J Med. 1997;337: 1512–23.
3. Jennette JC, Falk RJ. Renal involvement in systemic vasculitis. In: Greenberg A, Cheung AK, Coffman TM, Falk RJ, Jennette JC, eds. National Kidney Foundation nephrology primer, 2nd edn, Ch 27. San Diego, CA: Academic Press; 1998:200–7.
4. Jennette JC, Falk RJ, Andrassy K, et al. Nomenclature of systemic vasculitides: the proposal of an international consensus conference. Arthritis Rheum. 1994;37:187–92.
5. Jennette JC, Falk RJ. Anti-neutrophil cytoplasmic autoantibodies: discovery, specificity, disease associations and pathogenic potential. Adv Pathol Lab Med. 1995;8:363–77.
6. Savige J, Davies D, Falk RJ, et al. Antineutrophil cytoplasmic antibodies (ANCA) and associated diseases. Kidney Int 2000;57:846–62.
7. Franssen CF, Stegeman CA, Kallenberg CG, et al. Antiproteinase 3- and antimyeloperoxidase-associated vasculitis. Kidney Int. 2000;57:2195–206.
8. Jennette JC, Falk RJ. Pathogenesis of the vascular and glomerular damage in ANCA-positive vasculitis. Nephrol Dial Transplant. 1998;13(Suppl 1):16–20.
9. Herringa P, Brower E, Klok PA, et al. Autoantibodies to myeloperoxidase aggravate mild anti-glomerular basement membrane-mediated glomerular injury in the rat. Am J Pathol. 1996;49: 1695–706.
10. Xiao H, Heeringa P, Hu P, et al. Antineutrophil cytoplasmic autoantibodies specific for myeloperoxidase (MPO-ANCA) cause glomerulonephritis and vasculitis in mice. Am J Pathol. 2001; submitted.
11. Gayraud M, Guillevin L, le Toumelin P, et al. Long-term followup of polyarteritis nodosa, microscopic polyangiitis, and Churg-Strauss syndrome: analysis of four prospective trials including 278 patients. Arthritis & Rheumatism. 2001;44:666–75.
12. Jennette JC, Thomas DB, Falk RJ. Microscopic polyangiitis (microscopic polyarteritis). Semin Diagn Pathol 2001;18:3–13.
13. Hagen EC, Daha MR, Hermans J, et al. Diagnostic value of standardized assays for anti-neutrophil cytoplasmic antibodies in idiopathic systemic vasculitis. EC/BCR Project for ANCA Assay Standardization. Kidney Int. 1998;53:743–53.
14. Boomsma MM, Stegeman CA, van der Leij MJ, et al. Prediction of relapses in Wegener's granulomatosis by measurement of anti-neutrophil cytoplasmic antibody levels: a prospective study. Arthritis Rheum. 2000 Sep;43(9):2025–33.
15. Nowack R, Grab I, Flores-Suarez LF, et al. ANCA titres, even of IgG subclasses, and soluble CD14 fail to predict relapses in patients with ANCA-associated vasculitis. Nephrol Dial Transplant. 2001;16(8):1631–7.
16. Bacon PA. Therapy of vasculitis. J Rheumatol. 1994;21:788–90.
17. Duna GF, Galperin C, Hoffman GS. Wegener's granulomatosis. Rheum Dis Clin North Am. 1995;21:949–86.
18. Nachman PH, Hogan SL, Jennette JC, Falk RJ. Treatment response and relapse in ANCA-associated microscopic polyangiitis and glomerulonephritis. J Am Soc Nephrol. 1996;7:33–9.
19. Pusey CD, Rees AJ, Evans DJ, et al. Plasma exchange in focal necrotizing glomerulonephritis without anti-GBM antibodies. Kidney Int. 1991;40:757–63.
20. Jayne DR, Davies MJ, Fox CJ, et al. Treatment of systemic vasculitis with pooled intravenous immunoglobulin. Lancet. 1991; 337:1137–9.

21. Pusey CD, Gaskin G, Rees AJ. Treatment of primary systemic vasculitis. APMIS Suppl. 1990;9:48–50.
22. Jayne D, Gaskin G. Randomised trial of cyclophosphamide versus azathioprine in ANCA-associated systemic vasculitis. JASN. 1999;10:105A.
23. Stegeman CA, Cohen Tervaert JW, Sluiter WJ, et al. Association of chronic nasal carriage of Staphylococcus aureus and higher relapse rates in Wegener's granulomatosis. Ann Intern Med. 1994;120:12–17.
24. de Groot K, Reinhold-Keller E, Tatsis E, et al. Therapy for the maintenance of remission in sixty-five patients with generalized Wegener's granulomatosis. Methotrexate versus trimethoprim/sulfamethoxazole. Arthritis Rheum. 1996;39:2052–61.
25. Rostaing L, Modesto A, Oksman F, et al. Outcome of patients with antineutrophil cytoplasmic antibody-associated vasculitis following cadaveric kidney transplantation. Am J Kidney Dis. 1997;9:96–102.
26. Nachman PH, Segelmark M, Westman K, et al. Recurrent ANCA-associated small vessel vasculitis after transplantation: A pooled analysis. Kidney Int. 1999;56:1544–50.
27. Guillevin L, Lhote F, Amouroux J, et al. Antineutrophil cytoplasmic antibodies, abnormal angiograms and pathological findings in polyarteritis nodosa and Churg–Strauss syndrome: indications for the classification of vasculitides of the polyarteritis nodosa group. Br J Rheum. 1996;35:958–64.
28. Lhote F, Guillevin L. Polyarteritis nodosa, microscopic polyangiitis, and Churg–Strauss syndrome. Clinical aspects and treatment [review]. Rheum Dis Clin North Am. 1995;21:911–47.
29. Guillevin L, Lhote F, Leon A, et al. Treatment of polyarteritis nodosa related to hepatitis B virus with short term steroid therapy associated with antiviral agents and plasma exchanges. A prospective trial in 33 patients. J Rheumatol. 1993;20:289–98.
30. Naoe S, Takahashi K, Masuda H, Tanaka N. Kawasaki disease. With particular emphasis on arterial lesions [review]. Acta Pathol Jap. 1991;41:785–97.
31. Newburger JW, Takahashi M, Burns JC, et al. The treatment of Kawasaki syndrome with intravenous gammaglobulin. N Engl J Med. 1986;315:341–7.
32. Lagneau P, Michel JB. Renovascular hypertension and Takayasu's disease. J Urol. 1985;134:876–9.
33. Yoshimura M, Kida H, Saito Y, et al. Peculiar glomerular lesions in Takayasu's arteritis. Clin Nephrol. 1985;24:120–7.
34. Rapoport M, Averbukh Z, Chaim S, et al. Takayasu aortitis simulating bilateral renal-artery stenoses in patients treated with ACE inhibitors [letter]. Clin Nephrol. 1991;36:156.
35. Blank M., Tomer Y, Stein M, et al. Immunization with anti-neutrophil cytoplasmic antibody (ANCA) induces the production of mouse ANCA and perivascular lymphocyte infiltration. Clin Exp Immunol. 1995;102:120–30.

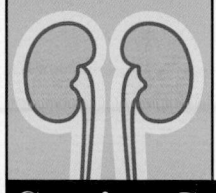

Chapter 27
Lupus Nephritis

J Stewart Cameron

INTRODUCTION AND DEFINITION

The importance of lupus nephritis[1-4] to practicing nephrologists is that it is a serious but usually treatable disease. The term 'lupus' (Latin: wolf) has been used for many centuries to denote any skin condition where one component is ulceration. Although Brooke first noted albuminuria in lupus in 1895, recognition of visceral involvement including renal disease was slow for the next decade or two. The modern era began in 1957 with the amazingly complete description by Kark, Muehrcke and colleagues of renal biopsy appearances of lupus nephritis[5].

Lupus is defined by its clinical picture, together with antibodies directed against one or more nuclear components, particularly double-stranded DNA[6]. It is best regarded as a syndrome in which a number of different patterns of immune disturbance may lead to a similar final common pathway and thus disorders with similar clinical pictures. The criteria of the American College of Rheumatology (ACR), revised in 1982 and modified slightly in 1997, have been applied widely to the diagnosis of lupus and have proved durable – although they were introduced originally only to distinguish the disease from other closely related clinical conditions (Table 27.1). The presence of four or more of the major criteria is usually taken as establishing the diagnosis with about 96% sensitivity and specificity.

Defining 'typical' or 'core' patients in this fashion excludes a considerable number of patients with 'lupus-like' disorders who should also be recognized and treated. Many patients with a clinical lupus syndrome but a negative antinuclear antibody (ANA) have low titers of anti-Ro antibody and rarely have significant renal disease, but often show a high incidence of antiphospholipid antibodies (APA) with associated thromboses and abortions, as well as inherited complement deficiencies.

ETIOLOGY AND PATHOGENESIS

Origins of autoimmunity

How autoimmunity and the lupus syndrome arise remains obstinately obscure[7,8]. In lupus there is a *generalized autoimmunity*, with autoantibodies directed against a variety of self components, but the role of the autoantibodies in generating organ damage is unclear. This contrasts with *organ-specific autoimmunity* (such as antiglomerular basement membrane (anti-GBM) nephritis), in which clearly pathogenetic autoantibodies are directed against a single self epitope.

Genetic factors

Genetic factors are important in lupus, with racial preponderance and familial clustering, and monozygotic twins showing 25% concordance. In addition, healthy relatives of patients with lupus may show antinuclear and other autoantibodies. Only weak major histocompatibility complex (MHC) associations have been noted, the strongest being with C4A or C4B null genes and low tumor necrosis factor (TNF) production. A few patients may show genetic deficiencies of complement components, and some studies have shown associations with FcγRIIIa receptor polymorphisms. Acquired complement deficiencies occur also, for example in complement receptor CR1 and a pathogenic role for poor immune clearance of complexes has been postulated. However in human lupus there is no evidence for genetic defects in the apolipoprotein-1 (APO-1)/fas receptor whose engagement leads to apoptosis, such as has been described in some forms of murine lupus.

Other etiologic agents

There is no convincing evidence that infective agents provoke human lupus. Hydralazine, procainamide, and occasionally other drugs, may precipitate a lupus syndrome which, however, rarely affects the kidney. Interaction of genetic and

The American College of Rheumatology criteria for the diagnosis of lupus
The presence of four or more of the following criteria gives 96% sensitivity and specificity for the diagnosis of lupus:
1. Malar rash
2. Discoid rash
3. Photosensitivity
4. Oral ulcers
5. Nonerosive arthritis
6. Pleuropericarditis
7. Renal disease (proteinuria and/or granular casts)
8. Neurologic disorder (fits or psychosis in the absenceof precipitating circumstances)
9. Hematologic disorder (hemolytic anemia,leukopenia/lymphopenia, thrombocytopenia)
10. Positive LE cell preparation, raised antiDNA antibody, anti-Sm present, false-positive antitreponemal test
11. Positive, fluorescent, antinuclear antibody test

Table 27.1 The American College of Rheumatology criteria for the diagnosis of lupus, revised 1982 and modified in 1997.

environmental factors is shown in hydralazine-induced lupus: three genetic factors (female gender, slow acetylator status, and HLA-DR4) plus exposure to hydralazine account for 98% of the risk.

Animal models of lupus nephritis

Spontaneous lupus has been reported in a number of strains of mice, such as the NZB B/W F1 hybrid and MRL-lpr. Both have primary defects that lead to B-cell proliferation, including defects in the fas/APO-1-ligand system, which has a role in apoptosis. It is assumed in these animals that defective apoptosis leads to defective clonal deletion. In addition, lupus can be provoked in mice by injecting autoantibodies against DNA or phospholipid, or by inducing graft versus host disease, and in rabbits by injection of peptides derived from the Sm-antigen.

Pathogenesis

Typically there are multiple autoantibodies in lupus directed against nucleic acids and proteins concerned with intracellular transcriptional and translational machinery[6]. The main targets are nucleosomes (DNA-histone) or even quaternary antigens on the chromatin itself, small nuclear ribonucleoproteins (snRNPs), and small cytoplasmic RNPs (scRNPs).

Polyclonal hyperactivity of the B-cell system or defects of T-cell autoregulation are likely primary events in lupus. One hypothesis is that some autoreactive T cells survive thymic deletion and persist into adult life in a state of suppression, with the emergence of clones of autoreactive cells and antibodies and tissue damage if this suppression fails. A second hypothesis is that presentation of self antigen (such as histone-derived peptides) to a mature immune system is capable of inducing germline mutations resulting in the production of new autoantibodies, that are not adequately suppressed. A variant of this hypothesis is that viral or bacterial peptides contain sequences that are similar or identical to those of native antigens with which they cross-react: so-called 'antigenic mimicry'. A third hypothesis is that there is nonspecific, polyclonal B-cell stimulation via superantigens, the resultant B-cell repertoire including pathogenetic autoantibodies that again fail to be suppressed.

Mediation of tissue injury

Patients with lupus nephritis most usually show antibodies directed against dsDNA, Sm, and C1q. But it has proved difficult to show that the DNA–antiDNA antibody system, so characteristic of lupus, has a direct role in pathogenesis.

Aggregates of immunoglobulin and complement components are present at sites of injury in the glomeruli, and in the tubules in about two-thirds of renal biopsies. Whether these are derived from circulating complexes or from *in situ* combination of antigen and antibody is still unclear. Deficiencies in the handling of immune complexes and other foreign material have been described. These are perhaps inherited in association with the MHC haplotype HLA-A1-B8-DR3 or FcγRIIIa receptor polymorphisms.

Anti-dsDNA antibody has been eluted from nephritic kidneys together with dsDNA and histone, but the mere presence of antibody does not prove it to be damaging. Infusions and transplacental transmission of antiDNA antibodies do not lead to nephritis in humans. Only in models in experimental animals is there direct evidence that murine or human antiDNA antibodies can penetrate cells and cause proteinuria.

In some instances dsDNA–anti-dsDNA antibody complexes fix to DNA receptors on cells, including endothelial cells. In others histones appear to mediate binding to both matrix and cells. Histones are present at sites of immune aggregates in murine and human lupus nephritis, but not in primary glomerulonephritis.

There is no reason to believe that the effector mechanisms of renal damage in lupus are different from those of primary glomerulonephritis. However the interstitial cellular infiltrates in lupus have an excess of CD8+ cytotoxic T lymphocytes over CD4+ compared to the usual mix of CD4+ helper T lymphocytes and monocytes seen in primary glomerulonephritis.

Immunologic findings in patients with and without nephritis

Why do only some patients with lupus develop clinically evident nephritis? We do not have an answer to this question, but those with nephritis usually have antibodies directed against dsDNA as well as ssDNA, and have at most low titers of anti-Ro and anti-La antibody. They also have high-avidity anti-DNA antibodies that activate complement strongly. Higher-avidity antiDNA antibodies also occur in proliferative more than in membranous lupus nephritis and cationic antibodies appear to be more pathogenetic. Antibodies directed against C1q are also more frequent in those with nephritis.

EPIDEMIOLOGY

Prevalence

Incidence, prevalence and mortality[1,4] are ten times higher in African American females (prevalence ~1 : 400) than in Caucasians, whereas it appears relatively rare in West Africans – except perhaps in urban areas. In the USA lupus is twice as frequent in Orientals compared to Caucasians, although there is a relatively low prevalence in mainland China, Taiwan, and Japan. On the other hand, lupus seems to be extremely common in the relatively small Chinese populations of both Singapore and Hong Kong. It is also more common in South Asians. There is some evidence that lupus and its associated nephritis are becoming more common.

Gender and age

Gender is the major risk factor for the development of lupus. The female : male ratio rises from 2 : 1 in prepubertal children up to 4.5 : 1 in adolescents to 8–12 : 1 in adults, falling back to 2 : 1 in patients over 60 years of age. These data are in accord with murine models of lupus where estrogens are precipitating factors in the emergence of lupus, whereas androgens protect. Lupus is rare before puberty.

CLINICAL MANIFESTATIONS

Renal manifestations of lupus[9]

Only 30–50% of unselected patients with lupus have abnormalities of urine or renal function early in their course[2,9], but up to 60% of adults and 80% of children may develop overt renal abnormalities later. Although in those with onset at more than 50 years of age, nephritis is distinctly less common (< 5% at onset).

The dominant feature in almost every patient with renal lupus is proteinuria (Table 27.2)[9]. Surprisingly, hypertension is not, overall, more common in those with nephritis but those with more severe nephritis are more commonly hypertensive. Renal tubular function is disturbed, which is not surprising in view of the findings of both immune aggregates in tubular basement membranes and interstitial nephritis. In a high proportion of patients, urinary excretion of light chains and β_2-microglobulin are both increased. Recently distal renal tubular acidosis has been emphasized as a manifestation of lupus. Bladder involvement may be prominent, often a severe immune interstitial cystitis[10].

Extrarenal manifestations of lupus

Overall those patients with lupus nephritis tend to have more alopecia and oral ulceration than those without, but have less arthritis, facial rash, and Raynaud's phenomenon[2]. The initial complaints are often nonspecific, with three-quarters of patients showing fever and malaise without weight loss.

A rash occurs in half to three-quarters of cases, usually the well-known 'butterfly' rash on the face; livedo reticularis may be seen on exposed areas in up to 15% of cases and may be associated with APA. The rash may be vasculitic with alterations in the nailbed capillaries and sometimes ulcerating lesions, especially around the ankles. Discoid lupus is unusual in patients with lupus nephritis, but photosensitivity is common. Some degree of hair loss is common, which amounts to patchy alopecia in a few cases. Oral ulceration is a presenting feature in 10% of patients.

Raynaud's phenomenon is common in young adults with lupus, affecting 20–30% and often preceding the clinical onset of other manifestations of disease. In some patients it is very severe with loss of digital tissue, as in scleroderma. Patients with renal disease rarely have severe Raynaud's, however, and overall it is a favorable feature in terms of survival.

The arthralgia of lupus is common, occurring in three-quarters of patients and is almost never deforming. Usually several joints are affected at once, often in the hands, but almost any joint may be a target; some myalgia is common in untreated patients at onset, often accompanied by weakness, but myositis is rare.

Neuropsychiatric involvement is one of the most serious extra-renal manifestations of lupus[11] and may be more common and run a more severe course in Orientals, and perhaps also African Caribbeans. It is apparent clinically in about one-third of patients, and is a presenting feature in about 10%. Mood and behavior disorders of a minor degree are common. They are difficult to interpret in the setting of an acute and disturbing illness but, especially if associated with persistent headache (sometimes migrainous), may be the prodrome of serious, overt, neuropsychiatric disorder.

Chorea may be seen, especially in children with neurologic lupus, sometimes in association with APA. In addition, cranial nerve palsies, for example ophthalmoplegias, brainstem lesions and hemiparesis may occur in addition to coma and frank psychosis. Cerebral bloodflow studies, positron emission

Clinical features of patients with evident lupus nephritis	
	%
Proteinuria	100
Nephrotic syndrome	45–65
Granular casts	30
red-cell casts	10
Microscopic hematuria	80
Macroscopic hematuria	1–2
Reduced renal function	40–80
Rapidly declining renal function	30
Acute renal failure	1–2
Hypertension	15–50
Hyperkalemia	15
Tubular abnormalities*	60–80
* usually without symptoms	

Table 27.2 Clinical features of patients with evident lupus nephritis

tomography scanning, and magnetic resonance imaging may show abnormalities additional to those revealed by computerized tomography, even in patients without obvious neuropsychiatric symptoms, but their significance is not yet clear.

Pleuritis and pericarditis affect about 40% of patients; these disorders are usually painful but sometimes symptomless effusions develop. Pericarditis with heart failure does occur but is rare. Endocarditis of the Libman–Sacks type has been associated by some with the presence of APA. It is often symptomless and difficult to diagnose except by echocardiography.

Pulmonary hypertension in lupus may be the result of multiple pulmonary emboli in association with APA, sometimes with vena caval thrombosis. However, it is associated clinically with Raynaud's phenomenon in about three-quarters of cases and may represent a similar vasospastic phenomenon in the lung. Treatment is ineffective and the outlook poor: heart–lung transplantation is possible in some cases. During the acute phase, as well as respiratory infections, acute, potentially fatal, pulmonary hemorrhage may be seen, albeit rarely. Acute, reversible hypoxemia is common, the pathogenesis of which is unclear. Chronic fibrosing alveolitis, a well-recognized feature of lupus, may be progressive and treatment is unsatisfactory.

Splenomegaly and lymphadenopathy are present in about one-quarter of patients with lupus, often with fever and weight loss although this group rarely develops severe nephritis.

Clinical hematologic abnormalities are common. Many patients have a normochromic, normocytic anemia at presentation. Occasional patients present with purpura, not from associated vasculitis but from thrombocytopenia. Thromboses present in about 12% of patients and their occurrence should prompt a search for APA and other procoagulant abnormalities. If a patient with lupus develops a nephrotic syndrome, there will be the additional thrombogenic potential of the alterations in platelet function and plasma coagulation factors that are seen in all nephrotics.

Thrombosis occurs in 5–15% of patients with lupus nephritis and may affect almost any vessel in the body. Venous thromboses occur most frequently, if an APA is present. Arterial thromboses are also seen, cerebral thrombosis being particularly common. Inferior vena caval thrombosis may be seen, and pulmonary embolism is common, perhaps causing pulmonary hypertension. Unilateral or bilateral renal venous thrombosis is common also, especially in lupus membranous nephropathy (WHO class V). A number of patients with a mixed picture of lupus and thrombotic microangiopathy have been described who may develop acute renal failure and who in general have a poor prognosis.

Laboratory investigations in lupus nephritis

Antinuclear antibodies

Antinuclear antibodies[6], particularly those against double-stranded DNA (present in up to 90% of untreated lupus) and the Smith (Sm) antigen, are strongly associated with the presence of nephritis. The Smith (anti-Sm) antibody is almost pathognomonic for the diagnosis of lupus. It is highly specific, but present only in some 30% of patients with nephritis, more in African-Caribbean patients than in Caucasians. Treatment may rapidly eliminate anti-dsDNA antibodies from the circulation while the fluorescent antinuclear antibody (FANA) test remains positive. The various patterns of FANA (diffuse, speckled etc.) are not reliable in distinguishing lupus from other ANA-positive diseases.

Hematology

Anemia of moderate degree is common, but a positive test for anti-red-cell antibodies (Coombs' test) can be obtained only in a minority of patients with lupus, and severe hemolytic anemias are not often seen. Leukopenia (caused by anti-white-cell antibodies) is common, and 50% of patients have a white-cell count below 5×10^9/L, while thrombocytopenia is found in about one-quarter of patients. The origins of the thrombocytopenia are complicated, resulting from accelerated platelet destruction after binding of antiplatelet antibody or APA and/or lysis after phagocytosis of circulating immune complexes.

Antiphospholipid antibodies and the 'lupus anticoagulant'

The double misnomer 'lupus anticoagulant' activity[12] is based upon the presence of APA, directed mainly against the β_2-globulin phospholipid-carrier-protein. These antibodies prolong phospholipid-dependent coagulation studies *in vitro* (activated partial thromboplastin time (APTT) and kaolin clotting time (KCT)) but *in vivo* are associated with thrombosis. The prolonged APTT and KCT are not corrected by mixing with normal plasma. The *in vitro* mechanisms are clear but the reason for thrombosis *in vivo* remains uncertain. APA can be detected in about one third to one half of patients with lupus nephritis, and have been associated with renal arterial, venous, and glomerular capillary thrombosis, as well as Libman–Sacks endocarditis and cerebral thrombosis. Prothrombotic risk factors other than APA include depressed release of plasminogen activator and possibly also of antagonists of plasmin, decreased plasma concentration of free protein-S, and raised von Willebrand factor concentrations.

As well as APA, true lupus anticoagulants may be present in the form of antibodies directed against factors leading to fibrin formation, such as factor VIII and IX, but also less commonly factors XI and XII. These lead to clinical bleeding as well as prolongation of clotting times, which are corrected on mixing with normal plasma.

It is important to note that despite the *in vitro* prolongation of clotting times, it is safe to do needle biopsies in the presence of APA. In contrast, prolongation of KCT, which reverses on mixing with normal plasma, is the action of a true anticoagulant and will require cover with fresh-frozen plasma.

DIAGNOSIS AND DIFFERENTIAL DIAGNOSIS

The diagnosis of lupus is usually easy but may, on occasion, be very difficult, especially in more unusual circumstances such as a middle-aged, nephrotic male or apparently idiopathic membranous nephropathy in a young woman. Thus it should be routine to screen *all* proteinuric patients for anti-nuclear antibodies. About 50% of patients with lupus are initially suspected of having a disease other than lupus, most commonly rheumatic fever, rheumatoid arthritis, and hemolytic anemia. The presence of four or more of the ARA criteria has a 96% sensitivity and specificity when applied to patients seen in rheumatology clinics where the criteria were originally defined. Differentiation from rheumatic fever is relatively easy, but in a child with chorea it may not be straightforward.

Nephritis has been reported in a minority of patients with mixed connective tissue disease; the differential diagnosis can be difficult clinically, but analysis of the antinuclear antibody for the anti-Ro and anti-La antibodies and the absence of anti-dsDNA antibodies should make the diagnosis clear.

Rheumatoid arthritis usually does not show systemic features but on occasion, proteinuria will be induced by one of the drugs used in its treatment and cause additional problems in diagnosis. Some of these patients go on to develop full clinical and immunologic lupus. The presence of erosions and a deforming arthritis makes lupus very unlikely, but does not exclude it.

Henoch–Schönlein purpura is much commoner in childhood than lupus, and on occasion differentiation may be difficult since the rash of lupus may be purpuric and affect the lower limbs only. A few patients with lupus may have IgA predominant in their renal biopsies with raised serum IgA concentrations. Lupus may on occasion be complicated by a vasculitis, which creates difficulties in differentiating it from other forms of vasculitis, especially when p-ANCA (anti-neutrophil cytoplasmic antibodies may seem to be present.

Immunologic tests and the diagnosis of lupus

Few clinicians are happy to make a diagnosis of lupus nephritis without some antinuclear antibodies in the serum, preferably those shown to react with dsDNA. 'Lupus-like' patients with negative antinuclear antibody tests generally present with little or no renal disease, although there are exceptions, and more than 80% of this 'fringe' have APA.

The proportion of positive ANA depends not only upon the population studied but upon the technique used[6]. The classic Farr assay detects only high-avidity anti-dsDNA antibodies; enzyme-linked immunosorbent assay (ELISA) also picks up low-avidity antibodies as does the *Crithidia lucilae* kinetoplast slide test. Correlations with the presence and severity of nephritis are best with high-avidity antibodies using the Farr assay, but for screening diagnosis, the ELISA assay has advantages since it will detect positives in some FANA-positive patients in whom the Farr assay is negative, but who do have lupus. Anti-Sm antibodies are almost entirely specific for lupus, but are found only in about 30% of patients and thus have a very low sensitivity.

Hypocomplementemia is found at presentation in more than three quarters of untreated, younger patients with lupus and is more common with evident nephritis. C4 and C1q tend to be more depressed than C3 suggesting complement activation via the classical pathway; this pattern is rare in membranoproliferative GN (MPGN) type I and poststreptococcal GN, but is common in MPGN type II and essential cryoglobulinemia (see Chapter 23). However, concentrations of properdin and factor B are also depressed, with activation of the alternative pathway. The C5b-9 complex is also found in the circulation in increased amounts. In the absence of active disease null C4 genes will confer concentrations of about half normal C4 in heterozygotes, and absent C4 in homozygotes.

The interpretation of antineutrophil cytoplasmic antibodies (ANCA) is difficult in the presence of antinuclear antibodies. However, the finding of multiple immunoglobulin deposition together with complement in the affected glomeruli and a proliferative/membranous pattern rather than a pauci-immune necrotizing glomerulonephritis, should cause no diagnostic difficulty.

Immune complexes can be detected in the serum of the majority of patients with lupus, especially those with nephritis, and the titer generally rises and falls with indices of clinical activity. However, their clinical utility is minimal since immune complexes can be detected in so many other conditions, and immune-complex detection is no longer in routine clinical use. Complement-based tests have been shown to measure not immune complexes, but anti-C1q autoantibodies.

PATHOLOGY[3,13]

Renal biopsy is worthwhile in all patients with lupus and abnormal urine. It provides prognostic information and influences initial treatment. The overriding characteristic of lupus nephritis is its variability between patients, within biopsies, and even within glomeruli.

Glomerular appearances

The World Health Organization (WHO) classification of lupus nephritis (see Figs 27.1–27.5), which is based on light microscopy, is widely accepted but allows only a broad judgment of severity. Class III (focal proliferative nephritis) is a particular source of difficulties since it covers such a wide range of appearances. Nevertheless, there is a remarkable similarity in the proportion of patients allocated to each class in different series; more than half show WHO class III (focal proliferative) or IV (diffuse proliferative) nephritis – severe forms that most clinicians would treat vigorously. The proportion of class V (membranous) biopsies is about the same in all series (10–15%).

On immunohistology, IgG is almost always the dominant immunoglobulin, IgG1 and IgG3 being especially prevalent, but a few patients have predominant IgA or IgM. Early complement components such as C4 and especially C1q are usually present along with C3. The finding of positivity for all three isotypes of immunoglobulin together with C3, C4, and C1q is called a 'full house' and is present in about one-quarter of patients with lupus and almost never in non-lupus disease. Other immune reactants such as complement components H, B, C5b-9, and properdin are present also in many patients. Fibrin, sometimes accompanied by cross-linked fibrin, is often present in class IV biopsies but rare in other classes.

Tubulointerstitial nephritis

In about 50% of patients with nephritis, less in those with class II and up to three-quarters of those with class IV,

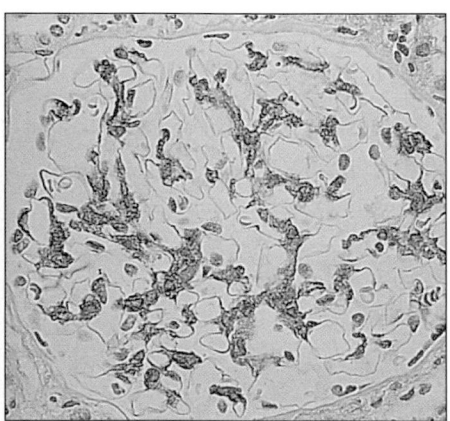

Figure 27.1 WHO class I lupus nephritis (minimal changes): present in <5% of biopsies (dependent upon biopsy policy in patients with mild or no renal disease). Light microscopy is normal, but immunoperoxidase shows extensive C1q (associated with IgG and C3) throughout the mesangial areas.

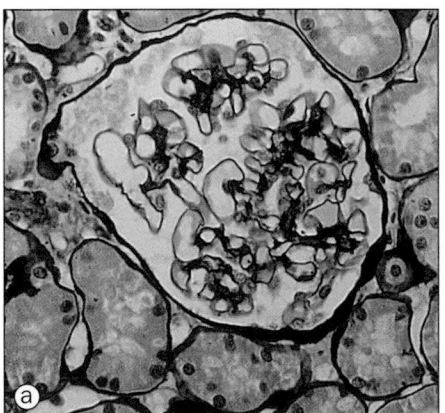
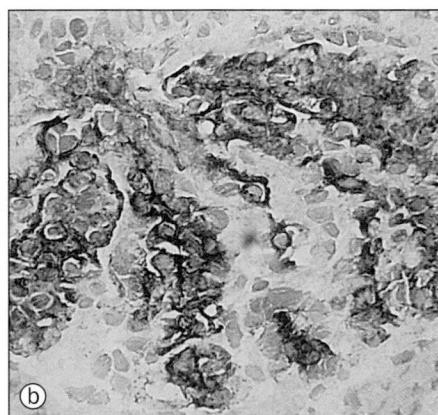

Figure 27.2 WHO class II lupus nephritis (mesangial disease): present in 10–25% of renal biopsies. (a) Mesangial expansion but little increase in tuft cellularity and the peripheral capillary walls are normal. (Silver methenamine stain.) (b) Extensive mesangial IgG deposits shown by immunoperoxidase; the aggregates are just beginning to invade peripheral capillary walls. This represents the most severe changes in this class.

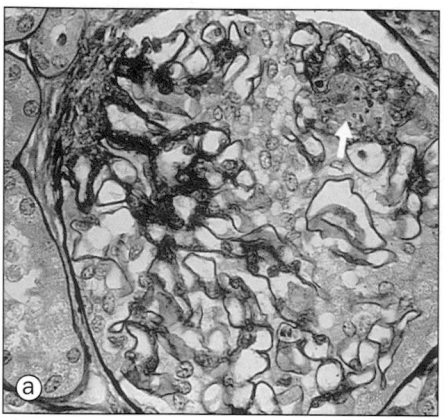 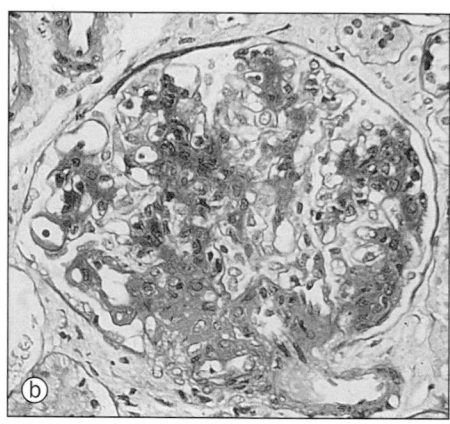 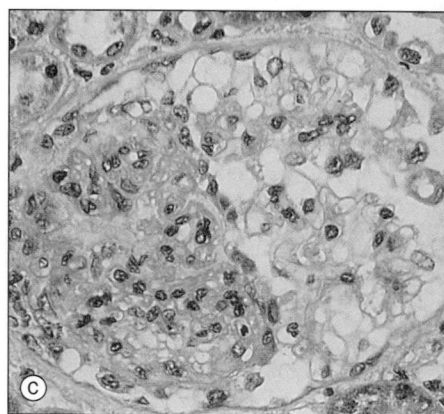

Figure 27.3 WHO class III lupus nephritis (focal proliferative): present in 20–35% of renal biopsies. (a) An area of focal necrosis containing cellular debris (arrow) is surrounded by a degree of epithelial cell proliferation (silver methenamine/hematoxylin eosin.) This is a mild example of class III nephritis. (b) A more severe example of class III: numerous areas of the tuft are affected by segmental capillary wall thickening and mesangial expansion, with cellular proliferation and infiltration. (PAS.) (c) A major focal and segmental lesion affecting almost half the glomerular tuft: another severe variant of class III (hematoxylin/lissamine green).

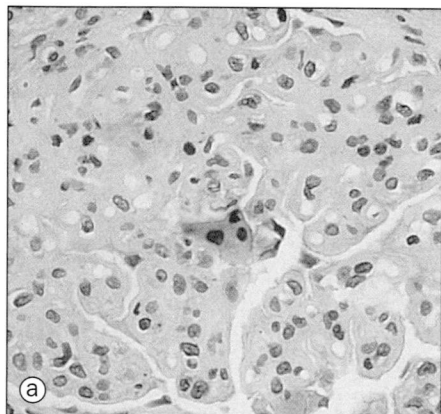 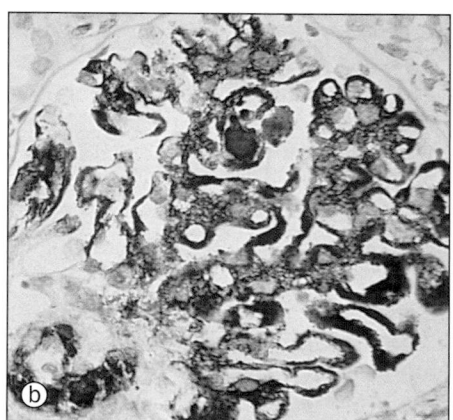 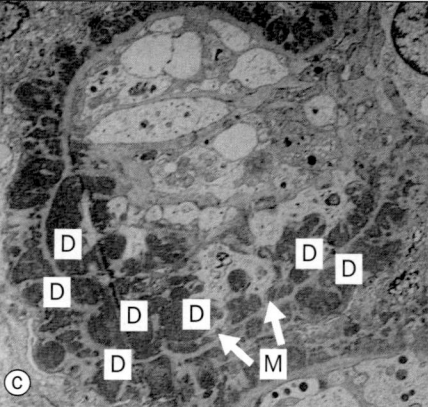

Figure 27.4 WHO class IV lupus nephritis (diffuse proliferative): present in 35–60% of biopsies. (a) The tuft is increased in size by both a diffuse increase in matrix and an excess of cells; capillary walls are irregularly thickened (hematoxylin/eosin). (b) Dense, irregular aggregates of IgG along the peripheral capillary walls by immunoperoxidase. (c) Electron microscopy shows the immune aggregates as electron-dense masses (D) at both subendothelial and subepithelial sites, with the lighter capillary basement membrane (M) (arrows) between them.

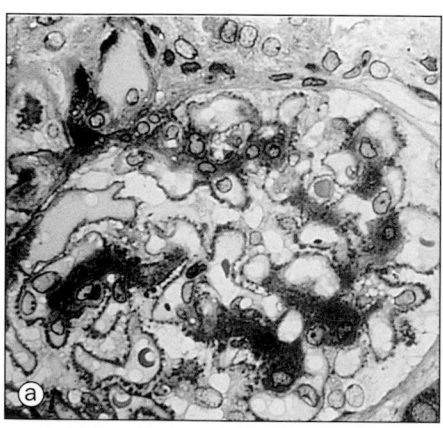 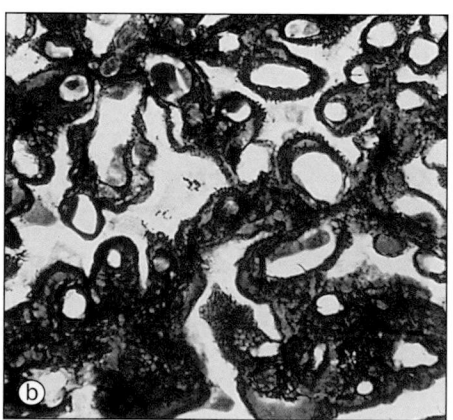 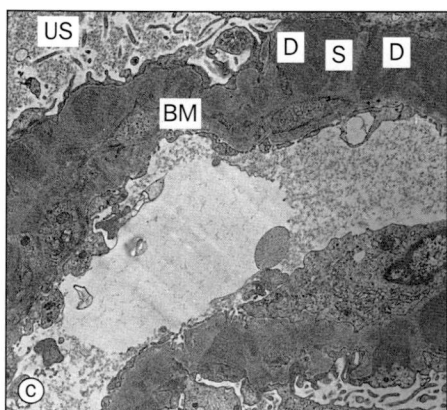

Figure 27.5 WHO class V (membranous): present in 10–15% of biopsies. (a) The predominant aggregates are along the outside of the capillary wall. Note that there are also abundant dark-blue, mesangial aggregates, as well as those along the capillary wall (class Vb). Focal and diffuse proliferative lesions are absent. (b) Silver methenamine staining shows the silver positive 'spikes' along the peripheral capillary wall protruding between the immune aggregates. (c) Electron microscopy of a capillary loop and adjacent urinary space (US) shows electron-dense immune aggregates (D) on the outer surface of the basement membrane (BM), separated by 'spikes' (S) of exuberant basement membrane-like material, mainly laminin. The immune aggregates in class V membranous lupus nephritis are typically more irregular in size and position than those commonly found in idiopathic membranous nephropathy.

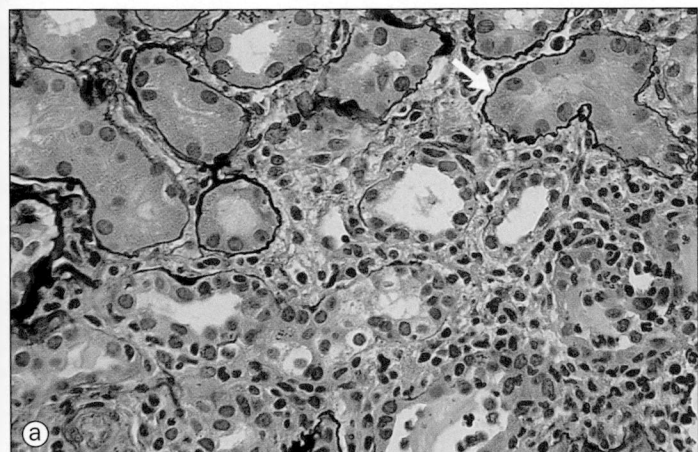

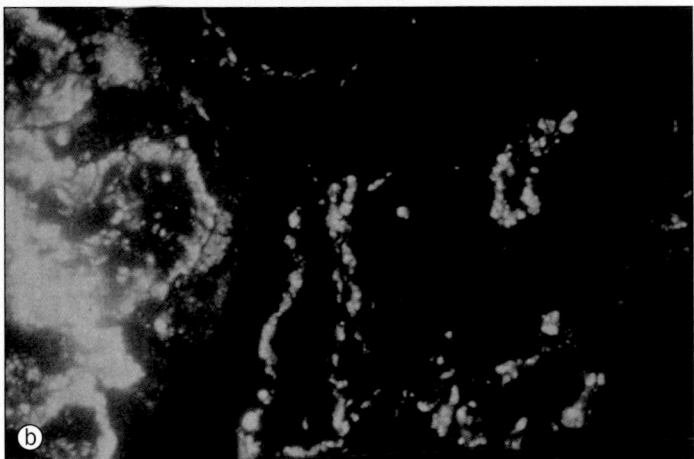

Figure 27.6 Interstitial lupus nephritis. (a) Interstitial infiltrate invading and destroying tubules ('tubulitis'). The tubular basement membrane (TBM), stained black with silver (arrow), is digested (see the lower half of figure(a)) and lymphocytes together with macrophages invade the tubules. (Silver methenamine/hematoxylin.) (b) Immunofluorescence showing aggregates of C3 in the TBM (right) as well as within the glomerulus (left). Such TBM aggregates are common in lupus nephritis, being found in 60–65% of biopsies overall and with increasing frequency from class II (20%) through to class IV (75%).

immune aggregates are present in the tubular basement membrane (TBM). In an occasional patient, linear tubular immunofluorescence is seen, suggestive of anti-TBM antibodies. The interstitial infiltrate is mainly T lymphocytes (both CD4+ and CD8+) and monocytes, with only a few B cells, plasma cells, and natural killer cells. Among the T lymphocytes, are present. Infiltration and invasion of tubules (tubulitis) is frequently present (see Fig. 27.6)[14] in active disease. In more chronic disease the interstitium is expanded with variable amounts of collagen. In a few patients an acute tubulointerstitial nephritis is seen in the absence of glomerular disease and may present as acute renal failure.

Intrarenal vessels

Vascular immune aggregates, hyaline, and non-inflammatory necrotizing lesions, and true vasculitis with lymphocytic and monocyte infiltration of the vessel wall, may all be seen and,

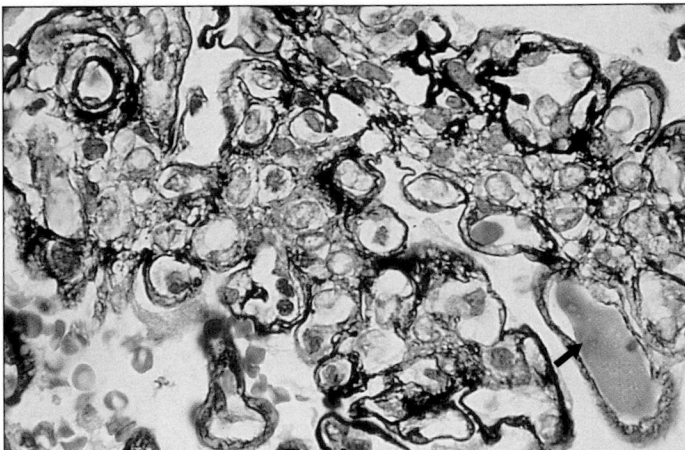

Figure 27.7 Vascular damage in lupus nephritis. 'Thrombus' (arrow) occludes a glomerular capillary loop in this class IV biopsy. Such a 'thrombus' contains platelets and cross-linked fibrin as well as immunoglobulins and thus has some characteristics of true thrombus. Note also the subepithelial aggregates, spike formation, and 'double contouring' of the capillary walls, all typical of class IV and active class III biopsies. (Silver methenamine/hematoxylin.)

more rarely, intrarenal arteriolar thrombi (see Fig. 27.7)[15]. All these vascular changes are signs of a poor prognosis. Occasionally, patients show overt thrombotic microangiopathy. Correlations have been shown between the presence of APA and intraglomerular thrombi.

Other glomerular appearances

Amyloidosis is rare in lupus. This is consistent with the fact that acute phase proteins such as amyloid-A and C-reactive protein do not rise during acute flares of activity in the disease. Dense deposit disease has occasionally been reported in the context of lupus.

Transformation of histologic appearances

Serial biopsies show that transformation of WHO classes is quite frequent. A particularly common transformation is one from diffuse proliferative glomerulonephritis (class IV) to a predominant membranous (class V) pattern under successful treatment. Under these circumstances, proteinuria may become massive as renal function improves.

Inapparent renal disease in lupus

Patients without clinical manifestations of nephritis may have significant glomerular disease on renal biopsy. There have been few follow-up studies on such patients, but one study showed that the majority remain without clinical nephritis for some years. However, it is equally obvious that all patients with clinically evident nephritis must go through a period of absent or occult disease before the disease becomes evident; how many of these patients run a subclinical course for a prolonged period is not known.

Clinicopathologic correlations

While nephritis that is histologically more severe has a tendency to more severe clinical manifestations, renal histology

Glomerular Disease

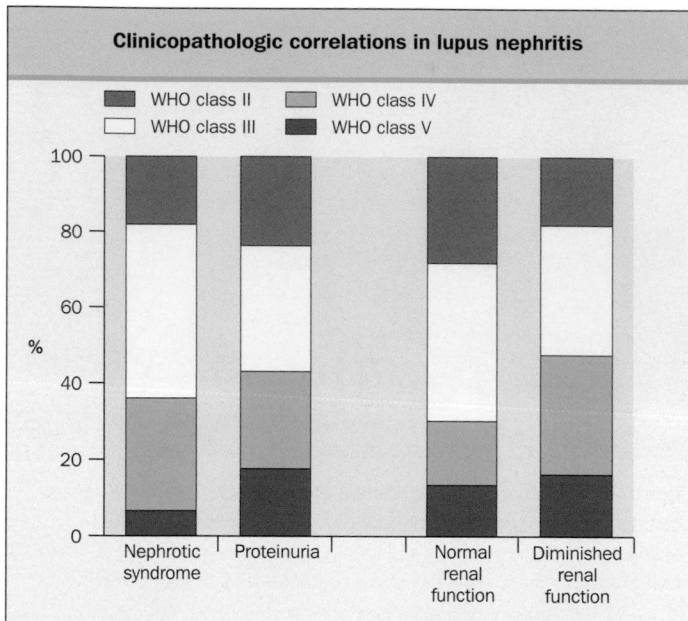

Figure 27.8 Clinicopathologic correlations in lupus nephritis.
Correlations between the presence of a nephrotic syndrome, proteinuria, and normal or diminished renal function with the WHO class on renal biopsy. The clinical picture has almost no value in predicting the biopsy appearances.

Table 27.3 Survival in lupus and lupus nephritus			
	5 Year survival (weighted mean of published series) %		
Period	All lupus	Lupus nephritis	Class IV nephritis
1953–1969	49	44	17
1970–1979	82	67	55
1980–1989	86	82	80
1990–1995	92	82	82

Five-year actuarial survival for lupus, lupus nephritis, and WHO class IV nephritis over the past 40 years.

Table 27.3 Survival in lupus and lupus nephritus

cannot be predicted with any certainty from the clinical picture (see Fig. 27.8). In *untreated* patients, WHO biopsy class is a powerful determinant of outcome. However, this is no longer true if patients with more severe nephritis are given more active treatment (see below). Interstitial changes (both in cells and interstitial volume) correlate well with glomerular filtration rate (GFR) at the time of biopsy, as well as with outcome. Titers of anti-dsDNA antibody were similar in our own patients in all histologic groups, but other researchers have noted significant, though not clinically useful, differences. By the time a renal biopsy is done the patient will almost certainly have received some immunosuppressive treatment, which will alter the serologic results.

The group at the US National Institutes of Health (NIH) have popularized a histologic scoring system for disease 'activity' versus 'chronicity' to generate a numeric assessment of the biopsies. Others, however, have been unable to replicate its prognostic utility.

NATURAL HISTORY

Outcome and mortality in treated patients in recent years

The clinical course of lupus can no longer be considered separately from the results of treatment. Forty or 50 years ago, few patients with severe grade IV nephritis survived more than a year or two, and half of those with even less severe forms of nephritis used to die within 5 years (see Table 27.3). There has now been marked improvement in the outcome for patients with class IV biopsies, which today differs little from lupus nephritis as a whole.

There seems little doubt that this improvement has been the result of better management of lupus nephritis and this has led to almost all patients with the disease receiving treatment, including those with the mildest forms. However, the early data of Ropes[16] must not be forgotten: in the 1960s she studied 68 unbiopsied patients with lupus and proteinuria (some nephrotic) who were left without treatment, and in 16 (28%) cases the proteinuria became intermittent or disappeared spontaneously.

In most patients today, there is a gratifying response to early treatment, followed by relatively quiescent disease under continuing immunosuppression that can be tapered off eventually without further relapse. Another common pattern is the quiescent patient who suddenly relapses. The frequency of relapse depends not only on the underlying disease but on the intensity and duration of immunosuppression.

Since lupus is a multisystem disease, the outlook does not of course depend only upon what happens to renal function, especially now that this is treatable by dialysis and transplantation. Also there are many accessory factors such as the socioeconomic circumstances of the family and the comprehension of treatment goals by the patient. These goals must be adhered to over many years, even when the patient is apparently well but perhaps suffers side-effects of treatment. Measures to deal with these psychosocial problems may be as important as specific treatments in determining survival.

Although long-term results are now very encouraging compared with 20 years ago (Table 27.3), many questions remain unresolved.
- Will reduced renal function evolve eventually into renal failure?
- What is the significance of persistent proteinuria in the absence of disease activity?
- How long should treatment continue and what should it be?
- On what grounds can treatment be stopped safely?

The causes of death in lupus are much more varied than in primary glomerulonephritis, in which renal failure is the dominant cause. End-stage renal disease (ESRD) now affects 8–15% of patients with lupus nephritis, and fatal infections are the usual cause of death in this group. Infection also remains the commonest reported cause of early death in those without ESRD, although retrospective reports may not reflect current practice. Extra-renal disease is the next most common cause of early death, particularly affecting the CNS or lung. But overall almost half of all lupus deaths are the result of excess cardiovascular mortality, often later in the course of the disease and particularly from premature myocardial ischemia.

Outcome in relation to clinical, histologic, and laboratory findings

There has been more controversy than agreement as to which features might be associated with a poorer outcome in lupus nephritis[1,3,17,18]. Factors influencing outcome in some series but not others are: age at onset of > 55 years, childhood onset, Black race, raised plasma creatinine, and hypertension. Indices of clinical activity, number of ACR criteria present at onset and the number of clinical relapses also predict outcome.

Today there is little difference in outcome between different WHO classes of nephritis in *treated* patients, although extensive subendothelial deposits and tubulointerstitial changes point to poorer prognosis as do the number of macrophages and T cells in the interstitium. Crescents have also been related to a poorer prognosis, as in other forms of nephritis, but extensive crescentic disease is uncommon in lupus.

Vascular lesions within the biopsy and intraglomerular capillary thrombi have been associated with unfavorable outcomes also, although the latter observation has been contested. Calculation of activity and chronicity indices has allowed the NIH group to identify groups of high and low risk for a poor outcome and also has permitted therapeutic decisions, especially when and when not to use aggressive treatment although these data are not supported by all other analyses.

Correlations between complement concentrations and levels of circulating anti-dsDNA antibody and outcome have been reported but are not useful in practice. The principal useful predictor amongst laboratory tests is anemia, with thrombocytopenia, hypocomplementemia, and a raised DNA-binding at onset all correlated with a poorer outcome.

TREATMENT[19-39]

Despite a half-century of clinical inquiry, the useful data upon which to base recommendations for the treatment of lupus nephritis remain pathetically small[19]. Two quite distinct therapeutic problems emerge:

- The *induction treatment* of severe, acute life-threatening disease, often affecting many systems and usually near the onset of the disease; here the threat of the disease is paramount.
- There follows the *maintenance treatment* and long-term management of chronic, more or less indolent disease, during which protection from the side-effects of treatment becomes more and more important.

The evidence for treating all but the mildest types of lupus nephritis with corticosteroids is very strong, but no prospective trial directly comparing a corticosteroid-treated group with one not so treated has ever been performed – nor is such a trial likely to be mounted.

In most patients with absent or trivial urine abnormalities, the biopsy appearances will be bland, the outlook good, and treatment unnecessary. Whether treatment with corticosteroids at this point might prevent subsequent evolution of severe disease has never been tested. There is equally little evidence that early treatment alters subsequent evolution of the disease in those with definite but minor urine abnormalities, normal renal function and mild histopathologic appearances (WHO class II). Nor is their clear evidence whether the outcome of membranous nephropathy (WHO class V) improves following treatment, although most clinicians do treat patients with this pattern at least with corticosteroids. Certainly, a proportion of such patients may slowly develop renal failure.

Therefore, it is in those groups with focal proliferative nephritis of varying severity (WHO class III), or severe diffuse proliferative nephritis (WHO class IV), that immunosuppression seems to have most to offer.

The acute phase: induction treatment
Corticosteroids
High-dose oral corticosteroids (starting dose: 60 mg/24 h) carry a heavy penalty in terms of side effects. Thus many clinicians believe a few (1–3) 'pulse' intravenous methylprednisolone infusions (0.5–1.0 g) combined with low-dose oral prednisolone (10–20 mg/day) can reduce the incidence of these side effects, particularly the altered facial appearance. Side effects following intravenous injection of high doses of corticosteroids are more common in children and adolescents, and include: cardiac arrhythmias or even cardiac arrest if given through central venous lines; unpleasant flushing sensations; acute hypertension; and very occasionally acute psychosis. However the only controlled trial comparing 'pulse' and oral corticosteroids was with small numbers of patients with mainly nonrenal lupus.

Cytotoxic agents
Today, most physicians use cytotoxic agents in both the acute and maintenance phases of the treatment of severe lupus nephritis[19,20], a strategy reinforced by results of recent meta-analyses (see below), although there are contrary views[17,18,21]. The choice of agent and the route of administration, however, remain controversial[19].

Cyclophosphamide has the advantage for the induction phase that it is a much more powerful inhibitor of B cells than is azathioprine, and the resynthesis of autoantibodies is reduced to normal levels rapidly and efficiently. Therefore most clinicians prefer it for induction therapy. Additional benefit from intravenous rather than oral administration during the acute phase is unproven[20,21] and undoubtedly carries a penalty in side effects in that leukopenia is deliberately induced. In spite of this, intravenous cyclophosphamide has become virtually the standard initial management for severe nephritis, although often using a regimen less aggressive than that carefully evaluated by the NIH group (0.75–1 g/m^2 monthly), and therefore of uncertain benefit. In addition it does not seem logical to use a drug intravenously that was specifically developed for oral use, which has to be extensively metabolized before it is active so that (unlike methylprednisolone) there is no immediate effect. Since the patient is usually in hospital at this point, compliance should not be an issue.

Plasma exchange

Although there is an obvious rationale for plasma exchange in lupus, no role in acute severe lupus nephritis has been defined except perhaps in patient with vasculitis and/or cryo-globulinemia. Two controlled trials in severe lupus nephritis[22] showed no benefit from the addition of thrice-weekly plasma exchange over conventional, combined cytotoxic and corticosteroid therapy, even when synchronized with plasma exchange to minimize antibody rebound. Other groups have used a more intensive course of exchange, one plasma volume daily for 7–10 days, but it is unknown if this extra treatment confers benefit.

Practical treatment guidelines for the *acute phase of lupus nephritis* are shown in Figure 27.9.

The chronic phase: maintenance treatment

Usually the acute disease will be under control after 12 weeks or less, although occasionally patients may have a stormy course and require several courses of 'pulse' methylpred-nisolone. The balance of benefit between strategies to avoid relapses or smoldering disease activity and the many side effects of the drugs are poorly evaluated, despite a number of controlled trials and a large amount of anecdotal information.

Corticosteroids

Corticosteroids remain the backbone of treatment in the maintenance as well as the acute phase; there are no studies of other treatments without prednisolone. To minimize the side effects of long-term corticosteroids, the dosage should be limited to prednisolone 5–15 mg/day. Daily and alternate-day regimens have not been formally compared in lupus. Monthly 'pulses' of methylprednisolone have been used also, but again the toxicity and benefits of this regimen have never been investigated.

Cytotoxic agents

Meta-analyses are unequivocally in favor of an additional clinical benefit of a cytotoxic agent during the maintenance phase when used in combination with corticosteroids[23,24]. Further, the long-term follow-up of the NIH trials have shown less progression of renal scarring at 10–15 years in those groups treated with a cytotoxic agent than in those treated with prednisolone alone[25] (Fig. 27.10). However, in these studies it was not possible to distinguish any difference between outcomes of the (rather small) groups receiving the various cytotoxic drugs used (cyclophosphamide, azathio-prine or both), or the route of administration. Nevertheless only a group treated with intravenous cyclophosphamide showed improved survival in contrast to a group of (partially historic) controls treated only with prednisolone[26,27] but this difference in outcome did not become apparent until more than 5 years' follow-up[27].

The use of oral cyclophosphamide for longer than about 12 weeks should always be avoided because of bladder but also gonadal toxicity. Therefore, regular monthly, then bimonthly intravenous cyclophosphamide (0.75–1 g/m²) has been advocated for up to 2 years because the medium- and long-term results are superior to those obtainable with prednisolone alone. However, it has become evident that the intravenous

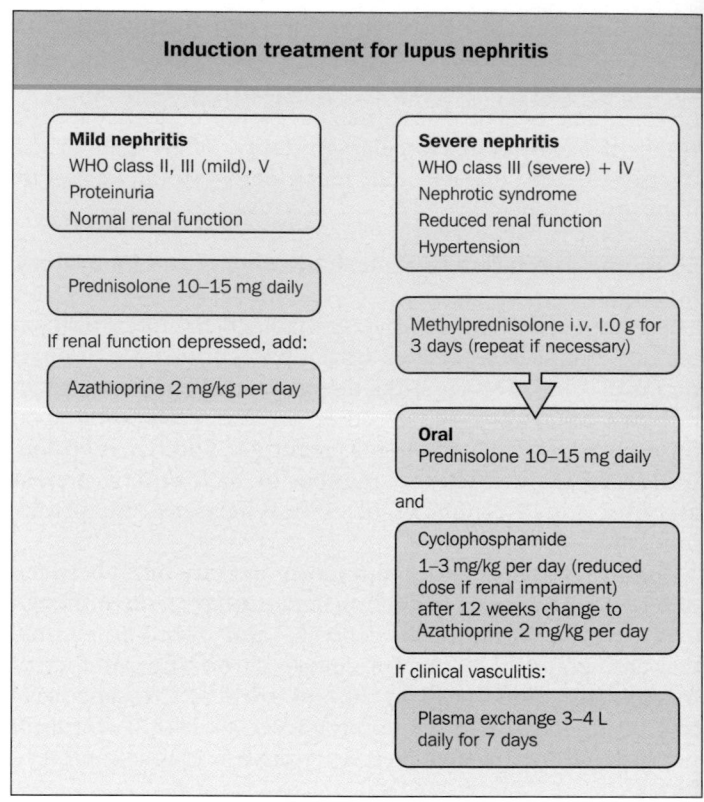

Figure 27.9 Induction treatment for lupus nephritis.

cyclophosphamide regimen, like prolonged daily oral treatment, carries a considerable dose- and age-dependent risk of gonadal damage with late menarche and early menopause being regular findings[28]. Relapse is common[29] and the very long-term outcome in terms of stable remission still unclear. There is an increased risk of infection compared to corticosteroids alone.

Gonadal damage could in theory be limited by giving the pulse timed so that a developing follicle is not present, but pregnancy cannot be contemplated during such treatment, although it may be possible at a later date in those who do not become sterile. The oncogenic risk of such regimens may not be evident for many years and, apart from the bladder, this risk remains whatever route of administration is used. However, a major advantage of the intravenous regimen is that in non-compliant patients it permits low corticosteroid dosage with acceptable effects on appearance, and the treatment can be given under observation. A recent controlled trial showed that combined treatment with monthly pulses of both intravenous cyclophosphamide and methylprednisolone together carried long-term advantages over either treatment alone[30].

Azathioprine in doses of 2–2.5 mg/kg/24 h has proved remarkably safe in the very long term[20], although macrocy-tosis is very common and higher doses will induce leukopenia. Previously we used this agent during the acute phase of the disease but in the past decade we have used oral cyclophos-phamide initially and then transferred patients to azathioprine after 12 weeks' induction (see Fig. 27.9).

There is evidence that the addition of azathioprine does not increase infections; which mostly depend upon corticosteroid

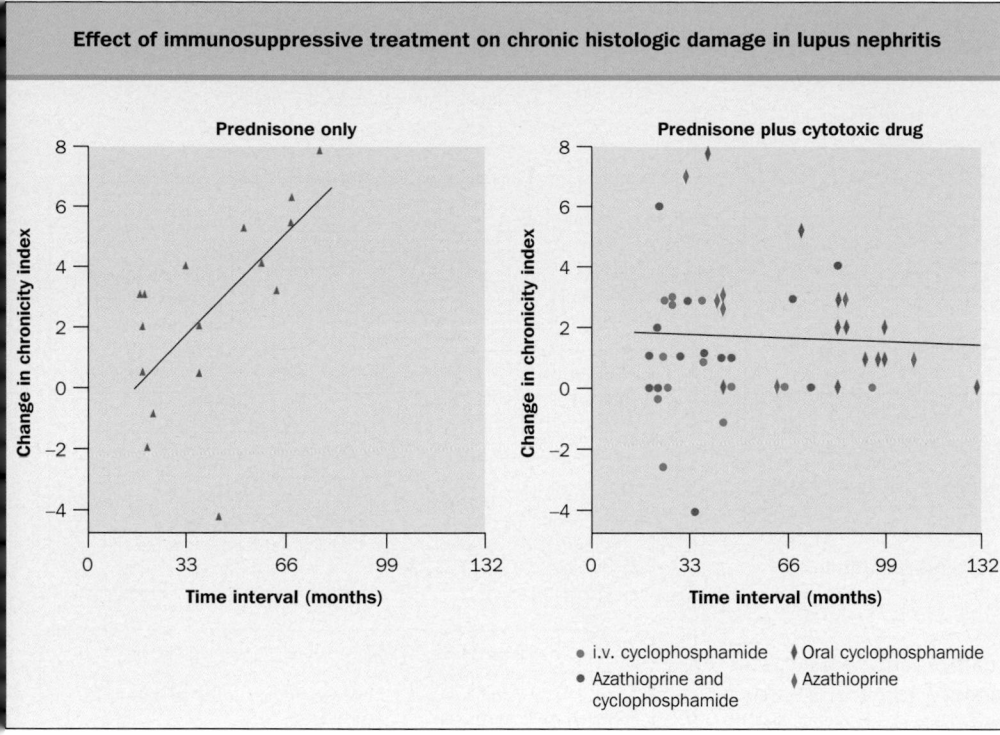

Figure 27.10 Effect of immunosuppressive treatment on chronic histologic damage in lupus nephritis. Combined analysis from NIH trials of prednisone plus cytotoxic agents versus prednisone alone. Change in chronicity index occurs (glomerular and interstitial fibrosis plus sclerosis) in individual patients, as shown by repeat biopsies 24–132 months apart. Patients receiving prednisone alone show a steady increase in the chronicity index, whereas there is an insignificant change in chronicity index in those receiving a cytotoxic drug in addition. Various cytotoxic therapies were given including intravenous and oral cyclophosphamide; oral azathioprine; and oral azathioprine plus cyclophosphamide. There was no difference in the data between any of these groups.

dosage. Both azathioprine and cyclophosphamide almost certainly have a steroid-sparing effect. Azathioprine has only a very small oncogenic potential; pregnancy during maintenance azathioprine can be encouraged and is safe. Pancreatitis and hepatotoxicity are very rare. Long-term results as good or better than the best obtainable with cyclophosphamide by whatever route can be achieved using initial intravenous methylprednisolone and 12 weeks' oral cyclophosphamide, followed by long-term combined azathioprine and corticosteroids. In practice a choice of cytotoxic agents is useful[31]. In the author's view[1,20] there is no evidence, as yet, that intravenous cyclophosphamide offers a better risk/benefit ratio in the long-term than azathioprine (Fig 27.11) and this suggestion is upheld in the only small controlled trial comparing the two treatments in the long term[32].

Mycophenolate mofetil has been used in lupus nephritis during the past five years or so[33], first in small series and then in larger controlled trials[34], some of which are ongoing. Results have been encouraging, with results comparable to the best obtained using any of the regimens outlined above. Its precise role in the treatment of lupus nephritis remains to be determined, however, and long term results are not yet available. Nevertheless, it seems at the time of writing to present a viable and less toxic alternative cytotoxic agent in the long term, and it may be of use in treatment of acute lupus as well.

Chlorambucil has been advocated as maintenance treatment also, but it has never been subjected to any controlled trials in lupus nephritis and its gonadal effects and oncogenic potential are, if anything, greater than those of cyclophosphamide.

Cyclosporine might be expected to benefit patients with lupus because of its powerful effect on helper T-cell clonal expansion through inhibition of interleukin-2 synthesis (Chapter 85). Limited evidence suggests that a dose of ~ 5 mg/kg/24 h (chosen to avoid nephrotoxicity) produces a good

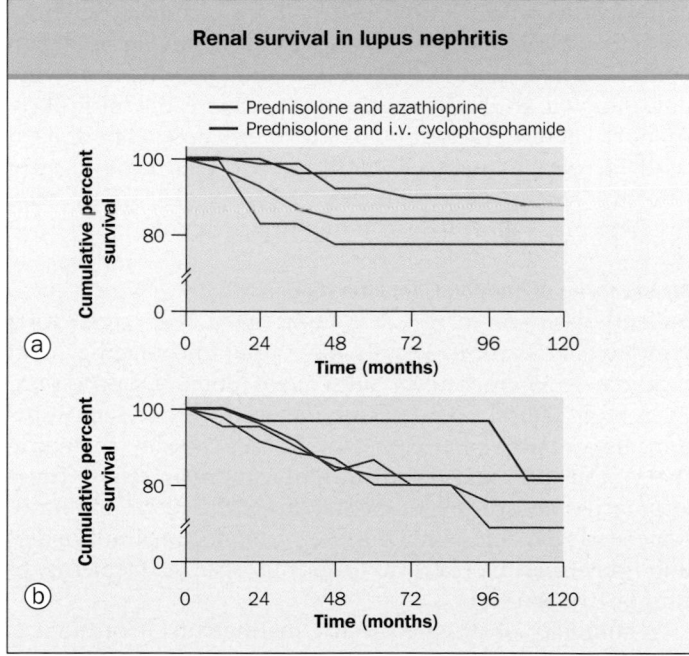

Figure 27.11 Renal survival in lupus nephritis. (a) Renal survival in lupus nephritis in three series of patients treated with azathioprine and the NIH trial data for patients treated with i.v. cyclophosphamide; there was no statistical difference in the outcomes. (b) Renal survival in class IV lupus nephritis treated with azathioprine compared favorably with NIH data for i.v. cyclophosphamide. Again there is no statistical difference in the outcomes using the different treatment regimens at 0.05 level. All patients in all studies received background maintenence prednisolone treatment.

response in some patients although relapse often follows withdrawal of treatment. There is no effect in reducing anti-dsDNA antibody levels. Cyclosporine does not appear to be useful in

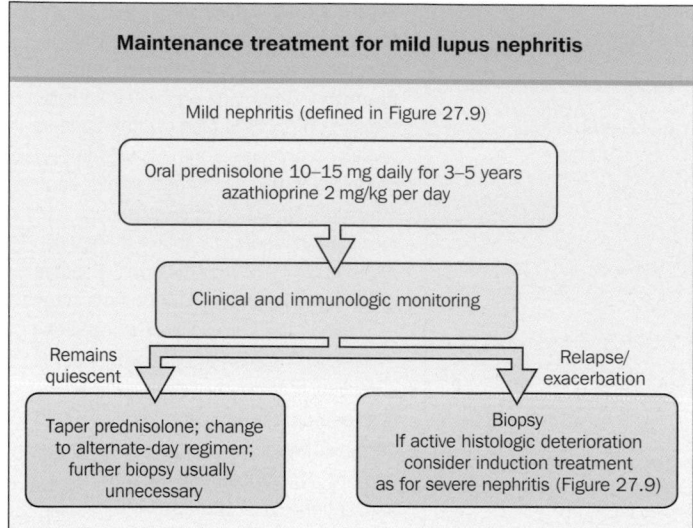

Figure 27.12 Maintenance treatment for mild lupus nephritis.

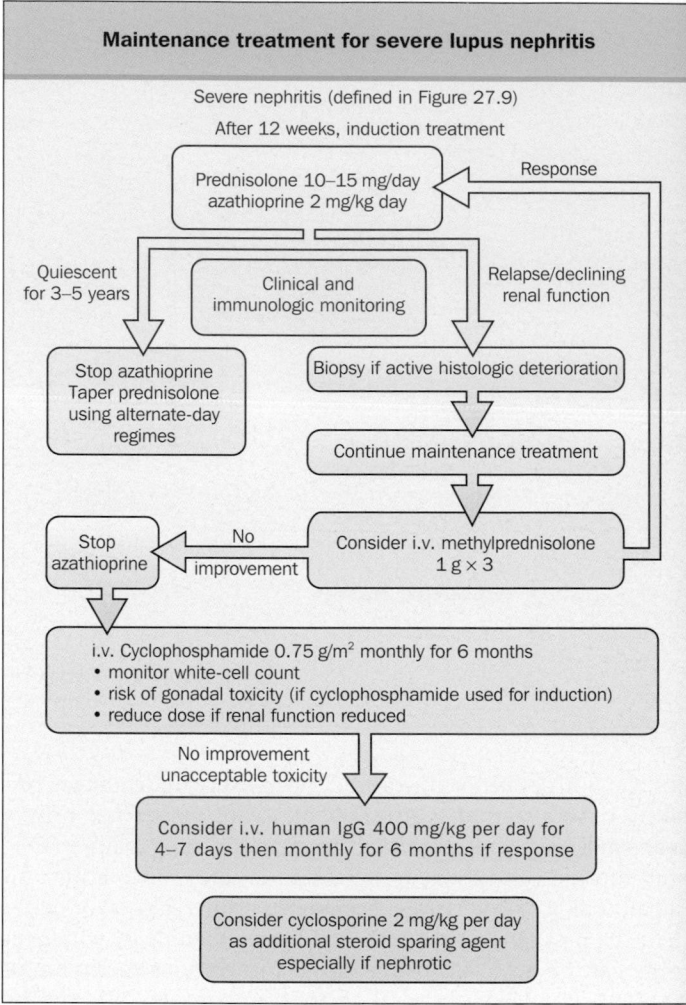

Figure 27.13 Maintenance treatment for severe lupus nephritis.

acute lupus but can have a role in the maintenance phase as a steroid-sparing agent and to reduce massive proteinuria[35], for example in membranous lupus nephritis.

Intravenous immunoglobulin[36,37] has been used with encouraging results in a number of small series, including those patients resistant to conventional treatment, and in one small controlled trial. Modification of anti-idiotype networks by the anti-idiotypic antibodies in the preparation is the most likely mode of action[36]. Various preparations and dosages have been used for periods up to 6 months or 1 year. Relapse after improvement is seen frequently. Transient decline in renal function may follow its use in nephrotic patients.

Newer forms of immunologic intervention

Patients with severe resistant lupus have been given total lymphoid irradiation. Results have been encouraging, with minimal requirements for subsequent immunosuppression. Even more radical approaches have been used in very resistant disease with major treatment side effects, including marrow ablation and reconstitution using stem cells[38]. These approaches are still experimental as are the newer immunologic strategies including the use of monoclonal antibodies and molecular blockers to interrupt specific elements of immune recognition[39].

A summary of disease-specific maintenance treatment is given in Figures 27.12 and 27.13. General renoprotective measures, such as the use of angiotensin-converting enzyme (ACE) inhibitors and lipid-lowering drugs, should be used in addition in long-term progressive lupus nephritis, especially if there is profuse proteinuria and hyperlipidemia.

Serologic tests in monitoring effects of specific treatment

While persisting anti-dsDNA antibody may be associated with subsequent relapses, a number of patients maintain elevated levels for years without relapse; and there is a fine balance between undertreatment and overtreatment. The main value of anti-dsDNA antibody levels is that normal values usually permit safe reduction of treatment during the

chronic phase. Likewise, complement concentrations are of limited value during the acute phase in severe nephritis; clinical and biochemical data are almost always sufficient.

When can treatments for lupus nephritis be stopped?

The goal of long-term management in patients with lupus nephritis is suppression of disease with minimum side effects of treatment. This balance is not easily achieved and requires close attention to detail in individual patients. Repeat renal biopsy may suggest whether a slow decline in renal function with proteinuria is the result of active nephritis, or of secondary sclerosis. Normal results from immunologic tests are a help in this distinction, but nevertheless in selected patients a repeat biopsy is a useful test to perform.

While occasionally patients will relapse more than 20 years from the onset of the disease when treatment is reduced, it is usually possible to stop treatment altogether after 5 years or so, even in patients with very severe lupus at onset, whose disease will have apparently 'burnt out', although some may relapse. Stable renal function, lack of proteinuria and normal immunologic tests are pointers to success. The very long-term outcome of a cohort of 110 patients first treated between 1963 and 1986 is shown in Figure 27.14.

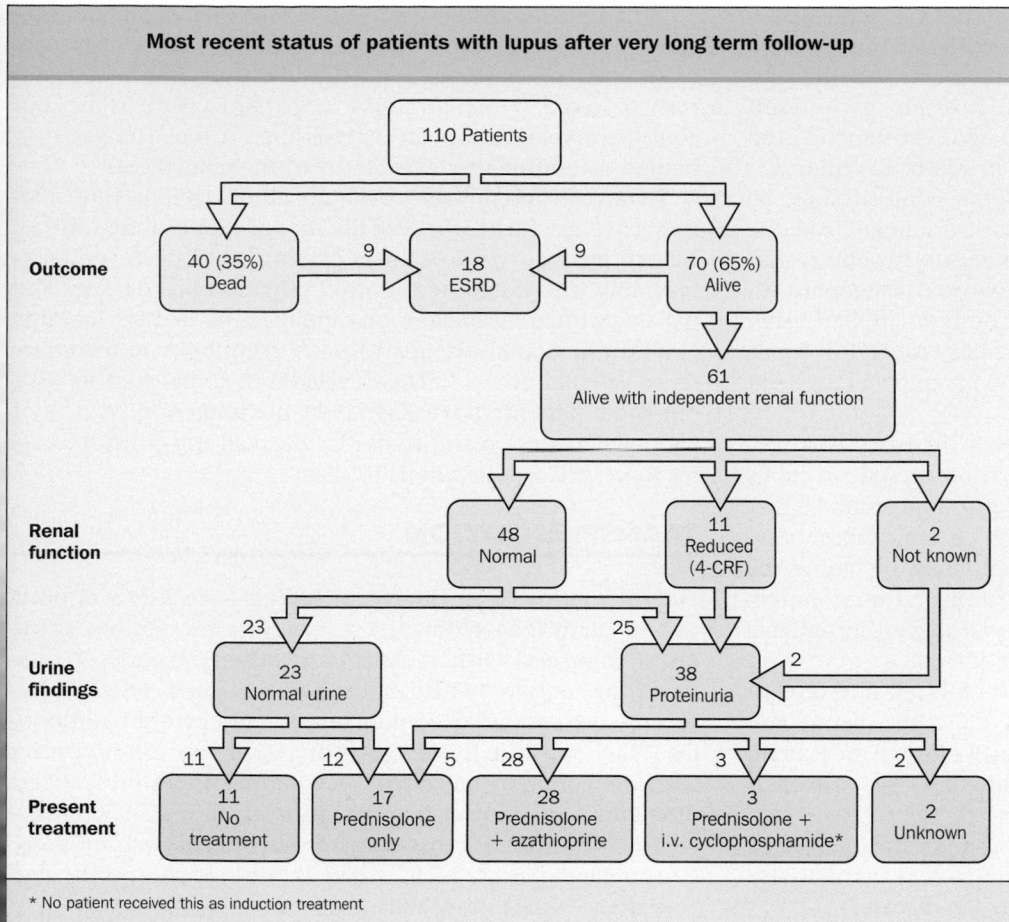

Figure 27.14 Most recent status of patients with lupus after very long-term follow-up. A cohort of 110 patients observed between 1963 and 1986 (mean age at diagnosis 15.4, range 10–32 years) (Adapted with permission from Bono, Cameron and Hicks[40]).

Antiphospholipid antibodies and thrombosis[12]

There is no evidence that *prophylactic anticoagulation* brings extra benefit even if the APA is of the IgG isotype, which is more likely to be of clinical significance than IgM APA. If thrombosis has occurred, *therapy* with warfarin is required as long as APA persists – disappearance of APA is uncommon. If IgG APA is present in high titer, the international normalized ratio must be maintained at 3.0 or above; re-thrombosis can occur at 2.0–2.5. Immunosuppression has little effect on APA. APA are associated also with second trimester abortions, and low-dose aspirin (75 mg/day) may be of benefit, although this has not been shown in controlled trials.

Other treatments

A number of other treatments have been used for lupus, mostly without overt nephritis, but have not made a major impact[1].

Indomethacin has been used but in view of the fall in GFR with nonsteroidal anti-inflammatory drugs and their potential for inducing interstitial nephritis, this has not proved popular. Antimalarials and androgens seem to be ineffective in lupus nephritis, either alone or as agents to reduce steroid dosage.

ω-3 unsaturated eicosapentanoic acid (EPA) has been shown to protect mice from lupus nephritis, with a reduction in anti-dsDNA antibody titers, while a high saturated-fat diet accelerates the disease. A controlled trial of EPA in human lupus showed favorable short-term effects on hematuria, blood lipids, and hemostatic parameters; anti-dsDNA titers were not affected. No benefit has yet been shown on nephritis. Effects on hemostasis and lipids are particularly attractive in view of the accelerated vascular disease reported in young women with lupus, which is a major cause of late morbidity and mortality.

Complications of lupus and its treatment[1,40–42]

Sepsis is the commonest early complication of treated lupus, and is related to the total dosage of corticosteroids and cyclophosphamide, but not azathioprine[40,41]. Infections are also more common in *un*treated lupus. Herpes zoster is particularly common in younger patients; early treatment with acyclovir should always be given to avoid dissemination. Pyogenic meningitis can be a major problem and *Cryptococcus* should be excluded in any lupus patients with meningitis. The C-reactive protein concentration is useful (but not specific) in distinguishing relapse of lupus from infection, since there is usually only a minor rise with exacerbations of disease. Bacterial endocarditis is rare but also presents obvious problems in diagnosis. With improvements in the survival of patients with lupus, accelerated atherogenesis has emerged as a major cause of later mortality. Myocardial infarction has been reported in very young patients in the absence of vasculitis. Possible risk factors for atheroma in lupus include hyperlipidemia, corticosteroids and hypertension even in children, and in a minority, the added vascular risks of ESRD[42].

Ischemic necrosis of bone is a common complication, affecting 15–20% of patients. Total corticosteroid dosage is the predominant risk factor, but it may present in patients who have never received corticosteroids, possibly as a result of microthromboses in association with APA. The femoral head is the commonest site of involvement in adults; in children it is the femoral condyle. Almost any other bone site may be involved, the next most frequent being the humeral head, the border of the scapula, and the carpus or tarsus. In some unfortunate patients, multiple sites may be involved. Osteoporosis[1], as judged by X-ray densitometry is common in Caucasian women treated long-term with corticosteroids for lupus (~40%), but clinical fractures are rare (3% in our own long-term series[40]).

The incidence of neoplasia is modestly increased in lupus. Risk factors are the immune dysregulation present in lupus and the added effect of chronic immunosuppression. Either might be mediated by direct damage to chromosomes, or by facilitation of oncogenic viruses. Lymphomas, including the intracerebral site, are the principal form of tumor noted. Carcinoma of the cervix is commoner also, even in patients who have not received cytotoxic therapy.

Growth retardation is inevitable in children and adolescents treated long-term with corticosteroids. The main correlation is with the duration of daily corticosteroid treatment, emphasizing the need to use alternate-day corticosteroids wherever possible in children and adolescents.

Pancreatitis is a rare but well-known complication of treated lupus. Lupus itself, corticosteroid therapy, and perhaps also azathioprine are all capable of inducing the disease.

Cataracts are frequent after years of prednisolone treatment, affecting 20–30% of patients. They are usually symptomless, although occasionally lens removal and replacement may be necessary. The procedure is safe even in the presence of immunosuppression. Steroid-induced diabetes mellitus has been described although it is significantly less common than following transplantation. Raised intracranial pressure may appear and complicate yet further neurologic and psychiatric assessment. Proximal myopathy is underdiagnosed and a Cushingoid appearance and hirsutism are common, forming a major disincentive for adolescent girls and young women to take corticosteroids, compliance in this major group of patients therefore being poor. This may, on occasion, lead to relapses, with complications from untreated disease and further acute treatment.

End-stage renal disease and renal replacement therapy[43,44]

Today, no more than 10–15% of patients with lupus develop ESRD[40], and lupus provides only 1–2% of all patients with ESRD. Many patients have inactive disease by the time they reach ESRD but another group develop irreversible renal failure quite rapidly, may have active disease and suffer a higher mortality and morbidity.

Patients with ESRD from lupus nephritis will sometimes show recovery of renal function sufficient to allow dialysis to be stopped, in some cases indefinitely. Thus, one should not rush to renal transplantation in patients with lupus, but consider a year or two on dialysis first. A renal biopsy may help to determine the reversibility of the renal disease.

Some patients continue to require immunosuppression after they have reached ESRD; usually prednisolone alone suffices. Nevertheless, survival of lupus patients on dialysis compares favorably with outcome for other primary renal diseases and patients with lupus make good candidates for dialysis, whether CAPD or hemodialysis, apart from susceptibility to thrombosis of vascular access[28]. This is related in some cases to APA, but some patients have Raynaud's phenomenon with poor peripheral perfusion and veins may be small and difficult to use for successful arteriovenous fistulae.

TRANSPLANTATION

Transplantation[43,44] in lupus (including from living donors) can be performed with only a few extra precautions being taken compared with recipients in other categories. Cross-matching donors with lupus patients may be difficult, because their sera may contain anti-lymphocyte autoantibodies. These are usually of IgM isotype, of low affinity, react with the common leukocyte CD45 antigen and present few problems. Some however are of IgG isotype, and so will register in conventional cross-matches but their target antigens, even if they include MHC antigens, are not allospecific and they do not affect graft outcome.

As is the case during dialysis, thrombosis may be a problem post-transplantation, especially in patients with APA. Both renal transplant arterial and venous thrombosis have been reported. Anticoagulation should be considered in patients with circulating APA of IgG isotype in high titers. Lupus disease activity lessens post-transplant, presumably because of the immunosuppressive regimens used.

The striking feature of transplantation in lupus remains the very low rate of recurrence of lupus nephritis[44], even in patients with active disease at the time of receiving a transplant. The incidence is no more than 1 : 100, and even in those in whom recurrence has been clearly identified, it very rarely causes graft loss. In many reports of supposed recurrence, although electron-dense immune aggregates were present in glomeruli of the allograft, glomerular IgG – the hallmark of lupus nephritis – was not detected.

Immunosuppression usually does not need to be modified in patients with lupus, although cyclosporine monotherapy is best avoided because this drug is not a powerful suppressant of lupus and relapse has been described in this context. There is no difference in the number and severity of rejections in recipients with lupus compared with recipients in other categories and, with current immunosuppressive regimens, there seems to be no higher incidence of infections.

REFERENCES

1. Cameron JS. Systemic lupus erythematosus. In: Nielson EG, Couser WG, eds. Immunologic Renal Disease, 2nd edition. Philadelphia: Lippincott-Raven; 2001:1057–104.
2. Wallace DH, Hahn BH. Dubois' lupus erythematosus, 4th edn. Baltimore: Lea & Febiger;1993.
3. Lewis EJ, Schwartz MM, Korbet SM (eds) Lupus nephritis. Oxford University Press, Oxford 1999.
4. Ruiz-Arastorza G, Khamashta M, Castellino G, Hughes GRV. Systemic lupus erythematosus. Lancet. 2001;357:1027–32.
5. Muehrcke RC, Kark RM, Pirani CL, Pollak VE. Lupus nephritis: a clinical and pathological study based on renal biopsies. Medicine (Baltimore).1957;36:1–146.
6. Hahn BH. Antibodies to DNA. N Engl J Med. 1998;338:1359–68.
7. Davidson A, Diamond B. Autoimmune diseases. N Engl J Med. 2001;345:340–50.
8. Goodnow CC. Pathways for self-tolerance and the treatment of autoimmune diseases. Lancet. 2001;357:2115–21.
9. Cameron JS. Clinical manifestations of lupus nephritis. In Lewis EJ, Schwartz MM, Korbet SM (eds) Lupus nephritis. Oxford: Oxford University Press; 1999:159–84.
10. De Arriba G, Velo M, Barrio V, et al. Association of interstitial lupus cystitis with systemic lupus erythematosus. Clin Nephrol. 1992;39:287–8.
11. West SG. Neuropsychiatric lupus. Rheum Clin N Am. 1994;20:129–58.
12. Kashgarian M. Lupus nephritus: lessons from the path lab. Kidney Int. 1994;45:928–38.
13. Asherson RA, Cervera R, Piette J-C, et al. The antiphospholipid syndrome. Boca Raton: CRC Press; 1996.
14. Hill GS, Delahousse M, Nochy D, et al. Proteinuria and tubulointerstitial lesions in lupus nephritis. Kidney Int. 2001;60:1893–903.
15. Appel GB, Pirani CL, D'Agati V. Renal vascular complications of systemic lupus erythematosus. J Am Soc Nephrol. 1994;4:1499–515.
16. Ropes MW. Observations on the natural history of disseminated lupus erythematosus, Medicine (Baltimore). 1964;43:387–91.
17. Donadio JV, Hart GM, Bergstralh EJ, et al. Prognostic determinants in lupus nephritis: a long-term clinicopathologic study. Lupus. 1995;4:109–15.
18. Gruppo Italiano per lo Studio della Nefrite Lupica (GISNEL). Lupus nephritis: prognostic factors and probability of maintaining life-supporting renal function 10 years after the diagnosis. Am J Kidney Dis. 1992;19:473–9.
19. Adu D. The evidence base for the treatment of lupus nephritis in the new millennium. Nephrol Dial Transplant. 2001;16:1536–8.
20. Cameron JS. What is the role of long-term cytotoxic agents in the treatment of lupus nephritis? J Nephrol. 1993;6:172–6.
21. Donadio JV, Glassock RJ. Immunosuppressive drug therapy in lupus nephritis. Am J Kidney Dis. 1993;21:239–50.
22. Lewis EJ, Hunsicker LG, Lan S-P, et al. for the lupus nephritis collaborative study group. A controlled trial of plasmapheresis therapy in severe lupus nephritis. N Engl J Med. 1992;326:1373–9.
23. Felson DT, Anderson J. Evidence for the superiority of immunosuppressive drugs and prednisone over prednisone alone in lupus nephritis. N Engl J Med. 1984;311:1528–33.
24. Bansal VK, Beto JA. Treatment of lupus nephritis: a meta-analysis of clinical trials. Am J Kidney Dis. 1997;29:193–9.
25. Balow JE, Austin HA, Muenz LR, et al. Effect of treatment on the evolution of renal abnormalities in lupus nephritis. N Engl J Med. 1984;311:491–5.
26. Austin HA III, Klippel JH, Balow JE, et al. Therapy of lupus nephritis. Controlled trial of prednisone and cytotoxic drugs. N Engl J Med. 1986;314:614–19.
27. Steinberg AD, Steinberg SC. Long-term preservation of renal function in patients with lupus nephritis receiving treatment that includes cyclophosphamide versus those treated with prednisolone alone. Arthritis Rheum. 1991;34:945–50.
28. Boumpas DT, Austin HA III, Vaughan EM, et al. Risk for sustained amenorrhea in patients with systemic lupus erythematosus receiving intermittent pulse cyclophosphamide therapy. Ann Intern Med. 1993;119:366–9.
29. Ioannidis JPA, Boki KA, Katsordia ME, et al. Remission, relapse, and re-remission of proliferative lupus nephritis treated with cyclophosphamide. Kidney Int. 2000;57:258–64.
30. Illei GG, Austin HA, Crane M, et al. Combination therapy with pulse cyclophosphamide plus pulse methylprednisolone improves long-term outcome without adding toxicity in patients with lupus nephritis. Ann Intern Med. 2001;135:296–8.
31. Ponticelli C. Treatment of lupus nephritis: the advantages of a flexible approach. Nephrol Dial Transplant. 1997;12:2057–9.
32. El-Fattah M, El-Tayeb M, Abd El-Kader A, et al. Intravenous pulse cyclophosphamide versus sequential therapy with azathioprine in treatment of severe lupus nephritis: a prospective study. Afr J Nephrol. 2000;4:17–24.
33. Adu D, Cross J, Jayne DRW. Treatment of systemic lupus erythematosus with mycophenolate mofetil. Lupus. 2001;10:203–8:
34. Chan TMS, Li FK, Tang CSO, et al. for the Hong Kong-Guangzhou nephrology study group. Efficacy of mycophenolate mofetil in patients with diffuse proliferative lupus nephritis. N Engl J Med. 2000;343:1156–62.
35. Tam LS, Li EK, Leung KC, et al. Long-term treatment of lupus nephritis with cyclosporin A. Q J Med. 1998;91:573–80.
36. Kazatchkine MD, Kaveri SV. Immunomodulation of autoimmune and inflammatory diseases with intravenous immune globulin. N Engl J Med. 2001;345:747–55.
37. Rauova L, Lukac J, Levy Y, et al. High-dose intravenous immunoglobulins for lupus nephritis - a salvage immunomodulation. Lupus. 2001;10:209–13.
38. Traynor AE, Schroeder J, Rosa RM, et al. Treatment of severe systemic lupus erythematosus with high-dose chemotherapy and haemopoietic stem-cell transplantation: a phase I study. Lancet. 2000;356:701–7.
39. Balow JE, Boumpas DT, Austin HA III. New prospects for treatment of lupus nephritis. Semin Nephrol. 2000;20:32–9.
40. Bono L, Cameron JS, Hicks JA. The very long-term prognosis and complications of lupus nephritis and its treatmernt. Q J Med. 1999;92:211–18.
41. Ginzler E, Diamond H, Kaplan D, et al. Computer analysis of factors influencing frequency of infection in systemic lupus erythematosus. Arthritis Rheum. 1978;21:37–44.
42. Font J, Ramos-Casals M, Cervera R, et al. Cardiovascular risk factors and the long-term outcome of lupus nephritis. Q J Med. 2001;94:19–26.
43. Nossent HC. End-stage renal disease in the patient with SLE. In Lewis EJ, Schwartz MM, Korbet SM. Lupus nephritis. Oxford: Oxford University Press; 1999:284–304.
44. Thervet E, Anglicheau D, Legendre C. Recent issues concerning renal transplantation in systemic lupus erythematosus. Nephrol Dial Transplant. 2001;16:12–14.

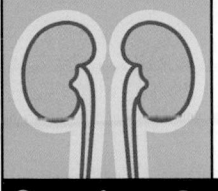

Section 5 Glomerular Disease

Chapter 28	Glomerular Diseases Associated with Infection
	Bernardo Rodríguez-Iturbe, Emmanuel A. Burdmann Vuddhidej Ophascharoensuk, and Rashad S Barsoum

INTRODUCTION

Glomerulonephritis (GN) may occur in a variety of diseases caused by bacterial, viral, fungal and helminthic pathogens (Table 28.1). Some infection-related glomerulonephritides are subclinical and transient; others are chronic and lead to end-stage renal disease (ESRD). This chapter discusses the pathogenesis of the major histological patterns of glomerular disease associated with infections and will focus on specific characteristics and management of renal disease associated with individual infectious syndromes.

GENERAL CHARACTERISTICS OF GLOMERULAR DISEASES ASSOCIATED WITH INFECTION

The majority of renal disease associated with infection is immune complex-related (Table 28.2). Antigen load, charge and size and the characteristics of the host antibody response and efficiency of disposal of the nephritogenic immune complexes, are factors that define the characteristics of the renal lesion. Therefore, the duration and severity of the infection, the effectiveness of treatment and the existence of comorbid conditions are, to a large extent, responsible for the histological appearance and course of GN. Not surprisingly, pathologic patterns of glomerular damage and their corresponding clinical manifestations vary in different stages of the natural history of some infectious diseases. For example, the initial, serum sickness-like, clinical presentation of hepatitis B may be associated with self-limited acute mesangial proliferative GN, while the chronic carrier state may be associated with membranous nephropathy in children and with membranoproliferative (mesangiocapillary) GN (MPGN) in adults. Alternatively, different infectious diseases, such as visceral bacterial abscesses and hepatitis C viral infection, may present with nephrotic syndrome resulting from histologically similar MPGN.

The histological patterns and the most typical infectious disease associated with them are shown in Table 28.2. Mesangial proliferative GN is usually acute and self-limited. Microscopic hematuria and non-nephrotic proteinuria are present in association with deposits of IgG, IgM and C3. Serum complement may be transiently decreased. Acute typhoid fever and acute malaria (*Plasmodium falciparum*) are typical examples of infections causing mesangial proliferative GN. Diffuse

Some infectious agents associated with renal disease

A. Bacterial. *Streptococcus* (group A, S. viridans), *Staphylococcus* (*aureus*, *epidermidis*), *Salmonella* (*typhi, paratyphi*), *Escherichia coli, Leptospira, Treponema pallidum, Neisseria* spp, *Mycobacterium leprae, Yersinia enterocolitica, Coxiella burnetii, Brucella abortus, Listeria monocytogenes*

B. Viral. Hepatitis A, B and C, human immunodeficiency virus, varicella-zoster, mumps. Influenza, Epstein–Barr, Cocksackie and ECHO

C. Fungus. *Histoplasma capsulatum*, candida

D. Protozooal. *Plasmodium falciparum, malariae, vivax* and *ovale*; *Trypanosoma, Toxoplasma*

E. Helminthic. *Schistosoma mansoni* and *haematobium, Wuchereria bancrofti, Trichinella spiralis*, filaria (*Onchocerca volvulus*, Loa Loa)

Table 28.1 Some infectious agents associated with renal disease.

proliferative GN is also acute and self-limited if the infection is eradicated. IgG, IgM and C3 deposits are prominent in the mesangium and glomerular capillaries and electron dense deposits are present in mesangium, subendothelial and subepithelial locations. The immune complexes deposited in the glomeruli may or may not contain bacterial antigens and cryoglobulins may be present. The clinical presentation is the acute nephritic syndrome and typical examples of this histological type are poststreptococcal GN, and GN resulting from bacterial endocarditis and pneumococcal pneumonia. MPGN is the usual pattern of GN resulting from chronic infections. The clinical presentation is frequently that of the nephrotic syndrome with microscopic hematuria, and variable degrees of hypertension. Complement may be low or normal. Immunoglobulins and C3 deposits are usually found and, if liver disease is present (as in *Schistosoma mansoni* infection), IgA may be a predominant component of the immune deposits. Hepatitis C virus, *S. mansoni* and *P. malariae* infections are usually associated with MPGN. Membranous nephropathy (MN) is associated with chronic infections. Infection-related MN generally presents as the nephrotic syndrome; hepatitis B viral infection in children and acquired syphilis are typical infections resulting in this form of GN.

Infections may also be associated with renal disease via mechanisms that do not involve immune complexes (Table 28.2). Focal segmental glomerulosclerosis with glomerular collapse ('collapsing glomerulopathy') may occur with human

Major renal syndromes associated with infection				
Type	Time course	Clinical presentation	Other	Examples
Mesangial proliferative IgM, C3 dominant IgA dominant	Acute Acute or chronic	Subclinical, microhematuria, non-nephrotic proteinuria	Coexistent liver disease is frequent in IgA dominant cases	Acute typhoid fever, acute malaria
Diffuse proliferative IgM; IgG, C3 C3 only	Acute	Renal dysfunction, hypertension, proteinuria, edema	Occasionally with crescents or thrombi	Endocarditis-associated GN Poststreptococcal GN
Membranoproliferative Type I (± cryoglobulinemia)	Chronic	Nephrotic or non-nephrotic, GFR depressed	Occasionally with sclerosis	Hepatitis C virus-associated GN, shunt nephritis, schistosomal GN (class III), quartan malaria nephropathy
Membranous	Chronic	Nephrotic syndrome	Occasionally with mesangial deposits	Hepatitis B virus-associated GN, syphilis
Vasculitis	Acute or chronic	Hypertension, renal dysfunction, systemic symptoms		Hepatitis B virus-associated vasculitis, HIV-associated vasculitis, vasculitis associated with poststreptococcal GN
Focal glomerulosclerosis	Acute or chronic	Nephrotic syndrome, GFR depressed		HIV infection
Amyloid	Chronic	Nephrotic syndrome		Leprosy, kala-azar, schistosomiasis
Hemolytic uremic syndrome	Acute	Acute renal failure, low platelets, anemia		*Escherichia coli* 0157:H7 infection, shigellosis
Interstitial nephritis	Acute	Acute renal failure, microhematuria		Epstein–Barr virus, Legionnaires' disease, leptospirosis, kala-azar, Hanta virus

Table 28.2 Major renal syndromes associated with infection.

immunodeficiency virus (HIV) or parvovirus B19 infection and usually presents as a sudden, massive nephrotic syndrome with rapid progression to chronicity. Vasculitis may develop in association with viral (especially hepatitis B virus and HIV) or bacterial (rarely streptococcus) infections; the hemolytic uremic syndrome from verotoxin-producing *Escherichia coli* or *Shigella* species) (see Chapter 31); and amyloidosis from chronic infections such as tuberculosis, leprosy and schistosomiasis. Interstitial nephritis manifested as acute renal failure may be associated with several viral (especially Epstein–Barr virus) or bacterial (especially *Legionella*) infections and also may be due to antibiotic therapy. Certain viruses, especially within the Hanta virus family, can also induce a hemorrhagic fever–renal failure syndrome in which infection of the interstitial capillaries and tubules leads to an acute renal failure (see Chapter 15).

PATHOGENESIS OF INFECTION-RELATED GLOMERULAR DISEASE

GN results from both humoral and cell-derived mediators released in response to immune complexes localizing in glomeruli. Immune complex formation consisting of an bacterial or viral antigen and its corresponding antibody may occur in the circulation, and be subsequently deposited in the glomeruli or, alternatively, may occur *in situ*, within the glomerulus. The formation of circulating immune complexes and their nephritogenic potential has been best studied in acute and chronic serum sickness. The deposition of circulating complexes occurs upon reaching an appropriate antigen : antibody ratio that favors precipitation and their pathogenic potential depends on the characteristics of the immune complex (quantity, size, charge, complement fixing capacity, etc.) and the efficiency of their removal by the mononuclear

phagocytic system. If the clearance of immune complexes is defective or if the capacity of the phagocytic system is overwhelmed, the immune complexes are deposited in the mesangium and subendothelial areas. The *in situ* formation of complexes occurs when the antigen is 'planted' in the glomerular basement membrane (GBM). This mechanism may occur in conditions of antigen excess, in which the immune complexes are easily dissociable. Penetration of the antigen and antibody across the filtration barrier is favored by charge-dependent attraction; therefore, cationic antigens that are attracted by the GBM polyanion (negatively charged heparan sulfate in the basement membrane and the sialoproteins in the podocytes) penetrate readily to subepithelial locations where they are joined by the antibody.

Deposited or locally formed immune complexes activate the complement system, resulting in the generation of the chemotactic factor C5a and the expression of chemokines and leukocyte adhesion molecules that stimulate leukocyte infiltration, as well as proliferation and matrix expansion by glomerular cells. Whereas clearance of the immune complexes with resolution of injury may occur, progression to ESRD may also result if the infection is not controlled and the immune process continues. In the event extensive nephron loss occurs, renal disease may progress even if the infection is controlled (see Chapter 66).

Several studies suggest that infection-related GN, as well as immune complex-associated GN, may occur more frequently and have worse prognosis in conditions in which there is difficulty clearing the infection and/or immune complexes. These conditions include HIV infection, infections acquired in the neonatal period (when tolerance is often induced such as is observed with hepatitis B virus infection), chronic liver disease and chronic alcoholism (increased infection risk and reduced clearance of immune complexes).

BACTERIAL INFECTIONS

Poststreptococcal glomerulonephritis
History and epidemiology
The observation of dark scanty urine in the convalescent period of scarlet fever is more than two centuries old. The postulate that the disease had an allergic, serum-sickness-like etiology, made by Bela Schick nearly a century ago, was a landmark observation that opened the field of immune-mediated renal disease.

Poststreptococcal glomerulonephritis (PSGN) is decreasing in frequency in the United States, Central Europe and other industrialized countries; nevertheless, sporadic cases appear worldwide, often in alcoholic patients, and recurrent epidemics are reported from certain regions where communities have crowded housing and poor hygienic conditions. The observation that epidemics of PSGN occur in some areas (such as the Red Lake Indian Reservation in Minnesota, Port of Spain in Trinidad and Maracaibo in Venezuela) but not in others with similar socioeconomic characteristics has suggested a potential genetic predisposition although none has been identified. PSGN is more common in males (2 : 1) and usually affects children 2–14 years old, but cases have been reported in small children and patients more than 40 years of age. Only certain 'nephritogenic' strains of group A *Streptococcus pyogenes*, and rarely group C (*S. zooepidemicus*)[1], result in GN. In the tropics and southern United States, PSGN usually follows streptococcal impetigo of M types 47, 49, 55 and 57. Throat infections with streptococcus types 1, 2, 4 and 12 are also nephritogenic. The risk of nephritis in epidemics may range from 5% in throat infections to as high as 25% in M type 49 pyoderma. The risk for PSGN is reduced by early antibiotic treatment and is likely one reason for the declining incidence in industrialized nations.

Pathogenesis
Several putative nephritogenic streptococcal antigens have been studied over the years. The two major antigens currently investigated are nephritis-associated plasmin receptor (NAPLr) that was identified as glyceraldehyde-3-phosphate dehydrogenase (GAPDH) and a cationic (pK > 8.0) streptococcal antigen, which was identified as the erythrogenic exotoxin B precursor, zymogen[2]. GAPDH and zymogen have been identified in renal biopsies of acute PSGN and antibody titers to both these antigens have been demonstrated in the vast majority of convalescent sera. GAPDH and zymogen when injected intravenously have affinity for glomeruli and a streptococcal extract, likely containing GAPDH, injected into rabbits induced histologic features of PSGN and is also capable of activating the alternative complement pathway 2. According to the current paradigm, persistent streptococcal infection results in antigenemia and the development of circulating immune complexes that primarily deposit in the subendothelial and mesangial locations to initiate an inflammatory cascade with local complement activation and the recruitment of neutrophils and monocytes/macrophages. Subepithelial immune deposits ('humps') develop due to the presence of cationic antigens (e.g., zymogen) and/or the dissociation of immune complexes in the subendothelial space with transit and reformation on the outer aspect of the

GBM. A role for cell-mediated immunity is supported by the presence of CD4 ('helper') T-lymphocytes. Cytokines (interleukin-6, tumor necrosis factor-α (TNF-α) and vasoactive mediators (platelet activating factor) also contribute to the local inflammation and injury[3].

Several issues remain unresolved. First, it remains unknown if disease is due to the deposition of circulating immune complexes or to the *in situ* deposition of antigen followed by antibody. Second, immune complex disease should result in activation of the classical complement pathway, yet in most cases C4 levels are normal and only C3 is found in the deposits. This potentially could be explained by the presence of antigens (such as GAPDH) that activate the alternative pathway. In addition, in occasional cases C3Nef IgG antibodies) have been demonstrated in sera that are capable of activating the alternative complement pathway. More recently, the lectin complement pathway has been shown to be activated in PSGN, likely as a result of the presence of N-acetyl glucosamine residues in the bacterial cell wall[4]. Finally, a role for autoimmune mechanisms is suggested by the presence of rheumatoid factors (especially IgG-rheumatoid factor) and cryoglobulins in the serum of one-third of patients in the first week of the disease. Anti-IgG deposits have been shown in one-third of the renal biopsies and in the eluate from the kidney in a fatal case. Anti-IgG reactivity may result from the loss of sialic acid from autologous IgG due to streptococcal neuraminidase (sialidase) or from binding of the Fc fragment of IgG to type II Fc-receptors in the streptococcal wall.

Pathology
Renal biopsy shows a diffuse endocapillary GN with proliferation of mesangial and endothelial cells (Fig. 28.1). Glomerular and interstitial infiltration of monocytes and lymphocytes is present, and occasional biopsies show vasculitis of the intrarenal arteries. Glomerular accumulation of neutrophils, and rarely eosinophils, is common and is termed 'exudative' GN. Glomerular immune deposits of C3 (100% of the cases), IgG (62%), IgM (76%), properdin and the terminal membrane attack complex C5b–C9 (MAC, 85% of the cases, usually co-deposited with C3) have been shown in glomerular capillary loops and in the mesangium. A seminal work by Sorger[5] described three patterns of immunofluorescence in the glomeruli and their clinical correlations: the mesangial pattern of irregular and heavy immune deposits, the 'starry-sky' pattern of deposits scattered in mesangium and in capillary walls and the 'garland' pattern formed by gross deposits in the capillary loops (Fig. 28.1). The 'garland' pattern is clinically relevant because it is associated with heavy proteinuria, and a large number of electron dense subepithelial immune deposits. Heavy proteinuria results in a higher incidence of chronic renal disease. Ultrastructural studies demonstrate the subepithelial 'humps' which are typical although not pathognomonic of PSGN, as they may also be observed in post-infectious GN of other etiologies (classically endocarditis-associated GN secondary to *Staphylococcus*), cryoglobulinemia and lupus nephitis.

GN resolves by apoptosis of the excess cells, a mechanism that is stimulated by streptococcal erythrogenic toxin B. Residual renal injury is common, and biopsies years later

Glomerular Disease

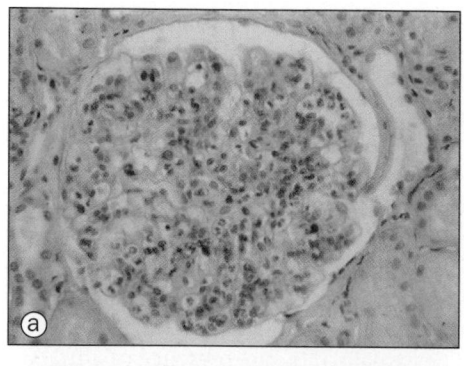
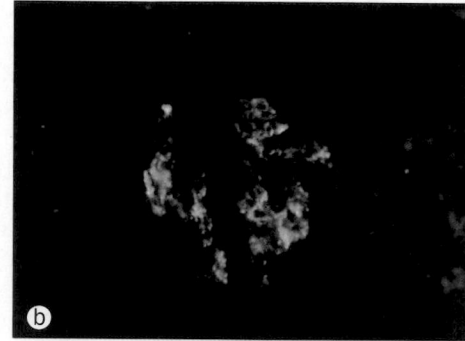
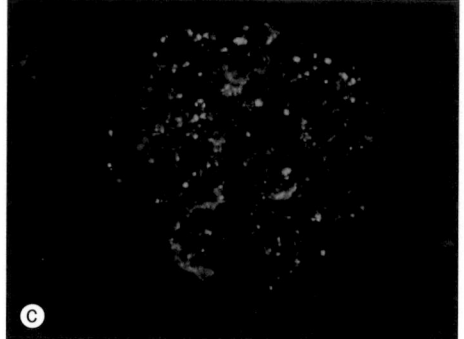
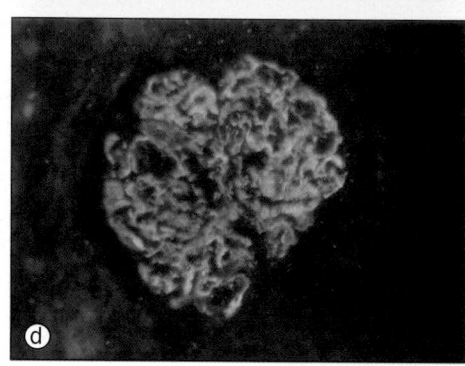
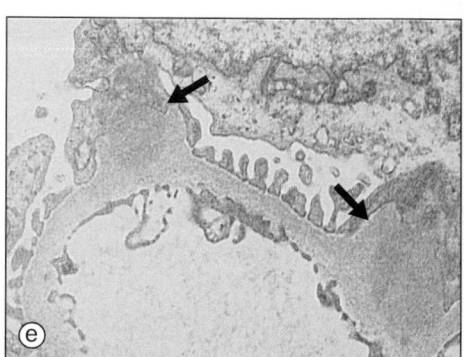

Figure 28.1 Poststreptococcal glomerulonephritis. (a) A diffuse proliferative and exudative glomerulonephritis can be seen by light microscopy. Immunofluorescence showing the (b) 'mesangial' (c) 'starry sky' and (d) 'garland' patterns. (e) Electron microscopy demonstrates large subepithelial 'humps' (arrows) beneath effaced foot processes. ((e) with permission L. de Moura).

show variable degrees of focal glomerulosclerosis and mesangial expansion even in the absence of clinical disease. The significance of these changes is undetermined.

Clinical manifestations

Most patients give a history of a previous streptococcal infection. The incubation period is classically longer after skin infections (several weeks) than after throat infections (2 weeks) (Fig. 28.2). However, the infection is often resolved at presentation. The acute nephritic syndrome is observed in the vast majority of overt cases. Hypertension is found in 80% of patients. Edema occurs in 80–90% of cases and is the chief complaint in 60%; yet, ascites is distinctly unusual. Hematuria is universal and in 30% of cases is macroscopic. The clinical picture is usually uncomplicated in children but in the elderly patient with PSGN, congestive heart failure and early mortality may occur in 43% and 25% of the patients, respectively[6]. The nephrotic syndrome may occur at the onset in 2% of the children and 20% of adults. A rapidly progressive course, resulting from extracapillary crescent formation, occurs in less than 1% of the patients. Azotemia occurs in 25–40% of the children and in as many as 83% of the adults.

Positive cultures for streptococcus are obtained in 10–70% of the cases during epidemics and in about 20–25% of sporadic cases. While historically antistreptolysin O (ASO) titers were reported to be positive in 60–80% of patients with PSGN following throat infections, in a recent study only 33% had elevated ASO titers at presentation[7]. Anti-DNAse B titers are elevated in 73% of the post-impetigo cases. The streptozyme panel (which measures antibodies to four antigens, anti-DNAse B, antihyaluronidase, ASO and antistreptokinase) is more sensitive, and is positive in more than 80% of subjects. Antibody titers to GAPDH and zymogen are the most sensitive (>85%) and specific but are not clinically available[2,7].

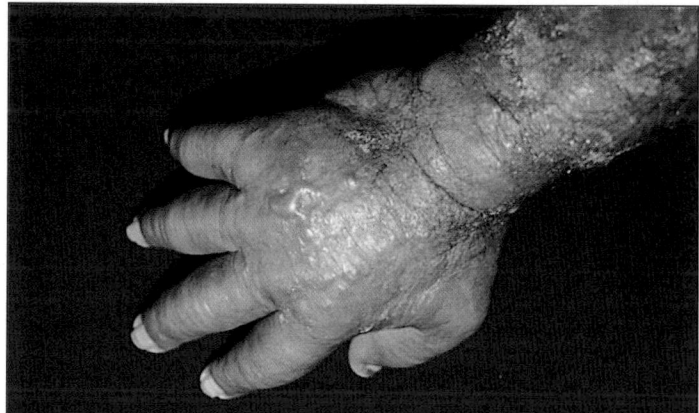

Figure 28.2 Acute erysipelas in a patient. (Courtesy of J Antonio, São Jose de Rio Preto, Brazil.)

Serum C3 levels are depressed in 90% of patients in the first week of disease and return to normal in the vast majority within 2 months. C4, a measure of classical complement pathway activation, is usually normal or near normal. The terminal complement complexes (C5b–C9) are elevated in samples taken within 30 days from onset and return to normal with the improvement of GN. Serum IgG and IgM are elevated in 80% of the cases and in contrast with another poststreptococcal disease, rheumatic fever, IgA is normal. Cryoglobulins and elevated rheumatoid factor are present in up to one-third of patients, and rare patients may have low titers of anti-DNA and antineutrophil cytoplasmic antibodies (ANCA).

It is important to note that subclinical disease, manifested by microscopic hematuria and fall in serum complement, occurs four to five times more frequently than clinically overt disease and prospective studies in families have shown that 38% of the siblings of index cases of sporadic PSGN develop the disease[8]. Occasionally, whole families have various manifestations of PSGN; it is thus important to inquire about a history of streptococcal infections and signs of nephritic syndrome among family members.

Management

Renal biopsy is not routinely indicated in PSGN but may be required to confirm the diagnosis when it occurs in association with other conditions (e.g., sickle cell anemia), or presents unusual clinical features, such as nephrotic proteinuria, depressed C3 levels lasting for more than a month (suggests lupus or hypocomplementemic MPGN), or increasing azotemia (suggests crescentic GN).

Management of PSGN includes treatment of any persistent streptococcal infection (1.2 million units of benzathine penicillin or 200 000 units oral penicillin every 6 h for 7 to 10 days) and the treatment of the acute nephritic syndrome. The latter includes restriction of fluid and sodium intake and the use of loop diuretics to treat circulatory congestion. Oral nifedipine is usually sufficient to control hypertension but parenteral hydralazine may be required. Nitroprusside is needed in exceptional cases with hypertensive encephalopathy. Pulmonary edema may require the use of oxygen and tourniquets. Dialysis (either hemodialysis or peritoneal dialysis) is required in 25–30% of adults but seldom in children.

Anecdotal reports suggest that patients with superimposed crescentic GN may benefit from pulse methylprednisolone therapy, but a complete recovery may be expected in less than half of the cases.

The clinical manifestations of acute GN last usually less than 2 weeks. The immediate prognosis of PSGN is excellent in children but some series have reported an early mortality of 15–20% in elderly patients because of the higher incidence of cardiovascular complications[6]. While symptomatic GN resolves within a few weeks, mild proteinuria (< 500 mg/day) may persist for several months and microscopic hematuria for up to one year without worsening the long-term prognosis.

The long-term prognosis is worse in adults compared to children, and also for patients with persistent severe proteinuria. The prognosis of subclinical PSGN is excellent. However, other issues are more controversial: in most studies in which the follow-up extends from 10–15 years, the incidence of proteinuria is 4–13%, but the range extends from 1.4 to 46%. The incidence of hypertension ranges from values similar to those in the general population to 42%. Despite these discrepancies, which may reflect population differences and dissimilar characteristics of the studies, some conclusions may be derived from the meta-analysis of the available data. Taken collectively, the studies of long-term follow up of PSGN indicate that progression to ESRD occurs in less than 1% of the cases followed for one to two decades after the acute attack. A significantly worse long-term prognosis has been reported in alcoholic patients with PSGN and in a specific outbreak of PSGN resulting from consumption of cheese contaminated with S. zooepidemicus in which 30% of the adults had impaired renal function in the 2-year follow up (with ESRD in 10%)[9].

Endocarditis-associated glomerulonephritis

Infective endocarditis with 'embolic nonsuppurative GN' was noted more than 90 years ago by Lohlein. In subsequent years the embolic component was questioned and the immune complex etiology was emphasized. In the 1970s and 1980s immune complex GN was observed primarily in patients with rheumatic or congenital heart disease with subacute bacterial endocarditis caused by Streptococcus viridans. With the more rapid recognition and treatment of subacute bacterial endocarditis and the virtual eradication of rheumatic heart disease, the endocarditis causing nephritis is now more frequently acute, the bacteria responsible is usually Staphylococcus aureus, and the infection more commonly is observed in intravenous drug abusers or in subjects with prosthetic heart valves or central venous lines.

One-third of patients with bacterial endocarditis develop azotemia and the risk increases with age, a history of hypertension, thrombocytopenia and prosthetic valve infection[10]. Several renal syndromes may be observed. In a recent survey of 62 of 354 patients with infective endocarditis in whom renal tissue was available for study, biopsy and autopsy material reported GN in 26%, of which many cases were characterized by vasculitis without glomerular immunoglobulin deposition. Other pathologies included localized infarcts in 31%, half of which were septic; and interstitial nephritis, mostly attributable to antibiotics, in 10%. Cortical necrosis was found in 10% of the cases, all of them at necropsy[11].

Pathogenesis and pathology

The pathogenesis of endocarditis associated-GN involves the deposition of immune complexes containing bacterial antigens in glomeruli, a mechanism similar to that proposed for PSGN. Cryoglobulins (of the polyclonal or type III type) are present in 50% of subjects and may be found in glomeruli. Some bacteria (classically methicillin-resistant Staph. aureus) express 'superantigens' that can also activate T cells directly and lead to a polyclonal gammopathy and immune complex GN[12].

The most common glomerular pathology is diffuse proliferative GN. Less commonly, membranous nephropathy and MPGN type I may be found. Widespread deposition of IgM, IgG and C3 and electron dense subendothelial, mesangial and subepithelial deposits (which resemble poststreptococcal 'humps'), are usually evident. In subacute endocarditis, focal segmental proliferative lesions with fibrinoid necrosis or capillary thrombi and mesangial immune deposits may be present. Tubulointerstitial cellular infiltration and variable degrees of atrophy and fibrosis may be seen. Intense eosinophilic infiltration should suggest another diagnosis such as acute interstitial nephritis, secondary to antibiotics[11].

Clinical manifestations and diagnosis

The clinical picture includes fever, arthralgias, anemia, leukocytosis, increased sedimentation rate and purpura. Classic findings in endocarditis, such as Osler's nodes, Janeway lesions and splinter hemorrhages are seldom seen. The renal manifestations usually are microscopic hematuria and mild proteinuria, with or without mild azotemia. A rapidly progressive clinical course may be present when the renal disease is characterized by crescentic GN. Nephrotic syndrome is unusual.

Abnormal serological tests include decreased C3 and C4 levels (consistent with activation of the classical complement pathway), high titers of rheumatoid factor, circulating immune complexes and type III cryoglobulins[13]. These serologic findings are observed in 50% of subjects with subacute bacterial endocarditis and in higher percentages in patients with endocarditis-associated GN, although complement levels may be normal in superantigen-mediated GN[12]. Cytoplasmic ANCA (cANCA) have been reported in rare cases with subacute endocarditis and GN.

The differential diagnosis includes antibiotic-associated interstitial nephritis and embolism. Embolism may originate from the left side of the heart, or from the right if the foramen ovale is patent. Microscopic or large emboli may occlude small or large vessels, the latter observed with fungal or *Haemophilus* endocarditis. Large emboli may produce flank pain; hematuria and pyuria while the microemboli produce local infarcts and microabscesses that give the kidney the classic 'flea-bitten' appearance. Typically urinary cultures are positive, and imaging studies may show focal abscesses or infarcts. Interstitial nephritis is often associated with fever, eosinophilia, and eosinophiluria. Unfortunately, endocarditis-associated GN may also present with fever, and eosinophiluria can complicate crescentic nephritis of any etiology[14]. Hence, biopsy may be required.

Antibiotic treatment for 4–6 weeks usually results in complete eradication of endocarditis with correction of serological abnormalities but microscopic hematuria, proteinuria and elevation of serum creatinine may persist for months after eradication of the infection. Normalization of C3 levels during therapy correlates with a good outcome. In cases with crescentic GN 'pulse' steroid therapy has been used in addition to effective antibiotic therapy but the value of this treatment is undefined and carries the risk of exacerbating the infection. The overall mortality of bacterial endocarditis is 20% and increases to 36% in the patients who develop renal failure[10].

Shunt nephritis

Atrioventricular (AV) shunts may become infected in about 30% of cases. GN may develop in 0.7–2% of the infected AV shunts in an interval of time ranging from 2 months to many years after insertion[15]. The infective organisms are usually *S. epidermidis* and *Staph. aureus* and less frequently *Propionibacterium acne*, diphtheroids, *Pseudomonas* and *Serratia* species. In contrast with AV shunts, ventriculoperitoneal shunts are rarely complicated with GN.

The clinical picture includes insidious low-grade fever, arthralgia, weight loss, anemia, skin rash, hepatosplenomegaly, hypertension and signs of increased intracranial pressure. The renal manifestations are microscopic hematuria and proteinuria, frequently massive and with the full nephrotic syndrome in 25% of the cases. Serologic findings include leukocytosis, elevated sedimentation rate, high rheumatoid factor titers, cryoglobulinemia and depressed serum C3, C4 and CH50 levels[15].

Renal histology is typically MPGN type I but a mesangial proliferative pattern may occasionally be present. There are IgM, IgG and C3 deposits in the glomerular capillary and mesangium. The pathogenesis of these lesions involves the deposition of bacterial immune complexes and activation of both the classic and alternative complement pathways.

Treatment requires antibiotic therapy and the prompt removal of the infected AV shunt; the latter is usually replaced by a ventriculoperitoneal shunt. Delay in diagnosis and in removal of the shunt worsens the prognosis of the renal lesion. In the event that dialysis is required, hemodialysis is the preferred modality since peritonitis is a frequent complication of chronic peritoneal dialysis and this complication carries the risk of meningitis in patients with a ventriculoperitoneal shunt.

Glomerulonephritis associated with other bacterial infections

Osteomyelitis and intra-abdominal, pelvic, pleural and dental abscesses can be associated with GN. A common feature in these conditions is that infection is usually present for several months before it is properly diagnosed and treated. The clinical presentation of renal disease may vary from mild urinary abnormalities to rapidly progressive GN but the most frequent presentation is the nephrotic syndrome. Unlike other infection-associated GN, complement levels are often normal. A polyclonal gammopathy is frequently present, which may relate to the fact that many of the organisms (especially methicillin-resistant *Staph. aureus*) contain superantigens[12]. Renal histology reveals MPGN, diffuse proliferative or mesangial proliferative GN (Fig. 28.3). Crescents may be present. Treatment is directed to eradicate the existing infection. Complete recovery of renal function may be expected only if treatment is started early.

Congenital and secondary (or early latent) syphilis may be associated with GN[16]. In congenital syphilis, patients present with anasarca 4–12 weeks after birth. Nephrotic syndrome may occur in 8% of the patients and it may be the primary clinical manifestation (as opposed to the more classic triad of rhinitis, osteochondritis and rash). In acquired syphilis, renal involvement occurs in 0.3% of all patients and adults may also present with the nephrotic syndrome or occasionally with an acute nephritic picture with red cell casts, hypertension and azotemia. Serologic tests for syphilis are positive (RPR, VDRL, and FTA antibodies). Membranous nephropathy is the most common form of renal pathology in children and adults. However, other histological patterns can be observed, particularly in adults, including diffuse proliferative GN, with or without crescents, MPGN and mesangial proliferative GN. *Treponema* antigens have been identified in the immune deposits. The glomerular disease generally responds to the treatment of syphilis, although complete remission may not occur for 4–18 months.

Acute typhoid fever (*Salmonella typhi* infection) is characterized by fever, splenomegaly and gastrointestinal symptoms[17]. Severe cases may develop shock and acute renal failure as a part of disseminated intravascular coagulation or hemolytic–uremic syndrome but these complications are rare. Overt manifestations of GN occur in 2% of the cases but microscopic hematuria and mild proteinuria may be present in 25% of the cases (Fig. 28.4). Diagnosis requires the culture of the organisms from blood or stools or rising antibody titers in the Widal test. A specific type of GN resulting from salmonella infection is that occurring in patients with schistosomiasis and coexisting salmonella infection of the urinary tract (see later).

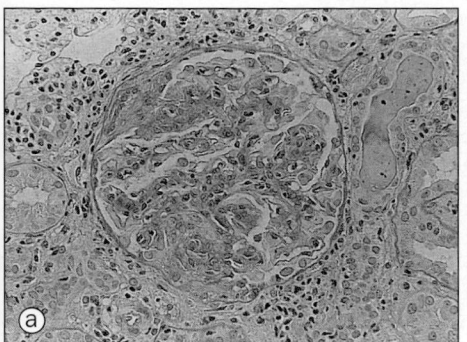
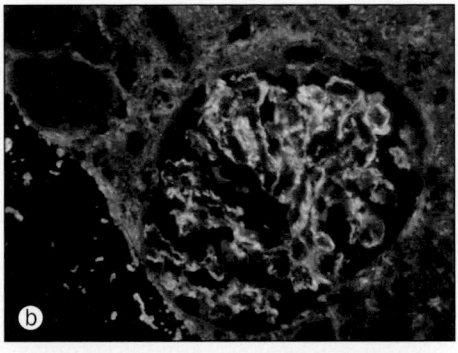

Figure 28.3 Glomerulonephritis associated with infection from methicillin-resistant *Staphylococcus aureus*.
(a) A membranoproliferative glomerulonephritis with early crescent formation is seen by light microscopy. (b) Immunofluorescence demonstrates IgG in a capillary wall and a mesangial pattern. (Courtesy of M Kobayashi, Ibaraki, Japan.)

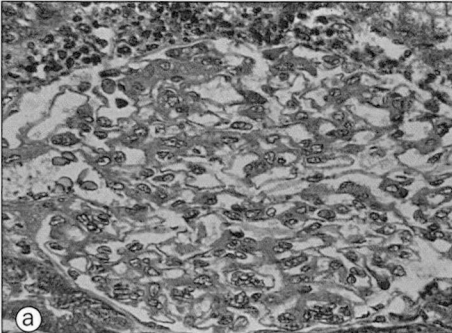
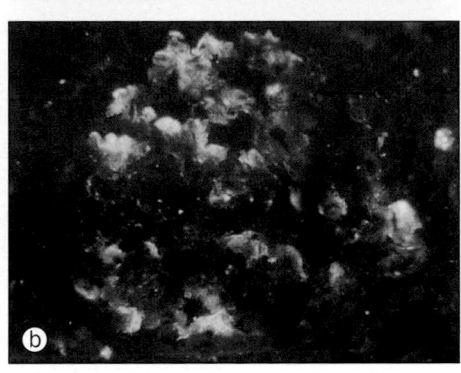

Figure 28.4 Glomerulonephritis in typhoid fever. (a) A mesangial proliferative nephritis. (b) Granular deposition of *Salmonella typhi* Vi antigens in the capillary wall. (Courtesy of V. Boonpucknavig, Bangkok, Thailand.)

Leprosy (*Mycobacterium leprae* infection) may be associated with GN, with interstitial nephritis, or with amyloidosis[18]. GN is manifested clinically in less than 2% of the patients but may be present in 13–70% of renal biopsies. It remains controversial whether GN is more common in lepromatous leprae than in tuberculoid leprae. Urinary abnormalities consistent with GN often accompany the episodes of erythema nodosum leprosum. The clinical manifestations are usually nephrotic syndrome, less frequently acute nephritic syndrome and, more rarely, rapidly progressive GN. The most commonly observed lesions are MPGN and diffuse proliferative GN. Immunofluorescence demonstrates IgG, C3, IgM, IgA and fibrin deposits. Response of glomerular disease to treatment of leprosy is variable. Prednisolone (40–50 mg/day) has been used in short courses to treat erythema nodosum leprosum associated with acute renal failure. AA amyloidosis was very frequent in the early investigations, but is reported in approximately 2% of the cases of leprosy in recent studies and is much more common in lepromatous leprosy than in tuberculoid leprosy. Other renal abnormalities associated with leprosy include interstitial nephritis and tubular functional defects without histological lesions.

Acute pneumonia due to *Strep. pneumoniae* infection may be associated with microhematuria and proteinuria. Most of the cases reported correspond to the preantibiotic era when effective treatment was unavailable. GN in pneumococcal infection is immune complex-mediated, with mesangial proliferative or diffuse proliferative histology, and with immunofluorescent and electron dense deposits similar to that observed with poststreptococcal GN. Pneumococcal antigen (particularly type 14) has been demonstrated in the immune deposits and the bacterial capsular antigen is capable of activating the alternative complement pathway. Rarely, pneumococcal pneumonia can also be associated with hemolyticuremic syndrome due to unmasking of the Thomsen–Friedenreich antigen in glomeruli by pneumococcal neuraminidase which then elicits an immune response[19].

Gastroenteritis due to *Campylobacter jejuni* may be associated with mesangial proliferative or diffuse proliferative GN. There are also reports of GN with other bacterial infections including those due to *E. coli*, *Yersinia*, *Meningococcus* and *Mycoplasma pneumoniae*.

VIRAL INFECTIONS

Hepatitis-associated glomerulonephritis

GN has been reported in association with infection with hepatitis A virus (HAV), hepatitis B virus (HBV) and hepatitis C virus (HCV). Patients with HAV infection may rarely present with the nephrotic syndrome resulting from immune complex mesangial proliferative GN[20] or with severe acute renal failure. The renal outcome of these patients is good. In view of their considerable epidemiological importance, HBV- and HCV-associated GN will be discussed in detail.

Hepatitis B virus-associated renal disease

Acute HBV infection may be associated with a short-lived serum sickness-like syndrome: urticaria or maculopapular rash, neuropathy, arthralgia or arthritis, microscopic hematuria and non-nephrotic proteinuria[21]. Renal biopsy, if performed, shows a mesangial proliferative GN and the clinical picture resolves spontaneously as the hepatitis improves. Acute HBV infection may resolve uneventfully, but in 10% of adults and in the majority of children, HBV is not eradicated and the patients become chronic carriers (defined as persistence of HBsAg positive serology 6 months after onset). The prevalence of the carrier state is high in Asia and Africa where HBV is passed at birth (vertical transmission) or shortly

Association of hepatitis B infection with membranous nephropathy			
Presence of hepatitis B virus antigen (HBsAg)	North America Western Europe Australia	Eastern Europe, South America	Asia, Africa
General carrier rate (%)	0.1–1	1–5	>5
Frequency in membranous nephropathy (%)			
Children	20–64	80	80–100
Adults	<5	15–20	30–45
(Adapted from Johnson and Couser[21].)			

Table 28.3 Association of hepatitis B infection with membranous nephropathy.

thereafter (horizontal transmission). In Europe and the United States the prevalence is lower and most carriers acquire the infection as adults as a consequence of drug abuse, blood transfusions, or sexual relations.

HBV carriers present the most important renal syndromes associated with HBV infection: membranous nephropathy (MN), polyarteritis nodosa (PAN) and MPGN[21].

Membranous nephropathy

The association between MN and the carrier state of HBsAg is well established, particularly in children, in whom this presentation is the most common (Table 28.3). Typically, the patient is 2–12 years of age, almost always male, with nephrotic syndrome, microscopic hematuria and normal renal function. History and clinical evidence of hepatitis is often missing and hepatic enzymes may be normal but HBsAg and anti-HBc antibodies are present. HBeAg has been found in 80% of the cases and liver biopsy reveals chronic persistent hepatitis. The clinical course in children is usually favorable, resolving spontaneously, frequently in association with the appearance of anti-HBe antibodies in circulation. In contrast, resolution is uncommon in adults, who have more severe pathologic changes in the liver (chronic active hepatitis or cirrhosis) and often progress to chronic renal disease[22].

Circulating immune complexes are present in the majority of patients and C3 and C4 levels are depressed in 20–50%. Renal pathology demonstrates membranous nephropathy with granular deposits of IgG, IgM and C3 in the capillary wall. Electron microscopy shows subepithelial as well as mesangial and subendothelial immune deposits, in contrast with idiopathic MN in which the mesangial and subendothelial locations are frequently absent. Viral-like particles have been identified in various areas of the glomeruli.

The pathogenesis of the HBV-related MN is thought to be due to passive trapping of immune complexes or to the formation of *in situ* immune complexes involving HBeAg and anti-HBe antibody. Since anti-HBe antibodies are cationic, charge-driven penetration into the basement membrane would favor the otherwise inaccessible subepithelial location.

Membranoproliferative glomerulonephritis

MPGN is the most common glomerular lesion in adult patients with HBV infection. HBsAg and anti-HBc antibodies are universally present. At the time of presentation, patients often have no history of liver disease but they have abnormal transaminases. However, liver biopsies, if performed, often show chronic active or chronic persistent hepatitis and occasionally cirrhosis. Hypertension is present in 54% of the cases and renal failure in 20%. Microscopic hematuria is frequently present[21].

The pathogenesis of HBV-MPGN involves mesangial and subendothelial deposition of immune complexes. Unlike HBV-MN in which the immune complex deposition appears to be due to HBeAg and anti-HBe antibodies, in HBV-MPGN the immune complexes are of the larger HBsAg and anti-HBs antibodies and are localized in the mesangial and subendothelial space. Renal histology is similar to MPGN type I with prominent subendothelial deposits and mild proliferation. Occasionally, histology resembles type III cryoglobulinemia, with coexisting subepithelial and mesangial deposits.

Treatment of HBV-associated glomerulonephritis

Treatment is recommended for both HBV-MN and HBV-MPGN in adults. In general, the response rate is greater for HBV-MN than HBV-MPGN, as in the former clinical remission generally occurs with clearance of HBeAg and the appearance of anti-HBe antibodies, whereas in the latter, remission correlates with actual cure of the viral infection (disappearance of HBsAg and development of anti-HBs antibodies). Interferond (IFN-α) (5 million units daily for 6 months) resulted in seroconversion in 8 of 15 patients (from HBeAg to anti-HBe) with clinical remission of their nephrotic syndrome; however, all responding patients had HBV-MN[23]. Recently, lamivudine (100 mg orally once daily for 52 weeks) has been used as initial treatment of chronic hepatitis B and has been reported to induce disappearance of HBeAg and HBV DNA levels and improve the hepatic disease[24]; since it is well tolerated it may be useful in the treatment for the GN. Steroid treatment is contraindicated because it is ineffective and may delay or prevent seroconversion and accelerate the progression of liver disease.

The prevailing view has been that treatment is not required for children with HBV-MN. The reasons for this opinion was that the majority of children are likely to undergo spontaneous remission and that steroids do not offer additional benefit. However, the only controlled trial of children with MN reported that sustained resolution of proteinuria was significantly more frequent in treated children than in controls[25]; in addition, there have been reports that HBV-MN, even in children, can occasionally progress to ESRD. Therefore a definite recommendation is difficult to make at the present time and it seems reasonable to evaluate individual cases and prescribe treatment when proteinuria is severe or there is evidence of progression of renal disease.

Polyarteritis nodosa (PAN)

HBV-related vasculitis (HBV-PAN) is observed primarily in adult males who acquire HBV infection from drug use or transfusion, and is usually observed during the convalescent phase of a mild attack of hepatitis. It is almost never observed in children and is rare in areas of the world where HBV infection is acquired in birth or childhood, such as in Asia[26].

The typical patient with HBV-PAN presents with signs of serum sickness preceding and during a mild or asymptomatic attack of hepatitis. Unlike HBV-associated serum sickness, which resolves spontaneously with clearing of the HBsAg, in these patients the disease progresses to involve numerous organs. Arteritis of small and medium size arteries may be manifested by symptoms of myocardial ischemia, mesenteric angina, Churg–Strauss pulmonary syndrome with asthma and eosinophilia, cerebral ischemia or mononeuritis multiplex. Renal vasculitis is manifested by microhematuria, nephrotic or non-nephrotic proteinuria, renin-dependent hypertension and renal failure.

The pathogenesis of HBV-associated PAN is thought to be the deposition of HBsAg-antiHBs immune complexes in the arterial wall that results in a subsequent inflammatory reaction with the activation of complement[21]. The vessels often show a predominance of IgM and HBsAg, suggesting that the injury is mediated by HBsAg/IgM complexes. Serologic tests reveal HBsAg and anti-HBc antibodies. Serum complement is frequently normal and occasionally reduced and ANCA are negative.

Diagnosis requires circulating HBsAg in association with either biopsy or angiographic evidence of vasculitis. Biopsy of the kidney, skeletal muscle, peripheral nerve and even testicle have been used to demonstrate vascular lesions, which are typically panmural and showing different stages of development. Variable degrees of fibrinoid necrosis, fibrin deposition and leukocyte infiltration are present in individual lesions. HBsAg, IgM and occasionally IgG are deposited in the vessel wall. Angiographic studies demonstrating narrow segments and saccular or fusiform aneurysms in celiac or renal arteries have higher diagnostic yield than biopsies.

Liver biopsy demonstrates chronic active or persisting hepatitis or, rarely, acute hepatitis. The renal biopsy, in addition to the arteriolar lesions, may show relatively preserved glomeruli with variable degrees of collapse in the glomerular tuft likely resulting from ischemic changes. In contrast with idiopathic microscopic polyangiitis, necrotizing lesions with crescent formation are rare. Mesangial proliferative, diffuse proliferative, MPGN or membranous nephropathy have all been reported.

The treatment of HBV-PAN historically involves both steroids (typically 'pulse steroids') and cytotoxic agents (classically cyclophosphamide) and this is associated with a marked increase in short-term survival; however, long-term studies demonstrated accelerated progression of liver disease in these patients. Recent studies suggest that excellent long-term results may be obtained with a short course of steroids (prednisone 1 mg/kg/day for 2 weeks) and plasma exchange (9–12 exchanges over 3 weeks) followed by IFNα therapy and/or lamivudine[26,27].

Hepatitis C virus-associated renal disease
Cryoglobulinemic MPGN and MPGN type I secondary to HCV infection

A full description of HCV-associated MPGN is provided in Chapter 23. Briefly, the disease is observed in adults with longstanding HCV infection (> 10 years) and is primarily seen in southern Europe, the United States, and Japan. Approximately 50% of patients present with systemic symptoms of cryoglobulinemia (especially the triad of purpura, weakness, and arthralgias) and 50% present with strictly renal manifestations (typically nephrotic or non-nephrotic proteinuria, microhematuria and mild renal dysfunction). Occasional patients manifest signs of a severe vasculitis, including rapidly progressive GN (RPGN). HCV RNA and anti-HCV antibodies are positive, liver function tests are frequently mildly abnormal (75%) and complement levels (C3, C4) are low. Renal histology shows MPGN, occasionally with cryoglobulins. Chronic disease is usually treated with interferon-α (3 to 5 mU three times weekly for 12 to 18 months)[28] or Pegylated interferon-α-2b (1 μg/kg weekly for 48 weeks)[29]. Ribavirin (0.6–1.0 g/day orally for 6 months) is often added if the GFR is normal. A clinical response is observed during treatment in 60–70% of cases, but relapse is common. If there are signs of severe vasculitis or rapid progression, antiviral agents are often held and the renal disease is treated with 'pulse' methylprednisolone with or without cyclophosphamide and plasma exchange. Interferon-α is generally not administered until the prednisone dose is reduced to 20 mg/day or less and the patient is off cytotoxic therapy, as there is data that efficacy may be retarded when cytotoxic therapy is used or prednisone doses are high (> 20 mg/day).

Other HCV-associated glomerulonephritis

HCV infection may be associated with other glomerular diseases with or without cryoglobulinemia. Patients with membranous nephropathy (HCV-MN) have been described in which HCV antigens have been identified in the subepithelial immune deposits. The association has been reported in Spain, Japan and the United States, especially in renal transplant patients. The clinical and histologic findings are similar to that observed in idiopathic MN except that HCV RNA and anti-HCV antibodies are positive. Treatment of the nontransplant patient is with IFN-α; in the transplant patient symptomatic management is preferred due to the risk for rejection with interferon therapy. Other reported associations include fibrillary GN, focal glomerulosclerosis (especially in African Americans), and thrombotic microangiopathy with anticardiolipin antibodies (especially following renal transplantation).

Human immunodeficiency virus-associated renal disease

HIV infection is associated with a number of renal syndromes, including HIV nephropathy, HIV-associated immune complex GN, thrombotic microangiopathies (hemolytic–uremic syndrome and thrombotic thrombocytopenic purpura), HIV-associated vasculitis, and electrolyte disorders. A variety of drugs used in the management of HIV infection can also cause renal dysfunction (e.g., pentamidine and sulfonamides) or nephrolithiasis (e.g., indanavir). HIV nephropathy is discussed in detail in Chapter 21 and the nephrotoxicity of HIV related drugs is presented in Chapter 15.

HIV-associated nephropathy is observed primarily (> 90%) in subjects of African descent, primarily male, and usually with a CD4 count of < 200/mm³. Clinically, patients present with severe nephrotic syndrome with rapid progression to renal failure over 2–6 months. Renal biopsy is that of focal segmental glomerulosclerosis with visceral epithelial cell prominence, shrunken glomerular tufts, and an enlarged Bowman's space ('collapsing glomerulopathy'). Tubules are focally enlarged resulting in a 'microcystic' appearance, and interstitial infiltration and fibrosis are prominent.

Glomerular Disease

Several trials have now provided strong evidence that ACE inhibitors can slow progression in HIV nephropathy. Additionally, there are case reports showing remission of nephrotic syndrome with antiretroviral therapy[30]. Remission of nephrotic syndrome has also been reported in some cases with prednisone or cyclosporine, but the long-term prognosis may not be improved.

HIV-associated immune complex GN is manifested by MPGN, mesangioproliferative GN, membranous nephropathy and IgA nephropathy. It is more frequently encountered in patients from Caucasian origin and it is caused by immune complexes composed of HIV gp120 or p24 and reactive antibodies. IgA nephropathy may result from the glomerular deposition of circulating idiotypic IgA directed against HIV-immunoglobulin complexes. The coexistence with co-morbid conditions such as hepatitis explains many of the cases in which cryoglobulinemia is present.

Other

Cytomegalovirus (CMV) was originally thought to be a cause for both IgA nephropathy and for 'transplant glomerulopathy', but subsequent studies demonstrated that this was not the case. However, there have been several rare reports in both adults and neonates of an immune complex GN with diffuse proliferative changes and granular immune deposits containing CMV antigens. CMV infection can also involve the kidneys in renal transplant patients, and is generally manifested by tubular cells and macrophages in the interstitium with characteristic intracytoplasmic, 'owl-like' inclusions; while there is some evidence this may be a cause of tubular dysfunction, there is no evidence that this results in glomerular injury.

Parvovirus B19 infection is a cause of aplastic crisis in patients with sickle cell disease and has been implicated in rare cases of nephrotic syndrome that sometimes develop 3 days to 7 weeks after the aplastic crises[31]. Histology during the acute phase shows diffuse proliferative or MPGN, and later as a collapsing focal segmental glomerulosclerosis, with similarities to heroin nephropathy and HIV-nephropathy. A few cases of GN have been associated with acute parvovirus B19 infection in adults who do not have sickle cell disease; clinically helpful signs include the presence of a transient rash, arthralgias or arthritis, and anemia. There is also serologic evidence for increased antibodies to parvovirus B19 in collapsing glomerulosclerosis[32] and its DNA has been demonstrated in kidney tissue of focal segmental glomerulosclerosis[33].

Other viruses, particularly causing upper respiratory infections, may result in transient proteinuria and a mesangial proliferative histology[34]. This has suggested the mild proteinuria often present with acute febrile illnesses may not always represent alterations in glomerular permeability due to changes in intrarenal hemodynamics from fever, but rather due to undiagnosed, transient and mild GN. Mumps, for example, can be associated with transient microscopic hematuria and non-nephrotic proteinuria with normal renal function in up to 25% of the patients. Biopsy reveals mesangial proliferative GN with IgM, IgA and C3 deposits and mumps antigens in mesangium. Measles may infrequently be associated with endocapillary proliferative GN and viral antigen was identified in the glomeruli. Anecdotal reports suggest that measles infection may result in remission of the nephrotic syndrome in minimal change disease. Varicella infection can rarely be associated with nephrotic syndrome and similar biopsy changes as those described with mumps. Varicella antigens have been demonstrated in the capillary walls and mesangium. Adenovirus and influenza A and B infections may also be associated with transient microhematuria, proteinuria and complement depression in 3% of the cases. Biopsy findings include MPGN with immune deposits, predominantly C3 and to a lesser degree, IgM and IgG. Upper respiratory infections with Coxsackie virus B-5 and A-4 strains are sometimes associated with microhematuria and mild proteinuria and diffuse proliferative GN. Dengue hemorrhagic fever may be caused by four serotypes of the family Flaviviridae. The clinical manifestations, reflecting increased vascular permeability include muscular pains, gastrointestinal symptoms, and in severe cases, bleeding manifestations and shock. Acute renal failure may accompany the severe cases and in some less severely ill patients acute endocapillary GN with mesangial proliferation may develop and may be manifested by microhematuria and proteinuria. Intense granular deposits of IgG, IgM and C3 in mesangial areas, and to a lesser degree in capillary walls, are usually present.

Mild renal abnormalities can also be observed with acute Epstein–Barr virus (EBV) infection, with microhematuria and proteinuria in 10–15% of cases. Acute interstitial nephritis is probably the most common renal complication but diffuse proliferative and MPGN may also occur. Replicating EBV virus was localized not only to infiltrating macrophages, but also to proximal tubular cells that were shown to express the CD21 receptor for EBV. It was posited that EBV might be a major cause of chronic interstitial nephritis[35].

PARASITIC INFECTIONS

Malaria-associated renal disease

Malaria is a major world health problem, with 300 to 500 million cases and 1.5–2.7 million deaths each year (Fig. 28.5). About 90% of the cases occur in tropical African countries[8,36]. Fluid and electrolyte disturbances and acute renal failure are common, especially with *P. falciparum*. Here we discuss the acute transient and chronic progressive GN that may result from malaria.

Infected red cells show increased fragility, enhanced hemolysis, and increased endothelial adhesion due to the presence of knob-like protrusions; these altered cell membrane proteins may predispose to autoantibody formation. Antigen-monocyte interactions occur with increased expression of intracellular adhesion molecule-1 and CD14, interaction with T helper 1 (Th1) and Th2 cytokines and secretion of TNF-α. Infected red cells express surface antigens (Pf155/RESA) that favor Th2 lymphocyte responses. *P. falciparum* also activates the alternative pathway of complement and the intrinsic coagulation cascade[36].

Acute transient GN may occur in *P. ovale* and *P. vivax* infections and in *P. falciparum* infections. In the latter, acute nephritic and nephrotic syndromes are occasionally seen. Mesangial proliferation, finely granular deposition of IgM and C3 and electron-dense deposits are present (Fig. 28.6). Patients

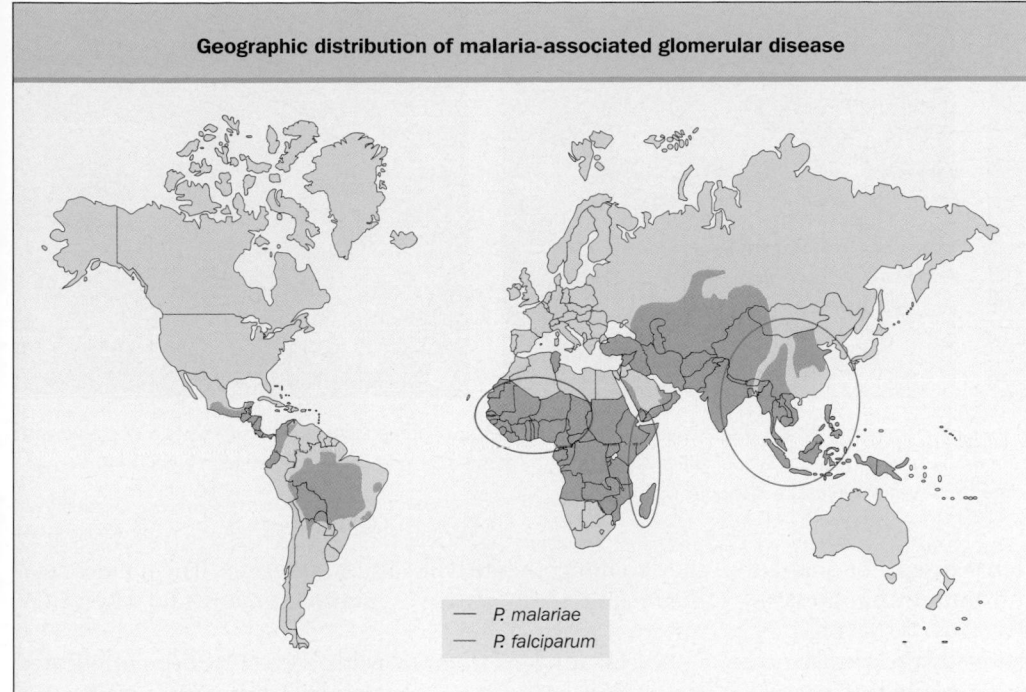

Figure 28.5 Geographic distribution of malaria-associated glomerular disease. Although malaria is endogenous to many areas of the world (shaded orange), the major areas where malaria-associated glomerular disease has been reported (ringed) and their respective species are shown.

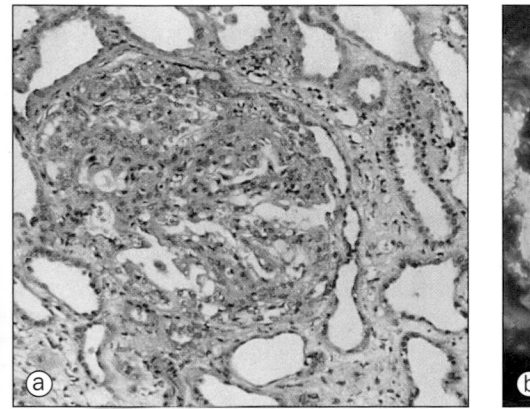
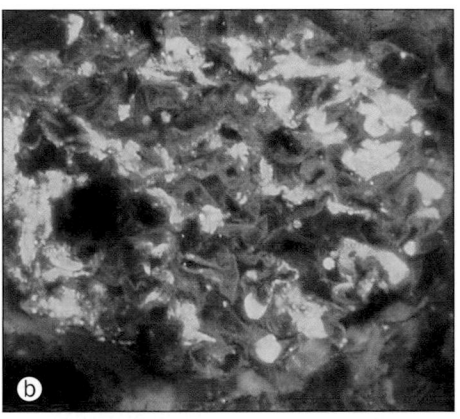
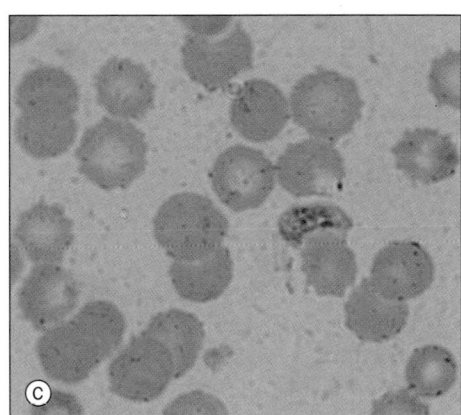

Figure 28.6 Glomerulonephritis associated with *Plasmodium falciparum* malaria. (a) Light microscopy shows a mesangial proliferative GN. (b) Immunofluorescence may reveal *P. falciparum* antigens in a mesangial pattern. (c) Peripheral blood smear confirms acute *P. falciparum* infection, with banana-shaped gametocytes and multiple ring forms in erythrocytes. ((a) reprinted with permission from Barsoum[37]; (b) and (c) courtesy of V Boonpucknavig.)

present with microscopic hematuria, mild proteinuria and often hypocomplementemia (low C3 and C4 levels) and circulating immune complexes.

Chronic GN is characteristic of *P. malariae* infections and is observed primarily in West Africa and Nigeria. The clinical syndrome is nonspecific, apart from the clinical features of quartan malaria. The patients are usually children, (peak age 6–8 years) or young adults, with heavy proteinuria and overt nephrotic syndrome. Serum complement is normal, cholesterol is normal because of the associated nutritional deficiency and hypertension is a late finding. Mesangial proliferation, doubled contoured glomerular capillaries with coarsely granular IgG, IgM and C3 deposits and subendothelial electron dense material and intramembranus lacunae (due to reabsorption of immune complexes) are typical biopsy characteristics of

quartan malaria nephropathy (Fig. 28.7). Crescent formation is rare. The reason why this chronic nephropathy is observed with *P. malariae* and not with *P. falciparum* may relate to the mechanism of infection. *P. falciparum* may infect all red blood cells (RBCs), so the symptoms are often severe and the patient is more likely to seek medical attention early. In contrast, *P. malariae* only infects senescent RBCs and the clinical manifestations are often more subdued and infection more indolent. *P. malariae* infection also results in a Th2 response as opposed to *P. falciparum* infection, which is mediated primarily by a Th1 response. Because parasitemia is more prolonged the host may have more time to stimulate humoral and cell-mediated responses and patients also have liver congestion and splenomegaly ('tropical splenomegaly'). Despite successful treatment of the malaria, chronic renal failure develops in

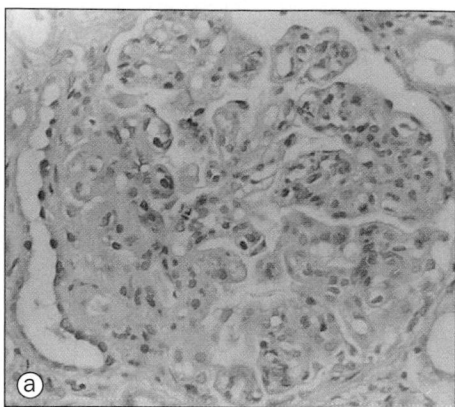 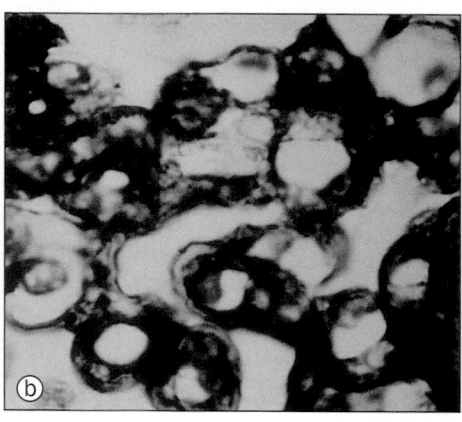 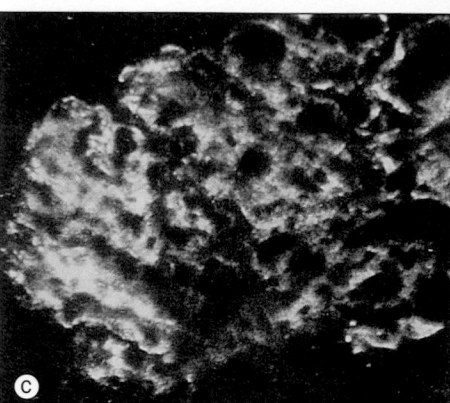

Figure 28.7 Quartan malarial nephropathy. (a) Light microscopy shows a sclerosing membranoproliferative glomerulonephritis. (b) This is associated with a double contour of the basement membrane shown by silver stain. (c) Malarial antigens detected by glomerular immunofluorescence in a child with quartan malarial nephropathy. ((a) and (b) reprinted with permission from Barsoum[37].)

3–5 years. The progressive course of renal disease of quartan malaria is unmodified by steroids and immunosuppressive agents. The progression to chronicity may be favored by genetic factors, yet undefined, and possibly by the coexistence of malnutrition, EBV infection and autoimmune reactivity.

Renal disease associated with schistosomiasis

Schistosomiasis results primarily from three species, *Schistosoma mansoni* present in Africa, Saudi Arabia, Brazil, Venezuela and West Indies, *S. japonicum* present primarily in Asia, and *S. haematobium* present in Africa, Arabia and a small focus in India. *S. haematobium* primarily involves the lower urinary tract, whereas *S. mansoni* and *S. japonicum* are associated primarily with hepatosplenic schistosomiasis.

S. haematobium infestation infects the lower urinary tract and is a cause of bladder granulomata, chronic cystitis and bladder stones, uroepithelial tumors, and bladder neck obstruction. Glomerular disease, if it results, is usually due to reflux nephropathy, although rare cases of immune complex GN have been reported. *S. haematobium* infection may be responsible for up to 20% of the patients on chronic dialysis in Egypt. It is discussed in more detail in Chapter 56.

Most glomerular disease from schistosomiasis occurs in patients with chronic hepatosplenic *S. mansoni* infection[38]. As the host slowly eliminates the antigen the response results in a granulomatous reaction in which the cytokine production, and particularly TGF-α, play a pre-eminent role. The prevalence of occult or subclinical glomerular pathology has ranged from 12 to 40% in autopsies of patients with hepatosplenic *S. mansoni* infections. Clinical evidence of glomerular disease is less frequent, occurring in approximately 15%. When it occurs, overt glomerulopathy invariably progresses to ESRD unless the patient dies of other complications of hepatic fibrosis and portal hypertension.

Most patients are 20–40 years old and present with proteinuria, with or without the nephrotic syndrome, microhematuria and a firm enlarged liver and spleen. Liver function tests, including transaminases are often normal. Polyclonal gammopathy is seen in most cases. Rheumatoid factor activity and anti-DNA antibodies are detected in 5–10% of the cases, particularly when associated with salmonella infection, but

they do not correlate with clinical severity[41]. The incidence of rheumatoid seropositivity is multiplied many fold when HCV infection is associated.

Several antigens from the worm's gut have been implicated in the pathogenesis of the glomerular disease[37]. Of these a glycoprotein (cathodal antigen) and a proteoglycan (anodal antigen) have been detected as free antigens as well as in immune complexes in the circulation. These antigens have also been localized in immune deposits in mesangial, and less commonly in subendothelial and intramembranous locations. The presence of liver fibrosis is likely critical as it results in impaired hepatic clearance of schistosomal antigens and immune complexes. Evidence of autoimmune reactivity (positive rheumatoid factor titers, false positive VDRL) has also been reported in some of these patients but what role, if any, autoimmunity plays in the progression to chronicity is yet undefined.

Glomerular lesions have been classified into five categories by the African Association of Nephrology, as shown in Table 28.4. It is assumed that class I (mesangial proliferative), III (membranoproliferative) (Fig. 28.8) and IV (focal segmental glomerulosclerosis) result from the deposition of immune complexes and represent different stages of the disease and correlate with clinical manifestations. Class III glomerulopathy is present in 15–20% of the patients with schistosomal hepatic fibrosis. IgA is detected in the glomerular deposits in parallel with the severity of proteinuria and mesangial proliferation. Impaired hepatic clearance as well as increased mucosal synthesis of IgA have been documented in those patients[38].

Class II (diffuse proliferative/exudative) is thought to be due to co-infection with salmonella strains, usually *S. paratyphi* (Africa) and *S. typhimurium* (Brazil). The mechanism of this association is likely related to the presence of salmonella receptors in the tissues of adult schistosomes. C3 and salmonella antigens have been found in the capillary walls and the mesangium. In these patients the clinical presentation is frequently suggestive of acute poststreptococcal GN since they present with acute nephritic syndrome. Manifestations of salmonella-related toxemia (fever, exanthema) and the absence of hypertension should arouse the suspicion of salmonella infection.

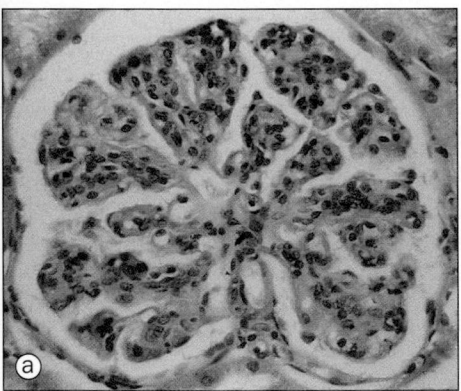
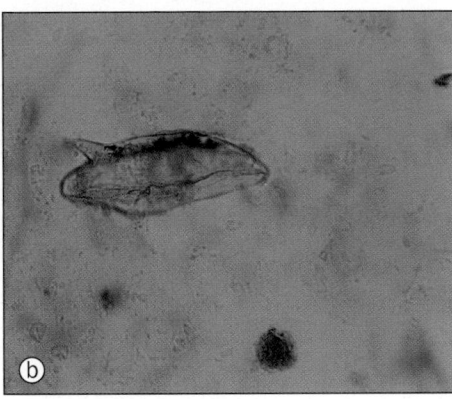

Figure 28.8 Schistosomiasis.
(a) Membranoproliferative glomerulonephritis in a patient with hepatosplenic schistosomiasis. (Courtesy of L de Moura, São Pablo, Brazil.) (b) *Schistosoma mansoni* eggs identified in a fecal specimen.

Table 28.4 Classification of schistosomal glomerulonephritis.

	Classification of schistosomal glomerulonephritis			
Class	Pathology	Immunofluorescence	Associations	Response to antischistosomal therapy
I	Mesangial proliferative	IgM, C3, IgA (late)		?
II	Diffuse proliferative	C3	*Salmonella typhi* coinfection	Responds to treatment of *Salmonella typhi* infection
III	Membranoproliferative	IgG, C3, IgA (late)		No
IV	Focal and segmental	IgM, IgG (occasionally IgA)		No
V	Amyloid			No
(Adapted from Barsoum[38].)				

Diagnosis is confirmed by identifying *S. mansoni* eggs in the stools of a patient with renal biopsy findings consistent with the diagnosis of schistosomal glomerulopathy. Concomitant HCV infection may modify the clinical syndrome in several ways. Impairment of hepatocellular function is more prominent, with significant elevation of transaminases, which is unusual in 'pure' hepatosplenic schistosomiasis. Rheumatoid factor activity is profoundly increased in the majority of the cases; cryoglobulins may be present and serum C4 levels are persistently depressed. Mesangial matrix expansion and interposition are more pronounced; cryoglobulinemic hyaline thrombi may be seen in the glomerular capillaries, and evidence of intrarenal vasculitis may be seen.

Other glomerular disorders associated with hepatic fibrosis, such as secondary IgA nephropathy and hepatic glomerulosclerosis, may be considered in the differential diagnosis. However, in both these conditions the renal lesions are relatively mild, presenting mainly with microhematuria but rarely with significant proteinuria or impaired renal function. The glomerular deposits are mostly mesangial, in contrast with those seen in schistosomiasis where subendothelial and intramembranous deposits may also be present.

Antischistosomal therapy (praziquantel or oxamniquine) and immunosuppressive therapy are ineffective for the renal lesion. Treatment of schistosomiasis does not improve the established renal disease[39]; however, treatment of coexisting salmonella infection often results in the improvement of class II glomerulopathy.

Other parasitic infestations

Renal involvement has been reported in filarial infections. *Onchocerca volvulus* infection ('river blindness') is associated usually with MPGN, Loa Loa infections induce membranous nephropathy or proliferative glomerulonephritides, and *Wuchereria bancrofti* and *Brugia malayi* may induce mesangial, mesangiocapillary or diffuse proliferative GN. Microfilariae have been found in the glomerular capillaries. Except in the case of onchocercosis, filarial antigens have not been demonstrated in glomeruli. Antifilarial treatment does not improve the nephrotic syndrome and treatment with the antifilarial drug diethylcarbamazine may exacerbate proteinuria. Visceral leishmaniasis ('kala-azar') frequently presents with microhematuria and interstitial nephritis or diffuse proliferative or membranous nephropathy. The pathogenesis of interstitial nephritis is uncertain. Trichinosis may occasionally present with MPGN, manifested clinically with microhematuria and non-nephrotic proteinuria. Immune deposits are present in mesangium and capillary walls but specific antigens have not been demonstrated in the glomeruli. GN has also been rarely reported with trypanosomiasis and with congenital toxoplasmosis.

REFERENCES.

1. Balter S, Benin A, Pinto SW, et al. Epidemic nephritis in Nova Serrana, Brazil. Lancet. 2000;355:1776–80.
2. Yoshizawa N. Acute glomerulonephritis. Intern Med. 2000;39: 687–94.
3. Soto HM, Parra G, Rodríguez-Iturbe B. Circulating levels of cytokines in poststreptococcal glomerulonephritis. Clin Nephrol. 1997; 47:6–12.
4. Oshawa I, Ohi H, Endo M, et al. Evidence of lectin complement pathway activation in postreptococcal glomerulonephritis. Kidney Int. 1999;56:1158–60.
5. Sorger K. Postinfectious glomerulonephritis. Subtypes, clinico-pathological correlations and follow-up studies. Veröff Pathol. 1986;125:1–105.
6. Melby PC, Musik WD, Luger AM, et al. Poststreptococcal glomerulonephritis in the elderly: report of a case and review of the literature. Am J Nephrol. 1987;7:235–40.
7. Parra G, Rodríguez-Iturbe B, Batsford S, et al. Antibody to strepto-coccal zymogen in the serum of patients with acute glomerulo-nephritis. Kidney Int. 1998;54:509–17.
8. Rodríguez-Iturbe B, Rubio L, García R. Attack rate of poststrepto-coccal nephritis in families. A prospective study. Lancet. 1981;1: 401–3.
9. Pinto SWL, Sesso R, Vasconcelos E, et al. Follow-up of patients with epidemic poststreptococcal glomerulonephritis. Am J Kidney Dis. 2001;38:249–55.
10. Conlon PJ, Jefferies F, Krigman HR, et al. Predictors of prognosis and risk of acute renal failure in bacterial endocarditis. Clin Nephrol. 1998;49:96–101.
11. Majumdar A, Chowdhary S, Ferreira MAS, et al. Renal patholog-ical findings in infective endocarditis. Nephrol Dial Transplant. 2000;15:1782–7.
12. Yoh K, Kobayashi M, Yamaguchi N, et al. Cytokines and T-cell responses in superantigen-related glomerulonephritis following methicillin-resistant Staphylococcus aureus infection. Nephrol Dial Transplant. 2000;15:1170–4.
13. Agarwal A, Clemens J, Sedmark DD, et al. Subacute bacterial endocarditis masquerading as type III essential mixed cryoglobu-linemia. J Am Soc Nephrol. 1997;8:1971–6.
14. Nolan C, Anger MS, Keller SP. Eosinophiluria – a new method of detection and definition of the clinical spectrum. N Engl J Med. 1986;315:1516–19.
15. Haffner D, Schinderas F, Aschoff A. The clinical spectrum of shunt nephritis. Nephrol Dial Transplant. 1997;12:1143–8.
16. Hunte W, Ghraoui F, Cohen RJ. Secondary syphilis and nephrotic syndrome. J Am Soc Nephrol. 1993;3:1351–5.
17. Chugh KS, Sakhuja V. Glomerular disease in the tropics. Am J Nephrol. 1990;10:437–50.
18. Nakayama EE, Ura S, Fleury RN, Soares V. Renal lesions in leprosy: a retrospective study of 199 autopsies. Am J Kidney Dis. 2001; 38:26–30.
19. Krysan DJ, Flynn JT. Renal transplantation after Streptococcus pneumoniae-associated hemolytic uremic syndrome. Am J Kidney Dis. 2001;37:E15.
20. Zikos D, Grewal KS, Craig K, et al. Nephrotic syndrome and acute renal failure associated with hepatitis A virus infection. Am J Gastroenterol. 1995;90:295–8.
21. Johnson RJ, Couser WG. Hepatitis B infection and renal disease: clinical immunopathogenetic and therapeutic considerations (Editorial review). Kidney Int. 1990;37:663–76.
22. Lai KN, Lai FM-M. Clinical features and natural course of hepatitis B-related glomerulopathy in adults. Kidney Int. 1991;40: S40–5.
23. Conjeevaram HS, Hoofnagle JH, Austin HA, et al. Long-term outcome of hepatitis B virus-related glomerulonephritis after therapy with interferon alfa. Gastroenterology. 1995;109: 540–6.
24. Dienstag JL, Schiff ER, Wright TL, et al. Lamivudine as the initial treatment for chronic hepatitis B in the United States. N Engl J Med. 1999;341:1256–63.
25. Lin CY. Treatment of hepatitis B virus-associated membranous nephropathy with recombinant alpha-interferon. Kidney Int. 1995;47:225–30.
26. Guillevin L, Lhote F, Cohen P, et al. Polyarteritis nodosa related hepatitis B virus. A prospective study with long-term observation of 41 patients. Medicine (Baltimore). 1995;74:238–53.
27. Erhardt A, Sagir A, Guillevin L, et al. Successful treatment of hepatitis B virus associated polyarteritis nodosa with a combina-tion of prednisolone, alpha interferon and lamivudine. J Hepatol. 2000;33:677–83.
28. Johnson RJ, Gretch DR, Couser WG, et al. Hepatitis C virus-asso-ciated glomerulonephritis. Effect of alpha-interferon therapy. Kidney Int. 1994;46:1700–4.
29. Lindsay KL, Trepo C, Heintges T, et al. A randomized, double-blind trial comparing pegylated interferon alfa-2b to interferon alfa-2b as initial treatment of chronic hepatitis C. Hepatology. 2001;34:395–403.
30. Ifudu O, Rao TK, Tan CC, et al. Zidovudine is beneficial in human immunodeficiency virus associated nephropathy. Am J Nephrol. 1995;15:217–21.
31. Wierenga KJJ, Pattison JR, Brink N, et al. Glomerulonephritis after human parvovirus infection in homozygous sickle-cell disease. Lancet. 1995;346:475–6.
32. Moudgil A, Nast CC, Bagga A, et al. Association of parvovirus B19 infection with idiopathic collapsing glomerulopathy. Kidney Int. 2001;59:2126–33.
33. Tanawattanacharoen S, Falk RJ, Jennette JC, Kjopp JB. Parvovirus B19 in kidney tissue of patients with focal segmental glomerulo-sclerosis. Am J Kidney Dis. 2000;35:1166–74.
34. Smith MC, Cooke JH, Zimmerman DM, et al. Asymptomatic glomerulonephritis after nonstreptococcal upper respiratory infections. Ann Intern Med. 1979;91:697–702.
35. Becker JL, Miller F, Nuovo GJ, et al. Epstein–Barr virus infection of renal proximal tubular cells: possible role in chronic interstitial nephritis. J Clin Invest. 1999;104:1671–2.
36. Barsoum RS. Malarial nephropathies. Nephrol Dial Transplant. 1998;13:1588–97.
37. Barsoum RS. Schistosoma glomerulopathies (Editorial Review). Kidney Int. 1993;44:1–12.
38. Barsoum R, Nabil M, Saady G, et al. Immunoglobulin A and the pathogenesis of schistosomal glomerulopathy. Kidney Int. 1996;50:920–8.
39. Sobh MA, Moustafa FE, Sally SM, et al. A prospective, randomized therapeutic trial for schistosomal specific nephropathy. Kidney Int. 1989;36:904–7.

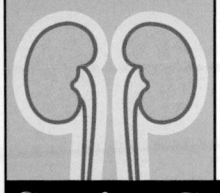

Chapter 29

Renal Amyloidosis and Glomerular Diseases with Monoclonal Immunoglobulin Deposition

Pierre M Ronco, Pierre Aucouturier, and Bruno Moulin

INTRODUCTION

Because the renal plasma flow represents 20% of the total plasma flow and the glomerulus is the renal filtering unit continuously exposed to plasma proteins, the glomerulus is the first structure in the body in which abnormal proteins or proteins with a peculiar affinity for constituents of the capillary wall (particularly of the glomerulus) become deposited. This chapter covers the glomerular protein deposition diseases in which intrinsic abnormal properties of the deposited protein are most likely responsible for renal pathogenicity. These diseases include amyloidosis, nonamyloid monoclonal immunoglobulin deposition disease (MIDD), and other plasma cell dyscrasia-related glomerulopathies. In most cases, the nephritogenic protein is a monoclonal immunoglobulin subunit, which makes it possible to establish correlations between protein structure and pathogenicity.

Since the first description of immunoglobulin amyloidosis by Glenner and associates in 1971[1], the spectrum of glomerular diseases with deposition or precipitation of monoclonal immunoglobulin components has expanded dramatically. These diseases can be classified into two categories by electron microscopy (Table 29.1). The first category includes diseases with fibril formation, mainly amyloidosis, and diseases with microtubule formation, including cryoglobulinemic kidney (Chapter 23) and immunotactoid glomerulonephritis. The second category is characterized by nonorganized electron-dense granular deposits. They are localized along basement membranes in most tissues, especially in the kidney, and define a disease now called MIDD. Deposits are most often made of isolated monoclonal light chains (light-chain deposition disease, LCDD), but the light chains may also be associated with monoclonal heavy chains (light- and heavy-chain deposition disease, LHCDD) or even be replaced by the heavy chains (heavy-chain deposition disease, HCDD), a newly described entity.

RENAL AMYLOIDOSIS

General characteristics of amyloidosis

Definition

Amyloidosis is a general term for a family of diseases defined by morphologic criteria. The diseases are characterized by the deposition in extracellular spaces of a proteinaceous material with well-defined morphologic and ultrastructural features. Amyloid deposits are 'typically composed of a felt-like array of 7.5–10 nm wide rigid, linear, nonbranching, aggregated

Glomerular diseases with tissue deposition or precipitation of monoclonal immunoglobulin components	
Immunoglobulin deposits	**Glomerular disease**
Organized	
Fibrillar	Amyloidosis (AL, AH)
Microtubular	Cryoglobulinemia; immunotactoid glomerulonephritis
Nonorganized: granular	Monoclonal immunoglobulin deposition disease (MIDD): light-chain, heavy-chain, and light plus heavy chain deposition diseases (LCDD, HCDD, LHCDD)

Table 29.1 Glomerular diseases with tissue deposition or precipitation of monoclonal immunoglobulin components.

fibrils of indefinite length'[1]. One amyloid fibril is made of two twisted 3-nm wide filaments, each having a regular anti-parallel β-pleated sheet configuration. The β-sheets are perpendicular to the filament axis. The numerous hydrogen bonds involving most amide functions of the peptide backbones make them highly stable.

Amyloid precursor-based classification

Amyloidoses include conditions as different as Alzheimer's disease and other neurodegenerative disorders, familial peripheral neuropathies, and systemic or localized complications of tumoral or inflammatory diseases (see Table 29.2). They differ essentially by the nature of the precursor protein that yields the main component of fibrils and are classified accordingly. The propensity for forming amyloid seems related to the ability of this precursor to adopt a β-pleated sheet conformation, either through native secondary structure or because of transconformational properties. The amyloidogenic potential is enhanced by an overproduction (such as in Down's syndrome, AA- and AL-amyloidosis) or an impaired clearance (such as in β_2-microglobulin-related amyloidosis) of the precursor, or by genetically transmitted mutations.

Renal amyloidoses essentially include immunoglobulin light chain (AL) and systemic secondary (AA) amyloidoses. Other precursors, such as transthyretin, fibrinogen and lysozyme, are responsible for rare familial cases.

Other components of all amyloid fibrils

In addition to the unique 'pseudocrystalline' stacking of β-sheets described above, several components are shared by all types of amyloid. Glycosaminoglycans (GAGs) have been

Classification of the most frequent amyloidoses			
Type	**Precursor protein**	**Involved organs**	**Associated clinical syndrome**
AL (AH)	Immunoglobulin light chain (heavy chain)	Systemic (mostly kidneys, liver, heart, spleen, vessels, lungs, gastrointestinal tract, nerves, tongue)	Systemic amyloidosis (multiple organ involvement); rarely, localized amyloidosis (orbital, for instance)
$A\beta_2m$	β_2-Microglobulin	Systemic (mostly musculoskeletal system, heart, synovium)	Hemodialysis-associated amyloidosis
AA	SAA apolipoprotein	Systemic (mostly spleen, liver, kidneys)	Systemic secondary amyloidosis; familial Mediterranean fever
$AapoA_1$	Apolipoprotein A_1	Nerves	Peripheral neuropathy
ATTR	Transthyretin	Nervous system, kidneys, thyroid, heart	Familial amyloid polyneuropathy; senile systemic amyloidosis
AGel	Gelsolin	Systemic (vessels)	Finnish hereditary systemic amyloidosis
$A\beta$	β-Amyloid precursor protein	Brain	Alzheimer's disease; Down's syndrome
APrP	Prn P	Brain	Creutzfeld–Jakob disease and other spongiform encephalopathies
ACys	Cystatin C	Brain and other tissues	Iceland-type hereditary amyloid angiopathy
AIAPP	Islet amyloid polypeptide	Pancreas	Insulinoma, type II diabetes
ACal	Procalcitonin	Thyroid	Thyroid medullary carcinoma

Table 29.2 Classification of the most frequent amyloidoses.

found tightly associated to amyloid fibrils. GAGs are polysaccharide chains made of repeating hyaluronic acid/hexosamine units normally linked to a protein core; as such they are proteoglycans, which are important constituents of extracellular matrices. Proteoglycans, mostly of the heparan sulfate type, might induce and stabilize the β-pleated amyloid structure.

Another constituent of all amyloid deposits is the serum amyloid-P component (SAP). SAP is a β-pleated calcium-dependent lectin. In the presence of calcium, SAP is remarkably resistant to proteolytic digestion, suggesting that coating of amyloid fibrils with SAP could result in their protection from catabolism. The high affinity of SAP towards amyloid was exploited for diagnosing, locating, and monitoring the extent of systemic amyloidosis using scintigraphy with ^{123}I-labeled SAP. The knowledge of SAP-binding properties offers the opportunity for designing competitive inhibitors for the treatment of amyloidoses.

Other proteins such as apolipoproteins E and J were also found associated with several amyloids and might play a role in fibrillogenesis.

General mechanisms of fibrillogenesis

The amyloidoses are diseases of protein conformation, in which a particular soluble innocuous protein transforms and aggregates into an insoluble fibrillar structure that deposits in extracellular spaces of certain tissues. Fibrillogenesis may be the consequence of several mechanisms of processing the amyloid precursor, including partial proteolysis and conformational modifications. In systemic secondary AA-amyloidosis, removal of the C-terminal part of an apolipoprotein acute phase reactant, SAA, yields a 5–10 kDa fibril-forming

fragment. Phagocytic cells, in particular macrophages, thus play a central role in this disease by providing the intra-lysosomal processing of the precursor. In AL-amyloidosis, partial proteolysis of immunoglobulin light chains has been demonstrated but may well occur after fibrillogenesis.

Amyloidogenesis seems to involve a nucleation-dependent polymerization process[2]. Formation of an ordered nucleus is the initial and limiting step, followed by thermodynamically favorable addition of monomers, leading to elongation of the fibrils. Amyloid fibril formation from native proteins might occur via a conformational change leading to a soluble partially folded intermediate, whose subsequent ordered self-assembly would lead to fibril formation[3].

Pathology

Amyloidoses affecting the kidney are usually systemic. Vital organs such as the heart, liver, and gut are the targets of fibril deposition in most cases, and although impairment of renal function is frequently the first manifestation, involvement of those organs (particularly of the heart) is indicative of severe prognosis. The diagnosis is based upon well-defined pathologic criteria, which in many cases can be achieved with biopsies of easily accessible tissues such as the rectal submucosa, the accessory salivary glands, the skin, or the subcutaneous abdominal fat. In spite of this, renal amyloidosis is frequently demonstrated after a renal biopsy performed in a patient presenting with unexplained glomerulopathy.

The unique conformation of fibrils is responsible for peculiar tinctorial properties. By light microscopy, the deposits are extracellular, eosinophilic, and metachromatic. After Congo red staining, they appear faintly red (Fig. 29.1a) and show the

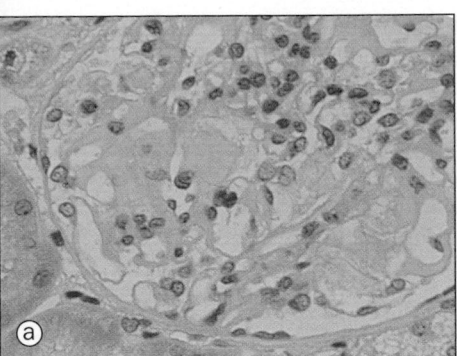 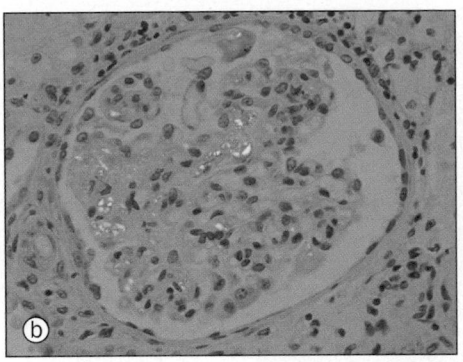 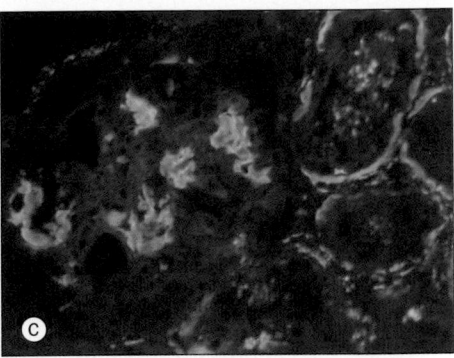

Figure 29.1 Amyloidosis. (a) Amyloid deposits in a renal glomerulus (Hematoxylin–eosin, ×312). (b) Congo red staining. Apple-green birefringence under polarized light (×312). (c) Immunofluorescence with anti-κ antibody. Note glomerular and tubular deposits (×312). (Courtesy of Dr Béatrice Mougenot.)

characteristic apple-green birefringence under polarized light (Fig. 29.1b). Metachromasia is also observed with Crystal violet, which stains the deposits red. The use of other stains such as Thioflavine T has been proposed, but the results lack specificity. Treatment with permanganate before the Congo red procedure may help to discriminate AA fibrils, which are sensitive to permanganate oxidation, from AL amyloid, which is resistant. However, permanganate treatment may be inconclusive because of the small size of the deposits, difficult to interpret because of only partial sensitivity, or conflict with the immunostaining with anti-AA and anti-light-chain antibodies.

In the kidney, the earliest lesions are located in the mesangium (see Fig. 29.1a), along the glomerular basement membrane, and in the blood vessels. Within the mesangium, deposits are primarily associated with the mesangial matrix, and subsequently increase irregularly by spreading from lobule to lobule then invading the whole mesangial area. Amyloid deposits may also infiltrate the capillary basement membrane or be localized on both sides of it. When subepithelial deposits predominate, spikes similar to those seen in membranous nephropathy may be observed. Advanced amyloid typically produces a nonproliferative, noninflammatory glomerulopathy, which is responsible for a marked enlargement of the kidney. The amyloid deposits replace the normal glomerular architecture, with a consequent loss of cellularity. When glomeruli become massively sclerotic, the deposits may be difficult to demonstrate by Congo red staining, and electron microscopy may then be helpful. The latter is also required at very early stages, which may not be detected by light microscopy examination in patients presenting with the nephrotic syndrome. The media of the blood vessels is prominently involved at early stages. Vascular involvement may predominate, and occasionally occurs alone, particularly in AL-amyloidosis. Deposits may also affect the tubules and the interstitium, leading to atrophy and disappearance of the tubular structures and to interstitial fibrosis.

Because of the heterogeneity of amyloidotic diseases, which results in specific diagnostic and therapeutic strategies adapted to the type of protein deposited within tissues, immunofluorescence with specific antisera should be routinely performed (Figs 29.1c and 29.2). Immunohistochemical classification of amyloid type is possible in most cases. However, immunofluorescence with sera directed against immunoglobulin chains

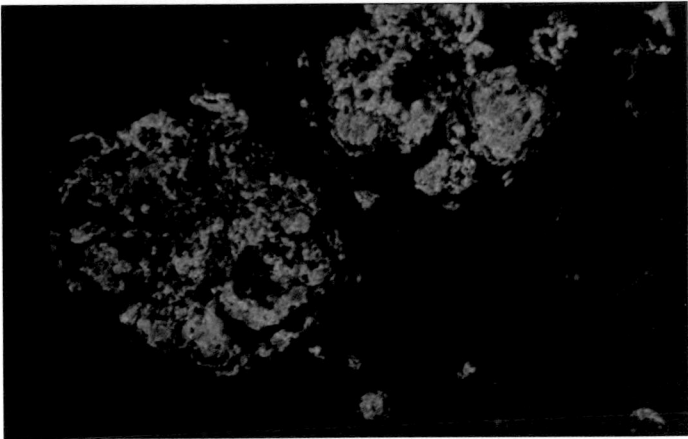

Figure 29.2 Portuguese-type hereditary amyloidosis. Heavy glomerular deposits of transthyretin are identified by specific antibodies (immunofluorescence, ×312). (Courtesy of Dr Béatrice Mougenot.)

may be more difficult to interpret than that with anti-AA antiserum, perhaps because of the absence or inaccessibility of light chain epitopes.

By electron microscopy, amyloid deposits are characterized by randomly oriented, nonbranching fibrils with an 8–15 nm diameter (Fig. 29.3).

Immunoglobulinic amyloidosis (AL and AH)

Free immunoglobulin subunits, mostly light chains, secreted by a single clone of B cells, are the cause of the most frequent and severe amyloidosis affecting the kidney. Studies on the mechanisms of AL-amyloidogenesis are made particularly difficult by the unique degree of structural heterogeneity of the precursor: each monoclonal light chain is different from all others, so each patient is a unique case. An immunoglobulin light chain typically includes two globular domains of 105 to 110 amino acid residues, exhibiting the classical 'β-barrel' conformation. The C-terminal region (which is the constant domain, C) is encoded by a single gene for κ chains and by four expressed genes for λ-chains. The N-terminal region (which is the variable domain, V) is encoded by two gene families, V and J and results from complex somatic rearrangement and mutation events occurring in the course of B-cell differentiation. This generates a high degree of diversity. The

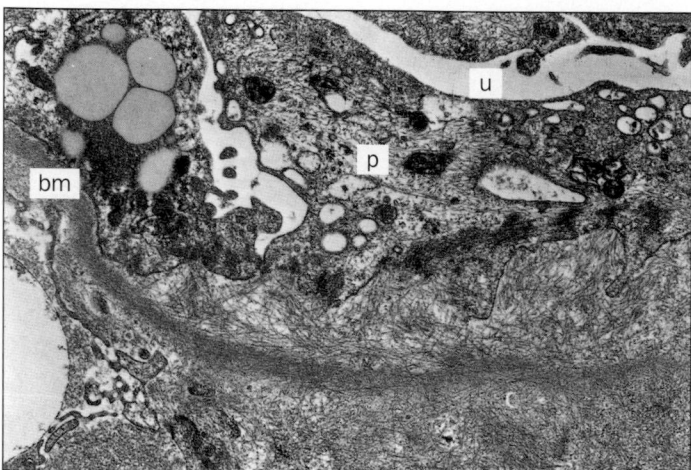

Figure 29.3 Electron micrograph of amyloid deposits invading glomerular basement membrane. Randomly oriented fibrils are located on both sides of the basement membrane (bm) and the lamina densa is attenuated (×10 000). p, podocyte; u, urinary space. (Courtesy of Dr Béatrice Mougenot.)

expressed $V\kappa$ and $V\lambda$ genes may be classified into four and six expressed variability subgroups, respectively, according to their sequence homology.

The involvement of an immunoglobulin heavy chain in amyloidosis is exceptional. In one case of AH-amyloidosis, the pathogenic IgG heavy chain had an internal deletion of half the molecule so that the V domain was directly joined to the C-terminal end of the heavy chain C domain, thus strikingly resembling a light chain[4].

Pathogenesis
There is experimental evidence that determinant factors are borne by the precursor light chain . The striking over-representation of the λ isotype, which is two- to fourfold more frequent than the κ isotype, is the most evident difference. A homology family of light chain variable regions, the $V_{\lambda VI}$ variability subgroup, is observed only in amyloid-associated monoclonal immunoglobulins and is over-represented in AL-amyloidosis.

Amyloidogenicity is frequently associated with certain physicochemical features such as the presence of low-molecular-mass light chain fragments in the patients' urine, and low isoelectric point (pI). Together with light chain isotypy, these parameters might allow prediction of the amyloidogenic/nonamyloidogenic character of a monoclonal light chain, although light chains with high pI may also be amyloidogenic. Directed mutation studies have suggested that light chains that are amyloidogenic *in vivo* are less thermodynamically stable than those that are nonamyloidogenic.

A potent analysis of nearly 200 light-chain sequences from defined pathologic conditions identified 12 positions in κ-chains and 12 in λ-chains where certain residues were significantly associated with amyloidosis[5]. Four structural risk factors were shown to define most fibril-forming κ light chains[6]. These findings suggest that it is feasible to predict fibril propensity by analysis of primary structure. However, environmental factors may also play some role. For example, the kidney contains

high concentrations of urea that were shown to enhance fibril formation by reducing the nucleation lag time[7].

The tropism of organ involvement may also be influenced by the germ line gene used for the light chain variable region (V_L). Patients expressing monoclonal light chain of the $V_{\lambda VI}$ subgroup are more likely to present with dominant renal involvement, whereas those with other λ light chains seem to develop dominant cardiac and multisystem disease[8]. Patients with κ light chains are more likely to have dominant hepatic involvement.

Analysis of the structure of extracted AL-amyloid fibrils revealed that the V domain is the main but not the exclusive component. The most common pattern is that of a protein made up of the V region and of a part of the C region. However, most studies were performed from necropsy organs, where proteases released by tissue damage might have participated, after the patient's death, in the C-domain digestion. The question of whether proteolysis plays a role in AL-fibrillogenesis has not yet been fully answered.

The three-dimensional structure of an AL-amyloidosis-associated urinary λ-chain dimer, protein Mcg, has been extensively studied by X-ray crystallography. The combination of complementarity-determining regions (CDR) from both subunits of the Mcg dimer mimics a normal antigen-binding site with affinities towards certain hapten-like compounds. Other light chains from patients with AL-amyloidosis were found to bind the hapten DNP-lysine, which does not occur with those from patients without amyloidosis. Amyloidogenic light chains also appear to have high dimerization constants. Antibody-like behavior of the light chains might, therefore, be implicated in their pathogenicity. Specific affinity of a light chain towards an extracellular structure might create a nucleus that could lead to elongation of a fibril.

From these results, it appears that structural factors govern the propensity of a particular light chain to form fibrils, but organ-specific environmental factors are also likely to be involved.

Epidemiology
The incidence of AL-amyloidosis is 9 per million per year in the USA[9]. Among systemic amyloidoses with predominant renal involvement, AL-amyloidosis is probably becoming more frequent than AA-amyloidosis since the widespread use of effective antimicrobial agents. Epidemiologic parameters of primary amyloidosis and myeloma are not significantly different. The median age at diagnosis is 64 years in patients without an immunoproliferative disorder[9], with a slight predominance of male patients. Amyloid deposits are found in approximately 10% of all patients with myeloma, and in 20% of those with pure light-chain myeloma. Less than one out of four patients with AL-amyloidosis is considered to have an overt immunoproliferative disease, which usually is a multiple myeloma, although other forms such as Waldenström's macroglobulinemia are not exceptional. In fact, the true incidence of myeloma depends on the criteria used for its diagnosis.

Clinical manifestations
The main clinical symptoms at presentation are weakness and weight loss (Table 29.3)[9]. Except for bone pain, there is

Features at presentation in AL-amyloidosis

Features	Percentage
Initial symptoms	
Fatigue	62
Weight loss	52
Pain	5
Purpura	15
Gross bleeding	3
Physical findings	
Hepatomegaly	24
Palpable spleen	5
Lymphadenopathy	3
Macroglossia	9
Laboratory findings	
Increased plasma cells (bone marrow ≥ 6%)	56[a]
Anemia (hemoglobin < 10 g/dL)	11
Elevated serum creatinine (≥ 1.3 mg/dL)(> 155 µmol/L)	45
Elevated alkaline phosphatase	26
Hypercalcemia (> 11 mg/dL)(> 2.75 mmol/L)	2
Proteinuria (≥ 1.0g/24 h)	55
Urine light chain	73[b]
—κ-chain	23
—λ-chain	50

A comparison of the prevalence of clinical syndromes according to the presence or the absence of myeloma is given in Table 29.4. (With permission from Kyle and Gertz[9].)
[a] 15% of patients having a myeloma.
[b] Of 429 patients.

Table 29.3 Clinical and laboratory features at presentation in 474 patients with proven AL-amyloidosis.

Syndromes at diagnosis in 229 patients with proven AL-amyloidosis

Syndromes	Without myeloma (182 patients) (%)	With myeloma (47 patients) (%)
Nephrotic syndrome	37	13
Carpal tunnel syndrome	21	38
Congestive heart failure	23	23
Peripheral neuropathy	20	6
Orthostatic hypotension	16	4

(With permission from Kyle and Greipp[10].)

Table 29.4 Syndromes at diagnosis in 229 patients with proven AL-amyloidosis.

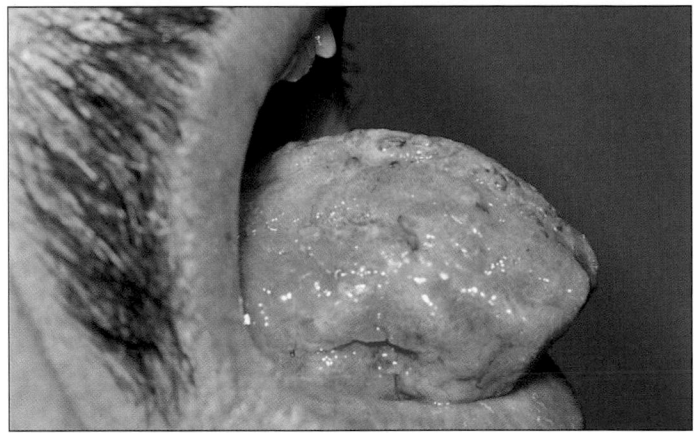

Figure 29.4 Macroglossia in a patient with AL-amyloidosis. (Courtesy of Dr S Aractinji.)

no difference in the incidence of initial symptoms in patients with and without myeloma. Nephrotic syndrome, orthostatic hypotension, and peripheral neuropathy are more frequent in patients with AL-amyloidosis without myeloma than in those with associated myeloma (Table 29.4)[10]. Renal insufficiency occurs usually in the presence of marked kidney enlargement and is usually not associated with hypertension. Proteinuria, mainly albumin, occurs in the absence of microscopic hematuria. When present, the hematuria should prompt examination for a bleeding lesion in the urinary tract.

AL-amyloidosis may infiltrate almost any organ other than the brain and, therefore, it can be responsible for a wide variety of clinical manifestations. Restrictive cardiomyopathy is found at presentation in up to one-third of patients and causes death in about one-half. Infiltration of the ventricular walls and the septum may be recognized by echocardiography. Amyloid may also induce arrhythmias and the sick sinus syndrome. Amyloid deposits in the coronary arteries may result in angina pectoris and myocardial infarction. Involvement of the gastrointestinal tract is also common and can cause motility disturbances, malabsorption, hemorrhage, or obstruction.

Macroglossia (Fig. 29.4) may interfere with eating and obstruct airways. Abnormalities of hepatic function remain generally mild. Hyposplenism, usually associated with splenomegaly, is occasionally found. Peripheral nerve involvement is usually responsible for a painful sensory polyneuropathy followed later by motor deficits. Autonomic neuropathy causing orthostatic hypotension, lack of sweating, gastrointestinal disturbances, bladder dysfunction, and impotence may occur alone or together with peripheral neuropathy. Orthostatic hypotension is one of the major hampering complications of AL-amyloidosis, some patients being bedridden. Skin involvement may take the form of purpura, characteristically around the eyes (Fig. 29.5), ecchymoses, papules, nodules, and plaques, occurring usually on the face and upper trunk. AL-amyloidosis may also infiltrate articular structures and mimic rheumatoid or an asymmetric seronegative synovitis. Infiltration of the shoulders may produce severe pain and swelling ('shoulder-pad' sign).

A rare but potentially serious manifestation of AL-amyloidosis is an acquired bleeding diathesis that may be associated with increased fibrinolysis or with deficiency of factor X and sometimes also factor IX. These factor deficiencies, that are partially linked to hepatic amyloid infiltration and nephrotic syndrome, may increase the thrombin time and the prothrombin time, but measurement of factor activity is necessary

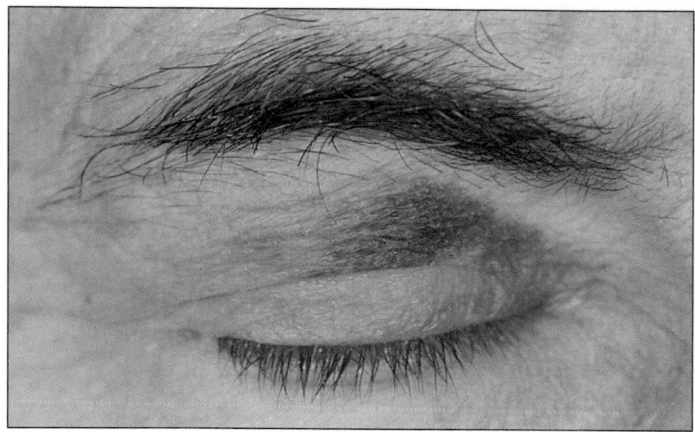

Figure 29.5 Skin involvement in AL-amyloidosis. Noninfiltrated purpuric macule of the superior eyebrow, very typical of AL-amyloidosis. (Courtesy of Dr S Aractinji.)

to detect milder forms. In both AL and AA types, widespread vascular deposits may also be responsible for bleeding, as manifested by spontaneous purpura. These bleeding complications should be systematically sought before any biopsy of a deep organ.

On average, monoclonal light chains can be detected by immunoelectrophoresis in 73% of the urine samples, and the λ isotype is twice as frequent as the κ[7], contrasting with the 1 : 2 ratio of λ to κ observed in patients with multiple myeloma alone. With the use of more sensitive immunochemical techniques, a monoclonal immunoglobulin is found in the serum and/or the urine in nearly 90% of patients. It is, however, worth noting that, even under such conditions, there is no detectable monoclonal immunoglobulin in serum and urine of some patients.

A distinction between 'primary' and myeloma-associated AL-amyloidosis may be useful for inclusion of patients in prospective therapeutic trials. However, from a pathophysiologic point of view, they represent two ends of a single entity. This conclusion is also supported by the fact that similar cytogenetic lesions (14q32 translocation) occur in patients with 'primary' amyloidosis and multiple myeloma[11]. The intrinsic pathogenicity of the precursor free light chain is highly variable, and expression of the disease occurs in the context of very different tumor masses. Whatever the hematologic status, the amyloid disease is responsible for the predominant symptoms in most patients. In AL-amyloidosis, the clinical 'malignancy' is conferred by the pathogenic monoclonal light chain rather than the underlying hematologic disease.

Treatment and outcome

AL-amyloidosis is among the most severe complications of plasma cell proliferative disorders. Cardiac involvement responsible for congestive heart failure and arrhythmia account for at least 40% of deaths. The only potentially efficient therapeutic tools to date are chemotherapies directed at the plasma cell clone to reduce light-chain production. In a prospective randomized study of 220 patients with AL-amyloidosis in which three treatment regimens were compared – melphalan and prednisolone, melphalan and prednisolone

plus colchicine, and colchicine alone – the median survival after randomization was 18 months, 17 months, and 8.5 months for the three groups, respectively ($P < 0.001$), excluding a beneficial effect of colchicine[12]. Alkylating cytotoxic therapy with melphalan and prednisone is, therefore, of significant, albeit rather limited, benefit in AL-amyloidosis when patients are examined as a whole. It was particularly advantageous for patients without major cardiac involvement. Among patients with the nephrotic syndrome analyzed in a previous study by the same group, a normal serum creatinine and no echocardiographic evidence of heart amyloidosis were associated with a high response rate (39%), as defined by a 50% reduction in proteinuria without an increase in serum creatinine. It is, however, essential to balance the potential benefits and risks of chemotherapy since a significant proportion of patients (about 25% of the responders) died as a result of dysmyelopoiesis or acute leukemia related to prolonged exposure to melphalan.

Based on promising results in myeloma patients, including both response rates and survival compared with conventional chemotherapies, high-dose melphalan (HDM) treatment with autologous bone marrow or blood stem cell transplantation (SCT) is being attempted in AL-amyloidosis[13,14]. HDM/SCT results in durable hematologic remissions (defined as absence of a monoclonal protein in serum and urine together with a bone marrow biopsy showing less than 5% plasma cells without clonal dominance) in a substantial proportion of patients (54/115 at 1 year). Such responses are associated with clinical improvement, decreased amyloid-related organ dysfunction, and prolonged survival (60% of 152 patients at 4 years). Survival is significantly influenced by whether or not hematologic complete remission is evident at 1 year and patients have evidence of amyloid cardiomyopathy at the time of treatment. However, toxicity from treatment is high (overall peritransplant mortality, 14%), particularly for those patients with clinically significant cardiac involvement[14]. Moreover, selection of patients for HDM/SCT plays a significant role in survival since the median survival was 45.6 months in 234 out of 1288 patients who met eligibility criteria for HDM/SCT but were treated with conventional alkylating agent therapy[15]. Randomized clinical trials are therefore warranted to evaluate HDM/SCT versus standard chemotherapy in selected groups of patients with AL-amyloidosis.

The results of chemotherapy in amyloidosis are difficult to document because there is no easy way to measure the amount of amyloid in a given patient. Resolution of the nephrotic syndrome does not necessarily reflect the disappearance of amyloid deposits, and the progressive deposition of amyloid can occur in the presence of improved clinical and laboratory findings. Scintigraphy after the injection of ^{123}I-labeled SAP may be helpful for monitoring the extent of systemic amyloidosis, but it is available in a rather limited number of centers. Because the tumor mass is frequently very low, effects of antitumor chemotherapies are better evaluated by the rate of excreted monoclonal immunoglobulin. Free monoclonal light chains, when detectable, are the most sensitive markers of the proliferative disorder. Since they are rapidly cleared from the blood, it would be suitable to follow the level of daily urinary excretion of light chains, while remembering that they usually account for a small proportion of protein in the urine. Nephelometric techniques, that allow measurement of very small concentrations of immunoglobulin free light chains, are promising.

Dialysis and transplantation

Most studies of the clinical course and outcome of patients on dialysis include both AL- and AA-amyloidosis. The patient's survival rate is low, but it compares favorably with that of patients not requiring dialysis: from 66 to 72% at 1 year, it falls to 30–44% at 5–6 years. No difference in survival was observed at any time between patients with AL- and AA-amyloidosis. The survival rate of patients treated with continuous ambulatory peritoneal dialysis (CAPD) is similar to that of patients on hemodialysis.

Cardiac amyloid is the most important predictor of poor survival in patients with AL-amyloidosis undergoing dialysis[16], and cardiac deaths represent the main cause of mortality in such patients. The management of patients with AL-amyloid on hemodialysis is also often complicated by permanent hypotension, gastrointestinal hemorrhage, chronic diarrhea, and difficulties in the creation and maintenance of vascular accesses. It has, therefore, been suggested that CAPD could have several advantages over hemodialysis in the management of end-stage renal amyloidosis, including avoiding vascular access and deleterious effects on blood pressure. However, it may induce protein loss in the dialysate and thus enhance malnutrition.

Little information is available regarding the outcome of AL-amyloid patients after renal transplantation, essentially because the series published so far include mainly patients with AA-amyloidosis (see below). However, the prognosis of patients with presumed AL-amyloidosis does not seem to differ from that of the patients with AA-amyloidosis. Recurrence of the deposits may occur in the graft.

Epidemiology and specific features of AA-amyloidosis

Epidemiology

An important epidemiologic aspect of AA-amyloidosis is the changing spectrum of underlying diseases. Pyogenic and granulomatous infections, especially tuberculosis, account for far fewer cases than in older series (10–20%). This is because of the efficacy of antibiotic treatments for bacteria, which shows that amyloidosis can be efficiently prevented when its cause is suppressed. In contrast, the prevalence (about 70%) of amyloid linked to autoimmune inflammatory diseases, such as rheumatoid arthritis, has increased dramatically. Amyloid-associated inflammatory bowel diseases remains stable at 5–10%. AA-amyloidosis in patients with Hodgkin's disease is rarely seen, in parallel with better control of the hematologic disease.

Clinical manifestations

There are a number of clinical manifestations of AA-amyloidosis (Table 29.5)[17,18]. The main target organ by far is the kidney. Gastrointestinal disturbances including diarrhea, constipation, and malabsorption are the most common after kidney manifestations. In contrast with AL-amyloidosis, congestive heart failure, peripheral neuropathy, macroglossia, and carpal tunnel syndrome are infrequent. The reason for the differential distribution of AA and AL tissue deposits is not understood. The optimal method for diagnosing AA-amyloid remains controversial. Although kidney biopsy is positive in 100% of symptomatic patients, less invasive biopsy procedures should be preferred first.

Outcome, dialysis, and transplantation

Survival time of patients with AA-amyloidosis is longer than in AL-amyloidosis (Table 29.5). An elevated serum creatinine and a low serum albumin are strong adverse prognostic indicators. The main causes of death are dialysis, but not cardiac, complications.

Table 29.5 Characteristics of patients with secondary AA-amyloidosis.

Characteristics of patients with secondary AA-amyloidosis		
Characteristics	Series 1[a]	Series 2[b]
Number of patients	75	64
Age (years)	57 (18–81)	56 (14–80)
Male-to-female ratio	0.8	1.5
Presenting clinical syndrome (%)	Proteinuria/renal failure (65) Gastrointestinal disturbance (5) Hepatosplenomegaly (4)	Proteinuria/renal failure (91) Gastrointestinal disturbance (22) Goiter (9) Neuropathy/carpal tunnel (3)
Source of tissue for diagnosis (%)	Rectum (60) Kidney (15)	Rectum (50) Kidney (38) Stomach/small bowel (23) Marrow (19)
Causes of death (%)	Renal failure (49) Bronchopneumonia (19) Cardiac disorder (11)	Uremia/dialysis complications (68) Sepsis (9) Cardiac disorder (9)
Survival	~40% at 3 years	~40% at 3 years (median 24.5 months)

[a] From Browning et al.[17]
[b] From Gertz and Kyle.[18]
(With permission Browning et al.[17] and Gertz and Kyle[18].)

Series of renal transplantation in AA-amyloidosis mostly concern patients with rheumatic diseases and come from Scandinavia. Amyloid deposits recur in about 10% of the grafts. Infection is the main cause of early deaths.

Familial Mediterranean fever

Familial Mediterranean fever represents both a particular type of AA-amyloidosis and the most frequent cause of familial amyloidosis. Interestingly, colchicine has proved to be efficient both in the prevention and treatment of this type of amyloidosis. Familial Mediterranean fever is usually transmitted as an autosomal recessive disorder and occurs most commonly in Sephardic Jews and Armenians. It is caused by mutations of the gene (MEFV) encoding a protein called pyrin or marenostrin[19]. Clinically there are two independent phenotypes. In the first, brief, episodic, febrile attacks of peritonitis, pleuritis, or synovitis occur in childhood or adolescence and precede the renal manifestations. In the second, renal symptoms precede and may be the only manifestation of the disease for a long time. The attacks are accompanied by dramatic elevations of acute-phase reactants, including serum amyloid A protein, which leads to amyloid deposition. In this context, AA-amyloid is responsible for severe renal lesions with prominent glomerular involvement, leading to end-stage renal disease (ESRD) at a young age, and for early deaths. Colchicine can prevent the development of proteinuria, may occasionally reverse the nephrotic syndrome, and may prevent the decline in renal function in patients with non-nephrotic proteinuria. It is less effective in preventing progression in patients with nephrotic syndrome or renal insufficiency. The minimal daily dose of colchicine for prevention of amyloidosis is 1 mg, and patients with clinical evidence of amyloidotic kidney disease and kidney transplant recipients should receive daily doses of 1.5–2 mg.

Other syndromes of inherited periodic fever with AA-amyloidosis

The recent identification of genes responsible for syndromes of periodic fever with amyloidoisis has opened the way to a molecular diagnosis of hereditary AA-amyloidosis. These syndromes include the tumor necrosis factor receptor-associated periodic syndrome (TRAPS), the hyperimmunoglobulinemia D and periodic fever syndrome (HIDS), and the Muckle–Wells syndrome/familial cold urticaria (MWS/FCU).

Summary and therapeutic prospects

Clinical experience of familial Mediterranean fever and infection-related AA-amyloidosis demonstrates that it is possible to prevent and treat AA-amyloidosis efficiently. Although isolated amyloid fibrils are stable in vitro, AA amyloid deposits exist in a state of dynamic turnover. It has been shown that outcome is favorable in AA amyloidosis when the SAA concentration is maintained below 10 mg/L[20]. These findings support therapeutic strategies to decrease the supply of amyloid fibril precursor proteins. Well-conducted trials of colchicine are warranted in rheumatic causes of AA-amyloidosis. Rheumatic patients may also benefit from immunosuppressive therapy, the efficacy of which needs to be demonstrated in further prospective randomized studies.

New therapeutic approaches in AL- and AA-amyloidosis are resulting from the increasing knowledge of the mechanisms of fibrillogenesis. It is first possible to prevent amyloid fibril deposition in experimental models. RAGE, a receptor for advanced glycation end-products, is also a receptor for the amyloidogenic form of serum amyloid A. Amyloid deposition that occurs in the spleen of mice injected with amyloid-enhancing factor and silver nitrate is inhibited by a soluble form of RAGE, or by blocking antibodies[21]. Small sulfated compounds can interfere with experimental mouse AA-amyloidosis, probably by competing with the interaction between the amyloid precursor and proteoglycans. Amyloid fiber assembly can be inhibited by BiP, a molecular chaperone that prevents aggregation of light chains, and by a synthetic peptide that is identical to a major light-chain binding site for BiP[22]. Inhibition of SAP binding to amyloid fibrils is also an attractive goal.

A second feasible therapeutic approach is removal or dissolution of amyloid fibrils. A new anthracycline, 4′-iodo-4′-deoxy-doxorubicin, was shown to inhibit and reverse AL-amyloid formation[23] and to disrupt the fibrillar structure of transthyretin amyloid, but only a minor proportion of patients with AL-amyloid respond to this drug. An anti-light chain monoclonal antibody having specificity for an amyloid-related epitope induced a rapid dissolution of mouse amyloidomas formed by subcutaneously injected amyloid from patients with AL-amyloidosis[24]. This antibody could be directed toward a β-pleated sheet conformational epitope expressed on amyloid fibrils.

MONOCLONAL IMMUNOGLOBULIN DEPOSITION DISEASE (MIDD)

History and definition

It was known from the late 1950s that nonamyloidotic forms of glomerular disease 'resembling the lesion of diabetic glomerulosclerosis', could occur in multiple myeloma. The presence of monoclonal light chains in these lesions was recognized more than 20 years later, and Randall and associates, published the first description of LCDD in 1976[25].

Monoclonal heavy chains were found together with light chains in the tissue deposits from some patients, thus defining LHCDD. The first deposits containing monoclonal heavy chains in the absence of detectable light chains (HCDD)[26], and two series of similar patients were reported later[27,28].

In clinical and pathologic terms, LCDD, LHCDD, and HCDD are similar and may therefore be referred to as MIDD. They differ from amyloidosis in that the deposits lack affinity for Congo red and do not have a fibrillar organization. The distinction also relates to different pathophysiology of amyloid, which implicates one-dimensional elongation of a pseudocrystalline structure, and MIDD, which would rather involve a one-step precipitation of immunoglobulin chains.

Pathogenesis

MIDD is characterized by kidney deposition of monoclonal immunoglobulin subunits, but at variance with amyloidosis, deposition induces a dramatic accumulation of extracellular matrix that is responsible for glomerular and tubular basement membrane thickening and for nodular glomerulosclerosis.

Renal Amyloidosis and Glomerular Diseases with Monoclonal Immunoglobulin Deposition

That light-chain deposition involves unusual light-chain properties is supported by the absence of detectable monoclonal free light chain in the serum and urine in 15–30% of LCDD patients, the recurrence of the disease in the transplanted kidney, the biosynthesis of abnormal light chains by bone marrow plasma cells, and the fact that discrete changes in the V_L sequence were responsible for light-chain deposition in a mouse experimental model[29]. However, light-chain deposition does not mean pathogenicity, as shown by Solomon and colleagues[30], who found that, after injection into mice, one-third (14/40) of light chains from patients with myeloma or AL-amyloidosis became deposited in basement membranes. Therefore, singular properties of light chain are most likely required for completion of the pathogenetic process leading to kidney fibrosis.

The following properties of light-chain variable domains may contribute to MIDD pathogenesis[29]. The first is the restricted usage of three κ germline genes, with an apparent over-representation of the rare $V_{\kappa IV}$ variability subgroup. Second, size abnormalities of light chains have been documented in about one-third of patients by bone marrow biosynthesis experiments. Third, unusual amino acid substitutions have been identified in primary structures of LCDD light chains, mostly in peptide loops corresponding to CDRs (complementarity determining regions, i.e., parts of the molecules normally implicated in antigen binding). In particular, molecular modeling experiments have underlined the presence of hydrophobic residues that could strongly modify the light-chain conformation, leading to its precipitation, or be responsible for hydrophobic interactions between V domains, or between V domains and extracellular matrix proteins. Fourth, when pathogenic light chains could not be detected in the serum and urine, they seemed to be N-glycosylated in all tested cases. Thus, glycosylation might increase the light-chain propensity to precipitate in tissues. However, as in AL-amyloidosis, extrinsic conditions may also contribute to aggregation of the light chain. The same light chain can form granular aggegates or amyloid fibrils depending on the environment, and different partially folded intermediates of this protein may be responsible for amorphous or fibrillar aggregation pathways[3].

A deletion of the first constant domain C_H1 was found in the deposited or circulating heavy chain in the 11 patients with HCDD where it was searched for[28,29]. A larger deletion also including the hinge and C_H2 domain was found in one case[26]. In the blood, the deleted heavy chain was associated with light chains, mostly of the λ isotype, or circulated in small amounts as a free unassembled subunit[27]. It is likely that the C_H1 deletion facilitates the secretion of free heavy chains that are rapidly cleared from the circulation by organ deposition. Deletion of the C_H1 is also found in heavy chain disease, a lymphoproliferative disorder with free HC secretion without corresponding renal tissue deposition, and in AH-amyloidosis in which deposits have a fibrillar organization. In heavy chain disease, however, the variable domain also is partially or completely deleted, which suggests that the V_H domain is required for tissue precipitation. Sequence analysis of two HCDD proteins did show unusual amino acid substitutions, that might change their physicochemical properties (e.g., charge, hydrophobicity) in the V_H[31].

Another common feature shared by LCDD and HCDD is the dramatic accumulation of extracellular matrix. Nodules are made of normal constituents (collagen type IV, laminin, fibronectin), and stain weakly for the small proteoglycans, decorin and biglycan[32]. A role for transforming growth factor β is supported by its strong expression in glomeruli of MIDD patients, and by in vitro experiments using cultured mesangial cells[33]. Incubation of mesangial cells with light chains from patients with LCDD induces cell changes, activation of platelet-derived growth factor-B and its receptor, production of monocyte chemoattractant protein-1 as well as increased expression of Ki-67, a proliferation marker, whereas light chains toxic to tubules have no effect[34]. Because of the similarities between MIDD- and diabetes-induced nodular glomerulosclerosis, including the strong periodic acid–Schiff reagent (PAS) reactivity of the lesions, it has been suggested that immunoglobulin chains might stimulate mesangial cells in a similar manner to advanced glycosylation end-products (AGE).

Epidemiology

MIDD is found in 5% of myeloma patients at autopsy, while the prevalence of AL-amyloidosis is about 11%. LCDD and HCDD may occur in a wide range of ages (31–79 years) with a slight male preponderance (Table 29.6). Twenty-two patients with HCDD have been reported so far, but the disease is most likely underdiagnosed.

Clinical manifestations

MIDD is a systemic disease with immunoglobulin chain deposition in a variety of organs leading to various clinical manifestations[29]. Light or heavy-chain deposition may be, however, totally asymptomatic.

Renal manifestations

Renal involvement is a constant feature of MIDD, and renal symptoms, mostly proteinuria and renal failure, often dominate the clinical presentation (Table 29.6)[28,29]. In 23–67% of LCDD patients, albuminuria is associated with the

Clinical manifestations and renal lesions in monoclonal immunoglobulin deposition disease		
Characteristics	LCDD/LHCDD	HCDD
Male/female ratio	1.4	0.8
Age (years)	55 (31–77)	57 (26–79)
Hypertension (%)	58	89
Renal failure (serum creatinine ≥ 130 µmol/L) (%)	90	85
Nephrotic syndrome (%)	38	32
Hematuria (%)	45	88
Nodular glomerulosclerosis (%)	31–100	100

Table 29.6 Clinical manifestations and renal lesions in monoclonal immunoglobulin deposition disease (MIDD). LCDD, HCDD, LHCDD, light-chain, heavy-chain, and light plus heavy-chain deposition diseases.

nephrotic syndrome. In 25%, the albumin loss is less than 1g/day, and these patients exhibit mainly a tubulointerstitial syndrome. Albuminuria is not correlated with the existence of nodular glomerulosclerosis, at least initially, and may occur in the absence of significant glomerular lesions as detected by light microscopy. Hematuria is more frequent than one would expect for a nephropathy in which cell proliferation is usually modest. The high prevalence, early appearance, and severity of renal failure are other salient features of LCDD. Renal failure occurs with comparable frequency in patients with either low or heavy protein excretion, and, therefore, may present in the form of a subacute tubulointerstitial nephritis or a rapidly progressive glomerulonephritis, respectively. The prevalence of hypertension is variable, but it must be interpreted according to associated medical history.

Extrarenal manifestations

Liver and cardiac involvement are the most common features of LCDD and LHCDD. Liver deposits are constant. They are either discrete and confined to the sinusoids and basement membranes of biliary ductules without associated parenchymal lesions or they are massive with marked dilatation and multiple ruptures of sinusoids, resembling peliosis. Hepatomegaly and mild alterations of liver function are the most usual symptoms, but patients may also develop life-threatening hepatic insufficiency and portal hypertension. Heart involvement also appears to be frequent and may be responsible for cardiomegaly and severe heart failure. As in the kidney and liver, monotypic light-chain deposits in the vascular walls and perivascular areas of the heart were seen in all autopsy cases when examined with immunofluorescence. Deposits may also occur along the nerve fibers and in the choroid plexus, as well as in the lymph nodes, bone marrow, spleen, pancreas, thyroid gland, submandibular glands, adrenal glands, gastrointestinal tract, abdominal vessels, lungs, and skin.

Extrarenal deposits are less common in patients with HCDD. They have been reported in the heart, synovial tissue, skin, striated muscles, pancreas, around the thyroid follicles, and in Disse's spaces (lymphatic channels) in the liver.

Hematologic findings

Myeloma is diagnosed in about 40% of the patients with LCDD or LHCDD, and in 25% of those with HCDD. MIDD, like AL-amyloidosis, is often the presenting disease that leads to the discovery of myeloma at an early stage. In some patients who presented with 'common' myeloma and normal-sized monoclonal immunoglobulin without kidney involvement, LCDD occurred when the disease relapsed after chemotherapy, together with immunoglobulin structural abnormalities. Because melphalan induces immunoglobulin gene mutations, the disease in these patients might result from the emergence of a variant clone induced by the alkylating agent. MIDD may complicate Waldenström's macroglobulinemia and chronic lymphocytic leukemia in rare cases. It often occurs in the absence of a detectable malignant process, even after prolonged (more than 10 years)

follow-up. A monoclonal bone marrow plasma cell population is then easily detectable by immunofluorescence examination.

It is worth noting that in 15–30% of patients with LCDD there is no detectable monoclonal immunoglobulin in serum and urine. Some patients, therefore, are affected with so-called nonsecretory myeloma or macroglobulinemia. However, true nonsecretion is very rare. In most patients, there is a secretion of abnormal immunoglobulin molecules that are either rapidly degraded postsynthetically or deposited in tissues.

Pathology

Light microscopy

Despite clinical manifestations that feature impairment of glomerular function in most cases, MIDD should not be considered a purely glomerular disease. In fact, tubular lesions may be more conspicuous than the glomerular damage. Tubular lesions are characterized by the deposition of a refractile, eosinophilic, PAS-positive, ribbon-like material along the outer part of the tubular basement membrane. The deposits predominate around the distal tubules, the loops of Henle, and, in some instances, around the collecting ducts whose epithelium is flattened and atrophied. Typical myeloma casts are only occasionally seen in pure forms of MIDD. In advanced stages, a marked interstitial fibrosis including refractile deposits is frequently associated with tubular lesions.

Glomerular lesions are much more heterogeneous. Nodular glomerulosclerosis is the most characteristic (see Fig. 29.6a); it is found in 30–100% of patients with LCDD. Expansion of the mesangial matrix was observed in all cases of HCDD, with nodular glomerulosclerosis in almost all of them. Mesangial nodules are composed of PAS-positive membrane-like material and are often accompanied by mild mesangial hypercellularity. The capillary loops stretch at the periphery of florid nodules and may undergo aneurysmal dilatation. Bowman's capsule may contain a material that is identical to that present in the center of the nodules. These lesions resemble diabetic nodular glomerulosclerosis, but some characteristics are distinctive: the distribution of the nodules is fairly regular in a given glomerulus, the nodules are often poorly argyrophilic, and exudative lesions as 'fibrin caps' and extensive hyalinosis of the efferent arterioles are not observed. In occasional cases with prominent endocapillary cellularity and mesangial interposition, the glomerular features mimic a lobular glomerulonephritis. Milder forms of LCDD simply show an increase in mesangial matrix and sometimes in mesangial cells, and a modest thickening of the basement membranes that are abnormally bright and rigid. Glomerular lesions may not be detected by light microscopy but require ultrastructural examination. These lesions may represent early stages of glomerular disease or be induced by light chains with a weak pathogenic potential. Their diagnosis would be unrecognized without the immunostaining results.

Arteries, arterioles, and peritubular capillaries all may contain PAS-positive deposits in close contact with their basement membranes. Deposits do not show the staining characteristics of amyloid, but they may be associated with Congo red-positive amyloid deposits in approximately 10% of patients[28].

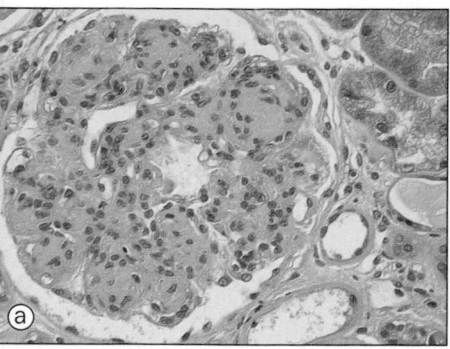
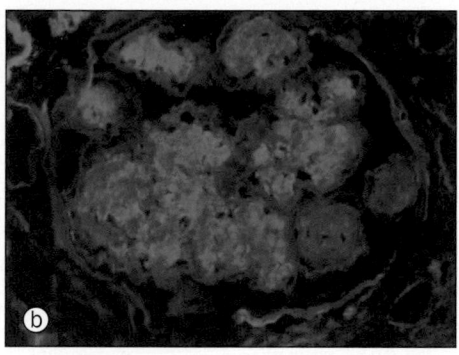
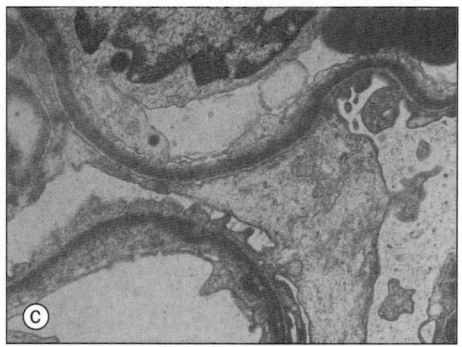

Figure 29.6 Light-chain deposition disease. (a) Nodular glomerulosclerosis with mesangial matrix accumulation (Masson's trichrome stain, ×312). (b) Bright staining of mesangial nodules and tubular basement membranes with anti-κ antibody (immunofluorescence, ×312). (c) Electron micrograph showing nonfibrillar, finely granular electron-dense material along the glomerular basement membrane (×3000). (Courtesy of Dr Béatrice Mougenot and Dr Laure-Hélène Noël.)

Immunofluorescence

A key step in the diagnosis of the various forms of MIDD is immunofluorescence examination of the kidney. All biopsy specimens show evidence of monotypic light chain (mostly κ) (Fig. 29.6b) and/or heavy chain (Fig. 29.7) fixation along tubular basement membranes. This criterion is required for the diagnosis of MIDD.

The tubular deposits stain strongly (see Fig. 29.6b) and predominate along the loops of Henle and the distal tubules, but they also often are detected along the proximal tubules. In contrast, the pattern of glomerular immunofluorescence displays marked heterogeneity. In patients with nodular glomerulosclerosis, deposits of monotypic immunoglobulin chains are usually found along the peripheral glomerular basement membranes and, to a lesser extent, in the nodules themselves (see Fig. 29.6b). The staining in glomeruli is typically weaker than that observed along the tubular basement membranes. This

may not be a function of the actual amount of deposited material, because several cases have been reported in which glomerular immunofluorescence was negative despite the presence of large amounts of granular glomerular deposits by electron microscopy. Local modifications of deposited light chains thus might change their antigenicity. In patients without nodular lesions, glomerular staining occurs mainly along the basement membrane, but it may involve the mesangium in some cases. A linear staining usually decorates Bowman's capsule. Deposits are frequently found in vascular walls and interstitium.

In patients with HCDD, immunofluorescence with anti-light-chain antibodies is negative despite typical nodular glomerulosclerosis. Monotypic deposits of γ, α, or μ heavy chain may be identified. Any γ subclass may be observed. Analysis of the kidney biopsy with monoclonal antibodies specific for the constant domains of the γ heavy chain allowed

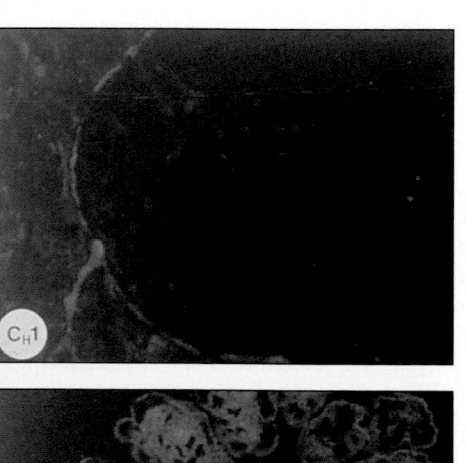
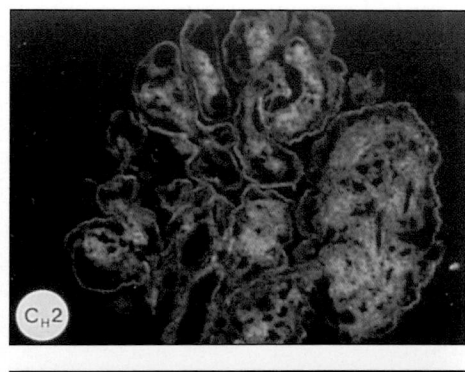
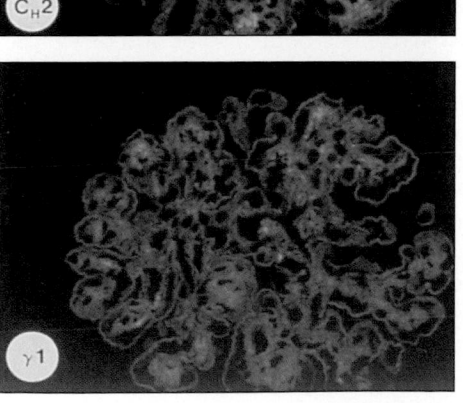

Figure 29.7 Heavy-chain deposition disease. Nodular glomerulosclerosis. Mesangial and capillary wall deposits stain with a monoclonal antibody specific for the γ1 isotype in the absence of detectable light chain (bottom right). Immunofluorescence with a panel of monoclonal antibodies directed to the various constant domains of the Ig heavy chain shows that the glomerular deposits are stained with anti-C$_H$2 and anti-C$_H$3, but not with anti-C$_H$1 antibodies (×312). (Courtesy of Dr Béatrice Mougenot.)

identification of a deletion of the C_H1 domain in all tested cases (see Fig. 29.7). In most cases of HCDD, especially when a γ1 or γ3 chain is involved, complement components including C1 could be demonstrated in a granular or pseudolinear pattern. Complement deposits were often associated with signs of complement activation in serum.

Electron microscopy

The most characteristic ultrastructural feature is the presence of finely to coarsely granular electron-dense deposits along the outer (interstitial) aspect of the tubular basement membranes. In the glomerulus, they predominate in a subendothelial position along the glomerular basement membrane and are located mainly along and in the lamina rara interna (see Fig. 29.6c). They can also be found in mesangial nodules, Bowman's capsule, and the wall of small arteries between the myocytes. Nonamyloid fibrils have been reported in a few patients with LCDD or HCDD.

Outcome and treatment

The outcome of pure MIDD is uncertain, mainly because extrarenal deposits can be totally asymptomatic or cause severe organ damage that leads to death. Survival from onset of symptoms varies from 1 month to 10 years whereas by comparison, the prognosis of a related disease, AL-amyloidosis, is much more homogeneous. Although renal prognosis is poor, patient survival can be substantial with 70 and 37% 5-year patient survival and renal survival, respectively[35]. The only predictor of renal patient survival seems to be the initial serum creatinine at the time of biopsy, whereas the presence of myeloma does not seem to influence renal or patient survival[28]. Outcomes in terms of renal and patient survival are significantly better in patients with pure MIDD, compared with those who present with myeloma cast nephropathy[28].

As in AL amyloidosis, treatment should be aimed at reducing immunoglobulin production. Chemotherapy is logical in patients with MIDD and myeloma. It is controversial in the absence of overt malignancy given the uncertain outcome of LCDD and the absence of reliable follow-up criteria, especially in patients without detectable monoclonal component. However, it has become general practice to treat patients with steroids plus melphalan or a cytotoxic agent, irrespective of the accompanying hematologic disease.

Whether appropriate treatment can result in sustained remission has long remained unclear. Clearance of the light-chain deposits has been demonstrated unequivocally in some patients after intensive chemotherapy with syngeneic bone marrow transplantation or blood stem cell autografting. Disappearance of nodular mesangial lesions and light-chain deposits was also reported after long-term chemotherapy. These observations are of paramount importance: they demonstrate that fibrotic nodular glomerular lesions are reversible, and they argue for intensive chemotherapy in patients with severe visceral involvement.

Kidney transplantation has been performed in a few patients with MIDD and ESRD. Recurrence of the disease is usually observed. Therefore, intensive chemotherapy should be performed before kidney transplantation.

Renal diseases associated with MIDD

Since the description of MIDD, it was expected that AL-amyloidosis and MIDD might coexist in a single patient. The first observations were reported in 1985. Since then, amyloid deposits have been found in one or more organs in about 7% of LCDD patients. Because amyloid deposits are focal, the true incidence of the association may be markedly underestimated. Although this association may result from peculiar light chains endowed with intrinsic properties that make them prone to form both fibrillar and nonfibrillar deposits depending on the environment[3], one cannot exclude the possibility that the coexisting diseases are induced by different variant clones.

The association of monoclonal light-chain deposits, mostly along renal tubule membranes, with typical myeloma cast nephropathy is more frequent than reported initially. It was found in 11 of 34 (32%) patients with MIDD[28]. Nodular glomerulosclerosis is, however, infrequent (< 10%), and some ribbon-like tubular basement membranes are seen in fewer than half of the patients. In addition, one-third of the patients do not have granular-dense deposits by electron microscopy. The lack of matrix accumulation in most of these patients who present with acute renal failure in the setting of a true myeloma may relate to insufficient time for the development of fibrosis or to a weaker sclerogenic effect of the light chain, if any. As discussed above, the presence of light-chain deposits along the tubular basement membrane is not sufficient to make a diagnosis of MIDD.

NONAMYLOID FIBRILLARY AND IMMUNOTACTOID GLOMERULOPATHIES

Definition

Fibrillary glomerulonephritis and immunotactoid glomerulopathy are recently described entities characterized, respectively, by fibrillar and microtubular deposits in the mesangium and the glomerular capillary loops (see Table 29.7). These deposits do not have a β-pleated sheet organization and, therefore, are readily distinguishable from amyloid by the larger thickness of fibrils and lack of Congo red staining. However, whether fibrillar and immunotactoid glomerulopathies are totally distinct entities is not clear from the literature and remains the subject of considerable debate.

For Korbet et al.[36], immunotactoid glomerulopathy is a unifying term for glomerular deposition of either amyloid-like fibrils (12–22 nm) or larger microtubules > 30 nm) in patients for whom an associated systemic disease including cryoglobulinemia and lymphoproliferative disorders has been excluded[28]. For others[37,38], the distinction between nonamyloid fibrillary glomerulonephritis and immunotactoid glomerulopathy may be of great clinical and pathophysiologic interest in the context of protein dyscrasias (see Table 29.7).

Pathology

In immunotactoid glomerulopathy, renal biopsy shows either membranous nephropathy (see Fig. 29.8) (often associated with segmental mesangial proliferation) or lobular membranoproliferative glomerulonephritis. By immunofluorescence, coarse granular deposits of IgG and C3 are observed along capillary basement membranes and in mesangial areas.

Immunopathologic and clinical characteristics of fibrillary and immunotactoid glomerulopathies			
Characteristics	Amyloidosis (AL-type)	Fibrillary glomerulonephritis	Immunotactoid glomerulopathy (GOMMID)[a]
Congo red staining	Yes	No	No
Composition	Fibrils	Fibrils	Microtubules
Fibril or microtubule size (nm)	8–15	12–22	>30
Organization in tissues	Random (β-pleated sheet)	Random	Parallel arrays
Immunoglobulin deposition	Monoclonal light chain (mostly λ)	Usually polyclonal (mostly IgG_4), occasionally monoclonal (IgGκ)	Usually monoclonal (IgGκ or IgGλ)
Glomerular lesions	Deposits spreading from the mesangium	Mesangial proliferation, membranoproliferative glomerulonephritis, crescentic glomerulonephritis	Atypical membranous nephropathy, membranoproliferative glomerulonephritis
Extrarenal manifestations (fibrillar deposits)	Systemic deposition disease	Pulmonary hemorrhage	Microtubular inclusions in leukemic lymphocytes
Association with lymphoproliferative disorder	Yes (myeloma)	Uncommon	Common (chronic lymphocytic leukemia, nonHodgkin lymphoma) but debated
Renal presentation	Severe nephrotic syndrome, absence of hypertension and hematuria	Nephrotic syndrome with hematuria, hypertension; rapidly progressive glomerulonephritis	Nephrotic syndrome with microhematuria and hypertension
Treatment	Melphalan + prednisolone; blood stem cell autograft	Corticosteroids ± cyclophosphamide (crescentic glomerulonephritis)	Treatment of the associated lymphoproliferative disorder

[a] GOMMID: glomerulopathy with organized microtubular monoclonal immunoglobulin deposits (see text)

Table 29.7 Immunopathologic and clinical characteristics of fibrillary and immunotactoid glomerulopathies.

Reviews[38,39] of all published cases analyzed with antilight chain antibodies have concluded that monotypic deposits occur in 50–80% of patients with immunotactoid glomerulopathy (see Fig. 29.8a,b), with both light-chain isotypes being represented. However, a circulating monoclonal immunoglobulin is detected only in a minority of patients, a finding reminiscent of MIDD. By electron microscopy, the distinguishing morphologic features of immunotactoid glomerulopathy are the presence of organized deposits of large, thick-walled microtubules, usually greater than 30 nm in diameter, at times arranged in parallel arrays (see Fig. 29.8c). A particular form of immunotactoid glomerulopathy termed 'glomerulonephritis with organized microtubular monoclonal immunoglobulin deposits' (GOMMID) has recently been described, often in the setting of chronic lymphocytic leukemia or related lymphoma[39]. Inclusions showing the same microtubular organization and containing the same IgG subclass and light-chain type as the renal deposits are then often detected in the cytoplasm of leukemic lymphocytes.

Mesangial proliferation and aspects of membranoproliferative glomerulonephritis are predominantly reported in series of fibrillary glomerulonephritis. Glomerular crescents are present in about 25% of the biopsy specimens. Immunofluorescence studies mainly show IgG deposits (of the γ_4 isotype in one series) with a predominant mesangial localization. Monotypic deposits containing mostly IgGκ are detected in no more than 15–20% of patients. By electron microscopy, fibrils are randomly arranged and their diameter varies between 12 and 22 nm. Of note, the fibril size alone is not sufficient to distinguish nonamyloidotic fibrillary glomerulonephritis from amyloid.

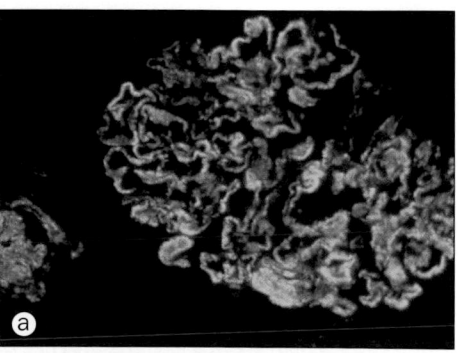 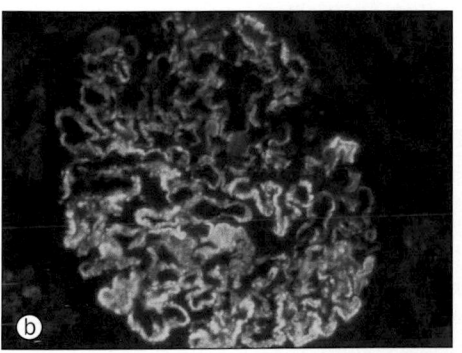 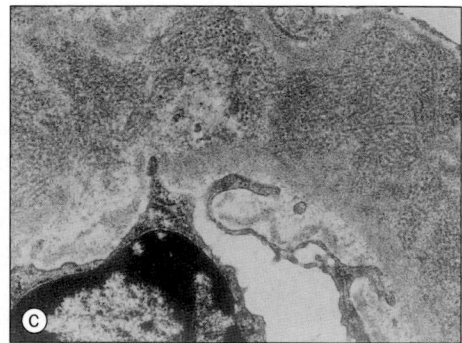

Figure 29.8 Immunotactoid glomerulopathy. (a,b) Atypical membranous nephropathy showing exclusive staining of the deposits with anti-γ (a) and anti-κ (b) antibodies (immunofluorescence, ×312). (c) Electron micrograph of glomerular basement membrane showing microtubular structure of the subepithelial deposits (uranyl acetate and lead citrate, ×12 000). (Courtesy of Dr Béatrice Mougenot.)

Pathogenesis

The cause of fibrillary glomerulonephritis is not known. Fibril formation is thought to be mediated by the deposition of abnormal polyclonal or monoclonal proteins or of immune complexes, which are then able to form either random fibrillary structures or more organized microtubular deposits in the mesangium and along the capillary wall of the glomerulus. The exclusive or prevailing presence of IgG_4 in the immune deposits of patients with fibrillary glomerulonephritis is of great interest. Although not monoclonal, this isotype-restricted homogeneous material made of highly anionic immunoglobulin may facilitate fibril formation. Amyloid P component has also been found in the fibrils. The recent description of fibrillar cryoprecipitates consisting of immunoglobulin–fibronectin complexes in the serum of a patient with fibrillary glomerulonephritis without evidence of systemic disease indicates that serum precursors can lead to the formation of fibrillary deposits.

The mechanisms of immunoglobulin deposition in lymphocytes and kidney of patients with immunotactoid glomerulopathy or GOMMID are also poorly understood. Analysis of monoclonal immunoglobulin both at the protein and mRNA levels has not disclosed size abnormalities in two patients. Whether crystallization in lymphocytes and the glomerulus results from unusual intrinsic physicochemical properties of the monoclonal immunoglobulin or from reactivity with a shared epitope remains to be established. These properties may also account for rapid disappearance of the immunoglobulin from the blood and its recurrence in renal grafts noted in several patients.

Clinical manifestations

The incidence of glomerulopathy with nonamyloid deposition of fibrillary or microtubular material in a nontransplant adult biopsy population is estimated at around 1% (equivalent to that of antiglomerular basement membrane (anti-GBM) disease). Despite a growing number of case reports, it is most likely underestimated because of the insufficient attention given to atypical reactions with histochemical stains for amyloid and the lack of immunoultrastructure studies of most biopsy specimens.

The age range extends from 10 to 80 years with a peak incidence between 40 and 60 years. On average, patients with immunotactoid glomerulopathy are older than those with fibrillary glomerulonephritis. Nonamyloid fibrillary glomerulonephritis occurs with the same frequency in males and females, while the male to female ratio is 2 : 1 in immunotactoid glomerulopathy.

Presenting renal manifestations include proteinuria, mostly in the nephrotic range, microhematuria, and hypertension. Renal insufficiency with rapid progression to ESRD occurs in approximately half of the patients followed for more than 2 years. Rapidly progressive glomerulonephritis is more frequently encountered in fibrillary glomerulonephritis, which seems more prone to superimposition of glomerular crescents.

Immunotactoid glomerulopathy and fibrillary glomerulonephritis differ also on the frequency of their association with plasma cell dyscrasia, which appears more frequently in patients with immunotactoid glomerulopathy. It is, however, difficult to assess precisely from the literature the respective prevalence of monotypic deposits and of circulating monoclonal immunoglobulin in each entity because studies of biopsies with anti-light-chain antibodies were often incomplete, urine and blood data were uncertain, and, even more, patients with dysproteinemias were excluded *a priori* from several series[36].

Although fibril deposition is almost always confined to the kidney, similar fibrillary deposits have been reported in the alveolar capillary membrane in patients presenting with a pulmonary–renal syndrome and in the skin of a patient with a leukocytoclastic skin vasculitis. These observations suggest that the pathologic process may be systemic in nature. Recurrence of fibrillary or immunotactoid glomerulopathies has also been mentioned in patients receiving a renal allograft.

Treatment

Treatment with combined corticosteroids and intravenous cyclophosphamide has achieved variable results in patients presenting with crescentic fibrillary glomerulonephritis. In those with immunotactoid glomerulopathy, especially in the GOMMID subgroup, corticosteroids and/or chemotherapy are associated with partial or complete remission of the nephrotic syndrome, with a parallel improvement of the hematologic disease when present.

Renal transplantation has been performed in only a few patients, and recurrent disease was evident in several of them[40].

GLOMERULAR LESIONS ASSOCIATED WITH WALDENSTRÖM'S MACROGLOBULINEMIA

In Waldenström's macroglobulinemia, symptomatic renal disease is much less common than in multiple myeloma. Glomerulonephritis with intracapillary thrombi of aggregated IgM, considered almost specific for Waldenström's macroglobulinemia, is the most frequent renal morphologic finding, but, it has become a rare entity probably because of the increased efficacy of chemotherapy. It is associated with variable degrees of proteinuria and normal or slightly altered renal function. It is characterized by PAS-positive, Congo red-negative endomembranous deposits that are sometimes so voluminous as to occlude the capillary lumens partially or completely. By immunofluorescence, thrombi and deposits stain with anti-IgM and with anti-κ. Some of these patients have cryoglobulinemia. Others have high amounts of circulating IgM, suggesting that hyperviscosity could favor IgM deposition in glomerular capillaries where ultrafiltration further increases the protein concentration. Treatment by intensive plasma exchange and alkylating agents is then indicated.

Renal amyloidosis, mostly of the AL type, is uncommon but may be found in patients presenting with massive proteinuria. Since renal biopsy may be hazardous in patients with Waldenström's macroglobulinemia, who frequently have increased bleeding time, it is wise to search for amyloid deposits first by a less invasive tissue biopsy.

REFERENCES

1. Glenner GG. Amyloid deposits and amyloidosis: the β-fibrilloses. N Engl J Med. 1980;302:1283–92.
2. Jarrett JT, Lansbury PT Jr. Seeding 'one-dimensional crystallization' of amyloid : a pathogenic mechanism in Alzheimer's disease and scrapie? Cell. 1993;73:1055–8.
3. Khurana R, Gillespie JR, Talapatra A, et al. Partially folded intermediates as critical precursors of light chain amyloid fibrils and amorphous aggregates. Biochemistry. 2001;40:3525–35.
4. Eulitz M, Weiss DT, Solomon A. Immunoglobulin heavy-chain-associated amyloidosis. Proc Natl Acad Sci USA. 1990;87:6542–6.
5. Stevens FJ, Myatt EA, Chong-Hwan C, et al. A molecular model for self-assembly of amyloid fibrils: immunoglobulin light chains. Biochemistry. 1995;34:10697–702.
6. Stevens FJ. Four structural risk factors identify most fibril-forming kappa light chains. Amyloid. 2000;7:200–11.
7. Kim Y-S, Cape SP, Chi E, et al. Counteracting effects of renal solutes on amyloid fibril formation by immunoglobulin light chains. J Biol Chem. 2001;276:1626–33.
8. Comenzo RL, Zhang Y, Martinez C, et al. The tropism of organ involvment in primary systemic amyloidosis: contributions of Ig V_L germ line gene use and clonal plasma cell burden. Blood. 2001;98:714–20.
9. Kyle RA, Gertz MA. Primary systemic amyloidosis: Clinical and laboratory features in 474 cases. Semin Hematol. 1995;32:45–59.
10. Kyle RA, Greipp PR. Amyloidosis (AL): clinical and laboratory features in 229 cases. Mayo Clin Proc. 1983;58:665–83.
11. Perfetti V, Coluccia AML, Intini D, et al. Translocation t(4; 14) (p16.3; q32) is a recurrent genetic lesion in primary amyloidosis. Am J Pathol. 2001;158:1599–603.
12. Kyle RA, Gertz MA, Greipp PR, et al. A trial of three regimens for primary amyloidosis: colchicine alone, melphalan and prednisone, and melphalan, prednisone, and colchicine. N Engl J Med. 1997;336:1202–7.
13. Comenzo RL, Vosburgh E, Falk RH, et al. Dose-intensive melphalan with blood stem cell support for the treatment of AL amyloidosis: one-year follow-up in five patients. Blood. 1996;88:2801–6.
14. Sanchorawala V, Wright DG, Seldin DC, et al. An overview of the use of high-dose melphalan with autologous stem cell transplantation for the treatment of al amyloidosis. Bone Marrow Transplant. 2001;28:637–42.
15. Dispenzieri A, Lacy MQ, Kyle RA, et al. Eligibility for hematopoietic stem-cell transplantation for primary systemic amyloidosis is a favorable prognostic factor for survival. J Clin Oncol. 2001;19:3350–6.
16. Gertz MA, Kyle RA, O'Fallon WM. Dialysis support of patients with primary systemic amyloidosis. A study of 211 patients. Arch Intern Med. 1992;152:2245–50.
17. Browning MJ, Banks RA, Tribe CR, et al. Ten years' experience of an amyloid clinic – a clinicopathological survey. Q J Med. 1985;215:213–27.
18. Gertz MA, Kyle RA. Secondary systemic amyloidosis: response and survival in 64 patients. Medicine (Baltimore). 1991;70:246–56.
19. Dode C, Pecheux C, Cazeneuve C, et al. Mutations in the MEFV gene in a large series of patients with a clinical diagnosis of familial Mediterranean fever. Am J Med Genet. 2000;92:241–6.
20. Gillmore JD, Lovat LB, Persey MR, et al. Amyloid load and clinical outcome in aa amyloidosis in relation to circulating concentration of serum amyloid a protein. Lancet. 2001;358:24–9.
21. Yan SD, Zhu H, Zhu A, et al. Receptor-dependent cell stress and amyloid accumulation in systemic amyloidosis. Nature Med. 2000;6:643–51.
22. Davis DP, Raffen R, Dul JL, et al. Inhibition of amyloid fiber assembly by both BiP and its target peptide. Immunity. 2000;13:433–42.
23. Gianni L, Bellotti V, Gianni AM, Merlini G. New drug therapy of amyloidoses: resorption of AL-type deposits with 4'-iodo-4'-deoxydoxorubicin. Blood. 1995;86:855–61.
24. Hrncic R, Wall J, Wolfenburger DA, et al. Antibody-mediated resolution of light chain-associated amyloid deposits. Am J Pathol. 2000;157:1239–46.
25. Randall RE, Williamson WC Jr, Mullinax F, et al. Manifestations of systemic light chain deposition. Am J Med. 1976;60:293–9.
26. Aucouturier P, Khamlichi AA, Touchard G, et al. Brief report: heavy-chain deposition disease. N Engl J Med. 1993;329:1389–93.
27. Moulin B, Deret S, Mariette X, et al. Nodular glomerulosclerosis with deposition of monoclonal immunoglobulin heavy chains lacking C_H1. J Am Soc Nephrol. 1999;10:519–28.
28. Lin J, Markowitz GS, Valeri AM, et al. Renal monoclonal immunoglobulin deposition disease: The disease spectrum. J Am Soc Nephrol. 2001;12:1482–92.
29. Ronco PM, Alyanakian MA, Mougenot B, Aucouturier P. Light chain deposition disease: a model of glomerulosclerosis defined at the molecular level. J Am Soc Nephrol. 2001;12:1558–65.
30. Solomon A, Weiss DT, Kattine AA. Nephrotoxic potential of Bence Jones proteins. N Engl J Med. 1991;324:1845–51.
31. Khamlichi AA, Aucouturier P, Preud'homme JL, et al. Structure of abnormal heavy chains in human heavy chain deposition disease. Eur J Biochem. 1995;229:54–60.
32. Stokes MB, Holler S, Cui Y, et al. Expression of decorin, biglycan, and collagen type i in human renal fibrosing disease. Kidney Int. 2000;57:487–98.
33. Zhu L, Herrera GA, Murphy-Ullrich JE, et al. Pathogenesis of glomerulosclerosis in light chain deposition disease. Am J Pathol. 1995;147:375–85.
34. Russell W, Cardelli J, Harris E, et al. Monoclonal light chain–mesangial cell interactions: early signaling events and subsequent pathologic effects. Lab Invest. 2001;81:689–703.
35. Heilman RL, Velosa JA, Holley KE, et al. Long-term follow-up and response to chemotherapy in patients with light-chain deposition disease. Am J Kidney Dis. 1992;20:34–41.
36. Korbet SM, Schwartz MM, Lewis EJ. Current concepts in renal pathology. The fibrillary glomerulopathies. Am J Kidney Dis. 1994;23:751–65.
37. Fogo A, Qureshi N, Horn RG. Morphologic and clinical features of fibrillary glomerulonephritis versus immunotactoid glomerulopathy. Am J Kidney Dis. 1993;22:367–77.
38. Alpers CE. Immunotactoid (microtubular) glomerulopathy: an entity distinct from fibrillary glomerulonephritis. Am J Kidney Dis. 1992;19:185–91.
39. Touchard G, Bauwens M, Goujon JM, et al. Glomerulonephritis with organized microtubular monoclonal immunoglobulin deposits. Adv Nephrol. 1994;23:149–75.
40. Pronovost PH, Brady HR, Gunning ME, et al. Clinical features, predictors of disease progression and results of renal transplantation in fibrillary immunotactoid glomerulopathy. Nephrol Dial Transplant. 1996;11:837–42.

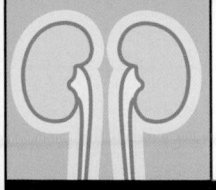
Chapter 30

Other Glomerular Disorders

Richard J Glassock

INTRODUCTION

This chapter will provide a description of several glomerular diseases, not necessarily related to each other. Although uncommon, each must be recognized and differentiated from other more common glomerular disorders in order to plan an appropriate course of therapy, to estimate the prognosis for progression to end-stage renal disease (ESRD), or to determine the risk for a recurrence in the transplanted kidney. Appropriately, emphasis will be placed on diagnosis and management.

MESANGIAL PROLIFERATIVE GLOMERULONEPHRITIS (WITHOUT IgA DEPOSITS)

Mesangial proliferative glomerulonephritis (mesPGN) encompasses a heterogeneous collection of disorders of diverse and largely unknown etiology and pathogenesis that have in common a histologic pattern by light microscopy of glomerular injury characterized by 'mesangial' proliferation (Fig. 30.1)[1–3]. As the name implies, it is noted for a diffuse and global increase in 'mesangial' or axial hypercellularity, often accompanied by an increase in mesangial matrix. Although the mesangial cells may be primarily involved in the proliferative response, other cells that are trafficking through the mesangial regions of the glomerulus but are normally not resident in the glomerulus may also contribute to the hypercellularity of the mesangial regions (e.g., monocytes).

For the purpose of this discussion, other forms of cellular proliferation that occur within the mesangial zones but are more focally and segmentally distributed will not be included. These focal and segmental forms of proliferative GN may be a part of the evolutionary stages of an initially 'pure' mesPGN but they very often signify the presence of systemic disease processes. These processes include systemic lupus erythematosus (SLE), Henoch–Schönlein purpura, infective endocarditis, microscopic polyangiitis, Goodpasture's disease, and IgA nephropathy. These topics are covered in other chapters. Occasionally, a lesion of focal and segmental proliferative GN is discovered in the absence of any recognizable multisystem disease process and in the absence of IgA deposits. Such patients have a clinical presentation, course, and response to treatment that is similar to that described for 'pure' mesangial proliferative GN, but they will not be discussed further in this section.

In 'pure' mesPGN, the peripheral capillary walls are thin and delicate without obvious deposits, reduplication, or necrosis. The visceral and parietal epithelial cells, while occasionally enlarged, have not undergone proliferation. Crescents, necrosis, and segmental sclerosis should be absent in the 'pure' disease. In addition, large deposits staining with periodic acid–Schiff or fuchsin in the mesangium should not be observed. The presence of these deposits suggests IgA nephropathy (see Chapter 24) or lupus nephritis (see Chapter 27), respectively. The tubulo-interstitium and vasculature are usually normal, unless reduced renal function or hypertension is present.

By immunofluorescence microscopy, the heterogeneity of the lesion is dramatically displayed and a variety of patterns is observed (see Table 30.1). Most commonly, diffuse and global IgM and C3 deposits are found scattered throughout the mesangium in a 'granular' pattern (so-called IgM nephropathy), but isolated C3, C1q, or even IgG deposits may also be seen[4]. If IgA is the predominant immunoglobulin deposited, then a diagnosis of IgA nephropathy can be made with confidence. Not uncommonly, no immunoglobulin deposits are found at all.

By electron microscopy, the number of 'mesangial' cells are increased, with an occasional infiltrating monocyte or polymorphonuclear leukocyte. The amount of mesangial matrix is commonly diffusely increased. Electron-dense deposits can be seen in many cases, particularly those with immunoglobulin (IgG, IgM, or IgA) deposits by immunofluorescence microscopy. Large mesangial or paramesangial electron-dense

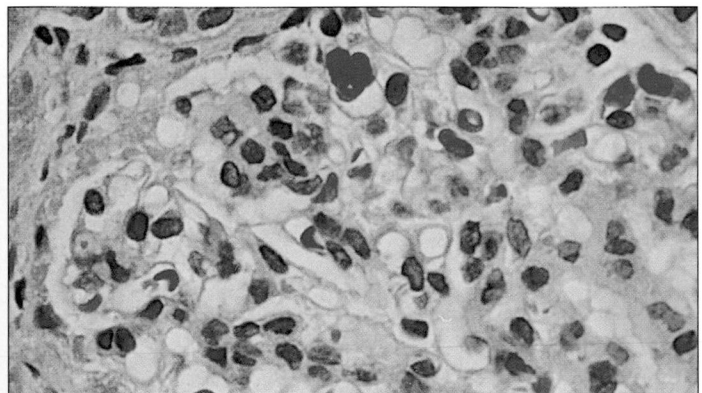

Figure 30.1 'Pure' mesangial proliferative glomerulonephritis. Note the increase in mesangial hypercellularity, the delicate peripheral capillary walls, and the absence of sclerosis or parietal epithelial cell proliferation (hematoxylin–eosin stain ×410). (Adapted with permission from Churg, Bernstein and Glassock[1].)

Immunofluorescence microscopy patterns in mesangial proliferative glomerulonephritis

Pattern	Associated disorders
Predominantly mesangial IgA deposits (± IgM C3)	IgA nephropathy
Predominantly mesangial IgG deposits (± IgM C3)	Often associated with systemic lupus
Predominantly mesangial IgM deposits (± C3)	IgM nephropathy
Mesangial C1q deposits (± IgG, IgM, C3)	C1q nephropathy
Isolated mesangial C3 deposits	Often associated with resolving poststreptococcal glomerulonephritis
Negative for immunoglobulin or complement deposits	'Idiopathic' mesangial proliferative glomerulonephritis

Table 30.1 Immunofluorescence microscopy patterns in mesangial proliferative glomerulonephritis

deposits suggest IgA nephropathy even if immunofluorescence microscopy is not available. Subendothelial and/or subepithelial deposits are not seen. If present, they suggest a postinfectious etiology or underlying lupus nephritis. Large numbers of tubulo-reticular inclusions and deposits of multiple immunoglobulin classes identified by immunofluorescence microscopy also suggest underlying lupus nephritis.

The clinical presentation of mesPGN is varied, although persistent or recurring microscopic or macroscopic hematuria with mild proteinuria is most common. Nephrotic syndrome with heavy proteinuria is a less frequent initial presentation but is seen more frequently in association with diffuse mesangial IgM deposits (IgM nephropathy) or C1q deposits (C1q nephropathy), see below. Pure mesPGN is a rather uncommon lesion (< 5–10%) in patients diagnosed as 'idiopathic' nephrotic syndrome[2,3]. Renal function and blood pressure are usually normal, at least initially. Serologic studies are generally unrewarding. Serum C3 and C4 complement components are normal. Assays for fluorescent antinuclear antibody (ANA), antineutrophil cytoplasmic autoantibody (ANCA), antiglomerular basement membrane (anti-GBM) autoantibody, and cryoimmunoglobulins are negative. Nevertheless, these studies should be performed in most patients to exclude known causes. Mesangial proliferative GN can also be a finding in 'resolving' postinfectious (poststreptococcal) GN. Isolated C3 deposits with scanty immunoglobulin deposits may be seen in this situation.

IgM nephropathy

IgM nephropathy[2] is characterized by diffuse glomerular deposits of IgM often accompanied by C3. Patients may present with hematuria and proteinuria, the latter in the nephrotic range in as many as 50% of patients. Persisting abnormalities and a poor 'response' to glucocorticoids is often seen. The etiology and pathogenesis is unknown.

C1q nephropathy

C1q nephropathy is characterized by diffuse deposits of C1q, often accompanied by IgG, IgM, or both[4]. C3 deposits are

observed less frequently. Nephrotic-range proteinuria, often with hematuria; is observed. Males predominate and African Americans are commonly affected. Serum C3 component and anti-DNA antibodies are normal. The response to treatment is poor and progression to ESRD may occur.

Mesangial proliferative GN associated with minimal change disease

Mesangial proliferative GN may also be a part of the minimal change disease/focal segmental glomerulosclerosis (FSGS) spectrum of lesions (see also Chapter 20). Distinct mesangial hypercellularity superimposed on a lesion of minimal change disease (diffuse foot process effacement) may point to a greater likelihood for glucocorticoid unresponsiveness and evolution to the FSGS lesion.

Natural history of mesangial proliferative GN

The natural history of mesPGN is quite varied, undoubtedly the result of pathogenetic and etiologic heterogeneity. Fortunately, in many patients, a benign course is pursued, especially if hematuria and scant proteinuria (< 1 g/day) are the principal features. Persisting nephrotic syndrome has a less favorable prognosis, and such patients may evolve into FSGS (see Chapter 20) and accompanying progressive renal insufficiency[3].

Treatment of mesangial proliferative GN

The treatment of mesPGN, unaccompanied by other underlying diseases such as SLE or IgA nephropathy, has not been well defined[2,3]. No prospective randomized controlled trials have been performed. As the prognosis for patients with isolated hematuria or hematuria combined with mild proteinuria is generally benign, no treatment other than management of hypertension is needed. For those patients with nephrotic syndrome, with or without impaired renal function, a more aggressive approach is often recommended, especially in the presence of diffuse IgM or C1q deposits, because many such patients will eventually progress to FSGS. As a result, even in the absence of controlled trials, an initial course of glucocorticoid therapy is justified in most patients with nephrotic-range proteinuria (e.g., prednisone 60 mg/day or 120 mg every other day for 2–3 months followed by lowered doses, on an alternate-day regimen, for 2–3 additional months). About 50% of patients so treated will experience a decrease in proteinuria to subnephrotic levels, and occasionally complete remissions will occur. However, relapses of proteinuria are common when glucocorticoids are tapered or discontinued. Such relapsing partially glucocorticoid-responsive patients might benefit from the addition of cyclophosphamide, chlorambucil, or even cyclosporine or mycophenolate mofetil to the regimen, although information on the therapeutic efficacy and safety of these agents in mesangial proliferative GN is quite limited and no randomized, prospective clinical trials have yet been conducted.

Patients with persistent treatment-unresponsive nephrotic syndrome will almost invariably progress to ESRD over a period of several years, often accompanied by the development of superimposed lesions of FSGS. While transplantation is not contraindicated, those patients who do progress to ESRD rapidly and who develop superimposed FSGS may have a high risk of recurrence of proteinuria and FSGS in the transplanted kidney.

GLOMERULONEPHRITIS WITH RHEUMATIC DISEASE

Several 'collagen–vascular' diseases other than SLE, may be complicated by GN (Table 30.2). This section will cover the glomerulonephritides that accompany rheumatoid arthritis, mixed connective tissue disease, dermatomyositis/polymyositis, acute rheumatic fever, scleroderma, and relapsing polychondritis.

Rheumatoid arthritis

A wide variety of glomerular, tubulo-interstitial, and vascular lesions of the kidney may complicate rheumatoid arthritis (Table 30.3). Renal abnormalities including abnormal urinalyses (hematuria, leukocyturia, proteinuria) and reduced renal function are quite common in patients with rheumatoid arthritis, particularly those with severe or long-standing disease. Membranous nephropathy (see Chapter 22) is the most common glomerular lesion encountered. This may be owing to the underlying disease itself or to its therapy (parenteral or oral gold or penicillamine). The presence of HLA-DR3 increases the risk of developing membranous nephropathy in a patient with rheumatoid arthritis, which itself is strongly associated with HLA-DR4.

The course of membranous nephropathy in association with rheumatoid arthritis, in the absence of drugs, is similar to the idiopathic disease, although spontaneous remissions appear to be less likely to occur. By comparison, membranous nephropathy associated with drugs used to treat rheumatoid arthritis is most likely to remit following discontinuance of the drug therapy[6]. Such remissions may take many months to occur. Nevertheless, 60–80% of patients with drug-induced membranous nephropathy in a setting of rheumatoid arthritis will remit within a year of discontinuance of treatment.

Amyloidosis is found in 5–20% of patients with rheumatoid arthritis undergoing renal biopsy. Such amyloidosis has the tinctorial and immunohistochemic properties of AA-amyloid,

and the serum amyloid A-associated protein is greatly increased in rheumatoid arthritis. However, an increase in the serum concentration of serum amyloid-associated protein is not sufficient for the induction of amyloidosis. Other factors, including a genetic predisposition, appear to play a role. Secondary amyloidosis in rheumatoid arthritis may also involve the heart, gastrointestinal tract, and nerves. Nephrotic syndrome and progressive renal failure are common. The use of nonsteroidal anti-inflammatory agents (NSAIDs) may also produce tubulo-interstitial nephritis, minimal change disease, and nephrotic syndrome. A severe, necrotizing polyangiitis may sometimes complicate the course of long-standing rheumatoid arthritis (rheumatoid vasculitis). The patients may have profound reduction in C3 levels, striking elevation of rheumatoid factors and marked polyclonal hypergammaglobulinemia. Renal involvement in rheumatoid vasculitis is relatively uncommon for poorly understood reasons.

Mixed connective tissue disease

Mixed connective tissue disease is characterized by features that overlap between SLE, scleroderma, and polymyositis. Typically, the serum of such patients contains high-titer auto-antibodies to extractable nuclear antigens (ribonucleoprotein-extractable nuclear antigen, U1 ribonucleoprotein antigen). Low titers of anti-double-stranded DNA antibody may also be found. Renal disease, originally thought to be quite rare, is found in 10–50% of patients, most frequently membranous nephropathy and mesangial proliferative GN[5]. Treatment with glucocorticoids is generally quite effective, but some patients may progress to chronic renal insufficiency. Patients with severe glomerulonephritis may respond to treatment regimens similar to those used in the treatment of lupus nephritis (see Chapter 27).

Collagen–vascular (rheumatic) diseases associated with glomerular lesions
Systemic lupus erythematosus
Rheumatoid arthritis
Mixed connective tissue disease
Rheumatic fever
Ankylosing spondylitis
Reiter's syndrome
Dermatomyositis/polymyositis
Scleroderma
Relapsing polychondritis
Systemic or renal limited polyangiitis (see Chapter 26)

Table 30.2 Collagen–vascular (rheumatic) diseases associated with glomerular lesions

Renal disease in rheumatoid arthritis
Glomerular lesions that may be complications of the disease
Membranous nephropathy
Mesangial proliferative GN (± IgA deposits)
Diffuse proliferative GN   Necrotizing and crescentic GN (rheumatoid vasculitis)
Amyloidosis
Glomerular lesions associated with agents used in the treatment of rheumatoid arthritis
Gold: membranous nephropathy, minimal change disease, acute tubular necrosis
Penicillamine: membranous nephropathy, crescentic GN, minimal change disease
Nonsteroidal anti-inflammatory agents: acute interstitial nephritis with minimal change disease, acute tubular necrosis
Cyclosporine: chronic vasculopathy and tubulo-interstitial nephropathy
Methotrexate: acute tubular necrosis
Azathioprine: acute interstitial nephritis

Table 30.3 Renal disease in rheumatoid arthritis

Polymyositis/dermatomyositis

These related 'collagen–vascular' diseases are characterized by inflammatory lesions in muscle, variably by skin lesions, and often include Raynaud's phenomenon. Occasionally, patients develop proteinuria and hematuria secondary to mesangial proliferative GN with IgM deposits. Acute renal failure may rarely supervene when severe muscle injury and myoglobinuria is present. Treatment with glucocorticoids may, at least in part, ameliorate the renal manifestations in concert with improvement in the muscle and skin manifestations.

Acute rheumatic fever

Acute rheumatic fever secondary to a pharyngeal infection with a 'rheumatogenic' strain of group A β-hemolytic streptococci is seldom accompanied by renal disease. Poststreptococcal GN and acute rheumatic fever almost never coexist because of the distinct difference between 'nephritogenic' and 'rheumatogenic' strains of streptococci. In addition, cutaneous streptococcal infections are never associated with acute rheumatic fever sequelae. Nevertheless, on rare occasions, mesangial proliferative GN has been associated with acute rheumatic fever[7]. It usually manifests with hematuria with scant proteinuria and often resolves with appropriate treatment and control of acute rheumatic fever.

Ankylosing spondylitis and Reiter's syndrome (seronegative spondyloarthropathies)

The seronegative spondylo- and oligo-articular arthropathies may from time to time be associated with mesangial IgA deposition. Clinical manifestations are usually mild and nonprogressive. Amyloidosis may complicate ankylosing spondylitis

Scleroderma (systemic sclerosis)

Scleroderma is a heterogeneous disorder of unknown etiology and pathogenesis characterized by uncontrolled expansion of connective tissue in the skin and other visceral organs. There is also a marked tendency to produce vascular thickening and narrowing. Clinical manifestations vary from increased connective tissue in localized patches of skin (morphea) to diffuse and generalized disease (systemic sclerosis). The latter pattern leads to thickening of the skin of the face and hands (telangiectasia), Raynaud's phenomenon, tendon friction rubs, and sclerodactyly. Visceral involvement in the systemic form causes interstitial pulmonary fibrosis, loss of esophageal and other gastrointestinal motility, restrictive cardiomyopathy, and renal disease. Limited forms of the disease (CREST syndrome: calcinosis, Raynaud's phenomenon, esophageal dysmotility, sclerodactyly, and telangiectasia) also occur but are seldom associated with renal disease. The disorder is seen more frequently in females, with an onset usually in young adults. Approximately 90% of patients will have a speckled pattern of fluorescent ANA; 20% will have detectable antibody to topoisomerase I (Scl-70). Anticentromere antibody is associated with the CREST syndrome. Anti-DNA polymerase is associated with a poor prognosis and a high prevalence of renal involvement. Rarely, the visceral abnormalities may occur in the absence of cutaneous lesions (scleroderma *sine* scleroderma).

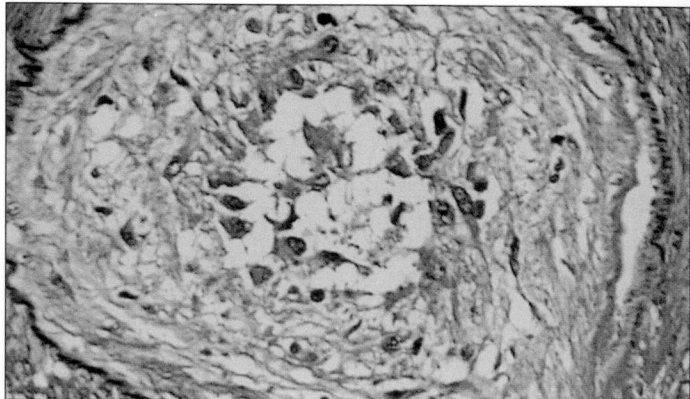

Figure 30.2 Systemic sclerosis. Note the thickening of this interlobular artery with a mucoid 'ground substance'. The internal elastic lamina is well preserved (van Gieson stain ×100). (Adapted with permission from Churg, Bernstein and Glassock[1].)

Renal involvement in scleroderma can be quite varied and may vary from a low-grade proteinuria and slight impairment of glomerular filtration rate (GFR) owing to a mild mesangial proliferative glomerulonephritis, to severe acute renal failure. The latter clinical phenomenon is referred to as scleroderma renal crisis and consists of severe (hyper-reninemic) hypertension, encephalopathy, heart failure, and acute renal failure. There is often an accompanying microangiopathic hemolytic anemia. Occasionally, acute renal failure may develop in the absence of hypertension. This last disease manifestation results from primary involvement of the arcuate and interlobular arteries (Fig. 30.2) and may be superimposed by lesions of malignant hypertension (such as fibrinoid necrosis of the afferent arterioles) and by ischemic glomerular changes such as wrinkling of the capillary wall and thickening of the basal lamina. The prognosis of scleroderma crisis has remarkably improved with the use of angiotensin-converting enzyme (ACE) inhibitors. In one study, ACE inhibitor treatment was associated with better patient survival at one year (75% versus 15%) and with significant preservation or recovery of renal function. Transplantation may be a reasonable treatment option, but progression of disease in other visceral organs may limit life expectancy.

Relapsing polychondritis

Polychondritis is a chronic relapsing disorder characterized by inflammation of cartilage (ear, nose, trachea, costal cartilage) and may be associated with crescentic GN, mesPGN, or membranous nephropathy. Destructive lesions of cartilage may lead to deformities (saddle nose, floppy ears) and the renal disease may be severe and progressive leading to renal failure. Aggressive management of progressive disease with steroids and cytotoxic agents is indicated to control both the systemic and renal manifestations.

GLOMERULONEPHRITIS ASSOCIATED WITH MALIGNANCY

Many malignant disorders and their treatment may be complicated by the development of glomerular lesions[8]. Furthermore, the treatment of glomerular disease with certain agents may give rise to neoplasia. Malignant neoplasms may also be associated with a wide variety of fluid, electrolyte, acid–base, divalent ion, tubulointerstitial, and vascular disorders, including direct invasion of the renal parenchyma by neoplastic cells.

The glomerular lesions commonly observed in association with neoplastic processes are listed in Table 30.4. Membranous nephropathy is the most common lesion. Approximately 7–10% of patients found to have membranous nephropathy by renal biopsy (most often for the evaluation of nephrotic syndrome) will be found to have an underlying malignancy. Most patients are adults over the age of 50; however, because of the rising frequency of malignancy with age, the association between membranous nephropathy and neoplasia may be more apparent than real. Some epidemiologic studies suggest that the prevalence of malignancy is no higher in patients with membranous nephropathy than in aged-matched controls. Notwithstanding these observations, remissions (albeit temporary) can be achieved by surgical removal or chemotherapy of the neoplastic disease, and relapses may develop with recurrence of tumor. Tumor neoantigens or antibodies have rarely been detected within the glomerular deposits, suggesting an immune pathogenesis. In about one third of patients, the neoplastic disorder is already evident before the development of glomerular lesions; in about one third it is discovered concomitantly with the onset of glomerular disease, and in about one third of patients, the neoplastic process is detected after the diagnosis of glomerular disease.

Less-frequent lesions observed in patients with neoplasia include minimal change lesion, FSGS, proliferative GN (including crescentic GN), thrombotic microangiopathy and amyloidosis. Minimal change disease may be associated with lymphoma (particularly Hodgkin's disease) and certain other cancers (pancreas, mesothelioma, prostate). Membranoproliferative GN (MPGN) may be associated with chronic lymphocytic leukemia and lymphoma. FSGS may also occasionally be encountered in patients with underlying malignancy, including leukemia and lymphoma. IgA deposits and crescentic GN may be associated with lung cancer. Vasculitis accompanied by crescentic GN, often resembling Henoch–Schönlein purpura, has been reported to occur with several malignancies, most notably lung cancer.

Systemic amyloidosis (AL type) may affect the kidney and produce nephrotic syndrome and renal failure in 10–15% of patients with multiple myeloma and rarely in association with Waldenström's macroglobulinemia (See Chapter 29). Carcinomas, including renal cell carcinoma, are also rarely complicated by amyloidosis, which is usually of the AA variety.

Thrombotic microangiopathies including hemolytic–uremic syndrome producing renal cortical necrosis or membranoproliferative glomerular lesions may be seen in association with disseminated cancer (carcinoma of the stomach) and mucin-producing carcinomas. It may also appear secondary to treatment with certain antineoplastic agents, especially mitomycin (mitomycin C).

Light-chain nephropathy, in which deposits of either κ or λ light chain are found in the glomerular capillaries and tubular-basement membranes, may occur in association with a variety of neoplastic lymphoproliferative states (see Chapter 29).

Major glomerular lesions associated with neoplastic disease	
Glomerular disease	Commonly associated malignancy
Membranous nephropathy	Gut, breast, and lung cancer
Minimal change disease	Hodgkin's lymphoma, pancreatic cancer, mesothelioma, prostate cancer
Focal segmental sclerosis	Leukemia, lymphoma
Membranoproliferative glomerulonephritis (GN)	Chronic lymphocytic leukemia, lymphoma (some associated with hepatitis C virus)
IgA nephropathy	Lung carcinoma
Crescentic GN/systemic angiitis	Lung carcinoma
Systemic amyloidosis AL type	Multiple myeloma, Waldenström's macroglobulinemia
AA type	Carcinoma (especially renal)
Cryoglobulinemic GN	Chronic lymphocytic leukemia (often hepatitis C associated)
Light chain nephropathy	Lymphoma, myeloma
Fibrillary (immunotactoid) GN	Lymphoma
Hemolytic uremic syndrome	Gastric cancer, mucin-producing cancer

Table 30.4 Major glomerular lesions associated with neoplastic disease

Interferon treatment, used in the management of certain malignancies, may rarely cause minimal change disease in association with interstitial nephritis. Finally, cyclophosphamide therapy of glomerular disease, particularly if prolonged high-dose therapy is involved, may result in a variety of malignancies including leukemias, B-cell lymphomas, and bladder cancers. Azathioprine increases the risk for papilloma virus associated-squamous cell carcinoma of the cervix and/or vulva.

CONGENITAL NEPHROTIC SYNDROME

According to the common usage of the term 'congenital' nephrotic syndrome, this disorder is defined as the presence of nephrotic syndrome at the time of birth or the discovery of nephrotic syndrome in infants less than 3 months of age. As such, congenital nephrotic syndrome can arise consequent to a number of disorders (Table 30.5).

Classic Finnish-type congenital nephrotic syndrome
The Finnish type of congenital nephrotic syndrome is the most common form, seen in about 1.2 per 10 000 live births in Finland. Congenital nephrotic syndrome is also observed in families of non-Finnish extraction. The Finnish form is an autosomal recessive disorder due to mutation of NHPS1 that codes for nephrin, a critical protein component of the slit-pore diaphragm of the visceral glomerular epithelial cell[9]. Loss of nephrin leads to increased glomerular permeability to plasma protein, chiefly albumin, and to marked visceral epithelial cell foot process effacement.

Causes of congenital nephrotic syndrome
'Classic' Finnish type
Diffuse mesangial sclerosis
With pseudohermaphroditism (Drash syndrome)
With microcephaly (Galloway–Mowat syndrome)
Idiopathic
Idiopathic (primary) focal and segmental glomerulosclerosis
Genetic disorders
Lowe's syndrome
Mucopolysaccharidoses
Nail–patella syndrome
Sialic acid storage disease
Congenital infections
Cytomegalovirus
Syphilis
Rubella
Toxoplasmosis
Hepatitis B

Table 30.5 Causes of congenital nephrotic syndrome

Children with the Finnish type of congenital nephrotic syndrome are born prematurely and often have a very large placenta. Such a placenta may give rise to a difficult delivery. Raised levels of α-fetoprotein occur in the amniotic fluid and are sometimes also observed in maternal plasma, which may be an indication of the development of congenital nephrotic syndrome *in utero*. These observations may lead to the consideration of early termination of pregnancy.

Children with congenital nephrotic syndrome may be markedly edematous at birth or develop severe anasarca within a few days of delivery. Ascites, delayed development, severe erythrocytosis, and spontaneous vascular thromboses are also common. Pathologically diffuse foot process effacement and cystic dilatations of the proximal tubule accompanied by mesangial sclerosis are commonly seen (see Fig. 30.3). Later, diffuse mesangial sclerosis is the most common pathology. The permeability abnormality due to nephrin deficiency responsible for the Finnish type of congenital nephrotic syndrome may cause alterations in podocyte attachment to the GBM leading to progressive capillary sclerosis.

Children with classic Finnish-type congenital nephrotic syndrome usually develop progressive renal failure within the first year of life. Aggressive therapy (see below) may permit some infants to survive long enough to receive a successful renal transplant. Other than transplantation, no treatments are effective. Interestingly, the disease may recur in the transplanted kidney in about 25% of patients, which has recently been shown to be mediated by an immune response to the nephrin in the normal transplanted kidney (similar to the situation in Alport syndrome; see Chapter 48).

Drash syndrome

Diffuse mesangial sclerosis and male pseudohermaphroditism (Drash syndrome) is a relatively uncommon cause of nephrotic

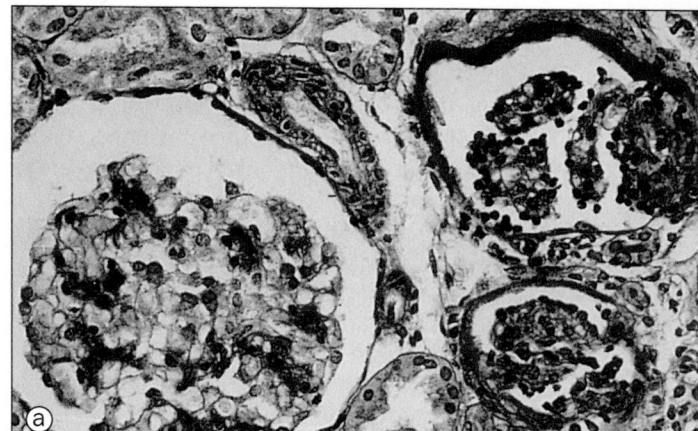

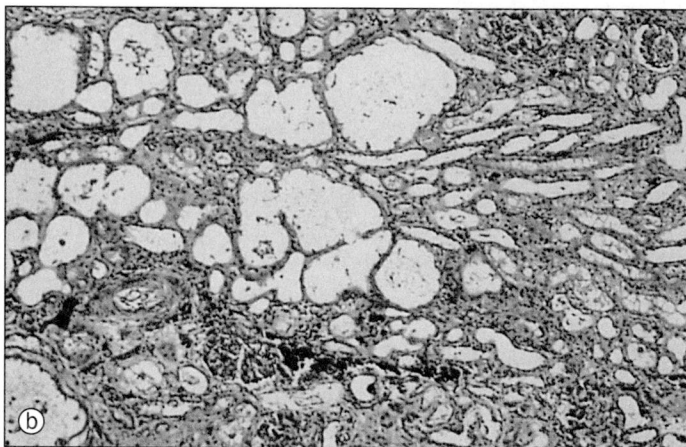

Figure 30.3 Congenital nephrotic syndrome Finnish type. (a) Diffuse mesangial thickening and partially collapsed glomeruli (periodic acid–Schiff ×260). (b) Microcystic dilatation of the tubules (hematoxylin–eosin stain ×150). (Adapted with permission from Churg, Bernstein and Glassock[1].)

syndrome in infants. Such patients have a high frequency of developing Wilms' tumors. Karyotyping will detect the abnormality in phenotypic females. The mutation responsible is on the Wilms' tumor suppressor gene (*WT-1*). The nephropathy almost invariably evokes progressive renal failure, and bilateral nephrectomies must be performed prior to renal transplantation to avoid the emergence of Wilms' tumor. There is no effective treatment. Diffuse mesangial sclerosis may also occur in the absence of systemic or developmental abnormalities. This 'idiopathic' form behaves in a similar fashion to the form associated with pseudohermaphroditism.

Galloway–Mowat syndrome

Galloway–Mowat syndrome is an autosomal recessive disorder that includes microcephaly, developmental retardation, seizures, hiatal hernia, and renal disease. The GBM abnormalities are similar to those found in the nail–patella syndrome (see Chapter 48). No treatment is successful and nearly all patients progress to ESRD within 3–5 years.

Infection-related congenital nephrotic syndrome

Several congenital infections may be associated with the development of nephrotic syndrome in early infancy. Most important among these infections are congenital syphilis and cytomegalovirus infection. Renal biopsy shows membranous nephropathy or proliferative GN, sometimes with immune deposits containing the microbial antigen. Treatment of the basic disease with appropriate antimicrobials or antiviral agents will often result in improvement.

Rare causes of congenital nephrotic syndrome
Recently an autosomal recessive steroid-resistant nephrotic syndrome has been associated with mutations in *NHPS2* which codes podocin. Mutations in *ACTN4* which codes the cytoplasmic protein, α-actinin 4, have been associated with a familial focal segmental glomerulosclerosis. Both of these mutations target podocyte proteins and likely alter podocyte function. A case of congenital membranous nephropathy has also been described in which antibodies to a podocyte antigen, neutral endopeptidase, were transferred by the mother (who lacked this antigen and was sensitized by the baby) to the baby during birth.

Management of nephrotic syndrome in infancy
In the past, most children with congenital nephrotic syndrome died within the first 6 months of life. However, increased survival is being observed with an aggressive regimen of daily intravenous albumin, early use of oral or intravenous diuretics, the use of ACE inhibitors or angiotensin receptor antagonists (the latter less effective in Finnish-type congenital nephrotic syndrome), as well as vitamin D supplements (along with magnesium and calcium), thyroxine replacement, anticoagulants (heparin and warfarin) and antibiotics (as indicated).

When severe nephrotic syndrome supervenes that produces a serious threat to the patient's life (from profound protein malnutrition), medical nephrectomy can be considered. This consists of high doses of ACE inhibitor plus high doses of an NSAID, such as indomethacin. However, if this approach is not successful, bilateral nephrectomy between 6 and 10 months of age with the institution of peritoneal dialysis could be attempted until the child reaches a size and weight (usually 8–9 kg) when renal transplantation can be performed.

OTHER UNCOMMON DISORDERS

Lipoprotein glomerulopathy
Lipoprotein glomerulopathy is believed to be caused by an abnormality in lipoprotein metabolism[10,11] and is characterized by extensive deposits of apolipoprotein E in the glomeruli, leading to greatly expanded capillaries filled with pale-staining mesh-like substance (Fig. 30.4). Clinically, heavy proteinuria with nephrotic syndrome may be present. Apolipoprotein E levels are increased in plasma in association with a type III hyperlipoproteinemia. The apolipoprotein E usually shows a heterozygous E2/E3 or E2/E4 phenotype, but homozygosity for apolipoprotein E2 has also been observed. Homozygous apolipoprotein E2 is also seen in familial type III hyperlipoproteinemia. Low LDL receptor binding and high heparin affinity may explain some of the pathogenetic processes in lipoprotein glomerulopathy. There are no apparent systemic manifestations. Familial cases have suggested a

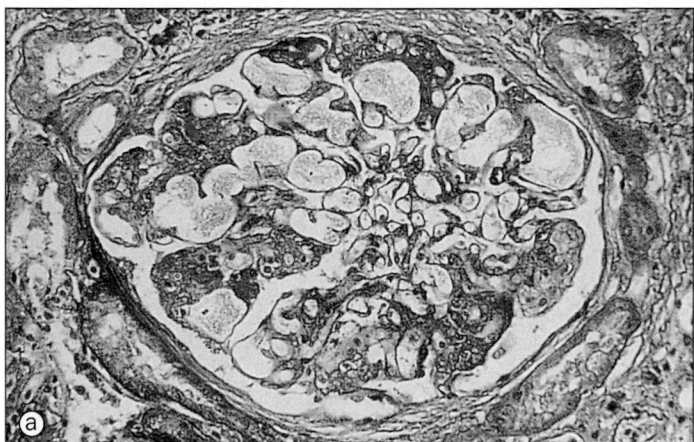

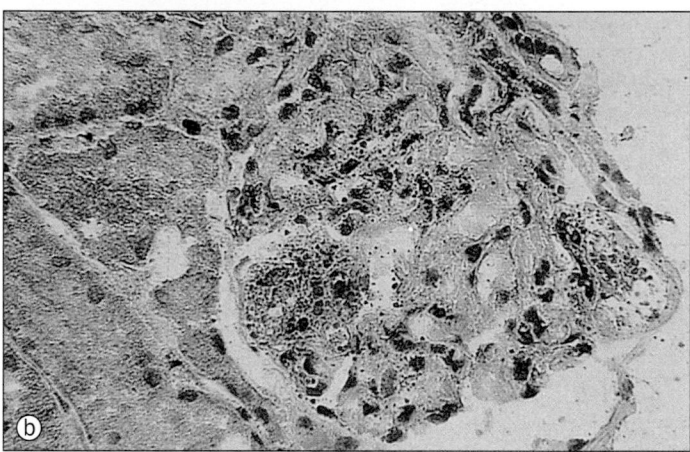

Figure 30.4 Lipoprotein glomerulopathy. (a) Dilated capillary lumina containing a pale-stained, mesh-like or granular substance (trichrome stain ×260). (b) The granules stain positively with oil red O and antilipoprotein E antisera. (oil red O ×260). (Adapted with permission from Churg, Bernstein and Glassock[1].)

hereditary abnormality. The disorder may recur in the renal transplant. Treatment is generally ineffective.

Lecithin cholesterol acyl transferase deficiency
Lecithin cholesterol acyl transferase (LCAT) deficiency is an autosomal recessive disorder. The genetic defect is located on chromosome 16q22. The clinical characteristics include corneal opacities (misty deposits), normocytic, normochromic anemia, premature atherosclerosis, and elevated low-density lipoproteins. Proteinuria (including the nephrotic syndrome), hypertension, and progressive renal failure are the main renal manifestations. By light microscopy, the glomeruli reveal foam cells, intimal hyperplasia, and thickening of the basement membrane with effacement of the foot processes (Fig. 30.5). Progressive renal failure is the rule; however, it is of slow and insidious onset and is usually first detected by the fourth decade of life. Treatment is generally ineffective.

Collagen III glomerulopathy
Collagen III glomerulopathy is a newly-described form that may be a *forme fruste* of nail–patella syndrome (see Chapter 48) since the glomerular abnormalities are similar[12].

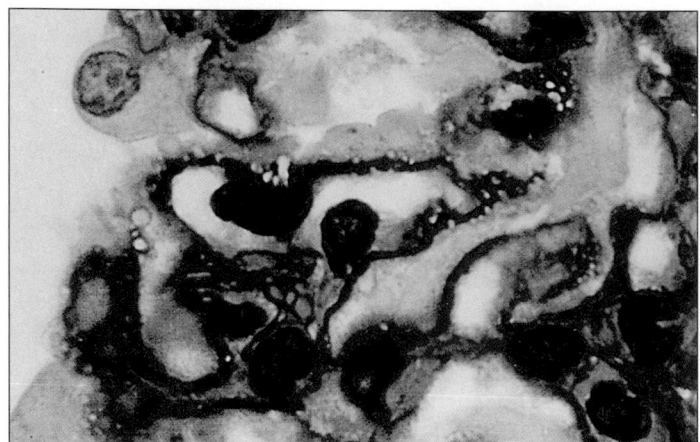

Figure 30.5 Lecithin cholesterol acyl transferase deficiency. Note the irregular thickened glomerular capillary walls containing clear vacuoles, which are characteristic of the lesion (periodic acid–Schiff ×1000). (Adapted with permission from Churg, Bernstein and Glassock[1].)

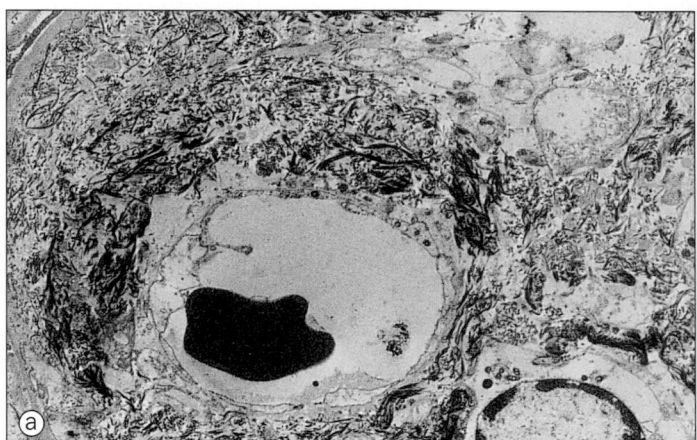

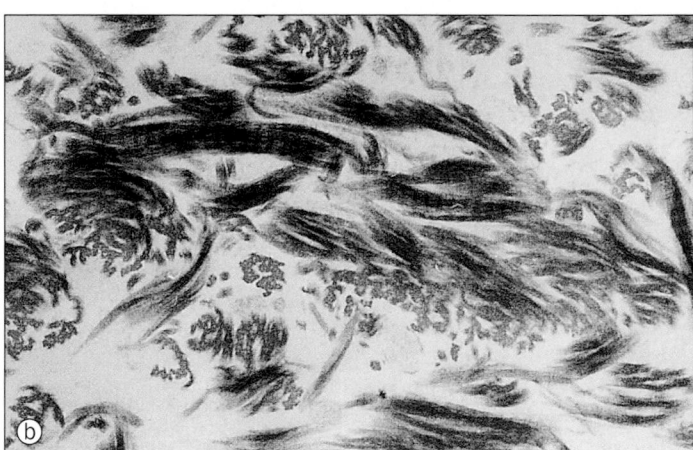

Figure 30.6 Electron microscopy of collagen III glomerulopathy (collagenofibrotic glomerulopathy). (a) Fine fibrils occur in the mesangial and subendothelial areas (×3000). (b) These fibrils are randomly oriented with typical periodicity and average 30 nm in diameter. The fibrils are strongly positive for staining with periodic acid–Schiff stain and react with anticollagen III antibodies (×15 000). (Adapted with permission from Churg, Bernstein and Glassock[1].)

Nevertheless, patients with collagen III glomerulopathy lack the typical skeletal abnormalities observed in the nail–patella syndrome. An autosomal recessive pattern is observed in pediatric patients. Clinically, patients present with proteinuria and slowly progressive renal failure. Patients may be of any age but males predominate. By light microscopy, the glomeruli are enlarged with a marked expansion of the mesangial matrix (Fig. 30.6). Conventional immunofluorescence microscopy is negative but antisera to collagen type III will strongly react with the glomerular deposits. Electron microscopy shows bundles of irregularly arranged fibrillar deposits (Congo-red negative) with periodicity characteristic of collagen. No treatment is effective and there are no data on recurrent disease.

Fibronectin glomerulopathy

Fibronectin glomerulopathy is a rare autosomal dominant fibrillary glomerular disease with onset usually in early adolescence with proteinuria, microhematuria, hypertension, and slowly progressive renal failure[13]. Most patients reach ESRD between the second and the sixth decade of life. The renal pathology usually reveals an enlarged, hyperlobular, and normocellular glomerulus with a homogeneous material (by periodic acid–Schiff stain) in the mesangium and subendothelium (Congo-red negative). Electron microscopy shows granular osmiophilic deposits, occasionally with scattered fibrils. Immunofluorescence is negative for antibody and complement components but will stain brightly using an antifibronectin antibody. The pathogenesis of the disease is unknown, although mice 'knocked out' for uteroglobin develop a similar lesion. However, preliminary studies in humans have not documented any linkage to the uteroglobulin gene but rather have tentatively localized the gene to chromosome locus 1q32. There is no known treatment.

Nephropathic cystinosis

Late-onset cystinosis is a variant of cystinosis in which the mutations in the *CTNS* gene result in a milder phenotype. These patients may present with glomerular disease during the teenage years. Nephrotic syndrome may occur and the glomerular lesions resemble FSGS except that crystals of cystine are found in glomerular and tubular epithelial cells[14]. Patients with cystinosis may also have blonde hair, photophobia, hypothyroidism, corneal deposits, rickets, and Fanconi syndrome (see also Chapter 50).

Miscellaneous storage diseases and other unusual lesions

A variety of diseases associated with storage of abdominal lipids or carbohydrates in tissue may provoke glomerular lesions; these include Hurler's syndrome (type I mucopolysaccharidoses), von Gierke disease (glycogen storage disease), Gaucher's disease, Refsum's disease, nephrosialidosis, and I-cell disease (mucolipidosis type II). Juvenile malabsorption of vitamin B_{12} with megaloblastic anemia (Imerslund syndrome) can be associated with glomerular proteinuria. Asphyxiating thoracic dystrophy (Jeune's syndrome) is associated with glomerular, tubular, and interstitial abnormalities. Hereditary osteolysis causing arthralgias and deformities of wrists and ankles can be accompanied by chronic GN. The nail–patella syndrome and Fabry disease are discussed in Chapter 48.

REFERENCES

1. Churg J, Bernstein J, Glassock R, eds. Renal disease: classification and atlas of glomerular disease. New York: Igaku-Shoin;1995:93.
2. Cohen AH, Border WA, Glassock R. Nephrotic syndrome with glomerular mesangial IgM deposits. Lab Invest. 1978;38:610–19.
3. Alexopoulos E, Papagianni A, Stangou M, et al. Adult onset idiopathic nephrotic syndrome associated with pure diffuse mesangial hypercellularity. Nephrol Dial Transpl. 2000;15:981–7.
4. Jennette C, Falk R. C1q nephropathy. In: Massry S, Glassock R, eds. Textbook of nephrology, 3rd edn. Baltimore, MD: Williams & Wilkins;1995:749–52.
5. Cohen IM, Swerdlin AHR, Steenberg S, Stone RA. Mesangial proliferative GN in mixed connective tissue disease. Clin Nephrol. 1980; 13:93–6.
6. Samuels B, Lee JC, Engleman EP, Hopper J. Membranous nephropathy in patients with rheumatoid arthritis: relationship to gold therapy. Medicine (Baltimore). 1978;57:319–27.
7. Whelton A. Nephrotoxicity of nonsteroidal anti-inflammatory drugs: physiological functions and clinical implications. Am J Med. 1999;106:13S–24S.
8. Geirsson AJ, Sturfelt G, Truedsson L. Clinical and serological features of severe vasculitis in rheumatoid arthritis: prognostic implications. Ann Rheum Dis. 1987;46:727–33.
9. Valenzuela OF, Reiser W, Porush JG. Idiopathic polymyositis and glomerulonephritis. J Nephrol. 2001;14:120–4.
10. Gibney R, Reinecke H, Bannayan G, Stein J. Renal lesions in rheumatic fever. Ann Intern Med. 1981;94:322–6.
11. Steen VD, Constantino JP, Shapiro AP, Medsger TA. Outcome of renal crisis in systemic sclerosis: relation to availability of angiotensin converting enzyme inhibitors. Ann Intern Med. 1991;114:249–50.
12. Alpers CE, Cotran RS. Neoplasia and glomerular injury. Kidney Int. 1986;30:465–73.
13. Penn I. Cancers in cyclosporine-treated versus azathioprine-treated patients. Transpl Proc. 1996;28:876–8.
14. Tryggvason, K. Unraveling the mechanism of glomerular ultrafiltration: Nephrin, a key component of the slit diaphragm. J Am Soc Nephrol. 1999;10:2440–5.
15. Patrakka J, Rhotsalainen V, Reponen P, et al. Recurrence of nephrotic syndrome in kidney grafts of patients with congenital nephrotic syndrome of the Finnish type: role of nephrin. Transplantation. 2002;73: 394–403.
16. Boute N, Gribouval O, Roselli S, et al. NHPS2, encoding the glomerular protein, podocin, is mutated in autosomal recessive steroid-resistant nephrotic syndrome. Nat Genet. 2000;24: 349–54.
17. Kaplan JM, Kim SH, North KN, et al. Mutations in ACTN4, encoding alpha-actinin-4, cause familial focal segmental glomerulosclerosis. Nat Genet. 2000;24:251–6.
18. Debiec H, Guigonis V, Mougenot B, et al. Antenatal membranous glomerulonephritis due to anti-neutral endopeptidase (NEP) antibodies. N Engl J Med. 2002;346:2053–60.
19. Savage JM, Jefferson JA, Maxwell AP, et al. Improved prognosis for congenital nephrotic syndrome of the Finnish type in Irish families. Arch Dis Child. 1999;80(5):466–9.
20. Saito T, Oikawa S, Sato H, et al. Lipoprotien glomerulopathy: Renal lipoidosis induced by novel apolipoprotein E variants. Nephron. 1999;83:193–201.
21. Ikeda K, Yokayama H, Tomosugi N, et al. Primary glomerular fibrosis: a new nephropathy caused by diffuse intraglomerular increase in atypical collagen III fibers. Clin Nephrol. 1990;33:155–9.
22. Strømf EH, Banfi G, Krapg R, et al. Glomerulopathy associated with predominant fibronectin deposits: a newly recognized hereditary disease. Kidney Int. 1995;48:163–70.
23. Pabico RC, Panner BJ, McKenna BA, Bryson MF. Glomerular lesions in patients with late onset cystinosis with massive proteinuria. Renal Physiol. 1980;3:347–54.

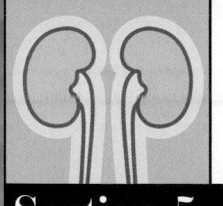

Chapter 31

Thrombotic Microangiopathies including Hemolytic–Uremic Syndrome

Roberto Pisoni, Piero Ruggenenti, and Giuseppe Remuzz

DEFINITION

Thrombotic microangiopathy (TMA) is characterized by an acute syndrome of microangiopathic hemolytic anemia, thrombocytopenia, and variable signs of organ injury due to platelet thrombosis in the microcirculation[1]. Depending on the distribution of the lesions – kidney or central nervous system – two pathologically identical but clinically distinct entities are described: hemolytic–uremic syndrome (HUS) and thrombotic thrombocytopenic purpura (TTP). The former usually affects young children, and is characterized by acute renal failure (ARF), and absent or minimal neurologic abnormalities. The latter occurs in adults, and is characterized by severe neurologic involvement in most cases, and variable renal involvement. In some patients, features of HUS and TTP may coexist and the disease is defined as HUS/TTP. The mechanisms behind the different organ involvement of TMA are not clearly understood.

PATHOGENESIS

Injury to the endothelium is an important and likely inciting factor of the events leading to microvascular thrombosis. This is suggested by data showing that most agents associated with TMA such as exotoxins, endotoxins, autoantibodies, immune-complexes, and certain drugs are toxic to endothelial cells.

Shiga toxin

Shiga toxins (Stx or verotoxins), named for their similarity to one of the *Shigella dysenteriae* type 1 bacteria, have a direct role in the pathogenesis of most cases of childhood HUS. They are released by certain strains of *Escherichia coli* (particularly O157:H7 serotype) and other bacteria. After oral ingestion of contaminated food or water, *E. coli* reaches the gut, closely binds to the gastrointestinal mucosa, and causes cell death. In non-Stx producing *E. coli* strains, this normally results in non-bloody diarrhea. Strains producing large amount of Stx may damage the mucosal vasculature, causing hemorrhagic colitis. Once the toxin reaches the systemic circulation, microvascular damage develops at target organs, giving rise to the clinical manifestations of HUS or, less frequently, TTP. Stx consists of a single subunit (A) that accounts for the cytotoxic effect, by inhibiting cellular protein synthesis and pentamers of subunit (B) that bind to specific glycolipid (Gb3) receptors on the cell surface, determining tissue specificity. It is suggested that in humans, the different organ involvement may reflect a different distribution of these receptors, which may vary with age. The microangiopathic process is then sustained and amplified by leukocyte adhesion to the injured endothelium, complement consumption, abnormal von Willebrand factor (vWf) release and fragmentation, and increased shear stress. A hypothetical pathway contributing to endothelial injury is shown in Figure 31.1. Endothelial injury induces subendothelial widening of the glomerular capillary wall due to the deposition of fibrin-like material, and myointimal proliferation, followed by narrowing or occlusion of the vascular lumen. In the narrowed lumen, blood flow becomes turbulent. Increased shear stress alters the processing of vWf multimers, which normally circulate in a coiled form, and induces platelet activation. Uncoiled vWf multimers become exposed to circulating proteases, with consequent abnormal fragmentation. vWf fragments bind activated platelets and contribute to further platelet activation and thrombi formation. Shear stress also influences endothelial nitric oxide synthesis and release, thus amplifying leukocyte activation.

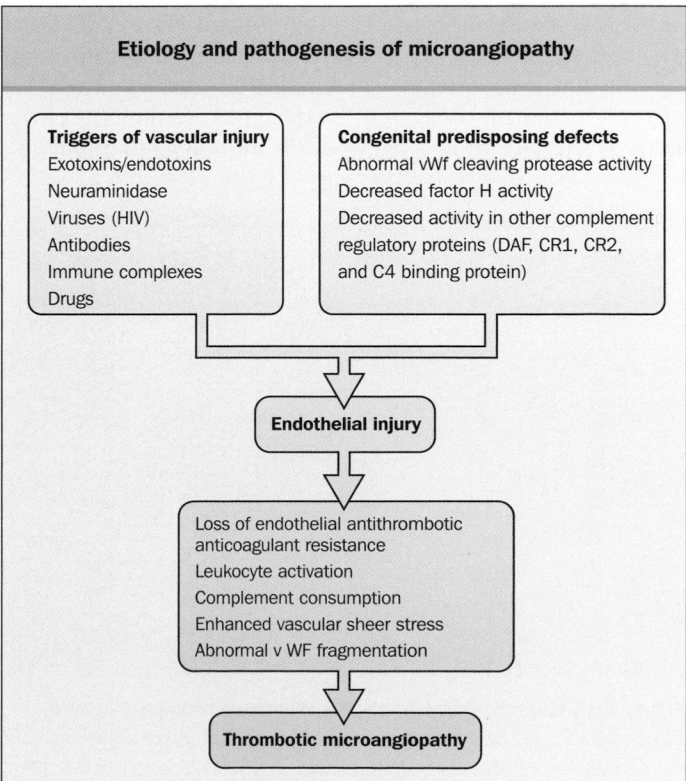

Figure 31.1 A suggested sequence of events leading to TMA in predisposed subjects exposed to triggers of endothelial injury.

Deficiency of vWf protease activity

Recent studies suggest that most patients with TTP have a specific pathogenetic defect characterized by inability to cleave unusually large vWf (ULvWf). Normally, ULvWf multimers are synthetized in endothelial cells, and rapidly degraded by a specific protease as soon as they are secreted in the circulation[2]. ULvWf multimers accumulate in patients with TTP and can attach to activated platelets, promoting their aggregation. This defect is due to inhibition (in idiopathic forms) or congenital absence (in familiar forms) of a specific circulating metalloprotease[3-5]. An inhibitory autoantibody, an IgG molecule that blocks the vWf-cleaving protease, has been found in a high percentage of patients with acute idiopathic, recurrent and ticlopidine/clopidogrel associated TTP. The congenital defect is inherited as an autosomal recessive trait and the gene encoding the protease, *ADAMTS13*, has been recently identified and cloned[6]. However, a deficiency of vWf-cleaving protease activity is not specific for TTP as it has been noted, although the reduction is less pronounced, in normal subjects and in diseases such as disseminated intravascular coagulation (DIC), idiopathic thrombocytopenic purpura, infection, acute inflammatory states, systemic lupus erythematosus (SLE), and malignancy[7].

Factor H abnormalities

Intrinsic abnormalities of the complement system may account for a genetic predisposition to the disease. Abnormalities in factor H, a plasma protein that inhibits the activation of the alternative pathway of complement, has been detected in several familial cases of TMA but also in patients with no familial history[8]. About 20 mutations, all heterozygous, have been found in factor H gene[9,10]. Since mutant factor H is functionally inactive but normally secreted, and as not all patients have a persistent reduction in complement C3, the diagnosis of factor H-related HUS cannot be excluded just on the basis of normal C3 and factor H serum concentrations. It is unclear how a deficiency in complement regulatory proteins may predispose to TMA. It is possible that the mutation is a predisposing factor and that an environmental insult (i.e., infection) then precipitates the disease; however, polymorphisms in other genes might be required to determine the HUS phenotype.

PATHOLOGY

The histologic lesions of TMA consists of vessel (capillaries and arterioles) wall widening on electron microscopy, with swelling and detachment of the endothelial cells from the basement membrane and the accumulation of fluffy material in the subendothelium (Fig. 31.2); intraluminal platelet thrombosis; and partial or complete obstruction of vessel lumina (Fig. 31.3). These lesions are similar to those seen in other renal diseases such as scleroderma, malignant nephrosclerosis, chronic transplant rejection, and calcineurin inhibitor nephrotoxicity[1]. In HUS, microthrombi are present primarily in the kidneys, while in TTP they mainly involve the brain. Thrombi may repeatedly form and resolve, producing intermittent neurologic deficits. In pediatric patients, particularly in those younger than 2 years of age, and in those with Stx-associated HUS, the glomerular injury is predominant (Figs 31.4 and 31.5). Thrombi and infiltration by leukocytes are common in the early phases of the disease and usually resolve after 2–3 weeks. Patchy cortical necrosis may be present in severe cases; crescent formation is uncommon. In idiopathic and familial forms, and in adults, the injury mostly involves arteries and arterioles (Fig. 31.6) with secondary glomerular ischemia and retraction of the glomerular tuft (Fig. 31.7). The prognosis is good in the patients with predominant glomerular involvement but it is more severe in those with predominant preglomerular injury. Focal segmental glomerulosclerosis may be a long-term sequela of acute cases of HUS and is usually seen in children with long-lasting hypertension and progressive chronic renal function deterioration.

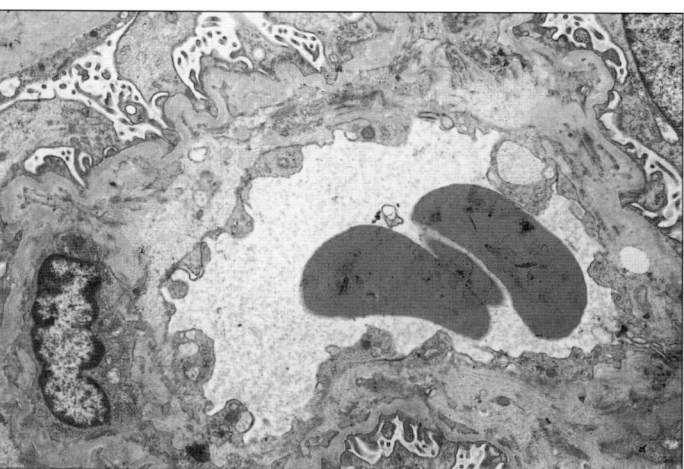

Figure 31.2 Electron micrograph of a glomerular capillary in HUS. The endothelium is detached from the glomerular basement membrane; the subendothelial space is widened and occupied by electron-lucent fluffy material and cell debris. Beneath the endothelium is a thin layer of newly formed glomerular basement membrane.

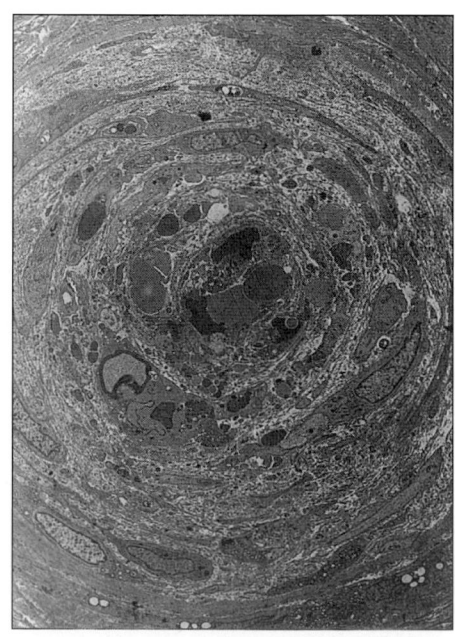

Figure 31.3 Electron micrograph of a renal arteriole in HUS. The vascular lumen is completely occluded by thrombi. There is marked intimal edema with consequent separation of myointimal cells.

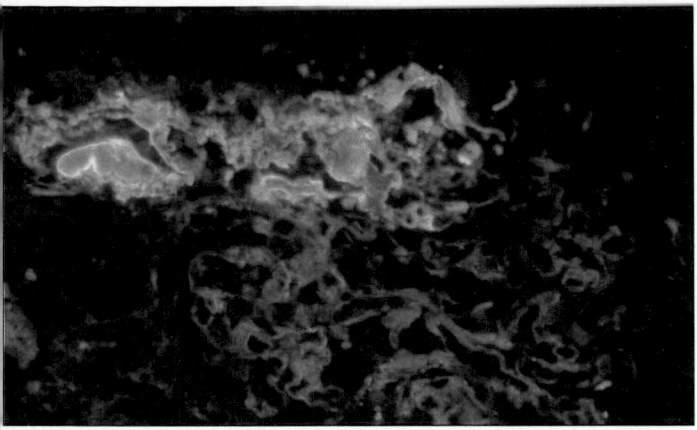

Figure 31.4 Glomerulus with its vascular pole from a patient with Stx-associated HUS. Strong staining with fluorescein-labeled antifibrinogen serum occurs in the glomerulus and in the arteriolar wall.

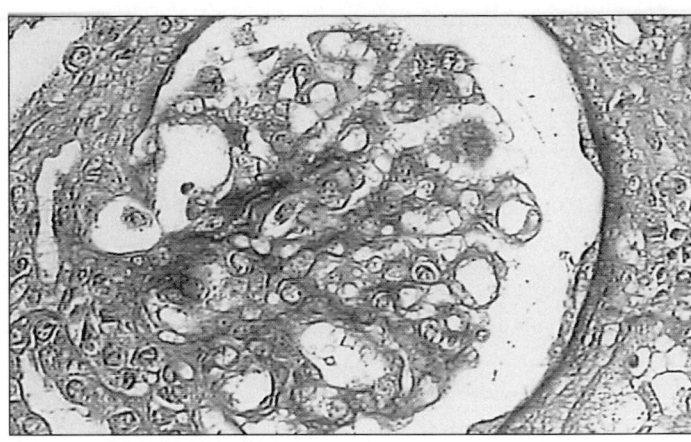

Figure 31.5 Glomerulus from a patient with Stx-associated HUS. A marked thickening of the glomerular capillary wall occurs with many double contours.

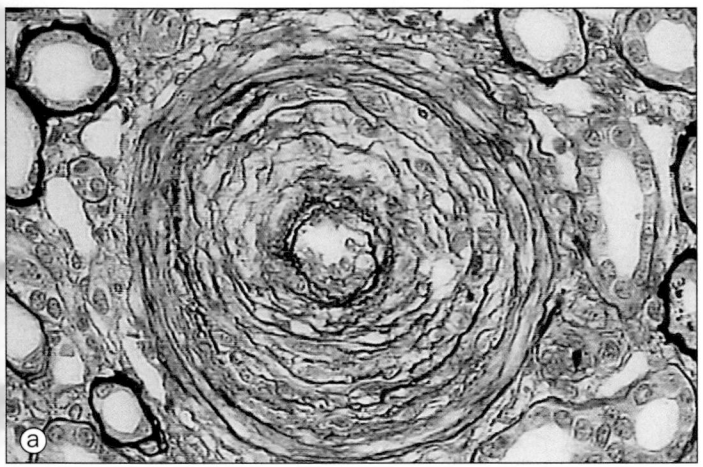

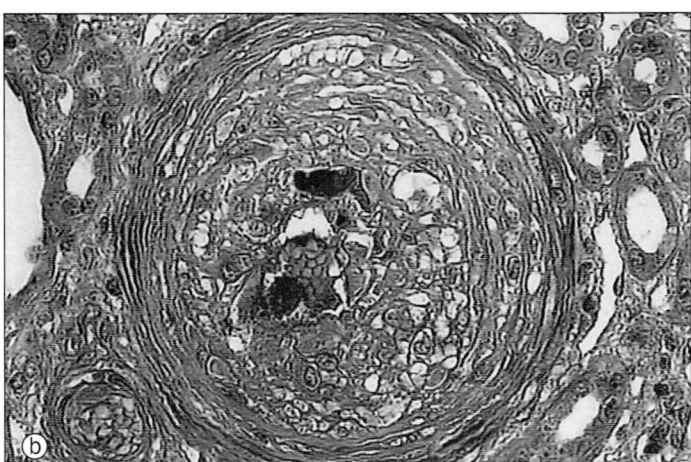

Figure 31.6 Interlobular artery in a case of HUS with severe vascular involvement. (a) The vascular lumen is almost completely occluded. Changes include myointimal proliferation and reduplication of the lamina elastica. (b) Thrombotic material and erythrocytes can be seen in the lumen and erythrocytes can be seen within the vascular wall.

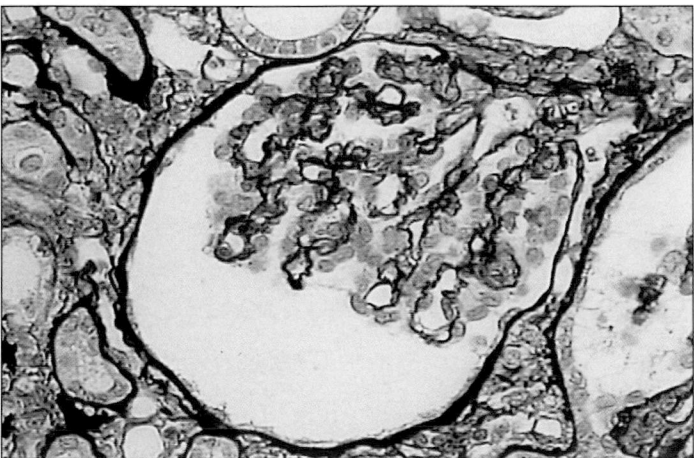

Figure 31.7 Glomerulus from a patient with atypical HUS with predominant vascular involvement. Severe ischemic changes have occurred. Note the shrinkage of the glomerular tuft and marked thickening and wrinkling of the capillary wall.

Clinical and laboratory findings

TMA is characterized by thrombocytopenia, often with purpura, but rarely with severe bleeding; microangiopathic hemolytic anemia; ARF that may be associated with anuria; neurologic deficits; and fever. Thrombocytopenia and hemolytic anemia are the key laboratory abnormalities. Thrombocytopenia is caused by platelet aggregation in the microcirculation while hemolytic anemia is due to mechanical fragmentation of erythrocyte during their passage through the narrowed vessels. Thrombocytopenia is usually more severe in TTP than in HUS. At the onset of TTP, platelet count may be below 20×10^9 cells/L. In HUS, values between 30×10^9 and 100×10^9 cells/L are frequent; however, normal values may also be detected. Anemia is usually severe with hemoglobin concentration less than 6.5 mg/dL in about 40% of cases. Hyperbilirubinemia (mainly indirect), reticulocytosis, circulating free hemoglobin, and low haptoglobin levels may be present. The serum lactate dehydrogenase (LDH) level is extremely high, reflecting hemolysis but also, in some

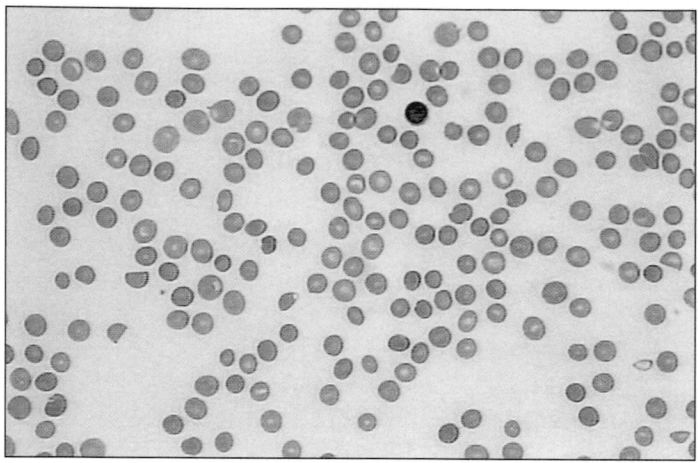

Figure 31.8 Peripheral blood smear from a patient with HUS. The presence of fragmented red blood cells with the appearance of a helmet is pathognomonic for microangiopathic hemolysis in patients with no evidence of heart valvular disease.

patients, diffuse tissue infarction. It is a useful parameter for both diagnosis and response to treatment. Fragmented red blood cells (schistocytes) with the typical appearance of a helmet in the peripheral smear (Fig. 31.8) and a negative Coombs' test (with the exception of neuraminidase associated TMA) are needed to confirm the microangiopathic nature of hemolysis. Stx-associated HUS is often associated with leukocytosis with a left shift, while leukocytes are usually normal in atypical HUS and TTP. Hypocomplementemia (low serum C3 levels) is occasionally present. Prothrombin (PT) and partial thromboplastin time (PTT), factor V, factor VIII, and fibrinogen are normal in most cases. ARF is usually associated with mild proteinuria (usually 1–2 g/day) and few red blood cells and casts on urinary sediment. Neurologic disturbances are commonly subtle (confusion and severe headache). Focal deficits are less frequent; seizure and coma may occur.

DIAGNOSIS AND DIFFERENTIAL DIAGNOSIS

The diagnosis of TMA is based on the above clinical and laboratory findings. The presence of known conditions associated with TMA including bloody diarrhea in young children, onset of symptoms in pregnancy or in the early postpartum period, and treatment with certain drugs, may be helpful in diagnosis. Renal biopsy is indicated when diagnosis is uncertain and thrombocytopenia is not severe. In case of thrombocytopenia, microangiopathic hemolytic anemia, and ARF, the differential diagnosis includes systemic vasculitis, malignant hypertension, and DIC. Vasculitis is usually characterized by other systemic symptoms such as cutaneous rash and arthralgias; the platelet count is usually normal and neurological involvement is predominantly peripheral rather than central. Patients with malignant hypertension have a history of high blood pressure, systolic/diastolic blood pressure above 210/130 mmHg at the time of evaluation, and typical retinal lesions. DIC is usually associated with sepsis, shock, and obstetrical complications; patients typically have

consumption of all the components of coagulation cascade, including platelets, fibrinogen, factor V, and factor VIII, with subsequent prolongation of PT and PTT.

DIAGNOSIS AND MANAGEMENT OF DIFFERENT FORMS OF TMA

Differentiation of the various forms of TMA is important to predict disease outcome and to establish the correct therapeutic approach (Fig. 31.9). Here we describe the main clinical characteristics of the different forms of TMA, with emphasis on therapeutic options based on different clinical presentations (Tables 31.1 and 31.2). Acquired forms are the most common. Toxins, autoantibodies, pregnancy, infections, systemic diseases, and drugs are associated with TMA that may present with the clinical feature of HUS and/or TTP.

Shigatoxin-associated HUS

Stx-associated HUS is the most frequent form of TMA[1]. It is associated with infection by certain strains of *E. coli* (mostly O157:H7 serotype) or *Shigella dysenteriae* that produce a powerful exotoxin (Shigatoxin or Stx, also referred to as verotoxin). It is also referred as D+ HUS because it is characterized by prodromal diarrhea followed by ARF. The overall incidence rate is estimated to be 2.1 cases per 100 000 persons/year, with a peak incidence in children younger than 5 years old (6.1/100 000 per year), though no age group is exempt. *E.coli* O157:H7 infection is most frequent in the warm summer months. Illness follows Stx *E.coli* infection a few days later. Abdominal cramps and nonbloody diarrhea are the typical presenting symptoms; diarrhea usually becomes bloody within a few days. Vomiting occurs in about 30–60% of cases and fever in 30%. Leukocytosis is usually present and a barium enema may show 'thumb-printing', suggestive of edema and submucosal hemorrhage, especially at ascending

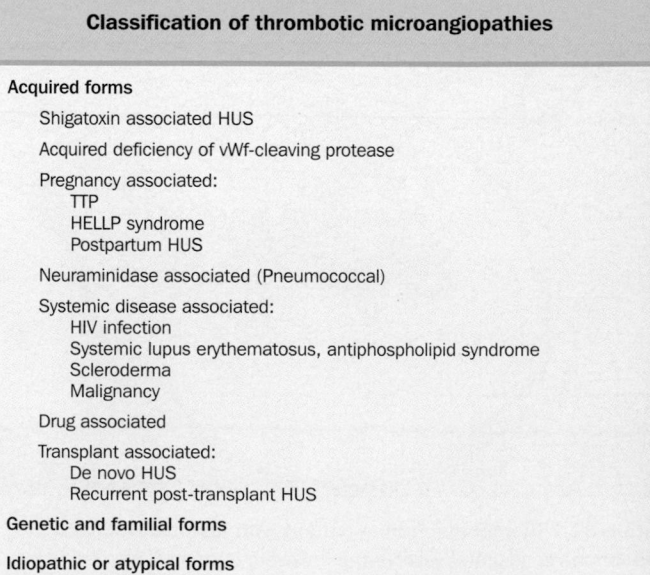

Classification of thrombotic microangiopathies

Acquired forms

Shigatoxin associated HUS

Acquired deficiency of vWf-cleaving protease

Pregnancy associated:
TTP
HELLP syndrome
Postpartum HUS

Neuraminidase associated (Pneumococcal)

Systemic disease associated:
HIV infection
Systemic lupus erythematosus, antiphospholipid syndrome
Scleroderma
Malignancy

Drug associated

Transplant associated:
De novo HUS
Recurrent post-transplant HUS

Genetic and familial forms

Idiopathic or atypical forms

Table 31.1 Classification of thrombotic microangiopathies.

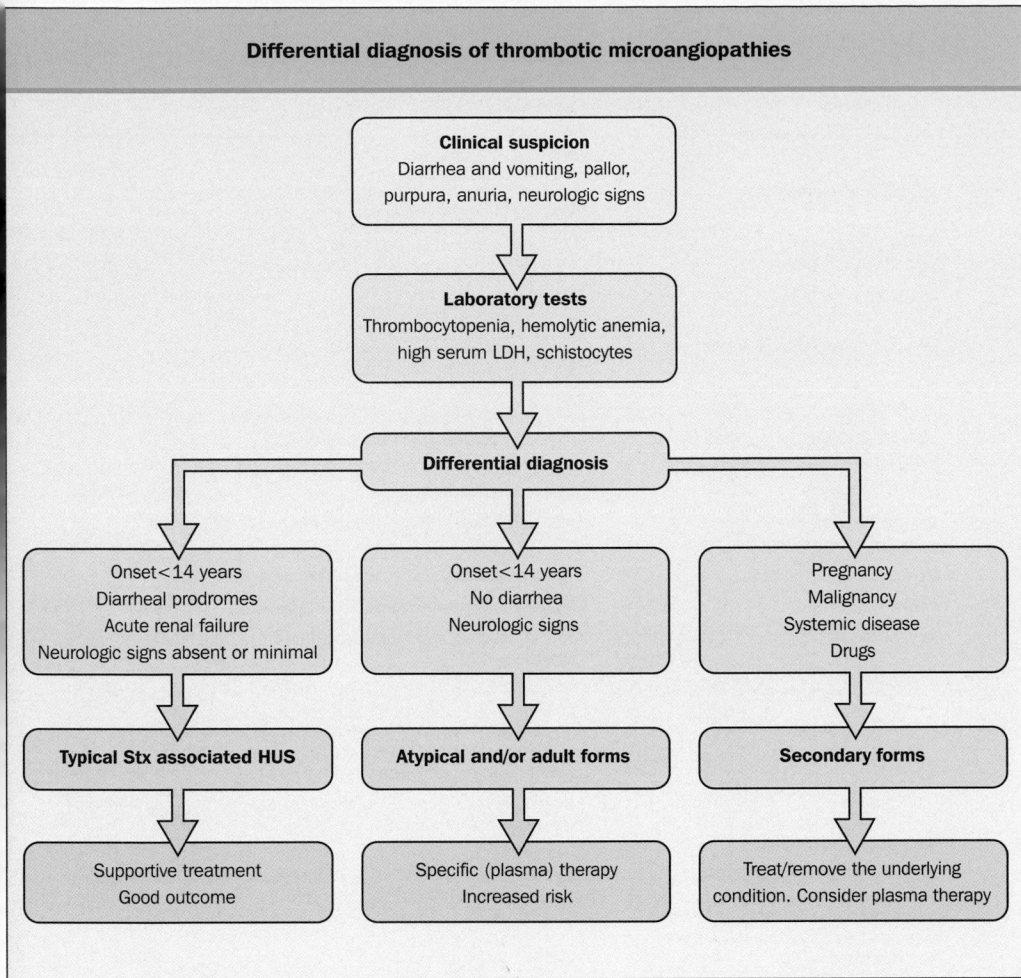

Differential diagnosis of thrombotic microangiopathies

Clinical suspicion
Diarrhea and vomiting, pallor, purpura, anuria, neurologic signs

Laboratory tests
Thrombocytopenia, hemolytic anemia, high serum LDH, schistocytes

Differential diagnosis

Onset<14 years
Diarrheal prodromes
Acute renal failure
Neurologic signs absent or minimal

Onset<14 years
No diarrhea
Neurologic signs

Pregnancy
Malignancy
Systemic disease
Drugs

Typical Stx associated HUS

Atypical and/or adult forms

Secondary forms

Supportive treatment
Good outcome

Specific (plasma) therapy
Increased risk

Treat/remove the underlying condition. Consider plasma therapy

Figure 31.9 Algorithm for the differential diagnosis of thrombotic microangiopathies. Patients with suggestive symptoms should be investigated for specific signs of microangiopathic hemolysis. In adults, secondary forms of the disease must be ruled out. Early diagnosis may help to establish the most appropriate therapy. In children, with Stx-associated HUS, supportive treatment is mandatory. Specific therapies should be considered only in adults and in atypical forms. In secondary forms, treating/removing the underlying disease is fundamental.

and transverse colon. HUS complicates enteric infection with *E. coli* O157:H7 infection in about 3–7% of sporadic cases and 20% or more of the epidemic form. HUS is usually diagnosed 6 days after the onset of diarrhea. Dialysis is required in 50% of cases, red blood cell transfusions in 75%, while neurologic signs including stroke, seizure and coma occur in 25%. Pancreatitis occurs in about 20% of cases. The outcome is usually good, with complete recovery in about 90% of patients. However, 3–5% of patients die during the acute phase, up to 5% have severe renal and extrarenal sequelae, and about 40% still have a low GFR at 10-year follow-up. Age under two years, severe gastrointestinal prodromes, elevated white cell count, anuria early in the course of the disease, and the presence of patched cortical necrosis or involvement of more than 50% glomeruli at renal biopsy are predictors of poor outcome. Anuria for more than ten days or need for dialysis in the acute phase, as well as proteinuria at 12 months follow-up, are associated with an increased risk of chronic renal failure in the long term. Diagnosis rests on detection of *E. coli* O157:H7 in stool cultures (it is shed for several weeks even after symptoms resolve). Serologic tests for antibodies to Stx and O157 lipopolysaccharide can be performed in research laboratories and tests are developing for rapid detection of *E. coli* O157:H7 and Stx in stools. Cattle represents the major natural reservoir of *E.coli* O157:H7. The most important route of HUS transmission is contaminated food (mainly undercooked ground beef including meat patties, roast beef, ham, turkey, cheese, potatoes, unpasteurized milk, and water). Secondary person-to-person contact is an important way of spreading in institutional centers, particularly day-care centers and nursing homes. In these cases, the most important preventive measure is hand washing.

Treatment

Supportive therapy
In children, Stx-associated HUS usually resolves spontaneously. Early diagnosis and improved supportive management of renal failure, anemia, hypertension, and fluid-electrolyte imbalance have played a major role in the significant reduction of mortality rate during the last decades. Early peritoneal dialysis prevents fluid overload, uremic symptoms, and may remove procoagulant substances from the plasma. Blood transfusions are often needed for symptomatic anemia. Bowel rest is important for the enterohemorrhagic colitis associated with D+ HUS. Antibiotics are contraindicated in case of *E. coli* O157:H7 infection where they increase the risk of HUS[11]. However, this does not apply to *E. coli* strains different from O157:H7 and other bacteria such as *Shigella dysenteriae* type 1. Antimotility agents are also contraindicated because they may exacerbate HUS by decreasing fecal excretion of *E. coli*. New agents targeted to prevent organ exposure to Stx are under investigation. The most promising are: Synsorb-PK,

Treatment options for thrombotic microangiopathy		
Treatment	Administration	Indications
Treatments of proven efficacy		
Plasma exchange	1-2 plasma volumes/day	1st line therapy in adult and atypical forms; life-saving in case of neurologic involvement; no risk of fluid overload
Plasma infusion	30-40 mL/kg on day 1, then 10-20 ml/kg/day	1st line therapy when exchange is not available; effective in the treatment or prevention of recurrence
Plasma cryosupernatant	See plasma exchange/infusion	2nd line therapy; may be effective in cases resistant to whole plasma exchange/infusion
Solvent detergent treated-plasma	See plasma exchange/infusion	Same indications of plasma exchange/infusion; may limit the risk of viral contamination
Other treatments		
Prednisone	Oral, 60-200 mg/day, tapered by 5 mg/week	May be effective in mild adult forms
γ globulins	IV 400 mg/kg/day	Unproven efficacy
Vincristine	1.4 mg/m² IV on day 1, than 1 mg every 4 days up to 4 doses	Unproven efficacy; might reduce the risk of recurrence
Antithrombotic agents (heparin, streptokinase)	IV	Unproven efficacy; increased risk of bleeding
Antiplatelet agents (aspirin, prostacyclin)	Oral or IV	Unproven efficacy; increased risk of bleeding
Vitamin E	Oral, 1000 mg/m²/day	May be effective in Stx-associated HUS; to be tested in controlled trials
Rescue treatments		
Bilateral nephrectomy		Life-saving in cases with refractory hypertension/thrombo-cytopenia, and hypertensive encephalopathy; restricted to patients with biopsy evidence of severe renal vascular involvement
Splenectomy		May be effective in patients with frequent relapses and requiring large amounts of plasma
Treatments under investigation		
Synsorb-PK	Oral, 0.5 g/kgx7 days; to be administered at the onset of diarrhea or when ingestion of contaminated food is suspected	May prevent/limit Stx absorption and the risk of Stx-associated HUS; under clinical investigation

Table 31.2 Treatment options for thrombotic microangiopathy.

a resin that binds Stx preventing its further absorption from the gut lumen; recombinant modified *E. coli* that efficiently adsorbs and neutralizes Stx; and Starfish, a carbohydrate ligand that can simultaneously bind two toxin molecules. Preliminary data show that early treatment (within 2 days from the onset of diarrhea) with Synsorb-PK significantly reduces the risk of HUS. Thus, in the future, oral administration of Synsorb-PK or recombinant modified *E. coli* might clear toxin from the gut while intravenous administration of Starfish might help to prevent toxin present in circulation from reaching target organs. Improved processing of cattle and animal products are also required to reduce the risk of *E. coli* O157:H7 or other pathogen infections.

Plasma therapy and other specific treatments
In children, the course of Stx-associated HUS is not affected by specific treatments aimed to prevent or limit the micro-angiopathic process. Long-term renal outcome and patient survival are not influenced by plasma therapy[12,13]. Steroids should be avoided because they increase the risk of colonic perforation in patients with active colitis. Heparin and antithrombotic agents increase the risk of bleeding; however, the effectiveness of tissue plasminogen activator is worth investigating. In adults with Stx-associated HUS, uncontrolled studies suggest that plasma therapy significantly lowers mortality rate and the risk of end-stage renal disease (ESRD)[14,15]. Thus, we suggest its use in adult patients in which renal and neurologic involvement are usually more severe and sequelae more frequent than in children.

Bilateral nephrectomy
In rare reports, when severe persistent thrombocytopenia, refractory hypertension, and major neurologic dysfunction exposed the patient to an imminent risk of death, bilateral nephrectomy induced complete clinical and hematological remission within two weeks[16]. It is possible that removing the kidneys eliminates a major site of vWf fragmentation, thus limiting platelet activation and further spread of microvascular lesions. This intervention should be considered only for patients in life threatening situations where all other therapeutic approaches failed (i.e., plasma-resistant or -dependent patients).

Acquired deficiency of vWf-cleaving protease
This is a recently defined form of TMA that include most cases previously described as idiopathic or sporadic TTP.

Recent studies showed that 70–90% of patients with a clinical diagnosis of acute TTP had an inhibitory autoantibody that resulted in a severe deficiency of a plasma metalloprotease that normally cleaves ULvWf. This form is reported in about 0.4 cases per 100 000 persons/year, with a peak incidence in the third decade, affecting women in about two-thirds of the cases. The clinical features are usually severe, characterized by an abrupt onset of neurologic abnormalities and purpura. Neurologic symptoms include confusion, headache, paresis, aphasia, dysarthria, visual problems, and coma. They are usually fleeting and fluctuating, and probably secondary to continuous thrombi formation and resolution. Fever is not frequently seen at onset but it is common during the illness. Proteinuria and microhematuria are common, renal function is depressed in several cases but severe renal insufficiency is rare. Although it is usually sporadic, recurrent episodes have been reported.

Supportive and plasma therapy

In the early 1960s, TTP was almost invariably fatal; now, because of earlier diagnosis, improved intensive care facilities and new techniques such as plasma therapy, survival rate is increased to 90%[17,18]. Plasma therapy is fundamental for the therapy of the acute episode of TTP. Theoretically, plasma infusion may induce remission of the disease by replacing the defective protease activity. When equivalent volumes of plasma are given, plasma infusion and exchange provide a similar response rate and survival. However, plasma exchange is preferred in situations such as renal or heart failure, when it is important to limit the amount of provided plasma. Plasma exchange, as compared to infusion, may also have the advantage of rapidly removing anti-vWf-cleaving protease antibodies. Usually one plasma volume (40 mL/kg body weight) is exchanged per day. Twice-daily exchanges may be required in refractory patients. Serum LDH and platelet count are the most reliable markers of response and plasma therapy should be continued until they remain normalized. Neurologic symptoms and serum LDH usually improve within 48 h of effective therapy while platelet count rises after several days. The outcome of renal function is unpredictable, and recovery is often incomplete with residual renal insufficiency and hypertension. Usually 7 to 16 daily exchanges are required to induce remission of the disease, but variability is wide and, occasionally, remission may occur after several months of plasma infusion or exchange. Patients who achieve remission must be monitored indefinitely with complete blood counts and serum LDH to screen for relapse of the disease. Relapsing episodes of TTP are separated by periods of 4 weeks or more (even months or years) of apparent recovery and must be distinguished from exacerbations of acute TTP, which are flare-ups of the same initial episode, usually secondary to overly aggressive tapering or interruption of therapy. Although relapses usually respond to plasma therapy, long-term prognosis is poor.

Plasma cryosupernatant

The use of the cryosupernatant fraction (i.e., plasma from which a cryoprecipitate containing the largest plasma vWf multimers, fibrinogen, and fibronectin has been removed)

instead of fresh frozen plasma was successful in a small number of patients who did not respond to repeated exchanges or infusion of fresh frozen plasma[19]. The rationale is that plasma cryosupernatant may provide the same beneficial factor(s) found in whole plasma (i.e., the defective/inhibited vWf protease) but does not contain those factors such as ULvWf multimers that may promote the formation of thrombi. However, results of the few small randomized studies did not find differences in efficacy between the cryosupernatant and whole plasma.

Other specific treatments

Corticosteroids might inhibit the synthesis of antiprotease antibodies. In one study, 30 out of 108 patients with mild forms of TTP recovered after corticosteroids alone but their vWf-cleaving protease activity were not tested[17]. Thus, the potential beneficial effect of corticosteroids needs to be tested with additional studies where response to treatment is evaluated in patients with circulating anti-vWf-cleaving protease antibodies. Vincristine has induced recovery in anecdotal cases, sometimes when other therapies have failed. There are also preliminary reports that suggest other cytotoxic agents such as cyclophosphamide and azathioprine may be effective in inducing remission for relapsing cases[20]. The effectiveness of immunoglobulins, which might inactivate platelet aggregating factor/s, has yet to be proved. Antiplatelet agents seem ineffective and should be avoided in the acute phase of TTP because of the risk of severe bleeding. They could be used in case of thrombocytosis during the recovery phase. However, two of these agents, ticlopidine and clopidogrel, trigger TTP. The effectiveness of prostacyclin is also unproved. Platelet transfusions are contraindicated in acute TTP, except in cases of life-threatening bleeding, because they may lead to new, or worse, neurologic symptoms, and ARF, probably due to new or expanding thrombi.

Splenectomy

Retrospective studies showed that splenectomy may increase mortality rate and disease duration in a small number of unselected patients with TTP refractory to plasma therapy[17]. However, splenectomy, by removing a major site of antibody production, might have a specific indication in those patients with autoantibodies against vWf-cleaving protease that persist in the circulation despite immunosuppressive therapy. Remission of the disease has been achieved after splenectomy with subsequent normalization of the protease activity in three patients but further studies on a large number of patients are needed to prove its effectiveness[3]. Preliminary evidence showed that splenectomy during hematological remission, might be beneficial in patients with chronic relapsing forms of TTP, reducing the relapse rate and the need for plasma therapy[21]. Thus, splenectomy might be considered in those patients with very disabling disease who require prolonged and frequent courses of plasma therapy.

Pregnancy-associated TMA

TMA associated with pregnancy may manifest as acute TTP; hemolysis, elevated liver enzymes, and low platelets (HELLP syndrome); and HUS[22].

Thrombotic thrombocytopenic purpura

Pregnancy-associated TTP usually develops during the antepartum period. Measurement of plasma antithrombin (AT) III activity may be a useful tool to differentiate TTP and pre-eclampsia. TTP is most likely before gestational week 28 and when AT III plasma activity is normal, while pre-eclampsia is most likely after week 34 of gestation, and is usually associated with decreased plasma AT III activity. The institution of plasma therapy significantly reduced maternal mortality rate to almost zero. Delivery is recommended for those patients with pregnancy-associated TTP who do not respond to plasma therapy and it is the treatment of choice for pre-eclampsia/HELLP syndrome. The role of other treatments often employed in idiopathic TTP remains unknown. When the disease persists, a course of plasma therapy is indicated. Between 28 and 34 weeks, the optimal treatment is controversial. Some authorities have held that delivery should always be considered as first line therapy whereas others believe that a course of plasma therapy can be reasonably attempted before inducing delivery if there is no evidence of fetal distress and plasma AT III activity is normal. There is no report of transmission of TTP to the infant.

The HELLP syndrome

The HELLP syndrome is a form of severe pre-eclampsia where there is evidence of microangiopathic hemolysis and liver injury in addition to hypertension and renal dysfunction. The syndrome is most common in white multiparous women with a history of poor pregnancy outcome. It usually occurs in the late third trimester, including the intrapartum period. Occasionally, after an uncomplicated pregnancy, symptoms may also arise within 24–48 h postpartum. Diagnosis is based on laboratory findings of hemolysis (defined as fragmented erythrocytes in the circulation and serum LDH ≥ 600 U/L), elevated liver enzymes (serum glutamicoxaloacetic transaminase > 70 U/L), and low platelets (platelet count $< 100 \times 10^3/mm^3$). Overt DIC is reported in 25% of cases. Intrahepatic hemorrhage, subcapsular liver hematoma, and liver rupture are rare but life-threatening complications. The maternal and perinatal mortality rates range from 0 to 24% and from 7.7 to 60%, respectively. Most of the perinatal deaths are related to abruptio placentae, intrauterine asphyxia, and extreme prematurity. As many as 44% of the infants are growth retarded. Delivery is the only definitive therapy. Hydralazine is the first-choice drug to control pregnancy-induced hypertension, and magnesium sulfate is used to prevent and treat convulsions. Both peritoneal dialysis and hemodialysis have been used to treat ARF. Platelet transfusions are needed for clinical bleeding or severe thrombocytopenia (platelet count $< 20\,000/\mu L$). In approximately 5% of patients with HELLP syndrome, symptoms and laboratory abnormalities do not improve after delivery. These more often include central nervous system abnormalities, associated with renal and cardiopulmonary dysfunction, and activation of coagulation. Uncontrolled studies suggest that plasma exchange may help recovery in patients with persistent evidence of disease 72 h or more after delivery. Plasma therapy is ineffective during pregnancy and may increase fetal and maternal risk when used to delay delivery. Preliminary evidence suggests that, postpartum, corticosteroids may hasten disease recovery and, antepartum, postpone delivery and reduce the mother's need of blood products.

Postpartum HUS

Postpartum HUS manifests within 6 months from normal delivery. The clinical course is usually fulminant. Supportive care including dialysis, transfusions, and careful fluid management, remains the most important form of treatment. Whether plasma therapy improves survival or limits renal sequelae has not been established. Antiplatelet agents, heparin, and antithrombotic therapy may enhance the risk of bleeding and have no proven efficacy.

Neuraminidase associated TMA

It is a rare but potentially fatal complication of pneumonia or, less frequently, meningitis by *Streptococcus pneumoniae*[1]. Neuraminidase is a protease produced by this bacteria that exposes a specific cryptic antigen, Thomsen–Friedenreich, present on platelets and endothelial cell surface, to preformed circulating IgM antibodies with subsequent platelet aggregation and endothelial injury. The clinical picture is usually severe with respiratory distress, anuria, neurological involvement, and coma. The outcome is strongly dependent on the effectiveness of antibiotic therapy. The role of plasma therapy is controversial. In theory, plasma should be contraindicated in the adult because it contains antibodies against the Thomsen–Friedenreich antigen that may accelerate polyagglutination and hemolysis[23]. However, in some cases, plasma therapy, in combination with corticosteroids, induced recovery. Antibiotics and leukocyte-poor erythrocyte preparations should be used.

Systemic disease-associated TMA

Antiphospholipid syndrome, scleroderma, malignant hypertension

Plasma therapy should always be attempted in TMA associated with systemic diseases even though its efficacy is poorly defined. In the antiphospholipid syndrome, oral anticoagulation remains the only treatment of proven efficacy to prevent and treat micro- and macrovascular thrombosis, even if concomitant thrombocytopenia may increase the risk of bleeding. Blood pressure control is fundamental in TMA associated with scleroderma crisis and malignant hypertension.

Human immunodeficiency virus-associated TMA

HUS and TTP are both possible complications of the acquired immune deficiency syndrome (AIDS) that may account for as much as 30% of hospitalized TMA cases in cities where AIDS is epidemic[24]. Plasma therapy is the only feasible approach in these forms although the prognosis is poor. Uncontrolled series show that the survival rate of human immunodeficiency virus infected patients with TTP and without AIDS is comparable to that of idiopathic TTP.

Malignancy associated TMA

TMA may spontaneously arise in patients with advanced cancer. It complicates almost 6% of cases of metastatic carcinoma with gastric cancer, which accounts for about 50% of all cases of malignancy associated TMA. The prognosis is extremely poor and most patients die within a few weeks. Therapy is minimally effective. Administration of blood products to correct symptomatic anemia often results in exacerbation of the syndrome, with rapid worsening of hemolysis, deterioration of renal function, and pulmonary edema.

Drug associated TMA

Different drugs have been associated with TMA[25], including mitomycin C (MMC), ticlopidine, clopidogrel, quinine, interferon, calcineurin inhibitors, and estrogen-containing oral contraceptives (Table 31.3). Discontinuing the offending drug is fundamental. The efficacy of plasma therapy is unclear; it seems ineffective with some drugs such as MMC and very important with others such as quinine.

Mitomycin and anticancer drugs

TMA, more commonly resembling HUS, is described in 2–10% of cancer patients treated with MMC. Disease manifestation is dose related since renal dysfunction rarely occurs in patients given a cumulative dose lower than 30 mg/m^2. Patients who develop MMC associated TMA usually are in remission from their malignancy, thus they significantly differ from the very ill patients who develop TMA as a complication of advanced tumor. The fatality rate is about 70% and median time to death is about 4 weeks. Patients surviving the acute phase often remain on chronic dialysis, or die later of recurrence of the tumor or metastases. The possibility of preventing the disease by giving steroids during mitomycin treatment has been suggested and needs to be confirmed in prospective controlled trials. Plasma exchange is usually attempted, but its effectiveness is unproved. Platinum- and bleomycin-containing combinations have also been reported to induce HUS.

Drug associated thrombotic microangiopathy

Drugs used in cancer therapy

    Mitomycyn C *
    Tamoxifen *
    Bleomycin *
    Cisplatin *
    Gemcitabine
    Deoxycorfomycin
    Methil-CCNU
    Daunorubicin
    Cytosine arabinoside
    Neocarcinostatin

Other drugs

    Ticlopidine/clopidogrel *
    Quinine *
    Interferon *
    Calcineurin inhibitors *
    OKT3 *
    Oral contraceptives
    Penicillin
    Rifampin (rifampicin)
    Metronidazole

* drugs most commonly involved in drug associated TMA

Table 31.3 Drug associated thrombotic microangiopathy.

Antiplatelet drugs

TMA has been reported in 1 case per 1600–5000 patients treated with ticlopidine. Neurologic abnormalities dominate the clinical picture and usually occur within a few weeks of treatment. The overall survival rate is 67% and is improved by early treatment withdrawal and plasma therapy. Generation of an autoantibody against vWF-cleaving protease may be involved in the pathogenesis of ticlopidine associated TTP. In seven patients who developed TTP 2–7 weeks after initiation of ticlopidine therapy, very low levels of vWF-cleaving protease were reported along with the appearance of IgG, that inhibited the vWF-cleaving protease activity[26]. This deficiency resolved after ticlopidine discontinuation and plasmapheresis therapy. Eleven cases have been reported during treatment with clopidogrel, a new anti-aggregating agent that has achieved widespread clinical use for its safety profile[27]. The disease occurred within 2 weeks of therapy in 10 patients. All patients had neurological involvement and were treated with plasma exchange: eight fully recovered, two had relapses that rapidly recovered after retreatment with plasma exchange, and one died. Half the patients were concomitantly treated with cholesterol lowering drugs and clinicians should be aware of this possible complication.

Quinine

Quinine is one of the most common drugs associated with TMA[28]. It is generally used to treat muscle cramps but it is also contained in beverages or nutrition health products (tonic water, and herbal preparations). TMA typically occurs in patients sensitized by prior exposure to quinine and rapidly follows re-exposure to the drug. Quinine-dependent antiplatelet, antierythrocyte, antigranulocyte, antilymphocyte, and antiendothelial antibodies may be involved in the pathogenesis of the disease. Predominant severe renal impairment is present and hemodialysis is required in most of cases. Despite a previous paper that reported a good outcome[29], a recent work has showed a high rate of death and chronic renal failure (4 and 7 out of 17 patients, respectively)[28]. Cessation of quinine and institution of plasma therapy should be provided as early as possible. Avoidance of future quinine use is necessary to prevent recurrences.

Interferon

Interferon-associated TMA is characterized by predominant renal impairment[25]. Recovery of the disease is common in cases of early discontinuation of the drug and prompt supportive therapy. However, kidney prognosis is usually poor, with chronic ESRD occurring in about 42% of cases. Because of the few cases reported, it is not possible to evaluate the effectiveness of specific therapies such as plasma exchange or infusion.

Organ transplantation-associated TMA

Post-transplant HUS is reported with increasing frequency. In renal transplants, HUS may develop for the first time in patients who have not previously had the disease (*de novo* post-transplant HUS) or may affect patients whose primary cause of ESRD was HUS (recurrent post-transplant HUS). Treatment of post-transplant HUS rests on relief of symptoms, removal of the inciting factor(s), and plasma therapy. No other approach has proved effective.

De novo *post-transplant HUS*

This form affects both renal and extrarenal transplant recipients, and is usually triggered by immunosuppressive drugs such as calcineurin inhibitors and OKT3, or less frequently, by virus infections (HIV, parvovirus B19) and, in renal transplant recipients, by acute vascular rejection[30,31]. A particular form of *de novo* post-transplant HUS may affects the recipients of bone marrow transplant (BMT), usually in cases of graft versus host disease (GVHD) or of intensive GVHD prophylaxis, including total body irradiation. Drug withdrawal or dose reduction and plasma therapy achieved high success rate (84%) in *de novo* cyclosporine or tacrolimus associated forms. A similar response rate, but in smaller studies, has been described with intravenous IgG infusion given with the rationale to neutralize hypothetical circulating cytotoxic or platelet agglutinating factors. Once remission is achieved, possible immunosuppression treatments may include a decreased dose of cyclosporine or tacrolimus, a change of cyclosporine to tacrolimus or vice versa, or the avoidance of calcineurin inhibitors by using mycophenolate mofetil. Recently, sirolimus therapy had a remarkably good outcome in 15 patients with cyclosporine or tacrolimus associated post-transplant HUS, with no patient requiring sirolimus withdrawal because of disease recurrence[32]. Monoclonal anti-interleukin-2 receptor antagonists may also be a valid option to maintain adequate immunosuppression while avoiding the toxic effects of calcineurin inhibitors. The outcome of *de novo* forms occurring in the setting of viral infection is strongly influenced by the response to the treatment of the underlying disease. The outcome of *de novo* forms complicating BMT is very poor, with a mortality rate closed to 90%. In addition to the severity of the microangiopathic process, infection, progressive graft-versus-host disease, or relapse of the underlying disease may account for these discouraging results.

Recurrent *post-transplant HUS*

The reported recurrence rate of HUS after transplantation is 25–50%. Patients with idiopathic and, above all, genetic forms of TMA are at high risk of post-transplant recurrence; in contrast Stx-associated HUS does not recur[33,34]. Older age at onset of HUS, short duration between HUS onset and ESRD, and transplant from living donors confer an increased risk of post-transplant recurrence[35]. Recurrent forms usually do not respond to any type of therapy and are associated with a graft loss in most of cases. Preliminary data suggest that patients with allograft loss because of recurrent HUS may be successfully retransplanted without the use of calcineurin inhibitors.

Genetic and familial forms of TMA

These forms are rare (fewer than 5% of reported cases), often familial. They present as HUS and/or TTP in different members of the same family and also in different episodes in the same patient. The rate of relapses is high. The outcome is poor with death, ESRD and permanent neurological deficits in most of cases[1]. Treatment is based on plasma therapy. Forms characterized by reduced factor H bioavailability, often with low serum C3 levels, are more common in children. The rate of recurrence after kidney transplantation alone is around 100%, occurring within one month after surgery in most of cases. We recently provided the evidence that combined kidney and liver transplantation protected the transplanted kidney from recurrence of the disease, by restoring the production of normal factor H[36]. Thus, in these cases, combined kidney and liver transplantation might be an effective way to gain independence from dialysis and improve life expectancy. Genetic counseling is very important if pregnancies are planned, because in families with recognized genetic mutations, affected offspring can be identified by amniocentesis or chorionic villus biopsy. Although more frequent in adults, the congenital complete lack of vWF-cleaving protease has been described also in a few patients with HUS. Plasma infusion, by supplying the missing enzyme, is the first-line treatment in this case. It is sufficient to achieve just a 5% of normal protease activity, through plasma therapy, in order to adequately degrade ULvWF.

Idiopathic or atypical TMA

These are forms of unknown etiology with poor outcome characterized by progressive course to ESRD and neurological involvement similar to TTP. Plasma therapy is indicated since may limit the risk of ESRD; uncontrolled studies also show its beneficial effect on mortality rate in adults[1,37]. Bilateral nephrectomy may be used as rescue therapy in the most severe cases.

REFERENCES

1. Ruggenenti P, Noris M, Remuzzi G. Thrombotic microangiopathy, hemolytic uremic syndrome, and thrombotic thrombocytopenic purpura. Kidney Int. 2001;60:831–46.

2. Furlan M, Robles R, Lammle B. Partial purification and characterization of a protease from human plasma cleaving von Willebrand factor to fragments produced by in vivo proteolysis. Blood. 1996;87:4223–34.

3. Furlan M, Robles R, Galbusera M, et al. von Willebrand factor-cleaving protease in thrombotic thrombocytopenic purpura and the hemolytic-uremic syndrome. N Engl J Med. 1998;339:1578–84.

4. Tsai HM, Lia ECY. Antibodies to von Willebrand factor-cleaving protease in acute thrombotic thrombocytopenic purpura. N Engl J Med. 1998;339:1585–94.

5. Veyradier A, Obert B, Houllier A, et al. Specific von Willebrand factor-cleaving protease in thrombotic microangiopathies: a study of 111 cases. Blood. 2001;98:1765–72.

6. Levy GG, Nichols WC, Lian EC. Mutations in a member of the ADAMTS gene family cause thrombotic thrombocytopenic purpura. Nature. 2001;413:488–94.

7. Mannucci PM, Canciani MT, Forza I, et al. Changes in health and disease of the metalloprotease that cleaves von Willebrand factor. Blood. 2001;98:2730–5.

8. Noris M, Ruggenenti P, Perna A, et al. Hypocomplementemia discloses genetic predisposition to hemolytic uremic syndrome and thrombotic thrombocytopenic purpura: role of factor H abnormalities. Italian Registry of Familial and Recurrent Hemolytic Uremic Syndrome/Thrombotic Thrombocytopenic Purpura. J Am Soc Nephrol. 1999;10:281–93.

9. Taylor CM. Complement factor H and the haemolytic uraemic syndrome. Lancet. 2001;358:1200–2.

10. Caprioli J, Bettinaglio P, Zipfel PF, et al. The molecular basis of familial hemolytic uremic syndrome: mutation analysis of factor H gene reveals a hot spot in short consensus repeat 20. J Am Soc Nephrol. 2001;12:297–307.

11. Wong CS, Jelacic S, Habeeb RL, Watkins SL, Tarr PI. The risk of the hemolytic-uremic syndrome after antibiotic treatment of Escherichia coli 0157:H7 infections. N Engl J Med. 2000;342:1930–6.

12. Rizzoni G, Claris-Appiani A, Edefonti A. Plasma infusion for hemolytic uremic syndrome in children: results of a multicenter controlled trial. J Pediatr. 1988;112:284–90.

13. Loirat C, Sonsino E, Hinglais N, et al. Treatment of the childhood hemolytic uremic syndrome with plasma. A multicenter randomized controlled trial. Pediatr Nephrol. 1988; 2:279–85.

14. Dundas S, Murphy J, Soutar RL, et al. Effectiveness of therapeutic plasma exchange in the 1996 Lanarkshire Escherichia coli O157:H7 outbreak. Lancet. 1999;354:1327–30.

15. Carter AO, Borczyk AA, Carlson JA, et al. A severe outbreak of Escherichia coli 0157:H7-associated hemorrhagic colitis in a nursing home. N Engl J Med. 1987;317: 1496–500.

16. Remuzzi G, Galbusera M, Salvadori M, et al. Bilateral nephrectomy stopped disease progression in plasma-resistant hemolytic uremic syndrome with neurological signs and coma. Kidney Int. 1996;49:282–6.

17. Bell WR, Braine HG, Ness PM, Kickler TS. Improved survival in thrombotic thrombocytopenic purpura-hemolytic uremic syndrome. Clinical experience in 108 patients. N Engl J Med. 1991;325:398–403.

18. Rock GA, Shumak KH, Buskard NA, et al. Comparison of plasma exchange with plasma infusion in the treatment of thrombotic thrombocytopenic purpura. N Engl J Med. 1991; 325:393–7.

19. Rock G, Shumak KH, Sutton DM, et al. Cryosupernatant as replacement fluid for plasma exchange in thrombotic thrombocytopenic purpura. Members of the Canadian Apheresis Group. Br J Haematol. 1996;94:383–6.

20. Allan DS, Kovacs MJ, Clark WF. Frequently relapsing thrombotic thrombocytopenic purpura treated with cytotoxic immunosuppressive therapy. Haematologica. 2001;86:844–50.

21. Hayward CP, Sutton DM, Carter WH Jr, et al. Treatment outcomes in patients with adult thrombotic thrombocytopenic purpura–hemolytic uremic syndrome. Arch Intern Med. 1994;154:982–7.

22. Weiner CP. Thrombotic microangiopathy in pregnancy and the postpartum period. Semin Hematol. 1987;24:119–29.

23. McGraw ME, Lendon M, Stevens RF, et al. Hemolytic uremic syndrome and the Thomsen Friedenreich antigen. Pediatr Nephrol. 1989;3:135–9.

24. Thompson CE, Damon LE, Ries CA, Linker CA. Thrombotic microangiopathies in the 1980s: Clinical features, response to treatment, and the impact of the human immunodeficiency virus epidemic. Blood. 1992;80:1890–5.

25. Pisoni R, Ruggenenti P, Remuzzi G. Drug-induced thrombotic microangiopathy: incidence, prevention and management. Drug Saf. 2001;24:491–501.

26. Tsai HM, Rice L, Sarode R, et al. Antibody inhibitors to von Willebrand factor metalloproteinase and increased binding of von Willebrand factor to platelets in ticlopidine-associated thrombotic thrombocytopenic purpura. Ann Intern Med. 2000;132:794–99.

27. Bennett CL, Connors JM, Carwile JM, et al. Thrombotic thrombocytopenic purpura associated with clopidogrel. N Engl J Med. 2000;342:1773–7.

28. Kojouri K, Vesely SK, George JN. Quinine-associated thrombotic thrombocytopenic purpura-hemolytic uremic syndrome: Frequency, clinical features, and long-term outcomes. Ann Intern Med. 2001;135:1047–51.

29. Gottschall JL, Neahring B, McFarland JG, et al. Quinine-induced immune thrombocytopenia with hemolytic uremic syndrome: Clinical and serological findings in nine patients and review of literature. Am J Hematol. 1994;47:283–9.

30. Remuzzi G, Bertani T. Renal vascular and thrombotic effects of cyclosporine. Am J Kidney Dis. 1989;13:261–72.

31. Abramowicz D, Pradier O, Marchant A, et al. Induction of thromboses within renal grafts by high-dose prophylactic OKT3. Lancet. 1992;339:777–8.

32. Ruggenenti P, Galli M, Remuzzi G. Hemolytic uremic syndrome, thrombotic thrombocytopenic purpura, and antiphospholipid antibody syndromes. In: Neilson EG, Couser WG, eds. Immunologic Renal Diseases, 2nd edn. 2001:1179–1208.

33. Miller RB, Burke BA, Schmidt WJ, et al. Recurrence of haemolytic-uraemic syndrome in renal transplants: a single-centre report. Nephrol Dial Transplant. 1997;12:1425–30.

34. Kaplan BS, Papadimitriou M, Brezin JH, et al. Renal transplantation in adults with autosomal recessive inheritance of hemolytic uremic syndrome. Am J Kidney Dis. 1997;30:760–5.

35. Ducloux D, Rebibou JM, Semhoun-Ducloux S, et al. Recurrence of hemolytic-uremic syndrome in renal transplant recipients: a meta-analysis. Transplantation. 1998;65:1405–7.

36. Remuzzi G, Ruggenenti P, Codazzi D, et al. Combined kidney and liver transplantation for familial haemolytic uraemic syndrome. Lancet. 2002;359:1671–2.

37. George JN. How I treat patients with thrombotic thrombocytopenic purpura-hemolytic uremic syndrome. Blood. 2000;96:1223–9.

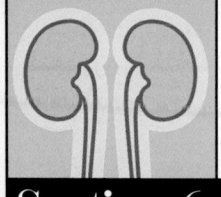

Chapter 32

Clinical Manifestations and Natural History of Diabetic Nephropathy

Jiten P Vora and Hisham A A Ibrahim

INTRODUCTION AND DEFINITIONS

Diabetic nephropathy is a leading cause of end-stage renal disease (ESRD) in Western societies. Diabetes is the single largest cause of ESRD in American and European adults, accounting for over one third of all patients beginning renal replacement therapy.

Type 1 diabetes is an autoimmune disease characterized by antibody and cell-mediated destruction of pancreatic islets. Circulating C-peptide is absent indicating failure of insulin production; all type 1 diabetics eventually require treatment with insulin. Type 1 diabetes may occur at any age but is common in childhood, usually presenting prior to the age of 30 years.

Type 2 diabetes is characterized by a combination of insulin resistance and qualitative or quantitative insulin deficiency. It may represent a component of the metabolic syndrome, comprising insulin resistance, obesity, type 2 diabetes, hypertension and hyperlipidemia. Whilst both insulin resistance and insulin deficiency are essential prerequisites, recent data demonstrates gradual decline in pancreatic β-cell function, culminating in supplemental insulin requirement in 40–50% of the patients. Type 2 diabetes is typically a disease of older adults although increasingly is seen in children.

Patients with type 2 diabetes comprise the largest and fastest growing single disease group requiring renal replacement therapy.

Diabetic nephropathy is a clinical syndrome characterized by persistent albuminuria (> 300 mg/24 h or > 200 μg/min), on at least two occasions separated by 3–6 months. This is equivalent to total proteinuria > 500 mg/24 h. Patients invariably develop associated hypertension, a progressive increase in proteinuria and a predictable and relentless decline in glomerular filtration rate (GFR).

EPIDEMIOLOGY

In UK general diabetic clinics, the overall prevalence of nephropathy is 4–8%, depending on the clinic's case mix.

Type 1 diabetic nephropathy

Traditionally, nephropathy is said to occur in 30–40% of patients with type 1 diabetes after 25–40 years with diabetes. Recent studies suggest a decline in this cumulative incidence to approximately 25%, which may reflect patient populations with consistently improved glycemic control over prolonged periods. This would reduce the incidence of all chronic microvascular complications, including renal disease[1,2].

Type 2 diabetic nephropathy

In type 2 diabetes, the cumulative incidence of nephropathy is similar to that seen in type 1, 25% at 20 years after diagnosis. Of these patients, 20% will develop clinically significant renal impairment over 10 years, requiring renal replacement therapy. Population-based studies also indicate a prevalence of nephropathy of 5–10% at the time of diagnosis of type 2 diabetes, probably reflecting previous prolonged periods of subclinical hyperglycemia.

Since type 2 diabetes is 10 to 15 times more common than type 1, the prevalence of type 2 diabetic nephropathy is substantially higher, with a cross-sectional prevalence of approximately 15%, which represents a large number of patients given the prevalence of type 2 diabetes. The rapid growth in the prevalence of type 2 diabetes in affluent countries is largely responsible for the increasing frequency of diabetic ESRD worldwide. Although typically a disease of adult life, the increasing incidence of type 2 diabetes in children in association with obesity is of particular concern.

While the contribution of type 2 diabetic nephropathy has been less in European populations compared to those of North America, there is also evidence of a continuing rise in the prevalence of ESRD caused by type 2 diabetic nephropathy in Europe[3].

Susceptibility to diabetic nephropathy

There is unequivocal evidence for the importance of glycemic control in predicting the risk of developing nephropathy in both type 1 and type 2 diabetes. In addition, there are genetic, gender, and age risk factors.

Ethnicity

The incidence of diabetes in those with newly diagnosed ESRD varies widely depending on the ethnic origin of the population. Studies of Pima Indians show a cumulative incidence of ESRD of 40% at 10 years and 61% at 15 years following the onset of proteinuria[4], compared to a cumulative incidence of 17% ESRD at 15 years following the onset of proteinuria in Caucasian type 2 diabetics. The incidence is also markedly increased in other Native American populations. For diabetes related ESRD, Mexican Americans have an incidence ratio of 6, while African Americans have a ratio of 4 compared to Caucasian populations[5]. In a Michigan based study, the incidence of diabetic ESRD was 2.6 fold higher among African Americans, with the excess risk occurring predominantly in the type 2 diabetic population; most of these patients with ESRD had type 2 diabetes, whereas most Caucasian patients

Diabetic Nephropathy

had type 1 diabetes[6]. The incidence of ESRD is significantly higher among South Asians and African-Caribbean populations within the UK, with a three- to four-fold higher acceptance rate onto renal replacement programs than Caucasians[7].

The causes for these ethnic differences in the incidence of renal disease in type 2 diabetic patients are multifactorial. Diabetes and hypertension are much more prevalent among South Asian and African-Caribbeans than Caucasians. Although there is an increased incidence of ESRD due to diabetes, there is also an increased incidence of glomerulonephritis and chronic pyelonephritis, with a five-fold increase in ESRD of uncertain cause associated with non-renal tuberculosis, suggesting a generalized increased susceptibility to renal disease[7]. In Native Americans with type 2 diabetes, those who become hypertensive after the diagnosis of diabetes are more likely to develop nephropathy compared to those subjects whose hypertension was diagnosed prior to diabetes. In the Caucasian population, hypertension does not uniformly herald a subsequent decline in renal function.

Among the Pima Indians, a strong familial clustering of nephropathy has also been reported: 14.3% of diabetic offspring if neither parent had proteinuria; 22.9% if at least one parent had proteinuria and 45.9% if both parents had nephropathy[8]. Despite this familial clustering, no gene has yet been clearly associated with susceptibility to diabetic nephropathy in the Pima Indian population.

Gender

Although type 1 diabetes is 1.5 times more common in females than males, males have a higher risk of developing diabetic nephropathy, with a male to female ratio of 1.7 : 1. Over 40 years, the cumulative incidence of nephropathy is 46% in males and 32% in females. The male-to-female incidence ratio for ESRD is 1.1 : 1.

In type 2 diabetes, there is also a male excess risk of developing nephropathy, with a male : female ratio as high as 5 : 1 in some studies.

Age at onset of diabetes

The highest long-term incidence of nephropathy is found in those who develop type 1 diabetes between the ages of 11 and 20 years. The median time between onset of proteinuria and ESRD is 14 years for those diagnosed under the age of 12 years, and 8 years for those diagnosed between the ages of 12 and 20 years.

A disproportionate increase in renal hypertrophy during the phase of puberty has been noted recently[9]. The full effect of age on the evolution of renal disease is unclear; but the pre-puberty duration of diabetes appears not to contribute, even though raised urinary albumin excretion rates (UAER) have been reported pre-pubertally, including in patients with diabetes of less than 5 years' duration.

In patients with type 2 diabetes, those diagnosed after the age of 50 years have a higher prevalence of microalbuminuria than those diagnosed before the age of 40 years.

Morbidity and mortality

After 40 years of diabetes, only 10% of those with proteinuria are alive compared to 70% of those without, the main cause of mortality being cardiovascular disease. The development of persistent proteinuria in patients with type 1 diabetes imparts a 50-fold increase in mortality. The risk of developing ischemic heart disease is estimated to be 15 times higher for patients with proteinuria compared to those with normoalbuminuria. By the age of 40 years, mortality from all causes is 20 to 40 times higher in proteinuric type 1 diabetics, while that for normoalbuminuric type 1 diabetics is twice that of a nondiabetic population. However, mortality is falling. After 10 years of persistent proteinuria, survival in the 1990s is 80% compared to 20% in the 1950s. For patients with type 2 diabetes with either microalbuminuria or proteinuria, the survival rate at 10 years is 30% compared to 55% for those with normoalbuminuria[10]. In type 2 diabetes, the United Kingdom Prospective Diabetes Study provides compelling evidence of the link between varying levels of proteinuria and mortality rates. Mortality rates for differing levels of proteinuria were: 1.4% per annum normoalbuminuria; 3.0% for microalbuminuria; 4.6% for macroalbuminuria and 19.2% in the presence of abnormal urea and creatinine.

CLINICAL MANIFESTATIONS AND NATURAL HISTORY

Renal dysfunction in type 1 diabetes

The natural history of renal involvement has been better defined in type 1 than in type 2 diabetes. Mogensen has identified five distinct stages of renal dysfunction (Figure 32.1)[11].

Stage 1

Stage 1 describes the renal hypertrophy and hyperfiltration that are present at the time of diagnosis of type I diabetes. UAER is elevated as is GFR, which is increased by 20% to 40% compared with age-matched controls. The renal plasma flow (RPF) is also elevated by 9–14%. Institution of insulin therapy produces a reduction of both GFR and UAER.

Stage 2

Stage 2 is clinically 'silent'. GFR remains elevated ('hyperfiltration') with normal UAER and blood pressure. It occurs during average glycemic control with conventional insulin regimens and typically lasts for 5–15 years. However, detailed renal morphometric studies during this phase have demonstrated early histologic changes, including a relatively nonspecific increase

Urinary albumin excretion rate (UAER)		
	Urinary albumin excretion rate	
Condition	24-hour (mg/day)	Overnight (µg/min)
Normoalbuminuria	<30	<20
Microalbuminuria	30–300	20–200
Overt nephropathy	>300	>200
Levels of 24-hour and overnight UAER diagnostic for microalbuminuria and overt diabetic nephropathy.		

Table 32.1 Urinary albumin excretion rate (UAER).

in basement membrane thickness but a more predictive increase in fractional mesangial volume (with increases in mesangial matrix) after 2–4 years. The hyperfiltration is related to the degree of hyperglycemia up to 250 mg/dL (14 mmol/L). Levels of glycemia higher than this are associated with a reduction in GFR. The pathogenetic role of hyperfiltration in the development of progressive renal dysfunction remains debatable. Data have been reported both supporting and refuting the influence of hyperfiltration on further renal dysfunction. Other factors implicated in the genesis of diabetic nephropathy, including the direct consequences of abnormal glucose control, are discussed in Chapter 33. Improvement in glycemic control during the second stage will invariably reduce the extent of hyperfiltration.

Stage 3

Stage 3 is microalbuminuria or incipient nephropathy and usually occurs after 6–15 years of diabetes. The GFR may still be elevated or may be reduced into the normal range. UAER during this stage is 20–200 µg/min (30–300 mg/24 h) (Table 32.1). The development of microalbuminuria is associated with a small but detectable increase in blood pressure although, at this stage, it usually remains within the conventional age-corrected normal ranges. Impairment of the normal nocturnal 'dipping' of blood pressure on 24-h ambulatory blood pressure monitoring has also been reported. There is also further progression of the histologic changes, with increases in basement membrane thickness and fractional mesangial volumes within the glomerulus, which will ultimately impinge on the filtration surfaces. In adolescents who develop microalbuminuria, those with initial hyperfiltration have a greater subsequent rate of decline in GFR (1.1 mL/min/year) compared without (0.8 mL/min/year). The rate of fall in GFR is positively correlated with glomerular basement membrane thickness, fractional mesangial volume and interstitial volume fraction[12].

Stage 4

Stage 4, established or overt nephropathy, invariably follows stage 3. By now, there are clear histologic changes, and hypertension is established in most patients. Proteinuria increases at the rate of 15% to 40% per annum. Nephrotic syndrome is common and may occur when GFR is normal although becomes more frequent as GFR declines. The GFR commences an inexorable decline, typically at a rate of approximately 10 mL/min/year. The rate of decline in GFR is strongly correlated with blood pressure levels.

Microscopic hematuria is seen in 66% of those with overt diabetic nephropathy and does not necessarily imply a glomerular disease other than DN, as was previously thought.

Stage 5

Stage 5, the development of ESRD, ensues within a median of 7 years from the development of persistent proteinuria, if therapeutic interventions are not undertaken.

Renal dysfunction in type 2 diabetes

Information available on the natural history of renal dysfunction in type 2 diabetes would suggest similarities with type 1 diabetes. Initially, it was thought that hyperfiltration was confined to type 1 diabetics, but it is now clear that hyperfiltration is present in many newly diagnosed type 2 diabetics compared to age-matched nondiabetic controls, with reversion towards normal following treatment. In newly diagnosed patients with type 2 diabetes, 30–40% have an elevated GFR[13]. GFR values are unrelated to blood pressure, prevailing glycemic control or lipid levels. The effective RPF is not raised; therefore, the filtration fraction (GFR divided by effective RPF) is also elevated in these patients. The increased filtration fraction implies an elevation in the glomerular capillary pressure (glomerular hypertension), which is thought to be an important factor in the development and progression of diabetic nephropathy.

Institution of effective therapy and the consequent improvement in glycemic control leads to a decrease in GFR. These changes are seen predominantly in the younger patients. Cross-sectional data indicate a persistent elevation in GFR in 25% of the younger patients with type 2 diabetes. Subsequent follow-up demonstrated a continuing decline in GFR in patients with hyperfiltration, while it remains stable in those with normal GFR. Hyperfiltration persists in approximately a third of the patient population compared to age-matched controls[13–15].

The course of GFR can be variable in type 2 diabetes. As in type 1, GFR remains stable in type 2 diabetes up to and possibly during the phase of microalbuminuria, or until hypertension intervenes or persistent proteinuria develops[13–15]. Hyperfiltration has been demonstrated in microalbuminuric compared with normoalbuminuric type 2 diabetics and nondiabetic controls (GFR 117 ± 24, 99 ± 15 and 98 ± 21 mL/min per 1.73 m², respectively)[14].

By comparison with type 1, the rate of decline in GFR in type 2 diabetics with established nephropathy has a wider range, with a mean of 5–10 mL/min/year but with a range of 1–20 mL/min/year. The rate of decline of GFR is still generally predictable in a given patient, unless a superimposed illness develops. The rate of decline correlates with blood pressure levels; in patients with type 2 diabetes, this correlation is particularly evident for the systolic blood pressure. Progressors are depicted by poorer glycemic control, higher blood pressures, higher initial albumin excretion rates, hypercholesterolemia, and smoking.

MICROALBUMINURIA

Definition and screening

Correct identification of incipient 'early' nephropathy by accurate measurement of microalbuminuria as UAER is crucial to strategies to modify the natural history of DN.

In a healthy population, the normal range for UAER is 1.5–20 µg/min, with a mean of 6.5 µg/min. UAER is known to increase with strenuous exercise, oral protein intake, fluid loading, urinary tract infection, and pregnancy. On avaerage, albumin excretion is 25% higher during the day than overnight, with a 40% day-to-day variation. Any definition must therefore apply to a standardized timed collection. An overnight urine sample is simpler and more convenient for patients to collect and will reduce the effect of many of these complicating

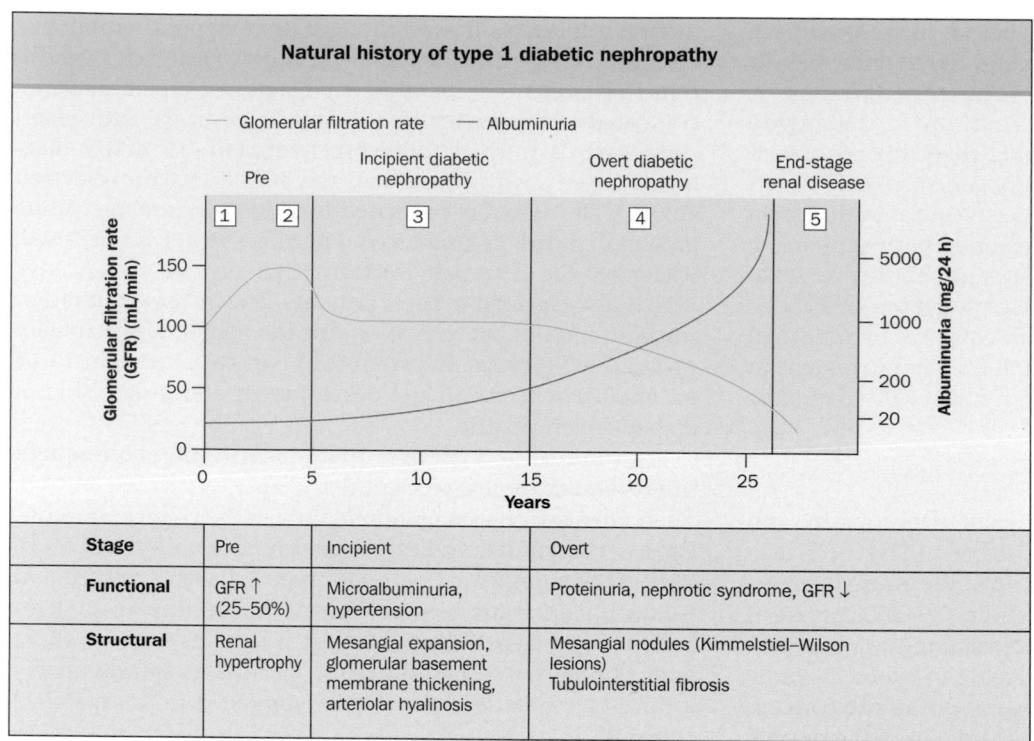

Figure 32.1 Natural history of type I diabetic nephropathy. Functional and structural manifestations of diabetic nephropathy. Numbers 1–5 indicate the stages of nephropathy defined by Mogensen[10].

factors. To make the diagnosis, two out of three consecutive collections within 3 months should be in the microalbuminuric range (Table 32.1).

To screen a large unselected diabetic population, measurement of the albumin:creatinine ratio (ACR, mg albumin : mmol creatinine) in an early morning urine sample is more practicable than collecting timed urine samples. In a mixed group of diabetics ACR > 2 predicts UAER > 30 μg/min with a sensitivity of 96% and a specificity of 99.7%. In females, ACR tends to be slightly higher than in males. A cut-off for microalbuminuria is often taken as ACR over 3.5 mg:mmol [50mg:g] for women and over 2.5 mg:mmol [35mg:g] in men. ACR values > 25 mg:mmol suggest persistent proteinuria.

Recently, a new system that utilizes reagent cartridges processed automatically (Bayer DCA 2000) has been marketed for immediate and quantitative detection of microalbuminuria, which on comparative testing with a routine laboratory-based method (immuniturbidimetric assay) was found to have a high sensitivity and specificity of approximately 92% and 100% respectively[16–17]. Its accuracy, ease of use and low cost would make it suitable for the clinic environment as the system could also be used for the immediate measurement of glycated hemoglobin (HbA$_{1c}$).

Screening recommendations

For early detection of nephropathy and the establishment of a successful prevention program, the recommendations are that all type 1 diabetics diagnosed for more than 5 years and over 12 years of age and all type 2 diabetics from diagnosis should have their urine screened for albumin yearly until the age of 70 years. If the morning ACR is raised, and a concurrent urinary tract infection excluded, three timed overnight urine collections should be arranged. Those with an elevated UAER should then be screened every 6 months (Fig. 32.2).

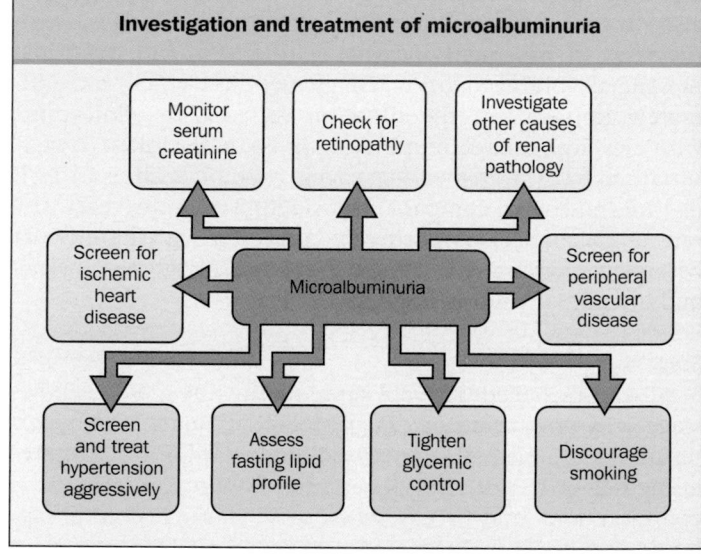

Figure 32.2 Investigation and treatment of microalbuminuria.

Microalbuminuria in type I diabetes

The prevalence of microalbuminuria in type 1 diabetics is approximately 20% (Table 32.2). The mean duration of diabetes for patients with microalbuminuria is 20 years; it is rarely detected with a disease duration of less than 5 years. The incidence of diabetic nephropathy, and the prevalence of microalbuminuria, is higher in those diagnosed under 20 years of age.

Microalbuminuria is now well recognized to represent the earliest clinically detectable phase of diabetic renal dysfunction, with a predictive value of > 80% for subsequent progression to overt nephropathy over 10–15 years. Prospective studies

Clinical Manifestations and Natural History of Diabetic Nephropathy

Prevalence and incidence of microalbuminuria and overt proteinuria in type 1 and type 2 diabetes		
	Type 1	Type 2
Prevalence		
Microalbuminuria (%): mean (range)	16 (9–21)	38 (15–60)
Overt proteinuria (%): mean (range)	15 (18–22)	15 (5–48)
At diagnosis (%): mean (range)	0	9 (5–20)
Incidence		
Overt proteinuria (%/year): mean (range)	1.2 (0–3)	1.5 (1–2)
Cumulative incidence of nephropathy (%/25 year): mean (range)	35 (28–34)	28 (25–47)

Table 32.2 Prevalence and incidence of microalbuminuria and overt proteinuria in type 1 and type 2 diabetes.

have shown that while only 0.5% of normoalbuminuric normotensive type 1 diabetic patients develop nephropathy over a 5-year follow-up period, 29% of normotensive patients with persistent microalbuminuria will become nephropathic. The GFR is normal or slightly elevated during the first 6 years of microalbuminuria before nephropathy develops, after which it declines by an average of 3.5 mL/min/year.

Epidemiologic studies have identified several putative risk factors for the development and progression of microalbuminuria in both type 1 and type 2 diabetes. These include glycemic control, genetic predisposition (including familial clustering, angiotensin converting enzyme (ACE) insertion/deletion (ID) polymorphism, and certain ethnic groups), male sex and age at diagnosis of type 1 diabetes, mean arterial blood pressure > 95 mmHg, smoking, hyperlipidemia, presence of retinopathy, and above median normoalbuminuria[18]. Patients with type 1 diabetes and microalbuminuria are characterized by increasing prevalence of hypertension and other microvascular complications, such as retinopathy (Table 32.3).

Microalbuminuria in type 2 diabetes
In a population of newly diagnosed patients with type 2 diabetes, UAER is, on average, two to three times higher than in age-matched controls. There is a poorer correlation with disease duration than in type 1 diabetes, possibly as a consequence of delayed diagnosis following the onset of type 2 diabetes. The prevalence of microalbuminuria at diagnosis is

5–20% (Table 32.2), although there is an initial decrease in UAER with treatment of diabetes. Cross-sectional studies in type 2 diabetes show a 15–60% prevalence of microalbuminuria depending on the racial origin of the patients. Pima Indians in the USA and Indo-Asians in the UK have a particularly high incidence of microalbuminuria[19]. In European cohorts, there is now agreement on a prevalence of approximately 25% to 30%. Compared to their normoalbuminuric counterparts, such patients are characterized by being older, with poorer glycemic control, higher mean blood pressure levels, hypercholesterolemia and smoking. In patients with type 2 diabetes, albuminuria can develop as a consequence of hypertension, cardiovascular disease, and diabetic or nondiabetic renal disease. Approximately 2% of a cohort of type 2 diabetic patients progress from normoalbuminuria to microalbuminuria per annum. Microalbuminuria in such patients predicts the development of nephropathy in approximately 10–40% at 10 years. In those patients likely to progress, there is a predictable increase in the UAER of 15–40% per annum, with a transition rate of microalbuminuria to overt nephropathy of 2.5% per annum. Modelling suggests that patients remain in a given stage of albuminuria for approximately 9–10 years. As mentioned above, GFR changes in type 2 patients with microalbuminuria can be variable, from a baseline of normal or high-normal values.

Recent studies have evaluated the course of microalbuminuria in type 2 diabetes during anti-hypertensive treatment. During a 2-year study period, blood pressure levels of 145/84 mmHg, using antihypertensive agents other than those interfering with the renin–angiotensin system, resulted in normalization of urinary albumin excretion in 20% of patients, whilst progression to overt nephropathy was observed in 15%. In such patients, a small but gradual overall reduction in albuminuria of approximately 10%, was seen over 2 years. Thus, the control of elevated blood pressure is an important factor in preventing the progression of microalbuminuria in type 2 diabetes.

Renal structure–function relationships in microalbuminuria
Diabetic patients with microalbuminuria have more advanced mesangial and matrix expansion with an increase in basement membrane thickness compared to normoalbuminuric individuals with prolonged duration of diabetes. Type 1 diabetics with microalbuminuria have an increased renal volume compared with normoalbuminuric controls. Generally, in type 1

Albuminuria in type 1 diabetics and the development of hypertension, retinopathy, and neuropathy				
Urine albumin excretion status	Prevalence of hypertension (>140/90 mmHg) (%)	Prevalence of proliferative retinopathy(%)[a]	Prevalence of diabetes-related blindness(%)	Prevalence of neuropathy(%)
Normoalbuminuria	20	12	1	21
Microalbuminuria	40	28	6	31
Macroalbuminuria	80	58	11	50
[a] Background retinopathy is found in over 90% of patients with nephropathy.				

Table 32.3 Albuminuria in type 1 diabetics and the development of hypertension, retinopathy, and neuropathy.

Diabetic Nephropathy

Decline of glomerular filtration rate in diabetics with varying rates of urinary albumin excretion		
	Rate of decline in glomerular filtration rate (mL/min per year)	
	Type 1	Type 2
Normoalbuminuria	1.2–3.6	0.96
Microalbuminuria	1.2–3.6	2.4
Overt nephropathy	9.6–12	5.4–7.2

Table 32.4 Decline of glomerular filtration rate in diabetics with varying rates of urinary albumin excretion.

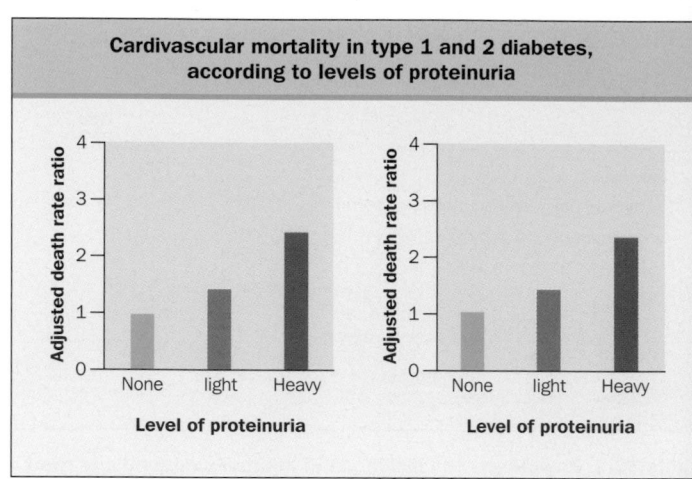

Figure 32.3 Cardiovascular mortality in type 1 and 2 diabetes, according to levels of proteinuria. Death rates adjusted for age, duration of diabetes, systolic blood pressure, serum cholesterol and smoking.

diabetic nephropathy, the renal structure is homogenous and the decline in GFR is the same as in age-matched controls until the development of overt nephropathy. However, patients with type 2 diabetes and microalbuminuria, show structurally heterogenous patterns with less than one third having 'typical' diabetic nephropathology[20]. Other subsets include up to a third of patients in whom renal histology may appear 'normal', and another third having 'atypical' changes with a preponderance of interstitial fibrosis and vascular hyalinosis. In addition, the rate of progression of nephropathy is variable in type 2 diabetic patients, with a subset of patients who have a rapid decline in GFR in line with increasing UAER; these patients have more advanced diabetic glomerulopathy than the remaining patients, whose GFR remains stable[21] (Table 32.4).

CONDITIONS ASSOCIATED WITH MICROALBUMINURIA AND PROTEINURIA

The distinction between microalbuminuria and proteinuria in diabetic nephropathy is tightly defined in clinical practice. Nevertheless, there is a continuum of risk for vascular complications associated with increasing urinary protein excretion, even within the currently accepted 'normal' range, with further increases as microalbuminuria increases to overt proteinuria. These complications include extrarenal microangiopathic complications of diabetes, and also cardiovascular disease.

Diabetic microangiopathy
There is compelling evidence in both type 1 and 2 diabetes that prevalence of proliferative retinopathy and blindness increases with progressive albuminuria. Peripheral neuropathy also increases, together with the risk of foot ulceration, with a prevalence of 21% in normoalbuminuria, 31% in microalbuminuria and 50% in those with macroalbuminuria (Table 32.3)[22,23].

Cardiovascular disease
In patients with both type 1 and 2 diabetes, as indeed in elderly nondiabetic individuals, abnormal albumin excretion rate, especially microalbuminuria, is a stronger predictor of cardiovascular morbidity and mortality, as discussed above. There is a significant excess mortality (relative risk 2.3) for

those with microalbuminuria compared to those with normoalbuminuria. In a study of patients with type 2 diabetes, there was a 28% mortality rate in those with microalbuminuria compared with 4% in the normoalbuminuria group over a 3–4-year period, or 70% at 10 years compared to 20% of normoalbuminuric patients[24]. In another study, 69% of microalbuminuric patients died in 10 years; 58% from cardiovascular or cerebrovascular disease and 7% from ESRD . The continuum of increasing cardiovascular mortality applies to both type 1 and 2 patients (Fig 32.3)[22]. Recent studies have also documented the continual variable effect of abnormal urinary albumin excretion on mortality with increasing cardiovascular mortality. Microalbuminuria is also associated with coronary heart disease, including silent myocardial ischemia, and left ventricular hypertrophy.

Microalbuminuria may represent the renal manifestation of generalized vascular endothelial dysfunction, which could underlie the link with cardiovascular disease. In both type 1 and type 2 diabetes, microalbuminuric patients have an unfavorable cardiovascular risk factor profile, with an increased incidence of hyperlipidemia, hypertension, obesity and insulin resistance. The positive correlation with UAER indicates that endothelial cell function and coagulation disorders deteriorate with the progression of nephropathy (Fig. 32.4).

Hypertension
Type 1 diabetics with overt nephropathy have an 80% prevalence of hypertension (> 140/90 mmHg) compared to 40% in those with microalbuminuria and 20% in those with normoalbuminuria (Table 32.3). Although blood pressure may remain below 140/90 mmHg until there is overt nephropathy, it begins to rise once UAER has increased into the microalbuminuric range, increasing by an average of 2.7 mmHg/year. This is commonly associated with an impairment of physiologic nocturnal dipping of blood pressure.

A significant increase in extracellular fluid volume with increased sodium retention, due to hyperinsulinemia with or

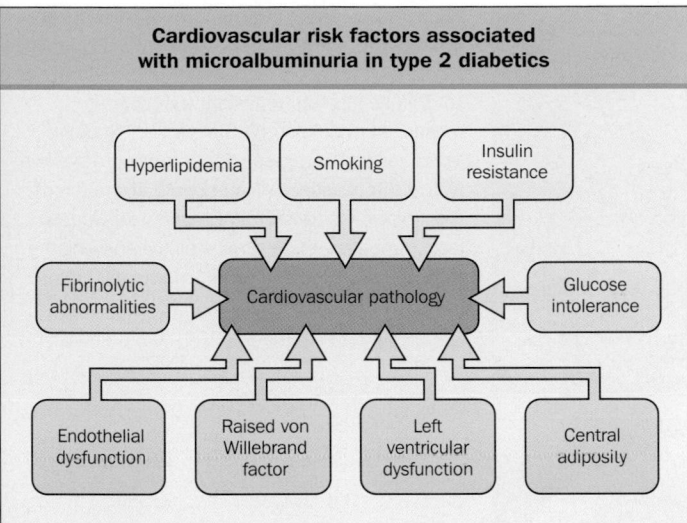

Figure 32.4 Cardiovascular risk factors associated with microalbuminuria in type 2 diabetics.

RENAL PATHOLOGY

Renal size
The kidneys of patients with diabetes are, on average, larger than those of nondiabetic control subjects. Following the onset of diabetes, kidney weight increases by an average of 15%, with parallel increases in the protein and RNA content of the kidney and an increase in DNA synthesis. These changes can be reversed with induction of early normoglycemia, but strict metabolic control after the establishment of renal hypertrophy has no effect on kidney size. In diabetics with microalbuminuria, renal volume continues to increase as UAER rises to the level of overt proteinuria. Thus, renal size remains increased until overt nephropathy is established.

In most patients with type 1 diabetes, there is a sustained increase in glomerular volume and glomerular capillary luminal volume. The initial glomerular enlargement is not accompanied by hyperplasia. Hypertrophy may be an expression of compensatory growth in the face of progressive glomerular loss. Although atrophic ischemic glomeruli are present, some of the non-functioning glomeruli fill up with material staining with periodic acid–Schiff (PAS), thus preserving their increased dimensions. These changes are accompanied by hypertrophy of the interstitium, which of course accounts for a large proportion of the overall renal weight.

In animal models, glomerular growth is prominent during the first 4 days following induction of diabetes. Glomerular capillary length and radial cross-sectional area of the capillary loop are responsible for the increase in glomerular size. Tubular growth then catches up and exceeds glomerular growth over the course of the first 6 weeks. The length of both the proximal and the distal tubules increases by approximately 20%. Whereas proximal tubular cells retain a normal appearance, the distal cells in the cortex and outer medullary strip appear laden with glycogen-like granules and show a marked reduction in the number of organelles and basal infoldings. These morphologic changes appear to precede the early hemodynamic alterations and may contribute to them.

Light microscopy
Nodular glomerular intercapillary lesions
Nodular glomerular intercapillary lesions in the diabetic kidney were described in 1936 by Kimmelstiel and Wilson[25] (Fig. 32.5c,d). They also related them to the clinical syndrome of profuse proteinuria and renal failure accompanied by arterial hypertension.

Early biopsy series confirmed similar histologic changes in the kidneys of patients with type 1 and type 2 diabetes. Reports that the characteristic changes have been found in the absence of diabetes have not withstood critical review. The nodules are located in the central regions of peripheral glomerular lobules as well-demarcated hard masses that are eosinophilic and PAS positive (Fig. 32.5c,d). They are irregular in size and distribution, both within and between glomerular loops, and are located away from the hilum. When not acellular, they contain pyknotic nuclei. Nodules appear to be of mesangial origin. It is suggested that they result from microaneurysmal dilatation of the associated capillary followed by mesangiolysis and laminar organization of the mesangial debris with lysis of the

without insulin resistance, is a significant factor in the rise in blood pressure. In type 2 diabetes, the prevalence of hypertension is 30–50% at onset of diagnosis of diabetes, increasing to 90% with the development of abnormal urinary albumin excretion. The increase in hypertension after the diagnosis of diabetes is related to albuminuria.

Hyperlipidemia
Hypertriglyceridemia typically develops once microalbuminuria has occurred. High-density lipoprotein cholesterol falls and there are variable increases in low-density lipoprotein (LDL) cholesterol and lipoprotein (a). Hydroxymethylglutaryl CoA reductase inhibitors (statins) are the drug therapy of choice if non-pharmacologic approaches to therapy are unsuccessful. Fibrate derivatives should also be used if hypertriglyceridemia is prominent. There is no definitive evidence yet that lipid lowering may reduce progression of diabetic nephropathy. However, small scale studies do suggest a reduction in abnormal urinary albumin excretion rate. Such an effect is also suggested by a meta-analysis of studies of lipid-lowering agents in renal impairment. There is strong evidence that lipid lowering has a role in primary and secondary prevention of coronary heart disease in diabetics, especially in patients with increased risk of mortality, such as those with increased urinary albumin excretion rates in both type 1 and 2 diabetes. Available data support a target LDL cholesterol of 120 mg/dL (3.0 mmol/L) in diabetes.

MANAGEMENT OF MICROALBUMINURIA

Once microalbuminuria is established, active management is required both to diminish UAER to minimize the risk of progression to overt nephropathy and to treat the associated cardiovascular risk factors. The treatment strategies presently available for treatment of microalbuminuria include glycemic control, early use of ACE inhibitors and optimum control of blood pressure (see Chapter 33).

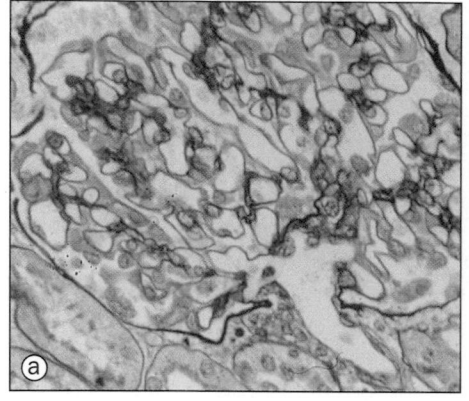
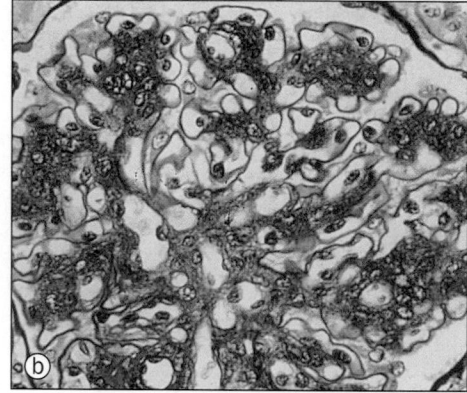
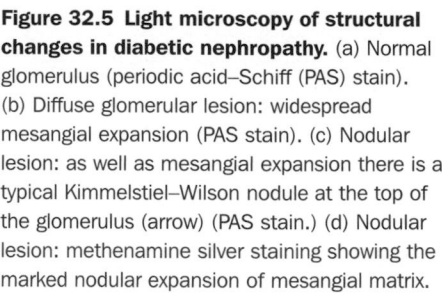
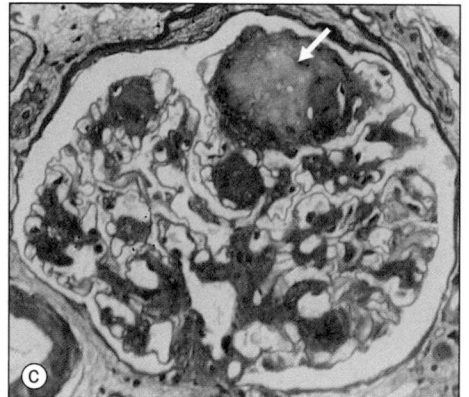
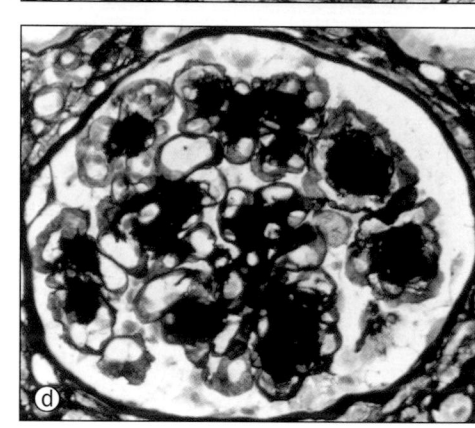

Figure 32.5 Light microscopy of structural changes in diabetic nephropathy. (a) Normal glomerulus (periodic acid–Schiff (PAS) stain). (b) Diffuse glomerular lesion: widespread mesangial expansion (PAS stain). (c) Nodular lesion: as well as mesangial expansion there is a typical Kimmelstiel–Wilson nodule at the top of the glomerulus (arrow) (PAS stain.) (d) Nodular lesion: methenamine silver staining showing the marked nodular expansion of mesangial matrix.

center of the lobule. Foam cells often surround the nodules, with distension of adjoining capillaries. When present, these appearances are pathognomonic for diabetes, but they are not a universal finding and are reported in only 12% to 46% of biopsies in both type 1 and type 2 diabetes.

Diffuse glomerular lesions

The diffuse glomerular lesion is more frequent than the nodular lesion, with an incidence of over 90% for patients with type 1 diabetes of over 10 years duration and an incidence of 25–50% in patients with type 2 diabetes. It comprises an increase of mesangial matrix extending to involve the capillary loops (Fig. 32.5b). In more severe disease, the capillary wall thickening and mesangial expansion lead to capillary narrowing and hyalinization, with accompanying periglomerular fibrosis. The distribution of the diffuse lesions is irregular, both among lobules of the same glomeruli and between different glomeruli.

Exudative lesions

The exudative lesions are highly eosinophilic, rounded homogeneous structures seen in the capsular space, overlying a capillary loop (fibrin cap) or lying on the inside of a Bowman's capsule (capsular drop). These lesions, containing proteins and some lipid material, are nonspecific; similar lesions are seen in a variety of nondiabetic renal conditions.

Arteriolar lesions

Arteriolar lesions are prominent in diabetes, with hyaline material progressively replacing the entire wall structure and involving both the afferent and efferent vessels. Whereas afferent arteriolar hyalinization occurs in other conditions, including hypertension, involvement of the efferent vessel is highly specific for diabetes. The changes can occur in the absence of hypertension. In nondiabetic kidneys transplanted into diabetic patients, the vascular changes occur as early as 2 years after grafting.

Tubules and interstitium

The tubules and the interstitium may show a variety of nonspecific changes. Common findings are tubular cell vacuolization, a decrease in the intercellular spaces normally present between the macula densa cells, and a significant increase in the contact area between them and the extraglomerular mesangial cells.

Immunopathology

In patients with type 1 diabetes, immunofluorescence microscopy may show linear staining of the glomerular basement membrane, Bowman's capsule, and outer aspect of the tubule for IgG and IgM, albumin and fibrinogen. These proteins probably reach such sites passively as the result of increased capillary permeability, rather than through more specific interactions. There are also increases of type IV and V collagen, laminin and fibronectin in the mesangium, and the presence of antigens normally expressed in fetal glomeruli only. Heparan sulfate proteoglycans are decreased, whereas levels of fibronectin do not differ from normal controls. The possibility of abnormalities in the contractile properties of the mesangium has been considered following the demonstration of increased amounts of actomyosin. Fibrin products, as well as IgG and complement components, have been found in the exudative lesions of the glomeruli and of the arterioles, suggesting a role for the coagulation process in the genesis of glomerulosclerosis.

Electron microscopy

Thickening of the glomerular basement membrane is a prominent feature in the kidneys of diabetic patients and can be evident within 2 years following the diagnosis (Fig. 32.6). There is an 80% increase in the area of the capillary wall found within months of the onset of type 1 diabetes. Excessive irregular thickening of the basement membrane is associated with nodular renal disease. In all stages of diabetic nephropathy, there are no electron-dense deposits. The foot processes of the epithelial cells remain discrete until renal function has declined to 20% of normal, when they become wider in cross-section with shortening of the filtration slits[26]. Eventually, podocyte fusion and effacement are noted. The fractional volume of the mesangium can be more than double that of controls. The nodules appear to comprise matrix components with their laminated periphery derived from expanded folded basement membrane. The exudative lesions appear on electron microscopy as finely granular electron-dense material. In arterioles, this material spreads from a subintimal location towards the media and then to its near replacement. The capsular drop corresponds to accumulation of this material between the epithelial cells and the basement membrane of Bowman's capsule, whereas the fibrin cap represents its presence along the endothelial side of the glomerular membrane.

Correlation of structure and function

Most of the data on the correlation of morphology and function comes from patients with type 1 diabetes. Unlike other chronic renal pathologies, relatively large kidneys persist with progressing renal failure. Hypertrophied glomeruli are probably a prerequisite for hyperfiltration. The increase in luminal volume and filtration surface is visible on light and electron microscopy. Nodular lesions are of little functional significance, while the degree of diffuse glomerulosclerosis, with changes in the mesangium and glomerular capillaries,

correlates with the clinical manifestations of worsening renal function. The extent of renal histologic changes may correlate poorly with varying degrees of urinary albumin excretion. However, with advancing renal disease, there is a more consistent correlation between glomerular basement membrane thickness and fractional mesangial volumes with UAER[27]. Mesangial volume correlates inversely with the capillary filtering area and is inversely associated with GFR. In patients with type 1 diabetes, mesangial fraction does not correlate with UAER under 30 µg/min; above this value, the mesangial volume is significantly increased. However, there are occasional patients with long-term type 1 diabetes who do not demonstrate abnormal urinary albumin excretion rate but do have marked abnormalities of renal histology.

Biopsy interpretation

Many of these histologic changes are nonspecific but when described simultaneously are highly suggestive of diabetes. The degree of efferent arteriolar hyalinization seen in diabetes is uncommon outside this condition. Nodular masses similar to diabetic nodules may be found in membranoproliferative glomerulonephritis (MPGN), but the nodules in MPGN are evenly distributed with characteristic loop changes and hypercellularity. Immunofluorescence findings and electron microscopy will establish the diagnosis. Nodules are also seen in amyloid, where they are unevenly distributed, and in light-chain deposition disease (see Chapter 29). In these conditions, specific stains and immunofluorescence findings, respectively, will clarify the diagnosis.

When there are no nodules seen, specific staining should be used to exclude amyloid. In membranous nephropathy, the thickening of the capillary loops and the degree of glomerular involvement are even, whereas this is rare in diabetes. In non-specific arteriosclerosis and in age-related changes, obsolete glomeruli tend to be reduced in size, whereas in diabetes large hyalinized glomeruli are seen. Interstitial inflammation and scarring are present in 10% to 40% of renal biopsies from patients with diabetes, although these changes may result from ischemia or papillary necrosis or may be secondary to glomerular disease rather than to recurrent infections.

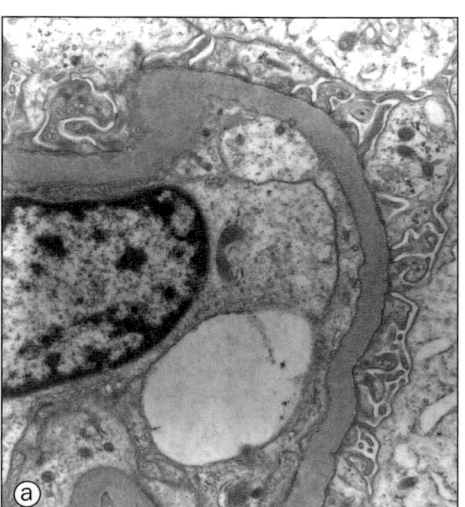
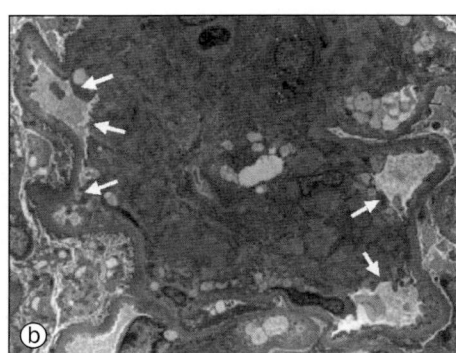

Figure 32.6 Electron microscopy of structural changes in diabetic nephropathy. (a) Glomerular basement membranes are diffusely thickened. (b) The expanded mesangium encroaches on the capillary spaces (arrows).

DIAGNOSIS AND DIFFERENTIAL DIAGNOSIS

When proteinuria develops in a diabetic, the clinical evaluation is directed at establishing a presumptive diagnosis of diabetic nephropathy, thus obviating the need for renal biopsy. Alternatively, atypical clinical and laboratory features may be identified that point to nondiabetic glomerular disease requiring identification by renal biopsy. The third possibility, particularly if azotemia develops with no more than low-grade proteinuria, is that there is a nonglomerular disease, most commonly renovascular disease or papillary necrosis. An approach to the evaluation of the proteinuric diabetic is shown in Figure 32.7.

The majority of diabetic patients with proteinuria and retinopathy will have diabetic nephropathy. With prolonged disease duration, most type 1 diabetics develop the typical histologic lesions of diabetic glomerulosclerosis, although only one third develop clinically apparent nephropathy. Studies of renal histopathology indicate that approximately one third of type 2 diabetics with proteinuria will demonstrate the classical diabetic glomerular changes and they usually have coexisting retinopathy; slightly under one third have nondiabetic renal disease or indeed, on light microscopy, demonstrate normal histology, while the rest will have a mixed picture of diabetic and nondiabetic renal changes, encompassing interstitial and vascular changes. Some 50% of patients in the latter group also have significant retinopathy. Nondiabetic renal disease superimposed on diabetic nephropathy occurs more frequently in type 2 than in type 1 diabetes. Figures for nondiabetic causes for proteinuria in type 2 diabetes range from 6% to 25%, depending on patient selection criteria. Proteinuria develops in only 4% of patients with type 1 diabetes within 10 years of diagnosis, so early-onset proteinuria should raise the suspicion of nondiabetic renal disease. Approximately, 8% of patients with type 2 diabetes have proteinuria at diagnosis, making the duration of known diabetes of less value in elucidating the cause of renal pathology.

Retinopathy and diabetic nephropathy have a concordance rate of 85–99% in type 1 and 63% in type 2 diabetes, making the absence of retinopathy a strong indication for renal biopsy, particularly in type 1 patients. In a series of 136 consecutive biopsies in both type 1 and type 2 diabetics, a 66% incidence of microscopic hematuria was noted. Other studies have shown 69% of type 1 diabetics with proteinuria and hematuria to have concomitant nondiabetic renal disease. While low-grade microscopic hematuria is common in diabetic nephropathy, macroscopic hematuria is not a feature of diabetic nephropathy, and red cell casts have only been found in 4% of biopsy-proven diabetic nephropathy. There is an increased incidence of renal papillary necrosis and tuberculosis in diabetes and, in the presence of modest proteinuria, these diagnoses should be considered. In type 2 diabetics, it is important also to consider renal artery stenosis.

Indications for renal biopsy (Fig. 32.7)

Therefore, in both type 1 and type 2 diabetes, but particularly in type 2, further investigations including a renal biopsy should be considered

- in the absence of retinopathy especially in type 1 diabetes;
- with sudden and rapid onset of proteinuria particularly with known disease duration of less than 5 years and/or abnormal evolution without transition through usual stages (e.g., the development of nephrotic syndrome without previous microalbuminuria);

Figure 32.7 Clinical evaluation of diabetic renal disease.

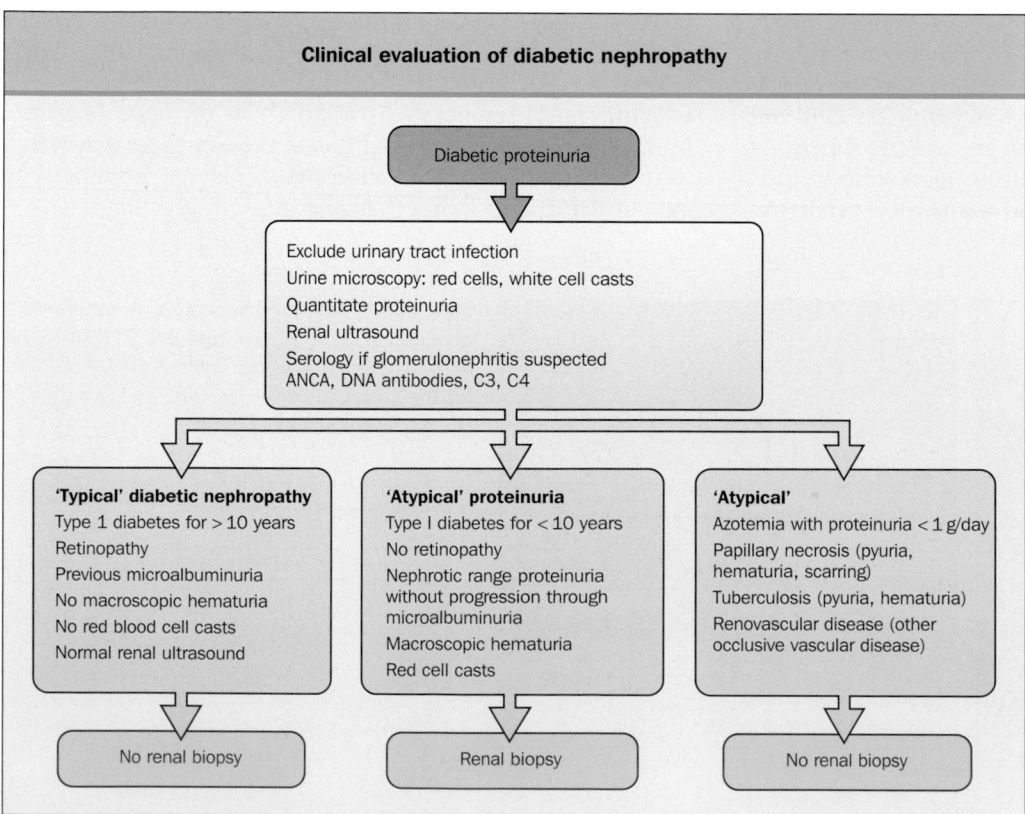

Clinical evaluation of diabetic nephropathy

Diabetic proteinuria

Exclude urinary tract infection
Urine microscopy: red cells, white cell casts
Quantitate proteinuria
Renal ultrasound
Serology if glomerulonephritis suspected
ANCA, DNA antibodies, C3, C4

'Typical' diabetic nephropathy
Type 1 diabetes for > 10 years
Retinopathy
Previous microalbuminuria
No macroscopic hematuria
No red blood cell casts
Normal renal ultrasound

'Atypical' proteinuria
Type I diabetes for < 10 years
No retinopathy
Nephrotic range proteinuria without progression through microalbuminuria
Macroscopic hematuria
Red cell casts

'Atypical'
Azotemia with proteinuria < 1 g/day
Papillary necrosis (pyuria, hematuria, scarring)
Tuberculosis (pyuria, hematuria)
Renovascular disease (other occlusive vascular disease)

No renal biopsy

Renal biopsy

No renal biopsy

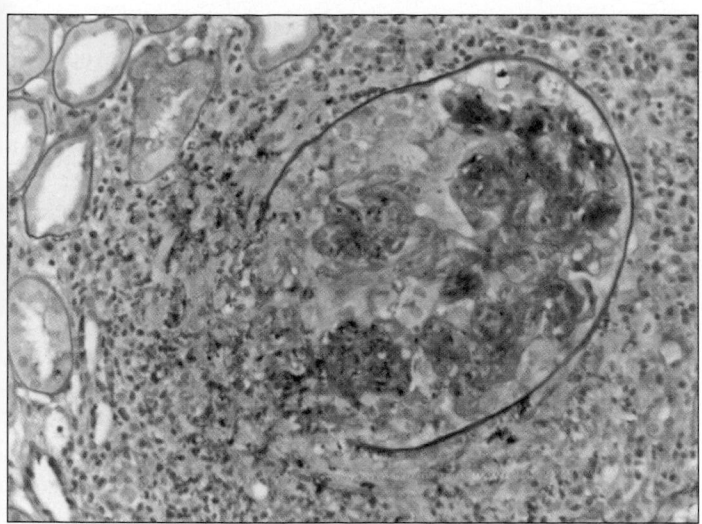

Figure 32.8 Glomerulonephritis superimposed on diabetic nephropathy. A glomerulus showing a cellular crescent with rupture of Bowman's capsule superimposed on nodular diabetic nephropathy. The patient, known to have diabetic nephropathy presented with rapidly deteriorating renal function and red cell casts in the urine.

- with macroscopic hematuria;
- with a urinary sediment suggestive of an active glomerulonephritis, such as red cell casts (Fig. 32.8);
- with a rapid decline of renal function or renal dysfunction without significant proteinuria, when renovascular disease has to be considered.

OTHER RENAL DISEASE IN DIABETICS

Glomerulonephritis

Almost every form of glomerular disease has been reported in association with diabetes. The incidence of nondiabetic causes for proteinuria in diabetes range from 4–25%, the latter figure relating particularly to the type 2 cohort. It is not clear whether most of these reports merely represent the coincidence of the two conditions rather than a specific association. Inevitably, the perceived incidence of nondiabetic glomerular disease will depend on the frequency with which renal biopsy is performed and the clinical criteria used to select patients for renal biopsy.

Membranous nephropathy

Membranous nephropathy is the glomerular disease most commonly reported in association with diabetes. In most cases patients present at the age of 40–60 years after 10 or more years of diabetes. In one series, only 25% of those with membranous nephropathy had retinopathy and most had nephrotic-range proteinuria. While the assocation of membranous nephropathy and diabetes may also be a coincidence of common conditions, it has been proposed that structural alterations of the glomerular basement membrane and its interactions with the podocyte may predispose to expression of a neoantigen initiating an autoimmune process at that site.

Renal papillary necrosis

At autopsy, 4.4% of diabetic kidneys showed evidence of papillary necrosis, though 50% of patients with papillary necrosis had diabetes. The incidence and severity of papillary necrosis is decreasing with early antibiotic treatment but tends to occur in those with long-standing diabetes. If initially unilateral, it will often affect the contralateral kidney over subsequent years and will eventually be bilateral in 65% of patients. Papillary necrosis is more common in females, especially when recurrent urinary tract infections occur. Presentation can be asymptomatic, following an indolent course with recurrent urinary tract infections and/or renal colic. Microscopic hematuria is frequent with renal papillary necrosis and sterile pyuria is typical. Modest proteinuria (< 2 g/24 h) is common. The urographic appearances are often characteristic (see Fig. 51.9).

Renovascular disease

Diabetics have an increased incidence of occlusive vascular disease. Renovascular disease is recognized with increasing frequency, especially in association with peripheral vascular disease. Typically, there may be renal impairment that develops in the context of microalbuminuria or mild proteinuria. Hypertension is common but is not a universal feature. When suspected, the diagnosis should be sought by duplex scanning, spiral computed tomography scanning or magnetic resonance angiography followed by conventional angiography. The problem of renovascular disease and its investigation is discussed further in Chapters 5, 39 and 63.

Autonomic neuropathy of the bladder

When diagnosed on urodynamic criteria, autonomic neuropathy of the bladder has a prevalence of 40% in long-standing diabetes (Table 32.5). Ultrasound scanning may lead to

Diabetic autonomic neuropathy of the bladder: clinical presentations and pathology		
Symptoms	**Signs**	**Pathology**
Asymptomatic	Decreased awareness of bladder distension ⇓ Micturition at progressively larger volumes	Destruction of proprioceptive afferent fibers
Loss of nocturia and decrease in daytime micturition frequency Weak stream after straining, dribbling, involuntary stream interruption, overflow incontinence	Weakened bladder contraction ⇓ Incomplete emptying, increased residual volume	Disruption of parasympathetic innervation to detrusor and efferent sympathetic innervation to trigone
Recurrent urinary tract infections	Functional incompetence of vesicoureteral junction plus incomplete relaxation of internal sphincter during micturition	Urethral sphincter dysynergy

Table 32.5 Diabetic autonomic neuropathy of the bladder: clinical presentations and pathology.

detection of a large residual volume, while urodynamic studies can characterize the nature of the bladder dysfunction. Patients should be advised to assist regular voiding in the absence of urge with suprapubic manual pressure. Intermittent self-catheterization may lead to a reduction in bladder volume and some recovery of detrusor function. Long-term catheterization may ultimately be the only solution.

Urinary tract infection

The incidence of asymptomatic bacteriuria in diabetic women is double that of a control nondiabetic population. Diabetic nephropathy only appears to be associated with an increase in symptomatic urinary tract infection during pregnancy.

Acute pyelonephritis

Acute pyelonephritis leads to perinephric abscesses with increased frequency in diabetics. Urine culture may be negative, with flank tenderness and pyrexia as the main signs. Infections with Gram-negative organisms are also more common in diabetes: 90% of cases of emphysematous pyelonephritis occur in patients with diabetes, predominantly females, where the parenchyma is most commonly infected by *Escherichia coli*.

Renal tuberculosis

Diabetics have an increased risk of developing renal tuberculosis. It should be suspected when there is azotemia with modest proteinuria especially if there is also sterile pyuria. Although renal imaging may be suggestive and a tuberculin test may be positive, the diagnosis requires culture of *Mycobacteria* spp. in the urine (see Chapter 54).

Contrast nephrotoxicity

Diabetic patients with established nephropathy are at increased risk of deterioration in renal function following the use of contrast media, although a lower incidence is reported using nonionic contrast. Patients with type 1 diabetes appear to be at greater risk than type 2 patients. Patients without pre-existing renal dysfunction would appear to be at minimal risk. Good hydration and avoidance of concomitant nonsteroidal anti-inflammatory agents or aminoglycosides will minimize the risk. The need to avoid treatment with metformin prior to and for 2 days following an investigation involving contrast has been recommended: it has been reported that metformin-induced metabolic acidosis can be provoked by the administration of contrast.

PREGNANCY AND DIABETIC NEPHROPATHY

In European populations, type 1 diabetes occurs in about 3 per 1000 pregnancies. During pregnancy, there is an increase in GFR and a decrease in the tubular absorption of protein. Most women with diabetic nephropathy have a gradual increase in proteinuria during the first two trimesters with a more rapid increase in the third. There is a significant increase in blood pressure and proteinuria, with nephrotic syndrome developing in 71% of pregnancies. All values return to those seen during the first trimester after delivery[28]. Whether pregnancy

causes a worsening of diabetic nephropathy or hastens progression to ESRD is still debated. In diabetic nephropathy, approximately 50% of patients will have an increase in serum creatinine and/or a decline in creatinine clearance during pregnancy. Long-term data in those with moderate renal impairment suggest no consistent adverse long-term effects of pregnancy on renal function, although differing changes in renal function were observed during pregnancy. After delivery renal function usually returns to baseline. For four out of five women with pre-existing moderate renal insufficiency, pregnancy does not lead to a long-term deterioration in renal function. Most support the view that pregnancy in type 1 diabetes does not increase the risk of subsequently developing nephropathy. Data are limited for pregnancy in the type 2 diabetic patient, but this situation is likely to develop more frequently with the earlier development of type 2 diabetes, including in early teens. The principles of aggressive management of all risk factors, particulary hypertension, are similar to those applicable to type 1 diabetes. Given the contraindications of use of oral hypoglycemic agents in those contemplating or already pregnant, the need for insulin therapy is universal.

The metabolic derangement of the diabetes itself, the renal dysfunction, and the frequently associated problem of hypertension can all adversely affect fetal growth and development and threaten the health of the mother.

Pregnancy outcome

Diabetic nephropathy, more than any other vascular complication, has the greatest impact on fetal outcome. The risk of preterm birth, stillbirth, neonatal death, and fetal distress are increased significantly among diabetic women with nephropathy (Table 32.6). Intrauterine growth retardation is more common in women with diabetic nephropathy, with

Pregnancy outcomes in diabetic nephropathy	
	Number (%)
Patients	57
Fetal death	4 (7)
Preterm (>34 weeks)	18 (32)
Small for gestational age	10 (17.5)
Large for gestational age	7 (12)
Major congenital abnormalities	6 (10.5)
Respiratory distress syndrome	12 (21)
Hypoglycemia	13 (23)
Hyperbilirubinemia	19 (33)
Death	1 (1.8)
Perinatal survival	52 (91)
(Adapted with permission from Reece et al.[28])	

Table 32.6 Pregnancy outcomes in diabetic nephropathy.

approximately 19% having babies small for gestational age compared to 2.2% for diabetic women without renal disease. The frequency of fetal growth retardation doubles in the first trimester if hypertension is also present. The perinatal mortality in this group can exceed 90% if the fetus is delivered after 36 weeks of gestation[28,29].

Management

Ideally, management should begin before the planned pregnancy with optimization of glycemic and hypertension control, and of medications. Oral hypoglycemic agents should be stopped prior to conception because of the possible teratogenic effects of currently available agents, and insulin commenced if required. ACE inhibitor therapy during pregnancy has been associated with fetal morbidity, including renal tubular dysplasia, anuria/oligohydramnios, growth retardation, hypocalvaria, intrauterine death and increased first-trimester loss. Discontinuation of ACE inhibitors and stabilization of the patient on alternative antihypertensive therapy prior to conception is recommended.

Further general management of pregnant women with pre-existing renal disease is discussed in Chapter 45.

REFERENCES

1. The Diabetes Control and Complications Trial Research Group. Effect of intensive therapy on the development and progression of diabetic nephropathy in the Diabetes Control and Complications Trial. Kidney Int. 1995;47:1703–20.

2. UK Prospective Diabetes Study Group [UKPDS]. Intensive blood glucose control with sulphonylureas or insulin compared to conventional treatment and the risk of complications in patients with type 2 diabetes. Lancet. 1998;352:837–53.

3. Rychlik I, Miltenberger-Miltenyi G, Ritz E. The drama of the continuous increase in end-stage renal failure in patients with type II diabetes mellitus. Nephrol Dial Transplant. 1998;13(Suppl. 8):6–10.

4. Nelson RG, Knowler WC, McCance DR, et al. Determinants of end-stage renal disease in Pima Indians with Type 2 (non-insulin-dependent) diabetes mellitus and proteinuria. Diabetologia. 1993; 36:1087–93.

5. Pugh JA, Stern MP, Eifler CW, Zapata M. Excess incidence of treatment of end-stage renal disease in Mexican Americans. Am J Epidemiol. 1988;127:135–44.

6. Harris MI. Non-insulin-dependent diabetes mellitus in black and white Americans. Diabetes Metab Rev. 1990;6:71–90.

7. Lightstone L, Rees AJ, Tomson C, et al. High incidence of end-stage renal disease in Indo-Asians in the UK. QJ Med. 1995;88:191–5.

8. McCance DR, Hanson RL, Pettitt DJ, et al. Diabetic nephropathy: a risk factor for diabetes mellitus in offspring. Diabetologia. 1995;38:221–6.

9. Lawson ML, Sochett EB, Chait PG, et al. Effect of puberty on markers of glomerular hypertrophy and hypertension in IDDM. Diabetes. 1996;45:51–5.

10. Chan JCN, Cheung C-K, Cheung MYF, et al. Abnormal albuminuria as a predictor of mortality and renal impairment in Chinese patients with NIDDM. Diabetes Care. 1995;18:1013–16.

11. Mogensen CE. How to protect the kidney in diabetic patients with special reference to IDDM. Diabetes. 1997;46(Suppl. 2):104–11.

12. Rudberg S, Østerby R. Decreasing glomerular filtration rate – an indicator of more advanced diabetic glomerulopathy in the early course of microalbuminuria in IDDM adolescents. Nephrol Dial Transplant. 1997;12:1149–54.

13. Vora JP, Dolben J, Dean JD, et al. Renal haemodynamics in newly presenting non-insulin-dependent diabetes mellitus. Kidney Int. 1992;41:829–35.

14. Vedel P, Obel J, Bang LE, et al. Glomerular hyperfiltration in microalbuminuric NIDDM patients. Diabetologia. 1996;39:1584–9.

15. Vora JP, Dolben J, Williams JD, et al. Impact of initial treatment on renal function in newly-diagnosed type-2 (non-insulin-dependent) diabetes mellitus. Diabetologia. 1993;36:734–40.

16. Poulsen PL, Mogensen CE. Clinical evaluation of a test for immediate and quantitative determination of urinary albumin-to-creatinine ration. Diabetes Care. 1998:21:97–8.

17. Collins AC, Vincent J, Newall RG, et al. An aid to the early detection and management of diabetic nephropathy: assessment of a new point of care microalbuminuria system in the diabetic clinic. Diabetic Med. 2001;18:928–32.

18. Parving H-H. Renoprotection in diabetes: genetic and non-genetic risk factors and treatment. Diabetologia. 1998;41:745–59.

19. Allawi J, Rao PV, Gilbert R, et al. Microalbuminuria in non-insulin-dependent diabetes: its prevalence in Indian compared with European patients. Br Med J. 1988;296:462–4.

20. Fioretto P, Mauer M, Brocco E, et al. Patterns of renal injury in NIDDM patients with microalbuminuria. Diabetologia 1996;39:1569–76.

21. Nosadini R, Velussi M, Brocco F, et al. Course of renal function in type 2 diabetic patients with abnormalities of albumin excretion rate. Diabetes. 2000;49:476–84.

22. K/DOQI clinical practice guidelines for chronic kidney disease: evaluation, classification and stratification. Part 7, Guideline 14: Association of Chronic kidney disease with diabetic complications. Am J Kidney Dis. 2001;39(Suppl. 2):S198–203.

23. Parving H-H, Hommel E, Mathiesen ER, et al. Prevalence of microalbuminuria, arterial hypertension, retinopathy and neuropathy in insulin-dependent diabetic patients. Br Med J. 1988;296:156–60.

24. Vora JP, Ibrahim HAA, Bakris G. Responding to the challenge of diabetic nephropathy: the historic evolution of detection, prevention and management. J Hum Hypertens. 2000;14:667–85.

25. Kimmelstiel P, Wilson C. Intercapillary lesions in glomeruli of kidney. Am J Pathol. 1936;12:83–97.

26. Bjørn SF, Bangstad HJ, Hanssen KF, et al. Glomerular epithelial foot processes and filtration slits in IDDM patients. Diabetologia. 1995;38:1197–204.

27. Osterby R. Microalbuminuria in diabetes mellitus – is there a structural basis? Nephrol Dial Transplant. 1995;10:12–14.

28. Reece EA, Coustan DR, Hayslett JP, et al. Diabetic nephropathy: pregnancy performance and fetomaternal outcome. Am J Obstet Gynecol. 1988;159:56–66.

29. Kitzmiller JL, Brown ER, Phillippe M, et al. Diabetic nephropathy and perinatal outcome. Am J Obstet Gynecol. 1981;141:741–51.

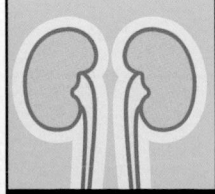

Chapter 33

Pathogenesis, Prevention, and Treatment of Diabetic Nephropathy

Mark E Cooper and Richard E Gilbert

INTRODUCTION

Diabetes is the leading cause of end-stage renal disease (ESRD) in the Western World and is a major cause of end-stage renal disease in Asia[1,2]. As many as 40% of type 1 and 5–10% of type 2 diabetic patients will develop ESRD from diabetic nephropathy (DN). Although type 1 diabetic subjects appear more prone to develop DN, approximately 50–60% of diabetic subjects receiving renal replacement therapy have type 2 diabetes due to the greater prevalence of this type of diabetes in the general population. The importance of this disease is emphasized by the fact that patients with ESRD secondary to DN have a 50% greater mortality rate on dialysis (Chapter 34). In this chapter we discuss the pathogenesis and management of DN; for a discussion on clinical manifestations and natural history, see Chapter 32.

PATHOGENESIS

The structural and hemodynamic changes that occur in diabetic nephropathy are described in detail in Chapter 32 (Fig. 33.1). One of the earliest changes is an increase in glomerular filtration rate (GFR), or 'hyperfiltration', and is observed in many type 1 diabetic subjects and a lesser percentage of type 2 diabetic subjects. This is paralleled by an increase in renal size. The next observable change is the development of microalbuminuria (see Chapter 32). Persistent microalbuminuria, as noted by repeated testing, is associated with changes in both glomerular structure (mesangial expansion and basement membrane thickening) and permeability, and thus is sometimes referred to as 'incipient nephropathy'. These changes occur in 30–50% of type 1 diabetic subjects within 5 to 10 years after onset of diabetes and may be present in 20 to 30% of type 2 diabetic subjects at initial diagnosis.

Diabetic subjects with persistent microalbuminuria are at marked increased risk for the development of overt DN, which is heralded by the development of proteinuria around 15 years after disease onset. This progresses to nephrotic syndrome, hypertension, and progressive renal insufficiency. Glomeruli show glomerular basement membrane (GBM) thickening, mesangial expansion eventually resulting in diffuse and/or nodular glomerulosclerosis ('Kimmelstiel–Wilson' lesions), afferent and efferent arteriolar hyalinosis, and tubulointerstitial fibrosis.

Genetic and environmental factors

Between 30–40% of patients with type 1 diabetes and 10–20% of those with type 2 diabetes develop nephropathy. Nephropathy may develop in some patients despite good glycemic control and it may fail to develop in others despite years of severe hyperglycemia. These findings suggest that nonmetabolic influences such as familial, ethnic and environmental factors may also contribute to the development of diabetic nephropathy.

The prevalence of nephropathy among diabetic patients varies between different racial and ethnic groups such that it is relatively increased in African Americans, Native Americans, Mexican Americans, Polynesians, Australian Aborigines, and urbanized Indo-Asian immigrants in the United Kingdom when compared with Caucasians. Although barriers to care seem likely to account for some of these inter-population differences, genetic factors are also likely to contribute. Familial clustering of diabetic nephropathy has been reported in both type 1 and in type 2 diabetes and in both Caucasian and non-Caucasian population. However, linkage between specific genes and the development of diabetic renal disease system has not been conclusively demonstrated although several studies have suggested a detrimental effect of the double deletion (DD) polymorphism of the ACE genotype on disease progression[3–5].

Natural history of type 1 diabetic nephropathy

Stage	Pre	Incipient	Overt
Functional	GFR ↑ (25–50%)	Microalbuminuria, hypertension	Proteinuria, nephrotic syndrome, GFR ↓
Structural	Renal hypertrophy	Mesangial expansion, glomerular basement membrane thickening, arteriolar hyalinosis	Mesangial nodules (Kimmelstiel–Wilson lesions), tubulointerstitial fibrosis

Figure 33.1 Natural history of type 1 diabetic nephropathy.

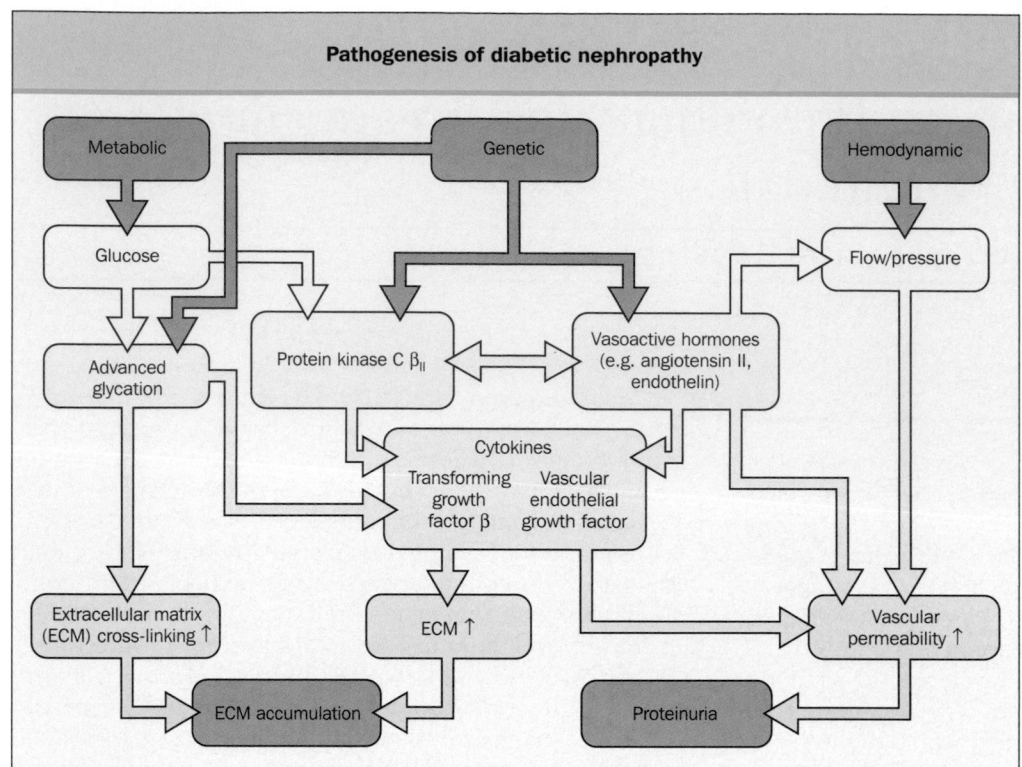

Figure 33.2 The pathogenesis of diabetic nephropathy involves both potential and proven interactions of metabolic, hemodynamic and genetic factors. (Adapted with permission from Cooper[2].)

In addition to genetic factors, shared environmental influences may also contribute to the familial and racial clustering of diabetic renal disease. For instance, tobacco smoking promotes both the onset and progression of diabetic nephropathy in addition to accelerating cardiovascular disease[6]. Intrauterine malnutrition may also predispose to the later development of renal disease, possibly because intrauterine malnutrition significantly reduces nephron number. It is hypothesized that this may, in turn, lead to compensatory glomerular hypertrophy and increased SNGFR with the acceleration of glomerular injury in the setting of further renal insult, such as diabetes[7].

The role of glucose control

Although the renal complications of diabetes had been described in the 18th century, it is only over the last 20 years that the mechanisms linking chronic hyperglycemia to the development of DN have begun to be unravelled (Fig. 33.2)[2]. Within 30 years of the discovery of insulin, studies by the Joslin clinic identified poor glycemic control and duration of disease as the two major risk factors for the development of DN. Indeed, the evidence for the role of tight glycemic control in retarding the development of DN is overwhelming. This includes:

1. Studies suggesting that with good glycemic control (reflected by an average HbA1C of 7.0%) only 9% of type 1 diabetic subjects will develop ESRD after 25 years as opposed to the historical prevalence of 40%[8]
2. Results from the Diabetes Control and Complications Trial (DCCT) which showed a remarkable reduction in progression from normoalbuminuria to microalbuminuria in type 1 diabetic patients with tight glycemic control[9]

3. Studies in which euglycemia following pancreas transplantation is associated with a regression of the diabetic changes within the glomeruli after 10 years[10]
4. Recent evidence from the United Kingdom Prospective Study (UKPDS) that reducing HbA1c by ~0.9% in type 2 diabetic subjects reduces the risk of development of microvascular complications including nephropathy[11].

The mechanisms by which hyperglycemia induces DN are complex and may involve not only effects of elevated glucose levels *per se*, but also the generation from the hyperglycemic state of glycated proteins and alcohol sugars (polyols)[2].

Pathogenesis of diabetic nephropathy: the hemodynamic changes

As discussed above, hyperfiltration is common in early diabetes. Diabetic subjects show an increased GFR response to amino acid infusion compared to non-diabetic controls, and this can be corrected with good glycemic control. The mechanism for the increased GFR is not completely elucidated, but may involve glucose-dependent effects on afferent arteriolar dilation, mediated by a range of vasoactive hormones and cytokines including insulin-like growth factor 1 (IGF-1), nitric oxide, prostaglandins and/or glucagon. It has been suggested that hyperfiltration may predict the development of DN, especially in type 1 diabetes, where a GFR of over 125 mL/min carries a 50% risk as compared to 5% in those with a GFR under 125 mL/min for the subsequent development of microalbuminuria over an 8-year period. However, not all studies have found an elevation in GFR to be a predictor of subsequent renal disease.

Experimentally, the hyperfiltration has been shown to be mediated by afferent arteriolar dilatation with an increase in glomerular hydrostatic pressure. Indeed, measures that reduce the glomerular pressure, such as systemic blood pressure reduction, low protein diet (which blocks the afferent arteriolar dilation), or angiotensin-converting enzyme (ACE) inhibitors (which blocks angiotensin II mediated constriction of the efferent arteriole) all reduce the development of glomerular damage and proteinuria[13].

Pathogenesis of diabetic nephropathy: renal hypertrophy
The early hyperfiltration response is associated with both glomerular and tubulointerstitial proliferation and hypertrophy. Kidney size may increase by several centimeters. Glomeruli enlarge with both an increase in capillary loop number and surface area. Most of the changes in the glomeruli are due to hypertrophy, whereas the tubular epithelial cells undergo both proliferation and an increase in cellular size.

Experimentally, diabetic renal hypertrophy can be largely prevented by intensified insulin therapy and resultant normoglycemia. The mechanisms by which elevated plasma glucose levels cause hypertrophy appears to be due to the stimulation of a variety of growth factors within the kidney, including IGF-1, epidermal growth factor (EGF), platelet-derived growth factor, and transforming growth factor-β (TGF-β). Proliferation and hypertrophy may also be initiated by the fall within the kidney of certain antiproliferative factors, such as SPARC, the secreted protein, acidic and rich in cysteine.

The role of TGF-β in diabetic renal hypertrophy has been most studied. Both glucose and glucose generated advanced glycation end products (AGEs) stimulate production of TGF-β in a variety of cell types. Although TGF-β is secreted in a latent form, hyperglycemia also induces the expression of thrombospondin, a potent activator of TGF-β. In turn, TGF-β stimulates protein synthesis (hypertrophy) in numerous cell types, but prevents cell proliferation and division due to the stimulation of proteins (cyclin kinase inhibitors) that block progression through the cell cycle. TGF-β is also expressed in glomeruli and the tubulointerstitium of both experimental and human DN. The role of TGF-β in mediating renal hypertrophy is further suggested by studies in which treatment of diabetic mice with neutralizing anti-TGF-β antibodies has been shown to attenuate diabetes related renal hypertrophy. This has also been shown to result in less renal extracellular matrix accumulation with preservation of renal function.

Pathogenesis of diabetic nephropathy: microalbuminuria and proteinuria
Early in the course of diabetes the GBM widens, and may reach three- to four-fold normal thickness. Glycation of the GBM appears to make it less prone to degradation, and there is also some evidence for increased type IV collagen synthesis. Structurally, the increased GBM thickness is associated with a loss of heparan sulfate proteoglycans, the principal negatively charged constituents in the GBM that provide the charge barrier to prevent proteins from escaping into Bowman's space. In addition, studies of the nephropathy in the Pima Indians have also shown that, despite increases in glomerular size, there is loss of the overlying glomerular epithelial cell (podocyte), a cell type important in restricting protein permeability.

The observation that tight glycemic control can retard the development of microalbuminuria is consistent with a role for hyperglycemia in this process. Experimentally, several studies suggest that this may be mediated by glucose induced AGEs and glucose induced activation of protein kinase C (see below). Furthermore, control of systemic and glomerular hypertension by antihypertensive agents, and most notably by ACE inhibitors, also confers protection, which suggests a role for angiotensin II (see below). Several groups are also examining a potential link between proteinuria and a family of newly described slit pore proteins including nephrin. It remains to be determined if changes in expression of this protein are linked to the development of albuminuria in diabetes.

Pathogenesis of diabetic nephropathy: mesangial expansion and nodule formation
The hallmark of DN is mesangial expansion, eventually culminating in the development of the Kimmelstiel–Wilson nodule. Several studies have shown that the mesangial expansion correlates better than GBM thickness with the subsequent development of renal failure. Histologically, the early lesion is characterized by variable increases in mesangial cell number with an increased deposition of several extracellular matrix components, including type IV and type V collagen, laminin, and fibronectin. Later, there is a general loss of mesangial cellularity, and the homogenous acellular nodules consist primarily of type VI collagen.

The mesangial expansion is mediated by both direct effects of glucose and glucose induced advance glycation end products (AGEs), as mesangial changes can largely be prevented in experimental models with tight glycemic control or with the use of AGE inhibitors such as aminoguanidine. As discussed above, the effects may be mediated by the prosclerotic cytokine, TGF-β, given its known propensity to stimulate mesangial matrix production. A direct effect of glucose to stimulate protein kinase C is also likely with experimental evidence suggesting that albuminuria can be reduced by protein kinase C inhibitors[14] (see below).

Pathogenesis of diabetic nephropathy: tubulointerstitial fibrosis
It is now recognized that the two most important structural changes that correlate with progression in DN are the degree of mesangial expansion and the severity of the tubulointerstitial disease. As in other renal diseases, the degree of tubulointerstitial fibrosis correlates not only with current renal function, but also with prognosis[15].

The potential mechanisms for the development of tubulointerstitial fibrosis are similar to those postulated for tubulointerstitial fibrosis that occurs with other progressive renal diseases and include release of growth factors and cytokines from the glomerulus and direct or indirect effects of proteinuria. An important mechanism may relate to renal ischemia induced by the progressive hyalinosis of the afferent and efferent arteriole.

Mechanisms by which hyperglycemia mediates DN
Direct effects of glucose: the role of protein kinase C (PKC)
A direct role for glucose in DN has been suggested by cell culture studies that have shown that glucose can induce

441

Diabetic Nephropathy

cell hypertrophy, extracellular matrix synthesis, and TGF-β production in a variety of cell types. Many of the adverse effects of hyperglycemia have been attributed to activation of PKC, a family of serine–threonine kinases that regulates diverse vascular functions, including contractility, blood flow, cellular proliferation, and vascular permeability. PKC activity, especially the membrane-bound form, is increased in the retina, aorta, heart, and glomeruli of diabetic animals, probably because of the *de novo* synthesis of diacylglycerol, a major endogenous activator of PKC. The observation that there is preferential activation of the βII isoform of PKC in diabetes led to the synthesis of an orally effective PKCβ-selective inhibitor, LY333531[14]. This inhibitor is a competitive, reversible inhibitor of PKCβ1 and PKCβII, with a 50-fold lesser effect on other PKC isoforms. In short and long term studies in diabetic rats, LY333531 ameliorated glomerular hyperfiltration, albuminuria, and renal TGF-β overexpression and extracellular matrix accumulation[16].

Effects of AGEs

Chronic hyperglycemia can lead to the nonenzymatic glycation of amino acids and proteins (Maillard or Browning reaction). Glucose nonenzymatically binds to amino residues to become glycated Schiff bases, with later 'rearrangement' to form a more stable but still reversible 'Amadori' products. Over time these products undergo rearrangement including crosslinking to become irreversible advanced glycation end products (AGEs) (Fig. 33.3). Both circulating and tissue proteins as well as lipids and nucleic acids may be glycated. A classic example is hemoglobin (Hb) that initially forms the Amadori product, HbA1C, but ultimately AGE-Hb is generated. Although primarily observed in diabetes, AGEs also accumulate in aging and in renal failure. The specific AGEs involved in diabetic complications and in particular renal disease have not been clearly determined.

AGEs have been shown to be increased in the sera of diabetic patients with nephropathy and have also been localized to glomeruli by immunohistochemistry in experimental diabetes (Fig. 33.4). AGEs bind to a variety of cell types, including the macrophage and mesangial cell. AGEs mediate a variety of cellular actions, including expression of adhesion molecules involved in mononuclear cell recruitment, cell hypertrophy,

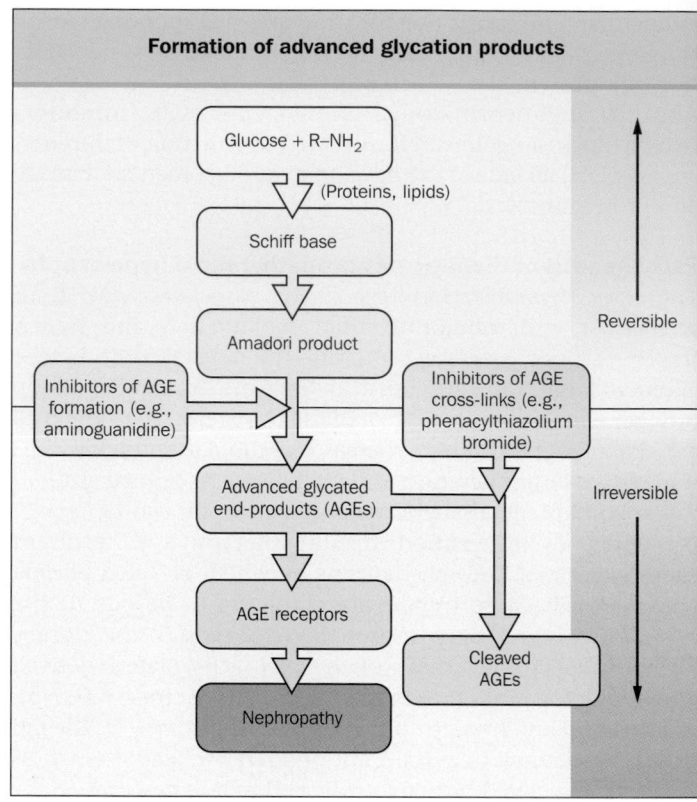

Figure 33.3 Mechanism of formation of advanced glycation endproducts (AGEs).

extracellular matrix synthesis, epithelial to mesenchymal transdifferentiation of tubular cells, and the inhibition of nitric oxide synthesis. AGEs injected *in vivo* induce albuminuria and glomerulosclerosis[17]. The first binding site and putative receptor to be cloned and known as RAGE has been localized to tubules, and to a lesser extent glomeruli. However, it is not known if RAGE and other putative receptors are predominantly involved in mediating these effects or whether they are also involved in the clearance of AGEs.

Administration of aminoguanidine, an inhibitor of AGE formation, to animals with diabetes reduces AGE deposition

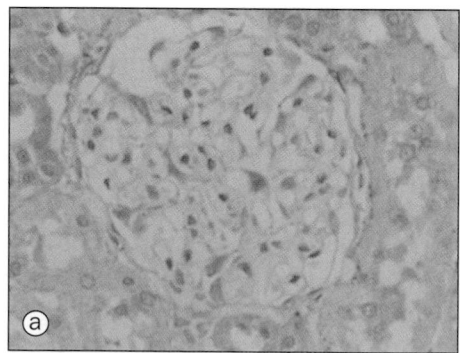
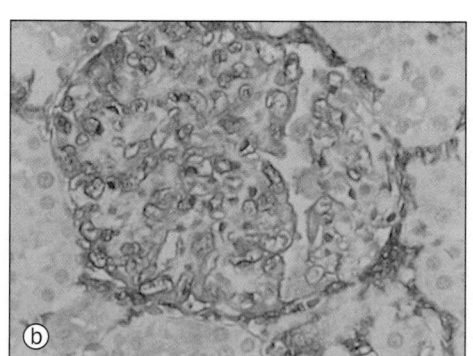
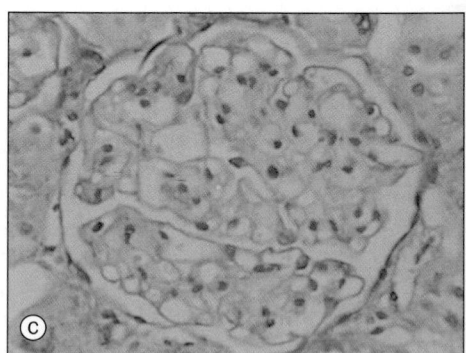

Figure 33.4 Immunohistochemical localization of advanced glycated endproducts (AGEs) in control (a), diabetic (b) and diabetic + aminoguanidine (c) treated rodents. Diabetes is associated with increased deposition of AGEs in the glomerulus which is prevented by aminoguanidine therapy.

(Fig. 33.4) and results in less mesangial matrix expansion, and albuminuria, but has inconsistent effects on GBM thickening. Aminoguanidine has also been reported to stabilize or improve diabetic retinopathy and neuropathy in experimental models and preliminary clinical studies suggest beneficial effects on retinopathy, lipids and proteinuria. Newer agents have also been developed, which may be more potent at blocking AGE formation. These agents, unlike aminoguanidine, may be more specific, without significant *in vivo* effects on NO synthase. Furthermore, phenacylthiazolium bromide (PTB) is a novel compound which cleaves covalent, AGE-derived protein cross-links, and provides a conceptual basis for the reversal of AGE-mediated tissue damage, which until now has been regarded as irreversible. Aminoguanidine and PTB related compounds such as ALT-711 are under investigation in a range of clinical conditions including diabetic nephropathy and various cardiovascular disorders.

Effect of sorbitol (the polyol pathway)

Hyperglycemia-induced generation of polyols has also been suggested to mediate some of the complications of diabetes. In tissues where glucose uptake is independent of insulin, such as in the lens, retina and kidney, chronic hyperglycemia results in increased tissue levels of glucose. The excess glucose is subsequently reduced to sorbitol by the reduced nicotinamide adenine dinucleotide phosphate (NADPH)-dependent enzyme aldose reductase, the first enzyme in the polyol pathway. Accumulation of sorbitol is accompanied by an increase in intracellular osmolality, a depletion of free myoinositol, loss of Na^+,K^+ ATPase activity, and increased consumption of the enzyme cofactors NADPH and NAD^+, leading to changes in cellular redox potential.

The role of polyols in diabetic complications has been assessed primarily by studies using aldose reductase inhibitors, such as sorbinil, tolrestat and ponalrestat. These agents have shown promise in preventing diabetic cataracts and in improving or stabilizing diabetic neuropathy (by improving nerve conduction velocity). Aldose reductase inhibitors also blunt hyperfiltration and have a mild effect on reducing albuminuria in both experimental and human diabetes. However, the beneficial effects of aldose reductase inhibitors on DN appear mild, and treatment with these agents may be associated with hypersensitivity reactions and liver function abnormalities. As such, it is unlikely that these agents will have a major role in the management of DN.

The renin–angiotensin system

A role for the renin–angiotensin system (RAS) has been strongly suggested by the observation that ACE inhibitors can slow the progression of DN in experimental animals. Zatz et al. reported that in rats with streptozotocin-induced diabetes, treatment with ACE inhibitors could reduce proteinuria and ameliorate glomerular changes in association with a reduction in glomerular hydrostatic pressure (Fig. 33.5)[13]. More recently, it has been shown that ACE inhibitors also reduce tubulointerstitial injury in experimental diabetes. Studies in man (to be reviewed below) have also suggested that ACE inhibitors may retard progression in microalbuminuric type 1 and type 2 diabetes.

Despite the evidence that the RAS is involved in DN, plasma renin activity is low in DN, although it may be inappropriately high for the increased extracellular volume and exchangeable sodium that accompany DN. This has raised the possibility that it may be activation of the intrarenal RAS that is critical

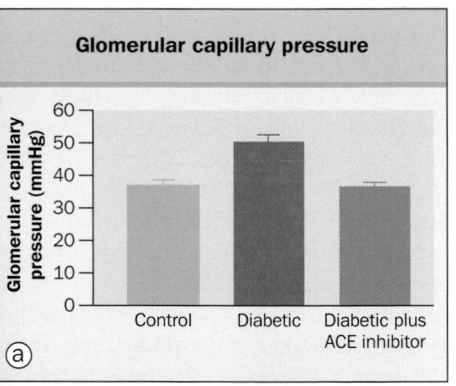

(a)

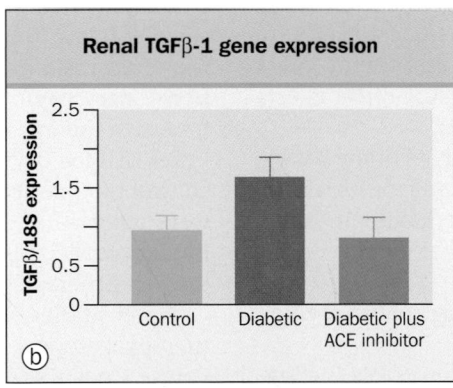

(b)

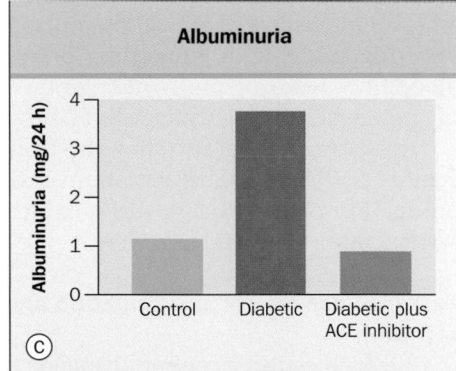

(c)

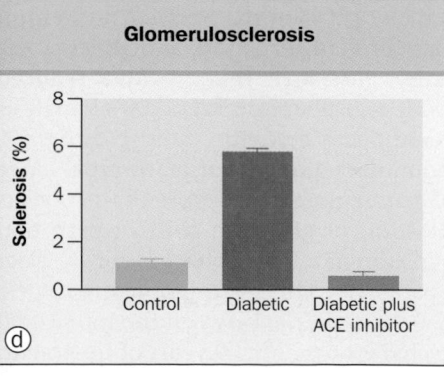

(d)

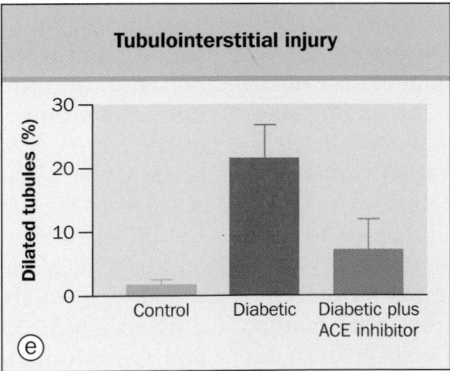

(e)

Figure 33.5 Reduction of glomerular pressure by ACE inhibitors in diabetic rats is associated with less glomerulosclerosis.
(Adapted with permission from Zatz, Dunn, Meyer, Brenner[13] and Gilbert and Cooper[15].)

Postulated mechanisms for the renoprotective effect of angiotensin-converting enzyme (ACE) inhibitors
Lower systemic blood pressure
Lower intraglomerular pressure
Increase renal bloodflow (counter ischemia secondary to intrarenal vasoconstriction)
Reduce proteinuria (average of 45% (range 40–50))
Natriuretic: secondary to inhibition of angiotensin II-induced solute transport across the proximal tubule, decrease in aldosterone production, decrease in tubuloglomerular feedback sensitivity, fall in filtration fraction and a decrease in peritubular osmotic pressure
Inhibit nonhemodynamic effects of angiotensin II on various cell types, resulting in less proliferation, hypertrophy, matrix expansion, and cytokine and growth factor synthesis
Inhibit macrophage activation, proliferation, and migration

Table 33.1 Postulated mechanisms for the renoprotective effect of angiotensin-converting enzyme (ACE) inhibitors.

for DN. Anderson et al. have identified sites of local activation of the RAS in both the glomerulus and renal vessels in rats with experimental diabetes[18]. In addition, prorenin levels (which may reflect increased synthesis) are elevated in patients with DN. Rats transgenic for murine renin also show an accelerated injury following the induction of diabetes.

The pathogenic mechanisms by which angiotensin II contributes to DN have not been fully delineated. In addition to its hemodynamic effects to increase systemic and glomerular pressure, to mediate proteinuria, and to induce renal vasoconstriction, angiotensin II also has nonhemodynamic effects and can mediate cell proliferation, hypertrophy, matrix expansion and cytokine (TGF-β) synthesis. Therefore, ACE inhibitors and angiotensin receptor antagonists (ATRA) could act by lowering systemic or glomerular pressure, improving renal blood flow, reducing proteinuria, or by blocking direct effects of angiotensin II to activate cells (Table 33.1).

Other vasoactive agents may also be involved in the pathogenesis of DN, including alterations in systemic or intrarenal production of endothelin, nitric oxide, the kallikrein–kinin system, and natriuretic peptides.

Extracellular matrix accumulation and degradation: role of TGF-β

As discussed earlier, a central histologic feature of DN is extracellular matrix accumulation in the mesangium and in the tubulointerstitium. Studies in experimental diabetes suggest that this is due to both increased synthesis as well as decreased degradation. Experiments *in vitro* suggest that the impaired degradation is due to reduced activity of matrix metalloproteinases and that these changes are attenuated by ACE inhibition. There is also evidence that glycation may make matrix components more resistant to degradation.

As well as its role in renal hypertrophy (discussed above), TGF-β has been shown to have a pivotal role in the extracellular matrix accumulation in DN. For example, in diabetic mice anti- TGF-β antibody can reduce extracellular matrix gene expression. Increased TGF-β expression in diabetes could

be a consequence of a direct effect of glucose or AGEs to increase its synthesis. Furthermore, inhibition of AGEs with aminoguanidine is associated with reduced TGF-β expression in diabetic tissues undergoing injury including the kidney. A role for angiotensin II is also suggested by the observation that angiotensin II can directly stimulate TGF-β production by mesangial and tubular epithelial cells. Furthermore, ACE inhibitors reduce renal gene expression of TGF-β and its receptors in diabetic rodents.

PREVENTION AND TREATMENT

The major therapeutic approaches that have been investigated include intensive glycemic control, antihypertensive treatment with a particular focus on agents that interrupt the RAS, and restriction of dietary protein. The evolution of DN can be considered as passing through several stages, best defined clinically in terms of urinary albumin excretion. The various interventions will be described in the setting of normoalbuminuria, microalbuminuria (incipient DN) and macroalbuminuria (overt DN).

Glycemic control in diabetes

In a prospective study it was shown that the rate of increase in albuminuria correlated with glycated hemoglobin over a mean period of approximately 10 years in both type 1 and type 2 diabetic subjects[19]. Indeed, there is now evidence that good glycemic control can slow progression particularly in the early phases of DN.

Normoalbuminuria

The importance of strict glycemic control in the prevention of microalbuminuria in type 1 diabetes was best shown in the DCCT in which patients were randomized to intensive insulin therapy (consisting of at least three injections per day or the use of an insulin pump) or conventional therapy (two injections per day)[9]. Over the 9-year period, patients on intensive therapy (mean HbA1c levels of 7.0%) had a 35–45% lower risk for developing microalbuminuria compared to the control group (mean HbA1c of 9%) (Fig. 33.6). Similar findings were reported in another study[20]. However, the number of hypoglycemic episodes was also increased in patients on the intensive therapies.

Fewer studies have examined the effect of intensive insulin therapy in type 2 diabetes. In a 6-year study of 110 relatively young (mean age of 50 years) nonobese Japanese patients, intensive insulin therapy reduced the risk of microalbuminuria by 62% and albuminuria by 100% in the primary prevention cohort[21]. In the secondary prevention cohort, as defined by the presence of retinopathy, intensive therapy also reduced microalbuminuria by 52% and albuminuria by 100%. Analysis of the HbA1c levels identified a glycemic threshold of 6.5% below which microalbuminuria did not worsen (normal range 4.8–6.4%). The UKPDS has explored over more than 10 years the effect of intensification of glycemic control with oral antidiabetic agents or insulin in a large cohort of newly diagnosed type 2 diabetic patients[11]. This treatment led to a 0.9% difference in HbA1c (7.0 versus 7.9%) between the intensified and conventionally treated groups. After 9 years of treatment,

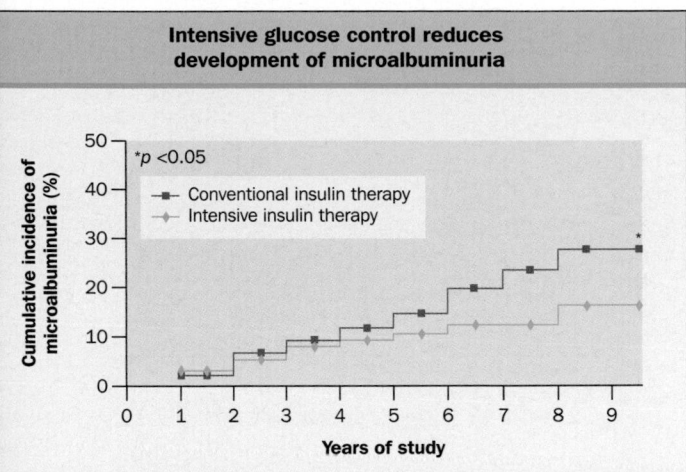

Figure 33.6 DCCT Trial. Intensive glucose control was associated with a decreased risk for the subsequent development of microalbuminuria in type 1 diabetes. (Adapted with permission from Diabetes Control and Complications Trial Research Group[9].)

there was a 25–30% decrease in the development of micro-albuminuria and proteinuria, and over a 50% decrease in the number of patients with a doubling of serum creatinine (Fig. 33.7).

Microalbuminuria and overt DN

The evidence that intensified insulin therapy slows progression of either type 1 or type 2 diabetic patients with microalbuminuria remains controversial. Only a small number of patients entering the DCCT had microalbuminuria at baseline, and although fewer patients progressed to frank albuminuria under intensive insulin treatment, it did not reach statistical significance[9]. A similar lack of statistical significance of intensified insulin treatment was reported by the Microalbuminuria Collaborative Study Group from the United Kingdom. However, several Scandinavian studies have reported slower progression to DN in microalbuminuric type 1 diabetic patients with intensive glucose control.

One reason why it may be difficult to show a benefit of glucose control in patients with incipient or established DN is that the frequent concurrence of hypertension may overshadow the benefits of intensive insulin therapy. Thus, it is of interest that a study from Guy's Hospital reported that intensive glycemic control is of benefit in DN provided blood pressure is well controlled[22]. However, these results must be interpreted with caution since these results were not obtained as part of a prospective study.

Antihypertensive therapy

Hypertension, defined as BP > 140/90, classically develops within 2 to 5 years after the onset of microalbuminuria, and is usually associated with volume expansion and salt-sensitivity. Numerous studies have shown that control of systemic hypertension has a major effect on reducing proteinuria and slowing progression to renal failure in both type 1 and type 2 diabetes (Fig. 33.8)[23].

A major question relates to the target BP one should achieve. The Modification of Diet in Renal Disease study of nondiabetic

Parameter	Therapy (years)	Risk reduction	p value	Favors intensive treatment	Favors conventional treatment
Microalbuminuria	0	0.89	0.24		
	3	0.83	0.043		
	6	0.88	0.13		
	9	0.76	0.00062		
	12	0.67	0.000054		
	15	0.70	0.033		
Proteinuria	0	0.79	0.37		
	3	0.68	0.12		
	6	0.90	0.61		
	9	0.67	0.026		
	12	0.66	0.036		
	15	0.58	0.12		
Twofold increase in plasma creatinine	0–3	0.67	0.37		
	0–6	0.42	0.12		
	0–9	0.40	0.61		
	0–12	0.26	0.026		
	0–15	1.25	0.036		

Intensive glycemic control in type 2 diabetes

Figure 33.7 The effect of intensive glycemic control on nephropathy in type 2 diabetics. (Adapted with permission from UK Prospective Diabetes Study (UKPDS) Group[11].)

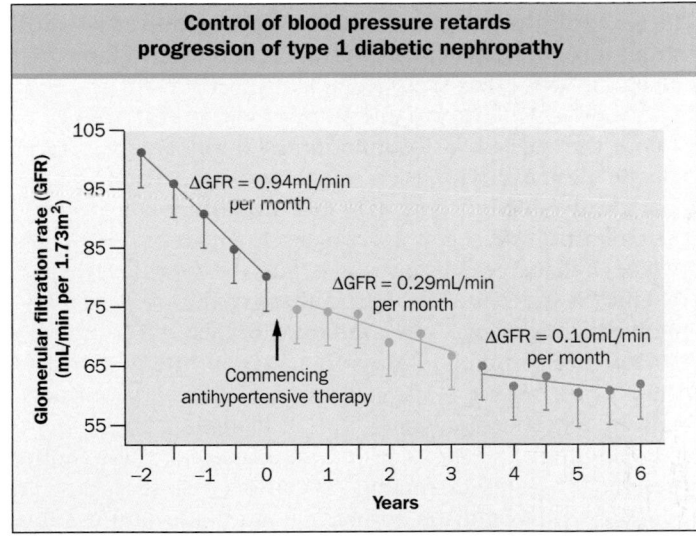

Figure 33.8 Control of systemic BP reduces the risk for progression in type 1 DN. (Adapted with permission from Parving, Andersen, Smidt, et al[23].)

patients with renal disease provided strong evidence that achieving a lower BP (BP 125/75 mmHg) was associated with a slower rate of progression in proteinuric patients compared to standard BP (140/90 mmHg) goals. These observations, as well as others, led the Sixth Joint National Committee to recommend a lower target for instituting antihypertensive therapy in diabetic subjects. Commencement of treatment at a BP of 130/85 and a goal BP of 125/75 in proteinuric patients was suggested[24].

Diabetic Nephropathy

A second question relates to whether certain antihypertensive agents confer specific renoprotective effects in DN. In this regard, the major issue has been whether additional benefit is achieved with ACE inhibitors or ATRA antagonists, including in patients who are normotensive.

ACE inhibitors in DN
Normoalbuminuria
The observation that ACE inhibitors slow progression in microalbuminuric type 1 diabetic patients[25] has led to consideration that it may be of benefit in diabetic patients prior to the development of microalbuminuria. However, in the EUCLID study, no evidence for a beneficial role for the ACE inhibitor, lisinopril, was observed in normoalbuminuric type 1 diabetic subjects, despite evidence that it reduced the development of retinopathy[26]. However, the lack of an observed effect may have been related to the short duration of only 2 years for the study. Indeed, a recent study over 3 years noted that the ACE inhibitor, perindopril, retarded the increase in albuminuria that is observed in the placebo treated group[27]. In an Israeli study[28] ACE inhibition was shown to retard the development of microalbuminuria in a cohort of type 2 diabetic subjects with or without hypertension. Whether this ultimately translates to long-term renoprotection remains to be determined.

Microalbuminuria associated with normal BP
The exciting observation by Brenner's group that ACE inhibitors lower glomerular pressure and prevent glomerular damage in diabetic rats independent of effects on systemic hypertension[12] led to a large number of clinical studies to explore the role of ACE inhibition in normotensive type 1 diabetic patients with early renal disease[25]. These studies have clearly documented that ACE inhibitors will decrease microalbuminuria and retard the development of proteinuria in type 1 diabetes. However, it is not always clear whether the effect is independent of BP in these studies, as most cases involved comparing ACE inhibitors to placebo, and as a consequence systemic BP was often lower in the ACE treated groups. In a recent meta-analysis of 12 placebo-controlled trials in 698 normotensive type 1 diabetic patients with microalbuminuria treated with ACE inhibitors, the majority for over 2 years, treatment was associated with a 60% reduction in progression to macroalbuminuria and a 3-fold increase in regression to normoalbuminuria[25].

The effect of ACE inhibitors on progression in normotensive microalbuminuric type 2 diabetic subjects has also been studied. Although many type 2 diabetic patients with microalbuminuria are hypertensive, a significant proportion will be normotensive (BP < 140/90 mmHg), particularly in the Asian population. Studies comparing ACE inhibitors to placebo have also suggested a benefit, particularly in decreasing the risk for developing proteinuria. In the study by Ravid et al., treatment with enalapril for 5 years was not only associated with a reduced risk for developing proteinuria, but was also associated with stabilization of renal function. In contrast, the placebo treated group had a 13% decline in renal function[29]. In another group of Indo-Asian normotensive and microalbuminuric type 2 diabetic subjects, Ahmad et al. reported that the reduction in

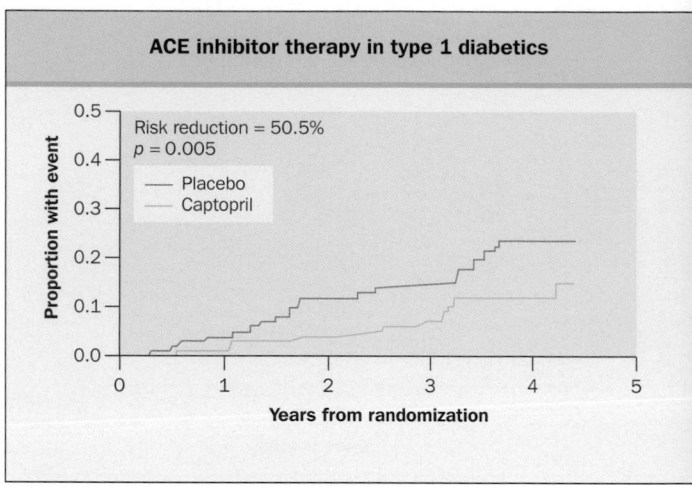

Figure 33.9 The Collaborative Study. Treatment with captopril was superior to placebo in reducing the risk for proteinuric type 1 diabetic subjects to progress to end-stage renal disease. (Adapted with permission from Lewis, Hunsicker, Bain and Rohde[30].)

albuminuria by enalapril occurred independently of a discernible difference in BP between the ACE inhibitor and placebo treated groups.

Microalbuminuric or proteinuric patients with hypertension
Most studies have shown that ACE inhibitors can reduce proteinuria of any etiology by 40–50%. As such, it is not surprising that most studies have documented that ACE inhibitors will reduce proteinuria in either type 1 or type 2 diabetic subjects as compared with standard antihypertensive therapy using diuretics and β-blockers. However, there is also evidence that, in addition to reducing proteinuria, ACE inhibitors may slow the deterioration of renal function. In the Collaborative Study, captopril treatment (25 mg three times daily) was compared to placebo in type 1 diabetic subjects with proteinuria (> 500 mg/day) and mildly impaired renal function (mean serum creatinine 1.3 mg/dL) (Fig. 33.9)[30]. Treatment was associated with a slowing of the deterioration of renal function over the 3-year period (11 vs 17 percent decline in creatinine clearance per year) and a 50% reduction in the proportion of patients reaching ESRD. Remission of nephrotic syndrome also occurred in 7 of 42 nephrotic patients on captopril but in only 1 of 66 controls, and was associated with lower BP in the captopril group[31].

In type 2 diabetic subjects with microalbuminuria and hypertension, ACE inhibitors have also been shown to be more potent at reducing proteinuria than conventional therapy (diuretic and β-blockers). ACE inhibitors appear to be superior to other antihypertensive agents in type 2 diabetic subjects with albuminuria, with in general most studies showing an advantage of ACE inhibitors particularly over dihydropyridine CCBs in reducing proteinuria and stabilizing renal function[32,33].

While the above studies clearly document the benefit of ACE inhibitors in normotensive and hypertensive microalbuminuric patients with type 1, and, to a lesser extent, type 2 diabetes, it is still unclear if the mechanism is independent of their BP lowering effects. For example, in the Collaborative

Study there was clearly less benefit in type 1 diabetic subjects with normal BP and relatively preserved renal function. A recent meta-analysis also could not show superiority of ACE inhibitors over other agents at maximum hypotensive doses. The concept of focusing on aggressive BP reduction rather than ACE inhibition *per se* is further suggested by a recent study by the Collaborative Study group[34]. Proteinuric type 1 diabetic subjects received either low or high dose ramipril. Patients on high dose had a BP that was 7 mmHg lower with a reduction in albuminuria whereas the low dose group had an increase in albuminuria. That study was unable to discern if the superior efficacy of the high dose ramipril group was related to lower blood pressure or to more effective blockade of the RAS.

The role for other antihypertensive agents and in particular AT1 receptor antagonists in the treatment of DN also has to be considered. Experimental studies suggest that ATRA may have similar beneficial effects as ACE inhibitors. Importantly, three recent landmark studies have demonstrated the utility of ATRA in hypertensive type 2 diabetic subjects with microalbuminuria (IRMA-2) or overt nephropathy (RENAAL, IDNT) (Table 33.2). In the RENAAL study[35] which involved a predominantly hypertensive type 2 diabetic population with macroproteinuria and impaired renal function, losartan was compared to conventional antihypertensive treatment which included a significant number of subjects receiving dihydropyridine calcium channel blockers (CCBs). Losartan treatment reduced the risk of progression to ESRD by 28% in association with a reduction in proteinuria of 35% (Table 33.2). The IDNT study, performed in a similar population to the RENAAL study, compared irbesartan to amlodipine or conventional treatment[36]. Irbesartan

was superior to both conventional or amlodipine therapy in reducing the number of subjects reaching the primary endpoint, a composite of doubling of serum creatinine, ESRD and mortality. These effects occurred in the context of a less than 4 mmHg blood pressure difference between conventional and irbesartan treatment and no difference in achieved blood pressure between amlodipine and irbesartan therapy. In the IRMA II study of hypertensive microalbuminuric type 2 diabetic patients[37] irbesartan reduced the development of overt proteinuria in a dose dependent manner with increased regression to normoalbuminuria in the ATRA treated group (Table 33.2).

With new targets for blood pressure in diabetic subjects particularly with proteinuria, various combinations of antihypertensive drugs are now being investigated to optimize blood pressure control. A number of antihypertensive drug classes have been shown to reduce proteinuria and/or cardiovascular events in high-risk populations[38]. While these agents have additive effects on BP reduction, it remains to be established if certain combinations such as ACE inhibitor/ATRA also confer additional renoprotection remains to be established. The candesartan and lisinopril microalbuminuria (CALM) study has demonstrated the ability of the combination of the ACE inhibitor, lisonopril and the ATRA , candesartan to reduce blood pressure and urinary albumin excretion in hypertensive, microalbuminuric type 2 diabetic subjects[39]. Similar benefits have now been reported by Parving's group in macroproteinuric subjects. As most patients have extracellular volume expansion, diuretics are also often required for adequate BP control and fixed combinations of

Study	n	Population	Design	F/u	BP	1° endpoint	2° endpoints
Studies evaluating angiotensin receptor antagonists in incipient and overt diabetic nephropathy							
RENAAL	1513	Type 2 diabetes Hypertension (97%) macroproteinuria	Losartan 50–100 mg (L) Placebo (P)	3.4 y	L 140/74 P 142/74	Composite of doubling of sCr, ESRD and death Risk reduction 16% ↓ L vs P Doubling of sCr: 25% ↓ ESRD: 28% ↓ Death: similar	Cardiovascular: similar Hospitalization for heart failure (HF): L vs P 32%↓
IDNT	1715	Type 2 diabetes Hypertension macroproteinuria	Irbesartan 300 mg (I) Amlodipine 10 mg (A) Placebo (P)	2.6 y	I 140/77 A 141/77 P 144/80	Composite of doubling of sCr, ESRD and death 20% ↓ I vs P 23% ↓ I vs A doubling of sCr 33% ↓ I vs P 37% ↓ I vs A ESRD 23% ↓ I vs both groups	Cardiovascular: similar Irbesartan 23% ↓hospitalization from HF vs Placebo
IRMAII	590	Type 2 diabetes Hypertension microalbuminuria	Placebo (P) Irbesartan 150 mg (I 150) Irbesartan 300 mg (I 300)	2 y	P: 144/83 I 150: 143/83 I 300: 141/83	Time to onset of overt nephropathy Hazard ratio I 150 vs P: 0.61, P = 0.08 I 300 vs P: 0.30, P < 0.001	Changes in level of albuminuria +2% P −24% I 150 −38% I 300 Regression to normoalbuminuria 21% P 24% I 150 34% I 300

Table 33.2 Studies evaluating angiotensin type 1 receptor antagonists in incipient and overt diabetic nephropathy.

Diabetic Nephropathy

	Management of type 1 diabetes	
Stage	**Assessment**	**Management**
Normoalbuminuric/ normotensive	Screen yearly for microalbuminuria; assess cardiovascular risk factors	Optimize glycemic control (target HbA1c <7%)
Persistent microalbuminuria/ normotensive	Close monitoring of lipids, blood pressure (BP), glycemic control, and urinary albumin excretion	Add angiotensin-converting enzyme (ACE) inhibitor or ATRA
Persistent microalbuminuria/ hypertensive	Follow urinary albumin excretion, creatinine clearance, BP	Titrate ACE inhibitor, aim for BP < 130/85 mmHg; consider addition of a diuretic or a low-sodium diet; perhaps add another antihypertensive
Proteinuria	Monitor urinary protein, BP, lipids, creatinine clearance	Aggressive BP control, aim for < 125/75 mmHg; possibly add lipid-lowering drugs, low-protein diet
Declining glomerular filtration rate (GFR)	Prepare for dialysis or transplant	Low-protein diet (0.8 g/kg daily); initiate dialysis when GFR is 10–12 mL/min (usually equating to a creatinine clearance of < 15 mL/min or a serum creatinine of > 6 mg/dL)

A similar strategy can be used in type 2 patients with increased emphasis on cardiovascular risk factors. In all diabetic patients with early or overt nephropathy, there should be continued and possibly increased surveillance for other diabetic micro- and microvascular complications.

Table 33.3 Management of type 1 diabetes.

agents which interrupt the RAS and diuretics are being used in this population. Bakris et al. have demonstrated a role for the combination of an ACE inhibitor and CCB in proteinuric diabetic patients.

An additional concern in relation to the choice of anti-hypertensive therapy relates to their role in providing cardioprotection[32]. Diabetic patients with persistent microalbuminuria are also at increased risk for all-cause mortality, especially from cardiovascular disease. Therefore, the monitoring of other cardiovascular risk factors in these patients is critical. In this regard, several studies suggest that ACE inhibitors may provide additional cardioprotective effects in hypertensive patients with either type 1 or type 2 DN. In the ABCD trial, in which cardiovascular endpoints were assessed, the hypertensive arm of the study was prematurely halted due to a possible superiority of the ACE inhibitor over the calcium channel antagonist in terms of cardiovascular events. In the FACET study involving 380 hypertensive type 2 diabetic subjects it was also shown that the ACE inhibitor, fosinopril, was associated with fewer cardiovascular events than amlodipine. In the Hypertension Optimal Treatment study which involved felodipine based antihypertensive treatment, aggressive blood pressure reduction particularly in the diabetic subgroup was associated with reduced cardiovascular mortality[40]. The HOPE study provides the most convincing evident that ACE inhibitors confer cardiovascular protection in diabetic subjects[33]. Indeed, a *post-hoc* analysis of those individuals in that study with renal disease including those with diabetic nephropathy confirmed that these agents are cardioprotective in this population. In both the RENAAL and IDNT studies, AII antagonist therapy, although not reducing the composite secondary end-point of cardiovascular mortality and morbidity, reduced the risk of hospitalization for heart failure by ~30%[36,41].

Dietary protein intake

In addition to its ability to ameliorate uremic symptoms, several studies involving small numbers of patients have suggested that protein restriction may also slow the progressive loss of renal function in patients with DN. Zeller et al., for example, reported that a low protein diet (0.6 g/kg/day) was associated with a 75% reduction in the rate of decline of the GFR in patients with type 1 DN as compared to patients on a 1.0 g/kg/day protein diet[42]. A meta-analysis of the various trials in diabetic subjects also concluded that there was a beneficial effect on glomerular filtration rate, creatinine clearance, and albuminuria with modest (0.5–0.85 g/kg/day) protein restriction[43]. In contrast, in the large, multicenter, Modification of Diet in Renal Disease study of nondiabetic patients with renal disease, the effects of dietary protein restriction were inconclusive, although subgroup analysis suggested that patients with heavy proteinuria did benefit. Although, a large, long-term prospective study would be needed to establish the safety, efficacy and compliance with protein restriction in diabetic nephropathy, the American Diabetes Association recommends that nonpregnant diabetic patients should restrict their protein intake to 0.8 g/kg ideal body weight/day[44].

Lipids

There are many theoretical reasons for lipids to accelerate renal injury including activation of cytokine-dependent pathways and stimulation of macrophage proliferation and recruitment. Several studies have suggested that HMG CoA reductase inhibitors retard the progression of incipient and overt diabetic nephropathy but these findings have not been universal[45,46].

Management strategies for the diabetic patient

Several scientific societies and expert panels have prepared consensus guidelines or position statements on the management of diabetic nephropathy. Some of the more important points include trying to optimize metabolic control, considering the use of ACE inhibitors in 'microalbuminuric' patients with conventionally defined 'normal' blood pressures, and aim to lower BP to less than 130/85 mmHg in nonproteinuric patients and greater than 125/75 if the patients are proteinuric, i.e., > 1 g/day[22].

A suggested algorithm for the management of type 1 DN, particularly if microalbuminuria is detected, is shown in Table 33.3. Although less definitive data is available in type 2 DN, a similar approach to management would seem to be appropriate in this population particularly with the recent findings of renoprotection with ATRA in hypertensive type 2 diabetic subjects with early or overt nephropathy. It is incumbent on clinicians to carefully monitor type 1 diabetes and type 2 diabetic patients for evidence of early renal disease. This involves regular screening for microalbuminuria, either by using the reliable urine dipstick methods, such as Micral 2, or by measuring the albumin/creatinine ratio in an early morning urine sample. In addition, excellent blood glucose and BP control are important, as is the judicious use of ACE inhibitors and/or ATRA in patients who develop persistent microalbuminuria. One must be cautious in using ACE inhibitors in diabetic patients with advanced renal impairment because of the risk of hyperkalemia. Nevertheless, reports from both the RENAAL and IDNT studies[35, 36] suggest that drugs which interrupt the renin angiotensin system were remarkably safe in patients with serum creatinines > 3.4 mg/dL (300 µmol/L) with a relatively low prevalence of significant hyperkalemia. Finally, it is likely that recent insights into the pathogenesis of this disease will result in a variety of new treatments with additional benefit in not only slowing but in possibly reversing the disease process.

REFERENCES

1. Mogensen CE, Keane WF, Bennett PH, et al. Prevention of diabetic renal disease with special reference to microalbuminuria. Lancet. 1995;346:1080–4.
2. Cooper ME. Pathogenesis, prevention and treatment of diabetic nephropathy. Lancet. 1998;352:213–19.
3. Parving H-H, Jacobsen P, Tarnow L, et al. The effect of deletion polymorphism of angiotensin converting enzyme inhibition: observational follow up study. Br Med J. 1996;313:591–4.
4. Bjorck S, Blohme G, Sylven C, Mulec H. Deletion insertion polymorphism of the angiotensin converting enzyme and progression of diabetic nephropathy. Nephrol Dial Transpl. 1997;12:67–70.
5. Schmidt S, Ritz E. Angiotensin I converting enzyme gene polymorphism and diabetic nephropathy in type II diabetes. Nephrol Dial Transpl. 1997;12:37–41.
6. Ritz E, Ogata H, Orth SR. Smoking: a factor promoting onset and progression of diabetic nephropathy. Diabetes Metab. 2000;26 Suppl 4:54–63.
7. Hoy WE, Rees M, Kile E, et al. A new dimension to the Barker hypothesis: low birthweight and susceptibility to renal disease. Kidney Int. 1999;56:1072–7.
8. Krolewski AS, Laffel LMB, Krolewski M, et al. Glycosylated hemoglobin and the risk of microalbuminuria in patients with insulin-dependent diabetes mellitus. N Engl J Med. 1995;332:1251–5.
9. Diabetes Control and Complications Trial Research Group. The effect of intensive treatment on the development and progression of long-term complications in insulin-dependent diabetes mellitus. N Engl J Med. 1993;329:977–86.
10. Fioretto P, Steffes MW, Sutherland DE, et al. Reversal of lesions of diabetic nephropathy after pancreas transplantation. N Engl J Med. 1998;339:69–75.
11. UK Prospective Diabetes Study (UKPDS) Group. Intensive blood-glucose control with sulphonylureas or insulin compared with conventional treatment and risk of complications in patients with type 2 diabetes (UKPDS 33). Lancet. 1998;352:837–53.
12. Rudberg S, Persson B, Dahlquist G. Increased glomerular filtration rate as a predictor of diabetic nephropathy: an 8-year prospective study. Kidney Int. 1992;41:822–8.
13. Zatz R, Dunn BR, Meyer TW, Brenner B. Prevention of diabetic glomerulopathy by pharmacological amelioration of glomerular capillary hypertension. J Clin Invest. 1986;77:1925–30.
14. Ishii H, Jirousek MR, Koya D, et al. Amelioration of vascular dysfunctions in diabetic rats by an oral PKC beta inhibitor. Science. 1996;272:728–31.
15. Gilbert RE, Cooper ME. The tubulointerstitium in progressive diabetic kidney disease: More than an aftermath of glomerular injury? [Review]. Kidney Int. 1999;56:1627–37.
16. Koya D, Haneda M, Nakagawa H, et al. Amelioration of accelerated diabetic mesangial expansion by treatment with a PKC beta inhibitor in diabetic db/db mice, a rodent model for type 2 diabetes. FASEB J. 2000;14:439–47.
17. Vlassara H, Striker LJ, Teichberg S, et al. Advanced glycation end products induce glomerular sclerosis and albuminuria in normal rats. Proc Natl Acad Sci USA. 1994;91:11704–8.
18. Anderson S, Jung FF, Ingelfinger JR. Renal renin-angiotensin system in diabetes: functional, immunohistochemical, and molecular biological correlations. Am J Physiol Renal Physiol. 1993;265:F477–86.
19. Gilbert RE, Tsalamandris C, Bach L, et al. Glycemic control and the rate of progression of early diabetic kidney disease: a nine year longitudinal study. Kidney Int. 1993;44:855–9.
20. Reichard P, Nilsson BY, Rosenqvist U. The effect of long-term intensified insulin treatment on the development of microvascular complications of diabetes mellitus. N Engl J Med. 1993;329:304–9.
21. Ohkubo Y, Kishikawa H, Araki E, et al. Intensive insulin therapy prevents the progression of diabetic microvascular complications in Japanese patients with non-insulin-dependent diabetes mellitus: a randomized prospective 6-year study. Diabetes Res Clin Pract. 1995;28:103–17.
22. Alaveras AEG, Thomas SM, Sagriotis A, Viberti GC. Promoters of progression of diabetic nephropathy - the relative roles of blood glucose and blood pressure control. Nephrol Dial Transpl. 1997;12:71–4.
23. Parving H-H, Andersen AR, Smidt VM, et al. Effect of antihypertensive treatment on kidney function in diabetic nephropathy. Br Med J. 1987;294:1443–7.
24. Joint National Committee on Prevention, Detection, Evaluation, and Treatment of High Blood Pressure. The sixth report of the Joint National Committee on Prevention, Detection, Evaluation, and Treatment of High Blood Pressure. Arch Intern Med. 1997;157: 2413–45.
25. The ACE Inhibitors in Diabetic nephropathy Trialist group. Should all patients with type 1 diabetes mellitus and microalbuminuria receive angiotensin-converting enzyme inhibitors? A meta-analysis of individual patient data. Ann Intern Med. 2001;134:370–9.
26. The EUCLID study group. Randomised placebo-controlled trial of lisinopril in normotensive patients with insulin-dependent diabetes and normoalbuminuria or microalbuminuria. Lancet. 1997;349:1787–92.
27. Kvetny J, Gregersen G, Pedersen RS. Randomized placebo-controlled trial of perindopril in normotensive, normoalbuminuric patients with type 1 diabetes mellitus. Q J Med. 2001;94:89–94.

28. Ravid M, Brosh D, Levi Z, et al. Use of enalapril to attenuate decline in renal function in normotensive, normoalbuminuric patients with type 2 diabetes mellitus – a randomized, controlled trial. Ann Intern Med. 1998;128:982–8.

29. Ravid M, Savin H, Jutrin I, et al. Long-term stabilizing effect of angiotensin-converting enzyme inhibition on plasma creatinine and on proteinuria in normotensive type II diabetic patients. Ann Intern Med. 1993;118:577–81.

30. Lewis EJ, Hunsicker LG, Bain RP, Rohde RD. The effect of angiotensin converting enzyme inhibition on diabetic nephropathy. N Engl J Med. 1993;329:1456–62.

31. Hebert LA, Bain RP, Verme D, et al. Remission of nephrotic range proteinuria in type I diabetes. Collaborative Study Group. Kidney Int. 1994;46:1688–93.

32. Cooper ME, Johnston CI. Optimizing treatment of hypertension in patients with diabetes. JAMA. 2000;283:3177–9.

33. Gerstein HC, Yusuf S, Mann JFE, et al. Effects of ramipril on cardiovascular and microvascular outcomes in people with diabetes mellitus: results of the HOPE study and MICRO-HOPE substudy. Lancet. 2000;355:253–9.

34. Lewis JB, Berl T, Bain RP, et al. Effect of intensive blood pressure control on the course of type 1 diabetic nephropathy. Collaborative Study Group. Am J Kidney Dis. 1999;34:809–17.

35. Brenner BM, Cooper ME, de Zeeuw D, et al. Effects of losartan on renal and cardiovascular outcomes in patients with type 2 diabetes and nephropathy. N Engl J Med. 2001;345:861–9.

36. Lewis EJ, Hunsicker LG, Clarke WR, et al. Renoprotective effect of the angiotensin-receptor antagonist irbesartan in patients with nephropathy due to type 2 diabetes. N Engl J Med. 2001;345:851–60.

37. Parving HH, Lehnert H, Brochner-Mortensen J, et al. The effect of irbesartan on the development of diabetic nephropathy in patients with type 2 diabetes. N Engl J Med. 2001;345:870–8.

38. Bakris GL, Williams M, Dworkin L, et al. Preserving renal function in adults with hypertension and diabetes: A consensus approach. Am J Kid Dis. 2000;36:646–61.

39. Mogensen CE, Neldam S, Tikkanen I, et al. Randomised controlled trial of dual blockade of renin-angiotensin system in patients with hypertension, microalbuminuria, and non-insulin dependent diabetes: the candesartan and Lisinopril microalbuminuria (CALM) study. Br Med J. 2000;321:1440–4.

40. Hansson L, Zanchetti A, Carruthers SG, et al., for the HOT Study Group. Effects of intensive blood-pressure lowering and low-dose aspirin in patients with hypertension: principal results of the Hypertension Optimal Treatment (HOT) randomised trial. Lancet. 1998;351:1755–62.

41. Brenner BM, Cooper ME, de Zeeuw D, et al., for the RENAAL study investigators. The losartan renal protection study – rationale, study design and baseline characteristics of RENAAL (Reduction of Endpoints in NIDDM with the Angiotensin II Antagonist Losartan). JRAAS. 2000;1:328–35.

42. Zeller K, Whittaker E, Sullivan L, et al. Effect of restricting dietary protein on the progression of renal failure in patients with insulin-dependent diabetes mellitus. N Engl J Med. 1991;324:78–84.

43. Pedrini MT, Levey AS, Lau J, et al. The effect of dietary protein restriction on the progression of diabetic and nondiabetic renal diseases-a meta-analysis. Ann Int Med. 1996;124:627–32.

44. American Diabetes Association and the National Kidney Foundation. Consensus development conference on the diagnosis and management of nephropathy in patients with diabetes mellitus. Diabetes Care. 1994;17:1357–61.

45. Park YS, Guijarro C, Kim Y, et al. Lovastatin reduces glomerular macrophage influx and expression of monocyte chemoattractant protein-1 mRNA in nephrotic rats. Am J Kidney Dis. 1998;31:190–4.

46. Tonolo G, Ciccarese M, Brizzi P, et al. Reduction of albumin excretion rate in normotensive microalbuminuric type 2 diabetic patients during long-term simvastatin treatment. Diabetes Care. 1997;20:1891–5.

47. Jandeleit-Dahm K, Cao ZM, Cox AJ, et al. Role of hyperlipidemia in progressive renal disease: Focus on diabetic nephropathy. Kidney Int. 1999;56:S31–S36.

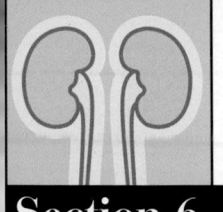

Section 6 Diabetic Nephropathy

Chapter 34 Management of End-stage Renal Disease in Diabetes

Susan J Carr

INCIDENCE OF END-STAGE RENAL DISEASE RESULTING FROM DIABETIC NEPHROPATHY

Diabetic nephropathy is the leading cause of end-stage renal disease (ESRD) worldwide[1]. There are marked differences in the reported incidence of ESRD caused by diabetes in different populations and a wide variation in the proportion of diabetic subjects with ESRD receiving renal replacement therapy.

Before 1975, fewer than 2% of the dialysis population in Europe carried the diagnosis of diabetic nephropathy[2]. However, since that time an increasing number of patients with ESRD resulting from diabetic nephropathy have been accepted for renal replacement therapy in Europe (Fig. 34.1). In the USA, 42% of patients starting dialysis in 1994–8 had diabetic nephropathy[3,4] compared with 20% in Europe[2,5] and 20% in Japan.

The risk of ESRD is higher in type 1 diabetics but, because of the higher prevalence of type 2 diabetes, most diabetics with ESRD worldwide have type 2 diabetes and the incidence of diabetic ESRD is higher in those at increased risk of type 2 diabetes, including women, older subjects, and certain racial groups, notably African Caribbeans, South Asians, Australian Aborigines, Hispanics, and native Americans. Although 40% of type 1 diabetics have previously been thought to develop nephropathy, more recent data suggest it is only 15–25%. The rate of progression of nephropathy does appear to be slower in type 2 diabetes (glomerular filtration rate (GFR) reducing by 5–6 mL/min per year) compared with type 1 diabetics (GFR reducing by 10 mL/min per year). However, as type 2 diabetics are older and have a lower baseline GFR they will usually develop ESRD within 10–12 years of diagnosis.

In the USA, the increased burden of ESRD owing to diabetic nephropathy results not only from the increased number of type 2 diabetics but also, possibly, from differences in the criteria for acceptance onto renal replacement therapy programs. The increased incidence of ESRD owing to diabetic nephropathy in certain racial groups has major implications for health care resources and planning in areas serving these populations.

PREDIALYSIS CARE FOR THE DIABETIC

A recent National Institutes of Health (NIH) consensus statement stressed the importance of early medical intervention in predialysis patients. Ideally patients should be referred at an early stage of their disease to a multidisciplinary diabetic nephropathy clinic comprising nephrologist, diabetologist, podiatrist, dietitian, and specialist renal and diabetes nurses.

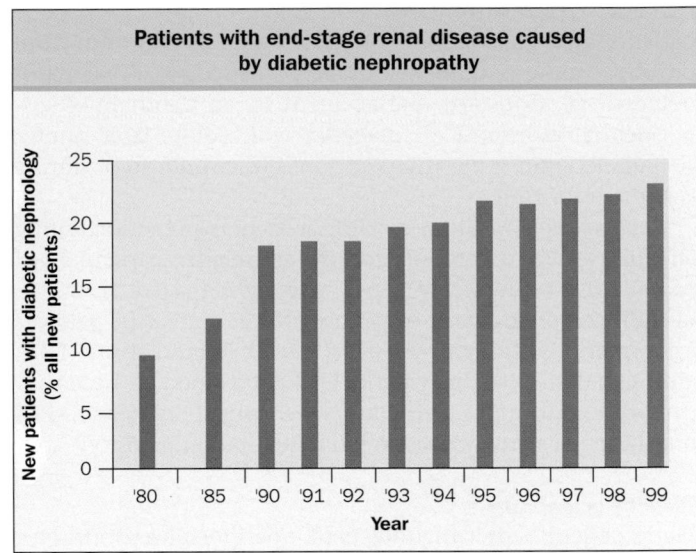

Figure 34.1 Diabetic nephropathy and end-stage renal disease. Patients with diabetic nephropathy as a percentage of all new patients accepted for renal replacement therapy in Europe 1980–1999. (Data are from the EDTA Registry, adapted with permission from van Dijk PCW, Jager K, de Charro F, et al[2].)

Initially attention will be directed towards delaying the rate of progression of renal disease, improving diabetic control, and preventing other diabetic complications (as described in Chapter 33). In view of the high death rate from cardiovascular disease in diabetic subjects, attention should focus on control of cardiovascular risk factors including smoking, hypertension, and hyperlipidemia.

As renal insufficiency progresses, attention must also be given to treatment of anemia, hyperparathyroidism, and nutritional status. Patients can be counseled regarding future dialysis with time for full consideration of the medical and social implications of treatment. Dialysis access can be organized in good time before it needs to be utilized, which is particularly important in diabetics. It may also be appropriate to consider some patients for predialysis transplantion.

There is a strong consensus (90% of nephrologists in a recent publication), although not truly evidence based, that diabetic subjects should initiate dialysis at an earlier stage than patients with other causes of ESRD – serum creatinine approximately 5.5 mg/dL (500 µmol/L) or GFR 10–20 mL/min[6]. This is a recommendation in the National Kidney Foundation Dialysis Outcomes Quality Initiative (DOQI) guidelines[7]. Patients with diabetes do appear to be more vulnerable to uremic symptoms, fluid retention, and hyperkalemia at an earlier stage than non-diabetic subjects (GFR 10–20 mL/min)[1,8]. A study of urea kinetic modeling in predialysis subjects showed that, although diabetic and nondiabetic subjects started dialysis at same K_t/V, the serum creatinine was lower in diabetic subjects[9,10].

THE DIABETIC PATIENT WITH END-STAGE RENAL DISEASE

Microvascular complications
Diabetic retinopathy
Diabetic retinopathy occurs in 97% of uremic diabetic patients and 25–30% are blind[11]. Visual loss results from proliferative retinopathy, cataracts, glaucoma, or vitreous hemorrhage. Constant management by an ophthalmologist is essential as almost all diabetics will require laser photo-coagulation and other interventions either prior to or during treatment for ESRD.

Regular heparinization and intermittent hypotension during HD may lead to a deterioration in retinopathy, particularly if proliferative retinopathy is not actively managed. However, overall, the progression of retinopathy is similar in patients undergoing peritoneal dialysis (PD) or hemodialysis (HD), although there is some evidence that good blood pressure control with continuous ambulatory peritoneal dialysis (CAPD) may be associated with less rapid deterioration in vision[12].

Diabetic neuropathy
Many patients suffer the effects of a peripheral sensorimotor neuropathy, or from gastroparesis or other bowel disturbances caused by autonomic neuropathy. These are very difficult to treat and respond poorly to conventional treatments[11]. Neuropathy is less likely to progress in renal transplant recipients. It also tends to be less severe in patients treated with PD, theoretically because of improved clearance of medium-sized molecules[11].

Many patients may also suffer from impotence caused by neuropathy, vascular disease, or medication, which may require specialist investigation and treatment.

Macrovascular complications
Peripheral vascular disease
Problems related to the diabetic foot are a major cause of hospital admission (Fig. 34.2a), and 50–70% of all nontraumatic amputations occur in diabetics. One UK study reported that 6.8% of diabetics receiving renal replacement therapy had a major amputation[13,14]. However, reports of the incidence of lower limb ischemia in diabetics on dialysis have conflicted: some studies reported increased rates and others lower rates. There is no reported difference between CAPD and HD[13]. The major contributory etiologic factors in diabetic foot problems are peripheral vascular disease, diabetic neuropathy, and stress caused by inappropriate footwear (Fig. 34.2b). Some studies have reported symptomatic deterioration in the lower limbs correlating with falls in blood pressure; therefore, care should be taken to avoid excessive ultrafiltration in diabetic patients on dialysis. In type 2 diabetics, better glycemic control is associated with fewer amputations[12].

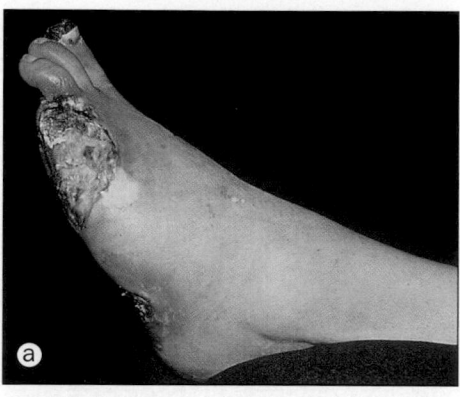

Figure 34.2 The diabetic foot. (a) Gangrenous ulcers in a diabetic caused by a combination of large and small vessel disease and neuropathy. (b) Prevention of diabetic foot complications.

Prevention of diabetic foot complications

Identification of patients at risk

Education about foot care

Regular examination of the feet at clinic

Provision of appropriate footwear

Provision of podiatry services

The treatment of this condition requires a multidisciplinary approach, ideally in a combined clinic with nephrologist, diabetologist, and podiatrist. At the first sign of lower limb ischemia, patients should be assessed by a vascular surgeon.

Cardiovascular disease
Cardiovascular disease is the major cause of death in patients with ESRD worldwide and is increased further in diabetics (Fig. 34.3)[4]. Diabetic patients with ESRD may have numerous risk factors for the development of atheromatous vascular disease, including hypertension, hyperlipidemia (especially if previously nephrotic), obesity, and smoking. Coronary heart disease is accelerated in diabetics and the protective effect of female gender lost. The death rate from cardiovascular disease increases with age in diabetic (and nondiabetic) subjects and is higher in type 2 diabetes[15]. EDTA Registry data[2] indicate that the difference in mortality between diabetics and nondiabetics due to myocardial ischemia and infarction is greatest in young diabetics with ESRD (Fig. 34.4).

Glycemic control has a major effect on macrovascular disease in diabetics with ESRD; HbA$_{1C}$ is an independent predictor of the presence of coronary artery disease on arteriography in uremic type 1 diabetics.

Blood pressure control
The optimal first line therapy in diabetics is not definitively established but trial evidence supports the use of angiotensin-converting enzyme (ACE) inhibitors, angiotensin receptor antagonists (ATRA), dihydropyridine calcium channel blockers, α-blockers, β-blockers and thiazide diuretics in diabetic subjects. In view of the proven beneficial effect of ACE inhibition on progression of renal disease and reduction in cardiovascular risk ACE inhibitors should be used as first line agents in suitable subjects. However, most diabetic subjects will require several agents to control the blood pressure

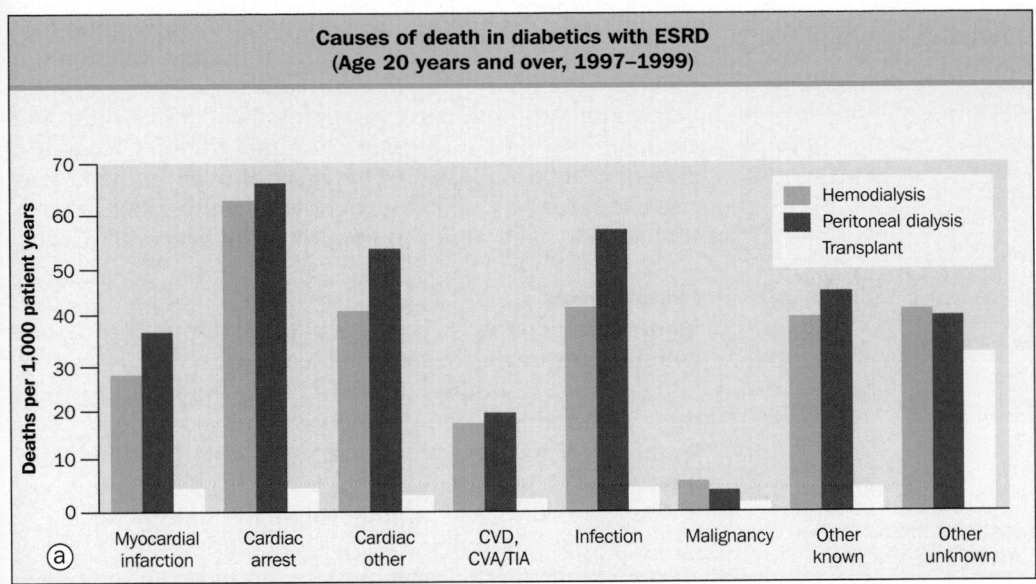

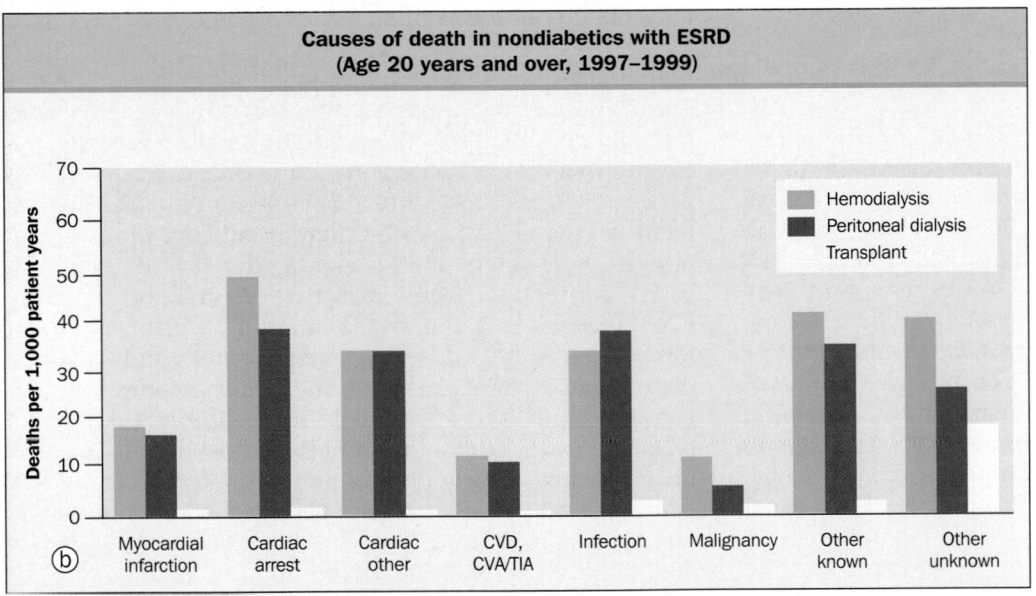

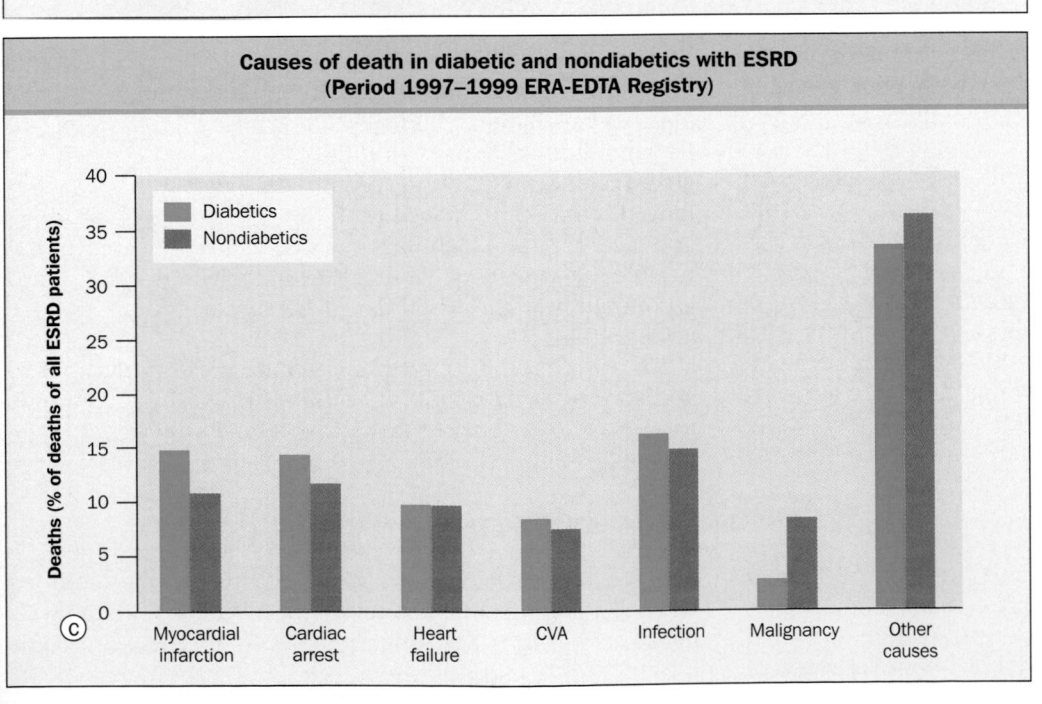

Figure 34.3 Cause of death in diabetic and nondiabetic subjects with end-stage renal disease. (a) Data from the USRDS 2001 Report, Causes of death in diabetics with ESRD, USA 1997–1999. (b) Data from the USRDS 2001 Report, Causes of death in non-diabetics with ESRD, USA 1997–1999. (c) Data from EDTA Registry Causes of death in diabetic and non-diabetic subjects with ESRD, Europe 1997–1999. (Adapted with permission from US Renal Data System, USRDS Annual Data Report[4].)

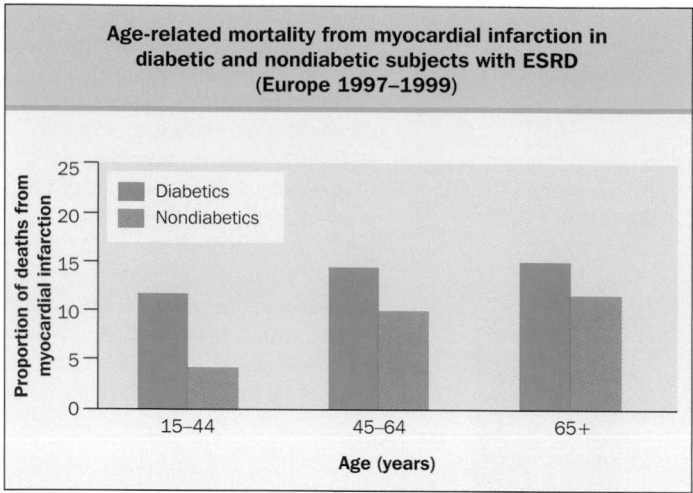

Figure 34.4 Age-related mortality from myocardial infarction in diabetic and nondiabetic subjects with end-stage renal disease.
(Reprinted from data supplied by the EDTA Registry adapted with permission from van Dijk PCW, Jager K, de Charro F, et al[2].

adequately and the presence of other medical conditions, particularly coronary heart disease, will also dictate the therapeutic regimen. Some diabetic subjects with impaired renal function have hyporeninemic hypoaldosteronism leading to an increased incidence of hyperkalemia, which may restrict the use of ACE inhibitors and ATRA. In this situation it may be possible with careful supervision to safely continue the use of an ACE inhibitor in the predialysis diabetic subject with a reduction in dietary potassium intake or improved control of acidosis. β-Blockers are used to treat hypertension in diabetic subjects (especially with cardiac disease) but care needs to be taken in subjects with poor warnings of hypoglycemia, and these agents are unsuitable in the presence of peripheral vascular disease.

Infection

The antibacterial function of leukocytes is impaired in diabetic subjects without ESRD. Diabetics with poor glycemic control demonstrate abnormalities in granulocyte adherence, chemotaxis, and phagocytosis. Diabetics may be at increased risk of staphylococcal infection as a result of increased skin and mucosal colonization with these organisms. Diabetics who inject insulin do have higher staphylococcal carriage rates than diabetic subjects receiving oral hypoglycemic agents, although the mechanism for this is unknown[16].

There is justification for screening diabetic subjects with ESRD for nasal staphylococcal carriage and treating carriers with topical mupirocin. Diabetics are more prone to urinary tract infections, pulmonary infections, and candidiasis. Foot ulcer infections often progress to septic gangrene and amputation.

Metabolic complications
Hyperparathyroidism
Diabetic patients undergoing dialysis develop secondary hyperparathyroidism at a slower rate than nondiabetics and this may predispose to adynamic bone disease[11] in which there is a reduced rate of bone turnover without an excess of

unmineralized osteoid. The reduced bone formation may lead to enhanced deposition of aluminum at the ossification front. Diabetics appear to accumulate aluminum more readily, perhaps due to prolonged gastrointestinal transit time, and are more susceptible to bone pain and fractures related to aluminum bone disease, which may also be unmasked by parathyroidectomy. Aluminum-containing phosphate binders should always be avoided in the diabetic patient with ESRD.

Hyperlipidemia
Many diabetic dialysis patients have cardiovascular disease and need treatment for hyperlipidemia as secondary prevention for cardiac disease. In view of the high incidence of cardiovascular disease in diabetics with renal failure, primary treatment of hyperlipidemia may be justified, but no study has addressed this specific issue.

Diabetics on CAPD become hypertriglyceridemic and have a small increase in cholesterol levels because of absorption of glucose from the dialysate. The tendency to hypertriglyceridemia may be lower when intraperitoneal insulin is used.

Malnutrition
The incidence of malnutrition on CAPD is higher in diabetics than in nondiabetics. Many studies have recognized the adverse effect of poor nutritional status on survival in dialysis patients[1,11,13], and early nutritional support (enteral or parenteral) is essential in diabetic dialysis patients who develop a severe intercurrent illness (e.g., a complicated episode of CAPD peritonitis). Many diabetics on dialysis, especially CAPD, become malnourished as a result of dialysate protein losses, diabetic gastroparesis leading to nausea and vomiting, diarrhea as a consequence of autonomic neuropathy, and continued urinary protein losses. The peritoneal protein loss is much greater in those with high peritoneal transport and in some patients hemodialysis may be preferred. The use of amino acid based PD fluids have been shown to provide some benefit but use is limited to one exchange a day to prevent development of metabolic acidosis[17].

Glycemic control
Control of blood glucose can be problematic in diabetic patients on dialysis. Hyperglycemia may be asymptomatic through lack of osmotic diuresis, and warnings of hypoglycemic attacks are often absent. Oral agents can cause prolonged hypoglycemia as a result of altered drug metabolism, and agents chosen should be those metabolized by the hepatic route, such as tolbutamide and gliclazide. Metformin is contraindicated in renal failure because of the risk of lactic acidosis.

The effects of exogenous insulin are prolonged in ESRD, and severe hypoglycemia may occur. However, long-acting insulins may still be used with careful monitoring in the diabetic patient with ESRD.

Psychologic and social care
Withdrawal from dialysis is a significant cause of death in diabetic subjects on dialysis[1,3,11]. Many patients become depressed when developing renal failure, which is often associated with deteriorating vision and limb problems. Many patients become

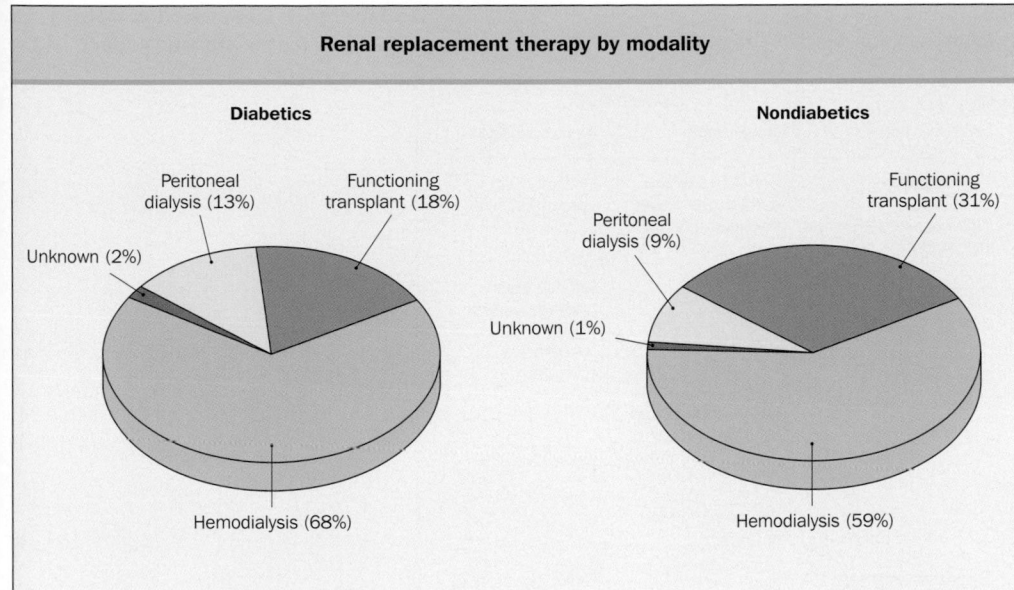

Figure 34.5 Renal replacement therapy by modality in diabetic and nondiabetic subjects. Data are combined: from USRDS (Adapted with permission from USRDS (United States Renal Data System)[3]; and from data from the EDTA Registry (1994) prepared by Dr E Jones.

unemployed, causing additional financial strain on families. The involvement of patient-support groups, a psychologist, and a liaison psychiatrist are valuable adjuncts to care.

FUTURE DIRECTIONS IN THERAPY

Diabetic subjects on dialysis (especially PD) have elevated levels of advanced glycosylation end-products (AGE) that fall sharply to within the normal range in the days following transplantation. There is no difference in level of AGE with hemodialysis or peritoneal dialysis. However, some studies show reduced formation of Amadori albumin and AGE products using icodextrin based instead of glucose based PD fluids[18,19]. It has been widely postulated that AGE are a major cause of tissue and organ damage in diabetes of long duration (see Chapter 33)[1,20,21]. If so, preventing the formation of AGE would be an attractive means of preventing diabetic microvascular complications. Aminoguanidine, a hydrazine compound, interferes with nonenzymatic glycosylation and reduces AGE formation. In animal studies, aminoguanidine has been shown to prevent microvascular complications, and intraperitoneal aminoguanidine to prevent glucose induced changes in the peritoneum.

DIALYSIS IN THE DIABETIC: PERITONEAL DIALYSIS OR HEMODIALYSIS

The management options for diabetic subjects with ESRD are similar to those for patients with other primary renal diseases, i.e., PD, HD, or transplantation. However, many diabetics are excluded from transplantation because of the presence of comorbid conditions, particularly vascular disease or advanced age. Selection of the mode of dialysis is based upon the particular requirements of the individual patient (medical, social, cultural), physician bias, and available national resources (Fig. 34.5) (see Chapter 75). The advantages and disadvantages of each technique are outlined in Table 34.1.

Peritoneal dialysis
Advantages
The initiation of PD with insertion of the catheter is generally straightforward and the technique simple for the patient to learn, although account may need to be taken of visual impairment in a diabetic. The use of PD maintains the patient's independence and encompasses fewer dietary restrictions than HD.

Maintenance of steady-state biochemical parameters and continuous removal of fluid and solutes on CAPD allow good control of circulating volume and blood pressure[13]. This avoids the episodes of intravascular fluid depletion and hypotension to which diabetics are particularly prone with HD because of cardiovascular disease and autonomic neuropathy. Residual renal function may be preserved for a longer period of time in diabetics on PD versus HD, leading to a reduction in the dose of dialysis required and contributing to the overall clearance of small- and medium-molecular-weight solutes and fluid removal[22]. There is no evidence that PD or HD adequacy in diabetics differs from that in nondiabetic subjects[13].

Automated peritoneal dialysis (APD)
The use of shorter, frequent dialysis exchanges can achieve greater ultrafiltration in relation to the amount of glucose absorbed especially in diabetic subjects. This technique in combination with a daytime dwell using icodextrin (or an amino acid-based PD fluid in malnourished patients) has been advocated to maximize ultrafiltration and reduced excess glucose absorption in diabetics[17].

Disadvantages
There are also disadvantages of PD in the diabetic. Technique survival is poor mainly because of infection and loss of ultrafiltration. Several of the problems with PD relate to the use of glucose as the osmotic agent. Ultrafiltration failure commonly results from high peritoneal transport of glucose in patients on PD. Hyperglycemia in diabetics may increase thirst and this leads to increased fluid consumption and fluid

Comparison of dialysis options for the diabetic patient				
	Peritoneal dialysis		Hemodialysis	
Parameters	Advantages	Disadvantages	Advantages	Disadvantages
Technique	Peritoneal access is easy	Low technique survival rate, high hospitalization rate, higher rate of infection	Better technique survival rate, lower hospitalization rate, lower infection rate	Difficulty with vascular access
Blood pressure	Good blood pressure control, slow ultrafiltration and fewer episodes of cardiovascular instability	–	–	Difficult blood pressure control, frequent hypotensive episodes
Biochemical parameters	Steady-state biochemical parameters, preservation of residual renal function for longer	–	Efficient solute and water extraction	–
Social factors	Maintains independence	–	Can be performed at home	–
Nutritional factors	Fewer dietary restrictions	Excessive weight gain, poor nutrition, hyperlipidemia	–	Difficulty with fluid and dietary restrictions

Table 34.1 Comparison of dialysis options for the diabetic patient.

overload. High glucose absorption leads to increased insulin requirement, obesity, and hyperlipidemia. Marked swings in blood glucose also occur in diabetic subjects when hypertonic dialysate is used to facilitate fluid removal.

New PD fluids have been developed and do ameliorate these problems to some extent but at present none can replace glucose as the primary osmotic agent. Glycerol-containing PD fluid resulted in hyperosmolarity in some diabetic subjects and has shown no advantages over glucose.

Icodextrin, a large-molecular-weight polymer has numerous advantages in diabetic CAPD patients and begins to offer an effective alternative to hypertonic glucose solutions[21,23]. Icodextrin as a single overnight dwell can reduce the nocturnal glucose load and provide improved ultrafiltration[17]. Animal studies have also shown suppressed peritoneal phagocyte function and reduction in tumor necrosis factor-α production by peritoneal macrophages which may lead to reduced peritoneal thickening and ultrafiltration failure. A further theoretical advantage is a reduction in the formation of advanced glycation end-products induced by heat sterilization of commercially available PD fluids[18,19]. There have been reports of hypersensitivity reactions with icodextrin, and care needs to be taken with glycemic monitoring as the Accutrend Sensor monitor tends to overestimate the glucose level in the presence of the maltose and glucose polymers in icodextrin. This is due to the enzyme reaction involved but there are no reported problems with other devices employing glucose oxidase, hexokinase or other kits using glucose dehydrogenase[24].

Peritonitis

Peritonitis is one of the major causes of morbidity in CAPD patients and has been reduced greatly by the use of disconnect systems[13]. Most studies report no increased risk of CAPD peritonitis in diabetics[13,14]. Data from the NIH CAPD Registry[13] showed peritonitis rates to be lowest for patients using a combination of intraperitoneal and subcutaneous insulin, compared with diabetics receiving intraperitoneal

insulin alone or diabetics who were not receiving insulin. There is an independent relationship between increasing age and peritonitis rate. In general, there is no increase in the severity of peritonitis episodes in diabetics or the number of episodes necessitating removal of the CAPD catheter[13]. Unfortunately, these registry data are based on CAPD techniques now superseded by double-bag or Y-set disconnect systems, leading to an improvement in peritonitis rates. It has also been shown that the peritonitis rate is lower in patients on APD, but only a minority in this report were diabetic[25].

Exit site infection

The NIH CAPD Registry[13] reported no increase in the incidence of CAPD exit site infections (Fig. 34.6) in diabetics but there was a significant increase in *Staphylococcus aureus* tunnel infections. Diabetic subjects have increased nasal carriage rates for *S. aureus*[16] especially in insulin-requiring patients (53 versus 35% for non-insulin requiring) and attempts to eradicate the nasal carrier state in diabetic subjects may reduce infection rates[13,16]. A recent study suggested antibiotic prophylaxis should be prescribed to all peritoneal dialysis patients who are *S. aureus* exit site carriers[26].

Blood glucose control in peritoneal dialysis

Diabetic subjects on CAPD may receive insulin by either subcutaneous (s.c.) or intraperitoneal (i.p.) routes. Administration of insulin s.c. leads to variable absorption, and i.p. administration of insulin has several theoretic advantages based upon the pharmacokinetics of insulin[21,27,28]. Unfortunately, there has been no direct comparison of i.p. insulin administration with conventional multiple daily s.c. injections of insulin.

When insulin is administered subcutaneously, there are relatively low portal insulin levels, which leads to increased hepatic glucose production and peripheral hyperinsulinemia. The presence of peripheral hyperinsulinemia leads to insulin resistance in the peripheral tissues and results in a more atherogenic lipid profile. Intraperitoneally administered insulin

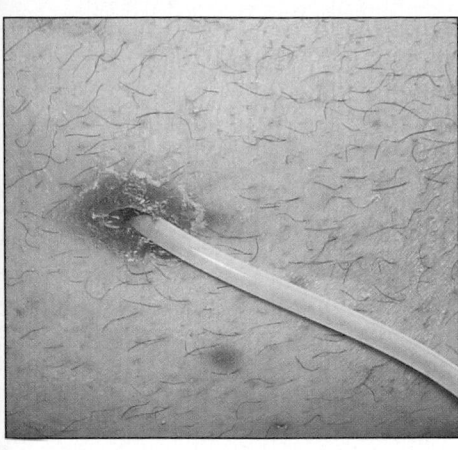

Figure 34.6 Exit site infection in continuous ambulatory peritoneal dialysis.

preferentially enters the portal circulation, thus mimicking more closely physiologic secretion of insulin. Consequently, it reduces endogenous glucose production, increases tissue insulin sensitivity, and is associated with a lipid profile of lower atherogenic potential[13,27]. Absorption of insulin i.p. is between 13 and 46% of the administered dose, absorption varying with dialysate volume, dwell time, and insulin concentration. In addition, 25% of the dose is lost through adsorption to the PVC dialysate bag and associated tubing. In general, a two to three times increased dose is required in patients changing to i.p. insulin when beginning CAPD (the conversion factor is less in those already established on CAPD as the insulin dose has already been increased to account for the dialysate carbohydrate load). It is usually recommended that the baseline dose is increased with hypertonic bags and the night-time dose reduced (to 10% of total daily dose).

Possible adverse effects of intraperitoneal insulin
Administration of insulin i.p. can give rise to a number of adverse effects[14,27,28].

Hepatic steatosis
The nature of the hepatic steatosis lesion is not fully understood and it has only been observed at autopsy. Liver function tests are typically normal.

Peritonitis
Data concerning a link between i.p. insulin and peritonitis are conflicting. There are reports of an increased incidence of peritonitis[14] although this concern is not borne out in published trials where patients were selected and undertook extensive training. Although i.p. insulin requirements generally increase in peritonitis there is a report of hypoglycemia arising in patients with peritonitis taking their usual dose of insulin. This occurs because of enhanced insulin absorption through the inflamed peritoneum, and blood glucose should be monitored closely.

The 'malignant omentum syndrome' is heralded by a sudden and marked change in insulin requirement. The peritoneal catheter becomes enveloped in omentum facilitating increased contact between peritoneal dialysate containing insulin and omental adipocytes. The adipocytes are able to bind and degrade insulin and thereby altering the patient's insulin requirements.

Despite the theoretic benefits of i.p. insulin, practical administration is often difficult. Patients may be blind or have extremely poor vision. They may also be reluctant to change their insulin regimen. At the present time it is not our practice to use i.p. insulin.

Hemodialysis
Advantages
In general, technique survival and hospitalization rates are better for patients receiving HD than PD. In addition, HD also provides more efficient solute and water removal and can be performed at home, maintaining patient independence.

Disadvantages
The major problem with HD in diabetics is the establishment and maintenance of vascular access. Diabetic patients usually need to start dialysis earlier in the course of renal failure, and a significant proportion as a uremic emergency requiring unplanned dialysis even if they were previously under nephrological care. These factors make the timely establishment of vascular access very difficult and often unsuccessful. In addition, patients with diabetes often have vascular calcification or atherosclerosis of the arterial tree, which make arteriovenous fistula formation very difficult (Fig. 34.7). The rate of fistula loss is significantly higher among diabetic subjects than in nondiabetics and the majority of studies have shown that the presence of diabetes is an independent risk factor for access-related morbidity. Many diabetic subjects are not therefore suitable candidates for primary arteriovenous fistula formation and require prosthetic grafts or temporary access with tunneled vascular catheters, with consequent risk of complications of the procedure: infection, thrombosis, inadvertent arterial puncture, and, later, vessel stenosis[12]. Diabetics on HD are often subject to interruptions in dialysis because of

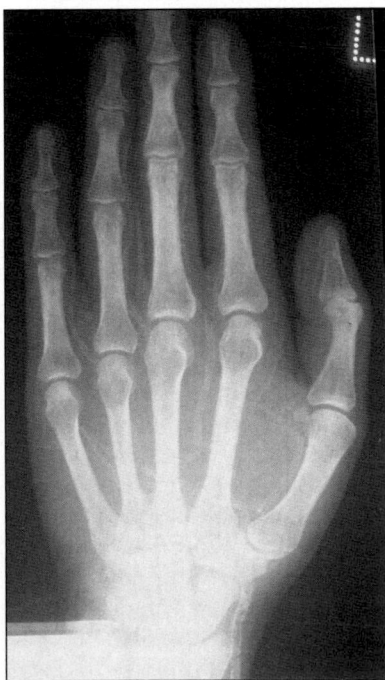

Figure 34.7 Vascular calcification in a diabetic. Extensive vascular calcification in the hand of a 38-year-old man on hemodialysis with a 25-year history of type 1 diabetes.

hypotensive episodes or limitations in bloodflow rates as a consequence of poor or temporary vascular access, leading to inadequate dialysis and failure to reach target weight[12].

Several studies have demonstrated poor blood pressure control in hemodialyzed diabetics. Hypertension in patients on HD is largely volume dependent and may often be controlled by attaining dry body weight. Many diabetics have a high intradialytic weight gain, which may result from noncompliance with dietary restrictions or from thirst initiated by hyperglycemia. However, even after correction of such factors, many diabetic patients on HD still require antihypertensive medication. One of the factors that makes achieving 'dry weight' difficult in diabetic subjects is the episodes of hypotension that occur frequently in diabetics during HD even when patients may appear volume overloaded. The factors that predispose to this are the presence of autonomic neuropathy and underlying cardiac dysfunction. Bicarbonate dialysate should be used, long-acting antihypertensive agents omitted on the morning of the dialysis session, and the use of sodium profiling or the administration of albumin considered in diabetics prone to episodes of hypotension[12]. As a result of the intermittent nature of HD, the dietary and fluid restrictions are more severe and often pose problems with compliance.

SURVIVAL AND CAUSES OF DEATH IN DIABETICS WITH END-STAGE RENAL DISEASE

The life expectancy of diabetics on renal replacement therapy has been poor because of the high incidence of comorbid conditions, especially vascular disease and the many complications of dialysis that may arise, particularly in diabetics. Many type 2 diabetics are elderly and age is a very important independent determinant of survival irrespective of renal disease or mode of therapy.

Data from Europe and USRDS reported reduced survival of diabetic subjects with ESRD[2,3,4]. Brunner quoted a 5-year survival rate in diabetic subjects of 30.2% compared with 62.2% in nondiabetic dialysis patients[2]. The life expectancy of diabetics on renal replacement therapy is improving steadily but remains inferior to that of patients with glomerulonephritis and hypertensive nephrosclerosis (Fig. 34.8).

The increased mortality probably results from the high prevalence of concomitant multisystem disease, especially vascular disease, and also the increased incidence of complications on dialysis.

In both EDTA and USRDS registry data[2,3,4] death due to malignancy is less common in diabetics; this is likely the result of the high probability of a diabetic dying from other causes. Data from the USRDS[3,4] shows mortality from all causes to be 1.5 times higher in diabetics with ESRD compared with nondiabetic subjects. Several studies have shown the prognosis to be worse when patients have evidence of severe pre-existing vascular disease before starting dialysis. Previous stroke, myocardial infarction, or peripheral vascular disease are independent predictors of lower survival in patients on renal replacement therapy. A recent European study demonstrated survival to be worse in type 2 than in type 1 diabetics with ESRD[15]: age, previous stroke, apoprotein A_1, and fibrinogen levels were independent predictors of death.

There is a higher incidence of withdrawal from dialysis reported in diabetics (Fig. 34.9) in the USA, Canada, and Australia. This withdrawal rate increases with age and possibly reflects a higher incidence of comorbid conditions in older diabetics that may reduce the quality of life for these individuals. There is marked national and racial variation in withdrawal from dialysis. In Italy, the incidence of withdrawal from dialysis was 0.5% in diabetics and 0.9% in nondiabetics, whereas in a study from Newcastle, UK, the incidence of withdrawal was 15% in diabetics and 7% in nondiabetics. These discrepancies may reflect different patterns of acceptance of diabetic and nondiabetic subjects onto dialysis programs in different countries. There is a marked racial variation in withdrawal from dialysis in that African-Caribbean subjects are at half to one third the risk of withdrawal from treatment, which may have a sociocultural explanation. The reasons for withdrawal from dialysis include failure to thrive, medical complications, and access failure. There were no discernible differences in these factors in the USRDS data for diabetics and nondiabetics[3].

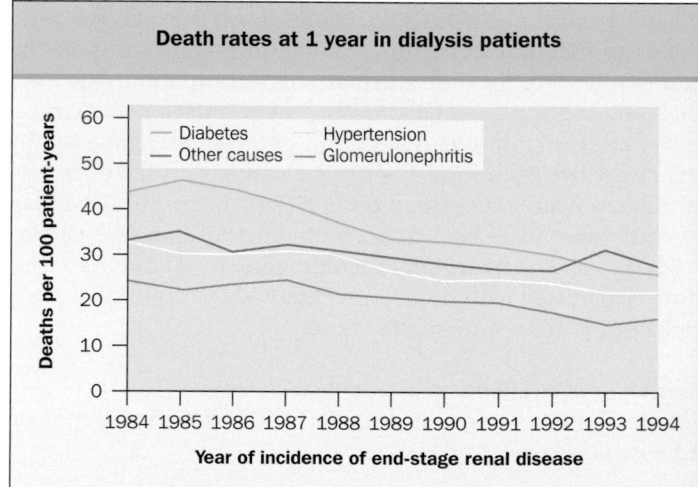

Figure 34.8 Mortality in dialysis patients with and without diabetes. Adjusted 1-year death rates for dialysis patients by diagnosis and year of incidence (1984–1994). (Adapted with permission from USRDS (United States Renal Data System)[3].)

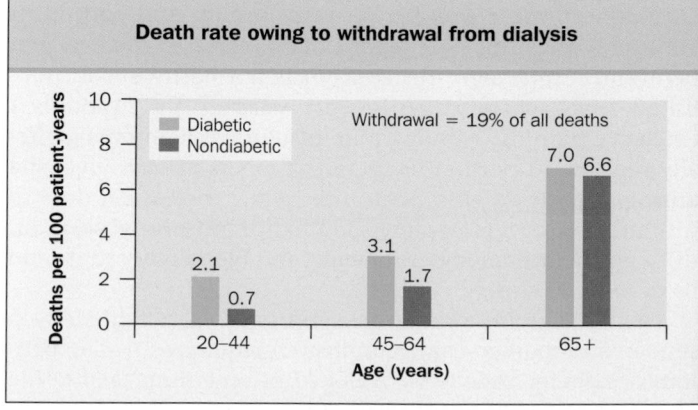

Figure 34.9 Death rate due to withdrawal from dialysis by age and diabetic status. Data from 1993–1995. (Adapted with permission from USRDS (United States Renal Data System)[3].)

Since cardiovascular disease is the major cause of death in diabetic subjects with ESRD, the identification of cardiovascular risk factors at an early stage of disease, and continuing active management of these risk factors on renal replacement therapy are of paramount importance.

OUTCOME OF DIALYSIS: PERITONEAL DIALYSIS VERSUS HEMODIALYSIS

A clear difference in outcome between PD and HD has not been observed. Younger patients with minimal comorbid conditions tend to have transplants and hence older patients who are unfit for transplantation remain on dialysis with a poorer outcome. The outcome of dialysis treatment is to a large extent determined by the extent of comorbid conditions. A significant difference in survival between PD and HD can only be adequately assessed by a randomized controlled trial of the two dialysis modalities. However, there has not been nor is there likely to be in the future such a trial because of the complexities and ethical issues involved.

Comparisons of survival between PD and HD are very difficult to interpret as patient selection biases will influence the number of patients entering each form of therapy. An analysis of the USRDS data using Cox's proportional hazards model showed a significantly higher mortality for diabetics on CAPD compared with HD. However, the excess mortality was accounted for by an increased risk of death in elderly subjects with severe cardiovascular or peripheral vascular disease[5,8,13]. Data from the Canadian Registry (1996) reported a 14% lower risk of death in diabetics on CAPD compared with HD for diabetics up to 64 years of age[8].

Reviews of data from the EDTA and USRDS Registries suggest that younger diabetic subjects (age 45–55 years) may survive longer on CAPD, whereas older diabetic subjects survive longer on HD[5]. Further analysis of these data showed that the increased death rate in elderly diabetic patients may have resulted from the presence of peripheral vascular disease in the CAPD patients. An age-adjusted analysis of data from the Michigan registry also suggests that younger diabetics (< 59 years) survive longer on CAPD and older diabetics longer on

HD: lower risk of death on CAPD versus HD is 38% for young patients and 19% for patients over 60[29].

In contrast, numerous smaller multicenter prospective studies of CAPD and HD have reported no significant difference between treatment modalities.

Generally, studies showing higher rates of survival on CAPD tend to include younger patients, who may gain from the benefits of CAPD, such as better blood pressure control and improved diabetic control using i.p. insulin. The higher mortality demonstrated in older diabetics on CAPD in these studies may be a reflection of increased comorbidity and possibly a physician selection bias of such patients for PD.

HOSPITALIZATION AND TECHNIQUE SURVIVAL

There have been many studies comparing hospitalization rates in dialysis patients[30]. Data from the USRDS identified an increase in hospitalization rate per patient-year at risk of 14% in PD compared with HD patients when data were adjusted for age, race, gender, and cause of ESRD[30]. The number of recorded hospital days was also higher in PD patients. The USRDS[4] has shown an age related increase in hospitalization for all ESRD patients, the most marked increases are in older patients on peritoneal and hemodialysis (Fig. 34.10). However, other smaller and single-center studies have reported no difference in admission rates in diabetics on CAPD or HD[30]. One confounding factor in many studies may be that many of the patients on PD have a higher comorbidity than those on HD.

The technique survival rate for CAPD is lower in both diabetics and nondiabetics compared with HD. The main reason for failure has been peritonitis and inadequate dialysis. However, the use of the Y-set and double-bag systems has led to a significant reduction in peritonitis rates and this should lead to increased technique survival on CAPD. A reduction in peritonitis rates should also lead to a reduction in CAPD failures owing to peritoneal membrane failure. Many patients also fail CAPD through inadequacy of dialysis.

The most frequent reasons for hospitalization in diabetics on HD are problems related to formation and maintenance of

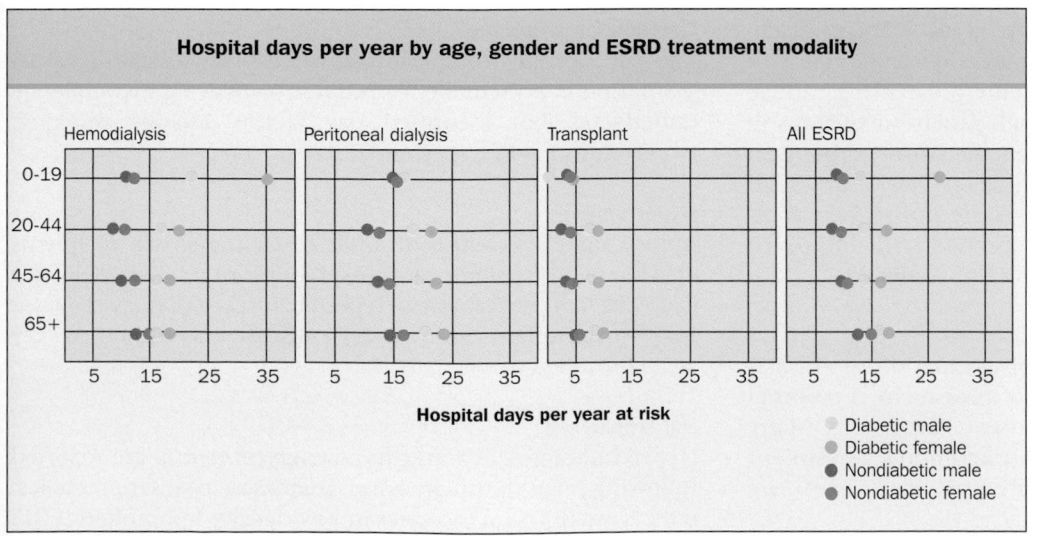

Figure 34.10 Hospitalization days per year by age, gender and ESRD treatment modality in diabetic and nondiabetic subjects. (Adapted with permission from US Renal Data System, USRDS Annual Data Report[4].)

Diabetic Nephropathy

vascular access, i.e., placement, thrombosis, and infection. In practice, both dialysis modalities have advantages and disadvantages and the choice of dialysis modality is based upon the particular requirements of the individual patient, the opinion of the nephrologist, and the available resources.

RENAL TRANSPLANTATION IN THE DIABETIC

Renal transplantation is a safe and effective treatment modality for diabetic subjects with ESRD. It offers both improved survival and rehabilitation compared with dialytic therapies[1,20].

Initially, diabetic subjects were considered unsuitable for renal transplantation because of the potential risk of post-transplant morbidity and mortality and the possible adverse effects of corticosteroids and other immunosuppressive agents. Since the mid-1980s, there has been a dramatic improvement in survival after renal transplantation mainly attributed to the reduction in early post-transplant cardiovascular death, better first-year graft survival, and a reduction in the number of patients who die with a functioning graft. However, many (> 50%) diabetic subjects are still precluded from renal transplantation as a result of advanced age or the presence of comorbid factors.

The majority of (but not all) recent studies have reported graft survival to be similar in diabetic and nondiabetic subjects at 1 and 5 years[31] but only when data are censored for patients who die with a functioning graft.

As expected, living donor graft survival is superior to cadaveric donor grafts in diabetics (80 versus 64%, 5-year survival) as in nondiabetics. The higher mortality rate seen in cadaveric graft recipients is probably a consequence of a higher cumulative burden of immunosuppression and comorbidities[3]. The introduction of improved immunosuppressive agents should further improve patient and graft survival both in the diabetic and nondiabetic population.

Survival of the diabetic transplant patient ranges from 45 to 75% at 5 years. This is significantly lower than that in nondiabetic renal transplant recipients and is a consequence of cardiovascular disease; 36% of diabetic transplant recipients die from cardiovascular disease[3,32].

There is also an increased risk of death from infection, cerebrovascular disease, and peripheral vascular disease compared with nondiabetic graft recipients. The presence of any vascular disease pretransplant has a significant effect on mortality in diabetic transplant recipients, especially pre-existing cardiac or peripheral vascular disease. Although patient survival is still suboptimal compared with nondiabetic transplant patients, it is still better than for diabetics remaining on dialysis, although selection bias means the populations are not strictly comparable. Transplantation is also associated with improved rehabilitation and a better quality of life than dialysis.

Pretransplant assessment

In view of the increased incidence of vascular disease in diabetics, a pretransplant cardiovascular assessment is essential in addition to the routine workup (see Chapter 86). Many diabetic subjects will also require an additional assessment of the peripheral arterial system to ensure iliac vessels are suitable for transplantation

Pretransplant cardiovascular disease

Widespread coronary artery disease, which is often asymptomatic, is common in diabetic dialysis patients and the cardiovascular mortality is particularly high in these patients post-transplantation.

There is evidence that this risk can be reduced in diabetics by aggressive investigation and intervention prior to renal transplantation. Manske et al. studied 151 consecutive diabetic renal transplant candidates who underwent coronary angiography and demonstrated that 31 (21%) had > 75% stenosis in one or more coronary arteries and yet the majority of patients had no symptoms of ischemic heart disease[33].

Of these patients, 26 were allocated to medical management or revascularization (angioplasty or bypass surgery). Cardiac end points occurred in 2 of 13 subjected to revascularization compared with 10 of 13 treated medically. These data suggest asymptomatic diabetic patients should be screened for the presence of occult cardiovascular disease to identify lesions suitable for revascularization. In view of the potential complications of coronary angiography and the resource implications of screening all diabetic patients who are potential transplant recipients, an alternative noninvasive screening test would be beneficial. Multiple gated acquisition scanning, dipyridamole thallium scanning, and dobutamine stress echocardiography have all been evaluated in diabetic subjects prior to transplantation, but the sensitivity and specificity of these investigations has been disappointing and to date no ideal noninvasive test has been identified.

Selected diabetic patients have acceptable outcome from coronary artery bypass grafting and this is probably preferable to angioplasty, which has a high restenosis rate in renal failure. One further problem is that following cardiac screening, patients may need to wait for a considerable time before transplantation takes place and may develop further asymptomatic lesions during this time (see Chapter 69).

It is unlikely that the high incidence of cardiovascular deaths can be explained entirely by occlusive coronary disease, and other factors such as left ventricular hypertrophy leading to impaired myocardial blood supply and altered myocardial oxygen demand may play an important role.

Post-transplantation in diabetics
Cardiovascular disease

The pathogenesis of cardiovascular disease following transplantation in both diabetics and nondiabetics is incompletely understood, but identified risk factors include smoking, hypertension, and hyperlipidemia.

Hypertension

Approximately 80–90% of adult renal transplant recipients develop hypertension post-transplantation[19,20]. This incidence is no different in diabetics. Hypertension is a major risk factor for post-transplant cardiovascular disease and should be very well controlled in the diabetic.

Hyperlipidemia

Hypercholesterolemia and hypertriglyceridemia are reported following renal transplantation. Increased total serum cholesterol is usually from increases in low-density lipoprotein (LDL)

cholesterol (74% of patients)[34]. Many patients also have elevated levels of triglyceride (29%) and very low-density lipoprotein (VLDL) cholesterol especially in the presence of proteinuria and graft dysfunction. High-density lipoprotein (HDL) cholesterol levels are normal or may be reduced in up to 10% of transplant recipients and the composition of HDL may be abnormal, leading to a reduced cardioprotective effect.

The patterns of hyperlipidemia do not generally differ in diabetics. There have been no controlled trials investigating whether reducing lipid levels influence cardiovascular mortality or morbidity in diabetic or nondiabetic transplant recipients. Therefore, any decisions to treat are based upon extrapolation from other populations. Given the very high incidence of cardiovascular death in diabetic transplant recipients, the use of diet and pharmacologic approaches to treat hyperlipidemia appears reasonable until evidence from clinical trials is available.

Infection

Diabetics are at increased risk of infection following transplantation. As well as the effects of immunosuppression, which are similar to those in nondiabetic patients, factors specific to diabetics include impaired chemotaxis, increased colonization, and the effects of hyperglycemia on host defenses. Cell-mediated immunity is essentially normal in diabetics. Diabetics are at increased risk of foot infections and fungal infections, especially candidiasis and mucormycosis. Urinary tract infection is more common in diabetic transplant recipients and is often associated with glycosuria and urinary stasis as a result of poor bladder emptying. In this situation, antibiotic prophylaxis is often required.

Diabetic control and continuing complications of diabetes

Glycemic control remains an important factor posttransplantation affecting the development of macrovascular disease and the development of recurrent disease. A number of factors result in altered blood glucose homeostasis. Corticosteroid therapy and cyclosporine alter blood glucose control and insulin requirements. Cyclosporine and, particularly, tacrolimus may lead to *de novo* diabetes. Improved renal clearance may also change insulin requirements posttransplantation.

Recurrent diabetic nephropathy

Lesions consistent with diabetic nephropathy develop in almost all grafts, with basement membrane thickening and mesangial expansion reported after 2 years and hyalinization of arterioles after 4 years. The development of nodular glomerulosclerosis is, however, rare in the transplant.

REFERENCES

1. Friedman EA. Dialytic therapy for the diabetic ESRD patient: comprehensive care essentials. Semin Dial. 1997;10:193–202.
2. van Dijk PCW, Jager K, de Charro F, et al. Renal replacement therapy in Europe: the results of a collaborative effort by the EDTA-ERA registry and six national or regional registries. Nephrol Dial Transpl. 2001;16:1120–9.
3. USRDS (United States Renal Data System). Annual Data Report 1997. Bethesda, MD: The National Institutes of Health, National Institute of Diabetes and Digestive Disease; April 1997.
4. US Renal Data System, USRDS Annual Data Report: Atlas of End-Stage Renal Disease in the United States. National Institutes of Health, National Institute of Diabetes and Digestive and Kidney Diseases, Bethesda, MD; 2001.
5. Mailloux L. Dialysis in diabetic nephropathy. In: Rose BD, ed. Up to date (CD-ROM). Wellesley, MA; 1998.
6. Ledebo I, Kessler M, van Biesen W, et al. Initiation of dialysis – opinions from an international survey: Report of the Dialysis Opinion Symposium at the ERA-EDTA Congress, 18 September 2000, Nice. Nephrol Dial Transpl. 2001;16:1132–8.
7. National Kidney Foundation dialysis outcomes quality initiative, clinical practice guideleines. I Initiation of Dialysis. Am J Kid Dis. 1997: 30(Suppl 2):S67–136.
8. Khanna R, Oreopoulos DG. Peritoneal dialysis for diabetics with failed kidneys: Long term survival and rehabilitation. Semin Dial. 1997;10:209–14.
9. Tatersall JE, Greenwood R, Farrington K. Urea kinetics and when to commence dialysis. Am J Nephrol. 1995;15:283–9.
10. Walker RJ. Early-start dialysis in diabetic nephropathy. Perit Dial Int. 1999;19(Suppl 2):S219–21.
11. Miles AMV, Friedman EA. Dialytic therapy for diabetic patients with terminal renal failure. Curr Opin Nephrol Hypertens. 1993; 2:868–75.
12. Woredekdal Y, Barth RH. Tiptoeing through a minefield: haemodialysis in the diabetic. Semin Dial. 1997;10:219–24.
13. Tzamaloukas AH, Yuan ZY, Balaskas E, Oreopoulos DG. CAPD in end stage patients with renal disease due to diabetes mellitus – an update. Adv Perit Dial.1992;8:185–91.
14. Khanna R. Peritoneal dialysis in diabetic end-stage renal disease. In: Gokal R, Nolph KD, eds. Textbook of peritoneal dialysis. Dordrecht, Netherlands: Kluwer Academic; 1994:639–59.
15. Koch M, Kutkuhn B, Grabensee B, Ritz E. Apolipoprotein A, fibrinogen, age, and history of stroke are predictors of death in dialysed diabetic patients: a prospective study of 412 patients. Nephrol Dial Transplant. 1997;12:2603–11.
16. Breen JD, Karchmer AW. *Staphylococcus aureus* infections in diabetic patients. Infect Dis Clin North Am. 1995;9:11–24.
17. Diaz-Buxo JA. Peritoneal dialysis prescriptions for diabetic patients. Adv Perit Dial. 1999;15:91–5.
18. Posthuma N, ter Wee PM, Niessen H, et al. Amadori albumin and advanced glycation end-product formation in peritoneal dialysis using icodextrin. Perit Dial Int. 2001;21(1):43–51.
19. Roob JM. Possible application of polyglucose (icodextrin) as a peritoneal dialysis fluid. Wien Klin Wochenschr. 2000;112 (Suppl 5):43–6.
20. Friedman EA. Management choices in diabetic end stage renal disease. Nephrol Dial Transplant. 1995;10(Suppl 7):61–9.
21. Bertoli M, Bonfante L, Gambaro G, et al. Peritoneal dialysis in diabetic subjects. Contrib Nephrol. 2001;131:51–60.
22. Rottembourg J, Issad N, Allouache M, et al. Clinical aspects of continuous ambulatory and continuous cyclic peritoneal dialysis in diabetic patients. Perit Dial Int. 1989;9:289–94.
23. Mistry CD, Gokal R. Optimal use of glucose polymer (Icodextrin) in peritoneal dialysis. Perit Dial Int. 1996;16(Suppl 1):S104–8.

24. Wens R, Taminne M, Devriendt J, et al. A previously undescribed side effect of icodextrin: overestimation of glycaemia by glucose analyser. Perit Dial Int. 1998;18(6):603–9.
25. Locatelli AJ, Marcos GM, Gomez MG, et al. Comparing peritonitis in continuous ambulatory peritoneal dialysis patients versus automated peritoneal dialysis. Adv Perit Dial. 1999;15:193–6.
26. Vychytil A, Lorenz M, Schneider B, et al. New strategies to prevent *Staphylococcus aureus* infections in peritoneal dialysis patients. J Am Soc Nephrol. 1998;9:669–76.
27. Chan E, Montgomery PA. Administration of insulin by continuous ambulatory peritoneal dialysis. Pharmacotherapy. 1993;13:455–60.
28. Zimmerman SW, Oxton LL, Bidwell D, Wakeen M. Long-term outcome of diabetic patients receiving peritoneal dialysis. Perit Dial Int. 1996;16:63–8.
29. Nelson CB, Port FK, Wolfe RA, Guire KE. Dialysis patient survival: evaluation of CAPD v HD using 3 techniques. Perit Dial Int. 1992;12(Suppl 1):144.
30. Habach G, Bloembergen WE, Mauger EA, et al. Hospitalization among United States dialysis patients: haemodialysis versus peritoneal dialysis. J Am Soc Nephrol. 1995;5: 1940–8.
31. Ekberg H, Christensson A. Similar treatment success rate after renal transplantation in diabetic and non-diabetic patients due to improved short and long-term diabetic patient survival. Transplant Int. 1996;9:557–64.
32. Raine AEG. Management of renal failure in Europe XXII, 1991. Cardiovascular mortality in patients on renal replacement therapy. Nephrol Dial Transplant. 1992;7(Suppl 2):7–35.
33. Manske CL, Wang Y, Rector T, Wilson RF, White CW. Coronary revascularization in insulin-dependent diabetic patients with chronic renal failure. Lancet. 1992;340:998–1002.
34. Kasiske BL. Risk factors for cardiovascular disease after renal transplantation. Miner Electrol Metab. 1993;19:186–95.

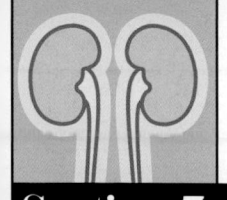

Chapter 35

Normal Blood Pressure Control and the Evaluation of Hypertension

William J Lawton and Gerald F DiBona

NORMAL BLOOD PRESSURE CONTROL

The regulation of pressure within the intravascular system is a complex interaction of a number of systems and mechanisms. The circulation is divided into several compartments: the high-pressure arterial circuit containing 13% of the blood volume, the capillary bed containing 7% of the blood volume, and the low-pressure venous bed containing 64% of the blood volume. The pulmonary circulation contains 9% and the heart 7% of the blood volume. Although the venous system stores and propels large volumes of blood and regulates cardiac output by venous return to the heart, in considering blood pressure (BP) control, attention is focused on the high-pressure arteries. The basic function of the circulation is to provide nutrients to peripheral tissues. Blood vessels in local tissue beds regulate blood flow in relation to local needs. Blood flow (Q) is defined by Ohm's law and varies directly with the change in pressure (P) across a blood vessel and inversely with the resistance R ($Q = P/R$). It can be seen that pressure varies directly with blood flow and resistance ($P = QR$). BP, or the tension or pressure of the blood within the arteries, exerted against the arterial wall, is produced by the contraction of the left ventricle (producing blood flow) and by the resistance of the arteries and arterioles. Systolic pressure, or maximum BP, occurs during left ventricular systole. Diastolic pressure, or minimum BP, occurs during ventricular diastole. The difference between systolic and diastolic pressure is the pulse pressure[1].

The inter-related systems that regulate and modulate the arterial BP include the heart, the blood vessels, the extracellular volume, the kidneys, the nervous system, numerous humoral factors and cellular events at the membrane and within the cell (Fig. 35.1). These multiple systems are intertwined in order to maintain adequate tissue perfusion and nutrition within recognized limits considered to be normal. Normal BP control can be related to cardiac output and the total peripheral resistance. Cardiac output is determined by the stroke volume (liters/minute) and the heart rate. As one example of the interaction of these multiple systems, the stroke volume is dependent in part on intravascular volume regulated by the kidneys as well as on myocardial contractility. The latter is, in turn, a complex function involving sympathetic and parasympathetic control of heart rate; intrinsic activity of the cardiac conduction system; complex membrane transport and cellular events requiring influx of calcium, which lead to myocardial fiber shortening and relaxation; and the effects of humoral substances (e.g., catecholamines) in stimulating heart rate and myocardial fiber tension.

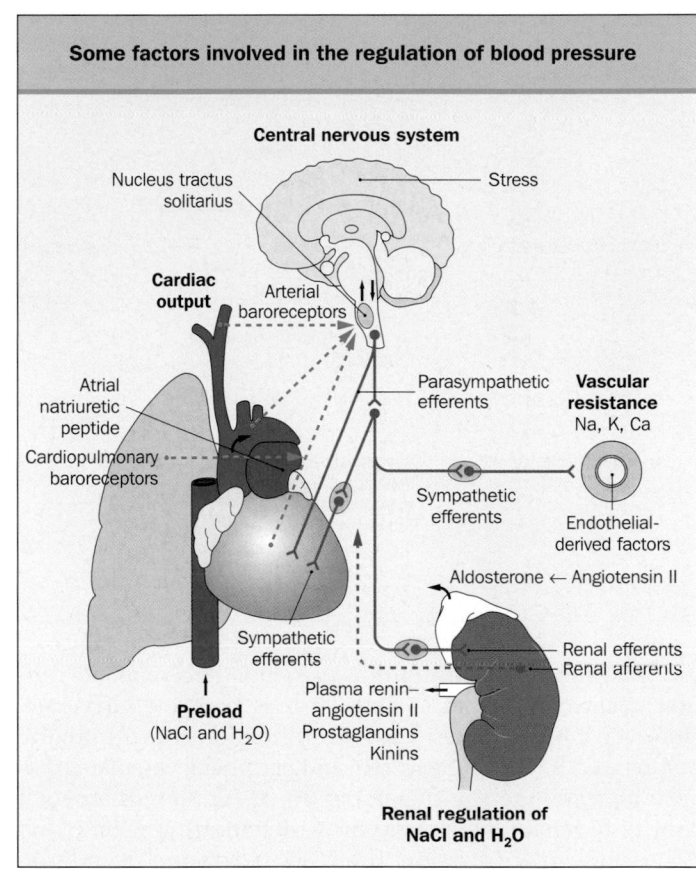

Figure 35.1 Some factors involved in the regulation of blood pressure.

The regulation of the total peripheral resistance also involves the complex interactions of several mechanisms. These include baroreflexes and sympathetic nervous system activity; response to neurohumoral substances and endothelial factors; myogenic adjustments at the cellular level, some mediated by ion channels and events at the cellular membrane; and intercellular events mediated by receptors and mechanisms for signal transduction[2]. As examples of some of these mechanisms, there are two major neural reflex arcs. Baroreflexes are derived from 'high-pressure' baroreceptors in the aortic arch and carotid sinus and 'low-pressure' cardiopulmonary baroreceptors in ventricles and atria. These receptors respond to stretch (high pressure) or filling pressures (low pressure) and send tonic inhibitory signals to the brainstem (nucleus tractus solitarius). If BP increases and tonic

Vasoactive substances		
Group	**Compound**	**Effect**
Catecholamines	Norepinephrine, epinephrine, dopamine	Adrenergic receptors (α_1, α_2, β_1, β_2) causing protein phosphorylation and increased intracellular calcium via G proteins linked to ion channels or second messengers (cyclic nucleotides, phosphoinositide hydrolysis)
Renin–angiotensin system	Angiotensin II	Angiotensin receptors (AT1, AT2, AT4) causing increased intracellular calcium and protein phosphorylation via second messenger, phosphoinositide hydrolysis, and activated protein kinases
		Aldosterone stimulation
Arachidonic acid products	Prostaglandins: prostaglandin E, prostacyclin, thromboxanes	
	Lipoxygenase enzyme products: leukotrienes,	
	HETEs (hydroxyeicosatetraenoates)	
Endothelial-derived factors	Endothelial-derived relaxing factor (nitric oxide)	Increased levels of cGMP cause activatation of protein kinases
	Endothelins (ET-1, ET-2, ET-3)	G proteins activate phospholipase C and L-type calcium channels
Kallikrein–kinin system	Bradykinin	
Natriuretic peptides (NPs)	Atrial, brain, and C-type NPs	Activation of three receptor types; further effects mediated by cGMP
Other substances	Acetylcholine, adenosine, insulin, neuropeptide Y, serotonin, sex hormones (estrogens, progesterone, androgens), glucocorticoids, other mineralocorticoids, substance P, vasopressin	

Table 35.1 Vasoactive substances that modulate blood pressure.

inhibition increases, inhibition of sympathetic efferent outflow occurs and decreases vascular resistance and heart rate. However, if BP decreases, less tonic inhibition ensues from the baroreflexes and both heart rate and peripheral vascular resistance increase, thereby increasing BP. In addition, the neural control of renal function produces alterations in renal blood flow; glomerular filtration rate (GFR); excretion of sodium, other ions, and water; and release of renin and other vasoactive substances. These, in turn, have effects on the regulation of intravascular volume, vascular resistance and BP[3].

Numerous vasoactive substances have major effects on blood vessels, the heart, the kidneys, and the central nervous system (CNS) and often serve to counterbalance one another. Some of these substances and membrane and cellular events are shown in Tables 35.1 and 35.2. As examples of the physiologic actions, norepinephrine (noradrenaline), via α-adrenergic mechanisms, is a potent vasoconstrictor. Epinephrine (adrenaline), via α- and β-adrenoceptors, increases heart rate, stroke volume and systolic BP. The renin–angiotensin system generates angiotensin II. Angiotensin II, in turn, constricts vascular smooth muscle; stimulates aldosterone secretion; potentiates sympathetic nervous system activity; leads to salt and water reabsorption in the proximal tubule; stimulates prostaglandin, nitric oxide and endothelin release; increases thirst; and is a growth factor. Aldosterone mediates changes in sodium channels in distal renal tubular epithelium, leading to

Cellular events linked to the activity of vasoactive substances
Membrane sodium transport: Na^+/K^+ ATPase; Na^+/Li^+ countertransport; Na^+–H^+ exchange; Na^+–Ca^{2+} exchange; Na^+–K^+–$2Cl^-$ transport; passive Na^+ transport
Potassium channels
Cell volume and intracellular pH changes
Calcium channels
Signal transduction via G proteins, cyclic nucleotides, inositol phosphates, protein kinases

Table 35.2 Cellular events linked to the activity of vasoactive substances.

sodium retention and potassium excretion. Prostaglandin E and prostacyclin act to counterbalance vasoconstriction by angiotensin II and norepinephrine. Two endothelial derived factors have opposite effects on the blood vessels: nitric oxide is a vasodilator whereas the endothelins are vasoconstrictors. The kallikrein–kinin system produces vasodilator kinins which, in turn, may stimulate prostaglandins and nitric oxide. Natriuretic peptides induce vasodilation, induce natriuresis, and inhibit other vasoconstrictors (renin–angiotensin, sympathetic nervous system, and endothelin).

Guyton and Hall have analyzed the temporal sequence for adjustment of BP. In their analysis, CNS mechanisms (e.g., baroreflexes) will provide regulation of the circulation within seconds to minutes. Other mechanisms, such as the renin–angiotensin–aldosterone system and fluid shifts, will occur over minutes to hours. Only the kidneys have the ability for long-term adjustments in BP, predominantly through regulation of extracellular volume (Fig. 35.2)[1].

DEFINITION OF HYPERTENSION

Concepts

In defining hypertension, three conceptual approaches have been used: relation to morbidity and mortality, excess over arbitrary cut-off points, and thresholds for therapeutic benefit. Schemes to define hypertension attempt to take into account these three approaches[4].

Blood pressure in relation to morbidity and mortality

The first approach defines hypertension by relating BP to the risk of morbidity and mortality. Numerous studies that correlate both the systolic and diastolic pressure with cardiovascular–renal complications demonstrate continuous risks from low or high BP values. The BP–risk relationship provides a rationale for treating hypertension. Analysis of levels at which the risk increases provides a system for the initiation of antihypertensive therapy. The relative risk of hypertension in relation to cardiovascular mortality shows the continuum of increased risk with progressively higher levels of pressures. An analysis has been made of 420 000 individuals from nine combined studies. The relative risk of stroke was increased nearly four-fold, and the risk of coronary heart disease was doubled for individuals with diastolic BP of 105 compared to 91 mmHg[5]. In a separate analysis of men screened for the MRFIT trial and grouped by seven BP categories, the mortality risk from coronary artery disease increased nearly seven-fold and mortality risk from strokes increased 19-fold when the highest level of BP is compared with the lowest (Table 35.3)[6].

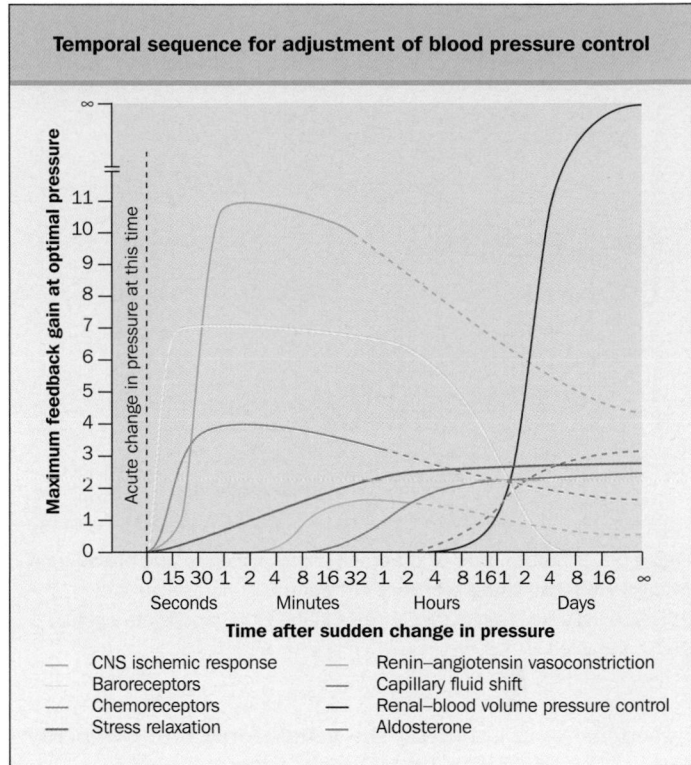

Temporal sequence for adjustment of blood pressure control

Figure 35.2 Temporal sequence for adjustment of blood pressure control. Degree of activity, expressed as feedback gain, of several arterial pressure control systems at various times after a sudden change in arterial pressure. Note the infinite gain of the renal-volume mechanism for pressure control. (Reproduced with permission.)

Elevation of blood pressure by arbitrary cut points

The second approach defines hypertension using the frequency distribution within a population. This statistical approach will arbitrarily designate values above a certain percentile as hypertensive. This method is used in defining

Blood pressure stratum	Number (%)	Ischemic heart disease mortality		Stroke mortality	
		Cumulative percentage	Relative risk	Cumulative percentage	Relative risk
Optimal	63 671 (18.2%)	1.4	1.00	0.10	1.00
Normal, not optimal	85 273 (24.5%)	1.9	1.31	0.19	1.73
High normal	77 248 (22.2%)	2.6	1.61	0.24	2.14
High blood pressure stage					
I	90 015 (25.9%)	4.1	2.33	0.45	3.58
II	24 744 (7.1%)	6.3	3.20	0.83	6.90
III	5783 (1.7%)	9.3	4.64	1.57	9.66
IV	1544 (0.4%)	12.6	6.88	3.05	19.19

Baseline blood pressure, degree of hypertension, and cause of mortality for men screened by the MRFIT trial

The trial contained 347 978 men who were free of myocardial infarction history at baseline. The cumulative percentage is the number dying in a 15-year period. The blood pressure strata are defined in Table 35.5. The relative risk was adjusted by the proportional-hazards regression model stratified by clinic and adjusted for baseline age, race, income, serum cholesterol, cigarettes smoked, and use of medication for diabetes mellitus. (Adapted with permission from Stamler.)

Table 35.3 Baseline blood pressure, degree of hypertension, and cause of mortality for men screened by the MRFIT trial.

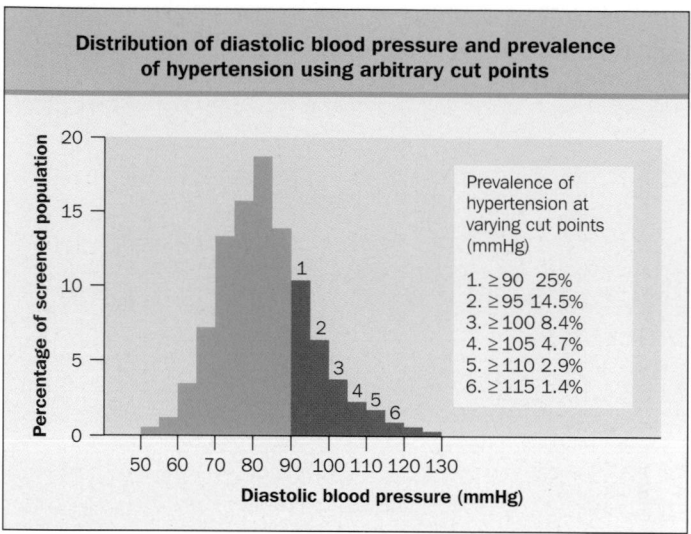

Figure 35.3 Distribution of diastolic blood pressure and prevalence of 'hypertension' using arbitrary cut points. At-home screen of 158 906 individuals aged 30–69 years in the HDFP Cooperative group, 1974. (Adapted with permission.)

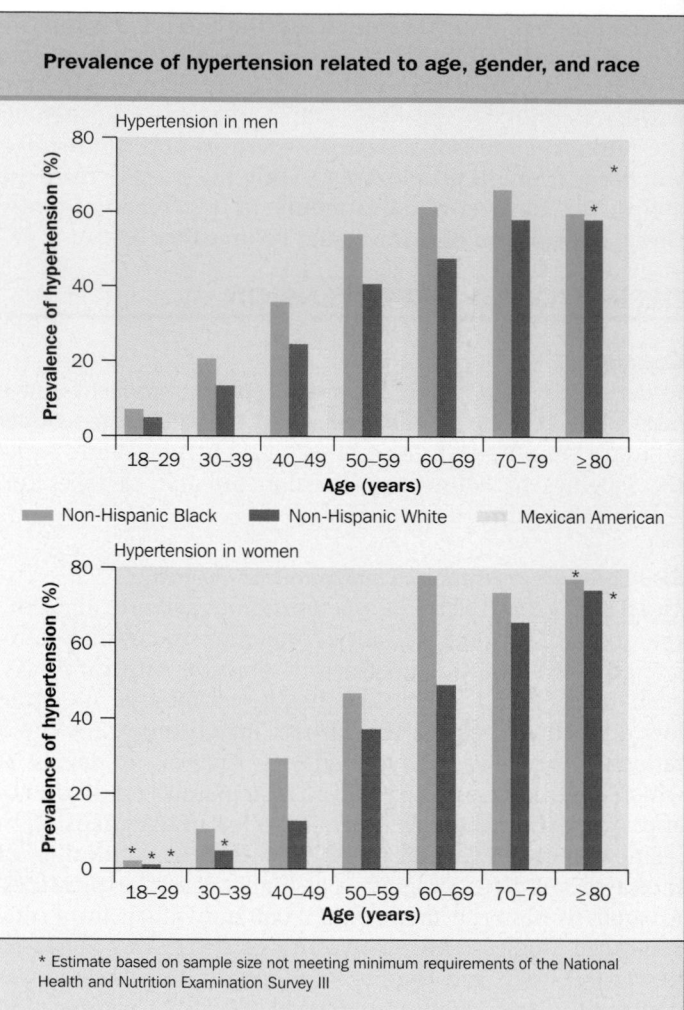

Figure 35.4 Prevalence of hypertension related to age, gender, and race/ethnicity. Data from a US population, aged 18 years of age and older. (Reproduced with permission.)

hypertension in children. The values for defining hypertension will vary depending on age, gender and race. This method is not helpful for determining a value for initiating antihypertensive treatment but is useful in epidemiologic studies, for example defining the prevalence of hypertension in various age groups. The frequency distribution of diastolic BP in a large population follows a nearly normal distribution skewed to the right (Fig. 35.3)[7]. The prevalence of hypertension in adults in the USA, as defined by a mean BP of 140/90 mmHg or higher, is 24% of the total population. Hypertension increases with age[8] and differs by gender and race (Fig. 35.4).

Threshhold of therapeutic benefit
The third concept for defining hypertension involves an understanding of data from randomized trials that have demonstrated reductions in mortality and morbidity. As a result of these clinical trials, consensus has been reached on intervention levels for moderate and severe hypertension but not for lower levels of hypertension. The HOT Study (Hypertension Optimal Treatment) showed benefits of lowering blood pressures to 138/83 mmHg[9].

Operational definitions
Classification by World Health Organization and Joint National Committee
The World Health Organization (WHO) has defined borderline hypertension as an arterial pressure of 140–160 mmHg systolic and/or 90–95 mmHg diastolic BP. Mild hypertension is defined as 140–180 mmHg systolic and/or 90–105 mmHg diastolic (Table 35.4 and Fig. 35.5)[10]. In the USA, the Joint National Committee (JNC) on detection, evaluation, and treatment of high BP have defined hypertension for individuals 18 years of age and older. For children, the JNC considers that BP at the 95th percentile or greater at each age is elevated.

Differences in the classification of pressure between the 1993 (JNC V) and 1997 (JNC VI) reports include the addition of an 'optimal blood pressure' category and the combination of stage IV (very severe hypertension) with stage III hypertension (Tables 35.5 and 35.6)[11,12].

The JNC VI report, in addition to stratifying patients by BP stage (level of pressure), now adds risk categories related to target organ disease and other risk factors. Target organ disease is defined as heart disease (left ventricular hypertrophy, angina, prior myocardial infarction, prior coronary revascularization, or heart failure), stroke or transient ischemic attack, nephropathy, peripheral arterial disease, or retinopathy. Major risk factors include smoking, dyslipidemia, diabetes mellitus, age older than 60 years, sex (men and postmenopausal women), and family history of cardiovascular disease in women under age 65 years or men under age 55 years. Recommendations for treatment are linked to the absence or presence of risk factors and target organ disease. The treatment of hypertension is further discussed in Chapters 37 and 38.

Classification of hypertension by blood pressure level

Classification	Blood pressure level (mmHg)	
	Systolic	Diastolic
Normotension	< 140 and	< 90
Mild hypertension	140–180 and/or	90–105
Borderline hypertension	140–160 and/or	90–95
Moderate and severe hypertension*	≥ 180 and/or	≥ 105
Isolated systolic hypertension (ISH)	≥ 140 and	< 90
Borderline ISH	140–160 and	< 90

* Risk to be indicated by reporting the actual values of systolic and diastolic blood pressures.
(With permission from the Guidelines Subcommittee of the WHO/ISH Mild Hypertension Liaison Committtee.)

Table 35.4 Classification of hypertension by blood pressure level.

Classification of blood pressure for adults

Category	Blood pressure level (mmHg)	
	Systolic	Diastolic
Optimal*	<120	<80
Normal	<130	<85
High-normal	130–139	85–89
Hypertension		
Stage I	140–159	90–99
Stage II	160–179	100–109
Stage III	≥180	≥110

* Unusually low readings should be evaluated for clinical significance
Classification is for those over 18 years of age, not taking antihypertensive drugs, and not acutely ill. A diagnosis of hypertension is based on the average of two or more readings taken at each of two or more visits after an initial screening. When blood pressure measurements for systolic (SBP) and diastolic (DBP) values fall into different categories, the higher category should be selected to classify the individual's blood pressure status. Isolated systolic hypertension is defined as SBP of 140 mmHg or greater and DBP below 90 mmHg and staged appropriately (e.g. 170/82 mmHg is defined as stage II isolated systolic hypertension). In addition to classifying stages of hypertension on the basis of average blood pressure levels, clinicians should specify presence or absence of target organ disease and additional risk factors. This is important for risk classification and treatment. (With permission from the National Heart, Lung, and Blood Institute.)

Table 35.5 Classification of blood pressure for adults.

Special definitions
Borderline hypertension

Despite lack of uniform agreement, borderline hypertension is most usefully defined as BP intermittently above 140/90 mmHg and decreasing to levels below this with rest. Estimates of borderline hypertension have ranged between 16% and 30% of the adult population. Although some individuals with borderline hypertension will progress to fixed hypertension, the frequency with which this occurs is not clear. Some estimates indicate only 12% develop sustained hypertension during a 20-year follow-up. However, weight gains of 15–20 lb (6.8–9.1 kg) in this group may be associated

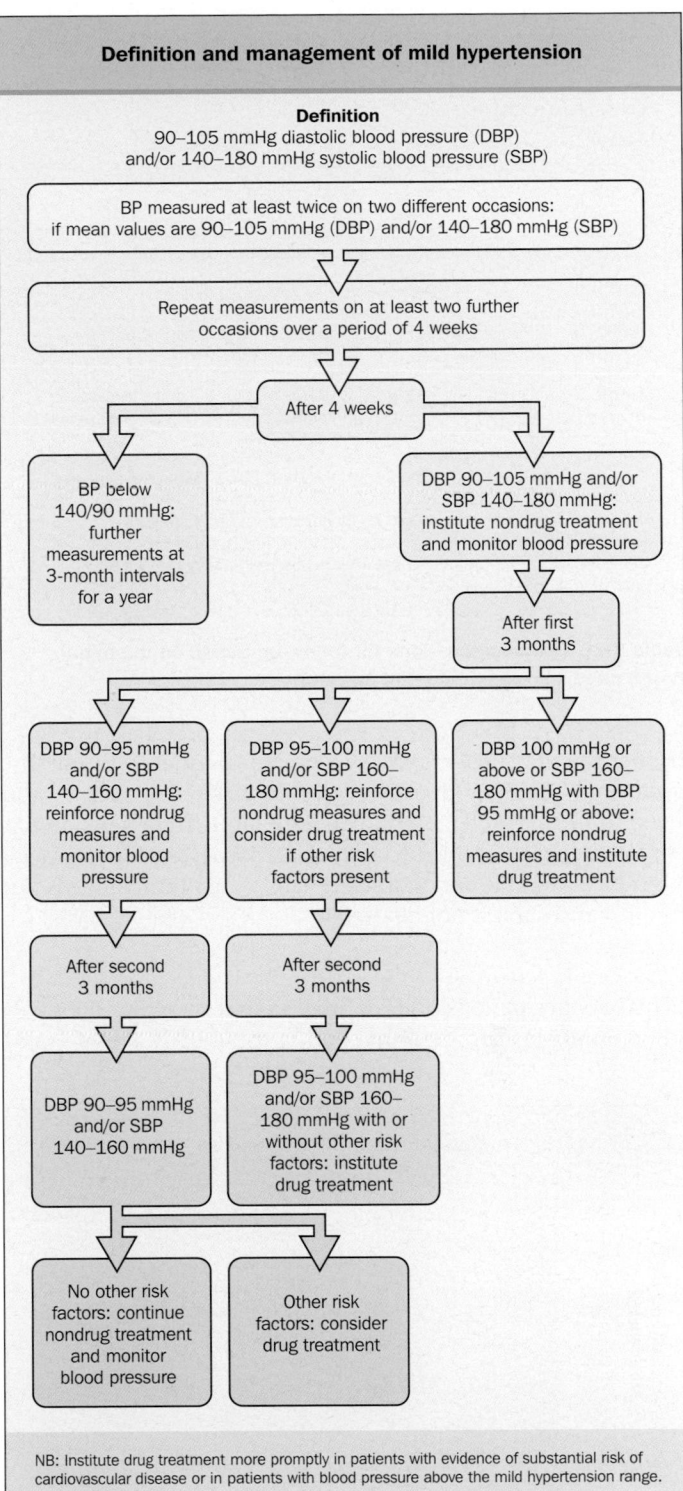

Figure 35.5 Definition and management of mild hypertension.
(Reproduced with permission.)

with a higher risk of developing fixed or sustained hypertension. Some of these individuals have been shown to have a high cardiac output and increased catecholamine turnover. Borderline hypertension may represent an exaggeration of normal physiologic responses to stress[13]. Individuals with

Recommendations for follow-up based on the initial blood pressure measurements for adults		
Initial blood pressure (mmHg)*		
Systolic	Diastolic	Follow-up recommended
<130	<85	Recheck in 2 years
130–139	85–89	Recheck in 1 year; provide information about lifestyle modification
140–159	90–99	Confirm within 2 months
160–179	100–109	Evaluate or refer to source of care within 1 month
≥180	≥110	Evaluate or refer to source of care immediately or within 1 week depending on clinical situation

* If systolic and diastolic categories are different, follow recommendations for the shorter time for follow-up
The schedule for follow-up should be modified according to reliable information about past blood pressure measurements, other cardiovascular risk factors, or target organ disease. (With permission from the National Heart, Lung, and Blood Institute.)

Table 35.6 Recommendations for follow-up based on the initial blood pressure measurements for adults.

borderline pressures may have a greater frequency of obesity, abnormal lipids, and other cardiovascular risk factors and need to be followed closely. The term labile hypertension has sometimes been applied to borderline hypertension. Since all high BP is variable and in a sense 'labile', the term labile is not helpful and should not be used.

White coat hypertension

White coat hypertension is defined as that seen in individuals in whom BP levels are normal during usual daily activities but hypertensive in a clinical setting. Normal pressures outside the physician's office have been determined by measurement with standard techniques or by ambulatory BP recordings. White coat hypertensives are more likely to be young women with a lower body weight, although this phenonomen can be seen at all ages including the elderly. The white coat phenonomen has also been more frequent when BP is taken by a physician rather than a nurse or technician. Estimates of white coat hypertension are approximately 20% of hypertensives. A clear separation of white coat hypertensives is presented by Pickering, when awake (ambulatory) pressures are compared with clinic systolic pressures (Fig. 35.6)[14].

The significance and prognosis of white coat hypertension is unclear. Some studies show that the office- or clinic-induced rise in BP is benign. Other studies show that white coat hypertension is characterized by increases in left ventricular mass index at levels intermediate between normotensives and persistent hypertensives (Fig. 35.7)[15]. White coat hypertensives have also been reported to have impaired diastolic function and higher levels of catecholamines, plasma renin activity, aldosterone and low-density lipoprotein cholesterol. There is also some evidence that subjects with white coat hypertension may be at increased risk for developing persistent hypertension[16]. Thus, each patient with white coat hypertension needs evaluation for cardiovascular risk factors and correction of these, if present, as well as continued follow-up.

Persistent hypertension

Persistent hypertension, also called sustained hypertension, defines individuals whose BP levels are elevated both inside and outside of the clinic setting, including at home, during usual daily activities. It should be noted that office BP readings are frequently higher in sustained hypertensives compared to their ambulatory BP.

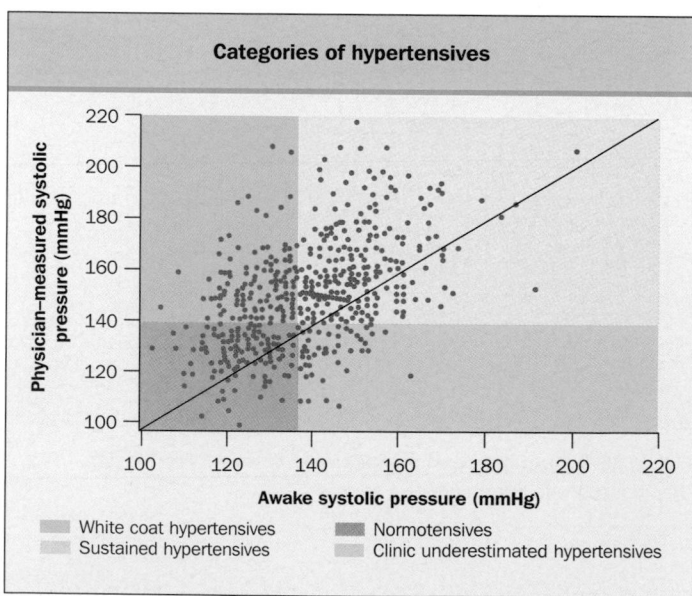

Figure 35.6 Categories of hypertensives, including 'white coat' hypertension, as defined by awake (ambulatory) blood pressure and blood pressure measured in a clinic setting. Data from 573 patients. (Reproduced with permission.)

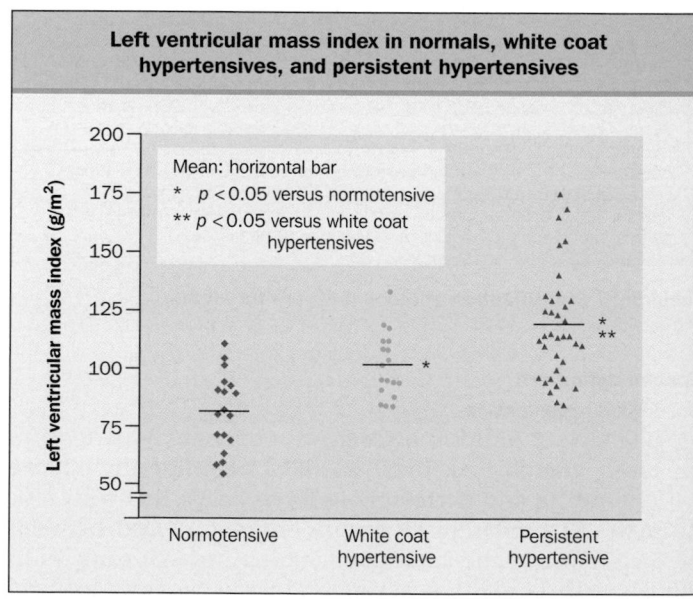

Figure 35.7 Left ventricular mass index in normals, white coat hypertensives and persistent hypertensives. (Reproduced with permission.)

Pseudohypertension

Pseudohypertension has been defined by Messerli as 'a condition in which the cuff pressure is inappropriately higher when compared to the intra-arterial pressure because of excessive atheromatosis and/or medial hypertrophy in the arterial tree'[17]. The presence of pseudohypertension can be suspected by the 'Osler maneuver'. This is performed by inflating the BP cuff above systolic pressure (detected by auscultation). If either the brachial or radial artery remain palpable, when pulseless, the patient is considered to be 'Osler maneuver positive'. In general, patients with pseudohypertension have intra-arterial diastolic BP measurements 10–15 mmHg below indirect BP cuff diastolic measurements. None of the definitions specifically address the systolic pressure. If a patient is suspected of having pseudohypertension, confirmation by intra-arterial pressure measurement may need to be considered and modification of goal BP considered during treatment (Fig. 35.8).

Isolated systolic hypertension

Isolated systolic hypertension (ISH) is defined as systolic BP of 140 mmHg or greater and diastolic BP below 90 mmHg (WHO and JNC VI). Others have defined ISH as systolic BP > 160 mmHg and diastolic < 90 mmHg. The prevalence of ISH increases with age and is approximately 25% in individuals 80 years of age. In the Framingham study, elevations in systolic BP determined a greater risk for both heart attacks and strokes compared to elevations of diastolic BP[18,19].

Accelerated malignant hypertension

Accelerated hypertension has referred to severe diastolic hypertension (usually above 120 mmHg) in the presence of grade III retinopathy (arteriosclerotic changes of arteriolar narrowing and nicking, plus hypertensive changes of flame-shaped hemorrhage and soft exudates). In the past, 'malignant' hypertension referred to severe diastolic hypertension and grade IV retinopathy (grade III plus papilloedema). Since the prognosis for untreated severe hypertension with grade III or IV retinopathy is so poor, there is little clinical rationale to use the two terms separately. 'Accelerated-malignant hypertension' is preferred for severe diastolic hypertension with fundoscopic findings as noted above and usually represents a hypertensive 'urgency', requiring treatment and decrease of BP within hours. Hypertensive 'emergencies' are clinical conditions in which severe hypertension must be lowered within minutes. 'Emergencies' include acute dissection of the aorta, acute left ventricle failure, intracerebral hemorrhage, and crises caused by pheochromocytoma, drug abuse, and eclampsia.

Hypertension in children

Hypertension in children is defined by average systolic and/or diastolic pressures on or above the 95th percentile for gender and age, measured on at least three occasions. The identification of causes of hypertension in children varies depending on the published series. Most prepubertal hypertension is thought to have renal causes, although some children may have BP levels above the 95th percentile because of an earlier growth spurt and large size. In postpubertal children, mild hypertension is likely to be primary hypertension,

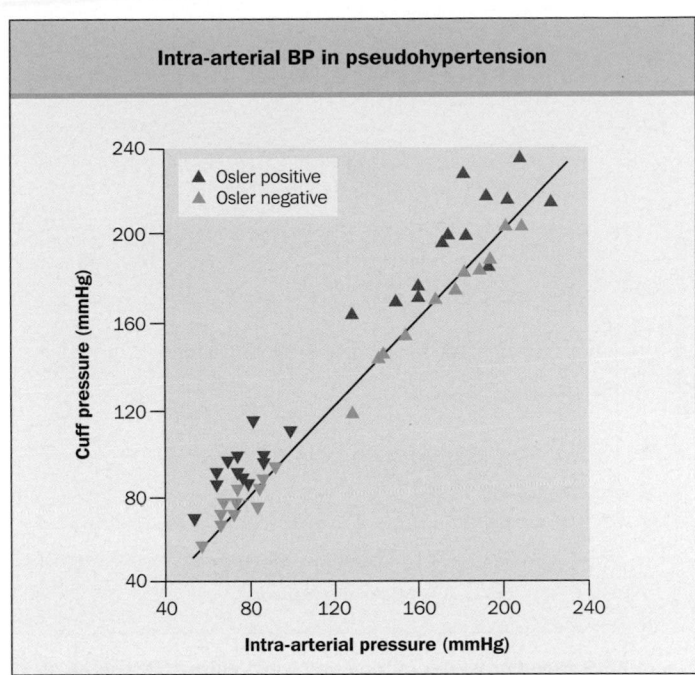

Figure 35.8 Comparison of intra-arterial and standard cuff BP in patients with pseudohypertension. Note the discriminant value of the Osler maneuver. (Reproduced with permission.)

while more severe hypertension is usually of renal cause. Primary aldosteronism and thyroid disease seem rare.

Hypertension in pregnancy

Hypertension may occur in over 5% of all pregnancies and, over 5 years, in approximately 5% of women taking oral contraceptives. One widely accepted classification uses terminology proposed by the American College of Obstetrics and Gynecology in 1972[20], and endorsed by the National High Blood Pressure Education Program Working Group in 1990. Useful definitions include the following: (1) Chronic Hypertension: Hypertension diagnosed before the twentieth week of gestation, or present before pregnancy, or persisting 6 weeks postpartum. (2) Pre-eclampsia: Elevated blood pressure that occurs after 20 weeks' gestation in a normotensive woman (usually a primigravida), and usually accompanied by edema and proteinuria. (3) Eclampsia: Seizures not due to other causes in a woman with pre-eclampsia. (4) Pre-eclampsia superimposed on chronic hypertension: Increases of blood pressure of 30/15 mmHg (systolic/diastolic) with the appearance of edema or proteinuria in a woman with chronic hypertension. (5) Transient hypertension: Blood pressure elevations during pregnancy or occurring in the first 24 h postpartum, with no other signs of pre-eclampsia or pre-existing hypertension; this may be due to latent chronic hypertension and usually recurs in other pregnancies.

Blood pressure in normal pregnancy usually falls during the first and middle trimester. Average sitting systolic pressures are between 100–105 mmHg, lying systolic pressure 115 mmHg, and diastolic pressure 55 mmHg (Fig. 35.9)[21]. Blood pressure then returns toward prepregnant levels during the third trimester. This reduction in blood pressure also occurs in women with pre-existing hypertension.

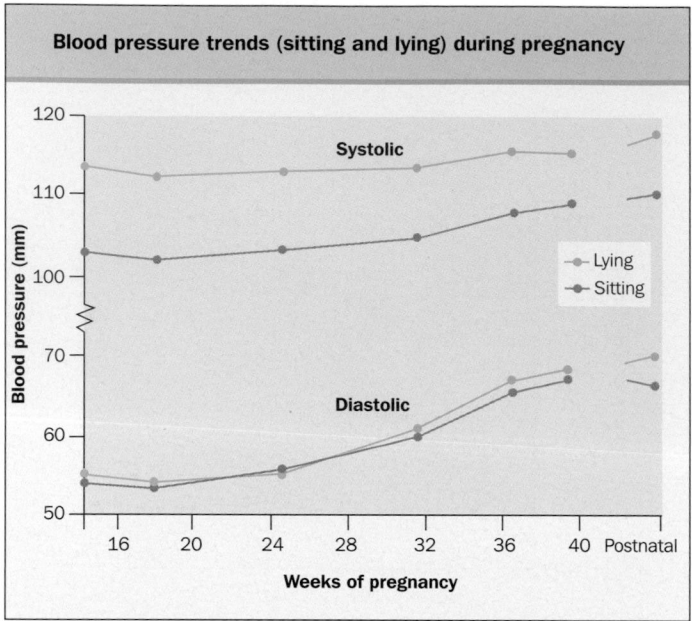

Blood pressure trends (sitting and lying) during pregnancy

Figure 35.9 Blood pressure (sitting and lying) during the course of pregnancy. (Reproduced with permission.)

Classification by cause of hypertension

Although a large number of causes are recognized for hypertension, the etiology in 90–95% of patients with hypertension is unknown. These patients are termed essential or primary. Although it is known that individuals with hypertensive relatives have an increased risk of developing hypertension, the estimate of the role of genetics is quite variable. Hypertension is considered to be a complex polygenic disease.

The most common causes of hypertension include patients with chronic renal disease and renovascular hypertension[22]. An often overlooked category is hypertension related to medication. Table 35.7 shows the more common causes of hypertension. Primary or essential hypertension occurs in 89–95% of hypertensives. The more common causes of secondary hypertension are renal parenchymal disease (2–6% of all hypertensives), renovascular hypertension (1–4%), all endocrine hypertension (1%, primary aldosteronism, pheochromocytoma, Cushing syndrome), drug induced (1%, including oral contraceptives) and coarctation of the aorta (0.1–1.0%).

Table 35.7 Common causes of secondary hypertension[2,22].

Common causes of secondary hypertension	
Condition/disorders	**Disease**
Renal disorders	Renal parenchymal disease: acute and chronic glomerular diseases, chronic tubulointerstitial disease, polycystic disease, obstructive uropathy
	Renovascular disease: renal artery stenosis caused by atherosclerosis and fibromuscular dysplasia; arteritis; extrinsic compression of the renal artery
	Other renal causes: renin-producing tumors, renal sodium retention (Liddle's syndrome)
Endocrine disorders	Adrenocortical disorders: primary aldosteronism, congenital adrenal hyperplasia, Cushing syndrome
	Adrenal-medullary tumors: pheochromocytoma (also extra-adrenal chromaffin tumor)
	Thyroid disease: hyperthyroidism, hypothyroidism
	Hyperparathyroidism: hypercalcemia
	Acromegaly
	Carcinoid tumors
Exogenous medications and drugs	Oral contraceptives, sympathomimetics, glucocorticoids, mineralocorticoids, nonsteroidal anti-inflammatory drugs, cyclosporine, tyramine-containing foods and monoamine oxidase inhibitors, erythropoietin, ergot alkaloids, amphetamines, herbal remedies, licorice (mimics primary aldosteronism), ethanol, cocaine and other illicit drugs, abrupt withdrawal of clonidine
Pregnancy	Pre-eclampsia, and eclampsia
Coarctation of the aorta	
Neurologic disorders	Sleep apnea
	Increased intracranial pressure: brain tumors
	Affective disorders
	Spinal cord injury: quadriplegia, paraplegia, Guillain–Barré syndrome
	Baroreflex dysregulation
Psychosocial factors	
Intravascular volume overload	
Systolic hypertension	Loss of elasticity of aorta and great vessels
	Hyperdynamic cardiac output: hyperthyroidism, aortic insufficiency, anemia, arteriovenous fistula, beri-beri, Paget's disease of the bone

EVALUATION OF HYPERTENSION

Proper measurement of blood pressure

There are three types of sphygmomanometer in use. The standard is a mercury manometer; the meniscus should be at 0 when there is no pressure in the cuff bladder. The second type of manometer in wide use is the aneroid manometer. As these can become inaccurate, they need to be calibrated against a mercury manometer. A Y-tube connecting the bladder to both the aneroid and mercury manometer is recommended. In addition, there are numerous semiautomatic electronic recording manometers. Some may be inaccurate and these also need to be checked against a mercury manometer. Both the aneroid and the electronic manometers should be checked against a mercury device at least twice a year.

Additional guidelines for BP measurement are shown in Table 35.8[23,24]. The cuff size is critical to avoid errors in measurement. If the cuff is too small, the BP will be falsely elevated.

Conversely, if the cuff is too large, BP may be falsely lowered. Recommendations for bladder dimensions have been published (Table 35.9)[23].

Variability of blood pressure

Variability with wake–sleep cycle and in office versus home blood pressure

It is well recognized that BP varies considerably in individual subjects and may vary during a single office or clinic visit, throughout the day–night cycle, and over time. This variation causes considerable difficulties in identifying individuals who are hypertensive, especially in terms of the classification schemes listed above. The source of the variability has been attributed to both biologic variation (variations of pressures within a given individual) and variation in the measurement itself. Errors in measurement can be minimized by attention to the proper technique for recording BP, as noted above. Biologic variation is addressed by repeated BP measurement

Table 35.8 Guideline for measurement of blood pressure.

Guideline for measurement of blood pressure	
Factors	**Important features**
Patient factors	Caffeine should not be taken for up to 1 h before the blood pressure measurement
	Cigarettes should not be smoked for at least 15 min prior to the blood pressure reading
	The standard measurement should be made with the patient seated comfortably, arm supported, and the cuff must be at the level of the heart; the arm should be bared
	On an initial examination, blood pressure should also be checked in the supine position after 5 min of rest, in the standing position after 2 min and in both arms in patients who are diabetic, over 65 years or receiving antihypertensive therapy. Use the higher value if the arms have differing blood pressures
	If sequential pressures are taken in the same position, at least 30 s must elapse between blood pressure readings
	In younger patients, less than 30 years of age, check blood pressure in one leg
	To establish a diagnosis of hypertension, obtain blood pressure readings on three different occasions, at least one week apart
Equipment	The length of the bladder with the cuff should encircle at least 80% of the arm
	The width of the cuff should be equal to two thirds of the distance from the antecubital space to the axilla and be 40% of the arm circumference. The best cuff for most adults is the 15 cm wide cuff with a bladder of 33–35 cm in length. The distal edge of the cuff should be 2.5 cm above the antecubital fossa
	In extremely obese patients, blood pressure may be more accurate when measured in the forearm, palpating and auscultating the radial artery
	For infants, ultrasound equipment may need to be used
Technique	The initial systolic blood pressure should be checked by palpating the disappearance of the radial or brachial pulse prior to auscultation, and the cuff then deflated
	The second blood pressure check requires cuff inflation 20–30 mmHg above the palpable systolic level
	Deflate the cuff at a rate of 2–4 mmHg per second
	Record the Korotkoff sound 1 (appearance of sound) as the systolic pressure and record the Korotkoff sound V (the last sound before complete disappearance of sound) as the more reproducible diastolic pressure. If the sounds do not disappear, record the muffled sound (phase IV) as the diastolic
	The sounds may be augmented by having the patient raise the arm, and by opening and closing the hand 10 times before inflating the pressure
	Do not stop between systolic and diastolic readings; deflate the cuff, wait at least 30 s and then reinflate. On each occasion, record at least two readings. If the readings vary by more than 5 mmHg, take additional readings until two are within 5 mmHg
	In children, the same standards apply for cuff size and Korotkoff sound V should be used. If the child is uncooperative, the systolic blood pressure may be determined by palpation

Accepted bladder dimensions for varying arm sizes			
Patient	Arm circumference range at midpoint (cm)	Bladder width (cm)	Bladder length (cm)
Newborn	≤6	3	6
Infant[a]	6–15	5	15
Child[a]	16–21	8	21
Small adult	22–26	10	24
Adult	27–34	13	30
Large adult	35–44	16	38
Adult thigh	45–52	20	42

[a] To approximate a bladder width to arm circumference ratio of 0.4 more closely in children, additional cuffs are available.
There is some overlap in the recommended ranges for arm circumference in order to limit the number of cuffs. It is suggested that the larger cuff is used if it is available. (With permission from Perioff et al.)

Table 35.9 Accepted bladder dimensions for varying arm sizes.

at a given visit (at least two pressures taken at least 30 seconds apart, or additional BP measurements if there is a 5 mmHg difference between repeated measures). In addition, in most patients with milder forms of hypertension, repeated measurements during different clinic visits over time are recommended to approach the 'true' BP.

Readings of BP at home, and outside the clinic or office setting, are recommended in order to assess the degree of hypertension and BP control during treatment. The instruments used at home must be checked against a standard mercury manometer on a regular basis. In addition, the techniques for correct BP measurement must be taught to the patient. Levels measured at home are generally lower than those measured in the clinic or office.

Biologic variation can be considered in two broad categories. The variability in BP that occurs during the day is related to physical and mental activity and emotional factors. The second consideration is diurnal variation. Sleeping is associated with a fall in BP, with an average decrease during sleep of 20%. This results from decreases in sympathetic activity; reductions in BP are also noted after hospital admission and bed rest. The normal diurnal pattern includes a rise in BP before awakening that has been associated with increased incidence of myocardial infarction, stroke, and sudden death in the first few hours after awakening. The usual pattern is for individuals to decrease their BP during sleep and these are referred to as 'dippers'. Some individuals fail to reduce their BP during sleep and these have been labeled 'non-dippers'. The failure to decrease BP during sleep has been associated with increased incidence of left ventricular hypertrophy.

Ambulatory blood pressure

Because BP varies throughout the day, over time, and with the setting when measured, home BP and ambulatory BP monitoring are available to enable hypertension to be defined more clearly. Home BP monitoring is advised for as many

patients as is practical. Home BP monitoring will help to identify white coat hypertension from persistent hypertension, identify individuals with borderline hypertension, and monitor response to therapy. The last includes identifying hypotension as well as hypertension. The instructions to each patient must be individualized, but home BP monitoring may be advised several times per day while the patient is awake. These BP values must be self-recorded and reviewed.

Ambulatory BP monitoring is recommended for certain indications beyond the information available from home BP recording. Ambulatory BP monitoring uses a noninvasive system. The BP is determined by auscultation using either oscillometry, which measures variations in pressure within the cuff, or by a microphone placed under the cuff and over the brachial artery. The ambulatory BP device can be programmed to record at frequent intervals during the daytime (e.g., every 10 min) and less frequently at night during sleep (e.g., every 30 min). The ambulatory BP equipment might not provide accurate readings in patients with large upper arms owing to obesity or increased musculature, and the equipment may be inaccurate during vigorous activity. The equipment generally records BP during a 24-h period. Although most patients adjust to the repetitive measurements throughout the day, some patients may have a 'startle response' with each BP recording. Most patients are able to sleep, although some have their sleep disturbed by the BP recording and, therefore, determination of nocturnal fall in BP is inaccurate. Indications for ambulatory BP are shown in Table 35.10[12].

There are disadvantages to using the ambulatory BP equipment. The monitoring equipment must be placed by trained personnel. Calibration of ambulatory BP equipment with a mercury manometer must be recorded at the beginning and end of the ambulatory BP session. Three to six readings must be taken at each time and the systolic and diastolic pressure measurements must both agree within 5 mmHg. The end calibration is critical to assure proper functioning of the ambulatory BP monitor throughout the 24-h period. The cuff inflation

Indications for ambulatory blood pressure
White coat hypertension
Evaluation of apparent drug resistance
Hypotensive symptoms
Autonomic dysfunction
Episodic hypertension
Evaluation of nocturnal decreases in blood pressure, as a prognostic factor for target organ disease (left ventricular hypertrophy, ischemic optic neuropathy)
Evaluation of blood pressure changes in patients with paroxysmal nocturnal dyspnea and nocturnal angina
Carotid sinus syncope
Pacemaker syndromes
Safety of withdrawing antihypertensive medication
Assess 24-hour blood pressure control on once daily medication
Borderline hypertension with target organ damage
Evaluation of antihypertensive drug therapy in clinical trials

Table 35.10 Indications for ambulatory blood pressure.

may interfere with activities, work, or sleep. The cuff may cause discomfort or skin irritation or it may malfunction and fail to deflate, causing pain and interruption of recording. The data correlating ambulatory BP with target organ disease are limited. Standards for assessment of data and their use in decisions for therapy are limited. In addition, equipment is expensive and its use is limited by lack of reimbursement by health insurance systems in a number of countries, including the USA and Belgium.

Risk factors for hypertension

A number of factors are known to be associated with an increased risk for hypertension. These need to be considered in evaluating individuals with hypertension, and modification of some of these factors may have a role in primary prevention for individuals at risk for developing hypertension. Individuals who are genetically at risk for hypertension, by virtue of one or both parents or first-degree relatives having hypertension, may have their risk heightened by the factors given below.

Age

As discussed above, the prevalence of hypertension rises from age 18 years to those above 80 years of age.

Race

The prevalence of hypertension is higher in African Americans compared to Caucasians and Hispanic Americans.

Gender

Between the ages of 18 and 64 years, men have a higher prevalence of hypertension.

Weight

A strong relationship exists between body weight and BP. Individuals with a higher body weight have an increased prevalence of hypertension. Those who are overweight have a two- to six-fold increased risk for developing hypertension compared with normal weight individuals. A common definition for overweight is body mass index over 27 kg/m².

Psychosocial stress

Acute stress activates neurohumoral mechanisms that lead to elevations of systolic and diastolic BP. Speculation has persisted that long-term stress may lead to the development of hypertension. Evidence indicates that the risk for hypertension is increased in individuals who are exposed to chronic stress at work, lack the ability to make decisions or regulate the exposure to stress, and/or lack social support. These factors may be more common in individuals within certain ethnic groups who have lower levels of income and education.

Physical activity

In general, an inverse association has been noted between level of activity and systolic or diastolic BP. The odds ratio for being hypertensive, if an individual is physically unfit or sedentary, compared with the most physically fit persons has ranged from 1.06 to 1.52.

Dietary factors

Considerable attention has been given to many dietary factors. The strongest association exists between sodium intake and BP. Most populations studied consume between 100 and 200 mmol sodium per day (2.5–5 g sodium or 6–12 g salt). In a recent study of 47 000 individuals, a difference of sodium intake of 100 mmol/day was associated with differences in systolic BP in the range 5–10 mmHg. Potassium has also been inversely associated with BP such that a 60 mmol/day (2.3 g/day) increased excretion of urinary potassium has been related to approximately 3 mmHg lower systolic BP. These data come from the INTERSALT study, which includes data from countries across four continents[25]. In addition, an inverse relationship has been identified between intake of calcium and BP. Also, societies that consume diets with low fat and low protein of animal origin plus a high fiber content tend to have lower BP and a low prevalence of hypertension. The relationship of dietary modification to treatment of hypertension is discussed in Chapter 37.

Behavioral factors

Increased alcohol consumption has been associated with hypertension in numerous studies. This relationship is seen with alcohol consumption of three drinks or more per day (approximately 40 g ethanol). This roughly corresponds to

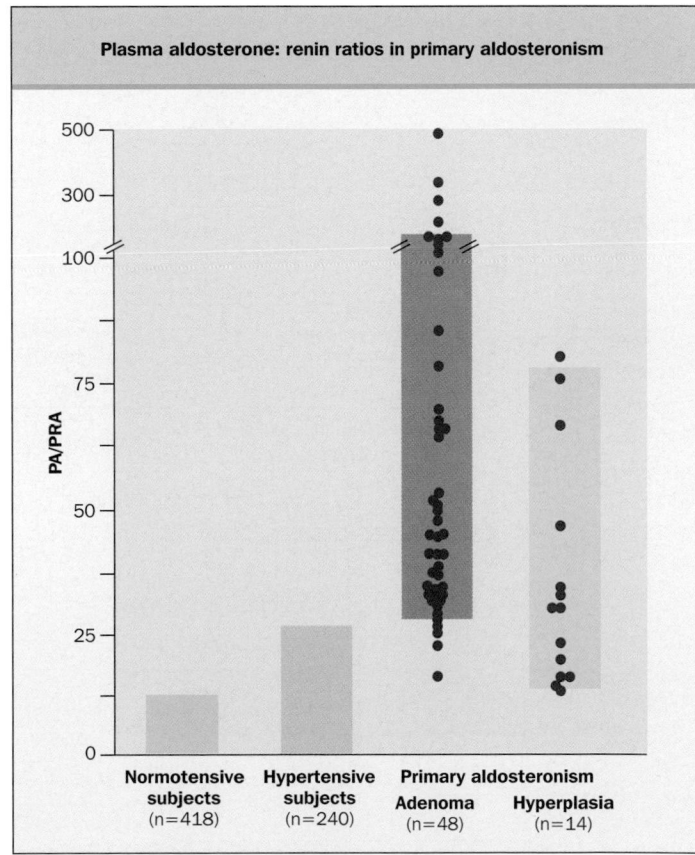

Figure 35.10 Plasma aldosterone : renin ratios in primary aldosteronism. PA, Plasma aldosterone; PRA, plasma renin activity. (Adapted with permission.)

Evaluation for primary versus secondary hypertension			
Classification	Medical history	Physical examination	Laboratory studies
General information and evaluation of target organs	Duration and course of hypertension Prior work-up and treatment Diet/lifestyle: salt intake, tobacco, caffeine	Evaluation of volume status, optic fundi, heart, lungs, peripheral vessels, and nervous system	Complete blood count, fasting glucose, lipid profile (includes HDL, LDL, cholesterol, triglyceride), uric acid Consider echocardiogram (ECG)
Primary (essential or idiopathic)	Familly history: hypertension, cardiovascular and renal diseases		
Secondary	Symptoms of target organ disease (related to eyes, central nervous system, cardiorespiratory, and peripheral vascular)	See Table 35.12	See Table 35.12

Table 35.11 Evaluation for primary versus secondary hypertension.

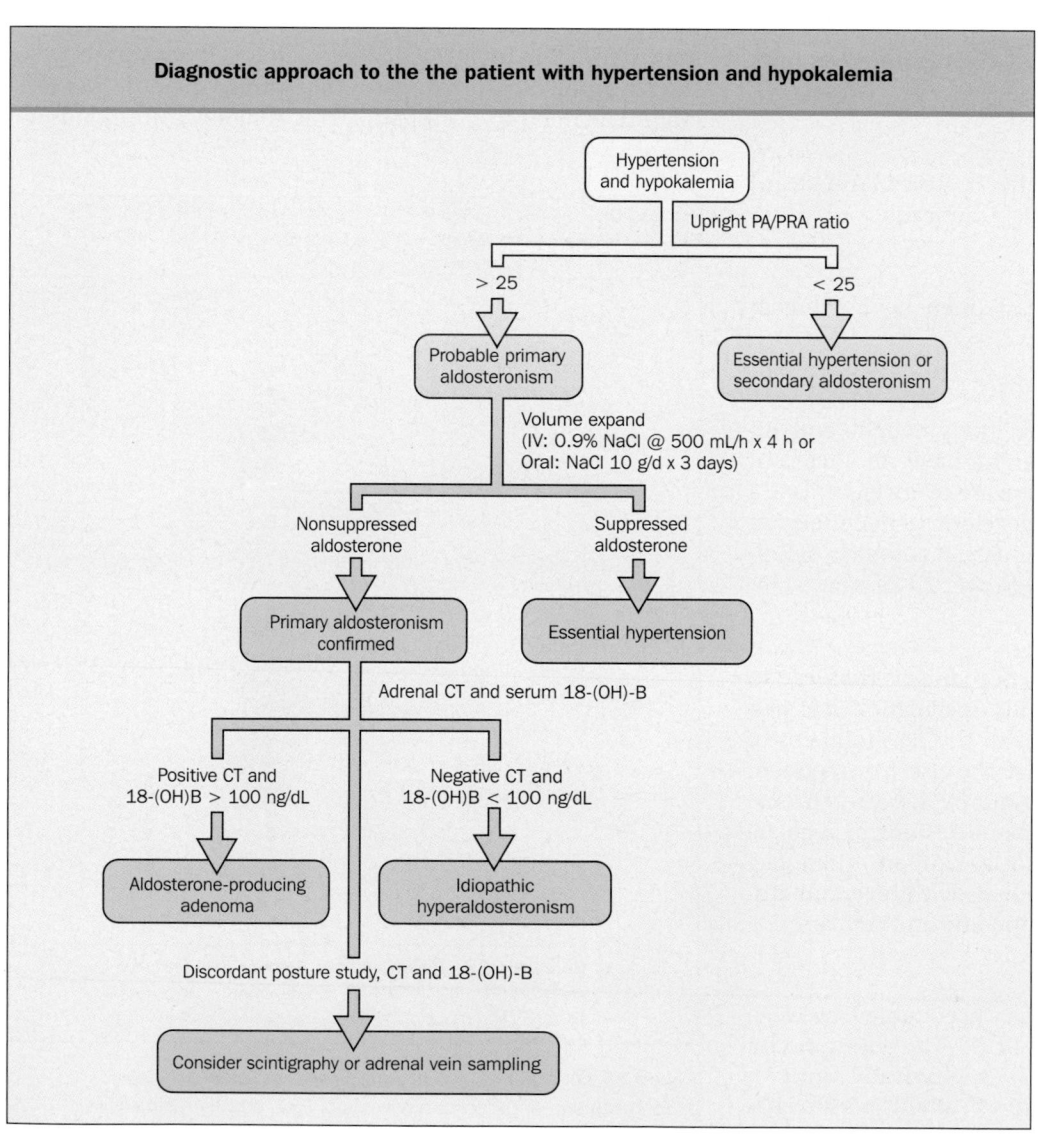

Diagnostic approach to the the patient with hypertension and hypokalemia

Figure 35.11 Diagnostic approach to the patient with hypertension and hypokalemia. PA, Plasma aldosterone concentration; PRA, plasma renin activity. (Adapted with permission.)

Evaluation of secondary hypertension			
Target organ/system	**Medical history**	**Physical examination**	**Laboratory studies**
Renal Parenchymal	History of renal disease (including glomerulonephritis, nephrotic syndrome, calculi, urinary tract infection) Symptoms include nocturia, frequency, dysuria, hesitancy, urgency, incomplete emptying, dribbling, hematuria, pyuria, flank pain	Tenderness in costovertebral angles; palpable kidneys	Blood urea nitrogen, serum creatinine; urinalysis, urine culture and sensitivity if indicated; 24-h urine for protein and creatinine clearance if indicated; consider microalbumin, or random urine protein/creatinine ratio
Renovascular hypertension		Epigastric bruit; other vascular bruits	Isotope renogram; renal ultrasound with duplex doppler flow study, consider aortogram with iodinated contrast, or magnetic resonance angiogram
Endocrine Primary aldosteronism	Muscle weakness, cramps		Serum potassium[a] Consider serum aldosterone/plasma renin activity ratio; consider 24-h urine aldosterone, Na, K, creatinine
Cushing syndrome		Body habitus: body fat, striae	Morning serum cortisol after dexamethasone suppression[a]
Pheochromocytoma	Headaches; vasomotor symptoms, (inappropriate sweating, pallor); cardiac symptoms ('awareness', tachycardia, palpitations)	Paroxysmal or intermittent hypertension (50% of patients)	Single voided urine for metanephrine and creatinine[a]; consider 24-h urine for catecholamines, vanillyl mandelic acid (VMA), metanephrines; if positive, proceed with magnetic resonance imaging or thin section CT of the adrenals
Carcinoid	Flushing		24-h urine 5HIAA excretion
Hyperthyroidism	Weight loss, tachycardia, palpitations, sweating, heat intolerance	Palpable thyroid	Total and free thyroxine
Hypothyroidism	Weight gain, dry skin, cold intolerance, hair loss		Thyroid-stimulating hormone (TSH), total and free thyroxine
Hyperparathyroidism	Nausea, vomiting		Serum calcium, intact parathyroid hormone
Acromegaly	Change in size of head, hands or feet (adult)	Appearance	
Medication	Review of prescribed and over-the-counter medications (especially oral contraceptives, nonsteroidal anti-inflammatory drugs, sympathomimetic agents ('cold and allergy' drugs), illicit or recreational drugs, including alcohol, herbal remedies)		
Pregnancy[b]			
Coarctation of the aorta	Onset or detection of hypertension in childhood or adolescence	Simultaneous palpation of radial and femoral arteries to detect pulse lag in femorals; leg blood pressure	Chest X-ray for heart size, configuration of aorta, rib notching; consider aortogram
Neurologic disorders Sleep apnea	Obesity; weight gain; daytime somnolence; snoring, poor sleep habits (frequent awakening, not rested on arising); early morning headache	Obesity; reduced airway in hypopharynx; redundant pharyngeal tissue	Formal sleep study (polysomnogram)
Increased intracranial pressure	Headache; neurologic symptoms	Papilledema	↑ CSF pressure
Affective disorders[b]			
Spinal cord injury[b]			
Psychosocial factors	Family and support structure, occupation, education, stressors		
Volume overload	Excess salt and water intake (may be iatrogenic with excess parenteral fluid)	Increased jugular venous distension, pulmonary crackles, presacral and peripheral edema, hepatomegaly	Chest X-ray
Systolic hypertension		Pseudohypertension (positive Osler's maneuver); cardiac and vascular examination (evaluate for aortic insufficiency, arteriovenous fistula)	

[a]Additional special diagnostic studies are covered elsewhere.
[b]Medical history, physical examination and laboratory tests are either obvious or beyond the scope of this discussion.

Table 35.12 Evaluation of secondary hypertension.

24 ounces of beer (720 mL), 10 ounces (300 mL) of wine, or 2 ounces (60 ml) of 100-proof whiskey per day. Nicotine causes a rise in both systolic and diastolic pressure that may last for 15–30 min. If BP is taken more than 30 min after a cigarette, smokers may have normal BP. However, the repeated pressor effects likely contribute to elevated pressure in individuals who typically smoke one pack per day. Caffeine will raise BP in individuals who do not take caffeine or use it infrequently. However, tolerance to caffeine develops and BP generally does not rise in individuals who regularly use caffeine[24].

Evaluation for primary versus secondary hypertension

The medical history, physical examination, and a limited number of laboratory tests provide critical information in deciding which individuals require further evaluation for secondary hypertension and target organ disease (Tables 35.11 and 35.12). If the history, physical examination, or screening laboratory studies suggest secondary hypertension, additional studies are generally warranted. If renal parenchymal disease is suspected, in addition to quantitative studies to assess glomerular filtration rate and/or proteinuria (Table 35.12), renal ultrasound is useful to evaluate renal size and echogenicity (to help assess chronicity) as well as evaluate for obstructive uropathy. Renal artery stenosis can be suspected by the presence of severe hypertension with abnormal renal function or with asymmetric renal size (see Chapter 39)[26]. If primary aldosteronism is suspected due to hypokalemia, the ratio of plasma aldosterone to plasma renin activity may be useful as presented by Weinberg and Fineberg[27] (Fig 35.10). If the ratio is elevated above 25–30 and plasma aldosterone is > 20 ng/dL, an algorithm for further evaluation has been proposed by Litchfield and Dluhy[28] (Fig 35.11). Further evaluation for other forms of secondary hypertension are listed in Table 35.12.

REFERENCES

1. Guyton AC, Hall JE. Dominant role of the kidneys in long-term regulation of arterial pressure and in hypertension: the integrated system for pressure control. In: Guyton AC, Hall JE, eds. Textbook of medical physiology, 9th edn. Philadelphia, PA: Saunders; 1996:221–34.
2. Izzo JL Jr, Black HR, eds. Hypertension primer, 1993. Dallas, TX: Council on High Blood Pressure Research; American Heart Association; 1993:3–94.
3. DiBona GF. Neural control of renal function: cardiovascular implications. Hypertension. 1982;13:539–48.
4. Roccella EJ, Bowler AE, Horan M. Epidemiologic considerations in defining hypertension. Med Clin North Am. 1987;71:785–801.
5. MacMahon S, Peto R, Cutler J, et al. Blood pressure, stroke, and coronary heart disease. Part 1, prolonged differences in blood pressure: prospective observational studies corrected for the regression dilution bias. Lancet. 1990;335:754–74.
6. Neaton JD, Kuller L, Stamler J, Wentworth DN. Impact of systolic and diastolic blood pressure on cardiovascular mortality. In: Laragh JH, Brenner BM, eds. Hypertension pathophysiology, diagnosis, and management, 2nd edn. New York: Raven Press; 1995:127–44.
7. Hypertension Detection and Follow-Up Program Cooperative Group. The hypertension detection and follow-up program: a progress report. Circ Res. 1977;40(Suppl. 1);I-106–9.
8. Burt VL, Whelton P, Roccella EJ, et al. Prevalence of hypertension in the US adult population: results from the Third National Health and Nutrition Examination Survey, 1988–1991. Hypertension. 1995;25:305–13.
9. Hansson L, Zanchetti A, et al. Effects of intensive blood-pressure lowering and low-dose aspirin in patients with hypertension: principal results of the Hypertension Optimal Treatment (HOT) randomised trial. Lancet. 1998;351:1755–62.
10. The Guidelines Subcommittee of the WHO/ISH Mild Hypertension Liaison Committee. 1993 Guidelines for the management of mild hypertension. Hypertension. 1993;22:392–403.
11. National Institutes of Health, National Heart, Lung and Blood Institute. The fifth report of the Joint National Committee on Detection, Evaluation, and Treatment of High Blood Pressure. NIH Publication No. 93–1088. Washington, DC: the National Institutes of Health, National Heart, Lung and Blood Institute; 1993.
12. National Institutes of Health, National Heart, Lung and Blood Institute. The sixth report of the Joint National Committee on Detection, Evaluation, and Treatment of High Blood Pressure. NIH Publication No. 98–4080. Washington, DC: the National Institutes of Health, National Heart, Lung and Blood Institute; 1997.
13. Kuchel O, Cuche JL, Hamet P, et al. Labile (borderline) hypertension: new aspects of a common disorder. Angiology. 1975;26:619–31.
14. Pickering TG. The ninth Sir George Pickering memorial lecture: ambulatory monitoring and the definition of hypertension. J Hypertens. 1992;10:401–9.
15. Cardillo C, DeFelice F, Campia U, Folli G. Psychophysiological reactivity and cardiac end-organ changes in white coat hypertension. Hypertension. 1993;21:836–44.
16. Bidlingymeyer I, Burnier M, Bidlingmyer M, et al. Isolated office hypertension: a prehypertensive state? J Hypertens. 1996;14:327–32.
17. Messerli FH, Ventura HO, Amodeo C. Osler's maneuver and pseudohypertension. N Engl J Med. 1985;312:1548–51.
18. Kannel WB, Wolf PA, Verter J, McNamara PM. Epidemiological assessment of the role of blood pressure in stroke: the Framingham study. JAMA 1970;214:301–10.
19. D'Agostino RB, Russell MW, Huse DM, et al. Acute ischemic heart disease: Primary and subsequent coronary risk appraisal: New results form the Framingham study. Am Heart J. 2000;139:272–81.
20. Hughes EO. Obstetric gynecologic terminology. Philadelphia: FA Davis; 1972:433–43.
21. MacGillivray I, Rose GA, Rowe B. Blood pressure survey in pregnancy. Clin Sci. 1969;37:395.
22. Kaplan NM. Clinical hypertension, 6th edn. Baltimore: Williams and Wilkins; 1994:1–109,423–36.
23. Perloff D, Grim C, Flack J, et al. Human blood pressure determination by sphygmomanometry. Circulation. 1993;88:2460–70.
24. National High Blood Pressure Education Program Working Group. Arch Intern Med. 1993;153:186–208.
25. Stamler J. THE INTERSALT study: background, methods, findings. Am J Clin Nutr. 1997;65(Suppl.):626S–42.
26. Mann SJ, Pickering TG. Detection of renovascular hypertension. State of the art: 1992. Ann Int Med. 1992;117:845–53.
27. Weinberger MH, Fineberg NS. The diagnosis of primary aldosteronism and separation of two major subtypes. Arch Intern Med. 1993;153:2125–9.
28. Litchfield WR, Dluhy RG. Primary aldosteronism. Endocrinol Metab Clin North Am. 1995;24:593–612.

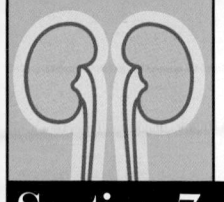
Chapter 36

Pathogenesis and Clinical Course of Essential Hypertension

John Kanellis, George L Bakris, Kiyoshi Kurokawa, and Richard J Johnson

INTRODUCTION

Essential (or primary) hypertension is defined as a blood pressure (BP) of > 140/90 mmHg without an identifiable cause. Several readings on different occasions and times are necessary to document the BP as being elevated, because of substantial variability in BP. This variability in BP results from a circadian rhythm that generates the most significant increase in BP in early morning hours (6:00–10:00). BP falls at bedtime, secondary to a decrease in sympathetic nervous system (SNS) tone and reduced activity of other neuroendocrine systems, an event that occurs with recumbency or sleep. Additionally, there are minute-to-minute variations in BP (Fig. 36.1). Transient elevations in BP, reaching 150 mmHg systolic, occur in the majority of normotensive patients in any given day[1]. However, BP that repeatedly is documented at 140/90 mmHg or greater is considered elevated. Blood pressure is classified according to severity (Table 36.1)[2].

Stages in hypertension have been adopted to allow a prognosis to be associated with different levels of BP elevation. The prognosis has been adapted from epidemiologic studies that demonstrate a linear relationship between the risk of cardiovascular events and sustained elevations of arterial pressure.

If only the systolic BP is elevated (systolic BP > 140 and diastolic BP < 90 mmHg), it is called 'isolated systolic hypertension'. BP that is either intermittently or slightly elevated is classified as 'borderline' and is further classified as 'white coat' hypertension if an elevation of > 20 mmHg systolic pressure is noted only in the physician's office. Further details on the method and interpretation of BP measurements, including the use of ambulatory BP monitoring, can be found in Chapter 35.

In the great majority of patients with hypertension, no identifiable cause can be found, and the hypertension is labeled as essential. In adults, over 90% of hypertension is considered essential (Table 36.2), whereas hypertension occurring in a child should alert the physician to search for a secondary cause. The major secondary causes include renal parenchymal disease, renal artery stenosis, adrenal hyperplasia or tumors

Classification of blood pressure

Level/degree of severity	Systolic (mmHg)	Diastolic (mmHg)
Optimal	< 120	< 80
Normal	< 130	< 85
High normal	130–139	85–89
Stage I	140–159	90–99
Stage II	160–179	100–109
Stage III	> 180	> 110

Table 36.1 Classification of blood pressure.

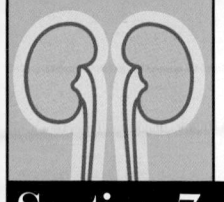

Diurnal variation in blood pressure (BP)

Figure 36.1 Blood pressure variability in a normotensive individual.
In most normal individuals, systolic blood pressure reaches 150 mmHg at least once per day. (Adapted with permission from Bevan, Honour and Stott[1].)

Major causes of hypertension

Cause	Percentage of hypertensives
Essential	90
Renal disease	3
Renovascular disease	2
Birth control pills	2
Primary aldosteronism	2
Coarctation of the aorta	0.2
Pheochromocytoma	0.1
All others	0.5

Table 36.2 Major causes of hypertension.

(such as primary aldosteronism), medications such as sympathomimetics, illicit drugs such as cocaine, and heavy alcohol use. A more complete list is provided in Table 35.12.

EPIDEMIOLOGY

High BP affects 20–25% of the population in the USA, and similar prevalence rates have been reported in other developed countries. This has led to controversy over whether elevated BP may simply represent the upper end of a normal Gaussian curve for arterial pressure. Epidemiologic studies suggest that BP does follow a general Gaussian pattern, but there is some skewing that could reflect hidden subpopulations at increased risk (see Fig. 35.3).

There are a number of known risk factors for the development of essential hypertension (Table 36.3). A genetic component is suggested by the observation that if both parents or a sibling are hypertensive the child has a 40–60% chance of developing hypertension when an adult. The risk is 80% if the sibling is a monozygotic twin. However, it has often been difficult to separate environmental from genetic factors in these studies. In addition, the inheritance patterns do not follow classic Mendelian genetics for a single gene locus. Most authorities believe that environmental factors may be involved in the hypertensive phenotype and that the susceptibility to develop hypertension may be polygenic, that is it requires the presence of multiple susceptibility genes. In this regard, an increased risk for hypertension has been noted with certain genetic polymorphisms of angiotensinogen, the endothelial nitric oxide synthase, and the β_2-adrenoceptor. Others have noted an association with certain α-adducin proteins associated with the actin cytoskeleton and sodium transport. Much attention is also focusing on genetically mediated alterations in the regulation or expression of sodium channels within the kidney. Studies examining subjects with essential hypertension have also identified gene polymorphisms which appear to be significantly associated with the salt-sensitivity phenotype. In this regard, polymorphisms of the angiotensin converting enzyme (ACE) and 11β-hydroxysteroid dehydrogenase type 2 (11βHSD2) have been found to be important[3].

There are other important risk factors for the development of hypertension (Table 36.3). Essential hypertension is uncommon in young adults but increases with age, with 65% prevalence in the population at age 65, and 75% at age 75. This age-related increase in prevalence of hypertension has been observed in most Western countries but has not been uniformly observed in all populations. Second, the prevalence of hypertension is greater in men, although the prevalence in women approaches that of men in the postmenopausal years. Certain racial groups are also at increased risk, particularly African Americans. Obesity, insulin resistance, gout, and sleep apnea are also associated with an increased risk, as are low socioeconomic status and increased stress at work. Certain physical features, such as elevated heart rate or an increased BP response to exercise, are also predictive[4].

As already suggested, the risk for development of hypertension is also related to diet. Studies support the view that both genetic and acquired factors may underlie the susceptibility to hypertension from dietary factors. Epidemiologic and interventional studies have strongly linked salt (NaCl) intake with hypertension. Populations with a high sodium content in their diet (> 4 g/day), such as observed in northern Japan and the southeastern USA, have a high prevalence of hypertension. Conversely, populations consuming a low-sodium diet, such as the Alaskan Eskimo or the Yanamamö Indians from the Amazon, have an almost negligible prevalence of hypertension. Diets low in calcium or potassium have also been associated with a higher prevalence of hypertension. Increasing potassium intake has been found to lower BP in both experimental and human studies. Obesity is perhaps the most salient risk factor for phenotypic expression of hypertension. The proportion of obese individuals as a function of the total population is continuing to grow in all Westernized societies. This parallels the incidence of hypertension in these societies.

Certain metabolic features are associated with the development of high BP. In addition to elevated glucose (insulin resistance), an elevated hematocrit is also associated with the development of hypertension. Several studies have also found elevated serum uric acid to predict the development of hypertension and to be present in 25% of untreated hypertensive subjects. The controversial issue regarding the role of hyperuricemia in the pathogenesis of hypertension, and whether or not it is an independent risk factor for hypertension will be discussed in more detail later in this chapter.

The cardiovascular and cerebrovascular morbidity and mortality increases linearly with increments in BP from 120/80 mmHg upward (Fig. 36.2)[5]. This increased risk is also dependent on age (increases with age), sex (greater in males), ethnic origin (greater in African Americans), and the presence of associated risk factors (diabetes, etc.). This increased cardiovascular morbidity and mortality results from an increased prevalence of both atherosclerotic and hypertensive (primarily pressure-related) diseases. Increased systolic, diastolic, and

Major risk factors for essential hypertension	
Type	**Risk factors***
Genetic	Family history
	Polymorphisms: adducin protein, endothelial nitric oxide synthase, angiotensinogen (AGT 235), β-adrenoceptor
	African American
Physical	Raised heart rate (> 83beats/minute)
	Obesity
	Age (> 70 years)
	Exaggerated blood pressure with exercise
	Increased emotional stress
	Heavy alcohol use
Metabolic abnormality (laboratory-assessed parameters)	Insulin resistance
	Raised uric acid level
	Raised hematocrit

* Low socioeconomic status is also a factor to be considered in the risk profile.

Table 36.3 Major risk factors for essential hypertension.

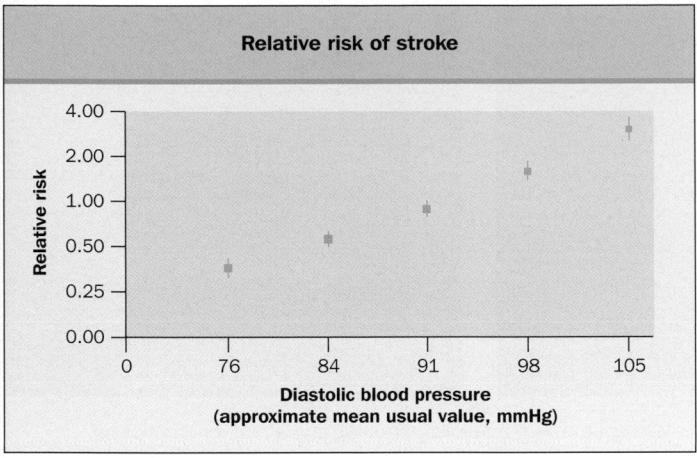

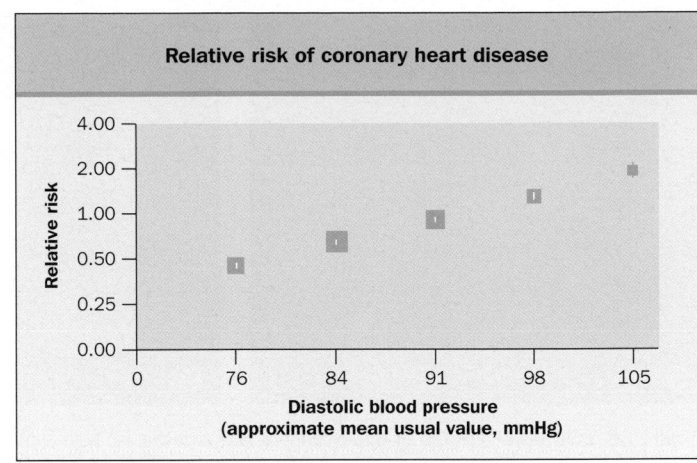

Figure 36.2 Relative risks for stroke (left) and coronary heart disease (right) increase with increased diastolic blood pressure. The stroke data are from seven prospective observational studies and 843 events; the coronary heart disease data are from nine studies and 4856 events. Size of squares are proportional to the number of events in each category; the vertical lines indicate 95% confidence intervals. (Adapted with permission from MacMahon, Peto, Cutler, et al[5].)

pulse pressure all confer risk. Moreover, the systolic BP is perhaps the more important determinant for the risk of the hypertensive complications, especially in relation to stroke and renal disease.

CLINICAL MANIFESTATIONS

Evaluation of a patient with hypertension should include:

- documenting an elevated blood pressure by examining the BP on repeated occasions in the office, work place, or home (with or without ambulatory BP monitoring);
- evaluating for secondary causes by a careful history and a physical and laboratory examination;
- assessment for risk factors for conditions that may contribute to development of hypertension (family history, alcohol intake, obesity, etc.);
- assessment for other conditions that may contribute to or are associated with vascular disease (diabetes, hyperlipidemia, hyperuricemia, smoking);
- evaluation for end-organ damage (retinal changes, left ventricular hypertrophy, renal damage, peripheral vascular and coronary artery disease, etc.).

Chapter 35 gives guidelines on BP measurement and for evaluation of secondary causes.

The medical history should include questions related to the history and duration of hypertension in the patient. A family history of hypertension and cardiovascular and renal disease should be sought. The history should seek to identify risk factors (obesity, diabetes, physical activity, alcohol, smoking, diet, emotional or work-related stress, over-the-counter and prescribed medications, etc.) and any hypertension-related morbidity.

Symptoms directly related to the hypertension should also be sought. Hypertension *per se* is usually asymptomatic. On rare occasions, some patients may complain of headache (classically occipital and pulsatile), although most studies have not been able to document a strong relationship unless the person has stage III hypertension. Hypertensive encephalopathy may

rarely occur and is defined as stage III hypertension with mental status changes and/or seizures. In these patients with malignant hypertension, there may also be visual changes (from papilledema), and patients are at acute risk for myocardial infarction and congestive failure with pulmonary edema, dissection, stroke, and renal failure. Lastly, it should be noted that data from the Hypertension Optimal Treatment (HOT) trial demonstrate that those with hypertension whose blood pressure was controlled to diastolic pressures < 85 mmHg report better memory and generally feeling better than before their blood pressure was reduced.

Physical examination should include careful attention to the cardiovascular system. Remember the definition of hypertension is the product of stroke volume and heart rate. Therefore, measurement of BP in both arms and a careful cardiac examination including measurement of the pulse is mandatory. Attention should be focused on both the large vessels (by both palpation and listening for bruits) and the retina to grade the severity of disease in the microvasculature (Fig. 36.3).

Basic laboratory tests should include hematocrit, electrolytes, urea nitrogen and creatinine, calcium and phosphate, serum lipid profile (cholesterol and triglycerides), uric acid, and urinalysis, including a spot urine albumin : creatinine ratio for microalbuminuria. A chest X-ray and electrocardiograph should also be performed to assess the cardiac size and the presence of left ventricular hypertrophy, as well as to look for evidence of aortic dilatation (see Fig. 36.4).

Additional tests that may be helpful under certain circumstances include a 24-h urine collection to assess creatinine clearance and sodium and potassium levels. The latter is an indication of how much sodium and potassium the patient is ingesting, as the urinary excretion will correlate closely with intake if the patient is in steady state (the desirable values are < 100 mmol/L Na+ and > 100 mmol/L K+ in 24 h). Testing for microalbuminuria and performing echocardiography to look for concentric left ventricular hypertrophy (Fig. 36.5) may provide additional evidence for end-organ damage.

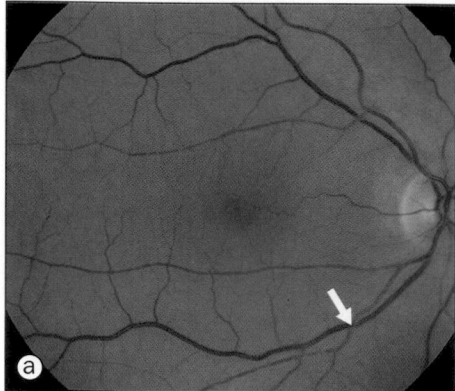
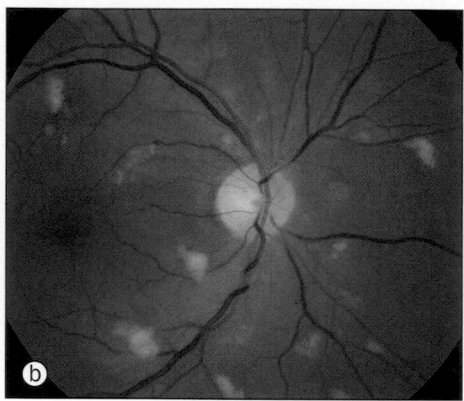
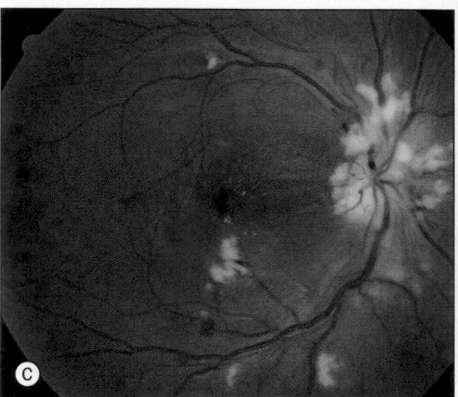

Figure 36.3 Different grades of hypertensive retinopathy. (a) Mild hypertensive retinopathy, with arteriolar narrowing and arteriovenous nicking. (b) Moderate hypertensive retinopathy, with cotton wool spots (nerve fiber layer infarcts) and arteriovenous nicking. (c) Malignant hypertension with papilledema, cotton wool spots, macular yellow exudates ('star formation' pattern), and retinal hemorrhages. (Courtesy of J. Kinyoun.)

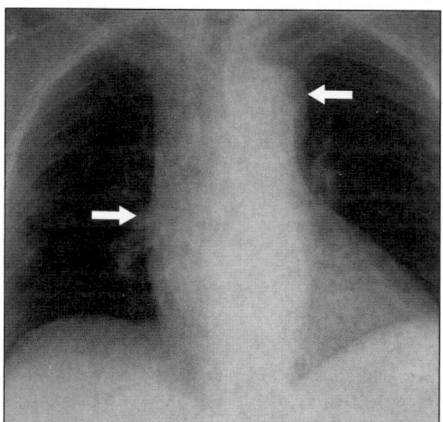

Figure 36.4 Chest X-ray film of aortic dilatation in a patient with essential hypertension. Dilatation of the aortic arch (arrow) and ascending aorta (noted by the mediastinal convexity, arrow) is present. (Courtesy of D. Godwin.)

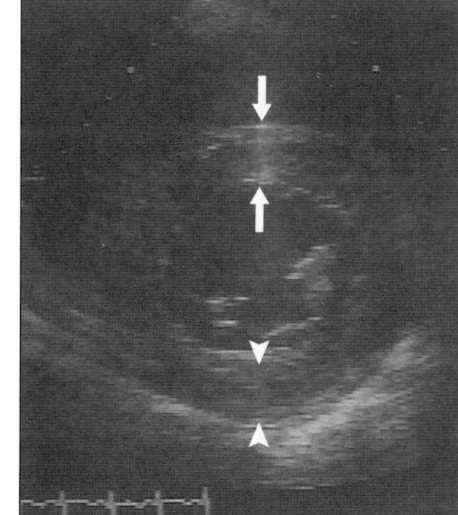

Figure 36.5 Echocardiogram showing concentric left ventricular hypertrophy. Septal thickness (between large arrows) and posterior wall thickness (between arrowheads) are increased (to 16 mm) in a patient with essential hypertension (normal is 11 mm or less). (Courtesy of A. Pearlman.)

If the examination or laboratory results suggest a secondary cause, then further studies such as aldosterone : renin ratios, renal arterial duplex studies, and urinary catecholamines should be performed, as discussed in Chapter 35.

PATHOGENESIS

The pathogenesis of essential hypertension is unknown, although a large number of hypotheses have been proposed[4–14]. In reviewing these hypotheses, at least three major areas need to be addressed: (i) the role of the sympathetic nervous system (SNS), (ii) the renin–angiotensin system (RAS), and (iii) the kidney, particularly as it relates to the handling of sodium. Other factors such as endothelin, nitric oxide, and the kallikrein–kinin system need to be considered as well. Recent animal studies by Mazzali et al.[15] have also rekindled interest in hyperuricemia as a possible cause of hypertension.

The sympathetic nervous system
Guyton et al. suggested that much of the short-term arterial pressure control is mediated by the central and autonomic nervous systems (see Fig. 35.2)[8]. High-pressure baroreceptors in the carotid sinus and aortic arch respond to acute elevations in pressure by causing a reflex vagal bradycardia and inhibition

of sympathetic output from the central nervous system (CNS); the opposite occurs when BP suddenly falls. Low-pressure cardiopulmonary receptors in the atria and ventricles likewise respond to increases in atrial filling by increasing heart rate (via inhibition of the cardiac SNS), increasing atrial natriuretic peptide (ANP) release, and inhibiting vasopressin release. These reflexes are largely controlled centrally, particularly in the nucleus tractus solitarius of the dorsal medulla. This vasomotor center also receives input from the limbus and hypothalamus in response to emotional or psychologic stress.

The consequences of SNS stimulation are peripheral vasoconstriction, an increase in heart rate, release of norepinephrine (noradrenaline) from the adrenals, and a resultant rise in systemic BP. The increase in SNS activity also has a role in mediating vascular hypertrophy and stiffness. Renal efferent sympathetics are also activated and cause intrarenal vasoconstriction, with a fall in renal blood flow and an increase in renal vascular resistance. The renal SNS directly stimulates sodium reabsorption and renin release from the juxtaglomerular apparatus.

Numerous studies have shown that the SNS is often hyperactive in essential hypertension, particularly in young or borderline hypertensive patients[4]. Many patients with newly diagnosed hypertension have elevated plasma norepinephrine levels, with increased heart rate and cardiac indices. These patients often show elevations of BP with stress, exercise, or emotion. Some of these patients also have elevated plasma renin levels, which may reflect β-adrenergic stimulation of renin secretion. Many of these patients have increased vascular reactivity, raised systemic vascular resistance, and low blood volume.

The mechanisms involved in the stimulation of the SNS in hypertension have been studied intensely. A defect in baroreceptor sensitivity has been postulated and may contribute to the increased BP variability noted in some hypertensive patients. The observation that some patients have an increase in SNS response to emotional or work-related stress also suggests this as a contributing factor. The SNS is increased in certain high-risk groups, such as African Americans, in obesity, in insulin resistance, and with the use of certain drugs (nicotine, alcohol, cyclosporine, cocaine, etc.) associated with hypertension. Furthermore, there may be a subset of patients in which compression of the lateral medulla by cranial nerves and/or vessels may result in increased SNS activity and hypertension; in some of these patients, selective decompression may ameliorate the hypertension. Finally, activation of the CNS/SNS may result from renal afferent sympathetics from hypertensive kidneys. Indeed, in several experimental models of hypertension, renal sympathectomy can cause a reduction in BP[16].

The renin–angiotensin system (RAS)

The RAS is one of the most important mechanisms by which the host regulates blood volume and pressure. Angiotensinogen, released primarily from the liver, is converted by renin to angiotensin I, which is further degraded in the presence of angiotensin-converting enzymes (ACE) or chymases (such as present in the human heart) to angiotensin II (AII) (Fig. 36.6). Most of the actions of AII are mediated by the AT_1 receptor and include stimulating vascular smooth muscle contraction and hypertrophy, increasing cardiac contractility, stimulation of the SNS in the central and peripheral nervous system, increasing thirst and vasopressin release, and stimulating aldosterone synthesis. Within the kidney, stimulation of the AT_1 receptor by AII also causes renal vasoconstriction (especially of the efferent arteriole and vasa rectae), a fall in renal blood flow, and an increase in renal vascular resistance. AII also increases sodium reabsorption, not only through aldosterone but also by direct effects on the proximal tubules and by increasing the sensitivity of the tubuloglomerular feedback response (see Chapter 2). In addition to the systemic RAS, there is evidence that a local RAS is present in blood vessels, the heart, and the kidney, where it may mediate local effects (such as tissue remodeling) independent of circulating renin or angiotensinogen levels.

The role of the RAS in essential hypertension is complex. Whereas plasma renin activity is elevated in 20% of patients, renin activity is either normal (50%) or low (30%) in the majority. However, in many of the patients with normal renin activity the plasma renin may be inappropriately high in relation to the total body sodium. This is indicated by the observation

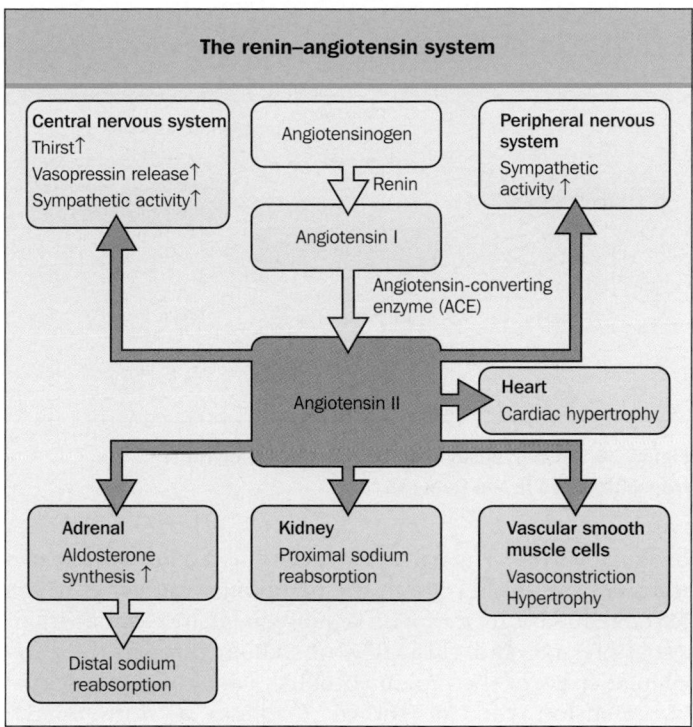

Figure 36.6 The renin–angiotensin system.

that saline depletion or infusion results in blunted changes in renin levels in these patients, and by the observation that BP in these patients frequently responds to ACE inhibitors[6]. Sealey and colleagues have suggested that the reason for the widely varying renin levels may be nephron heterogeneity within individual kidneys, in which there are some ischemic nephrons making excess renin and other hyperfiltering nephrons in which renin secretion is suppressed[6]. According to the authors, the increased renin release from the ischemic nephrons enters the circulation and then leads to AII generation, which causes inappropriate vasoconstriction and sodium reabsorption in the other, hyperfiltering nephrons. This results in sodium retention and the development of hypertension.

The role of the kidney in essential hypertension

Guyton et al. has noted that, while the SNS and RAS are important for short-term changes in BP, ultimately it is the kidney that is responsible for long-term blood volume and pressure control (see Fig. 35.2)[8]. Indeed, Dahl was the first to show that hypertension can be transferred from the hypertensive Dahl salt-sensitive rat to the nonhypertensive Dahl salt-resistant rat by transplantation of the kidney, and this has been subsequently verified in four other different genetic strains of rats with hypertension (Fig. 36.7)[17]. Patients with essential hypertension-associated renal failure have also been cured of their underlying hypertension by renal transplantation from a normotensive donor.

Most authorities believe that the mechanism by which the kidney causes hypertension involves impaired excretion of NaCl. Guyton proposed that the physiological abnormality involves an impairment in pressure-natriuresis (Fig. 36.8)[8]. A rise in systemic blood pressure is normally associated with a

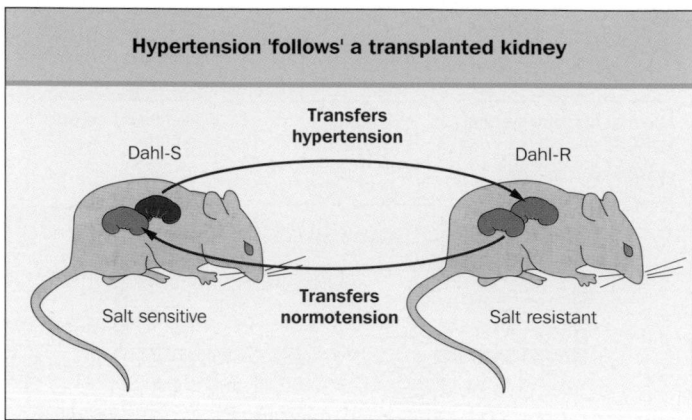

Figure 36.7 Hypertension can be transferred by renal transplantation in the Dahl rat.

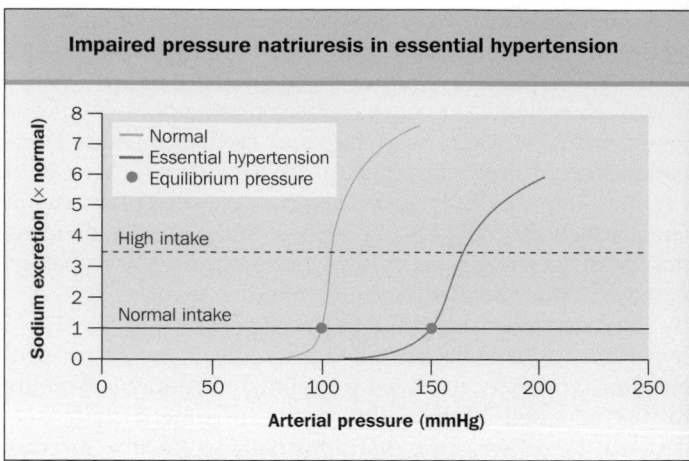

Figure 36.8 Essential hypertension is associated with impaired pressure natriuresis. Evidence suggests that in patients with essential hypertension there is a shift to the greater blood pressure values needed to maintain normal sodium excretion (the equilibrium pressure). (Adapted with permission from Guyton, Coleman, Cowley Jr., et al[8].)

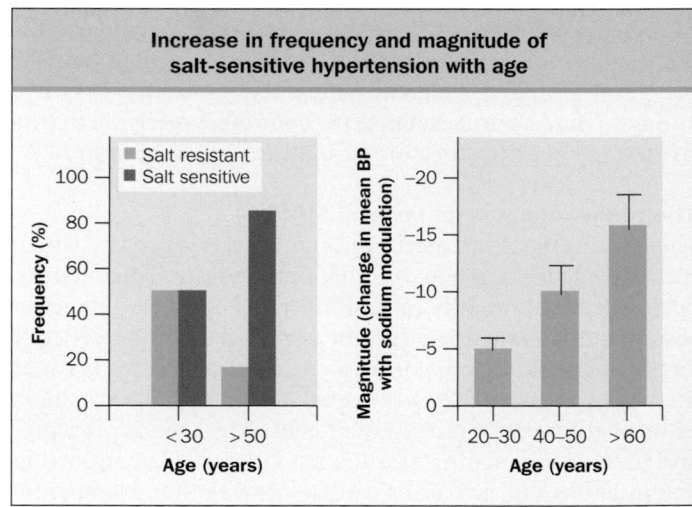

Figure 36.9 Salt sensitivity increases in both frequency and magnitude over time. (Adapted with permission from Weinberger and Fineberg[19].)

brisk natriuresis. The natriuresis occurs as a consequence of a transient rise in pressure in the peritubular capillaries in the juxtamedullary region, with a subsequent increase in interstitial pressure and a backflow of sodium through the paracellular space of the proximal tubule. Patients with essential hypertension can be shown to have a shift in the pressure–natriuresis curve, in which higher systemic pressures are required to excrete a salt load. Epidemiologic studies have also linked the relative sodium content in the diet with the prevalence of hypertension in various populations, and intervention studies with salt restriction or loading have shown that the BP response in many hypertensive patients is salt sensitive. In addition, several studies have demonstrated that salt loading of patients with essential hypertension results in some net total body sodium accumulation. Further evidence has been provided by the observation that three genetic diseases associated with hypertension in childhood (Liddle's syndrome, the syndrome of apparent mineralocorticoid excess, and glucocorticoid remediable aldosteronism) are also associated with increased reabsorption of salt by the kidney[7]. This has led many investigators to search for genetically mediated alterations in the regulation or transport of NaCl in the nephrons of hypertensive patients. Another possibility proposed by Brenner, is that a genetic reduction in nephron number may play the key initiating event. Over time, the hyperfiltration and increased glomerular pressure may damage the kidney and affect its ability to excrete salt[18].

However, the concept of a genetically mediated defect in the ability of the kidney to excrete salt does not readily explain certain observations. First, young hypertensive subjects appear to excrete salt normally or super-normally. Second, subjects with borderline or early hypertension may have low blood volume. Third, as many as 40% of hypertensives do not show a change in BP with salt loading (salt resistance), and this is primarily observed in younger patients. Fourth, with aging, salt sensitivity increases both in frequency and in degree such that by 70 years of age almost all hypertensive patients are salt sensitive (Fig. 36.9)[19]. In fact, it has been argued from meta-analyses that salt restriction is not important in either normotensives or in patients with hypertension under the age of 45[20]. All of these findings are most consistent with the possibility that the defect in sodium excretion in hypertensive patients is acquired.

Acquired renal injury as a mechanism for salt-sensitive hypertension

Early studies of essential hypertension documented the nearly universal presence of preglomerular arteriolar thickening ('arteriolosclerosis') and mild tubulointerstitial injury[21]. While some investigators suggested that these changes were secondary to hypertensive-induced renal injury, Goldblatt postulated that the renal preglomerular arteriolopathy might be a primary disease that is responsible for the development of hypertension[9]. Specifically, Goldblatt postulated that progressive arteriolar disease could reduce the lumen area, causing a reduction in renal blood flow and the development of renal ischemia with activation of the RAS and stimulation of sodium reabsorption[9]. Brezis and Epstein further showed that the most vulnerable region for renal ischemia is the region of

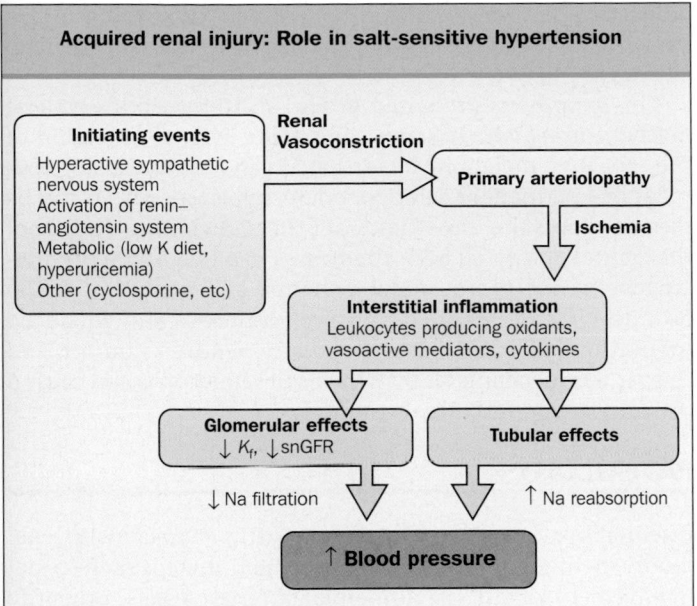

Figure 36.10 Hypothesis for the pathogenesis of essential hypertension. (Adapted with permission from Johnson, Herrera-Acosta, Schreiner and Rodriguez-Iturbe[14].)

the outer medulla[22]. Further studies by Cowley and colleagues showed that ischemia to the inner and outer medulla itself can cause hypertension[10].

The major problem with Goldblatt's hypothesis was that he lacked a mechanism by which primary renal arteriolar disease would develop. However, recent studies have demonstrated that preglomerular microvascular disease can be induced by a variety of means[14]. These studies have confirmed that the induction of microvascular disease can cause hypertension and have also elucidated a likely pathway for its development (Fig. 36.10). According to this pathway, the initiating stimulus is usually something that leads to transient renal vasoconstriction, such as a hyperactive SNS mediated by emotional stress, smoking, alcohol, medications (sympathomimetics, etc.), obesity, congenital brainstem compression (see above) or baroreceptor dysfunction. Activation of the RAS through either elevations in angiotensinogen (via genetic polymorphisms or oral contraceptives) or increased renin levels (secondary to activation of the renal SNS, renal ischemia, hypokalemia, or other mechanisms) would also lead to vasoconstriction. In turn, the vasoconstriction results in preglomerular arteriolar thickening and ischemia with tubular injury and an interstitial infiltration of macrophages and T cells. The infiltrating leukocytes generate oxidants that inactivate nitric oxide that is present within the kidney and many of the leukocytes also actively express AII. There is also a decrease in renal kallikrein and urinary prostaglandins as well as an increase in local vasoconstrictors (endothelin 1). The imbalance of vasoconstrictors and vasodilators may potentiate the preglomerular vasoconstriction, and in the glomerulus results in a fall in the ultrafiltration coefficient (K_f) and single nephron glomerular filtration rate (GFR), thereby leading to a decrease in sodium filtration. In addition, tubular reabsorption of sodium occurs due to the direct effects of AII and the local loss of nitric oxide. Sodium retention results, increasing the extracellular volume (ECV) and blood pressure.

As systemic blood pressure increases, the renal perfusion pressure across the fixed arteriolar lesion increases blood flow until the ischemia is relieved, allowing sodium handling to return to normal but at the expense of an increase in blood pressure and a shift in the pressure-natriuresis curve, thus fulfilling Guyton's hypothesis.

Evidence in support of this hypothesis can be found in experimental models in which salt-sensitive hypertension can be induced by measures that lead to an arteriolopathy and tubulointerstitial inflammation (such as by transiently administering AII, cyclosporine, or an inhibitor of nitric oxide synthesis)[14]. Furthermore, prevention of the tubulointerstitial inflammation or arteriolopathy with agents such as mycophenolate mofetil will block the development of salt sensitivity in some of these models[23]. Treatment of the arteriolopathy and tubulointerstitial injury with vascular remodeling agents such as vascular endothelial growth factor can also ameliorate the salt-sensitivity and reduce blood pressure in the cyclosporine model[24].

Potential role of hyperuricemia in the development of hypertension

Hyperuricemia (defined as > 7.0 mg/dL (0.4 mmol/L) in males and > 6.0 mg/dL (> 0.35 mmol/L) in women) has been found to predict the development of hypertension and to be present in 25–40% of hypertensive individuals[25]. Its role in hypertension has been debated, however, since uric acid is elevated in populations at risk for hypertension (such as in subjects with obesity, renal disease, and African Americans), and therefore hyperuricemia may only be a 'marker' for individuals at increased risk. However, recent studies have demonstrated that mild hyperuricemia causes hypertension and primary renal microvascular disease in rats[15]. The mechanism appears to be mediated through both the cyclo-oxygenase-2 and RAS pathways. A caveat is that evidence that uric acid is directly mediating hypertension and vascular disease is limited to animal studies. Indeed, the Joint National Commission VI does not currently recognize uric acid as a major cardiovascular risk factor[2]. Clinical studies will be required to determine the role of uric acid in mediating microvascular disease and hypertension in man.

How does salt retention lead to hypertension?

Whereas an acute infusion of saline administered to animals with experimentally induced hypertension will initially raise blood volume and cardiac output, the increase in cardiac output is transient and is replaced by a rise in the systemic vascular resistance, a process that Guyton et al. termed 'autoregulation'[8]. There are several potential mechanisms for this observation.

First, the normal response to a salt load is an inhibition of the SNS. However it is known that, in salt-sensitive hypertensive patients, the SNS is not inhibited but may even be activated with a salt load[16]. A possible explanation is that, in the setting of tubulointerstitial injury and intrarenal ischemia, the salt load will trigger an intense tubuloglomerular feedback signal with activation of the renal afferent SNS that subsequently triggers the CNS response. Indeed, there is evidence that renal afferent nerves activate CNS sympathetic activity in both experimental hypertension and chronic renal disease[16].

Hypertension

Second, parabiotic experiments have suggested that there may be circulating factors in salt-loaded animals with hypertension that are responsible for some of the increase in the peripheral vascular resistance. Circulating Na^+/K^+ ATPase inhibitors as well as nitric oxide synthase inhibitors have been documented in some patients with essential hypertension[12]. One of the Na^+/K^+ ATPase inhibitors has been identified as ouabain and is derived from the adrenals. Blaustein has suggested that these substances, which are presumably secreted in an attempt to facilitate sodium excretion, may have the adverse consequence of increasing intracellular sodium and thus facilitating sodium–calcium exchange in the vascular smooth muscle cell. This would lead to a rise in intracellular calcium and stimulate vascular smooth muscle contraction, vasoconstriction, and the rise in vascular resistance[12]. Vasopressin has also been implicated in African-American hypertensives since vasopressin V_{1A} receptor antagonists lower BP by as much as 10 mmHg in the presence of a high-salt diet and clonidine (suppression of SNS)[26].

A third mechanism is the loss of a vasodepressor substance. There is good evidence that a lipid-like vasodepressor factor, termed medullipin, is expressed by a subset of interstitial cells in the renal medulla and juxtamedullary region. Release of this factor into the circulation appears to depend on medullary blood flow and can be inhibited if activation of renal SNS or inhibition of nitric oxide[13] reduces blood flow. In these circumstances, there may be reduced circulating levels of this substance in the setting of tubulointerstitial injury and intrarenal ischemia.

Fourth, the increase in pressure associated with the saline load could cause increased tension in the peripheral vasculature, leading to microvascular rarefaction (which has been observed in forearms and nail beds of patients with essential hypertension), which could raise the peripheral vascular resistance. An increased pressure load on the vessels could also result in compensatory vascular hypertrophy, mediated by local growth factors and the local RAS. Indeed, there is certain evidence that AII, platelet-derived growth factor, and transforming growth factor-β are involved in these processes.

Finally, whereas the emphasis has been on how expansion of the blood volume with salt intake may affect BP, it is likely that an increased hematocrit (such as occurs with polycythemia vera, androgen use, or epoetin), which is also associated with hypertension, may involve the same general pathway.

The hypothesis presented in Fig. 36.10 provides a general mechanism by which various initiating events (activation of the SNS, RAS, metabolic factors, etc.) can lead to the development of a permanent salt-dependent hypertension. As can be seen, it adopts the hypotheses of others, including the role of the central and renal SNS, the role of the RAS and renin heterogeneity, the role of renal ischemia and medullary blood flow, the role of impaired pressure natriuresis and enhanced tubuloglomerular feedback, the role of nephron number, and the various mechanisms by which salt retention could cause a rise in systemic vascular resistance.

PATHOLOGY

Essential hypertension is associated with a characteristic renal biopsy (benign nephrosclerosis) in which there is preferential involvement of the preglomerular arterial vessels, primarily the afferent arteriole and interlobular artery. The classic arterial lesion, which is observed in 90% of biopsy cases[21], is termed arteriolosclerosis and consists of the replacement of smooth muscle cells of the afferent arteriole in the media by connective tissue (Fig. 36.11). Often there is also accumulation of hyaline material (plasma proteins) in the subintima (hyalinosis). In association with the arteriolar disease, there is often evidence of glomerular and tubulointerstitial ischemia, as evidenced by shrinkage of the glomerular tuft, tubular atrophy, and interstitial fibrosis. Occasionally biopsies show evidence of glomerulosclerosis and severe tubulointerstitial injury (termed decompensated nephrosclerosis)[27]. In cases of malignant hypertension, the arterial lesion is more of a proliferative arteriolopathy, occasionally with fibrinoid necrosis. Occasionally, concentric layers of connective tissue and cells may give an onion-skin appearance to the vessels.

NATURAL HISTORY

Onset and prevalence
Prior to the onset of hypertension, many patients display signs of increased SNS activity, for example, increased basal

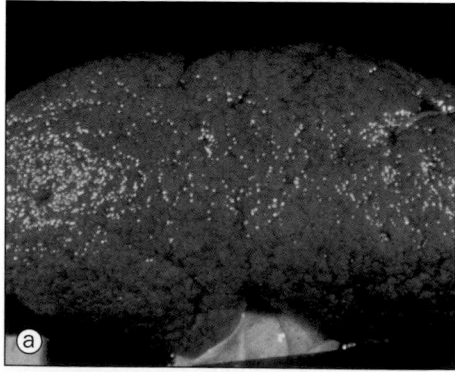 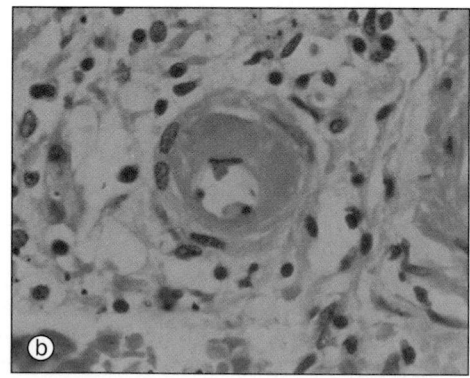 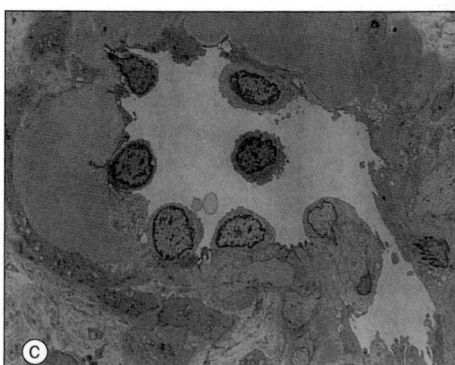

Figure 36.11 Renal biopsy findings in essential hypertension. (a) A granular pitted kidney of benign nephrosclerosis. (b) Arteriolosclerosis with subintimal hyalinosis. (c) Electron micrograph showing hyalinosis with the accumulation of insudative plasma proteins in the subendothelium of an arteriole. (Part (a) is courtesy of Harvard Medical School; parts (b) and (c) courtesy of C. E. Alpers.)

heart rate and increased BP response to stress or exercise. Other risk factors (obesity, insulin resistance, increased uric acid, etc.) may also be present (see above). These risk factors frequently are associated with high normal blood pressures that are a harbinger of frank hypertension, which develops later in the natural history of disease. Although once considered benign, borderline and white coat hypertension have now been shown to be associated with some end-organ disease (increased left ventricular thickness, microalbuminuria, etc.) and an increased risk for progressing to persistent hypertension.

The onset of essential hypertension usually begins after the age of 20, when the prevalence in the population increases progressively. By the age of 70, two-thirds of individuals will have hypertension which is often isolated systolic hypertension.

Cardiovascular and cerebrovascular consequences of hypertension increase linearly with increments in BP from 120/80 mmHg upward (see Fig. 36.2). This increased risk also increases with age and the presence of diabetes and is more prevalent in certain racial and ethnic groups, such as African Americans and Mexican Americans. The cardiovascular and cerebrovascular morbidity and mortality results from an increased frequency of both atherosclerotic and hypertensive changes in the vasculature. Atherosclerotic complications include myocardial infarction, thrombotic stroke, peripheral vascular disease, and aortic aneurysm; hypertensive complications include congestive heart failure, hemorrhagic stroke, aortic dissection, and cerebral aneurysms. In addition to an increased prevalence of hypertension, African Americans also have 80% greater stroke mortality and 50% greater heart disease.

Hypertensive heart disease often begins with concentric left ventricular hypertrophy associated with supernormal systolic function. Over time, impaired diastolic dysfunction may occur, as manifested by slow diastolic filling, which reflects decreased diastolic relaxation. This may progress to congestive heart failure. Nearly 90% of patients with heart failure have a history of hypertension.

Renal disease

Most patients with newly diagnosed essential hypertension will have either Stage 1 (GFR > 90 mL/min per 1.73 m^2) or Stage 2 renal disease (GFR 60–90 mL/min per 1.73 m^2) with elevated renal vascular resistance[28]. Despite relatively normal renal function, renal biopsy, if done, usually shows arteriolosclerosis and hyalinosis that preferentially involve the afferent arteriole and interlobular artery (see Fig. 36.11). Some patients have evidence of glomerulosclerosis or glomerular ischemia (capillary collapse with wrinkling of the basement membranes); tubular ischemia and tubulointerstitial fibrosis are also common.

Prior to the development of effective antihypertensive agents, proteinuria developed in up to 40% of patients and as many as 18% developed renal insufficiency over time. Currently, microalbuminuria is observed in 15–30% of patients, and fewer patients develop non-nephrotic, or, rarely, nephrotic-range proteinuria. The development of microalbuminuria is associated with salt sensitivity, with the loss of nocturnal dipping in BP, and with increased target organ damage (especially left ventricular hypertrophy).

An elevated serum creatinine develops in 10–20% of patients, and the risk is greater in African Americans, in the elderly, and in those with higher systolic BP (systolic BP > 160 mmHg)[29,30]. In 2–5%, progression to renal failure will occur over the subsequent 10–15 years (Figs 36.12 and 36.13). Despite the relative infrequency for hypertension to progress to end-stage renal disease, the large population of hypertensive patients means that hypertension remains the second most common cause of end-stage renal disease after diabetes in the USA. Furthermore, essentially all diabetic subjects have hypertension when they start dialysis. The risk for renal failure secondary to hypertension appears three-fold greater in African Americans[31].

Effect of antihypertensive therapy on the natural history of hypertensive cardiovascular disease and renal disease progression

According to a recent survey of 50 million people with hypertension in the USA, only 55% are on treatment and only 29%

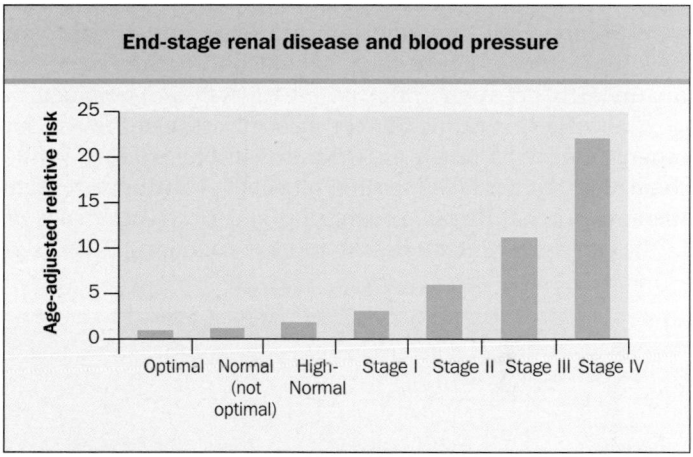

Figure 36.12 Incidence of end-stage renal disease related to baseline blood pressure in the MRFIT study. Mean follow-up was 16 years. (Adapted with permission from Klag, Whelton, Randall, et al[29].)

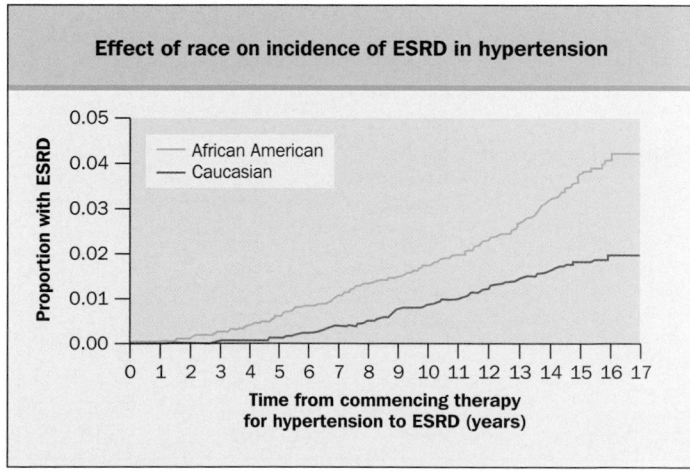

Figure 36.13 The rate of end-stage renal disease in African American and Caucasian hypertensive veterans. Kaplan–Meier estimates of the rates of end-stage renal disease in hypertensives. (Adapted with permission from Perry Jr., Miller, Fornoff, et al[30].)

have their BP under adequate (< 140/90 mmHg) control[2]. Although there has been significant reduction in the age-adjusted death rate for stroke and coronary artery disease since the early 1980s as a result of better BP control (and better treatment of other risk factors such as hyperlipidemia), heart disease and stroke remain the first and third leading causes of death in the USA. This emphasizes the importance of identifying and treating patients with hypertension.

Antihypertensive therapy has been shown to reduce cardiovascular and cerebrovascular complications in patients with moderate-to-severe hypertension (diastolic BP > 105 mmHg) and in patients with mild hypertension and associated cardiovascular risk factors (Table 36.4). The risk reduction has been most significant for stroke, but it has also been shown for congestive heart failure and myocardial infarction[32]. There are in addition, several epidemiological studies that have clearly shown a benefit in treating mild hypertension[33,34].

Antihypertensive therapy also reduces the risk for progression of renal disease[35,36] and may even be associated with some recovery of renal function in patients presenting with malignant or stage III hypertension. Lowering BP in subjects with mild-to-moderate hypertension and renal impairment can slow renal disease progression, provided the achieved BP on treatment is between 130–139 mmHg systolic. A reduction of 20 mmHg in systolic BP was shown to reduce the risk for progression by as much as two-thirds in one study[30]. While some older studies failed to show a benefit of antihypertensive therapy on renal disease progression in African Americans or in the elderly, recent studies are more encouraging. Results of

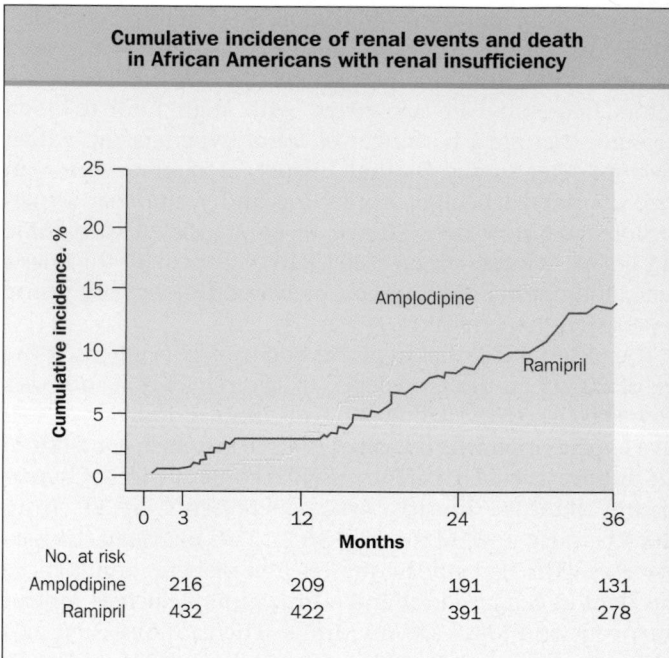

Figure 36.14 Antihypertensive treatment in African Americans with mild to moderate renal insufficiency. Initial therapy with an ACE inhibitor appeared to offer greater benefit than treatment with a calcium blocker. ACE inhibitor treatment was associated with a better outcome for all clinical end-points (proteinuria, decline in renal function, end-stage renal disease and death). (Adapted with permission from Agodoa, Appel, Bakris, et al[36].)

Table 36.4 Effect of antihypertensive therapy on stroke, coronary artery disease, congestive heart failure, and total and cardiovascular mortality.

Outcome in clinical trials according to first-line therapy for hypertension						
				Relative risk (95% confidence interval)		
Outcome	Drug regimen	Dose	No. of trials	0.4	0.7	1.0
Stroke	Diuretics	High	9			
	Diuretics	Low	4			
	β-blockers		4			
	Hypertension and Detection Followup Program (HDFP)	High	1			
Coronary heart disease	Diuretics	High	11			
	Diuretics	Low	4			
	β-blockers		4			
	HDFP	High	1			
Congestive heart failure	Diuretics	High	9			
	Diuretics	Low	3			
	β-blockers		2			
Total mortality	Diuretics	High	11			
	Diuretics	Low	4			
	β-blockers		4			
	HDFP	High	1			
Cardiovascular mortality	Diuretics	High	11			
	Diuretics	Low	4			
	β-blockers		4			
	HDFP	High	1			

Data are taken from a meta-analysis of randomized, placebo-controlled clinica trials in hypertension according to first-line therapy. The total numbers of participants was 24 294 (active treatment) and 23 926 (placebo). (With permission from Psaty et al.[32])

recently completed trials in African Americans[36] as well as other groups with nondiabetic renal disease[37], indicate that lowering systolic blood pressure to 130–139 mmHg, utilizing an ACE inhibitor as one of the blood pressure lowering agents, markedly slows disease progression reducing the risk of end-stage renal disease or death by as much as 55% (Fig 36.14). ACE inhibitors or angiotensin receptor antagonists are particularly attractive agents for patients with renal disease as they may confer benefits independent of their ability to lower BP. Several studies suggest that these agents slow progression more effectively than other agents with similar BP control, in both diabetics and nondiabetics (see Chapter 66).

Accumulating evidence suggests that lower BP goals than previously recommended are necessary in order to maximally reduce cardiovascular risk and preserve renal function. This is particularly true for subjects at higher risk (diabetics, renal disease) where the achieved BP may need to be even lower. Based on current evidence, achieved BP levels should be < 140 mmHg systolic in nondiabetics, and < 130/80–85 mmHg in diabetics and subjects with renal disease[38–40].

Can essential hypertension spontaneously remit?

In early, borderline hypertension, as many as 15–20% of patients may become normotensive spontaneously. Furthermore, in patients with established hypertension who have good BP control for 5 years under treatment, as many as 20–40% can be withdrawn from therapy successfully, especially if the BP is mild and if the patients are placed on salt restriction or weight reduction. This suggests that the processes that mediate hypertension are at times reversible.

REFERENCES

1. Bevan AT, Honour AJ, Stott FH. Direct arterial pressure recording in unrestricted man. Clin Sci. 1969;36:329–44.
2. The sixth report of the Joint National Committee on prevention, detection, evaluation, and treatment of high blood pressure. Arch Intern Med. 1997;157:2413–46.
3. Poch E, Gonzalez D, Giner V, et al. Molecular basis of salt sensitivity in human hypertension. Evaluation of renin–angiotensin–aldosterone system gene polymorphisms. Hypertension. 2001;38:1204–9.
4. Julius S, Schork MA. Predictors of hypertension. Ann N Y Acad Sci. 1978;304:38–58.
5. MacMahon S, Peto R, Cutler J, et al. Blood pressure, stroke, and coronary heart disease. Part 1, Prolonged differences in blood pressure: prospective observational studies corrected for the regression dilution bias. Lancet. 1990;335:765–74.
6. Sealey JE, Blumenfeld JD, Bell GM, et al. On the renal basis for essential hypertension: nephron heterogeneity with discordant renin secretion and sodium excretion causing a hypertensive vaso-constriction–volume relationship. J Hypertens. 1988;6:763–77.
7. Lifton RP. Molecular genetics of human blood pressure variation. Science. 1996;272:676–80.
8. Guyton AC, Coleman TG, Cowley AV, Jr., et al. Arterial pressure regulation. Overriding dominance of the kidneys in long-term regulation and in hypertension. Am J Med. 1972;52:584–94.
9. Goldblatt H. The renal origin of hypertension. Physiol Rev. 1947;27.
10. Cowley AW, Jr., Mattson DL, Lu S, Roman RJ. The renal medulla and hypertension. Hypertension. 1995;25:663–73.
11. Kurokawa K. Kidney, salt, and hypertension: how and why. Kidney Int Suppl. 1996;55:S46–51.
12. Blaustein MP, Hamlyn JM. Pathogenesis of essential hypertension. A link between dietary salt and high blood pressure. Hypertension. 1991;18:III184–95.
13. Muirhead EE. Renal vasodepressor mechanisms: the medullipin system. J Hypertens Suppl. 1993;11(Suppl)5:S53–8.
14. Johnson RJ, Herrera-Acosta J, Schreiner GF, Rodriguez-Iturbe B. Subtle acquired renal injury as a mechanism of salt-sensitive hypertension. N Engl J Med. 2002;346:913–23.
15. Mazzali M, Kanellis J, Han L, et al. Hyperuricemia induces a primary renal arteriolopathy in rats by a blood pressure-independent mechanism. Am J Physiol Renal Physiol. 2002;282:F991–7.
16. DiBona GF, Kopp UC. Neural control of renal function. Physiol Rev. 1997;77:75–197.
17. Dahl LK, Heine M. Primary role of renal homografts in setting chronic blood pressure levels in rats. Circ Res. 1975;36:692–6.
18. Mackenzie HS, Lawler EV, Brenner BM. Congenital oligonephropathy: The fetal flaw in essential hypertension? Kidney Int Suppl. 1996;55:S30–4.
19. Weinberger MH, Fineberg NS. Sodium and volume sensitivity of blood pressure. Age and pressure change over time. Hypertension. 1991;18:67–71.
20. Midgley JP, Matthew AG, Greenwood CM, Logan AG. Effect of reduced dietary sodium on blood pressure: a meta-analysis of randomized controlled trials. JAMA. 1996;275:1590–7.
21. Sommers SC, Relman AS, Smithwick RH. Histologic studies of kidney biopsy specimens from patients with hypertension. Am J Pathol. 1958;34.
22. Brezis M, Epstein FH. Cellular mechanisms of acute ischemic injury in the kidney. Annu Rev Med. 1993;44:27–37.
23. Rodriguez-Iturbe B, Pons H, Quiroz Y, et al. Mycophenolate mofetil prevents salt-sensitive hypertension resulting from angiotensin II exposure. Kidney Int. 2001;59:2222–32.
24. Kang DH, Kim YG, Andoh TF, et al. Post-cyclosporine-mediated hypertension and nephropathy: amelioration by vascular endothelial growth factor. Am J Physiol Renal Physiol. 2001;280:F727–36.
25. Rich MW. Uric acid: is it a risk factor for cardiovascular disease? Am J Cardiol. 2000;85:1018–21.
26. Bakris G, Bursztyn M, Gavras I, Bresnahan M, Gavras H. Role of vasopressin in essential hypertension: racial differences. J Hypertens. 1997;15:545–50.
27. Bohle A, Ratschek M. The compensated and the decompensated form of benign nephrosclerosis. Pathol Res Pract. 1982;174:357–67.
28. DOQI clinical practice guidelines for chronic kidney disease: evaluation, classification, and stratification. Kidney Disease Outcome Quality Initiative. Am J Kidney Dis. 2002;39:S1–231.
29. Klag MJ, Whelton PK, Randall BL, et al. Blood pressure and end-stage renal disease in men. N Engl J Med. 1996;334:13–18.
30. Perry HM, Jr., Miller JP, Fornoff JR, et al. Early predictors of 15-year end-stage renal disease in hypertensive patients. Hypertension. 1995;25:587–94.
31. Bakris GL, Mangrum A, Copley JB, et al. Effect of calcium channel or beta-blockade on the progression of diabetic nephropathy in African Americans. Hypertension. 1997;29:744–50.
32. Psaty BM, Smith NL, Siscovick DS, et al. Health outcomes associated with antihypertensive therapies used as first-line agents. A systematic review and meta-analysis. JAMA. 1997;277:739–45.
33. Mann JF, Gerstein HC, Pogue J, et al. Renal insufficiency as a predictor of cardiovascular outcomes and the impact of ramipril: the HOPE randomized trial. Ann Intern Med. 2001;134:629–36.

34. Staessen JA, Wang JG, Thijs L. Cardiovascular protection and blood pressure reduction: a meta-analysis. Lancet. 2001;358: 1305–15.

35. Walker WG, Neaton JD, Cutler JA, et al. Renal function change in hypertensive members of the Multiple Risk Factor Intervention Trial. Racial and treatment effects. The MRFIT Research Group. JAMA. 1992;268:3085–91.

36. Agodoa LY, Appel L, Bakris GL, et al. Effect of ramipril vs amlodipine on renal outcomes in hypertensive nephrosclerosis: a randomized controlled trial. JAMA. 2001;285:2719–28.

37. Jafar TH, Schmid CH, Landa M, et al. Angiotensin-converting enzyme inhibitors and progression of nondiabetic renal disease. A meta-analysis of patient-level data. Ann Intern Med. 2001;135:73–87.

38. Bakris GL. Maximizing cardiorenal benefit in the management of hypertension: achieve blood pressure goals. J Clin Hypertens (Greenwich). 1999;1:141–7.

39. Bakris GL, Williams M, Dworkin L, et al. Preserving renal function in adults with hypertension and diabetes: a consensus approach. National Kidney Foundation Hypertension and Diabetes Executive Committees Working Group. Am J Kidney Dis. 2000;36:646–61.

40. Green L. Implications of recent hypertension trials for the generalist physician: whom do we treat, and how? Curr Control Trials Cardiovasc Med. 2000;1:22–4.

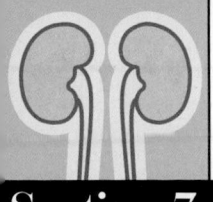

Chapter 37
Nonpharmacologic Treatment of Hypertension

Myron H Weinberger and Richard J Johnson

INTRODUCTION

Blood pressure is influenced by lifestyle, metabolic, and nutritional factors. While some of these components have been the subject of debate, the evidence regarding their relationship to blood pressure and their usefulness in treating uncomplicated forms of hypertension are often compelling and bear consideration before antihypertensive drug therapy is initiated. The most recent report of The Joint National Committee on Prevention, Detection, Evaluation and Treatment of High Blood Pressure (JNC VI) from the National High Blood Pressure Education Program has emphasized the role of nonpharmacologic therapy as an initial step in the treatment of essential hypertension for many, but not all, individuals[1]. Some lifestyle changes may be useful in the prevention of hypertension as well for individuals with 'high-normal' blood pressure levels. Unfortunately, lifestyle modifications are often both difficult to achieve and to maintain.

PREVENTION

The prevention of hypertension has been as elusive as the identification of the multiple causes for hypertension itself. Despite this obstacle, the importance of primary prevention has been underscored by the recognition that treatment of hypertension is expensive, that control of blood pressure in hypertensive individuals does not restore cardiovascular risk to normal, and by the fact that the majority of hypertensive individuals are not receiving adequate treatment. The challenge in preventing the development of hypertension is further compounded by the multifactorial nature of the abnormalities that may impact blood pressure control. It, therefore, becomes important to identify the factors influencing increases in blood pressure as well as those individuals who are most susceptible to these factors. One then needs to know how and when to take steps towards the prevention of a pathophysiologic event that has not yet occurred[1].

It is clear that hypertension occurs in families and has a genetic basis. With the exception of a few rare genetic abnormalities such as Liddle's syndrome, the brachydactyly syndrome (associated with sympathetic overactivity from neurovascular compression of the medulla), glucocorticoid-remediable aldosteronism, and other forms of congenital adrenal synthetic disorders, there are currently no clear-cut genetic markers that will identify those destined to become hypertensive. Therefore, we are left with family history of hypertension in first-degree relatives as a weaker marker. There also appear to be racial or demographic factors that are associated with differences in the prevalence of hypertension. For example, African American individuals have a higher prevalence of hypertension than is seen in Caucasian or Hispanic Americans. Certain physical characteristics, such as obesity, and lifestyle–behavioral factors (smoking, alcohol consumption, and dietary intake of sodium and potassium) are associated with hypertension. Environmental factors can also modulate the genetic or demographic susceptibility to develop high blood pressure. Finally, it is clear that blood pressure, particularly the systolic pressure, rises with age in most industrialized societies. However, this latter age-associated event is not an inevitable biologic event since there are many societies in the world in which it does not occur.

Another clue to the increased susceptibility for the development of hypertension is the blood pressure level itself. In fact, the Fifth report of the JNC acknowledged this fact by the creation of a new category of blood pressure designated 'high-normal' (130–139/85–89 mmHg)[2]. In earlier studies, these individuals were found to have an increased prevalence of early vascular damage and an increased risk for the development of 'fixed' hypertension. Recent reports from the Framingham Study indicate that 'high-normal' levels of blood pressure are associated with an increased risk for cardiovascular events when compared to those with 'normal' blood pressure (120–129/80–84) who were at greater risk than those with 'optimal' levels (< 120/< 80)[3]. Individuals with 'high-normal' levels of blood pressure have been the subjects of several studies that have examined the potential of preventing the rise in blood pressure often observed. These findings have now established the fact that lifestyle changes such as reduction in alcohol consumption or salt intake, weight loss, and increased intake of fruits, vegetables, and low-fat dairy foods can reduce the risk of developing fixed hypertension in such susceptible individuals. Therefore, for individuals with blood pressure levels between 130/85 and 160/100 mmHg in whom target organ damage, concomitant cardiovascular disease, or other cardiovascular disease risk factors are not present, treatment should begin with appropriate recommendations for lifestyle modifications[1]. Simultaneously, there must be an agreement with the patient to adhere to a careful schedule of follow-up in order to evaluate the success of such efforts as well as to determine the need for subsequent drug therapy if goal blood pressure is not reached by life-style modifications alone.

Weight loss

Obesity, indicated by a body mass index > 27 (weight in kilograms divided by height in meters squared), is epidemic in society, affecting 33% of the US adult population, and with other Western countries following close behind. Obese individuals have a three-fold increased prevalence of hypertension. Hypertension is also particularly common in patients with obesity and obstructive sleep apnea. Possible mechanisms for obesity-induced hypertension include overactivity of the sympathetic nervous system and the effect of hyperinsulinemia which may increase renal sodium reabsorption. An increase in upper-body fat, the so-called 'apple' shape, is a greater predictor of both hypertension and cardiovascular disease risk as compared to a predominant lower-body fat distribution ('pear' shape). In obese hypertensives or those with 'high–normal' blood pressure, weight loss of as little as 4–5 kg is often associated with a significant reduction in blood pressure. Weight loss is, in fact, one of the most effective nonpharmacologic interventions to reduce blood pressure (Fig. 37.1)[4]. It is not necessary for such individuals to reduce to their 'ideal' body weight in order to reap the beneficial effects on their blood pressure level. Unfortunately, not all obese hypertensives demonstrate a blood pressure reduction with weight loss. Moreover, recidivism (relapse with regain in weight) after successful weight reduction is a common and limiting factor. Notwithstanding these limitations, a trial of weight reduction is a worthwhile step in such individuals. Since many obese subjects are sedentary and since such a lifestyle is associated with increased blood pressure and cardiovascular risk, weight reduction should be accompanied by recommendations to increase physical activity unless contraindicated for other reasons.

Physical activity

A program of regular physical activity accomplishes many beneficial effects. It improves cardiovascular fitness, aids in weight loss, improves insulin sensitivity, and often lowers blood pressure. It is not clear that the beneficial effects of exercise on blood pressure can always be separated from these multifactorial effects. Nonetheless, a gradual, progressive program of increased physical activity is worthwhile for most subjects. Debate exists as to the amount, frequency, and intensity of exercise required for optimal beneficial effects. In general it is recommended that a goal of 30–45 min per day, 5 days per week be sought. For individuals in whom there is no evidence of cardiovascular disease or no other contraindications exist, the intensity of exercise should be sufficient to increase pulse rate to about 70% of predicted maximum. It should be noted, however, that blood pressure will rise during the exercise period, and this may reach unacceptably high levels in patients whose blood pressure is not well controlled. The program must also be individualized and realistic for a given individual if it is to have any hope of success and long-term adherence.

Alcohol consumption

Increased alcohol consumption is associated with elevation of blood pressure, hypertension, and an increased risk for stroke. For that reason, all subjects being evaluated for elevated

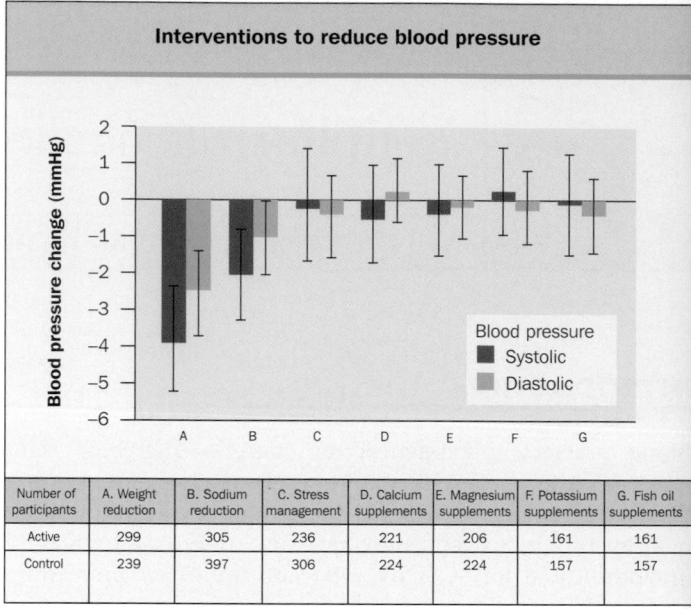

Figure 37.1 Interventions to reduce blood pressure. Net mean changes in systolic and diastolic blood pressure (baseline minus follow-up) with various interventions in patients with high–normal levels of blood pressure. (Adapted with permission from the Trials of Hypertension Prevention Collaboration Research Group[4].)

blood pressure levels should be asked about their typical consumption of alcohol-containing beverages. It appears that alcohol has a biphasic effect on blood pressure, lowering it slightly at relatively low levels of intake and causing a dose-dependent increase at higher levels. The optimal amount per day is 1 ounce (30 g) of ethanol (24 ounces of beer; 10 ounces of wine; 2 ounces of 100 proof or 2.5 ounces of 80 proof spirits). There appear to be racial, gender, and body weight differences in the susceptibility of blood pressure to alcohol intake that should be considered. Since the mechanism for the alcohol-related rise in blood pressure appears to be mediated by the sympathetic nervous system, abrupt cessation of heavy alcohol consumption can be associated with a 'rebound' increase in blood pressure immediately after withdrawal, which typically abates over a few days.

Salt intake

Few subjects in the area of blood pressure and hypertension have aroused as much emotional debate and controversy as the role of dietary salt (NaCl). Individuals on each side in the debate have amassed much support in favor of their contentions or against the other side. It is often difficult to separate fact from opinion and bias since the participants in the debate are very persuasive.

There is substantial epidemiologic evidence to indicate that the prevalence of hypertension and its associated cardiovascular consequences are directly related to the level of dietary salt intake in societies throughout the world in whom the intake is above a level of 50–100 mmol/day (Fig. 37.2)[5]. In societies where habitual intake is below that range, hypertension is rare (Fig. 37.3). This suggests that there is a threshold level of salt intake required for its pressor effect. However, it is

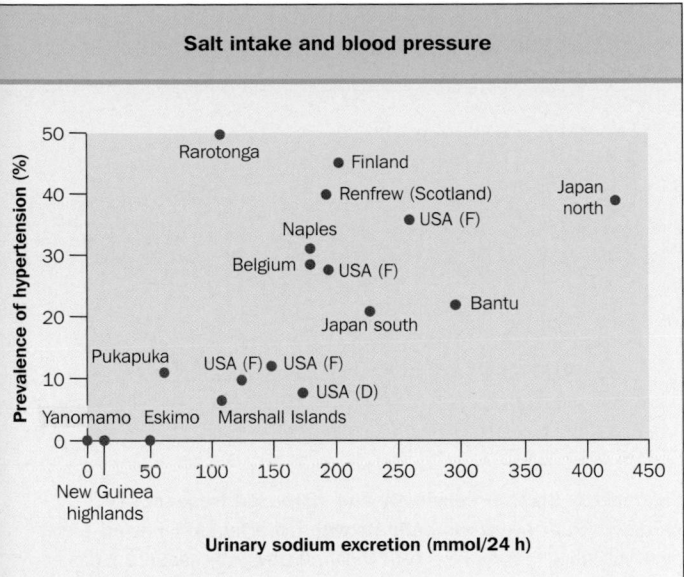

Figure 37.2 **Relationship of salt intake with frequency of blood pressure in different populations.** F = data from the Framingham Study; D = data from Dahl. (Adapted with permission from MacGregor[5].)

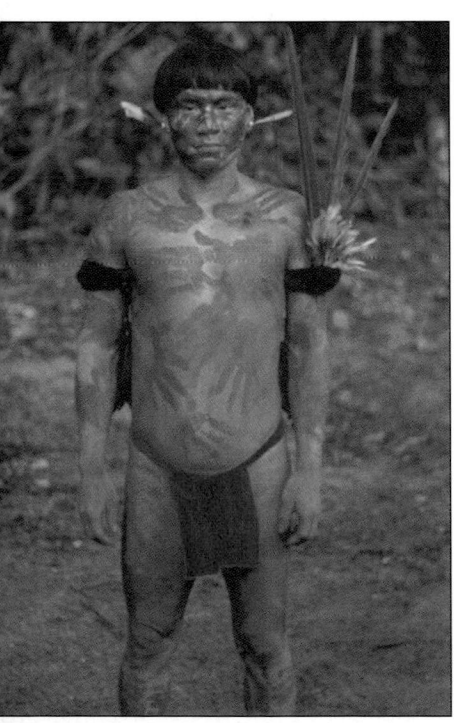

Figure 37.3 A Yanomamo Indian from southern Venezuela. This tribe of Indians ingests a low sodium (1 mmol/day) and high potassium (200–300 mmol/day) diet and has an almost complete absence of hypertension. (Courtesy of W. Oliver.)

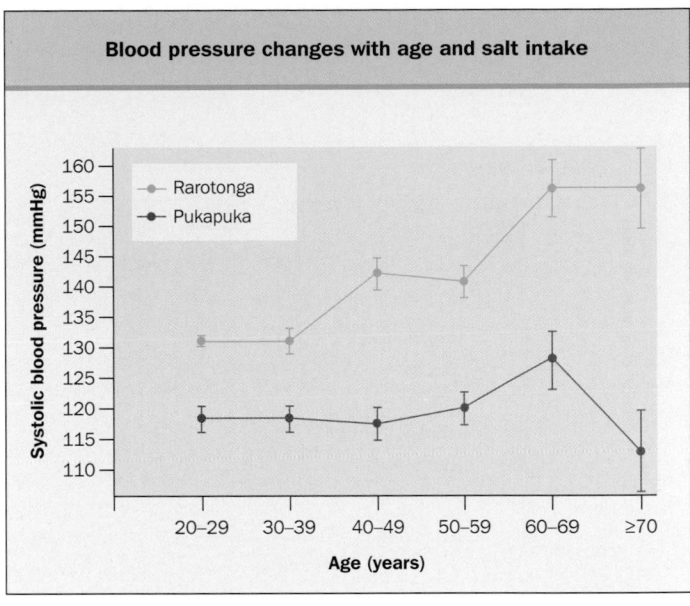

Figure 37.4 **Blood pressure changes with age and salt intakes.** The rise in systolic blood pressure with age correlates with a higher sodium intake in two Polynesian populations. In men of Rarotonga Island in Polynesia, where the sodium intake averages 130 mmol/day, (range 120–140 mmol/day), systolic blood pressure increases with age. In contrast, it remains constant in men from Pukapuka Island, in which the sodium intake averages 50–70 mmol/day (range 50–70 mmol/day). (Adapted from Prior et al.[6].)

we know that such age-related increases in blood pressure are most commonly observed in 'industrialized' societies; that is those featuring habitual salt intake in excess of 120 mmol/day[5]. By comparison, in societies in which the usual salt intake is much lower, such age-related increases in blood pressure have not been reported. Other cross-sectional studies, such as the Intersalt study, have also shown a correlation between urinary sodium excretion (reflecting dietary intake) and the age-related increase in blood pressure[6].

Recent studies have focused on identifying and distinguishing individuals whose blood pressure is modulated by salt intake ('sodium sensitive') and those in which blood pressure is not ('sodium resistant' individuals)[7]. Interestingly, 'sodium sensitivity' is best determined by demonstrating a decrease in blood pressure during periods of salt restriction as opposed to an increase in blood pressure with sodium chloride loading[8]. This presumably reflects the concept that sodium sensitive individuals have already had an increase in blood pressure during exposure to habitual salt excess.

'Sodium sensitivity' can be observed in both normotensive and hypertensive individuals. Epidemiologically, 'sodium sensitivity' is seen with increased frequency in certain demographic groups. These include:

- African Americans;
- elderly people;
- obese (not in all studies);
- insulin-dependent diabetic subjects;
- patients on cyclosporine;
- renal insufficiency.

clear that not all individuals are equally susceptible to this effect. Therefore, it is not surprising to find little, if any, correlation between salt intake and blood pressure in societies in which salt intake is above the threshold level, since those who are 'sensitive' to the salt effect may have already become hypertensive while those 'resistant' will not have an elevation of pressure at the same level of intake as their 'sensitive' cohorts. It is also evident that salt plays a role in the age-related increase in blood pressure (Fig. 37.4)[6]. From cross-sectional observations,

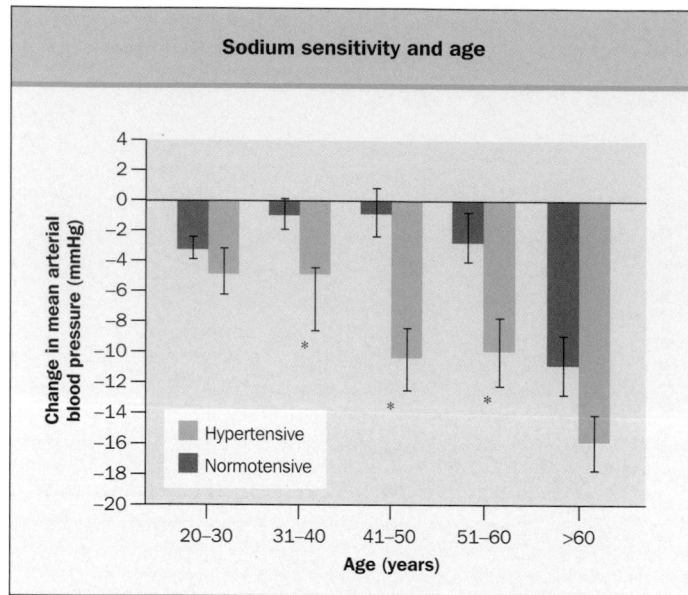

Figure 37.5 Increase in magnitude of sodium sensitivity with increasing age. Sodium sensitivity (determined by a standardized test evaluating the change in blood pressure from a volume-expanded to a contracted state) increases proportionately with age in both hypertensive and normotensive subjects (bars indicate SEM; * $P < 0.05$). (Adapted with permission from Weinberger and Fineberg[10].)

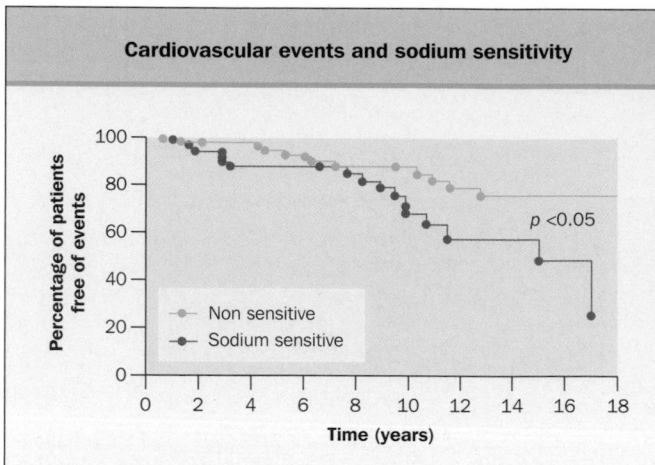

Figure 37.6 Sodium sensitivity and increased frequency of cardiovascular events in patients with hypertension. Kaplan–Meier plots indicating that patients with sodium-sensitive hypertension have an increased number of fatal and nonfatal cardiovascular events (such as angina pectoris, myocardial infarction, and heart failure) compared with patients with sodium-resistant hypertension. (Adapted with permission from Morimoto et al.[11].)

Characteristics of sodium-sensitive hypertension

Loss of nocturnal 'dipping' of blood pressure

Increased target organ damage

  Cardiovascular: increased incidence of left ventricular hypertrophy, cardiac 'events'

  Renal: increased microalbuminuria

Increased blood pressure response to nonsteroidal agents (NSAIDs)

Low plasma renin

Other changes

  Decreased vasodilators: fall in urinary dopamine, kallikrein, and nitrites

  Increased vasoconstrictor response: increased response to angiotensin II and norepinephrine (noradrenaline)

Table 37.1 Characteristics of sodium-sensitive hypertension.

Sodium sensitivity is observed in 75% of hypertensive African Americans compared to ~50% of Caucasian hypertensives[9]. Salt sensitivity increases with increasing age in both the normotensive and hypertensive population (see Fig. 37.5)[10], and is present in the vast majority of hypertensive subjects who are 60 years or older. Sodium sensitivity is also associated with a greater increase in blood pressure over a 10-year period or longer compared to sodium-resistant subjects, which is consistent with a role for sodium sensitivity in the age-related rise in blood pressure. Sodium sensitive hypertensive subjects also have a greater frequency of microalbuminuria and more cardiovascular events compared to sodium-resistant subjects (Fig. 37.6)[11]. Salt sensitivity in normotensives is associated with reduced survival in long-term follow-up studies[12].

The pathogenesis of sodium sensitivity has been studied. A variety of physiological abnormalities have been reported in salt-sensitive subjects including alterations in circulating levels of (or renal responses to) atrial natriuretic factor, kallikrein, prostaglandins, and nitric oxide (Table 37.1)[9]. Some but not all studies have reported that sodium-sensitive subjects have increased levels of norepinephrine (adrenaline) in plasma or urine. It has been suggested that salt loading increases catecholamine release or modifies adrenergic receptor binding, thereby enhancing the effect of circulating catecholamines to cause vasoconstriction by increasing α-adrenoceptor and blunting β-adrenoceptor responses. Indirect support for this concept has come from the finding that African Americans, a group in whom sodium sensitivity is commonly found, exhibit enhanced α-adrenergic responsiveness upon challenge with physical stress (cold applied to the forehead).

Sodium-sensitive subjects have also been shown to have reduced renin levels suggesting abnormal suppression of both renin and aldosterone[9]. It has been assumed that the diminished renin response represents increased sodium retention with extracellular volume expansion rather than a primary event. However, there is increasing evidence that a diminished renin response to changes in sodium and volume may exert a permissive effect on the sodium sensitivity of blood pressure[13]. Specifically, we found that sodium-sensitive individuals failed to increase their renin levels as well as salt-resistant individuals during sodium restriction, thus resulting in a greater blood pressure fall in sodium-sensitive individuals[13]. It is also known that renin responsiveness is blunted in African Americans and decreases with age in most individuals. This could explain why such subgroups more frequently demonstrate sodium sensitivity of blood pressure than do those in whom the renin response appears to be more vigorous.

Reduced dietary sodium and blood pressure			
Group	No. of trials	Relative decrease in blood pressure (mmHg) for a decrease in Na⁺ intake of 100 mmol/day mean (95% confidence intervals)	
		Systolic	Diastolic
Older hypertensives (>45 years)	17	6.3 (4.1–8.4)	2.2 (0.6–3.9)
Younger hypertensives (<45 years)	11	2.4 (0.4–4.4)	–0.1 (–1.6–1.4)
Normotensives	14	–0.2 (–1.5–1.0)	0.6 (–0.9–2.1)

A meta-analysis of randomized controlled trials. (Adapted with permission from Midgley et al.[15].)

Table 37.2 Effect of reduced dietary sodium on blood pressure.

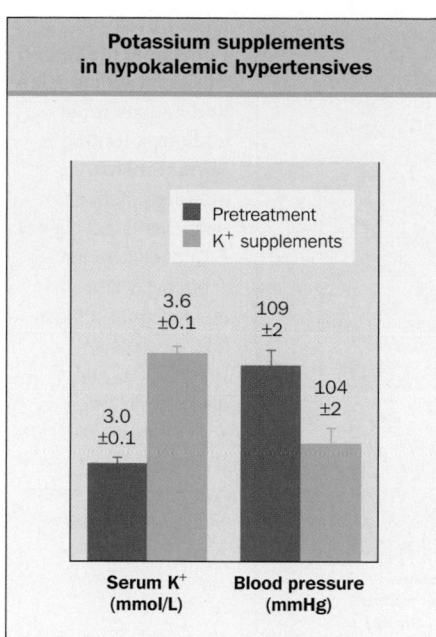

Potassium supplements in hypokalemic hypertensives

- Pretreatment
- K⁺ supplements

3.6 ±0.1

109 ±2

3.0 ±0.1

104 ±2

Serum K⁺ (mmol/L)   Blood pressure (mmHg)

Figure 37.7 Potassium supplementation lowers blood pressure in hypokalemic hypertensive patients. Treatment with potassium chloride (60 mmol/day potassium for 6 weeks) resulted in an increase in serum potassium and a decrease in mean arterial pressure in hypertensive patients taking thiazide diuretics. (Adapted from Kaplan et al. [17].)

In addition to the important role of genetic mechanisms in sodium sensitivity, there is also some experimental evidence that acquired renal microvascular and tubular injury may also play a role in the pathogenesis of sodium sensitivity[14]. Specifically, primary renal arteriolar disease, as originally proposed by Goldblatt, may result in renal ischemia and inflammation leading to alterations in vasoactive mediators that may limit sodium excretion (see Chapter 36). Further studies will be necessary to determine if such a mechanism may potentially explain some sodium sensitivity in man.

Given the relationship of sodium intake with hypertension in various populations, some experts have proposed that population-wide modest reduction in salt intake might prevent or delay development of hypertension in susceptible normotensive individuals and may reduce blood pressure in susceptible sodium-sensitive hypertensive subjects. Opponents have argued that only severe degrees of sodium restriction (i.e., levels of < 575 mg/day (25 mmol/day)) are effective in reducing blood pressure and that such levels are difficult to achieve and maintain, and that sodium restriction may also increase morbidity, especially in the setting of gastrointestinal illness.

Recent studies, however, suggest that a beneficial reduction in blood pressure can be achieved in sodium-sensitive hypertensives who reduce their dietary sodium intake to levels of 1.84–2.3 g/day (80–100 mmol/day). A meta-analysis suggests that the benefit of sodium restriction may be greatest in hypertensive subjects who are over 45 years of age (Table 37.2)[15]. A recent study demonstrated a graded reduction in blood pressure among those with blood pressure ranging from 120/80 through stage 1 hypertension (140–159/90–95) with modest reduction in sodium intake from 150 mmol/day to 100 mmol/day and 50 mmol/day in conjunction with a diet high in fresh fruits and vegetables and low-fat dairy products (DASH diet)[16]. In this study, no adverse effects of sodium restriction were reported. Furthermore, most individuals with simple instructions and avoidance of prepared and processed foods can readily achieve such levels, which are sufficiently modest that they are unlikely to be associated with adverse health effects. For these reasons, the JNC in its most recent report recommended a level of sodium of no more than 100 mmol/day (2.4 g sodium or 6 g sodium chloride).

Potassium intake

One of the confounding factors regarding the epidemiologic observations connecting levels of sodium intake in societies throughout the world to blood pressure has been the inverse relationship between the intakes of sodium and potassium. Typically, societies in which salt intake is high are relatively deficient in potassium (and calcium) consumption while in those groups who habitually consume little salt, the potassium (and calcium) intakes are quite high (see Fig. 37.3). These disparate groups also differ in other factors such as physical activity, the degree of industrialization (acculturation) of the society, as well as in racial and genetic characteristics. Therefore, interventional studies have been useful to clarify the effect of potassium intake on blood pressure.

In normotensive subjects with an average potassium intake > 1.95 g/day (50 mmol/day), further potassium supplementation appears to have no significant effect on blood pressure. However, among hypertensive individuals who are potassium deficient as the result of diuretic treatment or a low dietary potassium intake, potassium supplementation has been observed to lower blood pressure (Fig. 37.7)[17]. In a recent 8-week trial of subjects with 'high–normal' blood pressure, a diet with increased fruit and vegetable, a low-fat dairy content, and modestly lowered sodium content was found to reduce blood pressure[18]. It is not clear which of these components or combination thereof was responsible for this observation. Furthermore, some studies have found that potassium restriction can raise blood pressure in association with retention of sodium by the kidney (Fig. 37.8)[19]. The mechanism by which a low potassium diet leads to sodium retention is complex, as experimental and human studies have demonstrated that a low potassium diet has many effects on the kidney (Table 37.3). Experimental animal studies have also demonstrated that potassium supplementation has a protective effect on the occurrence of cardiovascular events in genetically hypertensive animals without having an effect on blood pressure. This

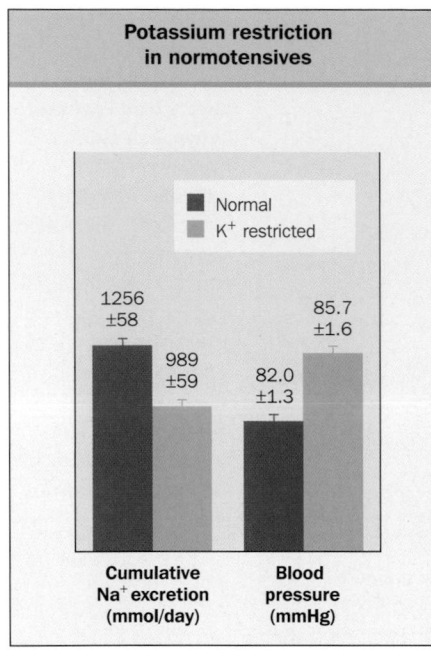

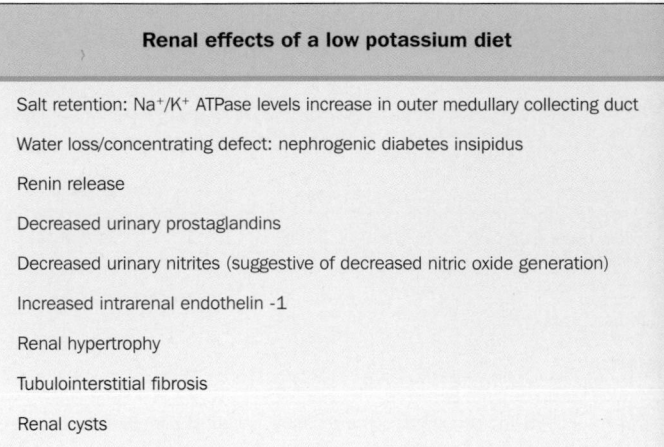

Figure 37.8
Potassium restriction raises blood pressure and causes renal sodium retention in normotensive subjects. Potassium restriction (780 mg/day (20mmol/day)) for 9 days resulted in an increased 24-h mean arterial pressure ($P < 0.001$) and a lower cumulative sodium excretion ($P < 0.001$) in normotensive subjects. (Adapted from Gallen et al.[19].)

Table 37.3 **Renal effects of a low potassium diet.**

benefit appears to derive from a direct effect on blood vessels. Overall, it appears to be beneficial to optimize potassium intake in hypertensive humans being careful to avoid the risk of hyperkalemia in subjects with renal impairment or in other susceptible individuals. If renal function is normal, optimal potassium intake is 80–120 mmol/day.

Calcium intake
Cross-sectional population surveys of self-reported nutrient intake suggest an inverse relationship between calcium intake and blood pressure. Interventional trials have been equivocal with respect to the effect of calcium supplementation on blood pressure. Meta-analyses have suggested a very modest effect in both normotensive and hypertensive subjects. Like the observations with salt intake, it appears that there are sub-groups in both normotensive and hypertensive populations who are 'calcium sensitive' in their blood pressure responses to calcium supplementation. African American and older subjects typically consume diets relatively deficient in calcium and have been identified as 'calcium sensitive' in terms of blood pressure responses. Curiously, these are the same subgroups that also have been frequently found to be 'sodium sensitive'. We conducted a study of randomized assignment to placebo or calcium supplementation (1200 mg/day (60 mmol/day)) with a crossover design in subjects who had been previously characterized in terms of the sodium responsive-ness of their blood pressure. We found that those who had demonstrated sodium sensitivity in an earlier study were likely to have a significant fall in blood pressure with calcium supplementation while those who were not sodium sensitive did not decrease their pressure with the added calcium. Moreover, it has been demonstrated that calcium has a natri-uretic effect, further suggesting a link between these nutrients. It is presently recommended that an adequate calcium intake be consumed[1] (1500–2000 mg/day including dietary intake) being careful not to increase the intake of saturated fat.

Magnesium intake
A weak inverse relationship has been reported between dietary magnesium intake and blood pressure, although the weight of evidence is minimal. Moreover, there have been few convincing interventional data to support a recommen-dation for magnesium supplementation for the reduction of blood pressure. Magnesium has been shown to influence cardiac function and rhythm; therefore, the JNC has recom-mended an adequate intake of magnesium pending more definitive information[1]. The optimal levels of intake of magnesium are not clearly established.

Dietary fats
There is little information to support the use of increased dietary fat intake for reduction of blood pressure. Scant evi-dence suggests that administration of omega-3 marine oils may reduce blood pressure slightly, but the amounts required for this effect were not tolerable by most subjects[1]. Moreover because of the enhancement of cardiovascular risk posed by dyslipidemia in hypertensive subjects, it is important to avoid dietary fats that can exacerbate lipid levels, particularly in the large subset of hypertensives who have an abnormality of one or more plasma lipid fractions.

Smoking
It appears that cigarette smoking raises blood pressure in some hypertensive subjects. Careful studies have demon-strated that the pressor effect of smoking is usually related to the initial cigarette of the day in habitual smokers. It has been suggested that cessation of smoking is associated with lower blood pressure in some individuals. However, the evidence to suggest an additive effect of smoking with hypertension in causing cardiovascular disease is overwhelming[1]. Therefore, cessation of smoking should be a compelling goal for all individuals who smoke.

Caffeine
Epidemiologic observations have failed to demonstrate a consistent relationship between caffeine consumption and blood pressure. In acute studies of caffeine-naive individuals, a small rise in blood pressure has been observed with the initial

caffeine consumption that is not sustained or enhanced by subsequent continued ingestion of caffeine-containing beverages[1]. Therefore, it is not likely that cessation of caffeine consumption will reduce blood pressure. A recent longitudinal study of medical students followed for 26 years indicates a greater prevalence of hypertension among heavy coffee drinkers[21]. These observations may not provide a causal role for coffee in the development of hypertension in these individuals since potential confounding factors were not excluded.

Relaxation, meditation, and biofeedback

Despite the modulation of blood pressure by stress and anxiety in both normotensive and hypertensive subjects, careful controlled trials of relaxation, meditation, or biofeedback have not shown significant or sustained reductions of blood pressure in hypertensive subjects[1]. There is abundant evidence that blood pressure declines during the active performance of such techniques, but this effect is evanescent and disappears when the exercise is ended. Furthermore, there is no beneficial effect of tranquilizer medications on blood pressure.

REFERENCES

1. The Joint National Committee on Prevention, Detection, Evaluation and Treatment of High Blood Pressure. The sixth report. Arch Intern Med. 1997;157:2413–46.
2. Joint National Committee on Detection, Evaluation and Treatment of High Blood Pressure. The fifth report. Arch Intern Med. 1993;153:154–83.
3. Vasan RS, Larson MG, Leip EP, et al. Impact of high-normal blood pressure on the risk of cardiovascular disease. N Engl J Med. 2001;345:1291–7.
4. Trials of Hypertension Prevention Collaboration Research Group. The effects of nonpharmacologic interventions on blood pressure of persons with high normal levels. JAMA. 1992;267:1213–20.
5. MacGregor GA. Sodium is more important than calcium in essential hypertension. Hypertension. 1985;7:628–37.
6. Prior IAM, Evans JG, Harvey HB, et al. Sodium intake and blood pressure in two Polynesian populations. N Engl J Med. 1968;279:515–20.
7. Rodriquez BL, Labarthe DR, Huang B, Lopez-Gomez J. Rise of blood pressure with age. Hypertension. 1994;24:779–85.
8. Kawasaki T, Delea CS, Bartter FC, Smith H. The effect of high-sodium and low-sodium intakes on blood pressure and other related variables in human subjects with idiopathic hypertension. Am J Med. 1978;64:193–8.
9. Weinberger MH. Salt sensitivity of blood pressure in humans. Hypertension. 1996;27:481–90.
10. Weinberger MH, Fineberg NS. Sodium and volume sensitivity of blood pressure: age and pressure change over time. Hypertension. 1991;18:67–71.
11. Morimoto A, Uzu T, Fujii T, et al. Sodium sensitivity and cardiovascular events in patients with essential hypertension. Lancet. 1997;350:1734–7.
12. Weinberger MH, Fineberg NS, Fineberg SE, Weinberger M. Salt sensitivity, pulse pressure, and death in normal and hypertensive humans. Hypertension. 2001;37:429–32.
13. Weinberger MH, Stegner JE, Fineberg NS. A comparison of two tests for the assessment of blood pressure responses to sodium. Am J Hypertens. 1993;6:179–84.
14. Johnson RJ, Herrera-Acosta J, Schreiner GF, Rodriguez-Iturbe B. Mechanisms of disease: subtle acquired renal injury as a mechanism of salt-sensitive hypertension. N Engl J Med. 2002;346:913–23.
15. Midgley JP, Mathew AG, Greenwood CM, Logan AG. Effect of reduced dietary sodium on blood pressure. A meta-analysis of randomized controlled trials. JAMA. 1996;275:1590–7.
16. Sacks FM, Svetkey LP, Vollmer WM, et al. Effects on blood pressure of reduced dietary sodium and the dietary approaches to stop hypertension (DASH) diet. N Engl J Med. 2001;344:3–10.
17. Kaplan N, Carnegie A, Risking P, et al. Potassium supplementation in hypertensive patients with diuretic-induced hypokalemia. N Engl J Med. 1985;312:746–9.
18. Appel LJ, Moore TJ, Obarzanek E, Vollmer WM. A clinical trial on the effects of dietary patterns on blood pressure. N Engl J Med. 1997;336:1117–24.
19. Gallen IW, Rosa RM, Esparaz DY, et al. On the mechanisms of the effects of potassium restriction on blood pressure and renal sodium retention. Am J Kidney Dis. 1998;31:19–27.
20. Weinberger MH, Wagner UL, Fineberg NS. The blood pressure effects of calcium supplementation in humans of known sodium responsiveness. Am J Hypertens. 1993;6:799–805.
21. Klag MJ, Wang N-Y, Meoni LA, et al. Coffee intake and the risk of hypertension. Arch Intern Med. 2002;162:657–62.

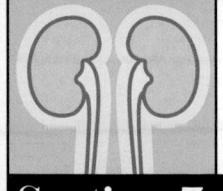

Chapter 38

Pharmacological Treatment of Hypertension

Jay Garg, Munawar Izhar, Renee Ellis, and George L Bakris

INTRODUCTION

Appropriate treatment of an asymptomatic disease associated with a high risk of cardiovascular and renal complications is difficult. This is apparent in the treatment of hypertension. Historically, awareness, detection and treatment of hypertension has been poor. Moreover, while the awareness of high blood pressure has improved, the percent of patients whose blood pressure is controlled to ≤ 140/90 mmHg has remained unchanged (Fig. 38.1).

This failure to achieve adequate blood pressure control is evidenced by a flattened downward trend in cardiovascular mortality and stroke as well as an increased incidence of heart failure[1]. This trend in mortality and heart failure, along with the increased incidence of end-stage renal disease (ESRD) (Fig. 38.2), suggests that we need to be more aggressive in achieving blood pressure control. Our ability to lower but inadequately achieve the recommended arterial pressure goals has led to more people living longer but with a substantially greater morbidity. In addition to increased morbidity associated with both ESRD and heart failure, the subsequent loss in productivity translates into a major financial burden to society. Inadequate arterial pressure lowering is more sobering in the context of recent data that support further blood pressure reduction (e.g., levels below 130/80 mmHg) in order to optimally preserve renal function in certain high-risk groups.

This chapter addresses the approach and pharmacologic management of patients with essential hypertension. Many of the concepts put forth are adopted from the report of the Joint National Committee (JNC VI) on Detection, Evaluation, Treatment and Prevention of High Blood Pressure, as well as the recommendations of the American Diabetes Association and the National Kidney Foundation. Mechanisms of antihypertensive drug action are reviewed and put into the context of rational antihypertensive drug combinations to maximally reduce blood pressure, minimize side effects, maintain organ function and reduce morbidity and mortality. High-risk populations for renal disease progression as well as new lower levels of blood pressure control are also discussed.

WHO SHOULD RECEIVE PHARMACOLOGICAL THERAPY?

The National Health and Nutrition Examination Survey (NHANES III) documented that many patients are either under-treated or not treated for their elevated blood pressure[1]. While lifestyle modifications, especially weight loss and reduced dietary sodium intake, significantly contribute to blood pressure reduction, most people fail to consistently follow such recommendations. Thus, antihypertensive agents are required to adequately reduce arterial pressure in most people.

A high systolic pressure (≥ 140 mmHg) in the absence of an elevated diastolic pressure is associated with a higher cardiovascular and renal event rate compared to diastolic hypertension[1,2]. Therefore, a more aggressive approach to the treatment of blood pressure, both diastolic and isolated systolic, is recommended to reduce cardiovascular and renal morbidity and mortality. In light of the NHANES III findings, this more aggressive approach to hypertension may appear unachievable. Nevertheless, increasing patient awareness, together with more diligent effort by physicians, may allow attainment of blood pressure within the recommended goals.

GOAL OF ANTIHYPERTENSIVE THERAPY

The goal of treating hypertension is to reduce morbid events, such as renal failure and stroke, as well as cardiovascular mortality. All mortality trials, to date, demonstrate that blood pressure needs to be reduced to levels < 140/90 mmHg in order to achieve this benefit[1-3]. However, previous studies call into question whether this level of pressure is low enough. In

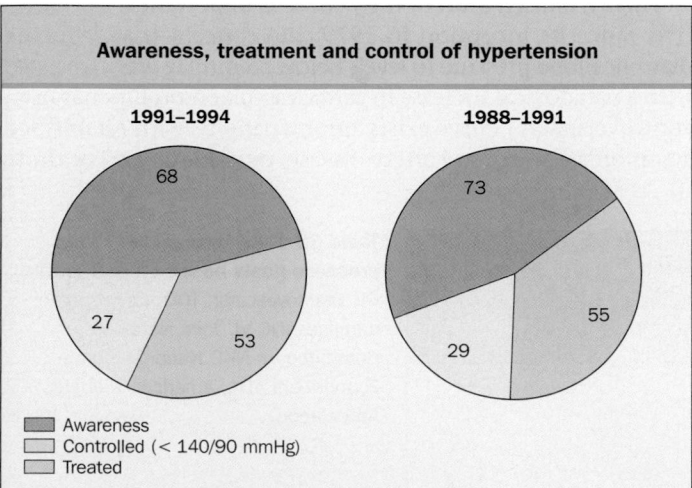

Figure 38.1 The awareness, treated and controlled percent of the population surveyed by NHANES over two distinct periods of time. Note that, hypertensive, there was no improvement in the number controlled or treated. (Adapted with permission[1].)

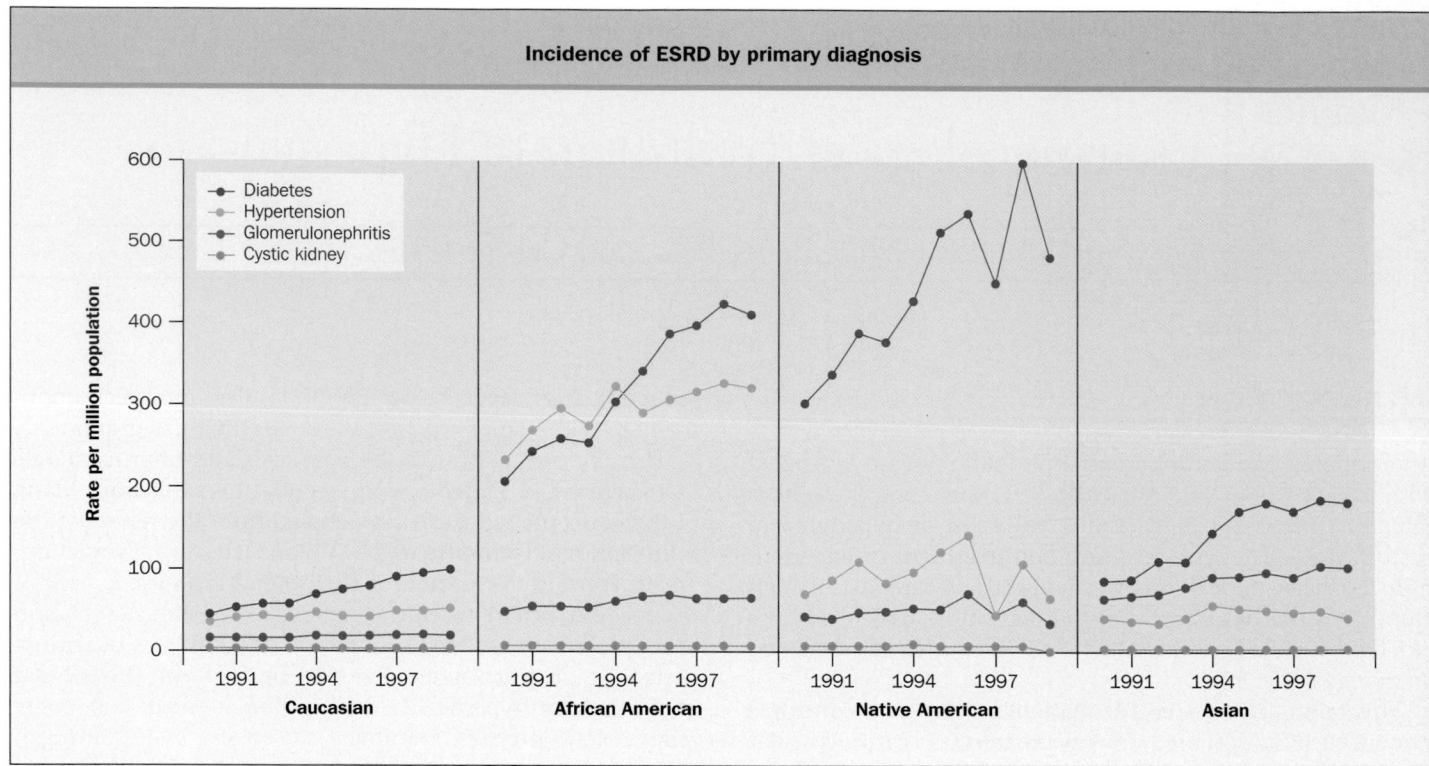

Figure 38.2 The incidence of ESRD by primary diagnosis adjusted for age and race.

3657 men and women, after adjustment for risk factors and clinical state, the group with lower arterial pressures had the greatest reduction in cardiovascular events[4]. In the Modification of Diet in Renal Disease (MDRD) trial, patients with renal insufficiency and proteinuria randomized to a mean arterial pressure of < 92 mmHg manifested significantly slower rates of decline in renal function compared to those randomized to mean pressures between 102–106 mmHg[5]. Moreover, the subgroup of African Americans randomized to the lower blood pressure in this trial had far better renal outcomes[6]. The African American Study of Kidney Disease trial, which compared two different blood pressure goals (low and usual) in this specific population, was recently completed and will definitively answer the question of whether further reductions in blood pressure to lower levels will optimally slow or stop progression of renal disease[7].

Evidence from post-hoc analyses of prospective studies, as well as retrospective studies among those with diabetes, supports the notion that arterial pressure should be reduced to levels well below 130/80 mmHg in order to maximally slow or prevent progression of nephropathy as recommended by the American Diabetes Association and the National Kidney Foundation[8,9]. A summary of the JNC VI recommendations as well as recommendations from other societies that define both the level to which blood pressure should be reduced as well as in whom these recommendations apply is presented in Table 38.1.

Finally, a discussion of the J curve is important for perspective. Since its inception in 1979, the concept that reducing diastolic blood pressure to levels below 85 mmHg was associated with a paradoxical increase in cardiovascular mortality has been controversial. A J curve exists among patients with established symptomatic coronary artery disease, unstable angina or those

Recommended blood pressure goals based on risk profile			
	JNC VI	NKF	ADA
No CV risk factors, no TOD, or clinical CV disease	< 140/90 mmHg		
No TOD or clinical CV disease and at least one CV risk factor (not diabetes)	< 140/90 mmHg		
TOD or clinical CV disease	< 130/85 mmHg		
Diabetes mellitus	< 130/85 mmHg	< 130/80 mmHg	< 130/80 mmHg
Nondiabetic renal disease	< 130/85 mmHg	< 130/85 mmHg	

Table 38.1 Recommended blood pressure goals based on risk profile.
CV, Cardiovascular; TOD, target organ damage; JNC VI, Joint National Commitee VI; NKF, National Kidney Foundation; ADA, American Diabetes Association.

High risk groups that require aggressive blood pressure reduction to protect against renal disease progression		
Patient groups	Desired BP goal	Data supporting agents in specific 'antihypertensive cocktail'
Patients with type 2 diabetes	< 130/80 mmHg	ACE inhibitors or angiotensin II receptor antagonists (ATRA)
Patients with renal insufficiency (>1.4 mg/dL)	< 130/85 mmHg	ACE inhibitors
Antihypertensive cocktail refers to the concept that more than one antihypertensive agent must be used to control blood pressure to the prescribed levels. Moreover, the agents selected should have complementary effects on mechanisms that reduce pressure		

Table 38.2 High risk groups that require aggressive blood pressure reduction to protect against renal disease progression.

who are in the immediate post myocardial infarction period[10]. However, a posthoc analysis of trials in kidney disease that have randomized subjects to different levels of blood pressure control (i.e., MDRD, African American Study of Kidney Disease and Hypertension (AASK) and the Appropriate Blood Pressure Control in Diabetes study) demonstrates no significant increase in cardiovascular events among those with renal insufficiency, proteinuria and diastolic blood pressures of below 85 mmHg compared to the group randomized to higher diastolic blood pressures[6]. Moreover, the absence of a J curve in the general population comes from the Hypertension Optimal Treatment trial. This trial did not have a higher cardiovascular event rate in the group randomized to a diastolic blood pressure of 80 mmHg[11]. Thus, each patient needs to be evaluated in the context of these observations.

The J curve should not serve as a deterrent for failing to adequately lower blood pressure to recommended levels. In the absence of any clear evidence of coronary disease or unstable angina, patients such as African Americans, who are at higher risk for renal disease, and those with diabetes or renal insufficiency should have their blood pressures aggressively reduced to levels recommended for these populations[1] (Table 38.2).

OVERVIEW OF ANTIHYPERTENSIVE DRUG MECHANISMS

The JNC has been updating its recommendations since the early 1970s. The current report (JNC VI) recommend tailoring therapy for individual groups of patients so as to reduce morbidity and mortality related to cardiovascular and renal causes by the least intrusive means possible. This tailored therapy approach is evidenced-based and considers individual patients based on their risk factor profile as well as their comorbidities[1].

There are three primary neurohumoral systems that maintain arterial pressure in humans. These neurohumoral systems include: (1) the sympathetic nervous system; (2) the renin–angiotensin–aldosterone system (RAS); and (3) arginine vasopressin in African Americans. Historically, many studies have described the state of the RAS system as a predictor of antihypertensive drug efficacy. For example, when the RAS is not activated, such as in African Americans and the elderly, antihypertensive agents that lower pressure by mechanisms that do not affect this system have been considered to have greater efficacy (i.e., calcium antagonists or diuretics).

This has led to the avoidance of certain antihypertensive agents such as angiotensin converting enzyme (ACE) inhibitors that may be clearly indicated but are not used because they 'don't lower blood pressure in these groups'. In fact, numerous studies attest to the antihypertensive efficacy of ACE inhibitors in African Americans when used in higher doses. Moreover, one ACE inhibitor, trandolapril, has a Food and Drug Administration (FDA) indication for use in African Americans to lower arterial pressure starting at double the normal initiating dose[12]. Additionally, a large prospective study failed to show any predictive value of the RAS system on antihypertensive drug response.

When the RAS is not activated, arginine vasopressin may be playing a key role in maintaining high blood pressure. A recent study demonstrated calcium antagonists lower blood pressure in African Americans, in part, through peripheral blockade of the vasopressin V_1 receptor[13].

In order to understand how to select and add-on antihypertensive medications for a given patient, the mechanisms by which a drug lowers pressure must be understood. The pharmacological mechanisms and sites of action for the seven different drug classes are shown in Fig. 38.3. The principal positive and adverse effects for each of the seven antihypertensive drug classes are summarized in Table 38.3.

SELECTION OF INITIAL DRUG THERAPY

The goal of lowering arterial pressure is to prevent the development of vascular disease and associated target organ injury (i.e., myocardial infarction, renal failure or stroke). For the purposes of this discussion, we will classify approaches to antihypertensive therapy in the uncomplicated and complicated patient.

Uncomplicated patients

An uncomplicated patient is one with an absence of comorbid conditions, such as dyslipidemia, obesity or surrogate markers of target organ disease. The JNC VI committee reviewed long-term, randomized, double-blinded controlled trials available up to 1997 and found that diuretics and, to a lesser extent, β-blockers, were the only classes of medications shown to reduce mortality from cardiovascular events in persons with uncomplicated hypertension. Thus, they are listed as the initial choice for blood pressure reduction in uncomplicated patients[1,14–16].

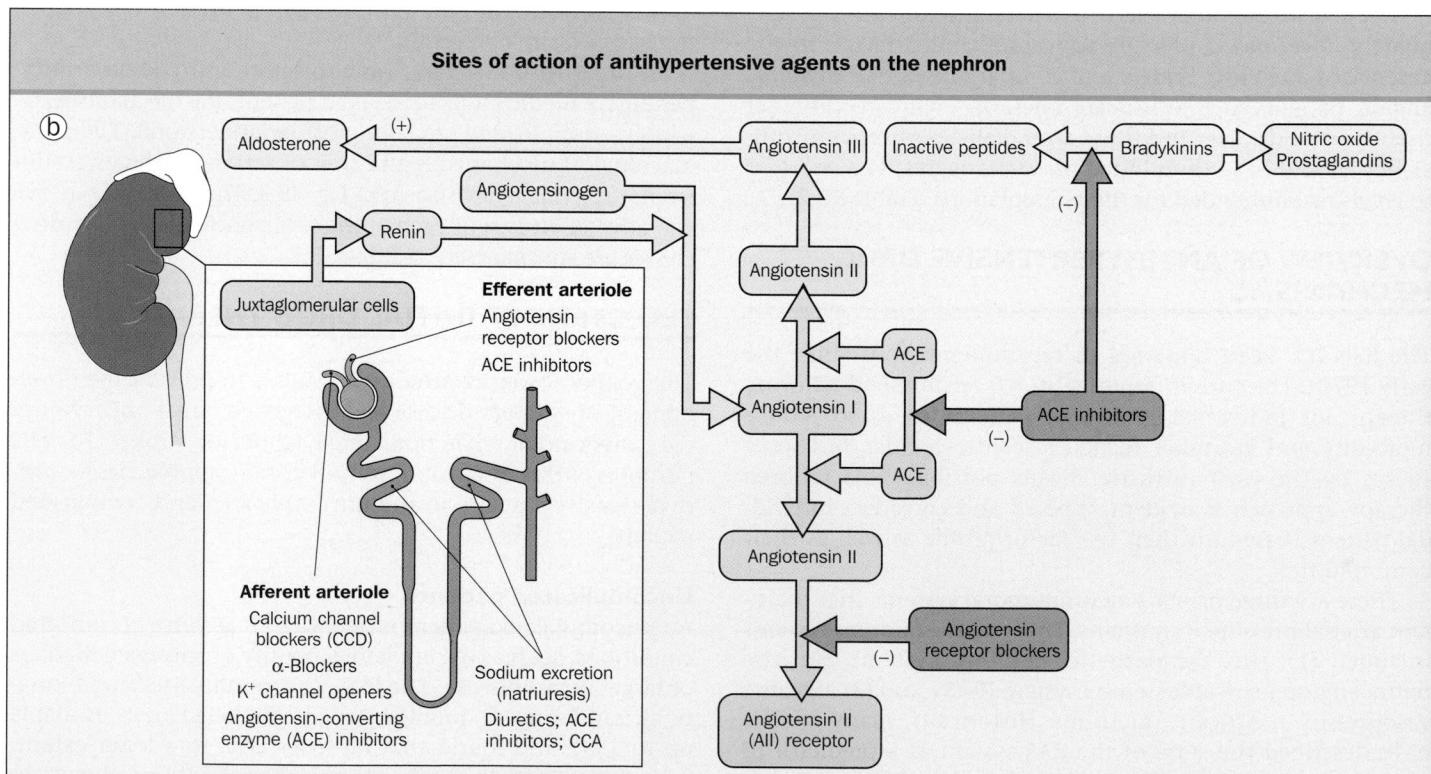

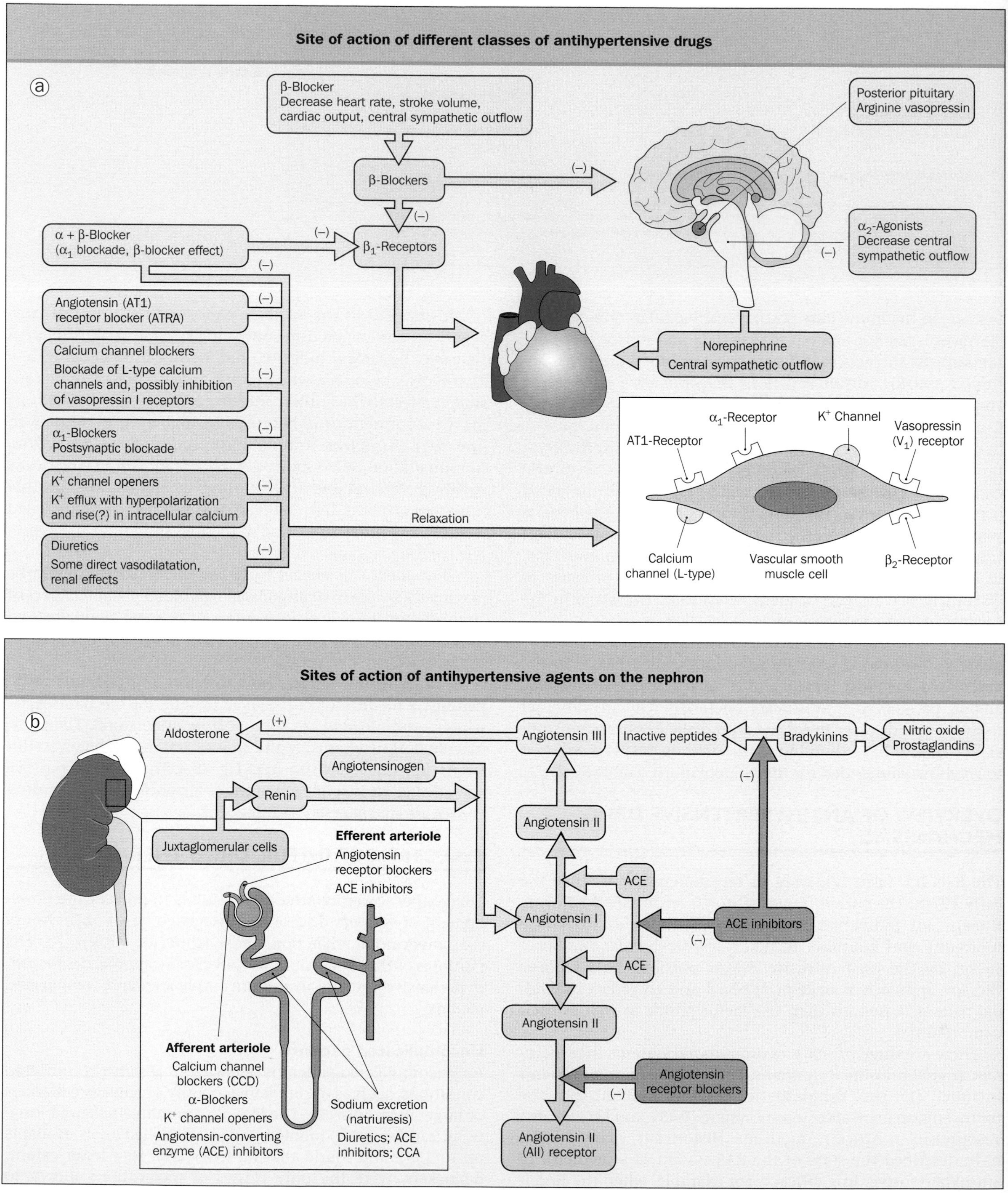

Site of action of different classes of antihypertensive drugs

(a)

β-Blocker
Decrease heart rate, stroke volume, cardiac output, central sympathetic outflow

β-Blockers

(−) → Posterior pituitary / Arginine vasopressin

(−) β₁-Receptors

α + β-Blocker (α₁ blockade, β-blocker effect) (−)

α₂-Agonists
Decrease central sympathetic outflow (−)

Angiotensin (AT1) receptor blocker (ATRA) (−)

Calcium channel blockers
Blockade of L-type calcium channels and, possibly inhibition of vasopressin I receptors (−)

Norepinephrine
Central sympathetic outflow

α₁-Blockers
Postsynaptic blockade (−)

K⁺ channel openers
K⁺ efflux with hyperpolarization and rise(?) in intracellular calcium (−)

Diuretics
Some direct vasodilatation, renal effects (−)

Relaxation

AT1-Receptor / α₁-Receptor / K⁺ Channel / Vasopressin (V₁) receptor
Calcium channel (L-type) / Vascular smooth muscle cell / β₂-Receptor

Sites of action of antihypertensive agents on the nephron

(b)

Aldosterone (+) ← Angiotensin III ← Inactive peptides ← Bradykinins → Nitric oxide / Prostaglandins

Angiotensinogen

Renin

Angiotensin II (−)

Juxtaglomerular cells

Efferent arteriole
Angiotensin receptor blockers
ACE inhibitors

Angiotensin I ← ACE ← ACE inhibitors (−)

ACE

Afferent arteriole
Calcium channel blockers (CCD)
α-Blockers
K⁺ channel openers
Angiotensin-converting enzyme (ACE) inhibitors

Sodium excretion (natriuresis)
Diuretics; ACE inhibitors; CCA

Angiotensin II

Angiotensin receptor blockers (−)

Angiotensin II (AII) receptor

Figure 38.3 Site of action and effects of different classes of antihypertensive agents. (a) Site of action by different classes of antihypertensive medications. (b) The effects of various antihypertensive agents on the nephron. (−) Inhibition of effect. (+) indicate potentiation of effect.

Common side effects associated with various classes of antihypertensive drugs	
Drug class	**Side effects**
ACE inhibitors	Cough, hyperkalemia
Angiotensin II receptor blockers (ATRA)	Much less frequent hyperkalemia compared to ACE inhibitors
Calcium channel blockers	
DHPCCAB	Pedal edema, headache
Non-DHPCCAB	Constipation (verapamil) Headache (diltiazem)
Diuretics	Frequent urination, hyperglycemia, hyperlipidemia, hyperuricemia
Central α-agonists	Sedation, dry mouth, rebound hypertension
α-Blockers	Pedal edema, orthostatic hypotension, dizziness
Central neuronal blockers (reserpine)	Depression, sedation, nasal congestion
β-Blockers	Fatigue, bronchospasm, hyperglycemia
[K+] Channel openers	Hypertrichosis(minoxidil); lupus-like reactions and pedal edema (hydralazine)

Table 38.3 Common side effects associated with various classes of antihypertensive drugs. DHPCCB, dihydropyridine CCB; Non-DHPCCB, non-dihydropyridine CCB.

Since 1997, there have been other trials with 'newer agents', most notably ACE inhibitors. The Heart Outcomes Prevention Evaluation (HOPE) study randomized over 9000 participants who were considered to be high-risk because of age and vascular disease and/or diabetes to either ramipril or placebo. Ramipril reduced the risk of cardiovascular events by 22%

overall[17]. Given that 'diseases of the heart' is the leading cause of death in the USA (accounting for 30% of deaths in 2000)[18], ACE inhibitors should be considered as an option for first-line therapy in hypertension. In addition, therapy with an ACE inhibitor resulted in 1.9 times better adherence than therapy with diuretics in a large group of hypertensive subjects[19].

Complicated patients

A complicated patient has comorbid conditions, such as diabetes and/or renal dysfunction, older age, a particular race, smoking, dyslipidemia, obesity, or evidence of surrogate markers of end-organ disease, such as left ventricular hypertrophy or microalbuminuria[1]. These comorbid conditions mandate tailoring antihypertensive therapy to optimally reduce cardiovascular risk and renal disease progression. The effects of various antihypertensive agents on these surrogate markers of target organ damage is shown in Table 38.4. Four prominent risk factors associated with a high cardiovascular mortality (left ventricular hypertrophy, microalbuminuria, dyslipidemia and renal dysfunction) in addition to the special populations of the elderly and the obese are discussed.

Left ventricular hypertrophy (LVH)

LVH results from chronic elevations in arterial pressure causing cardiac myocyte hypertrophy and remodeling of the coronary resistance vessels. This leads to perivascular fibrosis of the intramyocardial arteries and arterioles. Over time, these changes in the myocardium contribute to the development of ventricular wall stiffness and diastolic dysfunction[20].

LVH is an independent risk factor for predicting an adverse cardiovascular event[21]. In the Framingham study, there was a significant relationship between the presence of LVH and a high cardiovascular morbidity and mortality[22]. Previous studies have suggested that regression of hypertrophy is associated with improved prognosis in hypertensives[23,24]. In the Treatment of Mild Hypertension Study, although nutritional hygienic

Effects of different classes of antihypertensive agents on surrogate markers of cardiovascular disease									
	Central α-agonists	α-Blockers	α,β-Blocker	Vasodilator	β-Blockers	ACEI	ATRAs	CBBs	Diuretics
Metabolic									
Cholesterol	→	→	→	→	→*↑	→	→	→	→↑
(LDL)									
(HDL)	→	↑	→	→	→↓	→	→	→	→
Insulin resistance	→	↓	→↑	→↑	→↑	↓	↓	→	→↑
Glucose control	→	→	→	→	→↓	→↑	→	=↓→	→↓
Cardiovascular									
Left ventricular hypertrophy	↓	↓	↓	→↑	↓	↓	↓	↓	→↓
Renal									
Microalbuminuria	→	→	→↓	→↑	→↓	↓↓	↓↓	**↓→	→↓

Table 38.4 Pharmacologic effects by different classes of antihypertensive agents on surrogate markers of cardiovascular disease. HDL, High-density lipoprotein; LDL, low-density lipoprotein; ACEI, ACE inhibitor; ATRA, angiotensin II receptor antagonist; →, no effect; ↑, increase; ↓, decrease;. aOnly β-blockers with intrinsic sympathomimetic activity; only when used in high doses (e.g., 480 mg/day diltiazem, 480 mg/day verapamil, 90 mg/day nifedipine); bonly nonhydropyridine calcium blockers (CCBs, verapamil, diltiazem).

measures such as weight loss, reduced salt and alcohol intake and exercise, were effective by themselves to regress LVH, the presence of a diuretic added to the benefit[25].

There are pharmacological differences in the degree of LVH regression. A meta-analysis of randomized controlled trials revealed that ACE inhibitors were the most efficacious for regressing LVH followed by calcium channel blockers (CBBs), diuretics and β-blockers[20]. The Prospective Randomized Enalapril Study Evaluating Reversal of Ventricular Enlargement was recently completed. This study randomized participants with LVH confirmed by echocardiography to either enalapril or once-daily nifedipine with echocardiographic follow up at 6 and 12 months. Both agents significantly reduced left ventricular mass index and relative wall thickness, although there was no statistical difference between the two agents[26]. The most important factor responsible for left ventricular regression is prolonged reduction of systolic blood pressure. In contrast, direct vasodilators such as minoxidil and hydralazine, that work through opening [K+] channels, do not reduce LVH[20]. This is thought to result from profound sympathetic stimulation and subsequent increase in cardiac workload. Thus, if these agents are used to lower arterial pressure, they should always be used in the presence of a β-blocker to reduce sympathetic activity and a diuretic to counteract their effect on sodium retention. It should be noted that minoxidil has been implicated in the development of myocardial fibrosis and, hence, should be either avoided or used with agents such as spironolactone, ACE inhibitors or angiotensin II receptor blockers (ATRAs) in order to the reduce the risk of such a development[27,28].

ATRAs act by blocking AT1 receptors and are considered as substitute therapy if ACE inhibitors cannot be tolerated. The second Losartan Heart Failure Survival Study, found that there was no significant difference between losartan and captopril on all cause mortality[29]. The recently published Losartan Intervention for Endpoint reduction found that losartan was markedly superior to atenolol (a β-blocker) for reducing cardiovascular mortality in patients with hypertension and LVH[30]. Losartan was also found to significantly reduce the frequency for developing diabetes[30]. These studies suggest that ATRAs and ACE inhibitors should be first-line therapy for hypertensive subjects with LVH, especially if they have risk factors for development of diabetes.

Microalbuminuria

Microalbuminuria is not only a predictor of diabetic complications, such as diabetic nephropathy, but is also a powerful independent risk factor of cardiovascular disease (CVD) in those considered to be high-risk individuals (diabetic, obese, hypertensives)[31–34]. Microalbuminuria is defined as an abnormal urinary excretion rate of albumin between the range of 20 to 200 μg/min or 30 to 299 mg/day, which is below the detectable range with conventional dipstick methodology[35]. Although microalbuminuria has been identified as a risk factor for progression of renal disease, it is the magnitude of proteinuria that correlates with loss of renal function[33]. More importantly, numerous clinical studies have demonstrated that persons with both type 1 or type 2 diabetes and microalbuminuria have a higher CVD mortality[36,37]. Because of this,

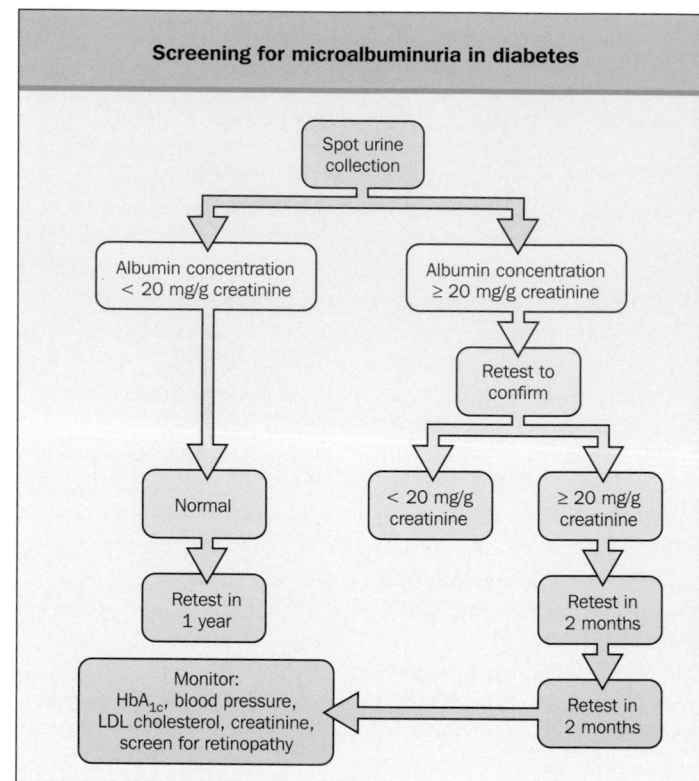

Figure 38.4 Screening for microalbuminuria in diabetes.

it should be measured in all people with diabetes (Fig. 38.4). Conversely, because of the low prevalence of microalbuminuria in the nondiabetic population and uncertainty of the significance of its modification in these groups, it is not advised that routine screening should be done in this population[38]. However, microalbuminuria prevalence among those with essential hypertension relates to both duration of blood pressure control, as well as associated lipid abnormalities, especially low-density lipoprotein levels. A recent analysis of the African American Study of Kidney Disease Trial illustrates this point. In this trial of 1094 African American individuals with hypertension and no diabetes, the strongest predictor of albuminuria at baseline was the level of low-density lipoprotein cholesterol[39]. Moreover, a recent meta-analysis of small clinical studies demonstrates decreases in microalbuminuria when HMG CoA reductase inhibitors are used to lower low-density lipoprotein levels[40]. A second related predictor was the duration of hypertension[39]. In this way, microalbuminuria may be the HbA1c of blood pressure control, since blood pressure reduction with all agents, except dihydropyridine calcium antagonists, direct acting vasodilators and central and peripheral sympathetic blockers, reduce albuminuria[41].

The merits of normalizing or reducing the level of microalbuminuria in diabetic subjects are unquestionable but there are still several unanswered questions in nondiabetic patients[38,42]. Because there are established renoprotective and cardiovascular-protective effects of lowering microalbuminuria in diabetic patients with antihypertensive regimens containing either an ACE inhibitor, ATRA, or non-dihydropyridine calcium channel blocker, one of these agents should be part of the antihypertensive regimen used in patients with micro-albuminuria[9,43,44]. The data are especially compelling for ACE inhibitors. These agents reduce albuminuria by reducing intra-glomerular pressure as well as decreasing glomerular membrane permeability. The substudy of HOPE, the Microalbuminuria, Cardiovascular, and Renal Outcomes (MICRO) HOPE, looked at whether the addition of the ACE inhibitor, ramipril, to the current regimen of patients with diabetes mellitus can lower the risk of cardiovascular events and overt nephropathy in patients with microalbuminuria. Out of 3577 participants with diabetes randomized to ramipril or placebo, 1140 were con-sidered to have microalbuminuria. Ramipril lowered the risk of the primary outcome (myocardial infarction, stroke, or car-diovascular death) by greater than 21%. Of 295 participants who developed an albumin/creatinine ratio of more than 36 mg/mmol, 117 (7%) participants on ramipril and 149 (8%) on placebo developed overt nephropathy (relative risk 24% (3–40%), $P = 0.027$). Ramipril lowered the risk of overt nephropathy in participants who did and did not have base-line microalbuminuria and led to a lower albumin/creatinine ratio[45].

ATRAs are thought to have similar renal benefits. In a recent study, 590 type 2 diabetics were randomly assigned to either irbesartan (150 or 300 mg/day) or placebo and followed for 2 years. The primary endpoint was the time from baseline to first detection of overt nephropathy (urine albumin excretion > 200 μg/min and at least a 30% increase from baseline on two consecutive visits). This endpoint occurred with signifi-cantly higher frequency in the placebo group compared to irbesartan (14.9 versus 9.7% and 5.2%, respectively, with 150 and 300 mg of irbesartan) and was not related to significant differences in blood pressure[46]. The effects of various classes of antihypertensive drugs on intrarenal hemodynamics and membrane permeability as it relates to development of albuminuria are summarized in Figure 38.5.

DIABETES

More than 11 million Americans have both diabetes and hypertension. In these patients, hypertension may account for up to 75% of all diabetes-mellitus related complications, including nephropathy and ESRD[47]. Additionally, a large number of these patients have cardiovascular events prior to progressing to ESRD. Reduction of hypertension has proven beneficial not only for reducing renal disease progression, but also for reducing cardiovascular morbidity and micro-angiopathic complications.

An important observation is that what is considered nor-motensive in people without diabetes is actually 'hyperten-sive' in diabetics. JNC VI recognized this fact by placing diabetics in the higher risk group and recommending a target blood pressure goal < 130/85 mmHg[1]. Both the National Kidney Foundation and the American Diabetes Association have recommended an even lower goal of 130/80 mm Hg or lower[8,9]. Analysis of data from a variety of studies found that the lower the blood pressure over a range of values, the greater the preservation of renal function[5,48] (Fig. 38.6). Additionally, in the Hypertension Optimal Treatment study, in which 1501 diabetic subjects were randomized to three different levels of

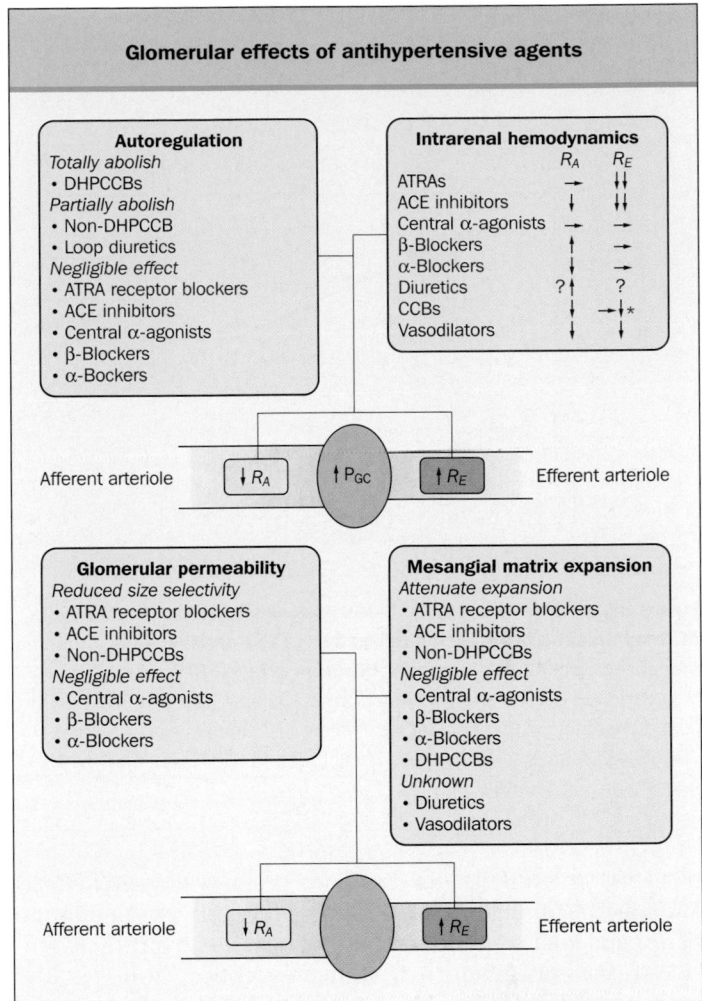

Figure 38.5 Glomerular effects of antihypertensive agents. *Some evidence exists to suggest a reduction of efferent arteriolar tone by verapamil.

diastolic blood pressure control (< 90 mmHg, < 85 mmHg and < 80 mmHg), those who achieved the lowest blood pressure goal experienced the lowest rate of cardiovascular events. Although there was only a 4 mmHg difference in the achieved diastolic blood pressure between the intensively treated group and the other groups, this resulted in a significantly lower car-diovascular event rate in the diabetes subgroup and a greater preservation of renal function[11].

The choice of the antihypertensive agents to use in diabet-ics, although important, is not a one-time decision since achieving this lower level of blood pressure requires an average of 3.2 different antihypertensive medications[9] (Fig. 38.7). JNC VI states that ACE inhibitors have a 'compelling' indication in type 1 diabetics with proteinuria and may have favorable effects in type 2 diabetics with proteinuria[1]. Clinical trials com-pleted since JNC VI was published have expanded the role of ACE inhibitors. In the HOPE trial, ramipril reduced the risk of the composite outcome (myocardial infarction, stroke, or death from any cardiovascular cause) by more than 21% in the dia-betic subpopulation[45]. Additional agents that can be added to ACE inhibitors are low-dose diuretics and/or calcium channel

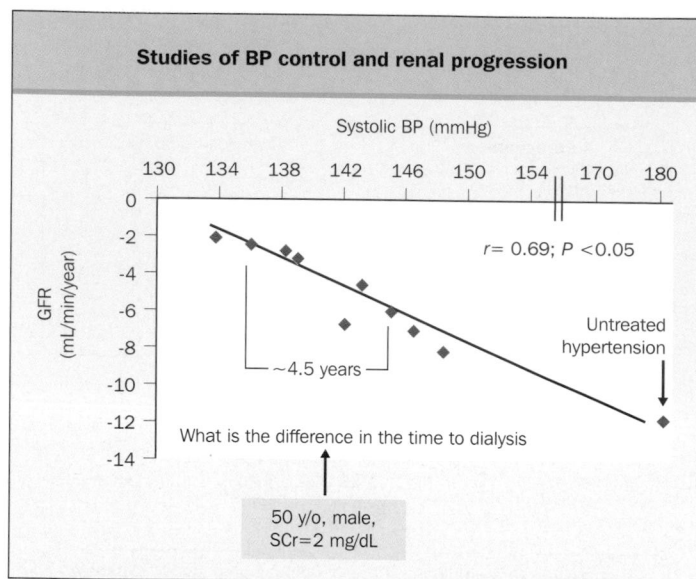

Figure 38.6 Achieved systolic blood pressure (SBP) in clinical trials of renal disease progression in relation to the calculated or measured decline in glomerular filtration rate (GFR)[47]. Given a linear progression in decline of kidney function, it is estimated that a man with a serum creatinine of 2 mg/dL (approximately 177 μmol/L) would require dialysis 4.5 years earlier if systolic blood pressure (SBP) was 145 mmHg rather than 135 mmHg.

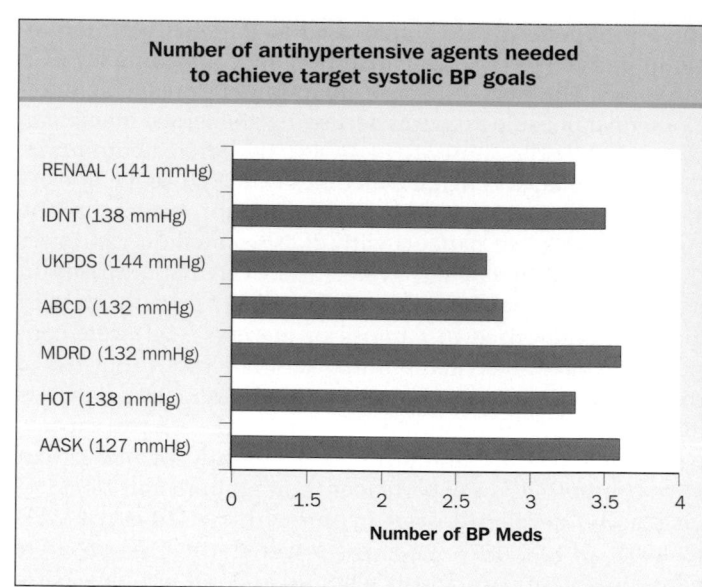

Figure 38.7 The number of antihypertensive agents used for intensive blood pressure goal. (Adapted with permission[5,11,62,85].)

blockers, which have additive blood pressure reducing effects and together antagonize side effects, such as hypokalemia and peripheral edema. β-Blockers also play a role in antihypertensive treatment, given their ability to reduce cardiovascular events and mortality. Their adverse metabolic effects in diabetics is the limiting aspect, but one β-Blocker, carvedilol, has demonstrated cardiovascular risk reduction with neutral metabolic effects. β-Blockers have additive blood pressure lowering properties if the patient has a baseline pulse rate > 84 beats/min. At pulse rates lower than this, there is little effect on blood pressure when used in combination with ACE inhibitors.

Any agent or group of agents that adequately lowers arterial pressure to levels < 130/80 mmHg will slow progression of nephropathy, but specific antihypertensive agents have properties that are more beneficial in those diabetics with nephropathy than other agents. Captopril reduced the risk of the combined endpoint of death, dialysis or transplantation in type 1 diabetics by 50% compared to other agents used to attain similar levels of blood pressure control[49]. Both the RENAAL and the IDNT showed that ATRAs reduced the risk of attaining the primary combined endpoint of doubling of serum creatinine, dialysis or transplantation or death compared to placebo, despite similar levels of blood pressure control (relative risk 16%, P = 0.02 and relative risk 19% P = 0.03, respectively)[50,51]. In addition, nondihydropyridine CBs reduce albuminuria and have additive antialbuminuric effects with ACE inhibitors independent of further reductions in blood pressure[52]. Thus, either an ACE inhibitor or ATRA should be first-line antihypertensive therapy in patients with diabetes, although other agents will undoubtedly need to be used. Although both classes of agents are well-tolerated, ATRAs have

a significantly lower incidence of cough and hyperkalemia compared to ACE inhibitors[53]. Figure 38.8 shows a recommended paradigm.

RENAL DYSFUNCTION

The available data show that aggressive blood pressure reduction (< 130/80 mmHg) is needed to maximally slow progression of renal disease, especially among patients with an elevated serum creatinine ≥ 1.4 mg/dL[1,2,5]. ACE inhibitors slow progression of diabetic nephropathy to a greater extent than other antihypertensive agents, assuming blood pressure reduction to levels around 140/90 mmHg. To assess the effect of ACE inhibitors in nondiabetic renal disease, a meta-analysis was performed which analyzed pooled individual-patient data. It was found that ACE inhibitors reduced the risk of ESRD and doubling of serum creatinine by 31% and 30%, respectively, adjusting for baseline variables, decrease in systolic blood pressure, and decrease in urinary protein excretion[54].

In spite of the evidence from many long-term clinical trials, there is a general fear by clinicians to use ACE inhibitors in such patients. This is because the initiation of ACE inhibitors often is followed by a rise in serum creatinine. While this may be a concern, it should only be worrisome if the serum potassium rises or if the creatinine continues to climb after a month of therapy (Table 38.5).

It is common to see reductions of 5–15 % in glomerular filtration rate in people within 1–4 weeks of ACE inhibitor initiation[55]. Long-term clinical trials have confirmed that this reduction in renal function plateaus within a month[55]. Moreover, after ACE inhibitors were discontinued following 10 years of therapy, GFR returned to baseline[56]. This return to baseline GFR has not been reported with other classes of antihypertensive agent studied. It should be noted that the rise in serum creatinine is most commonly seen in individuals that are

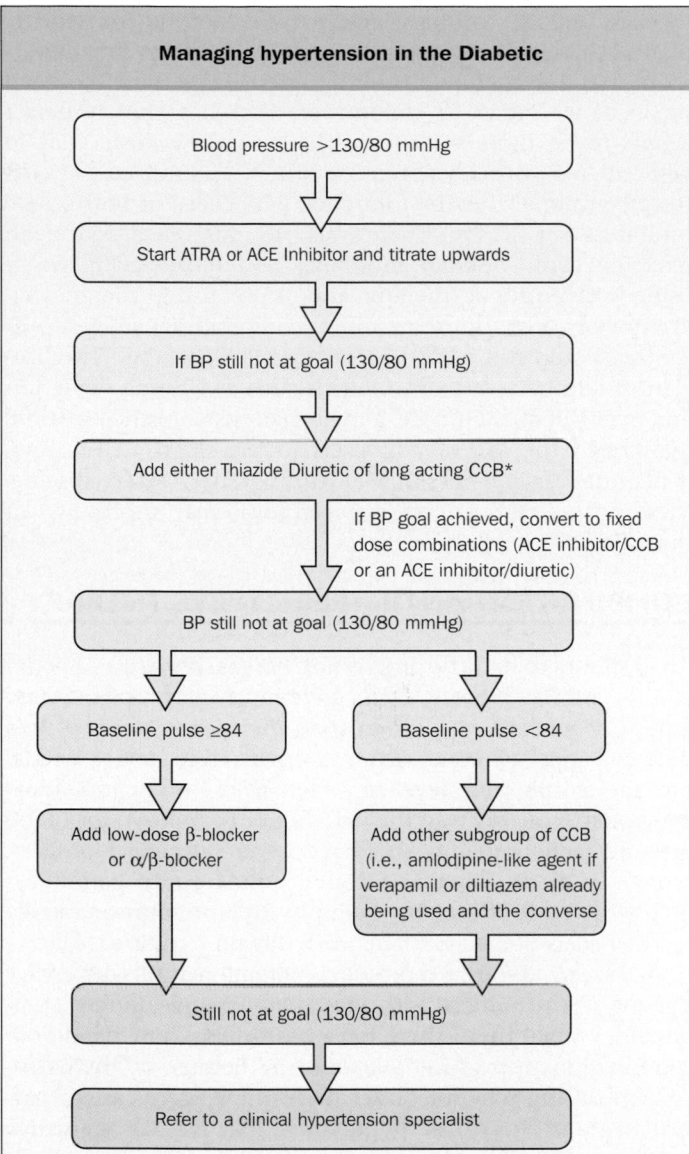

Figure 38.8 Clinical approach to managing hypertension in a diabetic patient. Everyone with diabetes mellitus, renal insufficiency, or both, should be instructed on lifestyle modifications as per the JNC VI However, initiate therapy if blood pressure (BP) is 130/85 mmHg. If BP is less than 15/10 mmHg above goal (i.e., 130/80 mmHg), then ACEs inhibitors can be used alone. Asterisk indicates that calcium channel blockers (non-dihydropyridine) have been shown to reduce cardiovascular mortality rates and progression of diabetic nephropathy independent of ACE inhibitor use. *If proteinuria present (> 300 mg per day), nondihydropyridine CBBs preferred.

over diuresed or volume depleted. However, because of the benefits of ACE inhibition in subjects with renal dysfunction, a rise in creatinine should be tolerated under certain circumstances. A review of 12 randomized clinical trials using ACE inhibitors in patients with pre-existing renal insufficiency found that a strong association existed between acute increases in serum creatinine of up to 30% that stabilized within the first 3–4 months of ACE inhibitor therapy and was with long-term preservation of renal function[57]. Thus, a useful clinical

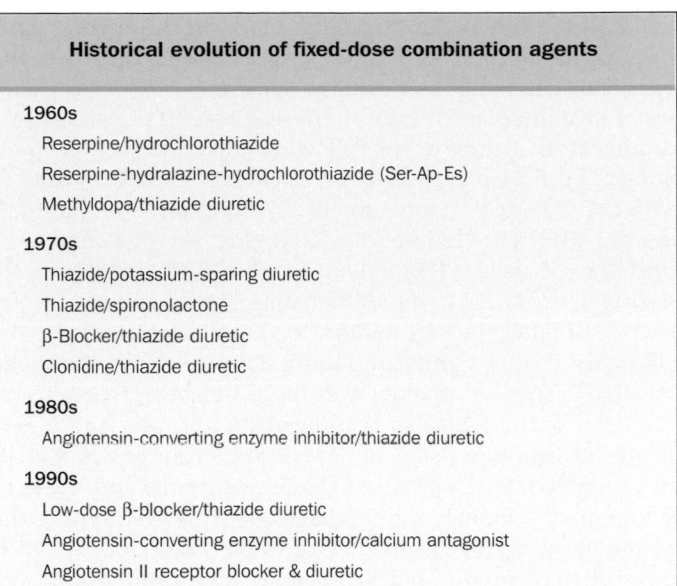

Table 38.5 Historical evolution of fixed-dose combination agents.

recommendation is that serum creatinine and potassium be checked within the first 7–14 days following initiation of an ACE inhibitor in anyone with a serum creatinine of ≥ 1.4 mg/dL, and a withdrawal of an ACE inhibitor in such patients should occur only when the rise in creatinine exceeds 30% above baseline within the first 3–4 months of therapy or if hyperkalemia develops (i.e., serum potassium levels of 5.6 mmol/L or greater) in a patient who is euvolemic[57].

Diuretics may need to be withdrawn or the dose significantly reduced for short periods of time to promote euvolemia. If the serum creatinine has risen greater than this amount, it should be rechecked within 1 week. If the creatinine continues to rise or hyperkalemia is present, then ACE inhibitors should be stopped and the patient assessed for bilateral renal arterial disease. Failure to follow this recommendation may lead to chronic irreversible renal failure.

Thus, while any class of antihypertensive agent may be used to achieve this new recommended lower level of blood pressure to preserve renal function, the following should be kept in mind. First, blood pressure will never be adequately controlled in patients with renal insufficiency without the use of a diuretic, usually a loop diuretic. Second, various combinations of medications will be needed to achieve blood pressure reduction, though these 'antihypertensive cocktails' should contain an ACE inhibitor. If side effects are noted with the ACE inhibitor, an ATRA may be substituted to ensure renal protection and blood pressure reduction. However, while animal studies clearly demonstrate similar efficacy between ACE inhibitors and ATRAs in regard to renal preservation, clinical trials have not yet demonstrated this effect in nondiabetic renal disease, although ATRAs may be the preferred class for treatment of diabetic nephropathy.

OBESITY AND THE METABOLIC SYNDROME

The metabolic syndrome is a condition that promotes atherosclerosis and increases the risk of cardiovascular events. The hallmark features include dyslipidemia, a prothrombotic state, insulin resistance, hypertension and abdominal obesity[58]. The National Cholesterol Education Program Adult Treatment Panel III states that to establish the diagnosis of metabolic syndrome, at least three of the following criteria need to be present: (1) a waist circumference > 102 cm (40 inches) for men or > 88 cm (37 inches) for women; (2) triglyceride levels ≥ 150 mg/dL; (3) HDL cholesterol < 40 mg/dL for men and < 50 mg/dL for women; (4) blood pressure ≥ 130/85 mmHg; or (5) fasting glucose ≥ 110 mg/dL[59]. Using similar criteria, it has been estimated that 50 million to 75 million people in the USA may exhibit significant manifestations of this syndrome by 2010[60]. These components are highly related. Hypertension has been well established as a metabolic disorder and is predictive of insulin resistance[61]. In addition, as many as 50% of hypertensives have comorbid insulin resistance and hyperinsulinemia[62]. Optimal management of hypertension in the metabolic syndrome through aggressive reduction of blood pressure may improve both cholesterol levels and insulin sensitivity. JNC VI discusses specific pharmacological therapy in this population of patients[1]. High-dose thiazide diuretics may worsen insulin resistance, and β-blockers may confer an increased risk of general side effects[63,64]. Conversely, ACE inhibitors reduce blood pressure through vasodilation, which may actually improve insulin resistance by increasing insulin-mediated glucose uptake. Because of this action, ACE inhibitors may improve insulin sensitivity and may be especially appropriate in those with the metabolic syndrome[65], a property also seen with ATRAs[66]. In addition, given the propensity for development of impaired glucose tolerance and increased cardiovascular risk in this population, trials with agents that benefit diabetics need to be considered when it comes to choosing an antihypertensive agent in those with the metabolic syndrome. Results from the HOPE study, which showed the benefit of ACE inhibitors in high-risk patients both with and without diabetes, along with the beneficial effects of ACE inhibitors on insulin-resistance, suggest that ACE inhibitors should be included in the antihypertensive regimen used in patients with the metabolic syndrome. ATRAs can be substituted if ACE inhibitors cannot be tolerated.

ELDERLY

Isolated systolic hypertension increases in prevalence as people age related to increasing arterial stiffness (and thus loss of arterial compliance) which leads to an increase in systolic blood pressure and actually a decrease in diastolic blood pressure[67]. The importance of treating isolated systolic hypertension in this age group was explored in a recent meta-analysis. Staessen et al. found that a 10 mmHg increase in systolic blood pressure was significantly and independently correlated with increases by nearly 10% in the risk of all fatal and nonfatal complications, except for coronary events. At any given level of systolic blood pressure, the risk of death rose with lower diastolic blood pressure, thereby suggesting that pulse pressure (difference between systolic and diastolic blood pressure) was an important predictor of cardiovascular risk. Antihypertensive therapy reduced the risk of stroke by 33% and of coronary events by 23%[68]. As for specific pharmacological recommendations, JNC VI states that diuretics be first-line therapy in this age-group, and there has been no evidence since its publication that has shown newer agents to be more effective[1]. The second Swedish Trial in Old Patients with Hypertension study randomized patients to conventional therapy (diuretics, β-blockers, or both), ACE inhibitors, or CCBs. There was no difference found in reducing cardiovascular morbidity and mortality in those using conventional therapy and those using the 'newer' agents[69]. As such, diuretics, unless comorbidities suggest otherwise, should still be considered first-line therapy. The clinician should be aware of problems such as volume depletion and hypokalemia. Of note, a meta-analysis published in 1998 questioned the use of β-blockers in the elderly, citing evidence that, except in subjects with coronary artery disease, these agents did not reduce cardiovascular morbidity or mortality[70].

COMBINATION ANTIHYPERTENSIVE THERAPY

An ideal way to halt the progression of renal disease and better control arterial pressure is to combine two complementary groups of medications. Lower than therapeutic doses of two different drugs are combined in a single pill to reduce arterial pressure to the same level as a higher dose of an individual component. In this way they are not only additive for blood pressure reduction, but also have lower side effect profiles. Moreover, many fixed-dose combinations act to counteract each other's side effects. For example, ACE inhibitors markedly reduce pedal edema associated with dihydropyridine CCBs.

In the early 1960s, fixed-dose combination antihypertensive therapy was introduced with a reserpine/thiazide diuretic combination. Since then, there have been many new fixed-dose combinations introduced (Table 38.5). Because of their convenient dosing schedule, once daily, these agents are of particular use in 'high-risk' populations that require aggressive reduction of blood pressure. Thus, the physician may now select agents with complementary modes of action that minimize side effects and maximize compliance in order to achieve better rates of blood pressure control. A detailed discussion of this topic is beyond the scope of this chapter but is reviewed elsewhere[71,72].

REFRACTORY HYPERTENSION

Failure to adequately reduce blood pressure may be a result of multiple factors including secondary causes of hypertension and noncompliance[1]. However, a very common cause of uncontrolled blood pressure is related to concomitant over-the-counter medications, the two most prevalent types being nonsteriod anti-inflammatory agents, such as ibuprofen, and sympathomimetics, such as a pseudoephedrine, in cold preparations. Additionally, oral contraceptive and steroid medications will blunt the antihypertensive effect of most agents. In prospective studies only CCBs and, to a lesser degree, diuretics, maintain their antihypertensive effects in the presence of these symptom relieving medications.

Sexual dysfunction

A common cause of refractory hypertension in males is non-compliance secondary to the development of impotence. Almost all medications have been implicated in causing impotence; however, the incidence is highest for the central α_2 agonists, diuretics and β-blockers. However, in most cases, with the exception of the central α_2 agonists and possibly β-blockers, the drug is only the indirect cause of the problem[73].

The primary problem of impotence relates to abnormal vascular homeostasis within the penile circulation dampens intrapenile blood pressure. Thus, when blood pressure is dramatically reduced and maintained at lower levels, there is a period of readjustment. In many cases, impotence resolves on its own but may take as long as 4–6 months[73]. Thus, all patients, including diabetics without neuropathy, should be encouraged to stay on their medications if arterial pressure is controlled because the problem should resolve.

MALIGNANT HYPERTENSION/ HYPERTENSIVE CRISES

Malignant hypertension' was the term originally used to classify patients who presented with severely elevated BP and signs or symptoms of acute target organ damage[74]. Such patients were unlikely to survive a year. The dramatic advancements in therapy and a correspondingly improved prognosis for afflicted patients have led to the evolution of the terms hypertensive urgency and hypertensive emergency. The terminology of malignant hypertension is now replaced by 'Hypertensive Crises'. Nearly all authorities[75] (including the authors of the JNC VI)[1] have accepted the revised terminology.

Hypertensive emergency, as defined by JNC VI, is a severely elevated blood pressure with signs and symptoms of acute end organ damage i.e., encephalopathy, intracranial hemorrhage, chest pain, myocardial infarction, aortic dissection, pulmonary edema, eclampsia, microscopic hematuria with acute renal failure. Patients must be hospitalized and treated immediately with parenteral drug therapy. The blood pressure should be reduced by 25% in 1–2 h and then towards a goal of 130–160/100 mmHg over the next several hours. A rapid drop in blood pressure should be avoided because it may precipitate cerebral or cardiac ischemia. Patients sometimes present with very high blood pressures, but without evidence of acute target organ damage; this situation is considered a 'hypertensive urgency' and need not be treated either in the hospital setting or using intravenous medication. A physician taking care of a patient with elevated blood pressures needs to be able to distinguish between these two situations, for two major reasons. The route of administration of drug therapy is different (parental therapy is typical for emergencies, whereas oral therapy can be given for urgencies), and hospitalization (usually in the intensive care unit) is almost always necessary for hypertensive emergencies, but rarely required for hypertensive urgencies.

The most common presentation of severe hypertension is that of an asymptomatic patient with Stage III hypertension (typically = 200/120 mmHg) who is seen for an unrelated complaint, with a normal physical examination and stable (if not normal) laboratory results. This patient is not having a hypertensive crisis, and requires only a prescription for an antihypertensive drug, and an appointment for follow-up within 24–48 h[76]. In such cases, every effort should be made to ensure that the patient is seen as scheduled, and that the blood pressure has been lowered out of a potentially dangerous range.

In most clinical settings, the typical antecedent history involves a hypertensive person who discontinued treatment or reduced therapy without having the blood pressure checked thereafter. In a large series from New York City, not having a primary care physician (available to refill antihypertensive medication prescriptions) was the single most important risk factor for presenting to a hospital Emergency Department with severely elevated blood pressure[77]. Occasionally, withdrawal of antihypertensive medications, especially drugs such as clonidine, or ingestion of substances that raise blood pressure, is responsible for hypertensive emergency. The Public Health data from Georgia suggests that nonadherence to chronic antihypertensive therapy (due to lack of a primary care physician or funds to pay for antihypertensive medications) is the primary reason for hypertensive emergencies in the USA today.

Hypertensive crises are more likely to occur in patients with certain forms of secondary hypertension, particularly renovascular disease or pheochromocytoma. Crises are rare in patients with mineralocorticoid excess states (e.g., primary hyperaldosteronism), perhaps because blood pressure rises more gradually or because renin secretion tends to be suppressed as a result of chronic volume expansion[78]. An evaluation for secondary causes of hypertension is a routine part of the care of a person with a hypertensive crisis and is typically undertaken after the patient is stable. The structural compensatory changes and the attendant functional shift of the autoregulatory range explain why chronically hypertensive patients can often tolerate very high blood pressures without problems, and why normotensive, or those with only a recent onset or rapidly-increasing blood pressure, can develop hypertensive crises at relatively lower blood pressure levels.

The organ systems that require special attention during the initial evaluation of the patient a hypertensive crisis include the neurological, ophthalmologic, cardiac, renal and peripheral vasculature. The patients with either new hemorrhages/exudates or papilledema represent a hypertensive crisis. High-grade retinopathy and hypertensive crises in general, are extremely unusual in patients with primary hyperaldosteronism. The presence of an abdominal bruit (with both a systolic and diastolic component) suggests the presence of renovascular hypertension[79]. The radiofemoral pulse delay due to a coarctation of the aorta should not be missed on clinical examination. Occasionally, palpation of a pheochromocytoma can initiate a typical episode and suggest the diagnosis. Assessment of renal function is crucial. It is important to compare the presenting serum creatinine with a recent measurement of the patient's renal function, because an acute deterioration in renal function in the presence of very elevated blood pressure is classified as a hypertensive crisis. The presence of gross or microscopic hematuria at presentation is consistent with acute renal damage due to very elevated blood pressures. Red cell casts and significant proteinuria generally mean that acute glomerulonephritis is the cause of the elevated blood pressure and subsequent crisis.

Treatment of hypertensive emergencies			
Medications	**Mechanism**	**Dose (onset of action)**	**Side effects**
Vasodilators			
Sodium nitroprusside	↑ Cyclic GMP Blocks cell [Ca^{++}]	0.25–10 µg/kg/min (Immediate)	Nausea, severe hypotension, Thiocyanate toxicity (check levels every 48 h especially in renal failure
Nitroglycerine	↑ Nitrate receptors	5–100 µg/min (2-5 min)	Headache, vomiting, methemoglobinemia, tachyphylaxis
Hydralazine	Opens [K$^+$] channels	10–50 mg I.V./I.M. every 4–6 h (15–30 min)	Hypotension, reflex sympathetic stimulation, exacerbaate angina, MI
Diazoxide	Direct acting	50–150 mg every 5 min or 15–30 mg/min (2–4 min)	Nausea, flushing, reflex sympathetic stimulation, exacerbate angina, MI
Fenoldopam	Dopamine (DA$_1$) receptor agonist	0.1–0.3 µg/kg/min (<5 min)	Tachycardia, headache, nausea, flushing
Nicardipine	CCB	5–15 mg every hour I.V. (1–5 min)	Hypotension, tachycardia, nausea, vomiting, phlebitis
Enalaprilat	ACE inhibitor	0.625–1.25 mg every 6 h (15–30 min)	Severe hypotension, delayed excretion in renal failure
Labetalol	α,β-blocker	20–80 mg I.V. bolus every 10 min or 0.5–2.0 mg/min Infusion (5–10 min)	Nausea, hypotension, asthma, CHF, formication
Treatment of hypertensive urgency			
Captopril	ACE inhibitor	25 mg every 1–2 h 15–30 min	Angioedema, acute renal failure
Clonidine	Central α$_2$ agonist	0.1–0.2 mg every 1–2 h 30–60 min	Hypotension, sedation, dry mouth
Labetalol	α,β-blocker	200–400 mg every 2–3 h 30–120 min	Heart block, bronchoconstriction, orthostatic hypotension
Nifedipine	CCB	Used frequently in hypertensive emergency however has potential for abrupt hypotension with risk for stroke, angina, myocardial infarction or sudden death	

Table 38.6 Treatment of hypertensive emergencies and urgencies.

Most authorities suggest that in most true hypertensive emergencies (with the exception of aortic dissection and some neurological crises), the mean arterial pressure should be reduced only 10–15% during the first hour. Gradually thereafter, a diastolic blood pressure target between 100 and 110 mmHg (or a reduction in 25% compared to the initial baseline, whichever is higher) is appropriate. Reduction of blood pressure to less than 90 mmHg diastolic, or even by as little as 35% of the initial mean arterial pressure, has been associated with major organ dysfunction, coma and death, even in recent years.

The goal in a hypertensive crisis is to lower the patient's blood pressure gradually over 6–24 h. An intravenously administered medication with a short duration of action is almost always used for this purpose, since the hypotensive effect of the drug can be promptly reversed if the response is excessive (Table 38.6). With a short-acting, intravenous drug, the clinician has much tighter control over both the rates of blood pressure decline and the ultimate blood pressure target. For many years, sodium nitroprusside was the standard intravenously administered drug for all hypertensive crises. Nitroprusside has an onset of action within 2–3 min, serum half-life of 1–2 min, may be easily titrated, is inexpensive, and has a long record of effectiveness in treating hypertensive crises of nearly all types. Limitations of nitroprusside therapy include the need for invasive monitoring (an arterial line is required in many hospitals), and its metabolic products (thiocyanate and cyanide), which contraindicate its use in pregnancy, and accumulate when nitroprusside is used in patients with renal or hepatic dysfunction. Nitroprusside is typically begun at 0.3 µg/kg/min, and increased by 0.2–1.0 µg/kg/min every 3–5 min until the blood pressure reaches the target range. Once the effective dose of nitroprusside has been found, an oral medication should also be started.

Two other drugs approved in the US in hypertensive crises are being increasingly used; neither has potentially toxic metabolites. Nicardipine, a dihydropyridine CCB, may have a special role in patients with coronary disease or after cardiac surgery[80]. Fenoldopam mesylate, a dopamine-1 agonist, was approved in 1997. The drug acts on receptors that are located in the renal and splanchnic arteries with lesser density in the coronary and cerebral arteries. However, intravenous fenoldopam does not cross the blood brain barrier and has no central nervous activity because it is a poorly lipid soluble molecule. In clinical trials against nitroprusside fenoldopam demonstrates beneficial renal effects (increased diuresis, natriuresis, and creatinine clearance) over nitroprusside[81]. Fenoldopam probably is most useful for blood pressure reduction in patients with renal impairment and those undergoing vascular surgery[82]. In addition, fenoldopam is not associated with any thiocyanate toxicity and is not degraded by light. Both nicardipine and fenoldopam are more expensive than nitroprusside but often can be given with just a blood pressure cuff to monitor the effects outside an ICU. The total cost of care may be lower with either of these than with nitroprusside, which in most hospitals is used only in an ICU with an arterial line in place. However, no outcome studies have yet had sufficient power to demonstrate the potential benefits of these agents against the time-tested standard, nitroprusside. The adverse effects are similar to any vasodilator, which include headache, flushing, dizziness, tachycardia or bradycardia. Of note, two important adverse effects were noted during the fenoldopam studies. One is the T wave flattening on the electrocardiogram in all leads except aVR without evidence of myocardial ischemia. It has been speculated that acute reductions in blood pressure might be responsible for this finding. This also occurs with nitroprusside. The second adverse effect is increased intraocular pressure, which has been attributed in part to diminished drainage of aqueous humor. Thus, cautious administration of fenoldopam, if at all, in patients with glaucoma or high intraocular pressures has been recommended. Fenoldopam is typically begun at 0.1 µg/kg/min, and increased at 20-min intervals by 0.1–0.2 µg/kg/min, with a maximum dose of 1.5 µg/kg/min.

There are several other drugs being investigated for use in hypertensive crisis but are not yet FDA approved for use in the USA. These include urapidil (an α-blocker which also interferes with both central and peripheral uptake of serotonin), intravenous felodipine (a dihydropyridine CCB), and lacidipine (a dihydropyridine CCB).

Other intravenously administered antihypertensive drugs are most useful only in specific clinical situations. Nimodipine (either oral or intravenous) has been associated with improved outcomes after subarachnoid hemorrhage, but its use in acute stroke is controversial. Its beneficial effects may be more related to preserving neurons in peril by limiting calcium influx into ischemic cells rather than to its hypotensive effects. The usual dose is 60 mg (two 30-mg capsules) every 4 h for 21 days after the neurological event. Nitroglycerin is useful in the setting of

angina pectoris, coronary artery bypass surgery, or neurosurgery, but is now being replaced in some hospitals by nicardipine. It has the disadvantages of being unstable in solution, adhering to intravenous line leading to tolerance during prolonged administration, and causing profound headaches. It is typically begun at 5 µg/min, and the dose increased every 3–5 min by 5–10 µg/min, as needed. Phentolamine is a nonselective α-antagonist and is very useful in pheochromocytoma and other catecholamine excess states. It is typically delivered in 2–5-mg 'minibolus' injections, in order to minimize precipitous falls in blood pressure.

The choice of drugs for the treatment of a hypertensive urgency is currently much broader than for emergencies, since almost all antihypertensive drugs lower BP effectively and reasonably rapidly (Table 38.6). The drug of choice should be effective, quick-acting, and unlikely to cause alterations in mental status or to produce hypotension. Nifedipine, clonidine, labetalol and captopril are often used. The dangers of short-acting nifedipine were highlighted in 1996[83]. The issue with nifedipine capsules is not that they are ineffective in lowering BP, but that their effects are somewhat unpredictable. The FDA declined to approve this approach to treatment. Several other dihydropyridine CCBs have been reported to be effective in treating hypertensive urgencies. As might be expected from their pharmacokinetics, both nicardipine and isradipine have a slightly longer onset of action and are less likely to cause the precipitous falls in blood pressure seen occasionally with nifedipine.

Although clonidine effectively controls blood pressure, there is a significant risk of hypertensive urgency in those patients who are nonadherent given the danger of 'rebound hypertension' associated with clonidine withdrawal. In Brazil, oral captopril is a common drug for hypertensive urgencies; it is typically given in a 12.5–25 mg dose, crushed to hasten absorption. ACE inhibitors must be used with caution, since either can cause or exacerbate renal impairment in the occasional patient with critical renal artery stenosis. Parenteral hydralazine has been reformulated, and typically is the first parental drug given in obstetrics for hypertensive urgencies. Minoxidil has been used effectively, when patients present with uncontrolled hypertension but already taking a diuretic and a β-blocker. Recent reviews suggest that each of these drugs is effective in approximately 85–95% of hypertensive urgencies with an approximate equal tolerability.

The unanswered question is whether it is really necessary to give any particular antihypertensive medication to most people with hypertensive urgency. Many Emergency Departments have 'standard operating procedures' which prohibit release of patients into the community with blood pressures in excess of 180/110 mmHg. Primarily medicolegal concerns, rather than medical and therapeutic principles, generate these policies.

HYPERTENSION IN PREGNANCY

General treatment recommendations for hypertension in pregnancy are discussed in Chapters 44 and 45. For hypertensive crises, the first choice of antihypertensive therapy is complicated, because there are two patients who must be considered, the mother and the baby. Drugs with teratogenic potential (e.g., nitroprusside, ACE inhibitors and ATRAs) are contraindicated. Although most obstetricians prefer $MgSO_4$ and methyldopa for inpatient and outpatient treatment of hypertension, respectively, parenteral hydralazine or labetolol is the typical drug chosen for initial treatment of pre-eclampsia.

SCLERODERMA RENAL CRISIS

Scleroderma renal crisis is defined as a new onset of accelerated hypertension and/or rapidly progressive renal failure and is deemed a medical emergency. It requires hospitalization and parenteral drug therapy, occurs in 10–25% of patients with scleroderma (systemic sclerosis), and is associated with diverse outcomes. Diffuse skin involvement, rapid progression of skin thickening, new onset anemia, disease duration of less than 4 years, presence of anti-RNA polymerase antibody, new cardiac events such as congestive heart failure and pericardial effusion and use of high glucocorticoids may be predictors of scleroderma renal crisis. When associated with thrombocytopenia, hyperreninemia and hemolytic anemia, it carries the poorest prognosis. The vascular changes of intimal proliferation, medial thinning and increased collagen deposition in the adventitial layer of the small renal arteries, result in decreased renal blood flow, hypertension and progressive renal impairment. Interestingly, many patients may initially present in a renal crisis as a manifestation of their disease. The mainstay of treatment is an ACE-inhibitor or an ATRA and additional agents (i.e., nondihydropyridine calcium channel blocker or other vasodilators, as necessary) to control blood pressure. This treatment slows the progression to ESRD[84]. The fact that scleroderma renal crisis is declining in frequency is consistent with the observation that renal disease has been superseded by cardiopulmonary complications as the leading cause of death in systemic sclerosis.

NEWER AGENTS: MOXONIDINE

Increased sympathetic tone, which controls arterial tone, has been associated with the development and maintenance of hypertension. The sympathetic nervous system can be modulated centrally with moxonidine, a second-generation centrally acting antihypertensive. It acts specifically at I1-imidazoline receptors within the vasomotor center to reduce synaptic drive to sympathetic neurons and has low affinity for α_2-adrenergic receptors[85].

Moxonidine in comparative drug studies is similar to enalapril in both diastolic and systolic blood pressure reductions[86]. It also appears to lower the early morning surges of blood pressure. This may be beneficial in the prevention of myocardial infarction and related coronary events that occur more frequently in early morning hours secondary to a catecholamine surge[85].

Moxonidine is a sympathoplegic agent, which reduces albuminuria and the development of glomerulosclerosis in a blood pressure-independent manner. Low-dose moxonidine caused a highly significant decrease in urinary albumin despite having little effect on blood pressure. The agent reduces central sympathetic activity, which reduces efferent sympathetic stimulation to the kidney. However, as promising as this appears, more clinical investigation needs to be performed[85]. The common adverse effects are headache, dizziness and tiredness, as well as causing a dry mouth like clonidine. However, unlike clonidine, there is no rebound hypertension when moxonidine is abruptly stopped[85].

DRUG CONTROVERSIES

α-Blockers
The ALLHAT trial compared doxazosin and chlorthalidone as primary antihypertensive agents. Because of an increased number of cardiovascular events including heart failure and strokes that occurred, the doxazosin arm of the study was terminated early. Specifically, users of doxazosin had a 25% increased risk of cardiovascular events and were two times more likely to be hospitalized. At present α-blockers should not be considered as a first line therapy, especially in those with risk factors for coronary artery disease[87].

Calcium channel blockers
A meta-analysis of randomized controlled trials evaluating health outcomes with CCBs compared to other first line therapies showed no significant differences in the reduction in systolic or diastolic blood pressures between these groups. Also, no significant differences were found for the outcomes of stroke and all-cause mortality. However, the odds ratios for the dihydropyridine CCBs versus other antihypertensive treatment were significantly higher for the outcomes of acute myocardial infarction, congestive heart failure and combined cardiovascular events. The etiology of these findings has been debated for some time and it has been postulated that CCBs may have proinflammatory effects, antifibrinolytic effects and may promote sympathetic activation, all of which are established cardiovascular risk factors[88].

More recently, a study compared irbesartan and amlodipine in patients with nephropathy due to type 2 diabetes and found that the risk of doubling the serum creatinine was 37% lower in the irbesartan group than in the amlodipine group. In addition, the serum creatinine concentration increased 21% more slowly in patients in the irbesartan group than in those in the amlodipine group. Proteinuria was reduced on average by 33% in the irbesartan group compared to 6% in the amlodipine group. Overall, the patients in the amlodipine group had worse renal outcomes than in those in the irbesartan group despite equal control of blood pressure within the amlodipine group[50]. Thus, therapeutic decisions should be tailored to the entire clinical picture, risks and benefits of the drug, and the patient's risk profile.

REFERENCES

1. The sixth report of the Joint National Committee on prevention, detection, evaluation, and treatment of high blood pressure. Arch Intern Med. 1997;157:2413–46.
2. Perry HM Jr, Miller JP, Fornoff JR, et al. Early predictors of 15-year end-stage renal disease in hypertensive patients. Hypertension. 1995;25:587–94.
3. Staessen JA, Wang JG, Thijs L. Cardiovascular protection and blood pressure reduction: a meta-analysis. Lancet. 2001;358: 1305–15.
4. Sowers JR, Farrow SL. Treatment of elderly hypertensive patients with diabetes, renal disease, and coronary heart disease. Am J Geriatr Cardiol. 1996;5:57–70.
5. Peterson JC, Adler S, Burkart JM, et al. Blood pressure control, proteinuria, and the progression of renal disease. The Modification of Diet in Renal Disease Study. Ann Intern Med. 1995;123:754–62.
6. Lazarus JM, Bourgoignie JJ, Buckalew VM, et al. Achievement and safety of a low blood pressure goal in chronic renal disease. The Modification of Diet in Renal Disease Study Group. Hypertension. 1997;29:641–50.
7. Wright JT Jr, Kusek JW, Toto RD, et al. Design and baseline characteristics of participants in the African American Study of Kidney Disease and Hypertension (AASK) Pilot Study. Control Clin Trials. 1996;17:3S–16S.
8. American Diabetes Association. Clinical practice recommendations 2002. Diabetes Care. 2002;25:S33–49.
9. Bakris G, Williams M, Dworkin L, et al. Preserving renal function in adults with hypertension and diabetes: a consensus approach. Am J Kidney Dis. 2000;36:646–61.
10. Farnett L, Mulrow CD, Linn WD, et al. The J-curve phenomenon and the treatment of hypertension. Is there a point beyond which pressure reduction is dangerous? JAMA 1991;265:489–95.
11. Hansson L, Zanchetti A, Carruthers SG, et al. Effects of intensive blood-pressure lowering and low-dose aspirin in patients with hypertension: principal results of the Hypertension Optimal Treatment (HOT) randomised trial. HOT Study Group. Lancet. 1998;351:1755–62.
12. Weir MR, Gray JM, Paster R, Saunders E. Differing mechanisms of action of angiotensin-converting enzyme inhibition in black and white hypertensive patients. The Trandolapril Multicenter Study Group. Hypertension. 1995;26:124–30.
13. Bakris G, Bursztyn M, Gavras I, et al. Role of vasopressin in essential hypertension: racial differences. J Hypertens. 1997;15:545–50.
14. Prevention of stroke by antihypertensive drug treatment in older persons with isolated systolic hypertension. Final results of the Systolic Hypertension in the Elderly Program (SHEP). SHEP Cooperative Research Group. JAMA. 1991;265:3255–64.
15. Bakris GL, Kusmirek SL, Smith AC, et al. Calcium antagonism abolishes the antipressor action of vasopressin (V1) receptor antagonism. Am J Hypertens. 1997;10:1153–8.
16. Soriano JB, Hoes AW, Meems L, Grobbee DE. Increased survival with beta-blockers: importance of ancillary properties. Prog Cardiovasc Dis. 1997;39:445–56.
17. Yusuf S, Sleight P, Pogue J, et al. Effects of an angiotensin-converting-enzyme inhibitor, ramipril, on cardiovascular events in high-risk patients. The Heart Outcomes Prevention Evaluation Study Investigators. N Engl J Med. 2000;342:145–53.
18. Minino A, Smith B. Deaths: preliminary data for 2000. National Vital Statistics Reports; 2000:49.
19. Monane M, Bohn RL, Gurwitz JH, et al. The effects of initial drug choice and comorbidity on antihypertensive therapy compliance: results from a population-based study in the elderly. Am J Hypertens. 1997;10:697–704.
20. Devereux RB. Do antihypertensive drugs differ in their ability to regress left ventricular hypertrophy? Circulation. 1997;95:1983–5.
21. Koren MJ, Devereux RB, Casale PN, et al. Relation of left ventricular mass and geometry to morbidity and mortality in uncomplicated essential hypertension. Ann Intern Med. 1991; 114:345–52.
22. Levy D, Garrison RJ, Savage DD, et al. Prognostic implications of echocardiographically determined left ventricular mass in the Framingham Heart Study. N Engl J Med. 1990;322:1561–6.
23. Muiesan ML, Salvetti M, Rizzoni D, et al. Association of change in left ventricular mass with prognosis during long-term antihypertensive treatment. J Hypertens. 1995;13:1091–5.
24. Verdecchia P, Schillaci G, Borgioni C, et al. Prognostic significance of serial changes in left ventricular mass in essential hypertension. Circulation. 1998;97:48–54.
25. Neaton JD, Grimm RH Jr, Prineas RJ, et al. Treatment of Mild Hypertension Study. Final results. Treatment of Mild Hypertension Study Research Group. JAMA. 1993;270:713–24.
26. Devereux RB, Palmieri V, Sharpe N, et al. Effects of once-daily angiotensin-converting enzyme inhibition and calcium channel blockade-based antihypertensive treatment regimens on left ventricular hypertrophy and diastolic filling in hypertension: the prospective randomized enalapril study evaluating regression of ventricular enlargement (preserve) trial. Circulation. 2001;104: 1248–54.
27. Mesfin GM, Piper RC, DuCharme DW, et al. Pathogenesis of cardiovascular alterations in dogs treated with minoxidil. Toxicol Pathol. 1989;17:164–81.
28. Kirsten R, Nelson K, Kirsten D, Heintz B. Clinical pharmacokinetics of vasodilators. Part I. Clin Pharmacokinet. 1998;34:457–82.
29. Pitt B, Poole-Wilson PA, Segal R, et al. Effect of losartan compared with captopril on mortality in patients with symptomatic heart failure: randomised trial – the Losartan Heart Failure Survival Study ELITE II. Lancet. 2000;355:1582–7.
30. Dahlöf B, Devereux RB, Kjeldsen SE, et al. Cardiovascular morbidity and mortality in the Losartan Intervention for Endpoint reduction in hypertension study (LIFE): a randomised trial against atenolol. Lancet. 2002;359:995–1003.
31. Mogensen CE. Microalbuminuria predicts clinical proteinuria and early mortality in maturity-onset diabetes. N Engl J Med. 1984;310:356–60.
32. Yudkin JS, Forrest RD, Jackson CA. Microalbuminuria as predictor of vascular disease in non-diabetic subjects. Islington Diabetes Survey. Lancet. 1988;2:530–3.
33. Keane WF, Eknoyan G. Proteinuria, albuminuria, risk, assessment, detection, elimination (PARADE): a position paper of the National Kidney Foundation. Am J Kidney Dis. 1999;33:1004–10.
34. Damsgaard EM, Froland A, Jorgensen OD, Mogensen CE. Microalbuminuria as predictor of increased mortality in elderly people. Br Med J. 1990;300:297–300.
35. Bigazzi R, Bianchi S, Campese VM, Baldari G. Prevalence of microalbuminuria in a large population of patients with mild to moderate essential hypertension. Nephron. 1992;61:94–7.
36. Stephenson JM, Kenny S, Stevens LK, et al. Proteinuria and mortality in diabetes: the WHO Multinational Study of Vascular Disease in Diabetes. Diabet Med. 1995;12:149–55.
37. Mathiesen ER, Ronn B, Storm B, et al. The natural course of microalbuminuria in insulin-dependent diabetes: a 10-year prospective study. Diabet Med. 1995;12:482–7.
38. Lydakis C, Efstratopoulos A, Lip GY. Microalbuminuria in hypertension: is it up to measure? J Hum Hypertens. 1997;11:695–7.
39. Garg JP, Bakris GL. Microalbuminuria: marker of vascular dysfunction, risk factor for cardiovascular disease. Vascular Biol. 2002.
40. Fried LF, Orchard TJ, Kasiske BL. Effect of lipid reduction on the progression of renal disease: a meta-analysis. Kidney Int. 2001;59: 260–9.

41. Tarif N, Bakris GL. Preservation of renal function: the spectrum of effects by calcium-channel blockers. Nephrol Dial Transplant. 1997;12:2244–50.

42. Bennett PH, Haffner S, Kasiske BL, et al. Screening and management of microalbuminuria in patients with diabetes mellitus: recommendations to the Scientific Advisory Board of the National Kidney Foundation from an ad hoc committee of the Council on Diabetes Mellitus of the National Kidney Foundation. Am J Kidney Dis. 1995;25:107–12.

43. Ravid M, Neumann L, Lishner M. Plasma lipids and the progression of nephropathy in diabetes mellitus type II: effect of ACE inhibitors. Kidney Int. 1995;47:907–10.

44. Ravid M, Lang R, Rachmani R, et al. Long-term renoprotective effect of angiotensin-coverting enzyme inhibition in non-insulin-dependent diabetes mellitus. Arch Intern Med. 1996;156:286.

45. Effects of ramipril on cardiovascular and microvascular outcomes in people with diabetes mellitus: results of the HOPE study and MICRO-HOPE substudy. Heart Outcomes Prevention Evaluation Study Investigators. Lancet. 2000;355:253–9.

46. Parving H, Lehnert H, Brochner-Mortensen J, et al. The effect of irbesartan on the development of diabetic nephropathy in patients with type 2 diabetes. N Engl J Med. 2001;345:870.

47. Remuzzi G, Ruggenenti P, Benigni A. Understanding the nature of renal disease progression. Kidney Int. 1997;51:2–15.

48. Bakris GL. Progression of diabetic nephropathy. A focus on arterial pressure level and methods of reduction. Diabetes Res Clin Pract. 1998;39(Suppl.):S35–42.

49. Lewis EJ, Hunsicker LG, Bain RP, Rohde RD. The effect of angiotensin-converting-enzyme inhibition on diabetic nephropathy. The Collaborative Study Group. N Engl J Med. 1993;329:1456–62.

50. Lewis EJ, Hunsicker LG, Clarke WR, et al. Renoprotective effect of the angiotensin-receptor antagonist irbesartan in patients with nephropathy due to type 2 diabetes. N Engl J Med. 2001;345:851–60.

51. Brenner BM, Cooper ME, de Zeeuw D, et al. Effects of losartan on renal and cardiovascular outcomes in patients with type 2 diabetes and nephropathy. N Engl J Med. 2001;345:861–9.

52. Bakris GL, Weir MR, DeQuattro V, McMahon FG. Effects of an ACE inhibitor/calcium antagonist combination on proteinuria in diabetic nephropathy. Kidney Int. 1998;54:1283–9.

53. Tarif N, Bakris GL. Angiotensin II receptor blockade and progression of nondiabetic-mediated renal disease. Kidney Int Suppl. 1997;63:S67–70.

54. Jafar TH, Schmid CH, Landa M, et al. Angiotensin-converting enzyme inhibitors and progression of nondiabetic renal disease. A meta-analysis of patient-level data. Ann Intern Med. 2001;135:73–87.

55. Bakris GL, Barnhill BW, Sadler R. Treatment of arterial hypertension in diabetic humans: importance of therapeutic selection. Kidney Int. 1992;41:912–19.

56. Hansen HP, Rossing P, Tarnow L, et al. Increased glomerular filtration rate after withdrawal of long-term antihypertensive treatment in diabetic nephropathy. Kidney Int. 1995;47:1726–31.

57. Bakris GL, Weir MR. Angiotensin-converting enzyme inhibitor-associated elevations in serum creatinine: is this a cause for concern? Arch Intern Med. 2000;160:685–93.

58. Grundy SM. Hypertriglyceridemia, atherogenic dyslipidemia, and the metabolic syndrome. Am J Cardiol. 1998;81:18B–25B.

59. Executive Summary of The Third Report of The National Cholesterol Education Program (NCEP) Expert Panel on Detection, Evaluation, and Treatment of High Blood Cholesterol In Adults (Adult Treatment Panel III). JAMA. 2001;285:2486–97.

60. Hansen BC. The metabolic syndrome X. Ann NY Acad Sci. 1999;892:1–24.

61. Lind L, Lithell H. Decreased peripheral blood flow in the pathogenesis of the metabolic syndrome comprising hypertension, hyperlipidemia, and hyperinsulinemia. Am Heart J. 1993;125:1494–7.

62. McLaughlin T, Reaven G. Insulin resistance and hypertension. Patients in double jeopardy for cardiovascular disease. Geriatrics. 2000;55:28–32, 35.

63. Efficacy of atenolol and captopril in reducing risk of macrovascular and microvascular complications in type 2 diabetes: UKPDS 39. UK Prospective Diabetes Study Group. Br Med J 1998;317:713–20.

64. Krentz AJ. Insulin resistance. Br Med J. 1996;313:1385–9.

65. Tillmann HC, Walker RJ, Lewis-Barned NJ, et al. A long-term comparison between enalapril and captopril on insulin sensitivity in normotensive non-insulin dependent diabetic volunteers. J Clin Pharm Ther. 1997;22:273–8.

66. Paolisso G, Tagliamonte MR, Gambardella A, et al. Losartan mediated improvement in insulin action is mainly due to an increase in non-oxidative glucose metabolism and blood flow in insulin-resistant hypertensive patients. J Hum Hypertens. 1997;11:307–12.

67. Staessen J, Amery A, Fagard R. Isolated systolic hypertension in the elderly. J Hypertens. 1990;8:393–405.

68. Staessen JA, Gasowski J, Wang JG, et al. Risks of untreated and treated isolated systolic hypertension in the elderly: meta-analysis of outcome trials. Lancet. 2000;355:865–72.

69. Hansson L, Lindholm LH, Ekbom T, et al. Randomised trial of old and new antihypertensive drugs in elderly patients: cardiovascular mortality and morbidity the Swedish Trial in Old Patients with Hypertension-2 study. Lancet. 1999;354:1751–6.

70. Messerli FH, Grossman E, Goldbourt U. Are beta-blockers efficacious as first-line therapy for hypertension in the elderly? A systematic review. JAMA. 1998;279:1903–7.

71. Villarosa IP, Bakris GL. The Appropriate Blood Pressure Control in Diabetes (ABCD) Trial. J Hum Hypertens. 1998;12:653–5.

72. Epstein M, Bakris G. Newer approaches to antihypertensive therapy. Use of fixed-dose combination therapy. Arch Intern Med. 1996;156:1969–78.

73. Jaffe A, Chen Y, Kisch ES, et al. Erectile dysfunction in hypertensive subjects. Assessment of potential determinants. Hypertension. 1996;28:859–62.

74. Keith N, Wagener H, Kernohan J. The syndrome of malignant hypertension. Arch Intern Med. 1928;41:141–53.

75. Kaplan N. Management of hypertensive emergencies. Lancet. 1994;344:1335–8.

76. Zeller K, Kuhnert LV, Matthews C. Rapid reduction of severe asymptomatic hypertension: a prospective controlled trial. Arch Intern Med. 1989;149:2186–9.

77. Shea S, Misra D, Ehrlich MH, et al. Predisposing factors for severe, uncontrolled hypertension in an inner-city minority population. N Engl J Med. 1992;327:776–81.

78. Oka K, Hayashi K, Nakazato T, et al. Malignant hypertension in a patient with primary aldosteronism with elevated active renin concentration. Intern Med. 1997;36:700–4.

79. Mann SJ, Pickering TG. Detection of renovascular hypertension. State of the art. Ann Intern Med. 1992;117:845–53.

80. Vincent JL, Berlot G, Preiser JC, et al. Intravenous nicardipine in the treatment of postoperative arterial hypertension. J Cardiothorac Vasc Anesth. 1997;11:160–4.

81. Shusterman NH, Elliott WJ, White WB. Fenoldopam, but not nitroprusside, improves renal function in severely hypertensive patients with impaired renal function. Am J Med. 1993;95:161–8.

82. Oparil S, Aronson S, Deeb GM, et al. Fenoldopam: a new parenteral antihypertensive: consensus roundtable on the management of perioperative hypertension and hypertensive crises. Am J Hypertens. 1999;12:653–64.

83. Grossman E, Messerli FH, Grodzicki T, Kowey P. Should a moratorium be placed on sublingual nifedipine capsules given for hypertensive emergencies and pseudoemergencies? JAMA. 1996;276:1328–31.

84. Chang YJ, Spiera H. Renal transplantation in scleroderma. Medicine (Baltimore). 1999;78:382–5.

85. Benedict CR. Centrally acting antihypertensive drugs: re-emergence of sympathetic inhibition in the treatment of hypertension. Curr Hypertens Rep. 1999;1:305–12.

86. Kuppers HE, Jager BA, Luszick JH, et al. Placebo-controlled comparison of the efficacy and tolerability of once-daily moxonidine and enalapril in mild-to-moderate essential hypertension. J Hypertens. 1997;15:93–7.

87. Major cardiovascular events in hypertensive patients randomized to doxazosin vs chlorthalidone: the antihypertensive and lipid-lowering treatment to prevent heart attack trial (ALLHAT). ALL-HAT Collaborative Research Group. JAMA. 2000;283:1967–75.

88. Pahor M, Psaty BM, Alderman MH, et al. Health outcomes associated with calcium antagonists compared with other first-line antihypertensive therapies: a meta-analysis of randomised controlled trials. Lancet. 2000;356:1949–54.

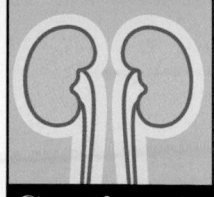

Chapter 39

Renovascular Hypertension

Stephen C Textor

INTRODUCTION

Renovascular hypertension remains among the most common of the secondary forms of hypertension and one that is most amenable to surgical or endovascular therapy. While reduced perfusion of the kidney can raise arterial pressure and eventually threaten the viability of the kidney, determining how often this occurs and under what circumstances evaluation and repair of the renal vasculature should be undertaken in a specific patient raises complex issues. These include identifying the best way to document the diagnosis and determining whether blood pressure control and stable renal function can be achieved with medical therapy alone or whether revascularization should be considered.

This chapter will examine these issues from the perspective of treating renovascular hypertension. In practice, this rarely can be separated entirely from consideration of preservation of renal function beyond an atherosclerotic lesion, which is discussed further in Chapters 63 and 64.

DEFINITION AND PREVALENCE

Renovascular hypertension is defined as a syndrome of arterial hypertension induced by reduced renal perfusion pressure secondary to a vascular lesion. It is important to distinguish this from the simple presence of an arterial stenotic lesion, which may or may not produce hemodynamic consequences related to blood pressure. In the final analysis, proof that a stenotic vascular lesion is causally related to hypertension depends upon a reduction in blood pressure after restoring the blood supply with renal revascularization. Recognition that renal artery lesions may not be hemodynamically important is critical to sorting through the complex literature of renovascular disease. Much of this literature is directed primarily towards identification of vascular lesions themselves, without addressing their functional significance.

Table 39.1 lists a variety of lesions that can produce the syndrome of renovascular hypertension by impairing renal blood supply. Many of these are rare but underscore the point that the final common pathway depends upon reduced renal perfusion pressure rather than upon a specific pathologic lesion.

Fibromuscular disease (FMD) of the renal arteries is most common among young females. Medial fibroplasia is the most prevalent of the subtypes observed. This diagnosis should be considered in anyone with early-onset, severe hypertension, but occasionally it is discovered only incidentally during

Lesions producing the syndrome of renovascular hypertension by impairing renal blood supply	
Type	**Lesions**
Two-kidney hypertension: implies contralateral (nonaffected) kidney is present	Unilateral atherosclerotic renal artery disease
	Unilateral fibrous and fibromuscular disease (FMD)
	Intimal fibroplasia
	Medial fibromuscular dysplasia
	Periarterial fibroplasia
	Renal artery aneurysm
	Arterial embolism
	Arteriovenous fistula (congenital and traumatic)
	Segmental arterial occlusion (traumatic)
	Pheochromocytoma compressing the renal artery
	Metastatic tumor (compressing the renal parenchyma)
One-kidney hypertension: implies total renal mass ischemia	Stenosis to a solitary functioning kidney
	Bilateral arterial stenosis
	Aortic coarctation
	Vasculitis (polyarteritis nodosa and Takayasu disease)

Table 39.1 Lesions producing the syndrome of renovascular hypertension by impairing renal blood supply.

angiography for other reasons. It is important to recognize because FMD responds well to either surgical or endovascular revascularization. These lesions often arise beyond the first several centimeters of the renal artery and may be associated with more distal branch disease (Fig. 39.1).

Atherosclerotic disease of the renal arteries (see Fig. 39.2) is the most common cause of renovascular hypertension[1]. These lesions most often arise in the first 1–2 cm of the renal artery and may comprise an extension of a large aortic plaque. It is essential to recognize that renal artery stenosis from atherosclerotic disease represents a manifestation of a systemic disease and that disease is commonly present in other vascular beds, including coronary, cerebrovascular, peripheral vascular, and aortic sites.

The prevalence of atherosclerotic renal artery disease appears to be increasing. This likely reflects demographic trends within the USA and other Western countries. Since the early 1970s, mortality rates from stroke and coronary artery disease have been falling steadily, associated with lengthening lifespans. The age group above 65 years is the most rapidly expanding group in the USA. As a consequence more people are surviving to ages when atherosclerotic vascular disease in the visceral abdominal organs can reach critical levels, producing renovascular hypertension when the kidney is affected.

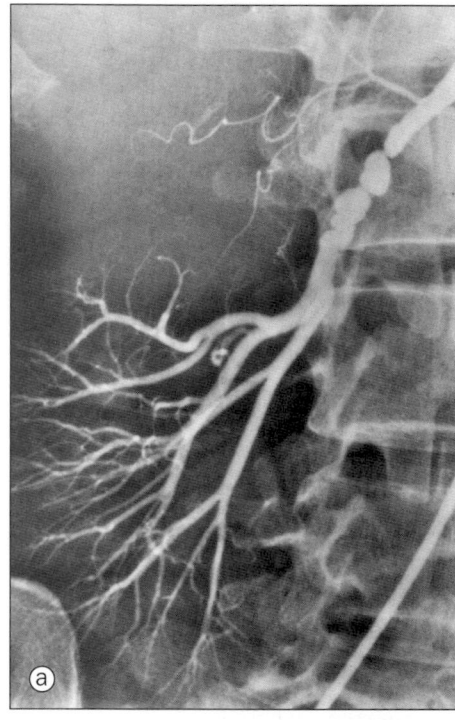
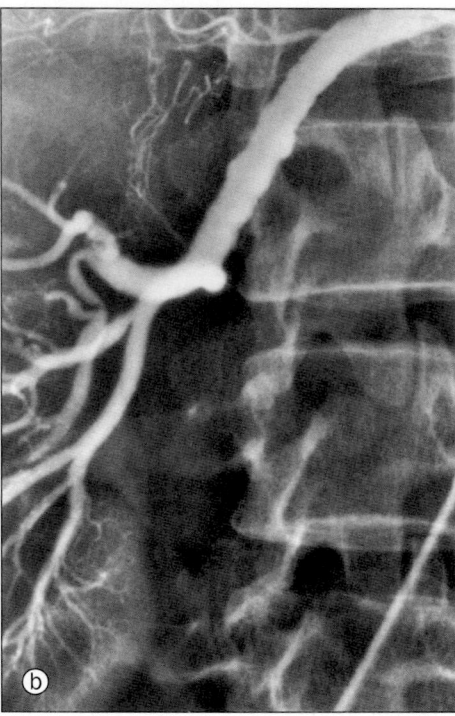

Figure 39.1 Fibromuscular dysplasia. (a) Selective renal arteriogram illustrating the 'beaded' appearance of fibromuscular dysplasia (FMD) with multiple webs characteristic of medial fibroplasia in a 39-year-old female. (b) Selective injection of the same renal artery after technically successful PTRA. (Figure courtesy of Michael McKusick, M.D., Mayo Clinic.)

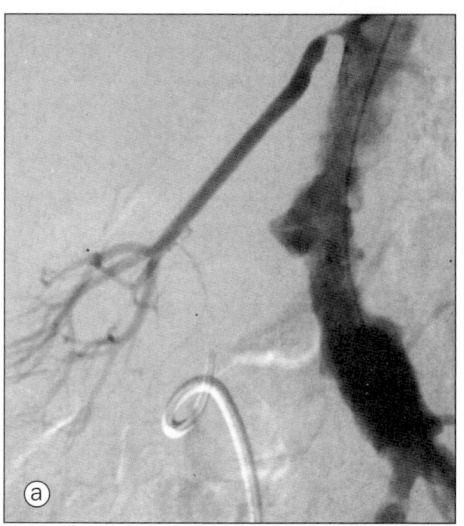
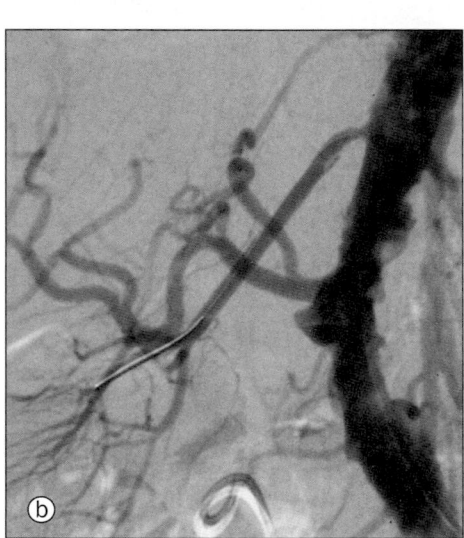

Figure 39.2 Proximal renal artery stenosis secondary to atherosclerosis. Before (a) and after (b) successful percutaneous angioplasty. (With permission from Textor SC, Canzanello VJ. Radiographic evaluation of the renal vasculature. Curr Opin Nephrol Hypertens. 1996;5:541–51.)

Hence, atherosclerotic renal artery stenosis is the single most common cause of secondary 'resistant' hypertension in patients above 50 years of age[2].

PATHOPHYSIOLOGY OF RENOVASCULAR HYPERTENSION

The simple presence of a vascular stenotic lesion does not establish its role in regulating arterial pressure. The cross-sectional area of the stenotic lesion must be severely reduced before any measurable change in either blood flow or perfusion pressure can be detected (Fig. 39.3), usually in the range of 72–80%[3]. Hence, lesions with luminal compromise below this level are unlikely to have hemodynamic significance.

When 'critical' levels of stenosis develop and reduce renal perfusion pressure, multiple mechanisms are activated within the kidney to restore renal blood flow. Central to this process

is the release of renin from the juxtaglomerular apparatus, leading to activation of the renin–angiotensin–aldosterone system. This is mediated in part by stimulation of neuronal nitric oxide synthase (NOS-1) and cyclo-oxygenase (COX)-2 in the macula densa. Blockade of the renin–angiotensin system (RAS) at the time of placement of an experimental renal artery lesion prevents the development of hypertension[3]. Without blockade of this system, systemic arterial pressures rise until renal perfusion is restored. Studies in experimental models and humans indicate that additional mechanisms contribute to long-term elevation of blood pressure in the presence of renal artery stenosis, including intrarenal activation of the sympathetic nervous system, impairment of nitric oxide generation, and release of endothelin, as well as hypertensive microvascular injury to the nonstenosed kidney[3].

Mechanisms responsible for sustained renovascular hypertension differ depending upon whether one or both kidneys

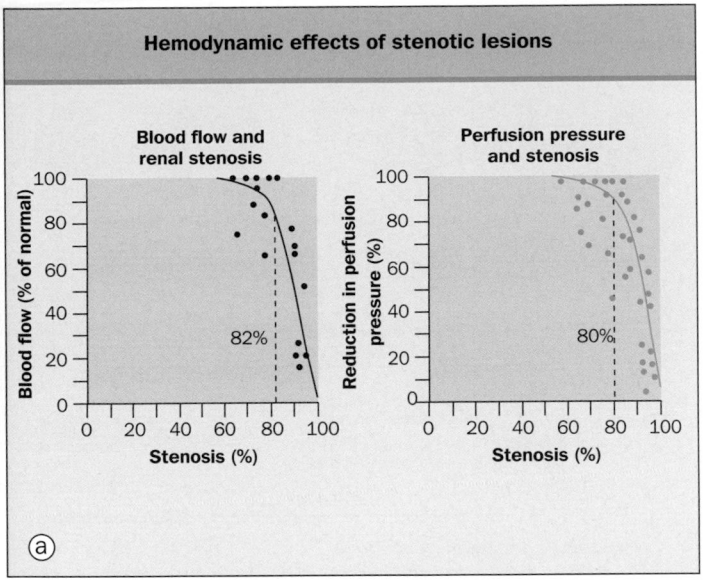

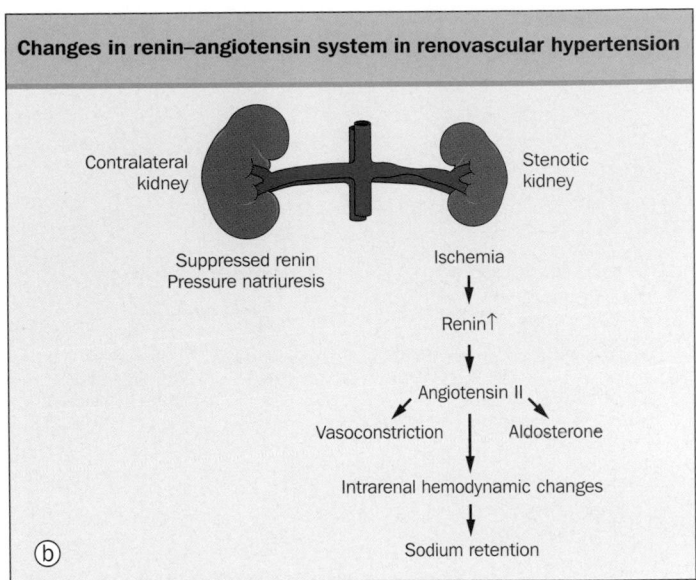

Figure 39.3 Hemodynamic effects of stenotic lesions. (a) Changes in blood flow and arterial pressure across a carefully quantitated arterial lesion are barely detectable until cross-sectional area diminishes by 75–80%. (b) When critical levels of renal artery stenosis occur, a sequence of steps activating the renin–angiotensin system, among others, leads to both elevation of arterial pressure and retention of sodium by the stenotic kidney. (With permission from Textor SC. Pathophysiology of renovascular hypertension. Urol Clin N Am. 1984;11:373–81.)

are affected by vascular lesions, either pathologic or created in animal models using clips. A nomenclature has evolved regarding this phenomenon, in which one clip is present with a normal contralateral or unclipped kidney (so-called 1-clip-2-kidney hypertension) as distinct from a situation in which the entire renal mass is affected with no 'contralateral' kidney (1-clip-1-kidney hypertension). Both of these situations depend upon impaired renal perfusion and initial activation of the RAS with sodium retention. However, the presence of a 'normal' contralateral kidney has important consequences, as it responds to elevated arterial pressures by excreting the excess sodium due to an intact pressure natriuresis mechanism (Chapter 2). (Fig. 39.4). Because the nonstenotic kidney effectively functions to eliminate the excess sodium, the level of perfusion to the stenotic side remains reduced, leading to sustained activation of the RAS.

By contrast, the model of 1-clip-1-kidney hypertension represents a model in which the entire renal mass is exposed to poststenotic pressures. There is no 'normal' or nonstenotic kidney to counteract elevated systemic pressures. As a result, sodium is retained and blood volume expanded, which eventually feedbacks to inhibit the RAS (Fig. 39.4). Therefore, hypertension is typically not angiotensin-dependent unless removal of volume is achieved that reduces renal perfusion pressure and activates the RAS.

Understanding the fundamental differences between these forms of renovascular hypertension has clinical implications. Many diagnostic studies used to establish the functional significance of renal artery lesions depend on comparisons of the physiological response of the two kidneys which may give a false impression if both kidneys are involved. Furthermore, diagnostic tests that depend on differences in physiological responses to alterations in sodium status (such as measuring renal vein renins following sodium depletion) may

be problematic, as high levels of angiotensin II and aldosterone stimulate sodium reabsorption in both the stenotic and nonstenotic kidney. This may account partly for the less frequent use of such tests in recent years.

Complicating the understanding of the pathophysiologic mechanisms of renovascular hypertension is the element of its 'natural history'. Rarely is it known at which point 'critical' levels of stenosis develop. In experimental models, the relative importance of pressor mechanisms, including measurable activation of the RAS, changes with time. Levels of circulating plasma renin fall, as does the responsiveness of blood pressure to short-term blockade of the renin system. Several mechanisms have been proposed to explain such changes, including a slowly developing pressor action of angiotensin II, a transition to alternate pressor mechanisms, and intrinsic renal injury to the nonstenotic kidney, which ultimately sustains hypertension despite reversal of the vascular lesion[4]. Experimentally, this translates into a time limit for reversibility of renovascular hypertension. From a clinical perspective, it is not yet known how to identify when revascularization will fail to benefit blood pressure with certainty. As a result, many of the diagnostic studies that depend upon 'lateralization' of effects have only modest predictive value when negative. As a general rule, they are reliable when positive, meaning that high-grade lateralization accurately predicts a benefit with revascularization. A negative test, however, may also be associated with a beneficial outcome in the majority of cases.

Relationship to 'ischemic nephropathy'

Activation of pressor mechanisms producing renovascular hypertension can occur without loss of renal size or function. However, the more common clinical scenario involves both increasing severity of hypertension and deteriorating renal function, often with loss of renal size. Hence, the decision to

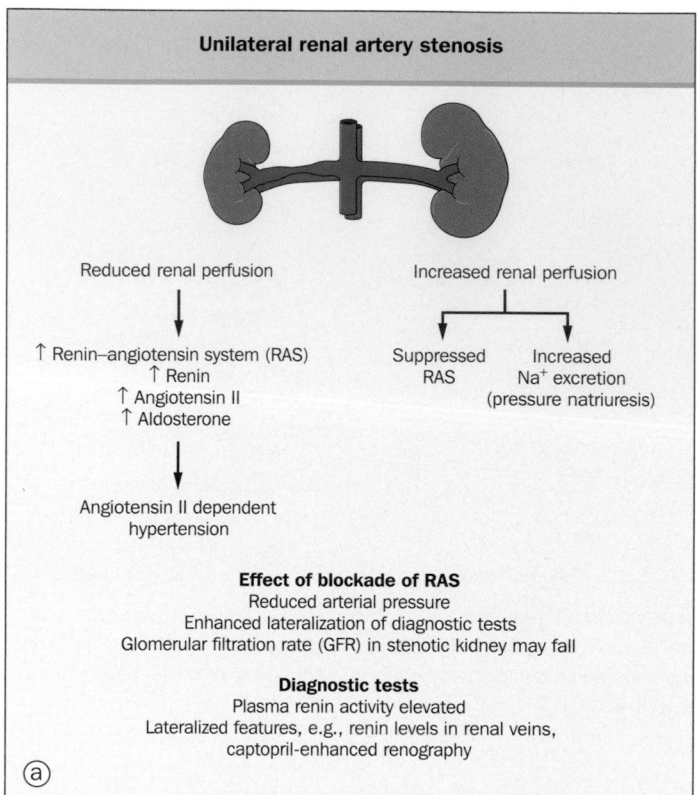

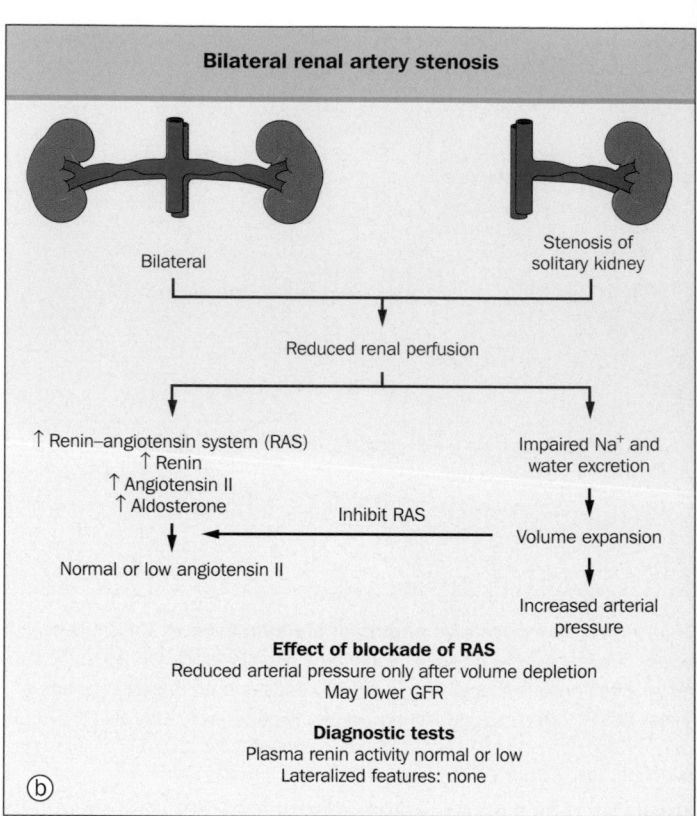

Figure 39.4 Pathogenesis of renovascular hypertension in 'one-kidney' versus 'two-kidney' model. (a) In unilateral stenosis with two kidneys, opposing forces between the stenotic kidney, which has reduced perfusion pressures, and the nonstenotic contralateral kidney, which has increased perfusion pressures, result in laboratory and clinical features of angiotensin-dependent hypertension. (b) In unilateral stenosis with a solitary functioning kidney (or in a patient with bilateral critical renal artery stenosis) reduced perfusion pressure to the stenotic kidney(s) in the absence of a normal kidney excreting sodium leads to sodium and volume retention, ultimately associated with hypertension without persistent activation of the renin–angiotensin system.

consider renal revascularization most commonly combines consideration of both the likelihood of salvage or 'preservation' of function and the benefits regarding blood pressure control. It should be emphasized that mechanisms underlying parenchymal renal damage may differ from those responsible for generating hypertension. Improved blood pressure control after revascularization may be achieved without appreciable benefits to the function of the kidney.

CLINICAL MANIFESTATIONS OF RENOVASCULAR HYPERTENSION

Renovascular disease leads to elevation of arterial pressure fundamentally indistinguishable from that resulting from other causes, particularly essential hypertension. In the 1970s, a cooperative study of renovascular hypertension compared clinical characteristics of patients with surgically proven renovascular hypertension with those of patients identified as having essential hypertension. Some of these were statistically more prevalent, such as the identification of an abdominal bruit, hypokalemia, absence of a family history of hypertension, etc. (Table 39.2). Studies of 'resistant hypertension' from the Netherlands indicate that clinical features of elevated cholesterol, azotemia, body mass index, and smoking offer positive clues[5]. In practical terms, none of these features is of sufficient sensitivity or specificity to offer

diagnostic precision. Recent reports indicate that renovascular hypertension may rarely be associated with nephrotic-range proteinuria. This may regress with correction of the vascular lesions[6]. Hence, the finding of proteinuria does not exclude this diagnosis.

The severity of renovascular hypertension may span a wide range. In humans, acute occlusion of a renal artery may only gradually produce a rise in pressure or it may produce accelerated-phase hypertension rapidly. Before the current era of antihypertensive agents, 30% of Caucasian patients appearing in an emergency department with accelerated-phase hypertension (defined as severe hypertensive retinopathy (see Chapter 36) with or without malignant hypertension) were ultimately found to have renovascular hypertension[7]. Patients with renovascular hypertension may have labile blood pressures, with loss of normal circadian patterns of blood pressure control. Syndromes of polydipsia and accelerated hypertension, sometimes attributed to the dipsogenic actions of angiotensin II, with hyponatremia and hypokalemia also have been observed. Current antihypertensive medications have changed the clinical presentation of renovascular hypertension. Most recent consensus documents regarding hypertension emphasize the need for effective population-wide blood pressure control, while limiting the number and expense of diagnostic studies. As a result, most patients with identified hypertension simply are treated and subjected to few laboratory investigations. For

Clinical characteristics of renovascular hypertension

Clinical features	Essential hypertension (%)	Renovascular hypertension (%)
Duration: under 1 year	12	24
Age of onset >50 years	9	15
Family history of hypertension	71	46
Grade 3 or 4 retinopathy	7	15
Abdominal bruit	9	46
Blood urea nitrogen >20 mg/L	8	16
Potassium <3.4 mmol/L	8	16
Urinary casts	9	20
Proteinuria	32	46

Clinical features that differ (p <0.05) between closely matched groups of 131 patients with essential and renovascular hypertension[34]. These features underscore the potential severity of hypertension in candidates for surgery, but none allows clinical discrimination with confidence. (With permission from Simon N, Franklin SS, Bleifers KH, Maxwell MH. Clinical characteristics of renovascular hypertension. JAMA. 1972;220:1209–18.)

Table 39.2 Clinical characteristics of renovascular hypertension.

those reaching acceptable blood pressure control without adverse effects, no further studies are performed. The introduction of orally active antihypertensive agents that block the RAS, beginning with captopril, improved medical therapy of renovascular hypertension. Initial studies indicated that satisfactory blood pressure control can be achieved in more than 86% of patients with renovascular hypertension, compared with less than 50% with previous available drugs[1]. In recent years, widespread application of angiotensin-converting enzyme (ACE) inhibitors and angiotensin receptor blockers (ATRA) for indications other than hypertension, e.g., congestive cardiac failure, diabetic nephropathy and other proteinuric renal disease increase the exposure of individuals with undetected renal artery stenosis to these drugs[8, 9]. Hence, many, if not most, cases of true renovascular hypertension are not detected (Fig. 39.5) unless hypertension becomes more difficult to treat or renal dysfunction ensues. One result of these changes has been the emergence of distinctive clinical syndromes that merit evaluation in patients at risk for renovascular hypertension. These are summarized in Table 39.3 and are discussed in further detail in Chapters 63 and 64. The overall result of these developments is that patients reaching consideration for evaluation and renal revascularization are a subset of the patient population with renovascular hypertension. This subset is characterized generally by more severe hypertension, declining renal function, propensity for rapid volume accumulation manifest as 'flash' pulmonary edema, and, occasionally, advanced renal failure.

Comorbid disease risk

Many of the entities leading to renovascular hypertension (Table 39.4) may appear as isolated lesions in the kidney. FMD may involve other vascular sites, particularly the carotid circulation. Both sites are involved in approximately 15% of

Identification of atherosclerotic renovascular hypertension

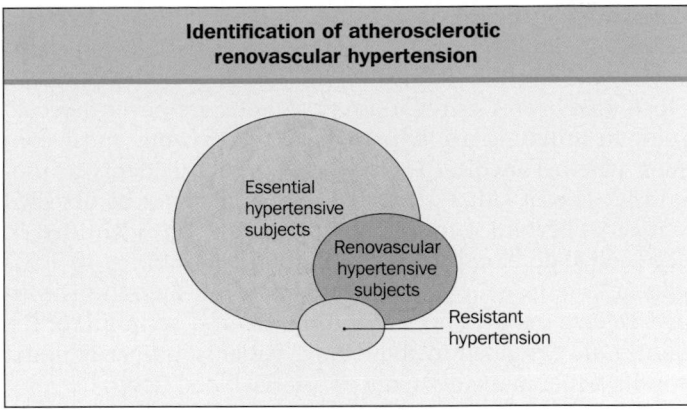

Figure 39.5 Identification of atherosclerotic renovascular hypertension. Venn diagram indicates that many patients with renovascular hypertension are indistinguishable from patients with essential hypertension. A subset develop problematic or 'resistant' hypertension, which brings them to clinical attention and consideration for renal revascularization.

Clinical syndromes associated with renovascular hypertension

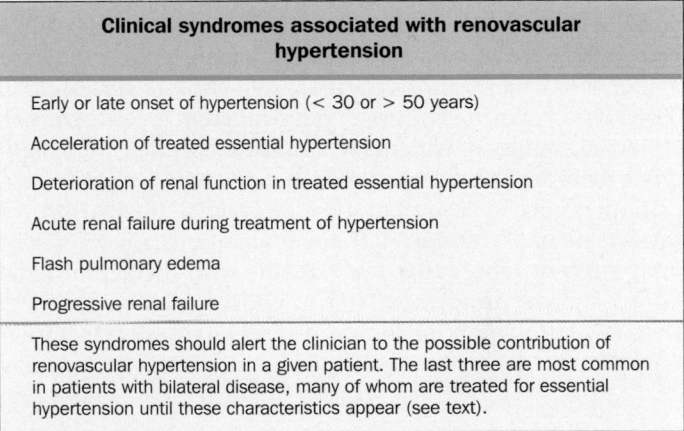

Early or late onset of hypertension (< 30 or > 50 years)

Acceleration of treated essential hypertension

Deterioration of renal function in treated essential hypertension

Acute renal failure during treatment of hypertension

Flash pulmonary edema

Progressive renal failure

These syndromes should alert the clinician to the possible contribution of renovascular hypertension in a given patient. The last three are most common in patients with bilateral disease, many of whom are treated for essential hypertension until these characteristics appear (see text).

Table 39.3 Clinical syndromes associated with renovascular hypertension.

patients. Hence, young patients presenting with spontaneous carotid artery dissection or occlusion should be considered at risk for FMD of the kidney and vice versa.

Atherosclerotic disease of the renal arteries is highly correlated with disease both in the coronary and peripheral vasculature. Series of patients undergoing coronary angiography indicate that between 20 and 30% of patients will have some degree of renal artery stenosis, the severity of which is generally correlated with the severity and extent of coronary disease. Series of patients undergoing evaluation for lower-extremity peripheral vascular disease may have identifiable renal artery stenoses in more than 50% of cases. Whether the renal artery lesions in such patients participate in progressive vascular disease and warrant revascularization when detected incidentally is controversial (see below). Follow-up of patients with incidentally detected renal artery lesions during coronary angiography indicates that the presence of renal artery lesions is an independent risk factor for mortality, which may reach 30% over 4 years in high-risk groups[10].

Hypertension

Disease progression

A central clinical issue in managing renovascular hypertension is the likelihood that vascular occlusion will progress. Since many cases of renal artery stenosis are never detected prior to initiating antihypertensive therapy, one must consider whether medical therapy assigns such patients to progressive loss of kidney function, which may not be detected until it is beyond recovery. Most of the lesions identified in Table 39.1 do not progress, although some forms of FMD appear to induce more severe hemodynamic limitations with age. Occasional instances of thrombosis and occlusion of the kidney are described in these latter patients, primarily under conditions of markedly reduced arterial blood flow.

Atherosclerotic lesions can progress to more severe stenosis. Factors regulating the severity and progressive nature of this process are not well understood. Retrospective studies using serial angiograms (obtained for other reasons) indicate rates of clinical progression approaching 40–50% over 4–5 years, with 16% of the most severe lesions producing total occlusion. Prospective studies using Doppler ultrasound in patients with incidentally detected renal artery lesions indicate that progression overall approaches 31% over 3 years, varying considerably by the degree of initial stenosis. In this series, 9/295 vessels (3%) produced total occlusion[11]. How often changes in apparent vascular stenosis translate into clinical worsening of either blood pressure control or renal function is controversial. Follow-up studies of patients with incidentally detected, high-grade renal artery stenosis (> 70%) treated without revascularization results in less than 10% later revascularization for intractable hypertension[12]. These observations are consistent with a recent report that few patients with incidental renal artery stenosis progressed later to end-stage renal disease[13]. Determining the rate of clinical disease progression is important because decisions regarding vascular intervention may depend heavily upon estimating the likelihood of losing renal parenchymal viability during medical therapy of renovascular hypertension.

DIAGNOSTIC STUDIES FOR RENOVASCULAR HYPERTENSION

Several 'screening' studies have been proposed to identify patients with renovascular hypertension. Some of these depend upon identifying activation of the RAS, such as renin–sodium profiling, and many depend upon side-to-side comparisons of kidneys, assuming that one kidney is unaffected. Under the best of circumstances, these studies are rarely more than 80% sensitive or specific. As a result, their value as predictors depends greatly on the pre-test probability of renovascular disease[14,15]. Furthermore, most of the functional tests related to activation of the RAS depend heavily upon the test conditions, including sodium intake and concurrent antihypertensive medications, many of which affect levels of plasma renin activity. As a result, many clinicians no longer use these tests extensively.

Fundamentally, the *sine qua non* of renovascular hypertension is identification of a stenotic vascular lesion affecting the renal arteries. Conventional angiography remains the reference standard to identify the anatomy of the renal vasculature but it is commonly performed only after a less invasive procedure has raised the level of probability that such a lesion is present. In many cases, angiography is performed at the same time as percutaneous transluminal renal angioplasty (PTRA) with or without stenting.

Various imaging methods of the renal vasculature provide different types of information regarding blood supply and parenchymal renal function (Table 39.4). Noninvasive vascular

Relative value of imaging methods for evaluating the renal vasculature					
Methods	Images of vessels	Tissue perfusion	Function (GFR)	Advantages	Disadvantages
Contrast angiography	+++	++	±	Nephrogram estimates volume of viable tissue; the gold standard	Risk of catheter-induced injuries and contrast nephropathy
Captopril renography	–	+++	++	Change in GFR might estimate reversibility of the lesion; widely available, noninvasive; totally normal renogram effectively excludes significant vascular disease	
Duplex ultrasound	++	++	–	Precise measurement of flow velocity, suitable for serial studies, relatively inexpensive	Produces little functional information, is not suitable for accessory vessels
Magnetic resonance angiography	++	++	±	Nontoxic in advanced renal failure	Accuracy limited to proximal vessels, produces little functional information, not suitable for accessory vessels
Spiral computed tomographic angiography	+++	+	±	Provision of three types of image, examination of venous structures, might be useful for evaluating transplant donors	High contrast requirement, demanding breath-holds

Table 39.4 Relative value of imaging methods for evaluating the renal vasculature. The available techniques vary in their ability to image the renal vessels, assess tissue perfusion, and measure GFR.

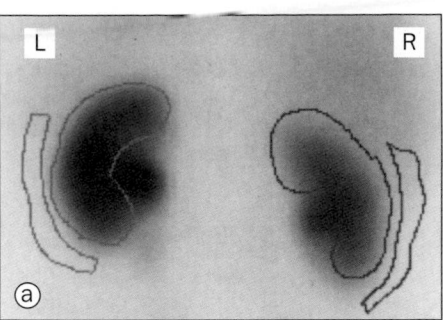

Figure 39.6 Captopril-enhanced renography.
(a) Scan in a patient with newly developing hypertension.
(b) Renogram demonstrates delayed arrival and excretion of isotope (MAG3) in the affected left kidney.

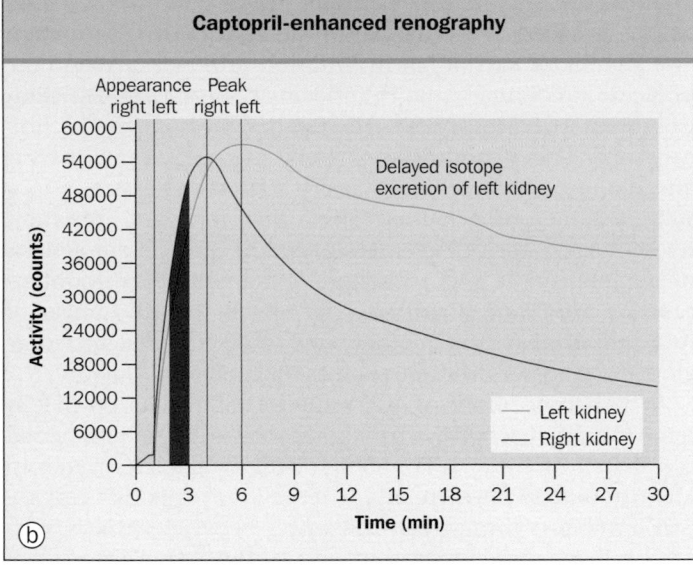

the size and excretory capacity of the kidney as well as emphasizing the role of angiotensin II in maintaining glomerular filtration rate (GFR). Some studies emphasize the potential for predicting benefit from renal revascularization based upon changes induced by the ACE inhibitor. This test has a high negative predictive value when completely normal. It may be argued that many intrinsic renal abnormalities may change these curves, particularly in the presence of reduced GFR (serum creatinine > 2.0 mg/dL). Several studies indicate that a completely normal captopril renogram effectively excludes the presence of hemodynamically significant renal artery stenosis[16]. This observation underscores the central issue related to noninvasive testing: the most important consideration is the negative-predictive value of the study. In effect, a clinician performs such a study as a prelude to further studies. A positive result will lead commonly to subsequent angiography. The real goal and merit of noninvasive testing is to allow the physician to discontinue further invasive testing. Hence, the practical value of such studies should be assessed by the degree of confidence that a negative study provides that no important lesion is being overlooked by not proceeding further.

Renal artery duplex scanning is applied widely to identify and to follow hemodynamic effects of vascular lesions serially. It is relatively inexpensive and requires no contrast. It is most effective in detecting lesions of the main renal artery near the origin. The reliability of this method depends upon the skill and dedication of the ultrasound technician, however, and upon the body habitus of the patient in many instances. Duplex ultrasound does not provide functional information regarding the kidney beyond the vascular lesion, although many important structural features including the size of the kidney and presence of ureteral obstruction may be determined.

Magnetic resonance angiography (MRA) offers the potential to provide both structural vascular imaging and functional information. Particularly with gadolinium contrast enhancement, the main renal arteries may be visualized with confidence in many patients (see Fig. 39.7). While expensive, MRA imaging offers the ability of examining the aorta and renal arteries with confidence in patients with significant renal failure without risk of contrast-induced nephropathy or atheroembolic complications associated with catheter-induced injuries.

studies most commonly employed include renography (usually captopril- or enalapril-enhanced renography), renal artery duplex ultrasound, or magnetic resonance angiography (MRA) (see Chapter 5). It should be emphasized that these methods provide different information and may differ in availability and reliability between institutions. Figure 39.6 illustrates an example of a captopril-enhanced renogram in a patient with renal artery stenosis. No direct image of the vessel is presented, but the study provides a view of the rate of isotope appearance and washout, reflecting the sequence of renal blood flow and filtration. The study provides functional information regarding

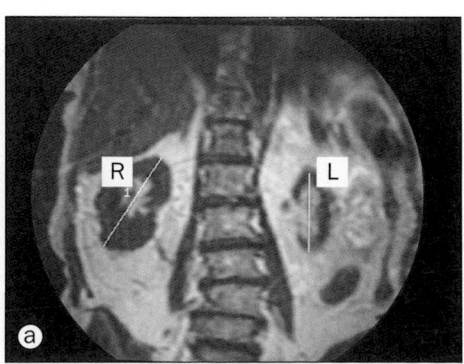

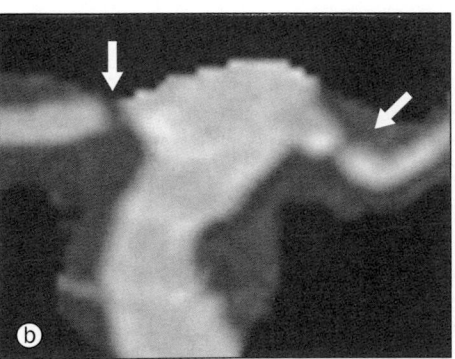

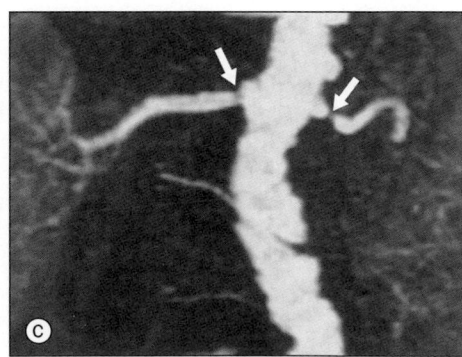

Figure 39.7 Magnetic resonance angiogram in renal failure. Angiogram of an elderly woman with renal failure (serum creatinine 2.5 mg/dL) and severe hypertension. (a) Severe discrepancy in kidney size with a small left kidney. (b) Gadolinium-enhanced aortography illustrating high-grade, bilateral renal artery stenotic lesions (arrows). (c) Extensive aortic and iliac disease, bilateral renal artery stenoses (arrows) and markedly diminished filtration on the left side.

Using these methods, clinicians now evaluate patients at risk for renovascular disease with greater confidence than ever before. It is prudent to determine exactly the question to be addressed with such studies beforehand: is there justification for proceeding further if the test is suggestive of vascular stenosis? Is the patient a candidate clinically for revascularization, and will a negative test allow conclusion of vascular studies? In some instances, it may be sufficient to answer the question, 'Is bilateral disease present?'.

MANAGEMENT OF PATIENTS WITH RENOVASCULAR HYPERTENSION

The overall goal of hypertension therapy is 'to reduce morbidity and mortality by the least intrusive means possible', as stated by the Joint National Committee (JNC VI). In renovascular hypertension, this means balancing the risks and benefits of many potential means of treating the disorder, ranging from medical therapy to surgical or endovascular repair.

Medical therapy

Most patients with renal artery stenosis and renovascular hypertension are treated initially with conventional antihypertensive medications (see Chapter 39)[17]. Before the introduction of calcium channel blockers and those that interrupt the RAS (ACE inhibitors and angiotensin receptor antagonists (ATRA)), acceptable levels of blood pressure (considered <160/90 mmHg at the time) could be achieved in a minority of such patients. Early studies with both captopril and enalapril indicated that regimens based upon ACE inhibition could achieve lower blood pressures more than 86% of the time, at least for several months. The later introduction of calcium channel-blocking agents, particularly the dihydropyridine class, allowed vascular smooth muscle dilatation regardless of the pressor stimulus. The effectiveness of these newer antihypertensive agents considerably reduces the clinical need to evaluate patients for renovascular hypertension. As will be discussed below, even successful renal revascularization rarely leads to withdrawal of all antihypertensive medications in the current era (so-called 'cure' of hypertension). Current definitions of satisfactory blood pressure control target levels below 140/90 mmHg. Most patients with atherosclerotic renovascular disease have pre-existing essential hypertension as a risk factor. For these reasons, most patients with successful renal revascularization remain candidates for antihypertensive drug therapy. Hence, it may be questioned whether the costs and risks of renal revascularization are warranted at all in patients whose blood pressures and kidney function are stable on an acceptable regimen of current antihypertensive medications. Such patients are unlikely to gain much with revascularization procedures.

Adverse consequences of medical therapy

Studies of 'critical' stenosis of the renal artery indicate that reduction of arterial pressures poses the potential for reduction of renal blood flow below levels needed to sustain glomerular filtration. Because of the gradient across the stenotic lesion, renal artery pressures may fall below those needed for autoregulation, considered to be about 60 mmHg

in humans. Such a reduction in blood flow can develop with many antihypertensive drugs, including β-blockers and sodium nitroprusside. Under these circumstances, rates of renal blood flow may fall so far as to allow complete occlusion, as discussed in Chapter 64. In this respect, antihypertensive agents acting by blockade or interruption of the RAS can prevent the effects of angiotensin II at the efferent arteriole. When preglomerular pressures are reduced for any reason, intrarenal activation of angiotensin II preserves transcapillary filtration pressures at the glomerulus, allowing continued urine formation despite marginal blood flow. Removal of angiotensin II under these conditions allows abrupt cessation of glomerular filtration and urine formation (see Fig. 39.8). Such a fall in filtration produces a syndrome of 'acute functional renal insufficiency', first described clinically with ACE inhibitors[18]. The fall in GFR is apparent clinically only under conditions whereby the entire renal mass is affected, e.g., bilateral renal artery stenosis or stenosis to a solitary functioning kidney. These principles are important for the nephrologist, because removal of the efferent actions of angiotensin II and reduction of transcapillary filtration pressure are primary pathways by which the advantages of ACE inhibition accrue in other renal diseases characterized by glomerular hyperfiltration, such as diabetic nephropathy.

Whether the effects of ACE inhibitors and ATRA on GFR in renovascular hypertensive patients are beneficial or detrimental is a matter of controversy. Some of the diagnostic studies to identify functionally important renal artery stenosis employ ACE inhibitors to magnify differences between kidneys, e.g., captopril-enhanced renography and captopril-stimulated renal vein renin determinations. It may be argued that identifying a fall in GFR with an ACE inhibitor allows early detection of critical stenotic lesions in time for renal revascularization. Conversely, some have proposed that administration of an ACE inhibitor to patients with renal artery stenosis poses the hazard of a 'pharmacologic nephrectomy', with the potential for inducing irreversible renal parenchymal injury through ischemia[19]. Although the fall in GFR induced by ACE inhibitors is usually reversible, occasionally patients do not recover renal function. Hence, ACE inhibitors must be recognized as a 'double-edged' sword in renovascular hypertension. They have unique properties, allowing more effective blood pressure control than previously possible, but at the same time, this class of medication has the potential for early loss of filtration pressure in patients with critical levels of renal artery stenosis.

Clinical experience with ACE inhibitors is reassuring in this regard. Monitoring studies both in clinical use and in large, prospective trials in patients at high risk for undetected renal artery stenosis, such as the trials of congestive cardiac failure, indicate that clinically important loss of glomerular filtration is not common. Most of these trials excluded patients with significant renal dysfunction, however. Postmarketing surveys of more than 15 000 prescriptions in the UK after the release of enalapril indicated few, but significant, adverse experiences. Most often, these were patients with pre-existing renal dysfunction who were taking potassium-sparing diuretics and had other known atherosclerotic disease[20,21]. Taken together, the clinician caring for patients with complex hypertension should recognize both hyperkalemia and rising creatinine values

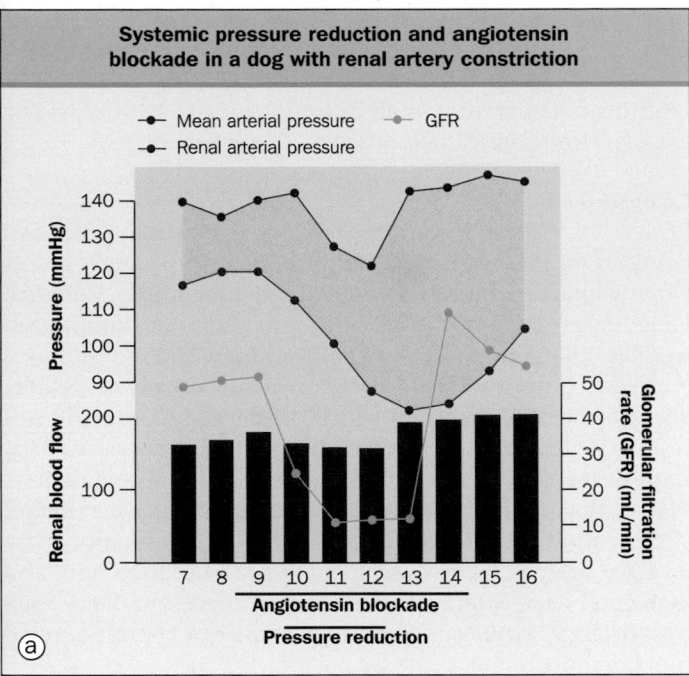

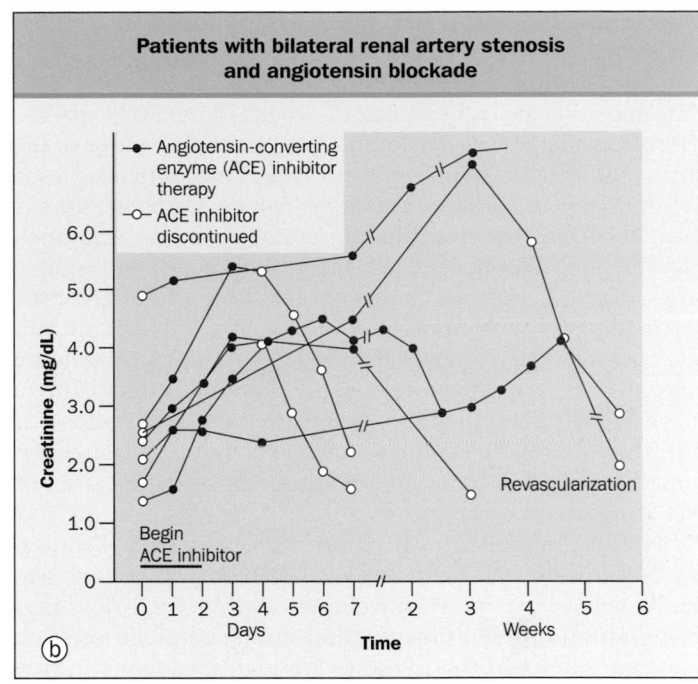

Figure 39.8 Systemic pressure reduction and angiotensin blockade in renal artery constriction. (a) In a dog with renal artery stenosis, arterial pressures were reduced with sodium nitroprusside and the intravenous angiotensin II antagonist Sar-1-Ala-8-angiotensin was used to block the renin–angiotensin system. Despite preservation of renal blood flow, GFR fell. Such a fall in GFR reflects its dependence upon angiotensin II at the efferent arteriole under these conditions. (b) In patients with bilateral renal artery stenosis or a stenotic solitary kidney, acute 'functional renal insufficiency' can develop during administration of ACE inhibitors. In most cases, discontinuing the ACE inhibitors is associated with rapid improvement of the renal function.

during treatment with ACE inhibitors or ATRA (Table 39.5) as a sign of potentially 'critical' renal artery stenosis, which may be considered for alternative therapy and/or renal revascularization.

Difficult to control hypertension and/or declining renal function during medical therapy

Further diagnostic and therapeutic maneuvers may be warranted in patients requiring more complex medical regimens (usually three drugs or more) whose blood pressures remain unsatisfactorily controlled. As noted above, these patients are likely to have associated cardiovascular disease and other comorbid risk. Such patients may benefit materially from renal revascularization regarding both level of blood pressure control and stabilization of renal function.

Renal revascularization for renovascular hypertension

Restoring the renal blood supply is a rational goal of treating hypertension related to renovascular disease. Few conditions are more rewarding to treat than hypertension in a young person with fibromuscular dysplasia where a permanent 'cure' is achievable. Revascularization offers such a patient relief from a lifelong regimen of antihypertensive medications and cardiovascular risk associated with high blood pressure. In practice, however, 'cures' are infrequent. More often, renal revascularization allows improved blood pressure control and stabilization of the kidney circulation. Most institutions are limited in available expertise regarding vascular intervention and tend to favor either surgical or endovascular intervention depending upon local experience.

Guidelines for limiting renal toxicity in administration of ACE Inhibitors	
Assessment points	**Risk factors**
Recognize predisposing condition	Widespread atherosclerotic disease
	Associated renal artery stenosis
	Impaired pretreatment renal function
	Solitary functioning kidney
	Activated renin–angiotensin system
	Low sodium intake
	Diuretic therapy
	Other volume losses: vomiting, diarrhea
	Vasodilator administration
	Low cardiac function: hypotension, hyponatremia
	Other agents affecting kidney function, e.g., nonsteroidal anti-inflammatory agents
Monitor effects of initiating ACE therapy	Serum creatinine: measure over the first days or weeks especially in high-risk subjects
	Serum potassium: withhold potassium supplements (?),withhold potassium-sparing agents (?)
Manage volume	Temporarily withhold diuretics
	Dose titrate both diuretics and ACE inhibitor
	Liberalize sodium intake/replace volume, consider rechallenge with ACE inhibitor after volume repletion

Table 39.5 Guidelines for limiting renal toxicity in administration of ACE Inhibitors.

Hypertension

Percutaneous renal transluminal angioplasty and stenting

In many institutions, PTRA is the method of choice for both fibromuscular and atherosclerotic lesions of the renal arteries. Fibromuscular lesions are located away from the orifice of the aorta and often respond well to PTRA alone. Atherosclerotic lesions vary in location and may not be separable from a plaque arising from within the aorta at the ostium. Such ostial lesions have lower rates of technical success with simple angioplasty. Recent developments favor the use of endovascular stents in such cases, with higher rates of both immediate and secondary patency achieved[22]. Although no stents are currently FDA-approved for use in the renal arteries, these have become a standard tool of the interventional radiologist for this purpose. The use of stents is expanding, although the long-term patency rates and incidence of restenosis are not yet known with certainty.

Table 39.6 summarizes 17 reported series assessing technical success and clinical effect of PTRA in patients with renovascular hypertension[23, 24]. When technically successful, PTRA offers stabilization of renal function and improved blood pressure control. Results in these studies are highly variable, in part depending upon definitions of blood pressure change and length of follow-up. 'Cure' of hypertension is unusual in any of these series, even in patients with FMD. It is more common in FMD than in patients with atherosclerotic disease of the renal arteries. More recent series (after 1989) generally acknowledge a higher rate of 'failure' with PTRA in FMD. Restenosis rates before the introduction of stents were 12 to 24% at 1 year, sometimes leading to repeat procedures. Antihypertensive medication requirements commonly fall but rarely disappear entirely in patients with atherosclerotic disease, presumably because of pre-existing essential hypertension. The overall benefits of PTRA may be overstated somewhat as a result of the convention of omitting patients from analysis for whom PTRA could not be achieved for technical reasons (10–20% of patients)[25–27].

Complications

Reviews of PTRA and stenting vary widely regarding the incidence of minor and major complications. These likely reflect varying practice between centers and individual operators. Large reviews emphasize this disparity, and are summarized in Table 39.7. Among those complications with greatest prevalence are contrast nephrotoxicity, which is usually reversible, and atheroembolism, from which patients commonly do not recover. Particularly in patients with a badly diseased aorta, some degree of atheroembolism is unavoidable. Recent reviews suggest that between 7.5 and 9% of individuals have a 'major' complication related to the procedure[28]. Occasionally these produce arterial dissection, including aortic dissection and segmental renal infarction. These may progress to overt renal insufficiency. While such occurrences are not common, renal function only rarely recovers.

Surgical revascularization for renovascular hypertension

Prior to introduction of PTRA, surgical revascularization was the standard treatment for renovascular hypertension. Procedures were developed in the 1960s that for the first time allowed vascular bypass to the kidneys with grafts to the aorta. A recent summary of results of surgical revascularization for renovascular hypertension is shown in Table 39.8[29]. Blood pressure responses were consistently better in patients

Technical success and clinical effect of percutaneous renal transluminal angioplasty (PTRA)		
	1989–1995	1981–1987
Patients	1359	691
Arteries	1664	–
Fibromuscular disease		
Cured	42.4	53
Improved	36.2	38.7
Cured plus improved	78.6	91.7
Failed	21.4	8.4
Atherosclerosis of renal arteries		
Cured	14.8	18.4
Improved	51.7	48.9
Cured plus improved	65.4	67.3
Failed	34.6	32.7
Summary of 17 reports of PTRA comprising more than 2000 patients, beginning in 1981. (Adapted with permission from Aurell M, Jensen G. Treatment of renovascular hypertension. Nephron. 1997;75:373–83; and Ramsey LE, Waller PC. Blood pressure response to percutaneoustransluminal angioplasty for renovascular hypertension: an overview of published series. Br Med J. 1990;300:569–72.)		

Table 39.6 Technical success and clinical effect of percutaneous renal transluminal angioplasty (PTRA).

Complications of percutaneous renal transluminal angioplasty (PTRA)	
Type	Complications
Total (63/691 (9.1%))	–
Fatal (3/691)	Cholesterol embolism
	Cerebral hemorrhage
	Bowel infarction
Most frequent	Cholesterol embolism
	Contrast-associated nephrotoxicity
	Renal artery dissection
	Renal artery thrombosis/occlusion
	Segmental renal infarction
	Hematoma at puncture site
Classified as 'indirect'	Cerebrovascular accident
	Myocardial infarction
	Anterior spinal artery thrombosis
	Brachial artery thrombosis
	Bowel infarction
Adapted from Ramsey LE, Waller PC. Blood pressure response to percutaneous transluminal angioplasty for renovascular hypertension: an overview of published series. Br Med J. 1990;300:569–72.	

Table 39.7 Complications of percutaneous renal transluminal angioplasty (PTRA).

Blood pressure outcome for surgical revascularization in renovascular hypertension		
Outcome	Fibromuscular disease (n = 575)	Atherosclerosis of renal arteries (n = 631)
Cured	62.3	37.4
Improved	26.9	46.9
Cured plus improved	89.1	84.3
Failed	10.8	15.7

A summary of results for over 1200 patients. Follow-up procedures and definitions of blood pressure 'cure' varied greatly between series. Surgical mortality was 1.3–5.8% in patients with stenosis from atherosclerosis, nil in those with fibromuscular disease. (Adapted with permission from Stanley JC. Surgical treatment of renovascular hypertension. Am J Surg. 1997;174:102–10.)

Table 39.8 Blood pressure outcome for surgical revascularization in renovascular hypertension.

with FMD compared with those with atherosclerosis and the former group had no surgical mortality in the procedure. Many developments have improved surgical outcomes, including preoperative screening of the coronary and carotid circulation in high-risk patients. Such procedures nonetheless involve major vascular surgery and carry considerable risk, cost, and morbidity. This is especially true in older patients with widespread comorbid disease risk. As a result, surgical intervention for renovascular disease commonly is reserved for patients refractory to medical therapy in whom PTRA fails or may not offer adequate therapy for associated aortic disease[30]. In many institutions, advances in medical therapy have made surgical revascularization no longer a first choice for blood pressure control. Revascularization now is undertaken both for improved blood pressure control and in the hope of 'preserving' renal function by restoring blood supply to compromised kidneys. As a result, surgical series now more commonly include patients with more advanced renal failure, combined renal and aortic disease, and widespread vascular disease. Despite these caveats, it must be emphasized that successful surgical revascularization offers durable restoration of kidney blood supply and long-term survival (81% at 5 years) against which newer techniques must be compared[31].

While restoration of blood flow and salvage of kidney function is the primary objective, occasional cases of renovascular hypertension present with either total occlusion or nonfunction of one kidney. In such cases, the pressor role of the nonfunctioning kidney may be relieved by nephrectomy. Results from a recent series indicate that improved blood pressures can be obtained in such instances without detectable loss of renal function. Estimates of renal function in this group were 11% in the removed kidney and 89% in the contralateral kidneys[32]. With the introduction of laparoscopic techniques for nephrectomy, such an approach may offer clinical benefits in selected cases with less morbidity than a standard operative nephrectomy.

Complications of surgical revascularization
In most cases, surgical revascularization requires comparable hospitalization and care to other aortic surgery. The primary immediate causes of morbidity and mortality are related to coronary and cerebrovascular events. In most cases, risk stratification and therapy for associated coronary and cerebrovascular diseases should be performed first.

Outcomes of renal revascularization
In many patients, successful renal revascularization leads to improved blood pressure control and reduced morbidity and mortality in the long term. Antihypertensive medication requirements fall, although rarely are they eliminated entirely. Most series report 'stabilization' of renal function, meaning that average serum creatinine levels do not change. This interpretation may be misleading. Some patients experience a marked improvement in renal function, while others have a clinically significant loss of renal function. In most series this occurs in up to 18–20% of patients treated either with PTRA or surgery. Although group average values do not change, a substantial number of patients experience adverse effects on renal function that must be considered before undertaking vascular intervention of any kind, particularly when blood pressure control is the primary concern[33]. The benefits of modestly improved blood pressure control should

Studies comparing medical treatment and PTRA			
Study	Number of subjects	Features	Outcome
Webster, et al.[25]	n = 55 Unilateral = 27		Lower BP in the PTRA group with bilateral renal artery stenosis. No difference in BP in the unilateral renal artery stenosis group. No difference in renal function or survival.
Plouin, et al.[26]	n = 49 All Unilateral	Multicenter, Evaluation with ambulatory BP monitoring at 6 months. No ACE inhibitors	No difference in BP. Fewer BP med requirements in PTRA group, but more complications. Crossover in med treatment: 7/26 (27%)
Van Jaarsveld et al.[27]	n = 106	Multicenter, office and automated BP, lateralization studies (scan, renal vein renin)	No difference in BP at 12 mos Crossover in med treatment: 22/50

Table 39.9 Three randomized prospective studies comparing medical treatment and PTRA (with and without stents)[25–27].

not be understated. Treatment trials in hypertension based upon blood pressure differences of 10–15 mmHg between treatment and placebo groups established major differences in cardiovascular end points, including overall mortality. Early series of medically treated versus surgically treated patients with renovascular hypertension underscored the high risks of uncontrolled blood pressure in the medical group.

There are few prospective data comparing medical therapy with renal revascularization in the current era. Most of the literature regarding endovascular procedures for renal revascularization are observational reports and frequently are limited by poorly standardized methods of blood pressure measurement and drug therapy. Three recent, prospective, randomized trials comparing medical therapy with angioplasty report only modest benefits attributable to PTRA. The major features of these prospective RCTs are summarized in Table 39.9[25–27]. These studies are small and are limited by patient selection, but do underscore the effectiveness of current drug regimens and the relative infrequency of 'cure' in patients with atherosclerotic renal arterial stenosis. All of these were limited in size and excluded many patients with progressive renal dysfunction, accelerated hypertensive disease or recent cardiovascular events.

The largest of these studies was published in 2000 as the DRASTIC study (Dutch Renal Artery Stenosis Intervention Cooperative Study Group). It included 106 patients with relatively resistant hypertension randomized either to medical therapy or PTRA. The lack of difference in blood pressure after 1 year between patients treated with PTRA and treated medically led the authors to conclude that 'angioplasty has little advantage over antihypertensive drug therapy…'[25]. This study was analyzed under 'intention to treat' statistical rules, in which 22/50 patients assigned to medical therapy (44%) crossed over to the PTRA arm due to uncontrolled blood pressure levels at 3 months. Despite their inclusion in the medical arm, many authorities reviewing these data might argue that this group offers compelling evidence of medical treatment failure in some instances and the benefit of renal revascularization for such individuals. The available data suggest that effective blood pressure control achieved by any means is the central determinant of cardiovascular outcomes.

An integrated approach to the patient at risk for renovascular hypertension

The aging demographics of the USA and other Western countries favor more patients developing critical levels of renal artery stenosis than ever before. Critical to the management of such patients is the recognition of distinctive clinical syndromes of renovascular disease, linking acceleration of hypertension with deteriorating renal function and, occasionally, episodic circulatory congestion ('flash' pulmonary edema). Many patients can be managed by medical means. It must be emphasized that evaluating such patients is an ongoing process that must be reviewed at regular intervals. When progressively more complex antihypertensive regimens become required and/or renal function deteriorates, consideration should be given to identification and correction of critical vascular lesions affecting the kidneys. Figure 39.9 is an algorithm

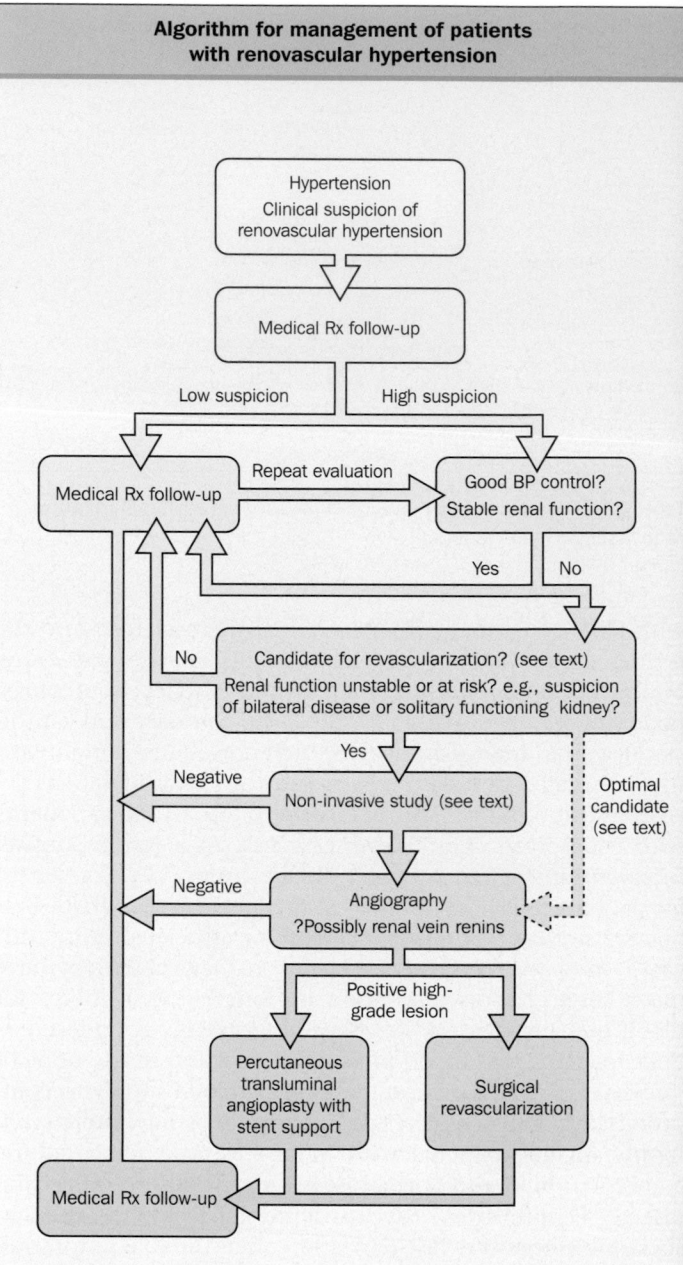

Algorithm for management of patients with renovascular hypertension

Figure 39.9 Clinical algorithm for management of patients with renovascular hypertension. Initiation of the algorithm depends on the index of suspicion for the possible role of renovascular disease in aggravating hypertension and/or declining renal function and the success of medical therapy (see text).

by which such patients can be managed. This scheme emphasizes the need to evaluate whether the patient is a candidate for renal vascularization based upon clinical features, including age, other diseases, and whether stable blood pressure and kidney function can be achieved using medical therapy. If the patient is not a candidate for revascularization, there is little to be gained from extensive diagnostic studies. Conversely, if blood pressure control and stable renal function are not achieved by a reasonable effort at medical therapy, one is justified in beginning a systematic evaluation of the renal vasculature with the objective of vascular intervention if a significant lesion is identified. Evaluation for surgery or angioplasty should be considered for patients resistant to therapy, either by virtue of inadequate blood pressure control or unstable renal function, and who are candidates for renal vascularization should a stenotic lesion be found. The latter is a highly individual judgement based upon comorbid disease risk, age, etc. If the patient is a candidate for further evaluation, a noninvasive study, such as MRA, may allow exclusion of a high-grade lesion or bilateral disease. In cases of atherosclerotic disease, invasive angiography should be limited mainly to patients in whom revascularization is anticipated, often at the same procedure. This approach limits the hazards of vessel intrumentation and contrast nephrotoxicity to a single procedure. With the introduction of stent-supported angioplasty, surgical reconstruction is often limited to patients with technically challenging vascular lesions and/or associated aortic disease needing additional reconstruction.

Even with successful revascularization, medical therapy and follow-up remain essential. Balancing the potential risks and benefits of medical therapy versus primary revascularization remains a complex challenge. This is particularly true in view of other causes of morbidity and mortality in patients with atherosclerotic vascular disease. Most often, management decisions are based upon considerations of preserving renal function and avoiding adverse effects of progressive vascular disease.

REFERENCES

1. Safian RD, Textor SC: Medical progress. Renal artery stenosis. N Engl J Med. 2001;344:431–42.
2. Anderson GH, Blakemen N, Streeten DH. The effect of age on prevalence of secondary forms of hypertension in 4429 consecutively referred patients. J Hypertens. 1994;12:609–15.
3. Textor SC. Pathophysiology of renovascular hypertension. Urol Clin N Am. 1984;11:373–81.
4. Romero JC, Feldstein AE, Rodriguez-Porcel MG, Cases-Amenos A. New insights into the pathophysiology of renovascular hypertension. Mayo Clin Proc. 1997;72:251–60.
5. Krijnen P, van Jaarsveld BC, Steyerberg EW, et al. A clinical prediction rule for renal artery stenosis. Ann Int Med. 1998;129:705–11.
6. Chen R, Novick AC, Pohl M. Reversible renin mediated massive proteinuria successfully treated by nephrectomy. J Urol. 1995;153:133–4.
7. Davis BA, Crook JE, Vestal RE, Oates JA. Prevalence of renovascular hypertension in patients with grade III or IV hypertensive retinopathy. N Engl J Med. 1979;301:1273–6.
8. Heart Outcomes Prevention evaluation study investigators. Effects of an angiotensin-converting enzyme inhibitor, ramipril, on cardiovascular events in high risk patients. N Engl J Med. 2000;342:145–53.
9. Lewis EJ, Hunsicker LG, Clarke WR, et al. Renoprotective effect of the angiotensin-receptor antagonist irbesartan in patient with nephropathy due to type 2 diabetes. N Engl J Med. 2001; 345:851–60.
10. Conlon PJ, Athirakul K, Kovalik E, et al. Survival in renal vascular disease. J Am Soc Nephrol. 1998;9:252–6.
11. Caps MT, Perissinotto C, Zierler RE, et al. Prospective study of atherosclerotic disease progression in the renal artery. Circulation. 1998;98:2866–72.
12. Chabova V, Schirger A, Stanson AW, et al. Outcomes of atherosclerotic renal artery stenosis managed without revascularization. Mayo Clin Proc. 2000;75:437–44.
13. Leertouwer TC, Pattynama PMT, van den Berg-Huysmans A. Incidental renal artery stenosis in peripheral vascular disease: a case for treatment? Kidney Int. 2001;59:1480–3.
14. Wilcox CS. Non-invasive evaluation of renovascular disease. Tech Vasc Intervent Radiol. 1999;2:60–4.
15. Mann SJ, Pickering TG. Detection of renovascular hypertension: state of the art 1992. Ann Int Med. 1992;117:845–53.
16. Wilcox CS. Ischemic nephropathy: noninvasive testing. Semin Nephrol. 1996;16:43–52.
17. Pohl MA. Medical management of renovascular hypertension. In: Novick A, Scoble J, Hamilton G, eds. Renal Vascular Disease. London: W.B.Saunders Co. Ltd., 1996;339–49.
18. Hricik DE, Browning PJ, Kopelman R, et al. Captopril-induced functional renal insufficiency in patients with bilateral renal-artery stenosis or renal-artery stenosis in a solitary kidney. N Engl J Med. 1983;308:377–81.
19. Jackson B, Matthews PG, McGrath BP, Johnston CI. Angiotensin converting enzyme inhibition in renovascular hypertension: frequency of reversible renal failure. Lancet. 1984;i:225–6.
20. Speirs CJ, Dollery CT, Inman WHW, et al. Postmarketing surveillance of enalapril II: investigation of the potential role of enalapril in deaths with renal failure. Br Med J. 1988;297:830–2.
21. Textor SC. Renal failure related to ACE inhibitors. Semin Nephrol. 1997;17:67–76.
22. van de Ven PJ, Kaatee R, Beutler JJ, et al. Arterial stenting and balloon angioplasty in ostial atherosclerotic renovascular disease: a randomised trial. Lancet. 1999;353:282–6.
23. Aurell M, Jensen G. Treatment of renovascular hypertension. Nephron. 1997;75:373–83.
24. Ramsay LE, Waller PC. Blood pressure response to percutaneous transluminal angioplasty for renovascular hypertension: an overview of published series. Br Med J. 1990;300:569–72.
25. Webster J, Marshall F, Abdalla M, et al. Randomised comparison of percutaneous angioplasty vs continued medical therapy for hypertensive patients with atheromatous renal artery stenosis. J Hum Hypertens. 1998;12:329–35.
26. Plouin PF, Chatellier G, Darne B, Raynaud A. Blood pressure outcome of angioplasty in atherosclerotic renal artery stenosis: a randomized trial. Hypertension. 1998;31:822–9.
27. van Jaarsveld BC, Krijnen P, Pieterman H, et al. The effect of balloon angioplasty on hypertension in atherosclerotic renal-artery stenosis. N Engl J Med. 2000;342:1007–14.
28. Leertouwer TC, Gussenhoven EJ, Bosch JP, et al. Stent placement for renal arterial stenosis: where do we stand? A meta-analysis. Radiology. 2000;21:78–85.
29. Stanley JC. Surgical treatment of renovascular hypertension. Am J Surg. 1997;174:102–10.
30. Hallett JW, Textor SC, Kos PB, et al. Advanced renovascular hypertension and renal insufficiency: trends in medical comorbidity and surgical approach from 1970 to 1993. J Vasc Surg. 1995;21:750–9.
31. Steinbach F, Novick AC, Campbell S, Dykstra D. Long-term survival after surgical revascularization for atherosclerotic renal artery disease. J Urol. 1997;158:38–41.
32. Kane GC, Textor SC, Schirger A, Garovic V. Predictors of cure in patients undergoing nephrectomy for pressor kidney. J Am Soc Nephrol. 2001;345:485A(Abstract).
33. Textor SC, Wilcox CS: Renal artery stenosis: a common, treatable cause of renal failure? Annu Rev Med. 2001;52:421–42.
34. Simon N, Franklin SS, Bleifer KH, Maxwell MH. Clinical characteristics of renovascular hypertension. JAMA. 1972;220:1209–12–18.

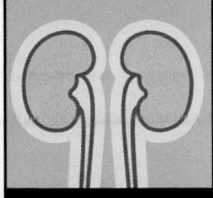

Chapter 40

Endocrine Causes of Hypertension

Mark Richards and Gary Nicholls

INTRODUCTION

The true incidence and prevalence of hypertension with pure endocrine etiology is unknown. In the past, endocrine forms of hypertension were thought to account for <1% of all cases of hypertension. However, many patients with an endocrine cause of hypertension are underdiagnosed because physicians do not consider this possibility due to perceived rarity of these conditions or because of limited access to the specialized tests for diagnosis. Recent reports have identified primary aldosteronism in 2–12% of newly diagnosed hypertension. Causes of endocrine hypertension are shown in Table 40.1.

Although endocrine hypertension often occurs in the absence of readily observed signs, symptoms (e.g., mineralocorticoid syndromes), or abnormality in routine biochemical tests, certain features should trigger a simple screen (Fig. 40.1) for these conditions. First, these include a positive family history of conditions with inherited forms, including pheochromocytoma, neurofibromatosis, multiple endocrine

---

Causes of endocrine hypertension

Pituitary
  Cushing's disease
  Acromegaly

Adrenal cortex
  Primary aldosteronism
  Pseudoaldosteronism
  Cushing's syndrome

Adrenal medulla
  Pheochromocytoma

Thyroid
  Hypothyroidism
  Hyperthyroidism

Renin-secreting tumors

Others
  Hyperparathyroidism?
  Endothelioma

Table 40.1 Causes of endocrine hypertension.

Screening for endocrine hypertension

Triggers for endocrine investigation in hypertension

Family history
Pheochromocytoma
Neurofibromatosis
Multiple endocrine neoplasia
Aldosteronism

Refractory hypertension: high blood pressure resistant to 2–3 drugs
Consider
  Iatrogenic source
  Compliance with medication
  Renal/renovascular disease
  Endocrine disorder
Measure
  Serum electrolytes – Na$^+$/K$^+$
  Dipstick/urinalysis
  Aldosterone/Plasma renin activity (PRA)
  Catecholamines
  ?Renal angiography

Hypokalemia: persistent? K$^+$ wasting? (i.e., >30 mmol/24 h excreted when plasma K$^+$ <3.5 mmol/L)
Consider
  Iatrogenic, diuretics, licorice
  Accelerated essential hypertension
  Aldosteronism
  Pseudoaldosteronism
  Cushing's syndrome
  Renin-producing tumor

Symptoms/signs
?Pheochromocytoma
  Hyperadrenergic: sweating
?Thyroid
  Change in:
    Temperature tolerance
    Weight
    Skin/hair
    Bowel habit
    Eyes
    Tremor
    Sweating
?Acromegaly
  Size of face/hands/feet
  Sweating
?Cushing's syndrome
  Striae, acne, central weight gain

Hyperglycemia
Diabetic nephropathy
Cushing's syndrome
Pheochromocytoma
Acromegaly

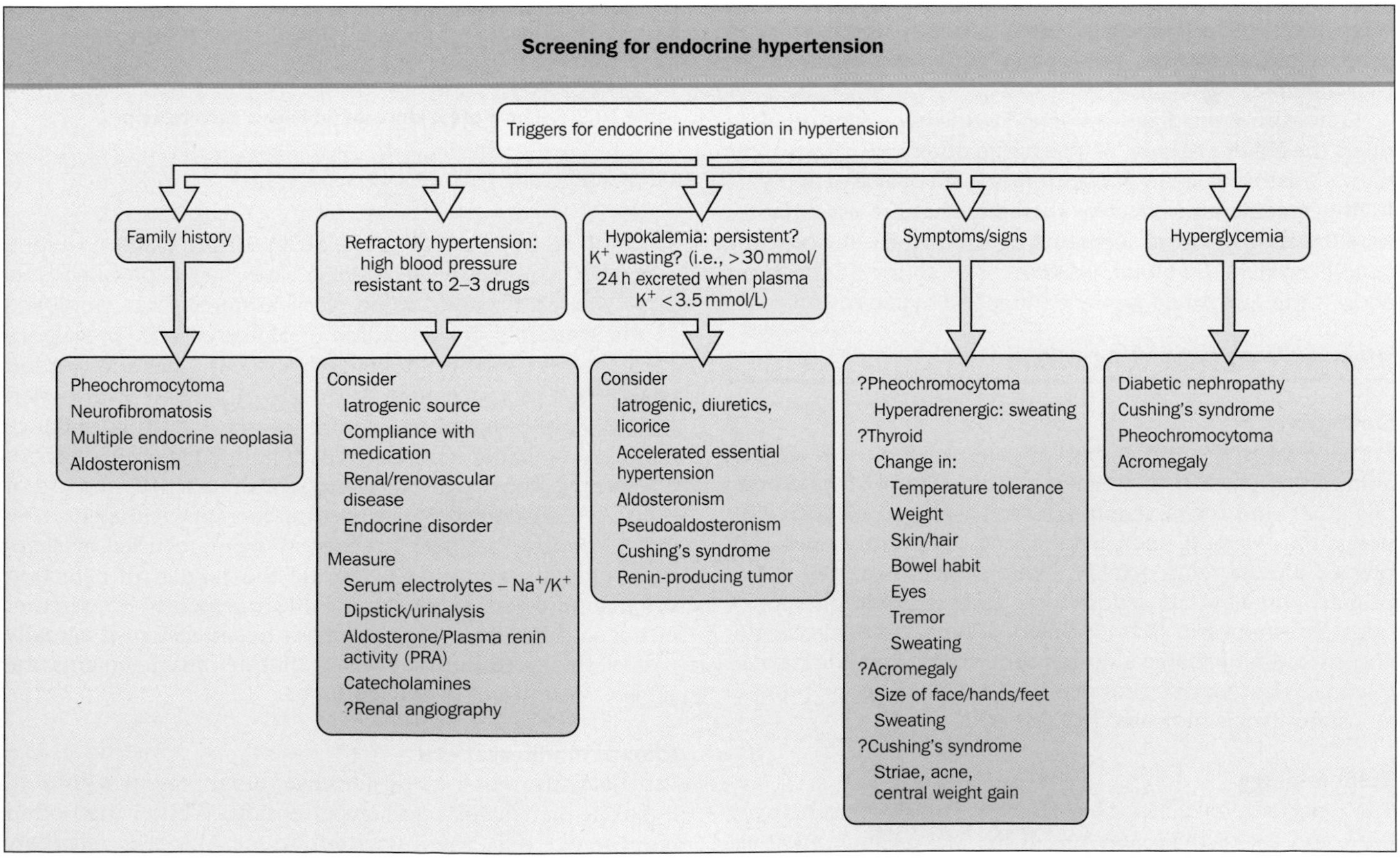

Figure 40.1 Clinical observations suggesting endocrine investigation in hypertension.

neoplasia and aldosteronism. Second, refractory hypertension (i.e., blood pressure that is resistant to administration of two or three antihypertensive drugs of different classes) should trigger consideration of secondary hypertension provided iatrogenic factors and noncompliance have been ruled out. The differential diagnoses will include renal and renovascular disease but, once these are excluded, a screen for endocrine hypertension should be employed.

Third, symptoms and signs may be present. If hypokalemia becomes sufficiently severe in potassium-wasting forms of hypertension, weakness, polyuria and, possibly, cardiac arrhythmia may ensue. Hyperadrenergic symptoms occur with pheochromocytoma. Changes in temperature tolerance, body weight, hair and skin condition, and bowel habit are clues in thyroid dysfunction or hypercortisolism. Thyroid disease, Cushing's syndrome and acromegaly are associated with typical changes in body habitus. Abnormal sweating occurs in pheochromocytoma, thyrotoxicosis, and acromegaly.

Fourth, hypokalemia and diabetes mellitus are hallmarks of endocrine pathologies in hypertension. Hypokalemia, although most commonly iatrogenic, is a feature common to primary aldosteronism, pseudoaldosteronism, renin-secreting tumor, Cushing's disease and accelerated hypertension of any cause. Therefore, concurrent high blood pressure and hypokalemia should prompt consideration of possible endocrine or other secondary causes of hypertension. Hyperglycemia, although most commonly reflecting insulin- or noninsulin-dependent diabetes, in the absence of any other endocrine abnormality is a common feature of Cushing's syndrome, pheochromocytoma (especially where epinephrine levels are increased), and acromegaly. Also, it is not uncommon in primary aldosteronism, presumably partly as a result of the hypokalemia.

Establishing the diagnosis of endocrine hypertension often offers the chance of cure, of altering an otherwise catastrophic natural history (e.g., in pheochromocytoma), and of applying highly specific and effective therapies that are essential for amelioration of other elements of the disease beyond the simple control of blood pressure. The following sections address the individual types of endocrine hypertension.

PRIMARY ALDOSTERONISM

Definition

Primary aldosteronism is most commonly due to an adrenal aldosterone-producing adenoma (APA; Conn's syndrome) (Fig.40.2)[4] and is characterized by hypokalemic alkalosis with potassium wasting, increased plasma aldosterone and suppressed plasma renin activity. Other causes associated with a primary increase in aldosterone level include idiopathic hyperaldosteronism (IHA), primary adrenal hyperplasia, glucocorticoid-remediable aldosteronism (GRA) and adrenal carcinoma. The relative prevalence of these forms of primary aldosteronism is indicated in Table 40.2.

Epidemiology

The reported prevalence of APA has previously been between 0.5% and 2% of hypertensives. At the Mayo Clinic, APA was found in 0.01% of 26 589 patients with hypertension seen in

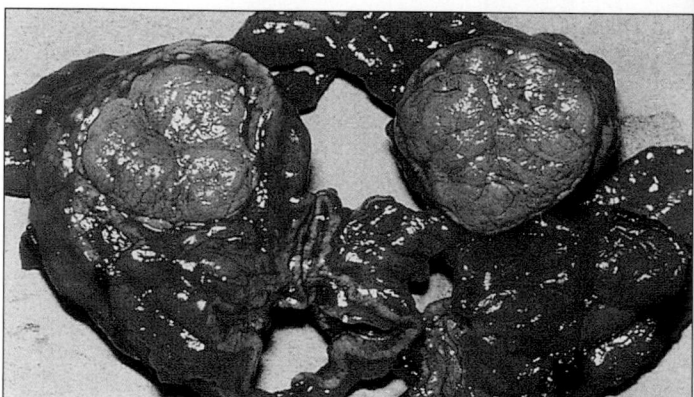

Figure 40.2 Conn's tumor. An aldosterone-producing adrenal adenoma with typical cholesterol-rich yellow appearance.

Relative prevalence of primary aldosteronism	
Forms	Percentage
Aldosterone-producing adenoma (APA)	57
Aldosterone-producing/angiotensin II responsive adenoma (AP-RA)	2.4
Idiopathic hyperaldosteronism (IHA) Familial hyperaldosteronism type II (FH-II)	37
Primary adrenal hyperplasia (PAH)	2.5
Glucocorticoid remediable aldosteronism (GRA aka familial hyperaldosteronism type I, FH-I)	<1
Adrenal carcinoma	<1

Table 40.2 Relative prevalence of primary aldosteronism.

1973–1975[9]. In contrast, at the SUNY Health Science Center, over 4000 consecutively referred cases had a prevalence of 2.7% when a diastolic value of >100 mmHg was employed as the threshold for selection[3,10]. However, this prevalence value has been further challenged in recent times and Gordon et al.[11] have proposed that up to 12% of patients with hypertension have primary aldosteronism and that, in accordance with Conn's earlier reports, frank hypokalemia occurs only in a minority. This controversy has continued with reports of primary aldosteronism accounting for approximately 10% of hypertensive patients screened[12,13] being rebuffed by skeptical commentary centered around the validity of detection through aldosterone–renin ratio measurements[14,15]. Whether or not so called 'low-renin essential hypertension' is actually part of the spectrum of primary aldosteronism remains the subject of controversy and research.

Clinical manifestations

Patients with primary aldosteronism often present with mild hypokalemic alkalosis and hypertension. While it had often been stated that the hypertension of APA was relatively benign and had minimal end organ damage (such as in the heart and retina), recent evidence has shown this is not true, and patients with APA have increased left ventricular hypertrophy and diastolic dysfunction compared to essential hypertension at similar levels of blood pressure[1]. Carotid atherosclerosis, hemorrhagic stroke and congestive heart failure all occur at similar or higher prevalence as in essential hypertension. Cardiac effects may partly reflect the recently recognized fibrotic actions of aldosterone[2,3].

Diagnosis and differential diagnosis

The diagnosis is considered particularly in the setting where spontaneous hypokalemia is associated with hypertension. However, hypokalemia may only occur in one-third of all primary aldosteronism. If hypokalemia is present in the absence of diuretic therapy, then potassium wasting should be proven by measurement of plasma potassium and simultaneous measurement of 24-h urinary potassium excretion. Excretion of over 30 mmol potassium per day in the presence of a plasma potassium of 3.5 mmol/L or less indicates potassium wasting.

Primary aldosteronism is characterized by increased plasma aldosterone with suppression of plasma renin activity, which suggests the utility of their measurement for diagnosis. However, single measurements of plasma aldosterone are of little diagnostic value as diurnal variation is significant and is usually preserved in the presence of primary aldosteronism. Drugs also interfere with aldosterone levels in that diuretics increase aldosterone while angiotensin converting enzyme (ACE) inhibitors and β-blocker agents tend to reduce it. Plasma potassium levels are an important determinant of aldosterone secretion, and hypokalemia may markedly reduce the biosynthesis of aldosterone, producing plasma levels within the normal range. Plasma aldosterone is therefore best measured after restoration of normokalemia.

Random single measurements of plasma renin activity are also of little value. Antihypertensive agents, such as ACE inhibitors, diuretics and vasodilators cause renin levels to rise, whereas β-adrenoceptor blockade inhibits renin release. Hence, representative measurements may require cessation of antihypertensive therapy, which may not always be practical or safe. In any case, 20–30% of patients with essential hypertension have relatively low renin activity in the absence of primary aldosteronism, and therefore the specificity of this test in isolation is poor.

The divergent changes of renin and aldosterone in primary aldosteronism make the aldosterone–renin ratio a more sensitive and robust method of screening for primary aldosteronism than random measurement of one or other alone, and it is now an established mainstay in diagnosis. The specific ratio that is diagnostic will depend on the laboratory because renin assays may vary with relation to the units of measurement and reference ranges. Although the ratio is less disturbed by drugs, diurnal rhythms, or posture, ideally the measurement should be made in the absence of potential confounding by drugs. Falsely elevated values may occur in renal failure, and false-positive values occur when renin is suppressed by β-blockers or when aldosterone is abruptly stimulated by potassium supplementation. As mentioned, 'low renin essential hypertension' remains a controversial entity and whether it constitutes a large reservoir of false-positive aldosterone–renin

ratios or is actually part of the spectrum of primary aldosteronism remains subject to debate. ACE inhibitors, and possibly calcium antagonists, may produce false-negative values by reducing aldosterone secretion in angiotensin II-responsive adenomas (in the case of ACE inhibitors), or by nonspecific interference in the secretory process (by calcium antagonists).

If an elevation in aldosterone/renin ratio is confirmed, further tests should investigate the autonomy of aldosterone secretion (Table 40.3). Elevation of plasma aldosterone in the setting of saline infusion, administration of fludrocortisone, and administration of captopril is consistent with primary aldosteronism. As volume expansion is already present, additional volume load in the form of saline infusion or induced by fludrocortisone should not produce further lowering of plasma aldosterone levels. However, false-negative results may occur with the saline infusion test because some adenomas do not show complete autonomy and may cause diurnal shifts in plasma aldosterone as well as changes in aldosterone levels in response to angiotensin II. Additional tests include measurement of the aldosterone/renin ratio 2 h after administration of 25 mg captopril, or the fludrocortisone suppression test. The latter requires an in-patient stay for 4 days with administration of 0.1 mg fludrocortisone by mouth every 6 h, together with supplemental sodium chloride and potassium. In Table 40.3, one potential sequence of tests for primary aldosteronism is offered.

Distinguishing the form of primary aldosteronism is also important and can be aided by imaging studies (see below) as well as by laboratory testing. IHA may be distinguished from

Tests for diagnosis of primary aldosteronism	
Test	**Comment**
Plasma K+ levels	In any hypertensive patient 2–3 plasma K+ levels should be checked taking care to avoid drugs that alter plasma K+ or artifactual effects from poor blood sampling technique, delayed handling, or processing of the sample (hemolysis). The possibility of primary aldosteronism should be considered regardless of sex, age, severity of hypertension, and the level of plasma K+ but is obviously more likely when hypokalemia is present
24-h K+ excretion	> 30 mmol/24 h when plasma K+ < 3.5 mmol/L indicates K+ wasting
Plasma aldosterone to renin ratio	Can be measured under random conditions but preferably is assessed in the morning when aldosterone is at its highest level and in the absence of all antihypertensive medications (especially spironolactone) for 2 weeks. This test should be performed in the evaluation of all patients with hypertension and hypokalemia. An elevated ratio (as defined by each individual laboratory) is highly diagnostic for hyperaldosteronism
Fludrocortisone test	Fludrocortisone increases the volume load; plasma aldosterone levels will remain elevated if primary aldosteronism exists
Computed tomography	Scan the adrenals
Adrenal secretion: adrenal vein sampling	Adrenal vein aldosterone and cortisol sampling can be used if imaging is negative or equivocal

Table 40.3 Tests for diagnosis of primary aldosteronism.

Hypertension

APA through the response of aldosterone to upright posture: aldosterone rises in most patients with IHA, whereas in APA there is normally no response or a fall in plasma aldosterone. However, a small subset of APA patients will show increase of aldosterone levels in response to upright posture. Patients with APA have better retention of the normal circadian rhythm of plasma aldosterone than those with IHA. Measurement of plasma aldosterone together with cortisol at 08.00 h, 10.00 h, 12.00 h and 16.00 h may help differentiate these two conditions. Plasma 18-hydroxycorticosterone (the final precursor in aldosterone synthesis) is more elevated in APA than in IHA.

Localizing aldosterone source by adrenal imaging or venous sampling

Computed tomography (CT) scanning detects hyperplasia and adenomas if the adenomas are 10 mm or greater diameter (Fig. 40.3). As nonfunctioning adrenal adenomas are relatively common ('incidentalomas' may be present in up to 2% of the general population), interpretation of such a finding requires initial firm biochemical diagnosis of primary aldosteronism. In addition, the sensitivity of CT scanning for adrenal adenomas is relatively poor (50–70%). As yet, no clear advantage of magnetic resonance imaging (MRI) over CT scanning has been demonstrated.

APA can be confirmed by a nuclear medicine scan that utilizes ^{131}I-labeled 6-iodomethylnorcholesterol to label the adenoma. Dexamethasone (0.5 mg every 6 h for 10 days) is started 4 days before administration of the tracer to suppress endogenous adrenocorticotropic hormone (ACTH). Concurrence of lateralization of scintigraphic uptake with CT findings confirms APA.

Where imaging is unhelpful or equivocal, demonstration of lateralization of aldosterone production from one adrenal gland can direct surgery. The left adrenal vein drains via the left renal vein and is relatively easy to find and cannulate. However, the variable anatomy of the right adrenal vein and its small size restricts the use of the procedure to tertiary centers with experienced radiologists. Plasma cortisol should always be measured in the adrenal vein samples as this will verify successful cannulation of the adrenal vein.

Genetic causes of primary aldosteronism

Primary aldosteronism may also have genetic causes. Glucocorticoid-remediable aldosteronism (GRA or familial hyperaldosteronism, type I(FH-I)) is an autosomal dominant syndrome caused by unequal crossing over of genetic material[5], leading to the fusion of the 5′ regulatory region of the 11-hydroxylase gene to the coding sequence for aldosterone synthase on chromosome 8q. Aldosterone synthase (18-oxidase) becomes abnormally expressed in the zona fasciculata under the control of ACTH. Genotyping can secure the diagnosis of GRA using reliable rapid polymerase chain reaction methods. Corticosteroids such as dexamethasone will suppress ACTH production, will therefore block the aldosterone production.

A second autosomal dominant form of familial primary aldosteronism has also been described, termed familial hyperaldosteronism type II (FH-II), and is diagnosed by demonstrating primary aldosteronism in a relative of a patient known

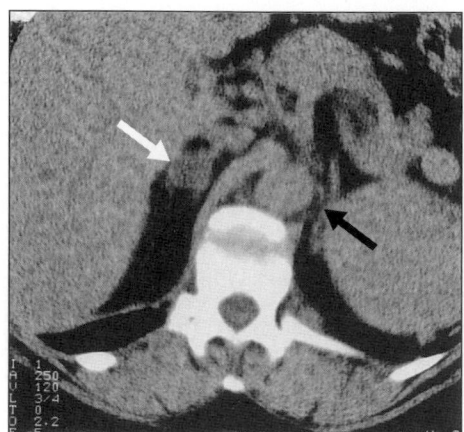

Figure 40.3 Computed tomography of the adrenal gland. A normal linear image of the left adrenal (black arrow) and expansion of the right adrenal, with a 2-cm aldosterone-producing adenoma (white arrow).

to have the condition, plus exclusion of FH-I. FH-II may demonstrate different biochemical and adrenal morphological features (both unilateral adenomas and bilateral hyperplasia) within the one pedigree[6]. Genetic linkage studies in a large kindred with FH-II has identified a locus on chromosome 7 corresponding to cytogenetic band 7p22. Future molecular elucidation of this genetic locus may offer insight into the etiology of primary aldosteronism[7].

Differential diagnosis

An array of rare syndromes produces endocrine hypertension that mimic primary aldosteronism. They are characterized by hypokalemia and hypertension with concomitant suppression of both renin and aldosterone. These include the syndrome of apparent mineralocorticoid excess (SAME I), Liddle's syndrome, congenital adrenal hyperplasia and licorice ingestion. These are discussed in more detail in Chapter 49. Cushing's syndrome may also present with hypokalemia and hypertension, and is discussed below.

Treatment

First-line treatment of primary aldosteronism due to APA is surgical removal of the adenoma. Pretreatment with spironolactone or amiloride should be performed in preparing the patient for adrenal surgery. Spironolactone blocks the renal action of aldosterone and also inhibits aldosterone synthesis. Amiloride acts in distal tubules on sodium/hydrogen exchange through a mechanism independent of aldosterone. Both drugs can control hypertension and correct hypokalemia in aldosteronism. Spironolactone is administered at 100–400 mg per day, and amiloride at up to 40 mg per day. A period of treatment of 4–6 weeks may be required before the full effect is apparent. Preoperative response to either of these drugs indicates the likely blood pressure response to surgery.

Removal of the adenoma is associated with correction of aldosterone levels and hypokalemia in all cases. Blood pressure is normal postoperatively in 50–75% of patients. Left ventricular hypertrophy is reversed. There is some evidence that residual hypertension, if present, is due to previous hypertension-induced microvascular structural changes in the kidney.

Where surgery is contraindicated or refused, long-term treatment with spironolactone or amiloride is effective. Over time, the dosage of spironolactone may possibly be reduced to 100–150 mg daily. Side effects reflect spironolactone's antiandrogen action. Dose-related gynecomastia and impotence may occur in males, while females may suffer menstrual disturbance.

Amiloride remains the only well-tried agent other than the aldosterone receptor antagonists. In contrast to spironolactone where approximately one-half of patients are controlled on monotherapy, adjunctive antihypertensive treatment is required in 75% of cases where amiloride is used. Experience with triamterene, another potassium sparing diuretic is very limited but it may be an adequate substitute when amiloride is not tolerated.

Response to calcium channel blockers (including nifedipine, nicardipine and amlodipine) is controversial but positive trials have been reported and cases of masking of aldosteronism by calcium channel blocker use have been documented. Therefore, they may be worth exhibiting as third-line treatment in refractory cases.

Newer agents for the treatment of primary aldosteronism are also being developed[16]. Canrenoate, a spironolactone metabolite, and eplerenone, a selective and competitive aldosterone receptor antagonist, have comparable efficacy to spironolactone but with minimal anti-androgen effects such as gynecomastia. A study comparing the efficacy of eplerone versus spironolactone in primary aldosteronism is in progress. Aldosterone synthesis inhibitors (trilostane and metyrapone) have been disappointing and are not a long-term option.

ACE inhibitors and angiotensin receptor antagonists (ATRA) are useful adjunctive treatment in the rare cases of angiotensin II responsive adenoma and adrenal hyperplasia where aldosterone secretion remains partially angiotensin II-dependent.

GRA constitutes a special entity. It is recognized by demonstration of reversal of the hypertension and biochemical abnormalities with 2–3 weeks of treatment with dexamethasone 1–2 mg daily. Plasma aldosterone may fall to very low levels within 2 days of commencing treatment. If successful, dexamethasone therapy should be continued indefinitely by using the smallest possible dose (0.25–0.5 mg daily).

Where adrenal cortical carcinoma is present, prompt surgical excision is indicated. Recurrence is common. Chemotherapy with mitotane, aminoglutethimide and fluorouracil has been used with metastatic disease, but benefit is inconsistent and usually brief.

CUSHING'S SYNDROME

Definition, epidemiology and clinical features
Cushing's syndrome results from sustained glucocorticoid excess, which may be pituitary dependent (Cushing's disease) or caused by an adrenal adenoma or carcinoma. Additional causes are iatrogenic glucocorticoid excess, the ectopic ACTH syndrome, or the ectopic corticotropin-releasing factor (CRF) syndrome. Chronic alcohol excess can result in a cushingoid appearance and altered cortisol metabolism. The clinical features in Cushing's disease relate to excessive cortisol production and, in addition in many patients, excess adrenal androgens. Features include central adiposity and muscle wasting, hirsutism, sexual dysfunction, plethoric facies and purple striae (Fig. 40.4), mental symptoms and skin abnormalities (acne, skin pigmentation, easy bruising). Androgen effects

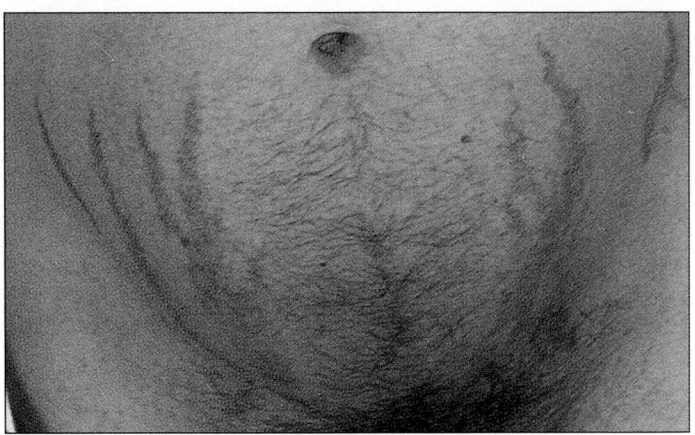

Figure 40.4 Striae and central obesity of Cushing's syndrome.

may be striking in adrenal adenoma or carcinoma. The ectopic ACTH syndrome, caused by bronchogenic carcinoma or other malignancy, is often a wasting disorder with hypokalemia.

The incidence of pituitary-based Cushing's disease is 5–25 per million of the population per year. Cushing's syndrome from adrenal tumors is less common (20% of the incidence of Cushing's disease)[17]. The prevalence of hypertension in Cushing's syndrome is approximately 80%[18]. The mechanism underlying raised blood pressure is unclear. There is an increase in total body sodium content, which enhances pressor responsiveness to angiotensin II and/or catecholamines. Renin substrate levels are elevated in Cushing's syndrome, but there is no strong evidence for a primary role of the renin-angiotensin system. Sympathetic overactivity has been claimed and may contribute to high cardiac output in Cushing's syndrome. Left ventricular hypertrophy is common and presumably results from both high blood pressure and raised levels of cortisol. Other factors which may contribute to the hypertension include a decrease in vasodilator prostaglandins and kallikrein production, direct effects of glucocorticoids through specific receptors on blood vessels, and mineralocorticoid effects of oversecreted adrenal hormones, such as deoxycorticosterone and corticosterone, in addition to cortisol.

Successful treatment of Cushing's syndrome results in normal blood pressure in the majority of patients[18,19]. Long-lasting exposure to increased cortisol with prolonged hypertension may result in persistent hypertension after successful treatment.

Diagnosis
Diagnosis of Cushing's syndrome requires documentation of cortisol oversecretion by measuring 24-h free cortisol excretion in urine, and/or lack of suppression of morning cortisol with low dose dexamethasone (1 mg) administered the night before. For equivocal results, the standard low-dose dexamethasone suppression test (0.5 mg every 6 h for eight doses) or, subsequently, the high-dose dexamethasone suppression test (2.0 mg every 6 h for eight doses) may be used to determine if plasma ACTH and cortisol levels can be suppressed, and endocrine consultation may be required for further testing. Once the biochemical diagnosis is secured, pituitary-based Cushing's disease must be differentiated from Cushing's

syndrome due to an adrenal-based adenoma or carcinoma, or from a benign lesion over-secreting ACTH such as carcinoid. Computer tomography, as well as special investigations such as bilateral inferior petrosal sinus sampling, may be required in some patients.

Treatment

Treatment of Cushing's syndrome is dependent on the underlying pathology. Trans-sphenoidal pituitary microsurgery in specialist centers is usually the treatment of choice for Cushing's disease. Surgical removal of an adrenal adenoma or carcinoma, or an ectopic ACTH or CRF-producing lesion, is otherwise required. Less commonly, pituitary irradiation, medical adrenalectomy (with mitotane), treatment with adrenal enzyme inhibitors or bilateral adrenalectomy is required. As mentioned above, successful and definitive treatment for Cushing's syndrome often normalizes blood pressure.

Antihypertensive drug treatment in Cushingoid patients could include any of the conventional drug groups, but thiazides can exacerbate hypokalemia, and β-blockers and centrally acting drugs should be used with caution to avoid precipitating depression. Potassium-sparing diuretics (amiloride or spironolactone) alone or in combination sometimes control blood pressure, reduce edema, and correct hypokalemia.

PHEOCHROMOCYTOMA

Definition and epidemiology

The term pheochromocytoma refers to a dusky tumor whose cells take on a brownish color when stained with chromium salts. The majority of such tumors arise within the adrenal glands (Fig. 40.5), but approximately 10% are extra-adrenal (paraganglioma). Whereas the majority of these tumors are benign, around 10% metastasize, particularly to bone, lungs, liver and regional lymph nodes. Histologic features are not specific for malignancy. The tumors can secrete a wide variety of hormones but most characteristically produce norepinephrine (noradrenaline), epinephrine and dopamine, with quite different patterns occurring in different patients. Few paragangliomas produce epinephrine. Very high dopamine production is frequently associated with malignancy or a large tumor mass.

The prevalence of pheochromocytoma varies widely between series. In the USA, the prevalence of pheochromocytoma in patients with sustained diastolic hypertension is probably somewhere between 0.05% and 0.1 %. However, it is likely that as many people die with unsuspected pheochromocytoma as die with a firm diagnosis, so the prevalence may be considerably higher[20].

Pheochromocytomas may be sporadic or familial. Whereas the former are usually unicentric and unilateral, familial pheochromocytomas are often multicentric and bilateral. Pheochromocytoma, often bilateral, may be part of a pluriglandular neoplastic syndrome (multiple endocrine neoplasia type II or III) (Table 40.4), the von Hippel–Lindau syndrome, neurofibromatosis, and other endocrinopathies.

Clinical features

Clinical manifestations relate primarily to the episodic or continuous overproduction of catecholamines. Symptoms may include headache, sweating, palpitations, anxiety, pallor, or upset in almost any bodily function[21] (Fig. 40.6). Hypertension or diabetes mellitus, with or without symptoms, may be the initial manifestation. Alternatively, pheochromocytoma may present as a tumor mass, usually an enlarging primary lesion in the abdomen or a paraganglioma in the neck, ear, thorax, or abdomen. Occasionally, a metastatic lesion may be the presenting sign. Physical examination may reveal labile (66%) or persistent (33%) hypertension, sometimes with reciprocal changes in blood pressure and heart rate when the tumor secretes norepinephrine predominantly (Fig. 40.7)[22]. The patient may have cool, mottled extremities and a low-grade fever with tachycardia and postural hypotension.

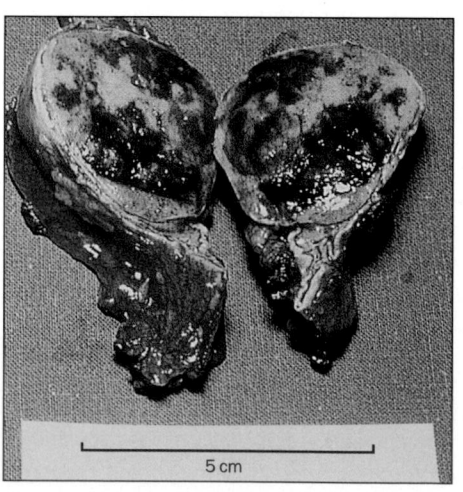

Figure 40.5 Large adrenal pheochromocytoma with areas of hemorrhagic necrosis.

5 cm

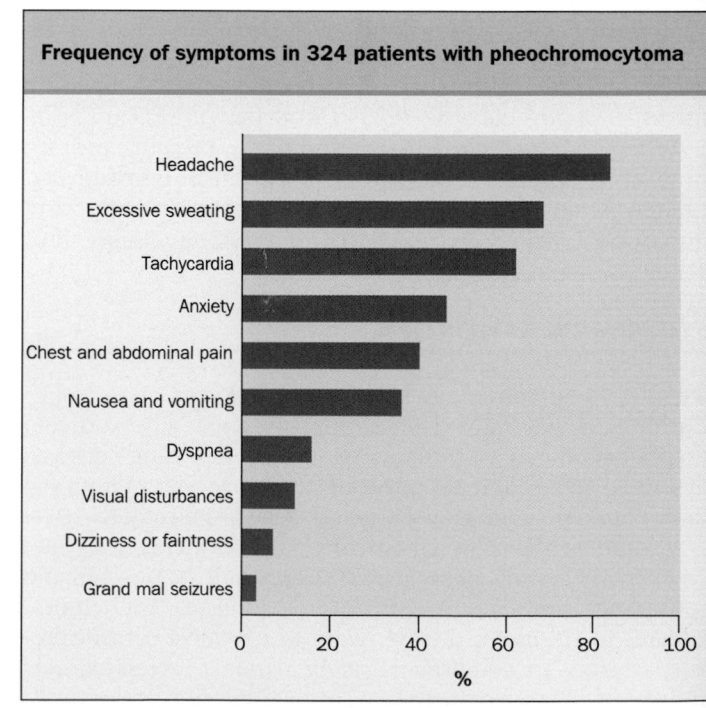

Frequency of symptoms in 324 patients with pheochromocytoma

Figure 40.6 Frequency of symptoms in 324 patients with pheochromocytoma. Adapted with permission.

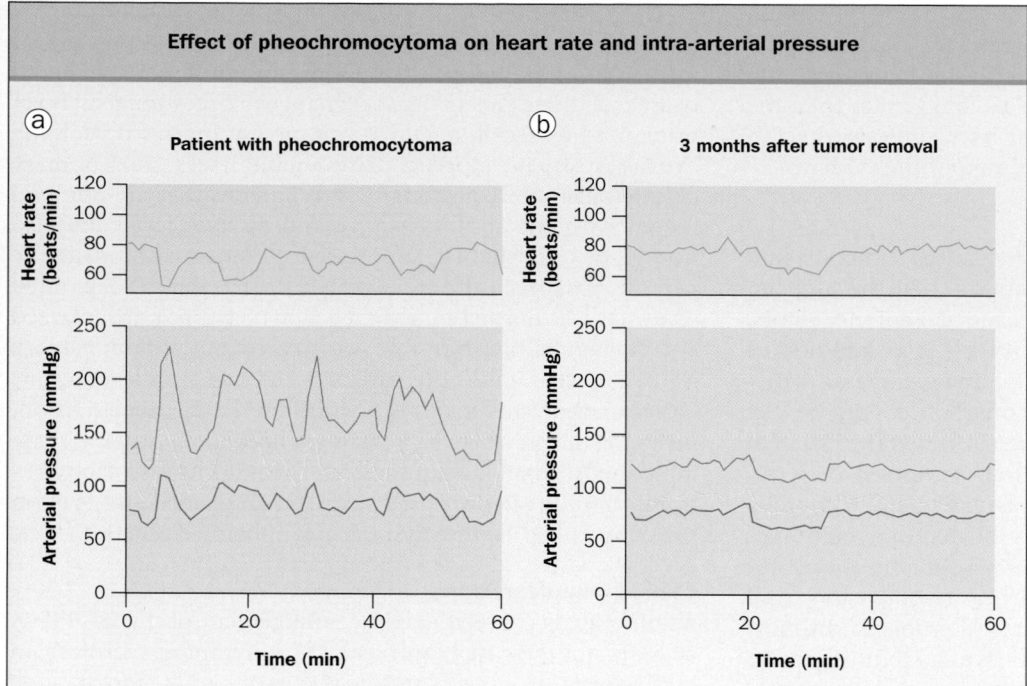

Figure 40.7 Effect of pheochromocytoma on heart rate and intra-arterial pressure. (Adapted with permission.)

The patient may also present as an emergency with severe hypertension with or without heart failure, and a variety of symptoms attributable to high plasma catecholamines. This can occur after minor or major trauma, at the time of delivery, or apparently spontaneously owing to sudden release of catecholamines from, or hemorrhage into, the tumor.

Diagnosis

Diagnosis of pheochromocytoma is based on clinical suspicion and requires biochemical confirmation with measurements of plasma or urine catecholamine levels or their metabolites. Typically plasma catecholamine levels are five- to ten-fold greater than normal. When catecholamine levels are not frankly elevated but rather are equivocal, a suppression test using clonidine (which suppresses plasma norepinephrine into the normal range if there is no pheochromocytoma but fails to do so in patients harboring a pheochromocytoma) is useful[23]. In patients with a familial predisposition to pheochromocytoma, measurements of plasma normetanephrine and metanephrine are reported to have high levels of sensitivity (97%) and specificity (96%) in detecting a tumor[24]. The same authors suggest that plasma free metanephrines provide the best single biochemical test for diagnosing or excluding a diagnosis of pheochromocytoma[25].

Once a biochemical diagnosis is secured, the lesion must be localized. A CT scan of the adrenal glands is successful in the vast majority of patients, but additional investigations may be required if no lesion is detected. Such investigations may include selective venous sampling from the great veins to detect where there is a 'step-up' in catecholamine levels, metaiodobenzyl-guanidine (MIBG) scanning, [111]indium-labeled octreotide scanning, measurements of plasma free metanephrines coupled with vena caval sampling, and positron emission tomographic scanning[26]. MIBG scanning of the remaining

Multiple endocrine neoplasia (MEN)		
Type	**Genetic locus**	**Gland affected**
MEN I	Chromosome 11	Parathyroid hyperplasia/adenoma
		Pancreatic islet cell hyperplasia/adenoma/carcinoma
		Pituitary hyperplasia/adenoma; rarely carcinoid, pheochromocytoma, lipomata
MEN II (also known as 'MEN IIA')	Chromosome 10	Medullary thyroid carcinoma
		Pheochromocytoma (bilateral in 50%)
		Parathyroid hyperplasia/adenoma; rarely cutaneous lichen amyloidosis
MEN III (also known as 'MEN IIB')	Chromosome 10	Medullary thyroid carcinoma
		Pheochromocytoma (commonly bilateral)
		Mucosal/gastrointestinal neuromas
		Marfanoid features/thickened 'bumpy' lips
Mixed syndromes	May occur in affected kindreds	Combinations of lesions from MEN I, II and/or III
Partial syndromes	May occur in affected kindreds	One or two features only of any of MEN I, II or III

All syndromes display autosomal dominant inheritance. Genetic (DNA polymorphism) testing identifies carriers of *MENII* and *MENIII* with >90% certainty.

Table 40.4 Multiple endocrine neoplasia (MEN).

adrenal gland after removal of a pheochromocytoma-containing adrenal needs cautious interpretation[27].

In the setting of renal failure, plasma catecholamine levels measured may be two to three times that observed in normal individuals owing to the presence in plasma of substances interfering with the assay system. However, diagnosis of a pheochromocytoma usually is not affected as, in this case, the plasma catecholamines are generally 10-fold greater than the 'normal' range. However, in equivocal cases, clinical suspicion and imaging studies provide essential supporting evidence.

Treatment

Once the tumor has been localized, the patient should be prepared for surgery with a cooperative approach by the surgeon, anesthesiologist, and physician. Blockade of α-adrenoceptors, usually with phenoxybenzamine, with the later addition of β-blockade if necessary to control blood pressure and tachycardia, should be implemented for some weeks prior to surgery. A laparoscopic approach to surgical removal of adrenal pheochromocytomas, through the transperitoneal or retroperitoneal route[28], is gaining acceptance[29]. This technique has also been utilized for hereditary bilateral pheochromocytoma where adrenal-sparing can avoid the need for adrenocortical replacement therapy[30]. Hypotension and hypoglycemia are potential postoperative problems. In most cases, surgical removal of pheochromocytoma returns plasma catecholamine levels to normal whilst restoring to normal previously suppressed central sympathetic outflow[31]. While blood pressure often improves with removal of the pheochromocytoma, in some patients, particularly in those whose hypertension was persistent as opposed to episodic, the blood pressure may remain elevated. These subjects will continue to require antihypertensive therapy. Follow-up should be for life since residual tumor may manifest symptoms years later. Family screening should also be considered, particularly where the pheochromocytoma is a component of a pluriglandular neoplastic syndrome.

For malignant pheochromocytoma, consideration should be given to aggressive surgical resection, particularly where there is a single metastatic lesion. Symptoms should be controlled with α- and β-blocking agents as needed, and radiation can be useful for bony metastases. Chemotherapy, usually with cyclophosphamide, vincristine, and dacarbazine should be considered for those with surgically inaccessible metastases producing symptoms that cannot be controlled by α- and β-blockade. Progression of malignant pheochromocytoma is extremely variable, with survival over decades in some cases. Median survival is approximately 5 years.

ACROMEGALY

Definition and epidemiology

Acromegaly is caused by excessive circulating growth hormone (GH) usually from a pituitary tumor. Acromegaly is rare with a prevalence of 40 cases per million. Hypertension appears to be more common in acromegaly than the general population with an estimated 35% of subjects with a diastolic pressure greater than 100 mmHg[32], and with higher frequencies in female and older patients. Uncertainty over the exact prevalence reflects variation in definitions of hypertension, and the stage of the disease. Acromegalic patients who have additional hypopituitarism or advanced cardiac disease may tend to have blood pressure reduction masking prior hypertension.

The pathogenesis of hypertension in acromegaly is complex but appears to be due to sodium and volume expansion associated with an inappropriate response of hormonal systems to counteract these effects. Total exchangeable sodium, total body water, and extracellular fluid volume are increased. Volume expansion should suppress plasma renin levels (as in primary aldosteronism) but, although levels are low, they are not consistent with the sodium status. Aldosterone levels are also normal or only slightly suppressed. Plasma atrial natriuretic peptide, which should be elevated in the volume-expanded state, remains normal in acromegaly. The kidneys are enlarged and glomerular filtration rate is increased, but sodium balance is not corrected unless the patient is cured of their acromegaly. Other mechanisms may also contribute to the hypertension, including the presence of circulating endogenous Na^+/K^+ ATPase inhibitors (digoxin-like substances), GH-induced vascular hypertrophy resulting in decreased vascular compliance, effects upon the sympathetic nervous system, and undefined genetic factors.

Clinical manifestations

Acromegaly is characterized by enlargement of the skull (Fig. 40.8), hands (Fig. 40.9) and feet. Other symptoms result from local effects of an expanding pituitary tumor and include visual field defects and headache. Signs and symptoms include headache (40%), excess sweating (50%), loss of libido (35%), amenorrhea (45%), carpal tunnel syndrome (25%), diabetes mellitus (19%) or visual field defects (5%)[32,34]. Thyroid enlargement occurs in 50% of subjects and thyrotoxicosis in 6%. Hirsutism occurs in 24% of women and galactorrhea in 10%. Increasing size of the feet or hands (ring size) in the adult may also be helpful clues.

Diagnosis

Clinical suspicion should be raised by symptoms and signs. Table 40.5 indicates appropriate tests. Elevated plasma GH, especially in response to an oral glucose tolerance test, is strongly suggestive of the diagnosis. Visual field assessment and MRI of the pituitary fossa are necessary to define the tumor and to exclude supratentorial extension. Most patients with acromegaly have a GH-secreting pituitary adenoma. Rarely, pancreatic or hypothalamic tumors release GH-releasing hormone with secondary GH excess. Breast and bronchial tumors can also produce growth hormone.

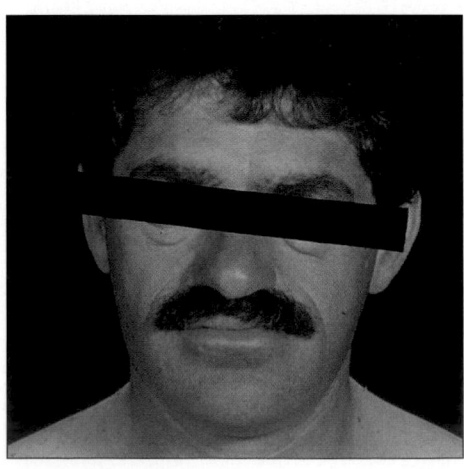

Figure 40.8 Facial features of acromegaly with enlargement of brow, nose, and jaw.

Tests for acromegaly
Plasma growth hormone
Plasma growth hormone responses to glucose tolerance test
Plasma insulin-like growth factor I
Lateral skull X-ray
Magnetic resonance imaging of the pituitary fossa
Visual field measurements
Assessment of other pituitary functions, e.g., thyroid function tests, thyroid-stimulating hormone, prolactin level, ACTH, and cortisol

Table 40.5 Tests for acromegaly.

Treatment

Trans-sphenoidal adenomectomy is the treatment of choice. Irradiation and drug therapy are valuable where complete removal of tumor tissue is not possible (in approximately one-third of cases) and where surgery is contraindicated. Dopaminergic agents, such as bromocriptine or cabergoline, and the somatostatin analog octreotide, reduce plasma growth hormone in acromegaly. Bromocriptine may induce tumor shrinkage and improves the diabetic state in the majority of patients. Irradiation therapy may not exert its full effect for months or years after initiation of treatment. Hypopituitarism may occur late after treatment and necessitate endocrine replacement for ACTH, thyroid stimulating hormone (TSH) and/or gonadotrophin deficiency. Hence, regular monitoring of pituitary function is required after treatment.

Management of hypertension in acromegaly

Surgical removal of the pituitary adenoma with normalization of GH levels may reduce blood pressure to some extent, but the majority of patients will continue to require antihypertensive therapy. For example, in one series[3] of 44 subjects undergoing surgery, only 14 had their diastolic pressure reduced to below 100 mmHg, and only five (11% of the total group) had diastolic pressures reduced to below 90 mmHg.

Antihypertensive treatment generally includes a diuretic given the volume-expanded state. Additional antihypertensive agents are frequently required, and both calcium channel blockers and ACE inhibitors have been reported to be useful. β-Blockers (e.g., propranolol) may also be used, although theoretically such agents may increase growth hormone concentration.

HYPOTHYROIDISM

Definition and epidemiology

Hypothyroidism is the clinical state resulting from deficient production of thyroid hormones, whether the cause is inadequate TSH secretion (from hypothalamic or pituitary lesions), or impaired functioning of the thyroid itself (loss or atrophy of the gland, autoimmune destruction, iodine deficiency, antithyroid agents, or hereditary defects in hormone synthesis)[35]. The true prevalence of hypertension in hypothyroidism

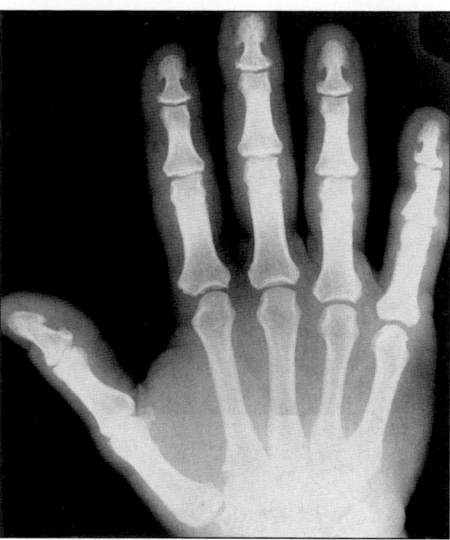

Figure 40.9 X-ray film of the hand in acromegaly. 'Arrow head' distal phalanges, expanded joint spaces, and increased soft tissue can be seen.

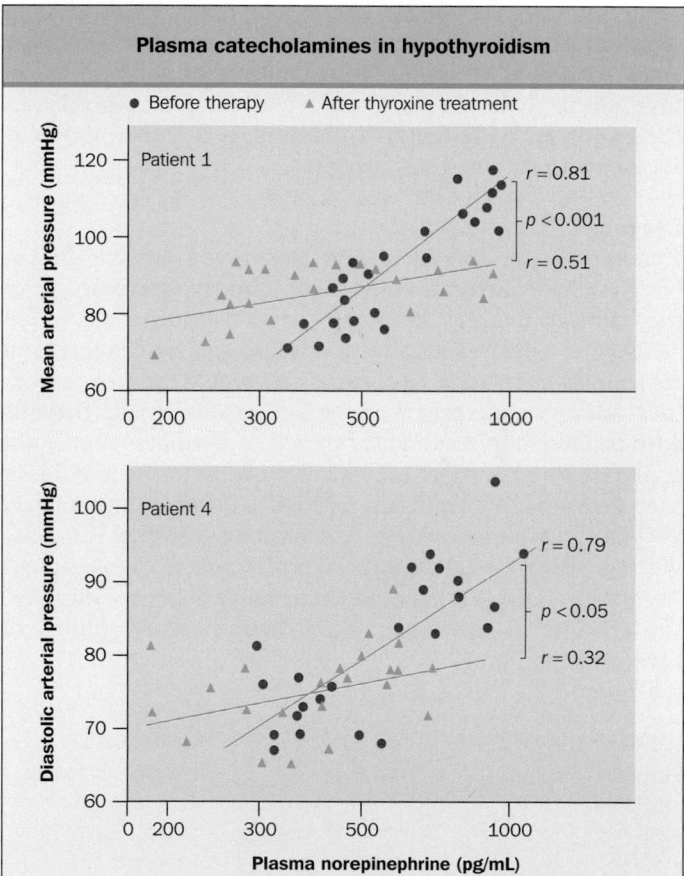

Figure 40.10 Plasma catecholamines in hypothyroidism.

is not known, but it is estimated that hypertension is 1.5 to 2 times more common in hypothyroid patients than in the general population[36].

The pathogenesis of the hypertension is multifactorial and is associated with both increased total body sodium and increased peripheral vascular resistance. Hypothyroid subjects also show higher plasma catecholamine levels, and the relationship between catecholamine level and blood pressure is more steep (Fig 40.10). The catecholamine levels of hypothyroid subjects also show more variability within a 24-h period, and this is also associated with more variability in blood pressure and heart rate during this period. This suggests 'underdamping' of swings in sympathetic activity in the hypothyroid state[37].

Hypertension develops despite a low cardiac output and reduced renin–angiotensin system activity and aldosterone levels. Thyroid replacement therapy corrects the electrolyte, hemodynamic, and hormone changes and cures the hypertension in most patients.

Clinical features

Any organ system can be affected in primary hypothyroidism; therefore, symptoms and signs can be protean. The onset of clinical abnormalities is usually gradual and diagnosis may not be made until gross hypothyroidism is established. Common clinical features include weakness, dry skin, lethargy, slow slurred speech, sensation of cold, thick tongue, facial puffiness (Fig. 40.11), coarse hair, failing memory, constipation and weight gain with reduced appetite. Coronary heart disease is common in patients with primary hypothyroidism. Whereas abnormal lipid metabolism may be the major etiologic factor, concomitant hypertension may accelerate the atherogenic process.

Diagnosis

Hypothyroidism should be considered as a possible underlying etiologic factor in any patient with hypertension. Since the clinical manifestations of hypothyroidism are often difficult to elicit, especially in the elderly, measurement of thyroid function tests, including TSH where the free thyroxine index is equivocal, should be considered. In patients with primary hypothyroidism in whom normotension is not achieved by full thyroxine-replacement therapy, it is likely that essential hypertension (which afflicts approximately 20% of the population) is a concomitant disorder. For those with gross or longstanding hypothyroidism, replacement thyroxine therapy should be cautious in order to minimize the chances of exacerbating or developing symptoms of myocardial ischemia.

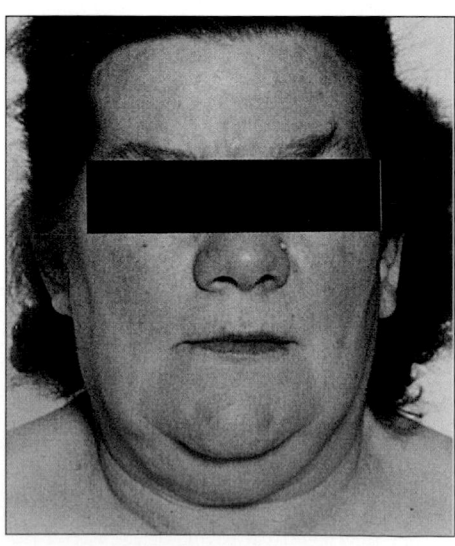

Figure 40.11
Hypothyroid facies.

HYPERTHYROIDISM

Definition and epidemiology

Hyperthyroidism and thyrotoxicosis may result from Graves' disease, and less commonly, toxic multinodular goitre, toxic adenoma, a high iodine intake, trophoblastic tumor and (rarely) excessive pituitary TSH secretion. Hypertension is common in hyperthyroidism, with a prevalence of 60% in toxic adenoma and approximately 30% in Graves' disease.

Clinical features

The clinical features depend upon the underlying cause of the hyperthyroidism, severity of the disorder, rapidity of onset, age of the patient, and concomitant disease. Abnormalities may be evident in the cardiovascular system (tachyarrhythmias, heart failure), skin (increased sweating, increasing pigmentation with vitiligo), eyes (lid lag, exophthalmos, etc.), nervous system (hypertension, nervousness, etc.), alimentary system (increased appetite yet weight loss, diarrhea, etc.), and muscles (proximal weakness), but any system may be affected.

Hypertension in hyperthyroidism is associated with elevated systolic blood pressure and normal or low diastolic pressure. It may be observed both in postpartum thyrotoxicosis and neonatal thyrotoxicosis. Unlike primary hypothyroidism, elevation of diastolic pressure is unusual unless there is concomitant essential hypertension.

The hemodynamic characteristics in hypertension of thyrotoxicosis are a raised cardiac output, increased myocardial contractility, tachycardia, decreased peripheral vascular resistance and an expanded blood volume. These indices return to normal in most patients on achieving the euthyroid state. Interestingly, catecholamine levels tend to be low (inversely to hypothyroid hypertension), and there is no heightened activity of the sympathetic system. The renin–angiotensin system tends to be activated and the aldosterone levels raised in hyperthyroidism and this may contribute to the development of systolic hypertension.

Suspicion of underlying hyperthyroidism should be particularly high in the elderly patient with hypertension and a high pulse pressure, particularly if there is also atrial fibrillation. Such patients are liable to develop cardiac failure, in which case the raised systolic arterial pressure will diminish, masking previous hypertension. Hypertension with a high pulse pressure, while typical of hyperthyroidism, may also be observed in some elderly essential hypertensives due to the loss of the compliance of the aorta with aging, and also in patients with coarctation of the aorta.

Diagnosis and treatment

Diagnosis of hyperthyroidism is confirmed by measuring thyroid function tests, including TSH. β-Blockers are often effective first-line therapy for hyperthyroidism associated hypertension. Treatment of hyperthyroidism, whether by antithyroid drugs, surgery, or radioiodine, will often normalize the raised systolic arterial pressure, although this is by no means invariable in the elderly where there may be concomitant essential hypertension.

RENIN-SECRETING TUMOR

Definition
Renin-secreting tumors are a rare cause of hypertension, and are usually due to juxtaglomerular cell tumors. Juxtaglomerular tumors are benign encapsulated tumors that consist of polygonal cells with cytoplasmic granules expressing renin; they average 1 cm in diameter but have been reported to be up to 6 cm in size. Only 30 cases have been reported since they were first described in 1967.

Clinical presentation
Patients usually present with severe hypertension with hypokalemia present in 90% and often with hyponatremia (likely due to angiotensin II-mediated thirst and/or stimulation of antidiuretic hormone). Significant proteinuria is present in approximately 50% of patients. Renal function and creatinine levels are usually normal. Clinically the patient may present as if they have malignant hypertension or severe renal artery stenosis.

Diagnosis and treatment
Patients presenting with severe hypertension, elevated plasma renin activity, and a dramatic response to agents that block the renin angiotensin system, should be considered candidates for a renin-secreting tumor (Fig 40.12). Renal angiography is indicated and may reveal the presence of a radiolucent, relatively avascular area (Fig. 40.13)[40], usually on the periphery of the renal silhouette; confirmation is provided by renal vein sampling documenting lateralization of renin. If angiography is negative despite lateralization of renin, renal CT will delineate most tumors greater than 10 mm in diameter. For angiography and renal ultrasound, the thresholds appear to be 15 mm and 20 mm, respectively.

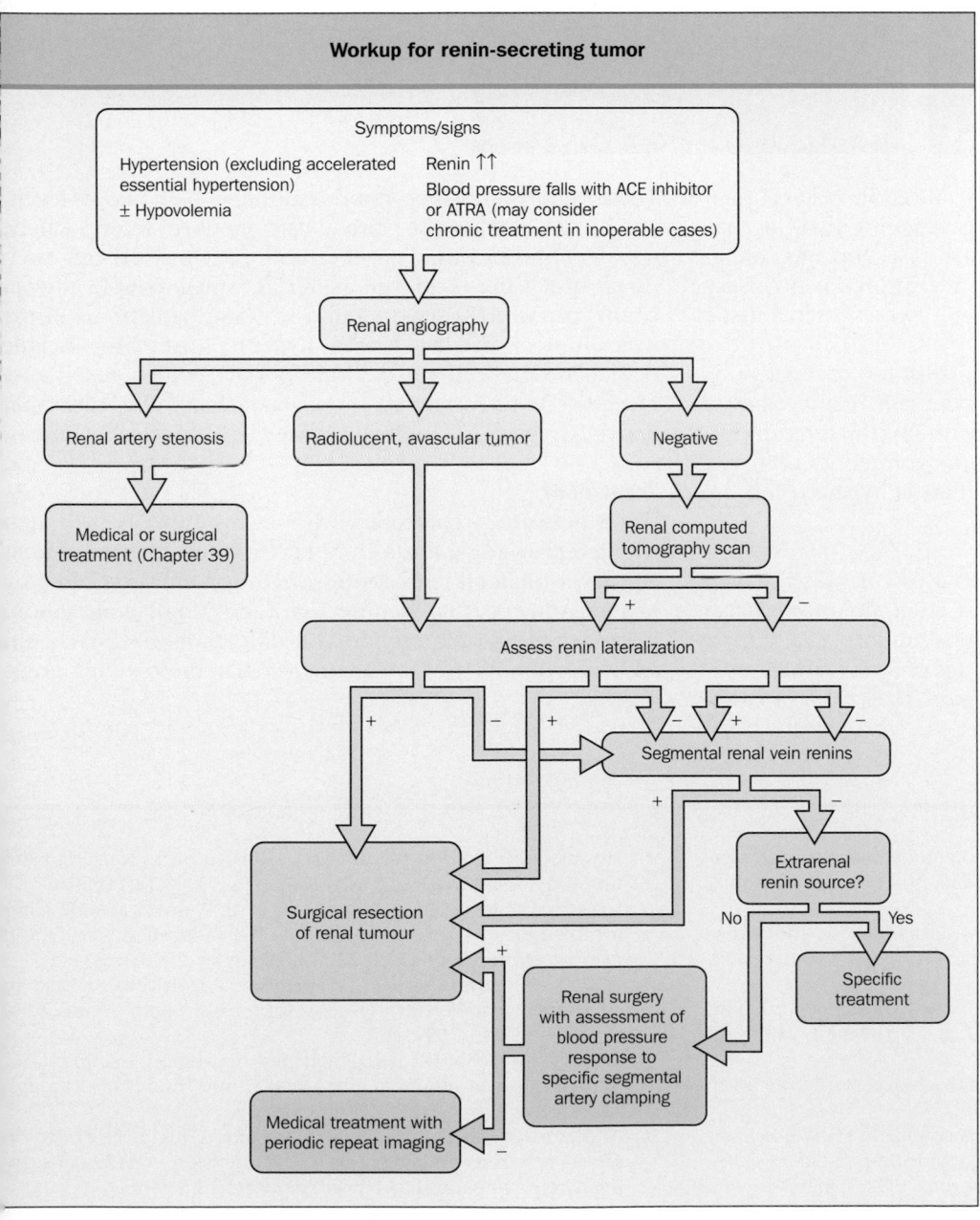

Figure 40.12 Diagnostic and management pathway for renin-secreting tumor.

Hypertension

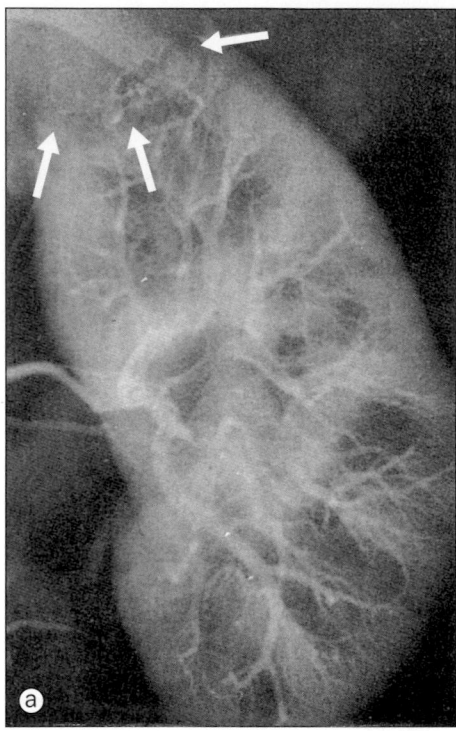 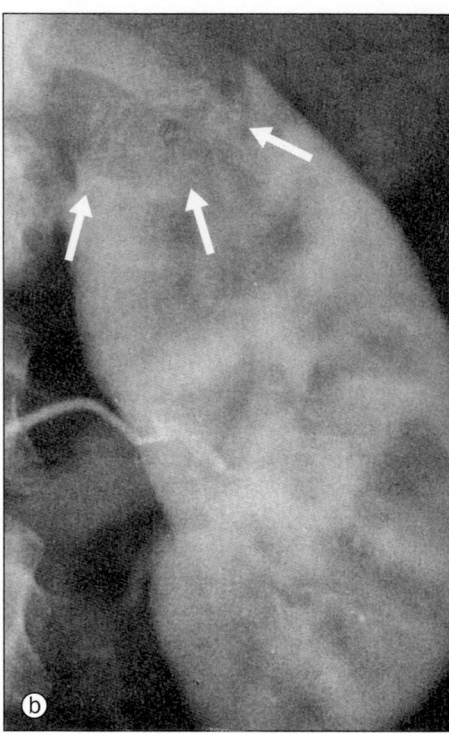

Figure 40.13 Renin-secreting tumor. Left renal angiography in (a) arterial and (b) nephrogram phases revealing a 2.5-cm juxtaglomerular cell tumor with a circumscribed and relatively avascular appearance at the upper pole (arrows). (Adapted with permission.)

If the CT scan is negative, but lateralization occurs, then selective segmental renal vein renin sampling may localize the tumor, guiding a limited renal resection. As juxtaglomerular cell tumors are benign, the minimum necessary surgery should be undertaken in order to preserve renal tissue and function.

Interestingly, whereas positive lateralization of renal veins is helpful, if no lateralization is shown, this may be due to damage to the contralateral kidney with increased renin production from this kidney. This is more commonly observed with larger tumors and a longer duration of hypertension.

Differential diagnosis

Both malignant hypertension and renal vascular disease may present as a high renin hypertension. Certain tumors may also produce renin. Nephroblastoma (Wilms' tumor) usually presents with abdominal mass before the age of 5 years and is associated with high blood pressure in more than 50% of cases.

These tumors can secrete renin resulting in high plasma levels. Renal carcinomas also rarely can produce renin. Rarely, extrarenal tumors may produce renin, such as oat cell carcinoma and cancers of the pancreas, small bowel, adrenal cortex, paraovarian region and ovary, and hamartoma of the liver. Tumors associated with hyper-reninism also include neuroblastoma and pheochromocytoma, which may cause increased renin secretion from juxtaglomerular cells that undergo hyperplasia in the presence of excess catecholamines.

Treatment

Blood pressure is controlled with ACE inhibitors, although AT1 receptor antagonists may be expected to have similar efficacy. Unilateral renal renin-secreting tumors are cured by nephrectomy, partial nephrectomy, or tumor enucleation. Intraoperative frozen section will differentiate benign renin secreting tumors from malignant renal tumors and guide surgery.

REFERENCES

1. Rossi GP, Sacchetto A, Pavan E, et al. Remodeling of the left ventricle in primary aldosteronism due to Conn's adenoma. Circulation. 1997;95:1471–8.
2. Weber KT, Janicki JS, Pick R, et al. Myocardial fibrosis and pathological hypertrophy in the rat with renovascular hypertension. Am J Cardiol. 1990;65:G1–7.
3. Young M, Fullerton M, Dilley R, Funder J. Mineralocorticoids, hypertension and cardiac fibrosis. J Clin Invest. 1994;93:2578–83.
4. Conn JW. Primary aldosteronism, a new clinical syndrome. J Lab Clin Med. 1955;45:3–17.
5. Lifton RP, Dluhy RG, Powers M, et al. A chimaeric 11-hydroxylase/aldosterone synthase gene causes glucocorticoid-remediable aldosteronism and human hypertension. Nature. 1992;355:262–5.
6. Stowasser M, Gordon RD. Primary aldosteronism: learning from the study of familial varieties. J Hypertens. 2000;18:1165–76.
7. Lafferty AR, Torpy DJ, Stowasser M, et al. A novel genetic locus for low renin hypertension: familial hyperaldosteronism type II maps to chromosome 7 (7p22). J Med Genet. 2000;37:831–5.
8. Walker BR, Edwards CRW. Hypermineralocorticoidism due to abnormal metabolism of cortisol. Curr Opin Endocrinol Diabetes. 1994;1:109–16.
9. Tucker RM, Labarthe DR. Frequency of surgical treatment for hypertension in adults at the Mayo Clinic from 1973 through 1975. Mayo Clinic Proc. 1977;52:549–55.
10. Anderson GH, Blakeman N, Streeten DHP. The effect of age on prevalence of secondary forms of hypertension in 4429 consecutively referred patients. J Hypertens. 1994;12:609–15.

11. Gordon RD, Stowasser M, Klemm SA, Tunny TJ. Primary aldosteronism and other forms of mineralocorticoid hypertension. In: Swales JD, ed. Textbook of hypertension. London: Blackwell Scientific; 1994:865–92.

12. Lim PO, Rodgers P, Cardale K, et al. Potentially high prevalence of primary aldosteronism in a primary-care population. Lancet. 1999;353:40.

13. Fardella CE, Mosso L, Gómez-Sánchez C, et al. Primary hyperaldosteronism in essential hypertensives: prevalence, biochemical profile and molecular biology. J Clin Endocrinol Metab. 2000;85:1863–7.

14. Montori VM, Schwartz GL, Chapman AB, et al. Validity of the aldosterone–renin ratio used to screen for primary aldosteronism. Mayo Clin Proc. 2001;76:877–82.

15. Kaplan NM. Caution about the overdiagnosis of primary aldosteronism. Mayo Clin Proc. 2001;76:875–6.

16. Lim PO, Young WF, MacDonald TM. A review of the medical treatment of primary aldosteronism. J Hypertens. 2001;19:353–61.

17. Orth DN, Kovacs WJ, DeBold CR. The adrenal cortex. In: Wilson JD, Foster DW, eds. Williams' textbook of endocrinology. Philadelphia: Saunders; 1992:489–619.

18. Atkinson AB. Cushing's syndrome. In: Robertson JIS, ed. Handbook of hypertension: clinical hypertension. Amsterdam: Elsevier; 1992:390–419.

19. Fallo F, Sonino N, Barzon L, et al. Effect of surgical treatment on hypertension in Cushing's syndrome. Am J Hypertens. 1996;9:77–80.

20. McNeil AR, Blok BH, Koelmeyer TD, et al. Phaeochromocytomas discovered during coronial autopsies in Sydney, Melbourne and Auckland. Aust NZ J Med. 2000;30:648–52.

21. Ross ZJ, Griffith DN. The clinical presentation of phaeochromocytoma. QJ Med. 1989;71:485–94.

22. Richards AM, Nicholls MG, Espiner EA, et al. Arterial pressure and hormone relationships in phaeochromocytoma. J Hypertens. 1983;1:373–9.

23. Bravo EL, Tarazi RC, Fouad FM, et al. Clonidine-suppression test. A useful aid in the diagnosis of pheochromocytoma. N Engl J Med. 1981;305:623–6.

24. Eisenhofer G, Lenders JWM, Linehan WM, et al. Plasma normetanephrine and metanephrine for detecting pheochromocytoma in von Hippel-Lindau disease and multiple endocrine neoplasia type 2. N Engl J Med. 1999;340:1872–9.

25. Lenders JW, Pacak K, Walther MM, et al. Biochemical diagnosis of pheochromocytoma. Which test is best? JAMA. 2002;287:1427–34.

26. Pacak K, Goldsteine DS, Doppman JL, et al. A 'pheo' lurks: novel approaches for locating occult pheochromocytoma. J Clin Endocrinol Metab. 2001;86:3641–6.

27. Burt MG, Allen B, Conaglen JV. False positive ^{131}I-metaiodobenzylguanide scan in the postoperative assessment of malignant phaeochromocytoma secondary to medullary hyperplasia. NZ Med J. 2002;115:18.

28. Atallah F, Bastide-Heulin T, Soulié M, et al. Haemodynamic changes during retroperitoneoscopic adrenalectomy for phaeochromocytoma. Br J Anaesth. 2001;86:731–3.

29. Duh Q-Y. Evolving surgical management for patients with pheochromocytoma. J Clin Endocrinol Metab 2001;86:1477–9.

30. Neumann HPH, Reincke M, Bender BU, et al. Preserved adrenocortical function after laparoscopic bilateral adrenal sparing surgery for hereditary pheochromocytoma. J Clin Endocrinol Metab. 1999;84:2608–10.

31. Grassi G, Seravalle G, Turri C, Mancia G. Sympathetic nerve traffic responses to surgical removal of pheochromocytoma. Hypertension. 1999;34:461–5.

32. Davies DL, Connell JMC, Reid R, Fraser R. Acromegaly: the effects of growth hormone on blood vessels, sodium homeostasis and blood pressure. In: Robertson JIS, ed. Handbook of hypertension: clinical hypertension. Amsterdam: Elsevier; 1992:545–75.

33. Nabarro JDM. Acromegaly. Clin Endocrinol. 1987;26:481–512.

34. Jadresic A, Banks LM, Child DG, et al. The acromegaly syndrome. QJ Med. 1982;51:189–204.

35. Larsen PR, Ingbar SH. The thyroid gland. In: Wilson JD, Foster DW, eds. Williams' textbook of endocrinology. Philadelphia: Saunders; 1992:357–487.

36. Bing RF. Thyroid disease and hypertension. In: Robertson JIS, ed. Handbook of hypertension: clinical hypertension. Amsterdam: Elsevier; 1992:576–93.

37. Richards AM, Nicholls MG, Espiner EA, et al. Hypertension in hypothyroidism: arterial pressure and hormone relationships. Clin Exp Hypertens. 1985;7:1499–514.

38. Robertson PW, Klidjian A, Harding LK, et al. Hypertension due to a renin-secreting renal tumour. Am J Med. 1967;43:963–76.

39. Lindop GBM, Leckie BJ, Mimran A. Renin-secreting tumours. In: Robertson JIS, Nicholls MG, eds. The renin–angiotensin system. London: Gower Medical; 1993:54.1–54.12.

40. Lam ASC, Bédard YC, Buckspan MB, et al. Surgically curable hypertension associated with reninoma. J Urol. 1982;128:572–5.

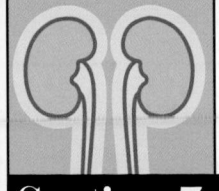

Chapter 41

Neurogenic Hypertension Including Following Stroke and with Spinal Cord Injury

John Amerena and Stevo Julius

INTRODUCTION

Although the autonomic nervous system is recognized for its importance in short-term control of blood pressure (BP), the nervous system is thought to play only a minor role in the pathophysiology of hypertension. However, there are a number of well-defined syndromes of secondary hypertension that are neurogenic and evidence for an important role for the nervous system in a large proportion of patients with essential hypertension is steadily accumulating.

HYPERTENSION AND CEREBRAL ISCHEMIC SYNDROMES

Definition and epidemiology

Hypertension is commonly associated with stroke, both as a cause of and as a response to cerebral ischemia. Hypertension is the major risk factor for stroke, and reduction of BP, particularly in the elderly, decreases the incidence of stroke by up to 40%. Nevertheless, only a small proportion of patients with hypertension have a cerebrovascular accident. Up to 80% of patients who suffer a stroke have significant elevation of BP at presentation or in the first 24 h; in two-thirds this is a *de novo* hypertension[1]. Severe hypertension is more common after cerebral hemorrhage than after cerebral infarction, but in both cases the BP usually falls spontaneously over several days and at 10 days two-thirds of patients are normotensive. Recent studies have suggested that a decrease in nocturnal blood pressure fall, perhaps due to pathological sympathetic activation, is associated with an unfavorable short- and long-term outcome after ischemic stroke[2,3] and that elevated 24-h blood pressure after acute stroke is associated with increased long-term mortality[4].

Pathogenesis

Hypertension following cerebral ischemia is probably mediated by the central nervous system and is not usually associated with bradycardia ('Cushing' reflex), as is sometimes seen after subarachnoid hemorrhage. Cerebral blood flow is tightly autoregulated; with changes in cerebral perfusion pressure matched by reciprocal changes in cerebral vascular resistance to maintain constant cerebral blood flow. A constant cerebral flow can been maintained between 60 and 150 mmHg in normotensive patients, but in patients with hypertension the autoregulatory curve is shifted to the right.

Autoregulation of the cerebral circulation is impaired in the elderly and in those with cerebral ischemia. With a cerebral infarct or hemorrhage there is a central area of infarct and necrotic tissue surrounded by a penumbra of ischemic but potentially viable brain, the survival of which is dependent on maintenance of cerebral blood flow. Within this area there is often a localized increase in pressure caused by edema or hemorrhage and a subsequent decrease in local blood flow. Local ischemia to the centers that regulate autonomic tone may activate the sympathetic nervous system as part of a global metabolic response to cerebral ischemia, thereby increasing blood pressure. The rise in systemic arterial BP may then act as a compensatory mechanism to maintain cerebral blood flow to the watershed areas of the brain.

Treatment

The timing and extent of antihypertensive treatment after a cerebrovascular insult remains debatable. If BP elevation is a compensatory mechanism to minimize neurologic damage, lowering BP may worsen outcomes by potentially increasing the extent of ischemia rather than decreasing it. There is now good evidence[2-4] that short-term and long-term elevation of BP after cerebrovascular events worsens outcomes; however, there is still controversy as to the threshold when antihypertensive treatment should be instituted after acute stroke, as BP values in excess of 200/115 mmHg have not been shown to be associated with a progression of symptoms[5]. Conversely, several papers have reported a deterioration in neurologic status with antihypertensive therapy[6].

After cerebral infarction, excessive lowering of BP in the acute setting may worsen outcomes, so antihypertensive therapy must be instituted judiciously. Elevated BP in this setting usually settles within 7 days but often is markedly elevated in the acute phase, and thus antihypertensive therapy with conventional agents should be considered. Several algorithms for initiation of antihypertensive treatment have been published[7,8] with the general recommendation that blood pressure lowering treatment be commenced if the systolic BP remains consistently above 180–200 mmHg and the diastolic BP greater than 120 mmHg (Fig. 41.1), particularly if anticoagulation is being used or thrombolytic therapy considered. After cerebral hemorrhage, more severe hypertension is common, but there is no evidence that lowering BP improves outcomes or reduces the risk of rebleeding, although intuitively this should be the case. The presence of comorbid conditions such as a dissecting aneurysm, myocardial infarction, congestive cardiac failure, or subarachnoid hemorrhage may mandate greater and more rapid BP lowering but at the potential expense of neurologic deterioration.

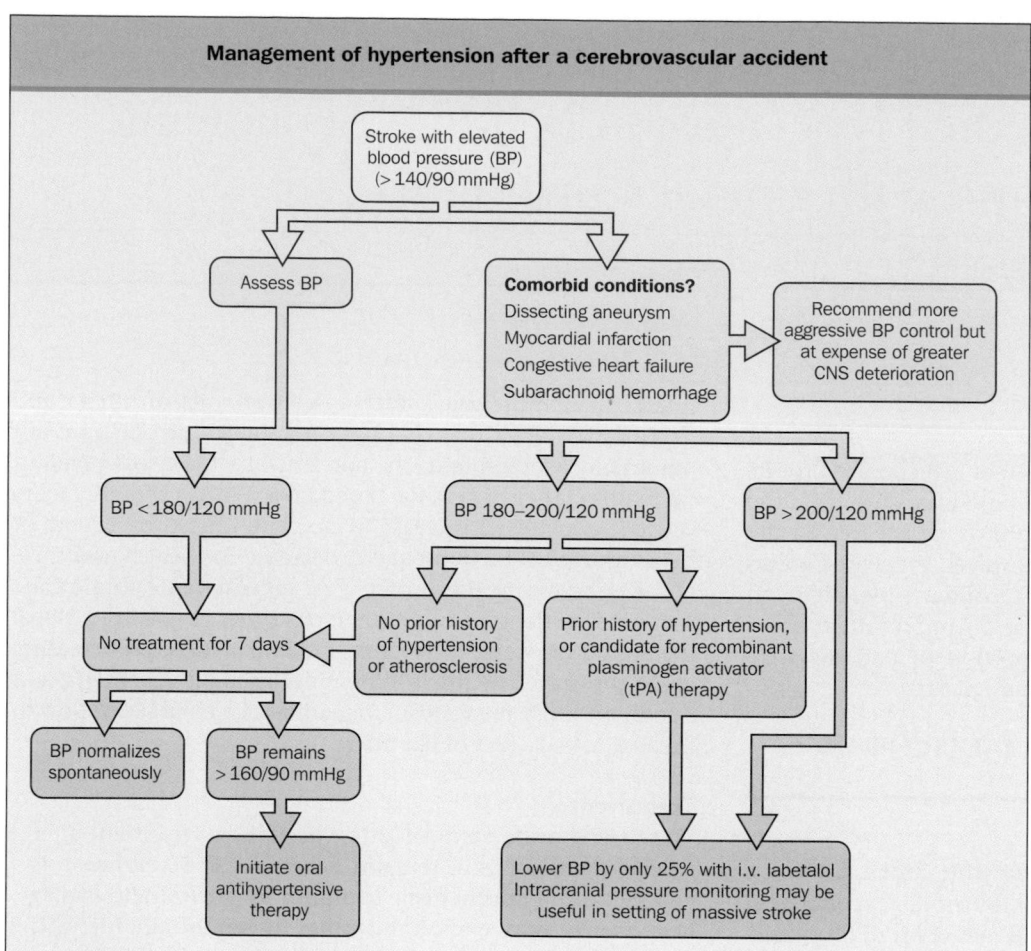

Figure 41.1 Management of hypertension after a cerebrovascular accident.

Management of hypertension after a cerebrovascular accident

Although there are no firm guidelines in this area, if it is decided that BP should be lowered after a cerebrovascular event, a conservative approach (see Fig. 41.1) would be to lower the mean arterial BP by no more than 25% in the first 24 h of treatment, as more than this may precipitate cerebral ischemia, particularly if cerebral autoregulation is disturbed. Reduction of BP in the immediate poststroke period is usually achieved with careful titration with intravenous labetalol (either as 10 mg intravenously every 10 min up to a total of 300 mg, or as an intravenous infusion at 1–2 mg/min). An alternative treatment is the use of intravenous vasodilators that have a short duration of action, such as nitroprusside and intravenous nitroglycerin (glyceryl trinitrate), which may be used to avoid prolonged falls in BP that could aggravate cerebral ischemia. However, these agents may increase intracranial pressure by cerebral vasodilatation or may cause a cerebral 'steal' phenomenon; intracranial pressure monitoring may be useful in these patients especially if the stroke is massive. Angiotensin-converting enzyme (ACE) inhibitors (enalapril), other β-blockers (esmolol) and calcium channel blockers (verapamil and nicardipine) have also been used intravenously after stroke but do not allow such smooth control. Transdermal clonidine can also be used but has the potential to depress the conscious state. Once neurologic and hemodynamic stability has been reached, a gradual transition to oral agents can be undertaken if BP remains elevated. Longer-term treatment with perindopril/indapamide after stroke has been shown to reduce the risk of secondary stroke and cardiovascular events. Blood pressure lowering reduced events irrespective of whether subjects had elevated blood pressure or were normotensive at entry into the study[9].

HYPERTENSION AFTER CAROTID ENDARTERECTOMY

Definition and epidemiology

Hypertension occurring in 20–60% of subjects after carotid endarterectomy is not uncommon. Hypertension is usually transient but can persist for days after surgery. Pre-existing hypertension and increasing severity of carotid stenosis increase the risk of postoperative hypertension, with studies suggesting that the presence of preoperative hypertension and/or a stenosis of more than 75% is associated with a 94% risk of postoperative hypertension[10]. When general anesthesia is used for surgery there is an increased risk of intra- and postoperative hypertension compared to regional anesthesia[11].

Pathogenesis

There may be several mechanisms that contribute to hypertension after endarterectomy. It was originally thought that transient denervation or stunning of the carotid baroreceptors could be the cause of hypertension in the postoperative period, but surgical techniques specifically designed to preserve baroreceptor innervation have not reported lower rates of postoperative hypertension[10] and baroreceptor function has not been demonstrated to change significantly following carotid endarterectomy.

The role of the brain in the genesis of postcarotid endarterectomy hypertension has been investigated. Ahn et al.[12] reported increased central and peripheral norepinephrine levels shortly after unclamping of the carotid artery, which they attributed to cerebral hypoperfusion and transient ischemia. Catecholamine levels correlated with changes in BP, but this association was not found in other studies. Studies in animal models have also suggested that an increase in central nervous system catecholamines resulting from transient ischemia plays some role in the development of hypertension after carotid endarterectomy. Defective autoregulation of cerebral blood flow in response to the transient underperfusion and hypoxia during cross-clamping may also contribute to postoperative hypertension.

Treatment

The onset of hypertension during or after carotid endarterectomy can cause hyperperfusion injury and cerebral hemorrhage due to a relative loss of cerebral autoregulation after the removal of arterial obstruction, thus making careful neurologic observations essential. However, while severe and labile hypertension in the immediate postoperative period is not uncommon, it is usually not associated with any adverse neurological events. It has been strongly recommended that BP be lowered if the systolic level exceeds 200 mmHg, but most clinicians would begin treatment once 170 mmHg was reached. Although there are no standardized guidelines for treatment of hypertension in the perioperative period after carotid endarterectomy, the principles are the same as for the treatment of hypertension after stroke (Fig. 41.1) and the same agents should be used.

NEUROGENIC ASPECTS OF ESSENTIAL HYPERTENSION

Definition and epidemiology

A strong neurogenic component is found in about 30% of young male patients with essential hypertension. These patients are characterized by a hyperkinetic circulation (fast heart rate, high cardiac output) and mild hypertension. In such patients, plasma catecholamines are elevated, norepinephrine (noradrenaline) turnover is increased, sympathetic overactivity is found by direct microneurography of the peroneal nerve, the increased cardiac output and heart rate can be abolished with pharmacologic blockade of autonomic receptors in the heart, and the elevation of BP can be abolished with a combined β-adrenergic and α-adrenergic blockade (Table 41.1). The autonomic dysfunction that occurs has numerous metabolic and hemodynamic effects on multiple organs (Fig. 41.2)[13], including weight gain due to decreased energy expenditure as a result of functional downregulation of β-adrenoreceptors (see below)[14]. Indeed, hypertension observed with obesity and with the sleep apnea syndrome is also associated with sympathetic nervous system overactivity.

The neurogenic component that characterizes early borderline hypertension
Hyperkinetic circulation
Tachycardia
High cardiac output
Low blood volume, high hematocrit
Increased sympathetic nervous system activity
Increased blood pressure response to stress or exercise
Increased plasma catecholamines and norepinephrine (noradrenaline) turnover
Blood pressure elevation can be corrected with combined α- and β-adrenergic blockers
Decreased parasympathetic nervous system activity
Less heart rate response to atropine
More heart rate variability as seen by spectral analysis
Activitation of the renin–angiotensin system
Increased circulating renin levels (?secondary to β-adrenergic stimulation)

Table 41.1 The neurogenic component that characterizes a subset (30%) of those with early borderline hypertension.

Early, borderline hypertensive patients with a hyperkinetic circulation have both an increase in sympathetic nervous system activity and a decrease in parasympathetic nerve activity. In these patients, sympathetic tone is increased and parasympathetic tone decreased, as demonstrated by a larger fall in heart rate and cardiac output after β-adrenergic blockade with a smaller increase after parasympathetic blockade with atropine compared with the effects seen in normal subjects (Fig. 41.3)[15].

These hyperkinetic patients are invariably young with a hemodynamic profile distinct from the normal cardiac output/high vascular resistance generally seen in more advanced hypertension. The question arises as to whether they will later develop classic essential hypertension and, if so, why the hemodynamic picture is different in the early versus later phase of hypertension. Evidence that the hyperkinetic state is a precursor of typical essential hypertension comes from epidemiologic observations and from longitudinal assessment of hemodynamic patterns in cohorts. In epidemiologic investigations, the hallmark of neurogenic hypertension, tachycardia, is a strong predictor of future hypertension[13]. When tachycardia is observed in patients with borderline hypertension, the rate of future hypertension is three to four times above average. That the hemodynamic picture in these patients evolves from 'hyperkinetic' to 'normokinetic' hypertension was first suggested by Eich et al.[16], but was later shown by Lund-Johansen and Omvik who followed a substantial group of patients over 20 years[17]. In the first decade of observation, the patients' hemodynamic picture changed from a hyperkinetic, low peripheral resistance pattern to one of normokinetic, high resistance; however, the average BP did not increase. In the second decade, the BP rose to levels that required antihypertensive medication in practically all patients.

Pathogenesis: transition from a hyperkinetic state to 'classic' essential hypertension

In the course of Lund-Johansen's observations, the stroke volume and heart rate decreased, the vascular resistance

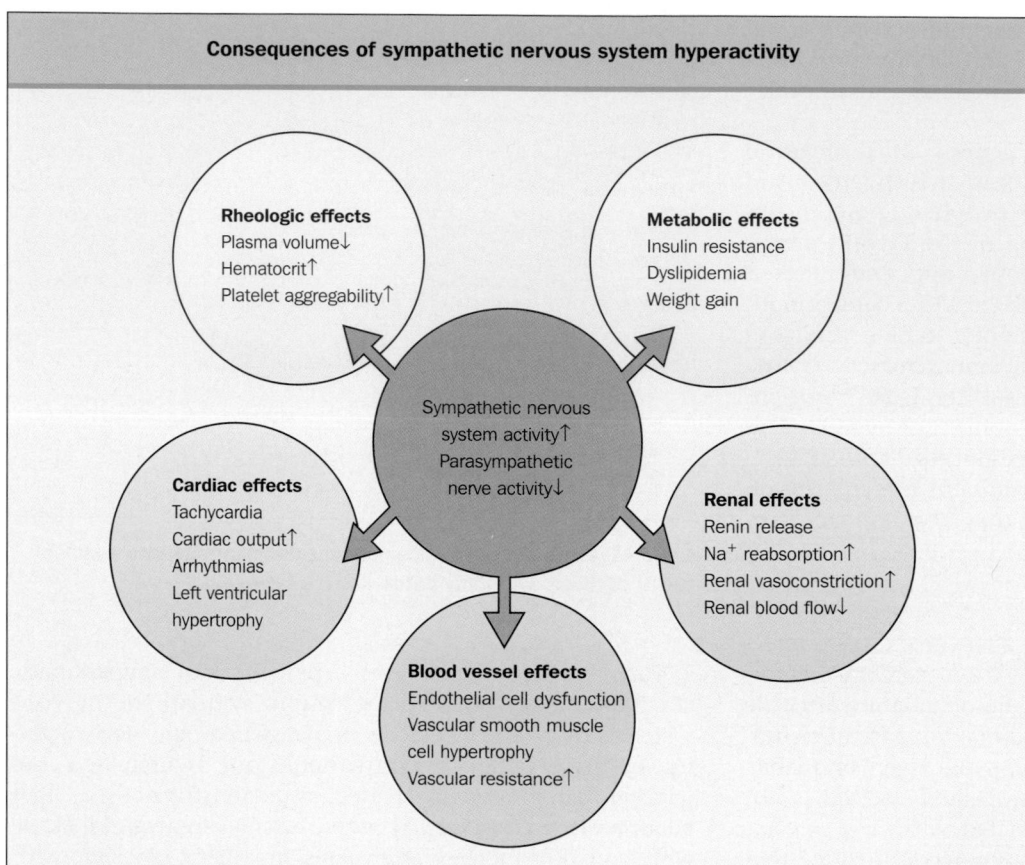

Figure 41.2 The consequences of sympathetic nervous system hyperactivity.

increased, and the hemodynamic picture of essential hypertension characterized by high peripheral resistance and normal cardiac output evolved. The mechanism of this hemodynamic transition is easily understood if one takes into consideration changes in the responsiveness of the heart and blood vessels in the course of hypertension (Fig. 41.4)[18]. A decreased chronotropic responsiveness of the heart to β-adrenergic stimulation has been repeatedly demonstrated in hypertension and it has been suggested that this mirrors a downregulation of β-adrenoceptors in response to prolonged and excessive sympathetic stimulation[13]. The decrease of stroke volume in the course of hypertension reflects a pressure-related increase in cardiac stiffness, which results in decreased diastolic filling of the heart. This has been documented in even very mild forms of hypertension[19]. As these changes lead to a progressive decrease in cardiac output (initially to normal range and subsequently to subnormal values), the vascular resistance steadily increases in the course of hypertension. This increase results from two pressure-induced consequences of hypertension: namely smooth muscle hypertrophy in resistance arterioles and endothelial dysfunction. Vascular hypertrophy amplifies vasoconstriction because at the same level of smooth muscle contraction a thicker wall encroaches more upon the lumen of the blood vessel. The same changes in vascular geometry limit the ability of the vessel to vasodilate. As hypertension advances, the vasodilatation is further limited by endothelial damage, which limits the release of the vasodilator nitric oxide. This potentiation of pressor responsiveness and limitation of vasodilatation cause a vicious circle in which higher pressure

enhances the hypertrophy and endothelial damage that, in turn, further aggravates vasoconstriction and accelerates hypertension. More recently upregulation of α₁-adrenoreceptors has been described in hypertensive patients, which in conjunction with downregulation of β-receptors could also promote the transition to high peripheral resistance seen in this population[20]. As the balance moves towards vasoconstriction and higher BP readings, less sympathetic tone is needed to maintain the same degree of BP elevation and the brain gradually resets sympathetic tone towards lower values. A decrease of sympathetic tone in the course of hypertension has been described and, ultimately, the initially neurogenic hypertension loses its pathognomonic clinical characteristics.

HYPERTENSION ASSOCIATED WITH SPINAL CORD INJURY (AUTONOMIC DYSREFLEXIA)

Definition and epidemiology

Hypertension is a common but underappreciated consequence of quadriplegia caused by cervical spinal cord transection. In this type of injury, central nervous control of BP is lost, as are centrally mediated reflex pressor responses to stimuli such as mental arithmetic. Centrally mediated responses to changes in peripheral hemodynamic conditions are also affected, and there is difficulty in BP maintenance with changes in posture[21]. Symptomatic orthostatic hypotension can be a problem in these patients but is not as severe as that seen in primary autonomic failure or diabetes, as the lack of reflex vasoconstriction is partially compensated for by increased release of vasopressin and aldosterone.

In quadriplegic patients, severe hypertension can be precipitated by stimulation of the skin by cold or noxious stimuli, spasm of skeletal muscle, and bladder or bowel contraction. The elevation in BP usually persists until the stimulus is removed and then slowly resolves.

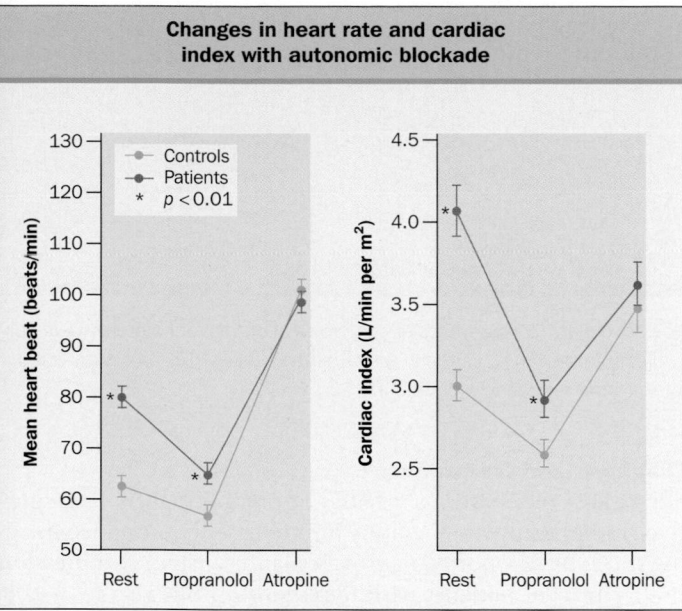

Figure 41.3 Changes in heart rate and cardiac index with autonomic blockade. Early hypertension is associated with increased sympathetic and decreased parasympathetic nervous activity. Patients with mild hypertension have a hyperkinetic circulation compared with controls; β-adrenergic blockade with propanolol resulted in a greater fall in heart rate (left) and cardiac index (right) compared with controls, indicating a higher baseline β-adrenergic tone. The addition of atropine, which blocks the parasympathetics, resulted in a lower increase in heart rate and cardiac index in hypertensive patients, indicating that they had a lower parasympathetic tone. At the end of the experiment, after the combined blockade of the autonomic control of the heart, the initial differences in the level of cardiac output and heart rate seen in hypertensives have been abolished, proving that the hyperkinetic state in these patients was of a neurogenic origin. (Adapted with permission from Julius, Pascual and London[15].)

Pathogenesis

This pressor response is partially mediated by peripheral afferent sympathetic nerves synapsing in the spinal cord, which can produce a generalized sympathetic discharge. However, since plasma catecholamines are not markedly elevated, and an excess sympathetic nervous discharge has not been documented by microneurography, other mechanisms must also contribute. The acute elevation of BP in this situation could be also explained by increased α-adrenoreceptor sensitivity, as it has been shown that intravenous norepinephrine (noradrenaline) elicits a greater pressor response in quadriplegic patients, without upregulation of receptor numbers. Unfortunately α-adrenergic blockade has been impressively unhelpful in treatment of pressor episodes in paraplegics, which may mean that subtherapeutic concentrations are reached in the synaptic cleft and/or that other vasoactive substances such as neuropeptide Y are contributing substantially to BP elevation.

Treatment

Agents that deplete sympathetic nerve terminals such as reserpine or guanethidine have generally been more successful in controlling BP surges in these patient[22]. Centrally acting sympatholytics such as clonidine and moxonidine may also be helpful. Other agents, such as angiotensin receptor antagonists or ACE inhibitors and calcium channel blockers, may lower systolic peaks but tend to increase postural symptoms. The repeated pressor episodes do not normally lead to chronic elevation of the BP and its long-term sequelae, although persistent hypertension has been reported in young paraplegics after ischemic upper spinal cord injury[22].

NEUROVASCULAR COMPRESSION SYNDROME

Definition and epidemiology

A type of neurogenic hypertension due to neurovascular compression of the brainstem was described in the early 1980s with clinical observations made in the course of neurosurgical procedures on patients with cranial nerve compression syndromes[23]. In a prospective study, 96% of the hypertensive patients undergoing microvascular decompression had obvious

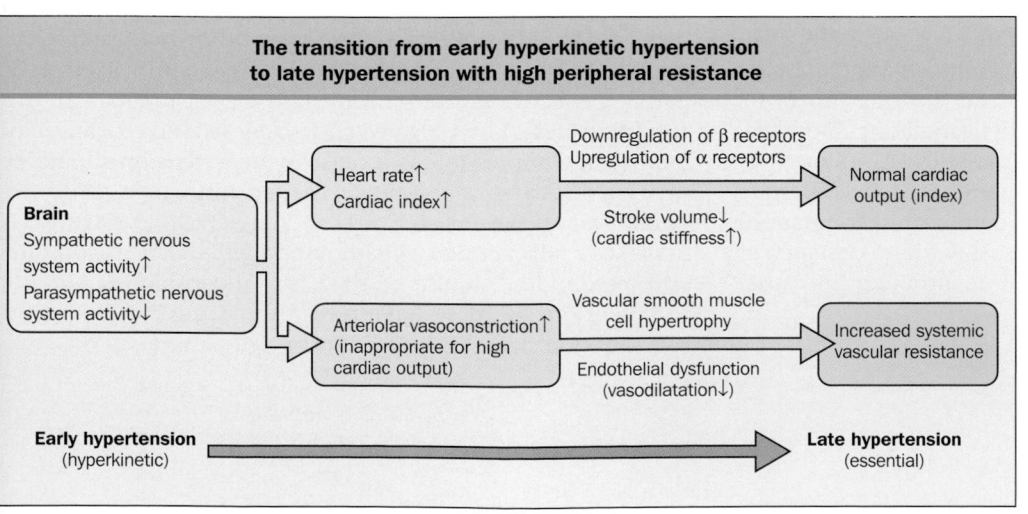

Figure 41.4 The transition from an early hyperkinetic hypertension to late hypertension with high peripheral resistance.

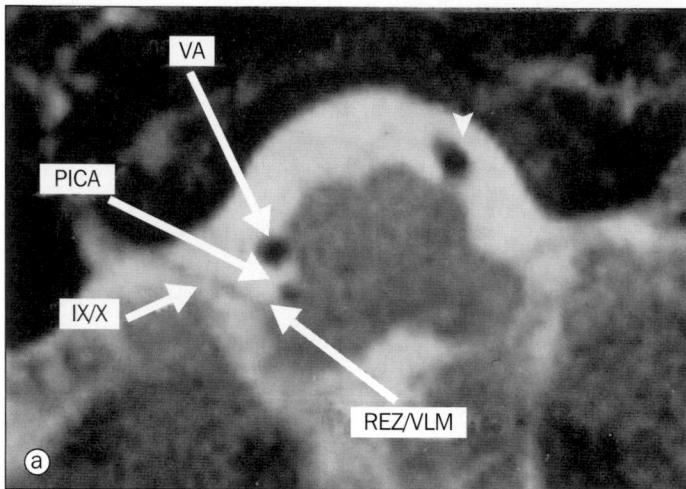
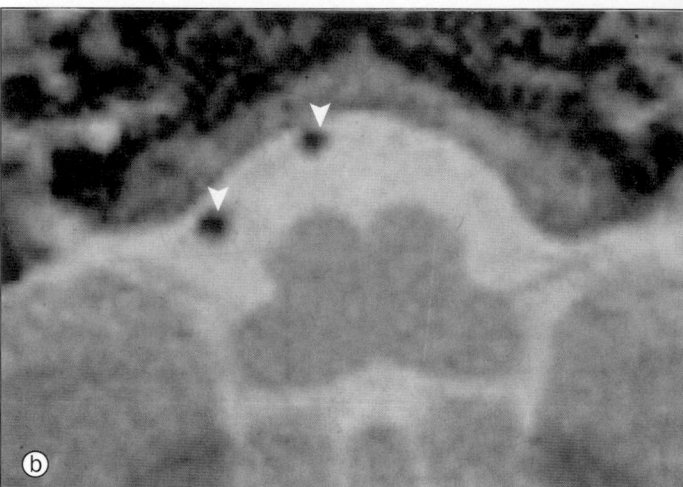

Figure 41.5 Neurovascular compression syndrome. (a) Patient with hypertension secondary to neurovascular compression of the ventrolateral medulla (VLM) by the posterior inferior cerebellar artery (PICA). (b) A normal case showing no compression. VA, vertebral artery (arrowheads); REZ, root entry zone; CN IX/X, cranial nerves IX and X; Axial T2 magnetic resonance imaging. (Courtesy of R. Naraghi, Friedrich-Alexander.)

compression of the left anterolateral medulla, most frequently with a loop of vertebral artery pressing into the medulla between the inferior olive and the root entry zone of the cranial nerves IX and X. In contrast only two of the normotensive patients had similar findings. Microvascular decompression caused significant and sustained lowering of the BP in almost 90% of the patients in whom the decompression was deemed adequate[23].

Pathogenesis

Janetta and coworkers[23] postulated that compression of the lateral brainstem may be a cause of essential hypertension, or at least be a major contributor to its maintenance. The assumed mechanism was that aging-related elongation and dilatation of central arteries could cause pulsatile compression of the brainstem, which could be further accentuated by the caudal sagging of the brain associated with advancing age. Compression of the root entry zones of cranial nerves IX and X in the lateral brainstem could disrupt sympathetic and vagal fibers in transit to the medullary centers of BP regulation and produce hypertension (see Fig. 41.5). Observations in humans that intraoperative manipulation of the brainstem causes acute hypertension have been experimentally validated by studies in rats, which have shown that pulsatile compression of the rostral ventrolateral medulla causes BP elevation that can be prevented by ganglionic blockade. However, this and similar experiments failed to induce sustained hypertension convincingly in animal models. Despite this, recent studies in humans have demonstrated enhanced sympathetic activity in some patients with neurovascular compression and essential hypertension, although the causal association is still speculative[24].

Diagnosis and treatment

Since these observations, a series of predominantly retrospective studies using angiography and magnetic resonance imaging (MRI) have reported neurovascular brainstem compression in 75–100% of patients with hypertension but also in 7–42% in patients with normal BP or secondary hypertension. When Watters et al. retrospectively evaluated 120 MRI scans for neurovascular brainstem compression in a study blinded to BP status, no significant difference was noted in the frequency of compression between hypertensive and normotensive patients (57 versus 55%)[25]. However, Naraghi and his coworkers recently reported that neurovascular compression was demonstrable in all 15 patients (aged 12–59 years) with hypertension associated with brachydactyly that they studied[26]. The onset of hypertension in this rare autosomal dominant condition is at an early age, which suggests that neurovascular compression may be the primary cause of the sustained and severe BP elevation seen in these patients.

While neurovascular compression of the lateral brainstem can produce hypertension, it is unlikely to be the underlying cause of 'essential' hypertension in the majority of hypertensive patients. Although there have been no reports of successful medical treatment of hypertension caused by brainstem compression, conventional antihypertensive therapy is likely to be partially effective as it is probable that most patients with this condition are not investigated and diagnosed. Investigation for brainstem compression as a cause of hypertension should be reserved for cases of resistant hypertension where other secondary causes have been ruled out. If a definitive diagnosis is made, centrally acting sympatholytic agents such as clonidine and moxonidine should be tried before considering surgical intervention, as there have only been scattered reports of surgical 'cure' apart from Jannetta's original observations[23].

REFERENCES

1. Britton M, Carlsson A, du Faire U. Blood pressure course in patients with acute stroke and matched controls. Stroke. 1986;17: 861–4.

2. Sander D, Winbeck K, Klingelhofer J, et al. Prognostic relevance of pathological sympathetic activation after acute thromboembolic stroke. Neurology. 2001;57(5):833–8.

3. Bhalla A, Wolfe CD, Rudd AG. The effect of 24h blood pressure levels on early neurologic recovery after stroke. J Intern Med. 2001;250(2):121–30.

4. Robinson TG, Dawson SL, Ahmed U, et al. Twenty four hour systolic blood pressure predicts long term mortality following acute stroke. J Hypertens. 2001;19(12):2127–34.

5. Britton M, Carlsson A. Very high blood pressures in acute stroke. J Intern Med. 1990;228:611–15.

6. Lavin P. Management of hypertension in patients with acute stroke. Arch Intern Med. 1986;146:66–8.

7. Brott T, Maccarthy EP. Antihypertensive therapy in stroke. In: Fisher M, ed. Medical therapy of acute stroke vol2. Marcel Decker: New York; 1989:117–41.

8. Kreiger D, Hacke W. The intensive care of the stroke patient. In: Barnett, Mohr Stein et al., eds. Stroke. Edinburgh: Churchill Livingstone; 1998.

9. Progress Collaborative Group. Randomised trial of a perindopril-based blood pressure lowering regimen among 6.105 individuals with previous stroke or transient ischemic attack. Lancet. 2001;358:1033–41.

10. Towne JB, Bernhard VM. The relationship of postoperative hypertension to complications following carotid endarterectomy. Surgery. 1980;88:575–80.

11. Scheinman M, Ascher E, Hingorani A, et al. Hemodynamic instability following carotid endarterectomy does not effect early discharge. Cardiovasc Surg. 1998;6(5):470–4.

12. Ahn SS, Marcus DR, Moore WS. Post carotid endarterectomy hypertension; association with elevated cranial norepinephrine. J Vasc Surg. 1989;9:351–60.

13. Julius S, Majahalme S. The changing face of sympathetic overactivity in hypertension. Ann Med 2000;32:365–70.

14. Julius S, Valentini M, Palatini P. Overweight and hypertension – a 2-way street? Hypertension. 2000;35:807–13.

15. Julius S, Pascual AV, London R. Role of parasympathetic inhibition in the hyperkinetic type of borderline hypertension. Circulation. 1971;44:413–18.

16. Eich RH, Cuddy RP, Smulyan H, Lyons RH. Hemodynamics in labile hypertension: a follow-up study. Circulation. 1966;34: 299–307.

17. Lund-Johansen P, Omvik P. Hemodynamic patterns of untreated hypertensive disease. In: Laragh JH, Brenner BM, eds. Hypertension: pathophysiology, diagnosis, and management. New York: Raven Press; 1990:305–27.

18. Julius S. Transition from high cardiac output to elevated vascular resistance in hypertension. Am Heart J. 1988;116:600–6.

19. Julius S, Jamerson K, Mejia A, et al. The association of borderline hypertension with target organ changes and higher coronary risk. Tecumseh Blood Pressure Study. JAMA. 1990;264:354–8.

20. Veglio F, Morra di Cella S, Schiavone D, et al. Peripheral adrenergic system and hypertension. Clin Exp Hypertens. 2001;23:3–25.

21. Mathias C. Role of sympathetic efferent nerves in BP regulation and in hypertension. Hypertension. 1991;18(Suppl. III):22–30.

22. Ho RM, Freed MM. Persistant hypertension in young spinal cord injured individuals resulting from aortic repair. Arch Phys Med Rehab. 1991;72:743–6.

23. Jannetta P, Segal R, Wolfson S. Neurogenic hypertension: etiology and surgical treatment. Ann Surg. 1985;201:391–8.

24. Morise T, Horita M, Kitagawa I, et al. The potent role of increased sympathetic tone in the pathogenesis of essential hypertension with neurovascular compression. J Hum Hypertens. 2000;14: 807–11.

25. Watters M, Burton B, Turner G, Cannard K. MR screening for brain stem compression in hypertension. Am J Neuroradiol. 1996;17:217–21.

26. Naraghi R, Schuster H, Toka HR, et al. Neurovascular compression at the ventrolateral medulla in autosomal dominant hypertension associated with brachydactyly. Stroke. 1997;28:1749–54.

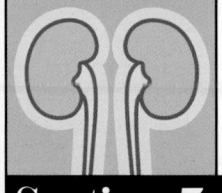

Chapter 42

Hypertension in African Americans

John M Flack and Hisham Alrefai

DEFINITION

African American men and women have an earlier onset, higher incidence and prevalence, greater severity, and excess cardiovascular-renal target organ damage (i.e., stroke, left ventricular hypertrophy (LVH), renal insufficiency) for any given blood pressure (BP) level compared with Caucasians. This observation has raised the question whether there should be race-specific BP levels for the diagnosis and treatment of hypertension. The sixth report of the Joint National Committee on Prevention, Detection, Evaluation, and Treatment of High Blood Pressure (JNC VI) indirectly addressed this issue[1]. This report recommended that a BP goal of < 130/85 mmHg be targeted for individuals with diabetes mellitus, renal dysfunction, and congestive heart failure, conditions that all disproportionately affect African Americans. However, no specific blood pressure treatment goals were put forth for African Americans. Recently, the American Diabetes Association and the National Kidney Foundation have suggested an even lower blood pressure threshold for the diagnosis of hypertension in persons with diabetes and/or renal dysfunction, that being a BP of > 130/80 mmHg. Because of the excess prevalence of these conditions among African Americans, these new therapeutic recommendations will impact the timing of initiation of therapy as well as the ultimate BP treatment goals in many African Americans.

EPIDEMIOLOGY

Hypertension affects approximately 25% of adults in the USA and is a leading cause of cardiovascular disease (CVD) morbidity and mortality[2]. The age-adjusted rate of hypertension is approximately 40% higher among African Americans than in Caucasians. Hypertension excess in African Americans is greatest at younger ages, particularly among women, and declines progressively with advancing age (see Fig. 35.4)[2]. Mean BP levels are higher in African American men compared with Caucasian men at all ages until 70 years of age, whereas in women the difference is apparent at all ages. The prevalence of stage III hypertension (systolic BP ≥ 180 and/or diastolic BP ≥ 110 mmHg) in the general population is much higher in African Americans than among Caucasians (8% versus 1%, respectively).

The risk of hypertension in African Americans varies by geography. Hypertension rates are higher for African Americans residing in the southeastern USA than for African Americans residing elsewhere. In the USA, the rates of hypertension are

also greater in rural than urban areas for African Americans, which is opposite to that observed in less developed countries[3]. Higher rates of hypertension in African Americans relative to majority reference populations have also been observed in many Latin American and Caribbean countries and in the UK. Nevertheless, in rural areas of Africa, hypertension rates have been documented in the single digits – rates that are far lower than observed even in US white populations – although much higher rates have been noted to occur in the urban areas. Cross-sectional studies have shown an escalating east:west prevalence gradient of hypertension risk being lowest in Africa, intermediate in the Caribbean, and highest in the urban Midwestern USA[4].

There is also an increased frequency of hypertension-related complications in African Americans (Fig. 42.1)[2]. Overall, African Americans have a higher prevalence of hypertension-related target organ damage (stroke, LVH, renal disease, and mortality)[5,6], which in part may relate to the onset of hypertension at an earlier age than in Caucasians. In addition to a threefold increase in cardiovascular mortality, African Americans have a marked (3–15-fold) increased risk for developing renal failure secondary to hypertension. This, coupled with the increased risk for diabetic nephropathy, is reflected by the finding that over 30% of patients with end-stage renal disease (ESRD) in the USA are African American despite the fact that African Americans constitute only 12% of the population. Although the absolute risk level for BP-related sequelae is

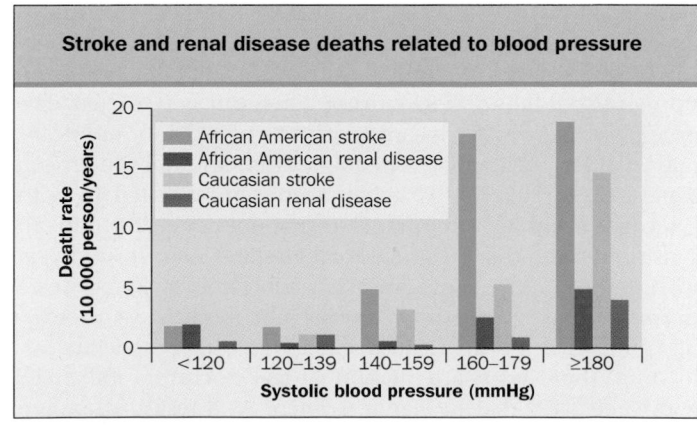

Figure 42.1 Male death rates from stroke and renal disease in African Americans and Caucasians at varying blood pressures. Men were screened for the Multiple Risk Factor Intervention Trial. (Adapted with permission from Flack et al.[5].)

higher in African Americans compared with Caucasians at a given BP level, the shape of the general relationship of BP to cardiovascular-renal complications across the entire range of BP differs little by race.

PATHOGENESIS OF HYPERTENSION IN AFRICAN AMERICANS

There are numerous theories for the excess prevalence of hypertension among African Americans, some of which are based on the notion that hypertension in African Americans is an entity distinct from that observed in the general population. However, it remains unclear whether hypertension in African Americans truly represents a distinct entity or rather represents an upward shift in the distribution of BP levels that leads to greater adverse clinical sequelae because of longer duration, greater severity, and more accompanying risk factors such as diabetes mellitus, cigarette smoking, and physical inactivity.

Table 42.1 lists physiologic characteristics of the African American hypertensive. None are unique to the African American hypertensive, but rather represent quantitative, not qualitative, differences between African Americans and other racial/ethnic groups. From an etiologic perspective, it is difficult to separate those characteristics that are primary or genetic factors from pressure-related target organ sequelae that have developed as a consequence of gene–environment interactions or from an overwhelming burden of environmental insults.

Several factors predispose to the increased frequency of hypertension in the African American population. These include lower socioeconomic status, a diet higher in sodium and lower in potassium and calcium, and an increased frequency of insulin resistance, obesity, and physical inactivity[7]. Physical inactivity, especially among African American women, is a contributor to the racial disparity in hypertension prevalence and incidence. Physical inactivity promotes not only hypertension but also risk factor clustering – obesity, diabetes mellitus, and dyslipidemia (raised cholesterol and triglycerides and/or low high-density lipoprotein (HDL) levels).

Salt sensitivity

Salt sensitivity is disproportionately manifest in African Americans, particularly among hypertensives. Salt sensitivity can be defined as a rise in BP occurring during salt administration and/or a fall in BP occurring when salt is restricted. The excess prevalence of salt sensitivity among African Americans may relate to the increased frequency of obesity in the African American population, as it has been demonstrated in both Caucasians and African Americans that obesity is linked to salt sensitivity[8] and that weight loss ameliorates salt sensitivity, at least among overweight Caucasian adolescents. Moreover, in normotensive salt-sensitive, overweight (body mass index > 32 kg/m²) African American women who undergo dietary salt loading, there is an attenuation of the nocturnal fall in BP compared with that in leaner women. As a result, there is a deleterious interaction between body size and dietary salt intake leading to a greater 24-h BP burden.

It has been speculated that the salt-sensitive hypertension in African Americans may have a genetic basis in which the

Physiologic characteristics associated with but not unique to hypertensive African Americans
Salt-sensitivity
Obesity
High prevalence of coexisting cardiovascular disease risk factors in addition to raised blood pressure (i.e., insulin resistance, diabetes mellitus, smoking, dyslipidemia)
Decreased renal vasodilator hormones (e.g., reduced urinary kallikrein excretion)
Increased urinary protein excretion
Suppressed renin levels; possibly increased intrarenal angiotensin II
Decreased renal natriuretic capacity
High renal vascular resistance
Reduced renal blood flow
Increased peripheral vascular resistance
Excess blood pressure-related target organ damage (i.e., left ventricular hypertrophy, stroke, renal insufficiency)
Increased frequency of the double deletion (DD) genotype of the angiotensin-converting enzyme (ACE-DD)

Table 42.1 Physiologic characteristics associated with but not unique to hypertensive African Americans.

kidney has a defect in its ability to excrete salt. In this regard, various studies have looked for mutations and/or alterations in the regulation of sodium transport in the nephron to account for the increased salt sensitivity. It is likely that a multiplicity of pathophysiological mechanisms either cause or contribute to the intermediate BP phenotype of salt sensitivity.

Possible mechanisms of excessive renal injury in African Americans

It has been hypothesized that African Americans have defective renal autoregulation, in which inappropriately low tone of the afferent (preglomerular) afferent arteriole leads to excessive transmission of systemic blood pressure to the renal glomerulus. Indeed, an exaggerated rise in glomerular filtration rate, consistent with vasodilation of the afferent glomerular arteriole, has been shown during dietary salt loading in African Americans when compared with Caucasians[9]. Furthermore, if excessive constriction of the efferent arteriole is also present as would occur with local activation of the renin–angiotensin system, then glomerular pressures would rise even further, leading to greater renal injury. A number of conditions can lead to abnormal renal autoregulation including high sodium diet, reduced renal mass, and diabetes mellitus[10]. Obesity also activates the tissue renin–angiotensin system. Thus, abnormal renal autoregulation may be a secondary, rather than primary phenomenon. Other renal abnormalities noted in hypertensive African Americans include higher renal vascular resistance and lower renal blood flow for the same degree of hypertension, when compared with Caucasians. Glomeruli from African Americans are larger than those observed in Caucasians and consequently may be predisposed to the development of glomerulosclerosis. These abnormalities may be related to a congenital reduction in nephron number, which has been linked to low birth weights[11]. Again, it is not clear if these racial differences represent primary or secondary phenomena.

Renin–angiotensin–aldosterone–kinin system

Hypertension in the African American has been characterized as a type of 'low-renin' hypertension. It has been assumed that plasma volume expansion in African Americans is a primary physiologic aberration[11] that results in secondary suppression of the renin system. However, plasma volume expansion has not been consistently demonstrated in African Americans. Moreover, in African Americans the relationship of circulating renin and plasma volume has been difficult to demonstrate.

We have proposed a different hypothesis, namely, that suppressed circulating renin levels represents overactivity of the vasoconstrictive, proliferative, antinatriuretic arm of the renin–angiotensin–aldosterone–kinin (RAAK) system and underactivity of the vasodilatory, antiproliferative natriuretic arm[12]. We have termed this imbalance 'RAAK system disequilibrium'. Certainly, angiotensin receptor antagonists or angiotensin-converting enzyme (ACE) inhibitors, which inhibit this negative feedback, result in an immediate, dose-related rise in circulating renin levels in both Caucasian and African American hypertensives, although it is less pronounced in African Americans. We postulated that intrarenal production of angiotensin II may be involved in both suppressing renin production and contributing to the pressure-related target organ damage in African Americans, particularly given the known involvement of the RAAK system in the pathogenesis of target organ injury. Activation of the local renin–angiotensin system, perhaps via reduced blood flow, renal ischemia, and/or obesity would lead to excessive tone of the efferent arteriole leading to further increases in intraglomerular pressure. Further, it has also been shown that hypertensive African Americans have lower urinary levels of various natriuretic and vasodilatory substances, including kallikrein, nitric oxide (NO) metabolites, and dopamine.

Endothelin

Endothelin-1, the main endothelin generated in the endothelium, can induce vascular smooth muscle cell contraction and stimulate cell hyperplasia and hypertrophy[13]. Endothelin stimulates angiotensin II synthesis while suppressing renin synthesis and has been linked to salt sensitivity in Italian hypertensives. Endothelin levels are elevated in hypertensive African Americans compared with normotensive and hypertensive African Americans and Caucasians[14]. In salt sensitive hypertension, such as in African American patients, the endothelin response is exaggerated as a response to increased sympathetic activity[15]. Thus, endothelin may have a role in hypertension and related target organ damage, particularly in salt sensitive African American hypertensives.

Transforming growth factor-β

TGF-β1 is a fibrogenic cytokine that may influence BP indirectly via stimulation of endothelin-1 from endothelial cells[16], by stimulation of renin from juxtaglomerular cells, and by inhibition of nitric oxide, a potent vasodilator[17]. TGF-β1 induces smooth muscle cell hypertrophy and vascular remodeling. TGF-β1 has been shown in an experimental model to cause progressive renal injury as manifested by matrix protein accumulation and interstitial fibrosis[18]. Angiotensin II also stimulates TGF-β1 synthesis. High serum levels of TGF-β1 have been found in hypertensive compared to normotensive individuals amongst both African Americans and Caucasians[19]. African normotensives have higher TGF-β1 levels than Caucasian normotensives suggesting that TGF-β1 is a plausible mediator of racial differences in target-organ injury. Salt has been shown to augment TGF-β1 expression. Amongst persons with renal disease, use of renin–angiotensin system modulators significantly lowers TGF-β1 levels[20,21].

CLINICAL MANIFESTATIONS

Virtually all forms of pressure-related target organ injury are more common in African Americans than in Caucasians, including renal insufficiency/ESRD, LVH, heart failure, retinopathy, and stroke. The risk of renal injury, as well as the risk for all other target organ damage, is directly related to the degree of BP elevation.

The increased risk for progression of renal disease in hypertensive African Americans has led some investigators to speculate that African Americans with hypertension and progressive renal disease may have renal lesions other than classic hypertensive (arteriolosclerotic) renal disease. In the African American Study for Kidney Disease and Hypertension (AASKD), however, the great majority of renal biopsies demonstrated classic but advanced hypertensive injury, with arteriolosclerosis of both the afferent arteriole and interlobular artery, focal and sometimes global glomerulosclerosis, and tubulointerstitial fibrosis (Fig. 42.2)[22].

DIFFERENTIAL DIAGNOSIS

In patients with hypertension and renal insufficiency, etiologies other than essential hypertension should be considered. Renovascular hypertension was once considered to have a

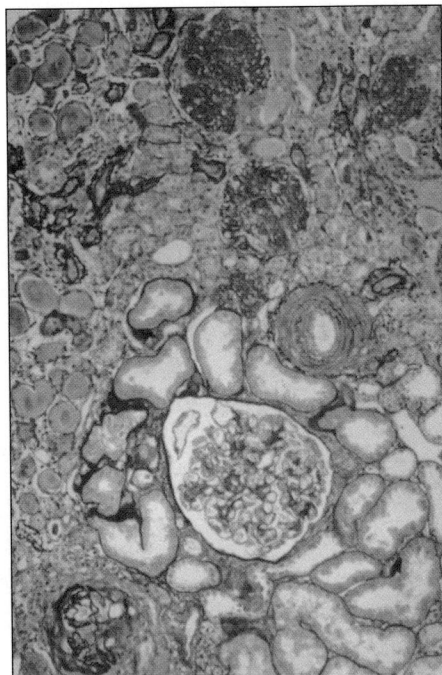

Figure 42.2 Renal histology in an African American with essential hypertension. Thickening of the interlobular artery with severe global glomerulosclerosis and patchy tubulointerstitial fibrosis is shown. (Adapted with permission from Fogo et al.[22].)

lower prevalence in African Americans than in Caucasians. However, recent data derived from renal artery duplex scanning from the Cardiovascular Health Study cohort (persons aged $\geq$ 60 years) has documented approximately an 8% prevalence of critical renal artery stenosis in both African Americans and Caucasians (K. Hansen, pers. comm.). Moreover, in a consecutive surgical series of hypertensive African Americans with critical renal artery stenosis, 13 of 23 (57%) patients with ischemic nephropathy experienced a greater than 20% decline in serum creatinine[23]. In these patients, a beneficial BP response to surgical revascularization was obtained in 74%, with a mean improvement in estimated glomerular filtration rate (GFR) from 34 to 43 mL/min per 1.72 m² ($P < 0.001$). Though presenting with more advanced disease at baseline, African Americans with critical renal artery stenosis experienced similar BP reductions as well as greater improvements in renal function from surgical revascularization than Caucasians. These data emphasize the need to consider renovascular hypertension in appropriately selected African American hypertensives.

NATURAL HISTORY

African Americans with hypertension have a higher absolute risk for cardiac mortality, stroke, and ESRD compared with their sex- and age-matched counterparts, in part because of a greater prevalence of 'severe' stage III hypertension, longer duration of BP elevations, frequent loss of the normal nocturnal dipping of BP, and their apparent increased target organ sensitivity to pressure-related injury at a given BP level.

TREATMENT

The observation that progressive renal injury occurs in the hypertensive African American, despite seemingly adequate BP control has raised the question of whether a lower target BP level may confer better renal protection. In the Modification of Diet in Renal Disease (MDRD) study, which included patients with many different renal diseases, a subset analysis documented a trend ($P = 0.11$) toward better renoprotection

in African Americans with a lower BP target (MAP 92 mmHg) compared with usual BP control (MAP 100 mmHg)[24]. The MDRD study also reported that a lower BP (< 125/75 mmHg) was associated with greater renoprotection in proteinuric (> 1 g/d) patients with renal insufficiency. Furthermore, a minimal target BP of 130/85 mmHg has been recommended to retard the progression of progressive renal dysfunction and to prevent ESRD in hypertensives with renal insufficiency[25].

What antihypertensive agents should be used in the African American hypertensive? First, all antihypertensive drug classes may provide clinically meaningful BP reductions in African American hypertensives[26]. Racial differences in BP response to selected antihypertensive agents are not of sufficient magnitude to justify the use of race as the sole, or even the predominant, factor in drug selection. Second, whereas all antihypertensive agents have some efficacy in the African American hypertensive, drug monotherapy is less likely to be effective among African Americans given their higher average pretreatment BP levels. Furthermore, among individuals with renal insufficiency, it takes an average of slightly more than four drugs to achieve BP normalization. Finally, salt sensitivity, which is characteristic of the African American hypertensives, presents another barrier to BP normalization. Salt intake in the USA is in excess of that required for normal physiologic functioning and can attenuate the BP-lowering effect of virtually all antihypertensive drugs, an effect that is particularly manifest in the highly salt sensitive African American hypertensive. This is especially true for antihypertensive drugs that inhibit or block the RAAK system (i.e., β-blockers, ACE inhibitors) and is less true for diuretics and calcium channel antagonists. Tables 42.2 and 42.3 list therapeutic considerations and recommendations for treating the African American hypertensive.

Diuretics

Diuretics are effective in African Americans and Caucasians and remain a favored drug class in the recent JNC VI report. In the setting of *ad libitum* (physiologically high) dietary sodium intake, diuretics retain a high proportion of their antihypertensive efficacy, an important pharmacologic characteristic in a highly salt sensitive population. These agents

Therapeutic considerations when treating African American hypertensive patients	
Risk factor	**Treatment factors**
High blood pressure (BP) levels	More monotherapy failures
Longer duration of hypertension	More short-term risk from rapid BP reduction; however, long-term benefits of BP normalization are greater
High burden of target organ damage	Need slow but aggressive BP control (< 130/85 mmHg); favor drugs with human data for target organ protection
Obesity	More likely to be salt sensitive; leading to higher BP medication requirements; lower sodium intake; titrate upward with angiotensin-converting enzyme (ACE) inhibitors
Glomerular hyperfiltration	Aggressive BP control; favor ACE inhibitors, possibly angiotensin type 1 receptor (AT1) antagonists
Reduced natriuretic capacity	More often need diuretics, especially in complex drug regimens; premium on reducing dietary sodium intake

Table 42.2 Therapeutic considerations when treating African American hypertensive patients.

Recommendations for the evaluation and treatment of hypertension in African Americans

Clinical/diagnostic evaluation	Action
Thorough, cost-efficient search for historical, biochemical, electrocardiogram/echocardiogram evidence of pressure-related target organ injury	The presence of pressure-related target organ damage portends a striking increase in absolute cardiovascular disease risk at a given blood pressure (BP) level and profoundly influences treatment initiation levels and the on-treatment target BP level
Avoid utilization of race as the sole, or even predominant, criterion for drug selection	The previously reported racial differentials are of insufficient magnitude to guide selection choices for individual patients; emphasize lifestyle modification in the context of cultural beliefs and preferences
Gradually lower BP over many weeks to months to the appropriate target	Give drugs for at least 6–8 weeks to manifest full BP-lowering effect after initiation of treatment and use dose titration; otherwise may risk greater drug-related side effects as well as inaccurate validation of the self-fulfilling prophecy that 'these drugs don't work'
Expect the overwhelming majority of patients with stage III hypertension (> 180/110 mmHg) ultimately to fail monotherapy	In this BP range it is still recommended to start with monotherapy, even though monotherapy failures are the rule; titrate the drug dose up over time and, ultimately, add a second agent if BP is not controlled.

are useful in complex antihypertensive drug regimens (more than two drugs), because they antagonize the sodium retention that occurs with vasodilator and/or sympatholytic drugs. Diuretics augment the BP-lowering efficacy of virtually all nondiuretic antihypertensive drug classes. Their absence in complex drug regimens is a common cause of therapeutic failure, particularly among individuals manifesting salt sensitivity and/or reduced renal function. It is critical to select the diuretic that is most appropriate for the level of kidney function. Thiazide diuretics are minimally effective when the GFR ≤ 45 mL/min per 1.73 m². Loop diuretics or metolozone are better choices when kidney function is reduced to below this level.

β-Blockers

β-Blockers lower BP in African Americans, though they are relatively less effective than monotherapy with either diuretics or calcium antagonists. As with other drugs that have their effects via the RAAK system, consumption of dietary sodium in amounts typical of many African Americans (and Caucasians), attenuates their BP-lowering efficacy. β-Blockers as well as combined αβ-blockers appear to be particularly efficacious in severe hypertensives, most often in combination with diuretics and/or other antihypertensive agents. However, the combination of a β-blocker with a calcium channel antagonist that lowers heart rate (such as verapamil or diltiazem), should be avoided.

Angiotensin-converting enzyme inhibitors

Based on the best available evidence, ACE inhibitors should be preferred agents in African Americans with diabetic and non-diabetic proteinuric renal disease. In a recent interim report from the African American Study of Kidney Disease (AASKD) study[27], initial therapy with ramipril, an ACE inhibitor, slowed the loss of renal function and reduced proteinuria more effectively than amlodipine, a dihydropyridine calcium antagonist, in nondiabetic African Americans with reduced kidney function. The difference was observed despite < 2 mmHg

difference in blood pressure and with both groups receiving a similar number (mean 2.75) of antihypertensive agents. The advantage of ACE inhibitors was most evident in patients with proteinuria. This observation replicates what has been observed in other studies of ACE inhibitors in non-African American populations with reduced kidney function. A desirable effect of ACE inhibitors is that they lower intraglomerular pressure, irrespective of whether they reduce systemic BP, thereby reducing hemodynamically-mediated renal injury.

ACE inhibitors have additional advantages. While ACE inhibitors do not affect fasting glucose levels, they do lessen insulin resistance and may lower the risk of developing diabetes mellitus[28], an effect of considerable potential importance in a diabetes-prone group such as African Americans. ACE inhibitors also lower the risk of both microvascular and cardiovascular complications, especially for the development of heart failure[28]. ACE inhibitors can also be safely combined with most other antihypertensive drugs.

However, the BP lowering effect of ACE inhibitors is relatively sensitive to the level of dietary sodium intake. The higher the level of sodium intake the less the blood pressure fall with these agents. The risk of both angioedema and cough, though low in absolute terms, is also higher in African Americans than Caucasians when prescribed these agents.

Angiotensin type I receptor antagonists

Angiotensin type 1 receptor antagonists (ATRAs) are a well-tolerated antihypertensive drug class that blocks activation of the AT1 receptor and, therefore, have the potential to block pathophysiologic consequences of angiotensin II. These agents are antiproteinuric, an important consideration in the renal-injury prone African American hypertensive. The ATRAs can be considered for ACE inhibitor-intolerant patients; however, similar to the ACE inhibitors, they should be avoided in patients with bilateral renal artery stenosis and used cautiously in patients prone to hyperkalemia. Two recently reported clinical trials of these agents in diabetic nephropathy are of particular importance to African Americans given the disproportionately high prevalence of this condition. The Irbesartan Diabetic Nephropathy Trial (IDNT) compared irbesartan, an ATRA, with amlodipine or placebo[29]. Amlodipine and irbesartan lowered BP to a similar degree but irbesartan provided greater renoprotection (30% less doubling of serum creatinine and lowered proteinuria to a greater degree). Heart failure incidence was also lower with irbesartan compared with the placebo and amlodipine groups. However, the rates of CVD death, nonfatal MI, and stroke tended to be higher in the irbesartan compared to the amlodipine group. The RENAAL study[30] compared the ATRA, losartan, to an antihypertensive regimen not containing ATRAs or ACE inhibitors. BP was lowered slightly more in the losartan group (140/74 versus 142/74 mmHg) and both proteinuria and the composite endpoint of doubling of serum creatinine, ESRD or death were also lower. There were fewer cases of new heart failure and a borderline significant trend toward fewer myocardial infarctions in the losartan group compared with placebo. Background therapy with calcium antagonists did not attenuate the benefits of losartan treatment. Similar clinical endpoint data for ATRAs in persons with nondiabetic renal insufficiency is not currently available.

Calcium antagonists

Calcium antagonists have long been considered a preferred monotherapy for achieving BP control in hypertensive African Americans. Monotherapy with these agents lowers BP to a similar degree as diuretics but is more effective than other antihypertensive drug classes in African Americans. The BP-lowering potency of the calcium antagonists, as with the diuretics, is minimally affected by physiologically high levels of dietary salt consumption[31]. Calcium antagonists reverse some of the excessive renal vasoconstriction seen in African American hypertensives. However, these agents, particularly the dihydropyridines, may disrupt renal GFR autoregulation, and in the setting of elevated systemic blood pressures, may lead to excess transmission of systemic pressures to the glomerulus especially in the absence of an ACE inhibitor. The calcium antagonists that lower heart rate, verapamil and diltiazem, do not disrupt renal GFR autoregulation. However, there is no long-term clinical endpoint data regarding renal outcomes with these rate-limiting calcium antagonists. The data with the calcium antagonists in the RENAAL trial suggested that, when an ATRA is used in combination with a dihydropyridine calcium antagonist, there is no attenuation of the clinical benefit attributable to the ATRA. Thus, calcium antagonists may be considered adjunctive drugs for the treatment of persons with reduced kidney function. Furthermore, as seen in the IDNT trial in persons with diabetic nephropathy, dihydropyridine calcium antagonists may have a more

favorable effect on nonrenal endpoints such as stroke and nonfatal MI, than ATRAs for similar levels of BP. Thus, in persons with diabetic nephropathy, and by extrapolation, in nondiabetics with reduced kidney function, calcium antagonists should be used primarily if administered in combination with ACE inhibitors or ATRAs.

α_1-Adrenoceptor antagonists

The α_1-adrenoceptor antagonists lower BP effectively in African Americans, although the dose required to achieve a given level of BP control appears to be slightly higher than in Caucasians. These agents may be useful in African Americans, both as monotherapy and in combination with other antihypertensive drugs because they not only lower BP but also improve glucose tolerance, lessen insulin resistance, and favorably impact all lipoproteins (lowering cholesterol and triglycerides and raising HDL). The α_1-adrenoceptor antagonists also favorably influence the fibrinolytic system. These agents can, however, cause orthostatic hypertension, especially in diabetics and when combined with either diuretics or sympatholytic drugs. In addition, the doxazosin arm of the Antihypertensive and Lipid-Lowering Treatment to Prevent Heart Attack Trial (ALLHAT) was discontinued because an interim analysis showed that, compared with chlorthalidone, the doxazosin group had higher rates of stroke, CVD events, and heart failure[32]. Interestingly, there was no difference between the doxazosin and chlorthalidone treatment arms on the primary endpoint of fatal or nonfatal MI. Systolic BP lowering was ~ 3 mmHg less with doxazosin. It seems more likely that doxazosin was not as effective as diuretics in lowering CV events as opposed to actually increasing the rate of these events. Thus, the most logical utilization of doxazosin in hypertension treatment is as an add-on drug.

Other antihypertensive agents

Central adrenergic inhibitors effectively lower BP in African Americans and may be used as first-line drug therapy; however, they are best reserved as add-on therapy. Typically, central adrenergic inhibitors are associated with bothersome side effects, such as dry mouth, depression, and orthostatic hypotension. Clonidine, however, may be the drug of choice for true hypertensive urgencies. Direct vasodilators such as minoxidil and hydralazine are not suitable for use as monotherapy. These drugs are most often reserved for use as adjunctive treatments for hypertension. Direct vasodilators activate the sympathetic nervous system leading to bothersome tachycardia and also promote profound salt and water retention necessitating that the patient be treated with a diuretic, usually a loop diuretic, and either a β-blocker or a rate-limiting calcium antagonist.

REFERENCES

1. The sixth report of the Joint National Committee on prevention, detection, evaluation, and treatment of high blood pressure (JNC VI). Arch Intern Med. 1997;157:2413–46.

2. Burt V, Whelton P, Roccella E, et al. Prevalence of hypertension in the US adult population. Results from the Third National Health and Nutrition Examination Survey, 1988–1991. Hypertension. 1995;25:305–13.

3. Cooper RS, Rotimi CN, Kaufman JS, et al. Hypertension treatment and control in sub-Saharan Africa: The epidemiological basis for policy. BMJ. 1998;316:614–17.

4. Cooper R, Rotimi C, Ataman S, et al. The prevalence of hypertension in seven populations of West African origin. Am J Public Health. 1997;87(2):155–6.

5. Flack JM, Neaton JD, Daniels B, Esunge P. Ethnicity and renal disease: lessons from multiple risk factor intervention trial and the treatment of mild hypertension study. Am J Kidney Dis. 1993;21 (Suppl)(4):31–40.

6. Levy D, Larson M, Vasan R, et al. The progression from hypertension to congestive heart failure. J Am Med Assoc. 1996;275:1557–62.

7. Liu K, Ruth KJ, Flack JM, et al. Blood pressure in young black and whites: relevance of obesity and lifestyle factors in determining differences – the CARDIA study. Circulation. 1996;93:60–6.

8. Flack JM, Grimm RH Jr, Staffileno B, et al. New salt-sensitivity metrics: variability-adjusted blood pressure change and urinary sodium to creatinine ratio. Ethn Dis. (in press).

9. Parmer J, Stone RA, Cervenka JH, et al. Renal hemodynamics in essential hypertension. Hypertension. 1994;24:752–7.

10. Palmer BF. Impaired renal autoregulation: implications for the genesis of hypertension and hypertension-induced renal injury. Am J Med Sci. 2001;321(6):388–400.

11. Mackenzie H, Lawler E, Brenner B. Pathogenesis and pathophysiology of essential hypertension. Congenital oligonephropathy: the fetal flaw in essential hypertension? Kidney Int. 1996;49: S30–4.

12. Flack JM, Mensah GA, Ferrario CM. Using angiotensin converting enzyme inhibitors in African American hypertensives: a new approach to treating hypertension and preventing target-organ damage. Curr Med Res Opin. 2000;16:66–79.

13. Battistini B, Chailler P, D'Orleans Juste P, et al. Growth regulatory properties of endothelins. Peptides. 1993;14(2):385–99.

14. Ergul S, Parish DC, Puett D, Ergul A. Racial differences in plasma endothelin-1 concentrations in individuals with essential hypertension. Hypertension. 1996;28:652–5.

15. Elijovich F, Laffer CL, Amador E, et al. Regulation of plasma Endothelin by salt in salt-sensitive hypertension. Circulation. 2001;16(103):263–8.

16. Kurihara H, Yoshizumi M, Sugiyama T, et al. Transforming growth factor-beta stimulates the expression of endothelin mRNA by vascular endothelial cells. Biochem Biophys Res Commun. 1989;159(3):1435–40.

17. Roberts AB, Vodovotz Y, Roche NS, et al. Role of nitric oxide in antagonistic effects of transforming growth factor-beta and interleudin-1 beta on the beating rate of cultured cardiac myocytes. Mol Endocrinol. 1992;6(11):1921–30.

18. Sanderson N, Factor V, Nagy P, et al. Hepatic expression of mature transforming growth factor beta 1 in transgenic mice results in multiple tissue lesions. Proc Natl Acad Sci USA. 1995;28(92):2572–6.

19. Suthanthiran M, Li B, Song JO, et al. Transforming growth factor-beta 1 hyperexpression in African American hypertensives: A novel mediator of hypertension and/or target organ damage. Proc Natl Acad Sci USA. 2000;28(97):3479–84.

20. Campistol JM, Inigo P, Jiminez W, et al. Losartan decreases plasma levels of TGF-beta 1 in transplant patients with chronic allograft nephropathy. Kidney Int. 1999;56(2):714–19.

21. Sharma K, Eltayeb BO, McGowan TA, et al. Captopril-induced reduction of serum levels of transforming growth factor beta-1 correlated with long-term renoprotection in insulin-dependent diabetic patients. Am J Kidney Dis. 1999;34(5):818–23.

22. Fogo A, Breyer J. Smith M, and the AASK Pilot Study Investigators. Accuracy of the diagnosis of hypertensive nephrosclerosis in African Americans: a report from the African American Study of Kidney Disease Trial. Kidney Int. 1997;51:244–52.

23. Deitch JS, Hansen KJ, Craven TE, et al. Renal artery repair in African Americans. J Vasc Surg. 1997;26(465):472.

24. Hebert L, Kusek J, Greene T, and the Modification of Diet in Renal Disease Study Group. Effects of blood pressure control on progressive renal disease in blacks and whites. Hypertension. 1997;30:428–35.

25. National High Blood Pressure Education Program, 1995. Update of the working group reports on chronic renal failure and renovascular hypertension. Arch Intern Med 1996;156:1938–47.

26. Grimm RH, Grandits GA, Flack JM. Are black and white hypertensives really different? ABC Dig Urban Cardiol. 1997;4:10–16.

27. Agodoa LY, Appel L, Bakris GL, et al. Effect of ramipril vs amlodipine on renal outcomes in hypertensive nephrosclerosis. JAMA. 2001;285:2719–28.

28. The Heart Outcomes Prevention Study Investigators. Effects of an angiotensin converting enzyme inhibitor, ramipril, on cardiovascular events in high-risk patients. N Engl J Med. 2000;342:145–53.

29. Lewis EJ, Hunsicker LG, Clarke WR, et al. Renoprotective effect of the angiotensin receptor antagonist irbesartan in patients with nephropathy due to type 2 diabetes. N Engl J Med. 2001;345(12):851–60.

30. Brenner BM, Cooper ME, Zeeuw D De, et al. Effects of losartan on renal and cardiovascular outcomes in patients with type 2 diabetes and nephropathy. N Engl J Med. 2001; 3435(12):861–9.

31. Weir MR, Hall PS, Berhrens MT, Flack JM. Salt and blood pressure responses to calcium antagonism in hypertensive patients. Hypertension. 1995;25:1339–44.

32. ALLHAT Collaborative Research Group. Major cardiovascular events in hypertensive patients randomized to doxazosin vs chlorthalidone: the antihypertensive and lipid lowering treatment to prevent heart attack trail (ALLHAT). JAMA. 2000;283(15):1967–75.

33. Battistini B, Chailler P, D'Orleans Juste P, et al. Growth regulatory properties of endothelins. Peptides. 1993; 14(2):385–99.

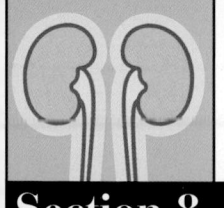

Chapter 43
Renal Physiology in Normal Pregnancy

Chris Baylis and John M Davison

INTRODUCTION

There are profound changes in renal function in normal pregnancy, which lead to marked alterations from the non-pregnant 'physiologic' norm. An appreciation and understanding of the mechanisms of these alterations are essential in order to recognize both normal and compromised pregnancies.

ANATOMY

The kidney volume increases by up to 70% in normal pregnancy because of increases in both vascular and interstitial fluid compartments. The most striking anatomical change is dilation of the calyces, renal pelvis, and ureter (more prominent on the right side), and by the third trimester about 80% of women show evidence of hydronephrosis[1] (Fig. 43.1). This may lead to collection errors in tests based on timed urine volume, which can be minimized by fluid loading. Another consequence of the ureteral dilation is urinary stasis, which predisposes pregnant women with asymptomatic bacteriuria, to develop ascending infection (acute symptomatic pyelonephritis). Very rarely the changes may be extreme and precipitate the 'overdistension syndrome,' hypertension or reversible acute renal failure[2].

SYSTEMIC HEMODYNAMICS

There are significant alterations in systemic hemodynamics in normal pregnancy. A plasma (and extracellular fluid) volume expansion occurs while red cell volume also increases leading to a large rise in blood volume which correlates with clinical outcome and birthweight. Interestingly, subsequent pregnancies tend to be more successful than the first, with bigger babies and larger plasma volume increases. Women with twins and triplets have proportionately greater increments and those with poorly growing fetuses, as in pre-eclampsia or where there is a history of poor reproductive performance, have correspondingly poor plasma volume responses. The rise in plasma volume (maximum increase ~1.25 L) takes place progressively up to 32–34 weeks, after which there is little further change. The plasma volume expansion has a hemodilutional effect, causing falls in hematocrit; the physiological 'anemia' of normal pregnancy[3].

Cardiac output is significantly increased by the 5th gestational week, initially caused by a 10–20% increase in heart rate (80–90 b.p.m.) with stroke volume enhanced by the 8th week.

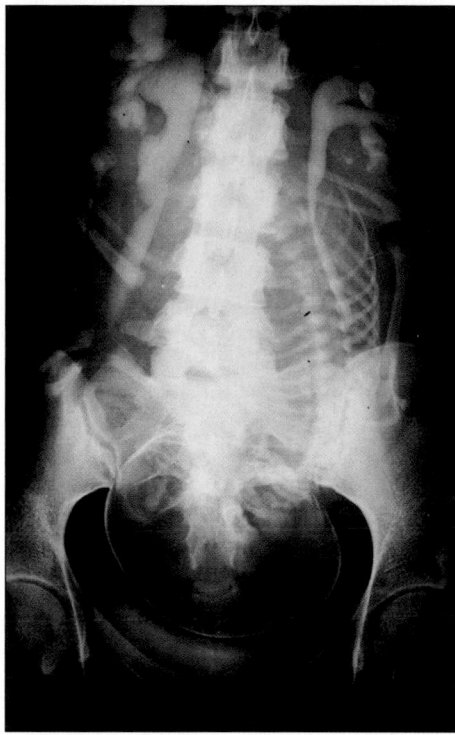

**Figure 43.1
Hydronephrosis in normal pregnancy.** Intravenous urogram at 36 weeks' gestation. Note bilateral hydronephrosis, more marked on the right side.

Maximal cardiac output increases of around 40–50% are well established by the 24th week. Left atrial and left ventricular end-diastolic dimensions increase, suggesting an associated increase in venous return. There is also a progressive increase in aortic valve orifice area. Despite the 40–50% rise in cardiac output, systemic blood pressure substantially *decreases* in normal pregnancy (see Fig 43.4 and Table 43.1 for representative values)[4]. The physiological fall in blood pressure results from a profound reduction in total peripheral vascular resistance of unknown cause, although the loss of responsiveness to vasoconstrictor agents (e.g., angiotensin II, arginine vasopressin, AVP) certainly contributes[5]. The combination of increased cardiac output and peripheral vasodilation means that organ blood flow increases in pregnancy, with the most dramatic changes occurring in the kidney and skin circulation throughout the gestation, and the uterus in the second part of the pregnancy[4]. In the third trimester the enlarged uterus compresses surrounding tissues and can influence hemodynamic measurements, so that attention should be paid to maternal posture. In the supine position, there is partial obstruction of the inferior vena cava and decreased venous return, reducing cardiac output and causing a fall in blood pressure, the

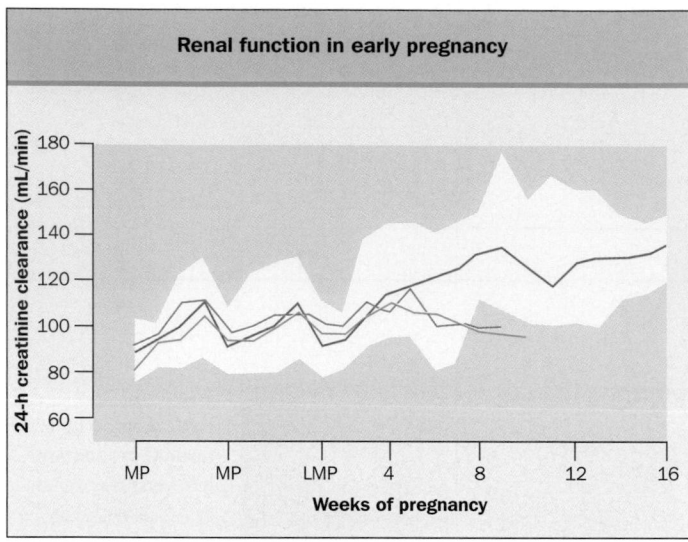

Figure 43.2 Renal function in early pregnancy. Changes in 24-h creatinine clearance measured weekly before conception and through to uncomplicated spontaneous abortion in two women. The solid line represents the mean and the stippled area shows the range for nine women with successful obstetric outcome. MP = menstrual period and LMP = last menstrual period. (Modified with permission from Sturgiss SN, Dunlop W, Davison JM[20–23].

Changes in some common indices during pregnancy		
	Nonpregnant	Pregnant
Hematocrit (vol/dL)	41	33
Plasma protein (g/dL)	7.0	6.0
Plasma osmolality (mosm/kg)	285	275
Plasma sodium (mmol/L)	140	135
Plasma creatinine (mg/dL (μmol/L))	0.8 (73)	0.5 (45)
Blood urea nitrogen (mg/dL)	12.7	9.3
Plasma urea (mmol/L)	4.5	3.3
pH units	7.40	7.44
Arterial P_{CO_2} (mmHg)	40	30
Plasma bicarbonate (mmol/L)	25	20
Plasma uric acid (mg/dL (μmol/L))	4.0 (240)	3.2 (190) early 4.3 (260) late
Systolic BP (mmHg)	115	105
Diastolic BP (mmHg)	70	60
Mean values (compiled from refs 7, 8, 15, 20, 23).		

Table 43.1 Changes in some common indices during pregnancy.

'supine hypotensive syndrome of pregnancy'. It is important to be aware of these postural effects when measuring blood pressure in late pregnant women[4].

RENAL HEMODYNAMICS

There are striking changes in renal hemodynamics in normal pregnancy with a rise in glomerular filtration rate (GFR) and consequent fall in serum creatinine detectable very early[6]. The creatinine clearance increases ~25% by 4 weeks after the last menstrual period and a robust early rise in GFR is invariably associated with a good obstetrical outcome (Fig. 43.2). Longitudinal studies in normal pregnant women show that GFR (measured by inulin or 24-h creatinine clearance) increases to a maximum of ~50% by mid-pregnancy, which is maintained until the last few weeks of the pregnancy when values begin to fall but remain above the nonpregnant level (Figs 43.2 and 43.4). These marked increases in GFR mean that serum creatinine falls to ~ 0.4–0.5 mg/dL (36–45 μmol/L) and values considered normal for nonpregnant conditions of 0.7–0.8 mg/dL (63–72 μmol/L) are a significant cause for concern in normal pregnancy (Table 43.1). The rise in renal plasma flow (RPF) of ~70% is slightly more pronounced than the increase in GFR (Fig. 43.3). Since the rise in RPF exceeds that of GFR in the first part of pregnancy, the filtration fraction (FF) declines (see below). At the end of pregnancy the RPF falls proportionally more than the GFR; i.e., FF increases to the non-pregnant value[7, 8].

A similar pattern of renal hemodynamic change occurs during pregnancy in some animals, including the rat in which

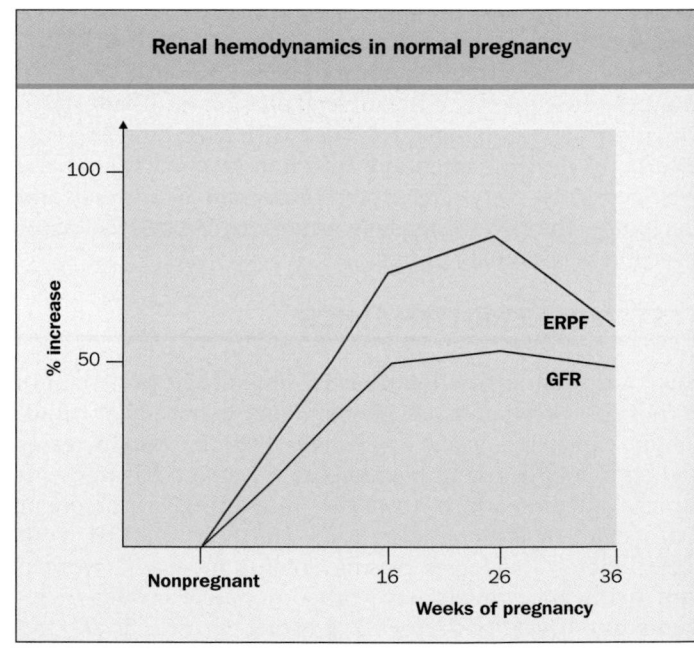

Figure 43.3 Renal hemodynamics in normal pregnancy. Relative changes in GFR and effective renal plasma flow (ERPF) during normal human pregnancy[7, 8, 15, 23].

GFR increases to a maximum of 30–40% above the virgin value by midterm, with a late return towards the non-pregnant value close to term (22 days). Glomerular micropuncture studies

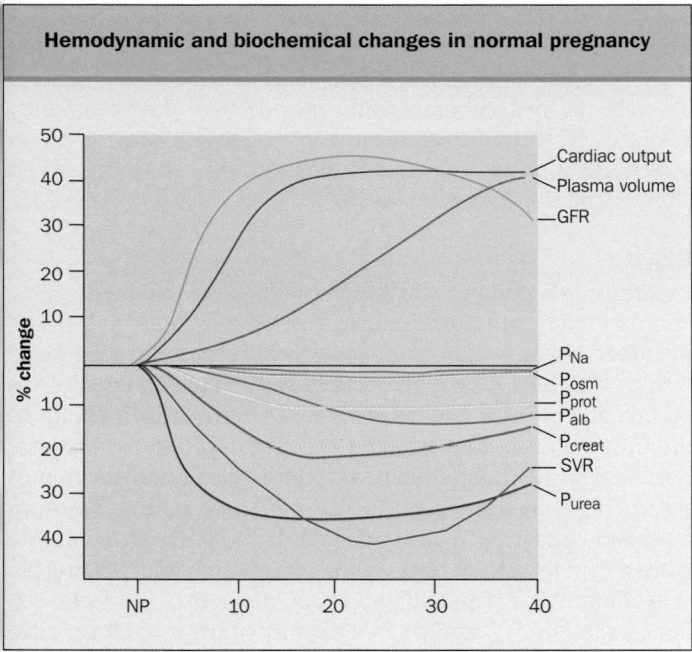

Hemodynamic and biochemical changes in normal pregnancy

Figure 43.4 Alterations induced by normal pregnancy. Increments and decrements in hemodynamic and biochemical parameters shown as % change from nonpregnant baseline. NP = Nonpregnant. 10–40 = weeks (gestation). SVR = systemic vascular resistance. GFR = glomerular filtration rate.

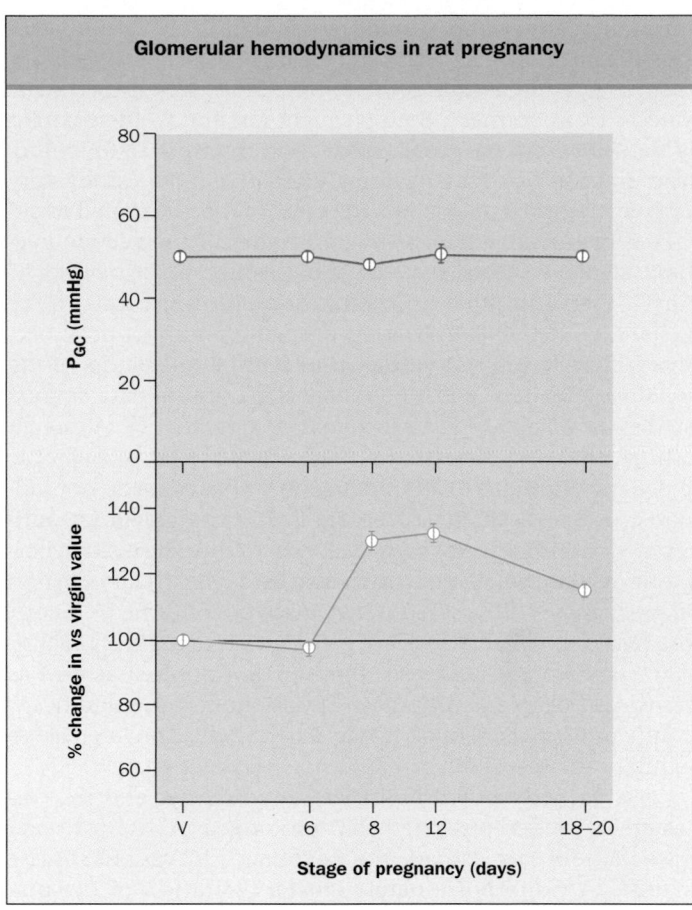

Glomerular hemodynamics in rat pregnancy

Figure 43.5 Glomerular hemodynamics in normal rat pregnancy. Summary of mean glomerular capillary blood pressure (P_{GC}; upper panel) and pre-glomerular arteriolar resistance (R_A; lower panel) in Munich Wistar rats in the virgin state and throughout normal pregnancy[9, 10].

have shown that the rise in GFR is paralleled by increases in single nephron GFR secondary to increased glomerular plasma flow[9]. Because the preglomerular and postglomerular resistance vessels dilate in parallel, glomerular plasma flow increases without a change in glomerular blood pressure. As shown in Figure 43.5, the glomerular blood pressure remains unchanged throughout the pregnancy despite serial, marked alterations in preglomerular vascular resistance. Similar conclusions have been reached using an indirect modeling approach in normal pregnant women[6, 8]. Whole kidney GFR, RPF, and plasma protein concentrations were measured and in addition, polydisperse neutral dextran was infused for determination of dextran sieving curves. This approach allows (with certain reasonable assumptions), modeling of glomerular hemodynamics in normal pregnant women. In pregnant women there is a fall in plasma protein concentration, which contributes slightly to the increased GFR. As in the rat, the majority of the gestational rise in GFR in normal women is due to increased RPF with no change in glomerular blood pressure. The constancy of glomerular blood pressure during sustained renal vasodilation has important implications for the long-term effects of pregnancy on renal function, discussed below.

The alterations in FF seen in pregnant women merit comment. It is often assumed that a change in FF reflects a change in glomerular blood pressure, but this is not always the case. GFR is determined by (a) a pressure which drives filtration at the glomerulus (the difference between transmural hydrostatic and colloid osmotic pressures); (b) water permeability of the glomerular wall; and (c) total glomerular capillary surface area available for filtration[7]. Glomerular wall water permeability is

very high, as is filtration pressure and thus filtration proceeds rapidly. In fact, in the normal rat, not all of the available filtration surface area is utilized so that filtration ceases (because transmural hydrostatic and colloid osmotic pressures equalize, thus the driving pressure is lost) before the end of the glomerulus. This state is known as filtration pressure equilibrium. When plasma flow increases (with no change in the other determinants of filtration) in an animal that remains at filtration pressure equilibrium, a proportional increase in GFR occurs with no change in FF. This is seen in the normal pregnant rat[9]. In contrast, FF falls during normal pregnancy in women as RPF is increasing[7]. Most likely this reflects the fact that humans are closer than rats to filtration pressure disequilibrium; a situation in which the entire glomerular capillary surface area available for filtration is used leaving a positive driving pressure at the end of the glomerulus. At filtration pressure disequilibrium, GFR becomes less dependent on plasma flow; thus an increase in plasma flow (with no change in the other determinants of filtration) leads to a disproportionately smaller rise in GFR, with a fall in FF (See ref. 11 for fuller explanation).

Despite the prolonged renal vasodilatation, the renal vasculature remains fully responsive to various stimuli during pregnancy. For example, in the rat the intrinsic renal autoregulatory ability remains intact[12] and the tubuloglomerular feedback component of renal autoregulation is reset to recognize the elevated GFR as normal[13]. Both pregnant rats and women exhibit a marked additional renal vasodilation in response to amino-acid infusion[14, 15], demonstrating substantial renal vasodilatory reserve in normal pregnancy. The cause of the gestational rise in GFR remains uncertain, although studies in the pseudopregnant rat have shown that the fetoplacental unit is *not* necessary[16], indicating that a maternal stimulus must initiate the gestational renal hemodynamic changes. A number of vasoactive factors have been evaluated as possible mediators of the renal vasodilation[9] and while there is no clinical data, animal studies have implicated a role for nitric oxide (NO)[17,18]. Although estrogen has been suggested as the hormone responsible for the pregnancy stimulus to NO production, animal data do not support this since estrogen levels are low in the gravid rat until term. A recent study has suggested a key role for the ovarian hormone, relaxin, which may signal increased renal NO production in pregnancy[19], although this remains to be confirmed. Of note, the renal vasodilatory signal of pregnancy is remarkably robust, since women with single kidneys (organ donors) as well as transplant recipients who have already undergone significant compensatory renal hypertrophy and vasodilation, are able to exhibit further increases in RPF and GFR in pregnancy[6, 20].

A large body of work, initiated by Brenner and his colleagues, has demonstrated that prolonged periods of renal vasodilation may damage the glomerulus in various disease states[21]. A disproportionately greater dilatation of the pre-glomerular resistance vessels leads to prolonged increase in glomerular blood pressure in a variety of progressive glomerulopathies, and the glomerular hypertension is believed to be the primary pathogenic stimulus[21]. As discussed above, normal pregnancy is also a state of chronic renal vasodilation; however, glomerular blood pressure remains normal. This may account for the findings that repetitive pregnancies in women and rats with normal renal function have no long-term, adverse effects on glomerular function or structure[22]. Pregnancy will increase the rate of loss of renal function in some women with underlying renal disease, but the available evidence suggests that this is not by a hemodynamically mediated action[6, 22].

RENAL TUBULAR FUNCTION IN PREGNANCY

There is an enormous plasma volume expansion in normal pregnancy and resultant small decrements in plasma concentration of many solutes (Fig. 43.4). Nevertheless, the large increase in GFR means that the filtered load of most plasma constituents will increase during pregnancy[6, 7]. Increments in excretion are seen for some substances but this is limited by increases in tubular reabsorption, preventing depletion. Often intake also increases, with net retention leading to positive balance for many of the key constituents. The renal handling of a number of solutes is altered in normal pregnancy.

Uric acid
Uric acid, an endpoint of purine metabolism, is freely filtered at the glomerulus, extensively reabsorbed in the proximal tubule with further downstream reabsorption and possibly

some active secretion, such that only ~10% of filtered load is excreted. Plasma uric acid concentration decreases during early pregnancy by ~25% (Table 43.1) which may reflect a decrease in net tubular reabsorption[23]. As the pregnancy advances fractional excretion of uric acid falls leading to an increasing plasma uric acid concentration, attaining levels close to the nonpregnant mean.

Glucose
Excretion of glucose increases soon after conception to approximately ten times above the nonpregnant value and remains high throughout pregnancy although the glycosuria is very variable[7]. The glycosuria is not related to changes in plasma glucose and reflects decreased tubular reabsorption. In the nonpregnant kidney there is usually complete reabsorption of glucose, mostly in the proximal tubule, where there is a very high capacity for glucose transport. This maximum transport capacity (T_{max}) is not usually reached until plasma glucose increases to values in excess of 200–300 mg/dL (11–17 mmol/L). The glucosuria of pregnancy is, however, due to a fall in T_{max} and/or the inability of the renal tubules to cope with the increased filtered glucose load and does not reflect a metabolic disturbance.

Water-soluble vitamins and amino acids
Nicotinic acid, ascorbic acid, and folic acid are all excreted in increased amounts during pregnancy[7], which emphasizes the need for adequate vitamin supplementation.

Urinary excretion of most amino acids increases in pregnancy, probably as a result of decreased tubular reabsorption[24]. There are three distinct patterns with glycine, histidine, threonine, serine, and alanine excretion increasing early and remaining elevated throughout pregnancy. Excretion of lysine, cystine, taurine, phenylalanine, valine, leucine, and tyrosine also increase in early pregnancy but later decline. Glutamic acid, methionine, and ornithine are excreted in slightly greater amounts than before pregnancy, isoleucine excretion is unchanged, and arginine excretion falls, consistent with falls in plasma arginine in normal pregnancy.

Acid–base balance
The generation of hydrogen ion increases in pregnancy due to an increased basal metabolism and greater food intake, despite which the blood concentration of hydrogen ions decreases, thus plasma pH increases (Table 43.1). This mild alkalemia is respiratory in origin, since pregnant women normally hyperventilate, leading to a primary fall in arterial P_{CO_2}, and secondary compensatory falls in plasma bicarbonate concentration (Table 43.1). A mild chronic respiratory alkalosis is a normal feature of pregnancy.

Potassium
Potassium excretion falls and there is a slow cumulative net potassium retention in pregnancy, which is distributed between the enlarging maternal tissues and the developing fetus. The fall in potassium excretion occurs in spite of the mild alkalosis and high aldosterone values of normal pregnancy and is at least partly due to the potent antimineralocorticoid action of progesterone[25] (see below).

Calcium

Calcium excretion increases two to three times during pregnancy due to the increased filtered load and despite some increase in tubular reabsorption. The increased calcium excretion in pregnancy predisposes to the formation of calcium stones but increased magnesium and citrate, acidic glycoproteins and nephrocalcin serve to inhibit calcium oxalate stone formation so that stone formation is not increased in normal pregnancy[26].

Protein

The increased total protein excretion in pregnancy should not be considered abnormal until it exceeds 500 mg in 24 h[6–8, 15]. This and the small increment in albumin excretion during the third trimester, continue into the puerperium, with truly non-pregnant levels not reattained until 5–6 months postdelivery. The gestational changes are related to alterations in glomerular perm- and charge-selectivity as well as tubular function.

Sodium

A massive, cumulative volume expansion occurs during pregnancy with an associated, gradual retention of sodium of ~900 mmol, distributed between the products of conception and maternal extracellular space. This positive sodium balance develops despite a ~30% increase in filtered load and reflects an increase in tubular reabsorption that allows net additional sodium retention of ~2–3 mmol/day[3]. Nevertheless, it is normal for sodium excretion to increase in pregnancy, reflecting the marked increase in sodium intake. Lithium clearance studies in women have indicated enhanced sodium reabsorption in the proximal tubule and distal nephron segments in late pregnancy, while animal studies have been contradictory[27]. The reason for the net renal sodium retention in pregnancy is not known and in fact sodium homeostasis in pregnancy represents a fascinating physiologic puzzle. As shown in Table 43.2 there are many factors operating to both increase and to decrease sodium excretion, and exactly how the normal balance of net retention is achieved remains a mystery. Several antinatriuretic systems are activated in normal pregnancy[28]. Renin, angiotensin and aldosterone levels are all markedly increased, and the renin–angiotensin system (RAS) can be appropriately regulated around these new 'set points', when changes occur in extracellular fluid volume. In addition to stimulating aldosterone release, physiologic levels of angiotensin II act directly on the proximal tubule to increase sodium reabsorption. However, a marked refractoriness develops to the vascular and possibly tubular actions of angiotensin II in normal pregnancy[28,29], which may nullify any net sodium retention by this mechanism. The high aldosterone levels of pregnancy will certainly promote renal sodium retention in the distal tubule and collecting duct. The very high levels of deoxycorticosterone (from 21-hydroxylation of progesterone) may also exert mineralocorticoid actions to promote sodium retention[27, 30]. Estrogens increase markedly during human pregnancy and may directly induce renal sodium retention and/or act indirectly by enhancing the conversion of progesterone to deoxycorticosterone[27, 30]. In addition to hormonal factors, the increased ureteral pressure and the fall in systemic blood pressure will both decrease sodium excretion.

Factors influencing sodium excretion during pregnancy		
Antinatriuretic	**Natriuretic**	**Uncertain or variable**
Aldosterone	GFR	Filtration fraction
Angiotensin II	Progesterone	Prostaglandins
Estrogen	ANP	AVP
Deoxycorticosterone	NO	Endothelin
Supine posture		Cortisol
Upright posture		Human placental lactogen (hPL)
Fall in blood pressure		Placental 'shunting'
Increased ureteral pressure		Kinins
		Sympathetic nerves

Table 43.2 Factors influencing sodium excretion during pregnancy.

The concentrations of several natriuretic agents also increase in pregnancy. Progesterone increases by 10–100 times and these levels exert a marked antimineralocorticoid action by competing with aldosterone for the mineralocorticoid receptor[27]. Plasma atrial natriuretic peptide (ANP) increases in pregnant women, although the increments are small relative to the marked intravascular volume expansion[31]. NO is also a potent natriuretic agent and NO production increases in the kidney of the normal rat during pregnancy[17, 18], although whether this also occurs in pregnant women is not known. In addition to circulating/ locally acting factors, the large increase in GFR leads to increased filtration of sodium (despite the small fall in plasma sodium concentration) which will also increase sodium excretion. Decreases in plasma albumin concentration and the increment in effective renal plasma flow during pregnancy will also enhance sodium excretion by inhibiting sodium reabsorption[9].

Despite the many conflicting stimuli, net sodium retention and marked plasma volume expansion is normal in pregnancy. In fact, there is a strong positive correlation between the maternal plasma volume expansion and a successful obstetric outcome[3, 32]. In the normal nonpregnant steady state plasma volume expansion and renal sodium retention cannot coexist. However, pregnancy is not a steady state, and the volume sensing and regulatory systems are dramatically readjusted throughout pregnancy to accommodate and maintain the volume expansion (see below).

OSMOREGULATION

There is a very early decrease in plasma osmolality by ~10 mosmol/kg below the nonpregnant norm, due to a reduction in plasma sodium and associated anions (Table 43.1). Whereas a fall in plasma osmolality of this magnitude would completely suppress antidiuretic hormone (AVP) release in nonpregnant individuals, in pregnancy the osmotic thresholds for AVP release (and thirst) are reduced to recognize the reduced plasma osmolality as normal[33]. Figure 43.6 demonstrates the resetting of the relationship between plasma AVP and plasma osmolality during normal pregnancy.

Pregnancy and Renal Disease

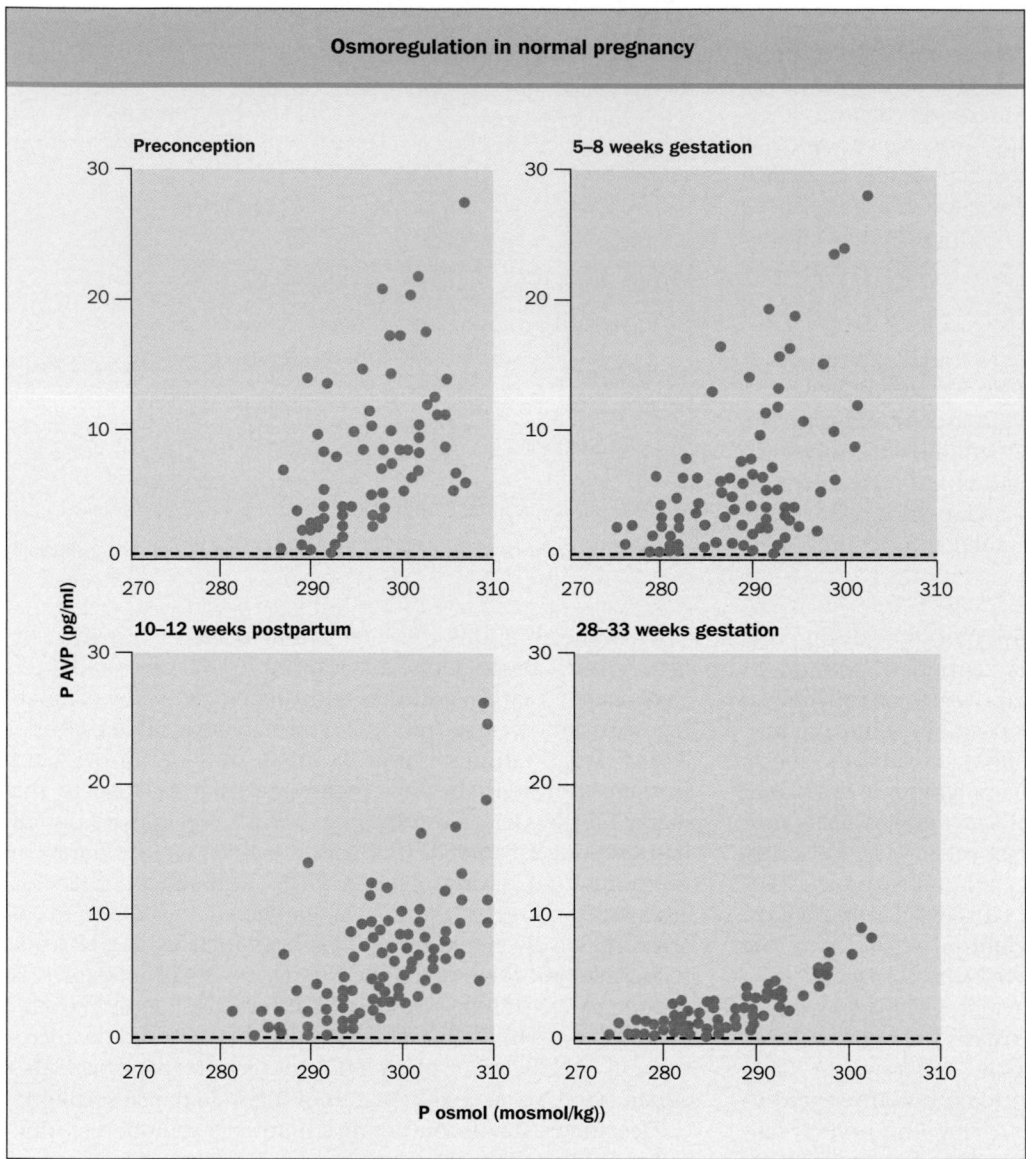

Osmoregulation in normal pregnancy

Figure 43.6 Osmoregulation in normal pregnancy. Relationship between plasma arginine vasopressin concentration (P AVP) and plasma osmolarity (POSMOL) during several 5% saline infusions in eight women before and during pregnancy. Each point represents an individual plasma measurement. There is a marked decrease in osmotic threshold for AVP release (abscissal intercept) during pregnancy. Values for the osmotic threshold for thirst (not shown) were always 2–5 mosmol/kg above AVP release thresholds and 10 mosmol/kg lower in pregnancy[7,31,33].

The placental hormone human chorionic gonadotrophin (which stimulates the release of ovarian relaxin[34]) may have a role in this reduction in the osmotic threshold for AVP release[33]. Plasma volume status is a separate, nonosmotic determinant of AVP release and this system is also reset, to recognize the massively expanded plasma volume as normal[33]. The metabolic clearance rate of AVP has increased four times by midpregnancy due to the release of cystine aminopeptidase (vasopressinase) from the placenta[33], so the rate of AVP production must also be accelerated. Despite these marked alterations, the urinary concentrating and diluting capacity remains good although there is a slight reduction in the maximum urine concentration in the second part of pregnancy[35].

VOLUME REGULATION

As discussed above, there is a continual sodium retention and cumulative volume expansion in pregnancy that reflects complex readjustments of the various volume regulatory systems. These readjustments also permit volume expansion without increases in blood pressure; in fact blood pressure falls

substantially as pregnancy proceeds (Table 43.1). What happens to volume perception/regulatory systems in pregnancy can be considered in terms of the 'effective circulating volume'; i.e., How the blood 'fills' the circulation[6,36,37]. The RAS is an antinatriuretic system activated by volume depletion, and the increase in plasma renin activity, angiotensin and aldosterone concentrations of normal pregnancy suggest an underfill or dehydration signal, despite the absolute increase in plasma volume. Schrier has suggested that the primary event in pregnancy is peripheral vasodilation that generates an underfill signal that then promotes renal sodium retention. In contrast, as discussed above, both osmotic and non-osmotic control of AVP release is reset in a manner indicating that the expanded volume of pregnancy is sensed as normal. The tubuloglomerular feedback system is suppressed by volume expansion in the nonpregnant state but is reset in pregnant rats to recognize the expanded volume and increased GFR as normal[13]. Plasma ANP increases slightly in late-pregnant women but this is unlikely to reflect a physiological response to volume expansion since even greater increases in ANP are seen in volume contracted, pre-eclamptic pregnancies[31].

REFERENCES

1. Brown MA. Urinary tract dilatation in pregnancy. Am J Obstet Gynecol. 1990;164:641–3.
2. Khauna N, Nguyn H. Reversible acute renal failure in association with bilateral ureteral obstruction and hydronephrosis in pregnancy. Am J Obstet Gynecol. 2001;184:239–40.
3. Brown M, Gallery EDM. Volume homeostasis in normal pregnancy and preeclampsia: physiology and clinical implications. Baillières Clin Obstet Gynaecol. 1994:8:287–310.
4. De Sweit M. The cardiovascular system. In: Chamberlain G, Broughton Pipkin F, eds. Clinical physiology in obstetrics, 3rd edn. Oxford: Blackwell Science; 1998:33–70.
5. Magness RR, Gant NF. Normal vascular adaptations in pregnancy. Potential clues for understanding pregnancy induced hypertension. In: Walker JJ, Gant NF, eds. Hypertension in pregnancy. London: Chapman & Hall Medical; 1997:5–26.
6. Lindheimer MD, Davison JM, Katz AI. The kidney and hypertension in pregnancy: Twenty exciting years. Semin Nephrol. 2001;21:173–89.
7. Sturgiss SN, Dunlop W, Davison JM. Renal haemodynamics and tubular function in human pregnancy. Baillières Clin Obstet Gynaecol. 1994;8:209–34.
8. Roberts M, Lindheimer MD, Davison JM. Altered glomerular permselectivity to neutral dextran and heteroporous membrane modeling in human pregnancy. Am J Physiol. 1996;270:F338–43.
9. Baylis C. Glomerular filtration and volume regulation in gravid animal models. Baillière's Clin Obstet Gynaecol. 1994;8:235–64.
10. Deng A, Engels K, Baylis C. Increased nitric oxide production plays a critical role in the maternal blood pressure and glomerular hemodynamic adaptations to pregnancy in the rat. Kidney Int. 1996;50:1132–8.
11. Baylis C. Glomerular filtration dynamics. In: Lote CJ, ed. Advances in renal physiology. London: Croom Helm; 1986: 33–83.
12. Reckelhoff JF, Yokota S, Baylis C. Renal autoregulation in mid-term and late pregnant rats. Am J Obstet Gynecol. 1992; 166:1546–50.
13. Baylis C, Blantz RC. Tubuloglomerular feedback activity in virgin and pregnant rats. Am J Physiol. 1985;249:F169–73.
14. Baylis C. Effect of amino acid infusion as an index of renal vasodilatory capacity in pregnant rats. Am J Physiol. 1988;254: F650–6.
15. Milne JEC, Lindheimer MD, Davison JM. Glomerular heteroporous membrane modelling in third trimester and post-partum before and during amino acid infusion. Am J Physiol. 2002; 282:F170–5.
16. Baylis C. Glomerular ultrafiltration in the pseudopregnant rat. Am J Physiol. 1982;243:F300–5.
17. Danielson LA, Conrad KP. Nitric oxide mediates renal vasodilation and hyperfiltration during pregnancy in chronically instrumented, conscious rats. J Clin Invest. 1995;96:482–90.
18. Baylis C, Engels K. Adverse interactions between pregnancy and a new model of systemic hypertension produced by chronic blockade of EDRF in the rat. Clin Exp Hypertens. 1992;B11:117–29.
19. Danielson LA, Sherwood OD, Conrad KP. Relaxin is a potent renal vasodilator in conscious rats. J Clin Invest. 1999;103:525–33.
20. Davison JM. Towards longterm graft survival in renal transplantation: pregnancy. Nephrol Dial Transpl. 1995;10(Suppl 1):85–9.
21. Brenner BM. Nephron adaptation to renal injury or ablation. Am J Physiol. 1985;249:F324–37.
22. Baylis C. Glomerular filtration rate (GFR) in normal and abnormal pregnancies. Semin Nephrol. 1999;9:133–9.
23. Dunlop W, Davison JM. The effect of normal pregnancy upon the renal handling of uric acid. Br J Obstet Gynaecol. 1977;84:13–21.
24. Hytten FE, Cheyne GA. The aminoaciduria of pregnancy. J Obstet Gynaecol Br Commonw. 1972;79:424–32.
25. Lindheimer MD, Richardson DA, Ehrlich EN, Katz AI. Potassium homeostasis in pregnancy. J Reprod Med. 1987;32:517–20.
26. Butler EL, Cox SM, Eberts EG, Cunningham FG. Symptomatic nephrolithiasis complicating pregnancy. Obstet Gynecol. 2000;96:753–6.
27. Atherton JC, Bielinska A, Davison JM, et al. Sodium and water reabsorption in the proximal and distal nephron in conscious pregnant rats and third trimester women. J Physiol. 1988; 396:457–70.
28. August P, Lindheimer MD. Pathophysiology of preeclampsia. In: Laragh JH, Brenner BM, eds. Hypertension: pathophysiology, diagnosis and management, 2nd edn. New York: Raven Press; 1995:2407–26.
29. Brown MA, Broughton-Pipkin F, Symonds EM. The effects of intravenous angiotensin II upon blood pressure and sodium and urate excretion in human pregnancy. J Hypertens. 1988;6: 457–64.
30. MacDonald PC, Cutter S, MacDonald SC, et al. Regulation of extra-adrenal steroid 21hydroxylase activity: increased conversion of plasma progesterone during estrogen treatment of women pregnant with a dead fetus. J Clin Invest. 1982;69:469–74.
31. Irons DW, Baylis PH, Davison JM. Atrial natriuretic peptide in preeclampsia: metabolic clearance, sodium excretion and renal hemodynamics. Am J Physiol. 1997;273:F483–7.
32. Chesley LC, Lindheimer MD. Renal hemodynamics and intravascular volume in normal and hypertensive pregnancy. In: Rubin PC, ed. Hypertension: hypertension in pregnancy. Amsterdam: Elsevier; 1988:10–38.
33. Lindheimer MD, Davison JM. Osmoregulation, the secretion of arginine vasopressin and its metabolism during pregnancy (mini-review). Eur J Endocrinol. 1995;132:133–43.
34. Randeva HS, Jackson A, Karteris E, Hillhouse EW. hCG production and activity during pregnancy. Fetal Mater Med Rev. 2001;12:191–208.
35. Gallery EDM, Gyory AZ. Urinary concentration, white cell excretion and acid–base status in normal pregnancy: alterations in pregnancy-associated hypertension. Am J Obstet Gynecol. 1979;135: 27–36.
36. Schrier RW. Pathogenesis of sodium and water retention in high-output and low-output cardiac failure, nephrotic syndrome, cirrhosis and pregnancy. Part 11. N Engl J Med. 1988;319:1127–34.
37. Durr JA, Lindheimer MD. Control of volume and body tonicity. In: Lindheimer MD, Roberts JM, Cunningham FG, eds. Chesley's hypertensive disorders in pregnancy, 2nd edn. Stamford CT: Appleton & Lange; 1999:103–66.

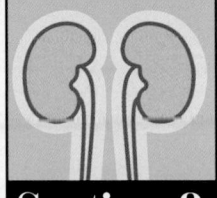

Chapter 44

Complications in the Normal Pregnancy

Mark A Brown and Lucy Bowyer

URINALYSIS

Pregnancy is the first occasion that most young women will have a urine microscopy and urinalysis. For this reason, a small percentage of pregnant women are found to have microscopic hematuria, proteinuria, or pyuria. The approach to each of these abnormalities is discussed below.

Hematuria

Definition
Hematuria in pregnancy is generally microscopic. There are very few studies defining the upper limit of normal red blood cell (RBC) excretion in pregnancy, but it appears that > 2500 RBC/mL urine is abnormal, as in nonpregnant women[1].

Epidemiology and etiology
Microscopic hematuria is common, detected at some stage during pregnancy in about 15–25% of women[2], and most of these cases are found before 30 weeks' gestation. In our clinic only 60% of those detected had persistent microscopic hematuria, mostly dysmorphic, and none had significant abnormalities on renal ultrasound or evidence of impaired renal function or connective tissue disease. Haematuria disappears in about three of four cases after delivery but hematuria secondary to glomerulonephritis persists through pregnancy, and can be further investigated postpartum. This group comprises about 6% of our antenatal population and reflects the utility of antenatal screening with urinalysis to detect underlying renal disorders. It is probable, although not well documented, that glomerulonephritis and pre-eclampsia are the most common causes of dysmorphic microscopic hematuria during pregnancy. Isomorphic hematuria is more likely to be due to bladder infection or bladder compression by the fetal head.

Macroscopic hematuria in pregnancy is most commonly the result of vaginal bleeding or urinary tract infection. Other less common causes include renal calculi, renal arteriovenous malformations, polycystic kidneys, placenta previa, and, rarely, both bladder and kidney neoplasms.

One retrospective study suggests that haematuria is associated with increased risks of pre-eclampsia, pregnancy-induced hypertension, and preterm labor[2], but we have not found this to be the case.

Differential diagnosis
The pregnant woman presenting with microscopic hematuria should be investigated first by urine culture to exclude infection. If there is no proteinuria, and blood pressure and serum creatinine are normal, further investigations can be safely delayed until postpartum review (usually about 3 months) when microscopy to determine RBC morphology, antinuclear antibody testing, and renal ultrasound can be performed. Intravenous urography (IVU) or computerized tomography (CT) scanning are preferable but are often not possible due to potential adverse effects of contrast in breast-feeding women.

When significant numbers of dysmorphic RBCs are present during pregnancy and blood pressure is normal, glomerulonephritis is the likely diagnosis, most commonly thin basement membrane disease and IgA nephropathy.

If hematuria is associated with renal angle pain or renal colic, ultrasound will exclude the presence of stone in only two-thirds of pregnant women with calculi but it will demonstrate other abnormalities such as polycystic kidneys and neoplasms.

In cases where isomorphic microscopic hematuria persists, we do not recommend cystoscopy during pregnancy. Such hematuria often disappears spontaneously after pregnancy and the likelihood of uroepithelial tumors is very low in this age group.

Treatment
The treatment of urinary infection and calculi is discussed elsewhere in this chapter. There is no specific treatment for glomerulonephritis during the pregnancy, provided renal function is normal and nephrotic syndrome is absent. In cases where renal function deteriorates, immunosuppression may be necessary depending upon the type of glomerulonephritis.

Proteinuria

The development of significant proteinuria in pregnancy warrants investigation and will most often be associated with pre-eclampsia.

Definition
Proteinuria is most commonly detected in pregnancy by dipstick urinalysis, but this method is notoriously unreliable with a significant proportion of false positives and false negatives. Dipstick is generally reliable for confirming either the absence of proteinuria or else the presence of true proteinuria (when dipstick readings are 3+ (>3 g/L) or 4+ (>20 g/L)). At intermediate levels, false-positive rates are as high as 50%[3]. Detection may be improved using an automated urinalysis device (Fig. 44.1), thereby reducing observer error[3].

Pregnancy and Renal Disease

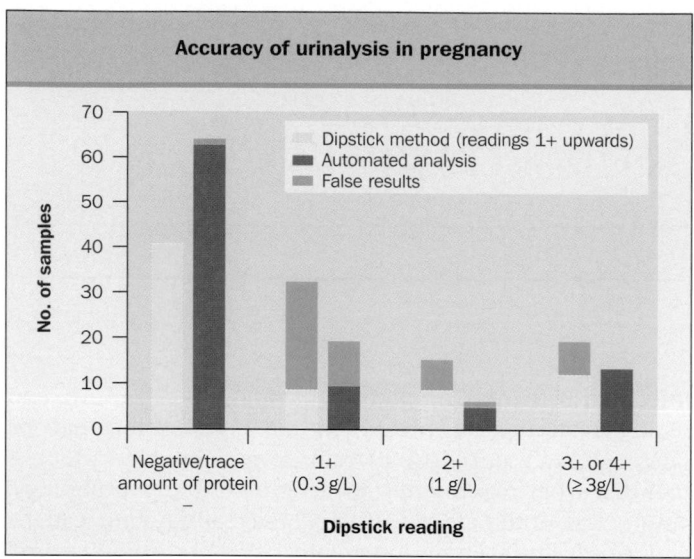

Figure 44.1 Accuracy of urinalysis in pregnancy. Urinalysis by the routine dipstick method and an automated method are compared with formal laboratory assay. The number of false results at three levels of proteinuria are indicated. (Adapted with permission from Brown and Buddle[6].

Proteinuria in pregnancy is generally defined as the excretion of >300 mg total protein per 24 h, though over 95% of pregnant women excrete less than 200 mg per day[4].

The 24-h urine collection remains the gold standard for quantitation, but is often impractical when a quick answer is required, as in pre-eclampsia. A reliable alternative is the protein to creatinine ratio[3]; a ratio >30 mg protein:mmol creatinine (~0.3 mg:mg) correlates well with protein excretion of >300 mg/24 h.

The 24-h urinary albumin excretion is similar in nonpregnant and normal pregnant women, with more than 20 mg/day being considered abnormal[5].

Differential diagnosis

Proteinuria arising *de novo* in pregnancy should be quantitated and further investigated according to the clinical situation. The course of pregnancy in women with proteinuria present before pregnancy is discussed in Chapter 45.

Persistent *de novo* proteinuria in pregnancy is most commonly associated with pre-eclampsia; this arises in the second half of pregnancy and will generally occur after the development of hypertension but proteinuria occasionally predates all other signs of pre-eclampsia. The presence of significant proteinuria in pre-eclampsia is an important finding as it is associated with increased maternal and fetal complication rates[6]. In the absence of urinary tract infection or pre-eclampsia, isolated proteinuria in the pregnancy of an otherwise asymptomatic woman usually reflects new-onset renal disease such as a primary glomerulonephritis, or an associated disease such as lupus or diabetes mellitus; much less commonly, other secondary causes of glomerulonephritis may occur.

We limit investigation of isolated non-nephrotic proteinuria during pregnancy to a renal ultrasound and the measurement of serum creatinine, electrolytes, albumin, and antinuclear antibodies. Renal biopsy is not indicated. Where underlying

renal disease has been unmasked by pregnancy, appropriate investigations can usually be delayed until the postpartum period. The exceptions to this rule are women with nephrotic syndrome and/or renal insufficiency in whom fetal viability is not yet assured and the pregnancy needs to be continued (earlier than 26 weeks of gestation). In these patients full investigation should be undertaken quickly, usually including renal biopsy to determine whether specific treatment (e.g., corticosteroids) will be of potential benefit.

Natural history

Proteinuria occurring as a complication of pre-eclampsia invariably recovers in the postpartum period, although this may take several months. We have also observed a number of women with *de novo* non-nephrotic proteinuria during pregnancy in whom the proteinuria disappears completely within a few months after delivery. This is perhaps mediated through glomerular hemodynamic changes during pregnancy.

Treatment

Proteinuria associated with pre-eclampsia has no specific treatment, other than to treat the complications of pre-eclampsia and effect appropriately timed delivery. For women with nephrotic syndrome, there is an inverse correlation between serum albumin and birth weight; as a result immunosuppression may be required (depending upon renal histology) to diminish urine protein loss. Angiotensin-converting enzyme (ACE) inhibitors are contraindicated in pregnancy because of their unwanted effects on the fetus.

Intravenous albumin has little role in managing nephrotic syndrome during pregnancy unless there is progressive deterioration in renal function. The pregnant woman with nephrotic syndrome is at high risk of venous thrombosis and should receive prophylactic heparin.

Pyuria

Isolated pyuria will uncommonly reflect an underlying renal disorder but more usually will be a feature of normal pregnancy requiring no further follow-up than to be certain that it disappears within the first 3 months postpartum.

Renal biopsy in pregnancy

Renal biopsy can usually be performed in the conventional prone position up to 20 weeks of gestation; thereafter it is best undertaken with the woman sitting. The relative and absolute contraindications to biopsy do not differ from the nonpregnant state (see Chapter 6). Renal biopsy is rarely required in pregnancy, but can be undertaken at any stage of pregnancy if the clinical situation demands. It is not indicated with isolated microscopic hematuria or non-nephrotic proteinuria if renal function is preserved. The most common indication is for nephrotic syndrome, not caused by pre-eclampsia and presenting early in pregnancy, or progressive renal impairment with proteinuria which is not apparently due to pre-eclampsia. Packham and Fairley reported the largest series of renal biopsies in pregnancy[7], with a complication rate of only 4.5% from 111 biopsies performed between 1967 and 1987. Only 8% of these biopsies were done for impaired renal function, and 12% for nephrotic syndrome. The remainder were done for combinations of hematuria, proteinuria, and hypertension. Although a large number of cases of glomerulonephritis were discovered from these biopsies, we believe that biopsy can still be reserved in most cases until after delivery.

URINE INFECTION

Definitions

In *asymptomatic bacteriuria* (ASB), there is persistent colonization of the urinary tract by a single species of bacteria in the absence of specific symptoms. It is now well recognized that ASB can lead to serious complications in pregnancy and that there is a definite cost benefit from screening[8,9].

The gold standard for diagnosis[10] is detection of $> 10^5$ organisms/mL, without epithelial cells, in a midstream urine specimen on two or more occasions, or from a single suprapubic aspiration. In practice, such bacteriuria is usually detected by routine urine culture early in pregnancy.

As many as 1–2% of pregnancies are complicated by *acute bacterial cystitis*, defined as an acute bladder infection by bacteria accompanied by symptoms such as frequency, dysuria, or strangury. While 10^5 organisms/mL define ASB, as few as 10^2 organisms/mL are sufficient to diagnose cystitis if accompanied by pyuria and characteristic symptoms.

In *acute pyelonephritis* there is urine infection in association with parenchymal renal infection, usually diagnosed on the clinical grounds of fever and loin pain.

Epidemiology

ASB affects 2–10% of all pregnant women. The prevalence is higher in women from lower socioeconomic groups and increases with age, parity, coexistent genital tract infection, and sickle cell trait. ASB is also more common in women with urinary tract abnormalities such as reflux nephropathy and neurogenic bladder, in diabetics, and in women who have had several previous urinary tract infections. The highest risk of infection is thought to be from the 9th to the 17th week of gestation, although this may simply reflect the stage at which routine screening usually takes place.

The overall incidence of acute pyelonephritis in pregnancy is approximately 1%, but among women with ASB it is much higher, up to 30%. It is thought that about 70% of women who develop acute pyelonephritis have preceding covert bacteriuria, but this is difficult to prove. With treatment of ASB it has been estimated that the incidence of pyelonephritis would be reduced by over 80%[8].

Pathogenesis

Certain women appear more prone to colonization of the urinary tract than others. Nonexpressors of the antibody to the O antigen of *Escherichia coli* are more susceptible. ASB will often predate pregnancy, some women being chronically colonized. Pregnancy is a state of relative urinary tract stasis; the calyces, pelves, and ureters dilate, particularly on the right, and there may be an element of vesicoureteral reflux because of anatomic displacement of the ureters. These factors contribute to ASB in pregnant women being at least twice as common as in nonpregnant women.

Organisms most commonly responsible for asymptomatic bacteriuria
Escherichia coli (> 70% of infections)
Klebsiella spp.
Proteus spp. (particularly in diabetic or urinary tract obstruction)
Enterococci
Staphylococci, especially *S. saprophyticus*
Pseudomonas
Streptococci

Table 44.1 Organisms most commonly responsible for asymptomatic bacteriuria.

The most common mechanism of infection is via the urethra from perineal bacteria (Table 44.1). Some strains of *E. coli* are particularly virulent and are associated with both ASB and pyelonephritis. They possess P fimbriae, which enable the bacteria to attach themselves to the uroepithelial cells with pili, allowing them to ascend the urinary tract from the perineum.

Clinical manifestations

Asymptomatic bacteriuria

A meta-analysis indicates that untreated ASB during pregnancy significantly increases rates of low birth weight and preterm delivery[11]; however, it is still unclear whether ASB is an independent risk factor for low birth weight or whether its association with low socioeconomic status is the predictor for low birth weight. The mechanism by which urinary tract infection (UTI) may cause premature labor is not yet fully understood but it is likely that proinflammatory cytokines secreted in response to bacterial endotoxins initiate labor.

Screening for asymptomatic bacteriuria

Most maternity units operate a policy of screening all pregnant women on at least one occasion, whether it be by dipstick urinalysis for leukocytes/nitrites or by direct urine culture. Both dipstick and urine culture were cost-saving compared with no screening when the prevalence of ASB is 2–6%[9]. However, it is not cost-beneficial to screen by primary urine culture when compared with the dipstick method except in populations with a prevalence of ASB above 9%[9].

Pyelonephritis

Pyelonephritis most commonly presents between 20 and 28 weeks of gestation with malaise, fever, loin pain, and rigors. Not all women will have had lower urinary tract symptoms, and pyelonephritis can also manifest in pregnancy as acute abdominal pain or be detected only after presentation with premature labor. Pyelonephritis is also more common in pregnant women with urologic abnormalities or diabetes, and more often affects the right kidney, probably because the ureter is generally more dilated on that side.

The diagnosis is usually made on clinical grounds. Definitive diagnosis requires positive urine culture, but this may take about 2 days and treatment should not be delayed. *E. coli* is the most common infecting organism (found in > 85% of cultures).

Pregnancy and Renal Disease

Bacteremia is a common and usually transient complication of pyelonephritis. However occasionally women become septicemic and may develop endotoxic shock, with sequelae including respiratory failure, disseminated intravascular coagulation (DIC) and acute renal failure (ARF). Pyonephrosis and perinephric abscess are rare complications but should be suspected when treatment fails.

Without treatment, the complications of pyelonephritis during pregnancy can be very severe. In the preantibiotic era, maternal mortality was 3–4%; death from pyelonephritis is now rare in developed countries but it still occurs.

Treatment
Asymptomatic bacteriuria

Antibiotic treatment of ASB significantly reduces the incidence of pyelonephritis in pregnancy. A systematic review also suggests treatment results in a significant reduction in the risk of preterm delivery[8].

In choosing treatment, the safety of the antibiotic in pregnancy must be taken into account (Table 44.2). In most cases treatment with amoxicillin/clavulanic acid, nitrofurantoin or a second-generation cephalosporin such as cefaclor is first line treatment. It was previously held that a longer course of therapy for ASB is required in pregnant women than in nonpregnant women but there is currently no good evidence as to whether a single dose or 4–7 day treatment course is necessary[12]. Some authorities now allow for a 3-day rather than 7-day course of antibiotics[13].

Without treatment, ASB will persist in 80% of women, and even with treatment 20% will still have ASB. Those with persistent colonization are difficult to treat, eradication being achieved in only 40% after a second course of antibiotics. The incidence of pyelonephritis following effective treatment is reduced from about 30% to 3%, comparing favorably with a 1% prevalence of pyelonephritis for the overall pregnant population.

Cystitis

Treatment of cystitis in the first instance should be for 7–10 days with an appropriate antibiotic (Table 44.2). It is very important, as for ASB, to obtain a follow-up urine culture to be certain infection has been eradicated.

Pyelonephritis

It is usual practice to admit pregnant women with pyelonephritis to hospital, although there has been a trial of successful outpatient management for milder cases[14]. Treatment may occasionally require resuscitation with intravenous fluids, but usually a short course of intravenous antibiotics followed by oral antibiotics, once the woman is afebrile, is adequate therapy.

It is desirable to choose an antibiotic that produces a high blood level that will concentrate in the renal parenchyma, most commonly a cephalosporin as first-line treatment. An aminoglycoside is a useful adjunct in more severe cases, used for 24–48 h while awaiting urine cultures, provided maternal renal function is satisfactory; the risk of fetal ototoxicity precludes its prolonged use and aminoglycosides are not recommended in the first trimester. The full duration

Safety of antibiotics commonly used to treat urine infection in pregnancy	
Category of drug	Antibiotic
A. Drugs taken by large numbers of pregnant women without any proven fetal harm	Amoxicillin, ampicillin
	Cefalexin, cephalothin
	Nalidixic acid
	Nitrofurantoin (care at term)
	Penicillins
B1. Drugs taken by a limited number of pregnant women without proven fetal harm; animal studies show no increase in fetal damage	Aztreonam
	Ceftazidime, cefotaxime, cefaclor
	Amoxicillin/clavulanic acid
	Floxacillin (flucloxacillin)
	Piperacillin
B2. As B1, but animal data is unavailable	Vancomycin
B3. As B1, but animal studies show an increase in fetal damage	Ciprofloxacin, norfloxacin, ofloxacin
	Imipenem, trimethoprim
C. Drugs whose pharmacologic effects are suspected of causing fetal harm	Sulfonamides
	Cotrimoxazole
	fusidic acid
D. Drugs which are proven to cause fetal harm	Tetracyclines
	Gentamicin & other aminoglycosides

Table 44.2 Safety of antibiotics commonly used to treat urine infection in pregnancy.

of treatment is generally at least 2 weeks and it is imperative to repeat urine culture a week after treatment to ensure eradication.

Renal ultrasound is generally not indicated during an initial infection, as urinary tract dilatation is likely to be present in any case and it is impossible to distinguish this from pathologic obstruction. However, if infection persists, ultrasound is indicated to help exclude pyonephrosis, perinephric abscess, and renal calculi. Ultrasound is safe in pregnancy and is preferred even though it is inferior to CT scanning for these purposes. If infection persists despite adequate antibiotic therapy and urinary tract dilatation is confirmed, percutaneous nephrostomy should be performed under ultrasound guidance; this is the only way to be certain urinary tract obstruction and/or pyonephrosis have been properly treated.

Finally, clinicians should remain alert for premature labor in the presence of pyelonephritis and institute appropriate treatment while aggressively treating the infection.

When more than two UTIs have occurred in pregnancy, prophylaxis is indicated with either nitrofurantoin 50 mg at night, or cefalexin 250 mg at night.

RENAL CALCULI

Epidemiology

Despite the fact that the physiologic state of pregnancy is an ideal environment for renal stone formation, the incidence of renal calculi remains similar in pregnant and nonpregnant

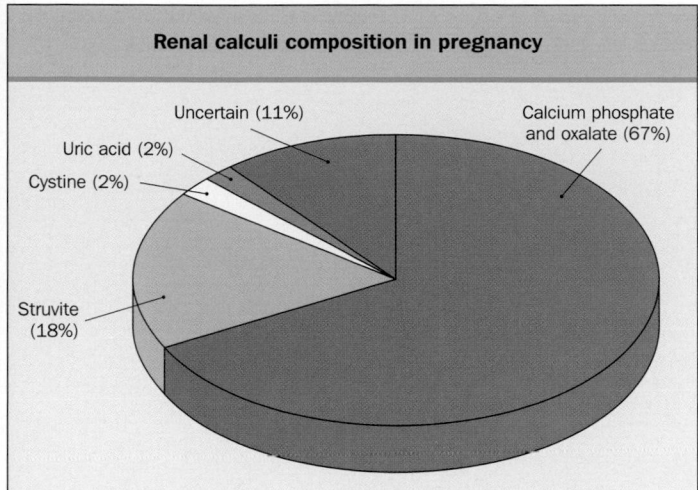

Figure 44.2 Composition of renal calculi in pregnancy.

women, in the range 0.03–1%. The incidence is higher in older women and those predisposed to dehydration.

Pathogenesis

The majority of stones are formed from calcium oxalate and calcium phosphate (Fig. 44.2). Struvite stones are the next most common, usually when the urinary tract is infected with organisms such as *Proteus* sp. Small proportions of renal stones are formed from uric acid or cystine.

Pregnancy is a physiologic state of relative urinary stasis as well as increased calcium and uric acid excretion; the fact that the incidence of renal calculi is not increased is probably because of the enhanced excretion of inhibitors of stone formation, such as magnesium, citrate, and the glycoprotein nephrocalcin.

Clinical manifestations

Renal colic is one of the commonest reasons for presentation with abdominal pain in the second and third trimester. However, clinical features of renal calculi may be more difficult to interpret because of the effects of pregnancy. Diffuse, poorly localized abdominal pain and lower urinary tract symptoms may occur and pregnant women with renal calculi are at greater risk of superimposed pyelonephritis. Fifty to eighty percent of stones will pass spontaneously during pregnancy, and 10–20% of women with calculi will have a concomitant UTI.

The diagnosis of renal calculi in pregnancy is made more difficult because of the accompanying physiologic hydronephrosis and the risks of radiation to the fetus if investigating the urinary tract. Ultrasound will detect hydronephrosis (usually as part of normal pregnancy) and will mostly detect calculi within the kidney, but it rarely finds ureteral stones. If symptoms persist and surgical intervention is being considered, a limited IVU is necessary. The risk of radiation to the fetus is well documented in the first trimester of pregnancy, but most renal colic presents in the second trimester beyond the risk period for fetal malformation secondary to radiation

and limited X-ray films can be performed. Total radiation dose received should be documented; it has been advised[15] that therapeutic abortion should be considered if dosage exceeds 5 cGy but a limited IVU (four films in total) will give an average dose of radiation to the fetus of around only 0.2 cGy. The pregnant woman should be given this information and the benefit of X-rays and subsequent therapy should be balanced against the potential harm to the fetus in each individual case.

The use of magnetic resonance imaging in the acute management of renal colic in pregnancy is not well documented.

Treatment

Initial management of renal calculi is conservative, with appropriate hydration, antiemetics, and analgesia. Calcium intake should not be limited in pregnancy. However, women in whom calcium oxalate stones form persistently can limit foods high in oxalate (such as spinach, rhubarb, and chocolate). Urine should always be cultured and appropriate antibiotics administered when a UTI is suspected.

Quantitation of urine calcium and urate is not necessary in pregnancy since specific pharmacological agents to modify excretion (including thiazides and allopurinol) are contraindicated. Investigation can be completed postpartum.

Urine output should be monitored, and renal function assessed. Surgical intervention is considered when stones cause persistent obstruction, deteriorating renal function, intractable pain or infection, and premature labor unresponsive to other treatment. Cystoscopy with ureteral stenting may be required in pregnancy, and there have been reports of ureteroscopic removal of stones[16,17]. Where pyelonephritis is persistent or renal function worsening, percutaneous nephrostomy may be necessary either as a temporary measure or for removal of the stone.

Lithotripsy is generally contraindicated during pregnancy because of the adverse effect of the shock waves upon the fetus; however, several centers are now using ureteroscopic laser lithotripsy in pregnancy[18]. Extracorporeal shockwave lithotripsy has been reported as an inadvertent procedure in six women in the first month of pregnancy, all of whom subsequently delivered normal infants[19].

Postpartum follow-up is important. A plain abdominal X-ray should be taken in the immediate postpartum period in women in whom it is suspected the stone has passed, followed by an IVU or renal CT scan 3 months later. This delay is necessary to eliminate confusion in interpreting the findings as calyceal and ureteral dilatation may persist that long after delivery. Women planning a further pregnancy should be assessed for idiopathic hypercalciuria or other causes of renal calculi after a minimum of 3 months postpartum.

HYPERTENSION IN PREGNANCY

Definitions

Hypertension during pregnancy can be considered as:
- arising *de novo* during pregnancy;
- already present prior to pregnancy;
- pre-eclampsia superimposed on chronic hypertension.

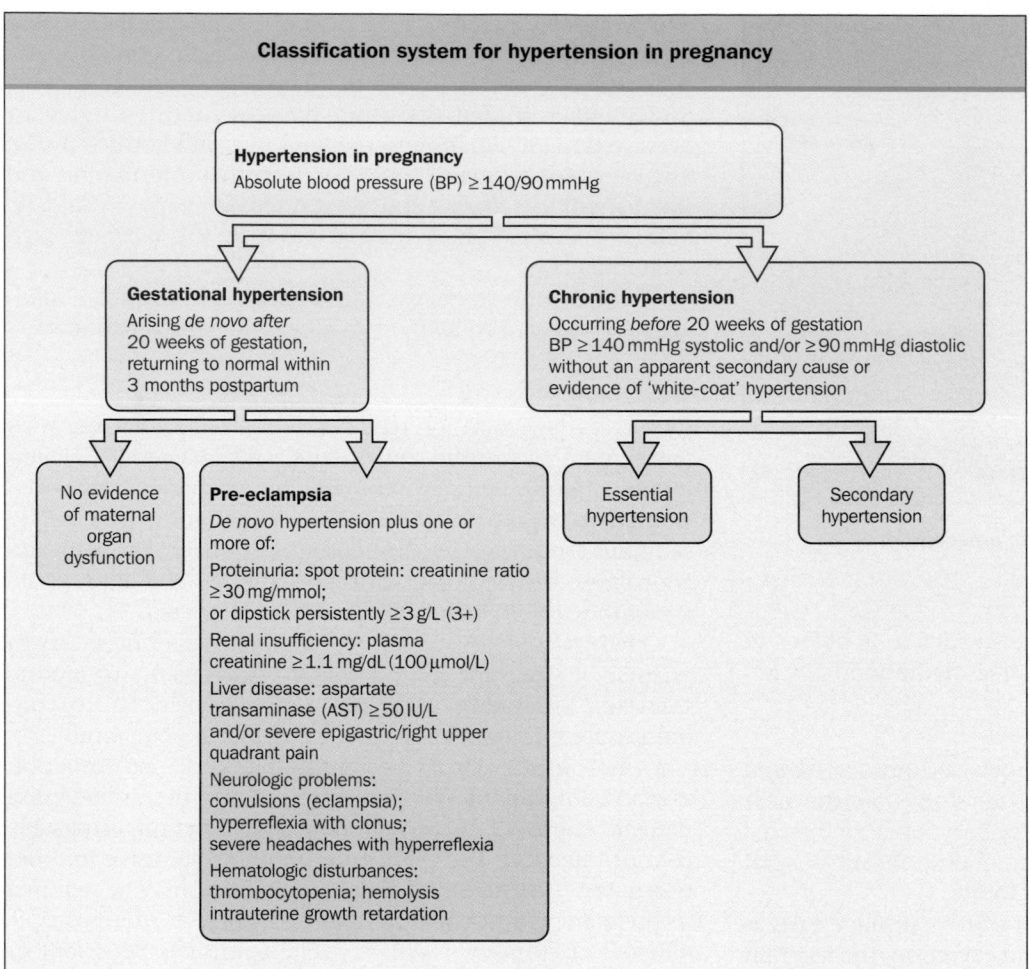

Classification system for hypertension in pregnancy

Figure 44.3 Classification system for hypertension in pregnancy.

Figure 44.3 gives a classification for hypertension in pregnancy.

Hypertension in pregnancy

Hypertension in pregnancy is defined as an absolute blood pressure >140/90 mmHg. It was previously considered that a rise in systolic blood pressure >25 mmHg and/or diastolic blood pressure >15 mmHg from preconception or first-trimester blood pressure values also constituted hypertension but this is no longer held to be correct[20].

The development of elevated blood pressure during pregnancy without evidence of maternal organ dysfunction is known as gestational hypertension. Pre-eclampsia is also hypertension developing in the second half of pregnancy, but this more serious disorder also includes accompanying evidence of maternal renal, cerebral, hepatic, or clotting abnormalities, or fetal growth restriction.

Pre-eclampsia

The traditional diagnosis of pre-eclampsia has been hypertension with proteinuria and edema developing after 20 weeks' gestation. However, edema accompanies two-thirds of both normal and pre-eclamptic pregnancies and is not a particularly useful sign. The detection of proteinuria in the past has also been quite unreliable, and insisting on the finding of proteinuria for this diagnosis ignores the protean manifestations of pre-eclampsia, discussed below. In practice, however, the majority of women with multisystem features of pre-eclampsia do have proteinuria.

Eclampsia

Eclampsia (convulsions) is now uncommon in developed countries, with a prevalence of around 0.3% of hypertensive pregnancies. In underdeveloped countries, eclampsia is much more common, with greater risks of maternal mortality and morbidity as well as perinatal mortality.

Epidemiology

Hypertension affects 10–12% of all pregnancies[21], and the distribution of causes in a population depends largely on the nature of the obstetric unit assessing that population; tertiary referral units will tend to have a higher proportion of severe pre-eclamptic cases. In general, essential hypertension comprises about 19%, secondary causes around 4%, pre-eclampsia 34%, and gestational hypertension the remainder of hypertensive disorders in pregnancy (Fig. 44.4). About one in four women with apparent essential hypertension early in pregnancy have 'white-coat' hypertension but until further data are gathered concerning the natural history of this disorder during pregnancy these women should be considered to carry the same pregnancy risks as those with confirmed essential hypertension.

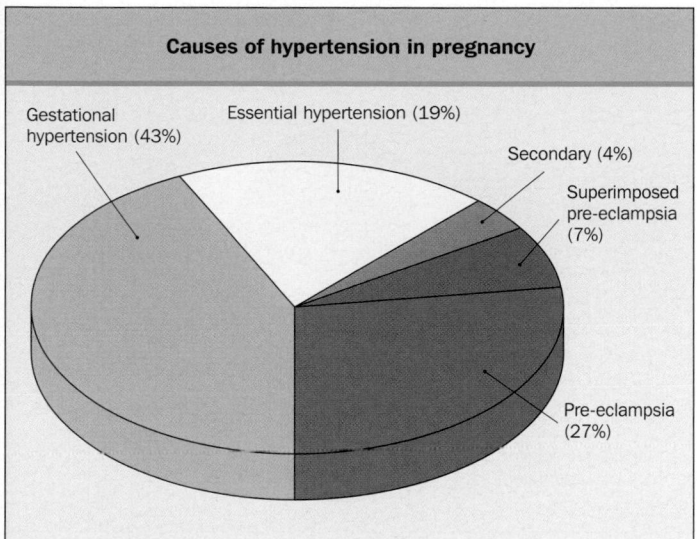

Figure 44.4 Causes of hypertension in pregnancy. (Adapted from Brown and Buddle[21].

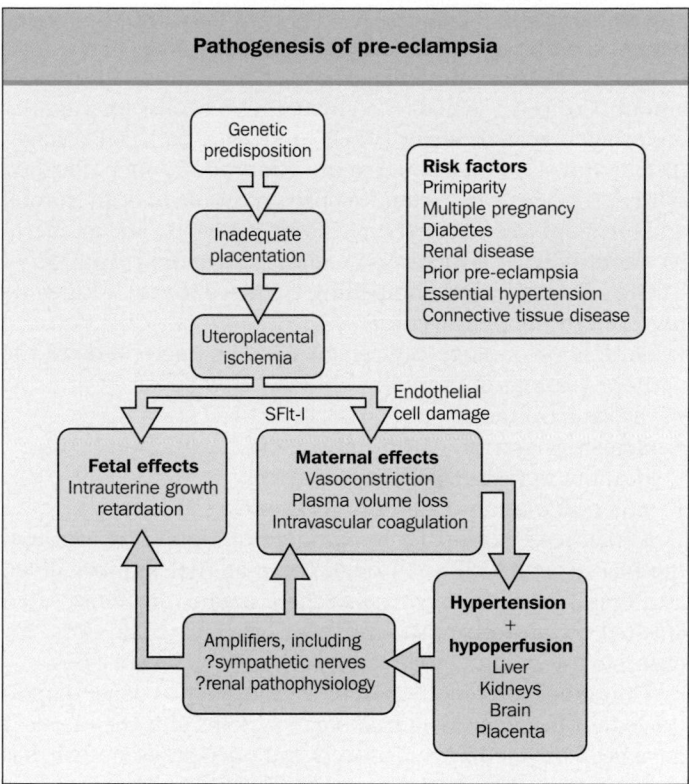

Figure 44.5 Proposed pathogenesis of pre-eclampsia. (Adapted from Brown MA. Pre-eclampsia: a case of nerves? Lancet. 1997; 349:297–8.)

PRE-ECLAMPSIA

Epidemiology

Pre-eclampsia does not follow any recognized racial patterns and there has been no specific human leukocyte antigens (HLA) consistently associated with this disorder. About two-thirds of cases occur in primigravidas, and pre-eclampsia is more common when this has occurred in a previous pregnancy, when there is a maternal or sororal family history of this disorder, and during multiple pregnancies. A recent study found that women who were the product of a pre-eclamptic pregnancy had about a three-fold increased risk of having a pre-eclamptic pregnancy themselves while men who were the product of a pre-eclamptic pregnancy had a two-fold increased chance of having a child who was the product of a pre-eclamptic pregnancy[22]. This possibly supports a recessive gene hypothesis. An intriguing observation is the reduced risk of pre-eclampsia in subsequent pregnancies but a return to the risks of the first pregnancy in women who have a new partner for subsequent pregnancies. This observation, combined with an increased likelihood of pre-eclampsia in women who have used barrier methods of contraception, raises the possibility of an impaired immunologic response to paternal antigens in such pregnancies. A similar explanation may lie behind the observation that the longer the sexual cohabitation prior to pregnancy, the lower the likelihood of pre-eclampsia.

Diabetes, essential hypertension, multiple pregnancy, connective tissue disorders, obesity, early pregnancy systolic blood pressure > 130 mmHg and Black race all increase the likelihood of developing pre-eclampsia. Smoking appears to reduce the likelihood of developing pre-eclampsia but babies of smokers tend to be small for gestational age. Activated protein C resistance (factor V (Leiden) mutation) and other inherited thrombophilias as well as hyperhomocysteinemia were thought to increase the risk for pre-eclampsia, but these findings have not been observed consistently. Underlying renal disease also increases that risk when there is pre-existing renal impairment, hypertension, or proteinuria. There is, however, no clear evidence that the risk is increased when microscopic hematuria is the only clinical manifestation of renal disease.

Pathogenesis

There appears little doubt that the placenta is the culprit in causing pre-eclampsia, with other maternal organs such as the kidney perhaps being amplifiers of the disease process (Fig. 44.5). In normal pregnancy, trophoblast cells invade the muscular coat of the spiral arterioles, converting them into capacitance vessels capable of carrying a greater blood flow through the placenta and, by minimizing their muscular coat, reducing their capacity for vasoconstriction. This process is impaired or lacking in pre-eclamptic women. Studies have shown that cytotrophoblasts normally upregulate their expression of receptors for cell adhesion molecules of the integrin, cadherin, and immunoglobulin superfamilies. This allows these cells to recognize vascular cells more readily, presumably enhancing the process of trophoblast invasion. In pre-eclampsia, there is a failure of such cytotrophoblasts to properly express receptors for these antigens[23]. Other studies have demonstrated placental production of cytokines such as tumor necrosis factor and interleukin-1, particularly in the presence of hypoxia. This may be determined by a candidate region on chromosome 4 but more recent interest has been focused on chromosome 2 as a candidate site for a genetic predisposition to pre-eclampsia[24]. Studies of candidate genes such as angiotensinogen, nitric oxide synthase and 5,10-methylenetetrahydrofolate reductase (*MTHFR*) have yielded conflicting results.

The net result of inadequate trophoblast invasion is reduced blood flow through the placenta. Recently it has been shown that placentas from pre-eclamptic women synthesise increased amounts of sFlt-l, which is a circulating receptor for vascular endothelial growth factor (VEGF) and acts as a VEGF antagonist. Serum sFlt-l is elevated in pre-eclamptic women. Purified sFlt-l also causes a pre-eclampsia like syndrome in both normal and pregnant rats with hypertension, proteinuria and glomerular endotheliosis, which can be reversed by administration of VEGF[25]. This provides compelling evidence that sFlt-l may be involved in the pathogenesis of pre-eclampsia.

Regardless of etiology pre-eclampsia is characterized by the pathophysiological triad of:

- vasoconstriction;
- platelet activation with intravascular coagulation (usually local but occasionally disseminated);
- maternal plasma volume contraction.

This triad leads to further impairment of blood flow through the placenta as well as through the maternal kidneys, liver, and brain. It is unknown why these organs are most often affected in pre-eclampsia and why other vascular beds, for example the gut, are unaffected even in very severe cases.

The clinical presentation of pre-eclampsia will depend upon the extent to which maternal organ systems and the placenta have been affected by this process, but once pre-eclampsia has begun it runs a progressive course until delivery. The mediators of this progression include sFlt-l but may also involve other placental toxins, pro-inflammatory factors, impaired maternal prostacyclin production or enhanced sympathetic nervous system activity.

Renal abnormalities in pre-eclampsia

There are several abnormalities of renal function and structure in pre-eclampsia (Fig. 44.6)[25].

Proteinuria

Both 'tubular' and 'glomerular' patterns of proteinuria have been reported in pre-eclampsia. Glomerular proteinuria is nonselective and may range from a few hundred milligrams per day to full-blown nephrotic syndrome. Proteinuria conveys a worse prognosis for both mother and fetus, but it appears that these risks are independent of the degree of proteinuria[27]. Therefore, women with mild proteinuria should be managed with the same caution as those with nephrotic range proteinuria. Measuring microalbuminuria has not yet proven useful in clinical management of pre-eclamptic women, nor in predicting which women with gestational hypertension will develop pre-eclampsia.

Proteinuria may be part of the general capillary leak of pre-eclampsia but glomerular endothelial swelling ('endotheliosis'), mesangial cell interposition, complement activation and deposition and subendothelial electron-dense deposits are prominent glomerular changes in pre-eclampsia. These are infrequently seen as renal biopsy is rarely performed in pre-eclampsia.

Decreased glomerular filtration rate

A fall in the glomerular filtration rate (GFR) may be partly caused by the decrease in renal blood flow (in turn caused by

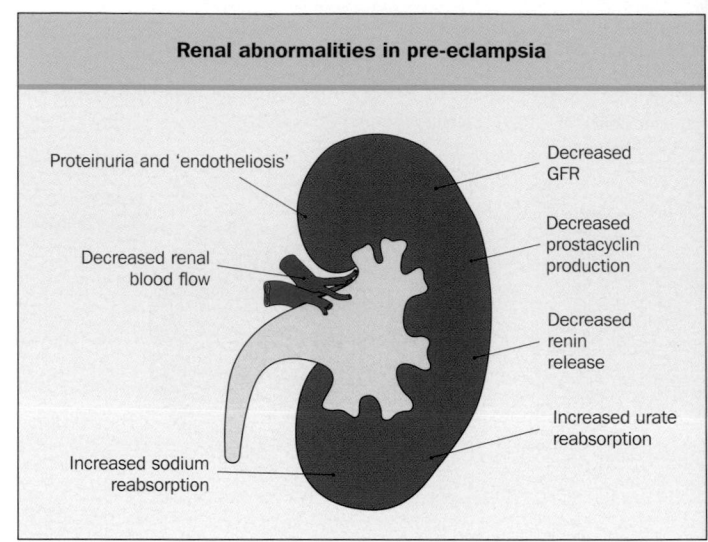

Figure 44.6 Renal abnormalities in pre-eclampsia.

vasoconstriction, plasma volume loss, and decreased cardiac output) but other factors, such as impaired placental production of the vasodilator relaxin or impaired renal prostacyclin or nitric oxide production or the glomerular morphologic changes themselves, may also be involved. A recent study showed a fall in GFR in 13 pre-eclamptic women who had no change in renal blood flow or oncotic pressure. Renal biopsies in these women showed reduced filtration surface area predominantly due to mesangial cell interposition and a reduced single nephron K_f.[28]

Acute tubular necrosis

Acute tubular necrosis is the most common cause of ARF in pre-eclampsia. If impaired GFR (i.e., serum creatinine $\geq 1\,mg/dL (\geq 90\,\mu mol/L)$) is not corrected by blood pressure control and plasma volume restoration, delivery is indicated if renal function continues to deteriorate.

Sodium retention

Avid sodium retention occurs in pre-eclampsia. This appears mainly to be caused by the decrease in filtered sodium but may also be a response to intravascular volume depletion. Oliguria in the absence of an elevated serum creatinine should not be an indication for delivery, as this may reflect the pronounced sodium and water retention of pre-eclampsia. If this is physiologic, it will resolve once the intravascular volume is restored and blood pressure controlled.

Renin

Plasma renin and aldosterone concentrations are reduced in pre-eclampsia, correlating inversely with the severity of the disorder. This has little direct clinical relevance; however it may be explained by the recent discovery of a mineralocorticoid receptor mutation (MRL810), which allows factors normally antagonistic to aldosterone, such as progesterone, to bind and activate this receptor leading to inappropriate sodium retention, hypertension and subsequent suppression of renin and aldosterone release[28].

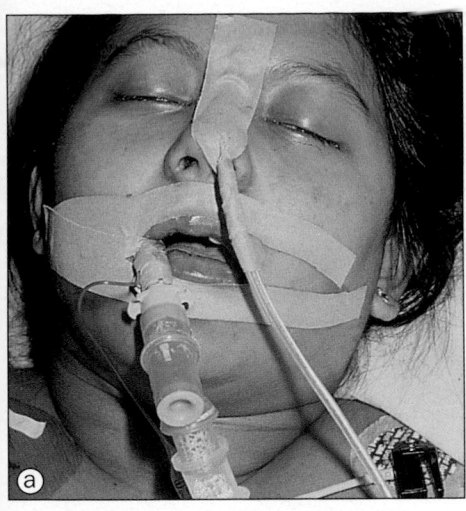
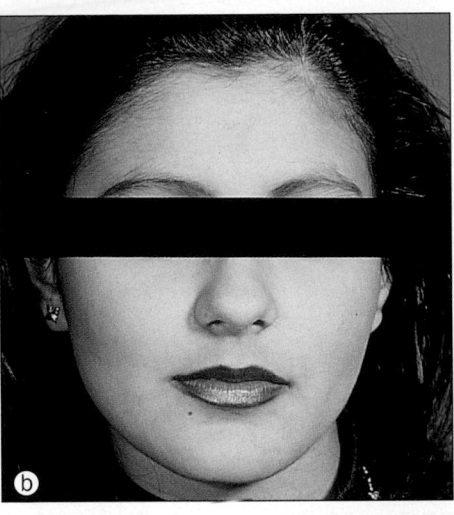

Figure 44.7 Clinical appearance of severe pre-eclampsia. (a) Marked facial edema occurs and intubation for treatment of acute pulmonary edema may be required. (b) Complete resolution of these features occurs postpartum.

Increased urate reabsorption

Hyperuricemia in pre-eclampsia results largely from renal urate retention though there may be some component of increased urate production, perhaps by the placenta. Plasma urate is a useful test in hypertensive pregnancies as it is generally elevated in pre-eclampsia. Values greater than 4.5 mg/dL (270 µmol/L) are indicative of pre-eclampsia. A concentration less than this should prompt review of the pregnant woman for another cause for hypertension, in particular, essential hypertension.

Clinical manifestations
Pre-eclampsia

Pre-eclampsia is detected initially in most cases by the presence of hypertension arising after the 20th week of pregnancy. It does not occur before the 20th week, except in the rare case of hydatidiform mole. Symptoms (Figs 44.7 and 44.8) are not always present, but may comprise severe headaches, convulsions, stroke, repeated visual scotomata (all manifestations of cerebral involvement), severe epigastric or right upper quadrant pain (reflecting hepatic ischemia with possible subcapsular hematoma of the liver or even liver rupture), oliguria, bleeding caused by DIC, lower abdominal pain caused by abruptio placenta, or reduced fetal movements associated with fetal demise.

In most cases, however, clinicians must search for evidence of maternal or fetal abnormalities in pre-eclampsia. Routine physical examination should include assessment of fetal growth and fetal heart rate, whether or not there is epigastric or right upper quadrant tenderness, and assessment of the reflexes, particularly detecting clonus as a warning sign of impending eclampsia.

In general, only a few laboratory tests are required for the full assessment of pre-eclampsia (Table 44.3). Fetal growth is best assessed by ultrasound, and fetal well-being by a combination of heart rate, cardiotocography, and ultrasonographic biophysical profile; it should be stressed that none of the assessments of fetal well-being provide any long-term certainty about fetal outcome.

Eclampsia

Eclampsia (convulsions) is not directly related to the level of blood pressure. Although some view this as a form of

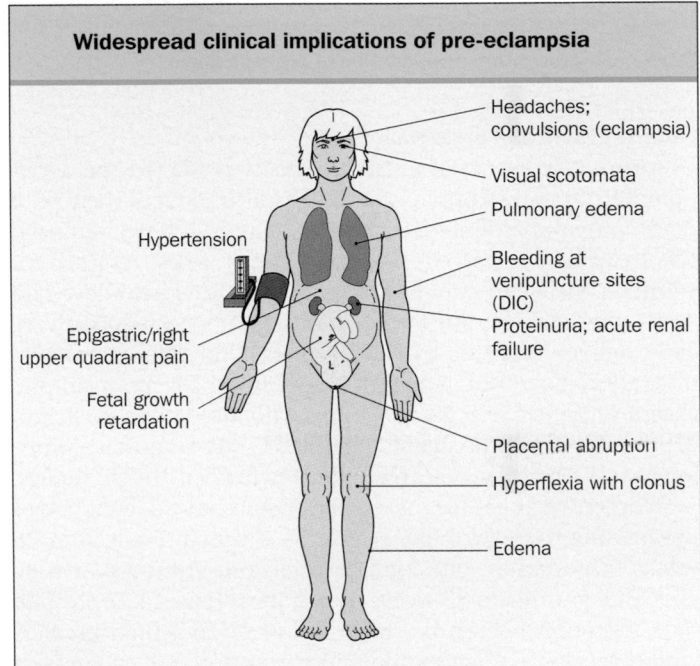

Widespread clinical implications of pre-eclampsia

Hypertension

Epigastric/right upper quadrant pain

Fetal growth retardation

Headaches; convulsions (eclampsia)

Visual scotomata

Pulmonary edema

Bleeding at venipuncture sites (DIC)

Proteinuria; acute renal failure

Placental abruption

Hyperflexia with clonus

Edema

Figure 44.8 The widespread clinical manifestations of pre-eclampsia. (Adapted from Brown MA[32].)

hypertensive encephalopathy, eclampsia may occur at relatively low levels of blood pressure and it has been reported in the absence of proteinuria. Importantly, about half the cases of eclampsia occur after delivery, though rarely more than 5 days postpartum.

HELLP syndrome

HELLP syndrome – hemolysis, elevated liver enzymes, low platelets – is a subcategory of pre-eclampsia. Although sometimes regarded as a separate entity, HELLP simply refers to a severe form of pre-eclampsia in which the hepatic and platelet abnormalities dominate. Clinicians should be careful to continue to look for all the other potential complications of pre-eclampsia in such women.

Laboratory investigation of pre-eclampsia	
Test	**Significance**
Hemoglobin	Hemolysis; bleeding
Hematocrit	>0.40 reflects plasma volume contraction
Platelets	$< 150 \times 10^9$ cells/L is abnormal, probably owing to increased platelet activation
Creatinine	Plasma level ≥ 1.1 mg/dL ($\geq 100\,\mu$mol/L) reflects impaired GFR
Uric acid	Plasma level ≥ 4.5 mg/dL ($\geq 270\,\mu$mol/L) is consistent with a diagnosis of pre-eclampsia
Aspartate transaminase (AST)	> 50 IU/L indicates hepatic dysfunction in pre-eclampsia
Proteinuria	A spot MSU protein:creatinine ratio >3 (mg protein: mg creatinine) (>30 mg: mmol) indicates increased protein excretion

Table 44.3 Laboratory investigation of pre-eclampsia.

Natural history and prevention

Unfortunately no set of tests has reliably predicted the development of pre-eclampsia. Low-dose aspirin reduces the risk of developing pre-eclampsia but approximately 100 women need this treatment to prevent one case[30] and it is best reserved for women considered at highest risk such as those who have had a previous fetal loss due to pre-eclampsia or who required very early delivery because of this disorder. Oral calcium supplementation does not reduce the likelihood of pre-eclampsia except in highly selected subgroups who are probably calcium deplete, but the antioxidants Vitamins C and E appear promising in this regard[31] and are the subject of further clinical studies.

Women with gestational hypertension have a 10% risk of progressing to develop pre-eclampsia if they present after 36 weeks of gestation, but a greater than one-third risk if they present e.g. prior to 32 weeks of gestation (Fig. 44.9). Despite several studies no test has been found so far which predicts which women with gestational hypertension will progress to the more severe disorder of pre-eclampsia.

In developing countries, pre-eclampsia remains one of the most common causes of maternal death and a common cause of death in young women. In the developed world, maternal mortality is now uncommon, although occasional cases still occur despite the best possible management. Perinatal mortality is of the order of 20–35 per 1000 cases in developed countries, with as many as one-quarter of babies being small for gestational age.

Treatment

The only definitive treatment for pre-eclampsia is delivery of the placenta. As the disorder may occur in the absence of the fetus (e.g., hydatidiform mole), it is removal of the placenta that is important. Therefore, pre-eclampsia that continues to worsen several days postpartum should prompt consideration of retained placental products.

Indications for delivery are generally:
- progressive evidence of maternal organ dysfunction: worsening renal or hepatic function, worsening

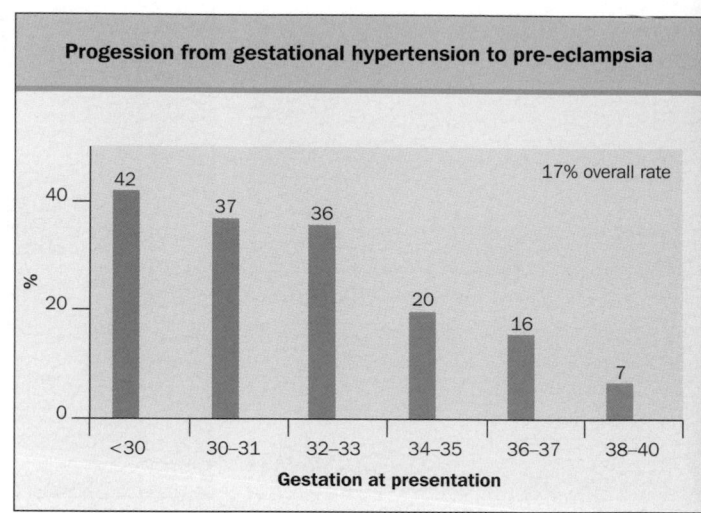

Figure 44.9 Progression from gestational hypertension to pre-eclampsia. Likelihood of progressing from gestational hypertension to pre-eclampsia according to gestation at diagnosis of gestational hypertension. Data are derived from a retrospective analysis of 416 women and a prospective analysis of 112 women presenting initially with gestational hypertension. The earlier the presentation with gestational hypertension, the more probable that pre-eclampsia will develop.

thrombocytopenia, development of neurologic symptoms or signs;
- inability to control blood pressure;
- inadequate fetal growth.

Antihypertensive medications are usually given if the systolic blood pressure is persistently >160 mmHg and/or diastolic pressure >90 mmHg (Table 44.4) though the choice of the exact blood pressure level at which treatment is required remains controversial. For such chronic treatment, several agents may be used including oxprenolol, labetalol, methyldopa, and clonidine as first-line agents. When additional treatment is required, hydralazine, nifedipine, or prazosin may be added. ACE inhibitors, angiotensin receptor antagonists and diuretics are generally avoided; the first two groups cause a fetal hypotension syndrome and the last reduces an already impaired maternal blood volume.

Blood pressure > 170/110 mmHg requires acute treatment in order to prevent maternal stroke and/or eclampsia. In this setting, intravenous hydralazine or intravenous labetalol are used most commonly. Oral or sublingual nifedipine is also useful.

Convulsions should be terminated with intravenous diazepam. Both phenytoin and magnesium sulfate have been used for convulsion prophylaxis, the latter now shown to be superior for prevention of recurrent convulsions after an initial eclamptic episode. Other studies suggest magnesium sulfate may also be superior to phenytoin for primary convulsion prophylaxis. In our view, convulsion prophylaxis should be reserved for pre-eclamptic women with clinical evidence of cerebral involvement. Withholding convulsion prophylaxis in the remainder is associated with an extremely low likelihood of fits and avoids the potential for drug toxicity in a large number of pregnant women. Ongoing international trials are designed to determine whether treatment of blood pressure alone offers as much convulsion prophylaxis as magnesium sulfate.

Common medications used in the treatment of hypertension in pre-eclampsia		
Type of hypertension	Drug	Treatment regimen
Acute	Hydralazine	5 mg bolus intravenous (i.v.) every 20–30 min to maximum of 20 mg then infusion at 5–10 mg/h
	Labetalol	50 mg i.v. every 20 min to maximum 300 mg
	Nifedipine	5–10 mg oral or sublingual capsules every 20 min to maximum 30 mg
	Diazoxide	Rarely used
Chronic		
First-line choice	Methyldopa	0.5–2 g/day oral
	Clonidine	0.2–0.8 mg/day oral
	Oxprenolol	80–480 mg/day oral
	Labetalol	0.2–1.2 g/day oral
	Atenolol	50–200 mg/day oral
Second-line choice	Hydralazine	25–200 mg/day oral
	Prazosin	1–10 mg/day oral
	Nifedipine SR	40–100 mg/day oral

Diuretics and propranolol are not recommended
ACE inhibitors and angiotensin receptor blockers are contraindicated
Ketanserin may prove useful in further studies

Table 44.4 Common medications used in the treatment of hypertension in pre-eclampsia.

Management of pre-eclampsia	
Clinical problem	Management
Assess indications for delivery	Always review whether an indication for delivery is present by clinical and laboratory monitoring
Control blood pressure (BP)	Acute treatment if BP ≥ 170/110 mmHg Chronic treatment if BP ≥ 160/90 mmHg
Eclampsia prophylaxis or treatment	Diazepam 10–20 mg intravenous (i.v.) to terminate convulsions
	Magnesium sulfate for persistent neurologic signs (also an indication for delivery): 4 g i.v. over 20 min then 1.5 g/h for 48 h
Volume expander therapy	500–1000 mL colloid over 4–6 h for persistent oliguria
	500 mL colloid in conjunction with parenteral antihypertensive therapy or before epidural anesthesia
Supportive therapies (sometimes required)	Platelet infusion if count < 20 to 40 × 10^9/L
	Fresh frozen plasma for microangiopathy or for reduced clotting factors
	Dialysis for established acute renal failure
Progressive decline in renal, hepatic or clotting function or of fetal growth	Delivery

Table 44.5 Management of pre-eclampsia.

Although pre-eclampsia is a volume-contracted state, the increased capillary permeability makes intravenous volume expansion a potentially harmful procedure, with the risk of pulmonary edema ever present. Therefore, volume expansion should be used only in selected settings, such as prior to parenteral treatment of acute severe hypertension (when rapid vasodilatation may occur) and as initial treatment in the persistently oliguric woman. No more than 1 L of colloid should be given in such women, usually over a 4–6-h interval. This will restore the average plasma volume deficit in most pre-eclamptic women, but careful observation is required for the possibility of pulmonary edema, particularly if oliguria persists. This latter setting would be one in which invasive hemodynamic monitoring would be warranted, an unusual requirement in the management of pre-eclampsia. There are a small number of reports indicating successful use of low-dose dopamine in the oliguric pre-eclamptic woman but this has never been subjected to proper study and in light of potential arrhythmic problems and recent data showing no benefit of dopamine in nonpregnant patients with ARF, we no longer advocate this treatment.

Platelet transfusion is generally given when the platelet count falls below 20 × 10^9/L but sometimes even at higher levels (e.g., 20–40 × 10^9/L) if hypertension is difficult to control and the risk of intracerebral hemorrhage is, therefore, high. Fresh frozen plasma is only indicated if there is accompanying microangiopathy and thrombocytopenia (when it may be difficult to differentiate pre-eclampsia from hemolytic–uremic syndrome, HUS) or when hepatic disease leads to impaired coagulation in pre-eclamptic women. The management of pre-eclampsia is summarized in Table 44.5.

Postpartum management

Recovery should be anticipated over 5–7 days in most women following delivery. Occasionally, patients may take up to 3 months for all the features to resolve, and a few patients will have proteinuria that takes up to a year to disappear completely.

Assessment of the pre-eclamptic woman several months postpartum is mandatory. Blood pressure should have returned to normal within 3 months and if not this should prompt a search for underlying essential or secondary hypertension. Urinalysis and urine microscopy should be normal, certainly by 12 months postpartum, and if this is not the case a primary underlying renal disease should be sought. There is no indication to evaluate all pre-eclamptic women for underlying renal disease. Provided a proper clinical history and assessment of the urine is made at the time of initial consultation in pregnancy, the likelihood of an underlying renal disease is < 2% and even so, the disorders discovered bear little or no relationship to the likelihood of pre-eclampsia[33].

Women with recurrent pre-eclampsia, or else severe early-onset disease (in whom recurrence is more likely) warrant special consideration and should be tested for underlying connective tissue, renal, and coagulation disorders (including protein C deficiency) but these tests are not required in women with a single episode of pre-eclampsia.

As a general rule, pre-eclampsia will recur in only about 5% of women in a subsequent pregnancy, though the likelihood of the more benign problem of gestational hypertension may be as high as 40% in subsequent pregnancies. Women who have presented at or before 28 weeks of gestation have at least a 25% risk of recurrence but some studies suggest

Pregnancy and Renal Disease

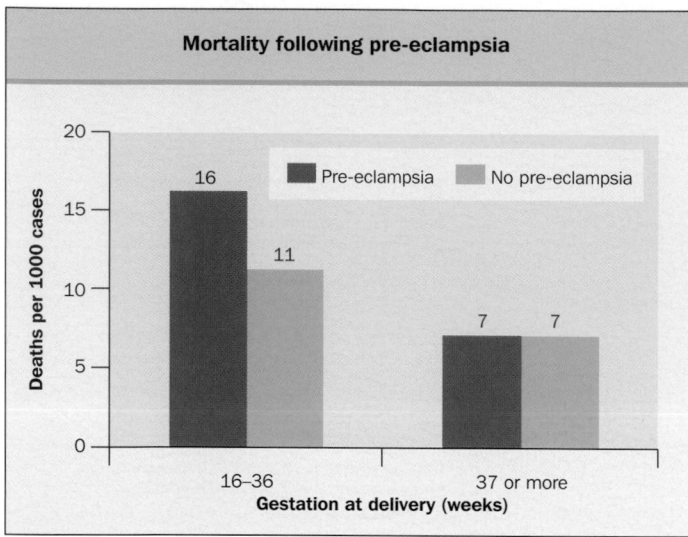

Figure 44.10 Mortality following pre-eclampsia. Mortality over 25 years follow up after first pregnancy in over 600 000 women from Norway. Women with pre-eclampsia had higher long-term mortality if they needed to be delivered prematurely but not if delivered at term. (Adapted from Irgens et al. [34].

that in such patients recurrence tends to present later in subsequent pregnancies.

The traditional view has been that pre-eclampsia is not associated with long-term health risks for the mother, though gestational hypertension, particularly when recurrent, predicts a greater likelihood of later essential hypertension. However, a recent study has shown that women who had pre-eclampsia and needed delivery prior to 37 weeks' gestation had greater overall mortality risk over 25 years and greater death rates from cardiovascular disease (Fig. 44.10). Women with pre-eclampsia needing premature delivery should therefore be advised about long-term cardiovascular risks and make every effort to modify risk factors such as weight, cholesterol, blood pressure, etc.

ACUTE RENAL FAILURE

Definition

There is no agreed definition of ARF in pregnancy. At one extreme ARF is oliguria with rapidly rising plasma creatinine and urea concentrations necessitating dialysis. Another definition is an acute 50% reduction in GFR, but it is important to remember that GFR is usually increased by about 50% in normal pregnancy, with a concomitant fall in serum creatinine. Consequently serum creatinine > 90 μmol/L (> 1.0 mg/L) in pregnancy will represent impaired GFR and if this occurs rapidly and is left untreated, severe ARF may ensue. This section will discuss dialysis-dependent ARF but from a practical point of view, acute renal insufficiency not yet requiring dialysis is of equal importance, as early treatment of this problem may preclude the need for dialysis.

Epidemiology

In the 1960s, ARF complicated 1 in 1500–5000 pregnancies and at least 20% of all cases of ARF occurred in association

with pregnancy[35]. At that time, there was a bimodal distribution of ARF, most occurring early in pregnancy following septic abortion; the remainder developed in the third trimester in association with obstetric hemorrhage or pre-eclampsia. With altered abortion laws, improved antepartum management, and a greater awareness of the potential for ARF in pre-eclampsia, this epidemiology has changed considerably. ARF necessitating dialysis now occurs in only about 1 of 20 000 pregnancies, so a typical primary care obstetric unit (with 2000–3000 unselected deliveries per year) will only see one case every 6–10 years; the incidence will, of course, be greater in tertiary referral centers but is still very low.

There are very few studies on the prevalence of acute renal insufficiency not requiring dialysis. In our unit, 7% of women with *de novo* hypertension in the second half of their pregnancy develop acute renal insufficiency, and only 0.4% of this hypertensive population have required dialysis[4]. Renal insufficiency or failure from other causes has been rare, highlighting the fact that the epidemiology of ARF in pregnancy will differ according to the nature of cases referred to a unit. While any of the causes of ARF may be encountered, antepartum hemorrhage and pre-eclampsia remain the most common causes in developed countries, septic abortion and acute pyelonephritis being predominant causes of ARF in developing countries. Obstructive uropathy is an uncommon cause of ARF in pregnancy.

Pathogenesis

Common to many of the disorders causing ARF in pregnancy are the prerenal elements of volume contraction and vasoconstriction, as well as intravascular coagulation, each abnormality tending to reduce renal perfusion and setting the scene for renal ischemia. The peptide relaxin, produced by the placenta, has been postulated as a factor augmenting GFR during pregnancy via production of endothelial cell nitric oxide. Failure to produce sufficient relaxin, in association with disorders causing placental dysfunction, may increase the risk for ARF in pregnancy though this hypothesis is yet to be proven.

It is generally believed that a pregnant woman is more likely to develop ARF than a nonpregnant woman exposed to the same set of conditions that threaten renal perfusion, although there are no confirmatory data for this view. The best explanation for this would be that many of the renal 'protective' mechanisms (e.g., increased prostacyclin production to enhance renal blood flow) are already activated maximally in normal pregnancy and may not be augmented in the setting of a prerenal problem.

It is also a common view that subsequent bilateral renal cortical necrosis is more likely than if ARF had developed outside of pregnancy. The risk of cortical necrosis is estimated at 20% when ARF follows septic abortion. This contrasts with a lower incidence of cortical necrosis (around 2%) following other causes of ARF in pregnancy[36]. Irreversible renal damage follows 10–25% of such cases of cortical necrosis, mostly following pre-eclampsia or antepartum hemorrhage[37]. Since septic abortion is now an uncommon problem in developing countries, cortical necrosis is a less common sequela of obstetric ARF than was reported in the past, although this risk remains higher in developing countries where opportunities to prevent ARF are fewer.

Antepartum hemorrhage

In antepartum hemorrhage, volume contraction is sufficient cause for ARF, but this is compounded in many patients by accompanying intravascular coagulation, which further reduces renal blood flow.

Pre-eclampsia

Pre-eclampsia is already a volume-contracted and vaso-constricted state with the added possibility of intrarenal coagulation or DIC. Again, renal cortical hypoperfusion with acute tubular necrosis is the major mechanism of ARF in pre-eclampsia, though this is made worse by the common lesion of glomerular 'endotheliosis' with swollen glomerular endothelial cells, which may also reduce filtering capacity.

Sepsis

In septic conditions in pregnancy, ARF is probably the result of cytokine-induced changes in vascular permeability and a loss of effective renal plasma flow, sometimes with accompanying hemolysis or DIC or, as in pyelonephritis, an acute interstitial nephritis.

Acute fatty liver of pregnancy

In acute fatty liver of pregnancy (AFLP), the mechanism of ARF is less certain, but there appears to be an overlap with pre-eclampsia; the pathophysiology leading to ARF is probably similar to that seen in pre-eclampsia.

Clinical manifestations and differential diagnosis

Most cases of ARF in pregnancy are associated with oliguria and the clinical manifestations in the mother are the same as for ARF in general (see Chapter 14). However, the clinical setting in which the ARF occurs is quite different from that in the general medical wards and there is the added concern of fetal death as the fetus does not survive in an environment of prolonged uremia. The following are some clinical features that should be considered in the differential diagnosis of ARF in pregnancy.

Pre-eclampsia

Pre-eclampsia is characterized by de novo hypertension in the second half of pregnancy with evidence of maternal organ system dysfunction, usually of kidneys, liver, brain, or coagulation systems. In the HELLP variant, liver dysfunction and thrombocytopenia dominate the clinical presentation.

Acute fatty liver of pregnancy

AFLP classically presents in the third trimester with nausea, vomiting, and jaundice. Marked elevation of plasma aspartate transaminase and alanine transferase, bleeding, thrombocytopenia, hypoglycemia, hyperuricemia, and renal failure may soon accompany this. In some patients, hypertension and proteinuria are also present; although these are thought to accompany pre-eclampsia, it is more likely that these disorders are a spectrum of one disease process. When appropriate stains are used, fatty infiltration can be demonstrated in liver biopsy samples from most patients with pre-eclampsia[38].

Hemolytic–uremic syndrome

HUS typically presents in the postpartum period but has been reported to occur as early as the first trimester and can occur at any time during pregnancy. HUS is generally an oliguric condition, often with hypertension, and is characterized by microangiopathic hemolysis and thrombocytopenia. Coagulation studies are usually normal, unlike cases of severe pre-eclampsia or AFLP. In practice, it can be difficult to distinguish HUS from pre-eclampsia without renal biopsy, which often has to be delayed until thrombocytopenia is resolving. Many consider these two disorders to be slightly different manifestations of endothelial cell dysfunction, and from a practical point of view it is not important to distinguish them initially as treatment will be similar once microangiopathy, thrombocytopenia, and renal failure are apparent. If renal failure is progressive, biopsy becomes more important to guide ongoing therapy (e.g., use of plasma infusion/exchange or prostacyclin, as discussed in Chapter 31).

Obstructive uropathy

Obstructive uropathy is uncommon in pregnancy. It will most commonly occur in a twin pregnancy with polyhydramnios but has been reported with other unusual causes such as uterine leiomyomas. Generally, there are no specific clinical clues in these patients; rather renal failure is discovered when serum creatinine is measured because a pregnant woman is progressively unwell or, at the other end of the spectrum, she is oliguric. However, the diagnosis of pathologic urinary tract obstruction in pregnancy can be challenging. Ureteral dilatation is part of normal pregnancy, more common on the right, and may reach up to 8 cm renal pelvic dilatation as part of normal pregnancy. Therefore, ultrasound diagnosis of obstructive uropathy is very difficult. Clinicians implicating urinary tract obstruction as the cause of ARF in pregnancy should first search for other disorders causing the ARF. If no other cause is found, renal failure is progressive, and delivery cannot be effected immediately, then percutaneous nephrostomy is required; the diagnosis is confirmed as the serum creatinine falls. In practice it is rare to reach this situation.

Natural history

The likelihood of renal insufficiency progressing to become established dialysis-dependent ARF in pregnancy has not been studied systematically. In our unit, where progressive renal insufficiency is an indication for delivery, 6% of our pre-eclamptic population with progressive renal insufficiency still required dialysis, though fortunately none remained dialysis dependent.

Recovery from dialysis-dependent ARF is far more likely in pre-eclamptics or those with AFLP or antepartum hemorrhage, as the pathophysiologic changes of these disorders resolve quickly following delivery. Recovery is much slower following HUS or thrombotic thrombocytopenic purpura (TTP), and chronic renal impairment is more likely. Chronic renal failure is, of course, more likely when any of these episodes of ARF occur on a background of chronic renal insufficiency.

Pregnancy and Renal Disease

Maternal mortality

Maternal mortality reports range from zero in Italy[40] to 44% in tropical Africa, intermediate figures being obtained from Pakistan (23%), Romania (15%), South Africa (5%), and Ethiopia (34%). Even in developed countries such as the USA 13% of patients with HELLP syndrome die[41], and 9% of pregnant women with ARF died between 1981 and 1998 in a French nephrology unit[42]. Many of these figures have been derived from data gathered over many years and are unlikely to reflect current trends in management, as highlighted in data from Italy in which maternal mortality from obstetric ARF was 31% in the 1950s and 1960s but no deaths were seen in the period 1988–1994[40]. Fetal mortality rates are much higher but vary enormously depending on the availability of perinatal care.

Treatment

The key issue in treatment of ARF in pregnancy is restoration of fluid volume deficits, and in later pregnancy, delivery of the baby and placenta, as this is likely to remove the stimulus for ARF as quickly as possible. This is relatively easy when ARF develops late in pregnancy, but when fetal viability is uncertain and the maternal condition stable, dialysis and specific treatment of the underlying condition are employed.

Treatment of pre-eclampsia/HELLP syndrome is considered above and HUS in Chapter 31. The latter has been treated using fresh frozen plasma and plasma exchange when ARF develops in the peripartum setting, but maternal and fetal outcomes remains poor. In one small study 2 of 11 women died and four of the remainder had chronic renal failure[43].

Pyelonephritis should be treated early and aggressively (initially with intravenous antibiotics) in pregnancy. Volume deficits from antepartum hemorrhage or hyperemesis should be corrected quickly, the general rule being that the pregnant woman will not tolerate volume deficits at all well compared with her nonpregnant state.

Both peritoneal dialysis and hemodialysis have been used in pregnancy with limited success. Peritoneal dialysis requires dialysis catheter insertion under direct vision high in the abdomen and has the potential advantage of maintaining fairly constant maternal hemodynamics without threatening uteroplacental blood flow, but it does carry the risk of peritonitis. Hemodialysis is likely to be required more frequently than usual and has the risk of impairing uteroplacental perfusion if sudden fluid shifts occur. Neither method is superior and there is only limited experience with continuous venovenous hemofiltration in pregnancy. There is no clear evidence to determine at what level of renal failure dialysis should be instituted in pregnancy, but many nephrologists advising keeping the plasma urea below at least 15 mmol/L (BUN 42 mg/dL) in order to maintain the best 'milieu' for the baby.

REFERENCES

1. Gallery ED, Ross M, Gyory AZ. Urinary red blood cell and cast excretion in normal and hypertensive human pregnancy. Am J Obstet Gynecol. 1993;168:67–70.
2. Stehman-Breen C,Miller L, Fink J, Schwartz SM. Pre-eclampsia and premature labour among pregnant women with hematuria. Paediatr Perinat Epidemiol. 2000;14:136–40.
3. Saudan PJ, Brown MA, Farrell T, Shaw L. Improved methods of assessing proteinuria in hypertensive pregnancy. Br J Obstet Gynaecol. 1997;104:1159–64.
4. Kuo VS, Koumantakis G, Gallery ED. Proteinuria and its assessment in normal and hypertensive pregnancy. Am J Obstet Gynecol. 1992;167:723–8.
5. Brown MA, Wang MX, Buddle ML, et al. Albumin excretory rate in normal and hypertensive pregnancy. Clin Sci. 1994;86: 2541–50.
6. Brown MA, Buddle ML. Hypertension in pregnancy: maternal and fetal outcomes according to laboratory and clinical features. Med J Aust. 1996;165:360–5.
7. Packham D, Fairley KF. Renal biopsy: indications and complications in pregnancy. Br J Obstet Gynaecol. 1987;94:935–9.
8. Smaill F. Antibiotic for asymptomatic bacteriuria in pregnancy. The Cochrane database of systematic reviews (Issue 4). 2001.
9. Rouse DJ, Andrews WW, Goldenberg RL, Owen JO. Screening and treatment of asymptomatic bacteriuria of pregnancy to prevent pyelonephritis: a cost-effectiveness and cost-benefit analysis. Obstet Gynecol. 1995;86:119–23.
10. Kass EH. The role of asymptomatic bacteriuria in the pathogenesis of pyelonephritis. In: Quinn EL, Kass EH, eds. Biology of pyelonephritis. Boston, MA: Little, Brown; 1960:399–412.
11. Romero R, Oyarzun E, Mazor M, et al. Meta-analysis of the relationship between asymptomatic bacteriuria and preterm delivery/low birth weight. Obstet Gynecol. 1989;73:576–82.
12. Villar J, Lydon-Rochelle MT, Gulmezoglu AM, Roganti A. Duration of treatment for asymptomatic bacteriuria during pregnancy. Cochrane Database of Systematic Reviews (Issue 4) 2001.
13. Locksmith G, Duff P. Infection, antibiotics and preterm delivery. Semin Perinatol. 2001;25:295–309.
14. Millar LK, Wing DA, Paul RH, Grimes DA. Outpatient treatment of pyelonephritis in pregnancy: a randomized controlled trial. Obstet Gynecol. 1995;86:560–4.
15. Swanson SK, Heilman RL, Eversman WG. Urinary tract stones in pregnancy. Surg Clin N Am. 1995;75:123–42.
16. Ulvik NM, Bakke A, Hoisaeter PA. Ureteroscopy in pregnancy. J Urol. 1995;154:1660–3.
17. Scarpa RM, de Lisa A, Usai E. Diagnosis and treatment of ureteral calculi in pregnancy with rigid ureteroscopes. J Urol. 1996;155: 875–7.
18. Carringer M, Swartz R, Johanson JE. Management of ureteric calculi during pregnancy by ureteroscopy and laser lithotripsy. Br J Urol. 1996;77:17–20.
19. Asgari MA, Safarinejad MR, Hosseini SY, Dadkhah F. Extracorporeal shock wave lithotripsy of renal calculi during early pregnancy. BJU Int. 1999;84:615–17.
20. Levine RJ, Ewell MG, Hauth JC et al. Should the definition of preeclampsia include a rise in diastolic blood pressure of ≥ 15 mmHg to a level ≥ 90 mmHg in association with proteinuria? Am J Obstet Gynecol. 2000;183:787–92.
21. Brown MA, Buddle ML. What's in a name? Problems with the classification of hypertension in pregnancy. J Hypertens. 1997;15: 1049–54.
22. Esplin MS, Fausett MB, Fraser A, et al. Paternal and maternal components of the predisposition to preeclampsia. N Engl J Med. 2001;344:867–72.

23. Zhou Y, Damsky CH, Fisher SJ. Preeclampsia is associated with failure of human cytotrophoblasts to mimic a vascular adhesion phenotype. One cause of defective endovascular invasion in this syndrome? J Clin Invest. 1997;99:2153–64.

24. Arngrimsson R, Sigurard ttir S, Frigge MI, et al. A genome-wide scan reveals a maternal susceptibility locus for pre-eclampsia on chromosome 2p13. Hum Mol Genet.1999;8:1799–805.

25. Maynard SE, Min J–Y, Merchan J, et al. Exess placental sFlt-l may contribute to endothelial dysfunction, hypertension and protein-uria in preeclampsia. J Clin Invest. 2003; 11 (in press)

26. Brown MA, Whitworth JA. The kidney in hypertensive pregnan-cies – victim and villain. Am J Kidney Dis. 1992;20:427–42.

27. Schiff E, Friedman SA, Kao L, Sibai BM. The importance of uri-nary protein excretion during conservative management of severe preeclampsia. Am J Obstet Gynecol. 1996;175:1313–16.

28. Lafayette RA, Druzin M, Sibley R, et al. Nature of glomerular dys-function in pre-eclampsia. Kidney Int. 1998;54:1240–9.

29. Geller DS, Farhi A, Pinkerton N, et al. Activating mineralocorti-coid receptor mutation in hypertension exacerbated by preg-nancy. Science. 2000;289:119–23.

30. Knight M, Duley L, Henderson-Smart DJ, King JF. Anti-platelet agents for preventing and treating pre-eclampsia. Cochrane data-base of systematic reviews (issue 2). 2000. CD000492.

31. Chappell LC, Seed PT, Briley AL, et al. Effect of antioxidants on the occurrence of pre-eclampsia in women at increased risk: a randomised trial. Lancet. 1999;354:810–16.

32. Brown MA. Pregnancy-induced hypertension: pathogenesis and management. Aust NZ J Med. 1991;21:257–73.

33. Brown MA, Reiter L, Whitworth JA. Hypertension in pregnancy: the incidence of underlying renal disease and essential hyperten-sion. Am J Kidney Dis. 1994;24:883–7.

34. Irgens HU, Reisaeter L, Irgens LM, Lie RT. Long term mortality of mothers and fathers after pre-eclampsia : population based cohort study. Br Med J. 2001;323:1213–17.

35. Pertuiset N, Grunfeld JP. Acute renal failure in pregnancy. Baillière's Clin Obstet Gynaecol. 1994;8:333–51.

36. Prakash J, Tripathi K, Pandey LK, Gadela SR. Renal cortical necro-sis in pregnancy-related acute renal failure. J Ind Med Ass. 1996;94: 227–9.

37. Naqvi R, Akhtar F, Ahmed E, et al. Acute renal failure of obstetri-cal origin during 1994 at one center. Renal Failure. 1996; 18:681–3.

38. Minakami H, Oka N, Sato T, et al. Pre-eclampsia: a microvesicular fat disease of the liver? Am J Obstet Gynecol. 1998;159:1043–7.

39. Brown MA. Urinary tract dilatation in pregnancy. Am J Obstet Gynecol. 1991;164:641–3.

40. Stratta P, Besso L, Canavese C, et al. Is pregnancy related acute renal failure a disappearing entity? Renal Failure. 1996;18: 575–84.

41. Sibai BM, Ramadan MK. Acute renal failure in pregnancies com-plicated by hemolysis, elevated liver enzymes, and low platelets. Am J Obstet Gynecol. 1993;168:1682–7.

42. Hachim K, Badahi K, Benghanem M, et al. Obstetric acute renal failure. Experience of the nephrology department, Central University Hospital, Casablanca. Nephrologie. 2001;22:29–31.

43. Egerman RS, Witlin AG, Friedman SA, Sibcui BM. Thrombotic thrombocytopenic purpura and hemolytic uremic syndrome in pregnancy review of 11 cases. Am J Obstet Gynecol. 1996;175:950–6.

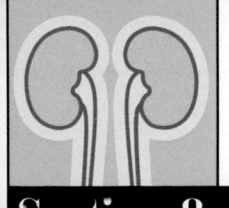

Chapter 45

Pregnancy with Pre-Existing Renal Disease

David K Packham, Kenneth F Fairley, and Priscilla Kincaid-Smith

INTRODUCTION

The effect and outcome of pregnancy in women with pre-existing renal disease has long been a subject of conflicting reports and opinions[1]. Until well into the 20th century, the failure to differentiate pre-eclampsia from chronic hypertension and renal disease and the grouping of these conditions into a broad category of 'nephritic toxemia', precluded the collecting of meaningful data. This was despite the very early observation of Lever in 1843 that the proteinuria of eclampsia resolved postpartum, whereas that of 'Bright's disease' persisted after pregnancy, i.e., the two conditions were separate and distinct.

From 1940 onwards, reports of pregnancy in women with pre-existing renal disease not only documented increased fetal loss and maternal complications but suggested that the pregnancy itself had a deleterious effect on remote renal prognosis. Proteinuria, impaired maternal renal function, and/or hypertension preceding pregnancy were identified as adverse prognostic features. These studies pre-dated the development of percutaneous renal biopsy and, as a result, histologic data were unavailable and the distinction between chronic nephritis and pre-eclampsia could be made only after prolonged postpartum observation. In addition, these early reports pre-dated the development of effective antihypertensive drug therapy in pregnancy and the substantial improvements in antenatal and perinatal care made since the 1970s.

Differentiating pre-eclampsia from pre-existing renal disease

Accurate distinction between pre-eclampsia and pre-existing renal disease is crucial in evaluating the effect and outcome of pregnancy in pre-existing renal disease. Naturally, there is no difficulty if renal disease is diagnosed prior to pregnancy, but a common clinical dilemma is the distinction between the two conditions in the pregnant patient with proteinuria and hypertension.

Clinical information directs the differential diagnosis (Table 45.1). In pre-eclampsia, hypertension typically accompanies proteinuria and it virtually never manifests before 20 weeks of gestation. Hematuria is not a feature of pre-eclampsia and the urine sediment is bland. Serum uric acid may also be discriminatory: in pre-existing renal disease with normal function, uric acid is typically < 4.5 mg/dL (270 µmol/L), but in pre-eclampsia it rises progressively, and often steeply, to above 8.5 mg/dL (500 µmol/L). Retrospective information comes

Differential diagnosis of pre-eclampsia and primary renal disease in pregnancy		
	Pre-eclampsia	Primary renal disease
During pregnancy		
Proteinuria	After 20 weeks of gestation	May occur before 20 weeks
Hematuria	–	May occur
Casts	Rarely seen	Usually seen
Hypertension	After 20 weeks of gestation	May occur before 20 weeks
Uric acid	> 4.5 mg/dL (270 µmol/L)	< 4.5 mg/dL (270 µmol/L)
Postpartum		
Proteinuria and hypertension	Resolves usually by 3 months (maximum 12 months)	Persists

Differentiation can be inferred from clinical features, but a definitive diagnosis requires a renal biopsy.

Table 45.1 Differential diagnosis of pre-eclampsia and primary renal disease in pregnancy.

from the postpartum natural history: proteinuria and hypertension will usually resolve completely in pre-eclampsia by 3 months. Pre-eclampsia occurring in second and subsequent pregnancies with the same partner also suggests underlying renal disease. A gold standard, renal histology, does exist but a reluctance to perform renal biopsy in pregnancy has encouraged categorization on clinical grounds. Clinical criteria are not always definitive; it has been stated that in half of the patients where mild pre-eclampsia is diagnosed, the true diagnosis might be essential hypertension or a variety of renal disorders[2]. More recent studies have confirmed the high incidence of underlying renal disease in severe pre-eclampsia or severe gestational proteinuria and confirmed that onset before 30 weeks' gestation was the best predictor of underlying renal disease[3].

The characteristic histology of pre-eclampsia is glomerular endotheliosis (tuft enlargement owing to endothelial cell swelling with cytoplasmic vacuolation) accompanied by capillary wall thickening. The nature of the capillary wall thickening has been widely discussed. Basement membrane thickening and sub-endothelial cell and mesangial cell interposition have all been described. If it is decided to defer renal biopsy until after delivery, the timing of the biopsy is crucial since histologic appearances can change rapidly in the postpartum period. Substantial subendothelial deposits are present in patients who undergo a biopsy during pregnancy or at delivery but these were found to be rare in biopsy specimens taken only 6 days postpartum[4].

GENERAL PRINCIPLES IN PREDICTING PREGNANCY OUTCOME

For every woman with renal disease considering pregnancy, there are two questions that need to be addressed to help the patient to make informed decisions. First, what will be the influence of the renal disease on the pregnancy and its outcome, particularly fetal morbidity and mortality? Renal disease is associated with placental failure, intrauterine growth retardation (IUGR), and the early delivery of babies small for gestational age, but these risks are not uniform in women with renal disease. Second, what effect will the pregnancy have on the natural history of the renal disease? Not only should the immediate effects during the pregnancy be considered but also the remote effects on the risk of progression of the renal disease.

There are general principles, based on clinical parameters, that can broadly predict the risk for all women with renal disease, including renal transplant recipients (Table 45.2). However, specific renal diseases do have some influence on outcome (Table 45.3). In addition, interstitial and vascular lesions, on renal biopsy, are associated with worse fetal outcome[5,6].

RENAL BIOPSY IN PREGNANCY

The place for renal biopsy in pregnancy is controversial. Our own published experience is that the procedure is safe and carries no additional risk over biopsy in nonpregnant patients[7]. Our rate of complications is much lower than other

General clinical principles predicting risk of pregnancy for women with renal disease
The great majority of women with preserved renal function at conception (judged by normal serum creatinine) do well with acceptable, although not normal, fetal and maternal outcome
Many of these women will manifest the increase in glomerular filtration rate (GFR) in the first trimester that is typical of normal pregnancy. Failure to make this increase is an adverse prognostic sign
Proteinuria, hypertension, and raised serum creatinine are independent risk factors for worse outcome and their effects are additive
Pre-existing proteinuria will very commonly increase during the pregnancy and reverse postpartum
Nephrotic syndrome worsens fetal outcome
Pregnancy does not provoke nephrotic relapses of minimal change disease
Hypertension often worsens and *de novo* hypertension is reported in 20% of pregnant women with renal disease
Primary renal disease in general carries less risk than renal involvement in those with multisystem disease (such as lupus or vasculitis)
Prognosis is worse in those women whose renal disease is first identified in pregnancy compared with those who embarked on pregnancy with known renal disease

Table 45.2 General clinical principles predicting risk of pregnancy for women with renal disease.

published series, probably because we biopsy the lateral edge of the kidney and not the lower pole[8]. The decision whether to biopsy, will always need to be made on the basis of risk/benefit of the procedure and in conjunction with the patient. Broadly speaking, we believe renal biopsy to be indicated before 30 weeks' gestation, in women whose underlying renal disease is not known but who present with signs of progressing renal disease, or nephrotic range proteinuria, in the absence of other signs of pre-eclampsia. An active urine

Table 45.3 Pregnancy outcome in primary glomerulonephritis.

Pregnancy outcome in primary glomerulonephritis				
	Percentage with complications			
Outcome	IgA nephropathy	Focal segmental glomerulosclerosis	Membranous nephropathy	Non-IgA mesangial proliferative glomerulonephritis
Fetal outcome				
Fetal loss	30	45	24	12
Intrauterine growth retardation	–	–	–	–
Preterm delivery	22	–	43	–
Histologic association with poor fetal outcome	Vascular lesions	–	–	Vascular lesions
Maternal outcome				
New hypertension	52	50	46	33
Increase in proteinuria	62	–	55	52
Temporary increase in serum creatinine	26	44	9	3
Permanent increase in serum creatinine	2	13	–	–
Histologic association with deterioration	Focal segmental lesions	–	Crescents	Focal segmental lesions
The risk of fetal and maternal complications in women with biopsy-proven primary glomerulonephritis and normal serum creatinine. (Data summarized from reference 5.)				

sediment with a high erythrocyte count (> 500 000/mL) or erythrocyte casts, suggests crescents are very likely to be present and is an indication for renal biopsy. Diagnosing such women enables appropriate treatment to both protect maternal renal function and, where possible, prolong pregnancy to ensure fetal survival.

PREGNANCY IN PRE-EXISTING RENAL DISEASE WITH NORMAL RENAL FUNCTION

The uncertainty of assessing the risks of pregnancy in pre-existing renal disease with normal renal function results in part from the difficulty in comparing published information. Reports have included women with renal impairment as well as preserved renal function and have variable lengths of follow-up. They may also include patients from previous eras when obstetric and neonatal practice were different from the modern era. However, four large series report on more than 900 pregnancies in women with primary glomerulonephritis (GN) of whom more than 95% had normal or slightly elevated serum creatinine levels (< 1.4 mg/dL (125 µmol/L))[5,9–11]. They show considerable concordance in the risk for both fetal loss and maternal complications (Table 45.4).

Whether the pregnancy itself causes permanent deterioration in renal function in women with primary GN who would otherwise have retained normal renal function still remains controversial. A study of 360 women showed no difference in long-term renal function between those who had pregnancies and those who did not[11]. In all series, a small number of women progressed to end-stage renal disease (ESRD), but this has usually been regarded as coincidental to pregnancy. However, ESRD does occur in a small minority of patients and its considerable implications require a critical appraisal of the available data before counseling women with pre-existing renal disease who may wish to become pregnant. The largest series of pregnancies in women with primary GN and normal renal function, as evidenced by serum creatinine[5], was analyzed for each of the recognized histologic categories of primary GN and showed clearly that fetal mortality and maternal morbidity varied considerably between groups. The findings are discussed here and summarized in Table 45.3.

IgA nephropathy

In IgA nephropathy (IgAN), there was fetal loss in 30% of the pregnancies and prematurity in 22%[12]. Maternal renal function declined during pregnancy in 26% of cases, and in 2% this did not improve postpartum. Hypertension developed in 52% of the pregnancies and in 13% this was irreversible. Increased proteinuria was recorded in 62% of the pregnancies. Fetal loss in pregnancies taking place after biopsy diagnosis, that is, where the patient was known to have renal disease before the pregnancy, was lower (16%) than in those in which biopsy was performed either during or following the pregnancy (36%). These findings are consistent with other published series.

Histologic features on biopsy are also predictors of pregnancy outcome[13]. Patients with superimposed focal and segmental proliferative lesions had a significantly worse maternal complication rate of renal impairment, hypertension, and

Pregnancy outcome and renal impairment			
Outcome		Renal impairment indicated by serum creatinine levels	
	Normal	> 1.4 mg/dL	> 2.0 mg/dL
Fetal outcome			
Fetal loss	23	22	36
Intrauterine growth retardation	–	–	50
Preterm delivery	–	60	80
Maternal outcome			
Hypertension	41	60	>80
Increase in proteinuria	40	60	>80
Temporary increase in serum creatinine	10.5	44	50
Permanent increase in serum creatinine	3.5	–	–
Accelerated decline to end-stage renal disease (ESRD)	–	20–50 (10% ESRD within 1 year)	>80

The percentage risk of fetal and maternal complications in women with pre-existing renal disease according to the degree of renal impairment. (Data summarized from references 5, 9–11, 29, 30 published 1980–1996.)

Table 45.4 Pregnancy outcome and renal impairment.

proteinuria. Since segmental proliferation, including crescent formation, is a feature of some cases of IgAN in non-pregnant individuals, it is not possible to confirm that pregnancy itself induced these changes in IgAN.

Jungers et al. reported that 9% of women with IgAN reached ESRD within 12 months of pregnancy[14]. Our own series included two patients (one of whom had pre-existing mild renal impairment) who followed a similar course and another three women who developed reversible renal impairment in pregnancy only to progress subsequently to ESRD 3, 4, and 7 years postpartum; others report 10% of patients reaching ERSD within 5 years. This is much worse than the natural history of IgAN in nonpregnant women, particularly as these patients had no adverse prognostic signs. Certainly our experience of an irreversible decline of renal function in 2% of cases and a permanent increase in blood pressure in 13% over the short period of a pregnancy cannot be regarded as part of the natural history of IgAN, nor can the severe hypertension that developed in relation to pregnancy in 20 patients.

Membranous nephropathy

In membranous nephropathy, we found that 24% of pregnancies resulted in fetal loss, 43% in premature delivery, and 33% in a live birth after 36 weeks of gestation. Maternal renal function declined during pregnancy in 9%, and in 46% hypertension developed. In 55%, proteinuria increased significantly during pregnancy. In 30%, nephrotic-range proteinuria was recorded in the first trimester. Presence of nephrotic-range proteinuria during the first trimester correlated with both poor fetal and poor maternal outcome[15].

Membranous nephropathy in women is usually a benign disorder that rarely progresses to renal failure. In addition, crescents are extremely rare whereas we found crescents in

Pregnancy and Renal Disease

three biopsies performed in pregnancy at the time of deterioration in renal function, suggesting that crescents contributed to the deterioration in renal function. The clinical feature which points to crescent formation is an increasing urinary erythrocyte count. Crescents are nearly always present with a urinary erythrocyte count above 10^6/mL.

Focal segmental glomerulosclerosis

A major consideration in pregnancy in women with primary focal segmental glomerulosclerosis (FSGS) is distinguishing between this lesion and focal, segmental lesions occurring as a complication of pre-eclampsia[16]. However, our diagnosis was based on biopsies in early pregnancy before pre-eclampsia developed, or on biopsy prior to or following pregnancy. In our series, fetal loss was high (45%), with a 35% incidence of stillbirth or neonatal deaths[5]. Maternal complications were also considerable: 13% of women suffered an irreversible decline in renal function and almost half showed some decline in renal function in pregnancy (44%). Hypertension developed in over half the patients and was severe in 45%. Comparison with other series is complicated by the use of the nonspecific nomenclature 'focal sclerosis' in those series: focal sclerosis occurs in a wide variety of renal diseases and the inclusion of such patients together with those having true primary FSGS might improve the apparent outcome.

Membranoproliferative glomerulonephritis
Type I

Membranoproliferative glomerulonephritis (MPGN) has become increasingly rare since the early 1970s and published series tend to include pregnancies taking place over a long time interval during which substantial improvements in obstetric and neonatal care have been made. Nevertheless, a poor pregnancy outcome was uniform in the reported series. While this condition is becoming increasingly uncommon in Western countries, it remains common in the developing world and it is likely that any more definitive studies are more likely to emerge from that area.

Type II: dense deposit disease

Our experience is that Type II MPGN has a more benign pregnancy prognosis than Type I. Of 14 pregnancies in seven women with Type II disease, all were successful and in none could an adverse effect of pregnancy on the course of the GN be identified. However, in all of these pregnancies the women exhibited clinical features that we associate with a stable course, namely: absence of recurrent macroscopic hematuria, low urinary erythrocyte and leukocyte counts, and the absence of heavy proteinuria. Acute renal failure associated with crescent formation has been described in pregnancy in MPGN Type II.

Diffuse non-IgA mesangial proliferative glomerulonephritis

Information on pregnancy outcome in diffuse non-IgA mesangial proliferative GN is limited, which probably reflects a reluctance to perform renal biopsies in cases of isolated microscopic hematuria. It has also been reported that a high proportion of patients with diffuse mesangial proliferative GN without mesangial IgA deposits have thin glomerular basement membranes on electron microscopy[17], suggesting that many women in the one large reported series[5] would now be diagnosed as having thin membrane nephropathy.

Our series of 168 pregnancies in 91 women had a late fetal loss rate of 12%[5]. Although less than that seen for other histologic patterns of GN, this appears high for a relatively benign condition. However, within our series, the renal disease presented for the first time on pregnancy in all but 6% of women, and a worse prognosis might be anticipated in such women compared with those diagnosed prior to pregnancy. A second factor, which correlated strongly with late fetal loss, was the presence of severe vascular lesions on renal biopsy. Given that a high proportion of these biopsies were performed during pregnancy, it is not possible to ascertain whether these changes predated pregnancy or were themselves pregnancy induced.

Maternal outcome in these patients was better than that in other histologic groups of GN. Only 3% of women developed a reversible decline in renal function; 33% developed reversible hypertension, and 52% developed reversible increases in proteinuria. Others have reported no difference in outcome between IgA nephropathy and non-IgA diffuse mesangial proliferative GN. This is not our experience and we believe that non-IgA mesangial proliferative GN diagnosed prior to pregnancy, and in the absence of significant vascular lesions on biopsy, carries a benign prognosis for pregnancy. Prospective data in pregnancy with an established diagnosis of thin membrane nephropathy can now be awaited with interest.

Systemic lupus erythematosus

Systemic lupus erythematosus most clearly exemplifies the need to analyze available data in renal disease according to the presence or absence of clinical and histologic features shown to influence pregnancy outcome. The presence of active nephritis and the lupus anticoagulant adversely influence outcome, as does the identification of lupus for the first time in the pregnancy.

Lupus anticoagulant (antiphospholipid antibodies)

The presence of a circulating lupus anticoagulant carries a substantial pregnancy risk factor for women with or without lupus in the absence of renal disease. It is associated with first and second trimester fetal loss in up to 40% of pregnancies. Following one such failed pregnancy, the risk of further fetal loss in a subsequent pregnancy is very high; in our experience around 80%. Thrombosis in renal and placental vessels is a feature of the antiphospholipid syndrome as also seen in pregnant women with renal disease (Figs 45.1 and 45.2). These thromboses led to our use of heparin and dipyridamole in pregnancy in patients with underlying renal disease. A controlled trial has shown that whereas only 42% of women with the antiphospholipid syndrome have living infants, this percentage is increased to 71% by administering 5000 units of unfractionated heparin subcutaneously from early pregnancy ($P < 0.01$)[18].

Maternal autoantibodies

Maternal autoantibodies known as anti-SSA/Ro and anti-SSB/La are typically found in Sjögren's syndrome and systemic

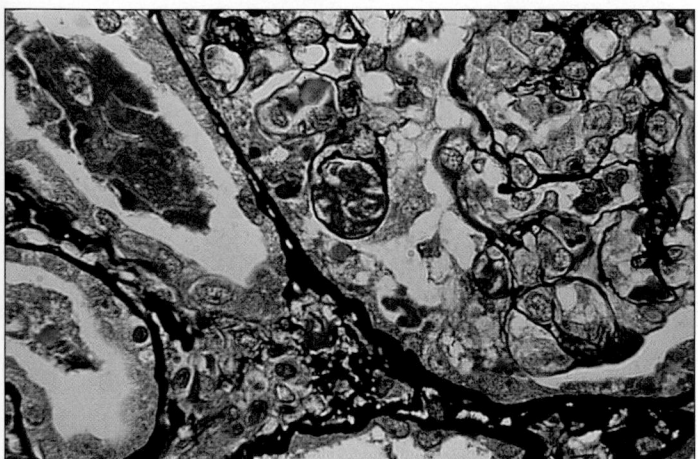

Figure 45.1 Glomerular fibrin deposition in pregnancy. Renal biopsy during pregnancy from a patient with reflux nephropathy showed fibrin thrombi (stained red) in a glomerular capillary lumen. Fibrin thrombi are not seen in reflux nephropathy except during pregnancy.

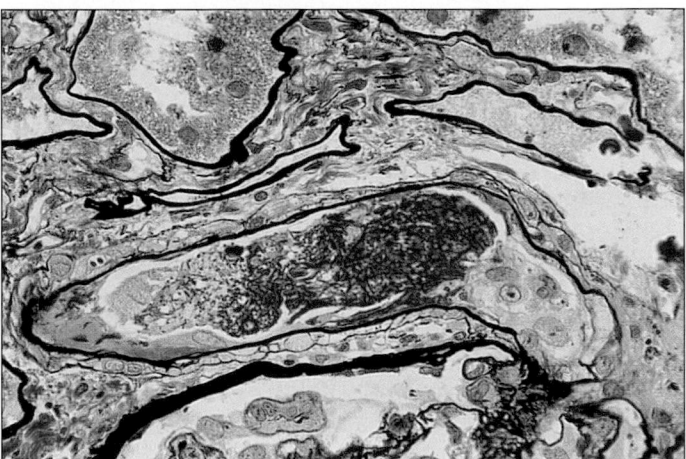

Figure 45.2 Arterial fibrin deposition in pregnancy. A fibrin thrombus in an interlobular artery in a patient with severe pre-eclampsia.

lupus. They are almost universally present when the rare complication of fetal congenital heart block occurs but are also present in up to half of women with a healthy fetus. More commonly these antibodies are associated with a transient neonatal lupus.

Lupus nephritis

In a series of 64 pregnancies in 41 women with biopsy-proven lupus nephritis[19], total fetal loss was 34% and perinatal mortality was 19%. However, those diagnosed prior to pregnancy had a 13% perinatal mortality compared with 33% for those diagnosed by renal biopsy during pregnancy or in the post-partum period. Overall fetal loss was 57% in patients with lupus anticoagulant and only 23% in those without. There was no perinatal mortality in women with membranous lupus nephritis compared with a perinatal mortality of 24% in those with diffuse proliferative lupus nephritis. Overall, maternal complications were impairment of renal function (11%), hypertension (44%), and increased proteinuria (50%); they were all more likely to occur in women diagnosed during pregnancy or in the postpartum period. There were no maternal deaths and no patient progressed to ESRD, but others have reported a maternal death rate of 3.4%[20] and an 8% incidence of ESRD[21].

Deterioration in renal function in pregnancy occurs in two-thirds of women with active lupus nephritis at the time of conception but in only one-third or less of those who have been in remission for at least 6 months at conception. Lupus nephritis should, therefore, be actively treated before pregnancy with the aim of inducing remission, ideally confirmed on renal biopsy, before pregnancy is undertaken. Maintenance therapy is then continued throughout pregnancy and in the postpartum period. For many women, this will require low-dose prednisolone and occasionally, azathioprine. Women may be reluctant to take treatment through conception and pregnancy for fear of inducing fetal damage, and the relative safety of medication and the risks of relapse in pregnancy to both mother and fetus must be strongly emphasized.

Flares may still develop in pregnancy and can cause diagnostic difficulty, especially in the differentiation from pre-eclampsia. Lupus flares will usually be accompanied by hypocomplementemia and a rise in anti-DNA antibody titers; there will also be hematuria and an active urine sediment. By comparison, in pre-eclampsia, proteinuria occurs with no other urine abnormality and complement is typically normal or raised. Whether flares of lupus are more likely to occur in the postpartum period remains controversial. It is less common than previously thought, especially if maintenance therapy is continued. We do not recommend a routine postpartum increase in corticosteroids.

Vasculitis

In contrast to lupus, which is a disease predominantly of women in their childbearing years, systemic vasculitis occurs in a substantially older age group and as much in men as in women As a consequence, there is little recorded experience of pregnancy in women with vasculitis and renal involvement. Available information suggests a very poor prognosis for both fetus and mother.

Diabetic nephropathy

Reported fetal outcome in women with diabetic nephropathy is generally good probably reflecting the careful monitoring of pregnancy and early treatment of hypertension. A systematic review of the literature between 1981 and 1996 reports a 5% perinatal mortality rate and preterm delivery in 22%[22]. This is similar to an earlier report where, excluding therapeutic abortions, fetal loss was 6%, with a 36% incidence of prematurity[23]. Later outcome is, however, also important; of concern is one series in which 20% of children had psychomotor retardation at later follow-up[24].

The situation regarding maternal complications is less encouraging. In one report, 32% of women had a decrease in renal function during pregnancy; in 58% there was an increase in blood pressure, and 13% had a progressive course[23]. Up to 80% of women may have increased proteinuria and many become nephrotic. While pregnancy did not seem immediately to accelerate the rate of decline in renal function, 8 of 29 mothers were on dialysis within 1 to 9 years postpartum of whom half died during the follow-up period. More recent pooled data found that of 185 patients available for long-term follow up (mean 35 months), 17% developed ESRD and 5% died as a result of renal failure[22]. If advising whether a diabetic woman with nephropathy should become pregnant, it should be remembered that these women are at risk of serious morbidity or even mortality while their children are still young. These women represent a group requiring specialized care and counseling before, during, and after pregnancy.

Reflux nephropathy

Reflux nephropathy is predominantly a disease of girls and young women. Those who progress to ESRD usually do so within their childbearing years. Fetal loss is reported in 14% of pregnancies[25,26]. As in other renal diseases, fetal loss and maternal complications are clearly related to renal function. Patients with plasma creatinine > 1.3 mg/dL (115 µmol/L) have a 24% fetal loss compared with 9% in those with normal plasma creatinine. Only 2% of pregnant women with reflux nephropathy and normal renal function had a deterioration in renal function, compared with 17% where renal function was impaired. Pregnancy itself is clearly associated with a more rapid deterioration in renal function than could be expected in women with initial serum creatinine > 2 mg/dL (180 µmol/L).

Polycystic kidney disease

Renal failure usually develops in the fourth or fifth decade of life; consequently, relatively few women with autosomal dominant polycystic kidney disease begin pregnancy with impaired renal function. Where renal impairment already exists, patients are presumed to continue in a similar manner to other women with renal impairment from alternative causes. Where renal function is preserved, pregnancy does not appear to be attended by excess fetal or maternal risk provided maternal hypertension, the single most important risk factor for maternal complications, is absent[27].

PREGNANCY AND PRE-EXISTING RENAL IMPAIRMENT

Pregnancy in women with pre-existing renal impairment is attended not only by an increased fetal and maternal complication rate but also by considerable likelihood of deterioration in renal function. An early report from our unit described 9 of 11 babies surviving in patients with renal impairment, but six of nine mothers died or developed ESRD soon after pregnancy[28]. However, subsequent improvements in obstetric and neonatal care might be expected to be associated with improved fetal and maternal outcome. Studies describing the outcome of 126 pregnancies in women with serum creatinine > 1.4 mg/dL (125 µmol/L)[29,30,31] are summarized in Table 45.4.

Fetal outcome
Moderate renal impairment
In women with serum creatinine between 1.4 and 2 mg/dL (125 and 180 µmol/L) fetal loss (excluding first-trimester

spontaneous or therapeutic abortions) is 22%, with up to 60% premature deliveries. However, an improving outcome in recent years is encouraging and presumably reflects increasing expertise in obstetric and neonatal care: Jungers et al. reported 28% fetal loss in pregnancies before 1984 and only 12% fetal loss in deliveries since 1985[31].

Uncontrolled blood pressure is the strongest independent risk factor for fetal loss. Fetal death is increased ten-fold in women with mean arterial pressure > 105 mmHg compared with those with normal values.

Severe renal impairment
The situation is still less favorable in women who embark on pregnancy with more severe renal impairment: serum creatinine > 2 mg/dL (180 µmol/L). Not only is there a fetal loss rate of 36%, but preterm delivery occurs in 80% of cases and IUGR in 50%. Mean live birth weight is reported as 1500 g.

Even here, there is some evidence of encouraging recent improvements. In one small series there was only one live birth among six pregnancies before 1984, but seven in nine occurring subsequent to 1985[31].

Maternal outcome
In moderate and severe renal impairment, maternal outcome worsens. Pre-eclampsia is superimposed in 60–80% of pregnancies especially if there was pre-existing hypertension. A rise in serum creatinine of 20–30% in the third trimester is very common and failure to return to prepregnancy values postpartum is a strong predictor of accelerated progression to ESRD. Accelerated progression occurs in 20–50% of women and 10% may reach ESRD within 12 months of pregnancy. There is no specific threshold for worsening prognosis but serum creatinine > 2 mg/dL (180 µmol/L) carries a high risk and for values above 3 mg/dL (270 µmol/L) accelerated deterioration in maternal renal function is virtually inevitable. A recent report of 14 pregnancies in 11 women with diabetic nephropathy and serum creatinine of 1.4 mg/dL before pregnancy or in the first trimester, showed an accelerated progression of renal disease in 45%[32]. Therefore, despite acceptable fetal survival rates, the likelihood of deterioration in renal function in pregnancy in patients with serum creatinine > 1.4 mg/dL (125 µmol/L) or blood urea nitrogen (BUN) > 25 mg/dL (urea 9 mmol/L) is high. Since renal function may remain stable for many years in patients with such levels of renal function if they do not become pregnant, we believe that a conservative approach in pregnancy counseling is appropriate in women with pre-existing renal impairment.

NEPHROTIC SYNDROME IN PREGNANCY

The management of nephrotic range proteinuria in pregnancy is determined by the underlying pathology. In late pregnancy (more than 30 weeks' gestation), nephrotic range proteinuria is most likely to occur as part of the clinical spectrum of pre-eclampsia and management will be directed to appropriate treatment of maternal complications and early delivery. However, prior to 30 weeks' gestation, the incidence of underlying renal disease has been shown in biopsy studies already described, to be high. In women where an underlying pathology has not been previously established, we believe that appropriate management should include renal biopsy, allowing targeted and appropriate therapy. For example, minimal change nephropathy might be expected to respond to corticosteroid therapy whilst an active lupus nephritis might require a more vigorous immunosuppressive regimen, for example with corticosteroids and azathioprine, although cyclophosphamide should be avoided.

PREGNANCY IN WOMEN ON MAINTENANCE DIALYSIS

Fertility is much reduced in women undergoing dialysis and in those who do become pregnant only a small minority have successful outcomes. Up to 1980, the European Dialysis and Transplant Association (EDTA) reported only 115 pregnancies among 13 000 women of childbearing age; of these only 16 (23%) ended successfully. There is, however, encouraging evidence of improving outcome[33]: while only 21% of such pregnancies before 1990 resulted in a live birth, 52% after 1990 were successful. Nevertheless, IUGR and preterm delivery are the norm, with very low birthweight babies usually requiring neonatal intensive care. A greater success rate of pregnancy in patients treated with continuous ambulatory peritoneal dialysis (CAPD) compared with hemodialysis has been reported[33]. CAPD has theoretical advantages, particularly a more consistent biochemical milieu and less hypotension, but the number of patients is still too small to provide conclusive evidence for the superiority of this technique.

Maternal complications are very common. Three maternal deaths have been reported in the 222 pregnancies recorded by the National Registry for Pregnancy in Dialysis Patients (NPDR). Hypertension may be severe. Severe hypertension (> 170/110 mmHg) was reported in more that half the pregnancies and there were five Intensive Care Unit admissions for accelerated hypertension[34]. Until the advent of epoetin, up to a third of patients required transfusion in pregnancy. The potential beneficial effects of epoetin on the course of pregnancy, and indeed fertility, remain to be assessed. However, when a dialysis patient becomes pregnant, an aggressive approach to management is justified to see whether by optimizing the milieu the pregnancy can be sustained. The management is discussed below.

PREGNANCY AFTER RENAL TRANSPLANTATION

Fertility is usually restored in women following successful renal transplant and for many young women with ESRD this will be one of the most important improvements in quality of life that will encourage them to go forward for transplantation. Davison has reviewed pregnancy outcome for 1569 pregnancies in 1009 transplant recipients[35]. In 38% the pregnancy ended in spontaneous or therapeutic abortion in the first trimester. Most proceeding beyond the first trimester were successful, although perinatal mortality was higher than that in the general population at 8%. The incidence of congenital abnormalities at 3% was no higher than expected and the few follow-up data on children born from transplant

recipients do not suggest an increased rate of developmental abnormalities. In 15% of pregnancies, maternal renal function deteriorated towards ESRD. Chronic rejection accounted for most of these cases[35].

However, within that overall summary there is substantial variation in fetal and maternal risk that parallels closely that described above for women with pre-existing renal disease (Table 45.4). For transplant recipients with normal serum creatinine, no proteinuria, and well-controlled hypertension, the risk of maternal complications is small and fetal loss is only 4%. However, if renal impairment predates pregnancy in patients with a renal transplant, the maternal outcome parallels that of women without transplant with renal impairment who become pregnant. Deterioration in serum creatinine is frequent when pre-pregnancy creatinine is > 2 mg/dL (180 µmol/L) and persists in 15% of cases postpartum. In order to assess whether pregnancy might interfere with the natural history of the patient's graft, the EDTA registry set up a case-control study that analyzed 53 pairs of transplant recipients and their matched controls. This study detected no differences in serum creatinine between pregnant and nonpregnant groups at 12 months postpartum. Whether the natural history of the grafts in those women who show apparently reversible deterioration during pregnancy is affected in the long term requires further study.

Maternal complications other than impairment in renal function are also increased. The estimated prevalence of preeclampsia is 30%. Hypertension in pregnancy in women with renal transplants is more than three times that of the general population and may be severe.

IMMUNOSUPPRESSIVE AGENTS IN PREGNANCY

Maintenance immunosuppressive therapy is required for substantial numbers of women with renal disease who become pregnant, including renal transplant recipients and those with lupus nephritis or other immune disease. Women should be advised of the relative risks of these agents in pregnancy and the benefits of continuing to take them.

Corticosteroids
While high-dose corticosteroids have been implicated in increased risk of fetal cleft palate and osteoporosis, there is no evidence that low dose (< 15 mg prednisolone daily) has any adverse fetal effects. Dose adjustment is not usually required. Prednisolone is however only detected at low levels in cord blood, whereas dexamethasone is present in cord blood at substantially higher concentrations and is, therefore, the preferred corticosteroid for therapy intended to increase fetal lung maturity.

Azathioprine
Extensive experience in transplant recipients indicates that azathioprine is a very safe agent in pregnancy with no known adverse fetal effects.

Cyclophosphamide
Cyclophosphamide may produce both male and female infertility, especially in cumulative doses above 200 mg/kg. When cyclophosphamide is given for treatment of lupus or vasculitis,

Pregnancy and Renal Disease

sperm or oocyte storage should be offered where appropriate to young men and women before therapy is initiated. Cyclophosphamide is also teratogenic and should be avoided in the first trimester. Evidence that it is damaging to the fetus beyond the first trimester is scanty, but it should be avoided if possible and only used for major flares of disease where organ function is threatened. Women should be advised not to become pregnant within 1 year of treatment with cyclophosphamide.

Chlorambucil
Less evidence is available for therapy with chlorambucil than for cyclophosphamide, but it also appears to be teratogenic and it should likewise be avoided in pregnancy.

Cyclosporine
There is now wide experience with thousands of successful pregnancies over more than 15 years in renal transplant recipients taking cyclosporine in maintenance dosage of 5 mg/kg daily or less. There is no evidence of adverse fetal effects other than a high proportion of babies who are small for gestational age, which may represent the effects of pregnancy with mild renal impairment and hypertension rather than the effect of cyclosporine. Monitoring of drug levels should continue as usual through pregnancy, but dose adjustments are not usually required.

Tacrolimus
With the increasing use of tacrolimus as a primary immunosuppressant, a growing number of reports have been published of pregnancies occurring in mothers receiving tacrolimus. The largest of these (100 pregnancies in 84 women with a variety of organ transplants, including kidney), reported favorable outcomes with complications to mother and fetus similar to conventional immunosuppression[36].

Mycophenolate
There are as yet insufficient data on the use of mycophenolate in pregnancy. Therefore mycophenolate should be discontinued before pregnancy, switching if appropriate to azathioprine.

Sirolimus
Sirolimus should not be used in pregnancy. It should be discontinued at least 6 weeks before conception is planned, substituting cyclosporine or tacrolimus as appropriate.

OKT3 and polyclonal antibodies
OKT3, an immunoglobulin, crosses the placenta as do polyclonal antibodies, such as ATG. Their effect on the developing fetus is not known. However, the NPDR has reported the treatment of five women with OKT3 during pregnancy, with four surviving infants[37].

MECHANISMS BY WHICH DETERIORATION IN RENAL FUNCTION MIGHT OCCUR IN PREGNANCY

Hyperfiltration
In normal pregnancy, in both humans and experimental animals, there is increased renal perfusion and glomerular filtration rate (GFR), but glomerular pressure does not rise. However in intrinsic renal disease, some increase in glomerular pressure may occur in pregnancy; this may theoretically be a mechanism for acceleration of renal disease during pregnancy. Whether the duration of such increases is sufficient to provoke progressive disease when renal mass is reduced is controversial. Brenner has suggested that the development of progressive renal insufficiency, in conjunction with sclerosis of residual glomeruli, is caused by hyperfiltration of the renal remnant. It has been argued that sustained increases in GFR are necessary for the 'Brenner hypothesis' to hold true and that human gestation is too short for such changes to occur, even with repetitive pregnancies. However, if renal disease prepregnancy had already resulted in increased or maximal single nephron perfusion, then the increased GFR of pregnancy could only be achieved by increasing effective transglomerular capillary pressure or decreasing the glomerular filtration coefficient. If such changes occurred in pregnancy, even in the absence of systemic arterial hypertension, intrarenal hypertension may be present throughout. Such intrarenal hypertension, which would result in increased transcapillary hydrostatic pressure, has been postulated as being the initiator and mode of progression of a variety of glomerulopathies. A further effect of the postulated combination of increased transglomerular capillary pressure and reduced filtration coefficient would be increased proteinuria, which itself may engender further glomerular damage by causing increased mesangial uptake of plasma proteins. It is interesting to speculate that pregnancy-associated lesions – focal and segmental hyalinosis and sclerosis, and active crescents – may be stimulated by increased proteinuria.

Focal and segmental hyalinosis
We have described the appearance of focal and segmental hyalinosis during pregnancy and their disappearance after pregnancy in patients with various forms of GN[5]. They are particularly common in IgAN, in which 67% of biopsies taken during pregnancy show segmental hyalinosis compared with only 9% of biopsies from nonpregnant women. These lesions may be a thrombotic manifestation[13].

Crescents
We have demonstrated the development of crescents adjacent to the subendothelial deposits of pre-eclampsia (Fig. 45.3), linking crescent formation to this specific glomerular lesion. The development of crescents was accompanied by increased proteinuria, severe hypertension, and deterioration in renal function. A reluctance to perform renal biopsy during pregnancy may be obscuring the importance of similar lesions in patients with pre-existing renal disease. For example, crescents are an extremely uncommon finding in membranous nephropathy, but were detected in three biopsies performed in pregnant women with this diagnosis. Biopsies performed after pregnancy might be expected only to show the end result of glomerular damage by crescent formation (i.e., glomerular sclerosis).

Hypercoagulable state
Pregnancy is a 'hypercoagulable state', which may account for the tendency for women in pregnancy to develop intravascular

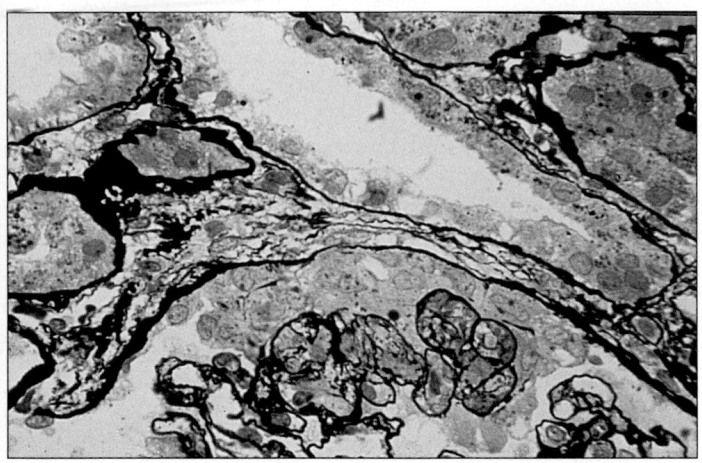

Figure 45.3 Crescent formation in pre-eclampsia. Renal biopsy from a patient with IgA nephropathy during an episode of pre-eclampsia in late pregnancy. Note that the crescent has developed in relation to fibrinoid subendothelial deposits (stained red), which are typical of pre-eclampsia.

coagulation and glomerular fibrin deposition. There is morphologic evidence of the participation of intravascular coagulation in the pathogenesis of glomerular and vascular lesions[38]. Deterioration in renal function during pregnancy has been recorded together with the development of active crescents in association with fibrinoid deposits. Although

such lesions have been recorded infrequently, this may well reflect the scarcity of data on renal biopsies performed during pregnancy and in the very early postpartum period. Frank fibrin may appear in glomerular capillaries during pregnancy both in mild disease such as thin membrane nephropathy and in more advanced disease such as reflux nephropathy (Fig. 45.1). Fibrin is found in blood vessels in biopsies in pre-eclampsia (see Figs 45.2 and 45.3) and may, therefore, be a factor in deterioration of renal function in renal disease. The lesions of focal and segmental hyalinosis, which appear so frequently during pregnancy, may also have a thrombotic basis.

ADVICE TO PATIENTS WITH RENAL DISEASE WISHING TO BECOME PREGNANT

Women with pre-existing renal impairment should be cautioned on the risks associated with pregnancy. The broad categories of risk summarized in Table 45.4 provide the basis for the management strategy and advice given (see Fig. 45.4).

For those with pre-existing renal disease and normal renal function it is rarely necessary to caution against pregnancy. The need for careful monitoring and a discussion of increased maternal morbidity is appropriate but the risk of irreversible decline in renal function is small. A decision regarding pregnancy will usually be arrived at by the patient and her partner after considering these factors and other social factors such as pre-existing family size.

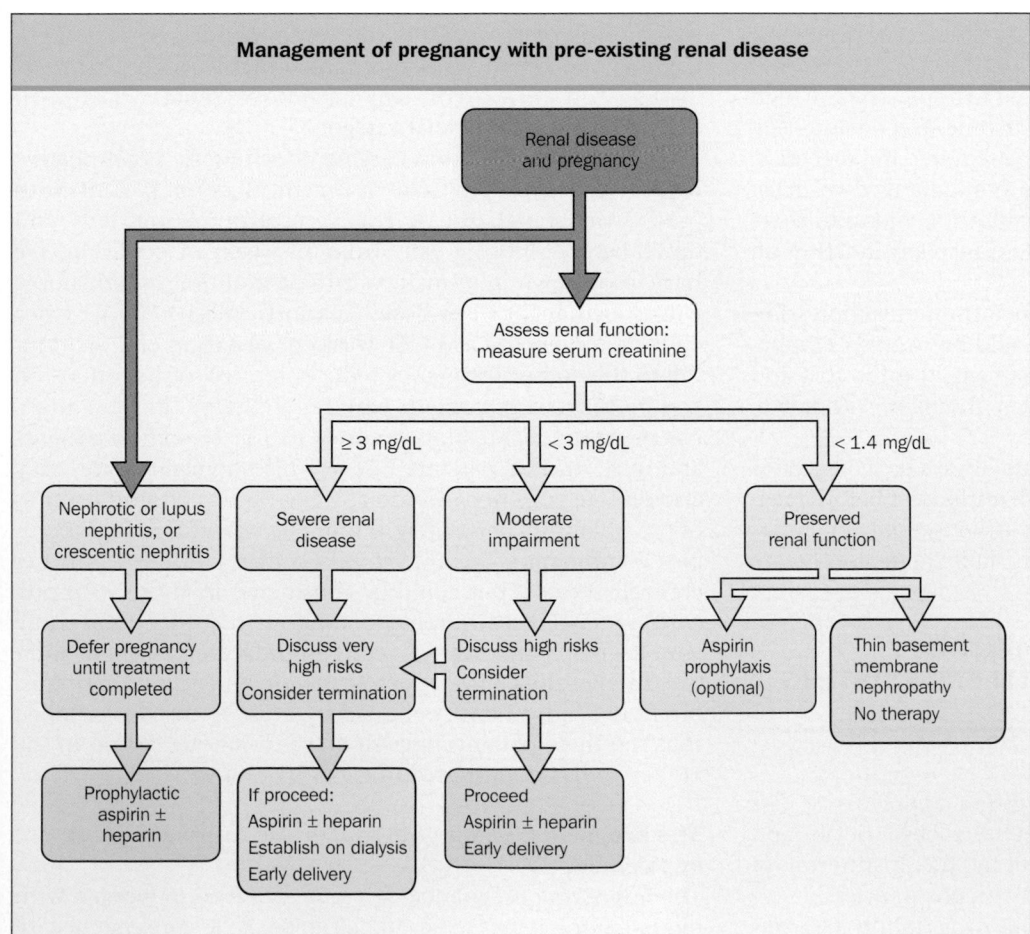

Figure 45.4 Management strategy for pregnancy in women with pre-existing renal disease.

The exceptions are those women who despite normal renal function have an active, crescentic GN or are nephrotic. In both these circumstances, pregnancy should be delayed until appropriate treatment has been given. The success of this approach is now generally accepted in diffuse proliferative lupus nephritis, but our experience suggests that a similar approach may be indicated in other forms of GN, particularly IgAN with crescents on biopsy. Nephrotic syndrome is a major risk factor for poor fetal outcome and attempts should be made to reduce proteinuria and improve hypoalbuminemia prior to pregnancy.

For women with pre-existing renal impairment, fetal complication rates remain far higher than in the general population and prematurity is so common as to be almost the norm. Deterioration in renal function can be expected in 30–60% of patients, and women should be apprised of the risk of requiring dialysis either during pregnancy or relatively soon after delivery.

For some women with chronic renal disease, pregnancy will carry a high risk and a more appropriate and safer time for pregnancy may be later in the natural history of the renal disease when the woman has had a successful renal transplant. However, if the renal disease is very slowly progressive, most commonly reflux nephropathy, such a delay may take the woman beyond her childbearing years. Adoption may be an alternative parenting option, but in many countries adoption agencies look unfavorably on women with chronic renal disease as adopting parents and this choice may not be available. As a consequence, women are sometimes tempted to embark on very high-risk pregnancies with pre-existing poor renal function as their one chance of having a child; they need most careful medical and social support.

Women already on dialysis will need to appreciate the high risk of early fetal loss, the uncertain outcome, and the intensity of therapy and monitoring that will be required in pregnancy.

Women with renal transplants are encouraged to delay pregnancy until 2 years after transplantation, and until there has been at least 12 months of stable transplant function on maintenance therapy.

The need to continue maintenance immunosuppression and treatment for blood pressure should be strongly emphasized. Angiotensin-converting enzyme (ACE) inhibitors and angiotensin receptor antagonists (ATRA) should be withdrawn, if possible before conception.

Women with lupus nephritis should always be screened for lupus anticoagulant and anti-SSA/SSB antibodies before pregnancy, and the risks of positivity discussed (see above). Lupus nephritis should be treated to obtain stable remission before pregnancy.

MANAGEMENT AND TREATMENT IN PREGNANCY IN WOMEN WITH PRE-EXISTING RENAL DISEASE

Clinical monitoring

Optimal pregnancy outcome for mother and fetus is best ensured by close co-operation between obstetrician and nephrologist. This is best achieved by the institution of combined clinics for those with high-risk pregnancies.

We review patients at 12–15 weeks of gestation and perform tests of renal function, including creatinine clearance,

urinary protein excretion, and careful urine microscopy. A failure of the expected increase in creatinine clearance over pre-pregnancy levels at this stage indicates an increased likelihood of complications later in pregnancy. Subsequently, patients are monitored frequently with special attention to blood pressure, weight gain, and proteinuria. Uterine artery Doppler sonography may be a useful adjunct to monitoring and we have seen very abnormal uterine artery wave forms at 20 weeks of gestation that have improved rapidly with treatment.

Before 28–30 weeks of gestation, any sudden deterioration in the monitored biochemical and clinical indices may well prompt renal biopsy. However, the widespread use of aspirin in 'high-risk' pregnancies (see below) may increasingly preclude this approach.

From 26 weeks of gestation, hemoglobin, hematocrit, platelet count, and uric acid levels are added to the regular biochemical and clinical testing, and selected patients may also require regular liver function tests. From 28 weeks, clinical and biochemical screening is usually on a weekly basis.

Antithrombotic and antiplatelet treatment

Following a study in 1985 showing that aspirin and dipyridamole commencing at 12–14 weeks of gestation considerably improved outcome in women with underlying renal disease, aspirin entered widespread use[39]. Unfortunately, there has been no other controlled trial of aspirin in women with underlying renal disease to confirm its benefit. The role of aspirin in the general prevention of pre-eclampsia remains controversial, with conflicting evidence from controlled trials[40]. However, aspirin is still recommended in very high-risk pregnancies and it is appropriate that women with renal disease and those with any degree of renal impairment should be regarded in that category[40].

Except for cases of thin basement membrane nephropathy, who receive no prophylactic treatment, all of our patients with pre-existing renal disease receive aspirin 75 mg daily and dipyridamole 400 mg daily from 12 weeks of gestation. We have also shown in a small controlled trial that dipyridamole with subcutaneous low-dose heparin (7500–10 000 IU twice daily) commencing at 14–16 weeks of gestation and continuing to the end of pregnancy reduces the risk of hypertension and proteinuria in patients with renal disease. In these high-risk pregnancies, fetal loss occurred in 5 of 11 control patients and in no treated patients[41]. Severe histological features may also resolve with heparin therapy even when clinical features of pre-eclampsia persist (Fig. 45.5). The role of this more complex combination therapy requires confirmation with further controlled trials, but could be considered in those with pre-existing renal disease and a poor obstetric history, or in those who develop complications early in their pregnancy. As indicated above, the value of heparin in women with the antiphospholipid syndrome is supported by a randomized controlled trial and these patients have similar thrombotic lesions in the kidney to those illustrated in Figs 45.1 and 45.2.

The pregnant patient with moderate-to-severe renal impairment

The improving pregnancy outcome achieved in women with moderate-to-severe renal impairment is a consequence of intensive management[33]. The mother must be protected from

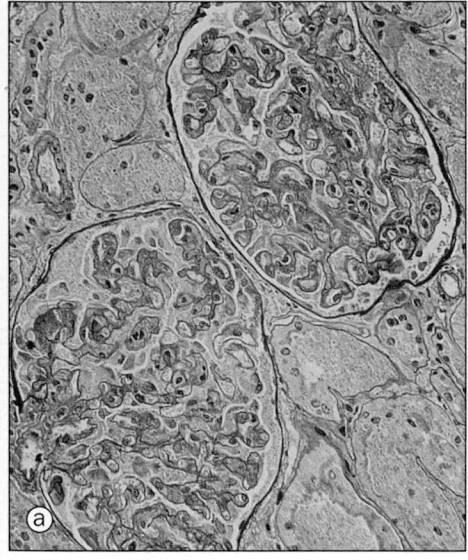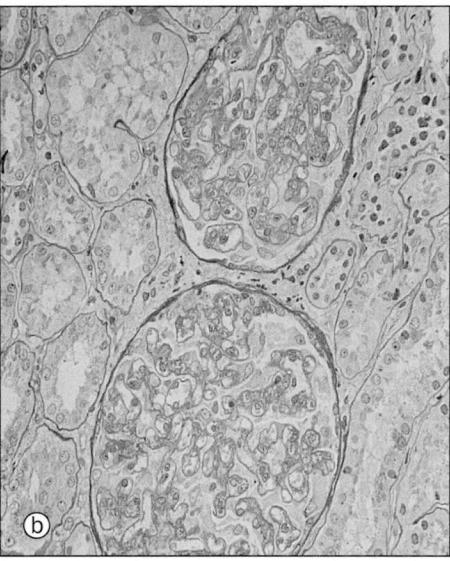

Figure 45.5 Effect of heparin in pre-eclampsia. (a) Renal biopsy at 27–30 weeks of gestation in severe pre-eclampsia. (b) Biopsy after 18 days of heparin therapy. The histologic abnormalities resolved despite continuation of the pregnancy and persisting proteinuria and hypertension.

Management of pregnancy with severe renal impairment		
Treatment area	Target	Strategy
Aspirin	Prophylaxis	75 mg daily from 12 weeks of gestation
Blood pressure	Diastolic 80–90 mmHg	Avoid ACE inhibitors, ATRA diuretics First line: methyldopa, β-blockers Second line: calcium channel blockers, α-blockers
Anemia	Maintain hemoglobin > 11 g/dL	Iron and folate supplements; start or increase epoetin
Metabolic acidosis	Maintain serum bicarbonate > 24 mmol/L	Sodium bicarbonate supplements
Calcium	Maintain normocalcemia	Diet, calcium carbonate, vitamin D analogs
Nutrition	Ensure high-class protein intake	Daily intake 1 g/kg + 20 g for fetal growth

Table 45.5 Management of pregnancy with severe renal impairment.

the risks of uncontrolled hypertension and severe pre-eclampsia. The internal milieu for the fetus must also be optimized since it is fetal loss caused by IUGR and death that has led to the poor outcome in these patients. The management of these patients is summarized in Table 45.5.

Blood pressure treatment
Target diastolic blood pressure should be < 80 mmHg throughout pregnancy. ACE inhibitors and ATRA are contraindicated in pregnancy as they produce fetal cardiac complications that may be fatal; ideally, they should be discontinued before conception. Early experience showed that diuretics were safe but some avoid them as this may aggravate the volume contraction seen in pre-eclampsia. The widest experience in pregnancy is with the use of methyldopa, β-blockers and labetalol. However, there is also increasing experience with calcium channel blockers, and we would not normally change an established successful antihypertensive regimen at the beginning of pregnancy. However, if additional treatment is required as blood pressure rises throughout pregnancy, methyldopa should be first choice.

Anemia
Iron and folate supplements will be required. In patients with severely impaired renal function or those on dialysis, epoetin should be initiated or increased to maintain hemoglobin levels above 11 g/dL.

Nutrition
Maintenance of adequate protein and calorie intake is important. A daily intake of 1 g/kg of high-class protein is recommended, with an additional 20 g daily for fetal growth. Adequate calories providing at least 35 kcal/g protein must be ensured for full utilization of protein.

Metabolic acidosis
Metabolic acidosis must be avoided, and oral supplementation with sodium bicarbonate may be required.

Hypocalcemia
Hypocalcemia is common as a result of fetal calcium demands. As well as optimizing dietary intake, increasing doses of oral calcium carbonate and vitamin D may be needed.

Dialysis
Dialysis should be initiated in the woman whose renal function deteriorates in pregnancy. The threshold for dialysis is usually serum creatinine 3.5–4 mg/dL (320–360 µmol/L) and BUN 50 mg/dL (urea 18 mmol/L), or even lower if acidosis, fluid overload, or blood pressure cannot be controlled. Pregnant women already on dialysis will require intensification of the regimen in order to maintain BUN below 40 mg/dL (urea 14 mmol/L) to avoid polyhydramnios.

Pregnancy and Renal Disease

Hemodialysis regimens should be increased to at least five sessions weekly with bicarbonate buffer and slow ultrafiltration to minimize volume contraction and hypotension.

Peritoneal dialysis exchange volumes may need reducing to avoid discomfort and an increase to five or six exchanges daily may be necessary. It has been proposed that peritoneal dialysis is superior to hemodialysis for pregnancy outcome, but this is not established and continuation of the woman's dialysis regimen at conception is recommended.

Intensification of dialysis is usually sufficient to control acidosis but oral bicarbonate may still be needed. Care should be taken to avoid hypercalcemia at the end of hemodialysis if dialysate with a supraphysiologic ionized calcium concentration is in use. Dialysis regimens in pregnancy are shown in Table 45.6.

Management of late pregnancy

Intensive monitoring of fetal well-being and the closest interaction between nephrologist and obstetrician are necessary to maximize the chance of a successful outcome. There is a high incidence of premature labor. Nonsteroidal anti-inflammatory agents have been advocated as effective in reducing premature contractions but are associated with premature closure of the ductus arteriosus and fetal anuria and are not recommended. Early operative delivery is often required if there is evidence of fetal compromise.

Postpartum management

For women with independent renal function, the postpartum period also requires careful management. Blood pressure can usually be reduced or brought to normal under close supervision. Proteinuria will usually lessen and third-trimester elevations in serum creatinine may improve. However, in more severe renal impairment, a trend of decline in renal

Dialysis regimens in pregnancy	
Regimen	
Pre-dialysis pregnancy	Institute dialysis if serum creatinine rises above 3.5–4.0 mg/dL, BUN
Pregnancy on dialysis	Intensify dialysis to maintain BUN < 50 mg/dL
Hemodialysis	5 treatments per week, bicarbonate buffer, avoid hypotension
Peritoneal dialysis	1.5 L exchange volumes, 4–5 exchanges per day
Metabolic acidosis	Oral sodium bicarbonate if predialysis serum bicarbonate < 24 mmol/L
Serum calcium	Avoid end-dialysis hypocalcemia or hypercalcemia by modifying dialysate calcium

Table 45.6 Dialysis regimens in pregnancy.

function established in late pregnancy may continue relentlessly. Women in whom dialysis is initiated during pregnancy may rarely become dialysis independent.

The pregnant transplant recipient

Maintenance immunosuppressive regimens using calcineurin inhibitors, azathioprine and corticosteriods should continue unchanged, but mycophenolate and sirolimus should be stopped, ideally before conception. Blood pressure is managed along the lines defined above.

The transplant kidney does not obstruct the birth canal and presents no restriction to vaginal delivery. Operative delivery is however more common because of the increased incidence of IUGR requiring pre-term delivery.

REFERENCES

1. Jungers P, Chauveau D. Pregnancy in renal disease. Kidney Int. 1997;52:871–85.
2. Chesley LC. Diagnosis of pre-eclampsia. Obstet Gynecol. 1985; 65:423–53.
3. Murakami S, Saitoh M, Kubo T, et al. Renal disease in women with severe pre-eclampsia or gestational proteinuria. Obstet Gynecol. 2000;96:945–96.
4. Packham DK, Matthews DC, Fairley KF, et al. Morphometric analysis of pre-eclampsia in women biopsied in pregnancy and post partum. Kidney Int. 1988;34:704–11.
5. Packham DK, North RA, Fairley KF, et al. Primary glomerulonephritis and pregnancy. Q J Med. 1989;70:537–53.
6. Abe S, Amagasaki Y, Konishik, et al. The influence of antecedent renal disease on pregnancy. Obstet Gynecol. 1985;153:508–14.
7. Packham DK, Fairley KF. Renal biopsy: indications and complications in pregnancy. Br J Obstet Gynaecol. 1987;94:935–9.
8. Fraser IR, Fairley KF. Renal biopsy as an outpatient procedure. Am J Kid Dis. 1995;25,26:876–77.
9. Katz A, Davidson J, Hayslett J, et al. Pregnancy in women with kidney disease. Kidney Int. 1980;18:192–206.
10. Surian M, Imbasciati E, Cosci P, et al. Glomerular disease in pregnancy. Nephron. 1984;36:101–5.
11. Jungers P, Houllier P, Forget D, et al. Influence of pregnancy on the course of primary chronic glomerulonephritis. Lancet. 1995;346:1122–4.
12. Packham DK, North RA, Fairley K.F, et al. IgA glomerulonephritis and pregnancy. Clin Nephrol. 1998:30:15–21.
13. Packham DK, Whitworth JA, Fairley KF, Kincaid-Smith P. Histological features of IgA glomerulonephritis as predictors of pregnancy outcome. Clin Nephrol 1988;30:22–6.
14. Jungers P, Forget D, Houllier P, et al. Pregnancy in IgA nephropathy, reflux nephropathy and focal glomerular sclerosis. Am J Kidney Dis. 1987;9:334–9.
15. Packham DK, North R, Fairley KF, et al. Membranous glomerulonephritis and pregnancy. Clin Nephrol. 1987;28:256–64.
16. Kida H, Takeda S, Yokoyama H, et al. Focal glomerular sclerosis in pre-eclampsia. Clin Nephrol. 1985;24:221–7.
17. Kincaid-Smith P. Unexplained haematuria. Br Med J. 1991; 302:177.
18. Rai R, Cohen H, Dave M, Regan L. Randomised controlled trial of aspirin and aspirin plus heparin in pregnant women with recurrent miscarriage associated with phospholipid antibodies (or antiphospholipid antibodies). Br Med J. 1997; 314:253.
19. Packham DK, Lam SS, Nicholls K, et al. Lupus nephritis and pregnancy. Q J Med. 1992;83:315–24.
20. Cameron JS, Hicks J. Pregnancy in patients with pre-existing glomerular disease. Contrib Nephrol. 1984;37:149–56.
21. Bobrie G, Loite F, Houllier P, et al. Pregnancy in lupus nephritis and related disorders. Am J Kidney Dis. 1987;9:339–43.

22. Reece EA, Leguizamon G, Homko C. Pregnancy performance and outcomes associated with diabetic nephropathy. Am J Perinatol. 1998;15:413–21.

23. Imbasciati E, Pardi G, Capetta P, et al. Pregnancy in women with chronic renal failure. Am J Nephrol. 1986;6:193–8.

24. Kimmerle R, Zass RP, Cupisti S, et al. Pregnancies in women with diabetic nephropathy: long-term outcome for mother and child. Diabetologia. 1995;38:227–37.

25. El Katib M, Packham DK, Becker GJ, Kincaid-Smith P. Pregnancy-related complications in women with reflux nephropathy. Clin Nephrol. 1994;41:50–4.

26. Jungers P, Houllier P, Chauveau D, et al. Pregnancy in women with reflux nephropathy. Kidney Int. 1996;50:593–9.

27. Chapman AB, Johnson AM, Gabow PA. Pregnancy outcome and its relationship to progression of renal failure in autosomal dominant polycystic kidney disease. J Am Soc Nephrol. 1994;5:1179–85.

28. Kincaid-Smith P, Fairley KF, Bullen M. Kidney disease and pregnancy. Med J Aust. 1967;2:1155–9.

29. Hou S, Grossman S, Madias N. Pregnancy in women with renal disease and moderate renal insufficiency. Am J Med. 1985;78:185–94.

30. Jones DC, Hayslett JP. Outcome of pregnancy in women with moderate or severe renal insufficiency. N Engl J Med. 1996;335:226–32.

31. Jungers P, Chauveau D, Choukroun G, et al. Pregnancy in women with impaired renal function. Clin Nephrol. 1997;47:281–8.

32. Purdy LP, Hautsch CE, Molitch ME, et al. Effect of pregnancy on renal function in women with moderate to severe diabetic renal insufficiency. Diabetic Care. 1996;19:1067–74.

33. Hou SH. Pregnancy in women on haemodialysis and peritoneal dialysis. Baillière's Clin Obstet Gynaecol. 1994;8:481–500.

34. Okundaye Ibm Abrinko P, Hov S. A registry for pregnancy in dialysis patients. Am J Kidney Dis. 1998;31:766–73.

35. Davison JM. The effect of pregnancy on kidney function in renal allograft recipients. Kidney Int. 1985;27:74–9.

36. Kainz A, Harabacz I, Cowlrick I et al. Review of the course and outcome of 100 pregnancies in 84 women treated with Tacrolimus. Transplantation. 2000;70:1718–21.

37. Eisenberg JA, Armenti UT, McGrory CH, et al. Use of muromonals – CD3(OKT3) during pregnancy in female transplant recipients. Am Soc Trans Phys 1997;20:108 (abst).

38. Kincaid-Smith P. Participation of intravascular coagulation in the pathogenesis of glomerular and vascular lesions. Kidney Int. 1975;7:242–53.

39. Beaufils M, Uzan S, Donslmoni R, et al. Prevention of pre-eclampsia by early antiplatelet therapy. Lancet. 1985;1:840–2.

40. Paller MS. Hypertension in pregnancy. J Am Soc Nephrol. 1998;9:314–21.

41. Kincaid-Smith P, North RA, Fairley KF, et al. Prevention of pre-eclampsia in high risk women with renal disease: a prospective randomised trial of heparin and dipyridamole. Nephrology. 1995;1:297–300.

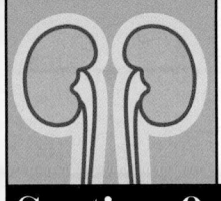

Chapter 46

Autosomal Dominant Polycystic Kidney Disease

Deirdre A O'Sullivan and Vicente E Torres

INTRODUCTION AND DEFINITION

Autosomal dominant polycystic kidney disease (ADPKD) is a multisystem disorder characterized by multiple, bilateral renal cysts associated with cysts in other organs such as liver, pancreas and arachnoid membranes. Noncystic, extrarenal manifestations of ADPKD include mitral valve prolapse, intracranial aneurysms and hernias. It is a genetic disorder, expressed in an autosomal dominant pattern, with 100% penetrance but variable expression. ADPKD is a genetically heterogeneous disease. Sonographic diagnostic criteria for individuals with a known family history of ADPKD include: two cysts arising unilaterally or bilaterally for individuals less than 30 years of age, two cysts in each kidney for individuals 30–59 years of age, and at least four cysts in each kidney for those over the age of 60[1]. These criteria may not apply to patients with *PKD2* mutations (see below). As many as one-third of ADPKD patients with *PKD2* mutations younger than 30 years of age may have less than two renal cysts detectable by ultrasound[2]. Very rarely, ADPKD will present in infancy as large echogenic kidneys without distinct, macroscopic cysts and is another exception to these criteria. Because of the possibility of clinical presentation in infancy, the term autosomal dominant polycystic kidney disease is preferred to adult polycystic kidney disease and the latter has been abandoned. Although benign renal cysts are common over the age of 50, multiple bilateral cysts are not. Therefore, an underlying inherited disease should be considered in patients with normal renal function who have multiple bilateral renal cysts.

ETIOLOGY AND PATHOGENESIS

Genetics

Identification of the genes responsible for ADPKD has provided a major breakthrough in the study of this disease[3–6]. *PKD1* is the gene responsible for 85–90% of clinically detected cases of ADPKD. A second gene, in the long arm of chromosome 4, *PKD2*, has been identified. Though it has not been mapped, a third gene for ADPKD exists as evidenced by the absence of linkage to *PKD1* and *PKD2* in certain families with ADPKD phenotype. In addition, a genetically distinct form of autosomal dominant polycystic liver disease (ADPLD) without kidney involvement has been mapped to chromosome 19[7].

The intron–exon sequences of the *PKD1* and *PKD2* genes are illustrated in Fig. 46.1[8]. Though *PKD2* is a larger gene, the open reading frame of *PKD1* is larger than *PKD2*. Approximately 75% of the *PKD1* gene is duplicated at least three times on chromosome 16. These duplicated segments are designated homologous genes. The *PKD1* gene contains three long polypyrimidine tracts within introns 1, 21 and 22 which may predispose to triple helix formation, erroneous repair and mutations during transcription. The mutations of both *PKD1* and *PKD2* are unique and dispersed over the entire gene. Most mutations identified so far are frameshift or nonsense mutations giving rise to truncated proteins.

The proteins encoded by *PKD1* and *PKD2* have been named polycystin 1 and polycystin 2 respectively and their structure predicted by their gene sequence has been determined by computer modeling[3–6] (Fig. 46.1). Polycystin 1 is predicted to contain a large N-terminal extracellular region, multiple transmembrane domains and a C-terminal cytoplasmic tail. This structure suggests that polycystin 1 may play a role in cell–cell or cell–matrix interactions. A region of polycystin 1 shares strong sequence homology to the receptor for egg jelly (REJ) module of the sea urchin. Binding of this receptor by egg-jelly glycoprotein results in an acrosomal reaction, an ion channel event. This suggests that polycystin 1 may also play a role in the regulation of an ion channel.

Polycystin 2 contains an N-terminal cytoplasmic domain, six transmembrane domains and a C-terminal cytoplasmic tail. The region that extends from the second transmembrane domain to the C-terminus has similarity to a voltage-activated calcium channel. Experiments using a two-hybrid system or co-immunoprecipitation have demonstrated that polycystin 1 and polycystin 2 can physically interact and suggest that the two may function through a common signaling pathway[9].

Using antibodies directed against its nonduplicated portion, polycystin 1, has been identified in various tissues such as the kidney, liver, pancreas, mammary ducts, intestinal crypts, myocardium, vascular smooth muscle of elastic and distributive arteries and certain endothelial cells[10–13]. In the kidney, staining is confined to the epithelial cells, with both cytoplasmic and cell surface associated localizations. Expression appears to be more intense in fetal than adult tissues. Transient expression is observed during development in the ureteric bud, S-shaped bodies, elongating nephron and proximal tubules. In adult kidneys most staining is found in distal tubules and increases in regenerating proximal tubules following acute tubular necrosis. In polycystic kidneys, there is strong staining of the cyst epithelium and less consistently in the noncystic tubules. However, 20–30% of cysts do not stain. The pattern of polycystin 2 expression in the developing kidney is similar to that observed for polycystin 1. In adult tissue, the pattern of expression is

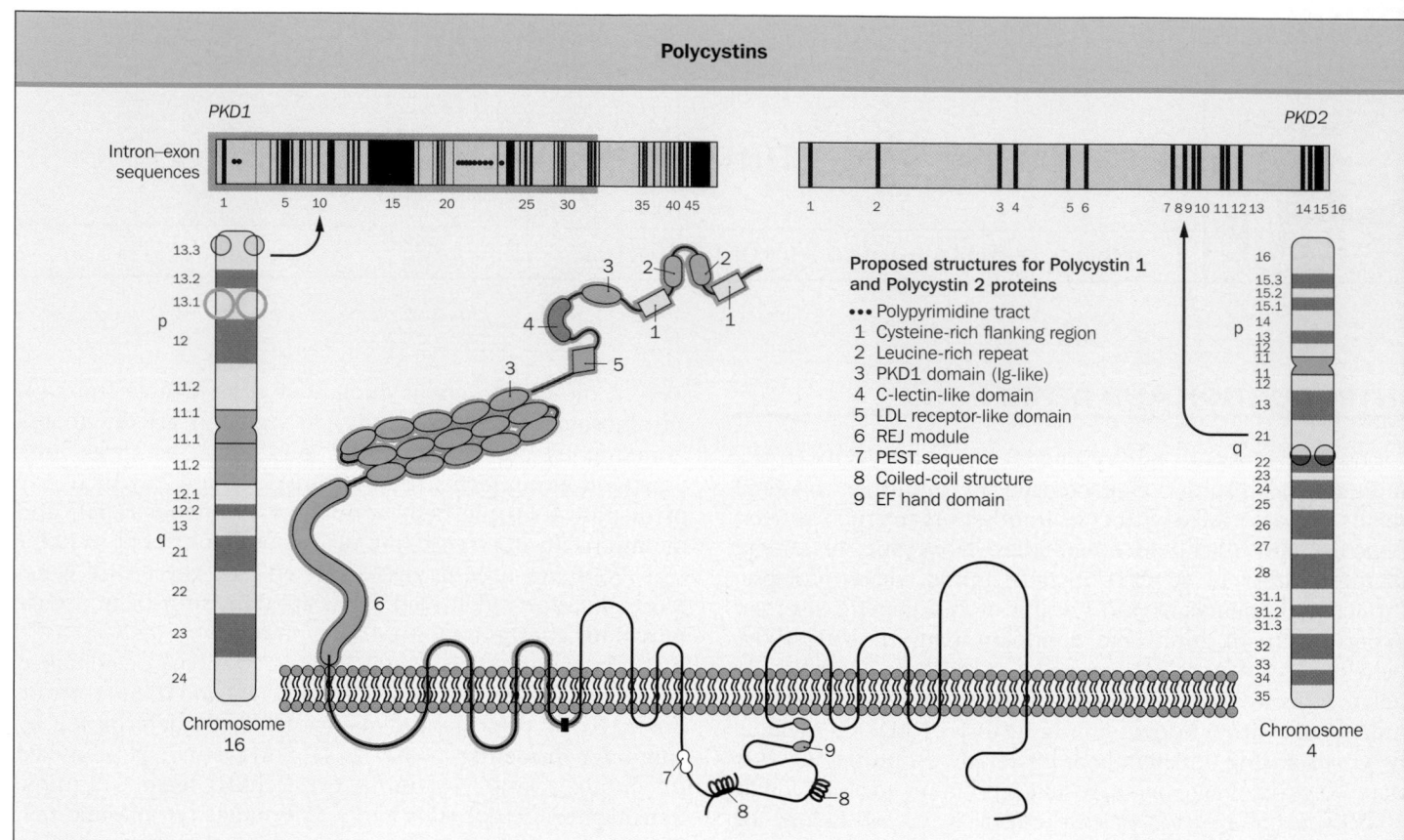

Figure 46.1 Polycystins: genes, mRNAs and proteins. Diagrammatic representation of chromosome 16 (left) and chromosome 4 (right). Intron-exon sequences of *PKD1* (upper left) and *PKD2* (upper right). Diagram of proposed structural features of the polycystin 1 and polycystin 2 proteins (center).

confined to the loop of Henle, distal convoluted tubule and collecting duct. Cellular localization is basolateral in the loop of Henle and distal convoluted tubule. In polycystic kidneys polycystin 2 is expressed strongly, but as with polycystin 1 a small percent of cysts do not stain.

Though ADPKD is caused by an inherited germ-line mutation, only a small percentage of nephrons develop cysts. These observations can be explained by a two-hit tumor suppressor model of cystogenesis[14,15]. It has been demonstrated that the epithelial cells lining the cysts arise from clonal expansion of a single cell. Analysis of the PKD gene in these cells has demonstrated loss of heterozygosity with deletion of the wild type allele in 20–30% of cysts. Also consistent with a two-hit mechanism are the mild cystic phenotype in heterozygote mice with a single copy of *PKD1* or *PKD2*, the severe fetal cystic changes in homozygote null mice and the intermediate cystic phenotype in *PKD2*[WS25/WS25] and *PKD2*[WS25/-] mice (*PKD2*[WS25] is an unstable allele that results in an increased rate of somatic mutations by intragenic homologous recombination). On the other hand, recent reports of transheterozygous mutations of *PKD1* and *PKD2* (for example, somatic mutations of *PKD2* in cells carrying a germline *PKD1* mutation) in cyst-derived cells and the observation that the overexpression of *PKD1* as a transgene also results in the development of a cystic phenotype suggests that other genetic mechanisms, in addition to the two-hit inactivation of *PKD1* or *PKD2*, may result in cyst formation[16–18].

Epithelial cells lining the cysts have a unique phenotype with an increased nuclear to cytoplasmic ratio, decreased microvilli on the apical surface, reduced basolateral folding, persistent expression of vimentin, clusterin, and PAX2, increased expression of proto-oncogenes c-myc, c-fos, and c-ras, and mislocalization of epidermal growth factor receptor to the apical membrane. These features, consistent with an immature phenotype, suggest that cyst cells manifest an intermediate state of cell differentiation[19]. Cyst epithelial cells appear to have an accelerated rate of proliferation and turnover since (1) cell number is increased in tubule walls early on; (2) cells express proliferative cell nuclear antigens; (3) apoptosis, or programmed cell death, is higher in cells lining cysts as evidenced by nuclear fragmentation detected by DNA analysis[20]; and (4) cyst fluid and urine of patients with ADPKD contain sloughed epithelial cells and cellular debris. Despite this, these cells are nonneoplastic and do not proliferate in nude mice.

Cysts arise from focal dilatation of existing renal tubules. As they grow, they dissociate from the parent tubule and eventually become isolated, fluid-filled sacs. They can arise from any segment of the nephron. Proximally-arising cysts are nongradient cysts and distally-derived cysts are typically gradient cysts with low sodium and high urea concentrations. Given that the majority of cysts are dissociated from their parent tubule and that the cyst lining epithelium originally was absorptive, the question arises as to how fluid accumulates within the

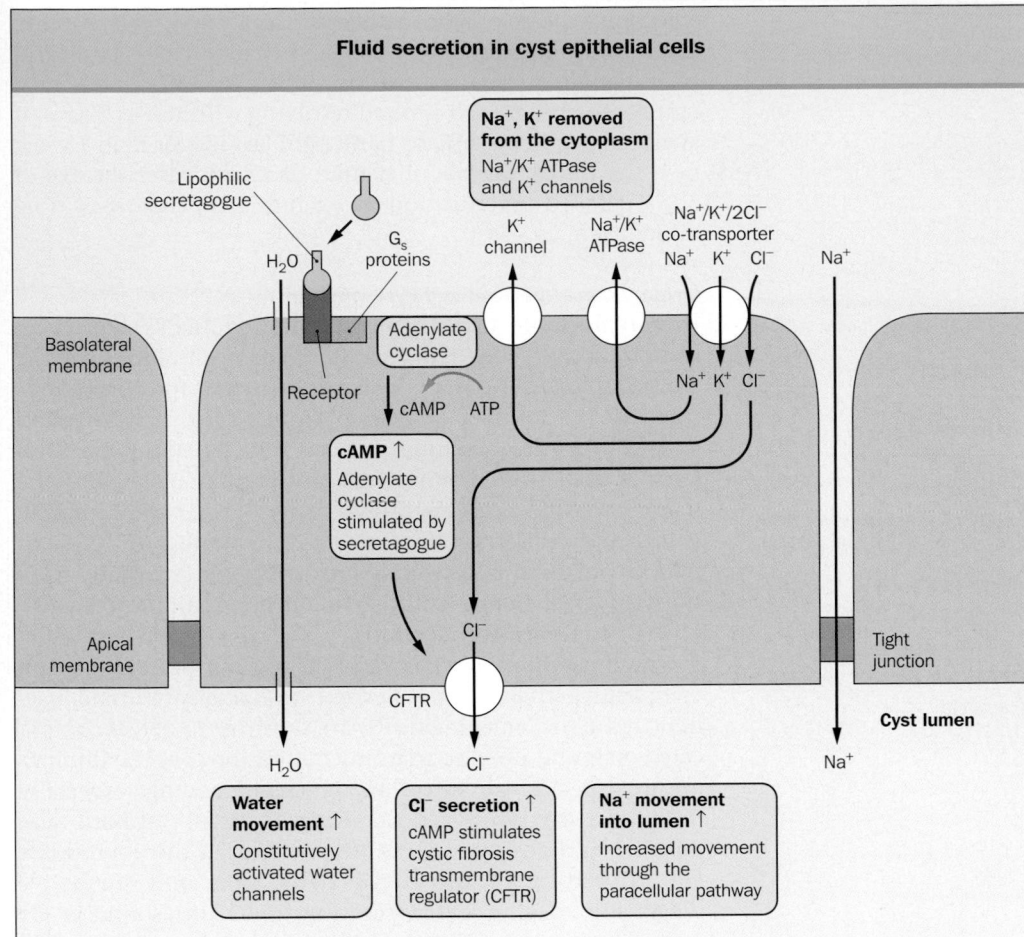

Figure 46.2 Mechanism of fluid secretion in cyst epithelial cells. Relative to normal tubular cells, cyst cells have decreased apical Na channels and increased apical Cl⁻ channels. The basolateral Na⁺/K⁺/2Cl⁻ cotransporter is activated, creating a favorable electrochemical gradient for movement of Na⁺ through paracellular channels into the cyst lumen. Intracellular cAMP stimulates Cl⁻ secretion by apical CFTR Cl⁻ channels. An endogenous lipophilic secretogogue present in polycystic kidneys is one of several agonists that may activate adenylate cyclase to form cAMP and thereby increase and activate Cl⁻ channels in the apical plasma membranes. This cAMP-dependent loss of Cl⁻ from the cytoplasm promotes entry of Cl⁻ from the interstitium via Na⁺/K⁺/2Cl⁻ cotransporters. The accompanying Na⁺ and K⁺ are removed from the cell by the Na⁺-K⁺-ATPase and K⁺ channels on the basolateral membrane. Water moves via constitutively activated water channels and follows Cl⁻ transport rather than Na⁺. (From Martinez JR, Grantham JJ. Polycystic kidney disease: etiology, pathogenesis and treatment. Disease-a-month. 1995;41:697–765.)

cysts (Fig. 46.2). It has been established that fluid secretion into cysts may be mediated by a cyclic-AMP (c-AMP)-dependent chloride channel known as the cystic fibrosis transmembrane regulator (CFTR)[19]. Application of c-AMP or its derivatives causes immediate fluid secretion in ADPKD-derived cysts *in vitro*. Organic osmolytes such as amino acids, sorbitol, glycerophosphorylcholine and betain have been identified in cyst fluid and may contribute to fluid accumulation, but the mechanism by which these osmolytes accumulate within cysts has not been established.

Epidemiology

ADPKD affects approximately 1 in 400 to 1 in 1000 individuals when ascertainment is complete, making it one of the most common hereditary diseases[21]. In the United States, approximately 400 000 people are affected and about 1800 begin hemodialysis each year. Given its inheritance pattern on an autosome, it has an equal gender distribution but males appear to manifest slightly more severe disease. ADPKD occurs worldwide and in all races. The disease may be less common in Africa. In the US ADPKD may be less common but more severe in African Americans than Caucasians.

CLINICAL MANIFESTATIONS

ADPKD is a multisystem disorder. Multiple renal and extrarenal manifestations of ADPKD have been described which

cause significant complications. Familiarity with these associated manifestations is essential so that they can be readily recognized and intervened upon to limit morbidity and mortality to the ADPKD patients.

Renal manifestations

There are a number of clinical features resulting from renal damage that can be identified (see Table 46.1).

Pain and renal size

Renal size increases with age and renal enlargement eventually occurs in 100% of patients with ADPKD. The severity of structural abnormality correlates with the manifestations of ADPKD such as pain, hematuria, hypertension and renal insufficiency[21]. Massive renal enlargement can lead to compression of local structures, resulting in such complications as inferior vena cava compression and digestive symptoms. Episodes of acute pain are seen frequently but chronic, severe pain is rare. Potential etiologies for acute flank pain include cyst hemorrhage, infection, stone or rarely tumor and these must be investigated thoroughly. A small subset of ADPKD patients with renal enlargement and structural distortion will develop chronic flank pain without specifically identifiable etiology. Patients with chronic flank pain are at risk for narcotic and analgesic dependence and a psychological evaluation and an understanding and supportive attitude on the part of the physician is essential in avoiding this.

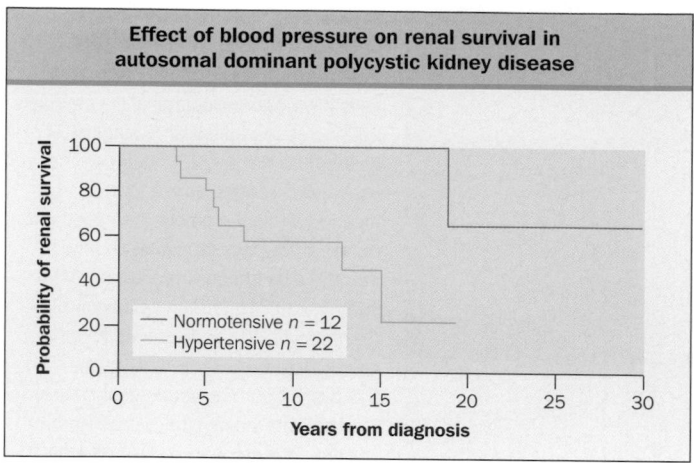

Figure 46.3 Patients with polycystic kidney disease and hypertension at diagnosis have less probability of renal survival than those with normal blood pressure. (From Iglesias CG, Torres VE, Offord KP, et al. Epidemiology and ADPKD, Olmsed County, Minnesota: 1935–1980. Am J Kidney Dis. 1983;2:630–9.)

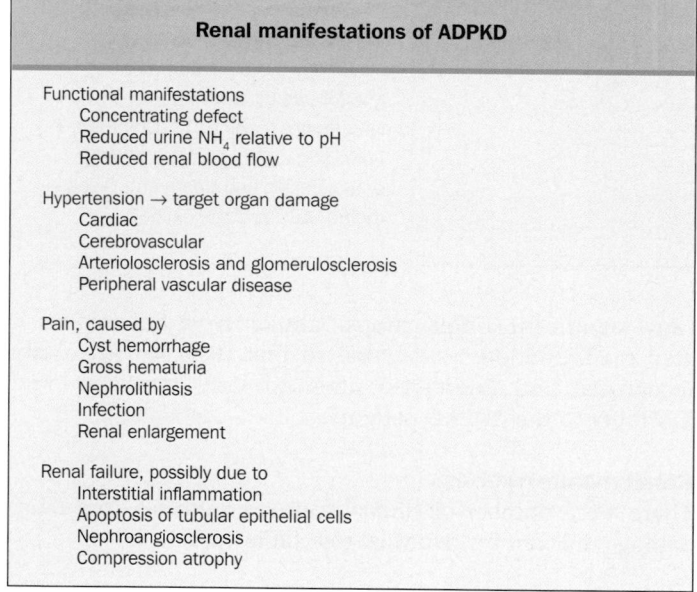

Table 46.1 Renal manifestations of ADPKD.

Reassurance, lifestyle modification and avoidance of aggravating activities may be helpful. If the kidneys are significantly distorted by large cysts decompression can be considered.

Hematuria and cyst hemorrhage

Gross hematuria may be the initial presenting symptom of ADPKD. It occurs in up to 42% of ADPKD patients at some time during the course of the disease. Many will have recurrent episodes. Differential diagnosis of hematuria in ADPKD patients includes cyst hemorrhage, stone, infection or tumor. Cyst hemorrhage is a frequent complication. If the cyst communicates with the collecting system then gross hematuria is observed. Frequently, the cyst does not communicate with the collecting system and flank pain without hematuria occurs. It can present with fever, raising the possibility of cyst

infection. Occasionally, a hemorrhagic cyst will rupture resulting in a retroperitoneal bleed that can be significant, potentially requiring transfusion. In the majority of patients, cyst hemorrhage is self-limited resolving within 2 to 7 days. If symptoms of hematuria or flank pain last longer than 1 week or if the initial episode of hematuria occurs after the age of 50, a detailed investigation to exclude neoplasm should be undertaken.

Urinary tract infection and cyst infection

Urinary tract infection (UTI) is common in ADPKD but it may have been overestimated because of the occurrence of sterile pyuria in many of these patients. Urinary tract infections occur in the form of cystitis, pyelonephritis, cyst infection and perinephric abscesses. As in the general population females are affected more frequently than males and the majority of infections are caused by *Escherichia coli*, *Klebsiella*, *Proteus* and other enterobacteriaciae. The route of infection in pyelonephritis and cyst infection is usually retrograde from the bladder, therefore cystitis should be promptly treated to prevent complicated infections.

The imaging modality of choice has not been defined in comparative studies. Computerized tomography (CT) and magnetic resonance imaging (MRI) are sensitive to detect complicated cysts and provide anatomic definition, but the findings are not specific for infection. Nuclear imaging, especially indium-labeled white cell scanning, is useful but both false negative and positive results are possible. In the appropriate clinical setting of fever and flank pain and suggestive diagnostic imaging, cyst aspiration under ultrasound or CT guidance should be undertaken to culture the organism and assist in selection of antimicrobial therapy.

Nephrolithiasis

The frequency of renal stone disease is increased, occurring in approximately 20% of patients. The majority of stones are uric acid and/or calcium oxalate in composition. Uric acid stones are more common in stone formers with ADPKD than without ADPKD. Urinary stasis thought secondary to distorted renal anatomy may play a role in the pathogenesis of nephrolithiasis. Predisposing metabolic factors include decreased ammonia excretion, low urinary pH and low urinary citrate concentration[22].

Stones can be difficult to diagnose in ADPKD by imaging studies due to the presence of cyst wall and parenchymal calcification. The distorted anatomy can cause difficulty localizing stones to the collecting system on plain films. Intravenous urography (IVU) has the advantage of specifically localizing stone material to the collecting system and can assist in the determination of stone composition. IVU can also detect perycaliceal tubular ectasia, found in 15% of ADPKD patients. CT scanning is more sensitive in detecting small or radiolucent stones and for differentiating stones from tumor, clot and cyst wall or parenchymal calcification.

Hypertension

Hypertension is an important complication of ADPKD associated with significant morbidity and mortality. Hypertension is present in at least 75% of ADPKD patients before the onset of renal failure and the prevalence increases with age. There is a statistical correlation between renal size and prevalence of hypertension in ADPKD. The most widely accepted hypothesis involves reduced renal blood flow, increased intrarenal angiotensin effect, increased filtration fraction and abnormal renal handling of sodium resulting in intravascular volume expansion with resultant hypertension. Evidence for activation of the intrarenal renin–angiotensin system in ADPKD includes: (1) partial reversal of the reduced renal blood flow, of the increased renal vascular resistance and of the increased filtration fraction by acute or chronic administration of angiotensin-converting enzyme (ACE) inhibitors; (2) a shift of immunoreactive renin from the juxtaglomerular apparatus to the walls of the arterioles and small arteries; (3) detection of renin in the epithelium of dilated tubules and cysts; and (4) the association of double dominant (DD) ACE gene polymorphism with worse renal outcome.

Recent studies have shown that nitric oxide (NO) endothelium-dependent vasorelaxation is impaired in small subcutaneous resistance vessels from ADPKD patients with normal- or near-normal renal function before the development of hypertension as compared to healthy control subjects. Furthermore, the decrease of renal plasma flow in response to the intravenous infusion of a competitive inhibitor of NO synthase has been found to be significantly reduced in ADPKD patients compared to normal controls or subjects with essential hypertension. The interactions between angiotensin II and NO at the level of endothelium are of key importance in determining whether end organ damage develops in response to the hemodynamic stress of hypertension, an imbalance between the generation of angiotensin II and that of NO may be responsible for the severity of the renal vascular lesions observed in ADPKD[23].

Unrecognized hypertension can lead to target organ damage that has been shown to significantly impact the life expectancy in ADPKD. The presence of hypertension and nephroangiosclerosis have been associated with increased risk for and a faster decline in renal function (Fig. 46.3). Proteinuria and microalbuminuria correlate with elevated mean arterial pressure and are independent risk factors for accelerated decline in renal function. Hematuria, a risk factor for the progression of renal failure in ADPKD, is more common in hypertensive patients. Left ventricular hypertrophy (LVH) occurs early in the course of ADPKD and may be a consequence of higher nocturnal blood pressures reported in young ADPKD patients. Valvular heart disease is also common in ADPKD and may be aggravated by hypertension. Hypertension may be a risk factor for intracranial aneurysm (ICA) rupture and may contribute to morbidity associated with rupture.

Renal failure

End-stage renal disease (ESRD) is not inevitable in ADPKD. Up to 77% of patients are alive with preserved renal function at age 50, and 52% at age 73. Fifty percent of ADPKD patients have reached ESRD by the ages of 57 to 73 years. *PKD1* is associated with a 15-year earlier onset of ESRD than *PKD2*. The influence of environmental factors as well as genetic background is demonstrated by intrafamilial variability in the severity of disease. Once renal insufficiency has begun, the rate of decline in renal function is linear, with a loss of approximately 5.0–6.4 mL/min/year on average in patients with moderate renal failure. Males tend to progress to renal failure more rapidly and require renal replacement therapy at a younger age than females. Other risk factors for renal failure include black race, diagnosis of ADPKD before the age of 30 years, first episode of hematuria before the age of 30 years, onset of hypertension before the age of 35, hyperlipidemia, low HDL, DD ACE polymorphism and sickle cell trait[24]. The location of the *PKD1* and *PKD2* mutations may also influence the clinical outcome. Patients with mutations in the 5′ region of *PKD1* were found to have significantly more severe disease than the patients with 3′ mutations (18.9% vs. 39.7% with adequate renal function at 60 years)[25,26].

The mechanism by which ADPKD causes renal failure is incompletely understood. An adverse association between renal volume and progression of renal failure has been recognized in younger patients, suggesting that compression of normal renal parenchyma by expanding cysts plays a role. However, cyst decompression does not improve renal function or delay the progression to renal failure. Hyperfiltration was also thought to play a role though ADPKD patients who have undergone unilateral nephrectomy for urologic emergencies show no difference in the slope of decline in renal function than controls. Histologically, ADPKD is characterized by advanced vascular sclerosis of afferent and interlobular arteries even in the absence of hypertension, and interstitial fibrosis[27]. Angiotensin II may play a role in the pathogenesis of interstitial inflammation and interstitial fibrosis. It has been shown to potentiate the mitogenic effects of epidermal growth factor and stimulate renal tubule cell synthesis of osteopontin, a strong chemotactic factor for macrophages, and of transforming growth factor-β, which in turn stimulates the synthesis of collagen type IV and metalloproteinase inhibitors which inhibit degradation of extracellular matrix.

Extrarenal manifestations
Polycystic liver disease

Polycystic liver disease (PLD) is the most common extrarenal manifestation of ADPKD[28]. It is associated with both *PKD1* and non-*PKD1* genotypes. In addition, PLD also occurs as a genetically distinct disease in the absence of renal cysts. Developmentally, liver cysts arise from a ductal plate abnormality with abnormal development and differentiation of the bile ducts.

PLD refers to any liver cysts in the presence of ADPKD. In the absence of renal cystic disease, PLD should be suspected when 4 or more cysts are present in the hepatic parenchyma. the number of cysts can help distinguish PLD from simple hepatic cysts. The majority of simple cysts are solitary and no more than three cysts are present in those with multiple cysts. The liver in PLD contains multiple microscopic or macroscopic cysts that result in hepatomegaly (Fig. 46.4), but typically there is preservation of normal hepatic parenchyma and liver function. Other pathologic findings in PLD include biliary hamartomas, biliary fibroadenomas, cystic dilatation of peribiliary glands and dilatation of intra- and extrahepatic bile ducts.

Hepatic cysts are exceedingly rare in children with ADPKD. Frequency increases with age; cysts are identified in 20% of

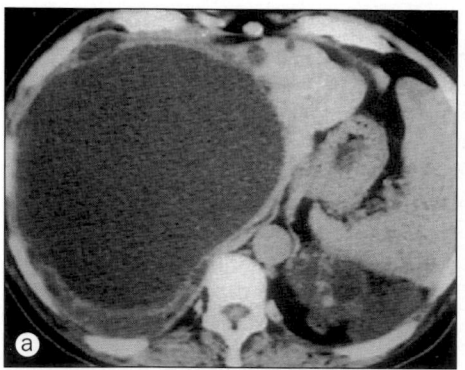 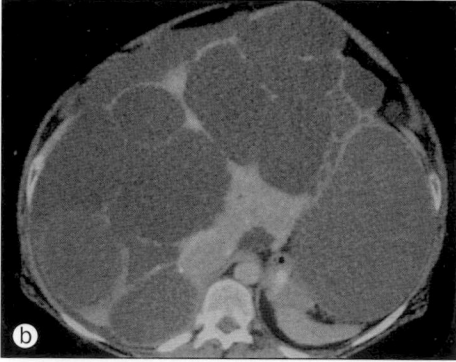 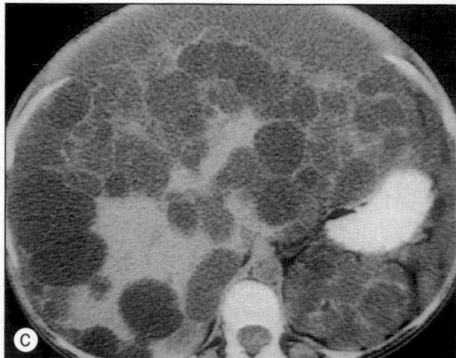

Figure 46.4 Variable presentation of symptomatic polycystic liver disease. (a) Hepatomegaly caused by a very large, isolated, dominant cyst. (b) Hepatomegaly caused by several large cysts. (c) Hepatomegaly caused by multiple smaller cysts throughout the hepatic parenchyma.

patients in the third decade and 75% by the seventh decade. Females develop more cysts, at an earlier age than men. Women who have multiple pregnancies or who have used oral contraceptive agents or estrogen replacement therapy post-menopausally have worse disease suggesting a direct role of estrogen exposure in hepatic cyst growth.

Typically, PLD is asymptomatic. Reported symptoms have become more frequent as the lifespan of ADPKD patients is pro-longed with dialysis and transplantation. Symptoms result from mass effect or from complications related to the cysts themselves. Symptoms typically caused by massive enlarge-ment of the liver or by mass effect from a single or a limited number of dominant cysts include dyspnea, orthopnea, early satiety, gastroesophageal reflux, mechanical low back pain, uterine prolapse, and even rib fracture. Other complications caused directly by mass effect include hepatic venous outflow obstruction, inferior vena cava compression, portal vein com-pression or bile duct compression presenting as obstructive jaundice. Hepatic venous outflow obstruction is an uncom-mon condition caused by severe extrinsic compression of the intrahepatic inferior vena cava and hepatic veins by cysts, in rare cases with superimposed thrombosis. Patients present with ascites. Obstruction of the intrahepatic inferior vena cava and hepatic veins should be relieved by cyst aspiration and alcohol sclerosis, laparoscopic fenestration or combined hepatic resec-tion and cyst fenestration. Prognosis is good, unless there is superimposed hepatic vein thrombosis. Symptomatic cyst com-plications include cyst hemorrhage which occurs less fre-quently than renal cyst hemorrhage, cyst infection and the rare occurrence of torsion or rupture of cysts. Hepatic cyst infection can be a serious complication and typically presents with localized pain, fever, leukocytosis, an elevated sedimen-tation rate and often elevated alkaline phosphatase. Enterobacteriaceae are the most common microorganisms causing cyst infection. Localization of the infected cyst by imaging techniques may be difficult. MRI may be the most sensitive technique to differentiate a complicated from an uncomplicated hepatic cyst.

Intracranial aneurysms

ICA occur in approximately 8% of the ADPKD population. There appears to be familial clustering, occurring in 5% of

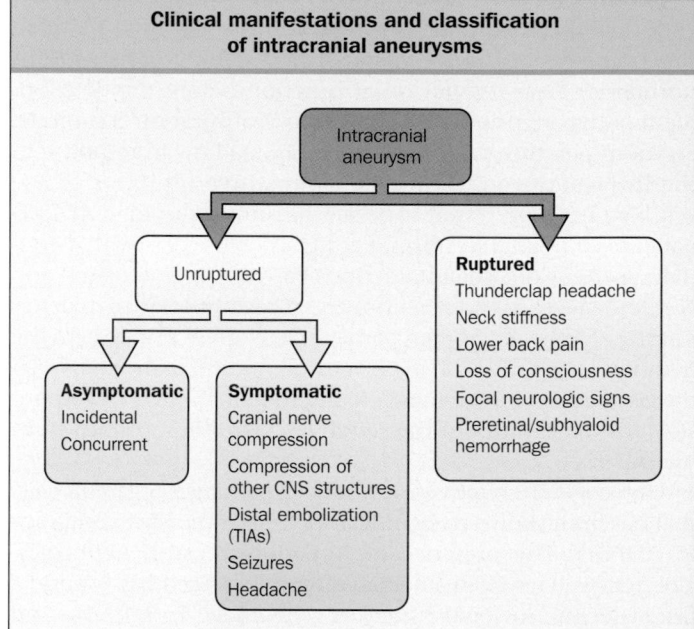

Figure 46.5 Intracranial aneurysms. Clinical manifestations and classification.

patients with a negative family history and 22% of those with a positive family history. The majority are asymptomatic. Focal findings such as cranial nerve palsy or seizure may result from compression of local structures by an enlarging aneurysm (Fig. 46.5). Yearly rupture rates increase with size, ranging from less than 0.5% for aneurysms less than 5 mm in diameter to 4% for aneurysms greater than 10 mm in diam-eter. Rupture carries a 35–55% risk of combined severe mor-bidity and mortality. The mean age at rupture is lower in the ADPKD population than in the general population (39 years versus 51 years) with a range of 15–69 years. Most patients have normal renal function and up to 29% will have normal blood pressure at the time of rupture.

Widespread screening is not indicated because most ICA found by presymptomatic screening are small, have a low risk of rupture and require no treatment. Indications for screening in patients with a good life expectancy include family history of ICA or subarachnoid hemorrhage (SAH), previous aneurysmal rupture, preparation for elective surgery with potential hemodynamic instability, high-risk occupations and significant anxiety on the part of the patient despite adequate information about the risks. Magnetic resonance angiography is the diagnostic imaging modality of choice for presymptomatic screening as it is noninvasive and does not require intravenous contrast material[29].

Other vascular abnormalities

In addition to intracranial aneurysms ADPKD has been associated with other vascular abnormalities such as thoracic aortic and cervicocephalic arterial dissections, intracranial arterial dolichoectasia, and coronary artery aneurysms (Fig. 46.6). Thoracic aortic dissection is seven times more common in the ADPKD population than in the general population by autopsy series but actual case reports are rare. In one series, 32 ADPKD patients underwent coronary angiography. Five had saccular or fusiform aneurysms and six had coronary ectasia in association with coronary atherosclerosis. Two had coronary aneurysms in the absence of atherosclerotic disease and presented with cardiac ischemia and thrombus in the aneurysm. Several cases reports describe abdominal aortic aneurysm in ADPKD patients. However, a prospective, sonographic study showed neither a wider aortic diameter nor a higher prevalence of abdominal aortic aneurysms in ADPKD patients versus unaffected kindred in any age group. Pathologically, tissues from arterial aneurysms and dissections demonstrate disruption of elastic tissue. Recent immunohistochemical studies demonstrated both, polycystin-1 and polycystin-2 expression in the myocytes of elastic and large distributive arteries, suggesting a direct pathogenetic role for ADPKD-related mutations in the arterial complications of this disease[13,30].

Valvular heart disease

Mitral valve prolapse is the most common valvular abnormality and has been demonstrated in up to 25% of ADPKD patients by echocardiography. Mitral insufficiency, tricuspid insufficiency and tricuspid prolapse also occur more frequently in ADPKD than in unaffected kindred. Aortic insufficiency has been reported in association with dilatation of the aortic root. Histologically, valvular tissue show myxoid degeneration with disruption of collagen as seen in Marfan and Ehlers–Danlos syndromes. Overall, the risk of valvular abnormalities is unclear; although the lesions may progress with time, they rarely require valve replacement. Screening echocardiography is not indicated unless a murmur is detected on physical examination.

Other associated conditions

Cyst formation has been described in such diverse organs as pancreas, and arachnoid membrane (Fig. 46.7), and less definitely in spleen, pineal gland, ovaries, seminal vesicles and testes. In addition, spinal meningeal diverticula have been described in these patients and may present with intracranial hypotension presumably due to cerebrospinal fluid leak. An association between ADPKD and colonic diverticula has been described but is controversial. These associated conditions are typically asymptomatic and require no intervention.

PATHOLOGY

Polycystic kidneys are diffusely cystic and enlarged but typically retain the reniform structure (Fig. 46.8). Size varies from normal to weighing greater than 4000 g. The outer and cut surfaces show numerous spherical cysts of varying size, which are distributed evenly between cortex and medulla. The collecting system typically is distorted.

Microscopically, polycystic kidneys demonstrate advanced sclerosis of preglomerular vessels, interstitial fibrosis and tubular epithelial hyperplasia, even in patients with normal renal function or early renal failure[27]. Sclerosis involves both afferent arterioles and interlobular arteries. This is more prominent in ADPKD than in patients with glomerular disease and comparable renal function, and may be attributable to hypertension and the activation of the renin–angiotensin system demonstrated in ADPKD. Interstitial fibrosis is also prominent even in early disease. It is associated with an interstitial infiltrate of macrophages and lymphocytes.

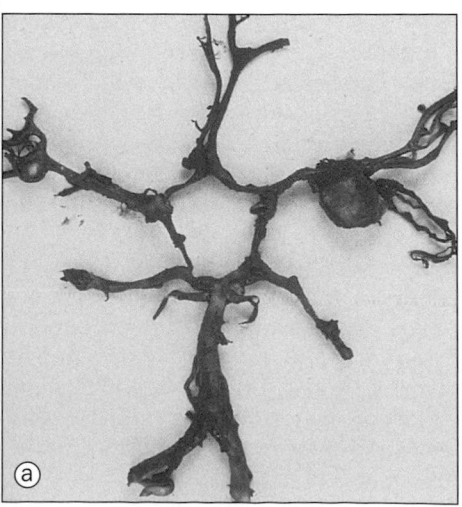 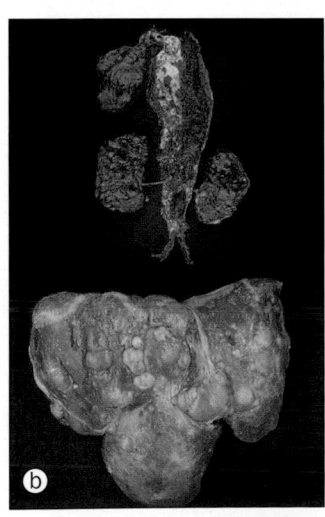

Figure 46.6 Vascular manifestations of ADPKD. (a) Gross specimen demonstrating bilateral aneurysms of the midddle cerebral arteries. (b) Gross specimen demonstrating a thoracic aortic dissection extending into the abdominal aorta in a patient with autosomal dominant polycystic kidney and liver disease.

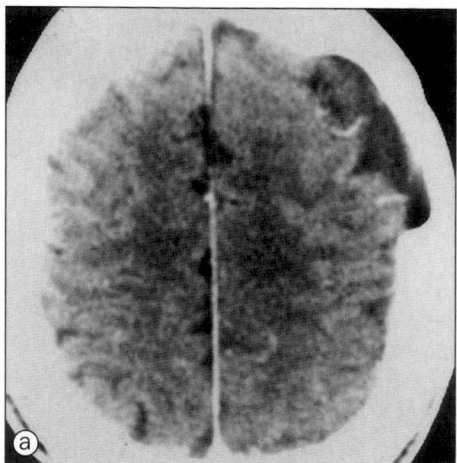
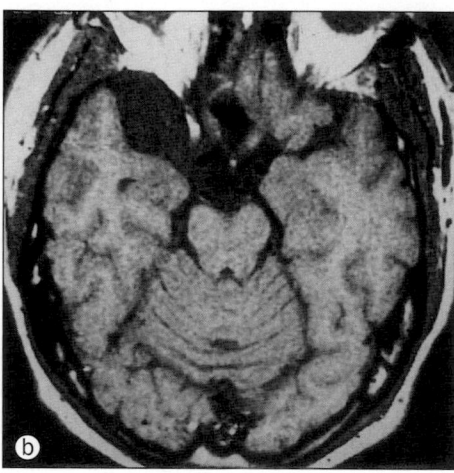

Figure 46.7 Extrarenal manifestations of ADPKD. Arachnoid cysts demonstrated by CT (a) or MRI (b).

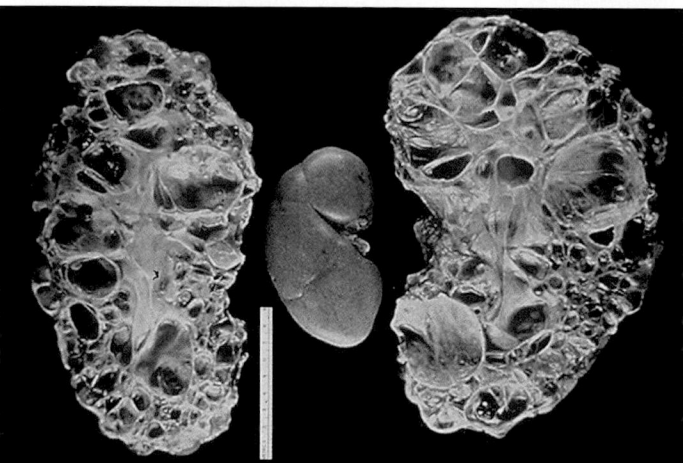

Figure 46.8 Markedly enlarged polycystic kidneys from a patient with ADPKD in comparison to a normal kidney in the middle.

There is hyperplasia of the tubular epithelium lining the cysts including flat nonpolypoid hyperplasia, polypoid hyperplasia and microscopic adenomas[31] (Fig. 46.9). Increased rates of apoptosis parallel the enhanced epithelial cell proliferation observed on the polycystic kidneys[20].

Despite the frequency of hyperplastic lesions and microscopic adenomas, the incidence of renal cell carcinoma is not increased.

DIAGNOSIS AND DIFFERENTIAL DIAGNOSIS

Presymptomatic screening of patients at risk for ADPKD is by ultrasound, or identification of the genes for ADPKD by linkage or direct mutational analysis. Diagnostic ultrasonographic criteria for individuals known to be at 50% risk by positive family history include: two cysts either unilateral or bilateral in patients less than 30 years of age, two cysts in both kidneys in patients 30–59 and at least four cysts in each kidney patients over the age of 60[1]. Presymptomatic screening by ultrasound before age 20 may not be conclusive and is not generally recommended. In addition, these criteria may not be sufficiently sensitive in *PKD2* patients younger than 30 years of age[2]. Genetic diagnosis by linkage analysis requires

participation of other family members with and without the disease. It allows for prenatal diagnosis and is important in the evaluation of young, living, related kidney donors with indeterminate diagnosis by imaging studies. Recent improvements in methodology have allowed direct mutation analysis of the *PKD1* and *PKD2* genes in the research setting. The analysis of the *PKD1* gene is hampered by the size, complexity, and large duplication of the gene in the three homologous genes. Recently, clinical testing of the *PKD1* and *PKD2* genes by DHPLC analysis has become available, but the detection rate for disease-causing mutations is not yet known[32]. Only individuals who have been properly informed about the advantages and disadvantages of screening should be offered presymptomatic screening. If ADPKD is diagnosed, the patient can receive appropriate genetic counseling and risk factors such as hypertension can be identified and intervention instituted early. If ADPKD is absent the patient is reassured. The disadvantages of presymptomatic screening relate to insurability and employability. Recommendations will change when more effective therapy for the disease becomes available.

Renal cystic disease can be a manifestation of many other systemic diseases, which are discussed further in Chapter 47. These should be kept in mind when renal cystic disease is detected but the presentation is not typical. In these cases the establishment of the correct diagnosis depends on the appropriate identification of the extrarenal manifestations of these diseases. For example, tuberous sclerosis complex (TSC) is an autosomal dominant disorder characterized by renal angiomyolipomas, renal cysts and renal cell carcinoma. The coexistence of renal cysts and angiomyolipomas is pathognomonic for TSC. However, renal cysts can occur in the absence of angiomyolipomas, particularly in the first year of life. In these cases, the kidneys mimic ADPKD radiographically.

Von Hippel–Lindau (VHL) is also an autosomal dominant disorder manifest as retinal and/or central nervous system hemangioblastomas, renal cysts, renal cell carcinoma, pancreatic cysts, pheochromocytomas and papillary cystadenomas of the epididymis. Renal cysts are usually multiple and bilateral and are usually, but not always associated with multiple solid tumors. In the absence of solid tumors, the appearance of the kidneys in VHL may mimic that of ADPKD.

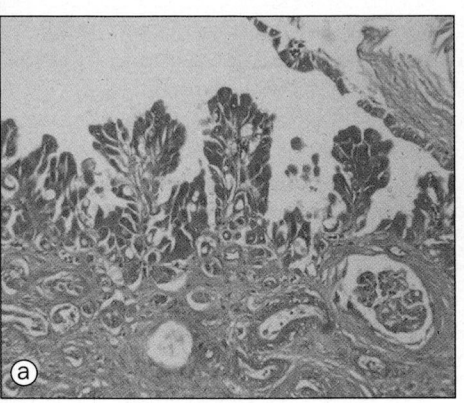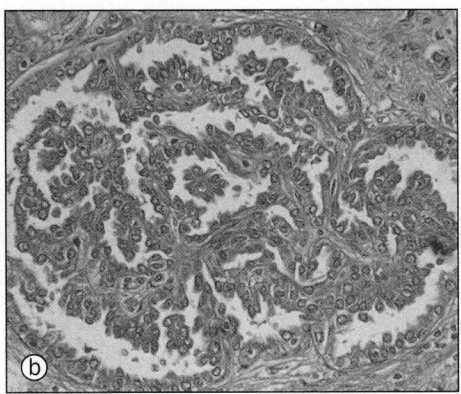

Figure 46.9 Renal cyst histology in ADPKD.
(a) Papillary hyperplasia of cyst epithelium.
(b) Papillary microscopic adenoma in an ADPKD kidney (original magnification × 200). (Dunn, Portis, Elbahnasy, et al[35].)

Orofaciodigital syndrome type 1 is a rare X-linked dominant disorder which is lethal in males. Affected females may have kidneys that are indistinguishable from ADPKD. Liver cysts may also be present. The correct diagnosis should be suggested by the extrarenal manifestations including oral anomalies such as hyperplastic frenula, cleft tongue, cleft palate or lip and malposed teeth, facial anomalies such as broad nasal root with hypoplasia of nasal alae and malar bone, and digital anomalies.

Simple renal cysts are the most commonly encountered of the renal cystic diseases. Typically, these cysts are unilocular, often located in the renal cortex, and occur more frequently with advancing age. They are typically asymptomatic, but rarely can cause abdominal or flank-pain, microscopic or macroscopic hematuria, and have been reported to cause renin-dependent hypertension. They are benign and usually require no intervention.

Acquired cystic disease of the kidney refers to cystic degeneration of the renal parenchyma that occurs in ESRD (see Chapter 73). It has been defined as five or more cysts per kidney occurring in the uremic patient in the absence of inherited renal cystic disease. The prevalence of acquired renal cystic disease as well as the size and number of renal cysts increases with duration of uremia and dialysis. Clinically, the patients are typically asymptomatic but occasionally complications such as hematuria, hemorrhage into cysts, cyst rupture with retroperitoneal hemorrhage, cyst infection and development of adenoma or adenocarcinomas can occur.

NATURAL HISTORY

ADPKD is a heterogeneous disease with significant variability in clinical presentation occurring between families. Even within the same family, significant variability in clinical presentation can occur. The natural history of renal insufficiency in ADPKD is as variable as the clinical presentation[21]. ESRD occurs in 50% of patients by the age of 57–73, depending on the clinical series. Risk factors for progressive renal failure include *PKD1* genotype, male gender, diagnosis before age 30, first episode of hematuria before age 30 and onset of hypertension before age 35[24]. Hyperlipidemia and low HDL may also worsen patient outcomes. Even though the degree of structural abnormality and renal size correlates with worse renal function in ADPKD, surgical decompression of renal cysts does not have a beneficial effect on preserving renal function. Once renal failure begins, renal function tends to decline linearly with time.

TRANSPLANTATION

Transplantation has become the treatment of choice for ESRD in ADPKD. Several studies have demonstrated no difference in patient or graft survival between ADPKD patients and other ESRD populations. The 1997 United States Renal Data System (USRDS) data shows a 1-year survival probability for cadaveric transplants in ADPKD of 87% versus 85% overall, and at 5 years 68% in ADPKD versus 59% overall. Living donor transplants also have graft survival no different to non-ADPKD populations. Because of the genetic nature of the disease, living-related transplantation has only recently been widely practiced in the ADPKD population. The number of living, related transplants for ADPKD increased from 12% in 1990 to 22% in 1995. In 1999, 30% of kidney transplants for ADPKD patients were from living donors.

Complications after transplant are no greater in the ADPKD population than in the general population and specific complications directly related to ADPKD are rare. One study showed a higher rate of cyst infection following transplantation relative to before transplantation though the difference was not statistically significant. No significant increase in the incidence of symptomatic mitral valve prolapse, aortic aneurysm rupture, hepatic cyst infection or native cancers was observed. Another study showed a higher rate of diverticulosis and perforation in ADPKD than controls but the association with colonic diverticulosis remains controversial.

Though practiced routinely in the past, pretransplant nephrectomy has fallen out of favor. Nephrectomy is an extensive procedure often with prolonged convalescence. In addition, native kidneys contribute to the maintenance of hemoglobin levels and assist in fluid management in ESRD. Indications for nephrectomy include a history of infected cysts, frequent bleeding, severe hypertension or massive renal enlargement with extension into the pelvis. There is no evidence for an increased risk of renal cell carcinoma developing in native ADPKD kidneys after transplantation so pretransplant nephrectomy is not indicated as cancer prophylaxis.

TREATMENT

Despite significant advances in the understanding of the genetics of ADPKD and the mechanism of cyst growth, no treatment specifically directed toward disease exists as yet.

Current therapy is therefore directed toward the renal and extrarenal complications of the disease in an effort to limit morbidity and mortality.

Flank pain

Causes of flank pain which may require intervention such as infection, stone or tumor, should be excluded. Nonopioid agents are preferred and care should be taken to avoid long-term administration of nephrotoxic agents such as combination analgesics and nonsteroidal anti-inflammatory drugs. Tricyclic antidepressants are helpful as in other chronic pain syndromes, with a generally well-tolerated side-effect profile. Narcotic analgesics should be reserved for the management of acute episodes of pain as chronic use can lead to physical and psychological dependence. Splanchnic nerve blockade with local anesthesia or steroids has been shown to result in pain relief prolonged beyond the duration of the local anesthetic.

When conservative measures fail, therapy can be directed toward cyst decompression with either cyst aspiration and sclerosis, surgical cyst decompression or laparoscopic cyst decompression. Cyst aspiration, under ultrasound or CT guidance is a relatively simple procedure; to prevent the reaccumulation of cyst fluid, sclerosing agents such as 95% ethanol or acidic solutions of minocycline are commonly used. There is a success rate of greater than 90% in benign renal cysts using 95% ethanol. Minor complications include microhematuria, localized pain, transient fever, and systemic absorption of the alcohol. More serious complications such as pneumothorax, perirenal hematoma, arteriovenous fistula, urinoma and infection are rare. Complications from aspiration of centrally located cysts are more common and the morbidity of the procedure is proportional to the number of cysts treated.

If multiple cysts are contributing to pain, laparoscopic or surgical cyst fenestration through lumbotomy or flank incision may be of benefit. Surgical decompression is effective in 80–90% of patients at one year and 62–77% have sustained pain relief for greater than 2 years (Fig. 46.10). Surgical intervention does not accelerate the decline in renal function, as once thought, but does not appear to preserve declining renal function either (Fig. 46.10). Laparoscopy is equally as effective as open surgical fenestration in short-term follow-up for patients with limited disease and there is a shorter, less

complicated recovery period compared to open surgery. Previous abdominal surgery with possible adhesion formation is a relative contraindication to the procedure[33].

There are a number of novel interventions for the management of pain in ADPKD whose roles have not yet been fully defined. Laparoscopic renal denervation has been used in combination with cyst fenestration and may be considered, particularly in polycystic kidneys without large cysts. Laparoscopic and retroperitoneoscopic nephrectomy and arterial embolization have been used to treat symptomatic polycystic kidneys in ADPKD patients with ESRD[34–36].

Cyst hemorrhage

Episodes of cyst hemorrhage are self-limiting and respond well to conservative management with bedrest, analgesics and adequate fluid intake to prevent obstructing clots. Rarely, bleeding is more severe with extensive subcapsular or retroperitoneal hematoma causing significant decrease in hematocrit and hemodynamic instability. This requires hospitalization, transfusion and investigation by CT or angiography. In cases of unusually severe or persistent hemorrhage, segmental arterial embolization can be successful. If not, surgery may be required to control bleeding.

Urinary tract and cyst infection

Since the great majority of upper tract infections begin as cystitis, prompt treatment of symptomatic cystitis and asymptomatic bacteriuria is indicated to prevent retrograde seeding of the renal parenchyma. Antibiotics that require glomerular filtration, such as highly polar aminoglycosides are not effective for upper tract infection in advanced renal insufficiency. Cyst infection is often difficult to treat despite prolonged therapy with an antibiotic to which the organism is susceptible. Treatment failure occurs because certain antibiotics do not penetrate the cyst epithelium and achieve therapeutic concentrations within the cysts. With gradient cysts, the epithelium lining the cyst has functional and ultrastructural characteristic of the distal tubule epithelium. Penetration is via tight junctions, allowing only lipid soluble agents access. Nongradient cysts, which are more common, allow solute access via diffusion, suggesting that water soluble agents should gain entry to the cysts. However,

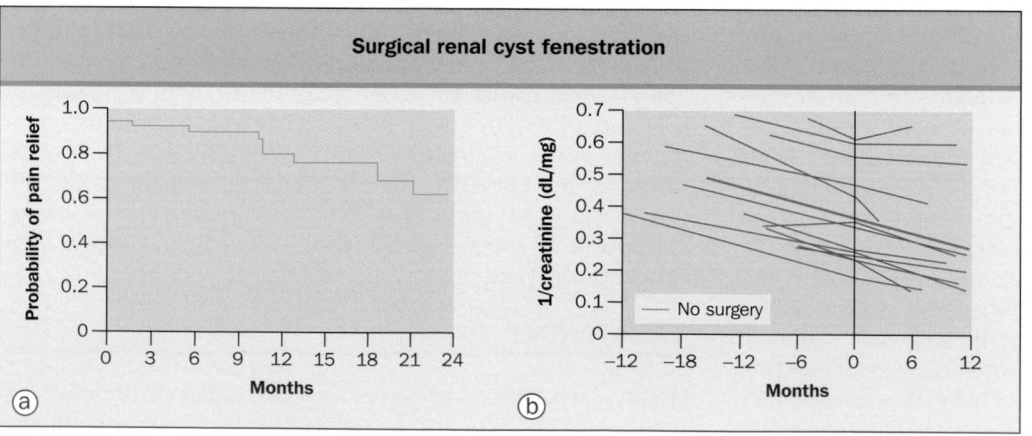

Figure 46.10 Surgical cyst fenestration for symptomatic ADPKD. Effects on relief of pain (a) and rate of decline of renal function (b). (From Elzinga LW, Barry JM, Torres VE, et al. Cyst decompression surgery for autosomal dominant polycystic kidney disease. J Am Soc Nephrol. 1992;2:1219–26.)

kinetic studies indicate that these agents penetrate non-gradient cysts slowly and irregularly, giving rise to unreliable drug concentrations within the cysts. Lipophilic agents have been shown to penetrate both gradient and nongradient cysts equally and reliably and have pK_a that allows for favorable electrochemical gradients into acidic cyst fluid. Therapeutic agents of choice include trimethoprim-sulfamethoxazole, fluoroquinolones, both of which have shown favorable intracystic therapeutic concentration gradients at physiologic pH in gradient and nongradient cysts, and chloramphenicol.

If fever persists after 1–2 weeks of appropriate antimicrobial therapy, percutaneous or surgical drainage of infected cysts should be undertaken. If fever recurs after stopping antibiotics, complicating features such as obstruction, perinephric abscess or stone should be excluded. If no such complicating features are identified, the antibiotic course should be extended and may require several months to fully eradicate infection.

Nephrolithiasis

Treatment of nephrolithiasis in patients with ADPKD is not different from that in patients without ADPKD. Potassium citrate is the treatment of choice in the three conditions associated with ADPKD, uric acid lithiasis, hypocitraturic calcium oxalate nephrolithiasis and distal acidification defects. Extracorporeal shock wave lithotripsy and percutaneous nephrostolithotomy are reported to be 82% and 80% successful, respectively, without significant complication[22].

Hypertension

Poorly controlled hypertension accelerates the decline in renal function and aggravate extrarenal complications. The optimal antihypertensive agent of choice in ADPKD has not clearly established. ACE inhibitors or angiotensin, receptor antagonists increase renal blood flow and may be the agents of choice in patients with preserved renal function. Calcium channel blockers also increase renal blood flow. In addition, ACE inhibitors and calcium channel blockers have a low side effect profile and may reduce vascular smooth muscle proliferation and the development of atherosclerosis. Two small prospective studies of hypertensive of ADPKD patients with preserved renal function have failed to demonstrate a beneficial effect of ACE inhibitors on the rate of decline of renal function[37,38]. On the other hand, a historical prospective nonrandomized study of 33 ADPKD patients treated with ACE inhibitors or diuretics showed that the rate of decline of renal function was significantly higher in those receiving diuretics[39].

Renal failure

Therapeutic intervention aimed at slowing the progression of renal failure in ADPKD include control of hypertension, treating hyperlipidemia, dietary protein restriction, control of acidosis and prevention of hyperphosphatemia. A subgroup analysis of the MDRD trial, however, showed no beneficial effect on renal function in ADPKD of strict compared to standard blood pressure control, and only a slight beneficial effect of borderline significance of a very low protein diet. Since these interventions were introduced at a late stage of the disease (glomerular filtration rate of 13–55 mL/min per 1.73 m²) these results do not exclude a beneficial effect of earlier interventions.

Actuarial data indicate that ADPKD patients do better on dialysis than patients with renal failure from other causes, particularly for age over 47 years. Females also appear to do better than males. The good outcome in ADPKD may be due to higher endogenous erythropoietin production and better maintenance of hemoglobin. Rarely, hemodialysis can be complicated by intradialytic hypotension if there is IVC compression by a medially-located renal cyst. Despite renal size, peritoneal dialysis can usually be performed in ADPKD patients, though they are at increased risk for inguinal and umbilical hernias, which require surgical repair.

Polycystic liver disease

Most cases of PLD are asymptomatic and require no treatment. When symptomatic, therapy is directed toward reducing cyst volume and hepatic size. Noninvasive measures include avoiding ethanol, other hepatotoxins and, possibly, cAMP agonists (for example caffeine) as the latter have been shown to stimulate fluid secretion by the cysts in vitro. Histamine H2 blockers and somatostatin have been suggested to reduce secretion of secretin and secretory activity of cyst walls. Estrogens likely contribute to cyst growth but the use of oral contraceptive agents and postmenopausal estrogen replacement therapy are contraindicated only if the liver is significantly enlarged and the risk of further hepatic cyst growth outweighs the benefits of estrogen therapy. Rarely, symptomatic PLD may require invasive measures to reduce cyst volume and hepatic size. Options include percutaneous cyst aspiration and sclerosis, laparoscopic fenestration or open surgical fenestration[28]. Cyst aspiration is the procedure of choice if symptoms are caused by one or a few dominant cysts or by cysts that are easily accessible to percutaneous intervention. To prevent the reaccumulation of cyst fluid, sclerosis with minocycline or 95% ethanol is often successful. Laparoscopic fenestration can be considered for large cysts which are more likely to recur after ethanol sclerosis or if several cysts are present that would require multiple percutaneous passes to treat adequately. Partial hepatectomy with cyst fenestration is an option as PLD often spares a part of the liver with adequate preservation of hepatic parenchyma and liver function (Fig. 46.11). Rarely, no segments are spared. In these patients liver transplantation may be necessary.

When a hepatic cyst infection is suspected, any cyst with unusual appearance on an imaging study should be aspirated for diagnostic purposes. The best management is percutaneous cyst drainage in combination with antibiotic therapy. Long-term oral antibiotic suppression or prophylaxis should be reserved for relapsing or recurrent cases. Antibiotics of choice are trimethoprim–sulfamethoxazole and the fluoroquinolones, which are effective against the typical infecting organisms and concentrate in the biliary tree and cysts.

Intracranial aneurysm

Ruptured or symptomatic ICA requires surgical clipping of the neck of the aneurysm. Asymptomatic aneurysms measuring less than 5 mm, diagnosed by presymptomatic screening,

Hereditary and Congenital Diseases of the Kidney

Hepatic resection in ADPKD

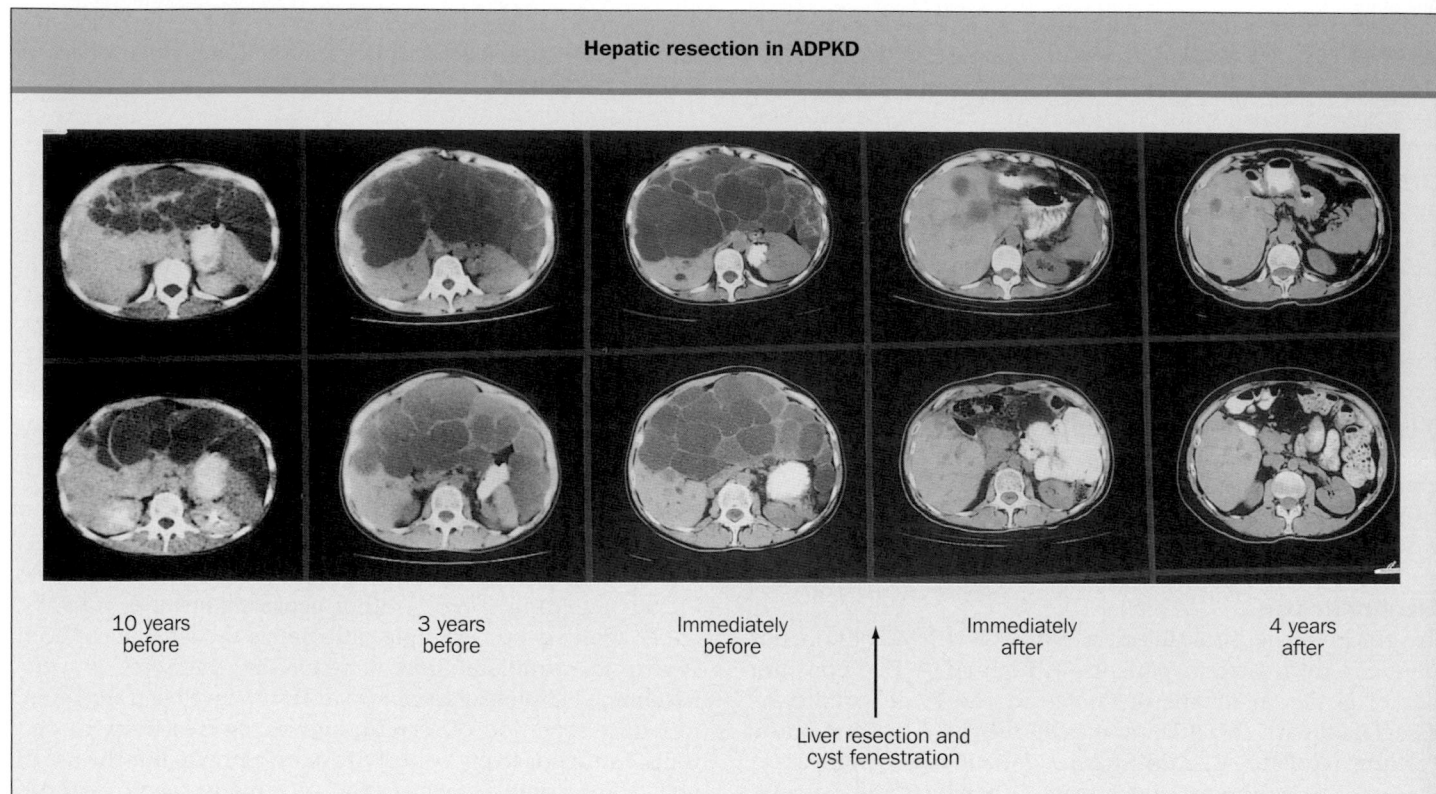

| 10 years before | 3 years before | Immediately before | Immediately after | 4 years after |

Liver resection and cyst fenestration

Figure 46.11 Hepatic resection in ADPKD. CT scans of the abdomen. Ten years before (column 1), 3 years before (column 2), immediately before (column 3), immediately after (column 4) and 4 years after (column 5) liver resection and cyst fenestration demonstrating long-term, sustained reduction in liver size after the procedure. (From Que F, Nagorney DM, Gross JB, Torres VE. Liver resection and cyst fenestration in the treatment of severe polycystic liver disease. Gastroenterology. 1995;108:487–94.)

can be observed initially and followed at yearly intervals. If the size increases, surgery is indicated. Definitive management of aneurysms between 6 and 9 mm remains controversial. Surgical intervention is usually indicated for all unruptured aneurysms 10 mm in diameter or greater. For patients with high surgical risk or with technically difficult lesions endovascular treatment with detachable platinum coils may be indicated.

REFERENCES

1. Ravine D, Gibson RN, Walker RG, et al. Evaluation of ultrasonographic diagnostic criteria for autosomal dominant polycystic kidney disease 1. Lancet. 1994;343:824–7.
2. Nicolau C, Torra R, Badenas C, et al. Autosomal dominant polycystic kidney disease types 1 and 2: assessment of US sensitivity for diagnosis. Radiology. 1999;213:273–6.
3. Hughes J, Ward CJ, Peral B, et al. The polycystic kidney disease 1 (PKD1) gene encodes a novel protein with multiple cell recognition domains. Nat Genet. 1995;10:151–60.
4. Consortium TIPKD. Polycystic kidney disease: the complete structure of the PKD1 gene and its protein. Cell. 1995;81:289–98.
5. Consortium TAP. Analysis of the genomic sequence for the autosomal dominant polycystic kidney disease (PKD1) gene predicts the presence of a leucine-rich repeat. Hum Mol Genet. 1995;4:575–82.
6. Mochizuki T, Wu G, Hayashi T, et al. PKD2, a gene for polycystic kidney disease that encodes an integral membrane protein. Science. 1996;272:1339–42.
7. Reynolds DM, Falk CT, Li AR, et al. Identification of a locus for autosomal dominant polycystic liver disease, on chromosome 19p13.2–13.1. Am J Hum Genet. 2000;67:1598–604.
8. Torres V: New insights into polycystic kidney disease and its treatment. Curr Opin Nephrol Hypertens. 1998;7:159–69.
9. Qian F, Germino FJ, Cai Y, et al. PKD1 interacts with PKD2 through a probable coiled-coil domain. Nat Genet. 1997;16:179–83.
10. Griffin M, Torres V, Grande J, Kumar R. Immunolocalization of polycystin in human tissues and cultured cells. Proc Assoc Am Phys. 1996;108:185–97.
11. Geng L, Segal Y, Peissel B, et al. Identification and localization of polycystin, the PKD1 gene product. J Clin Invest 1996;98:2674–82.
12. Ibraghimov-Beskrovnaya O, Dackowski W, Foggensteiner L, et al. In vitro synthesis, in vivo tissue expression, and subcellular localization identifies a large membrane-associated protein. Proc Natl Acad Sci USA. 1997;94:6397–402.
13. Griffin MD, Torres VE, Grande JP, Kumar R. Vascular expression of polycystin. J Am Soc Nephrol. 1997;8:616–26.
14. Qian F, Watnick TJ, Onuchic LF, Germino GG. The molecular basis of focal cyst formation in human autosomal dominant polycystic kidney disease type 1. Cell. 1996;87:979–87.
15. Germino G. Autosomal dominant polycystic kidney disease: a two-hit model. Hosp Pract. 1997;32:81–102.

16. Pritchard L, Sloane-Stanley JA, Sharpe J, et al. A human *PKD1* transgene generates functional polycystin-1 in mice and is associated with a cystic phenotype. Hum Mol Genet. 2000;9:2617–27.

17. Koptides M, Mean R, Demetriou K, et al. Genetic evidence or a trans-heterozygous model for cystogenesis in autosomal dominant polycystic kidney disease. Hum Mol Genet. 2000; 9:447–52.

18. Watnick T, He N, Wang K, et al. Mutations of *PKD1* in ADPKD2 cysts suggest a pathogenic effect of trans-heterozygous mutations. Nat Genet. 2000;25:143–4.

19. Grantham JJ: The etiology, pathogenesis and treatment of autosomal dominant polycystic kidney disease: recent advances. Am J Kidney Dis. 1996;28:788–803.

20. Woo D: Apoptosis and loss of renal tissue in polycystic kidney diseases. N Engl J Med. 1995;333:18–25.

21. Gabow P: Definition and natural history of autosomal dominant polycystic kidney disease. In: Watson M, Torres V, eds. Polycystic kidney disease, vol 1. Oxford: Oxford University Press; 1996: 333–55.

22. Torres VE, Wilson DM, Hattery RR, Segura JW. Renal stone disease in autosomal dominant polycystic kidney disease. Am J Kidney Dis. 1993;22:513–19.

23. Wang D, Iversen J, Strandgaard S. Endothelium-dependent relaxation of small resistance vessels is impaired in patients with autosomal dominant polycystic kidney disease. J Am Soc Nephrol. 2000;11:1371–6.

24. Johnson A, Gabow P. Identification of patients with autosomal dominant polycystic kidney disease at highest risk for end-stage renal disease. J Am Soc Nephrol. 1997;8:1560–7.

25. Rossetti S, Burton S, Strmecki L, et al. The position of the polycystic kidney disease 1 (PKD1) gene mutation correlates with the severity of renal disease. J Am Soc Nephrol. 2002;13:1230–7.

26. Hateboer N, Veldhuisen B, Peters D, et al. Location of mutations within the PKD2 gene influences clinical outcome. Kidney Int. 2000;57:1444–51.

27. Zeier M, Fehrenbach P, Geberth S, et al. Renal histology in polycystic kidney disease with incipient and advanced renal failure. Kidney Int. 1992;42:1259–65.

28. Torres V. Polycystic liver disease. In: Watson MT, Torres VE, eds. Polycystic kidney disease, vol 1. Oxford: Oxford Medical Publications; 1996:500–29.

29. Huston J, Torres V, Wiebers D, Schievink W. Follow-up of intracranial aneurysms in autosomal dominant polycystic kidney disease by magnetic resonance angiography. J Am Soc Nephrol. 1996;7: 2135–41.

30. Torres VE, Cai Y, Chen X, et al. Vascular expression of polycystin 2. J Am Soc Nephrol. 2001;12:1–9.

31. Gregoire J, Torres V, Holley K, Farrow G. Renal epithelial hyperplastic and neoplastic proliferation in autosomal dominant polycystic kidney disease. Am J Kidney Dis. 1987;9:27–38.

32. Rossetti S, Strmecki L, Gamble V, et al. Mutation analysis of the entire *PKD1* gene: Genetic and diagnostic implications. Am J Hum Genet. 2001;68:46–63.

33. Segura JW, King BF, Jowsey SG, et al. Chronic pain and its medical and surgical management in renal cystic diseases. In: Watson M, Torres VE, eds. Polycystic kidney disease, vol 1. Oxford: Oxford University Press; 1996:462–80.

34. Ubara Y, Katori H, Tagami T, et al. Transcatheter renal arterial embolization therapy on a patient with polycystic kidney disease on hemodialysis. Am J Kidney Dis. 1999;34:926–31.

35. Dunn MD, Portis AJ, Elbahnasy AM, et al. Laparoscopic nephrectomy in patients with end-stage renal disease and autosomal dominant polycystic kidney disease. (see comments). Am J Kidney Dis. 2000;35:720–5.

36. Valente JF. Laparoscopic renal denervation for intractable ADPKD-related pain. Neph Dial Transplant. 2001;16:160.

37. Kanno Y, Suzuki H, Okada H, et al. Calcium channel blockers versus ACE inhibitors as antihypertensives in polycystic kidney disease. Q J Med. 1996;89:65–70.

38. Ecder T, Chapman A, Brosnahan G, et al. Effect of antihypertensive therapy on renal function and urinary albumin excretion in hypertensive patients with autosomal dominant polycystic kidney disease. Am J Kidney Dis. 2000; 35:427–32.

39. Ecder T, Edelstein C, Fick-Brosnahan G, et al. Diuretics versus angiotensin-converting enzyme inhibitors in autosomal dominant polycystic kidney disease. Am J Nephrol. 2001;21:98–103.

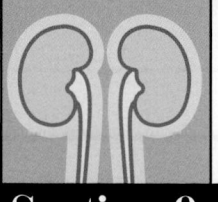
Chapter
47

Other Cystic Kidney Diseases

Lisa Guay-Woodford

INTRODUCTION

In addition to autosomal dominant polycystic kidney disease (ADPKD), there are numerous other disorders that share renal cysts as a common feature[1,2] (Table 47.1). These disorders may be inherited or acquired and their manifestations may be confined to the kidney or expressed systemically. They may present at a wide range of ages, from the perinatal period to old age (Fig. 47.1). The renal cysts may be single or multiple and their associated morbidity may range from clinical insignificance to progressive parenchymal destruction with resultant renal insufficiency.

The clinical context often helps distinguish these renal cystic disorders from one another. Echogenic, enlarged kidneys in a neonate or infant should raise suspicion about autosomal

Renal cystic disorders
Nongenetic
Developmental
Medullary sponge kidney
Renal cystic dysplasia
Multicystic dysplasia
Cystic dysplasia associated with lower urinary tract obstruction
Diffuse cystic dysplasia – syndromal and nonsyndromal
Acquired
Simple cysts
Hypokalemic cystic disease
Acquired cystic disease (in advanced renal failure)
Genetic
Autosomal dominant
ADPKD
VHL
TSC
Adult-onset medullary cystic disease
Autosomal recessive
ARPKD
Juvenile-onset nephronophthisis
Other rare syndromes associated with multiple malformations
X-linked
Orofaciodigital syndrome Type I

Table 47.1 Renal cystic disorders.

Age distribution of renal cystic disorders				
	Neonates	Infants/children	Adolescents	Adults

Autosomal dominant polycystic kidney disease (ADPKD)
Autosomal recessive polycystic kidney disease (ARPKD)
Nephronophthisis (NPH)
Medullary sponge kidney (MSK)
Tuberous sclerosis complex (TSC)
von Hippel–Lindau disease (VHL)
Simple cysts

Figure 47.1 Age distribution of renal cystic disorders.

recessive polycystic kidney disease (ARPKD), ADPKD, tuberous sclerosis complex (TSC), or one of the many congenital syndromes associated with renal cystic disease. Renal insufficiency in an adolescent suggests juvenile nephronophthisis-medullary cystic disease complex or ARPKD as possible etiologies. The finding of a solitary cyst in a 5-year-old may indicate a calyceal diverticulum, whereas this finding in a 50-year-old is most compatible with a simple renal cyst. Renal stones occur in ADPKD and medullary sponge kidneys. For those disorders with systemic manifestations, such as ADPKD, TSC, and von Hippel-Lindau disease, the associated extra–renal features may provide other important differential diagnostic clues.

AUTOSOMAL RECESSIVE POLYCYSTIC KIDNEY DISEASE

Introduction and definition
Autosomal recessive polycystic kidney disease (ARPKD) is an inherited malformation complex with varying degrees of renal collecting duct dilatation and biliary ductal ectasia[3].

Etiology and pathogenesis
Genetic basis of ARPKD
Studies in the 1970s subdivided ARPKD into four distinct phenotypes according to the age of presentation and the proportion of dilated renal collecting ducts. The ARPKD gene, *PKHD1*, has been mapped to the short arm of chromosome 6 (6p21) and to date, all phenotypic variants appear to result

611

from mutations in this single gene[4]. Recently, two groups have used complementary strategies to identify the *PKHD1* gene[5,6]. The genomic sequence includes at least 86 exons that are variably assembled into a number of alternatively spliced transcripts. The longest continuous open reading frame encodes a very large protein, fibrocystin, that is predicted to have a single transmembrane spanning domain near its carboxyl terminus. Several transcripts encode truncated products that lack the transmembrane domain and may be secreted polypeptides. The *PKHD1* gene products are members of a novel protein class and appear to belong to a superfamily of proteins involved in regulation of cell proliferation as well as cellular adhesion and repulsion.

Pathogenesis

ARPKD typically begins *in utero* and the renal cystic lesion appears to be superimposed on a normal developmental sequence. The tubular abnormality primarily involves fusiform dilatation of the collecting ducts and tubular obstruction has been excluded as a pathogenic mechanism.

The biliary lesion appears to involve defective remodeling of the ductal plate *in utero*. As a result, primitive bile duct configurations persist and progressive portal fibrosis evolves. The remainder of the liver parenchyma develops normally. The defect in ductal plate remodeling is accompanied by abnormalities in the branching of the portal vein. The resulting histopathologic pattern is referred to as congenital hepatic fibrosis.

The weight of the experimental evidence from human and animal model studies suggests that a maturational arrest in both renal and biliary tubuloepithelial differentiation underlies the pathogenesis of ARPKD.

Epidemiology

The estimated incidence of ARPKD is 1 per 20 000 live births and it appears to occur more frequently in Caucasians than in other ethnic populations[7].

Clinical manifestations

The clinical spectrum of ARPKD is variable and depends on the age at presentation (Fig. 47.2). The majority of cases are identified either *in utero* or at birth. The most severely affected fetuses have enlarged echogenic kidneys and oligohydramnios due to poor fetal renal output. These fetuses develop the 'Potter' phenotype, with pulmonary hypoplasia, a characteristic facies, and deformities of the spine and limbs. At birth, these neonates often have a critical degree of pulmonary hypoplasia that is incompatible with survival. Renal function, though frequently compromised, is rarely a cause of neonatal death. For those infants who survive the perinatal period, hypertension, renal failure, and portal hypertension usually evolve.

Hypertension usually develops in the first several months and ultimately affects 70–80% of patients. ARPKD patients have defects in both urinary diluting capacity and concentrating capacity. There is often hyponatremia, presumably resulting from defects in free water excretion. While net acid excretion may be reduced, metabolic acidosis is not a significant clinical feature.

Abnormal urinalyses are common in both infants and older children. Microscopic or gross hematuria, proteinuria and

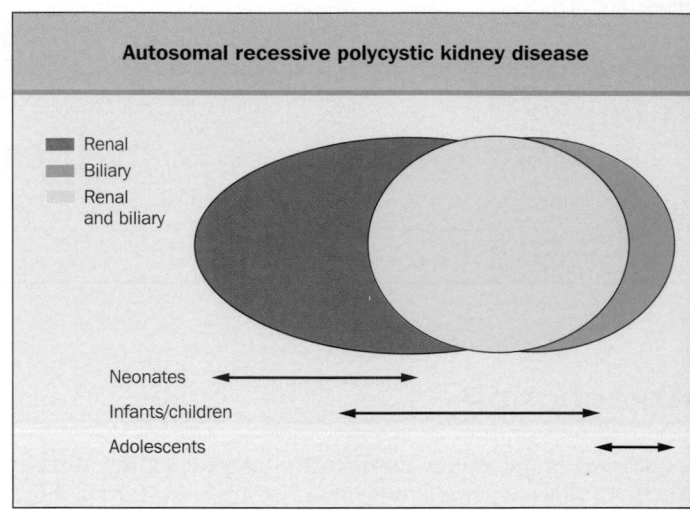

Figure 47.2 Correlation of clinical ARPKD phenotypes and age.

sterile pyuria have all been reported. Two retrospective studies report an increased incidence of urinary tract infections. In the first 6 months of life, ARPKD infants may have a transient improvement in their glomerular filtration rate (GFR) due to renal maturation. Subsequently, a progressive but variable decline in renal function occurs, with some patients not progressing to end-stage renal disease (ESRD) until adolescence or early adulthood. With advances in effective therapy for ESRD, prolonged survival is common and for many patients, the hepatic complications come to dominate the clinical picture.

Portal hypertension is frequently the predominant clinical abnormality in older children and adolescents with ARPKD. These children typically present with hepatosplenomegaly and bleeding esophageal or gastric varices, as well as hypersplenism with consequent thrombocytopenia, anemia, and leukopenia. Hepatocellular function is usually preserved. Ascending suppurative cholangitis is a serious complication and can cause fulminant hepatic failure.

Pathology

Kidney

The renal involvement is invariably bilateral and largely symmetric. The histopathology varies depending on the age of presentation and the extent of cystic involvement (Fig. 47.3a,b).

In the affected neonate, the kidneys can be 10 times normal size, but retain their reniform configuration. Dilated, fusiform collecting ducts extend radially through the cortex. In the medulla, the dilated collecting ducts are more often cut tangentially or transversely. Up to 90% of the collecting ducts are involved. There is little evidence of fibrosis.

In patients diagnosed later in infancy, the kidney size and extent of cystic involvement tend to be more limited. Cysts can expand up to 2 cm in diameter and assume a more spherical configuration. Progressive interstitial fibrosis is probably responsible for secondary tubular obstruction. In older children, medullary ductal ectasia is the predominant finding.

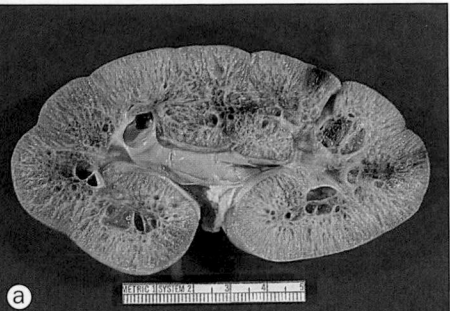
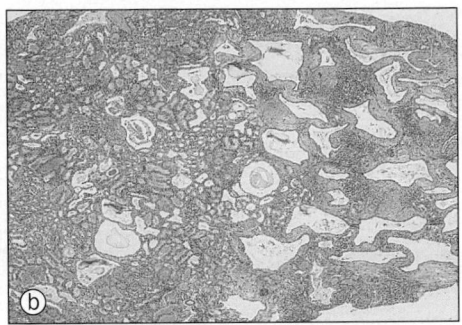
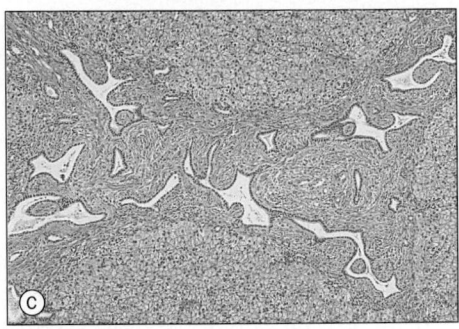

Figure 47.3 Pathologic features of ARPKD. (a) Cut section: ARPKD kidney from 1-year-old child reveals discrete medullary cysts and dilated collecting ducts. (b) Light microscopy: later-onset ARPKD kidney with prominent medullary ductal ectasia, H&E x 10. (c) Light microscopy: congenital hepatic fibrosis. There is extensive fibrosis of the portal area with ectatic, tortuous bile ducts and hypoplasia of the portal vein, H&E x 40.

Cysts are lined with a single layer of nondescript cuboidal epithelium. The glomeruli and nephron segments proximal to the collecting ducts are initially structurally normal, but are often crowded between ectatic collecting ducts or displaced into subcapsular wedges. The presence of cartilage or other dysplastic elements indicates a diagnosis other than ARPKD, such as cystic dysplasia or even ADPKD.

Liver
The liver in ARPKD can be either normal in size or somewhat enlarged. The hepatic parenchyma may be intersected by delicate fibrous septa, which link the portal tracts. Bile ducts are dilated (biliary ectasia) and marked cystic dilatation of the entire intrahepatic biliary system (Caroli's disease) has been reported. In neonatal ARPKD, the bile ducts are increased in number, rather tortuous in configuration, and often located around the periphery of the portal tract. In older children, the biliary ectasia is accompanied by increasing portal fibrosis and hypoplasia of the small portal vein branches (Fig. 47.3c). The portal fibrosis may be quite extensive, but the hepatocytes are seldom affected.

Diagnosis
Prenatal diagnosis
The diagnosis of ARPKD can be suggested by fetal sonography. Enlarged echogenic kidneys, oligohydramnios, and decreased urine in the bladder may become evident as early as the 16th week of gestation, but most often occur after the 20th week. However, these findings are not specific to ARPKD and may also be evident in ADPKD, glomerulocystic kidney disease, and Meckel syndrome. In families known to be 'at-risk' for ARPKD, the genetic mapping data and the absence of genetic heterogeneity has allowed for haplotype-based prenatal diagnosis[7]. The accurate diagnosis of ARPKD in previous affected sibling(s) is an absolute prerequisite for these genetic studies.

While the *PKHD1* gene is quite large and has a complex array of transcripts, the identification of this gene should lead to the development of a direct gene-based diagnostic test. Such a test could be applied to 'at-risk' pregnancies as well as aid in specific diagnoses for fetuses and children with less classic presentations of renal cystic disease.

Postnatal diagnosis
The sonographic findings vary with patient age and the severity of renal involvement. In ARPKD patients, the kidney size typically peaks at 1 to 2 years of age, then gradually declines relative to the child's body size, and stabilizes by 4 to 5 years.

Sonography in affected neonates reveals symmetrically enlarged, diffusely echogenic kidneys with poor demarcation from surrounding tissues as well as among the cortex, medulla, and renal sinus. With high-resolution sonography, the radial array of dilated collecting ducts may be imaged (Fig. 47.4a). As patients age, there is increased medullary echogenicity with scattered small cysts, measuring less than 2 cm in diameter. These cysts and progressive fibrosis can alter the reniform contour and ARPKD in older children may be mistaken for ADPKD. In adults with medullary ectasia alone, the cystic lesion may be confused with medullary sponge kidney. Contrast-enhanced CT scanning is useful in delineating the renal architecture in older children (Fig. 47.4b). In one small study, bilateral renal calcifications were evident in 50% of patients[8].

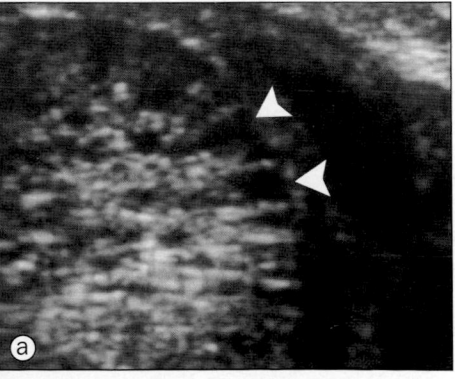
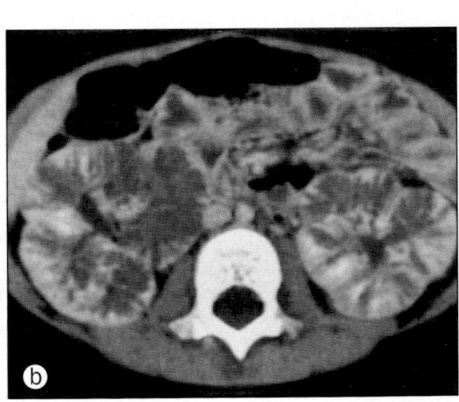

Figure 47.4 Radiologic findings associated with ARPKD. (a) ARPKD in a neonate. High resolution sonography reveals radially arrayed dilated collecting ducts (arrowheads). (b) ARPKD in a symptomatic 4-year-old girl. Contrast-enhanced CT shows a striated nephrogram and prolonged corticomedullary differentiation.

The liver may be either normal in size or enlarged. It is usually less echogenic than the kidneys. Prominent intrahepatic bile duct dilatation suggests associated Caroli's disease. With age, the portal fibrosis tends to progress and in older children, sonography typically reveals hepatosplenomegaly and a patchy increase in hepatic echogenicity.

Natural history

The estimated perinatal mortality is 30–50%. For those who survive the first month of life, the reported mean 5-year patient survival rate is 80–95%[9,10]. On average, those infants with serum creatinine values > 2.2 mg/dL (200 µmol/L) progress to ESRD within 5 years, but this is highly variable. In one study, the probability of survival without ESRD was 85% at 1 year, 76% at 5 years, and 63% at 15 years. Effective management of systemic and portal hypertension, coupled with successful renal replacement therapy, has allowed long-term patient survival. Therefore, the prognosis in ARPKD, particularly for those children who survive the first month of life, is far less bleak than popularly thought and aggressive medical therapy is warranted. In those patients with ESRD and severe portal hypertension, combined kidney and liver transplantation may be indicated.

Transplantation

Renal transplantation is the treatment of choice for ARPKD patients who develop ESRD. Native nephrectomies may be warranted in patients with massively enlarged kidneys to allow allograft placement. Living-related donors are preferable for pediatric transplant candidates[11]. Because ARPKD is a recessive disorder, either parent may be a suitable kidney donor.

Treatment

The survival of ARPKD neonates has improved significantly in the last decade because of advances in mechanical ventilation and other supportive measures for neonates. Aggressive interventions such as unilateral or bilateral nephrectomies and continuous hemofiltration have been advocated in neonatal management, but prospective, controlled studies have not been performed.

For those children who survive the perinatal period, careful blood pressure monitoring is required. Angiotensin converting enzyme (ACE) inhibitors, calcium channel blockers, β-blockers and loop diuretics are effective treatments. The management of ARPKD children with declining GFR should follow the standard guidelines established for chronic renal insufficiency in pediatric patients. Given the relative urinary concentrating defect, ARPKD children should be monitored for dehydration during intercurrent illnesses associated with fever, tachypnea, nausea, vomiting or diarrhea. In those infants with severe polyuria, thiazide diuretics may be used to decrease distal nephron solute and water delivery. Acid–base balance should be closely monitored and supplemental bicarbonate therapy initiated as needed.

Close monitoring for portal hypertension is warranted in all ARPKD patients. The severity of portal hypertension and its progression can be followed by serial ultrasound and Doppler flow studies. Hematemesis or melena suggests the presence of esophageal varices. Medical management may include sclerotherapy, variceal banding, or transjugular intrahepatic portosystemic shunt (TIPS). Surgical approaches such as portocaval or splenorenal shunting may be indicated in some patients. Although hypersplenism occurs fairly commonly, splenectomy is seldom warranted. Unexplained fever with or without elevated transaminase levels suggests bacterial cholangitis and requires meticulous evaluation, often including a percutaneous liver biopsy, to make the diagnosis and guide aggressive antibiotic therapy.

JUVENILE NEPHRONOPHTHISIS–MEDULLARY CYSTIC DISEASE COMPLEX

Introduction and definitions

Juvenile nephronophthisis and medullary cystic kidney disease share the same triad of histopathologic features: tubular basement membrane irregularities, tubular atrophy with cyst formation, and interstitial cell infiltration with fibrosis. These histopathologically similar disorders differ only in their mode of transmission and the age of onset. *Juvenile nephronophthisis* is an autosomal recessive disorder that presents in childhood, while *medullary cystic disease* is an autosomal dominant disorder that occurs in adults. The inclusive term juvenile nephronophthisis-medullary cystic disease complex has been used to describe these disorders. However, juvenile nephronophthisis is far more common than medullary cystic disease and has been reported both as an isolated renal disease and in association with retinitis pigmentosa, congenital hepatic fibrosis, oculomotor apraxia, and skeletal anomalies. Therefore, these entities will be considered separately.

AUTOSOMAL RECESSIVE JUVENILE NEPHRONOPHTHISIS

Etiology and pathogenesis
Genetic
Linkage studies have mapped the principal gene (*NPHP1*) for juvenile nephronophthisis (NPH) to the long arm of chromosome 2 (2q13). Approximately 85% of the cases of purely renal NPH have defects in *NPHP1*, which encodes a novel protein product called nephrocystin[12]. Large, homozygous deletions have been detected in 80% of affected members of NPH families and in 65% of sporadic cases[13]. At least two other genes are involved in the remaining families with purely renal NPH, as well as those families with NPH and associated retinal defects. These genes have yet to be identified. No significant clinical or pathologic differences are discernible between *NPHP1*-linked and unlinked families.

The renal histopathology is characterized by a chronic, sclerosing, tubulointerstitial nephropathy with sparse inflammatory cell infiltration and the development of medullary cysts late in the disease course. There is irregular thickening of the tubular basement membrane (TBM) with the absence of certain TBM components and the novel expression of α5 integrin by tubular epithelial cells[14]. These data suggest that altered cell–matrix interactions contribute to the pathogenesis of NPH. The role of the *NPHP1* gene product in this pathogenesis remains to be determined.

Clinical manifestations
Renal disease
NPH accounts for 6–15% of ESRD in children and adolescents[15].

Decreased urinary concentrating capacity is an invariable finding in NPH patients and usually precedes the decline in renal function. The mean age of onset is 4 years. Polyuria and polydipsia are common symptoms. Salt-wasting develops in most patients with renal insufficiency, and sodium supplementation is often required until the onset of ESRD. One-third of patients become anemic before the onset of renal insufficiency, probably due to a defect in the functional regulation of erythropoietin production by peritubular fibroblasts[15]. Growth retardation, out of proportion to the degree of renal insufficiency, is a common finding.

Progressive decline in renal function is typical of NPH. It may occur insidiously, such that 15% of affected patients are recognized only after ESRD has developed. There is no specific treatment. The disease is not known to recur in renal allografts.

Symptoms are usually detected after the age of 2 years, and ESRD develops by adolescence. Within a sibship, affected children have very similar clinical courses. Typical cases of autosomal recessive NPH have also been described in young adults and may represent a phenotypic variant of classic NPH. Children with an infantile variant develop symptoms in the first few months of life and rapidly progress to ESRD by 2 years of age. This disorder appears to be a distinct genetic entity, with a characteristic renal histopathology, and has not been reported in sibships with classic juvenile NPH[16].

Unlike patients with polycystic kidney disease or medullary sponge kidney, NPH patients rarely develop flank pain, hematuria, hypertension, urinary tract infections, or renal calculi.

Associated disorders
In 10–15% of NPH, there is an association with retinitis pigmentosa due to tapetoretinal degeneration (Senior-Loken syndrome) which presents with coarse nystagmus and early blindness. A late-onset form with blindness during childhood or adolescence has also been described. NPH associated with oculomotor apraxia and co-existing retinal degeneration (Cogan syndrome) has been reported in several kindreds. A subset of these cases has associated mental retardation. NPH has also been reported in patients with cone-shaped epiphyses of the bones, or cerebellar vermis aplasia, or coloboma of the eye (Joubert syndrome, type B). Congenital hepatic fibrosis occurs occasionally in NPH patients, but the associated bile duct proliferation is mild and qualitatively different from that found in ARPKD.

Pathology
There are no discernible differences in the renal lesions associated with NPHP1-linked and non-NPHP1 disease. In patients with ESRD, the kidneys are moderately contracted with parenchymal atrophy causing a loss of corticomedullary demarcation. Sometimes visible cysts of variable size are evident and are distributed in an irregular pattern at the corticomedullary junction and in the outer medulla. Up to 25% of NPH kidneys have no grossly visible cysts.

Microscopic examination initially reveals clusters of atrophic tubules with irregularly thickened TBM on electron microscopy. Reduced staining with anti-TBM antibodies suggests the absence of some normal antigenic component in the thickened TBM. Clusters of atrophic tubules typically alternate with either groups of viable tubules showing dilation or marked compensatory hypertrophy or groups of collapsed tubules. While this histopathologic pattern is not unique, the abrupt transition from one type of tubular profile to another is suggestive of NPH. Moderate interstitial fibrosis, usually without a significant inflammatory cell infiltrate, is interspersed among the atrophic tubules. Spherical, thin-walled cysts lined with a simple cuboidal epithelium may be evident at the corticomedullary junction, in the medulla and even in the papillae. Microdissection studies indicate that these cysts arise from loop of Henle, distal convoluted tubules, and collecting ducts. Glomeruli may be normal, although some may be completely sclerosed, others show periglomerular fibrosis and still others dilatation of Bowman's space (Fig. 47.5).

Diagnosis and differential diagnosis
In a child with NPH and renal insufficiency, renal sonography shows normal-sized or small kidneys with loss of corticomedullary differentiation and increased echogenicity. Sometimes cysts are detected in the medulla or at the corticomedullary junction. Thin-section CT may be more sensitive than sonography in detecting these cysts. Renal function scintigraphy may provide additional diagnostic information by identifying the characteristic concentrating defect in NPH patients.

The pathologic findings in NPH are not unique; hence in the early stages of the disease, neither renal imaging nor histopathology can confirm the clinical diagnosis of NPH. Fortunately, in the majority of suspected cases, molecular testing soon may replace renal biopsy in establishing the diagnosis of NPH. Hildebrant et al.[12] recently have developed an algorithm for gene-based diagnosis that addresses four critical diagnostic issues: (1) detection of the classic homozygous deletion of NPHP1, (2) detection of rare, smaller homozygous deletions of NPHP1, (3) testing for a heterozygous deletion, and (4) potential exclusion of linkage to NPHP1.

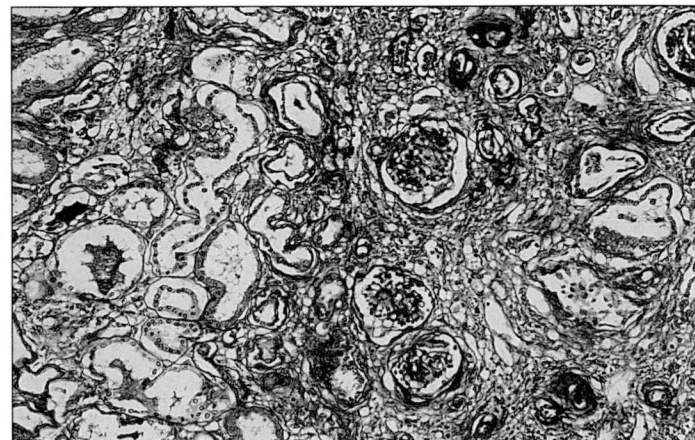

Figure 47.5 Renal pathology in juvenile nephronophthisis. Light microscopy: Tubulointerstitial nephropathy. Atrophic tubules with irregularly thickened basement membranes are surrounded by interstitial fibrosis. Dilated tubules are evident at the corticomedullary junction, H&E x 40.

AUTOSOMAL DOMINANT MEDULLARY CYSTIC KIDNEY DISEASE

Medullary cystic kidney disease is histopathologically indistinguishable from recessive NPH and occurs with male-to-male transmission in successive generations, suggesting an autosomal dominant mode of inheritance. Some patients have had phenotypically unaffected parents but an affected second or third degree relative, raising the possibility of variable penetrance. This disorder appears to be rare relative to recessive NPH. While the clinical manifestations of the two disorders are similar, medullary cystic kidney disease is distinguished by its dominant mode of inheritance, later age of onset, progression to ESRD in the third to fourth decade of life, and lack of associated extra-renal manifestations. Genetic linkage analyses indicate that defects in at least two genes can cause medullary cystic kidney disease, but the underlying genetic defects have not been determined. The diagnosis is ascertained on the basis of the family history and the sonographic finding of medullary cysts.

MEDULLARY SPONGE KIDNEY

Introduction and definition
Medullary sponge kidney (MSK) is a relatively common disorder characterized by dilated medullary and papillary collecting ducts that give the renal medulla a 'spongy' appearance[18].

Etiology and pathogenesis
MSK is likely the result of a developmental defect as evidenced by the occasional presence of embryonal tissue in the affected papillae and coexistence of other urinary tract anomalies. In addition, MSK occurs more frequently in individuals with other congenital defects, e.g., congenital hemihypertrophy, Beckwith–Wiedemann syndrome, Ehlers-Danlos syndrome, and Marfan's syndrome[18].

Fewer than 5% of cases are familial and a clear genetic basis for MSK has not been established.

Epidemiology
In the general population, the frequency of MSK may be underestimated because some affected individuals remain entirely asymptomatic. Up to 20% of patients with nephrolithiasis have at least a mild degree of MSK, but excretory urography in unselected patients indicates a disease frequency of 1 in 5000 individuals.

Clinical manifestations
Medullary sponge kidney disease is asymptomatic unless complicated by nephrolithiasis, hematuria, or infection. Symptoms typically begin between the fourth and fifth decade of life, but adolescent presentations have been reported[19]. In MSK patients, stones or granular debris are composed of either pure apatite (calcium phosphate) or a mixture of apatite and calcium oxalate. Several factors appear to contribute to stone-formation, including urinary stasis within the ectatic ducts, hypercalcuria, and hyperoxaluria. Hyperparathyroidism has also been reported in MSK.

Hematuria, unrelated to either coexisting stones or infection, may be recurrent. The bleeding is usually asymptomatic but with gross hematuria, clot formation may cause colic. Urinary tract infection may occur in association with nephrolithiasis or as an independent event. Of those patients with stones, infections are more likely to occur in females than in males. Decreased renal concentrating ability and impaired urinary acidification have been reported. In most patients, the acidification defect is not associated with systemic acidosis.

Pathology
The pathologic changes are confined to the renal medulla and papillae. Multiple spherical or oval cysts measuring 1–3 mm may be detected in one or more papillae. These cysts may be isolated or may communicate with the collecting system. The cysts are frequently bilateral and often contain spherical concretions composed of apatite. The affected pyramids and associated calyces are usually enlarged, and nephromegaly may result when many pyramids are involved. The renal cortex, medullary rays, calyces, and pelvis appear normal, unless complications such as pyelonephritis or urinary tract obstruction become superimposed.

Diagnosis
Plain films of the abdomen often reveal radio-opaque concretions in the medulla (Fig. 47.6a). The diagnosis is established by excretory urography (Fig. 47.6b). Retention of contrast media by the ectatic collecting ducts appears either as spherical cysts or more commonly, as diffuse linear striations. The latter impart a characteristic blush-like pattern to the papillae, the so-called 'bouquet of flowers' or 'paintbrush' appearance. CT is usually not necessary, but nonenhanced CT may help distinguish MSK from papillary necrosis or even ADPKD (Fig. 47.6c).

Natural history
With proper management of the clinical complications, the long-term prognosis is excellent. Progression to renal insufficiency is distinctly unusual.

Treatment
Asymptomatic patients in whom MSK is detected as an incidental finding require no therapy. Hematuria in the absence of stones or infection requires no intervention. If the tubular ectasia is unilateral and segmental, partial nephrectomy may alleviate recurrent nephrolithiasis and urinary tract infection. However, for the majority of patients who have bilateral disease, medical management is preferred.

Hypercalcuria is the predominant cause of nephrolithiasis in MSK. The mainstay of treatment is high-volume fluid intake, in order to increase urine output and reduce the precipitation of calcium salts in ectatic ducts. Patients with documented hypercalcuria may benefit from thiazide diuretics. If thiazides are poorly tolerated or contraindicated, inorganic phosphate therapy may be useful. To avoid struvite stone formation, oral phosphates should *not* be used in patients with previous urinary tract infections due to urease-producing organisms. Patients who form and pass stones recurrently may benefit

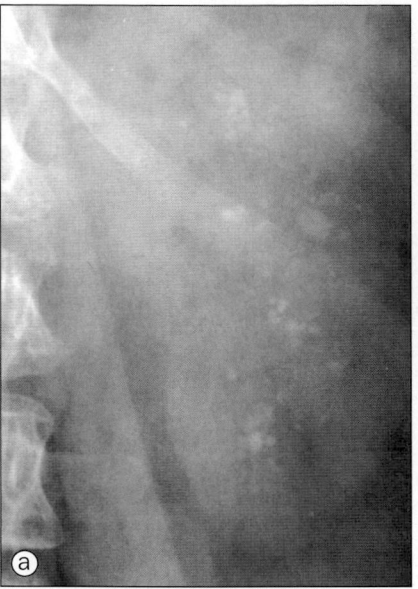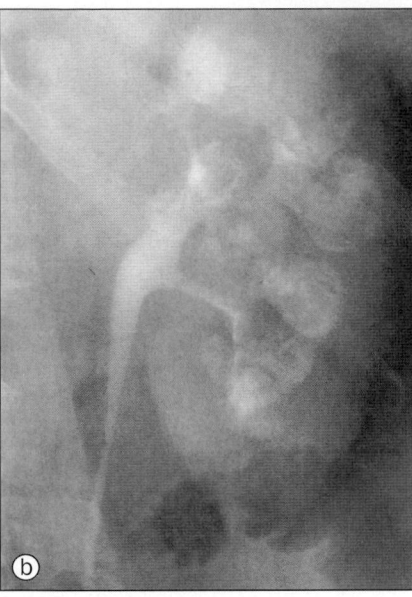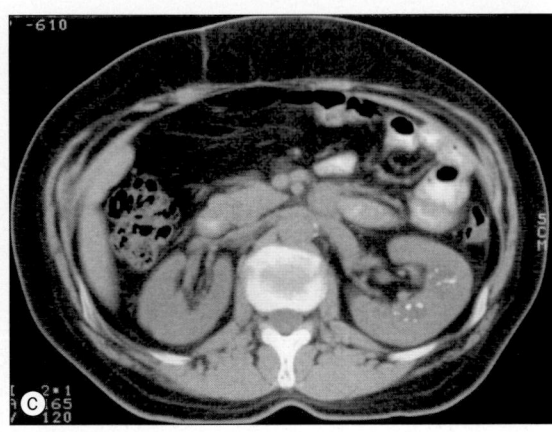

Figure 47.6 Radiologic findings associated with MSK. MSK in a 52-year-old symptomatic woman. (a) Preliminary film shows medullary nephrolithiases. (b) Ten-minute film from an excretory urography shows clusters of rounded densities in the papillae amidst discrete linear opacities (paintbrush appearance). (c) Nonenhanced CT reveals densely echogenic foci in the medulla.

from periodic lithotripsy. Urinary tract obstruction must be considered during acute episodes of renal colic and surgical intervention may be indicated.

Urinary tract infection should be treated with standard antibiotic regimens and for some patients, prolonged therapy may be warranted. Urease-producing organisms, such as coagulase-negative staphylococcus, are particularly problematic as urinary pathogens in MSK. Positive urine cultures, even with relatively insignificant colony counts, must be vigorously pursued.

TUBEROUS SCLEROSIS COMPLEX

Introduction and definition
Tuberous sclerosis complex (TSC) is an autosomal dominant disorder in which tumor-like malformations, called hamartomas, develop in multiple organ systems.

Etiology and pathogenesis
Genetic
TSC is genetically heterogeneous. At least two loci are involved, the first (TSC1) on chromosome 9q32-q34 and the second (TSC2) on chromosome 16p13, adjacent to the PKD1 gene[20,21]. Both the TSC1 and TSC2 genes have been identified and sequenced. The protein product of TSC2, called tuberin, has a region of homology to the GTPase activating protein, GAP3. GTPase activating proteins bind to Ras proteins, regulate their activity, and are involved in the control of cell proliferation and differentiation. The protein product of TSC1, which has been named hamartin, was more recently identified and its role in cell growth regulation is under investigation. Recent data from the *Drosophila* fly model suggest that the TSC1 and TSC2 gene products function together as negative regulators of the insulin signaling pathway[22].

The molecular defect in TSC appears to disrupt cell migration and differentiation in neural crest derivatives. The focal nature of TSC-associated disease and the variability of disease expression even within families have suggested that TSC1 and TSC2 function as tumor suppressor genes. The tumor suppressor gene paradigm was first proposed by Knudson, who hypothesized that two successive mutations are necessary to inactivate a tumor suppressor gene and cause tumor formation. The first mutation, inherited and therefore present in all cells, is necessary but not sufficient to produce tumors. A second mutation is required after fertilization to induce tumor transformation. The inactivating germline mutations identified in both TSC1 and TSC2 and the loss of heterozygosity detected in 50% of TSC2-associated hamartomas and ~10% of TSC1-associated hamartomas support the hypothesis that both TSC1 and TSC2 function as tumor suppressor genes. Contiguous deletions involving the TSC2 and PKD1 genes have been found in 22 of 27 TSC patients with renal cystic disease (Fig. 47.7), suggesting that PKD1 plays a significant cystogenic role in TSC2 disease[23].

Epidemiology
TSC affects 1 in 10 000 individuals. The disease penetrance is quite variable. Spontaneous mutations appear to occur at high frequency and are estimated to account for 60–70% of new cases.

Clinical manifestations
The most common clinical manifestations involve the central nervous system and the skin. Approximately 80% of affected individuals have seizures and 50% have mental retardation. In affected individuals over 5 years of age, the most common skin lesions are facial angiofibromas (Fig. 47.8), hypomelanotic macules, and ungual fibromas[24].

Heriditary and Congenital Diseases of the Kidney

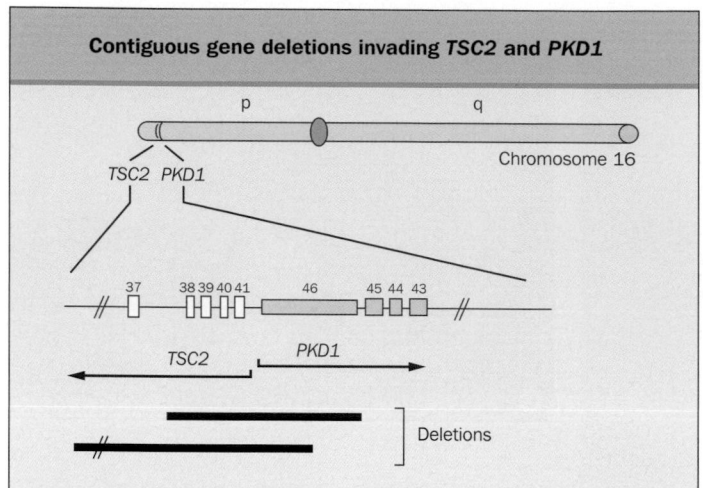

Figure 47.7 Contiguous gene deletions involving *TSC2* and *PKD1*.
The *TSC2* and *PKD1* genes lie immediately adjacent to one another on the tip of the short arm of chromosome 16. The arrows extend from the 3' end of each gene toward the 5' end and the exons of each respective gene are indicated by numbered boxes. The solid bars represent large deleted regions in two affected patients that disrupt the 3' end of each gene. Both patients fulfilled the definitive diagnostic criteria for TSC and had extensive renal cystic disease. (Modified from Sampson et al.[23], with permission.)

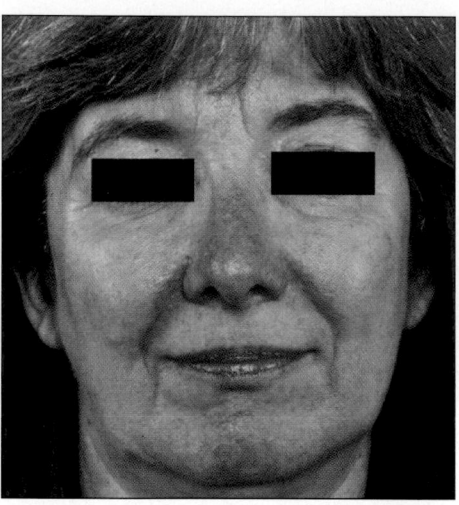

Figure 47.8 Facial angiofibromas in a 49-year-old patient with tuberous sclerosis complex.

Kidney involvement occurs frequently in TSC[24,25]. The principal manifestations include angiomyolipomas, cysts, and renal malignancies. Some of the malignant tumors originally thought to be renal cell carcinoma, are now regarded as malignant epithelioid angiomyolipomas[26]. Other renal neoplasms, interstitial fibrosis with focal segmental glomeulosclerosis (FSGS), glomerular microhamartomas, and peripelvic and perirenal lymphangiomatous cysts have been observed less often.

Renal angiomyolipomas
Angiomyolipomas are the principal form of hamartomas in TSC and occur very commonly, identified in 40 to 80% of patients at autopsy. While solitary angiomyolipoma are found in the general population, particularly among older women, angiomyolipomas in TSC patients are usually multiple and bilateral. Angiomyolipomas rarely occur before 5 years of age, but increase in frequency and size with age. The clinical manifestations relate to the potential for hemorrhage (gross hematuria, intratumoral or retroperitoneal hemorrhage), and to mass effects (abdominal or flank masses and tenderness, hypertension, renal insufficiency). Women tend to have more numerous and larger angiomyolipomas than men. Pregnancy appears to increase the risk of rupture and hemorrhage.

Renal cystic disease
Renal cystic disease is the earliest renal finding in TSC and may be the presenting manifestation in infants and children. In adults, renal cysts occur more frequently in men than in women[24]. The concurrence of cysts and angiomyolipomas, easily detected by CT, is strongly suggestive of TSC. In the absence of angiomyolipomas, the renal cystic disease may be radiographically indistinguishable from ADPKD.

Affected children frequently have early onset, severe hypertension, and a progressive decline in renal function that results in ESRD in the second or third decade of life. The majority of these patients have a contiguous TSC2-PKD1 gene syndrome[23]. Strict control of the hypertension may favorably impact the renal prognosis.

Renal carcinoma
Renal carcinoma reportedly occurs in TSC patients with a higher frequency and earlier age of onset than in the general population. Carcinoma is often bilateral and occurs more commonly in females, with a median age at diagnosis of 28 years. Between 19% and 50% of patients die of metastatic disease.

Pathology
Renal angiomyolipomas
Angiomyolipomas are hamartomatous structures composed of abnormal, thick-walled vessels, varying amounts of smooth muscle-like cells, and adipose tissue (Fig. 47.9a,b). These tumors can be locally invasive, extending into the perirenal fat or more rarely, the collecting system, renal vein, and even the inferior vena cava and right atrium. Lymph node and splenic involvement likely represent multifocal origin rather than metastases.

Renal cystic disease
The cysts in TSC develop from any nephron segment. When their number is limited and the size is small, they are predominantly cortical. In some cases, glomerular cysts predominate. The epithelial lining of the cysts is distinctive and appears to be unique to TSC. The cells are large and acidophilic and contain large hyperchromatic nuclei with occasional mitotic figures (Fig. 47.9c). Associated papillary hyperplasia and adenomas are common.

Renal neoplasms
Both benign and malignant epithelial tumors of the kidney, such as papillary adenomas and oncocytomas and renal cell

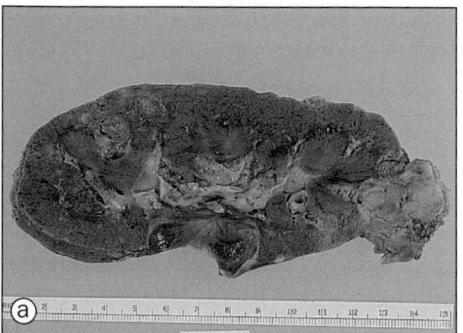
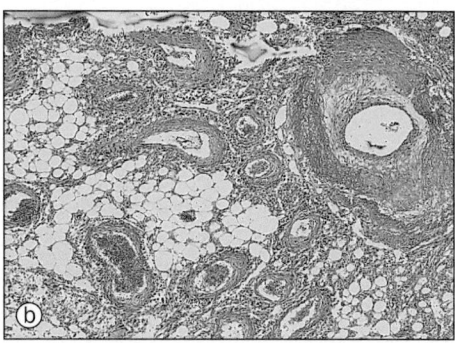
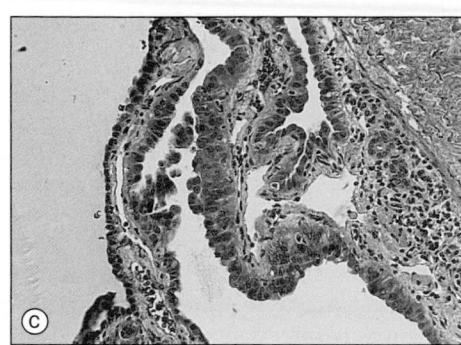

Figure 47.9 Renal pathology in TSC. (a) Cut section: Multiple angiomyolipomas in the kidney of a 60-year-old symptomatic woman. (b) Light microscopy: angiomyolipoma containing adipose tissue and spindle smooth muscle-like cells interspersed between abnormal vessels with thickened walls, H&E x 16. (c) Light microscopy: TSC cysts lined with a distinctive epithelia consisting of large, acidophilic cells with hyperchromatic nuclei, H&E x 65.

Clinical diagnostic criteria for TSC

Neurologic: (definite diagnosis: single with histologic confirmation; multiple with imaging studies or ophthalmoscopy)
 	
    Cortical tuber
    Subependymal glial nodule/giant cell astrocytoma
    Retinal hamartoma
 	
 Dermatologic: (definite diagnosis)
 	
    Facial angiofibromas
    Fibrous forehead plaque
    Ungual fibroma
    Shagreen patch (histologic confirmation)
 	
 Visceral: (presumptive diagnosis)*
 	
    Multiple renal angiomyolipomas
    Multiple cardiac rhabdomyomas
    Multiple renal cysts and an angiomyolipoma
    Pulmonary lymphangioleiomyomatosis and a renal angiomyolipoma
 	
 Suggestive
 	
    Hypomelanotic skin macules, enamel pits
    Hamartomatous rectal polyps
    Radiographic sclerotic bone patches and cysts
    Angiomyolipoma of kidney, liver, adrenal or gonads
    Thyroid adenoma (papillary or fetal type)
    Infantile spasms

*Individuals with only these findings have born children with TSC

Table 47.2 Clinical diagnostic criteria for TSC (Modified from Torres[24], with permission).

carcinomas as well as leiomyosarcoma have been identified in TSC patients. Recent data indicate that some cases of presumed TSC-associated carcinoma are actually malignant variants of epithelioid angiomyolipomas[26].

Diagnosis

TSC is a pleiotropic disease in which the size, number and location of the lesions can be variable, even among members of the same family. Specific clinical criteria have been defined to assist in the diagnosis of TSC (Table 47.2). Imaging is the mainstay for diagnosis of TSC-associated renal lesions. The presence of small cysts and fat-containing angiomyolipomas is strongly suggestive of TSC. Ultrasound (US) may be more sensitive than CT for detecting small angiomyolipomas because fatty tissue is highly echogenic. Conversely, CT may be superior for detecting small angiomyolipomas in a diffusely

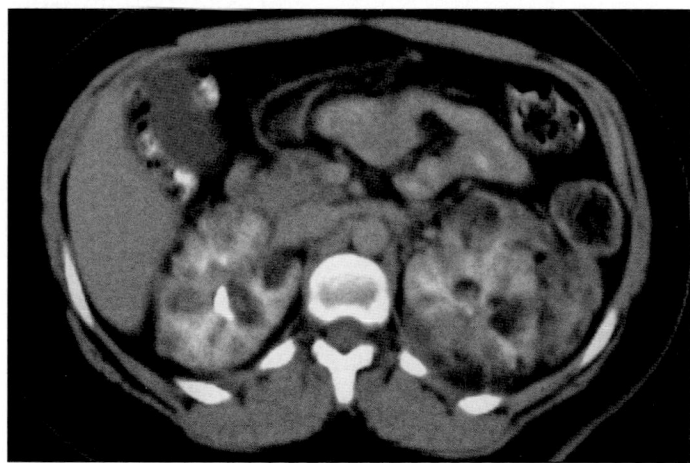

Figure 47.10 Radiologic findings associated with tuberous sclerosis complex. Contrast-enhanced CT showing bilateral angiomyolipomas in a 34-year-old symptomatic woman.

hyperechoic kidneys and differentiating small angiomyolipomas from perinephric or renal sinus fat (Fig. 47.10). Occasionally, the distinction between an angiomyolipoma and carcinoma cannot be reliably established by imaging and biopsy is indicated.

TSC-associated renal cysts can radiologically mimic simple cysts and, when numerous, ADPKD. In the absence of angiomyolipomas, TSC-related renal cystic disease is suggested by the absence of associated hepatic cysts. Although 10% of TSC patients have hepatic angiomyolipomas, hepatic cysts are rare.

Transplantation

ESRD in TSC may occur by different mechanisms including angiomyolipoma-related parenchymal destruction, polycystic kidneys, interstitial fibrosis and FSGS. As management of the central nervous system manifestations improves, renal failure will become a more important component of TSC clinical disease. Both dialysis and renal transplantation provide an adequate means of survival, but the risk of renal hemorrhage and malignant degeneration in TSC poses special problems. Therefore, it is advisable that patients with TSC and ESRD undergo bilateral nephrectomy when renal replacement therapy is initiated.

Treatment
Renal angiomyolipomas

Renal angiomyolipomas are benign lesions and often require no treatment. However, given the potential for growth and the development of complications, annual re-evaluation with US or CT is necessary. Most symptomatic angiomyolipomas measure > 4 cm in diameter and most of the angiomyolipomas measuring > 4 cm in diameter are symptomatic. Based on these observations, the current recommendation is to proceed with pre-emptive treatment either by surgery or embolization for angiomyolipomas that measure > 4 cm in diameter[27]. In addition to size and complications such as pain or hemorrhage, the inability to exclude an associated renal carcinoma is an indication for intervention. When an associated malignancy can not be excluded, renal-sparing surgery, such as enucleation or partial nephrectomy is preferred (see Ch. 59).

The increased frequency and size of the angiomyolipomas in women and the reports of hemorrhagic complications during pregnancy suggest that female sex hormones may foster growth of these lesions. It is prudent to caution patients with multiple angiomyolipomas about the potential risks of pregnancy and estrogen administration.

Renal cystic disease

The mainstay of treatment of the cystic disease associated with TSC is strict control of the hypertension. Surgical decompression of these cystic kidneys has been suggested, but no significant beneficial effect has been established.

Renal carcinoma

Renal carcinoma should be suspected in enlarging lesions with no fatty tissue demonstrable by imaging or when intra-tumoral calcifications are present. In these cases, biopsy is indicated. Because renal carcinoma is frequently bilateral in TSC, renal sparing surgery should be performed whenever possible.

VON HIPPEL-LINDAU DISEASE

Introduction and definition

Von Hippel-Lindau disease (VHL) is a dominantly-transmitted, tumor predisposition disorder associated with renal cancer as well as tumors of the eyes, brain, spinal cord, adrenal glands, pancreas, and epididymis[28,29]. VHL patients are more commonly seen by urologists and oncologists than nephrologists.

Etiology and pathogenesis
Genetic basis of VHL

The VHL gene has been mapped to the short arm of chromosome 3 (3p25-26). Mutations in the VHL gene have been demonstrated in both the germline of VHL patients as well as in sporadic clear cell renal carcinomas, implying that the VHL gene plays an important role in the pathogenesis of clear cell renal carcinoma.

As with TSC, VHL disease results from inactivation of a tumor suppressor gene via a 'two hit' mechanism. The VHL protein plays a pivotal role in regulating the rate of gene transcription. Loss of function of the VHL protein appears to cause unregulated cell growth and neoplastic transformation. The resulting VHL tumors (hemangioblastomas and renal cell

carcinomas (RCC)) are highly vascularized due in part to the overexpression of vascular endothelial growth factor (VEGF) within the tumors.

Clinical manifestations

VHL has a disease prevalence of 1 in 30 000–50 000 and is observed in all ethnic groups. VHL-associated disease appears to cluster into two disease complexes, based on the germline mutations. Deletions and protein-truncating mutations are associated with the VHL type 1 phenotype and those mutations that cause a single amino acid change are associated with VHL type 2 disease (Fig. 47.11)[28]. Type 1 mutations are associated with a disease complex characterized by retinal angiomas, spinal and cerebellar hemangioblastomas, pancreatic and renal cysts, and RCC. VHL type 2 is characterized by pheochromocytomas in addition to the other abnormalities described for VHL type 1.

RCC are typically multiple and bilateral. While RCC may present with hematuria or back pain, it is more often detected as an incidental imaging finding, or when VHL families are screened for occult renal disease. The mean age at presentation is 35–40 years, although patients have been diagnosed in adolescence. In VHL, men and women are equally affected

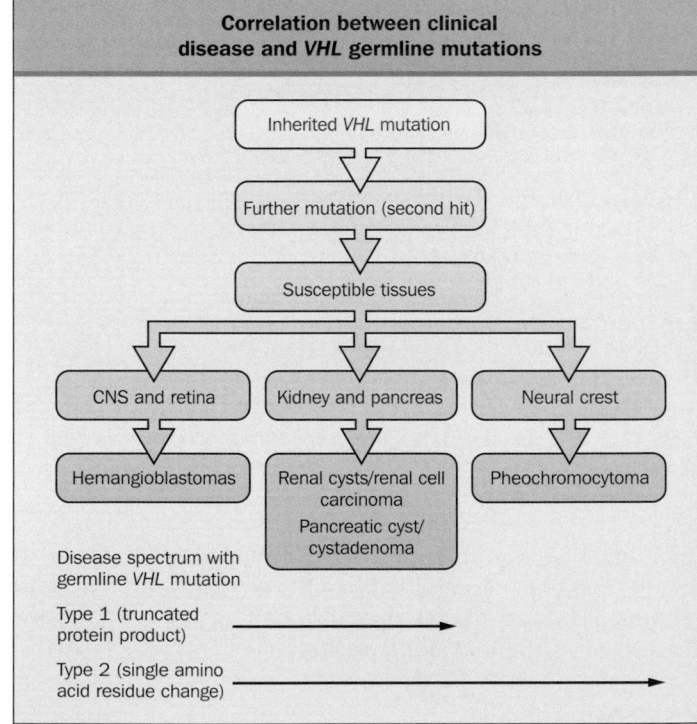

Figure 47.11 Correlation between clinical disease and VHL germline mutations. Following the second mutation event in the VHL gene, cystic disease and tumors develop in specific tissues. The type of VHL germline mutation correlates with the two overlapping disease complexes. VHL type 1 mutations produce truncated VHL proteins and disease characterized by CNS and retinal hemangioblastomas, pancreatic and renal cysts and RCC. VHL type 2 mutations produce intact VHL proteins with a single amino acid change and disease characterized by pheochromocytomas in addition to that described for VHL type 1. (Modified from Neumann and Zbar[29] with permission.)

with RCC, in contrast to the male predominance in sporadic RCC. VHL-associated RCC metastasizes to the lymph nodes, liver, lungs and bones and accounts for about 50% of VHL deaths.

Renal cysts are commonly bilateral and rarely multiple, simulating ADPKD. Deterioration of renal function due to cystic kidney disease has been reported in VHL, but is exceptional.

Pathology

VHL-associated renal tumors are clear cell carcinomas. Careful microscopic examination of cystic renal lesions often reveals small foci of carcinoma. Although RCC do metastasize, coincident tumors in the central nervous system are more likely to be hemangioblastomas.

Diagnosis

The minimal clinical criteria for the diagnosis of VHL in an individual known to be 'at-risk' include the presence of a single retinal or cerebellar hemangioblastoma, or RCC, or pheochromocytoma[30]. As many as 50% of patients from VHL families may show only one manifestation of the syndrome[28]. In presumed sporadic cases, the clinical diagnosis requires two or more retinal or CNS hemangioblastomas or a single hemangioblastoma and a characteristic visceral tumor.

With recent technological improvements, diagnostic techniques allow mutation detection in 100% of patients with definite VHL[28]. For those at-risk individuals who do not inherit the mutant gene, further clinical surveillance is not necessary. In proven gene carriers or those at-risk individuals who can not be evaluated at the molecular level, regular surveillance for occult disease manifestations is indicated. A comprehensive screening program includes gadolinium-enhanced magnetic resonance imaging (MRI) of the brain and spinal cord, detailed ophthalmologic examination, and an abdominal CT scan. For individuals with VHL type 2 mutations, surveillance for pheochromocytoma should include a 24-h urine collection for metanephrines and catecholamines, abdominal MRI, and m-iodobenzylguanidine (MIBG) scintigraphy.

Germline mutations in the VHL gene have been detected in some families who do not meet the clinical criteria for VHL. Such families should be considered to have VHL and be managed like typical VHL families.

Differential diagnosis

The differential diagnosis of VHL-associated renal lesions includes several conditions, most notably ADPKD and TSC (Table 47.3). Like VHL, ADPKD affects both sexes with a similar mean age at presentation. However, kidney involvement in VHL is characterized by a few bilateral cysts (Fig. 47.12a), RCC, normal kidney shape, normotension, and usually normal renal function. Cyst infection, a frequent finding in ADPKD, does not occur in VHL. RCC is an infrequent complication of ADPKD. Cysts in the liver are frequent in ADPKD and rare in VHL. Pancreatic cysts are rare in ADPKD, but can be numerous and scattered through the pancreas in VHL (Fig. 47.12a). The central nervous system in ADPKD is affected by arterial aneurysms, but in VHL the central nervous system is affected by tumors (Fig. 47.12b).

TSC should be considered in the differential diagnosis of multiple renal tumors. In both TSC and VHL, multiple renal cysts occur. However, the TSC-associated renal tumor is usually an angiomyolipoma and extrarenal lesions readily distinguish VHL and TSC.

Treatment

Surgery is the only accepted treatment of RCC in VHL patients. Optimal management requires surgical intervention before renal vein invasion and distant metastases occur because metastatic lesions respond poorly to chemotherapy and radiation. Nephron-sparing surgery is the procedure of choice when possible. Repeated surgical intervention may be required as tumors continue to develop. Laparoscopic

				Differential features of adult renal cystic disease			
	Simple cysts	ADPKD	MSK	VHL	TSC	Acquired cystic disease
Clinical onset (years)	> 40	30–40	20–40	30–40	10–30	chronic renal failure
Cysts	single/multiple	multiple	multiple	few, bilateral	multiple	multiple
Cyst infection	uncommon	common	common	uncommon	uncommon	uncommon
Tumors	no	rare	no	RCC, often bilateral	AML/RCC	common
BP	normal/ increased	increased	normal	normal/ increased	normal/ increased	normal/ increased
Renal function	normal	normal/ impaired	normal	normal	normal/ impaired	impaired/ESRD
Nephrolithiases	no	common	common	no	no	no
Liver cysts	no	common	no	rare	no	no
Pancreas cysts	no	few	no	multiple	no	no
CNS involvement	no	aneurysms	no	hemangioblastomas	seizures, mental retardation	no
Skin lesions	no	no	no	no	Fig. 47.8	no

Table 47.3 Differential features of adult renal cystic disease.

Heriditary and Congenital Diseases of the Kidney

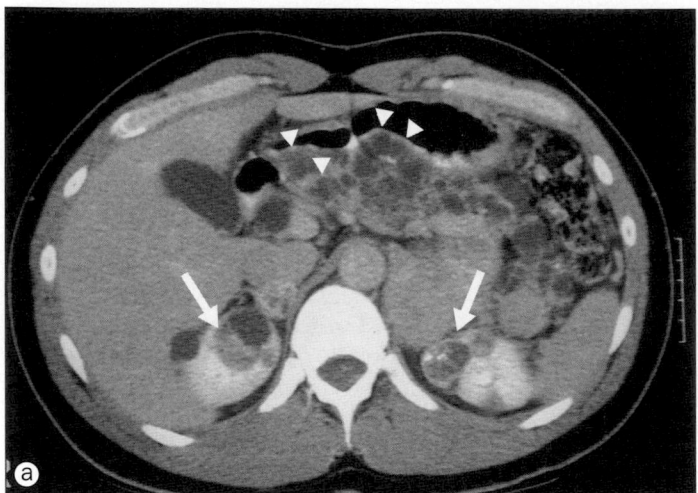

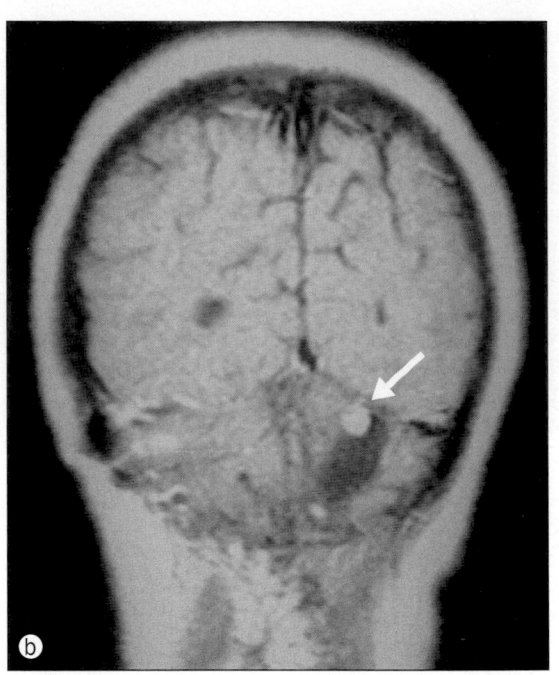

Figure 47.12 Radiologic findings associated with VHL. (a) Noncontrast CT shows massive cystic involvement of the pancreas (arrowheads) and bilateral renal cysts (arrows). (b) Contrast-enhanced MR image shows a right cerebellar hemangioblastoma with a small enhancing mass (arrowhead).

surgery may have a role in the future management of these patients.

Bilateral nephrectomy and renal transplantation may be an acceptable alternative to repeated nephron-sparing surgery in patients with VHL-associated RCC. It remains to be determined whether post-transplant immunosuppression enhances the growth of the retinal and central nervous system hemangioblastomas and other lesions found in patients with VHL.

SIMPLE CYSTS

Introduction and definition
Simple renal cysts are the most commonly acquired renal cystic lesion and are twice as common in men as in women. These cysts may be solitary or multiple. They occur rarely in children, but become increasingly common with age. In recent studies, unilateral cysts were detected in 1.7% of patients 30–49 years of age, 11.5% of patients 50–70 years of age, and 22–30% of patients over age 70 years[31].

Etiology and pathogenesis
Simple cysts probably arise from renal tubular diverticula, but the pathogenic mechanism is unknown. Focal tubular obstruction and renal parenchymal ischemia have both been suggested as etiologic processes. Less likely is the possibility that simple cysts arise from calyceal diverticuli, because these cysts are often found in the renal cortex and their frequency increases with age.

Clinical manifestations
Simple cysts are typically asymptomatic. Occasionally, patients with simple cysts present with hematuria, abdominal or back pain due to bleeding, a palpable abdominal mass, evidence of infection or obstruction of the collecting system. A significant association between simple cysts and systemic hypertension has been demonstrated, but a cause and effect relationship has not been established[32].

Pathology
Whether unilateral or bilateral, simple cysts are usually spherical in shape and unilocular. They may be solitary or multiple. On average, simple cysts measure 0.5–1.0 cm diameter, but 3–4 cm cysts are not uncommon. They protrude from the cortical surface and are overlapped at their margins by attenuated renal parenchyma. Simple cysts also occur at the corticomedullary junction or in the medulla. By definition, they do not communicate with the renal pelvis. The cyst walls are typically thin and transparent, but prior infection can cause thickening, fibrosis, and even calcification of the walls. They are lined with a single layer of flattened epithelium lining the cyst wall. This epithelial lining elaborates a cyst fluid that is essentially an ultrafiltrate of plasma.

Diagnosis
Most often, simple cysts are asymptomatic and are detected as incidental findings during abdominal imaging studies. Occasionally, they are discovered during radiological evaluation of palpable abdominal masses, pyelonephritis, or hematuria following abdominal trauma.

The critical clinical issue revolves around distinguishing single or multiple renal cysts from cysts associated with ADPKD, other cystic diseases, or renal cell carcinoma. This distinction can usually be made on the basis of patient age, family history, and renal imaging patterns[33]. The sonographic signature of simple cysts includes smooth walls, good sound transmission, and no intracystic debris. If the sonographic pattern is indeterminate, CT scanning should be performed. Benign cysts have homogeneous attenuation, no contrast enhancement, thin, smooth cyst walls, and no associated calcifications.

Treatment

Simple cysts associated with pain or renin-dependent hypertension can be punctured with ultrasound guidance, drained, and a sclerosing agent such as 99% ethanol instilled into the cyst cavity. Laparoscopic or retroperitoneoscopic cyst unroofing may be more appropriate for large cysts containing volumes in excess of a few hundred mL. Infection of simple cysts with Enterobactericeae, staphylococci, and *Proteus* has been reported. Operative or percutaneous drainage is often required for infected simple cysts.

SOLITARY MULTILOCULAR CYSTS

Solitary multilocular cysts are generally benign neoplasms that arise from the metanephric blastema[34]. These solitary cysts have also been designated multilocular cystic nephroma, benign cystic nephroma, and papillary cystadenoma. By definition, the cystic structures are unilateral, solitary, and multilocular. The cystic locules do not communicate each other or with the renal pelvis. These locules are lined with a simple epithelium and the interlocular septa do not contain differentiated renal epithelia structures. It is not certain whether a multilocular cyst represents a congenital abnormality in nephrogenesis, a hamartoma, a partially or completely differentiated Wilms' tumor, or a benign variant of Wilms' tumor.

A bimodal age distribution has been described, with approximately half the cases occurring in children less than 4 years of age and half the cases occurring in adults. As in Wilms' tumor, the childhood cases are equally distributed between the sexes. In contrast, multilocular cysts presenting in adulthood occur more commonly in women. The presence of an abdominal or flank mass is the most common clinical feature, as these cysts are typically quite large and often replace an entire pole. Associated hematuria, calculi, urinary tract obstruction, and infection occur in rare instances. Diagnosis can be made either by ultrasonography or CT (Fig. 47.13).

Partial nephrectomy is usually required. Tumors in children may contain blastema and incompletely differentiated metanephric tissue. These tumors, often referred to as partially differentiated cystic nephromas, have the same good prognosis as do ordinary multilocular cysts. In adults, associated foci of renal cell carcinoma or sarcoma must be excluded. The prognosis of solitary multilocular cysts is excellent.

RENAL LYMPHANGIOMATOSIS

Renal lymphangiomatosis is a very rare disorder that involves cystic dilatation of renal lymphatic channels. It has also been referred to as hilar, pericalyceal, paracalyceal, peripelvic or parapelvic lymphangiectasis[35]. The cystic phenotype is widely variable and the underlying pathogenesis is unclear. The dilatation may involve a single lymphatic channel or multiple channels. The lymphangiectasis may be unilateral or bilateral. It may be limited to the hilar region or may extend into the renal parenchyma to the corticomedullary junction. Occasionally, renal lymphangiomatosis may be very extensive and simulate ADPKD. The thin walled cysts are lined by lymphatic endothelium and the cyst fluid is quite distinct from

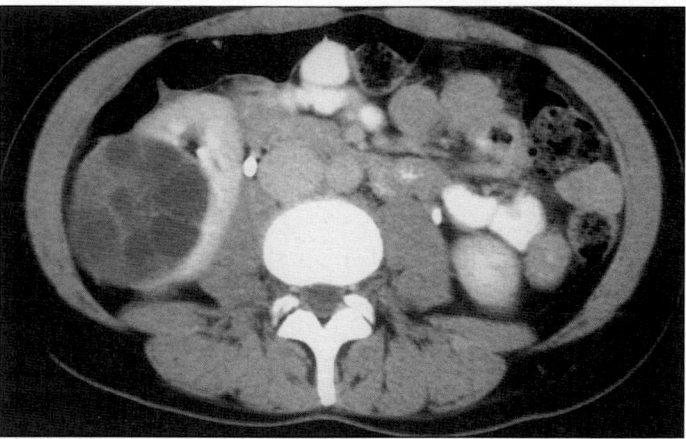

Figure 47.13 Solitary multilocular cyst. Contrast-enhanced CT shows a solitary, septated, and well-circumscribed renal cystic lesion in the right kidney.

that in ADPKD cysts, as it contains lymphatic constituents, such as albumin and lipid. Diagnosis can be made by ultrasonography or CT. Treatment is usually not required as renal lymphangiomas are most often asymptomatic. However, renal lymphangiomatosis may be complicated during pregnancy by large perinephric lymph collections and ascites[36].

OTHER CYSTIC CONDITIONS

Glomerulocystic kidney disease

Cystic glomeruli are evident in three different clinical contexts: (1) isolated glomerulocystic kidney disease (GCKD); (2) glomerulocystic kidneys associated with heritable malformation syndromes; and (3) glomerular cysts present in dysplastic kidneys[37]. Pathologically, the kidney architecture is normal, with no dysplastic elements in the cortex and no evidence of urinary tract obstruction. Cystic dilatation predominantly involves the Bowman's space and the initial proximal tubule.

GCKD can occur as a sporadic condition, a familial disorder, or as the infantile manifestation of autosomal dominant polycystic kidney disease. Familial hypoplastic GCKD, characterized by autosomal dominant inheritance, variable kidney size and function, and maturity onset diabetes of the young, is caused by mutations in the gene encoding hepatocyte nuclear factor (HNF)-1β[38].

Hypokalemic cystic disease

Renal cysts are often seen in association with chronic hypokalemia due to primary hyperaldosteronism or other renal potassium wasting disorders. Nearly 50% of patients with idiopathic adrenal hyperplasia and 60% of patients with adrenal tumors have been found to have renal cysts, which were distributed primarily in the renal medulla. These cysts typically regress following adrenalectomy[39].

Calyceal cysts

Calyceal cysts are not closed cysts but communicate directly with the collecting systems. They are described further in Chapter 52.

Hilar cysts

Hilar cysts are spherical accumulations of clear, fat droplet-containing fluid within the renal sinus. These cystic structures are not lined by epithelia. They are most commonly seen in debilitated patients and may represent atrophy of the renal sinus fat.

Perinephric pseudocysts

Perinephric pseudocysts are also unlined cavities. They typically occur under the renal capsule or in the perirenal fascia as a result of urine extravasation from a renal cyst following traumatic or spontaneous rupture[40]. Surgical intervention is indicated for associated urinary tract obstruction. Otherwise, treatment is directed to the underlying cause.

REFERENCES

1. Fick GM, Gabow PA. Hereditary and acquired cystic disease of the kidney. Kidney Int. 1994;46:951–64.
2. Levine E, Hartman D, Meilstrup J, et al. Current concepts and controversies in imaging of renal cystic diseases. Urol Clin No Am. 1997;24:523–43.
3. Guay-Woodford LM. Autosomal recessive disease: clinical and genetic profiles. In: Torres V, Watson M, eds. Polycystic Kidney Disease. Oxford: Oxford University Press; 1996:237–67.
4. Guay-Woodford LM, Muecher G, Hopkins SD, et al. The severe perinatal form of autosomal recessive polycystic kidney disease (ARPKD) maps to chromosome 6p21.1-p12: Implications for genetic counseling. Amer J Hum Genet. 1995;56:1101–7.
5. Ward C, Hogan M, Rossetti S, et al. The gene mutated in autosomal recessive polycystic kidney disease encodes a large, receptor-like protein. Nat Genet. 2002;30:259–69.
6. Onuchic L, Furu L, Nagasawa Y, et al. PKHD1, the polycystic kidney and hepatic disease 1 gene, encodes a novel large protein containing multiple IPT domains and PbH1 repeats. Am J Hum Genet. 2002;70:1305–17.
7. Zerres K, Becker J, Muecher G, et al. Haplotype-based prenatal diagnosis in autosomal recessive polycystic kidney disease (ARPKD). Am J Med Genet. 1998;76:137–44.
8. Lucaya J, Enriquez G, Nieto J, et al. Renal calcifications in patients with autosomal recessive polycystic kidney disease: prevalence and cause. Am J Radiol. 1993;160:359–62.
9. Zerres K, Rudnik-Schoneborn S, Deget F, et al. Autosomal recessive polycystic kidney disease in 115 children: clinical presentation, course and influence of gender. Acta Paediatr. 1996; 85:437–45.
10. Roy S, Dillon M, Trompeter R, Barratt T. Autosomal recessive polycystic kidney disease: long-term outcome of neonatal survivors. Pediatr Nephrol. 1997;11:302–6.
11. Warady B, Hebert D, Sullivan E, et al. Renal transplantation, chronic dialysis, and chronic renal insufficiency in children and adolescents. The 1995 Annual Report of the North American Pediatric Renal Transplant Cooperative Study. Pediatr Nephrol. 1997;11:49–64.
12. Hildebrandt F, Otto E, Rensing C, et al. A novel gene encoding an SH3 domain protein is mutated in nephronophthisis type 1. Nat Genet. 1998;17:149–53.
13. Konrad M, Saunier S, Heidet L, et al. Large homozygous deletions of the 2q13 region are a major cause of juvenile nephronophthisis. Hum Mol Genet. 1996;5:367–71.
14. Rahilly M, Fleming S. Abnormal integrin receptor expression in two cases of familial nephronophthisis. Histopathol. 1995; 26:345–9.
15. Ala-Mello S, Kivivuori S, Ronnholm K, Koskimies O, Siimes M. Mechanism underlying early anemia in children with familial juvenile nephronophthisis. Pediatr Nephrol. 1996;10:578–81.
16. Antignac C, Kleinknecht C, Habib R. Toward identification of a gene for familial nephronophthisis (autosomal recessive medullary cystic kidney disease). Adv Nephrol. 1995;24:379–93.
17. Heninger E, Otto E, Imm A, et al. Improved strategy for molecular genetic diagnostics in juvenile nephronophthisis. Am J Kidney Dis. 2001;37:1131–39.
18. Yendt E. Medullary sponge kidney. In: Gardner JKD and Bernstein J, eds. The Cystic Kidney. Dordrecht, Netherlands: Kluwer; 1990:379–91.
19. Ginalski J, Portmann L, Jaeger P. Does medullary sponge kidney really cause nephrolithiasis. Am J Roentgenol. 1990;155:299–302.
20. The European Chromosome 16 Tuberous Sclerosis Consortium. Identification and characterization of the tuberous sclerosis gene on chromosome 16. Cell. 1993;75:1305–15.
21. Slegtenhorst MV, Hoogt Rd, Hermans C, et al. Identification of the tuberous sclerosis gene TSC1 on chromosome 9q34. Science. 1997;277:805–8.
22. Potter CJ, Huang H, Xu T. Drosophilia Tsc1 functions with Tsc2 to antagonize insulin signaling in regulating cell growth, cell proliferation, and organ size. Cell, 2001;105:357–68.
23. Sampson J, Maheshwar M, Aspinwall R, et al. Renal cystic disease in tuberous sclerosis: role of the polycystic kidney disease 1 gene. Am J Hum Genet. 1997;61:843–51.
24. Torres V. Tuberous sclerosis complex. In: Torres V, Watson M. Polycystic Kidney Disease. Oxford: Oxford University Press; 1996:283–308.
25. Bernstein J, Robbins T. Renal involvement in tuberous sclerosis. Ann NY Acad Sci. 1991;615:36–49.
26. Pea M, Bonetti F, Martignoni G, et al. Apparent renal cell carcinomas in tuberous sclerosis are heterogeneous: the identification of malignant epithelioid angiomyolipoma. Am J Surg Pathol. 1998; 22:180–7.
27. Torres VE, King BF, McKusick MA, et al. Update on the tuberous sclerosis complex. Contrib Nephrol. 2001; 136:33–49.
28. Friedrich CA. Genotype-phenotype correlation in von Hippel-Lindau syndrome. Hum Mol Genet. 2001;10:763–7.
29. Neumann H, Zbar B. Renal cysts, renal cancer, and von Hippel-Lindau disease. Kidney Int. 1997;51:16–26.
30. Couch V, Lindor NM, Karnes PS, Michels VM. Von Hippel-Lindau disease. May Clin Proc. 2000;75:265–72.
31. Ravine D, Gibson R, Donlan J, Sheffield L. An ultrasound renal cyst prevalence survey: specificity data for inherited renal cystic diseases. Am J Kidney Dis. 1993;22:803–7.
32. Pedersen J, Emanian S, Nielsen M. Significant association between simple renal cysts and arterial blood pressure. Br J Urol. 1997;79:688–92.
33. Bosniak MA. The current radiological approach to renal cysts. Radiol. 1986;158:1–10.
34. Kissane J. Multilocular cystic renal lesions-malformations, benign neoplasms or differentiated Wilms' tumors. In: Gardner JKD, Bernstein J, eds. The Cystic Kidney. Dordrecht, Netherlands: Kluwer; 1990:413–36.
35. Androulakakis P, Kirayianis B, Deliveliotis A. The parapelvic renal cyst: a report of 8 cases with particular emphasis on diagnosis and management. Br J Urol. 1980;52:342–4.

36. Levine E, Grantham J. Radiology of cystic kidneys. In: Gardner JKD, Bernstein J, eds. The Cystic Kidney. Dordrecht, Netherlands: Kluwer; 1990:171–206.

37. Bernstein J. Glomerulocystic kidney disease – nosological considerations. Pediatr Nephrol. 1993;7:464–70.

38. Bingham C, Bulman MP, Ellard S, et al. Mutations in the hepatocyte nuclear factor-1b gene are associated with familial hypoplastic glomerulocystic kidney disease. Am J Hum Genet. 2001; 68:219–24.

39. Torres VE, Young WF, Offord KP, Hattery RR. Association of hypokalemia, aldosteronism, and renal cysts. N Engl J Med. 1990; 322:345–51.

40. Meyers M. Uriniferous perirenal pseudocyst: new observations. Radiol. 1975;117:539–45.

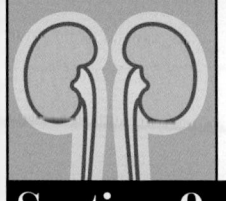

Chapter 48

Alport and Other Familial Glomerular Syndromes

Clifford E Kashtan

ALPORT SYNDROME

Introduction and definition

Alport syndrome (AS) is a generalized, inherited disorder of basement membranes due to mutations affecting specific proteins of the type IV (basement membrane) collagen family. The major features of AS are hematuria, progressive nephritis with proteinuria and declining renal function, sensorineural deafness and ocular abnormalities. The course of AS is gender-dependent: affected males typically have severe disease, while the manifestations of AS in women are usually mild. In 1902, Guthrie provided the first description of familial hematuria[1]. Later studies of Guthrie's family by Hurst[2] and Alport[3] revealed the progressive nature of the nephropathy, its association with deafness, and the poorer prognosis in affected males. In the 1970s, the glomerular basement membrane (GBM) was recognized as the site of the primary abnormality in AS[4–6]. Indirect evidence of abnormalities in type IV collagen[7,8] was followed by mapping of the major Alport locus to the X chromosome[9], cloning of a new type IV collagen gene (COL4A5) and its assignment to the same X-chromosomal region[10], and identification of the first COL4A5 mutations in patients with X-linked AS[11].

Etiology and pathogenesis

Type IV collagen

Genes and proteins

Type IV collagen is a major constituent of basement membranes. The type IV collagen family of proteins comprises six isomeric chains, designated $\alpha 1$–$\alpha 6$(IV)[12]. These chains show extensive sequence homology and share basic structural features, including a major collagenous domain of approximately 1400 residues containing the repetitive triplet sequence glycine (Gly)-X-Y, in which X and Y represent a variety of other amino acids; a C-terminal noncollagenous (NC1) domain of approximately 230 residues; and a noncollagenous N-terminal sequence of 15–20 residues. The collagenous domain of each chain contains approximately 20 interruptions of the collagenous triplet sequence, while each NC1 domain contains 12 completely conserved cysteine residues that participate in critical disulfide bonds.

Each type IV collagen molecule is a heterotrimer composed of three α-chains. Formation of these heterotrimers is initiated by C-terminal NC1 domain interactions, accompanied by folding of the collagenous domains into triple helices. There is evidence for at least three types of type IV collagen

heterotrimer: $\alpha 1(IV)_2$-$\alpha 2(IV)$, $\alpha 3(IV)$-$\alpha 4(IV)$-$\alpha 5(IV)$ and $\alpha 5(IV)_2$-$\alpha 6(IV)$. Type IV collagen triple helices form open, nonfibrillar networks, distinguishing type IV collagen from the interstitial collagens such as type I and type III which lack C-terminal NC1 domains in their mature forms and form fibrillar structures. Type IV collagen networks associate with laminin assemblies through interactions mediated by nidogen to form basement membranes.

The six type IV collagen genes are arranged in pairs on three chromosomes (Fig. 48.1). The five exons at the 3′ end of each gene encode the NC1 domain of the protein product, while most of the remaining exons encode the collagenous portion. The 5′ ends of each gene pair are adjacent to each other, separated by sequences of varying length that contain motifs involved in the regulation of transcriptional activity.

Tissue distribution

Several distinct type IV collagen networks appear to exist in basement membranes: a ubiquitous network comprising the $\alpha 1(IV)$ and $\alpha 2(IV)$ chains, and other networks, restricted in distribution, composed of $\alpha 3(IV)$, $\alpha 4(IV)$ and $\alpha 5(IV)$ chains, or $\alpha 5(IV)$ and $\alpha 6(IV)$ chains. GBM contains separate $\alpha 1/\alpha 2(IV)$ and $\alpha 3/\alpha 4/\alpha 5(IV)$ networks, while epidermal basement membranes contain separate networks of $\alpha 1/\alpha 2(IV)$ chains and $\alpha 5/\alpha 6(IV)$ chains. It is likely that these networks have different functional characteristics and interact differently with other matrix components and with adjacent cells.

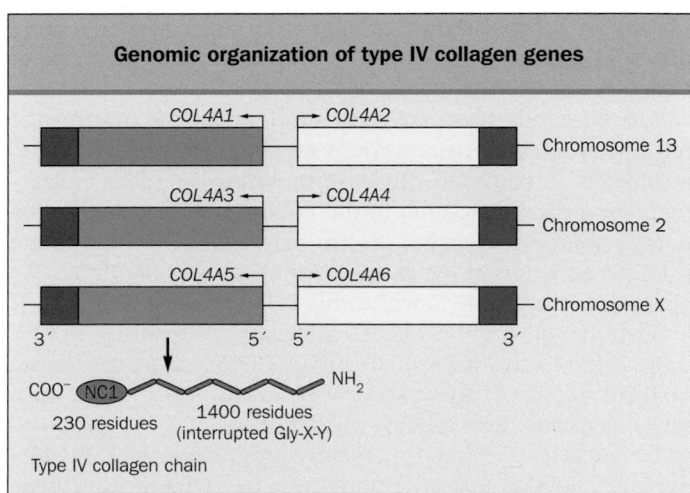

Figure 48.1 Genomic organization of type IV collagen genes.

Molecular genetics of Alport syndrome (AS)		
Inheritance	**Affected locus**	**Gene product**
X-linked (XLAS)	COL4A5	α5(IV)
X-linked + leiomyomatosis	COL4A5 + COL4A6	α5(IV) + α6(IV)
Autosomal recessive (ARAS)	COL4A3 COL4A4	α3(IV) α4(IV)
Autosomal dominant	COL4A3? COL4A4?	α3(IV)? α4(IV)?
Linkage of autosomal dominant AS to markers on chromosome 2, in the region of COL4A3 and COL4A4, has been reported. However, specific mutations causing autosomal dominant Alport syndrome have yet to be described.		

Table 48.1 Molecular genetics of Alport syndrome (AS).

Genetics

Three forms of AS have been established on a molecular genetic basis: an X-linked dominant form resulting from mutations at the COL4A5 locus, primarily affecting the α5(IV) chain; an autosomal recessive form arising from mutations at the COL4A3 locus or the COL4A4 locus, affecting the α3(IV) and α4(IV) chains, respectively; and an autosomal dominant form due to heterozygous mutations in COL4A3 or COL4A4 (Table 48.1).

X-linked Alport syndrome

X-linked Alport syndrome is the predominant form of the disease, accounting for approximately 80% of patients. Several hundred COL4A5 mutations have been described[13]. Mutations in COL4A6 have not been found in AS patients, except those with diffuse leiomyomatosis (see below), an observation consistent with the absence of α6(IV) from normal GBM.

Major rearrangements at the COL4A5 locus, predominantly deletions, account for approximately 10% of X-linked AS. A particular type of COL4A5 deletion is observed in families in which AS cosegregates with leiomyomatosis. All patients with the AS–leiomyomatosis complex have exhibited deletions of COL4A5 that extend upstream to involve the first two exons of COL4A6, with the deletion breakpoint occurring in the second intron of COL4A6[14]. The association between 5' deletions of COL4A6 and leiomyomatosis is not presently understood.

Missense mutations, splice-site mutations, and deletions of fewer than 10 base pairs account for the majority of COL4A5 mutations. A common missense mutation involves replacement of a glycine residue in the collagenous domain of the α5(IV) chain by another amino acid. Such mutations are thought to interfere with the normal folding of the α5(IV) chain into triple helices with other α(IV) chains.

Male patients with COL4A5 deletions consistently exhibit progression to end-stage renal disease (ESRD) during the second or third decade of life and have deafness. Most of the missense, nonsense and splicing mutations of COL4A5 described so far are also associated with early progression to ESRD and deafness. Several missense mutations of COL4A5 have been associated with late-onset (after the third decade) ESRD, and late development of deafness or normal hearing. The severity

of disease in a female heterozygous for a COL4A5 mutation probably depends on the nature of the mutation and the degree of inactivation of the X chromosome carrying the normal COL4A5 allele.

Autosomal recessive Alport syndrome

Autosomal recessive Alport syndrome arises from mutations affecting both alleles of COL4A3 or COL4A4[15,16]. Autosomal recessive AS should be suspected when an individual exhibits the typical clinical and pathologic features of the disease but lacks a positive family history, especially when a young female has findings indicative of severe disease such as deafness, renal insufficiency, and nephrotic syndrome. However, sporadic cases of AS may represent de novo mutations at the COL4A5 locus or a germline COL4A5 mutation in the proband's mother.

Phenotypic information in autosomal recessive AS is somewhat sparse, but patients with COL4A3 mutations appear to progress to ESRD before age 30 years and to have sensorineural deafness, regardless of gender.

Autosomal dominant Alport syndrome

Heterozygous mutations in COL4A3 or COL4A4 typically result in asymptomatic hematuria[15,16] but in some families may also be associated with progressive nephropathy, i.e., autosomal dominant Alport syndrome[17,18]. Autosomal dominant AS patients tend to have a slower course to ESRD than those with X-linked or autosomal recessive AS.

Type IV collagen in Alport basement membranes

The GBM and tubular basement membranes (TBM) of males with X-linked AS usually fail to stain for the α3(IV), α4(IV) and α5(IV) chains but do express the α1(IV) and α2(IV) chains (Fig. 48.2)[19]. The α6(IV) chain is not expressed in distal TBM or Bowman's capsule in males with X-linked AS whose basement membranes lack α5(IV) expression. Women who are heterozygous for X-linked AS mutations frequently

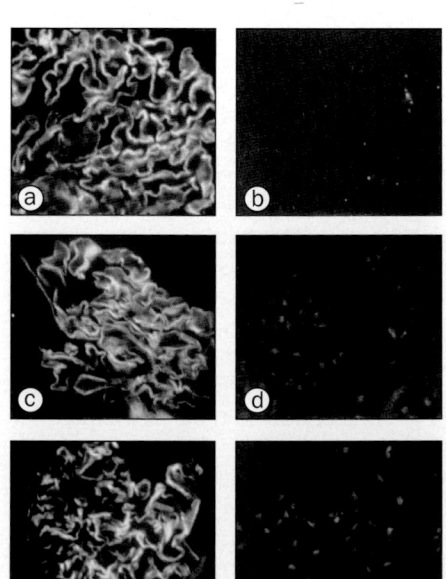

Figure 48.2 Immunohistochemistry of glomerular basement membrane (GBM) in a male with X-linked Alport syndrome. In a normal individual, GBM stains strongly for α3(IV) (a), α4(IV) (c) and α5(IV) (e). Staining of GBM of an affected male (b,d,f) is negative for each of these chains.

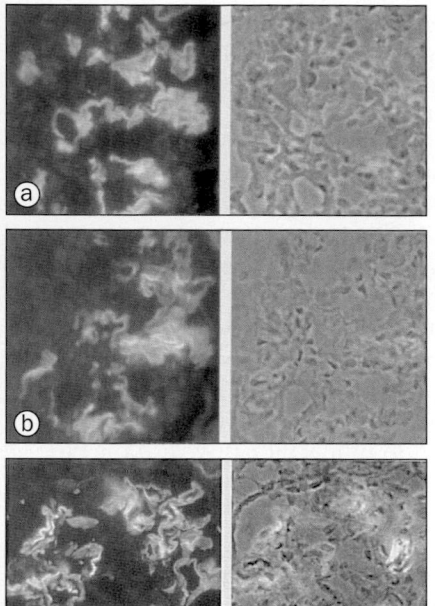

Figure 48.3 Immunohistochemistry of glomerular basement membrane (GBM) in a female with X-linked Alport syndrome. Mosaic staining is seen in (a) α3(IV), (b), α4(IV) and (c), α5(IV) chains (left). The location of GBM in the phase-contrast micrographs of the same sections (seen on the right) can be compared with the interrupted staining.

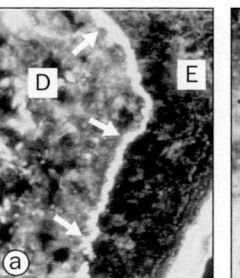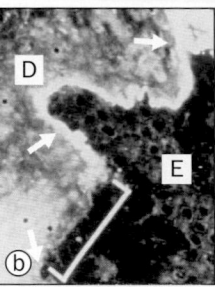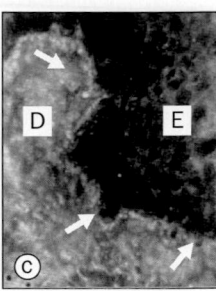

Figure 48.4 Immunohistochemistry of epidermal basement membrane (EBM) in X-linked Alport syndrome. (a) In a normal male, EBM shows strong staining for α5(IV) at the dermo-epidermal junction (arrow) between dermis (D) and epidermis (E). (b) In an affected female, EBM shows mosaic staining (arrows); the bracket identifies a length of EBM negative for α5(IV). (c) EBM staining for α5(IV) is absent in an affected male. (Reproduced with permission.)

exhibit mosaicism of GBM expression of the α3(IV), α4(IV) and α5(IV) chains, while expression of the α1(IV) and α2(IV) chains is preserved (Fig. 48.3). Most males with X-linked AS show no epidermal basement membrane (EBM) expression of α5(IV) or α6(IV), while female heterozygotes frequently display mosaicism (Fig. 48.4). Lens capsules of some males with X-linked AS do not express the α3(IV), α4(IV) or α5(IV) chains, while expression of these chains appears normal in other patients.

In patients with autosomal recessive AS, GBM shows no expression of the α3(IV), α4(IV) or α5(IV) chains, but α5(IV) and α6(IV) are expressed in Bowman's capsule, distal TBM and EBM (Fig. 48.5)[19]. Therefore, X-linked and autosomal recessive AS may be differentiated by immunohistochemical analysis. Basement membrane expression of type IV collagen α chains appears to be normal in patients with autosomal dominant AS.

These observations indicate that a mutation affecting one of the chains involved in the α3–α4–α5(IV) network can prevent GBM expression not only of that chain, but also of the other two chains as well. Similarly, a mutation involving the α5(IV) chain can interfere with basement membrane expression of α6(IV). It is likely that at least some mutations interfere with the formation of trimers; as a result, the normal chains that are prevented from forming trimers undergo degradation. Other mutations may allow formation of abnormal trimers that are degraded before deposition in basement membranes can occur.

Clinical manifestations
Renal defects
The cardinal finding of AS is hematuria. Affected males have persistent microscopic hematuria. Many also have episodic gross hematuria, precipitated by upper respiratory infections, during the first two decades of life. Hematuria has been discovered in the first year of life in affected boys, in whom it is probably present from birth. Boys who are free of hematuria during the first 10 years of life are unlikely to be affected.

Heterozygous females with X-linked AS may have intermittent hematuria, but about 10% of obligate heterozygotes never manifest hematuria. Hematuria appears to be persistent in both males and females with autosomal recessive AS. Approximately 50% or more of carriers of *COL4A3* or *COL4A4* mutations have hematuria[15,16].

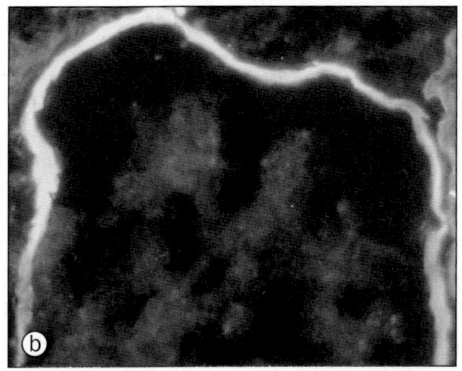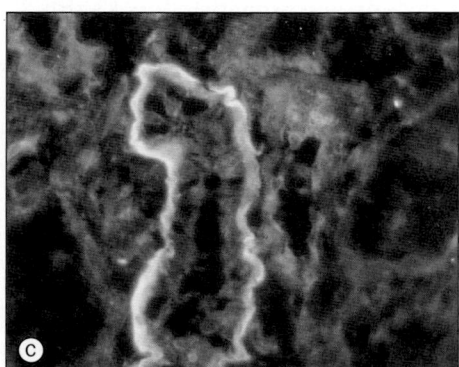

Figure 48.5 Immunohistochemistry of the kidney in a patient with autosomal recessive Alport syndrome. (a) Neither glomerular basement membrane (GBM) nor Bowman's capsule shows staining for α3(IV). (b,c) Staining for α5(IV) is negative in GBM but present in Bowman's capsule (b) and distal tubular basement membrane (c).

Proteinuria is usually absent early in life but develops eventually in males with X-linked AS and in both males and females with recessive disease. Proteinuria increases progressively with age and may result in the nephrotic syndrome. Significant proteinuria is infrequent in heterozygous females.

Hypertension also increases in incidence and severity with age. Similar to proteinuria, hypertension is much more likely to occur in affected males than in affected females with X-linked AS, but there are no gender differences in the autosomal recessive form.

ESRD develops in all affected males with X-linked AS. The rate of progression to ESRD is determined primarily by the nature of the underlying COL4A5 mutation[20]. Thus, the rate of progression is fairly constant among affected males within a particular family, but there is significant interkindred variability. Significant intrakindred variability in the rate of progression to ESRD has been reported in some families with missense COL4A5 mutations[20].

The prognosis in affected females with X-linked AS is generally benign, with most surviving into old age with minimal renal disease. Gross hematuria in childhood, nephrotic syndrome and diffuse GBM thickening observed by electron microscopy are features suggestive of progressive nephropathy in affected females[21]. Sensorineural deafness and anterior lenticonus are also indicative of an unfavorable outcome in affected women. Many women with progressive nephropathy maintain adequate renal function until late in life. Both males and females with autosomal recessive AS appear likely to progress to ESRD during the second or third decade of life.

Cochlear defects

Deafness is frequently but not universally associated with the Alport renal lesion, occurring in approximately 80% of males and 50% of females with the disease. In some families with the Alport nephropathy and apparently normal hearing, deafness may be a late and very slowly progressive phenomenon.

Hearing loss in AS is never congenital and usually becomes apparent by late childhood to early adolescence in boys with X-linked AS. Hearing impairment in members of families with AS is always accompanied by evidence of renal involvement. There is no convincing evidence that deaf males lacking renal disease can transmit AS to their offspring. In its early stages, the hearing deficit is detectable only by audiometry, with bilateral reduction in sensitivity to tones in the 2000–8000 Hz range. In affected males, the deficit extends progressively to other frequencies, including those of conversational speech. In females with X-linked AS, hearing loss is less common and tends to occur later in life. There do not appear to be gender differences in the incidence or course of deafness in autosomal disease.

Ocular defects

Ocular defects occur in 30–40% of AS patients[20]. The spectrum of ocular lesions appears to be similar in X-linked and autosomal recessive AS. Anterior lenticonus, which is virtually pathognomonic of AS, occurs in approximately 15% of X-linked AS males, and is almost entirely restricted to AS families with progression to ESRD before age 30 years and deafness[20]. Anterior lenticonus is absent at birth, usually appearing during the second to third decade of life, and is

bilateral in 75% of patients. Using oblique illumination, anterior lenticonus appears as a conical or spherical protrusion of the center of the anterior surface of the lens into the anterior chamber. On indirect illumination of the fundus, a dark disc is seen in the center of the pupillary region: the 'oil droplet in water' effect. Lens opacities may be seen in conjunction with lenticonus, occasionally resulting from rupture of the anterior lens capsule. Marked attenuation and fracturing of the anterior lens capsule have been demonstrated by light and electron microscopy.

Another common ocular manifestation of Alport syndrome is a maculopathy that consists of whitish or yellowish flecks or granulations in a perimacular distribution and occurs in 15–30% of patients. In contrast to lenticonus, there does not appear to be any correlation of maculopathy with the type of COL4A5 mutation[20]. The maculopathy does not appear to be associated with any visual abnormalities.

Corneal endothelial vesicles (posterior polymorphous dystrophy) have been observed in Alport patients and may indicate defects in Descemet's membrane, the basement membrane underlying the corneal endothelium. Recurrent corneal erosion in Alport patients has been attributed to alterations of the corneal epithelial basement membrane.

Leiomyomatosis

The association of AS with leiomyomatosis of the esophagus and tracheobronchial tree has been reported in approximately 20 families[14]. Affected females typically exhibit genital leiomyomas as well, with clitoral hypertrophy and variable involvement of the labia majora and uterus. Bilateral posterior subcapsular cataracts also occur frequently in affected individuals. Symptoms usually appear in late childhood and include dysphagia, postprandial vomiting, retrosternal or epigastric pain, recurrent bronchitis, dyspnea, cough, and stridor. All patients with the Alport syndrome–diffuse leiomyomatosis complex have been found to have deletions that encompass the 5' ends of COL4A5 and COL4A6.

Hematologic defects

An autosomal dominant syndrome of hereditary nephritis, deafness, and megathrombocytopenia, so-called Epstein syndrome, has been described in a handful of families. Families with Fechtner syndrome exhibit these features as well as leukocyte inclusions (May–Hegglin anomaly). Both Epstein and Fechtner syndrome arise from mutations in non-muscle myosin heavy chain IIA[22]. Basement membranes of these patients do not exhibit abnormalities in expression of type IV collagen α-chains. Therefore, Epstein and Fechtner syndromes are best considered as distinct forms of hereditary nephritis, rather than as variants of Alport syndrome.

Pathology

There are no pathognomonic lesions by light microscopy or direct immunofluorescence in AS. Indirect immunofluorescence of type IV collagen α-chain expression in renal and/or skin basement membranes can be diagnostic (see above).

Electron microscopy frequently reveals diagnostic abnormalities. The cardinal fine structural feature of the kidney in AS is the variable thickening, thinning, basket-weaving, and lamellation of the GBM (Fig. 48.6). This lesion occurs in most, but not all, patients with AS. The thick segments measure up to 1200 nm in depth, usually have irregular outer and inner contours, and are found more commonly in males than in females. The lamina densa is transformed into a heterogeneous network of membranous strands, which enclose clear electronlucent areas that may contain round granules of variable density measuring 20–90 nm in diameter. The altered capillary walls typically demonstrate variable degrees of epithelial foot process fusion.

Not all Alport kindreds demonstrate these characteristic ultrastructural features. Thick, thin, normal and nonspecifically altered GBM have all been described. Affected young males, heterozygous females at any age, and, on occasion, affected adult males may have diffusely attenuated GBM measuring as little as 100 nm or less in thickness, rather than the pathognomonic lesion. Although diffuse attenuation of GBM has been considered the hallmark of thin basement membrane nephropathy (as discussed elsewhere in this chapter), some patients with this abnormality are members of kindreds with a history of progression to renal failure. Therefore, the significance of an ultrastructural finding of thin GBM must be considered in the context of the family history, basement membrane expression of type IV collagen α-chains, and, if available, molecular genetic information.

Diagnosis and differential diagnosis

AS should be included in the initial differential diagnosis of patients with persistent microscopic hematuria once structural abnormalities of the kidneys or urinary tract have been excluded. The presence of diffuse thickening and multilamellation of the GBM, as demonstrated by electron microscopy, predicts a progressive nephropathy, regardless of family history. However, in a patient with a negative family history, electron microscopy cannot differentiate de novo X-linked from autosomal recessive AS. In some patients, the biopsy findings may be ambiguous, particularly females and young patients of either sex. Furthermore, families with progressive nephritis and COL4A5 mutations in association with GBM thinning have been described, indicating that the classic Alport GBM lesion is not present in all Alport kindreds.

It is not unusual to see a patient with hematuria and discover that multiple relatives also have hematuria, although none has ever undergone kidney biopsy. Who should undergo biopsy in such instances? The natural history of the Alport renal lesion suggests that older, male subjects are more likely to exhibit diagnostic ultrastructural GBM abnormalities. In families in which a firm diagnosis of AS has been established, evaluation of individuals with newly recognized hematuria can be limited to ultrasound of the kidneys and urinary tract to exclude coincidental tumor or structural anomalies of the urinary tract.

Absence of the α3, α4 and α5 chains of type IV collagen from GBM and distal TBM has not been described in any condition other than AS, making this a diagnostic finding on kidney biopsy (Table 48.2). Examination of skin biopsies by immunofluorescence for expression of α5(IV) in the epidermal basement membrane is an additional tool for diagnosing AS. However, apparently normal expression of type IV collagen α-chains in basement membranes does not exclude the diagnosis of AS. Heterozygous females frequently express α5(IV) mosaically. While mosaic expression of α5(IV) is diagnostic of the carrier state, a normal result does not exclude heterozygosity. A female member of an Alport kindred who does not have hematuria may still be a carrier but is less likely to exhibit detectable mosaicism than a female with hematuria.

A firm histologic diagnosis of AS cannot always be established, or it may not be possible to determine the mode of transmission, despite careful evaluation of the pedigree and application of the full range of histologic methods. In these situations, genetic analysis has the potential to provide information essential for determining prognosis and guiding genetic counseling. The inheritance of AS in a family can be determined by linkage analysis, which does not require identification of a particular mutation. However, genetic analysis for Alport syndrome is not yet widely available.

Other glomerular diseases which are typically sporadic will occasionally be familial and should be considered in the differential. These include focal segmental glomerulosclerosis, membranous nephropathy, and IgA nephropathy.

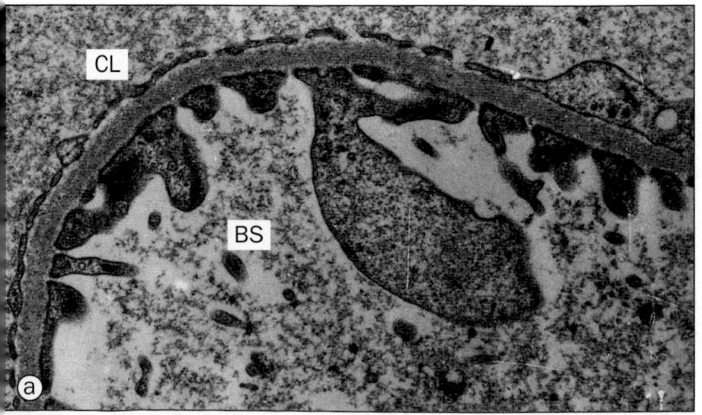
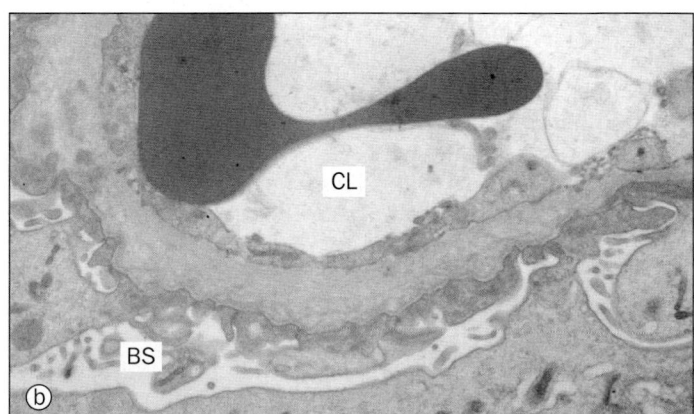

Figure 48.6 Renal biopsy in Alport syndrome. (a) A normal glomerular capillary wall is shown. (b) Glomerular capillary wall from a patient with Alport syndrome, at the same magnification. Note the thickening of the GBM, the splitting of the lamina densa into multiple strands and the marked irregularity of the epithelial aspect of the GBM in the patient with Alport syndrome. CL, capillary lumen; BS, Bowman's space.

Immunostaining for type IV collagen in Alport syndrome				
Type IV collagen group	Glomerular basement membranes	Bowman's capsules	Distal tubular basement membrane	Epidermal basement membrane
Normal (males and females)				
α3(IV)	Present	Present	Present	Absent
α4(IV)	Present	Present	Present	Absent
α5(IV)	Present	Present	Present	Present
X-linked (males)[1]				
α3(IV)	Absent	Absent	Absent	Absent
α4(IV)	Absent	Absent	Absent	Absent
α5(IV)	Absent	Absent	Absent	Absent
X-linked (females)[2]				
α3(IV)	Mosaic			Absent
α4(IV)	Mosaic			Absent
α5(IV)	Mosaic			Mosaic
Autosomal recessive (males and females)[1]				
α3(IV)	Absent	Absent	Absent	Absent
α4(IV)	Absent	Absent	Absent	Absent
α5(IV)	Absent	Present	Present	Present

[1] In some Alport syndrome (AS) kindreds, staining of basement membranes for type IV collagen chains is entirely normal. Therefore, a normal result does not exclude a diagnosis of X-linked or autosomal recessive AS.
[2] Some heterozygous females have normal basement membrane immunoreactivity for type IV collagen chains. Therefore, a normal result does not exclude the carrier state.

Table 48.2 Immunostaining for type IV collagen in Alport syndrome.

Natural history

Why is the Alport nephropathy progressive? The tissue pathology of AS arises from underexpression of the α3, α4, α5 and, possibly, α6, chains of type IV collagen. As a result, the networks formed by these chains are absent or are defective in structure and function. Anterior lenticonus most likely results from the inability of the lens capsule to maintain the normal conformation of the lens. Microhematuria, the first and invariable renal manifestation of AS, probably reflects GBM thinning and a tendency to develop focal ruptures because of defective expression of the α3(IV)–α5(IV) chains.

The inexorable development of GBM thickening, proteinuria, and renal insufficiency in males with X-linked AS and in both males and females with autosomal recessive AS are less readily explained, but some clues have been unearthed. AS is characterized by the accumulation of the α1(IV) and α2(IV) chains, along with types V and VI collagen, in the GBM[23]. These proteins appear to spread from their normal subendothelial location in GBM to occupy the full width of the GBM. As AS glomeruli undergo sclerosis, the α1(IV) and α2(IV) chains disappear from the GBM, but type V and type VI collagen persist and accumulate, perhaps as a compensatory response to the loss of the α3(IV), α4(IV) and α5(IV) chains. The Alport GBM exhibits increased susceptibility to proteolytic degradation *in vitro*[24], but the role of GBM proteolysis in progression of the Alport nephropathy remains to be defined.

Treatment

Is effective intervention possible? Clinical trials of therapy for the Alport nephropathy have not been conducted. The availability of canine[25] and murine[26] models of AS should allow the testing of genetic or pharmacologic therapies, in order to select promising treatments for human trials[27]. AS resembles other chronic glomerulopathies in that deterioration of glomerular filtration rate is closely correlated with fibrosis of the renal interstitium[28]. It is possible that therapies that interfere with interstitial fibrosis may be of benefit to AS patients, without correcting the primary abnormalities of type IV collagen expression. Cyclosporine appeared to stabilize renal function in a small, uncontrolled study of Alport males[29]; confirmatory studies will need to be published before this therapeutic approach can be recommended.

Transplantation

At present, renal transplantation is the only available treatment for AS. Allograft survival rates in patients with familial nephritis are equivalent to those in patients with other diagnoses. However, anti-GBM glomerulonephritis involving the renal allograft is a rare, but dramatic, manifestation of AS, occurring in 2–3% of transplanted male Alport patients. This is discussed further in Chapter 25.

Should women who are heterozygous for *COL4A5* mutations be allowed to serve as kidney donors? Clearly, those with proteinuria, hypertension, or renal insufficiency will not be allowed to donate, and the same should apply if any hearing loss is present. What about heterozygotes with hematuria but normal renal function and hearing? There is no long-term follow-up information on the impact of uninephrectomy in such women, although there does not seem to be a drastic decline in renal function over the first several years after transplant. The wishes of a heterozygous woman with asymptomatic microhematuria should be thoughtfully considered, but it must be assumed at this time that the risk to such an individual of ultimately developing significant renal insufficiency is substantially higher than it is for the usual kidney donor.

THIN BASEMENT MEMBRANE NEPHROPATHY: FAMILIAL AND SPORADIC

Introduction and definition

Isolated glomerular hematuria may occur as a familial or sporadic condition and is often associated with a renal biopsy finding of excessively thin GBM. The term 'benign familial hematuria' has been used to describe kindreds in which multiple individuals in several generations have isolated hematuria without progression to ESRD. More recently 'thin basement membrane nephropathy' (TBMN) has been used to identify both familial and sporadic isolated hematuria associated with attenuated GBM. It is likely that several disorders that differ at the molecular level can be associated with GBM thinning, and in some instances it is probably a normal variant. In general, the discussion that follows applies to both familial and sporadic TBMN.

Similar to AS, familial TBMN is an inherited GBM disorder manifested by chronic hematuria, but it differs clinically from

AS in several important respects: extrarenal abnormalities are rare; proteinuria, hypertension, and progression to ESRD are unusual; gender differences in expression of TBMN are not apparent; transmission is autosomal dominant. TBMN and early AS may be difficult to differentiate histologically, because diffuse GBM attenuation is characteristic of both. However, the GBM of TBMN patients remains attenuated over time, rather than undergoing the progressive thickening and multi-lamellation that is pathognomonic of AS.

Etiology and pathogenesis

TBMN is usually transmitted as an autosomal dominant condition. A negative family history may not be reliable, since patients are frequently unaware that they have relatives with hematuria. In one Dutch kindred with isolated hematuria[30], affected individuals were found to be heterozygous for a missense mutation in *COL4A4*. Following this initial report, familial TBMN has been localized to *COL4A4* in several other kindreds . Approximately 50% or more of heterozygous carriers of a *COL4A3* or *COL4A4* mutation exhibit hematuria[15,16]. However, linkage to *COL4A3* and *COL4A4* has been excluded in other families with isolated hematuria, indicating that TBMN is a genetically heterogeneous condition.

To date, immunohistologic studies of type IV collagen in GBM of patients with TBMN have failed to disclose any abnormalities in the distribution of any of the six chains. Immunohistologic evaluation of GBM type IV collagen may be useful in the differentiation of BFH from AS (see below).

Clinical manifestations

It has been estimated that 20–25% of patients referred to a nephrologist for evaluation of persistent hematuria will prove to have thin GBM on renal biopsy. Individuals with TBMN typically exhibit persistent microhematuria which is first detected in childhood. In some patients, microhematuria is intermittent and may not be detected until adulthood. Episodic gross hematuria, often in association with upper respiratory infections, is not unusual. The hematuria of TBMN appears to be life-long.

Overt proteinuria and hypertension are unusual in TBMN but have been reported. Some of these patients may have actually had AS, in which the predominant abnormality of GBM was attenuation rather than thickening and multilamellation. Other glomerular disorders, such as IgA nephropathy, may occur concurrently with TBMN, altering the expected natural history and histopathology of the condition.

Pathology

Light and immunofluorescence microscopy are unremarkable in typical cases of TBMN. Most patients exhibit diffuse thinning of the whole GBM and of the lamina densa (Fig. 48.7). GBM width is age and gender dependent in normal individuals. Both the lamina densa and the GBM increase rapidly in thickness between birth and age 2 years, followed by gradual thickening into adulthood. GBM thickness in adult men (373 ± 42 nm) exceeds that of adult women (326 ± 45 nm)[31].

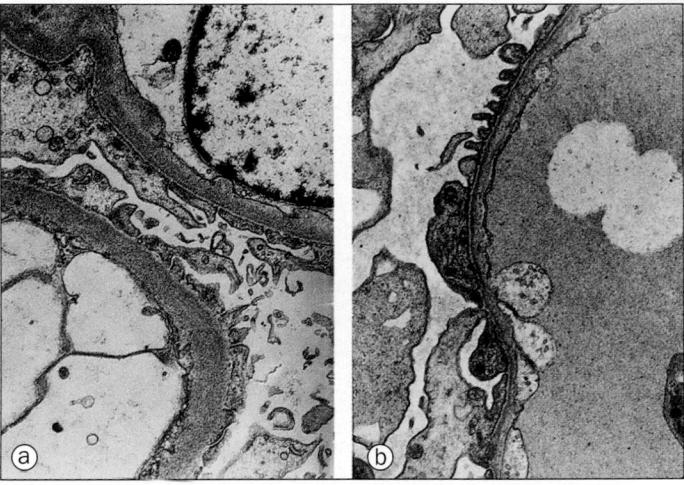

Figure 48.7 Thin basement membrane nephropathy. Electron micrographs of renal biopsies. (a) Normal glomerular capillary wall. (b) Thin basement membrane nephropathy at the same magnification. Note the diffuse and uniform attenuation of the GBM and the lamina densa. (Reproduced with permission of the Oxford University Press.)

Each electron microscopy laboratory should establish a consistent technique for measuring GBM thickness and determine its own reference range for GBM width to make comparisons with published data meaningful. When a laboratory has normal values for GBM width similar to those of Steffes et al.[31], a cut-off value of 250 nm will accurately separate adults with normal GBM from those with thin GBM. For children, the cut-off is in the range 200–250 nm. Intraglomerular variability in GBM width is small in thin GBM disease.

Diagnosis and differential diagnosis

If the patient's family history indicates autosomal dominant transmission of hematuria, if there is no history of chronic renal failure, and if kidney and urinary tract imaging are normal, a presumptive diagnosis of TBMN can often be made without kidney biopsy. When family history is negative or unknown, or there are atypical coexisting features such as proteinuria or deafness, renal biopsy may be very informative. A finding of thin GBM may be further characterized by examining the distribution of type IV collagen α-chains in the kidney. Normal distribution of these chains provides supportive, although not conclusive, evidence for a diagnosis of BFH. Marked variability in GBM width within a glomerulus in a patient with persistent microhematuria should raise suspicion of AS, although focal lamina densa splitting has been described in TBMN.

Treatment

Patients who are given a diagnosis of TBMN should be reassured but not lost to follow-up examination. The risk of chronic renal insufficiency appears to be small but real. Urinalysis and measurement of blood pressure and renal function are recommended every 1 to 2 years.

Heriditary and Congenital Diseases of the Kidney

FABRY DISEASE (ANDERSON–FABRY DISEASE)

Introduction and definition

Fabry disease comprises the clinical and pathologic manifestations of hereditary deficiency of the enzyme α-galactosidase A (αGal A), resulting in the intracellular accumulation of neutral glycosphingolipids with terminal α-linked galactosyl moieties (globotriaosylceramide, GL-3) (Fig. 48.8). Anderson[32] and Fabry[33] each described the characteristic skin lesions of this condition in 1898 and noted the association of proteinuria with the skin lesion, for which Fabry coined the term 'angiokeratoma corporis diffusum'.

Etiology and pathogenesis

Over 100 mutations causing Fabry disease have been identified in the gene for αGal A, which is located on the X chromosome[34]. Most of the described mutations are associated with the classic Fabry phenotype, in which there is multisystem involvement. Certain missense mutations have been identified in patients with a mild phenotype limited to cardiac abnormalities (see below)[26].

Clinical manifestations and pathology

Classic Fabry disease is a multisystem disorder, with prominent and potentially devastating involvement of the kidneys, heart, and peripheral and central nervous system. As expected for an X-linked disorder, clinical manifestations in heterozygous females tend to be mild. Severe Fabry disease in a female reflects extensive inactivation of the X chromosome carrying the normal αGal A allele.

Renal defects

The nephropathy of Fabry disease typically manifests as mild-to-moderate proteinuria, sometimes with microhematuria, beginning in the third decade of life. Nephrotic syndrome is unusual. Urinary oval fat bodies, exhibiting a Maltese cross configuration when viewed with a polarizing microscope, may be seen as a result of the large amounts of glycosphingolipid in the urine (Fig. 4.4b). Deterioration of renal function is gradual, with hypertension and ESRD developing by the fourth or fifth decade of life. Heterozygous women typically display mild renal involvement but may develop ESRD.

Light microscopy shows striking glomerular changes, with additional abnormalities of tubular epithelium and vessels. Glomerular visceral epithelial cells are enlarged and packed with small, clear vacuoles, which represent glycosphingolipid material that has been extracted during processing. Vacuoles may also be seen in parietal epithelial cells and the epithelial cells of the distal convoluted tubule and loop of Henle, but only rarely in mesangial cells, glomerular endothelial cells, or proximal tubular epithelial cells. With time, glomeruli exhibit segmental and global sclerosis. Vacuoles are also observed in endothelial cells and smooth muscle cells of arterioles and arteries.

Ultrastructural examination reveals abundant inclusions within lysosomes, particularly within visceral epithelial cells (Fig. 48.9). The inclusions ('myelin figures') are typically round, comprising concentric layers of dense material separated by clear spaces. The layers may be arranged in parallel ('zebra bodies').

Detachment of visceral epithelial cells from the underlying basement membrane may be observed. Inclusions are also observed in heterozygous females, although usually in smaller numbers than in affected males. Typical inclusions may be noted in excreted renal tubular cells.

The progression of the Fabry nephropathy to ESRD probably reflects two parallel processes. Visceral epithelial cell dysfunction, which results in proteinuria, is followed by visceral epithelial cell detachment and necrosis leading to capillary loop collapse and segmental sclerosis. Simultaneously, progressive impairment of arterial flow may develop, as enlarging endothelial cells impinge on vascular lumina, resulting in ischemic glomerular damage.

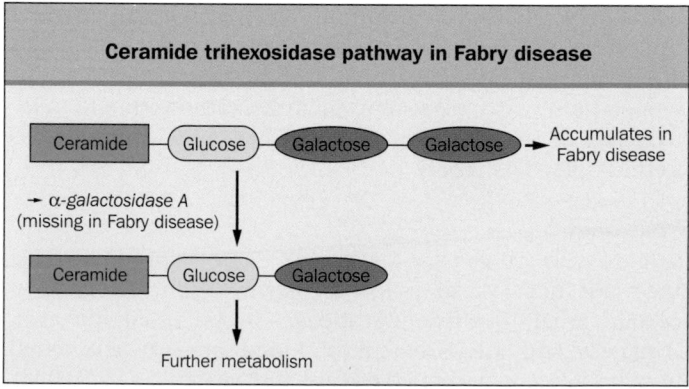

Figure 48.8 The ceramide trihexosidase pathway in Fabry disease. Alpha-galactosidase A deficiency leads to tissue accumulation of trihexosylceramide.

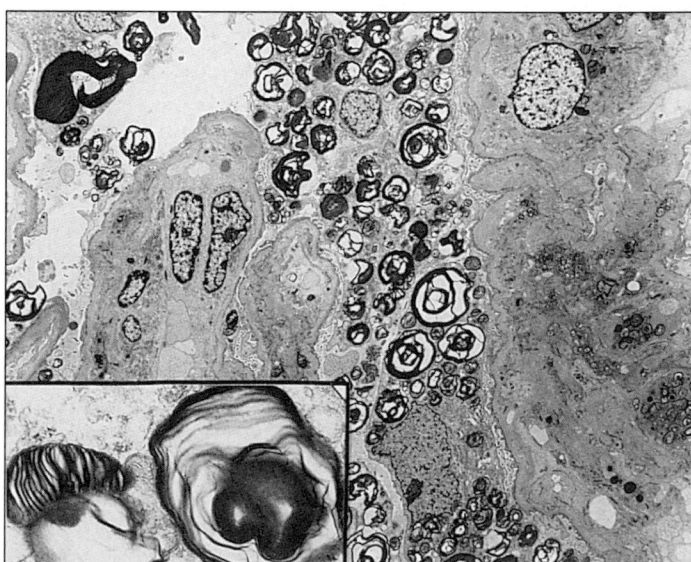

Figure 48.9 Electron micrograph of a renal biopsy in Fabry disease. Glycosphingolipid is deposited in cytoplasmic vacuoles in glomerular visceral epithelial cells. Insert: cytoplasmic vacuoles contain electron-dense material in parallel arrays (zebra bodies) and in concentric whorls (myelin figures). (Courtesy of J Carlos Manivel MD.)

Heart defects

Glycosphingolipid accumulation in coronary arterial endothelial cells and in the myocardium results in coronary artery narrowing, which may lead to angina, myocardial infarction, or congestive heart failure. Arrhythmias and valvular lesions have been identified. Certain missense mutations affecting αGal A may present as isolated left ventricular hypertrophy[35].

Nervous system

Autonomic dysfunction is a prominent feature of Fabry disease, commonly manifested by hypohidrosis, acral paresthesias and altered intestinal motility. Cerebrovascular symptoms tend to appear during the fourth decade of life and include hemiparesis, vertigo, diplopia, dysarthria, nystagmus, nausea and vomiting, headache, ataxia, and memory loss. The vertebrobasilar circulation is preferentially involved. Symptoms are often recurrent. Life-threatening intracerebral hemorrhage and infarction are not unusual. Dementia arising from glycosphingolipid accumulation in small cerebral blood vessels has also been described.

Skin

Angiokeratomas usually appear during the second decade of life, presenting as dark red macules or papules of variable size. Typical locations include the lower trunk, buttocks, hips, genitalia, and upper thighs. The number of lesions varies from none to 20–40. Histologically, angiokeratomas consist of dilated small veins in the upper dermis, covered by hyperkeratotic epidermis. Telangiectasias may be noted, especially behind the ears.

Eyes

Characteristic corneal opacities are common in both men and women with Fabry disease. These lesions, termed verticillata, are identified by slit-lamp examination and are whorls of whitish discoloration that radiate from the center of the cornea. Cataracts and dilated conjunctival or retinal vessels may be observed.

Lungs

Dyspnea and cough are common in men with Fabry disease, often with airflow limitation on spirometry. This may be a consequence of fixed narrowing of the airways owing to glycosphingolipid accumulation.

Diagnosis

When Fabry disease is suspected on clinical or pathologic grounds, the diagnosis may be confirmed by demonstration of reduced levels of αGal A in serum or urine.

Treatment

Efforts to reduce plasma and tissue GL-3 levels have been unsuccessful until recently. In a short-term trial, plasma, renal and cardiac GL-3 levels were reduced by recurrent infusion of recombinant human αGal A[36]. A longer trial will be needed to show that this form of therapy can alter renal and cardiac clinical outcomes.

Renal transplantation is an effective treatment for advanced Fabry nephropathy but does not ameliorate the extrarenal manifestations. Transplanted kidneys from cadaveric donors or unaffected living donors may exhibit glycosphingolipid inclusions, but these are generally infrequent and clinically insignificant. The use of Fabry heterozygotes as kidney donors should be avoided. Coronary artery and cerebrovascular disease are the major causes of death in patients with Fabry disease who have had renal transplants.

NAIL–PATELLA SYNDROME

Definition

Nail–patella syndrome (NPS) is an autosomal dominant disorder consisting of hypoplasia or absence of the patellae, dystrophic nails, dysplasia of the elbows and iliac horns, and renal disease.

Etiology and pathogenesis

The etiology of NPS was unknown until recently. Targeted disruption in mice of a transcription factor gene known as LMX1B resulted in skeletal defects (hypoplastic nails and absent patellae) as well as renal dysplasia[37]. The human homologue of LMX1B was found to map to chromosome 9q34, where the NPS gene is located, and mutations in LMX1B have been identified in patients with NPS[38]. While LMX1B appears to be important for normal limb and kidney development, the precise mechanisms for the renal effects of LMX1B mutations remain under investigation.

Clinical manifestations

Renal defects

Clinically apparent renal disease occurs in less than half of NPS patients. The nephropathy is usually benign, with an approximately 10% risk of progression to ESRD. The clinical signs of NPS nephropathy include microhematuria and mild proteinuria, and appear in adolescence or young adulthood. Some patients develop nephrotic syndrome and mild hypertension. The course of the nephropathy may differ substantially in related individuals.

Skeletal defects

The patellae are absent or hypoplastic in approximately 60% of patients with NPS (Fig. 48.10), and may be associated with effusions and osteoarthritis of the knees. In approximately 80% of patients, there are osseous processes projecting posteriorly from the iliac wings (iliac horns), which are pathognomonic (Fig. 48.11). Abnormalities of the elbows include aplasia, hypoplasia and posterior processes at the distal ends of the humeri.

Nails

Nail abnormalities occur in 80–90% of patients, and tend to be bilateral and symmetric. Fingernails are more commonly affected than toenails. The nails may be absent or dystrophic with discoloration, koilonychia, longitudinal ridges, or triangular lunulae.

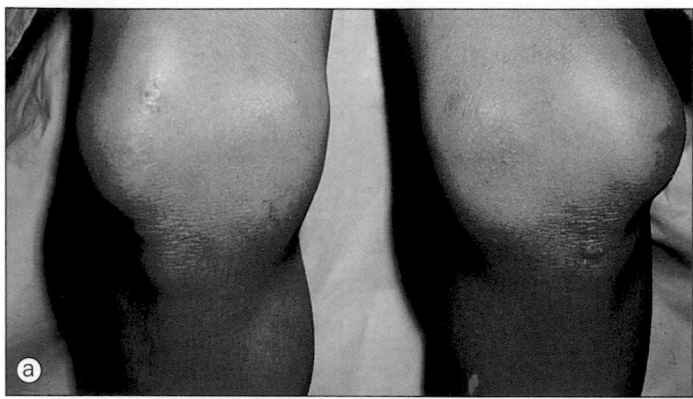

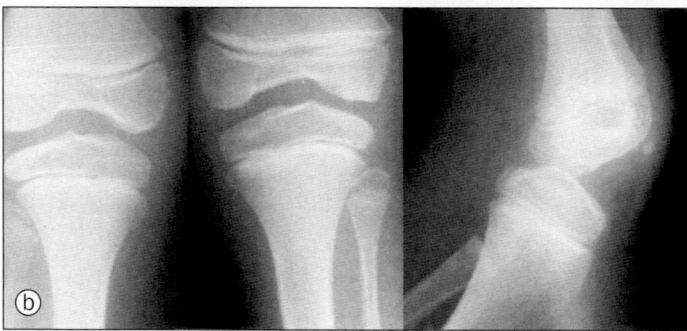

Figure 48.10 Nail–patella syndrome. Absence of the patellae: (a) clinical and (b) radiologic appearance. (Courtesy of R Vernier MD.)

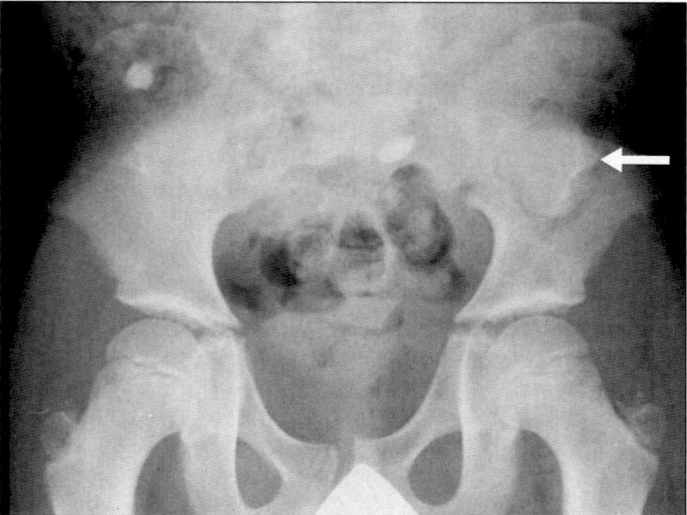

Figure 48.11 Nail–patella syndrome. Iliac horns (arrowed). (Courtesy of R Vernier MD.)

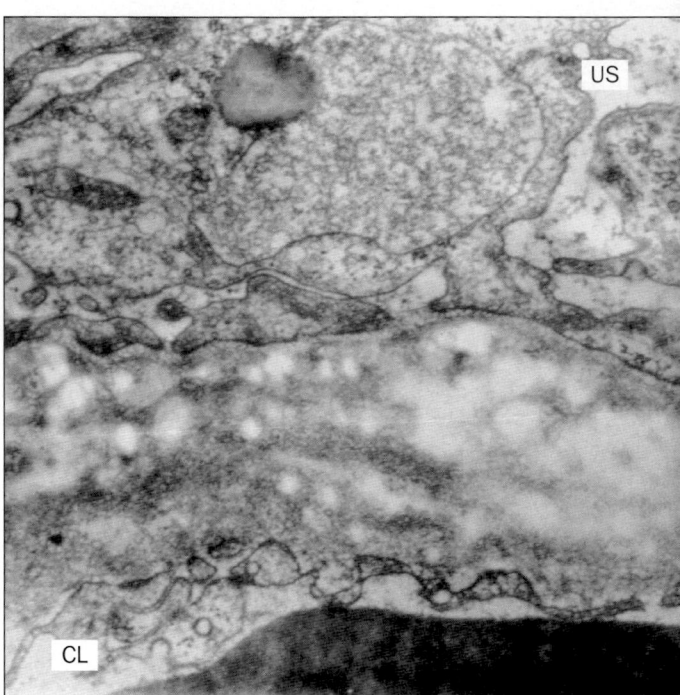

Figure 48.12 Electron micrograph of renal biopsy in nail–patella syndrome. The GBM appears 'moth-eaten' on routine staining. US, urinary space; CL, capillary lumen. (Courtesy of R Vernier MD.)

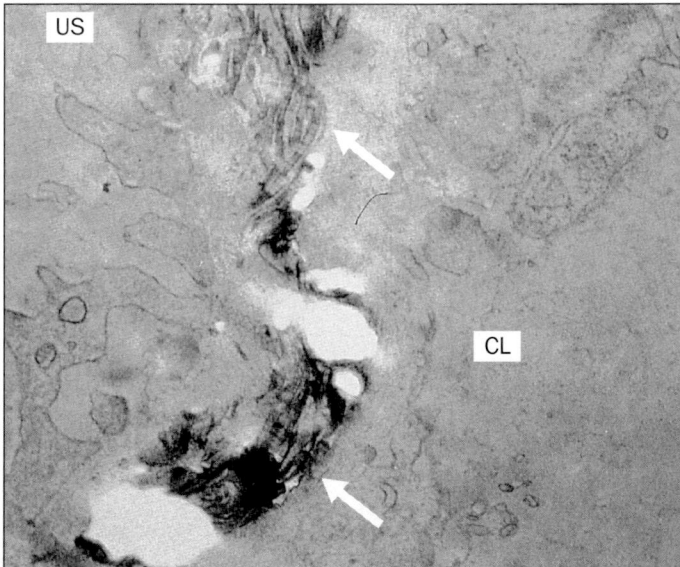

Figure 48.13 Electron micrograph of renal biopsy in nail–patella syndrome. US, urinary space; CL, capillary lumen. Staining with phosphotungstic acid reveals fibrillar collagen (arrows). (Courtesy of R Vernier MD.)

Pathology

There are no specific light or immunofluorescence microscopic features of the NPS renal lesion but, as demonstrated by electron microscopy, the GBM exhibits multiple irregular lucencies, giving it a 'moth-eaten' appearance (Fig. 48.12). Such lucencies may also be observed in the mesangium. These lucent areas sometimes appear to contain cross-banded collagen fibrils, which are better seen after staining with phosphotungstic acid (Fig. 48.13). The fibrils tend to be arranged in clusters, and the surrounding GBM is often thickened. These fibrils may be observed in the kidneys in the absence of clinically evident renal disease, but they have not been found in extraglomerular basement membranes.

Cross-banded fibrils of type III collagen have been seen in GBM of patients with glomerular disease who lack nail or skeletal abnormalities, sometimes as a familial condition with autosomal recessive inheritance ('collagen type III glomerulopathy, see Chapter 30). Collagen type III glomerulopathy and NPS appear to be distinct diseases. No published studies have established the collagen fibrils of NPS as type III collagen.

Treatment

There is no specific therapy for the nephropathy of NPS. Renal transplantation has been performed successfully, without apparent recurrence of the disease in the transplanted kidney. Because NPS is an autosomal dominant disorder, careful evaluation of potential living related kidney donors for features of the disease is essential.

REFERENCES

1. Guthrie LG. 'Idiopathic', or congenital, hereditary and familial hematuria. Lancet. 1902;1:1243–6.
2. Hurst AF. Hereditary familial congenital haemorrhagic nephritis occurring in sixteen individuals in three generations. Guy's Hosp Rec. 1923;3:368–70.
3. Alport AC. Hereditary familial congenital haemorrhagic nephritis. Br Med J. 1927;1:504–6.
4. Spear GS, Slusser RJ. Alport's syndrome: emphasizing electron microscopic studies of the glomerulus. Am J Pathol. 1972;69:213–22.
5. Hinglais N, Grunfeld J-P, Bois LE. Characteristic ultrastructural lesion of the glomerular basement membrane in progressive hereditary nephritis (Alport's syndrome). Lab Invest. 1972;27:473–87.
6. Churg J, Sherman RL. Pathologic characteristics of hereditary nephritis. Arch Pathol. 1973;95:374–9.
7. McCoy RC, Johnson HK, Stone WJ, Wilson CB. Absence of nephritogenic GBM antigen(s) in some patients with hereditary nephritis. Kidney Int. 1982;21:642–52.
8. Kashtan C, Fish AJ, Kleppel M, et al. Nephritogenic antigen determinants in epidermal and renal basement membranes of kindreds with Alport-type familial nephritis. J Clin Invest. 1986;78:1035–44.
9. Atkin CL, Hasstedt SJ, Menlove L, et al. Mapping of Alport syndrome to the long arm of the X chromosome. Am J Hum Genet. 1988;42:249–55.
10. Hostikka SL, Eddy RL, Byers MG, et al. Identification of a distinct type IV collagen α chain with restricted kidney distribution and assignment of its gene to the locus of X chromosome-linked Alport syndrome. Proc Natl Acad Sci USA. 1990;87:1606–10.
11. Barker DF, Hostikka SL, Zhou J, et al. Identification of mutations in the COL4A5 collagen gene in Alport syndrome. Science. 1990;248:1224–7.
12. Zhou J, Reeders ST. The α chains of type IV collagen. Contrib Nephrol. 1996;117:80–105.
13. Lemmink HH, Schröder CH, Monnens LAH, Smeets HJM. The clinical spectrum of type IV collagen mutations. Hum Mutat. 1997;9:477–99.
14. Antignac C, Heidet L. Mutations in Alport syndrome associated with diffuse esophageal leiomyomatosis. Contrib Nephrol. 1996;117: 172–82.
15. Boye E, Mollet G, Forestier L, et al. Determination of the genomic structure of the COL4A4 gene and of novel mutations causing autosomal recessive Alport syndrome. Am J Hum Genet. 1998; 63:1329–40
16. Heidet L, Arrondel C, Forestier L, et al. Structure of the human type IV collagen gene COL4A3 and mutations in autosomal Alport syndrome. J Am Soc Nephrol. 2001;12:97–106.
17. van der Loop FTL, Heidet L, Timmer EDJ, et al. Autosomal dominant Alport syndrome caused by a COL4A3 splice site mutation. Kidney Int. 2000;58:1870–5.
18. Ciccarese M, Casu D, Wong FK, et al. Identification of a new mutation in the α4(IV) collagen gene in a family with autosomal dominant Alport syndrome and hypercholesterolaemia. Nephrol Dial Transplant. 2001;16:2008–12.
19. Kashtan CE, Kleppel MM, Gubler MC. Immunohistologic findings in Alport syndrome. Contrib Nephrol. 1996;117:142–53.
20. Jais JP, Knebelmann B, Giatras I, et al. X-linked Alport syndrome: natural history in 195 families and genotype-phenotype correlations in males. J Am Soc Nephrol. 2000;11:649–57.
21. Grunfeld J-P, Noel LH, Hafez S, Droz D. Renal prognosis in women with hereditary nephritis. Clin Nephrol. 1985;23:267–71.
22. Heath KE, Campos-Barros A, Toren A, et al. Nonmuscle myosin heavy chain IIA mutations define a spectrum of autosomal dominant macrothrombocytopenias: May-Hegglin anomaly and Fechtner, Sebastian, Epstein and Alport-like syndromes. Am J Hum Genet. 2001;69:1033–45.
23. Kashtan CE, Kim Y. Distribution of the α1 and α2 chains of collagen IV and of collagens V and VI in Alport syndrome. Kidney Int. 1992;42:115–26.
24. Kalluri R, Shield CF, Todd P, et al. Isoform switching of type IV collagen is developmentally arrested in X-linked Alport syndrome leading to increased susceptibility of renal basement membranes to endoproteolysis. J Clin Invest. 1997;99:2470–8.
25. Zheng K, Thorner PS, Marrano P, et al. Canine X chromosome-linked hereditary nephritis: a genetic model for human X-linked hereditary nephritis resulting from a single base mutation in the gene encoding the α5 chain of collagen type IV. Proc Natl Acad Sci USA. 1994;91:3989–93.
26. Miner JH, Sanes JR. Molecular and functional defects in kidneys of mice lacking collagen α3(IV): implications for Alport syndrome. J Cell Biol. 1996;135:1403–13.
27. Tryggvason K, Heikkila P, Pettersson E, et al. Can Alport syndrome be treated by gene therapy? Kidney Int. 1997;51:1493–9.
28. Kashtan CE, Gubler MC, Sisson-Ross S, Mauer M. Chronology of renal scarring in males with Alport syndrome. Pediatr Nephrol. 1998;12:269–74.
29. Callis L, Vila A, Carrera M, Nieto J. Long-term effects of cyclosporine A in Alport's syndrome. Kidney Int. 1999;55:1051–6.
30. Lemmink HH, Nillesen WN, Mochizuki T, et al. Benign familial hematuria due to mutation of the type IV collagen α4 gene. J Clin Invest. 1996;98:1114–18.
31. Steffes MW, Barbosa J, Basgen JM, et al. Quantitative glomerular morphology of the normal human kidney. Lab Invest. 1983;49:82–6.
32. Anderson W. A case of 'angio-keratoma'. Br J Dermatol. 1898;10:113–17.
33. Fabry J. Ein Beitrag zur Kenntniss der Purpura haemorrhagica nodularis (Purpura papulosa haemorrhagica Hebrae). Arch Dermatol Syph. 1898;43:187–200.
34. Eng CM, Ashley GA, Burgert TS, et al. Fabry disease: thirty-five mutations in the alpha-galactosidase A gene in patients with classic and variant phenotypes. Mol Med. 1997;3:174–82.
35. Nakao S, Takenaka T, Maeda M, et al. An atypical variant of Fabry's disease in men with left ventricular hypertrophy. N Engl J Med. 1995;333:288–93.
36. Eng CM, Guffon N, Wilcox WR, et al. Safety and efficacy of recombinant human α-galactosidase A replacement therapy in Fabry's disease. N Engl J Med. 2001;345:9–16.
37. Chen H, Lun Y, Ovchinnikov D, et al. Limb and kidney defects in Lmx1b mutant mice suggest an involvement of LMX1B in human nail patella syndrome. Nat Genet. 1998;19:51–5.
38. Dreyer SD, Zhou G, Baldini A, et al. Mutations in LMX1B cause abnormal skeletal patterning and renal dysplasia in nail patella syndrome. Nature Genet. 1998;19:47–50.

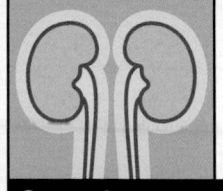

Section 9 Heriditary and Congenital Diseases of the Kidney

Chapter 49 Inherited Disorders of Sodium and Water Handling

Arvind Bagga and Michael J Dillon

INTRODUCTION

Renal tubular epithelial cells are adapted to maintain salt and water homeostasis. Their cell membranes contain specialized channels and transporters that are involved in regulation of fluid and solute balance. Inherited defects in these transporters account for many disorders of salt and water balance. This chapter will focus on inherited disorders of Na^+ and water handling localized to the loop of Henle and the distal nephron. Disorders of proximal tubule transport (see Chapter 50) and tubular acidification (see Chapter 11) are discussed elsewhere.

Molecular genetic studies have allowed greater precision in categorization of patients, with implications in terms of diagnosis, treatment, outcome and genetic counseling (Table 49.1). These conditions mostly present in childhood but they are of importance to adult nephrologists because many have lifelong clinical implications that will require future care. Furthermore, identification of single gene defects in cases of syndromic hypertension is providing new understanding of tubular physiology and the pathogenesis of essential hypertension.

PHYSIOLOGY OF SODIUM AND WATER REABSORPTION

Sodium reabsorption

Reabsorption of Na^+ occurs throughout the nephron. Approximately 60% of the filtered Na^+ and Cl^- are reabsorbed in the proximal tubule. The distal portions of the nephron reabsorb the remainder (thick ascending limb of loop of Henle 30%, distal convoluted tubule 7–8%, and collecting tubule 2%).

The reabsorption of Na^+ in the nephron is driven by the basolateral enzyme Na^+/K^+ ATPase, which through an energy-dependent step exchanges three intracellular Na^+ for two extracellular K^+. This maintains a concentration gradient

Table 49.1 Inherited single gene defects of sodium and water handling.

Inherited single gene defects of sodium and water handling			
Syndrome	Inheritance	Gene localization	Gene product
Neonatal Bartter syndrome	AR	15q	Na-K-2Cl cotransporter *NKCC2*
Neonatal Bartter syndrome	AR	11q	Renal potassium channel *ROMK*
Classic Bartter syndrome	AR	1p	Renal chloride channel *ClC-Kb*
Bartter syndrome with deafness	AR	1p	β-subunit of ClC-Kb *Barttin*
Gitelman syndrome	AR	16q	Na-Cl cotransporter *NCCT*
Liddle's syndrome	AD	16p	Epithelial sodium channel *ENaC*
Syndrome of apparent mineralocorticoid excess	AR	16q	11β-hydroxysteroid dehydrogenase type II
Glucocorticoid-remediable aldosteronism	AD	8q	Aldosterone synthase *CYP11B2*
Pseudohypoaldosteronism type 1	AD AR	4p 12p, 16p	Mineralocorticoid receptor ENaC
Gordon's syndrome	AD	12p 17q 1q	WNK1 WNK4 Not identified
Congenital adrenal hyperplasia	AR AR AR	6p 8q 10q	21 hydroxylase 11β-hydroxylase 17α-hydroxylase
Nephrogenic diabetes insipidus	X-linked AR	Xq 12q	AVP receptor 2 Aquaporin 2

AR, autosomal recessive; AD, autosomal dominant.

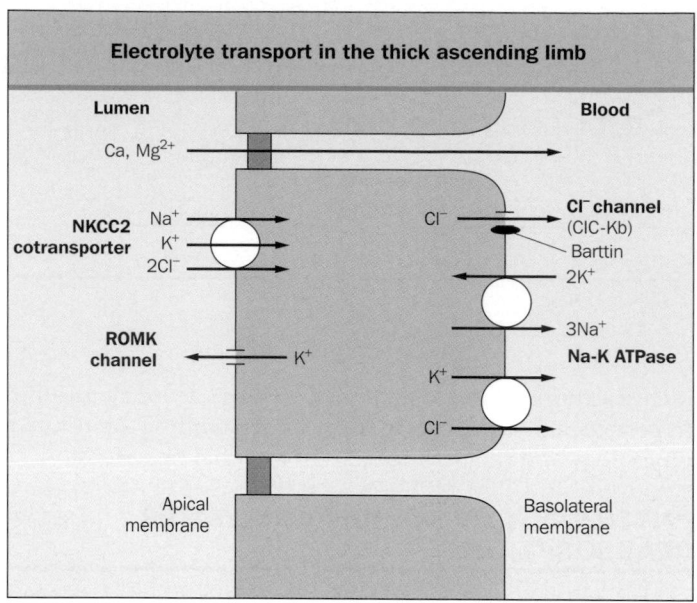

Figure 49.1 Electrolyte transport in the thick ascending limb of the loop of Henle. The furosemide-sensitive $Na^+/K^+/2Cl^-$ (NKCC2) co-transporter is driven by low intracellular Na^+ and Cl^- concentrations produced by the Na^+/K^+ ATPase pump, K^+/Cl^- cotransporter and the basolateral Cl^- channel (ClC-Kb). The β-subunit (barttin) is crucial for normal functioning of the ClC-Kb channels. Apical K^+ recycling via the low-conductance, ATP-sensitive renal medullary K^+ (ROMK) channel ensures the efficient functioning of the NKCC2 cotransporter.

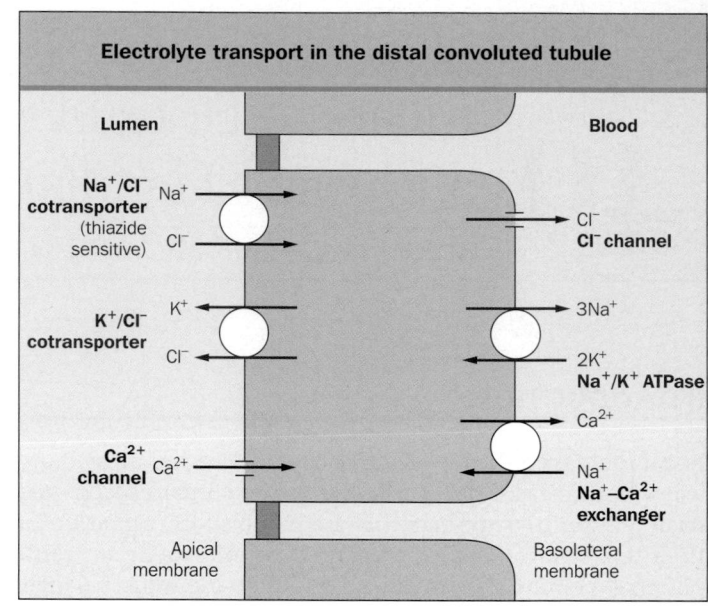

Figure 49.2 Electrolyte transport in the distal convoluted tubule. Reabsorption of Na^+ and Cl^- occurs across the apical membrane by the thiazide-sensitive Na^+/Cl^- cotransporter (NCCT) and these ions leave the cell through the Cl^- channels and via the Na^+/K^+ ATPase pump. Calcium ions enter the cell through the Ca^{2+} channels and exit via the Na^+/Ca^{2+} exchanger.

that enhances Na^+ transport from the tubular lumen to the cell. On the apical membrane, a number of transporters ensure Na^+, K^+, and Cl^- transport. Most Na^+ reabsorption in the proximal tubule results from active cotransport with organic solutes such as glucose and amino acids, or through the Na^+-H^+ exchanger.

The primary mediator of Na^+ uptake in the thick ascending limb of the loop of Henle is the furosemide (frusemide)-sensitive $Na^+/K^+/2Cl^-$ (NKCC2) cotransporter (Fig. 49.1). The levels of K^+ in the lumen of the loop of Henle are much lower than those of Na^+ and Cl^-. Therefore, K^+ entering the tubular cell from the lumen must be recycled to permit sustained NKCC2 activity. The renal outer medullary K^+ channel (ROMK) is an ATP-sensitive channel that 'recycles' reabsorbed K^+ back into the tubular lumen, ensuring efficient Na^+ and Cl^- uptake by NKCC2. The Cl^- channel, ClC-Kb, ensures Cl^- reabsorption from the tubular cell into the bloodstream. An accessory β-subunit, barttin, is necessary for normal functioning of these Cl^- channels.

In the distal convoluted tubule, the thiazide-sensitive apical Na^+/Cl^- cotransporter (NCCT) is the principal mediator of Na^+ and Cl^- reabsorption (Fig. 49.2). Amiloride-sensitive, epithelial Na^+ channels (ENaC) (Fig. 49.3) mediate Na^+ reabsorption in collecting tubules and collecting ducts. The mineralocorticoid hormone aldosterone regulates Na^+/K^+ balance in the distal nephron chiefly through its effect on the synthesis of ENaC. Figure 49.4 shows the sites of Na^+ reabsorption and the disorders resulting from abnormalities in specific transporters.

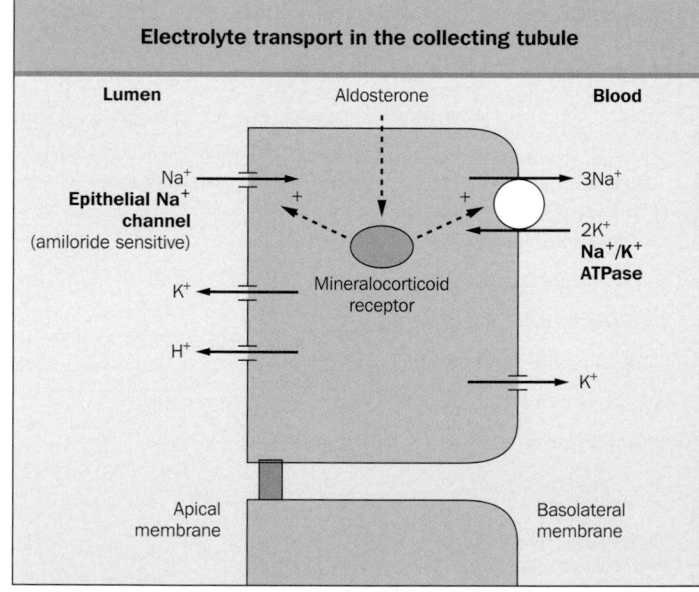

Figure 49.3 Electrolyte transport in the principal cell of the collecting tubule. Reabsorption of Na^+ occurs via the amiloride-sensitive epithelial Na^+ channel (ENaC). Its uptake is coupled to K^+ and H^+ secretion. Aldosterone increases the activity of ENaC and Na^+/K^+ ATPase, which increases Na^+ reabsorption and K^+ and H^+ secretion, resulting in hypokalemic alkalosis. Cortisol is also a ligand for the mineralocorticoid receptor but is normally removed by oxidation by 11β-hydroxysteroid dehydrogenase to cortisone.

Pathways and mediators of Na⁺ reabsorption

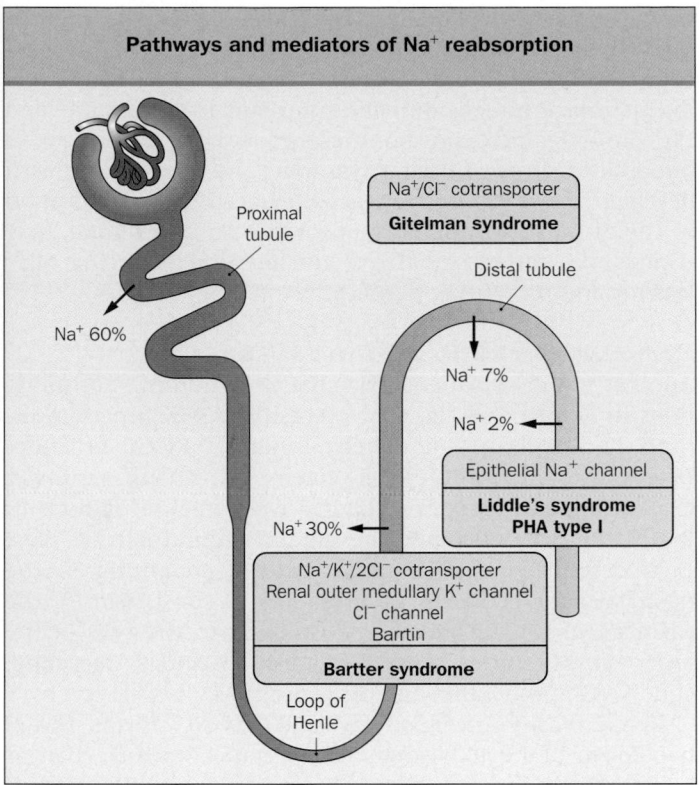

Figure 49.4 Pathways and mediators involved in Na⁺ reabsorption.
Almost 60% of the filtered Na⁺ is reabsorbed in the proximal tubule. The distal portions of the nephron reabsorb the remainder. The chief mediators involved in Na⁺ reabsorption and disorders resulting from their mutations are shown in boxes. PHA, pseudohypoaldosteronism.

Water reabsorption

Water is passively reabsorbed in the proximal tubule and thin descending limb of the loop of Henle. The ascending limb of the loop of Henle and the distal convoluted tubule are impermeable to water. Water reabsorption across the epithelial cells of the collecting tubules and ducts depends on the presence of the antidiuretic hormone arginine-vasopressin.

The aquaporins (AQP) are a family of membrane channel proteins that serve as selective pores through which water crosses cell membranes. AQP2, exclusively present in the principal cells of the collecting tubules and ducts, is the chief vasopressin-regulated water channel (Fig. 49.5).

DISORDERS OF SODIUM HANDLING

Inherited disorders of Na⁺ and water balance can be classified based on both their clinical presentation (Fig. 49.6) and pathogenesis. Sodium-wasting states associated with hypokalemic alkalosis are now separated clinically, biochemically, and genetically into classic Bartter syndrome, neonatal Bartter syndrome, and Gitelman syndrome.

Several loci controlling synthesis and regulation of mineralocorticoid activity have been implicated in single gene defects associated with hypertension (e.g., Liddle's syndrome, glucocorticoid-remediable aldosteronism (GRA), syndrome of apparent mineralocorticoid excess (AME), Gordon's syndrome, and deficiencies of the enzymes 11β-hydroxylase and 17α-hydroxylase).

Water reabsorption in the distal tubule

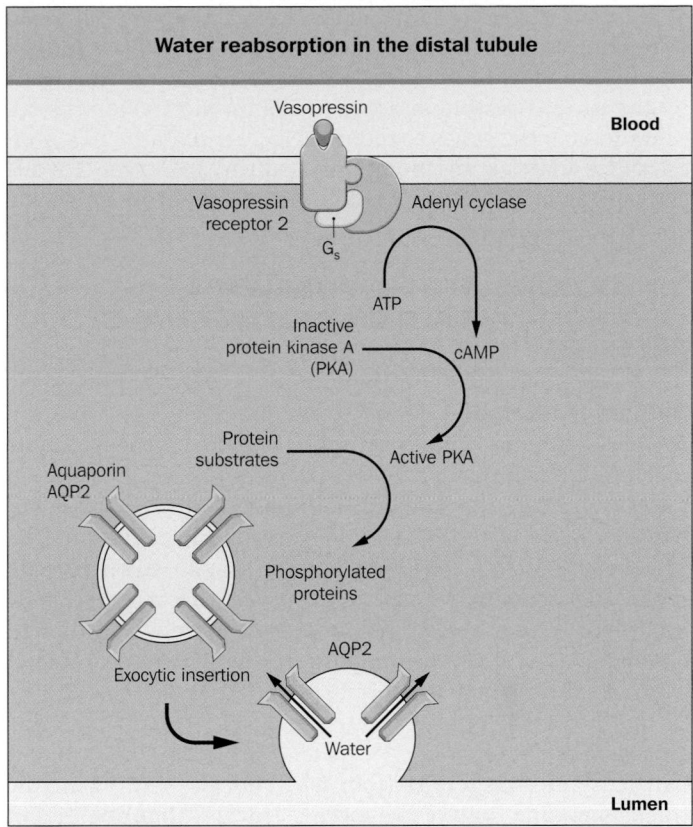

Figure 49.5 Water reabsorption in the distal tubule. The aquaporin AQP2, which is exclusively present in the principal cells of the collecting tubules and ducts, is the chief vasopressin-regulated water channel. Activation of cAMP-dependent protein kinase A mediates protein phosphorylation that triggers exocytic insertion of AQP2 channels into the apical membrane. These channels increase the water permeability of the apical membrane, facilitating water transport.

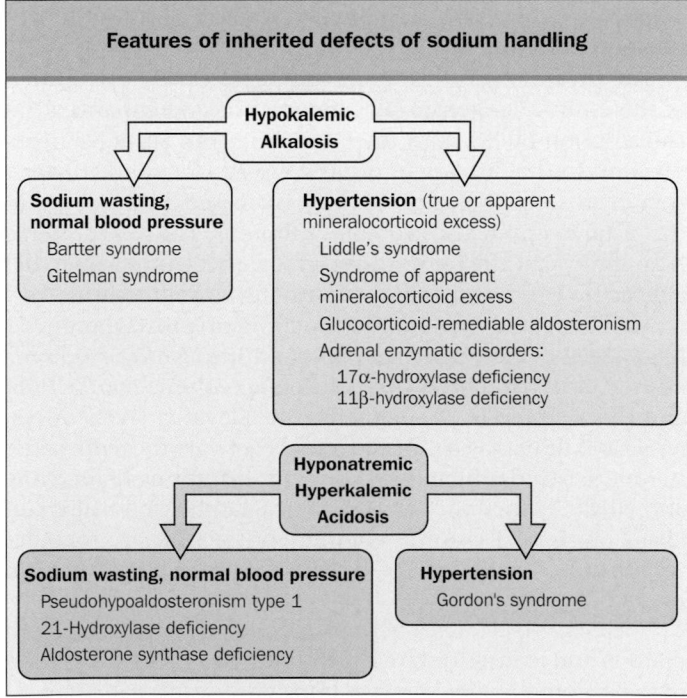

Figure 49.6 Features of inherited defects of sodium handling.

Heriditary and Congenital Diseases of the Kidney

By contrast, lack of mineralocorticoid activity or end-organ unresponsiveness to aldosterone action (e.g., due to 21-hydroxylase deficiency and pseudohypoaldosteronism (PHA) type 1) results in salt wasting and hyperkalemic metabolic acidosis. Mutations in the genes encoding ENaC are of particular interest, since inactivating mutations result in PHA type 1 while activating mutations cause Liddle's syndrome with a precisely converse phenotype.

CONDITIONS WITH HYPOKALEMIA, METABOLIC ALKALOSIS, AND NORMAL BLOOD PRESSURE

Bartter syndrome

Bartter syndrome comprises hypokalemia, hypochloremic metabolic alkalosis, and increased urinary Na^+, K^+, and Cl^- losses[1]. Plasma renin and aldosterone levels are elevated but blood pressure is normal. Children with Bartter syndrome are subdivided on clinical features into the 'classic' and 'neonatal' types. These conditions may occur sporadically but are usually inherited in an autosomal recessive manner. Although Gitelman syndrome has similarities with Bartter syndrome, it is genetically distinct and should be differentiated[2].

Pathogenesis

Bartter syndrome results from Na^+ and Cl^- wasting in the thick ascending limb of the loop of Henle[3]. Abnormalities in NKCC2, ROMK, ClC-Kb and its β-subunit (barttin) have been reported in patients with the Bartter phenotype (see Table 49.1 and Fig. 49.1).

Mutations affecting NKCC2

Bartter syndrome can be caused by mutations affecting NKCC2 in the thick ascending limb of the loop of Henle[4]. Frameshift, nonsense or missense mutations of the gene for NKCC2 have been found in affected patients. These mutant alleles cause loss in NKCC2 function leading to salt wasting in the loop of Henle.

The salt wasting with volume contraction leads to activation of the renin–angiotensin–aldosterone axis and enhanced Na^+ reabsorption by ENaC in the distal nephron. Since Na^+ reabsorption in the distal nephron is coupled to K^+ and H^+ secretion, hypokalemic alkalosis ensues. Increased fluid delivery to the distal nephron also promotes kaliuresis. The loop of Henle is an important site for K^+ reabsorption and it is probable that a defect in this segment also contributes to kaliuresis.

The increased systemic production of prostaglandin E_2 (PGE_2) seen in these patients is not specific to Bartter syndrome but secondary to chronic hypokalemia, volume contraction, and elevated levels of angiotensin II. Elevated levels of systemic and urinary PGE_2 independently activate the renin–aldosterone axis and inhibit ROMK activity, disrupting K^+ recycling and NKCC2 function. Elevated prostaglandin and kallikrein-kinin levels and chronic volume contraction are together responsible for the lack of hypertension despite very high plasma renin activity.

There is also evidence of impaired renal concentration and dilution and reduced distal Cl^- reabsorption. Increased excretion of urinary ammonium ions may impair the decrease in urine pH during ammonium chloride loading. Reduced Cl^- absorption in the loop of Henle inhibits the voltage-driven paracellular reabsorption of Ca^{2+} and Mg^{2+}, causing hypercalciuria and hypermagnesuria. Prostaglandins also contribute to urinary Ca^{2+} and Mg^{2+} losses by increasing bone resorption. Hypercalciuria is an important feature of Bartter syndrome and is associated with development of nephrocalcinosis. Enhanced Mg^{2+} reabsorption in the distal nephron, partly mediated by aldosterone, may compensate for proximal hypermagnesuria, reducing Mg^{2+} wasting and preventing significant hypomagnesemia.

Mutations affecting ROMK, ClC-Kb and Barttin

Another group of patients with Bartter syndrome has mutations in ROMK (see Fig. 49.1)[5]. Loss of ROMK function disrupts K^+ recycling and thereby inhibits NKCC2 function. Inactivating mutations of the gene for ClC-Kb also results in Cl^- wasting and features of Bartter syndrome[3]. Mutations in BSND, the gene encoding the subunit protein barttin, have been described in a group of patients presenting in the neonatal period[6]. Barttin is also a crucial constituent of the ClC-Ka and ClC-Kb membrane channels in the cells of the inner ear. Mutations in BSND abolish Cl^- and K^+ recycling, endolymph production and cause deafness.

Renal biopsy in 'neonatal' and 'classic' forms shows hyperplasia of the juxtaglomerular apparatus. Vacuolar changes in proximal tubular cells, tubular atrophy with marked cystic dilatation, and interstitial fibrosis may be observed as a consequence of chronic hypokalemia and hypercalciuria.

Clinical manifestations

Neonatal Bartter syndrome

Clinical features of neonatal Bartter syndrome include marked polyhydramnios (caused by intrauterine polyuria), premature delivery, postnatal polyuria, vomiting, failure to thrive, hypercalciuria and nephrocalcinosis. A variant with sensorineural deafness, motor retardation and early onset of renal failure has been described[6,7]. Some patients have salt craving. Urinary Cl^- excretion is markedly increased. Prenatal diagnosis of Bartter syndrome may be made by showing high levels of Cl^- in the amniotic fluid.

'Classic' Bartter syndrome

In 'classic' Bartter syndrome, symptoms begin during the first 2–3 years of life and are generally milder than in the neonatal form. They include polyuria, polydipsia and vomiting, recurrent episodes of dehydration, constipation and failure to thrive. Blood pressure is normal. Later findings include fatigue, recurrent carpopedal spasms and developmental delay. Nephrocalcinosis is usually not seen.

Diagnosis

The biochemical findings in neonatal and classic forms of Bartter syndrome are similar. The outstanding laboratory feature is hypokalemia, with blood K^+ levels of 1.5–2.5 mmol/L, and metabolic alkalosis. Elevated levels of renin and aldosterone are characteristic and reflect the extracellular fluid volume contraction. Occasionally, the levels of aldosterone may be inappropriately low because of severe hypokalemia but increase once treatment is started with K^+ supplements.

The fractional excretion of K^+, Na^+ and Cl^- is increased. Marked urinary excretion of PGE_2 is considered a distinguishing feature of neonatal Bartter syndrome but may not be present during early neonatal life.

Hyperuricemia may occur through extracellular fluid depletion; hypomagnesemia is reported in a few patients. Defects in urine concentration, dilution and acidification are present. The glomerular filtration rate (GFR) is normal in early stages but may reduce later.

Differential diagnosis

Conditions associated with persistent hypokalemic metabolic alkalosis can be differentiated on blood pressure and urinary Cl^- excretion (Fig. 49.7). The absence of hypertension distinguishes Bartter syndrome from renal artery stenosis, renin-secreting tumors and low-renin forms of hypertension (primary hyperaldosteronism, Liddle's syndrome, AME, GRA and salt-retaining forms of congenital adrenal hyperplasia). Chloride depletion occurs due to laxative abuse, cyclical vomiting, colonic adenoma. Similarly, excessive loss of Cl^- in sweat, as in cystic fibrosis, and dietary Cl^- deficiency may lead to Cl^- depletion. Urinary Cl^- in these cases is less than 10 mmol/L. Magnesium deficiency also causes urinary K^+ losses; serum and urinary magnesium levels are low in such cases.

Presence of high urinary Cl^- (> 20 mmol/L) with hypokalemic metabolic alkalosis suggests Bartter or Gitelman syndrome or diuretic use/abuse. The findings distinguishing Bartter from Gitelman syndrome are the presence of significant hypomagnesemia, hypermagnesuria and hypocalciuria in the latter (Table 49.2). Most patients with onset of symptoms in late childhood or adulthood have Gitelman syndrome. Most diuretics, other than potassium-sparing drugs and carbonic anhydrase inhibitors, may cause hypokalemic metabolic alkalosis. The metabolic derangement resulting from administration of loop diuretics mimics Bartter syndrome quite precisely. In adults, diuretics and their metabolites should be measured in the urine whenever diuretic consumption is suspected; testing may be necessary on several occasions to exclude this with certainty.

Most patients with 'neonatal' Bartter syndrome (marked clinical and biochemical abnormalities) show mutations of the genes encoding NKCC2 or ROMK; hypokalemia is less severe in the latter[7]. Patients with ROMK mutations, especially those born prematurely, often show mild salt wasting and a

Features differentiating Bartter and Gitelman syndromes

Feature	Neonatal Bartter syndrome	Classic Bartter syndrome	Gitelman syndrome
Age at onset	Neonatal period	Infancy/childhood	Childhood/later
Maternal hydramnios	Common	Rare	Absent
Polyuria, polydipsia	Marked	Present	Rare
Dehydration	Present	Often present	Absent
Tetany	Absent	Rare	Present
Growth retardation	Present	Present	Absent
Urinary calcium	Very high	Normal or high	Low
Nephrocalcinosis	Present	Rare	Absent
Serum magnesium	Normal	Occasionally low	Low
Urine prostaglandins	Very high	High or normal	Normal
Response to indomethacin	Good	Good	Rare

Table 49.2 Features differentiating Bartter and Gitelman syndromes. In addition to these clinical and laboratory features, molecular diagnosis is now possible (see text).

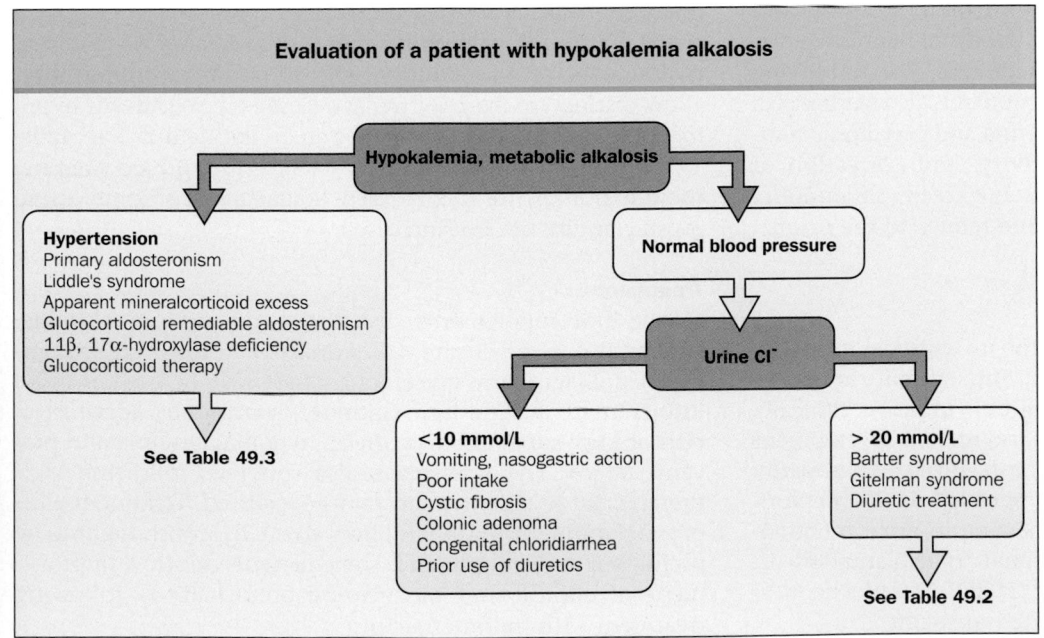

Figure 49.7 Evaluation of a patient with hypokalemia and metabolic alkalosis.

Evaluation of a patient with hypokalemia alkalosis

Hypokalemia, metabolic alkalosis

Hypertension
Primary aldosteronism
Liddle's syndrome
Apparent mineralcorticoid excess
Glucocorticoid remediable aldosteronism
11β, 17α-hydroxylase deficiency
Glucocorticoid therapy

Normal blood pressure

See Table 49.3

Urine Cl⁻

<10 mmol/L
Vomiting, nasogastric action
Poor intake
Cystic fibrosis
Colonic adenoma
Congenital chloridiarrhea
Prior use of diuretics

> 20 mmol/L
Bartter syndrome
Gitelman syndrome
Diuretic treatment

See Table 49.2

biochemical picture of PHA type 1 (hyponatremia, hyperkalemia and metabolic acidosis); hypokalemia and metabolic alkalosis manifest a few weeks later. Recently, mutations in the Barttin gene have been described in patients having neonatal Bartter syndrome and sensorineural deafness. Patients with the 'classic' Bartter syndrome show abnormalities of the gene for ClC-Kb (Fig. 49.1). However, the correlation between the genotype and phenotype is not perfect and overlap of features has been described, particularly with mutations of this gene[7].

Molecular diagnosis of Bartter and Gitelman syndromes is now possible. Mutations in NKCC2, ROMK, ClC-Kb, barttin and NCCT may be screened by single strand conformation analysis or polymerase chain reaction.

Erythrocytes from patients with Bartter syndrome show increased intracellular Na^+ (normal level 4.9–7.6 mmol/L) associated with reduced Na^+ efflux[8]. These abnormalities may represent a widespread defect in membrane electrolyte transport or more likely are secondary to chronic hypokalemia. The changes normalize following treatment with indomethacin and correction of hypokalemia. Measurement of erythrocyte intracellular Na^+ levels appears to have a diagnostic value in identifying children with Bartter syndrome and assessing response to therapy.

Treatment

Patients with the neonatal form of Bartter syndrome have marked fluid and electrolyte disturbances that need to be corrected carefully. Saline infusion may be required in the neonatal period. Potassium chloride supplementation is always necessary[9]. Addition of spironolactone or triamterene may be useful in correcting hypokalemia, but the effect of these drugs is usually transient. Angiotensin-converting enzyme (ACE) inhibitors have been used for correction of hypokalemia, with conflicting results. Magnesium deficiency may aggravate renal K^+ wasting and, if present, should be corrected.

The efficacy of long-term treatment with prostaglandin synthase inhibitors, such as indomethacin or ibuprofen, is well established[9]. They act by reducing cortical perfusion and decreasing delivery of Na^+ and Cl^- to the distal nephron, ameliorating many of the features of the disease. The amplifying effect of prostaglandins on the renal tubules is also neutralized. Treatment results in reduction of polyuria and polydipsia, restitution of normal growth and activity, and correction of hypokalemia; serum K^+, however, rarely exceeds 3.5 mmol/L. Plasma levels of renin and aldosterone reduce to the normal range.

Outcome

If not treated, patients may succumb to episodes of dehydration, electrolyte disturbance or intercurrent infection. With appropriate therapy, most children improve clinically and show catch-up growth; pubertal and mental development are usually normal. Chronic tubulointerstitial nephropathy owing to persistent hypokalemia, hypercalciuria and nephrocalcinosis may lead to progressive decline in renal function. There are anecdotal reports of renal transplantation in patients with end-stage renal disease (ESRD). The biochemical parameters return to normal following transplant.

Gitelman syndrome

Gitelman syndrome is an autosomal recessive condition also characterized by hypokalemic metabolic alkalosis, but with hypocalciuria and hypomagnesemia.

Pathogenesis

The similarity between the features of Gitelman syndrome and those caused by thiazide administration originally suggested the defect might be in the distal convoluted tubule. The condition has now been linked to inactivating mutations in the gene for NCCT (see Figs 49.2 and 49.4)[10]. Loss of NCCT function results in Na^+ and Cl^- wasting from this segment, leading to hypovolemia with secondary activation of the renin–aldosterone system. The resulting increase in collecting tubule Na^+ reabsorption is, however, counterbalanced by K^+ and H^+ excretion, causing hypokalemic alkalosis. The distal convoluted tubule normally reabsorbs only 7–8% of the filtered Na^+ and Cl^- load. The degree of volume contraction, stimulation of the renin–angiotensin system, and the amount of K^+ loss are, therefore, not substantial enough to stimulate PGE_2 production.

The reasons for the high levels of urinary Mg^{2+} and low levels of urinary Ca^{2+} are not clearly understood. Impaired Na^+ reabsorption across the luminal membrane and continued efflux of intracellular Cl^- through basolateral chloride channels may promote Ca^{2+} reabsorption in the cells of the distal convoluted tubule through the luminal voltage-activated Ca^{2+} channels. The reduced intracellular Na^+ concentration then facilitates Ca^{2+} exit via the Na^+/Ca^{2+} exchanger (see Fig. 49.2). This segment of the nephron also reabsorbs about 5% of filtered Mg^{2+}. Loss of function of the NCCT might inhibit Mg^{2+} absorption by a Na^+-dependent mechanism.

Clinical manifestations and diagnosis

Patients present with unexplained hypokalemia at a later age than those with 'classic' Bartter syndrome and are often asymptomatic. They occasionally manifest episodes of muscular weakness, cramps and tetany[2,3]. Polyuria and growth retardation are absent or mild; joint pains may occur as a result of chondrocalcinosis. There is no history of maternal hydramnios or prematurity. The important findings that allow distinction from Bartter syndrome are significant hypomagnesemia, hypermagnesuria and hypocalciuria (see Table 49.2). There is an increase in plasma renin and aldosterone, though not to the degree seen in Bartter syndrome; urine prostaglandins are not increased.

Treatment

Magnesium supplements, usually as magnesium chloride, which also compensate for urinary Cl^- loss, are recommended. Magnesium glycerophosphate may be used in those intolerant to magnesium chloride. Continuous administration of Mg^{2+} supplements corrects hypomagnesemia and prevents tetany. Hypokalemia is also corrected following Mg^{2+} therapy, but K^+ supplements may be required. Treatment with prostaglandin synthase inhibitors is usually not thought to be useful, but in our experience some patients do show improvement of clinical and biochemical abnormalities following treatment with indomethacin.

The long-term prognosis for renal function and growth is excellent. Therapy with Mg^{2+} supplements is required lifelong to reduce episodes of muscle weakness and tetany.

CONDITIONS WITH HYPOKALEMIA, METABOLIC ALKALOSIS, AND HYPERTENSION

Conditions with hypokalemia, metabolic alkalosis and hypertension all have true or apparent mineralocorticoid excess.

Liddle's syndrome (pseudohyperaldosteronism)

Liddle's syndrome is an autosomal dominant syndrome of hypertension and variable degrees of hypokalemic metabolic alkalosis. The patients resemble those with primary hyperaldosteronism, but levels of mineralocorticoid hormones are not increased. Renin and aldosterone are suppressed and there is no response to spironolactone[11]. However, triamterene and amiloride, aldosterone-independent inhibitors of distal Na^+ transport, correct hypertension, renal K^+ loss and hypokalemia[12].

Pathogenesis

Enhanced reabsorption of Na^+ due to constitutive overactivity of ENaC in the collecting tubule is the initiating mechanism. ENaC is a hetero-tetrameric protein comprising two α-, one β-, and one γ-subunit, each having intracellular N and C termini, two transmembrane domains, and a large extracellular loop. A gene on chromosome 12p encodes the α-units, while genes for β- and γ-subunits map to chromosome 16p. Heterozygous point mutations in the genes for β- or γ-subunits have been shown in Liddle's kindreds[13]. Both mutations lead to truncation of the intracellular C-terminal tails of the respective subunits, which then fail to bind to regulatory proteins. Failure of this binding prevents normal degradation of ENaC, resulting in enhanced Na^+ transport, volume expansion, hypertension and suppression of renin secretion[12].

Functional coupling of Na^+ reabsorption to K^+ and H^+ secretion in the distal nephron (see Fig. 49.3) results in hypokalemic alkalosis and decreased blood levels of aldosterone.

Clinical manifestations and diagnosis

Liddle's syndrome predominantly manifests in teenage children and adults although it can occur in early childhood. Clinical features include polyuria, increased thirst, failure to thrive and significant hypertension. Hypokalemic metabolic alkalosis with low blood levels of renin and aldosterone are characteristic. The severity of hypertension and hypokalemia is variable and the disease may often remain undiagnosed[12]. The original patient described by Liddle and coworkers developed ESRD necessitating renal transplantation[14], following which the blood pressure returned to normal and hypokalemia resolved.

Sodium restriction or correction of serum K^+ concentration does not increase aldosterone secretion; no improvement is seen after administration of spironolactone. Urinary mineralocorticoid metabolites are within normal limits.

This condition should be differentiated from primary hyperaldosteronism, AME, GRA (Table 49.3) and patients with 11β-hydroxylase (steroid 11β-mono-oxygenase) or 17α-hydroxylase (steroid 17α-mono-oxygenase) deficiency. Activating mutations of the mineralocorticoid (MR) receptor, presenting with similar features and exacerbation of hypertension during pregnancy and following administration of spironolactone have been reported recently[15].

Treatment

Therapy consists of sodium restriction and K^+ supplements. Triamterene directly inhibits apical Na^+ channels, resulting in increased urinary Na^+ and decreased K^+ excretion and resolution of hypertension. Amiloride also normalizes the blood pressure and K^+ levels. However, most patients continue to have growth retardation. Since the pathogenetic disorder is not correctable with age, lifelong therapy is required.

Table 49.3 Features of Liddle's syndrome, apparent mineralocorticoid excess (AME) and glucocorticoid remediable aldosteronism (GRA).

Features of Liddle's syndrome, apparent mineralocorticoid excess and glucocorticoid remediable aldosteronism			
	Syndromes with hypokalemia, metabolic alkalosis, and hypertension		
Feature	Liddle's syndrome	AME	GRA
Inheritance	Autosomal dominant	Autosomal recessive	Autosomal dominant
Chief features	Significant hypertension, polyuria, growth retardation	Low birth weight, early onset hypertension, polyuria, growth retardation	Significant hypertension, hemorrhagic stroke
Plasma aldosterone	Reduced	Reduced	Elevated
Plasma renin activity	Reduced	Reduced	Reduced
Urinary mineralocorticoid metabolites	Normal	Elevated ratios of THF + alloTHF to THE; free cortisol to cortisone	Elevated cortisol C-18 oxidation products
Response to:			
Glucocorticoids	No	Satisfactory	Satisfactory
Triamterene	Satisfactory	Satisfactory	Satisfactory
Spironolactone	No	Satisfactory	Satisfactory
THF, tetrahydrocortisol; THE, tetrahydrocortisone.			

Apparent mineralocorticoid excess

Pathogenesis

AME is an autosomal recessive condition resulting from deficiency of the type II (renal and placental) isoform of the enzyme 11β-hydroxysteroid dehydrogenase. Clinical features of this condition closely mimic those of Liddle's syndrome[16].

In normal conditions, aldosterone is the chief mineralocorticoid regulating electrolyte and water balance, through its effects on distal renal tubules and cortical collecting ducts. Following its binding to the MR, aldosterone increases synthesis of various proteins, chiefly Na+/K+ ATPase on the basolateral surface and ENaC on the apical surface. These proteins increase Na+ reabsorption and K+ secretion in the distal tubules (see Fig. 49.3). Cortisol is also a ligand for MR and shows potent salt-retaining activity. Cortisol is, however, normally metabolized by 11β-hydroxysteroid dehydrogenase to cortisone, which lacks such an action.

Deficiency of the enzyme 11β-hydroxysteroid dehydrogenase results in high intrarenal levels of cortisol, which bind to MR, resulting in Na+ retention and urinary K+ loss. The syndrome of AME, therefore, results from a loss of specificity of the MR. Loss of function mutations in the gene for the type II isoform (located on chromosome 16q) have been detected in all kindreds with AME[17,18]. The type II isoform of 11β-hydroxysteroid dehydrogenase is also expressed in high levels in the placenta, where it may protect developing tissues from the deleterious effects of cortisol. It has been speculated that low levels of placental 11β-hydroxysteroid dehydrogenase activity might be a risk factor for low birth weight and hypertension in later life.

Carbenoxolone and glycyrrhizic acid (glycyrrhizinic acid; found in licorice compounds) are potent inhibitors of this enzyme. Consumption of these agents may be associated with features similar to AME.

Clinical manifestations and diagnosis

The chief features of AME include polyuria, increased thirst, failure to thrive and early-onset hypertension. There is often a history of intrauterine growth retardation. Marked hypokalemia and metabolic alkalosis are present. Plasma renin and aldosterone levels are extremely low.

The diagnosis of AME is made by finding, on gas chromatography/mass spectroscopy, elevated urinary levels of hydrogenated metabolites of cortisol (tetrahydrocortisol plus allotetrahydrocortisol) compared with cortisone (tetrahydrocortisone). The ratio of urinary free cortisol to cortisone is also increased[19]. Heterozygotes may occasionally show hypertension, normal serum K+, suppressed plasma renin and aldosterone, and moderately elevated urinary cortisol to cortisone metabolite ratio. A variant of AME, called AME type II, has similar clinical features but a milder urinary steroid profile[20].

Treatment

Treatment with oral dexamethasone suppresses cortisol secretion, resulting in reduced Na+ reabsorption and amelioration of hypertension and hypokalemia. Urinary concentration of metabolites of cortisol and cortisone are only moderately affected. As in Liddle's syndrome, patients respond to treatment with K+ supplements combined with spironolactone,

triamterene or amiloride. Renal transplantation is followed by normalization of cortisol metabolism, biochemical abnormalities and hypertension[21].

Glucocorticoid-remediable aldosteronism

GRA is transmitted in an autosomal dominant fashion with complete penetrance. The most constant feature is hypertension, which may be moderate to severe; most patients have hypertension by the second decade of life. The risk of hemorrhagic stroke and ruptured intracranial aneurysms is high. Growth and sexual development are normal. Hypokalemia is characteristic, but serum K+ levels are occasionally normal.

Pathogenesis

Though cortisol and aldosterone both require 11β-hydroxylation of precursors, these steps are catalyzed by different isoenzymes: steroid 11β-hydroxylase (CYP11B1) and aldosterone synthase (CYP11B2), respectively (Fig. 49.8). The genes for

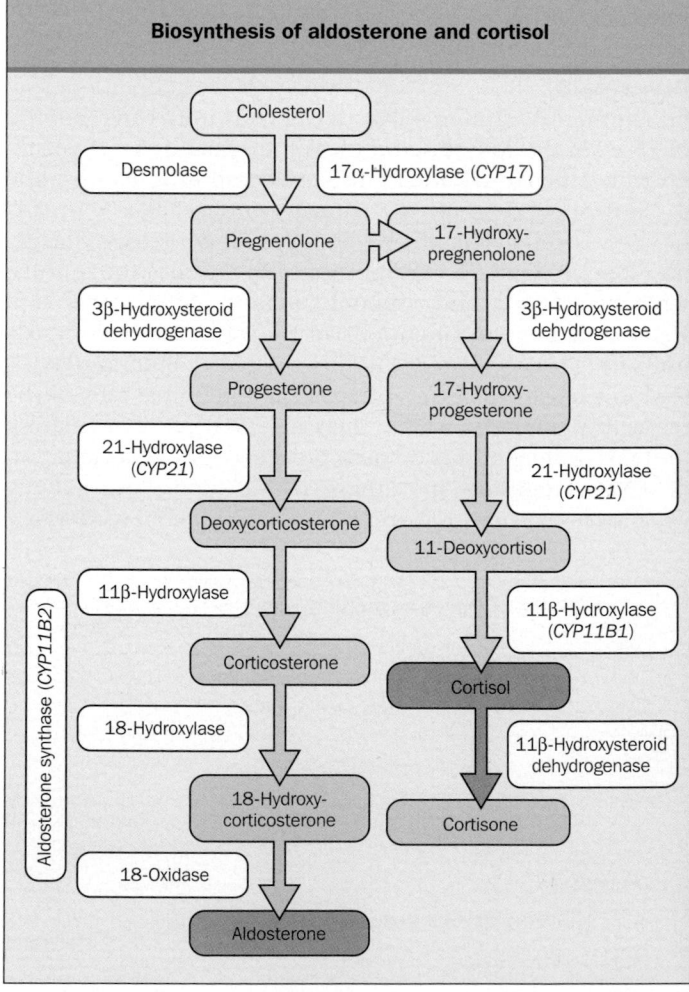

Figure 49.8 Biosynthesis of aldosterone and cortisol. Though cortisol and aldosterone both require 11β-hydroxylation of precursors, these steps are catalyzed by different isoenzymes: steroid 11β-hydroxylase (CYP11B1) and aldosterone synthase (CYP11B2), respectively. Aldosterone synthase also mediates two further conversions. Common enzyme deficiencies leading to derangement in salt and water balance are shown in boxes. Cortisol is converted peripherally by 11β-hydroxysteroid dehydrogenase to cortisone.

these isoenzymes are located close to each other on the long arm of chromosome 8. Unequal meiotic crossovers may produce hybrid genes by fusion of the promoter end of CYP11B1 with the coding sequence of CYP11B2[16]. CYP11B2 encoding aldosterone synthase will now be inappropriately regulated by adrenocorticotrophic hormone (ACTH) as is CYP11B1. Abnormal expression of this chimeric gene in the adrenal zona fasciculata has been shown by *in situ* hybridization.

Diagnosis
Overproduction and excretion of cortisol C-18 oxidation products is a unique feature of GRA.

The hybrid gene leads to increased synthesis and excess urinary secretion of aldosterone and hybrid sterols, 18-hydroxycortisol and 18-oxocortisol. The urinary ratios of 18-oxotetrahydrocortisol to tetrahydroaldosterone, and 18-hydroxycortisol to tetrahydroaldosterone are also increased.

Levels of plasma renin activity are reduced. Though the mean aldosterone levels are high, determination of serum aldosterone has poor sensitivity as a screening test. Hyperaldosteronism is increased by administration of ACTH and reduced by glucocorticoids. Dexamethasone leads to suppression of blood aldosterone levels. A level of aldosterone less than 4 ng/dL (110 pmol/L) after a dexamethasone suppression test is strongly suggestive of the diagnosis. Detection of the hybrid gene CYP11B1/CYP11B2 confirms the diagnosis[22].

Treatment
Treatment with low-dose dexamethasone is useful in reducing blood pressure and correcting electrolyte disturbances. Combination therapy with low doses of glucocorticoids and spironolactone or amiloride is occasionally necessary.

Incomplete phenotypes
Occasionally patients with Liddle's syndrome, AME or GRA either do not express the complete phenotype or may have mild clinical or biochemical features and are considered to have essential hypertension. Poor blood pressure control with conventional therapy should raise suspicion of an alternative diagnosis. Hypokalemia may not be present at the onset but develops after institution of diuretic treatment. These conditions should be considered in patients with early-onset hypertension, failure to thrive or an impressive family history. The response to specific treatment with potassium-sparing diuretics or glucocorticoids may suggest the diagnosis.

Adrenal enzymatic disorders
Inherited deficiency of 11β- or 17α-hydroxylase also causes mineralocorticoid excess with hypertension and hypokalemic metabolic alkalosis (see Fig. 49.8).

Deficiency of 17α-hydroxylase (CYP17) impairs normal production of cortisol and adrenal androgens, resulting in pseudohermaphroditism in genetic males and primary amenorrhea in females. Cortisol deficiency results in increased ACTH secretion and excessive production of deoxycorticosterone and corticosterone, low levels of renin and aldosterone, hypokalemia, metabolic alkalosis, and hypertension. Glucocorticoid replacement corrects the mineralocorticoid excess state.

Deficiency of 11β-hydroxylase (CYP11B1) also impairs cortisol production but results in excessive androgens. Genetic females show pseudohermaphroditism, while males have virilization. The cortisol deficiency results in high blood levels of ACTH, deoxycortisol and deoxycorticosterone; corticosterone levels are normal. Urine shows high levels of tetrahydro-11-deoxycortisol. Hypokalemia is variable. Treatment with glucocorticoids corrects hypertension and hypokalemia; renin levels increase but aldosterone remains low because of the biosynthetic defect.

CONDITIONS WITH HYPONATREMIA, HYPERKALEMIA, METABOLIC ACIDOSIS, AND NORMAL BLOOD PRESSURE

Conditions with hyponatremia, hyperkalemia, metabolic acidosis and normal blood pressure have features of mineralocorticoid deficiency, either because of a synthetic defect or because of end-organ resistance.

Pseudohypoaldosteronism
PHA is a state of renal tubular (and other tissue) unresponsiveness to the action of aldosterone[23]. PHA type 1 includes at least two major entities, with either renal or multiple target-organ defects; the former is more common. Differences between the two major types are shown in Table 49.4.

Renal PHA type I
The inheritance of renal PHA type 1 is autosomal dominant but may be sporadic. No mutations of genes for ENaC have been reported. Since aldosterone, acting through the MR, regulates ENaC activity in the kidney, the receptor gene has been screened for variants. Loss of function mutations of the gene for MR (located on 4p) have been identified[24].

Differential features of renal-limited and multisystem forms of pseudohypoaldosteronism type 1		
Feature	Renal-limited form	Multisystem form
Underlying defect	Mineralocorticoid receptor	Epithelial sodium channel
Affected organs	Kidney	Kidney, sweat, salivary glands, distal colon
Inheritance	Autosomal dominant	Autosomal recessive
Salt wasting	Variable	Severe
Blood renin, aldosterone	Very high	Very high
Sweat, salivary Na+	Normal	High
Need for Na+ supplements	1–3 years	Lifelong?
Improvement with age	Usually by 6–8 years	Rare
Response to carbenoloxone	Satisfactory	None

Table 49.4 Differential features of renal-limited and multisystem forms of pseudohypoaldosteronism type 1.

PHA type 1 is a salt-wasting syndrome often manifesting in the first few weeks of life with failure to thrive, hyponatremia, dehydration and hyperkalemic metabolic acidosis. Plasma renin and aldosterone levels are elevated. Urine Na^+ excretion is inappropriately high and K^+ excretion is low. Aldosterone metabolites are increased in the urine without evidence of biosynthetic block; the ratio of 18-hydroxytetrahydroaldosterone to tetrahydroaldosterone is normal.

Treatment with Na^+ supplements is followed by clinical and biochemical improvement. There is no response to treatment with mineralocorticoids. Therapy with carbenoxolone, which inhibits cortisol 11β-hydroxysteroid dehydrogenase and creates a situation akin to AME, is effective in some patients. With increasing age, the need for supplements diminishes because of compensatory increase of proximal tubular transport, development of salt appetite, and improved tubular response to mineralocorticoids. During stress (e.g., infections or diarrhea), patients may destabilize and show clinical and biochemical features characteristic of the disease.

Multiple end-organ PHA type I

Multiple end-organ PHA type 1 is a severe autosomal recessive disorder with multiple target-organ resistance to the action of mineralocorticoids and is associated with inactivating mutations of α-, β-, or γ-subunits of ENaC[25]. These effects of genetic inactivation of the Na^+ channel closely resemble the pharmacologic actions of the potassium-sparing diuretics, amiloride and triamterene on the distal tubule[13].

Clinical features

Symptoms start in early infancy with marked salt wasting and often life-threatening hyperkalemia. The external genitalia are normal. Markedly elevated levels of Na^+ are found in urine, sweat, saliva and feces. Excess Na^+ in the sweat and bronchial secretions encourages infections in the skin and lower respiratory tract. The urine 17-ketosteroids are normal.

Differential diagnosis

Hyponatremia, hyperkalemia, severe hypovolemia and elevated plasma-renin activity may also be found in subjects with defects in aldosterone synthesis: aldosterone synthase deficiency, salt-wasting forms of congenital adrenal hyperplasia, and adrenal hypoplasia. Clinical and biochemical features often help to distinguish these conditions from PHA. Patients with aldosterone synthase deficiency characteristically show elevated urinary excretion of 18-hydroxycorticosterone metabolites. Those with salt-losing forms of congenital adrenal hyperplasia and adrenal hypoplasia have additional clinical and biochemical features that may aid in diagnosis (see below). Estimation of renin and aldosterone profiles is also useful in differentiating patients with PHA from those with defects of aldosterone biosynthesis (Fig. 49.9).

Treatment

Sodium chloride supplements, initially in vast quantities, are required lifelong. Dietary K^+ restriction and ion-exchange resins are necessary in many patients; infants may require dialysis during episodes of life-threatening hyperkalemia. Prophylactic antibiotics are used to prevent skin sepsis.

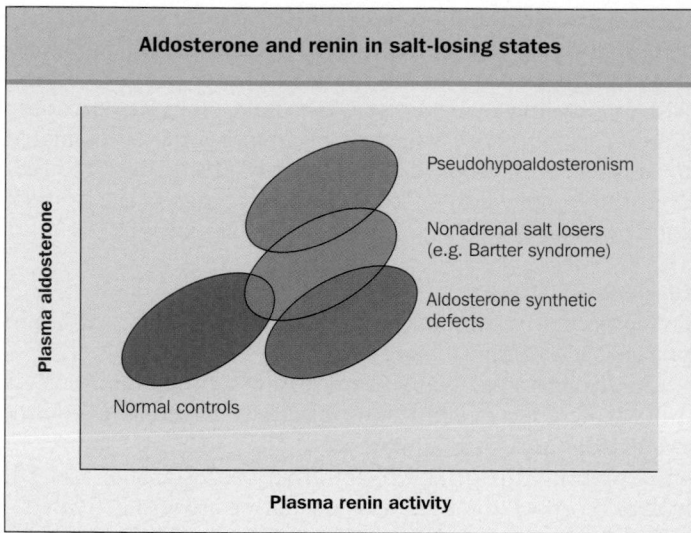

Figure 49.9 Aldosterone and renin in salt-losing states. Logarithmic plot of plasma aldosterone (PA) and renin activity (PRA) in patients with salt-losing states. Patients with pseudohypoaldosteronism (PHA) show high PA and PRA; those with defects in aldosterone synthesis have high PRA but inappropriately low PA. Intermediate levels of PA with similarly increased PRA values are found in subjects with salt-wasting disease but a normal renin–aldosterone axis, such as those with Bartter syndrome. These patients have hypokalemia, separating them from those with PHA or aldosterone biosynthetic defects, who manifest hyperkalemia.

Therapy with carbenoxolone, indomethacin (which reduces salt loss but worsens hyperkalemia) or carbonic anhydrase inhibitors (which temporarily reduce serum K^+ but increase acidosis) is not helpful.

Aldosterone biosynthetic defects

Patients with defects in aldosterone biosynthesis show salt wasting with hyponatremia, hyperkalemia, hypovolemia, and elevated plasma renin activity.

The enzymes cholesterol desmolase, 3β-hydroxysteroid dehydrogenase and 21-hydroxylase are required for synthesis of cholesterol and aldosterone in the adrenal cortex (see Fig. 49.8). Deficiency of any of these enzymes results in lack of both aldosterone and cortisol. Reduced levels of cortisol result in loss of feedback inhibition of ACTH, hence congenital adrenal hyperplasia. Deficiencies of the enzymes cholesterol desmolase and 3β-hydroxysteroid dehydrogenase are rare. Deficiency of 21-hydroxylase is the most common inherited cause of aldosterone deficiency.

Aldosterone synthase deficiency, however, results in selective deficiency of aldosterone without compromising glucocorticoid production. There is, therefore, normal negative feedback inhibition by cortisol and no adrenal hyperplasia.

Deficiency of 21-hydroxylase

Mutations in the gene encoding 21-hydroxylase (CYP21) result in two major forms of the disease: a virilizing form and the more common salt-wasting type.[26] Patients with signs only of androgen excess are said to have the virilizing form. Female infants show varying degrees of pseudohermaphroditism, whereas affected males have normal or precocious sexual development. The salt-wasting type presents with hyponatremia, hyperkalemia and moderate to severe volume depletion.

The diagnosis of 21-hydroxylase deficiency should be suspected in any newborn with genital ambiguity, salt wasting or hypotension. Blood levels of progesterone, 17-hydroxyprogesterone and dehydroepiandrosterone are raised several fold above normal. Increased quantities of pregnanetriol (chief urinary metabolite of 17-hydroxyprogesterone) and 17-ketosteroids (metabolites of adrenal androgens) are found in the urine. Blood levels of aldosterone are low or normal, but plasma renin activity is very high. Measurement of urine 17-ketosteroids, and plasma dehydroepiandrosterone and renin activity are useful for monitoring adequacy of treatment.

Patients with electrolyte imbalance and shock require resuscitation with intravenous fluids and salt supplements. Replacement therapy with oral hydrocortisone and 9α-fludrocortisone is required long term. Some amelioration of the tendency to salt wasting may be seen with age, because of the ability of children to regulate their dietary salt intake and maturation of proximal tubular function.

Reconstructive genital surgery may be required in females with genital ambiguity. Fetal DNA analysis and demonstration of elevated 17-hydroxyprogesterone in amniotic fluid allows prenatal detection of affected female infants. Treatment of the mother with dexamethasone from early in gestation reduces virilization of genitalia of the affected female fetus.

Aldosterone synthase deficiency

Three successive steps are required for conversion of deoxycorticosterone to aldosterone: 11β-hydroxylation, 18-hydroxylation, and 18-oxidation (see Fig. 49.8). The enzyme aldosterone synthase (CYP11B2) mediates all these steps. A genetic defect in the CYP11B2, therefore, impairs production of mineralocorticoids without affecting cortisol synthesis.

Children with aldosterone synthase deficiency show failure to thrive, intermittent episodes of fever and dehydration, vomiting, and poor feeding. Salt supplements and 9α-fludrocortisone are required, sometimes in high doses initially. A positive salt balance is necessary for normal growth.

CONDITIONS WITH HYPERKALEMIA, METABOLIC ACIDOSIS, AND HYPERTENSION

Gordon's syndrome (chloride shunt syndrome)

Gordon's syndrome is an autosomal dominant disorder of hypertension, hyperkalemia and hyperchloremia with normal GFR[27]. The condition has also been referred to as PHA type 2, perhaps inappropriately, since it is very different in its mechanisms to other forms of PHA.

Pathogenesis

The pathogenesis of the syndrome is unknown, though increased tubular absorption of Cl⁻ is proposed. Recent studies in kindreds of Gordon's syndrome show linkage to chromosomes 1q, 12p and 17q. Gain-of-function mutations encoding two novel kinases, WNK1 and WNK4, which localize to the distal convoluted tubule and cortical collecting ducts, have been identified[28]. Increased expression of these

kinases may promote salt reabsorption and dissipate the electrical gradient normally produced by Na⁺ reabsorption, which provides the driving force for normal K⁺ and H⁺ secretion. Linkage to chromosome 17q is also described in patients with 'familial' essential hypertension, suggesting some pathophysiologic relationship of Gordon's syndrome to essential hypertension.

Clinical manifestations and diagnosis

Hyperkalemia may be present from birth but, as in GRA, hypertension may not present until later in life. Patients show hyperchloremic metabolic acidosis with a normal GFR; plasma renin and aldosterone are reduced to variable degrees. Inconstant features include short stature, intellectual impairment, muscle weakness, hypercalciuria and renal stones. Occasionally, the phenotype may be mild and the patients remain undiagnosed.

Treatment

Treatment with hydrochlorthiazide or furosemide (frusemide) results in complete reversal of clinical and biochemical abnormalities. Sodium bicarbonate may be required to correct acidosis.

NEPHROGENIC DIABETES INSIPIDUS

Diabetes insipidus (DI) can occur as a result of several mechanisms. Congenital nephrogenic DI (NDI) is a rare polyuric disorder identified by the failure to concentrate urine despite normal or elevated levels of vasopressin. GFR and solute excretion rate are normal.

Pathogenesis

More than 90% of patients have X-linked recessive NDI mutations in the AVPR2, the gene at Xq28 coding for the vasopressin receptor (AVPR). These mutations usually result in intracellular trapping of the receptor, which cannot reach the plasma membrane. Occasionally, the receptor may be expressed on the cell surface but is unable to bind vasopressin or to trigger an appropriate cAMP response[29]. In less than 10% of the families, congenital NDI has an autosomal recessive inheritance and mutations have been identified in AQP2, the gene for aquaporin, located on chromosome 12q13. These mutations lead to misrouting of AQP2 mutant proteins. An autosomal dominant form of NDI, also caused by mutation in AQP2, has been reported[30]. Reduced expression of AQP2 may result in acquired NDI secondary to lithium or demeclocycline therapy, hypokalemia, ureteral obstruction and chronic renal failure.

Clinical features

Manifestations of congenital NDI appear within the first weeks of life. Males with AVPR2 mutations show marked polyuria and excessive thirst; these features are often not recognized in early infancy. Unless the condition is suspected early, children have recurrent episodes of severe hypernatremic dehydration, occasionally complicated by convulsions[31]. Delayed development and mental retardation are possible consequences of these episodes. Cranial computed tomography scans may, occasionally, show dystrophic calcification in the basal ganglia and the cerebral cortex.

A reduced intake of calories because of the large quantities of water that are drunk leads to growth failure beginning in early childhood. Increased urine volumes may result in dilatation of the lower urinary tract. Renal cortical damage, because of recurrent episodes of severe dehydration, may result in impairment of renal function. Heterozygous females may show variable degrees of polyuria and polydipsia.

The onset and severity of clinical features of autosomal recessive NDI are similar to those of the X-linked form.

Diagnosis

Episodes of dehydration are marked by hypernatremia, hyperchloremia, and, occasionally, elevated levels of urea and creatinine. Polyuria with low urine osmolality (< 200 mmol/kg) and hypernatremia plasma Na^+ > 150 mmol/L, plasma osmolality > 300 mmol/kg is highly suggestive of either vasopressin deficiency (central DI) or resistance to its action (NDI). Central DI is more common than NDI. Primary polydipsia resembles true DI in that compulsive water drinking results in polyuria with low urine osmolality; however, the plasma osmolality in primary polydipsia is normal or borderline low.

To confirm the lack of renal concentrating ability and distinguish NDI from central DI and primary polydipsia, a vasopressin test is performed. Desamino-8-D-arginine vasopressin (DDAVP) is administered nasally (5–10 μg in neonates and infants, 20 μg in children) or by an intramuscular injection (0.4–1.0 μg in infants and young children, 2 μg in older children). Hourly urine collection is done over the next 6 h. Following administration of DDAVP, patients with NDI fail to show a rise of urine osmolality, which remains below 200–300 mmol/kg (normal > 800 mmol/kg). Those with central DI and primary polydipsia concentrate urine appropriately.

Persistence of polyuria for years may result in a washout of the medullary counter-current concentration mechanism. Several days of treatment with DDAVP may be required to elicit an appropriate response in these patients. Where the diagnosis of primary polydipsia is strongly suspected, supervised reduction of fluid intake over several days may restore normal sensitivity to DDAVP.

Differential diagnosis

Patients with central DI show hypernatremia with inappropriately dilute urine, no primary renal disease and a rise in urine osmolality on administration of vasopressin or its analogs. Central DI usually results from posterior pituitary neuronal damage, which may be secondary to tumors (craniopharyngioma, optic glioma, metastasis), Langhans' cell histiocytosis, trauma (e.g., fracture of base of skull), or infections (meningitis, encephalitis). Deficiency of vasopressin may also be familial, with an autosomal dominant inheritance. Mutations of AVP-NP II, the gene for vasopressin–neurophysin II, located on chromosome 20p, have been reported[32]. The onset of vasopressin deficiency, in the familial form, is usually delayed and may not be apparent until after the first few years of life. Central DI may also occur with the syndrome of DI, diabetes mellitus, optic atrophy and deafness (DIDMOAD, or Wolfram syndrome), which is autosomal recessive. A Wolfram gene has recently been mapped to chromosome 4p16.1, but there is evidence for locus heterogeneity.

Many patients with central or nephrogenic DI have a partial defect in vasopressin secretion or action. They are, therefore, able to concentrate urine to varying degrees following DDAVP administration, making precise diagnosis difficult. Measurement of levels of plasma vasopressin in relation to plasma osmolality following an osmotic stimulus, such as fluid restriction, allows differentiatin in these patients. Patients with severe or partial central DI always show subnormal vasopressin levels relative to plasma osmolality. In contrast, the values from patients with NDI or psychogenic polydipsia are always within or above the normal range.

Magnetic resonance imaging of the brain produces a 'bright spot' on T1-weighted images of the posterior pituitary in normal individuals and also those with NDI or primary polydipsia. This signal is absent in most patients with central DI.

The differential response of clotting factors and urine osmolality to DDAVP is useful in differentiating X-linked (AVPR2 abnormalities) from autosomal recessive (AQP2 mutations) NDI. Patients with AQP2 abnormalities show normal increases in factor VIII and von Willebrand factor after DDAVP infusion; this response is absent in those with an AVPR2 defect.[31] Sequencing of AVPR2 and AQP2 is useful in identification of the molecular defect underlying NDI.

Congenital NDI should also be differentiated from secondary forms of NDI (see Table 8.11).

Treatment

Appropriate management of patients with NDI prevents episodes of dehydration, allowing normal physical growth and development. Patients must have adequate water intake to prevent dehydration. The renal solute load is minimized by restriction of dietary protein and Na^+ (20–25 mg/kg (≈1 mmol/kg) per day). Adequate energy and nutrients, depending on the age, should be provided to promote normal growth and development.

Thiazide diuretics, such as hydrochlorothiazide (1–2 mg/kg, q.12 h), when combined with reduction of salt intake are effective in reducing urine output. Thiazides may result in electrolyte disturbances, chiefly hypokalemia; supplemental K^+ may be needed. Prostaglandin synthase inhibitors also reduce urine volume and free water clearance in children with NDI. The agent most commonly used, indomethacin (1 mg/kg, q.12 h), is effective especially when combined with hydrochlorothiazide. Indomethacin may, however, reduce GFR and cause gastrointestinal side effects. Combination of the potassium-sparing diuretic amiloride (0.1–0.2 mg/kg, q.8–12 h) with hydrochlorothiazide is also effective in reducing urine volume and increasing osmolality.

REFERENCES

1. Bartter FC, Pronove P, Gill J, MacCardle R. Hyperplasia of the juxtaglomerular complex with hyperaldosteronism and hypokalemic alkalosis. Am J Med. 1962;33:811–28.
2. Gitelman HJ, Graham JB, Welt LG. A new familial disorder characterized by hypokalemia and hypomagnesemia. Trans Assoc Am Physic. 1966;79:221–35.
3. Shaer AJ. Inherited primary renal tubular hypokalemic alkalosis: a review of Gitelman and Bartter syndromes. Am J Med Sci. 2001;322:316–32.
4. Simon DB, Karet FE, Hamblan JM, et al. Bartter syndrome, hypokalemic alkalosis with hypercalciuria, is caused by mutations in the Na$^+$-K$^+$-2Cl$^-$ co-transporter NKCC2. Nat Genet. 1996;13:183–8.
5. International Collaborative Study Group for Bartter-like Syndromes. Mutations in the gene encoding the inwardly-rectifying renal potassium channel, ROMK, cause the antenatal variant of Bartter syndrome: evidence for genetic heterogeneity. Hum Mol Genet. 1997;6:17–26.
6. Birkenhager R, Otto E, Schurmann MJ, et al. Mutations of BSND causes Bartter syndrome with sensorineural deafness and kidney failure. Nat Genet. 2001;29:310–14.
7. Peters M, Jeck N, Reinalter S, et al. Clinical presentation of genetically defined patients with hypokalemic salt-losing tubulopathies. Am J Med. 2002;112:183–90.
8. Uchiyama M, Shah V, Daman-Willems C, Dillon MJ. Erythrocyte sodium transport in Bartter's syndrome. Acta Paediatr Scand. 1988;77:873–8.
9. Dillon MJ, Shah V, Mitchell MD. Bartter syndrome: 10 cases in childhood. Results of long term indomethacin therapy. Q J Med. 1979;48:429–46.
10. Simon DB, Nelson-Williams C, Bia MJ, et al. Gitelman variant of Bartter syndrome, inherited hypokalemic alkalosis, is caused by mutations in the thiazide-sensitive Na$^+$-Cl$^-$ co-transporter. Nat Genet. 1996;12:24–30.
11. Liddle GW, Bledsoe T, Coppage WS. A familial renal disorder simulating primary aldosteronism but with negligible aldosterone secretion. Trans Assoc Am Physic. 1963;76:199–213.
12. Palmer BF, Alpern RJ. Liddle's syndrome. Am J Med. 1998;104:310–19.
13. Rossier BC, Pradervand S, Schild L, Hummler E. Epithelial sodium channel and the control of sodium balance: Interaction between genetic and environmental factors. Annu Rev Physiol. 2002;64:877–97.
14. Botero-Velez M, Curtis JJ, Warnock DG. Liddle's syndrome revisited – a disorder of sodium reabsorption in the distal tubule. N Engl J Med. 1994;330:178–81.
15. Geller DS, Farhi A, Pinkerton N, et al. Activating mineralocorticoid receptor mutation in hypertension exacerbated by pregnancy. Science. 2000;289:119–23.
16. White PC. Abnormalities of aldosterone synthesis and action in children. Curr Opin Pediatr. 1997;9:424–30.
17. Stewart PM, Krozowski Z, Gupta A, et al. Hypertension in the syndrome of apparent mineralocorticoid excess due to mutations of the 11β-hydroxysteroid dehydrogenase type 2 gene. Lancet. 1996;347:88–91.
18. White PC. 11beta-hydroxysteroid dehydrogenase and its role in the syndrome of apparent mineralocorticoid excess. Am J Med Sci. 2001;322:308–15.
19. Palermo M, Delitala G, Mantero F, et al. Congenital deficiency of 11beta-hydroxysteroid dehydrogenase (apparent mineralocorticoid excess syndrome): diagnostic value of urinary free cortisol and cortisone. J Endocrinol Invest. 2001; 24:17–23.
20. Li A, Tedde R, Krozowski ZS, et al. Molecular basis for hypertension in the "type II variant" of apparent mineralocorticoid excess. Am J Hum Genet. 1998;63:370–9.
21. Palermo M, Delitala G, Sorba G, et al. Does kidney transplantation normalise cortisol metabolism in apparent mineralocorticoid excess syndrome? J Endocrinol Invest. 2000;23:457–62.
22. Yokota K, Ogura T, Kishida M, et al. Japanese family with glucocorticoid-remediable aldosteronism diagnosed by long-polymerase chain reaction. Hypertens Res. 2001;24:589–94.
23. Dillon MJ, Leonard JV, Buckler JM, et al. Pseudohypoaldosteronism. Arch Dis Child. 1980;55:427–34.
24. Geller DS, Rodriaguez Soriano J, Boado AV, et al. Mutations in the mineralocorticoid receptor gene causes autosomal dominant pseudohypoaldosteronism type 1. Nat Genet. 1998;19:279–81.
25. Chang SS, Grunder S, Hanukoglu A, et al. Mutations in subunits of the epithelial sodium channel cause salt wasting with hyperkalemic acidosis, pseudohypoaldosteronism type 1. Nat Genet. 1996;12:248–53.
26. Speiser PW. Congenital adrenal hyperplasia owing to 21-hydroxylase deficiency. Endocrinol Metab Clin North Am. 2001;30:31–59.
27. Gordon RD. The syndrome of hypertension and hyperkalemia with normal GFR. A unique pathophysiological mechanism for hypertension? Clin Exp Pharmacol Physiol. 1986;13:329–33.
28. Wilson FH, Disse-Nicodeme S, Choate KA, et al. Human hypertension caused by mutations in WNK kinases. Science. 2001;293:1107–12.
29. Knoers NV, Deen PM. Molecular and cellular defects in nephrogenic diabetes insipidus. Pediatr Nephrol. 2001;16:1146–52.
30. Mulders SM, Bichet DG, Rijss JP, et al. An aquaporin-2 water channel mutant, which causes autosomal dominant nephrogenic diabetes insipidus, is retained in the Golgi complex. J Clin Invest. 1998;102:57–66.
31. Bichet DG, Oksche A, Rosenthal W. Congenital nephrogenic diabetes insipidus. J Am Soc Nephrol. 1997;8:1951–8.
32. Heppner C, Kotzka J, Bullmann C, et al. Identification of mutations of the arginine vasopressin-neurophysin II gene in two kindreds with familial central diabetes insipidus. J Clin Endocrinol Metab. 1998;83:693–6.

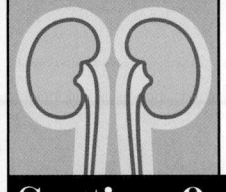

Chapter 50

Fanconi's Syndrome and Other Proximal Tubule Disorders

John W Foreman

INTRODUCTION

The proximal tubule is responsible for the reabsorption of the bulk of a number of solutes, including glucose, amino acids, bicarbonate, and phosphate. A number of disorders, mainly heritable, that affect proximal tubule reabsorption are described in this chapter, but renal tubular acidosis and familial forms of hyperphosphaturia are discussed in Chapters 11 and 10, respectively.

Most nonelectrolyte solutes are reabsorbed in the proximal tubule via specific transport proteins that cotransport them in conjunction with sodium (Fig. 50.1). The driving force for this solute transport is the electrochemical gradient for sodium entry maintained by the enzyme, Na^+/K^+ ATPase. Most disorders of isolated solute reabsorption are related to defects in specific transport proteins, while disorders affecting multiple solutes, such as Fanconi's syndrome, are probably secondary to defects in energy generation, Na^+/K^+ ATPase activity, or dysfunction of cellular organelles involved with membrane protein recycling.

FAMILIAL GLUCOSE-GALACTOSE MALABSORPTION AND HEREDITARY RENAL GLUCOSURIA

Definition

Renal glucosuria refers to the appearance of readily detectable glucose in the urine when the plasma glucose is in a normal range. When the plasma glucose is in a physiologic range, virtually all the filtered glucose is reabsorbed in the proximal tubule. Filtered glucose enters the proximal tubule via two specific carriers (SGLT1 and SGLT2) coupled to sodium and exits the cell via another sugar transporter, GLUT2 (Fig. 50.2). However, when the plasma level exceeds the physiologic range, the filtered load exceeds the capacity of these carriers and glucose begins to appear in the urine; this is termed the renal threshold.

Etiology and pathogenesis

Familial glucose-galactose malabsorption is a rare autosomal disorder that is due to mutations in the gene coding for the brush border sodium-glucose cotransporter, SGLT1 that is found in the intestinal cell and the S3 segment of the proximal renal tubule cell. The disorder is characterized by the neonatal onset of life-threatening diarrhea from the intestinal malabsorption of glucose and galactose that resolves rapidly with the removal of the offending sugars and their dipeptide,

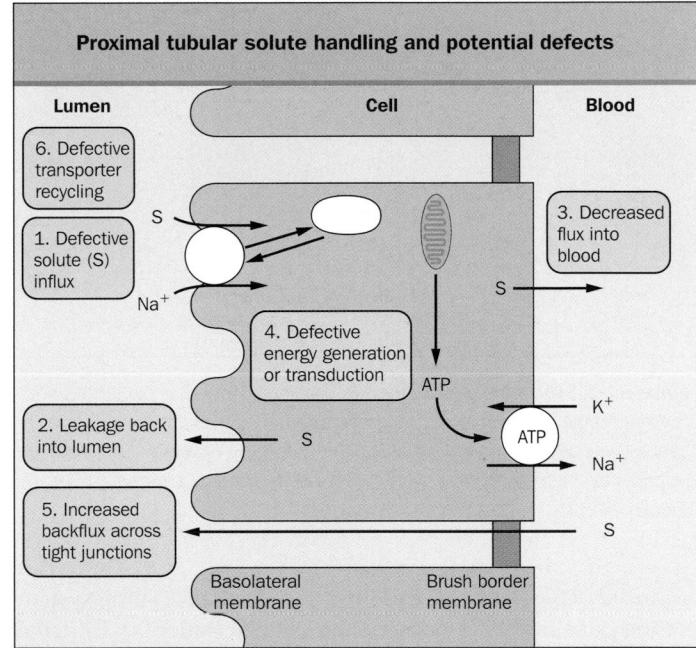

Figure 50.1 Defects and potential defects in proximal tubular solute handling. Solute uptake by the brush border membrane from the lumen is coupled to Na^+ influx. The favorable electrochemical driving force for luminal Na^+ is maintained by the Na^+/K^+ ATPase pump. Transported solute is then either used by the cell or returned to the blood across the basolateral membrane. Fanconi's syndrome could arise because of a defect in one of six areas, shown.

lactose, from the diet. These patients frequently also have a mild renal glucosuria.

Hereditary renal glucosuria occurs with an incidence of 1/20000 and appears to be inherited as an autosomal recessive trait. Putatively this disorder is due to a mutation in SGLT2 glucose transporter found in the early portion of the proximal tubule. To date no mutation has been identified. Renal glucosuria has been divided into three types based on the reabsorption patterns observed during glucose infusion studies (Fig. 50.3), although this separation has been called into question[1]. In type A, there is lowering of both the threshold and the maximal rate of tubular reabsorption of glucose. In type B, the maximal rate of glucose reabsorption is normal, but the threshold is low and there is exaggerated splay in the tubular reabsorption versus filtered load curve. In type 0, described by Brodehl et al., there is virtually no reabsorption of filtered glucose, with the clearance of glucose nearly the same as that

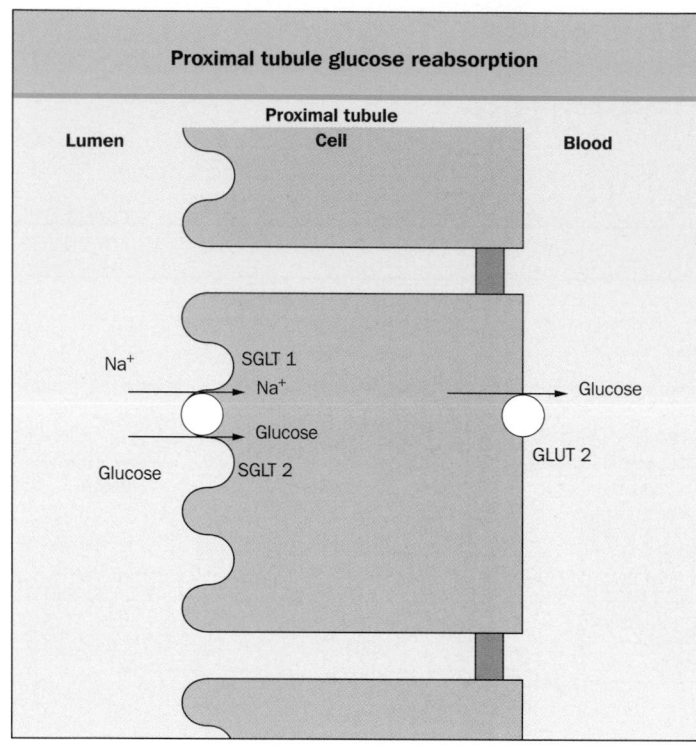

Figure 50.2 Proximal tubule glucose reabsorption. Glucose enters the proximal tubule cell coupled to Na^+ reabsorption from the lumen via a high capacity, low affinity transporter (SGLT2) in the early proximal tubule and a low capacity, high affinity transporter (SGLT1) in the late proximal tubule. Glucose exits the cell via the transporter GLUT2.

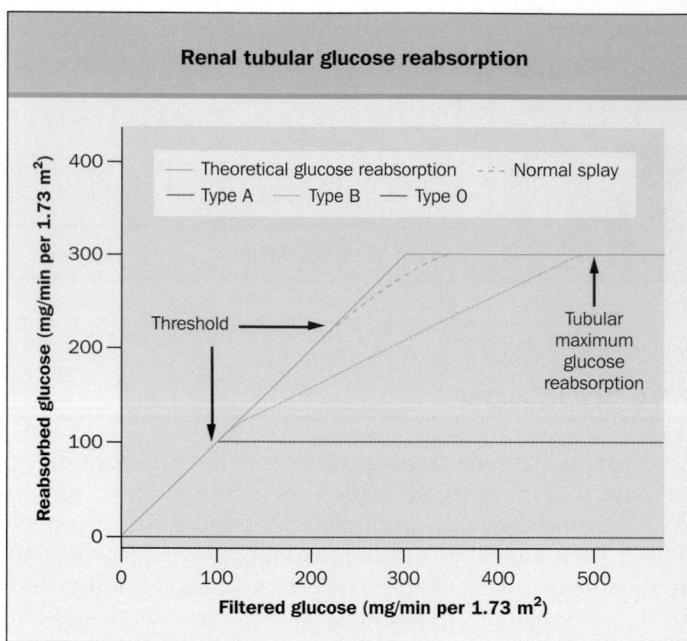

Figure 50.3 Renal glucose titration curves. The observed normal reabsorption curve follows the theoretical renal tubular glucose reabsorption until near the maximal reabsorption rate (T_mG) when the observed rate deviates from the theoretical rate (splay). The point of deviation is the threshold. Stylized titration curves for types A, B, and 0 renal glucosuria are shown. (Adapted with permission from Brodehl et al.[1].)

Inherited aminoacidurias		
Disease	**Clinical findings**	**Urine amino acids**
Cystinuria	Urolithiasis	Cystine, lysine, ornithine, arginine
Hartnup disease	Rash, neurologic disease	Neutral amino acids
Iminoglycinuria	None	Proline, hydroxyproline glycine
Lysinuric protein intolerance	Hyperammonemia, vomiting, diarrhea	Dibasic amino acids

Table 50.1 Inherited aminoacidurias.

of inulin[1]. These authors call into question this typing system as their data and that of others suggest that patients with renal glucosuria have rates of glucose reabsorption that vary from virtually no reabsorption to nearly normal rates, rather than three distinct types.

Natural history
Patients with familial glucose-galactose malabsorption appear to grow and develop normally with removal of the offending sugars from the diet. The clinical course of hereditary renal glucosuria is benign and is not a precursor to diabetes mellitus.

AMINOACIDURIAS

Like glucose, amino acids are nearly completely reabsorbed in the proximal tubule by a series of specific carriers. A number of heritable disorders resulting in the incomplete reabsorption of a specific amino acid or a group of amino acids have been described (Table 50.1)[2].

Cystinuria
Definition
Cystinuria is characterized by the excessive secretion of cystine and the dibasic amino acids ornithine, lysine and arginine[3].

Etiology and pathogenesis
These four amino acids share a transport system on the brush border membrane of the proximal tubule. Because of

cystine's relative insolubility when its urine concentration exceeds 250 mg/L (1.0 mmol/L), patients with cystinuria have recurrent renal calculi.

Cystinuria is an autosomal recessive trait with a disease incidence of 1/20000[4]. There appear to be three genetic types, based on *in vitro* studies of intestinal transport and amino acid excretion in the heterozygote. This has little clinical relevance except that type II and III heterozygotes have increased urinary cystine and dibasic amino acid excretion but not to a stone-forming range. The most common form is type I, and the defect is in the gene, SLC3A1, carried on the short arm of chromosome 2. Type III is much less common, and at least one more gene involved in cystine transport, SLC7A9 carried on the long arm of chromosome 19, has been identified. It is

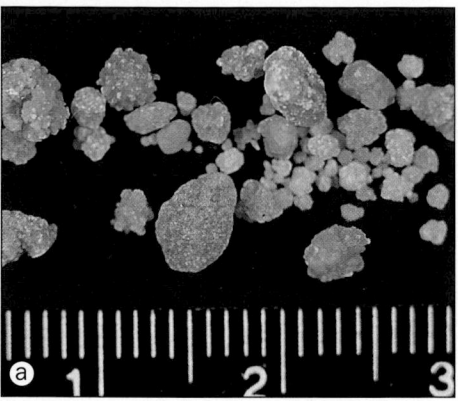 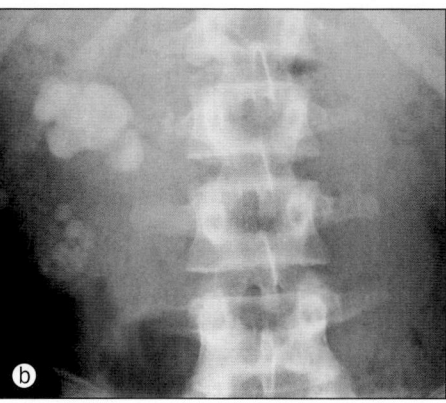 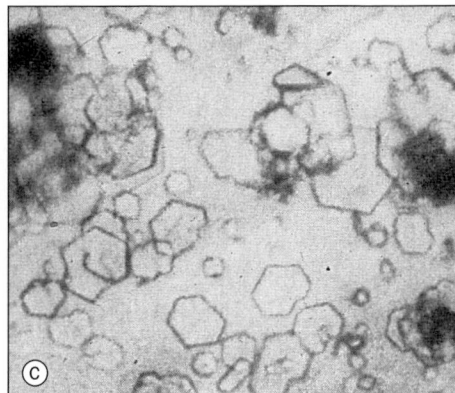

Figure 50.4 Cystinuria. (a) Both rough and smooth cystine calculi. (b) Plain radiograph of a cystine calculus in the right renal pelvis and further multiple parenchymal calculi. (c) Urine microscopy showing characteristic flat hexagonal crystals.

unclear whether Type II represents a third gene defect or is an extreme phenotype of Type III.

Clinical manifestations
Cystine stones are typically yellow-brown (Fig. 50.4a) and are radio-opaque (Fig. 50.4b). Cystine crystals appear as microscopic, flat hexagons in the urine (Fig. 50.4c) and this is a clue to the diagnosis.

Diagnosis
Patients can be screened for cystinuria with the cyanide–nitroprusside test, but type II and III heterozygotes may also give a positive result. The definitive test is to quantify cystine and dibasic amino acid excretion in a 24-h urine specimen. Homozygotes excrete more than 118 mmol cystine/mmol creatinine (250 mg/g).

Treatment
The aim of therapy in cystinuria is to lower the urine cystine concentration to below 300 mg/L (1.25 mmol/L). The first step is to increase the fluid intake. However, because most patients with cystinuria excrete 0.5–1 g cystine/d, a urine output of 2–4 L/d is needed to achieve this goal. Cystine solubility increases in alkaline urine, but the urine pH must be above 7.5 to be effective. In patients with recurrent stone disease, thiols, such as penicillamine, are extremely useful through the formation of a more soluble mixed disulfide of the thiol and cysteine from cystine. The thiols also reduce the overall excretion of cystine through an unknown mechanism. Penicillamine should be started at 250 mg/d and gradually increased (max 2 g/d) over 3 months to achieve a urine cystine concentration below 300 mg/L in conjunction with a high fluid intake. Thiola is equally effective and is better tolerated than penicillamine; it should also be started at a low dose and slowly increased (maximum 2 g/d). Captopril can be useful (an effect resulting from its thiol structure not its angiotensin-converting enzyme (ACE) inhibitor effect) but the dose range (75–150 mg/d) may be limited by its hypotensive effects.

Hartnup disease
Hartnup disease is an autosomal recessive trait characterized by a neutral aminoaciduria that probably arises from a defect in a specific carrier for neutral amino acid transport present in both the intestine and the proximal renal tubule. Preliminary studies suggest that the gene responsible for Hartnup disease resides on the short arm of chromosome 5. From newborn screening programs, the genetic defect is more common than originally thought, as most individuals with the aminoaciduria never manifest any symptoms. Individuals who became symptomatic with Hartnup disease have pellagra-like clinical features including a photosensitive dermatitis, ataxia, and psychotic behavior. These symptoms appear to be secondary to niacin deficiency that is in part due to inadequate intestinal absorption of tryptophan, the precursor for niacin synthesis. However, most individuals who inherit the Hartnup transport defect are asymptomatic, so there must be other environmental or genetic factors that lead to disease. Nicotinamide supplementation leads to clearing of the skin disease and, on occasion, some of the neurologic problems. The renal loss of neutral amino acids appears to have little clinical importance.

Iminoglycinuria
Iminoglycinuria is a benign heritable defect in the reabsorption of proline, hydroxyproline, and glycine, suggesting a common carrier for these three amino acids.

Lysinuric protein intolerance
Lysinuric protein intolerance is associated with recurrent bouts of hyperammonemia after a protein load, resulting from the decreased renal and intestinal dibasic amino acid transport.

Other aminoacidurias
Rare individuals have been described with abnormalities in the excretion of other amino acids. These usually occur in association with mental retardation.

HEREDITARY DEFECTS IN URIC ACID HANDLING

Hereditary renal hypouricaemia

Hereditary renal hypouricemia is a rare autosomal recessive disorder characterized by very low serum uric acid levels (< 2.5 mg/dL (< 150 µmol/L) in adult males and < 2.1 mg/dL (< 125 µmol/L) in adult women) and increased uric acid clearance, ranging from 30–150% of the filtered load. In the normal kidney, uric acid is both reabsorbed and secreted in the proximal tubule by two different uric acid/anion exchange transporters and a voltage sensitive pathway. The defect in renal hypouricemia is unknown, but thought to be secondary to a defect in reabsorption that leads to increased uric acid excretion and hypouricemia. Most patients are asymptomatic and found incidentally when low serum uric acid is noted during routine serum chemistry evaluation. Approximately a quarter of patients with renal hypouricemia have had renal stones, but only a third of these were uric acid stones. A few patients have also had hypercalciuria in addition to the hyperuricosuria. Most patients require no treatment, but if they are having uric acid stones, they should maintain a high fluid intake. Urine alkalinization and allopurinol can be used for patients with persistent uric acid stones.

Familial juvenile hyperuricemic nephropathy

This rare hereditary condition, usually autosomal dominant, is characterized by hyperuricemia associated with a tubular defect in uric acid excretion[6]. These children develop progressive renal insufficiency with interstitial fibrosis and glomerulosclerosis. The hyperuricemia is due to renal underexcretion of uric acid rather than over production. Medication aimed at lowering serum uric acid levels has been unsuccessful at preventing the progression of renal failure. Isosthenuria and hypertension are common. The pathogenesis of this disorder is unknown, but may be related to a defect in renal blood flow or a mutation in the proximal tubule anion exchanger. The gene has been linked to chromosome 16p 12 in one family[7].

FANCONI'S SYNDROME

Introduction and definition

In the 1930s, de Toni, Debre, and coworkers and Fanconi independently described several children with the combination of renal rickets, glucosuria, and hypophosphatemia. This clinical entity is now called Fanconi's syndrome and refers to a global dysfunction of the proximal tubule leading to excessive urinary excretion of amino acids, glucose, phosphate, bicarbonate, and other solutes handled by this nephron segment. These losses lead to the clinical problems of acidosis, dehydration, electrolyte imbalance, rickets, osteomalacia, and growth failure. Numerous disorders, ranging from inborn errors of metabolism to exogenous toxins, are associated with Fanconi's syndrome (Table 50.2).

Etiology and pathogenesis

The sequence of events leading to Fanconi's syndrome is incompletely defined and probably varies with each cause. Possible mechanisms include widespread abnormality of most

Causes of Fanconi's syndrome
Inherited causes
Cystinosis
Hereditary fructose intolerance
Tyrosinemia
Wilson's disease
Lowe's syndrome
Glycogenosis
Mitochondrial cytopathies
Idiopathic
Acquired causes
Heavy metal poisoning: lead, cadmium
Drugs: *cisplatin*, *Ifosfamide*, *gentamicin*, azathioprine, valproic acid (sodium valproate), suramin, streptozocin (streptozotocin), ranitidine
Other poisonings: glue sniffing, diachrome, Chinese medicine
Dysproteinemias: multiple myeloma, Sjögren's syndrome, light-chain proteinuria, amyloidosis
Other: Neprotic syndrome, renal transplantation, mesenchymal tumors

Table 50.2 Causes of Fanconi's syndrome. Commoner causes are shown in *italics*.

or all the proximal tubule carriers, for example a defect in sodium binding to the carrier or insertion of the carrier into the brush border membrane; 'leaky' brush border membrane or tight junctions; inhibited or abnormal Na^+/K^+ ATPase pump; or impaired mitochondrial energy generation (see Fig. 50.1). An abnormality in energy generation has been implicated in a number of disorders, including hereditary fructose intolerance, galactosemia, mitochondrial cytopathies, and heavy metal poisoning, as well as in a number of experimental models of Fanconi's syndrome. Abnormal subcellular organelle function, such as the lysosome in cystinosis or the megalin-endocytic pathway in Dent's disease (Fig. 50.5) is also a cause of Fanconi's syndrome.

Fanconi's syndrome can be inherited or acquired (see Table 50.2). In adults, the most common causes of persistent Fanconi's syndrome are an endogenous or exogenous toxin, such as a heavy metal or a dysproteinemia; in children, the most common persistent cause is an inborn error of metabolism, such as cystinosis. Specific causes of Fanconi's syndrome are discussed after a general description of the clinical manifestations and treatment of the syndrome.

Clinical manifestations of Fanconi's syndrome

Fanconi's syndrome gives rise to a number of abnormalities (Table 50.3).

Aminoaciduria

Aminoaciduria is a cardinal feature of Fanconi's syndrome. Virtually every amino acid is found in excess in the urine, hence the term 'generalized aminoaciduria'. There are however no clinical consequences because the losses are trivial in relation to the dietary intake.

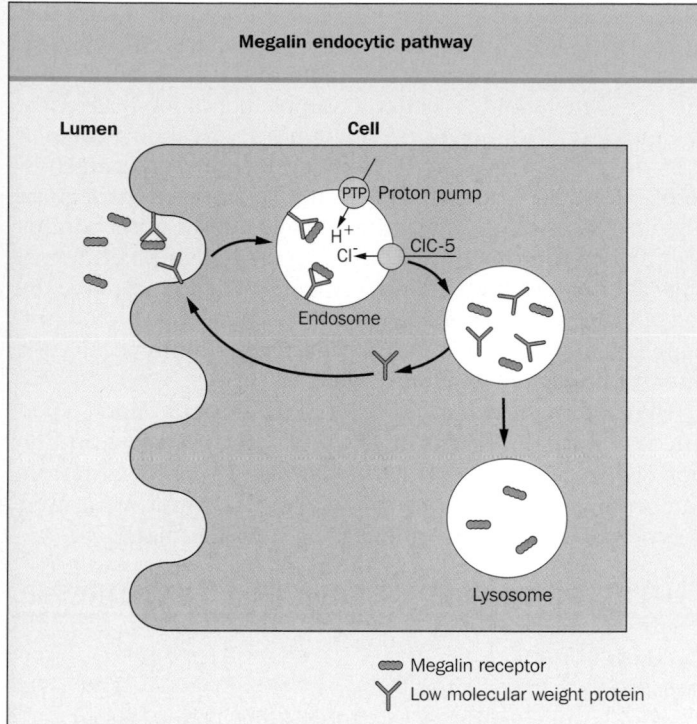

Megalin endocytic pathway

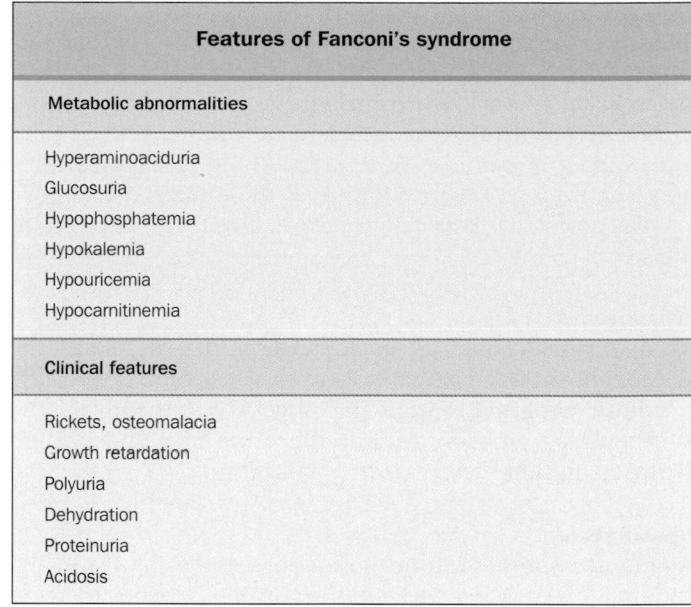

Features of Fanconi's syndrome
Metabolic abnormalities
Hyperaminoaciduria
Glucosuria
Hypophosphatemia
Hypokalemia
Hypouricemia
Hypocarnitinemia
Clinical features
Rickets, osteomalacia
Growth retardation
Polyuria
Dehydration
Proteinuria
Acidosis

Table 50.3 Features of Fanconi's syndrome.

Figure 50.5 Megalin-endocytic pathway. Low molecular proteins in the luminal fluid bind to megalin and are endocytosed. The recycling of megalin and further catabolism of these proteins are dependent on acidification of the vesicle by a proton pump. The ClC-5 chloride channel provides an electrical shunt for efficient functioning of the proton pump. This endocytosis pathway may also play a role in membrane transporter recycling and disruption of this pathway could interfere with absorption of other luminal solutes.

Glucosuria

Glucosuria secondary to proximal tubule dysfunction is another of the cardinal features of Fanconi's syndrome and occurs because of impaired tubular reabsorption of glucose. It is often one of the first diagnostic clues. Like aminoaciduria, it rarely causes symptoms.

Hypophosphatemia

Hypophosphatemia secondary to an impairment in phosphate reabsorption is a common finding in Fanconi's syndrome. Assessment of tubular phosphate handling can be made by measuring the maximum phosphate reabsorption in relation to the glomerular filtration rate (T_mP/GFR) on fasting urine and blood samples. Elevated parathyroid hormone (PTH) and low vitamin D levels also may play a role in the phosphaturia of Fanconi's syndrome, although these hormonal abnormalities are not always present. A few patients have impaired conversion of 25-hydroxyvitamin D to 1,25-hydroxyvitamin D. Metabolic acidosis, another feature of Fanconi's syndrome, may also impair the conversion of 25-hydroxyvitamin D to 1,25-hydroxyvitamin D. The hypophosphatemia, especially if accompanied by hyperparathyroidism and low 1,25-hydroxyvitamin D levels, often leads to significant bone disease, presenting with pain, fractures, rickets, or growth failure.

Hyperchloremic metabolic acidosis

Hyperchloremic metabolic acidosis, another feature of Fanconi's syndrome, is a result of impaired bicarbonate reabsorption by the proximal tubule (proximal RTA). This impaired reabsorption can lead to the loss of more than 30% of the normal filtered load. As the serum bicarbonate falls, the filtered load falls and excretion drops such that the serum bicarbonate usually remains between 12–18 mmol/L. Occasionally, there is an associated defect in distal acidification, usually in association with long-standing hypokalemia or nephrocalcinosis. Ammoniagenesis is usually normal or increased, because of the hypokalemia and acidosis, unless there is an associated impairment in GFR.

Natriuresis and kaliuresis

Natriuresis and kaliuresis are common in Fanconi's syndrome and can give rise to significant, even life-threatening, problems. These electrolyte losses are, in part, related to impaired bicarbonate reabsorption, with the subsequent urinary excretion of sodium and potassium ions with the bicarbonate. In some cases, sodium and potassium losses are so great that metabolic alkalosis and hyperaldosteronism result, simulating Bartter syndrome in spite of the lowered bicarbonate threshold. The clearance of potassium may be twice that of the GFR, and the resulting hypokalemia can cause sudden death.

Polyuria and polydipsia

Polyuria, polydipsia, and frequent bouts of severe dehydration are common symptoms in young patients with Fanconi's syndrome. The polyuria is mainly related to the osmotic diuresis from the excessive urinary solute losses, but in some patients, there is an associated concentrating defect, especially in patients with prolonged hypokalemia.

Growth retardation

Growth retardation in children with Fanconi's syndrome is multifactorial. Hypophosphatemia, disordered vitamin D metabolism, and acidosis contribute to growth failure as do chronic hypokalemia and extracellular volume contraction. Glucosuria and aminoaciduria probably do not play a role. However, even with correction of all these metabolic abnormalities, most patients fail to grow, especially those with cystinosis.

Hypouricemia

Hypouricemia, caused by an impairment in renal handling of uric acid, is often present in Fanconi's syndrome, especially in adults. Urolithiasis from the uricosuria has only rarely been reported probably because the urine flow and pH are increased, inhibiting uric acid crystallization.

Proteinuria

Proteinuria, another feature of Fanconi's syndrome, is usually minimal, except when Fanconi's syndrome develops in association with the nephrotic syndrome. Typically, only low-molecular-weight proteins (2000–30 000 Da) are excreted, for example enzymes, immunoglobulins, light chains, and hormones.

Treatment of Fanconi's syndrome

Therapy, whenever possible, should be directed at the underlying causes, which are discussed below, for example, avoidance of the offending nutrient in galactosemia, hereditary fructose intolerance, or tyrosinemia; treatment of Wilson's disease with penicillamine and other copper chelators; or treatment of heavy metal intoxication by chelation therapy. In these cases, resolution of Fanconi's syndrome usually is complete.

In other instances, therapy is directed at the biochemical abnormalities secondary to the renal solute losses and at the bone disease that is often present in these patients. The proximal RTA usually requires large doses of alkali for correction. Some patients benefit from hydrochlorothiazide to minimize the volume expansion associated with these large doses of alkali. Potassium supplementation is also commonly needed, especially if there is a significant RTA. The use of potassium citrate, lactate, or acetate will correct not only the hypokalemia but also the acidosis. A few patients will require sodium supplementation along with potassium. Again, the use of a metabolizable anion will aid in the correction of the acidosis. Rarely, patients may need sodium chloride supplementation. Usually these patients have alkalosis when untreated as a result of large urinary sodium chloride losses, which lead to volume contraction that overrides the RTA. Magnesium supplementation may be required. Adequate fluid intake is essential. Correction of hypokalemia and its effect on the concentrating ability of the distal tubule may lessen the polyuria.

Bone disease is multifactorial, including hypophosphatemia, decreased synthesis of calcitriol in some patients, hypercalciuria, and chronic acidosis. Both low and normal plasma levels of calcitriol have been reported. Hypophosphatemia should be treated with 1–3 g/d of oral phosphate with the goal of normalizing serum phosphate levels.

Many patients will require supplemental vitamin D for adequate treatment of the rickets and osteomalacia. It is unclear whether standard vitamin D (calciferol (ergocalciferol)) or a vitamin D metabolite is better for supplementation. Currently, the majority of clinicians use a vitamin D metabolite, such as 1,25-dihydroxycholecalciferol (calcitriol) or dihydrotachysterol. These metabolites obviate the concern of inadequate vitamin D hydroxylation by the proximal tubule mitochondria and reduce the risk of prolonged hypercalcemia because of their shorter half-life. Vitamin D therapy will also improve the hypophosphatemia and lessen the risk of hyperparathyroidism. Supplemental calcium is indicated in those with hypocalcemia after starting supplemental vitamin D.

Hyperaminoaciduria, glucosuria, proteinuria, and hyperuricosuria usually do not lead to clinical difficulties and do not require specific treatment. Carnitine supplementation, to compensate for the urinary losses, may improve muscle function and lipid profiles, but the results are mixed.

INHERITED CAUSES OF FANCONI'S SYNDROME

Cystinosis

Definition

Cystinosis, or cystine storage disease, is characterized biochemically by excessive intracellular storage, particularly in lysosomes, of the amino acid cystine[8].

Three different types of cystinosis can be distinguished, based on the clinical course and the intracellular cystine content. Benign or adult cystinosis is associated with cystine crystals in the cornea and bone marrow only and the mildest elevation in intracellular cystine levels; there is no renal disease. Infantile or nephropathic cystinosis is the most common form and is associated with the highest intracellular levels of cystine and the earliest onset of renal disease. The intermediate or adolescent form has intracellular cystine levels in between those of the infantile and adult forms and later onset of renal disease.

Etiology and pathogenesis

Nephropathic cystinosis is transmitted as an autosomal recessive trait localized to the short arm of chromosome 17, with an estimated incidence of 1/200 000 live births. CTNS, a novel gene mapped to chromosome 17p13, codes for a lysosomal membrane protein, cystinosin, which mediates the transport of cystine from the lysosome[9]. A number of mutations have been described in this gene in children with nephropathic cystinosis; the most common being a large 57 kb deletion. Both the benign and intermediate forms of cystinosis are also associated with mutations in this gene. However, in these patients, the mutations still result in some functional transport protein leading to lower intracellular cystine levels and slower onset of renal disease in the intermediate form and no renal disease in the benign form.

Clinical manifestations

The first clinical symptoms and signs in nephropathic cystinosis are those of Fanconi's syndrome and usually appear in the latter half of the first year of life. Subtle abnormalities of tubular function can be demonstrated earlier in families with

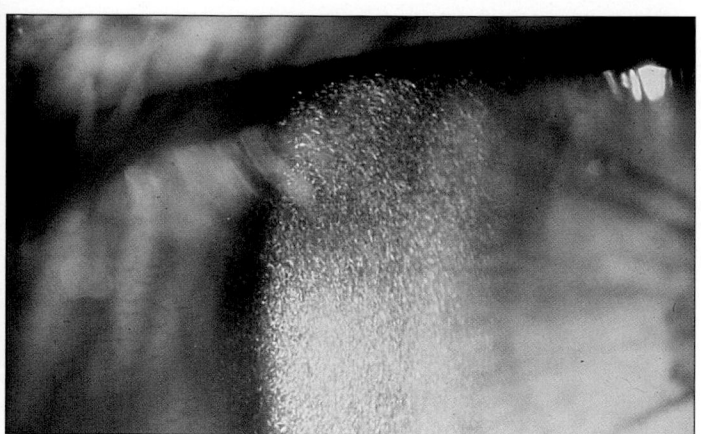

Figure 50.6 Corneal opacities in cystinosis. Tinsel-like refractile opacities in the cornea of a patient with cystinosis under slit lamp examination. (With permission from Foreman[10].)

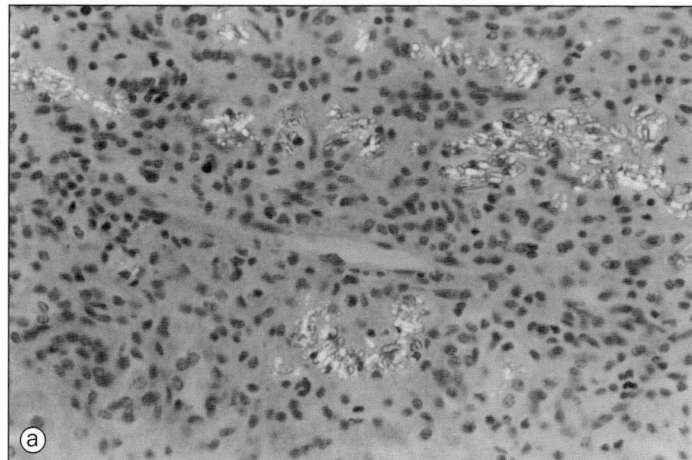

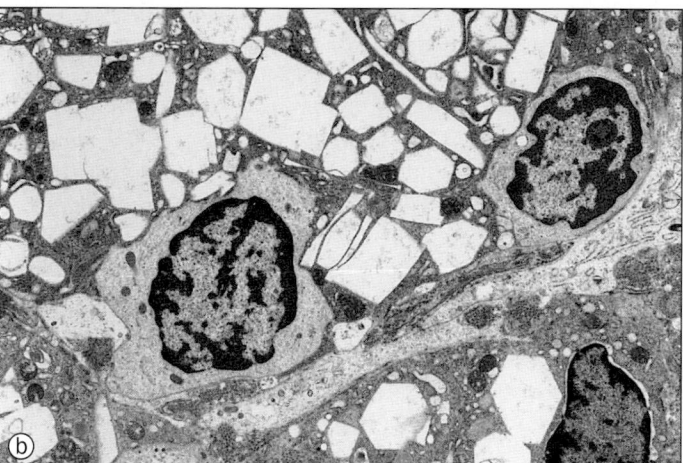

Figure 50.7 Cystine crystals. (a) Crystals in the kidney are seen in a photomicrograph of an alcohol-fixed nephrectomy specimen, taken through incompletely crossed polarizing filters. Birefringent crystals are evident in tubular epithelial cells and free in the interstitium. (With permission from Schnaper et al.[11].) (b) Electron micrograph of a renal biopsy showing hexagonal, rectangular, and needle-shaped crystals in macrophages within the interstitium (x3000). (With permission from van't Hoff et al.[12].)

index cases, but there always is a delay between birth and the first symptoms. Rickets is common after the first year of life, along with growth failure. The growth failure occurs before the GFR declines and despite correction of electrolyte and mineral deficiencies. The GFR invariably declines and end-stage renal disease (ESRD) occurs by late childhood. Nephrocalcinosis is relatively common and a few patients have developed renal calculi. Photophobia is another common symptom that occurs by 3 years of age and is progressive. Older patients with cystinosis may develop visual impairment and blindness. Children with cystinosis usually have fair complexions and blond hair, but dark hair has been observed in some. Cystinosis has been observed in African Caribbeans but is less common than in Caucasians. The diagnosis is based on the demonstration of elevated intracellular levels of cystine, usually in white blood cells or skin fibroblasts. A slit lamp demonstration of corneal crystals is strongly suggestive of the diagnosis (Fig. 50.6)[10]. A prenatal diagnosis can be made with amniocytes or chorionic villi.

Common late complications of cystinosis include hypothyroidism, splenomegaly and hepatomegaly, decreased visual acuity, swallowing difficulties, and corneal ulcerations. Less commonly, older patients have developed insulin-dependent diabetes mellitus, myopathy and progressive neurologic disorders. Cortical atrophy has also been noted in some patients.

Pathology
The morphologic features of the kidney in cystinosis vary with the stage of the disease. Early in the disease, cystine crystals are present in tubular epithelial cells, interstitial cells and, rarely, in glomerular epithelial cells (see Fig. 50.7a)[11,12]. A swan-neck deformity or thinning of the first part of the proximal tubule is an early finding, but is not unique to cystinosis. Later, there is pronounced tubular atrophy, interstitial fibrosis, and abundant crystal deposition with giant cell formation of the glomerular visceral epithelium, segmental sclerosis, and eventual glomerular obsolescence. Electron microscopy studies have demonstrated intracellular crystalline inclusions consistent with cystine (see Fig. 50.7b). Peculiar 'dark cells,' unique to the cystinotic kidney, have also been observed.

Treatment
Until recently, treatment of infantile cystinosis has been limited to vitamin D therapy and replacement of the urinary electrolyte losses followed, in due course, by the management of the progressive renal failure (Table 50.4). Cysteamine has now been shown to lower tissue cystine and to slow the decline in GFR, especially in children with a normal serum creatinine treated before 2 years of age (see Fig. 50.8)[13]. Cysteamine therapy also improves linear growth but not Fanconi's syndrome. The most common problems associated with cysteamine therapy are nausea, vomiting, and a foul odor and taste. Treatment should begin with a low dose of cysteamine, as the bitartrate (Cystagon™), soon after the diagnosis is made and increased over 4–6 weeks to 1.3 g/m² daily in four divided doses as close to every 6 h as possible. Slowly increasing the dose minimizes the risk of a serum sickness-like reaction. Leukocyte cystine levels should be checked every 3–4 months to monitor effectiveness and compliance, with the goal of achieving and maintaining a cystine level of below 1.0 nmol half-cystine/mg

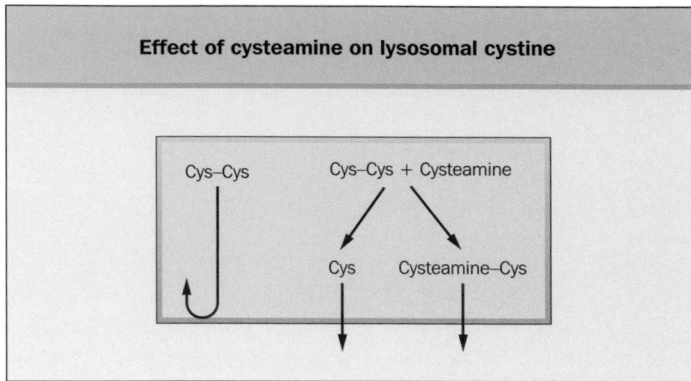

Effect of cysteamine on lysosomal cystine

Cys–Cys   Cys–Cys + Cysteamine

Cys   Cysteamine–Cys

Figure 50.8 Effect of cysteamine on lysosomal cystine. In cystinosis, the transporter for cystine (cys-cys) egress from the lysosome is defective. Cysteamine can easily enter the lysosome and combine with cystine, forming cysteine (Cys) and the mixed disulfide cysteamine–cysteine. Both of these compounds can exit the lysosome via a transporter other than the cystine carrier. (Reprinted with permission from Foreman.[10])

Treatment of cystinosis

Problem Therapy	Primary therapy
Removal of lysosomal cystine	0.325 g/m² Cystagon™ g 6 h to maintain leukocyte cystine level < 1nmoL half-cystine/mg protein
Correction of tubulopathy	
Dehydration	2–6 L/d fluid
Acidosis	2–15 mg/kg/d K⁺ citrate
Hypophosphatemia	1–4 g/d K⁺ phosphate
Rickets	0.25–1 µg/d calcitriol
Adjunct therapies	NaCl, carnitine, indomethacin, hydrochlorothiazide
Later therapies	
Growth failure	Growth hormone
Hypothyroidism	Thyroxine
Renal failure	Renal replacement therapy, ideally renal transplantation

Table 50.4 Treatment of cystinosis.

protein. Cysteamine eye drops have proved useful in depleting the cornea of cystine crystals but require very frequent administration to be effective.

Treatment of ESRD in these children poses no greater problems than with other children. Successful renal transplantation reverses the renal failure and Fanconi's syndrome but does not appear to improve the extrarenal manifestations of cystinosis. Cystine does not accumulate in the transplanted kidney, except in infiltrating immunocytes.

Galactosemia
Etiology and pathogenesis
Galactosemia is an autosomal recessively inherited disorder of galactose metabolism. It is most commonly the result of deficient activity of the enzyme galactose 1-phosphate uridyl transferase; this occurs with an incidence of 1/62 000 live births[14]. The gene for this enzyme is found on the short arm of chromosome 9. Deficiency of this enzyme leads to the intracellular accumulation of galactose 1-phosphate, with damage to the liver, proximal renal tubule, ovary, brain, and lens. A less frequent cause of galactosemia is a deficiency of galactose kinase, which forms galactose 1-phosphate from galactose. Cataracts are the only manifestation of this form of galactosemia. The pathogenesis of the symptoms of galactosemia is not clear. Accumulation of galactose 1-phosphate subsequent to the ingestion of galactose can inhibit a number of pathways for carbohydrate metabolism, and there is some correlation of its level with clinical symptoms. Defective galactosylation of proteins has also been postulated. Formation of galactitol from galactose by aldose reductase has been proposed as a pathogenetic mechanism and this is probably responsible for the cataract formation.

Clinical manifestations
Affected infants ingesting milk containing lactose, the most common source of galactose in the diet, rapidly develop vomiting, diarrhea, and failure to thrive. Jaundice from unconjugated hyperbilirubinemia is common, along with severe hemolysis. Continued intake of galactose leads to hepatomegaly and cirrhosis. Cataracts appear within days after birth, although they often are detectable only with a slit lamp. Mental retardation may develop within a few months. Fulminant *Escherichia coli* sepsis has been described in a number of infants, which may be a consequence of inhibited leukocyte bactericidal activity.

In addition to these clinical findings, galactose intake leads within days to hyperaminoaciduria and albuminuria. Raised urine sugar excretion is principally a result of galactosuria and not glucosuria. There seems to be little or no impairment in glucose handling by the renal tubule. Galactosemia should be suspected whenever there is a urinary reducing substance that does not react in a glucose oxidase test. The diagnosis can be confirmed by demonstrating deficient transferase activity in red blood cells, fibroblasts, leukocytes, or hepatocytes.

Treatment
Galactosemia is treated by eliminating galactose from the diet. Acute symptoms and signs resolve in a few days. Cataracts will also regress to some extent. However, even with early elimination of galactose, developmental delay, speech impairment, ovarian dysfunction, and growth retardation are a common outcome in galactosemia. Profound intellectual deficits are rare even in infants treated late.

Hereditary fructose intolerance
Etiology and pathogenesis
Hereditary fructose intolerance (HFI) is another disorder of carbohydrate metabolism associated with Fanconi's syndrome[15]. It is inherited as an autosomal recessive trait with an incidence estimated to be 1/20 000. It is caused by a deficiency of the B isozyme form of the enzyme fructose 1-phosphate aldolase, which cleaves fructose 1-phosphate

into D-glyceraldehyde and dihydroxyacetone phosphate. Deficient activity of aldolase B leads to tissue accumulation of fructose 1-phosphate and reduced levels of ATP. The gene for aldolase B resides on the long arm of chromosome 9.

Clinical manifestations

Symptoms of HFI appear at weaning when fruit, vegetables, and sweetened cereals that contain fructose or sucrose are introduced. Children with this disorder experience nausea, vomiting, and symptoms of hypoglycemia shortly after ingesting fructose, sucrose, or sorbitol. These symptoms may progress to convulsions, coma, and even death, depending on the amount consumed. Young infants, when exposed to fructose, may have a catastrophic illness, with severe dehydration, shock, acute liver impairment, bleeding, or acute renal failure. Concomitant serum biochemical findings after fructose ingestion are a fall in glucose, phosphate, and bicarbonate with a rise in uric acid and lactic acid. Chronic exposure to fructose leads to failure to thrive, hepatomegaly, jaundice, hepatic cirrhosis, and nephrocalcinosis. Children with HFI learn to avoid sweets and as a result have few dental caries.

Diagnosis

The diagnosis should be suspected when symptoms develop following the ingestion of fructose. Confirmation can be made either by a carefully applied fructose tolerance test or by assaying the activity of fructose 1-phosphate aldolase in a liver biopsy specimen.

Treatment

Treatment of HFI involves strict avoidance of foods containing fructose and sucrose. Most patients develop a strong aversion to such foods, making this interdiction easy. The greatest risk occurs during infancy before affected individuals learn to avoid fructose.

Glycogenosis

Most patients with glycogen storage disease and Fanconi's syndrome have an autosomal recessive disorder characterized by heavy glucosuria and glycogen storage in the liver and kidney, known as the Fanconi–Bickel syndrome, or a renal glucose-losing syndrome because the glucose losses can be massive[16]. The defect appears to be deficient activity of the sugar transporter, GLUT2 (Fig. 50.2). GLUT2 facilitates sugar exit from the basolateral side of the proximal tubule and intestinal cell and sugar entry and exit from the hepatocyte and pancreatic β-cell. A few patients with type I glycogen storage disease have mild Fanconi's syndrome, but not Fanconi–Bickel syndrome. The therapy of this disorder is directed at the renal solute losses, treatment of rickets, which can be quite severe, and frequent feeding to prevent ketosis. Uncooked cornstarch has been shown to lessen the hypoglycemia and improve growth.

Tyrosinemia

Definition

Hereditary tyrosinemia type I, also known as hepatorenal tyrosinemia, is a defect of tyrosine metabolism affecting the liver, kidneys, and peripheral nerves[17].

Etiology and pathogenesis

The cause of hereditary tyrosinemia type I is a deficiency of fumarylacetoacetate hydrolase (FAH) activity. It is an autosomal recessive disorder carried on the long arm of chromosome 15. Decreased or absent FAH activity leads to accumulation of maleylacetoacetate (MAA) and fumarylacetoacetate (FAA) in affected tissues. These compounds can react with free sulfhydryl groups, reduce intracellular levels of glutathione, and act as alkylating agents. MAA and FAA are not detectable in plasma or urine but are converted to succinylacetoacetate and succinylacetone. The latter is structurally similar to maleic acid, a compound that causes Fanconi's syndrome experimentally in rats and may be the cause of Fanconi's syndrome in humans affected with tyrosinemia.

Clinical manifestations

The liver is the major organ affected and this may be evident as early as the first month of life. Such infants usually have severe disease and die in the first year of life. All children will eventually develop macronodular cirrhosis and many will develop hepatocellular carcinoma. Acute, painful peripheral neuropathy and autonomic dysfunction can also occur in tyrosinemia. Proximal renal tubule dysfunction is evident in all patients with tyrosinemia, especially those presenting after infancy. Nephromegaly is very common and nephrocalcinosis may be seen. Glomerulosclerosis and impaired GFR may be seen with time.

Diagnosis

The diagnosis should be suspected with elevated plasma tyrosine and methionine levels together with their p-hydroxy metabolites. The presence of succinylacetone in blood or urine is diagnostic of hereditary tyrosinemia type I.

Treatment

The institution of a diet low in phenylalanine and tyrosine dramatically improves the renal tubule dysfunction. Nitrotrifluorobenzoylcyclohexadione (NTBC), which inhibits the formation of MAA and FAA, dramatically improves the renal and hepatic dysfunction[17]. Liver transplantation has been successfully used to treat patients with severe liver failure and to prevent the development of hepatoma. Liver transplantation leads to rapid correction of Fanconi's syndrome.

Wilson's disease

Definition

Wilson's disease is an inherited disorder of copper metabolism that affects numerous organ systems[18]. It has an overall incidence of 1/30 000. Approximately 40% of patients present with liver disease, 40% with extrapyramidal symptoms, and 20% with psychiatric or behavioral abnormalities.

Etiology and pathogenesis

Wilson's disease is a defect in a P-type copper-transporting ATPase in the liver. It impairs biliary copper excretion and the incorporation of copper into ceruloplasmin. These abnormalities cause excessive intracellular accumulation of copper in the liver, with subsequent overflow into other tissues such as brain, cornea, and renal proximal tubule. The gene for this enzyme has been localized to chromosome 13q14.3.

Hereditary and Congenital Diseases of the Kidney

Clinical manifestations

Excessive storage of copper in the kidney leads to renal tubule dysfunction in most patients and full-blown Fanconi's syndrome in some. Hematuria also has been noted. Renal plasma flow and GFR decrease as the disease progresses, but death from extrarenal causes occurs before the onset of renal failure. Fanconi's syndrome usually appears before the onset of hepatic failure. Hypercalciuria with the development of renal stones and nephrocalcinosis also has been reported. Besides proximal tubular dysfunction, abnormalities in distal tubular function, decreased concentrating ability, and distal RTA have also been observed.

Pathology

Histologically, the kidney in untreated Wilson's disease shows either no alterations on light microscopy or only some flattened proximal tubule cells without recognizable brush borders. Electron microscopy shows loss of the brush border, disruption of the apical tubular network, electron-dense bodies probably representing metalloproteins in the subapical region of tubule cell cytoplasm, and cavitation of the mitochondria with disruption of the normal cristae pattern. Rubeanic acid staining shows intracytoplasmic copper granules. The copper content of kidney tissue is markedly elevated.

Diagnosis

The diagnosis of Wilson's disease should be suspected in children and young adults with unexplained neurologic disease, chronic active hepatitis, acute hemolytic crisis, behavioral or psychiatric disturbances, or the appearance of Fanconi's syndrome. In such patients, the presence of Kayser–Fleischer rings is an important clue in making the diagnosis. Serum ceruloplasmin levels are decreased in 96% of patients with Wilson's disease. A markedly increased urinary copper level is also useful in making the diagnosis, especially if it increases significantly with D-penicillamine. Liver copper levels are increased in untreated patients.

Treatment

Treatment with D-penicillamine reverses the renal dysfunction and may reverse the hepatic and neurologic disease, depending on the degree of damage before the onset of therapy. Recovery, however, is quite slow. Trientine can also chelate copper and is indicated in patients who cannot tolerate D-penicillamine. Tetrathiomolybdate is a very potent agent in removing copper from the body and has been used in some patients with neurologic disease to prevent the immediate worsening of symptoms that can occur with penicillamine. Zinc salts, which induce intestinal metallothionein and blockade of intestinal absorption of copper, are useful in maintenance therapy. Liver transplantation has been successful in some patients but should be reserved for those with liver failure.

Lowe syndrome

Lowe syndrome (oculocerebrorenal syndrome) is characterized by congenital cataracts and glaucoma, severe mental retardation, hypotonia with diminished-to-absent reflexes,

and renal abnormalities[19]. Fanconi's syndrome is followed by progressive renal insufficiency. ESRD usually does not occur until the third to fourth decade of life.

Lowe syndrome is transmitted as an X-linked recessive trait mapped to Xp24–26. In spite of this inheritance pattern, Lowe syndrome has occurred in a few females. This gene codes for a phosphatidylinositol bisphosphate phosphatase localized in the Golgi complex.

Light microscopy of the kidney is normal early in the disorder, with endothelial cell swelling and thickening and splitting of the glomerular basement membrane seen by electron microscopy. In the proximal tubule cells, there is shortening of the brush border and enlargement of the mitochondria, with distortion and loss of the cristae.

The only treatment is symptomatic therapy.

Dent's disease

Definition

Dent's disease is an X-linked recessive disorder characterized by low molecular weight proteinuria, hypercalciuria, nephrolithiasis, nephrocalcinosis, and rickets.[20] In addition, affected males often have aminoaciduria, phosphaturia, and glucosuria. Renal failure is common and may occur by late childhood. Hemizygous females usually have only proteinuria and mild hypercalciuria. X-linked recessive nephrolithiasis, X-linked recessive hypophosphatemic rickets, and Japanese idiopathic low molecular weight proteinuria have similar features and all are now known to be part of the clinical spectrum of a defect in the renal ClC-5 chloride channel.

Etiology and pathogenesis

All of these disorders are caused by a mutation in the CLCN5 gene located on chromosome Xp11.22 leading to inactive ClC-5 chloride channel function. The ClC-5 chloride channel spans the membrane of pre-endocytic vesicles just below the brush border of the proximal tubule. There it facilitates the entry of Cl^- that is necessary for the active acidification of the vesicles by a proton pump (Fig. 50.5). Lack of this Cl^- channel interferes with protein reabsorption from the tubule and cell surface receptor recycling, which may explain the phosphaturia, glucosuria, and aminoaciduria.

Mitochondrial cytopathies

Definition

Mitochondrial cytopathies refers to a diverse group of diseases related to abnormalities in mitochondrial DNA that lead to mitochondrial dysfunction in various tissues[21].

Clinical manifestations

Most of the mitochondrial cytopathies present with neurologic disorders such as myopathy, myoclonus, ataxia, seizures, external ophthalmoplegia, stroke-like episodes, and optic neuropathy. Other manifestations include pigmentary retinitis, diabetes mellitus, exocrine pancreatic insufficiency, sideroblastic anemia, sensorineural hearing loss, pseudoobstruction of the colon, hepatic disease, cardiac conduction disorders, and cardiomyopathy. These various manifestations tend to group together in specific syndromes and reflect specific mutations in mitochondrial DNA (Table 50.5).

Mitochondrial cytopathies
MERRF: myoclonic epilepsy with ragged red fibers
NARP: neuropathy, ataxia, and retinitis pigmentosa
MELAS: mitochondrial encephalopathy, lactic acidosis, and stroke-like episodes
LHON: Leber hereditary optic neuropathy
Leigh disease: maternally inherited Leigh disease (somnolence, blindness, deafness, peripheral neuropathy, degeneration of brainstem)
Pearson syndrome: pancytopenia, exocrine pancreatic deficiency, hepatic dysfunction
Kearns-Sayre syndrome: ophthalmoplegia, pigmentary retinopathy, heart block, ataxia
Alpers' disease: intractable epilepsy, liver disease, neuronal degeneration

Table 50.5 Mitochondrial cytopathies.

The most common renal manifestation associated with mitochondrial cytopathies is Fanconi's syndrome, although a number of patients have been described with focal segmental glomerulosclerosis and steroid resistant nephrotic syndrome. All of the patients with renal abnormalities have had extrarenal disorders, mainly neurologic disease. Most patients present in the first months of life and die soon afterwards.

Diagnosis

A clue to these disorders is elevated serum or cerebrospinal fluid lactate levels, especially if associated with an altered lactate/pyruvate ratio, suggesting a defect in mitochondrial respiration. The presence of 'ragged red fibers,' a manifestation of abnormal mitochondria, in a muscle biopsy is another clue, especially with large abnormal mitochondria on electron microscopy of muscle tissue.

Treatment

There is little to offer these patients in terms of definitive therapy. Low complex III activity can be treated with menadione or ubidecarone. Deficient complex I activity may be treated with riboflavin and ubidecarone. Ascorbic acid has been used to minimize oxygen free radical injury. High-lipid, low-carbohydrate diet has been tried in cytochrome c oxidase deficiency.

Idiopathic Fanconi's syndrome

A number of patients develop the complete Fanconi's syndrome in the absence of any known cause. Traditionally, these cases have been called the adult Fanconi's syndrome because it was thought that only adults were affected. However, it is clear that children may be affected and a more proper designation is idiopathic Fanconi's syndrome. All of the features of Fanconi's syndrome may not be present when the patients are first seen but do appear with time. Idiopathic Fanconi's syndrome can be inherited in an autosomal dominant, autosomal recessive, or even an X-linked pattern. However, most cases occur sporadically, without any evidence of genetic transmission. The prognosis is quite variable and some develop chronic renal failure 10 to 30 years after the onset of symptoms. A few patients have undergone renal transplantation and in some of these Fanconi's syndrome has recurred in the allograft without evidence of rejection, suggesting an extrarenal cause for the idiopathic Fanconi's syndrome.

Renal morphologic descriptions of such cases are scanty. In some reports, no abnormalities were found and in others tubular atrophy with interstitial fibrosis were interspersed with areas of tubular dilatation. Markedly dilated proximal tubules with swollen epithelium and grossly enlarged mitochondria with displaced cristae have also been noted.

ACQUIRED CAUSES OF FANCONI'S SYNDROME

Numerous substances can injure the proximal renal tubule (see Table 50.2) and this injury can range from an incomplete Fanconi's syndrome to acute tubular necrosis and renal failure. The extent of the tubular damage is quite variable and is dependent on the type of toxin, the amount ingested, and the host. A careful history of possible toxin exposure is therefore important in patients with tubular dysfunction.

Heavy metal intoxication

A major cause of proximal tubular dysfunction is heavy metal intoxication, principally lead and cadmium. In lead poisoning the renal tubular dysfunction, mainly aminoaciduria and mild glucosuria and phosphaturia, is usually overshadowed by the involvement of other organs, especially the central nervous system. Fanconi's syndrome associated with cadmium poisoning is associated with severe bone pain, giving rise to the name 'itai-itai' (ouch-ouch) disease for its occurrence in Japanese patients affected by industrial contamination of the soil.

Tetracycline

Outdated tetracycline causes a reversible Fanconi's syndrome even in therapeutic doses. Recovery is rapid when the degraded drug is stopped. The compound responsible for the tubule dysfunction is anhydro-4-tetracycline formed from tetracycline by heat, moisture, and a low pH.

Cancer chemotherapy agents

A number of cancer chemotherapy agents have been associated with Fanconi's syndrome and renal tubule dysfunction, especially cisplatin and ifosfamide. The nephrotoxicity of both is dose dependent and often irreversible. Besides the usual manifestations of Fanconi's syndrome, cisplatin toxicity is characterized by hypomagnesemia, caused by hypermagnesuria, which can be extremely severe, persistent, and difficult to treat. Ifosfamide is more commonly associated with hypophosphatemic rickets. Chloroacetaldehyde, a metabolite of ifosfamide, appears experimentally to cause Fanconi's syndrome. Both ifosfamide and cisplatin can cause an irreversible reduction in GFR.

Other drugs and toxins

Exposure to a wide range of toxins may give rise to Fanconi's syndrome, often in association with a reduced GFR, including methyl 3-chromone (diachrome), 6-mercaptopurine, toluene (glue sniffing), and Chinese herbal medicines. There have also been anecdotal reports associating Fanconi's syndrome with valproic acid (valproate), suramin, Lysol, gentamicin, streptozocin (streptozotocin), and ranitidine.

Dysproteinemias

Dysproteinemia from multiple myeloma, light chain proteinuria, Sjögren's syndrome, and amyloidosis is sometimes associated with Fanconi's syndrome, which appears to be correlated with specific light chains or light chain fragments (Bence–Jones proteins) that crystallize within the tubular cells.

Glomerular disease

Nephrotic syndrome has rarely been associated with Fanconi's syndrome. Most of these patients have focal segmental glomerulosclerosis and the occurrence of Fanconi's syndrome heralds a poor prognosis.

After acute tubular necrosis

Tubular dysfunction during recovery from acute renal failure from any cause can occur, whether or not a known tubular toxin was originally implicated.

Postrenal transplant

Fanconi's syndrome has appeared rarely after renal transplantation. The pathogenesis probably is multifactorial, for example sequelae of acute tubular necrosis, rejection, nephrotoxic drugs, ischemia from renal artery stenosis, and residual hyperparathyroidism.

REFERENCES

1. Brodehl J, Oemer BS, Hoyer PF. Renal glucosuria. Pediatr Nephrol. 1987;1:502–8.
2. Foreman JW, Segal S. Aminoacidurias. In: Gonick HC, Buckalew VM Jr., eds. Renal Tubular Disorders: Pathophysiology, Diagnosis, and Management. New York: Marcel Dekker; 1985:131–57.
3. Ng CS, Streem SB. Contemporary management of cystinuria. J Endourology. 1999;13:647–51.
4. Goodyer P, Boutros M, Rozen R. The molecular basis of cystinuria: an update. Exp Nephrol. 2000;8:123–7.
5. Sperling O. Chapter 198 Hereditary renal hypouricemia. In: Scriver CR, Beaudet AL, et al. eds. The Metabolic and Molecular Bases of Inherited Disease, 8th edn. New York: McGraw-Hill; 2001:5069–85.
6. Puig JG, Miranda ME. Hereditary nephropathy associated with hyperuricemia and gout. Arch Int Med. 1993;153:357–65.
7. Kamatani N, Moritani M, Yamanaka H, et al. Localization of a gene for familial juvenile hyperuricemic nephropathy causing underexcretion-type gout to 16p 12 by genome-wide linkage analysis of a large family. Arthritis Rheum. 2000;43:925.
8. Thoene JG. Cystinosis. J Inherit Metab Dis. 1995;18:380–6.
9. Town M, Jean G, Cherqui S, et al. A novel gene encoding an integral membrane protein is mutated in nephropathic cystinosis. Nat Genet. 1998;18:319–24.
10. Foreman JW. Fanconi syndrome and cystinosis. In: Barratt TM, Avner ED, Harmon WE eds. Pediatric Nephrology, 4th edn. Philadelphia, PA: Lippincott; 1999:543.
11. Schnaper HW, Cottel J, Merrill S, et al. Early occurrence of end-stage renal disease in a patient with infantile nephropathic cystinosis. J Pediatr. 1992;120:576.
12. van't Hoff WG, Ledermann SE, Waldron M, Trompter RS. Early-onset chronic renal failure as a presentation of infantile cystinosis. Pediatr Nephrol. 1995;9:483–4.
13. Schneider JA, Clark KF, Greene AA, et al. Recent advances in the treatment of cystinosis. J Inherit Metab Dis. 1995;18:387–97.
14. Segal S. Galactosemia unsolved. Eur J Pediatr. 1995;154:S97–S102.
15. Cox TM. Aldolase B and fructose intolerance. FASEB J. 1994;8: 62–71.
16. Manz F, Bickel H, Brodehl J, et al. Fanconi-Bickel syndrome. Pediatr Nephrol. 1987;1:509–18.
17. Holme E, Lindstedt S. Diagnosis and management of tyrosinemia type I. Curr Opin Pediatr. 1995;7:726–32.
18. Schilsky ML. Wilson disease: genetic basis of copper toxicity and natural history. Semin Liver Dis. 1996;16:83–95.
19. Charnas LR, Bernadini I, Radar D, et al. Clinical and laboratory finding in the oculocerebrorenal syndrome of Lowe, with special reference to growth and renal function. N Engl J Med. 1991;324: 1318–25.
20. Thakker RV. Pathogenesis of Dent's disease and related syndromes of X-linked nephrolithiasis. Kidney Int. 2000;57: 787–93.
21. Niaudet P, Roetig A. Renal involvement in mitochondrial cytopathies. Pediatr Nephrol. 1996;10:368–73.

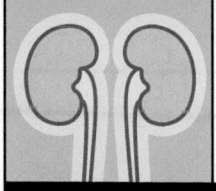

Section 9 Hereditary and Congenital Diseases of the Kidney

Chapter 51

Sickle Cell Disease

Jan C ter Maaten, Rijk O B Gans, and Paul E de Jong

INTRODUCTION AND DEFINITIONS

Sickle cell disease is an autosomal recessive inherited disorder, predominantly of the African American race. The gene for sickle hemoglobin (HbS) results in the replacement of the normal glutamine by valine in the β-globin subunit, thereby changing the configuration of the hemoglobin molecule and enhancing the aggregation of hemoglobin molecules. This aggregation decreases the pliability of the red cells and may distort their shape to a characteristic crescentic or sickle shape. This event results in premature destruction of red cells (hemolysis) and frequent, widespread vaso-occlusive episodes with subsequent organ damage. Sickle cell anemia occurs in those homozygous for HbS. Sickle cell trait occurs in those heterozygous for HbS.

Sickle cell nephropathy describes the structural and functional abnormalities of the kidney in sickle cell disease.

SICKLE CELL DISEASE

Epidemiology

Sickle cell disease was first recognized in West Africa. The high prevalence of HbS in this region likely represents a survival benefit since the presence of sickle cell trait protects against malaria. Nowadays, sickle cell disease is a worldwide health problem because HbS has spread throughout Africa, around the Mediterranean, to the Middle East and India, as well as to the Caribbean, North America, and Northern Europe. The prevalence of the sickle cell gene is approximately 8% in African Americans, around 25% in some areas in equatorial Africa, Greece, Saudi Arabia, and India, and even up to 50% in local West African areas.

Restriction enzyme techniques have identified several hemoglobin S haplotypes, mutations of the HbS molecule, which have probably arisen independently of each other. There are four major types in Africa – the Benin, Senegal, Cameroon, and Bantu (or Central African Republic) – and one Asian haplotype.

Pathogenesis
Genetics

Sickle cell disease comprises a group of heterogenous disorders that share the presence of the gene for HbS either homozygous (i.e., sickle cell anemia, HbSS) or double heterozygous (i.e., the combination of HbS with another abnormal hemoglobin)[1,2]. Sickle cell anemia is the most common form. The most common double heterozygous disorders are the combinations of hemoglobin S with hemoglobin C (HbSC) or β-thalassemia (HbS-thal). Subjects with the latter may also produce reduced amounts of normal β-chains (HbS-β+-thal), but not always (HbS-β0-thal). Subjects with a sickle cell trait or carrier state are heterozygous for hemoglobin S only.

Pathophysiology

The characteristic pathophysiologic feature in sickle cell disease is the episodic vaso-occlusive episodes, which can be triggered by several factors including infection, hypoxia, volume depletion, hypothermia, acidosis, and hyperosmolality. The common denominator is the occurrence of inflammation and/or cellular stress.

The two key processes in the pathophysiology of vaso-occlusion are adhesive interactions between the sickle red cells and the endothelium and the subsequent polymerization of HbS.

Sickle cell adherence

Sickle cells have enhanced adherence to the endothelium compared with that of normal red cells. This is further increased by endothelial cell activation, which may occur through stimulation by many infective and inflammatory agents, including proinflammatory cytokines such as tumor necrosis factor-α (TNF α), interleukin 1 β (IL-1 β) and interferon-γ (IFNγ). These induce the expression of cellular adhesion molecules on endothelial cells. In addition, inflammatory stress may induce a procoagulant state by increasing the release of von Willebrand factor, thrombospondin and other proteins

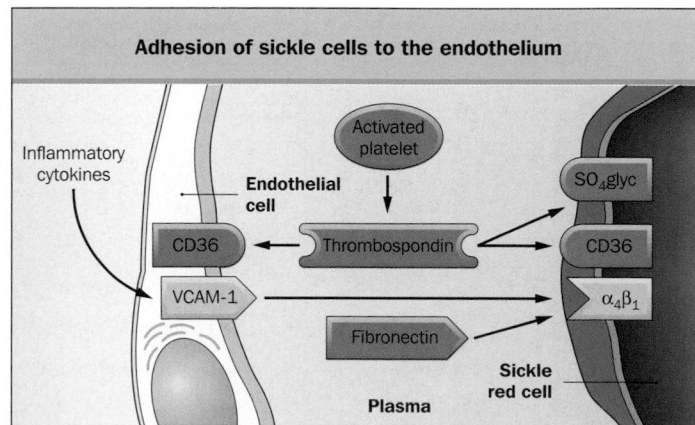

Figure 51.1 Principal interactions responsible for the adhesion of a sickle red cell to the microvascular endothelium. Thrombospondin acts as a bridging molecule by binding to CD36 on the surface of an endothelial cell and to CD36 or sulfated glycans (SO4glyc) on a sickle reticulocyte. Vascular cell adhesion molecule 1 (VCAM-1) on endothelial cells can bind directly to the $\alpha_4\beta_1$-integrin on the sickle reticulocyte. (Adapted with permission from Bunn[3].)

Hereditary and Congenital Diseases of the Kidney

which contribute to the adhesion process (Fig. 51.1). The adhesive interaction between sickle red cells and endothelium delays the capillary transit time, allowing polymerization of HbS and the sickling of red cells to occur.

Polymerization of HbS

When HbS polymerizes, the hemoglobin molecules adhere to each other and aggregate into chain-like formations[3].

Polymerization changes the shape of the red cell, increases its rigidity, and, thus, causes sickling of red cells (Fig. 51.2). Polymerization is a dynamic event and depends primarily on three independent variables: the degree of cellular hypoxia, the intracellular hemoglobin concentration, and the presence or absence of hemoglobin F (fetal hemoglobin)[3]. Deoxygenation of HbS causes a change in the conformation of the β-globin subunits that promotes the interaction of HbS molecules. The

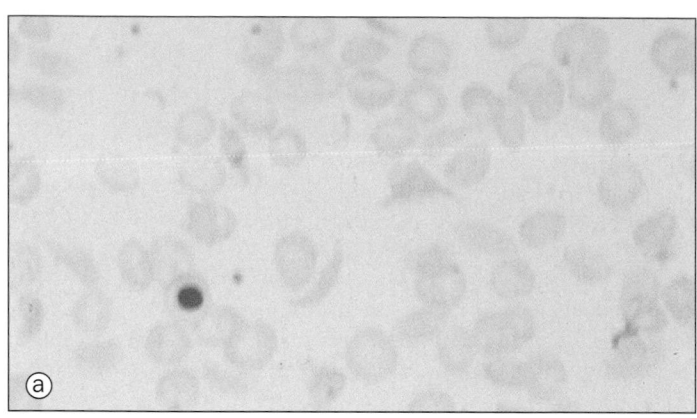

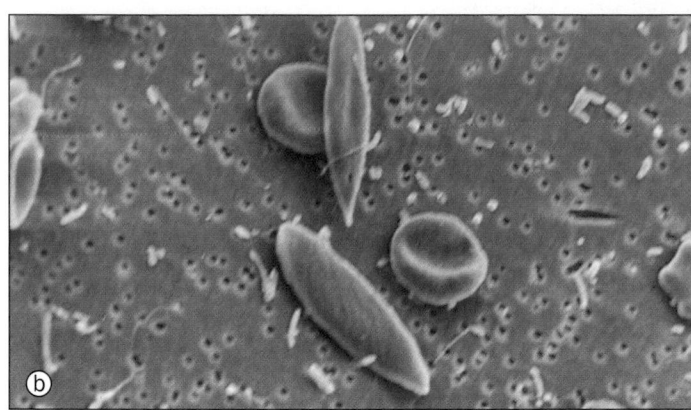

Figure 51.2 Sickle cells. (a) Characteristic sickle-shaped erythrocytes in peripheral blood film of a patient with homozygous sickle cell anemia. (b) Electron micrograph showing two normal and two sickle-shaped erythrocytes (Courtesy of Dr Sally C Davies).

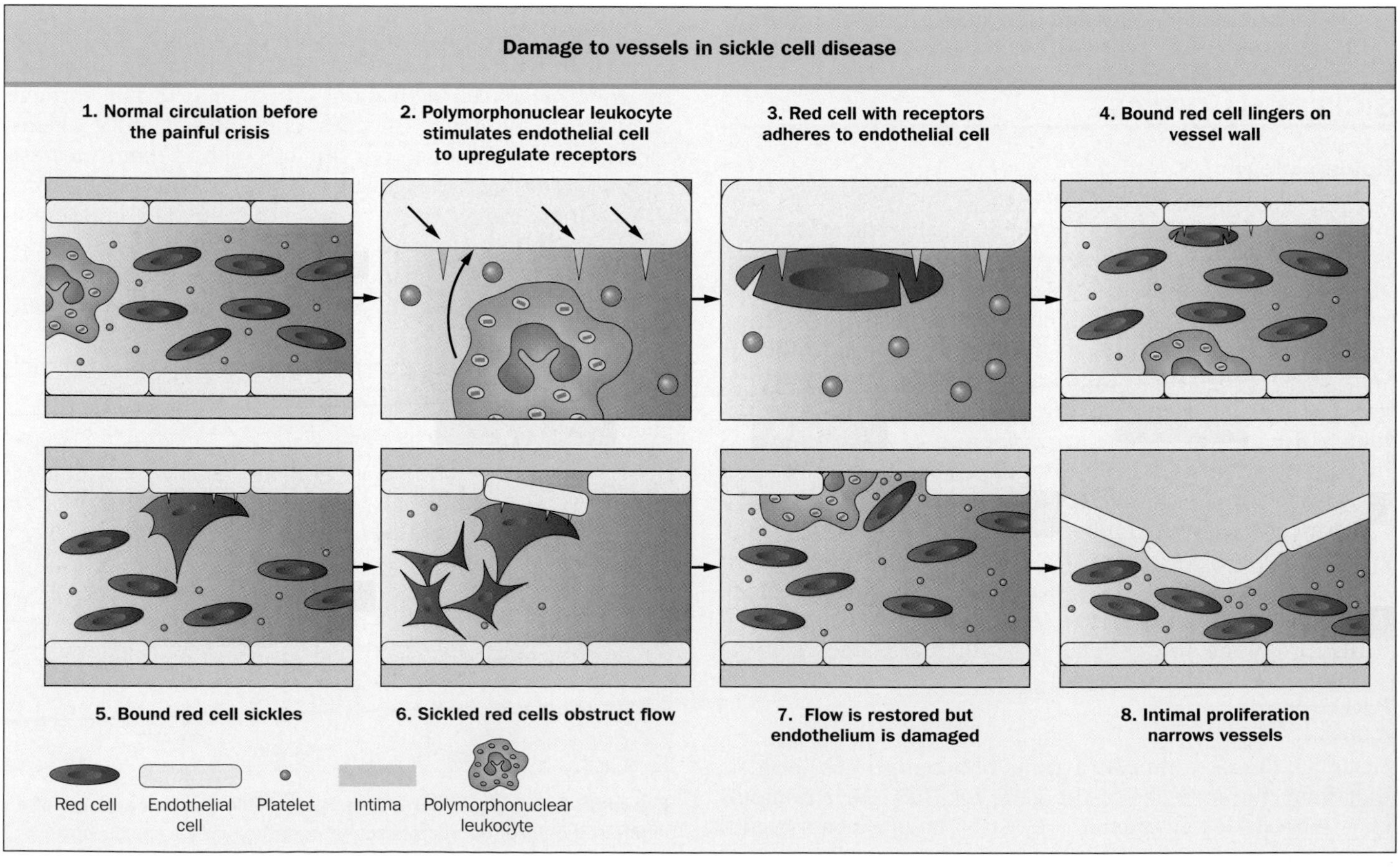

Damage to vessels in sickle cell disease

1. Normal circulation before the painful crisis

2. Polymorphonuclear leukocyte stimulates endothelial cell to upregulate receptors

3. Red cell with receptors adheres to endothelial cell

4. Bound red cell lingers on vessel wall

5. Bound red cell sickles

6. Sickled red cells obstruct flow

7. Flow is restored but endothelium is damaged

8. Intimal proliferation narrows vessels

Red cell   Endothelial cell   Platelet   Intima   Polymorphonuclear leukocyte

Figure 51.3 Possible pathophysiologic mechanisms of damage to vessels in sickle cell disease. Inflammation activates the endothelium and stimulates the upregulation of adhesion molecules and adherence of sickle cells to the endothelium. This promotes the sickling of red cells, increases the blood viscosity, and causes sludging in the microcirculation (eventually with microvascular thrombosis and infarction). After restoration of blood flow, vascular remodeling may contribute to persistent impairment of tissue blood flow. (Adapted with permission from Platt[4].)

intracellular hemoglobin concentration in red cells can increase through cellular dehydration caused by membrane transport lesions, especially activated potassium/chloride cotransport and calcium-activated potassium efflux. The presence of HbF decreases the polymerization tendency by reducing the concentration of HbS.

Possible mechanisms of vaso-occlusion and ensuing vessel damage are shown in Figure 51.3[4].

Clinical manifestations

The clinical manifestations of sickle cell disease show an individual and age-dependent variation (Fig. 51.4). A chronic low-grade hemolytic anemia always occurs and predisposes to gallstones. The most prevalent clinical problem is periodic crises of bone pain. During the first years of life, it presents as the hand–foot syndrome and in the course of life it can result in avascular necrosis of the heads of femur and humerus. Other important disabling problems are stroke resulting from occlusion of major cerebral vessels, the acute chest syndrome, priapism, and chronic leg ulceration.

Patients with sickle cell disease are prone to infections because of functional asplenia early in life as a result of splenic sequestration, recurrent splenic infarction, and consequent autosplenectomy. Ordinary bacterial infections can be fatal in these patients. Bacterial isolates during invasive bacterial infections show *S. pneumoniae* (38%), *Salmonella* species (33%), *H. influenzae* (14%), *E. coli* (11%) and *Klebsiella* species (4%)[5].

S. pneumoniae and *H. influenzae* occur predominantly before 5 years of age, *Salmonella* increases almost linearly with age, and *Klebsiella* and *E. coli* predominate in patients over 10 years of age. Pneumococcal infections carry a high morbidity and mortality in the early years of life, necessitating vaccination or prophylaxis[1].

Fever is a cause of concern in patients with sickle cell disease. Common complications accompanying fever are painful crisis and acute chest syndrome[6]. Bacteremia is not always confirmed. The cause of fever often remains unclear and is presumed to be of viral origin or related to infections due to atypical organisms. Nevertheless, early antibiotic treatment is recommended pending microbiologic information.

There are remarkable differences in clinical severity and outcome of disease. Sickle cell trait is a rather benign condition. Patients with HbSS tend to have a more severe disease than those with HbSC. Likewise, subjects with HbS- β+-thal do better than those with HbS-β0-thal. The Bantu haplotype is associated with the highest frequency of organ damage. However, the severity of disease may also differ among subjects with an identical genotype. In part, these differences can be explained by the amount of HbF present, since HbF may protect against clinical severity. In addition, endothelial factors probably play an important role. It has been shown that the degree of adherence between sickle red cells and endothelial cells correlates with the clinical severity of disease. Also, a relation has been found between circulating activated endothelial cells of microvascular origin and the onset of painful sickle cell crises[7].

Natural history

Life expectancy is reduced in sickle cell disease especially in subjects with symptomatic disease. In a prospective study of the clinical course of sickle cell disease, mortality resulted from overt organ failure, predominantly renal, in 18% of cases and from acute sickle crisis, presenting with pain, acute chest syndrome, or stroke, in 33% (Table 51.1)[8]. An increased risk of early death is associated with low levels of HbF, renal failure, the acute chest syndrome, and seizures.

Treatment

Management of sickle cell disease is primarily directed at the relief of symptoms and prevention of complications, whereas newer treatments are being devised that target the pathophysiology of the disease[9]. Daily oral penicillin among children from 2 or 3 years of age until 5 years of age is effective in reducing both the infection rate and the mortality related to pneumococcal infection[10]. Vaccination against pneumococcus is recommended for children at 2 years of age, with booster doses at 5 years of age[9], although protection from current vaccines is imperfect. Empiric antibiotic treatment of choice in adults with fever is amoxicillin (amoxycillin).

Sickle cell crises are managed with oxygen therapy, red cell transfusions, and analgesia.

SICKLE CELL NEPHROPATHY

Pathogenesis

The hallmark of sickle cell nephropathy is the combination of an impaired renal concentrating capacity with a normal diluting capacity[11,12].

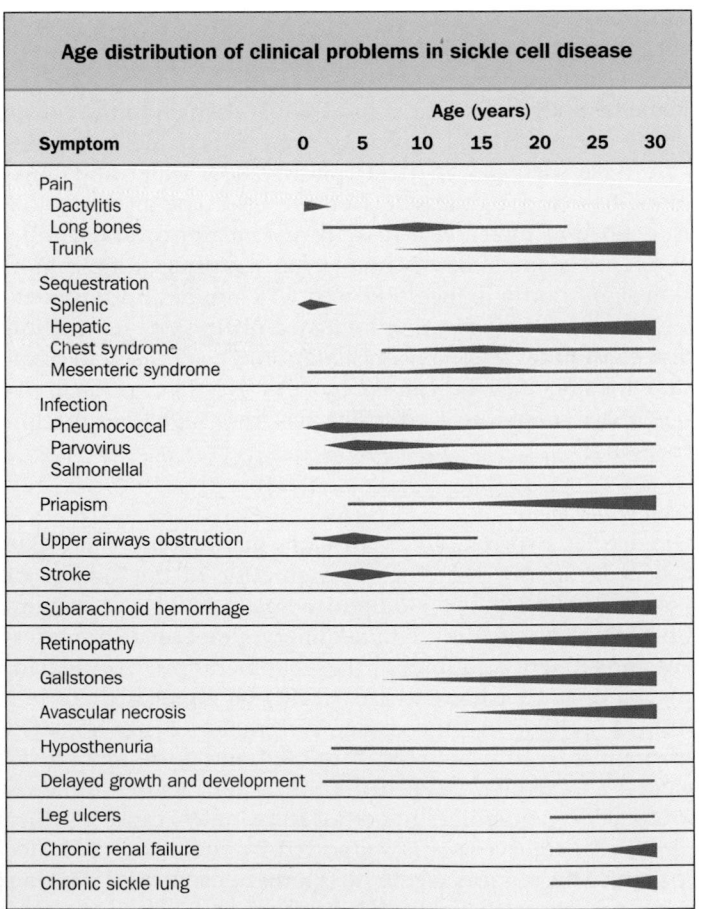

Figure 51.4 Age distribution of clinical problems in sickle cell disease. (Adapted with permission from Davies and Oni[1].)

Hereditary and Congenital Diseases of the Kidney

Causes of death in sickle cell disease	
Circumstances of death	No of patients
Patients without evidence of chronic renal failure, heart failure or chronic debilitating stroke	
Pain episode	45
Chest syndrome	9
Stroke	15
Infection	13
Perioperative death	14
Cancer	4
Gastrointestinal bleeding	3
Suddenly at home	10
Trauma	14
Miscellaneous	7
Circumstances not known	37
Patients with clinically diagnosed chronic organ failure	
Chronic renal failure	22
Chronic congestive heart failure	11
Chronic debilitating stroke	5

Circumstances of death in 209 patients with sickle cell disease who were 20 years of age or older at the time of death. (Adapted with permission from Platt et al.[8].)

Table 51.1 Causes of death in sickle cell disease.

Concentrating capacity

The defect in concentrating capacity results from loss of the countercurrent exchange mechanism in the inner renal medulla through loss of the vasa recta and long loops of Henle of the juxtamedullary nephrons (Fig. 51.5). The vasa recta of the juxtamedullary nephrons present an ideal setting for the sickling of red cells. The renal medulla is relatively hypoxic and hyperosmotic, the blood viscosity is increased in the medullary circulation, and medullary blood flow is slow. Studies in transgenic sickle cell mice have demonstrated distension and congestion of the vasa recta under hypoxic conditions. This environment facilitates the sickling of erythrocytes, formation of intravascular microthrombi, and obstruction of blood flow through the vasa recta. The loss of vasa recta has been confirmed by microradioangiographic studies (Fig. 51.6)[13]. Histologic examination of the medulla shows edema, focal scarring, and interstitial fibrosis resulting in tubular atrophy. Ischemic infarction in the vasa recta sometimes causes papillary necrosis. The concentration defect is found to be reversible in young children when sickling is prevented after multiple transfusions of normal blood, but it becomes irreversible thereafter. Adults with sickle cell anemia cannot concentrate the urine above 450 mmol/kg H_2O. This relates to the interstitial osmolality at the transition of the outer and inner medulla, at the tips of the short loops of Henle of the cortical nephrons. Subjects with sickle cell trait or hybrid sickling disorders show intermediate concentrating defects. Maximal osmolality varies from 400 to 900 mmol/kg H_2O in sickle cell trait and from 400 to 700 mmol/kg H_2O in HbSC, further declining with aging.

Diluting capacity

The diluting capacity is normal as a result of the intact reabsorptive function of the superficial loops of Henle of the cortical nephrons. These are supplied by peritubular capillaries, which present a less ideal setting for the sickling of red cells than the vasa recta. In contrast to the diluting capacity, the free water reabsorption, or capacity to generate negative free water balance, is impaired by defective trapping of solute in the inner medulla.

Other tubular abnormalities

Defects in urinary acidification and potassium excretion are other distal nephron function abnormalities[14]. These may only become overt when there is an increased supply of acid and potassium, for example during rhabdomyolysis. The exact causes of these defects are unknown, but they likely reflect failure to maintain the necessary energy-requiring hydrogen ion and electrochemical gradients along the collecting ducts owing to the impaired medullary blood flow and hypoxia. The impaired potassium excretion is aldosterone independent.

In contrast to the functional abnormalities of the distal nephron, proximal tubular function is enhanced. Reabsorption of phosphate and β_2-microglobin and secretion of uric acid and creatinine in the proximal tubule are increased. Therefore, creatinine clearance overestimates glomerular filtration rate (GFR) considerably. The cause of the enhanced proximal function is not clear, but it probably represents a secondary compensatory mechanism to correct for defects in medullary function.

Renal hemodynamics

Renal hemodynamics show remarkable changes in the course of the disease (Fig. 51.7). Young subjects with sickle cell disease have increases in renal plasma flow (RPF) and renal blood flow and, to a lesser extent, in GFR. The increased RPF is ascribed to increased release of vasodilator prostaglandins as a result of medullary ischemia, since prostaglandin inhibition significantly reduces RPF and GFR. Studies in transgenic sickle cell mice suggest that increased nitric oxide production also contributes to renal vasodilatation. The decrease in filtration fraction may be caused by selective damage of juxtamedullary nephrons, which have the highest filtration fractions.

Glomerular injury

Glomerular hypertrophy is an early manifestation of sickle cell nephropathy. Histologic examination of the kidneys of young children shows glomerular enlargement and congestion, especially in the juxtamedullary glomeruli. Both afferent and efferent arterioles of these glomeruli may be dilated. In young adult patients with sickle cell anemia, there is a distinct pattern of glomerular dysfunction, with impaired glomerular permselectivity, increased ultrafiltration coefficient, glomerular hyperfiltration, and proteinuria[15,16]. Prolonged glomerular hyperfiltration may cause further glomerular injury. This is supported by the common histologic finding of focal segmental glomerulosclerosis (FSGS) in adult patients with sickle cell disease (Fig. 51.8)[17]. Two consecutive patterns of FSGS have been described: a 'collapsing'

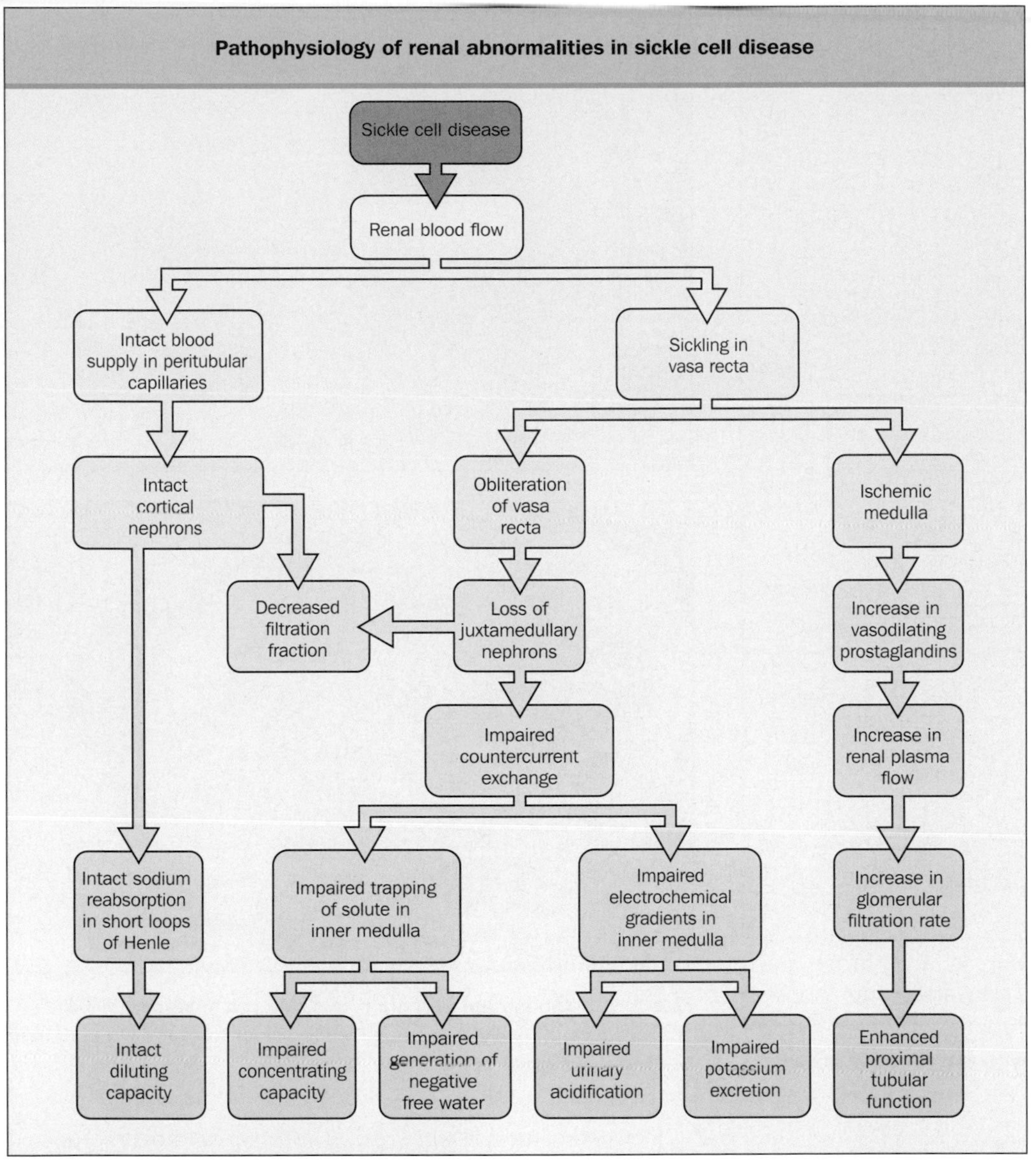

Pathophysiology of renal abnormalities in sickle cell disease

```
                    Sickle cell disease
                            │
                            ▼
                     Renal blood flow
                    ┌───────┴───────┐
                    ▼               ▼
           Intact blood         Sickling in
           supply in peritubular  vasa recta
           capillaries      ┌───────┼───────────┐
                    │       ▼       ▼           ▼
                    ▼   Obliteration      Ischemic
              Intact    of vasa          medulla
              cortical  recta                │
              nephrons     │                 ▼
                 │ │       ▼            Increase in
                 │ │   Loss of         vasodilating
                 │ └─► juxtamedullary  prostaglandins
                 │     nephrons             │
                 │   Decreased              ▼
                 │   filtration ◄──         Increase in
                 │   fraction              renal plasma
                 │         │                flow
                 │         ▼                   │
                 │    Impaired                 ▼
                 │    countercurrent      Increase in
                 │    exchange            glomerular
                 │     ┌────┴────┐        filtration rate
                 │     ▼         ▼             │
                 ▼                             ▼
           Intact sodium  Impaired    Impaired      Increase in
           reabsorption   trapping    electrochemical  glomerular
           in short loops of solute   gradients in    filtration rate
           of Henle       in inner    inner medulla
              │           medulla
              ▼            │ │         │ │             │
           Intact        ▼  ▼         ▼  ▼            ▼
           diluting  Impaired Impaired Impaired Impaired  Enhanced
           capacity  concen-  genera-  urinary  potassium proximal
                     trating  tion of  acidifi- excretion tubular
                     capacity negative cation             function
                              free
                              water
```

Figure 51.5 Pathophysiology of renal abnormalities in sickle cell disease.

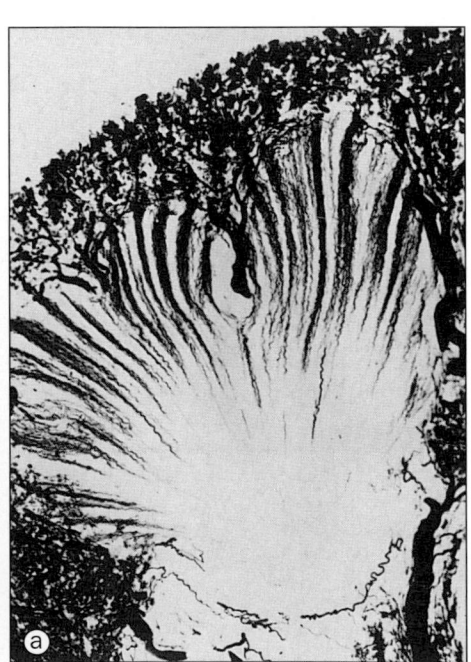
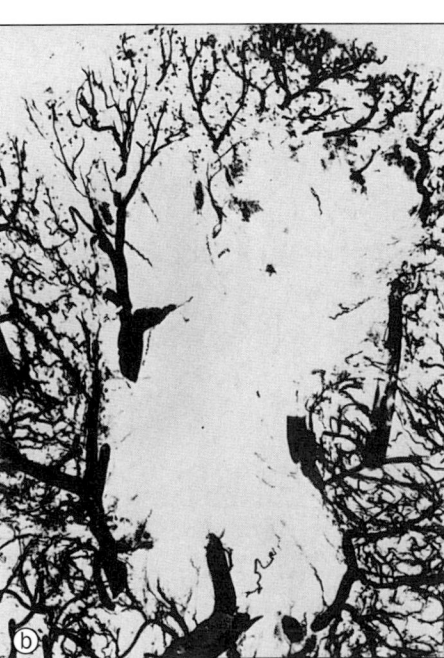

Figure 51.6 Microradioangiography showing loss of vasa recta in sickle cell nephropathy. (a) Kidney from a control subject, showing normal vasa recta. (b) A patient with sickle cell anemia, with the absence of the vasa recta. (Adapted with permission from Statius van Eps et al.[13].)

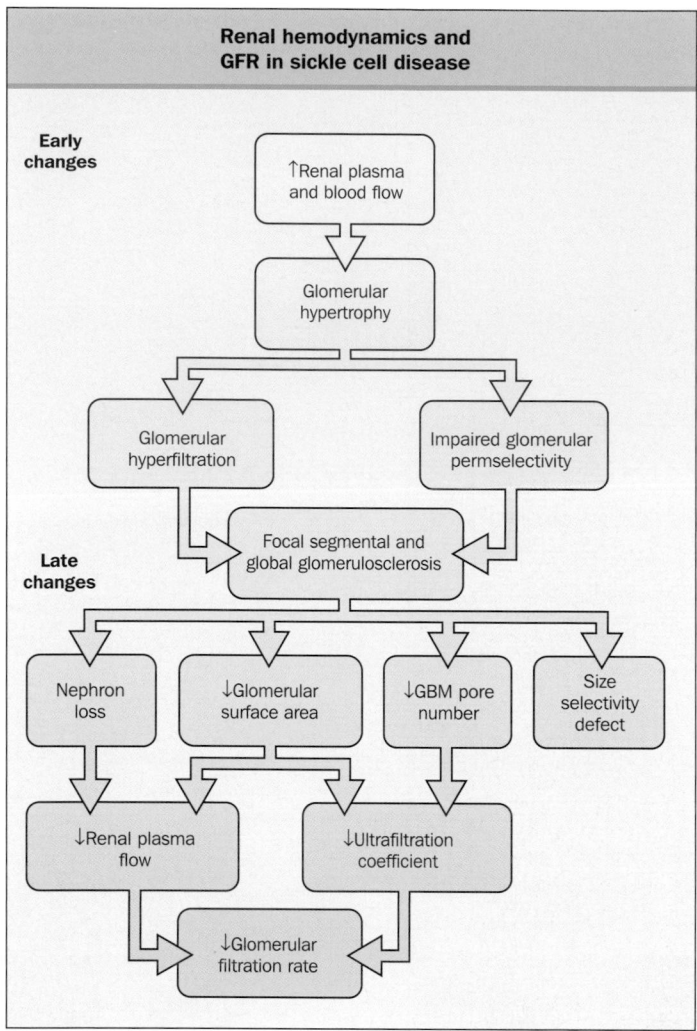

Figure 51.7 Renal hemodynamics and glomerular filtration in sickle cell nephropathy.

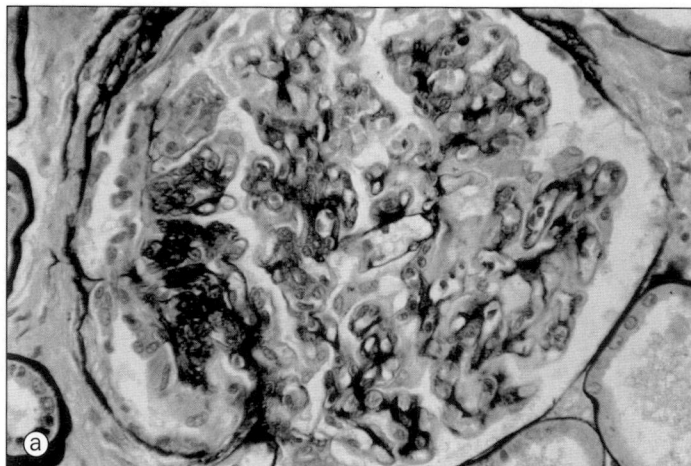

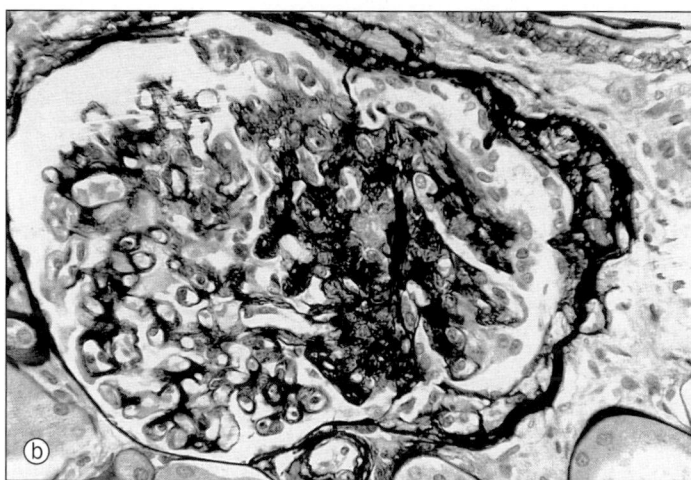

Figure 51.8 Glomerular pathology in sickle cell nephropathy. Mild (a) and moderate (b) perihilar focal segmental glomerulosclerosis. (Courtesy of Dr Charles Jennette.)

and an 'expansive' pattern[18]. The initial 'collapsing' pattern has been attributed to progressive obliteration of glomerular capillaries by red blood cell sickling in maximally hypertrophied glomeruli. The 'expansive' pattern is characterized by an expansive sclerosis with increased mesangial matrix and further capillary obliteration; it is ascribed to sustained or increasing hyperfiltration[18].

In older subjects, progressive ischemia and fibrosis with obliteration of glomeruli can be found. Glomerular function studies show a decrease in glomerular basement membrane pore number and a size selectivity defect in subjects with renal insufficiency[19]. Ultimately, a combined decrease in ultrafiltration capacity and RPF can result in end-stage renal disease (ESRD)[15].

Hormones in sickle cell nephropathy

There is relative *erythropoietin* deficiency in sickle cell disease i.e., erythropoietin levels do not increase to the expected level for the degree of anemia, perhaps due to the right-shifted hemoglobin-oxygen dissociation curve. In addition, erythropoietin levels fall with the decline in renal function, probably as a result of renal damage due to the sickling process.

Elevated values of *renin* and *aldosterone* have been reported in some studies, both under standard and volume-depleted conditions, although in general normal values are found in sickle cell anemia[11].

Hormone-infusion studies have helped to localize sites of action in the kidney. Failure of low-dose infusion of *atrial natriuretic peptide [ANP]* to increase natriuresis in sickle cell anemia[20], suggests that ANP at this dosage exerts its natriuretic effect in the long loops of Henle of the juxtamedullary nephrons. Whereas, *insulin* induces a similar sodium retention in patients with sickle cell anemia and normal subjects[20], suggesting its antinatriuretic effect is probably localized at a distal tubular site other than the long loops of Henle.

CLINICAL MANIFESTATIONS OF SICKLE CELL NEPHROPATHY

The presentation of the clinical manifestations of sickle cell nephropathy shows an age-dependent pattern. The frequency and etiology of the renal abnormalities associated with sickle cell anemia, sickle cell trait and the most common double heterozygous disorders (HbSC and HbS-thal) are listed in Table 51.2).

Type of renal disease	Frequencies in subsets of sickle cell disease			Etiology
	Sickle cell anemia	Sickle cell trait	HbSC and HbS-thal	
Impaired concentrating capacity	Irreversible defects in all adults	Intermediate defects in all adults nephrons	Intermediate defects in all adults	Loss of vasa recta of juxtamedullary
Impaired urinary acidification	Almost all, during acid loading	Rare	At least 30%, during acid loading	Incomplete form of distal renal tubular acidosis
Impaired potassium excretion	Almost all, during potassium loading	Rare	Unknown; probably at least 30%	Aldosterone-independent
Hematuria	Common	3–4%	Common	Infarction, extravasation of blood in renal medulla
Proteinuria	Up to 50–60% with increasing age	Rare	20–25%	Glomerular hyperfiltration + impaired permselectivity
Nephrotic syndrome	Approximately 4%	Rare	0–4%	FSGS most common
Chronic renal failure	4.2–4.6%	Rare	~ 2.4%	See Figure 51.7
Renal carcinoma	Rare	Absolutely rare, relatively frequent	Rare	Possible genetic predisposition

Table 51.2 Frequencies and etiology of renal abnormalities associated with sickle cell disease.

Hematuria

Hematuria is a common clinical manifestation in sickle cell anemia and the hybrid sickling disorders and occurs in 3–4% of subjects with sickle cell trait at some time. There is often persistent microscopic hematuria with episodic gross hematuria. The hematuria may follow relatively minor trauma. Hematuria occurs more often in males and is usually unilateral, originating from the left kidney in 80% of patients.

Pathogenesis
Sickling
The main mechanism of hematuria probably relates to the sickling of erythrocytes in the vasa recta and microthrombotic infarction and extravasation of blood in the renal medulla. Histologic examination typically shows severe stasis in peritubular capillaries of the cortex and, especially, the medulla, and extravasation of blood into the collecting system.

Papillary necrosis
Papillary necrosis is a frequent cause of hematuria in sickle cell anemia, hybrid sickling disorders, and sickle cell trait (Fig. 51.9). The incidence of papillary necrosis varies from 23–67% in several studies of selected patients with sickle cell disease[21]. This complication results from obliteration of vasa recta, with medullary necrosis and fibrosis. The large analgesic consumption by these patients because of their bone pain may also contribute to papillary necrosis. The most common presenting symptom is painless macroscopic hematuria. Other presentations are renal colic caused by the passage of blood clots or necrotic papillae, microscopic hematuria, symptoms of urinary tract infection, and, rarely, acute renal failure. Papillary necrosis may also be asymptomatic and it is frequently an incidental finding during radiography.

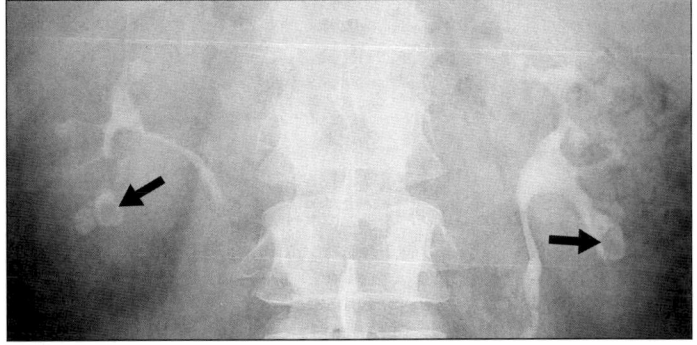

Figure 51.9 Papillary necrosis in sickle cell disease. Intravenous urography shows abnormal calyces with filling defects (arrows).

Nutcracker phenomenon
The left-sided predominance of hematuria has been attributed to the so-called nutcracker phenomenon, compression of the left renal vein between the aorta and the superior mesenteric artery, thereby increasing the pressure in the renal vein. This may especially contribute to the development of hematuria in sickle cell patients, because the increased renal vein pressure could lead to a relatively increased anoxia in the renal medulla, thereby increasing the likelihood of sickling in the left kidney.

Clinical manifestations
Painless macroscopic hematuria often presents after physical activity or minor renal trauma or is associated with hypoxic challenges, for example airplane flights. It usually is accompanied by a substantial fall in hematocrit. Bleeding typically remits spontaneously within a few days.

Hereditary and Congenital Diseases of the Kidney

Diagnosis and differential diagnosis

Urinalysis can exclude the presence of myoglobinuria and rhabdomyolysis, which can mimic hematuria. Rhabdomyolysis can be provoked during strenuous exercise and dehydration and may also occur during severe sickle cell crises. The coexistence of hematuria with leukocyturia or pyuria is not unusual and does not necessarily indicate a urinary tract infection, even in combination with flank pain. Infection must be confirmed by examination of the urinary sediment and urine cultures.

The presence of HbS has been reported in 50% of African American with ESRD caused by autosomal dominant polycystic kidney disease (ADPKD), whereas HbS was present in only 7.5% of African American patients with other causes of ESRD. In addition, patients with ADPKD and HbS had an earlier onset of ESRD[22].

Recently, renal medullary carcinoma has been recognized as a specific entity in sickle cell nephropathy[23-25]. It is a very aggressive form of renal cell carcinoma that appears to uniquely affect patients with sickle cell trait or HbSC, especially occurring in teenagers and young adults. The tumors tend to be metastatic at the time of diagnosis, with a reported mean survival from the time of surgery of only 15 weeks. The tumors are resistant to chemotherapy. Possibly, only early recognition may improve prognosis. One should consider hematuria as a potentially ominous harbinger of malignancy, particularly in young patients with sickle cell trait.

An additional work-up is indicated for patients with severe or prolonged hematuria, which is resistant to conservative therapeutic measures.

Ultrasound examination will be normal unless there is papillary necrosis or a coincidental cause of hematuria such as polycystic kidney disease, renal calculus, or tumor. Intravenous urography used to be the method of choice to diagnose papillary necrosis but may provide confounding information because blood clots in the renal pelvis may cause radiocontrast translucencies resembling neoplasm, calculus, or hemangioma. Ultrasound is, therefore, preferred.

The presence of von Willebrand's disease has occasionally been described in subjects with sickle cell trait and gross hematuria.

Cystoscopy is not routinely required but is indicated if the episode of hematuria is atypical: for example, a first episode of macroscopic hematuria in a patient over the age of 40 years or an episode that persists for more than 2 weeks. Cystoscopy may also be required to lateralize the source of the bleeding if surgical intervention is considered (see below).

Renal arteriography only rarely identifies the bleeding source, but when it does so, can be followed by embolization. However, the optimal approach in any institution depends on local experience with specific investigations.

Treatment

The therapeutic strategy for hematuria depends on the severity and duration of a specific bleeding episode. Bleeding will stop in most patients spontaneously or after a period of bed rest, although it may occasionally last for weeks or months. Approximately half of the patients will have recurrent episodes.

Initial therapeutic measures include bed rest and interventions aimed at retardation of the sickling process in the anoxic renal medulla. A high urine flow rate should be induced by intravenous fluid administration and diuretics (to further reduce medullary tonicity especially in subjects with sickle cell trait) and the urine alkalinized by administration of sodium bicarbonate by mouth or by vein, with a target of urine pH 8. Blood transfusion with normal HbA is indicated if anemia becomes severe; this may also decrease the sickling process. If necessary, bladder irrigation is performed for removal of blood clots.

Hyperbaric oxygen therapy may be helpful but has not been formally evaluated. Irrigation of the pelvicalyceal system with silver nitrate has also been described. The antifibrinolytic agent, ε-aminocaproic acid, may be effective, but unfortunately will sometimes lead to the formation of large blood clots and obstruction in the urinary collecting system. Therefore, this therapy should be used with care, starting at a low dose, $1 \text{ g}/1.73 \text{ m}^2$ body surface area orally, 3 times daily, increasingly cautiously until the bleeding subsides.

Unilateral nephrectomy has occasionally been necessary in patients with persistent, life-threatening hematuria refractory to a conservative approach. Full evaluation for another cause of hematuria, including cystoscopy to exclude a bladder lesion and to establish which kidney is the source of bleeding, is required before proceeding with nephrectomy.

Urinary tract infection

Subjects with sickle cell disease have an increased susceptibility to bacterial infections; even low-grade bacteremia with a common organism may be fatal. In addition to the impaired immunity that is a consequence of autosplenectomy, there is opsonic antibody deficiency, which predisposes to bacterial infections. The relative incidence of urinary tract infections is not exactly known. However, the incidence of asymptomatic bacteriuria during pregnancy and the puerperium appears to be twice as high in women with sickle cell disease or trait than in women without sickle cell disease and requires appropriate therapy (see Chapter 44).

Pyelonephritis and urosepsis, like any other infection, may precipitate a sickle cell crisis. One should especially be aware of this possibility in young children, who often do not complain of urinary tract symptoms. Most common organisms isolated include *Escherichia coli*, *Klebsiella* spp., and other Gram-negative Enterobacteriaceae. Invasive bacterial infections with *E. coli* occur especially in females after the age of 15 years suggesting a greater chance of urinary tract infections in relation to sexual activity[5].

Acute renal failure

Acute renal failure (ARF) defined as a doubling of serum creatinine, has been reported in 10.3% of patients hospitalized with sickle cell anemia[26].

Etiology

A prerenal cause of ARF will be found in more than half of patients, especially volume depletion in the setting of sickle cell crisis. Patients with sickle cell disease are prone to ARF caused by volume depletion because of impaired urine-concentrating capacity; it is therefore typically nonoliguric. A less frequent prerenal cause is congestive heart failure.

Typical intrinsic renal causes of ARF are rhabdomyolysis, sepsis, and drug nephrotoxicity. Less common are renal vein thrombosis and the hepatorenal syndrome (caused by hemosiderosis-induced hepatic failure). Both exertional and nontraumatic rhabdomyolysis have been reported in patients with sickle cell disease. The latter especially occurs during a sickle cell crisis and has been ascribed to intravascular sickling and muscle ischemia. Rhabdomyolysis is a common finding in patients who develop multiorgan failure during severe sickle cell crises, in addition to the acute chest syndrome, which further contributes to ARF.

The most typical postrenal cause of ARF is urinary tract obstruction by necrotic papillae or blood clots.

Treatment

Treatment and recovery of renal function depends on the specific underlying pathology. Metabolic acidosis may be prominent and should be actively corrected with sodium bicarbonate. Patients with volume depletion have a favorable outcome after fluid replacement[26]. Renal function may recover in the patients with sepsis and rhabdomyolysis, although temporary renal function replacement therapy may be necessary. ARF as a part of multiorgan failure during a severe sickle cell crisis may show a dramatic improvement with aggressive red cell transfusion therapy, although some renal function loss may persist.

Proteinuria and the nephrotic syndrome

Proteinuria has been reported in 17–33% of subjects with sickle cell disease in several studies using semiquantitative or dipstick measurements. The prevalence of proteinuria is lower in subjects with coinheritance of sickle cell anemia and α-thalassemia than in those with sickle cell anemia and intact α-globin genes (13 versus 40%)[27]. The 'renoprotective' effect of α-globin gene microdeletions could be related to a lower mean corpuscular volume or lower erythrocyte hemoglobin concentration in these sickle erythrocytes. The frequency of proteinuria increases with age (56% in subjects ≥ 40 years[28]) and its presence is associated with renal impairment.

The nephrotic syndrome has been estimated to occur in 4% of patients with sickle cell anemia[29]. The eventual development of renal failure appears virtually inevitable once the patient has nephrotic syndrome.

Pathology

The most common pathologic lesion is FSGS[17,18], which is also the major lesion in the subjects who develop renal failure. Another specific pathologic lesion is a form of membranoproliferative glomerulonephritis (MPGN) with mesangial expansion and basement membrane duplication[2]. The general absence of immune complexes and electron-dense deposits discriminates this entity from idiopathic MPGN. It has been proposed that this form of MPGN is caused by intracapillary red cell fragmentation. Fragments of red cells become lodged in isolated capillary loops and are continuously phagocytosed by mesangial cells. As a result the mesangium expands and lays down new basement membrane material[14,29].

Patients may become hepatitis C positive from multiple blood transfusions, which may also be associated with MPGN. Occasionally, other causes have been reported, such as poststreptococcal glomerulonephritis, minimal change disease, and immune complex-mediated glomerulonephritis. Glomerulonephritis has also been described in association with aplastic crises in parvovirus infection[30]. Renal vein thrombosis should be considered when nephrotic syndrome develops in sickle cell disease, but its incidence is not exactly known.

Treatment

Theoretically, dietary protein restriction may reduce hyperfiltration and retard the development of renal failure in those with FSGS, but this has not been evaluated specifically in sickle cell disease.

Short-term treatment with angiotensin-converting enzyme (ACE) inhibitors significantly reduces the degree of proteinuria without affecting blood pressure or renal hemodynamics[17]. More prolonged ACE inhibition reduces proteinuria with a slight decrease in blood pressure[31]. However, it remains to be established whether long-term treatment with ACE inhibitors *or angiotensin II receptor antagonist* delay the development of progressive renal failure.

Prevention of hyperfiltration can, theoretically, also be obtained with nonsteroidal anti-inflammatory drugs (NSAIDs), but these drugs reduce RPF and GFR in sickle cell anemia[11] and are not recommended.

Sodium and acid–base disturbances
Distal tubular function

Distal tubular function abnormalities are impaired potassium excretion and impaired urinary acidification caused by an incomplete form of distal tubular acidosis. However, hyperkalemia and metabolic acidosis are not present under normal circumstances and may only become manifest during potassium or acid loading, with mild renal insufficiency or volume depletion, and during rhabdomyolysis[11,12]. Hyperkalemia may also develop more readily during treatment with NSAIDs, ACE inhibitors, β-blockers, potassium-sparing diuretics, or heparin.

Urine pH does not fall below 5 during acid-loading tests unless maximal acidifying stimuli are used. The titratable acid and hydrogen ion excretion is reduced, whereas the ammonium excretion is either normal or decreased. Metabolic acidosis developing during renal insufficiency or intercurrent diseases in sickle cell disease requires active treatment with sodium bicarbonate because acidosis stimulates the sickling process. Plasma bicarbonate should be monitored routinely and oral sodium bicarbonate supplements given to keep it within the reference range.

Proximal tubular function

Proximal tubular function abnormalities modify solute handling, producing increased reabsorption of phosphate and increased secretion of uric acid. Hyperphosphatemia may develop easily when renal function declines, necessitating dietary phosphate restriction and the use of phosphate binders early in renal insufficiency. The increased uric acid secretion protects patients with sickle cell disease against the increased uric acid production resulting from hemolysis. However, the incidence of hyperuricemia and risk of gout increases with age as renal function declines.

Hypertension
Epidemiology
The prevalence of hypertension in patients with sickle cell anemia is approximately 2–6%, which is significantly lower than in age- and sex-matched control subjects[11,32]. However, blood pressure levels in patients with sickle cell anemia are higher than in matched subjects with β-thalassemia and similar levels of anemia. Hypertension in sickle cell anemia especially occurs in the presence of advanced renal failure.

Pathogenesis
It is not yet clear whether this relative hypotension compared with control subjects relates to the pathologic renal medullary condition in sickle cell disease or to other mechanisms. The kidney in sickle cell disease has a normal overall capacity for sodium conservation, despite a tendency to lose sodium and water through the medullary defect[11,32]. This sodium conservation in sickle cell disease may follow stimulation of the renin–angiotensin–aldosterone system, which has been described in some but not all studies. The relative hypotension may be related to general vasodilatation because skeletal vascular resistance is reduced in sickle cell patients. Increased production of vasodilatory prostaglandins or nitric oxide may be involved. Systemic vasodilatation and increased flow is a compensatory mechanism for microcirculatory flow disturbances and intermittent microvascular occlusion[33]. Finally, reduced vascular reactivity has been demonstrated in sickle cell patients and may protect against blood pressure elevation[32].

Treatment
The antihypertensive treatment of choice is an ACE inhibitor, because of the potential beneficial effects on the progression of proteinuria and renal failure, and because of the reported increments in plasma renin activity. However, the risk of hyperkalemia is increased.

An alternative therapeutic option is a calcium channel blocker, but it is not yet known whether these drugs reduce proteinuria in sickle cell disease. Loop diuretics are less effective in patients with sickle cell disease because of the specific medullary defect.

Chronic renal failure
Epidemiology
In a prospective, 25-year longitudinal study, chronic renal failure (CRF) developed in 4.2% of 725 patients with sickle cell anemia and in 2.4% of 209 patients with HbSC[34]. The patients with sickle cell anemia were much younger at the time of the diagnosis of renal failure than those with HbSC (median age 23.1 and 49.9 years, respectively). However, in another study in 368 patients with sickle cell anemia with an overall prevalence of CRF of 4.6%, the prevalence of CRF clearly increased with age[28]. Probably, the prevalence of CRF will increase even more in the future with further improved medical care and longer life expectancy.

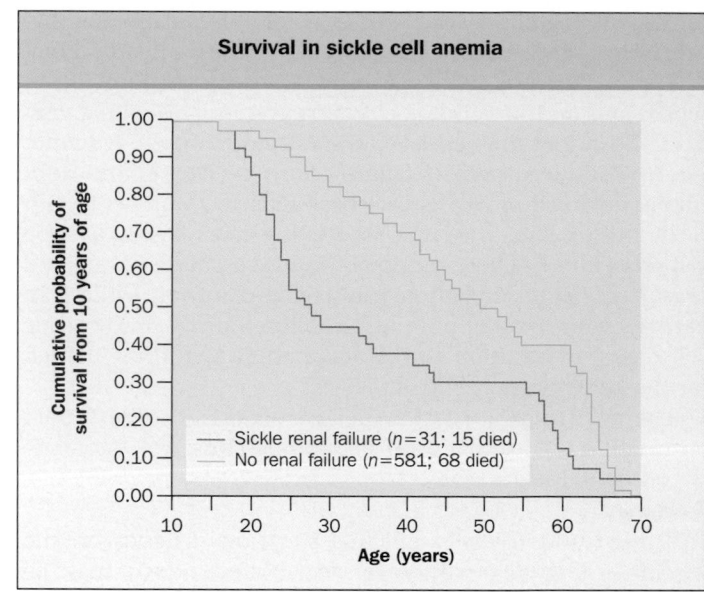

Figure 51.10 Survival in sickle cell anemia in the presence and absence of renal failure. (Adapted with permission from Powars et al[34].)

Predictors of CRF are hypertension, proteinuria, hematuria, increasingly severe anemia, the nephrotic syndrome, and inheritance of the Bantu, or Central African Republic, β-globin gene cluster haplotype[34]. Apart from an apparent genetic predisposition, the presence of glomerular capillary hypertension and prolonged glomerular hyperfiltration seem to be very important in the development of renal failure.

Natural history
Patients with sickle cell anemia and CRF have an increased mortality compared to patients without renal failure (Fig. 51.10). Median survival in sickle cell anemia from the diagnosis of CRF, despite dialysis, was only 4 years, despite renal replacement therapy, and the median age at the time of death was 27 years[34]. The patients with renal failure were also prone to other manifestations of sickle-induced vasculopathy and nonrenal organ failure, such as cerebrovascular accidents, chronic restrictive lung disease, and leg ulcers.

Treatment
To delay the development of progressive renal failure, it is important to control hypertension and to avoid the use of nephrotoxic drugs, especially NSAIDs. Although plausible, it remains to be established whether the reduction of the degree of proteinuria with either ACE inhibitors or a low protein diet retards the progression of renal failure.

The response to erythropoietin therapy is poor, even when high doses are used over long treatment periods[35]. Erythropoietin treatment predominantly results in the release of hemoglobin S containing reticulocytes, with only a modest increase in the more stable hemoglobin F. A marked increase in hemoglobin levels, although unexpected, may precipitate sickle cell crisis. Routine use of erythropoietin is therefore not recommended, but it can be tried on an individual basis with higher doses than needed in other forms of ESRD. As an alternative, supportive red cell transfusion may be given regularly to these subjects. Excessive iron accumulation should be prevented in patients undergoing regular transfusions, who are at risk for hemochromatosis, although organ dysfunction caused by tissue iron overload seems less predictable in sickle cell disease than in thalassemia major. Metabolic acidosis is also prominent and requires correction with sodium bicarbonate supplements.

ESRD in sickle cell disease has been treated successfully with hemodialysis, peritoneal dialysis, and transplantation. So far, hemodialysis has been used relatively more frequently than peritoneal dialysis in patients with sickle cell disease. Sickle cell crises are not common despite the potential for hypotension, hypoxemia, and cytokine release during hemodialysis. The 30-month survival of a group of 77 patients who were predominantly treated with hemodialysis was 59%, a figure comparable to the survival rates in other groups of patients with multisystem disorders receiving dialysis.

TRANSPLANTATION

Renal transplantation is an appropriate form of renal replacement therapy for those with sickle cell nephropathy who develop ESRD. After kidney transplantation, 1- and 3-year patient survivals are 90.5 and 75.0%, respectively; 1- and 3-year graft survivals are 82.5 and 53.8%, respectively[36]. These outcomes compare unfavorably to kidney transplantation for most other patient groups. Compared with other transplant patients, the adjusted mortality risk in transplanted patients with sickle cell disease is higher at 1 year (RR = 2.95) and at 3 years (RR = 2.82)[37]. Nevertheless, transplantation likely confers a survival advantage in patients with sickle cell disease; there is a trend toward improved survival in transplant recipients compared to dialysis-treated patients with sickle cell disease on the transplant waiting list[37].

In sickle cell disease, perioperative risks such as severe crisis and massive sickling can be reduced by preoperative transfusions of normal blood, thereby reducing the proportion of HbS. After transplantation, hematocrit values increase and are even higher than in patients with sickle cell disease and normal renal function. Sickle cell crisis may occur after transplantation but it is not yet clear whether the increase in hematocrit values enhances the risk of a crisis. Standard immunosuppressive therapy does not increase the risk of sickle cell crisis. However, caution is warranted with the use of antilymphocyte antibodies because the onset of a crisis has been related to this therapy in a few patients, perhaps as a consequence of increased cytokine release. Occasionally, the recurrence of hyposthenuria and sickle cell nephropathy after transplantation has been described.

REFERENCES

1. Davies SC, Oni L. Management of patients with sickle cell disease. Brit Med J. 1997;315:656–60.
2. Serjeant GR. Sickle-cell disease. Lancet. 1997;350:725–30.
3. Bunn HF. Pathogenesis and treatment of sickle cell disease. N Engl J Med. 1997;337:762–9.
4. Platt OS. Easing the suffering caused by sickle cell disease. N Engl J Med. 1994;330:783–4.
5. Magnus SA, Hambleton IR, Moosdeen F, Serjeant GR. Recurrent infections in homozygous sickle cell disease. Arch Dis Child. 1999;80:537–41.
6. Wierenga KJJ, Hambleton IR, Wilson RM, et al. Significance of fever in Jamaican patients with homozygous sickle cell disease. Arch Dis Child. 2001;84:156–9.
7. Solovey A, Lin Y, Browne P, et al. Circulating activated endothelial cells in sickle cell anemia. N Engl J Med. 1997;337:1584–90.
8. Platt OS, Brambilla DJ, Rosse WF, et al. Mortality in sickle cell disease. Life expectancy and risk factors for early death. N Engl J Med. 1994;330:1639–44.
9. Steinberg MH. Management of sickle cell disease. N Engl J Med. 1999;340:1021–30.
10. Gaston MH, Verter JI, Woods G, et al. Prophylaxis with oral penicillin in children with sickle cell anemia. N Engl J Med. 1986;314:1593–9.
11. Jong PE de, Statius Eps LW van. Sickle cell nephropathy: new insights into pathophysiology. Kidney Int. 1985;27:711–17.
12. Allon M. Renal abnormalities in sickle cell disease. Arch Int Med. 1990;150:501–4.
13. Statius Eps LW van, Pinedo Veels C, Vries CH de, Koning J de. Nature of concentrating defect in sickle cell nephropathy, micro-radioangiographic studies. Lancet. 1970;i:450–2.
14. Pham PT, Pham PT, Wilkinson AH, Lew SQ. Renal abnormalities in sickle cell disease. Kidney Int. 2000;57:1–8.
15. Guasch A, Cua M, Mitch WE. Early detection and the course of glomerular injury in patients with sickle cell anemia. Kidney Int. 1996;49:786–91.
16. Schmitt F, Martinez F, Brillet G, et al. Early glomerular dysfunction in patients with sickle cell anemia. Am J Kidney Dis. 1998;32:208–14.
17. Falk RJ, Scheinman J, Phillips G, et al. Prevalence and pathologic features of sickle cell nephropathy and response to inhibition of angiotensin-converting enzyme. N Engl J Med. 1992;326:910–15.
18. Bhathena DB, Sondheimer JH. The glomerulopathy of homozygous sickle hemoglobin (SS) disease: morphology and pathogenesis. J Am Soc Nephrol. 1991;1:1241–52.
19. Guasch A, Cua M, You W, Mitch WE. Sickle cell anemia causes a distinct pattern of glomerular dysfunction. Kidney Int. 1997;51:826–33.
20. Maaten JC ter, Serné EH, Statius Eps LW van, et al. Effects of insulin and atrial natriuretic peptide on renal tubular sodium handling in sickle cell disease. Am J Physiol. 2000;278:F499–F505.
21. Vaamonde CA. Renal papillary necrosis in sickle cell haemoglobinopathies. Semin Nephrol. 1984;4:48–64.
22. Yium J, Gabow P, Johnson A, et al. Autosomal dominant polycystic kidney disease in blacks: clinical course and effects of sickle-cell hemoglobin. J Am Soc Nephrol. 1994;4:1670–4.
23. Saborio P, Scheinman JI. Sickle cell nephropathy. J Am Soc Nephrol. 1999;10:187–92.
24. Davis CJ Jr, Mostofi FK, Sesterhenn IA. Renal medullary carcinoma. The seventh sickle cell nephropathy. Am J Surg Pathol. 1995;19:1–11.
25. Bruno D, Wigfall DR, Zimmerman SA, et al. Genitourinary complications of sickle cell disease. J Urol. 2001;166:803–11.
26. Sklar AH, Perez JC, Harp RJ, Caruana RJ. Acute renal failure in sickle cell anemia. Int J Artif Organs. 1990;13:347–51.
27. Guasch A, Zayas CF, Eckman JR, et al. Evidence that microdeletions in the a globin gene protect against the development of sickle cell glomerulopathy in humans. J Am Soc Nephrol. 1999;10:1014–19.

28. Sklar AH, Campbell H, Caruana RJ, et al. Population study of renal function in sickle cell anemia. Int J Artif Organs. 1990; 13:231–6.

29. Bakir AA, Hathiwala SC, Ainis H, et al. Prognosis of the nephrotic syndrome in sickle glomerulopathy: a retrospective study. Am J Nephrol. 1987;7:110–15.

30. Wierenga KJJ, Pattison JR, Brink N, et al. Glomerulonephritis after human parvovirus infection in homozygous sickle-cell disease. Lancet. 1995;346:475–6.

31. Foucan L, Bourhis V, Bangou J, et al. A randomized trail of captopril for microalbuminuria in normotensive adults with sickle cell anemia. Am J Med. 1998;104:339–402.

32. Hatch FE, Crowe LR, Miles DE, et al. Altered vascular reactivity in sickle hemoglobinopathy. A possible protective factor from hypertension. Am J Hypertens. 1989;2:2–8.

33. Maaten JC ter, Serné EH, Bakker SJL, et al. Effects of insulin on glucose uptake and leg blood flow in patients with sickle cell disease and normal subjects. Metabolism. 2001;50:387–92.

34. Powars DR, Elliott-Mills DD, Chan L, et al. Chronic renal failure in sickle cell disease: risk factors, clinical course, and mortality. Ann Intern Med. 1991;115:614–20.

35. Ataga KI, Orringer EP. Renal abnormalities in sickle cell disease. Am J Hematol. 2000;63:205–11.

36. Bleyer AJ, Donaldson LA, McIntosch M, Adams PL. Relationship between underlying renal disease and renal transplantation outcome. Am J Kidney Dis. 2001;37:1152–61.

37. Ojo AO, Govaerts TC, Schmouder RL, et al. Renal transplantation in end-stage sickle cell nephropathy. Transplantation. 1999;67: 291–5.

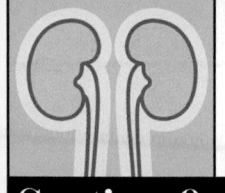

Chapter
52

Congenital Abnormalities of the Renal Tract

Guy H Neild

INTRODUCTION

This chapter discusses malformations of the urinary tract that can result in renal problems and renal failure. The most serious conditions involve bladder outflow obstruction and many can now be detected antenatally[1]. With the advances of molecular medicine, there has been rapid progress in genetics and developmental biology. What is becoming clearer is that malformations of the ureter, bladder, and urethra can be associated with primary renal malformations (renal dysplasia). This is a change from the still popular view that renal scarring and damage is all secondary to the outflow problem, and ureteral reflux.

Clinical principles

Congenital renal tract abnormalities may present in one of five settings:
- antenatal diagnosis by fetal ultrasound screening[1]
- failure to thrive in an infant or young child

- investigation of urinary tract infection
- an incidental finding in a child or adult
- an adult with abnormal urinalysis, stones, hypertension, or renal insufficiency.

The identification of these problems always poses the following questions:
- What is the cause?
- What is the natural history?
- Is surgical intervention required?

The details of antenatal and pediatric management of these patients are beyond the scope of this chapter, which focuses on their management in adolescence and adult life.

DEVELOPMENT OF THE URINARY TRACT

The urinary tract develops from the cloaca and intermediate mesoderm in parallel with the early differentiation of the metanephric blastema (future kidney) (Fig. 52.1)[2–4]. At the

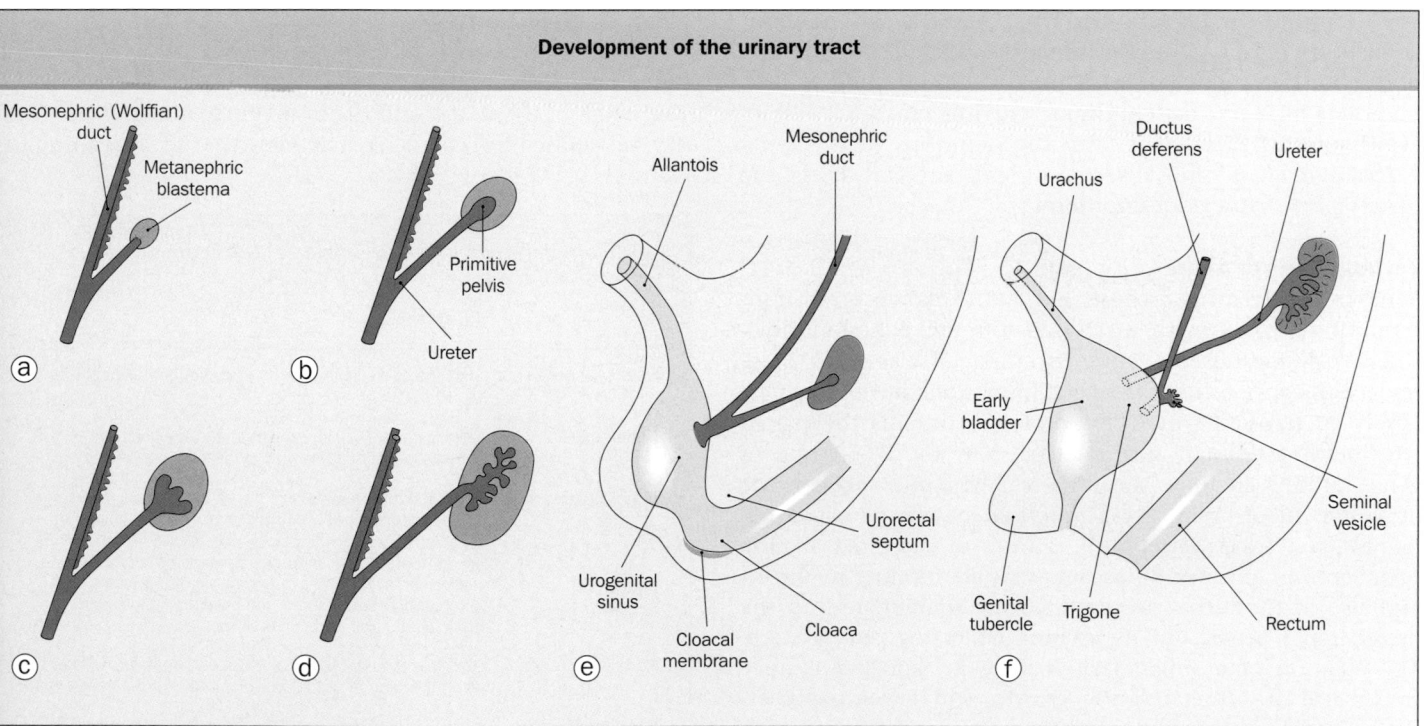

Figure 52.1 Development of the urinary tract. Growth and development of the ureter, pelvis, and calyces are shown in (a)–(d). (a) The metanephric kidneys first become detectable as small areas in the mesoderm close to the aorta. A small epithelial cell bud is surrounded by undifferentiated mesenchymal stem cells. (b) A primitive pelvis appears, which then divides to form the divisions of the calyces, shown in (c)–(d). As the fetus grows there is ascent of the kidney due to the continuous rostral growth. (e) Growth and development of the bladder and outflow tract during weeks 5–6. (f) Growth and development of the bladder and outflow tract during weeks 8–9.

5th week of fetal life, the mesonephric (Wolffian) duct connects to the allantois and the cloaca. By the 6th week, the urorectal fold appears and divides this cavity, which separates the urinary system (urogenital sinus) from the rectum. Growth of the anterior abdominal wall between the allantois and the urogenital membrane is accompanied by an increase in size and capacity of this bladder precursor. The allantois remains attached to the apex of the fetal bladder and extends into the umbilical root, although it loses its patency and persists as the urachal remnant, the median umbilical ligament, which connects the bladder to the umbilicus. By the 7th week, there is a separate opening of the mesonephric duct into the bladder at what will become the vesicoureteral opening and the area known as the trigone. The distal part of the primitive urogenital sinus will form the definitive urogenital sinus. In females this gives rise to the entire urethra and the vestibule of the vagina. In males it gives rise to the posterior urethra while the anterior urethra is formed from the closure of the urethral folds.

In the 6-week embryo, the mesonephric and paramesonephric (Müllerian) ducts run in parallel. By 7 weeks, in the male, the latter starts to regress and the Wolffian duct will eventually develop into the epididymis and the caudal part of the vas deferens. In the female, the Müllerian ducts fuse to become the uterovaginal cord, which opens into the urogenital sinus and will develop into the vagina[4].

As the urogenital tracts develops, there is simultaneous development of the fetal kidney. The primitive epithelial ureter first buds off from the mesonephric duct and makes contact with the metanephric mesenchyme. Under the influence of signals from the ureter, the mesenchyme condenses and proliferates around the ureteral tip, while there is simultaneous elongation and branching of the ureteral tip. The branching of the bud determines the structure of the collecting system. The branching process continues with the epithelial system eventually differentiating into the nephrons of the renal parenchyma. In the absence of the ureteral bud, the metanephric kidney does not form.

Pathogenesis of maldevelopment

Renal development is orchestrated by the expression of transcription factors, growth/survival factors, and adhesion molecules[3,5,6]. Mutations of genes encoding all classes of these molecules cause urinary tract malformations in mice[3,7]. One family of transcription factor proteins contains the paired DNA-binding domain and is encoded by the PAX group of genes. Studies in mice show these PAX genes regulate the development of brain, eyes, lymphoid system, musculature, neural crest, and vertebrae[8,9]. PAX-2 is expressed in the metanephros, and in cell lineages that are forming nephrons and also in those that are destined to differentiate into the ureter, renal pelvis, and branching collecting duct system. The ablation of a single PAX-2 allele in 'knock-out' mice causes impaired metanephric growth and fewer nephrons than normal, as well as megaureter, a finding consistent with gross vesico-ureteral reflux (VUR)[9]. WT1, which is mutated in a proportion of Wilms' tumours, is another transcription factor whose mutation is associated with abnormal urinary tract development. Primary VUR, the commonest of all

malformations leading to renal failure, maps to a locus on chromosome 1[10], and is not associated with PAX-2 or WT1.

Renal abnormalities have also been reported in angiotensin II knock-out mice and angiotensin type 2 receptor gene null mutant mice display congenital anomalies of the kidney and urinary tract. These include unilateral agenesis, unilateral megaureter and hydronephrosis, pelvic-ureteral junction obstruction, and mimic a range of abnormalities found in man[11]. Administration of angiotensin-converting enzyme (ACE) inhibitors in pregnancy is associated with renal tubular dysplasia.

RENAL MALFORMATIONS

Congenitally abnormal kidneys may be large or small, cystic or irregular in outline, and absent or misplaced.

Large kidneys

Enlarged kidneys resulting from congenital problems are usually hydronephrotic or cystic. Wilms' tumor must also be considered. The differential diagnosis in adults of enlarged kidneys, both congenital and acquired, is shown in Figure 5.7 and the differential diagnosis of cystic kidney disease is discussed further in Chapters 46 and 47.

Irregular kidneys

Irregularity of the renal outline may result from fetal lobulation or a 'dromedary hump' (see Fig. 5.3), neither of which have any functional implications. Much more important is the diagnosis of renal dysplasia, although in adults the etiology may have been complicated by scarring owing to ureteral reflux and infection.

Renal dysplasia

The range of dysplastic and other malformations of the kidney are defined in Table 52.1. The view that renal scarring in

Definitions of renal dysplasia and malformation	
Term	**Characteristics**
Renal agenesis	Absence of the kidney or an identifiable metanephric structure
Renal aplasia	Severe dysplasia with an extremely small kidney, sometimes identifiable only by histologic examination
Renal dysplasia	Abnormal differentiation of the renal parenchyma with the development of abnormal structures including primitive ducts surrounded by collars of connective tissue, metaplastic cartilage, a variety of nonspecific malformations such as preglomeruli of the fetal type, and reduced branching of the collecting ducts with cystic dilatations and primitive tubules
Renal hypoplasia	Significantly reduced renal mass and nephron number without evidence of maldevelopment of the parenchyma
Renal multicystic dysplasia	Severe cystic dysplasia with extremely enlarged kidney full of cystic structures. It occurs as an isolated renal lesion in response to ureteral atresia, and urethral obstruction. 10% have a family history

Table 52.1 Definitions of renal dysplasia and malformation.

congenital abnormality of the renal tract is all secondary to obstruction and vesicoureteral reflux resulting from outflow problems no longer dominates our approach to this problem[12,13]. It is clear that abnormalities of the ureter, bladder, and urethra are often associated with renal dysplasia. All types of renal dysplasia may also occur as isolated developmental anomalies. Renal dysplasia, while typically producing small irregular kidneys, may sometimes be cystic or multicystic renal dysplasia.

Differential diagnosis of scarred kidneys: dysplasia versus reflux

A practical clinical problem is the differential diagnosis of scarred, asymmetric kidneys. The differential diagnosis is influenced by the age of the patient, but opinion has also changed gradually since the 1960s.

Children

Progressive scarring and renal failure was considered to be chronic parenchymal infection (chronic pyelonephritis) and as such was a consequence of VUR. However, in the 1990s, there was some retreat from the paradigm of the primary role of infection, and emphasis placed on scarring as a result of reflux and the progressive nature of the glomerular lesion associated with glomerular hypertension (or hyperfiltration): so-called reflux nephropathy[14-17].

Currently, the emphasis is changing again to the concept that the gross scarring is a consequence of renal dysplasia, and that the reflux is a secondary feature (Fig. 52.2). Grossly scarred kidneys with normal caliber ureters are more likely caused by primary dysplasia, and there may be no evidence of VUR.

Although dysplasia typically affects the whole kidney, it may be segmental. Ask–Upmark kidney is a term used for segmental hypoplasia associated with accelerated hypertension that typically presents in adolescents.

Adults

With older patients, the differential diagnosis of scarred or 'lumpy, bumpy' kidneys widens. Whereas in the 1970s, this appearance was often attributed to analgesic nephropathy, today it is often designated as reflux nephropathy. In older patients, multiple scarring from atheromatous arterial disease and embolization of the kidney is an increasingly important cause of renal failure. The diagnosis can, in theory, be best made by the radiologic features of an intravenous urogram (IVU), but, in practice, patients often have advanced renal insufficiency and are unable to excrete enough radiocontrast to delineate the anatomy of the calyces and pelvis and their relationship to the scarring. With urologic conditions, there will be distortion and clubbing of calyces, whereas with other conditions the calyceal pattern should be normal (except for examples of papillary necrosis) (Fig. 52.3). Scarring is best demonstrated by [99]Tm-labeled dimercaptosuccinic acid (DMSA) renogram.

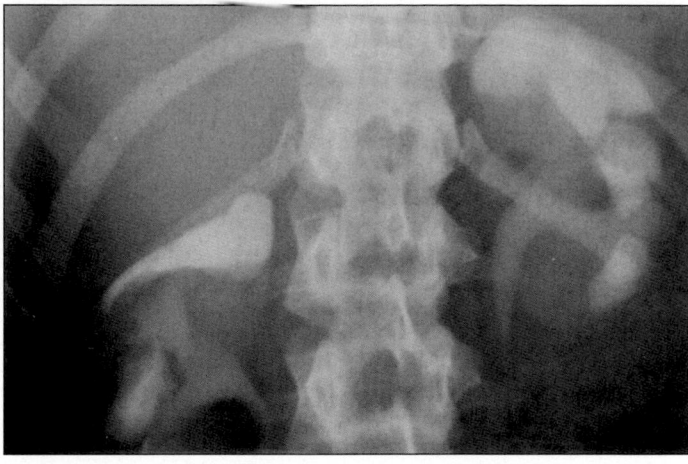

Figure 52.2 Renal dysplasia. Gross bilateral scarring in a 20-year-old woman who has been assessed since the age of 2. Progressive scarring has been observed in the absence of urinary tract infections and obstruction. This probably represents primary renal dysplasia.

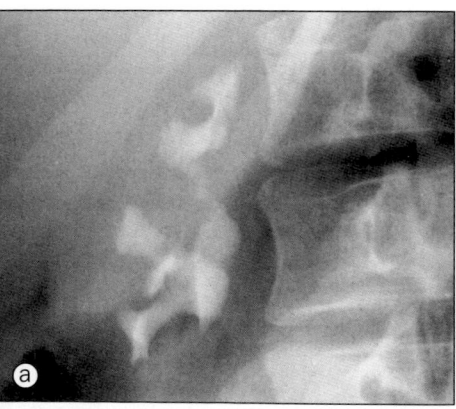 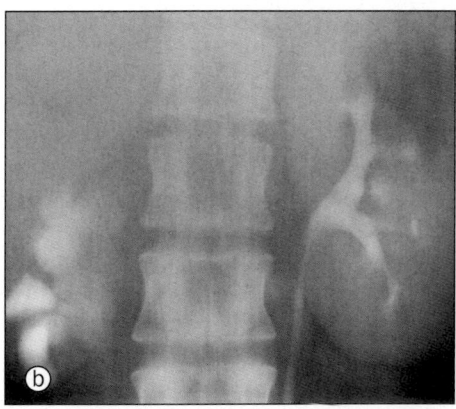 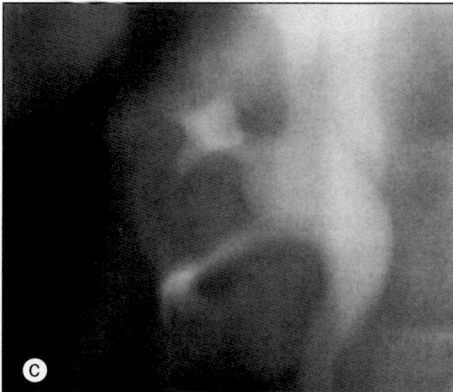

Figure 52.3 Differential diagnosis of 'lumpy bumpy' kidneys from the intravenous urogram appearance. (a) Sickle cell disease: papillary necrosis. Missing papillae leave a round hole in the medulla and give a 'clubbed' appearance. Otherwise, the calyceal architecture is relatively well preserved. (b) Reflux nephropathy. There is gross scarring and distortion of the calyceal pattern, giving rise to clubbed appearance of the dilated calyces. With reflux there is a predilection for scarring of the upper and lower poles, whereas with papillary necrosis or analgesic nephropathy changes are less predictable. (c) Analgesic nephropathy: the uniformly small shrunken kidney has relative preservation of the calyceal pattern. A plain film showed areas of calcification in both kidneys.

Absent kidneys

Unilateral renal agenesis

Complete absence of one kidney occurs in 1 in 500 to 1000 births. Typically there is no ureter and the ipsilateral half of the bladder trigone is missing. The remaining kidney is usually hypertrophic, but it may be ectopic, malrotated, or hydronephrotic with a megaureter (Fig. 52.4). The more severe the dysplasia of the remaining kidney, the earlier the presentation. The ipsilateral testis and seminal tract are usually absent, and in 10% of cases the adrenal gland is also missing. Girls can have an absent fallopian tube, ovary, or malformation of the vagina/uterus. Other associations include imperforate anus and malformations of the vertebrae and cardiovascular system. Agenesis could result from failure in formation of either the metanephros or the ureteral bud; however, when it is associated with cloacal abnormalities the latter is more likely.

Bilateral renal agenesis

Bilateral renal agenesis is lethal. It is associated with pulmonary hypoplasia and a characteristic facial appearance (Potter facies) caused by intrauterine compression, which is a consequence of oligohydramnios.

Misplaced kidneys

Renal ectopia, malrotation, and crossed fused kidneys

The starting position of the fetal kidney is deep in the pelvis. Kidneys that fail to ascend properly and, therefore, remain lower than usual occur in 1 in 800 births. During development and ascent of the kidney, the renal pelvis comes to face more medially. The most common anomaly is for the pelvis to face forwards. The more ectopic the kidney the more severe the rotation and abnormal the appearance (Fig. 52.5). This is best visualized on an IVU, except when the kidney overlies the pelvic bone and may be impossible to see. In this case, or if one is simply looking for the kidney, a DMSA renogram is best. Symptoms and complications are caused by associated reflux or pelvi-ureteral junction (PUJ) obstruction.

Horseshoe kidney

If both kidneys are low they may join at the lower pole and are usually drained by two ureters (Fig. 52.6). They lie lower than normal and further ascent is prevented by the root of the inferior mesenteric artery. This occurs in 1 in 400–1800 births and is more common in males (2 : 1). Patients present, if at all, with complications of reflux, obstruction, or stone formation.

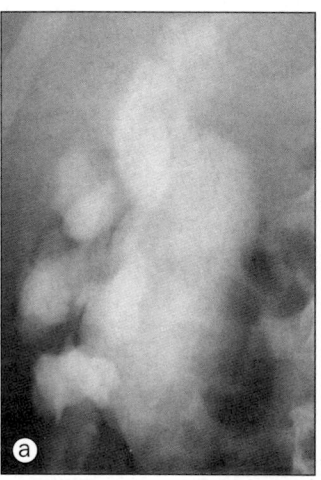
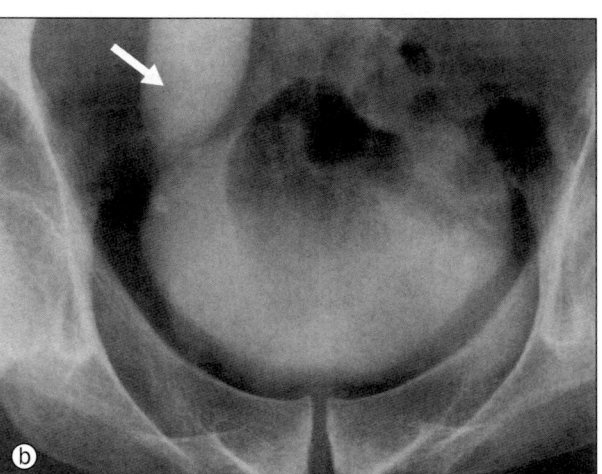

Figure 52.4 Megaureter and hydronephrosis. Intravenous urogram in a 50-year-old male showing a right megaureter and hydronephrosis. There was left renal agenesis. His GFR was 70 mL/min, and he had never had a urine infection or urinary tract symptoms. (a) Despite the grossly dilated appearance of the calyces, there was no evidence of obstruction on dynamic scans. (b) There is a single dilated megaureter (arrow). A micturating cystogram showed no evidence of reflux.

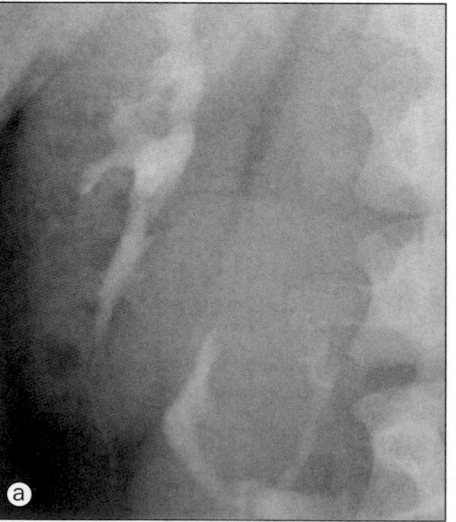
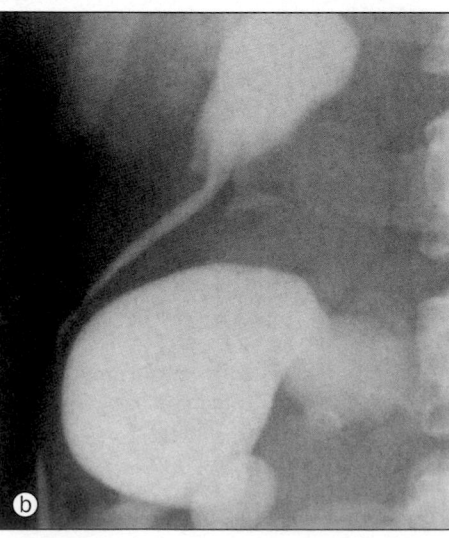

Figure 52.5 Crossed ectopia visualized by intravenous urography. (a) A relatively normal right kidney and a crossed ectopic left kidney. (b) A crossed left kidney with pelvi-ureteric junction obstruction. After furosemide (frusemide), the upper kidney washed out completely whereas the appearance in the lower kidney did not change. It is often impossible to tell from the intravenous urogram whether the kidneys are fused and this may require an isotopic DMSA renogram.

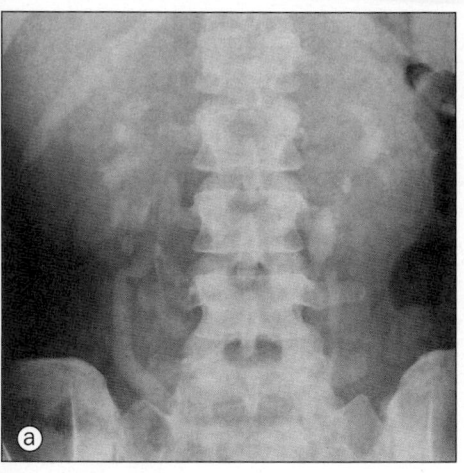

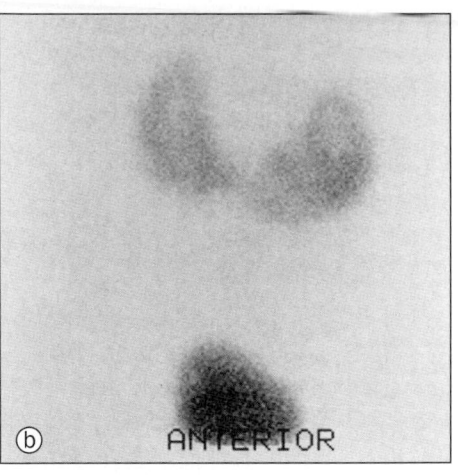

Figure 52.6 Horseshoe kidney. (a) Intravenous urogram soon after pregnancy in a 25-year-old woman shows not only the horseshoe kidney joining in the midline but also dilated ureters following her pregnancy. (b) Dimercaptosuccinate (DMSA) scan showing a horseshoe kidney.

Calyceal abnormalities

Hydrocalyx and hydrocalycosis

Dilated calyces are usually caused by obstruction. More focal dilatation can also be caused by congenital infundibular stenosis, extrinsic compression from vessel or tumor, stones, or tuberculosis. If obstruction is excluded, then the appearance is likely to be a congenital abnormality and can be an incidental finding.

Megacalycosis

In megacalycosis, there is bizarre dysplasia of the calyceal system with an increase in the number of calyces. There is no obstruction and it results from malformation of renal papillae. It is congenital, usually unilateral, and an incidental finding. It is much more common in males (6 : 1) and occurs only in Caucasians.

Bilateral disease is confined to males, and segmental, unilateral disease to females, which suggests an X-linked partially recessive gene with reduced penetrance in females. There may be an associated ipsilateral segmental megaureter, usually affecting the distal third.

Calyceal diverticulum (calyceal cyst)

Calyceal diverticulum is a cavity, peripheral to a minor calyx that is not a closed cyst but is connected to the calyx by a narrow channel. It is usually an incidental finding in 5 per 1000 IVUs and is best seen on a delayed film (Fig. 52.7). If present, symptoms relate to stones or infection within the cavity.

Bardet–Biedl syndrome

Multiple calyceal clubbing and calyceal diverticula are the characteristic feature of the renal dysplasia seen in Bardet–Biedl syndrome (formerly known as Laurence–Moon–Biedl syndrome)[18]. This autosomal recessive condition is characterized by retinitis pigmentosa, dysmorphic extremities (sometimes with polydactyly), obesity, and hypogonadism. Calyceal malformation is associated with parenchymal dysplasia; renal failure in early adult life is common.

Pelvi-ureteral junction obstruction

Pelvi-ureteral junction [PUJ] obstruction is one of the most frequent causes of obstructive uropathy in children. The

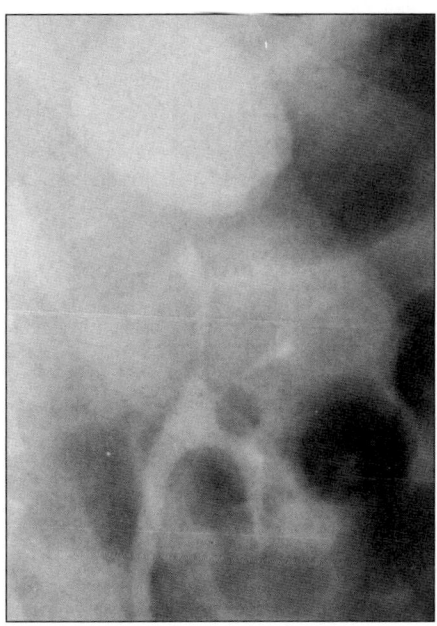

Figure 52.7 Calyceal cyst. Intravenous urogram showing an upper pole calyceal cyst. The plain abdominal film showed a group of five round stones in the floor of the cyst.

condition is usually congenital but can have an acquired mechanical basis caused by stenosis or external compression from adhesions, aberrant lower pole vessels, or kinking of the most proximal ureter. Associated abnormalities are common, and up to 50% of infants have another urologic abnormality, such as contralateral PUJ, contralateral renal dysplasia and multicystic kidney disease, minor degrees of VUR, and contralateral renal agenesis.

Older children can present with an abdominal mass or with pain in the flank, hematuria secondary to mild trauma, or urinary tract infection (UTI). Hypertension is unusual but can occur temporarily after surgical correction.

Diagnostic procedures have to differentiate between significant obstruction (Fig. 52.8) that requires surgical correction and congenital ectasia of the renal pelvis, in which case surgery is not indicated. Indications for surgical intervention include impairment of renal function, pyelonephritis, renal stones, and pain. Kidneys with good function can generally be left alone and surgery is only indicated when function is clearly shown to deteriorate[19].

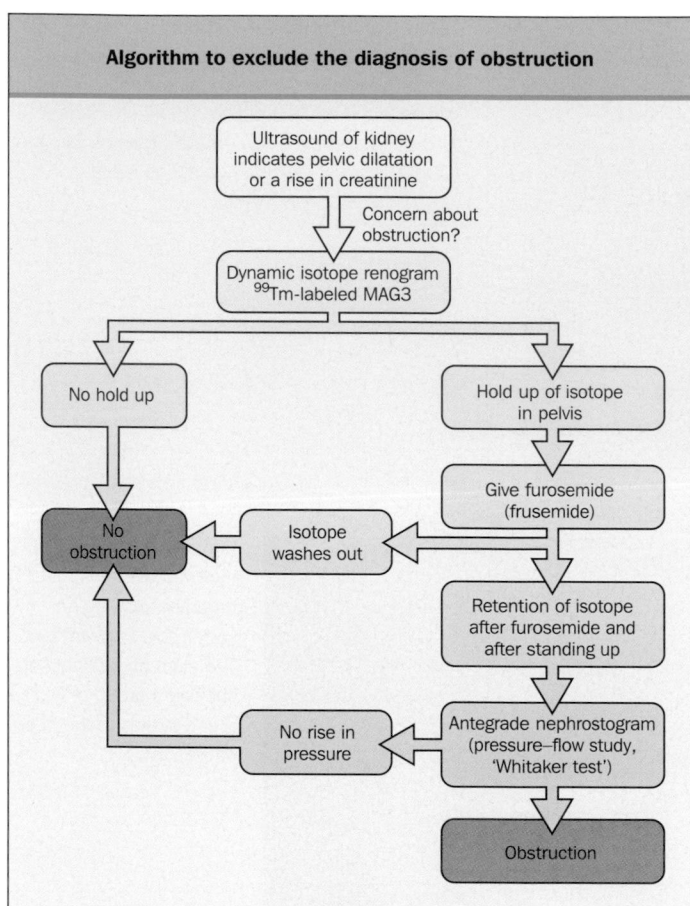

Algorithm to exclude the diagnosis of obstruction

Ultrasound of kidney indicates pelvic dilatation or a rise in creatinine

Concern about obstruction?

Dynamic isotope renogram ^{99}Tm-labeled MAG3

No hold up

Hold up of isotope in pelvis

Give furosemide (frusemide)

Isotope washes out

No obstruction

Retention of isotope after furosemide and after standing up

No rise in pressure

Antegrade nephrostogram (pressure–flow study, 'Whitaker test')

Obstruction

Figure 52.8 Algorithm to exclude the diagnosis of obstruction.

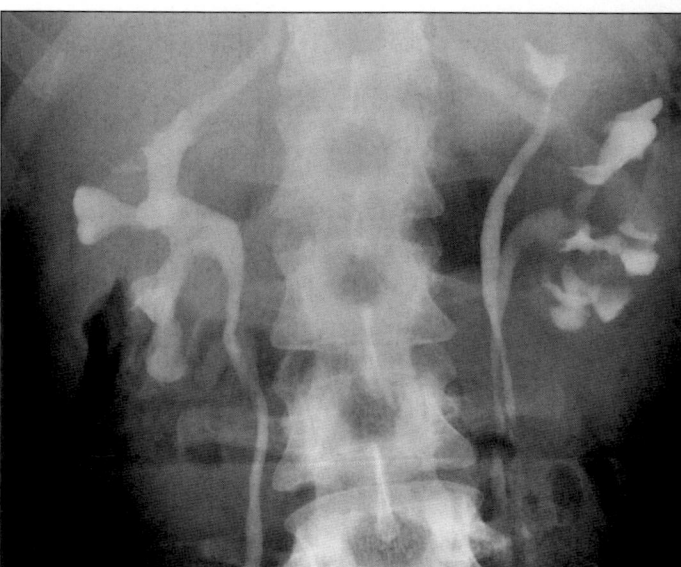

Figure 52.9 Duplex kidney. Intravenous urogram shows a duplex left kidney. The lower pole is scarred and shows evidence of reflux damage. The two ureters entered the bladder separately, with the lower pole ureter in the abnormal location. The right kidney also shows features of reflux, with clubbing of the calyces and some scarring.

URETERAL ABNORMALITIES

Duplex ureters

Duplication of the ureter and the renal pelvis is a common anomaly, with an incidence of approximately 1 in 150 births; unilateral duplication is six times more frequent than bilateral. It is more common in girls. If duplication has been detected in a patient, the likelihood of another sibling with duplication rises to 1 in 8.

Pathogenesis

If the ureteral bud bifurcates after its origin from the mesonephric duct but arises at a normal site, an incomplete ureteral duplication with a Y-ureter will develop[2]. Complete ureteral duplication occurs if there are two ureteral buds, one in the normal location and the other in a low position. The normal bud ends in a correct site on the trigone in the bladder and is nonrefluxing. The lower bud, representing the ureter of the lower pole of the kidney ends in the bladder as a lateral orifice with a short submucosal tunnel. The lower pole ureter is, therefore, often associated with VUR, and scarring of the lower pole can result.

If there are two ureteral buds, one with a normal location and one with a high position, the upper ureter is incorporated into the developing bladder, ending more distally and medial

to the normal one. Thus the upper pole ureter ends ectopically and as a consequence of either obstruction or dysplasia there is often severe scarring of the upper pole moiety.

Clinical manifestations

In most adult patients, ureteral reduplication is asymptomatic and causes no long-term problems. Children with ureteral duplication often have VUR. The spontaneous disappearance of reflux is less common in duplicate ureters than in patients with a single ureter[20]. Duplex ureters are best diagnosed by IVU and cystoscopy. PUJ obstruction of the lower pole moiety can occur.

Associated conditions such as ectopic ureters or ureterocele (see below) usually cause problems in early life and, therefore, have been dealt with by adolescence. Upper pole scarring is associated with an ectopic ureter, lower pole scarring with VUR (Fig. 52.9).

Ectopic ureters

Ectopic ureters are almost always associated with ureteral reduplication and 10% are bilateral. There is a female-to-male ratio of 7 : 1. The ectopic ureter comes from the upper pole and inserts into the bladder more distally and towards the bladder neck or it opens into the upper urethra. In the female, the ureter may end in the urethra, vagina, or vulva and patients present with incontinence, UTIs, or a persistent vaginal discharge, particularly if the external sphincter is damaged, for example during labor.

Ectopic ureters are rare in males and present as UTI. Usually there is a single ureter associated with a dysplastic kidney, which ends in the posterior urethra, ejaculatory duct, seminal vesicle, or vas. Males are usually continent as the ureter is proximal to the external sphincter.

Ectopic ureters are best visualized by an IVU, although a small dysplastic kidney may be missed. A micturating cystourethrogram (MCUG) shows reflux into the lower pole of the kidney in 50% of patients.

Ureterocele

Ureterocels are cystic dilatations of the terminal segments of the ureter and are caused by maldevelopment of the caudal ureter. They occur more commonly in females (4 : 1), almost exclusively in Caucasians, and 10% are bilateral.

Ectopic ureters and those with ureteroceles frequently (80%) drain the upper pole and are often associated with dysplastic or nonfunctional renal tissue. They usually present in childhood with infection; when large they can obstruct the bladder neck or even the contralateral ureter. In adults, they commonly present with stones in the lower ureter. The treatment of simple ureteroceles is surgical excision with reimplantation of the ureter, or simple incision if they subtend a well-functioning moiety. There are usually no medical sequelae.

Megaureter

Isolated dilatation of the ureter does not necessarily imply obstruction. There are three broad groups of conditions with widely dilated ureters.

- Obstruction of the ureter itself. This may be intrinsic (e.g., stone) or extrinsic (e.g., retroperitoneal fibrosis); it is obviously not associated with reflux.
- Bladder outflow obstruction, with secondary ureteral obstruction. Examples would include a neuropathic bladder or posterior urethral valves; it may or may not be associated with reflux.
- A dilated but nonobstructed ureter for which there is no apparent cause. This often occurs without reflux and there can be normal renal function; sometimes this is caused by an adynamic segment of the lower ureter (see Fig. 52.4).

Pathogenesis

In the normal ureter there is a characteristic helical orientation of muscle fibers. When the megaureter is secondary to bladder outflow obstruction, there is muscular hyperplasia and hypertrophy of the ureteral wall. In megaureters for which there is no apparent cause, a variety of abnormalities of muscle orientation are described, or even absence of muscle fibers at the proximal end of the undilated segment. By electron microscopy, there is an increase in collagen between the muscle bundles at the level of the obstructing segment[21]. Obstruction appears to be caused by a failure of peristalsis through the distal ureteral segment.

Clinical manifestations

Most cases of megaureter associated with obstruction present in childhood with severe infections, often complicated by septicemia. In such cases, there is a high incidence of other congenital abnormalities. In less severe cases or when there is no obstruction, patients can present with abdominal pain, loin pain, hematuria, and UTI. Renal stones can form easily in the dilated systems. The exclusion of obstruction is often only established by an antegrade pressure–flow study (Whitaker test)[22].

Treatment

A definite diagnosis (is there obstruction or not) must be made (see Fig. 52.8). The current view is that patients with nonobstructed asymptomatic disease should be managed conservatively and most do very well with this approach.

BLADDER AND OUTFLOW DISORDERS[23]

Prune belly syndrome

The prune belly syndrome occurs in males and consists of absence of the muscles of the anterior abdominal wall, bizarre malformations of the urinary tract with gross dilatation of the bladder and ureters, and bilateral undescended testes[24,25]. If diagnosed early, renal outcome is related to the degree of renal dysplasia. There are incomplete forms of the syndrome ('pseudo-prune'). Rarely, a similar megacystis/megaureter may be seen in either sex.

Pathogenesis

No gene defect or unifying hypothesis has emerged to explain these features. The incidence varies from 1 in 30 000 to 1 in 50 000. There are a few familial cases and the condition has been reported in twins, but there is 100% discordance reported in identical twins, which is a powerful argument against a genetic basis. There is evidence for a primary, localized arrest of mesenchymal development. This is supported by the lack of prostatic differentiation: the epithelial element in the prostate is absent or hypoplastic. Ultrastructure studies of the ureter show massive replacement of smooth muscle with fibrous and collagen tissue and the absence of nerve plexuses.

A nearly identical syndrome can occur as a consequence of fetal urethral obstruction, including urethral atresia.

Clinical manifestations

The prognosis is dependent on the degree of renal dysplasia and injury. Three groups can be distinguished. In group I, complete urethral obstruction causes stillbirth or neonatal death (20%); in group II, acute, early presentation requires diversion and reconstruction (20%); in group III, good health and renal function exist despite urologic appearances (60%).

There is complete absence or incomplete formation of the rectus abdominis and other muscles, which leads to the wrinkled abdominal wall of the prune infant. This gives way to a fairly smooth 'pot belly' in later life (Fig. 52.10). Reconstructive surgery is not normally required. The patients grow up physically active and strong but cannot sit up directly from a supine position. Abnormalities of the thoracic cage, such as pectus excavatum, are common.

Although true outflow obstruction is sometimes present, the gross and irregular dilatation of the urinary tract that is characteristic of this syndrome is primarily caused by a developmental defect with a variable degree of smooth muscle aplasia leading to aperistaltic ureters (Fig. 52.11). Urodynamics are often difficult to interpret because of gross VUR but typically there is a low-pressure bladder. With late presentation, some patients have detrusor instability.

Differential diagnosis

In severe cases of megacystis/megaureter with gross impairment of renal function (often with dysplastic kidneys), the

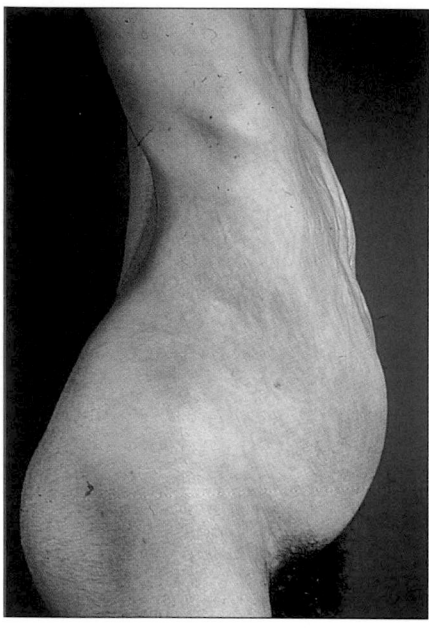

Figure 52.10 Prune belly syndrome. Note the lax abdominal musculature leading to a 'pot-bellied' appearance. There is also marked thoracic cage deformity. (Courtesy Mr CRJ Woodhouse.)

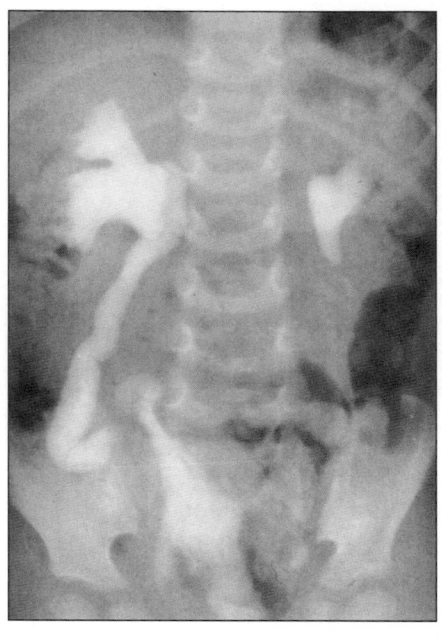

Figure 52.11 Prune belly syndrome. Typical intravenous urogram appearance of a patient with prune belly syndrome and good renal function. Often the ureters are extremely dilated and tortuous.

differential diagnosis includes posterior urethral valves, renal dysplasia with or without multiple congenital defects, neuropathic bladder, and nephrogenic diabetes insipidus.

Natural history

Once any outflow obstruction is dealt with, usually in infancy, the renal function should remain stable in spite of the frightening radiologic appearances. In those patients followed in our unit for up to 40 years, renal deterioration and hypertension have been rare. In the small number who have progressed, recurrent infection, hypertension, and proteinuria have been warning signs of impending trouble.

Renal scarring should be assessed by isotopic DMSA scans, and renal function followed by serial isotopic glomerular filtration rate (GFR) measurements. Life-long attention to blood pressure, UTIs, and stones is necessary.

Treatment

In all children, even with good renal function, there should be a careful search for obstruction, beginning with the urethra and working up to the PUJ, but often no obstruction is found and no surgery is required. In many others, the floppy bladder is not anatomically obstructed but bladder emptying is improved by urethrotomy ('functional obstruction'). In infancy, there is debate about the need for reconstructive surgery. There is certainly a group of patients born with severely compromised renal function who do require reconstruction after stabilization by early diversion[26].

The current view is that the testes should be brought down to the scrotum in infancy. It is hoped that earlier surgery will produce proper germ cell development and thus preserve fertility, but so far no prune patient has been shown to be fertile.

Bladder exstrophy (ectopia vesicae)

Classical exstrophy is the failure of the anterior abdominal wall and bladder to close, but there is a range of defects from

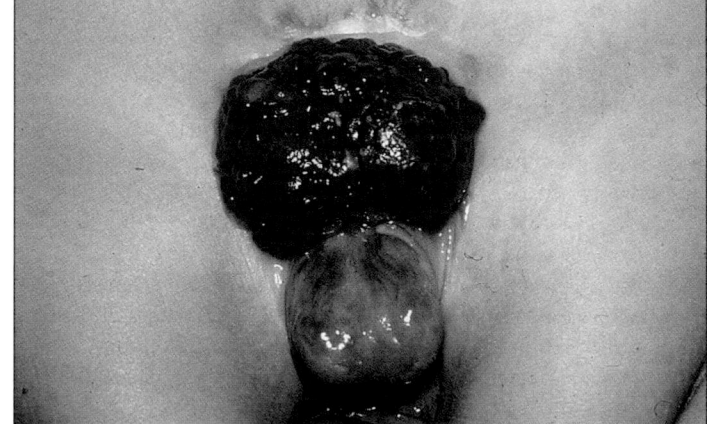

Figure 52.12 Bladder exstrophy. The entire length of the penis is also open (epispadias). (Courtesy Mr CRJ Woodhouse.)

epispadias of an otherwise normal penis to major cloacal abnormalities (Fig. 52.12).

Pathogenesis

Failure of growth of the lower abdominal wall between the allantois and the urogenital membrane, coupled with breakdown of the urogenital membrane leaves a small, open bladder plate, a low-placed umbilical root and diastasis of the pubic bones. The genital tubercle is probably placed lower in these patients so the cloacal membrane ruptures above it, leading to a penis with an open dorsal surface that is continuous with the bladder plate. A midline closure defect causes a failure of fusion of the lower anterior abdominal wall, including the symphysis pubis, lower urinary tract, and external genitalia. There are rare reports of a familial incidence. The condition occurs in 1 in 10 000 to 1 in 50 000 births. The male-to-female ratio is 2 : 1.

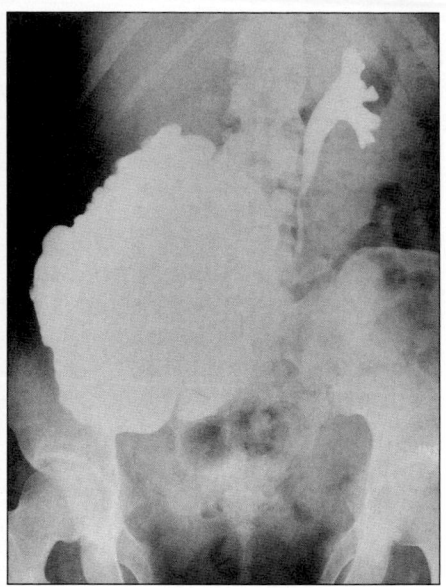

Figure 52.13 Cystography in bladder exstrophy. A 26-year-old female with bladder exstrophy who has a continent Mitrofanoff system using the colon to create a reservoir. There is reflux into the left kidney. There is also reflux into the right kidney but the kidney is obscured by the full reservoir. Her glomerular filtration rate is 130 mL/min.

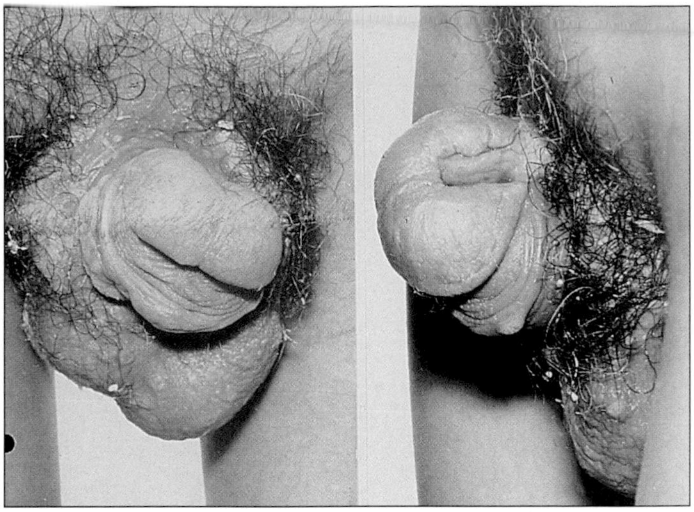

Figure 52.14 Epispadias. Result of multiple surgery to close the epispadias and lengthen the penis. (Courtesy Mr CRJ Woodhouse.)

Clinical manifestations

In severe cases, the bladder mucosa lies exposed on the lower abdominal wall with the bladder neck and urethra laid open. The prostate and testes are normal. Most patients have normal kidneys at birth (although many reports do not record the state of the kidneys at birth). In one series, 33% had dilated ureters at presentation, but an IVU was usually normal after diversion. However, in another series, one-third of patients were said to have unilateral renal agenesis[27]. Renal function may be preserved after the diversion although reflux is common (Fig. 52.13).

Other congenital abnormalities are only rarely present. More severe cloacal abnormalities are associated with imperforate anus and either high or low rectal atresia.

Natural history

Long-term renal outcome depends on the bladder. In the long term (up to 25 years), the kidneys survive much better with a well-functioning bladder: 13% of those with a good bladder had significant renal damage, compared with 82% with ileal conduits, 22% with non-refluxing colonic conduits and 33% with uretero-sigmoidostomy[28]. Today the bladder is augmented (enterocystoplasty, ileocystoplasty, caecocystoplasty) or replaced by bowel (intestinal reservoir). In a study of 53 such patients, who were followed for more than 10 years, renal function deteriorated (fall in GFR of 20% or more) in only 10 (20%)[29].

Treatment

When the infant is born, the three urological treatment goals are to close the abdominal wall, to establish urinary continence and preserve renal function, and to reconstruct cosmetically acceptable genitalia.

The aim of initial surgery is to convert the patient's defect to a complete epispadias (Fig. 52.14). At 4 years of age, reconstruction of the bladder neck and correction of the epispadias can be performed. If the bladder is small, intestinal augmentation is required. Patients may be able to void, but many have to use catheters. Incontinence may be a long-term problem.

Neuropathic bladder

In childhood, the most common cause of a neuropathic bladder is myelomeningocele. A neuropathic bladder may also be seen without associated neurologic or other obvious causes (Table 52.2). The principal consequences are incontinence, infection, and reflux with upper tract dilatation and subsequently renal failure. Early urodynamic assessment is essential (Fig. 52.15).

Three different patterns of bladder behavior are seen: contractile, intermediate, and acontractile.

Contractile behavior

An overactive detrusor (hyperreflexia) can produce some bladder emptying (incontinence). Unfortunately, 95% of patients have sphincter dyssynergia (inability to relax urethral sphincter), which results in no relaxation and incomplete emptying of the bladder. Patients with incomplete lesions may have some control of the distal sphincter and normal anal and sacral reflexes. Ironically, although this latter group has the least neurologic deficit they have the worst bladder situation generating high pressures and great risk of renal injury. The bladder becomes progressively hypertrophic, fibrotic, and poorly compliant.

Intermediate behavior

These patients have some detrusor activity but not sufficient to empty the bladder. Their bladders are poorly compliant and they have no voluntary control of their sphincters, so any rise in bladder pressure tends to cause incontinence or the high intravesical pressures lead to renal injury.

Acontractile behavior

In about 25% of patients, there is no detrusor activity and so the bladder overflows when it is sufficiently full. This is not usually associated with renal failure.

Myelodysplasia

Myelodysplasia refers to a group of neural tube anomalies that primarily affect the lumbar and sacral segment of the

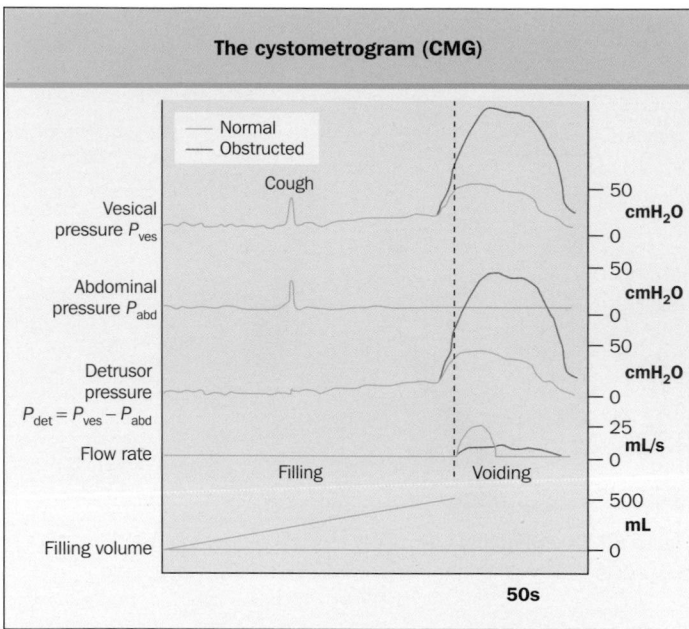

The cystometrogram (CMG)

Figure 52.15 Urodynamics: the cystometrogram (CMG). The vesical pressure is measured simultaneously with the abdominal pressure via the rectum; the detrusor pressure is the difference. A cough is used as a marker to show that the system is working. Normally during filling, the first desire to void is at a detrusor pressure of < 10 cmH$_2$O. This point is noted. Normally, the voiding pressure should be < 40 cmH$_2$O (and is lower in women). Detrusor instability is an unstable (spontaneous) contraction occurring with a detrusor pressure > 15 cmH$_2$O. Higher pressure can cause incontinence. When combined with radiologic imaging (VCMG) the following are all recorded: bladder neck, closed/open; bladder pressure, end-filling; voiding detrusor pressure; bladder stability; compliance; flow rate, maximum; sensation, first; volume, voided/residual. (Courtesy Professor M Craggs.)

Causes of neuropathic bladder	
Area affected	**Causes**
Cerebral	Cardiovascular accident/cerebral palsy, encephalopathy, trauma, Parkinson's disease, dementia
Spinal	Isolated (no other neurologic features), trauma, multiple sclerosis, compression, spina bifida, spinal dysraphism, tethered cord, sacral agenesis, sacral teratoma
Peripheral nerve	Pelvic surgery, diabetes

Table 52.2 Causes of neuropathic bladder.

incomplete tubularization of the neural tube, with inadequate mesodermal invagination and subsequent arrest of vertebral arch formation.

The incidence of myelodysplasia varies from 1 in 1000 to 5 in 1000 live births, but there are wide geographic variations. Monozygotic twins are often discordant for spina bifida, but siblings are at increased risk (1 : 10–20) and children of affected parents have a 4% chance of having a similarly affected child. Myelomeningocele accounts for over 90% of myelodysplastic infants. Folic acid supplements taken during the last trimester reduce the incidence of myelodysplasia by 50%.

Clinical manifestations

All causes of tethered cord can produce a variable neurologic deficit. During development, some children develop progressive neurologic disturbance with bladder dysfunction, bowel dysfunction, scoliosis, and a syndrome of pes cavus and limb growth failure.

Bladder dysfunction
Neuropathic bladder can be an isolated problem with abnormal urodynamic studies but a normal neurologic examination[30].

Bowel dysfunction
Bowel dysfunction is often present and needs to be treated accordingly. There may be severe constipation and overflow incontinence. The antegrade continent enterostomy procedure has been developed to improve the management. The appendix is brought out to the abdominal surface and thus the colon can be irrigated antegradely with saline.

Intelligence
Patients with myelomeningocele may have some intellectual impairment, especially those who have required ventriculoperitoneal shunting for associated hydrocephalus. Manual dexterity may also be affected. These are very important issues in long-term management.

Natural history
About 14% of patients have renal complications at birth and are at high risk in the next few years. Ultimately, about 50% will develop upper tract problems, although these can take up to 30 years to occur (Fig. 52.16). In one prospective study,

spinal cord and are the most common cause of neurogenic bladder dysfunction in children. Spina bifida means the defective fusion of the posterior vertebral arches. Meningocele implies that the meninges extend beyond the confines of the vertebral canal with no neural elements contained inside. A myelomeningocele has neural tissue protruding with the meningocele. Spinal dysraphism (symptomatic spina bifida occulta) defines a group of structural anomalies of the caudal end of the spinal cord that do not result in an open vertebral canal but are associated with incomplete fusion of the posterior vertebral arches. Sacral agenesis is a rare anomaly in which part or all of two or more vertebral bodies are absent. It occurs early in fetal development when there is failure of ossification of the lowest vertebral segments. The only known teratogen is insulin. Sacral agenosis occurs in 1% of children born to insulin-dependent mothers. Partial sacral agenesis can be associated with an anterior meningocele.

Pathogenesis
Normally, the neural tube forms as the neural folds close over and fuse, starting in the cervical region and progressing caudally. It is believed that the embryologic defect is an

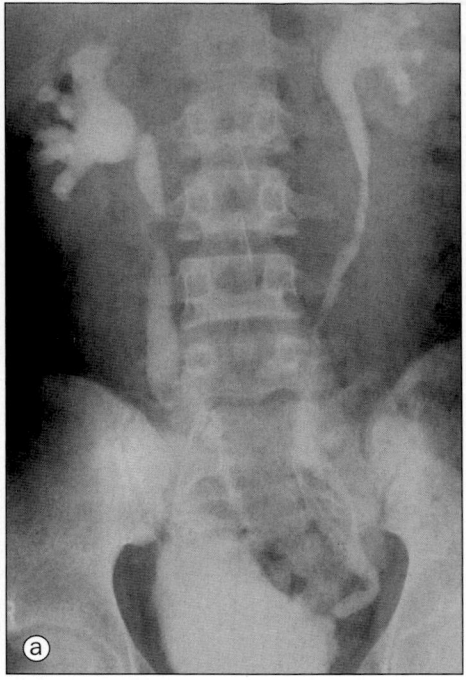 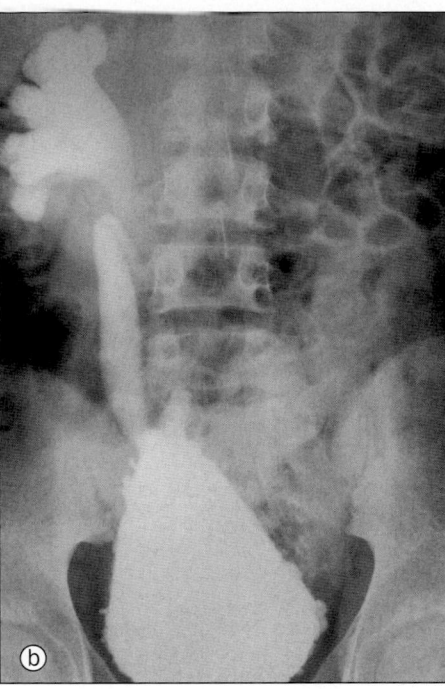

Figure 52.16 Sacral spina bifida with neuropathic bladder. (a) Intravenous urogram shows evidence of a previous hydronephrosis and subsequent scarring of the right kidney. The architecture of the left kidney is well preserved. (b) Micturating cystogram. The typical tapering hypertrophied, trabeculated bladder giving the characteristic 'fir cone' appearance. Note the gross reflux on the right side. This is probably helping to protect the left kidney by acting as a 'pop-off' mechanism. This is analogous to the protection that can occur in boys with posterior urethral valves.

renal outcome could be predicted by the urodynamic findings, with worst outcomes related to increased bladder wall thickness, the degree of reflux, urethral pressures above 70 cm H_2O, and reduced bladder capacity. VUR occurs in 3–5% of newborns with detrusor hypertonicity or dyssynergia. Without treatment, this figure increases to 30–40% by the age of 5 years[31].

Treatment

The management of the bladder depends on the urodynamic findings. In the 1970s, clean intermittent self-catheterization (CISC) was introduced[32], but before that urinary diversion was the usual treatment. Today, when reflux and hydroureter are present, the management is principally with CISC and anticholinergic drugs that increase bladder compliance[33].

Bladder neck obstruction

Congenital bladder neck obstruction is rare and is usually caused by a neuropathic bladder, posterior urethral valves (PUV), or an ectopic ureterocele.

Posterior urethral valves

Posterior urethral valves (PUV) is the most common cause of severe subvesical obstruction in the male infant (although in the newborn it accounts for only 10% of cases of hydronephrosis). As a consequence, bilateral hydronephrosis and megaureters occur. Obstruction is caused by a diaphragm that extends from the floor to the roof of the urethra at the apex of the prostate. Valves appear as mucosal folds in the posterior urethra below the verumontanum. There is dilatation of the proximal urethra, and bladder wall hypertrophy and trabeculation. Above the valves there is dilatation of the prostatic urethra, which undermines the bladder neck. The valves only obstruct flow in one direction, and therefore a catheter can be passed without difficulty.

Pathogenesis

The urethra develops in two parts: differentiation of the urogenital sinus part (posterior urethra) and tubularization of the urethral plate (anterior urethra). Early obstruction during renal development can result in severe renal dysplasia.

Clinical manifestations

Most cases of PUV are now detected antenatally by ultrasound. Half of all patients present before the age of 1 year. Infants present with a palpably distended bladder and enlarged kidneys, abnormal urine stream, or failure to thrive owing to renal failure. At diagnosis, 30–50% of children have VUR. Children with less severe disease present with poor stream, hematuria, incontinence, acute UTI, or renal failure; however, late presentation is also associated with worse outcome[34].

There are three abnormal features that can help to protect the kidney. These all act to reduce the high pressures generated during voiding. They are massive unilateral reflux, usually with ipsilateral renal dysplasia; large bladder diverticulum; and urinary extravasation, often with urinary ascites. These protective mechanisms are referred to as 'pop off' mechanisms (see Fig. 52.16)[35]. Ultrasound can show the bladder thickening, dilated system, and dilatation of the posterior urethra. A specific diagnosis should be documented by videocystometrogram (VCMG: see below).

Natural history

In the 1960s, 25% of children died within the first 12 months and 25% died later in childhood, including renal 'death' (i.e., end-stage renal disease (ESRD)). By the late 1990s, the early mortality was less than 5%, and after 15-year follow-up only 15–20% of patients had reached ESRD[36].

The bladder may become stretched, resulting in poor emptying, or unstable, leading to poor compliance, unsuppressed detrusor contractions, and high storage pressure. Both these situations are exaggerated by progressive polyuria. It is not uncommon for such patients to have a daily urine volume of 5 L. Urodynamic follow-up studies suggest that instability decreases with time; bladder capacity increases but there are unsustained voiding contractions. The prognosis correlates with the nadir creatinine value. Despite adequate early treatment, many children develop chronic renal insufficiency owing to renal dysplasia[34,37].

Treatment

Bladder diversion should be avoided. The question of 'undiversion' of ileal conduits is discussed below. Bladder instability and poor bladder compliance must be treated, irrespective of whether they are causing symptoms. Boys with substantial residual volumes can be managed by CISC. However, there is often poor compliance with this either because of urethral discomfort or because previous urethral surgery has made the passage of catheters difficult. Compliance is a particular problem with adolescents who are continent and for whom renal failure is too abstract a concept. Continence often improves spontaneously at puberty but can be helped by imipramine.

Urethral diverticulum

Urethral diverticulum usually occurs in boys and is rare. It may present with UTI, obstruction, or stones. There are two types: anterior or posterior. The former can be associated with anterior urethral valves and obstruction.

GENERAL MANAGEMENT OF CONGENITAL TRACT ABNORMALITIES

The principles of management of congenital tract abnormalities are shown in Table 52.3. The most important part of the management is ensuring that the patient, their family, and the primary care physician knows what can and must be done. The first thing to make clear is the necessity of long-term follow-up at no more than annual intervals. ESRD commonly occurs when a patient is lost to follow-up, often presenting later with accelerated hypertension and rapid loss of renal function.

Clinical evaluation

By the time the adolescent is passed on to an adult physician it should be assumed that the urinary tract is not obstructed and further surgery is not required. Nevertheless, it is the responsibility of the nephrologists and urologists who care for these children to review this aspect from time to time.

Symptomatic UTI is common and must be treated promptly. Increase in frequency or severity of infections must lead to investigations to find the cause. The blood pressure must be monitored regularly and kept normal. Finally, renal function must be monitored, proteinuria assessed, and the cause of any deterioration identified. As in any other renal condition, the remnant kidney function may decline inexorably, and this is associated with increasing proteinuria and hypertension. As with other renal conditions, function is usually stable when there is little or no proteinuria. Deterioration in the absence of proteinuria must alert the physician to the likelihood of obstruction or some other cause of acute-on-chronic renal failure, such as a nephrotoxic drug.

Management of congenital renal tract abnormalities
Educate and explain to encourage compliance
Review urological status
Find cause of urinary tract obstruction and treat
Control blood pressure
Monitor renal function and proteinuria
Treat acidosis
Prevent bone disease
Check for stones
Intermittent clean self-catheterization for chronic retention
Maintain bladder storage pressure below 40 cmH$_2$O

Table 52.3 General principles of management of congenital renal tract abnormalities.

Monitoring patients with congenital renal tract abnormalities	
Baseline measurements	**Reason for test**
Radiology	
Abdominal X-ray	Exclude stones
Ultrasound of kidneys	Baseline
Ultrasound of bladder postmicturition	Assess residual volume
Urine flow rate	Ensure adequacy
Nuclear medicine	
Glomerular filtration rate (GFR):^{51}Cr-labeled EDTA (ethylenediamine tetraacetic acid)	Baseline
Dynamic isotope scan with ^{99}Tm-labeled MAG3 or DTPA	Assess outflow obstruction/holdup
Static isotope scan with ^{99}Tm-labeled (DMSA)	Assess scarring and divided function
Biochemistry	
24-h urine protein	Baseline

Table 52.4 Monitoring patients with congenital renal tract abnormalities. Routine investigations for assessment of clinical status.

A number of routine investigations should be performed to document the current situation and to act as a reference point for the future (Table 52.4). If the bladder empties completely with an adequate flow rate (15 mL/s) no problems should arise. If there is any doubt about the condition of the bladder, urodynamic investigations are necessary. If the clinical situation changes, further investigations are required. An increase in UTIs might suggest a stone or increase in residual urine. With an unexpected decline in renal function, obstruction has to be excluded all over again.

It is helpful and important for the patient to keep a '24-h urine volume diary' every 1–2 years. Patients are asked to write down the time that they voided and measure and record the volume passed. It is best to ask them to do this on two consecutive days, then one can determine the maximum bladder capacity and the total 24-h urine volume. This should be done before urodynamic investigations, as results can be misleading if bladder is not filled to capacity.

Exclude obstruction

Obstruction must always be excluded if there is a change in renal function. The possibility of obstruction may be raised by a routine ultrasound (see Fig. 52.8) and should be pursued with a MAG3 scan to exclude obstruction (Fig. 52.17).

In patients with conduits, obstruction can be excluded by infusing contrast into the loop (loopogram) and demonstrating reflux up the ureter.

Rarely, in patients with large bladders or in transplant recipients, the kidney may become obstructed when the bladder reaches a certain volume. This can be investigated by filling the bladder by a catheter and performing a ^{99}Tm-labeled MAG3 scan, initially with the bladder full. If there is no excretion, the bladder volume can be reduced in 100 mL increments until there is flow down the ureter (Fig. 52.18).

Urodynamics

Any urodynamic investigation should start with a free urine flow rate. Provided that the flow rate is normal and the bladder empties completely (leaving no residual volume on post micturition ultrasound), it can be assumed that there is no significant bladder outflow obstruction.

Complete investigation of abnormalities of bladder and urethral function requires synchronous recordings of intravesical and intrarectal pressures taken during bladder filling and emptying (see Fig. 52.15). Combined with radiologic imaging, the study is known as a VCMG.

Surgical correction of the urinary tract

A normal bladder acts as a low-pressure, good-volume urine reservoir that is continent, sterile, and empties freely and completely. Any other form of urine reservoir aims to recreate such an environment. When this is not achieved in either a natural or reconstructed bladder, complications such as sepsis and renal dysfunction can occur.

A variety of conduits and continent reservoirs have been developed to replace unusable bladders. Ileal conduit diversion has been most widely used for native kidneys, although deterioration in renal function commonly occurs secondary to long-term complications including urosepsis, renal calculi, and, most commonly, stenosis leading either to obstruction or to reflux with ureteral dilatation. There is an overall complication rate of 45%, but with a high index of suspicion and an aggressive diagnostic and therapeutic approach, many of these problems can be detected and treated early, with resultant good long-term function of native kidneys. Similar results may be obtained when renal transplants are performed in these patients[38]. Other forms of urinary diversion that are continent and, therefore, more socially acceptable to patients are now widely used in general urological practice and are being encountered in renal transplantation (see Figs 52.13 and 52.19). These include augmented bladders draining via the urethra and augmented or intestinal bladders draining via continent stomas.

Undiversion of conduits

The only certain improvement with undiversion is cosmetic. Initially, undiversion was undertaken because of poor results

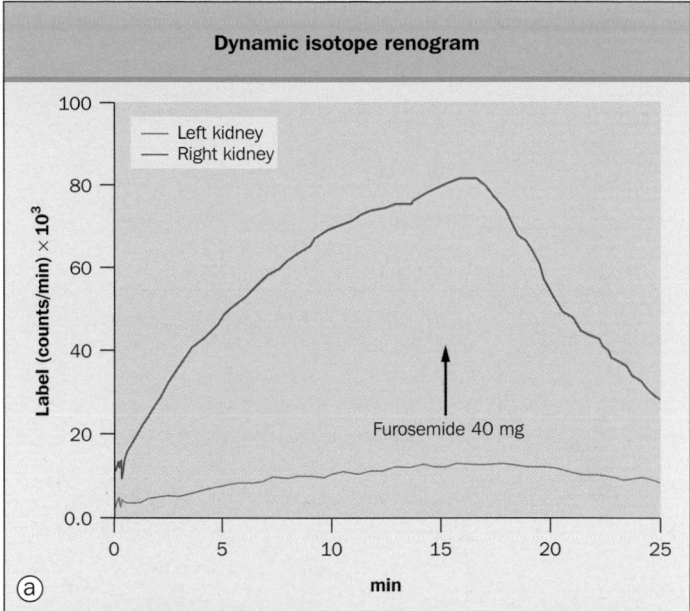

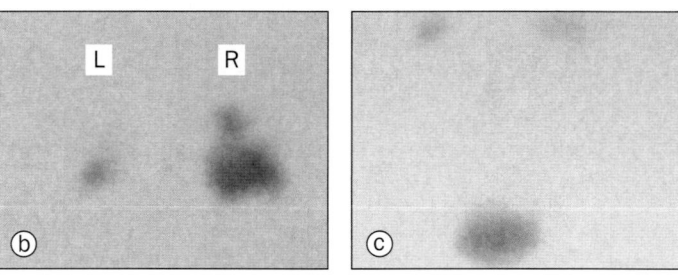

Figure 55.17 Dynamic ^{99}Tm-labeled MAG3 isotopic renogram.
(a) Time-activity curve showing accumulation of isotope in right kidney, which washes out with furosemide, thus excluding significant obstruction. (b) Images from the same study, showing hold-up of isotope in dilated right renal pelvis, which (c) washes out after furosemide, excluding significant obstruction.

or complications from conduits. Short-term results of undiversion are very promising and the major indications today would be convenience and cosmetic appearance (Fig. 52.19). Long-term results, however, are not available.

Before considering undiversion, four factors must be considered:
- Is there residual obstruction?
- What is the function of the bladder?
- What is the function of the sphincters?
- What is the normal 24-h urine output?

In particular, the bladder storage pressure must be considered, as one must achieve a low-pressure reservoir. This is a particular problem when patients are polyuric. The potential capacity of the bladder will often have to be reassessed following a period of bladder cycling, when the bladder is repeatedly filled via a suprapubic catheter and the volume, voiding capacity, and residual volume are determined. If the native bladder is not of sufficient volume and compliance, some form of augmentation will be required.

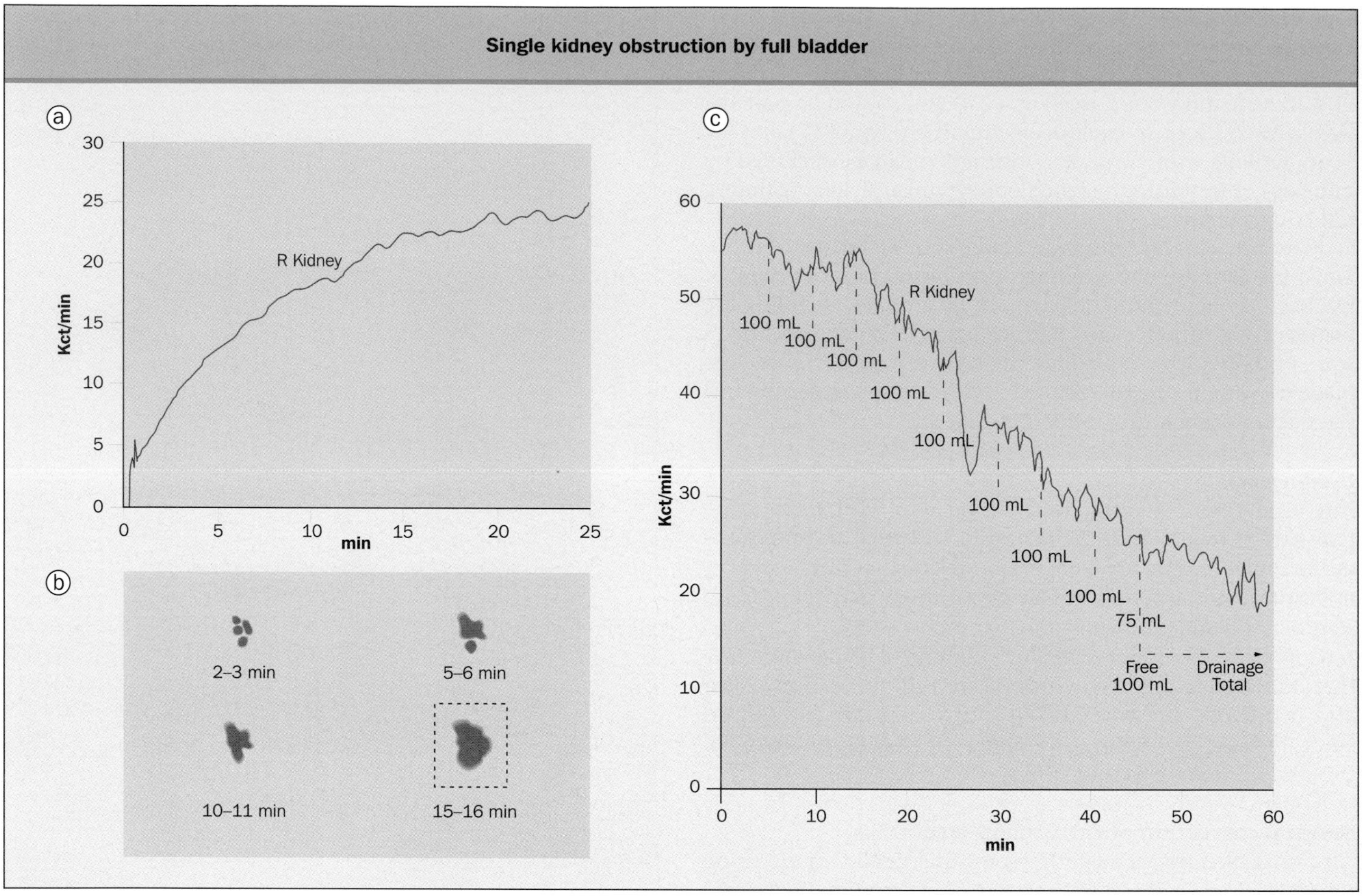

Single kidney obstruction by full bladder

(a)

[Graph showing Kct/min (y-axis, 0–30) vs min (x-axis, 0–25) with rising curve labeled "R Kidney"]

(b)

[Isotope scan images labeled: 2–3 min, 5–6 min, 10–11 min, 15–16 min]

(c)

[Graph showing Kct/min (y-axis, 0–60) vs min (x-axis, 0–60) with declining curve labeled "R Kidney", annotated with 100 mL increments: 100 mL (×8), 75 mL, Free 100 mL, Drainage Total]

Figure 52.18 Dynamic isotope scan (MAG3) starting with bladder full in a patient with solitary right kidney. (a) Rising curve of tracer accumulating in kidney and showing no excretion. (b) Accumulation of isotope in hydronephrotic pelvis without excretion to bladder. (c) 100 mL increments of fluid removed from bladder; after 400 mL removed kidney begins to drain.

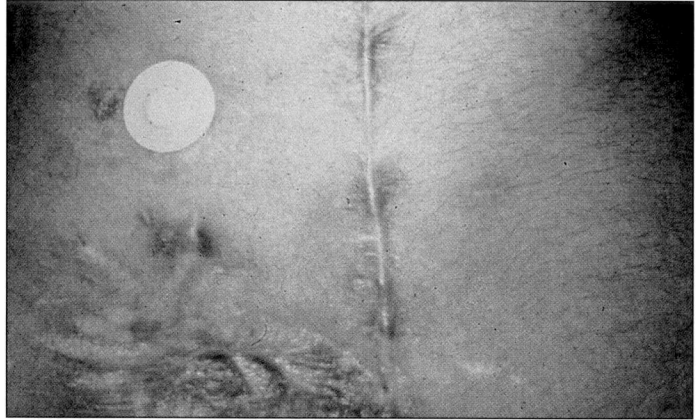

Figure 52.19 Mitrofanoff stoma. A patient born with bladder exstrophy who has had a successful renal transplant for the past 11 years. Her kidney is plumbed into a colonic reservoir and she catheterizes herself through a continent Mitrofanoff stoma, which in the picture is covered by a small piece of plaster.

COMPLICATIONS

Urinary tract infections (to treat or not to treat)

Symptomatic UTIs are common. Risk factors include stagnation of urine, stones, foreign bodies (stents, catheters), previous infections, and renal scarring. UTIs must be treated promptly after a urine culture (midstream or catheter specimen) has been taken. Recurrent UTIs, particularly after a period of stability, must lead to further investigations to exclude stones or obstruction, including abdominal X-ray, renal ultrasound, and postmicturition bladder ultrasound.

Asymptomatic UTIs often do not require treatment (except during pregnancy). For patients with urinary diversions, it is important to get a catheter specimen of urine, since urine taken from a bag is invariably infected.

Sometimes it is appropriate to give prophylactic antibiotics to eradicate infection. They should be chosen according to the known sensitivities of the organism. Tetracycline and oxytetracycline are contraindicated as they are toxic to damaged tubules and cause an acute-on-chronic renal failure. Doxycycline, however, can be used. Nitrofurantoin and nalidixic acid are avoided if GFR is reduced below 50 mL/min as they are both renally excreted and toxic in renal failure. Quinolones should not be used as a regular prophylactic antibiotic, if possible, because of the risk of inducing resistance. Attempts to sterilize the urinary tract, when foreign bodies such as stones remain, are unlikely to be successful.

If prophylactic antibiotics are no longer effective at preventing infection, it is advisable to stop all antibiotics and give the patient a supply of antibiotics to treat symptoms him/herself at home as they occur.

Hypertension and glomerular hyperfiltration

If renal function is declining and proteinuria and hypertension are present, glomerular hyperfiltration is likely, although all other causes of renal dysfunction must be excluded. It is our practice to treat such patients with angiotensin antagonists (ACE inhibitors and angiotensin II receptor antagonists). In our experience, patients with primary VUR (with normal caliber ureters) respond very well, with reduction of proteinuria and stabilization of renal function. In patients with secondary VUR (dilated ureters), ACE inhibitors have little or no effect on proteinuria and only a modest effect in stabilizing renal function.

Hypertension is common in the presence of scarred kidneys, but it is usually controlled easily with one to two drugs. Patients in whom chronic renal failure is secondary to obstruction tend to have volume contraction and, therefore, often have normal blood pressure or only mild hypertension. ACE inhibitors are preferred for patients who have evidence of hyperfiltration with proteinuria and progressive renal failure, but β-blockers and calcium channel blockers are also effective at lowering blood pressure.

Stones

Magnesium ammonium phosphate (struvite) and calcium phosphate stones form in the presence of infected urine, as these salts are poorly soluble in alkaline urine. In 90% of patients, the infecting organism is *Proteus sp.*[39], but other urea-splitting organisms (including some staphylococci and *Pseudomonas*) also generate ammonia.

Stones, usually calcium phosphate, are common in conduits because of the alkaline environment and occur in 5–30% of ileal conduits.

Stones must be suspected if UTIs recur or become more frequent, if renal function suddenly deteriorates, or if there is an unexplained sterile pyuria.

Tubular dysfunction

In patients whose renal failure is secondary to obstruction, there is significant tubular injury. This may cause problems, in particular with urinary concentration, acidification, and sodium reabsorption.

Polyuria

Nocturia is one of the most significant symptoms in the assessment of patients in whom obstruction or tubular dysfunction is suspected. Overfilling of the bladder or reservoir is an important cause of intermittent upper tract obstruction and deteriorating function. The 24-h urine volume diary is a simple way to assess this.

Salt depletion

Patients with tubular damage may have a salt-losing tendency. Patients typically have a cool periphery and constricted hand veins with no peripheral edema. Increasing salt intake can relieve cramps, improve renal function, and reduce hyperuricemia, but at the cost of increasing blood pressure. With patients who are salt depleted, it is important to give sodium chloride as it is the chloride anion that is deficient and responsible for the reduction in circulating volume.

Acidosis

There is often a metabolic acidosis disproportionate to the degree of renal impairment. This is secondary both to a proximal tubular failure of bicarbonate reabsorption and a distal tubular failure to secrete hydrogen ions. It is our practice to give sufficient sodium bicarbonate to correct the plasma bicarbonate into the normal range.

Bone disease

In addition to the typical bone disease of progressive renal failure, acidosis contributes significantly to osteomalacia. Growing children are particularly vulnerable to osteomalacia, and great care must be taken to correct acidosis and manage bone disease carefully.

Urinary diversions

Uretero-sigmoidostomy

Fortunately, it is now rare to meet a patient who still has an uretero-sigmoidostomy, which was widely used as a technique for urinary diversion until the 1970s. The ureters were anastomosed directly into the sigmoid colon with no disruption of bowel continuity. This technique was most commonly used in patients with bladder exstrophy. Although patients start with normal renal function, there is frequently deterioration in function. In one series of 25 patients, significant renal damage occurred in 50%. Stones, infection, and ureteral strictures are common, and patients remain at risk of colonic carcinoma with a 10% incidence of carcinoma at 20-year follow-up. However, this diversion is probably best known for the hyperchloremic, hypokalemic acidosis that occurs. Once the urine is in contact with the colonic mucosa, the urinary sodium exchanges for potassium, and the chloride for bicarbonate, and large quantities of ammonium ions are produced by the action of the fecal bacteria on urinary ammonia. Ammonium ions are absorbed both with chloride and in exchange for sodium. The severe acidosis is a consequence of the ammonium ion retention and stool loss of bicarbonate. Patients are managed with large doses of oral sodium bicarbonate, which is titrated to keep the plasma bicarbonate in the normal range (> 22 mmol/L).

Ileal conduits

Unlike the sigmoidostomy in which urine enters a reservoir, the ileal conduit is free flowing, with rapid urinary transit and no reservoir. Therefore, metabolic complications are much

Hereditary and Congenital Diseases of the Kidney

Long-term complications of urinary diversion
Pyelonephritis and scarring
Calculi
Obstruction
Strictures
Bladder mucus causing obstruction
Cancer at intestinal–ureteral anastomosis
Hyperchloremic acidosis
Delayed linear growth in children
Effects of intestinal loss from gastrointestinal tract, e.g., vitamin B$_{12}$ deficiency
Complications related to abnormal pelvic anatomy, e.g., in pregnancy
Psychologic and body image problems

Table 52.5 Long-term complications of urinary diversion.

less common, although again the bowel can exchange sodium and chloride for potassium and bicarbonate[40,41]. There are a number of other complications of ileal and colonic conduits that can lead to progressive loss of renal function (Table 52.5).

Enterocystoplasty and intestinal urinary reservoirs

In a study of 53 patients with bladder exstrophy, who were followed for more than 10 years and had serial isotopic GFRs, renal function deteriorated (fall in GFR of 20% or more) in only 10 (20%)[29]. Loss of function was caused principally by chronic retention with or without infection in poorly compliant patients who did not catherise regularly. Patients must also be checked regularly to ensure that anastomotic stenoses and high pressure reservoirs do not occur.

END-STAGE RENAL DISEASE AND TRANSPLANTATION

This group of patients presents two important problems at ESRD. First, because of multiple abdominal operations, continuous ambulatory peritoneal dialysis (CAPD) is often impossible. If there is any doubt, CAPD should be attempted. Second, the bladder/urinary reservoir must be suitable for renal transplantation. If a bladder has just destroyed two perfectly good native kidneys, it is likely to do the same to a transplant kidney. Most patients will be maintained on hemodialysis, but it is frequently difficult to establish a good arteriovenous fistula because of chronic hypovolemia and venoconstriction. Patients on dialysis will often continue to pass 1 litre or more of urine per 24th, and they also remain at risk of serious UTI and pyelonephritis.

Transplantation
Pretransplant assessment

Transplantation into the abnormal lower urinary tract requires careful evaluation and follow-up. Thorough preoperative assessment of bladder function is essential. Patients considered to have normal bladders require at least a postmicturition bladder ultrasound examination and urinary flow rate.

All patients with abnormal bladders or reservoir must have a full video cystometrogram (VCMG), to ensure that the bladder reservoir is large and adequately compliant. If the bladder is small or has not been used for some time, bladder 'cycling' may be required, which involves periodically filling and distending the bladder via a suprapubic catheter. A study of urodynamics before transplantation indicated that poor bladder function as shown by small bladder volumes was a predictor of graft loss even in patients with previously normal bladder function[42].

Intermittent self-catheterization is safe and effective for a patient with a poor flow rate who fails to empty the bladder. This however is only possible with a normal urethra and a co-operative patient. When this is not practical we would attempt to establish suprapubic drainage via a continent stoma, for example a Mitrofanoff stoma (see Fig. 55.19). If a conduit is to be used then a loopogram and endoscopy must ensure that it is in good condition. We do not remove native kidneys unless they are causing recurrent urinary tract infection.

Transplant outcome

We have assessed renal transplant outcome during a 15-year period (1985–1999) in 127 renal transplants performed in patients who had ESRD as a consequence of urological abnormalities. The patients fall into two broad groups: (1) those with 'normal' bladders and normal caliber ureters and (2) those with 'abnormal' bladders and dilated ureters, or some form of continent or incontinent urinary diversion. The bladder was considered normal if urine flow rate was > 15 mL/s, and there was no residual volume seen on ultrasound after voiding. Since 1997, tacrolimus has replaced cyclosporine as our routine calcineurin inhibitor. A total of 57 patients with abnormal bladders had 64 transplants, including one patient who had three transplants during this period. In 47 cases, the ureters were transplanted into unaugmented bladder, in the remaining 17 cases there was some form of augmentation or diversion. Results are compared with 63 transplants in 57 patients, who had renal failure from primary vesicoureteral reflux or renal dysplasia and whose bladder function was considered to be normal.

There was no difference in actuarial graft survival in the two groups at 10 years with both groups having 60% of grafts functioning, although longer follow-up is showing an advantage for normal bladders with a kidney half-life of 29–33 years, compared with 16 years for the abnormal bladders. Actuarial patient survival at 10 years is 88% in both groups. Renal function is better in the group with normal bladders. At latest follow up, the abnormal, unaugmented bladder group (n = 24) have been followed 93 (76) months (mean (median)) and have a plasma creatinine of 180 (160) µmol/L, while the normal bladder group (n = 35) have been followed 84 (75) months and have a creatinine concentration of 154 (131) µmol/L. Poorer outcome is associated with higher voiding pressures and residual volumes.

Management

We routinely use double-J ureteral stents for all our transplants. Adequacy of urinary drainage must be assessed frequently, even when renal function seems to be good. Three months after transplant, when the ureteral stent has been removed, we perform as a baseline

- ^{51}Cr-EDTA glomerular filtration rate (GFR)
- ultrasound of kidney and bladder post micturition
- dynamic isotope scan (^{99}Tm-MAG3), and
- static isotope scan (^{99}Tm-DMSA).

The GFR is repeated at 6 months and then annually. Ultrasound and ^{99}Tm-MAG3 are repeated at 1 year, and then when indicated. Twenty-four hour urine collections for protein are done at 6 months and then annually, although we now prefer to measure the protein:creatinine ratio on all random urine samples from the outpatient clinic. If there is renal dysfunction, imaging tests are repeated and, if there is a change from baseline, renal biopsy is performed to exclude an immunologic cause of graft dysfunction. If there is a documented deterioration in renal function in the absence of rejection or cyclosporine toxicity, the DMSA scan is repeated and the bladder reassessed urodynamically[43].

Complications

UTIs must be detected and treated early and recurrent infections may require long courses of antibiotics or even removal of the native tracts. All our patients with urological problems receive prophylactic antibiotics for the first 6 months.

We have previously reported that symptomatic urinary tract infections were common in the first 3 months after transplantation (63%); fever and systemic symptoms occurred in 39% with normal bladders and 59% with abnormal bladders. Urinary tract infection directly contributed to graft loss in patients with abnormal bladders, but caused no consequences in those with normal bladders[38].

If UTIs recur, then a cause must be sought with ultrasound of kidney and bladder. A plain abdominal X-ray is essential to look for stones in native or transplant kidneys and the bladder, or urinary diversion. If there is a residual volume after double micturition then the patient must be instructed to perform intermittent clean self-catheterization. With these measures good results are obtained.

ACKNOWLEDGMENTS

I would like to thank all my colleagues who have helped in the preparation of this chapter and contributed material from their clinical practice, in particular Drs MJ Kellett and J Bomanji, Professor M Craggs and Messrs CRJ Woodhouse and PJR Shah.

REFERENCES

1. James CA, Watson AR, Twining P, Rance CH. Antenatally detected urinary tract abnormalities: changing incidence and management. Eur J Pediatr. 1998;157(6):508–11.
2. Rascher W, Meyer-Schwickerath M, Olbing H. Congenital abnormalities of the urinary tract. In: Cameron JS, Davison AM, Grunfeld J, Kerr D, Ritz E, eds. Textbook of Clinical Nephrology. Oxford: Oxford University Press; 1998:2543–63.
3. Cuckow PM, Nyirady P, Winyard PJ. Normal and abnormal development of the urogenital tract. Prenat Diagn. 2001;21(11):908–16.
4. Mundy AR. Embryology TDFM. In: Fitzpatrick JM, Neal DE, George NJR, eds. Scientific Basis of Urology. Manila, Phillipines: Isis Medical Media; 1999:407–20.
5. Woolf AS, Winyard PJ. Advances in the cell biology and genetics of human kidney malformations. J Am Soc Nephrol. 1998;9(6): 1114–25.
6. Woolf AS, Winyard PJ. Molecular mechanisms of human embryogenesis: developmental pathogenesis of renal tract malformations. Pediatr Dev Pathol. 2002;5(2):108–29.
7. Bassuk JA, Grady R, Mitchell M. Review article: The molecular era of bladder research. Transgenic mice as experimental tools in the study of outlet obstruction. J Urol. 2000;164(1):170–9.
8. Dressler GR, Wilkinson JE, Rothenpieler UW, et al. Deregulation of Pax-2 expression in transgenic mice generates severe kidney abnormalities. Nature. 1993;362(6415):65–7.
9. Torres M, Gomez PE, Dressler GR, Gruss P. Pax-2 controls multiple steps of urogenital development. Development. 1995; 121(12):4057–65.
10. Feather SA, Malcolm S, Woolf AS, et al. Primary, nonsyndromic vesicoureteral reflux and its nephropathy is genetically heterogeneous, with a locus on chromosome 1. Am J Hum Genet. 2000;66(4):1420–5.
11. Pope JC, Brock JW, Adams MC, et al. How they begin and how they end: classic and new theories for the development and deterioration of congenital anomalies of the kidney and urinary tract, CAKUT. Am J Ther. 2001;8(4):275–89; 10(9): 2018–28.
12. Risdon RA, Yeung CK, Ransley PG. Reflux nephropathy in children submitted to unilateral nephrectomy: a clinicopathological study. Clin Nephrol. 1993;40(6):308–4.
13. Hiraoka M, Hori C, Tsukahara H, et al. Congenitally small kidneys with reflux as a common cause of nephropathy in boys. Kidney Int. 1997;52(3):811–16.
14. Cotran RS. Nephrology forum. Glomerulosclerosis in reflux nephropathy. Kidney Int. 1982;21(3):528–34.
15. Bhathena DB, Weiss JH, Holland NH, et al. Focal and segmental glomerular sclerosis in reflux nephropathy. Am J Med. 1980; 68(6):886–92.
16. Kincaid SP, Becker G. Reflux nephropathy and chronic atrophic pyelonephritis: a review. J Infect Dis. 1978;138(6):774–80.
17. Brenner BM, Meyer TW, Hostetter TH. Dietary protein intake and the progressive nature of kidney disease: the role of hemodynamically mediated glomerular injury in the pathogenesis of progressive glomerular sclerosis in aging, renal ablation, and intrinsic renal disease. N Engl J Med. 1982;307(11):652–9.
18. O'Dea D, Pafrey PS, Harnett JD, et al. The importance of renal impairment the natural history of Bardet-Biedl syndrome. Am J Kidney Dis. 1996;27(6):776–83.
19. Koff SA, Campbell KD. The nonoperative management of unilateral neonatal hydronephrosis: natural history of poorly functioning kidneys. J Urol. 1994;152(2, part 2):593–5.
20. Lee PH, Diamond DA, Duffy PG, Ransley PG. Duplex reflux: a study of 105 children. J Urol. 1991;146(2, part 2):657–9.
21. Ehrlich RM, Brown WJ. Ultrastructural anatomic observations of the ureter in the prune belly syndrome. Birth Defects Orig Artic Ser. 1977;13(5):101–3.
22. Whitaker RH, Johnston JH. A simple classification of wide ureters. Br J Urol. 1975;47(7):781–7.
23. Woodhouse CRJ. Long-Term Paediatric Urology. Oxford: Blackwell Scientific Publications; 1991:116–59.
24. Woodhouse CR, Ransley PG, Innes WD. Prune belly syndrome–report of 47 cases. Arch Dis Child. 1982;57(11):856–9.

25. Burbige KA, Amodio J, Berdon WE, et al. Prune belly syndrome: 35 years of experience. J Urol. 1987;137(1):86–90.

26. Woodard JR, Parrott TS. Reconstruction of the urinary tract in prune belly uropathy. J Urol. 1978;119(6):824–8.

27. Hurwitz RS, Manzoni GA, Ransley PG, Stephens FD. Cloacal exstrophy: a report of 34 cases. J Urol. 1987;138(4, part 2):1060–4.

28. Husmann DA, McLorie GA, Churchill BM. A comparison of renal function in the exstrophy patient treated with staged reconstruction versus urinary diversion. J Urol. 1988;140(5, part 2): 1204–6.

29. Fontaine E, Leaver R, Woodhouse CR. The effect of intestinal urinary reservoirs on renal function: a 10-year follow-up. BJU Int. 2000;86:195–8.

30. Johnston LB, Borzyskowski M. Bladder dysfunction and neurological disability at presentation in closed spina bifida. Arch Dis Child. 1998;79(1):33–8.

31. McLorie GA, Perez MR, Csima A, Churchill BM. Determinants of hydronephrosis and renal injury in patients with myelomeningocele. J Urol. 1988;140(5, part 2):1289–92.

32. Lapides J, Diokno AC, Silber SJ, Lowe BS. Clean, intermittent self-catheterization in the treatment of urinary tract disease. J Urol. 1972;107(3):458–61.

33. Edelstein RA, Bauer SB, Kelly MD, et al. The long-term urological response of neonates with myelodysplasia treated proactively with intermittent catheterization and anticholinergic therapy. J Urol. 1995;154(4):1500–4.

34. Tejani A, Butt K, Glassberg K, et al. Predictors of eventual end stage renal disease in children with posterior urethral valves. J Urol. 1986;136(4):857–60.

35. Rittenberg MH, Hulbert WC, Snyder HM, Duckett JW. Protective factors in posterior urethral valves. J Urol. 1988;140(5):993–6.

36. Smith GH, Canning DA, Schulman SL, et al. The long-term outcome of posterior urethral valves treated with primary valve ablation and observation. J Urol. 1996;155(5):1730–4.

37. Parkhouse HF, Barratt TM, Dillon MJ, et al. Long-term outcome of boys with posterior urethral valves. Br J Urol. 1988;62(1):59–62.

38. Crowe A, Cairns HS, Wood S, et al. Renal transplantation following renal failure due to urological disorders. Nephrol Dial Transplant. 1998;13(8):2065–9.

39. Dretler SP. The pathogenesis of urinary tract calculi occurring after ileal conduit diversion. I. Clinical study. II. Conduit study. 3. Prev J Urol. 1973;109(2):204–9.

40. McDougal WS. Metabolic complications of urinary intestinal diversion. J Urol. 1992;147(5):1199–1208.

41. Silverman SH, Woodhouse CR, Strachan JR, et al. Long-term management of patients who have had urinary diversions into colon. Br J Urol. 1986;58(6):634–9.

42. Kashi SH, Wynne KS, Sadek SA, Lodge JP. An evaluation of vesical urodynamics before renal transplantation and its effect on renal allograft function and survival. Transplantation. 1994;57(10): 1455–7.

43. Cairns HS, Spencer S, Hilson AJ, et al. 99mTc-DMSA imaging with tomography in renal transplant recipients with abnormal lower urinary tracts. Nephrol Dial Transplant. 1994;9(8):1157–61.

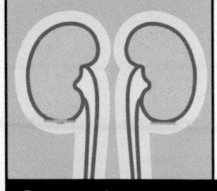

Chapter 53

Urinary Tract Infections in Adults

Thomas Hooton

DEFINITION

Urinary tract infection (UTI) in adults can be categorized into six groups: young women with acute uncomplicated cystitis, young women with recurrent cystitis, young women with acute uncomplicated pyelonephritis, adults with acute cystitis and conditions that suggest occult renal or prostatic involvement, complicated UTI, and asymptomatic bacteriuria (Table 53.1)[1]. A discussion of UTI in pregnancy is provided in Chapter 44 and of vesicoureteral reflux in children in Chapter 61.

A complicated UTI is one that is associated with a condition that increases the risk of serious complications or treatment failure. Distinction between uncomplicated and complicated UTIs is important mainly because of implications regarding pre- and post-treatment evaluation, type and duration of antimicrobial treatment, and the extent of evaluation of the urinary tract that is required. It is not always possible, however, to classify patients definitively as having complicated or uncomplicated infections when they first present, and the distinction is sometimes made only when a patient has a poor response to treatment. Patients with certain complicating conditions, such as those presented in Table 53.1, are at greatly increased risk for serious complications of UTI and warrant special concern. These conditions only serve as guidelines for the clinician who must decide, based on limited clinical information, whether to embark on a more extensive evaluation and treatment course when confronted with a patient with UTI.

EPIDEMIOLOGY

Acute uncomplicated UTIs are among the most common medical conditions, with several million episodes of acute cystitis and at least 250 000 episodes of acute pyelonephritis occurring annually in the USA. One recent survey estimated that as many as 11 million women in the USA had at least one treated UTI in 1995, and that the cost for evaluating and managing UTIs was US$1.6bn[2]. In a prospective study of young sexually active women, the incidence of cystitis was approximately 0.5 per person-year[3]. Acute uncomplicated cystitis may recur in 27–44% of healthy women, even though they have normal urinary tracts[4]. The incidence of symptomatic UTI in adult men less than 50 years of age is much lower than in women, ranging from 5 to 8 per 10 000 men annually. Incidence data are not available for postmenopausal women and older men.

Complicated UTIs encompass an extraordinarily broad range of infectious entities (Table 53.1). The incidence of

---

Categories of urinary tract infection in adults

Acute uncomplicated cystitis in young women

Recurrent acute uncomplicated cystitis in young women

Acute uncomplicated pyelonephritis in young women

Acute uncomplicated cystitis in adult with following condition suggesting possible occult renal or prostatic involvement but without other known complicating factors:

  Male sex

  Elderly

  Pregnancy

  Recent urinary tract instrumentation

  Childhood urinary tract infection

  Recent antimicrobial use

  Symptoms for more than 7 days at presentation

  Diabetes mellitus

Complicated urinary tract infection[a]

  Obstruction or other structural factor: urolithiasis, malignancies, ureteral and urethral strictures, bladder diverticuli, renal cysts, fistulae, ileal conduits, and other urinary diversions

  Functional abnormality: neurogenic bladder, vesicoureteral reflux

  Foreign bodies: indwelling catheter, ureteral stent, nephrostomy tube

  Other conditions: renal failure, renal transplantation, immunosuppression, multidrug-resistant uropathogens, hospital-acquired (nosocomial) infection, prostatitis-related infection, upper tract infection in an adult other than a young healthy woman, other functional or anatomic abnormality of the urinary tract

Asymptomatic bacteriuria

[a]This is a selected list of complicating factors[1]. Some factors complicate urinary tract infections through several mechanisms

Table 53.1 Categories of urinary tract infection in adults.

---

nosocomial UTI, one of the most common types of complicated UTI, is approximately 5/100 admissions in a university tertiary care hospital, with catheter-associated infections accounting for 88% of the infections. More than 1 million nosocomial UTIs occur each year in the USA, and catheter-associated bacteriuria is the most common source of Gram-negative bacteremia in hospitalized patients[5].

Asymptomatic bacteriuria is defined as the presence of two separate consecutive clean-voided urine specimens both with $\geq 10^5$ colony-forming units (cfu)/mL of the same uropathogen in the absence of symptoms[6]. Asymptomatic bacteriuria is found in approximately 5% of young adult women[7], but rarely in men aged below 50 years. The prevalence increases to 21%

of ambulatory women and 12% of ambulatory men older than 65, and to 53% of elderly women and 37% of elderly men who are institutionalized. Asymptomatic bacteriuria may be persistent or transient and recurrent, and many patients have had previous symptomatic infection or develop symptomatic UTI soon after having asymptomatic bacteriuria. Asymptomatic bacteriuria is generally assumed to be a benign condition although, as discussed below, it may lead to serious complications in some clinical settings.

PATHOGENESIS

Uncomplicated infection

Most uncomplicated UTIs in healthy women result when uropathogens (typically *Escherichia coli*) present in the rectal flora enter the bladder via the urethra after an interim phase of periurethral and distal urethral colonization. In the male, colonizing uropathogens may also come from a sex partner's vagina or rectum. Hematogenenous seeding of the urinary tract by potential uropathogens such as *Staphylococcus aureus* is the source of some UTIs, but this is more likely to occur in the setting of persistent bloodstream infection or urinary tract obstruction.

Many host genetic, biologic, and behavioral factors predispose young healthy women to uncomplicated UTI (Table 53.2)[8]. Important risk factors include sexual intercourse, use of spermicide products, and a history of previous recurrent UTI[3,9]. Nonsecretors of ABH blood group antigens have an increased risk of recurrent cystitis, and women with the P_1 blood group phenotype have an increased risk for recurrent pyelonephritis. The host's inflammatory and immunologic responses also help determine the clinical consequences of UTI.

In addition to these and other host factors that modulate UTI risk, certain strains of *E. coli* have a selective advantage for colonization and infection (Table 53.2)[10]. P-fimbriated strains of *E. coli* are associated with acute uncomplicated pyelonephritis, and their adherence properties may stimulate epithelial and other cells to produce cytokines and other proinflammatory factors that are responsible for some of the inflammatory response[10]. Other virulence determinants include adherence factors (type 1, S, Dr fimbriae), toxins (hemolysin), aerobactin,

and serum resistance[10]. Bacterial virulence determinants associated with cystitis and asymptomatic bacteriuria have been less well characterized[7,10].

The large difference in UTI prevalence between men and women is thought to result from a variety of factors, including the greater distance between the usual source of uropathogens (the anus and the urethral meatus) the drier environment surrounding the male urethra, the greater length of the male urethra, and the antibacterial activity of prostatic fluid. Risk factors associated with UTIs in healthy men include intercourse with an infected female partner, homosexual intercourse, and lack of circumcision, although these factors are often not present in men with UTI. Most uropathogenic strains infecting young men are highly virulent, suggesting that the urinary tract in healthy men is relatively resistant to infection.

Complicated infection

The initial steps leading to uncomplicated UTI discussed above probably also occur in most individuals who develop a complicated UTI. Factors that predispose individuals to complicated UTI generally do so by causing obstruction and/or stasis of urine flow, facilitating entry of uropathogens into the urinary tract by bypassing normal host defense mechanisms, providing a nidus for infection that is not readily treatable with antimicrobials, or compromising the host immune system (see Table 53.1)[1]. UTIs are more likely to become complicated in the setting of impaired host defense, as occurs with indwelling catheter use, vesicoureteral reflux, obstruction, neutropenia, and immune deficiencies. Diabetes mellitus, in particular, is associated with several syndromes of complicated UTI, including renal and perirenal abscess, emphysematous pyelonephritis and cystitis, papillary necrosis, and xanthogranulomatous pyelonephritis[11]. Uropathogen virulence determinants appear to be of much less importance in the pathogenesis of complicated UTIs compared with uncomplicated UTIs. However, infection with multidrug-resistant uropathogens is more likely with complicated UTI.

ETIOLOGIC AGENTS

The spectrum of etiologic agents is similar in uncomplicated upper and lower UTI, with *E. coli* the causative pathogen in 70–95% and *Staphylococcus saprophyticus* in 5% to more than 20% (Table 53.3). *S. saprophyticus* may be a less common cause of acute pyelonephritis[12]. Occasionally, other Enterobacteriaceae such as *Proteus mirabilis*, *Klebsiella* spp., or enterococci are isolated from such patients. Group B streptocococci also appear to cause occasional episodes and, rarely, *Pseudomonas aeruginosa*, *Citrobacter* spp., or other uropathogens cause uncomplicated UTI.

Unlike the narrow and predictable spectrum of causative agents in uncomplicated infection, a broad range of bacteria can cause complicated infections, and many are resistant to multiple antimicrobial agents. Although *E. coli* is the predominant uropathogen in complicated UTI, uropathogens other than *E. coli*, including *Citrobacter* spp., *Enterobacter* spp., *P. aeruginosa*, enterococci, and *S. aureus*, account for a relatively higher proportion of cases compared with uncomplicated UTIs (Table 53.3)[1]. The proportion of infections caused by fungi,

Factors modulating risk for acute uncomplicated urinary tract infections in women	
Host determinants	Uropathogen determinants
Behavioral: sexual intercourse, use of spermicidal products, recent antimicrobial use, suboptimal voiding habits **Genetic:** enhanced epithelial cell adherence, antibacterial factors in urine and bladder mucosa, nonsecretor of ABH blood group antigens, P_1 blood group phenotype, previous history of recurrent cystitis **Biologic:** estrogen peak in premenopausal, estrogen deficiency in postmenopausal, inflammatory and immunologic response	*Escherichia coli* virulence determinants: P, S, Dr, and type 1 fimbriae: hemolysin; aerobactin; serum resistance

Table 53.2 Factors modulating risk for acute uncomplicated urinary tract infections in women.

Bacterial etiology of urinary tract infections		
	Urinary tract infection (%)	
Organisms	Uncomplicated	Complicated
Gram-negative organisms		
Escherichia coli	70–95	21–54
Proteus mirabilis	1–2	1–10
Klebsiella spp.	1–2	2–17
Citrobacter spp.	<1	5
Enterobacter spp.	<1	2–10
Pseudomonas aeruginosa	<1	2–19
Other	<1	6–20
Gram-positive organisms		
Coagulase-negative staphylococci (*S. saprophyticus*)	5–20 or more	1–4
Enterococci	1–2	1–23
Group B streptococci	<1	1–4
Staphylococcus aureus	<1	1–2
Other	<1	2
(Data for complicated infections from Nicolle[1].)		

Table 53.3 Bacterial etiology of urinary tract infections.

especially *Candida* species, is increasing. Patients with chronic conditions, such as spinal cord injury and neurogenic bladder, are relatively more likely to have polymicrobic and multidrug-resistant infections.

CLINICAL SYNDROMES

Acute uncomplicated cystitis in young women

Women with acute uncomplicated cystitis generally present with acute onset of symptoms including dysuria, frequency, urgency, and/or suprapubic pain. Acute dysuria in a young sexually active woman is usually caused by acute cystitis, acute urethritis from *Chlamydia trachomatis*, *Neisseria gonorrhoeae*, or herpes simplex virus infections, or vaginitis caused by *Candida* spp. or *Trichomonas vaginalis*[4]. A distinction between these three entities can usually, but not always, be made with a high degree of certainty with data from the history and physical examination and simple laboratory tests. Pyuria is present in almost all women with acute cystitis, as well as in most women with urethritis caused by *N. gonorrhoeae* or *C. trachomatis*, and its absence strongly suggests an alternative diagnosis. Hematuria is common in women with UTI but not in women with urethritis or vaginitis.

The definitive diagnosis of UTI is the presence of significant bacteriuria, the traditional standard for which is $\geq 10^5$ uropathogen/mL of voided midstream urine. Recent studies, however, have shown that up to one-third of patients with cystitis have lower colony counts, which are missed using the traditional definition. The Infectious Disease Society of America consensus definition of cystitis is $\geq 10^3$ cfu/mL (sensitivity 80% and specificity 90%)[13]. Urine cultures are generally not necessary in women with uncomplicated cystitis since the causative organisms are predictable and the culture results become available only after therapeutic decisions have been made.

E. coli in patients with uncomplicated UTI are often resistant to sulfonamides and amoxicillin (amoxycillin). Moreover, there has been an increase in resistance to trimethoprim and trimethoprim–sulfamethoxazole (cotrimoxazole) among outpatient urinary strains in the USA and Europe, which is cause for concern[14]. Recent data have led to speculation that resistant strains may enter new environments by contaminated products ingested by community residents[15]. The prevalence of *E. coli* resistance to nitrofurantoin is generally < 5%, although nitrofurantoin is inactive against *Proteus* spp. and some *Enterobacter* and *Klebsiella* strains. Fluoroquinolones remain active against almost all *E. coli* strains causing uncomplicated cystitis although resistance is increasing in certain areas of the world.

Three-day regimens are recommended for the treatment of acute uncomplicated cystitis because of comparable efficacy, better compliance, lower cost, and lower frequency of adverse reactions than with longer regimens. Single-dose regimens, while highly effective in most women (especially trimethoprim–sulfamethoxazole and fluoroquinolones), are somewhat less effective than longer regimens[16]. Higher cure rates generally have been observed with trimethoprim–sulfamethoxazole and fluoroquinolones than with β-lactams regardless of the site of infection and duration of treatment. Fosfomycin tromethamine (fosfomycin trometamol) a single-dose regimen for uncomplicated cystitis, is less effective than 7- to 10-day regimens of ciprofloxacin or trimethoprim–sulfamethoxazole but is comparable to a 7-day regimen of nitrofurantoin.

Optimal management of acute uncomplicated cystitis is summarized in Figure 53.1 and Table 53.4. Trimethoprim or trimethoprim–sulfamethoxazole in a 3-day oral regimen should be considered the first-line agent for uncomplicated cystitis in women who can tolerate this agent and in areas where resistance is infrequent[17]. Fluoroquinolones are reasonable first-line agents in women who are known or suspected of having antimicrobial-resistant organisms, who are allergic or otherwise do not tolerate more conventional regimens, or who live in areas where resistance to trimethoprim–sulfamethoxazole is over 10%. Nitrofurantoin does not appear to be as effective in short-course regimens as trimethoprim–sulfamethoxazole or fluoroquinolones and, therefore, should be used in regimens of 7 days or longer. Broad-spectrum oral cephalosporins (such as cefixime, cefpodoxime, cefprozil, and cefaclor) demonstrate *in vitro* activity against most uropathogens causing uncomplicated cystitis, but clinical data are sparse. Amoxicillin–clavulanate (coamoxiclav) is approved for treatment of UTI but has a high rate of gastrointestinal side effects, which may be less common with use of short-course treatment regimens and the new twice-daily formulations.

Routine post-treatment cultures in asymptomatic women are not indicated because of the considerable costs necessary to detect a single case of asymptomatic bacteriuria, and because the benefit of detecting and treating asymptomatic bacteriuria in healthy women has been demonstrated only in pregnancy and prior to urologic instrumentation or surgery[6]. In women whose infection persists or recurs within 2 weeks, a urine culture and antimicrobial susceptibility testing should be performed and a longer course of therapy, usually with a fluoroquinolone, should be used. In those women whose infection resolves but recurs after 2 weeks, the approach should be the same as with sporadic infections.

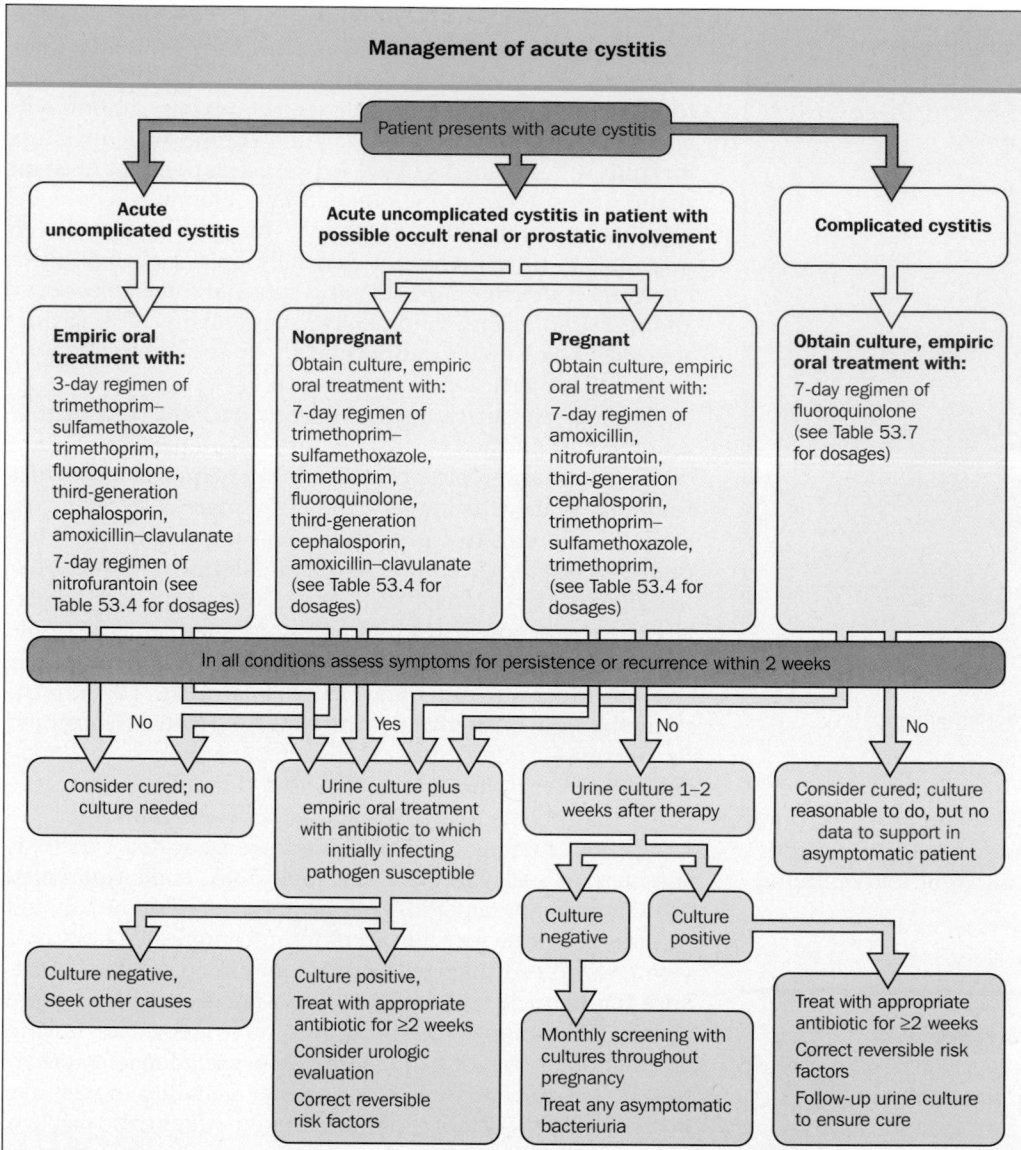

Figure 53.1 Algorithm for management of acute cystitis.

Management of acute cystitis

Patient presents with acute cystitis

Acute uncomplicated cystitis

Acute uncomplicated cystitis in patient with possible occult renal or prostatic involvement

Complicated cystitis

Empiric oral treatment with:

3-day regimen of trimethoprim–sulfamethoxazole, trimethoprim, fluoroquinolone, third-generation cephalosporin, amoxicillin–clavulanate

7-day regimen of nitrofurantoin (see Table 53.4 for dosages)

Nonpregnant

Obtain culture, empiric oral treatment with:

7-day regimen of trimethoprim–sulfamethoxazole, trimethoprim, fluoroquinolone, third-generation cephalosporin, amoxicillin–clavulanate (see Table 53.4 for dosages)

Pregnant

Obtain culture, empiric oral treatment with:

7-day regimen of amoxicillin, nitrofurantoin, third-generation cephalosporin, trimethoprim–sulfamethoxazole, trimethoprim, (see Table 53.4 for dosages)

Obtain culture, empiric oral treatment with:

7-day regimen of fluoroquinolone (see Table 53.7 for dosages)

In all conditions assess symptoms for persistence or recurrence within 2 weeks

No — Yes — No — No

Consider cured; no culture needed

Urine culture plus empiric oral treatment with antibiotic to which initially infecting pathogen susceptible

Urine culture 1–2 weeks after therapy

Consider cured; culture reasonable to do, but no data to support in asymptomatic patient

Culture negative — Culture positive

Culture negative, Seek other causes

Culture positive, Treat with appropriate antibiotic for ≥2 weeks
Consider urologic evaluation
Correct reversible risk factors

Monthly screening with cultures throughout pregnancy
Treat any asymptomatic bacteriuria

Treat with appropriate antibiotic for ≥2 weeks
Correct reversible risk factors
Follow-up urine culture to ensure cure

Oral regimens for acute uncomplicated cystitis

Table 53.4 Oral antimicrobial agents for acute uncomplicated cystitis or cystitis in patient with possible accult renal or prostatic involvement.
Duration of therapy depends on the clinical setting (see text and Fig. 53.1).

Drug	Dose (mg)	Interval	Comment
Trimethoprim–sulfamethoxazole	160/800	q12 h	Widely used in pregnancy, although not an approved use
Trimethoprim	100	q12 h	Widely used in pregnancy, although not an approved use
Fluoroquinolones			Avoid fluoroquinolones if possible in pregnancy, nursing mothers, or in persons <18 years old
Ciprofloxacin	100–250	q12 h	
Levofloxacin	250	q24 h	
Ofloxacin	200	q12 h	
Trovafloxacin	100	q24 h	
Cefpodoxime proxetil	100	q12 h	Data are sparse
Cefixime	400	q24 h	Data are sparse, may be less effective in infection caused by *Staphylococcus saprophyticus*
Nitrofurantoin			May be less active against *Proteus* spp.; should not be used in short courses. Avoid in conditions other than pregnancy with possible occult renal involvement
Monohydrate/macrocrystals (Macrobid)	100	q12 h	
Macrocrystals	50	q6 h	
Amoxicillin	250	q8 h	Used only when causative pathogen is known to be susceptible or for empiric treatment of mild cystitis in pregnancy
Amoxicillin–clavulanate	500/125	q12 h	

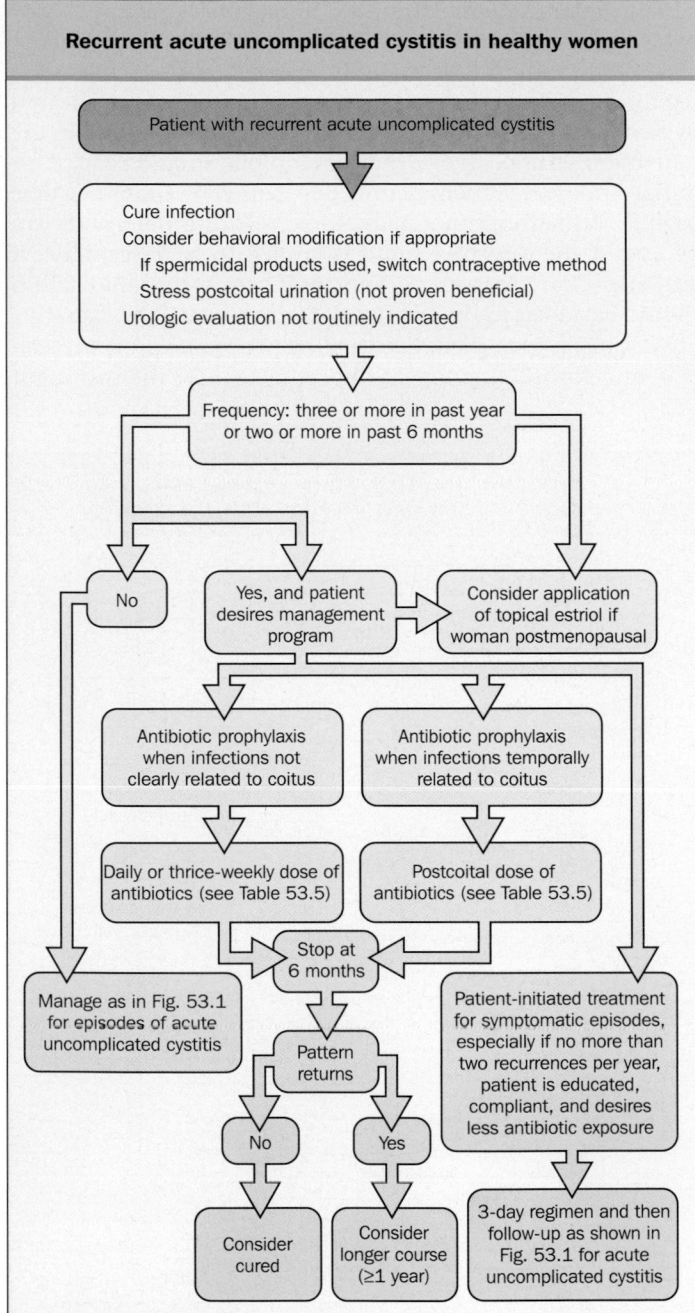

Figure 53.2 Management strategies for recurrent acute uncomplicated cystitis.

Prophylaxis for recurrent acute uncomplicated cystitis

Drug	Dose (mg)	Frequency
Continuous prophylaxis		
Trimethoprim–sulfamethoxazole	40/200	Daily
Trimethoprim–sulfamethoxazole	40/200	Thrice weekly
Trimethoprim	100	Daily
Nitrofurantoin	50 or 100	Daily
Cefaclor	250	Daily
Cefalexin (cephalexin)	125 or 250	Daily
Norfloxacin (other fluoroquinolones are likely to be as effective)[a]	200	Daily
Postcoital prophylaxis		
Trimethoprim–sulfamethoxazole	40/200	–
Trimethoprim–sulfamethoxazole	80/400	–
Nitrofurantoin	50 or 100	–
Cefalexin	250	–
Ciprofloxacin[a]	125	–
Norfloxacin[a]	200	–
Ofloxacin[a]	100	–

[a] Women should cautioned about pregnancy when fluoroquinolones are being used.

Table 53.5 Antimicrobial prophylaxis regimens for women with recurrent acute uncomplicated cystitis. (See text and Fig. 53.2 for management strategy).

Antimicrobial prophylaxis is highly effective in reducing recurrent UTI in women (see Fig. 53.2 and Table 53.5). Prophylaxis should be considered for women who experience three or more infections over a 12-month period, or whenever the woman feels her life is being adversely impacted by frequent recurrences. Several approaches have been shown to be effective in the management of recurrent uncomplicated UTIs, including continuous prophylaxis, postcoital prophylaxis, or intermittent self-treatment (which is not really a prophylaxis method). In postmenopausal women with recurrent UTI, intravaginal estriol has been demonstrated to be effective, presumably by normalizing the vaginal flora, which reduces the risk of coliform colonization of the vagina[18]. This offers an alternative for such women to the antimicrobial strategies discussed above (see Fig. 53.2).

Acute uncomplicated pyelonephritis in women

Acute pyelonephritis is suggested by fever, chills, flank pain, nausea/vomiting, fever (>38°C) and costovertebral angle tenderness. Cystitis symptoms are variably present. Symptoms may vary from a mild illness to a sepsis syndrome with or without shock and renal failure. Pyuria is almost always present but leukocyte casts, specific for UTI, are infrequently seen. Gram stain of the urine sediment may aid in differentiating Gram-positive and Gram-negative infections, which can influence empiric therapy. A urine culture, which should be performed in all women with acute pyelonephritis, will have $\geq 10^4$cfu/mL uropathogens in up to 95% of patients[13].

Pathologically, the kidney shows a focal inflammatory reaction with neutrophil and monocyte infiltrates, tubular damage,

Recurrent acute uncomplicated cystitis in women

Most episodes of recurrent cystitis in healthy women are reinfections, which, in many cases, are caused by the initially infecting strain persisting in the fecal flora[18]. Women with recurrent cystitis may benefit from modification of certain behavioral factors (see Fig. 53.2), such as increasing fluid intake and ensuring postcoital micturition, although this has not been proven. Women with frequent recurrent UTIs who do not wish to change their method of contraception and who do not benefit from behavioral modification suggestions should be offered antimicrobial management. Many women use cranberry juice to prevent UTIs, but data supporting its use are few.

and interstitial edema (see Fig. 53.3). Although imaging studies are generally not performed, the infected kidney is often enlarged and contrast computed tomography (CT) shows decreased opacification of the affected parenchyma, typically in patchy, wedge-shaped or linear patterns (see Fig. 53.4).

The availability of effective oral antimicrobials, especially the fluoroquinolones, allows for initial oral therapy in appropriate patients or, in those requiring parenteral therapy, the timely conversion from intravenous to oral therapy and reduced need for hospitalization. Indications for admission to hospital include inability to maintain oral hydration or take medications, uncertain social situation or concern about compliance, uncertainty about the diagnosis, and severe illness with high fevers, severe pain, and marked debility. Outpatient therapy has been shown to be safe and effective for selected patients, who can be stabilized with parenteral fluids and antibiotics in an urgent-care facility and sent home on oral antibiotics under close supervision.

The management strategy for acute uncomplicated pyelonephritis is shown in Figure 53.5. There are many effective parenteral (see Table 53.6) and oral (see Table 53.7) regimens for use in patients with acute uncomplicated pyelonephritis. For those patients who can be managed in the outpatient setting, an oral fluoroquinolone should be used for initial empiric treatment of infection caused by Gram-negative bacilli[17]. Trimethoprim–sulfamethoxazole or other agents can be used if the infecting strain is known to be susceptible. If enterococci are suspected from the Gram stain, amoxicillin should be added to the treatment regimen until the causative organism(s) is identified. Cefixime, cefpodoxime proxetil, cefaclor, or cefprozil also appear to be effective for the treatment

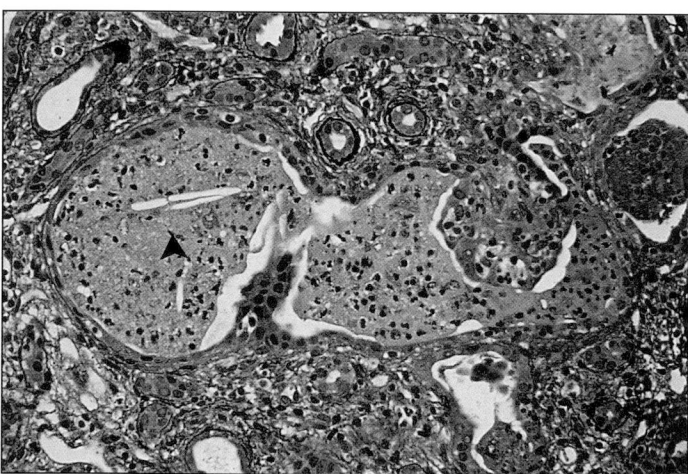

Figure 53.3 Acute pyelonephritis. Renal tissue shows a dilated tubule with neutrophils enmeshed in proteinaceous debris ('pus' casts) (arrowhead) with adjacent interstitial inflammation. (Courtesy of C Alpers.)

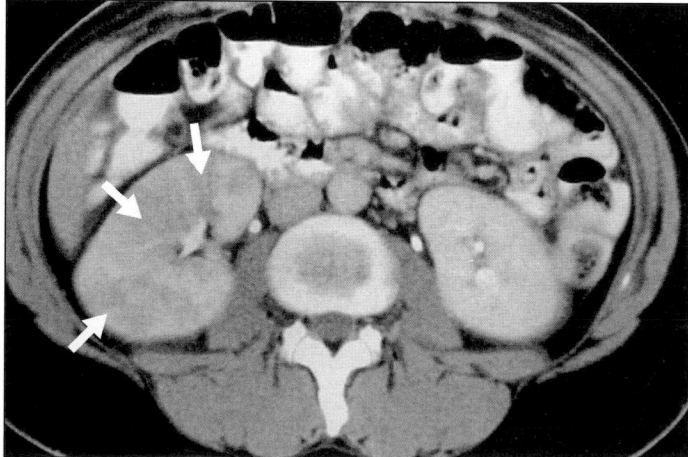

Figure 53.4 Acute pyelonephritis. Contrast computed tomography scan shows areas of lower density owing to infection and edema (arrows). (Courtesy of W Bush.)

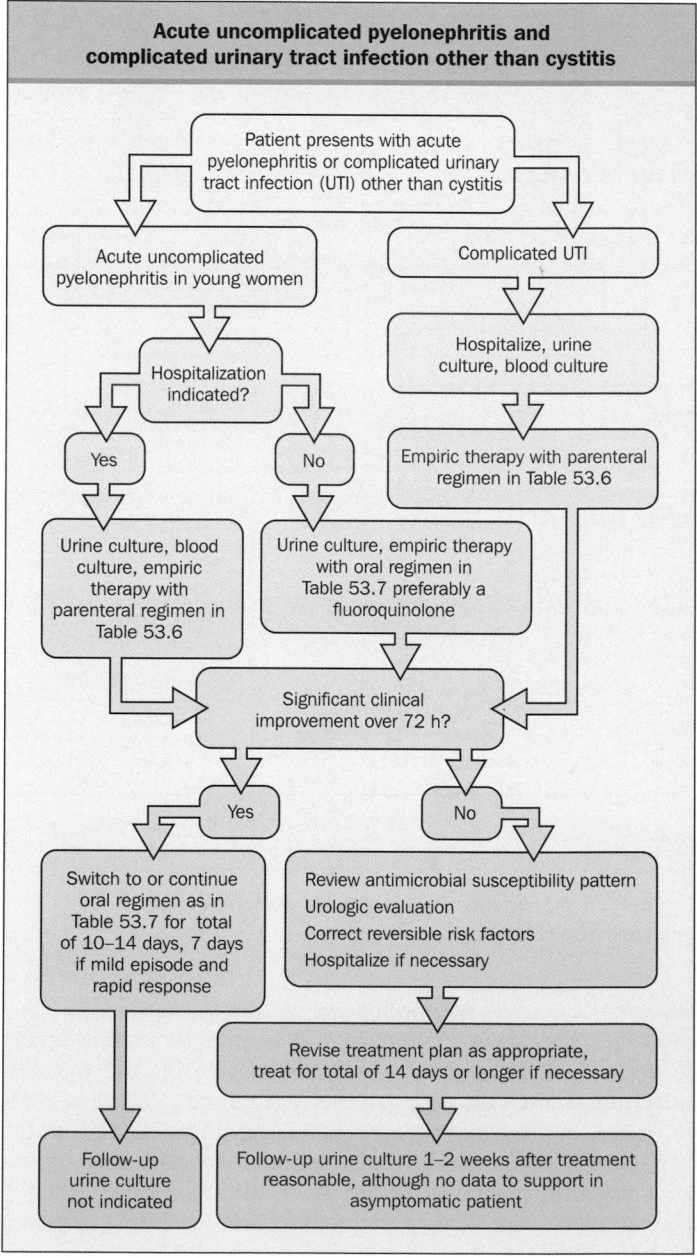

Figure 53.5 Management algorithm for acute uncomplicated pyelonephritis and complicated urinary tract infection other than cystitis.

Parenteral regimens for acute uncomplicated pyelonephritis and complicated urinary tract infection

Drug	Dose (mg)	Interval
Ceftriaxone	1000–2000	q24 h
Cefepime*	1000–2000	q12 h
Fluoroquinolones**		
Ciprofloxacin	200–400	q12 h
Levofloxacin	250–500	q24 h
Ofloxacin	200–400	q12 h
Gentamicin (± ampicillin)	3–5 mg/kg body weight	q24 h
	1 mg/kg body weight	q8 h
Ampicillin (+ gentamicin)	1000	q6 h
Trimethoprim–sulfamethoxazole***	160/800	q12 h
Aztreonam	1000	q8–12 h
Ampicillin–sulbactam*	1500	q6 h
Ticarcillin–clavulanate*	3200	q8 h
Piperacillin–tazobactam*	3375	q6–8 h
Imipenem–cilastatin*	250–500	q6–8 h

* Recommended if *Staphylococcus aureus* coverage desirable, such as for treatment of a renal or perirenal abscess or when the Gram stain suggests *S. aureus* infection.
** Avoid, if possible in pregnancy.
*** Widely used in pregnancy, although not an approved use.

Table 53.6 Parenteral regimens for acute uncomplicated pyelonephritis and complicated urinary tract infection. Duration depends on clinical setting (see text and Fig. 53.5).

of acute uncomplicated pyelonephritis, although published data are sparse. Nitrofurantoin should not be used for the treatment of pyelonephritis since it does not achieve reliable tissue levels.

For hospitalized patients, ceftriaxone is an effective and inexpensive agent if the Gram stain is not suggestive of infection caused by Gram-positive pathogens. If enterococci are suspected based on the Gram stain, ampicillin plus gentamicin, ampicillin-sulbactam or piperacillin–tazobactam are reasonable broad-spectrum empiric choices. Trimethoprim–sulfamethoxazole should not be used alone for empiric therapy for pyelonephritis in areas with a high prevalence of resistance to this combination. Patients with acute uncomplicated pyelonephritis can often be switched to oral therapy at 24–48 h, although longer intervals of parenteral therapy are occasionally indicated.

Six-week regimens are no more effective than 14-day regimens for uncomplicated pyelonephritis and cause more side effects[19]. Although there are few published data demonstrating that regimens shorter than 14 days are as effective as longer regimens, one recent study demonstrated superiority of a 7-day ciprofloxacin regimen over a 14-day trimethoprim–sulfamethoxazole regimen. The difference was accounted for entirely by the higher rate of resistance to trimethoprim–sulfamethoxazole compared with ciprofloxacin among the uropathogens[12]. In general, for those mild-to-moderately ill patients who have a rapid response with resolution of fever and symptoms soon after initiating treatment, treatment can be discontinued at 7 to 10 days. Of note, however, β-lactam regimens shorter than 14 days have been associated with unacceptably high failure rates. Routine post-treatment urine cultures in asymptomatic patients are not cost effective, but cultures should be performed if symptoms recur. Recurrent infections are treated with a second 2-week course, but in patients whose infection persists with the same strain as the initial infecting strain, complicating factors should be looked for and corrected if found.

Acute cystitis in healthy adults with possible occult renal or prostatic involvement

Episodes of acute cystitis in healthy individuals other than young women are more likely to involve occult renal or prostatic infection (see Table 53.1) and may respond poorly to short-course therapy. Some patients, such as those with diabetes or pregnancy, warrant special attention because of the serious complications that can occur if treatment is inadequate. Symptoms, signs, and laboratory findings in this group

Oral regimens for acute uncomplicated pyelonephritis and complicated urinary tract infection

Drug	Dose (mg)	Interval	Comment
Fluoroquinolones			Preferred for empiric treatment, avoid if possible in pregnancy, nursing mothers, or in persons <18 years old
Ciprofloxacin	500	q12 h	
Levofloxacin	250–500	q24 h	
Ofloxacin	200–300	q12 h	
Trimethoprim–sulfamethoxazole	160/800	q12 h	Widely used in pregnancy, although not an approved use
Cefpodoxime proxetil	200	q12 h	Data are sparse
Cefixime	400	q24 h	Data are sparse, may be less effective in infection caused by *Staphylococcus saprophyticus*
Amoxicillin	500	q8 h	Used only when the causative pathogen is known to be susceptible or in addition to a broad-spectrum agent when empiric coverage against enterococci is desirable

Table 53.7 Oral regimens for acute uncomplicated pyelonephritis and complicated urinary tract infection. Duration depends on clinical setting (see text and Figs. 53.1 and 53.5)

are the same as in uncomplicated cystitis. Urethritis must be excluded in dysuric sexually active men with a urethral Gram stain or a first-voided urine specimen wet mount evaluation for urethral leukocytosis.

The management approach to patients in this category is shown in Figure 53.1. Empiric use of the agents discussed previously for uncomplicated cystitis in women are suitable for the treatment of UTIs in these patients. Nitrofurantoin generally should be avoided because of poor tissue penetration, except for the treatment of mild cystitis in pregnancy. The recommended duration of treatment is at least 7 days. A pretreatment urine culture should be obtained routinely in patients in this category, whereas the need for a post-treatment culture is less certain, except in pregnant women (see Fig. 53.1). In men, early recurrence of UTI with the same species suggests a prostatic source of infection and warrants a 4- to 6-week regimen of either a fluoroquinolone (preferable) or trimethoprim–sulfamethoxazole.

Complicated infections

In addition to the classic signs of cystitis and pyelonephritis, complicated UTIs may also be associated with nonspecific symptoms such as fatigue, irritability, nausea, headache, abdominal or back pain, or other vague symptoms, especially in patients at the extremes of age and patients with neurologic disease. Signs and symptoms may occasionally be insidious and exist for weeks to months before diagnosis. Complicated UTI, like uncomplicated UTI, is generally associated with pyuria and bacteriuria, although these may be absent if the infection does not communicate with the collecting system. Because of the diverse spectrum of causative uropathogens and their unpredictable susceptibility profile, a urine culture should always be performed in patients with suspected complicated UTI. As with uncomplicated UTI, a colony count threshold of $\geq 10^3$cfu/mL should be used to diagnose complicated UTI except when urine cultures are obtained through a catheter, in which a level of $\geq 10^2$cfu/mL is evidence of infection[13].

The wide variety of underlying conditions (see Table 53.1), diverse spectrum of possible etiologic agents (see Table 53.3), and paucity of controlled clinical trials with stratification according to specific complicating factors make generalizing about antimicrobial therapy difficult. The management strategy for complicated cystitis is shown in Figure 53.1 and for complicated infections other than cystitis in Figure 53.5. Attempts must be made to correct any underlying anatomic, functional or metabolic defect, since otherwise antibiotics alone will often not be successful[1]. For empirical therapy in patients with mild-to-moderate illness who can be treated with oral medication, the fluoroquinolones provide the broadest spectrum of antimicrobial activity, cover most expected pathogens and achieve high levels in the urine and urinary tract tissue. Exceptions are sparfloxacin, grepafloxacin, trovafloxacin, and moxifloxacin, which, in contrast to other fluoroquinolones, may not achieve sufficient concentration in urine to be effective for complicated UTI. If the infecting pathogen is known to be susceptible, trimethoprim–sulfamethoxazole or other agents are reasonable therapeutic choices. For initial treatment in more seriously ill, hospitalized patients, several parenteral antimicrobial agents are available (see Table 53.6). In contrast to uncomplicated UTI, S. aureus is relatively more likely to be found in complicated UTIs and, if suspected, the therapeutic regimen should have activity against this pathogen.

The antimicrobial regimen can be modified when the infecting strain has been identified and antimicrobial susceptibilities are known. Patients who are given parenteral therapy can be switched to oral treatment after clinical improvement. At least 10–14 d of therapy is generally recommended, but longer therapy may be indicated in patients in whom an underlying complicating factor delays clinical response. By comparison, many patients in this category who have mild cystitis can be successfully treated with a 7-day regimen.

Catheter-associated infections

The incidence of bacteriuria associated with indwelling catheterization is 3–10%/d of catheterization, and the duration of catheterization is the most important risk factor for the development of catheter-associated bacteriuria. Catheter-associated bacteriuria is the most common source of Gram-negative bacteremia in hospitalized patients. Complications of long-term catheterization (> 30 d) include almost universal bacteriuria, often with polymicrobial and antibiotic-resistant flora, and (in addition to cystitis, pyelonephritis, and bacteremia as seen with short-term catheterization) frequent febrile episodes, catheter obstruction, stone formation associated with urease-producing uropathogens, local genitourinary infections, fistulae formation, and bladder cancer. An increase in mortality risk has been reported with catheter-associated bacteriuria, but it is difficult to distinguish the role of the catheter since most deaths occur in patients who have severe underlying disease.

Most episodes of catheter-associated bacteriuria are asymptomatic and do not require routine screening or treatment, since treatment does not reduce the complications of bacteriuria and can lead to antimicrobial resistance. Symptomatic infections, often polymicrobial and caused by multidrug-resistant uropathogens, warrant broad-spectrum therapy as described above. Since bacteria may be sequestered and protected from antibiotics in a biofilm on the catheter surface, it is reasonable to replace the catheter during antibiotic therapy, although there are few data to support this recommendation[5].

Preventive measures are indicated to reduce the morbidity, mortality, and costs of catheter-associated infection. Effective strategies include avoidance of a catheter when possible and, when the catheter is necessary, sterile insertion, prompt removal, and strict adherence to a closed collecting system[5,20]. Although randomized trials have not been performed, intermittent catheterization appears to result in lower rates of bacteriuria compared with long-term indwelling catheterization and condom catheterization. Prophylactic systemic antimicrobial agents are generally not recommended but may be useful in patients at high risk for serious complications if UTI occurs, such as pregnant women or patients undergoing urologic surgery who are undergoing short-term catheterization. Prophylaxis has also been demonstrated to be beneficial in patients undergoing renal transplantation and requiring indwelling catheterization.

Spinal cord injury

Spinal cord injury alters the dynamics of voiding and often requires the use of bladder drainage with catheters. The diagnosis of UTI in patients with spinal cord injuries is often problematic and is based on the combination of symptoms and signs, which are often nonspecific, pyuria, and significant bacteriuria, with uropathogens often present in quantities > 10^5cfu/mL. Fluoroquinolones are the empiric oral agents of choice in patients with mild-to-moderate infection, although many uropathogens, even in the outpatient setting, are resistant to this class of antibiotic and parenteral antibiotics may be needed.

Treatment of asymptomatic bacteriuria in patients with spinal cord injuries has not been shown to be beneficial and increases the risk of infection with antimicrobial-resistant uropathogens[21]. Likewise, antibiotic prophylaxis is generally not recommended except for selected outpatients with frequent symptomatic UTIs for whom there are no correctible risk factors.

Prostatitis

Prostatitis symptoms are experienced by approximately 50% of adult men but are caused by acute or chronic bacterial infection in a minority[22]. The most common organisms causing bacterial prostatitis are Gram-negative bacilli, including *E. coli*, *Proteus* spp., *Klebsiella* spp., *P. aeruginosa*, and, less commonly, enterococci and *S. aureus*. The pathogenesis of prostatitis is believed to be related to reflux of infected urine from the urethra into the prostatic ducts. Prostatic calculi, commonly found in adult men, may provide a nidus for bacteria and protection from antibacterial agents.

Acute bacterial prostatitis is rare. Patients present with dysuria, frequency, urgency, obstructive voiding symptoms, fever, chills, and myalgias. The prostate is tender and swollen. Prostatic massage is contraindicated in men in whom the diagnosis of acute prostatitis is being considered, because of the risk for precipitating bacteremia. The patient will usually have pyuria and a positive urine culture. Patients who are severely ill require hospitalization and parenteral antibiotics, but many patients can be treated in the outpatient setting with oral fluoroquinolones. The duration of treatment is recommended to be at least 30 d to help to prevent the development of chronic bacterial prostatitis[22]. Abscess formation may rarely occur.

Chronic bacterial prostatitis is characterized by recurrent UTIs with the same uropathogen with intervening asymptomatic periods. The prostate typically is normal to palpation during asymptomatic periods. Chronic bacterial prostatitis is characterized microscopically by the presence of ≥ 10 leukocytes/high-power field in expressed prostatic secretions or postmassage voided urine in the absence of significant pyuria in first-voided and midstream urine specimens, and a uropathogen colony count that is at least 10-fold higher in the expressed prostatic secretions or postmassage voided urine compared with the first-voided midstream urine. In addition, macrophage-laden fat droplets (oval fat bodies) are usually prominent in the prostatic secretions. Cure rates, which historically have been low, are now up to 90% with the fluoroquinolones, which are the antibiotics of choice. The optimal duration of treatment is unknown, but most authorities

recommend at least 1–3 months. Some patients require long-term, low-dose suppressive therapy to prevent symptomatic UTIs. Surgical intervention is only rarely considered and is associated with high morbidity.

Renal abscess

Renal cortical and corticomedullary abscesses and perirenal abscesses occur in 1–10 per 10 000 hospital admissions[23]. Patients usually present with fever, chills, back or abdominal pain, and costovertebral angle tenderness but may have no urinary symptoms or findings if the abscess does not communicate with the collecting system, as is often the case with a cortical abscess. Bacteremia at the time of diagnosis is more common with corticomedullary and perirenal abscesses. The clinical presentation may be very insidious and nonspecific, especially with perirenal abscess, and the diagnosis may not be made until admission to a hospital or at autopsy. CT is recommended to establish the diagnosis and location of a renal or perirenal abscess (Fig. 53.6). Empiric antibiotic therapy should be broad and cover *S. aureus* and other uropathogens causing complicated UTI (see Fig. 53.5 and Table 53.6) and modified once urine culture results are known.

A renal cortical abscess (renal carbuncle) is usually caused by *S. aureus*, which reaches the kidney through the hematogenous route. Treatment with antibiotics is usually effective, and drainage is not required unless the patient is slow to respond. A renal corticomedullary abscess, in contrast, usually results from ascending UTI in association with an underlying urinary tract abnormality, such as obstructive uropathy or vesicoureteral reflux, and is usually caused by common uropathogenic species such as *E. coli* and other coliforms. Such abscesses may extend deep into the renal parenchyma, perforate the renal capsule, and form a perirenal abscess. Treatment with antimicrobial agents without drainage is usually effective if the abscess is not very large and if the underlying urinary tract abnormality can be corrected. Aspiration of the abscess may be necessary in some patients, and nephrectomy may occasionally be required in patients with diffuse renal involvement or with severe sepsis. Perirenal abscesses usually occur in the setting of obstruction

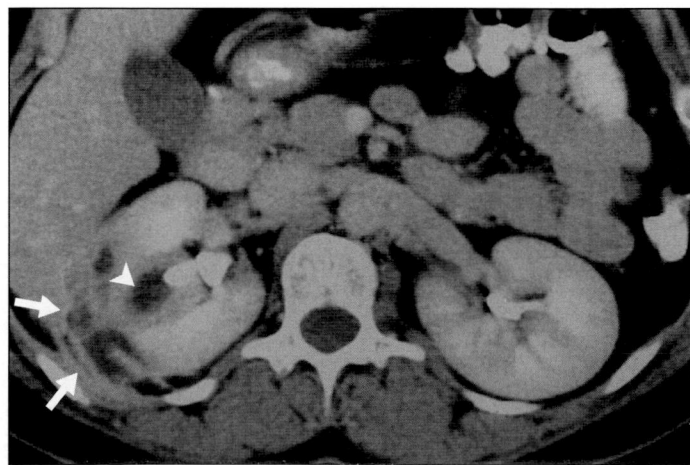

Figure 53.6 Renal abscess. Contrast computed tomography shows an abscess in the medulla of the kidney (arrowhead) with penetration and extension into the perinephric space (arrows). (Courtesy of L Towner.)

or other complicating factors (see Table 53.1) and result from ruptured intrarenal abscesses, hematogenous spread, or spread from a contiguous infection. Causative uropathogens are those commonly found in complicated UTIs (see Table 53.3), including *S. aureus* and enterococci; polymicrobic infections are common. Anaerobes or *Mycobacterium tuberculosis* may be causative. A previously high mortality rate has been lowered with earlier diagnosis and therapy. In contrast to the other types of abscess, drainage of pus is the cornerstone of therapy and nephrectomy is sometimes indicated.

Papillary necrosis

Over 50% of incidents of papillary necrosis occur in diabetics, almost always in conjunction with a UTI, but the condition also complicates sickle cell disease, analgesic abuse, and obstruction. Renal papillae are vulnerable to ischemia because of the sluggish blood flow in the vasa recta, and relatively modest ischemic insults may cause papillary necrosis. The clinical features are those typical of pyelonephritis. In addition, passage of sloughed papillae into the ureter may cause renal colic, renal insufficiency or failure, or obstruction with severe urosepsis. Papillary necrosis in the setting of pyelonephritis is associated with pyuria and a positive urine culture. Causative uropathogens are those typical of complicated UTI. The retrograde pyelogram is the preferred diagnostic procedure. Radiologic findings include an irregular papillary tip, dilated calyceal fornix, extension of contrast material into the parenchyma, and a separated crescent-shaped papilla surrounded by contrast, called the 'ring sign' (see Fig. 51.9). Broad-spectrum antibiotics are indicated. Papillae obstructing the ureter may require removal with a cystoscopic ureteral basket or relief of obstruction by insertion of a ureteral stent.

Emphysematous pyelonephritis

Emphysematous pyelonephritis is a fulminant, necrotizing, life-threatening variant of acute pyelonephritis caused by gas-forming organisms, including *E. coli*, *K. pneumoniae*, *P. aeruginosa*, and *P. mirabilis*[24]. Up to 90% of cases occur in diabetics, and obstruction may be present. Symptoms are suggestive of pyelonephritis, and a flank mass may be present. Dehydration and ketoacidosis are common. Pyuria and a positive urine culture are usually present. Gas is usually detected by a plain abdominal radiograph or ultrasound (see Fig. 53.7). CT is the diagnostic modality of choice, however, since it can better localize the gas than ultrasonography. Accurate localization of gas is important since gas may also form in an

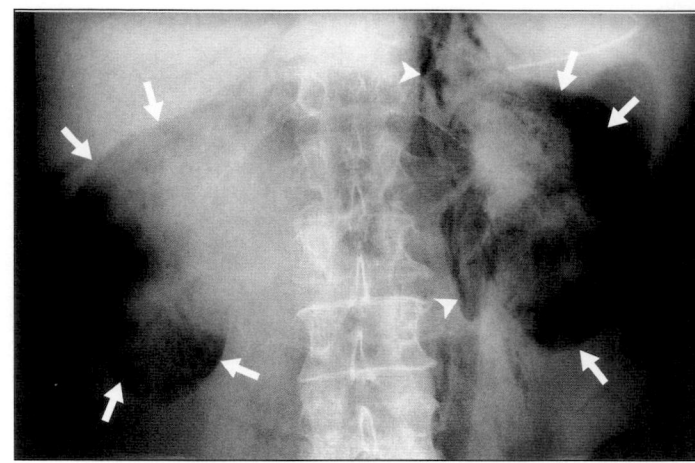

Figure 53.7 Emphysematous pyelonephritis. A plain radiograph in this febrile diabetic subject revealed diffuse gas formation throughout both kidneys (outlined by arrows), and gas dissecting in the left retroperitoneal space (arrowheads). (Courtesy of W Bush, University of Washington.)

infected obstructed collecting system or renal abscess; while serious, these conditions do not carry the same grave prognosis and are managed differently. Emergency nephrectomy in conjunction with broad-spectrum antibiotics is the treatment of choice. Medical treatment is associated with a mortality rate of 60–80%, which is lowered to 20% or less with surgical intervention[8].

Renal malacoplakia

Malacoplakia is a chronic granulomatous disorder of unknown etiology involving the genitourinary, gastrointestinal, skin, and pulmonary systems[25]. It is characterized by an unusual inflammatory reaction to a variety of infections and is manifested by the accumulation of macrophages containing calcified bacterial debris called Michaelis–Gutmann bodies (Fig. 53.8). The underlying disorder appears to be a monocyte–macrophage bactericidal defect. The diagnosis is made by histologic examination of involved tissue. Genitourinary malacoplakia, most commonly involving the bladder, is usually associated with Gram-negative UTI. Patients with renal malacoplakia generally have fever, flank pain, pyuria and hematuria, bacteriuria, and if both kidneys are involved, renal insufficiency. CT scanning usually shows enlarged kidneys with areas of poor enhancement, and the condition may be indistinguishable from other infectious or

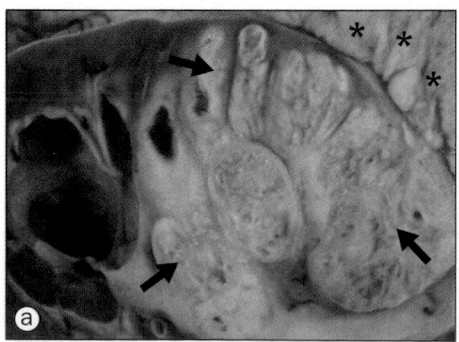
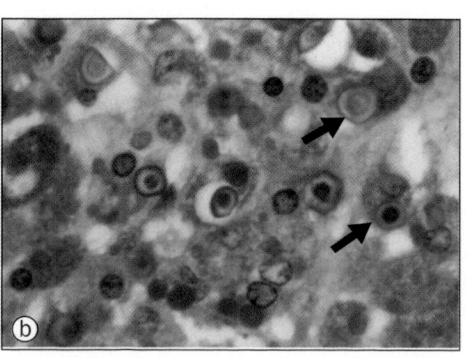

Figure 53.8 Renal Malacoplakia.
(a) Malacoplakia involving most of the kidney (arrows) with extension through the capsule (asterisks). A small portion of normal kidney is present that is associated with hydronephrosis secondary to obstruction by the malacoplakia. (b) The kidney tissue shows many macrophages containing intracytoplasmic inclusions (arrows identify two particularly well-demarcated macrophages with Michaelis-Gutmann bodies). (Courtesy of Luan Truong, Baylor College of Medicine and Neil Sheerin, Guy's Hospital.)

neoplastic lesions. Occasionally the malacoplakia may extend through the renal capsule into the perinephric space simulating a renal carcinoma (Fig. 53.8). Treatment consists of therapy with a fluoroquinolone, correction of any underlying complicating conditions if possible, and improvement of renal function. Nephrectomy is recommended for advanced unilateral disease. When the disease is bilateral or occurs in a transplanted kidney, the prognosis is very poor.

Xanthogranulomatous pyelonephritis

Xanthogranulomatous pyelonephritis is a poorly understood, uncommon, but severe chronic renal infection associated with obstruction of the urinary tract[23]. It is characterized by replacement of renal parenchyma with a diffuse or segmental cellular infiltrate of lipid-laden macrophages called foam cells. The process may also extend beyond the renal capsule to the retroperitoneum. Its pathogenesis appears to be multifactorial, with infection complicating obstruction and leading to ischemia, tissue destruction, and accumulation of lipid deposits. Patients with xanthogranulomatous pyelonephritis are characteristically middle-aged women and have chronic symptoms such as flank pain, fever, chills, and malaise. Flank tenderness, a palpable mass, and irritative voiding symptoms are often present. The urine culture is usually positive with *E. coli*, other Gram-negative bacilli, or *S. aureus*. CT generally shows an enlarged nonfunctioning kidney, a large calculus, low-density masses (xanthomatous tissue) and, in some cases, involvement of adjacent structures (Fig. 53.9). It may be difficult to distinguish from neoplastic disease. Broad-spectrum antimicrobials are indicated, but total or partial nephrectomy is usually necessary for cure.

ASYMPTOMATIC BACTERIURIA

Asymptomatic bacteriuria, as noted above, is a common and generally benign infection[6]. Pyuria is often present, especially in the elderly, and is a predictor for subsequent symptomatic UTI in some groups[7]. Causative uropathogens are the same as those causing UTIs in the same population. Treatment for asymptomatic bacteriuria is generally not warranted. However, patients at high risk for serious complications may warrant a more aggressive approach to diagnosis and treatment, including pregnant women, renal transplant recipients, patients undergoing urologic surgery or surgery involving a prosthetic device, and neutropenic patients. Some authorities also advise treatment of asymptomatic bacteriuria found in patients with anatomic or functional abnormalities of the urinary tract, diabetics, and patients with urea-splitting bacteria, such as *P. mirabilis*, *Klebsiella* spp., and others[6]. Evidence-based guidelines for screening and treatment of asymptomatic bacteriuria in these populations are needed.

UROLOGIC EVALUATION

Urologic consultation and evaluation of the urinary tract should be considered in patients who present with symptoms or signs of obstruction, urolithiasis, flank mass, or urosepsis. Similarly, such an evaluation should be considered for those

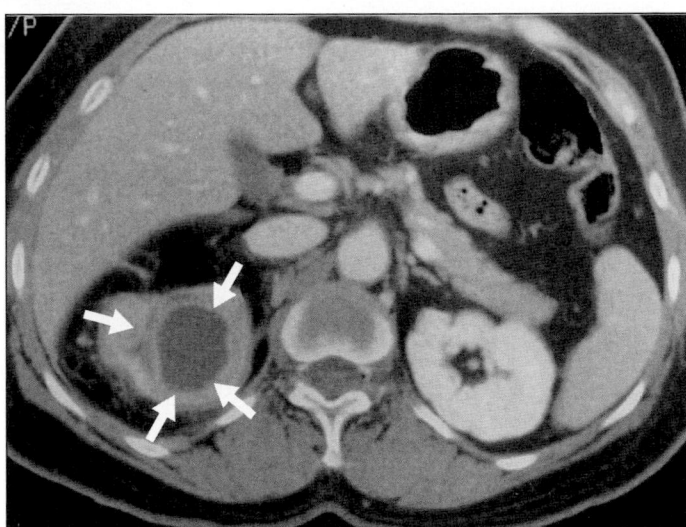

Figure 53.9 Xanthogranulomatous pyelonephritis. Contrast computed tomography scan with the inflammatory mass outlined by arrows. Pathologic diagnosis confirmed xanthogranulomatous pyelonephritis. (Courtesy of W Bush, University of Washington.)

patients with presumptive uncomplicated or complicated UTI who have not had a satisfactory clinical response after 72 h treatment to exclude the presence of a complicating factor. Contrast-enhanced CT scanning of the kidneys is the most effective imaging modality in adult patients with renal infection because of its superior resolution and sensitivity in detecting renal abnormalities and perirenal fluid collections[26]. Spiral (helical) CT may be superior to conventional CT[27]. Non-contrast spiral CT appears to be a rapid, safe, and sensitive method for evaluating patients with suspected renal stones. Renal ultrasound is useful for detection of stones and abscesses and is often more readily accessible than CT. However, it is less sensitive than CT for detection of many of the conditions present in patients with complicated UTI. The role of magnetic resonance imaging remains to be determined. Radionuclide imaging procedures have no role in the evaluation of adults with UTI, although they are very useful in children with pyelonephritis. A plain abdominal radiograph may be used to detect gas in the urinary tracts of diabetics with suspected pyelonephritis, but it is not as sensitive or specific as CT.

Studies of the value of excretory urography and of cystoscopy in women with recurrent cystitis have demonstrated that significant abnormalities that influence subsequent management of UTIs are very uncommon[4]. Therefore, routine urologic evaluation of patients with recurrent cystitis results in unnecessary expense and potential toxicity. Likewise, routine urologic investigation of young women with acute pyelonephritis is generally not cost effective and has a low diagnostic yield, although it is reasonable to obtain such an evaluation after two episodes of pyelonephritis or if any complicating factor (see Table 53.1) is identified with any of the recurrences. A urologic evaluation is probably not necessary in a man who has had a single UTI with no obvious complicating factors and whose infection responds promptly to treatment.

REFERENCES

1. Nicolle LE. A practical guide to the management of complicated urinary tract infection. Drugs. 1997;53:583–92.
2. Foxman B, Barlow R, D'Arcy H, et al. Urinary tract infection: self-reported incidence and associated costs. Ann Epidemiol. 2000;10:509–15.
3. Hooton TM, Scholes D, Hughes JP, et al. A prospective study of risk factors for symptomatic urinary tract infection in young women. N Engl J Med. 1996;335:468–74.
4. Hooton TM, Stamm WE. Diagnosis and treatment of uncomplicated urinary tract infection. Infect Dis Clin North Am. 1997;11:551–81.
5. Stamm WE, Hooton TM. Management of urinary tract infections in adults. N Engl J Med. 1993;329:1328–34.
6. Zhanel GG, Harding GKM, Guay DRP. Asymptomatic bacteriuria: which patients should be treated? Arch Intern Med. 1990;150:1389–96.
7. Hooton TM, Scholes D, Stapleton AE, et al. A prospective study of asymptomatic bacteriuria in young sexually active women. N Engl J Med. 2000;343:992–7.
8. Sobel JD. Pathogenesis of urinary tract infection: role of host defenses. Infect Dis Clin North Am. 1997;11:531–49.
9. Scholes D, Hooton TM, Roberts PL, et al. Risk factors for recurrent urinary tract infection in young women. J Infect Dis. 2000;182:1177–82.
10. Svanborg C, Godaly G. Bacterial virulence in urinary tract infection. Infect Dis Clin North Am. 1997;11:513–29.
11. Patterson JE, Andriole VT. Bacterial urinary tract infections in diabetes. Infect Dis Clin North Am. 1997;11:735–50.
12. Talan DA, Stamm WE, Hooton TM, et al. Comparison of ciprofloxacin (7 days) and trimethoprim-sulfamethoxazole (14 days) for acute uncomplicated pyelonephritis in women: a randomized trial. JAMA. 2000;283:1583–90.
13. Rubin UH, Shapiro ED, Andriole VT, et al. Evaluation of new anti-infective drugs for the treatment of urinary tract infection. Clin Infect Dis. 1992;15:S216–27.
14. Gupta K, Hooton TM, Stamm WE. Increasing antimicrobial resistance and the management of uncomplicated community-acquired urinary tract infections. Ann Intern Med. 2001;135:41–50.
15. Manges AR, Jonson JR, Foxman B, et al. Widespread distribution of urinary tract infection caused by a multi-drug-resistant Escherichia coli clonal group. N Engl J Med. 2001;345:1055–7.
16. Norrby SR. Short-term treatment of uncomplicated lower urinary tract infections in women. Rev Infect Dis. 1990;12:458–67.
17. Warren JW, Abrutyn E, Hebel JR, et al. Guidelines for antimicrobial treatment of uncomplicated acute bacterial cystitis and acute pyelonephritis in women. Clin Infect Dis. 1999;29:745–58.
18. Stapleton A, Stamm WE. Prevention of urinary tract infection. Infect Dis Clin North Am. 1997;11:719–33.
19. Stamm WE, McKevitt M, Counts GW. Acute renal infection in women: treatment with trimethoprim–sulfamethoxazole or ampicillin for two or six weeks. A randomized trial. Ann Intern Med. 1987;106:341–5.
20. Warren JW. Catheter-associated urinary tract infections. Infect Dis Clin North Am. 1997;11:609–22.
21. Cardenas DD, Hooton TM. Urinary tract infection in persons with spinal cord injury. Arch Phys Med Rehabil. 1995;76:272–80.
22. Brannigan RE, Schaeffer AJ. Prostatitis syndromes. Curr Opin Infect Dis. 1996;9:37–41.
23. Dembry LM, Andriole VT. Renal and perirenal abscesses. Infect Dis Clin North Am. 1997;11:663–80.
24. McHugh TP, Albanna SE, Stewart NJ. Bilateral emphysematous pyelonephritis. Am J Emerg Med. 1998;16:166–9.
25. Dobyan DC, Truong LD, Eknoyan G. Renal malacoplakia reappraised. Am J Kid Dis. 1993;22:243–52.
26. Kaplan DM, Rosenfield AT, Smith RC. Advances in the imaging of renal infection. Infect Dis Clin North Am. 1997;11:681–705.
27. Wyatt SH, Urban BA, Fishman EK. Spiral CT of the kidneys: role in characterization of renal disease. Part I: nonneoplastic disease. Crit Rev Diagn Imaging.1995;36:1–37.

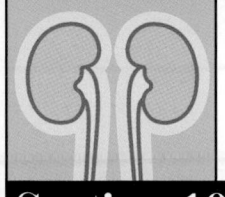

Chapter 54

Tuberculosis of the Urinary Tract

R Kasi Visweswaran and Suresh Bhat

INTRODUCTION AND DEFINITION

Tuberculosis is a multisystemic disease caused by *Mycobacterium tuberculosis*. Tuberculosis affects 15 to 20 million people worldwide, of which 8 to 10 million are infectious. Approximately 8 million people develop active disease annually from asymptomatically infected persons[1]. In developed countries, tuberculosis commonly affects older individuals and ethnic migrants, and most recently, individuals with human immunodeficiency virus (HIV) infection. When a tuberculin positive individual develops HIV, active disease is estimated to occur in 7–10% annually, which contrasts with the 5–10% per lifetime in the immunocompetent host[2].

Extrapulmonary tuberculosis occurs in approximately 15% of active cases in the non-HIV infected population[3]. Genitourinary tuberculosis (GUTB) is one of the more common forms of extrapulmonary tuberculosis and is almost always secondary to a symptomatic or asymptomatic primary lesion, most often in the lung. Renal involvement may also occur as a part of miliary tuberculosis.

ETIOLOGY

The tubercle bacillus, which was first identified by Robert Koch in 1882, is a nonmotile, nonsporing, strictly aerobic, straight or slightly curved rod-like bacillus that is weakly Gram positive, and acid and alcohol fast. Mycobacteria possess several unique features that help in their intracellular existence, including a cell wall that contains a lipid shell ('lipid barrier'), mycolic acid-derivatives that allow the organism to resist proteolysis and uptake into phagolysosomes, muramile dipeptide that stimulates both a T cell response that elicits the characteristic granuloma, and cell wall glycolipids (lipoarabinomannan) that inhibit macrophage function. This surrounding coat of inert lipids and surface proteins allow mycobacteria to survive inside phagocytes where they may remain dormant for years[4].

Other pathogenic mycobacteria may rarely cause clinical disease, usually in immunocompromised hosts; these include *M. avium-intracellulare*, and rarely M. *kansasi*, M. *bovis*, M. *fortuitum*, and M. *szulgai*. However, the vast majority of genitourinary tuberculosis is due to *Mycobacterium tuberculosis*[4].

PATHOGENESIS

The clinical and pathologic manifestations of tuberculosis vary depending on the virulence of the organism and the effectiveness of the host response. The host response may lead to complete containment of infection or result in an illness of varying severity. Evidence is accumulating that there are strain to strain differences that may determine whether an infected person develops primary tuberculosis, reactivation tuberculosis or a chronic asymptomatic infection. The clinical manifestations of tuberculosis represent not only the consequences of bacterial proliferation but also host destructive and reparative processes.

When an infected droplet with the size of 1–5 μm is deposited in the respiratory tract, tonsillar fossa, or the gastrointestinal tract, a primary focus develops in which there is formation of a nonspecific asymptomatic granuloma. The organisms from the primary focus drain to the regional lymph gland causing its enlargement, resulting in the 'primary complex'. This is often asymptomatic and self-limited.

However, the bacilli from the regional lymph node may reach the systemic circulation through the thoracic duct, where they undergo silent hematogenous dissemination, depositing in the glomerulus (Fig. 54.1). The high blood flow to the renal cortex, oxygen saturation in the glomeruli, and increased viscosity of blood toward the efferent arteriolar end of the glomerular capillary tuft favor the localization of bacteria in this location where they stimulate an inflammatory response, leading to the formation of granulomas. These granulomas in the cortex may heal forming a scar, remain dormant for many years, or rupture into the proximal tubule of the nephron as a result of proliferation of mycobacteria. The bacilli in the nephron are trapped at the level of the loop of Henle where they multiply. The relatively poor blood flow, hypertonicity, and high ammonia concentration in the renal medullary region may lead to weakening of immune responses locally and favor the formation of medullary granulomas, which contain macrophages. These granulomas (tuberculomas) may undergo coagulative necrosis (driven by macrophage production of cytokines), forming cheese-like caseous material and occasionally rupturing into the calyx[5].

The renal medulla is the most common site of involvement of clinical renal tuberculosis[6]. When this caseous focus ruptures into the collecting system, cavities and ulcers are formed, and involvement of renal papillae may lead to sloughing and papillary necrosis. Healing in the kidney occurs by fibrosis and scarring, resulting in strictures and obstruction. Dystrophic calcification of damaged structures may result in a nonfunctioning kidney called 'putty kidney' or 'cement kidney'. Spread of tuberculosis to contiguous structures may occur; ureteritis is common and may result in strictures and obstructive uropathy.

The bladder may develop hyperemia near the ureteric orifice followed by superficial ulcers and granulomatous changes involving all layers (pancystitis). Healing by fibrosis at the ureteric orifice results in a refluxing 'golf hole' ureter. Extensive fibrosis of the bladder wall results in a thick, small-capacity bladder ('thimble bladder'). Involvement of the genital tract is also common. In males with tuberculosis of the urinary tract, as many as 70–80% of patients have epididymitis, prostatitis, seminal vesiculitis, orchitis, or cold abscesses. In females, genital tract involvement is uncommon, but if present usually presents as salpingitis, that is often diagnosed during investigation for sterility.

While genitourinary tuberculosis usually results from hematogenous dissemination from a primary lung site, the urinary tract may also be primarily involved following instillation of Bacille-Calmette-Guérin (BCG) in the bladder as a part of treatment of superficial bladder carcinomas. Transplanted kidneys may also transmit tuberculosis to their recipients[7].

CLINICAL MANIFESTATIONS

Urinary tract tuberculosis may be asymptomatic or mimic other disorders. It may present with symptoms relating to the lower urinary tract, abdomen, genitalia, or general constitution. A high index of suspicion enables early diagnosis. Most patients are between 20 and 40 years of age with a male to female ratio of 2 : 1. Increased risk factors for tuberculosis include close contact with sputum smear-positive individuals, vagrancy, social deprivation, neglect, immunosuppression, HIV infection/AIDS, diabetes mellitus, renal failure, and other debilitating illnesses.

Nearly 25% of patients are asymptomatic and the diagnosis is made while investigating for other diseases, during surgery, or even at autopsy (Table 54.1). Another 25% may have asymptomatic urinary abnormalities, usually persistent asymptomatic pyuria or hematuria. Of the patients who are symptomatic, lower urinary tract symptoms such as frequency, urgency, dysuria, nocturia, frank pyuria, or hematuria occur in more than 75%. Increased frequency of micturition is one of the early symptoms and results from inflammation of the bladder and the acidic nature of the urine. The defect in the urinary concentrating mechanism explains the occurrence of nocturia.

Recurrent bouts of painless macroscopic hematuria is a symptom that draws the attention of the clinician to the diagnosis of urinary tuberculosis. Macroscopic hematuria occurs as a result of bleeding from the ulcerating lesions, inflammation of the urothelium, or rupture of blood vessel in the vicinity of a cavity. Colicky pain may occur as a presenting manifestation of urinary tuberculosis when associated with stone, clot, or acute obstruction.

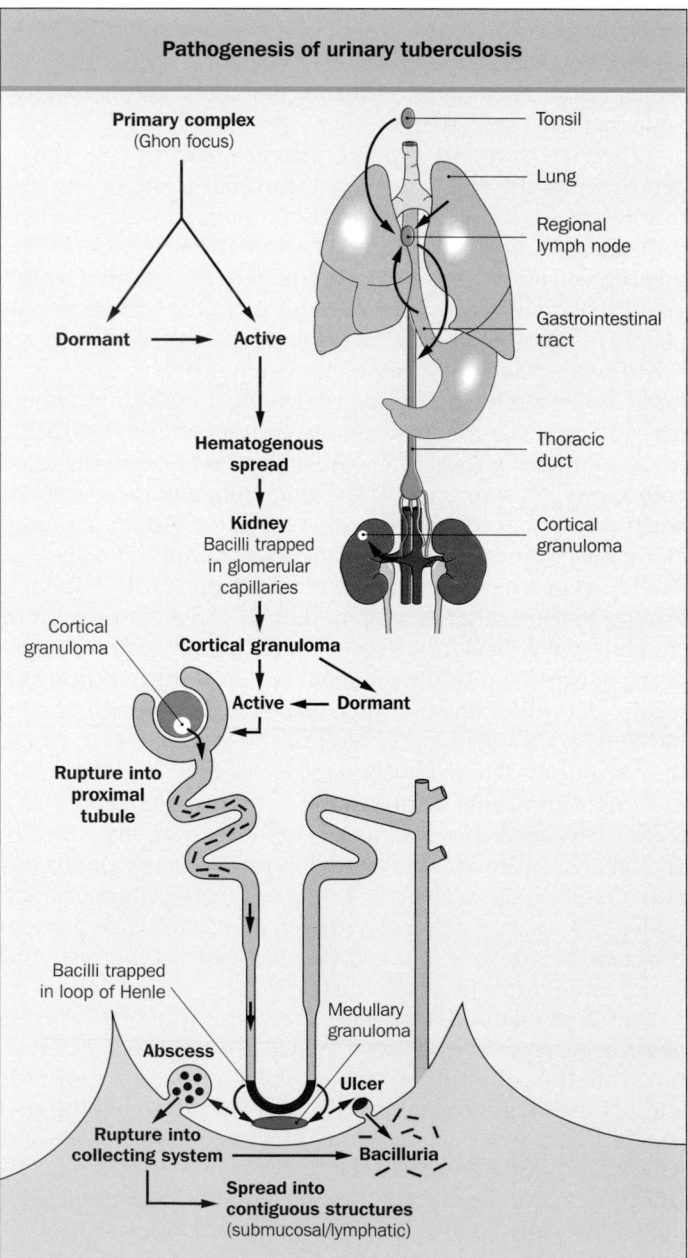

Figure 54.1 Pathogenesis of urinary tuberculosis.

Clinical features of urinary tuberculosis		
Features	Frequency (%)	Symptoms
Asymptomatic	25	Detected during autopsy, surgery, or during investigations for other diseases
Asymptomatic urinary abnormalities	25	Persistent pyuria, microscopic hematuria
Lower urinary tract symptoms (most common)	40	Frequency, urgency, dysuria, incontinence, nocturia, suprapubic pain, perineal pain
Male genital tract involvement	75	Epididymitis, hemospermia, infertility, reduced semen volume
Female genital tract involvement	<5	Amenorrhea, infertility, vaginal bleeding, pelvic pain
Constitutional symptoms	<20	Fever, reduced appetite, anorexia, weight loss, night sweats
Miscellaneous	–	Urolithiasis, hypertension, acute renal failure, chronic renal failure, abdominal colic, abdominal mass

Table 54.1 Clinical features of urinary tuberculosis.

In advanced diseases, frequency and urgency related to reduced bladder capacity ('thimble bladder') occur. Incomplete emptying, increased susceptibility to infection, and secondary vesicoureteral reflux may also occur. In chronic ureteric obstruction, enlargement of the kidney, infection, or perinephric collection of pus leads to a dull aching loin pain. Severe suprapubic pain with backache and dysuria suggests acute tuberculous cystitis. Episodes of pyuria, which may suggest secondary bacterial infection or drainage of a caseous focus into the collecting system, may also be a manifestation of renal tuberculosis. Persistence of pyuria after appropriate therapy should lead to an evaluation for urinary tuberculosis.

Long standing renal tuberculosis may result in mild proteinuria (< 1g/24 h) may be seen in up to 50% of lesions, while about 15% excrete more than 1 g of protein/24 h. Some patients may also develop amyloidosis with nephrotic syndrome.

Anemia is seen in less than 20% of patients with nonmiliary disease[8]. A few patients have nephrogenic diabetes insipidus. Renal tubular acidosis occurs as well, although its frequency has not been ascertained. Hyporeninemic hypoaldosteronism may potentially result from the tubulointerstitial injury secondary to obstructive uropathy[9]. Renal function is usually normal, but renal insufficiency may occur if large areas of both kidneys are extensively damaged.

During treatment, healing by fibrosis may lead to obstruction of one or both ureters, with hydronephrosis, parenchymal damage, and renal failure. Dehydration and/or salt depletion may occur as a result of tubulointerstitial damage, resulting in altered tubular function. Adrenal involvement may contribute to salt wasting. Oliguric acute renal failure caused by allergic interstitial nephritis may occur in those patients treated with intermittent rifampin (rifampicin) therapy.

Some patients may present with renal failure, pyuria, microscopic hematuria, and proteinuria, in whom the urine cultures for mycobacteria are repeatedly negative. These patients respond favorably to antituberculous chemotherapy combined with corticosteroids. The kidneys are normal sized and show typical diffuse interstitial nephritis with caseating granulomas containing the bacilli in 75% of the biopsies[10].

Hypertension is unusual in renal tuberculosis. Intimal proliferation of vessels near inflamed areas leads to segmental ischemia and renin release[11]. If associated with a nonfunctioning kidney, nephrectomy may help to improve the hypertension. Relief of obstruction, if any, may also help to lower the blood pressure. Nephrolithiasis may occur in 7–18% of patients. Secondary infection with *Escherichia coli* may be seen in 20–50% of patients.

As discussed above, genital involvement is common in males with urinary tuberculosis. Epididymitis may present with scrotal discomfort, mass, or a cold abscess that may rupture, leading to a nonhealing posterior scrotal sinus. Thickening of the vas deferens may result in the 'beaded vas'. Tuberculosis of the prostate may present with lower urinary symptoms and perineal pain. The prostate may be hard or boggy. Penile and urethral tuberculosis may present with strictures, fistulae, ulcers, or papillo-necrotic skin lesions. Hemospermia, reduction of semen volume, and infertility are other manifestations of genital involvement. Direct spread of M. tuberculosis to the sexual partner is possible.

In females, the association between genital and renal tuberculosis is rare, occurring in 5% of cases. The major manifestation of genital involvement in females is infertility resulting from adherent salpingitis. Secondary amenorrhea, vaginal bleeding, and pelvic pain caused by inflammation may be present.

Constitutional symptoms such as fever, weight loss, night sweats, fatigue, and anorexia occur in < 20% of patients and indicate active infection in other organs or secondary bacterial infection of the urinary tract. A careful examination to identify pulmonary, lymph node, or skeletal tuberculosis must be undertaken in all patients who present with constitutional symptoms. The chest X-ray may show evidence of active or healed tuberculous lesions in over 50% of cases.

PATHOLOGY

There are two major pathologic forms of urinary tuberculosis: ulcero-cavernous and miliary. In the early stages of the ulcero-cavernous form, the kidneys appear 'normal' or may show 'perinephritis'. Yellow nodules may be seen on the outer surface. On cut section, granulomas and ulcers in renal pyramid or medullary cavities may be seen. Larger cavities filled with caseous material communicating with the collecting system may also occur (Fig. 54.2). Other gross findings include multiple ulcers in the infundibular region of the calyces, calyceal stenosis with caliectasis, ulcers or strictures of the ureter with hydronephrosis, pyonephrosis, subcapsular collections or perinephric abscesses. The bladder may show ulcers or be grossly fibrotic and contracted. On microscopy, in early disease, neutrophilic infiltration with phagocytosis of the bacilli may be seen. Subsequent histologic features depend on the virulence of the organism and the cell-mediated immunity. In those with an effective cell-mediated response, granulomas, characterized by the presence of proliferation and macrophages with engulfed bacilli, are surrounded by epithelioid cells and Langhan's giant cells (Fig. 54.3). There is often a cuff of lymphocytes and plasma cells surrounding the lesion. Healing occurs by fibrosis and scarring. In those with less effective immune responses, caseating necrosis, characterized by amorphous and cheese-like eosinophilic material replacing the normal architecture of tissue, occurs. Later, this may calcify. This dystrophic calcification, unlike in other organs, suggests activity rather than healing. These changes may occur either in localized areas or extensively in one or both kidneys, ureters, bladder, prostate, or seminal vesicle.

The miliary form of tuberculosis is rare and is seen particularly in immunosuppressed individuals. The gross appearance of the kidney is characteristic, with the cortex studded with yellowish white, hard, pinhead-sized nodules that on microscopy show several coalescent granulomas with central caseation.

DIAGNOSIS AND DIFFERENTIAL DIAGNOSIS

In view of the wide spectrum of clinical manifestations and dormancy of the primary infection at the time of presentation, a high index of suspicion is necessary to diagnose genitourinary tuberculosis. Patients at risk include those with tuberculosis elsewhere, those who are immunosuppressed,

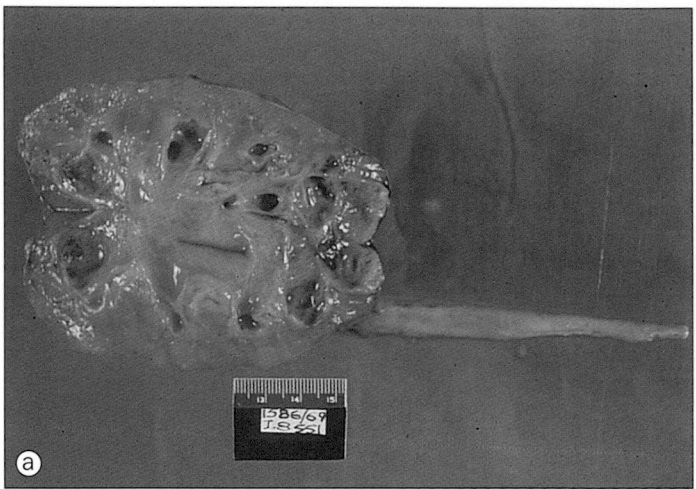

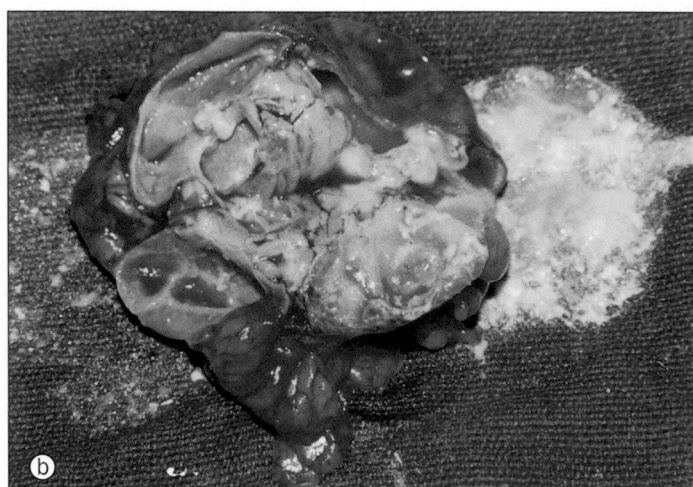

Figure 54.2 Ulcero-cavernous lesions. (a) A cut section of kidney showing areas of destruction in medulla and renal cortex. (Courtesy of Professor K Sasidhara.) (b) A cut section of kidney showing areas of cavitation and caseation necrosis (whitish chalky material).

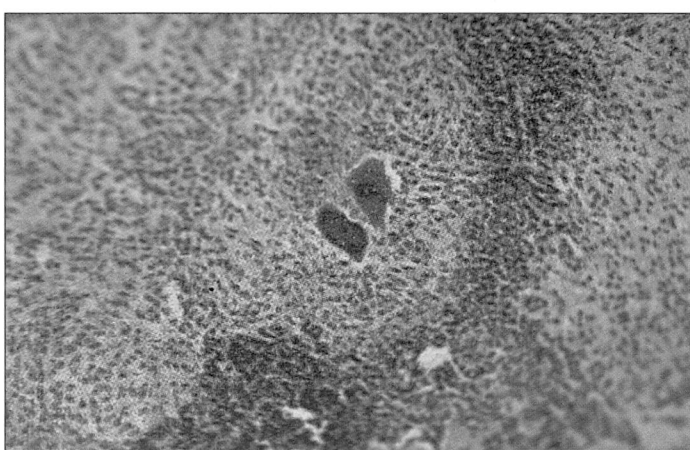

Figure 54.3 Tuberculous granuloma. The granuloma comprises Langhan's giant cells (two large cells in the center), surrounding epithelioid cells, and a rim of lymphocytes. (Courtesy of Dr Sathi Bai Panikker Kottayam.)

subjects recently exposed to infection in community/family, or the elderly.

Suspicion may also occur if there is sterile pyuria, which is present in 50% of patients. The tuberculin test (Mantoux test) is useful for proving infection, but not necessarily disease. A positive test only suggests prior exposure to the antigen and does not indicate active infection. A negative test in the absence of the immunosuppressed state rules out tuberculous infection.

Isolation of *M. tuberculosis* by urine culture is the definitive diagnostic test. Fully voided early-morning urine samples for 3–5 consecutive days are cultured on two standard solid mycobacterial culture media: the egg-based Lowenstein-Jensen medium and the agar-based Middlebrook 7H10 medium. These transparent media enable earlier visualization of microcolonies, which grow by 6–12 weeks. Sensitivity tests are performed to choose the optimum chemotherapeutic agents. Any tissue specimen submitted for mycobacterial culture should be macerated using sterile sand with a mortar and pestle before inoculation. It should be noted that direct demonstration of acid-fast bacilli in urine by Ziehl-Nielsen stain is not reliable for diagnosis because *M. smegmatis*, a saprophyte, may be easily mistaken for *M. tuberculosis*.

Rapid methods for diagnosis of tuberculosis are also available. Using the radiometric broth method for acid-fast bacilli isolation, a positive growth can be obtained in about 9 days. Serologic tests using the soluble antigen fluorescent antibody (SAFA) test, a sandwich adaptation of the solid-phase antibody competition test (SACT-SE), and the polymerase chain reaction (PCR) can be used for early diagnosis of tuberculosis[12]. Sonographically guided fine needle aspiration cytology is useful as a diagnostic tool in defining the granulomatous nature of sonographically visible lesion in patients with positive urine culture[13]. Histologic diagnosis is made by identifying the pathological triad of necrotic debris: caseous type, epithelioid histiocytes in loose aggregates and Langhans giant cells.

Imaging studies are essential to assess the extent and severity of involvement once a diagnosis of genitourinary tuberculosis is made. A plain radiograph may reveal calcification in the urinary or genital tract. Extensive dystrophic calcification in the kidney in some cases of advanced renal tuberculosis is described as 'cumulus cloud' calcification. Plain radiographs of chest and spine show active or healed tuberculous lesions in 60–70% of patients. Abnormalities in excretory urogram may be seen in 70–90% of patients. Minimal erosion of the tip of a calyx with spasticity, incomplete filling, distortion, infundibular stenosis, multiple ureteral strictures (Fig. 54.4), or nonvisualization of the kidney may be present. The renal pelvis, which may be dilated initially, may eventually be obliterated, leading to a distorted appearance, called 'hiked-up pelvis' (Kerrkink sign). Irregularities or narrowing of the ureter lead to hydroureteronephrosis (multiple strictures with beaded or corkscrew appearance of ureter followed by thickening and straightening of the whole ureter (Pipe-stem ureter)). Although the bladder may look normal initially, as the disease advances it becomes irregular and fibrosed, and refluxes. Antegrade or

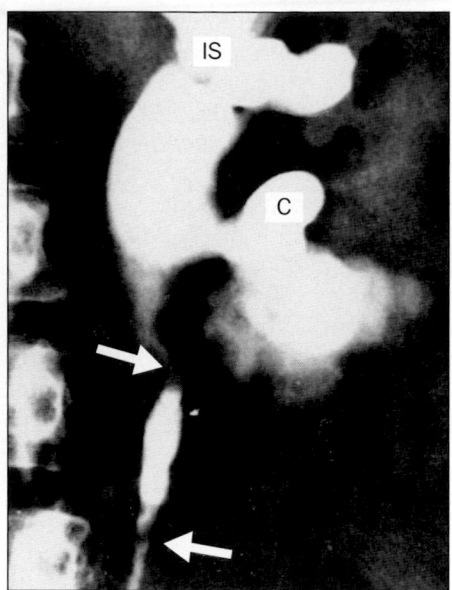

Figure 54.4 Multiple ureteric strictures. Strictures (arrows) associated with dilated lower ureter, infundibular stenosis (IS), and caliectasis (C) are seen in this intravenous urogram. (Courtesy of Professor K Sasidharan.)

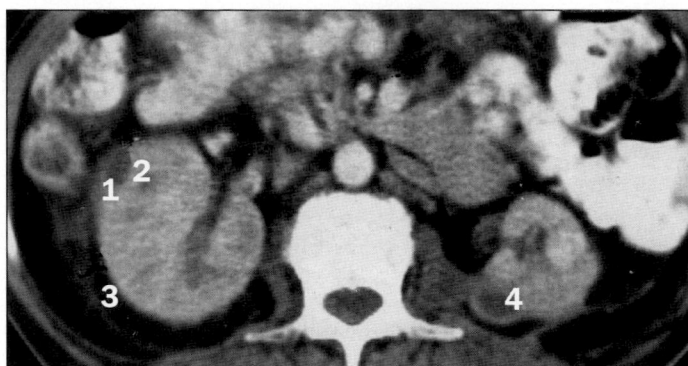

Figure 54.5 Renal tuberculosis. Computed tomography shows an enlarged left kidney with multiple cavities present bilaterally (marked 1, 2, 3 and 4). (Courtesy of Professor K Sasidharan.)

retrograde pyelography may be done to delineate the upper urinary tract, identify the number, length, or site of ureteric strictures, and to assist placement of a ureteric stent across the stenotic segment.

Ultrasound studies may be helpful to rule out obstruction. Computed tomographic scans are helpful to delineate renal structural damage (Fig. 54.5). Cystoscopy under general anesthesia with adequate muscle relaxation helps to visualize the mucosal lesions, the 'golf hole' ureteric orifice, or the efflux of toothpaste-like caseous material. Biopsy during the acute stage is avoided for fear of dissemination of tuberculosis.

In terms of differential diagnosis, tuberculosis mimics other diseases both clinically and radiologically. Chronic nonspecific urinary infections may be confused with renal tuberculosis. In about 20% of patients with renal tuberculosis, secondary bacterial infection may occur. Absence of response to usual antibiotics should arouse suspicion of urinary tuberculosis. Conditions causing recurrent painless hematuria such as IgA nephropathy and bilharziasis, are often misdiagnosed as tuberculosis in endemic areas. In interstitial cystitis, lower urinary symptoms similar to tuberculous cystitis may occur but the urinalysis does not show gross pyuria and tests for acid-fast bacilli are negative. Radiologically, chronic pyelonephritis, renal papillary necrosis, medullary sponge kidney, calyceal diverticulum, renal carcinoma, xanthogranulomatous pyelonephritis, and multiple small renal calculi have to be differentiated from tuberculosis. Of late, a few cases of pseudo-tuberculous pyelonephritis have been reported where caseating granulomas resembling tuberculosis were observed in the renal parenchyma but no mycobacteria or other micro-organisms were detected in the renal tissue or urine culture[14,15].

NATURAL HISTORY

The overall prognosis of tuberculosis of the urinary tract depends on the host resistance and the load and virulence of the organism. In many cases, foci in the urinary tract remain dormant indefinitely. Progression occurs through formation of tuberculous granuloma, caseation, ulceration, and dystrophic calcification. Most manifestations result from the complications, which can be prevented by timely chemotherapy and appropriate surgical intervention when indicated. With the advent of effective chemotherapeutic measures, the long-term complications/sequelae of tuberculosis have decreased significantly.

TREATMENT

In the pre-chemotherapy era, surgical removal of the diseased part/organ was the mainstay in management. With the advent of chemotherapeutic agents, patients are managed mainly by medical treatment. Surgery is reserved for correction of anatomic abnormalities and removal of infected or dead tissues and pus. Chemotherapy of tuberculosis can be planned adequately only after considering certain peculiarities of the mycobacteria. The tendency of the organism to remain dormant in many parts of the body poses a special problem, which is often not seen in other chronic infections. Three populations of organisms are believed to survive in the body in different environments (Fig. 54.6).

Curative therapy requires a combination of bactericidal drugs that will eradicate all three groups of mycobacteria. In addition to streptomycin, isoniazid, rifampin (rifampicin), and pyrazinamide, which are bactericidal, other bacteriostatic antituberculous drugs are also used (see Table 54.2). Fixed-dose combinations of antituberculous drugs incorporating two or more drugs in the same tablet have advantages, including increased compliance, administration of adequate dose, minimization of inadvertent medication errors, and avoidance of drug resistance. Genitourinary tuberculosis is more amenable to medical treatment because of the presence of far fewer organisms in the lesion compared with lesions in the lungs. Many of the drugs reach the kidneys, urinary tract, urine, and cavitary lesions in high concentration.

A short-course regimen is usually recommended. Treatment is started with daily rifampin 600 mg, isoniazid 300 mg, and pyrazinamide 1500 mg, in the morning. Unless the culture sensitivity indicates otherwise, pyrazinamide is discontinued

Subpopulations of *M. tuberculosis*		
Type of *M. tuberculosis*	**Type of lesion**	**Ideal bactericidal drug**
Group I Extracellular Neutral/alkaline pH Rapid multiplication	Cavitary lesions in medulla	Streptomycin Isoniazid Rifampin (Rifampicin)
Group II Intracellular Acidic pH Slow or intermittent multiplication	Macrophage	Pyrazinamide Rifampin (Rifampicin) Isoniazid
Group III Closed caseous lesion Neutral pH Slow or intermittent multiplication	Closed caseous lesions Cold abscess	Rifampin (Rifampicin)

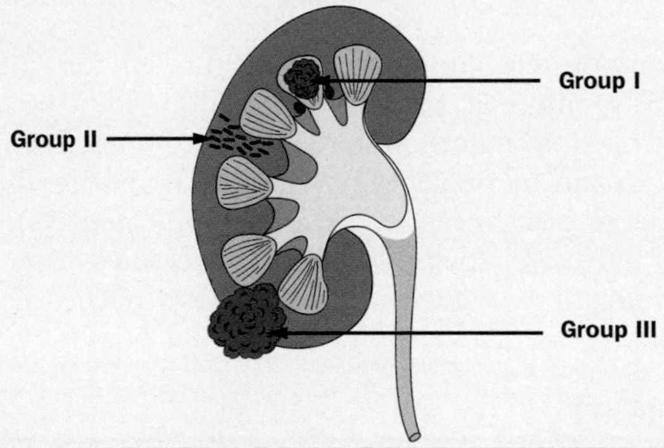

Figure 54.6 Subpopulations of mycobacteria in the kidney. The localization of three populations of *M. tuberculosis* and their drug susceptibility are shown.

after 2 months and isoniazid and rifampin (rifampicin) are continued for another 4 months. In instances where the patient is very sick with irritative bladder symptoms, streptomycin in daily doses of 1 g may be added during the first 2 months. However, if the patient is over 40 years of age, the daily dose of streptomycin may be reduced to 0.75 g with periodic monitoring for VIIIth cranial nerve involvement.

In situations where the probability of drug resistance is high, ethambutol in daily doses of 800–1200 mg may also be used in the first 2 months. Longer courses of antituberculous treatment ranging from 9 months to 2 years are useful in patients who do not tolerate pyrazinamide, those responding slowly to a standard regimen, those with miliary or central nervous system disease, and children with multiple site involvement.

Surgical treatment

The role of surgical treatment in urinary tuberculosis is limited. For ureteral strictures, timely introduction of stents across the narrow segment may help to avoid the need for major surgical procedures. Two broad types of surgical treatments are considered.

Reconstructive surgery involves the correction of obstruction to the ureter by pyeloplasty, uretero-ureterostomy, correction of reflux by ureteric reimplantation, and increasing the bladder capacity by augmentation cystoplasty, which involves anastomosing an isolated segment of bowel to the contracted bladder. *Ablative surgery* involves removal of the diseased parts together with the infected material containing the dormant organisms. The need for removal of a unilateral nonfunctioning kidney is controversial. Since prolonged antituberculous treatment for 18–24 months effectively sterilizes caseous and calcified masses

Antituberculous drugs					
Drug	**Dosage form**	**Dosage**	**Side effects**	**Mode of action**	**Remarks**
Isoniazid (INH)	Tablet:100 mg, 300 mg	5 mg/kg daily (oral) (maximum 300 mg/day)	Peripheral neuritis, hepatitis, hypersensitivity reactions	Bactericidal for groups I and II	Pyridoxine prophylaxis necessary
Rifampin (Rifampicin) (RIF)	Capsule or tablet: 150, 300, 450 mg	10 mg/kg daily (oral) (maximum 600 mg/day)	Hepatitis, febrile reactions, acute interstitial nephritis	Bactericidal for groups I, II, and III	
Pyrazinamide (PZM)	Tablet: 400, 500 mg	25 mg/kg daily (oral) (maximum 2 g/day)	Hepatotoxicity, hyperuricemia	Bactericidal for group II	Combination with aminoglycoside useful
Streptomycin (SM)	Powder for Injection: 1 g	15 mg/kg daily i.m. (maximum dose 1 g; dose to be reduced in those over 40 years of age)	Ototoxicity, nephrotoxicity	Bactericidal for group I	
Ethambutol (ETB)	Tablet: 100, 400 mg	15–25 mg/kg daily (oral) (maximum 2.5 g/day)	Optic neuritis (reversible), skin rash	Bacteriostatic for groups I and II	Used to inhibit development of resistant mutants; use with caution in renal failure
Thiacetazone (TZN)	Tablet: 150 mg	150 mg (oral) (not for intermittent therapy)	Skin rashes, exfoliative dermatitis, hepatic failure	Bacteriostatic and inhibits emergence of INH resistance	Not used in renal failure
Ciprofloxacin Ofloxacin	Tablet: 250, 500 mg Tablet: 200, 400 mg	500–1000 mg (oral) 400–500 mg (oral)	Hypersensitivity, drug interaction		Not used in children Not approved by FDA for tuberculosis
Capreomycin Kanamycin		15–30 mg/kg daily i.m.	Ototoxicity, nephrotoxicity	Bactericidal for group I	Avoided in older patient and in renal failure

Table 54.2 Antituberculous drugs. The main drugs are listed with dosage form, dosage, side effects, and mode of action.

of the tuberculous 'cement kidney', nephrectomy is advocated only if secondary sepsis, pain, bleeding, uncontrollable hypertension, or continued mycobacteriuria is present. Tuberculous abscesses can be aspirated under ultrasound or computer tomographic guidance and antituberculous drugs directly instilled into the cavity.

Treatment regimens in special situations
Standardized treatment regimens have been devised for a number of special situations[16].

Women during pregnancy and lactation
Most antituberculous drugs are safe for use during pregnancy. However streptomycin, which is ototoxic to the fetus, is avoided. If a four-drug schedule is indicated, streptomycin is replaced by ethambutol. There is no contraindication for the use of these drugs during breast-feeding and it is not necessary to isolate the baby from the mother. The baby should receive BCG immunization and isoniazid prophylaxis. Since rifampin interacts with oral contraceptive pills, women taking oral contraceptive while receiving rifampin should be advised to take a higher dose of estrogen or use alternative methods of contraception.

Treatment of patients with liver disorders
The usual short-term chemotherapy regimen can be used in patients with liver disorders if there is no evidence of chronic liver disease, hepatitis virus carrier state, past history of acute hepatitis, or excessive alcohol consumption. In chronic liver disease, isoniazid, rifampin and one or two non-hepatotoxic drugs (streptomycin and ethambutol) can be used for 8–12 months. Pyrazinamide is contraindicated. In those with acute hepatitis unrelated to tuberculosis or its therapy, it would be safer to defer the chemotherapy until the acute hepatitis has resolved. If immediate treatment of tuberculosis during acute hepatitis is mandatory, streptomycin plus ethambutol for a period of 3 months followed by isoniazid and rifampin for 6 months may be advised.

Treatment of patients with renal failure
In patients with renal failure, isoniazid, rifampin, and pyrazinamide, which are eliminated by the biliary route, can be given in normal dosages. Those receiving isoniazid should also be given pyridoxine to prevent peripheral neuropathy. Since streptomycin and ethambutol are excreted by the kidney, dosage modification of these drugs is necessary in renal failure. Streptomycin (15 mg/kg) is administered every 24–72 h for a creatinine clearance between 10–50 mL/min, and every 72–96 h for a creatinine clearance less than 10 mL/min to maintain a therapeutic peak level of 20–30 μg/mL. Monitoring for high pitched tinnitus, sense of fullness in the ears and audiography may be useful. For ethambutol, the dose is administered every 24–36 h if the creatinine clearance is between 10–50 mL/min and every 48 h if the creatinine clearance is below 10 mL/min. Periodic monitoring of visual acuity and ophthalmic examinations may identify toxicity early.

Treatment in AIDS
Even in patients with AIDS, short-term chemotherapy is sufficient. If the follow-up cultures are positive, prolonged therapy for up to 2 years may be needed based on the antibiotic sensitivity.

Monitoring of patients
After 2 months of intensive chemotherapy urine is cultured for *M. tuberculosis* for three consecutive days. If cultures are still positive, sensitivity is done and treatment modified accordingly. After completion of treatment all patients should have three consecutive early morning samples of urine for *M. tuberculosis* culture and this is repeated after 3 months and 1 year. Intravenous urography is repeated at the end of two months and at the completion of treatment to detect any evidence of obstruction. In cases of renal calcification patient should be evaluated yearly by three early morning samples of urine for AFB culture and plain X-ray abdomen for up to 10 years as calcification may harbor *M. tuberculosis* and may progress to destruction of the kidney[17].

REFERENCES

1. Raviglione MC, Srider DE, Kochi A. Global epidemiology of tuberculosis. JAMA. 1995;273:220–6.
2. Selwyn PA, Hartel D, Lewis VA, et al. A prospective study of the risk of tuberculosis among intravenous drug users with human immunodeficiency virus infection. N Engl J Med. 1989;370:546–7.
3. Schafer M, Kim D, Weiss J, et al. Extrapulmonary tuberculosis in patients with HIV infection. Medicine. 1991;70:384–96.
4. Ho JL, Rilay LW. Defenses against tuberculosis. In: Crystal RG, West JB, et al., eds. The Lung: Scientific Foundations, 2nd edn. Philadelphia: Lippincott-Raven; 1997:2381–91.
5. Turk JL. Granulomatous diseases. In: McGee JOD, Isacson PG, Wright NA, eds. Textbook of Pathology. Oxford: Oxford University Press; 1992:394–404.
6. Simon IIB, Weinstein AJ, Pasternak MS, et al. Genitourinary tuberculosis: clinical features in a general hospital population. Am J Med. 1977;63:410–14.
7. Mourad G, Soullilon JP, Chong G, et al. Transmission of mycobacterium TB with renal allografts. Nephron. 1985;41:82–5.
8. Wismia LG, Jukol S, Lopez SM de, et al. Renal function damage in 131 cases of urogenital tuberculosis. Urology. 1978;11:457–61.
9. De frongs RA. Hyperkalemia and hyporeninemic hypoaldosteronism. Kidney Int. 1980;17:118–34.
10. Mallinson WJW, Fuller RW, Levison DA, et al. Diffuse interstitial renal tuberculosis – an unusual cause of renal failure. Q J Med. 1981;50:137–48.
11. Marks LS, Poutasse EF. Hypertension from renal tuberculosis: operative cure predicted by renal vein renin. J Urol. 1973;109:149–52.
12. Schiuger NW, Rom WN. The polymerase chain reaction in the diagnosis and evolution of pulmonary infections. Am J Resp Crit Care Med. 1995;152:11–15.
13. Baniel J, Maunia A, Liamen G. Fine needle cytodiagnosis of renal tuberculosis. J Urol. 1999;146:689–91.
14. Casasole SV, Muntaner LP, Alonso UJ. Pseudotuberculous pyelonephritis. Arch Esp Urol. 1994; 47:172–4.
15. Hoorens AV, Niepen PV, Kauppens F, et al. Pseudotuberculous pyelonephritis. Associated with urolithiasis. Am J Surg Pathol 1993;17(3):314–16.
16. Maher D, Chaulet P, Spinaci S, Harries A. Standardised treatment regimens. In: Maher D, Chaulet P, Spinaci S, Harries A, eds. Treatment of Tuberculosis: Guidelines for National Programmes, 2nd edn. Geneva, Switzerland: WHO; 1997:25–31.
17. Gow GJ, Barbosa S. Genitourinary tuberculosis – A study of 1117 cases over a period of 34 years. Brit J Urol. 1984;56:449–55.

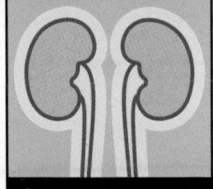
Chapter
55

Fungal Infection of the Urinary Tract

Jack D Sobel and Jose Vazquez

INTRODUCTION

Since the 1980s, there has been a marked increase in opportunistic fungal pathogens involving the urinary tract, of which *Candida* species are the most prevalent[1,2]. The kidney and urinary tract becomes infected as a result of hematogenous spread or from an ascending infection, usually in the presence of urinary obstruction. *Candida* species are common causes of ascending infection in catheterized and obstructed urinary tracts, particularly in diabetics. Patients receiving immunosuppressive therapy for renal transplantation are at risk of invasive fungal UTI caused by *Candida*, *Aspergillus* and *Cryptococcus* species. The acquired immunodeficiency syndrome (AIDS) is associated with mucosal *Candida* infections but not candiduria; however, disseminated histoplasmosis and cryptococcosis, both common complications of AIDS, frequently involve the urinary tract (Table 55.1).

Candida species are the main fungal species commonly associated with urethritis, cystitis, and pyelonephritis. Nevertheless, many species of fungi can cause prostatitis, epididymitis, chronic bladder inflammation or ulceration, and ureteral obstruction. In the absence of obstruction, fungal infections rarely cause renal insufficiency. Fungal infection should always be considered in the differential diagnosis of filling defects in the collecting system.

URINARY CANDIDIASIS

Epidemiology

Candida frequently exists as saprophytes on the external genitalia or urethra; however, yeast in measurable quantities are found in < 1% of clean voided urine specimens. *Candida* infections currently account for 5% of urine isolates in the general hospital and 10% of positive urinary cultures in tertiary-care centers[3]. Candiduria is especially common in the intensive care unit (ICU), and may represent the most common urinary infection in surgical ICU's[4]. Presently 10–15% of nosocomial UTIs are caused by *Candida* species[5–7]. Nosocomial candidiasis is also common in the neonatal and pediatric ICU[6]. Most positive cultures are isolated or transient and represent colonization rather than true infection; however, candiduria may lead to symptomatic UTR and/or fungemia.

Microbiology

C. albicans is the most common fungal species isolated from the urine and in one study was found in 446 (52%) of 861 patients with funguria[4]. *C. glabrata* accounts for 25–35% of infections whereas 8–28% of infections are due to *C. tropicalis*, *C. krusei*, and *C. parapsilosis*[4,7,8]. Unusual species are common in hospitalized patients, especially diabetics, with chronic indwelling bladder catheters. Mixed infections caused by more than one *Candida* species are not infrequent, as is concomitant bacteriuria.

Pathogenesis

Candida infections of the urinary tract generally occur in the presence of predisposing factors or in immunocompromised hosts (Table 55.2). Most infections are associated with the use of indwelling urinary devices including Foley catheters,

Urinary tract involvement by invasive mycoses				
Infection	Prostate	Bladder	Kidney	Penis/cutaneous
Blastomycosis	+++	±	+	+
Histoplasmosis	++	+	++	++
Coccidioidiomycosis	+	+	++	+
Aspergillosis	+	+	+++	+
Cryptococcosis	+++	+	+++	+
Candidiasis	+++	++++	++++	++

Table 55.1 Urinary tract involvement by invasive mycoses.

Risk factors for *Candida* urinary tract infection		
	Route	Risk factors
Renal candidiasis	Hematogenous (anterograde)	Neutropenia (prolonged), intravascular drug use, burns, recent surgery (abdominal, thoracic), systemic infection
Lower urinary tract infection (UTI)	Ascending (retrograde)	Foley catheter, female gender, extremes of age, instrumentation, diabetes mellitus, obstruction/stasis, recent antibacterial therapy, recent bacterial UTI, ureteral stent, nephrostomy tube, renal transplantation
Pyelonephritis	Ascending	Diabetes, obstruction/stasis, instrumentation, postoperative, nephrostomy tube, ureteral stent, nephrolithiasis

Table 55.2 Risk factors for *Candida* spp. urinary tract infection.

internal stents, and percutaneous nephrostomy tubes (Fig. 55.1). Diabetics have an increased overall risk of UTI for both bacterial and fungal infection[2,4]. *Candida* growth in urine is enhanced when urinary levels of glucose exceed 150 mg/dL (8.3 mmol/L). Diabetic females have higher perineal and periurethral *Candida* colonization rates. Diabetics also have impaired phagocytic and fungicidal activity of neutrophils; however, the dominant predisposing factor to candiduria is increased instrumentation, urinary stasis, and obstruction secondary to autonomic neuropathy.

Antibiotic therapy has a major role in predisposing to candiduria. No antibiotic appears exempt from this complication, although there is higher risk with either prolonged use or with broad-spectrum agents. By suppressing susceptible endogenous bacterial flora in the gastrointestinal and lower genital tract, antibiotic use results in the emergence of fungi colonizing these epithelial surfaces with ready access to the urinary tract especially in the presence of indwelling bladder catheters.

Most lower UTIs are caused by genital or perineal colonization with retrograde infection from an indwelling catheter. The upper urinary tract may rarely become involved via ascending infection and then usually only in the presence of urinary obstruction, reflux, or diabetes.

The majority of cases of renal candidiasis occur not as a result of ascending spread from the lower urinary tract, but as a consequence of hematogenous seeding of the renal parenchyma. *Candida* species express a tropism for the kidney. An autopsy study performed by Lehner documented that 90% of the patients dying with disseminated candidiasis had renal involvement, although renal infection (candidiasis) may occur as an isolated site of metastatic spread, especially following transient candidemia[9]. Autopsy studies demonstrated multiple abscesses in the renal interstitium, glomeruli, and peritubular vessels, with not infrequent papillary necrosis and, rarely, emphysematous pyelonephritis.

Clinical features

Most patients with candiduria are asymptomatic. Patients who have an indwelling bladder catheter most often are colonized rather than infected with a *Candida* species. Hospitalized candiduric patients with constitutional or systemic symptoms usually have another cause for their symptoms. However, patients with *Candida* cystitis may present with frequency, dysuria, urgency, hematuria, and pyuria. Cystoscopy reveals soft, pearly white, slightly elevated patches that resemble oral thrush, as well as hyperemia and inflammation of the bladder mucosa (Fig. 55.2). Most symptomatic patients with *Candida* cystitis are not catheterized and the converse also applies.

Ascending infection, although rare, may result in *Candida* pyelonephritis characterized by fever, leukocytosis, rigors, and costovertebral angle tenderness. Ultrasonography and computed tomography (CT) scanning are useful in diagnosing an intrarenal and perinephric abscess. Excretory urography may reveal ureteropelvic fungus balls with or without accompanying papillary necrosis. Ascending infection with *Candida* species uncommonly causes candidemia, with 3–10% of episodes of candidemia being secondary to candiduria[10]. When candidemia occurs it invariably complicates anatomic obstruction, manipulation, or a urologic procedure.

Fungal bezoars may develop anywhere in the urinary drainage system, but most commonly are found in the pelvis or upper ureters (Fig. 55.3). Fungal balls are rare and their presence is suggested by signs of ureteral obstruction associated with candiduria. When bilateral, they may induce obstruction sufficient to cause azotemia. Obstruction may be intermittent or passage of the fungal balls may result in renal colic or the passage of 'soft' stones. Excretory urography or retrograde

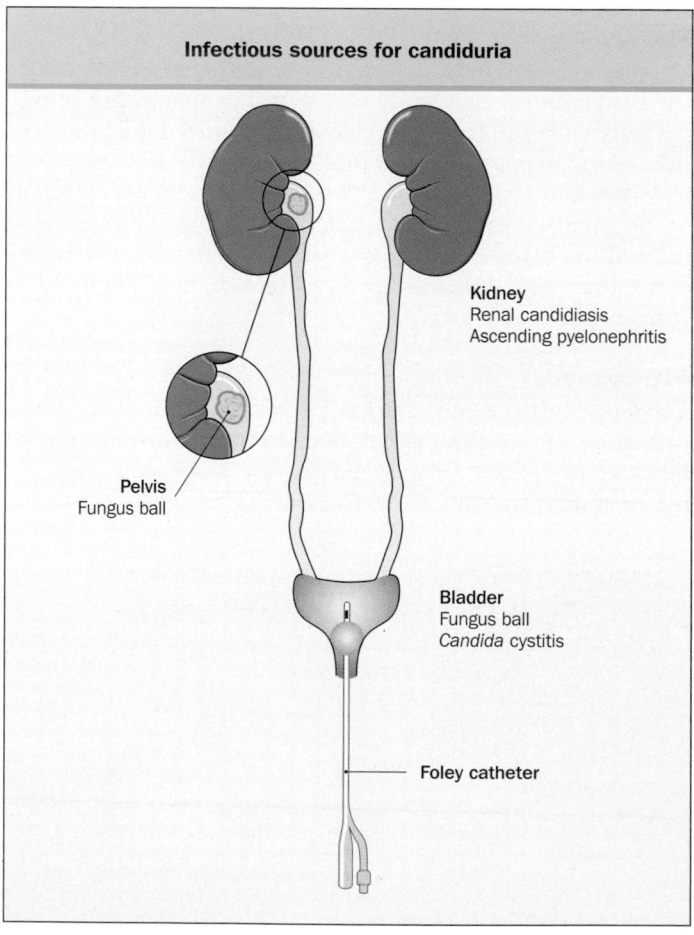

Infectious sources for candiduria

Kidney
Renal candidiasis
Ascending pyelonephritis

Pelvis
Fungus ball

Bladder
Fungus ball
Candida cystitis

Foley catheter

Figure 55.1 Infectious sources for candiduria. Candiduria may originate in the upper or lower urinary tract. Most infections occur by the ascending route, but not infrequently candiduria may be the result of hematogenous seeding of the kidneys.

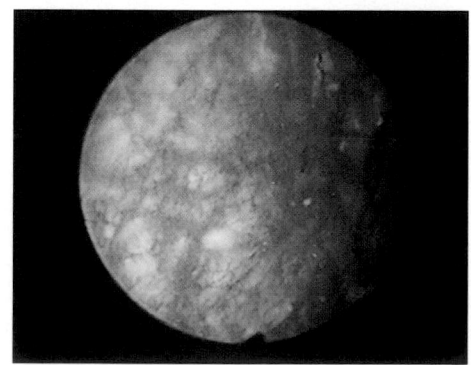

Figure 55.2 Macroscopic appearance of extensive cystitis caused by *C. krusei* as visualized on cystoscopy. Note the extensive hyperemia, exudative reaction resembling a 'snow storm'.

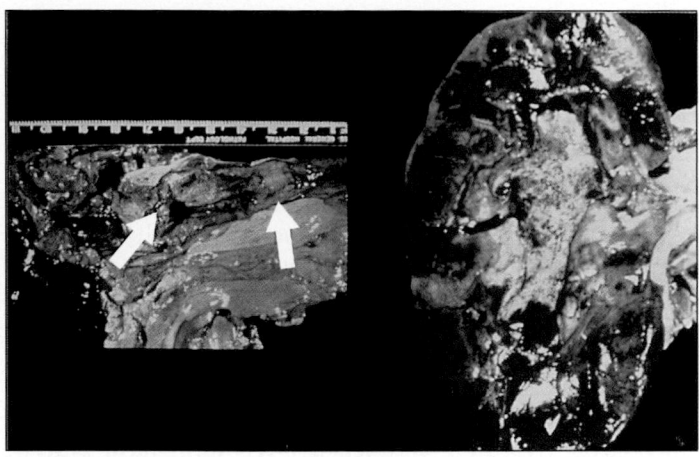

Figure 55.3 Fungal bezoars. Autopsy specimens showing large fungal bezoars in dilated renal pelvices (arrows).

pyelography reveals a filling defect in the collecting system. Fungal balls in the urinary tract have also been described with *Aspergillus*, *Penicillium* species and Zygomycetes.

Renal candidiasis secondary to hematogenous spread represents a systemic infection usually accompanied by fever and other constitutional manifestations of sepsis (Fig. 55.4). Positive blood cultures may be obtained; however, often when the diagnosis of renal candidiasis is considered, blood cultures are no longer positive, causing difficulty in diagnosis. Manifestations of disseminated candidiasis may include maculopapular skin rash and endophthalmitis. Most patients with candiduria secondary to renal candidiasis are febrile but lack other clinical manifestations that indicate renal involvement other than variable reduction in renal function. Accordingly, finding candiduria may be the only clue to the diagnosis of invasive and disseminated candidiasis[11].

Diagnosis
Isolation of *Candida* species from a urine sample may represent contamination, vulvovestibular or catheter colonization, or a superficial/deep infection of the lower or upper urinary tract. Contamination of the sample is common in women with vulvovaginal colonization. Contamination can usually be excluded by repeating the urine culture with special attention to proper collection techniques. Two consecutive positive isolates of *Candida* are essential before initiating antifungal therapy. Rarely, in hospitalized female patients, a bladder urine sample obtained with a straight catheter is necessary to determine the source.

Differentiating infection from colonization of the urinary tract is difficult, if not impossible, especially in patients with catheters. Clinical features are not specific, and in critically ill patients in intensive-care units, fever and leukocytosis may have other sources. The presence of pyuria in catheterized patients does not differentiate infection from colonization, as an indwelling catheter may itself lead to pyuria from mechanical irritation of bladder mucosa and because of concomitant bacteriuria. Quantitative urine colony counts are also not of value in the patient with an indwelling catheter. Fungal morphology (such as the presence of hyphae) is only helpful if hyphae or pseudohyphae are found within hyaline or granular casts (see Fig. 55.5).

In patients without catheters, there is greater likelihood for true infection in the presence of candiduria, particularly if urinary counts are > 10 000–15 000 cells/mL urine. However, renal candidiasis has rarely been reported with a colony count of < 10³ cells/mL. Therefore, considerable overlap occurs and quantitative cultures are not the final determinant in therapeutic decision-making; similarly, negative urine cultures cannot be used to exclude renal candidiasis.

After candiduria is deemed to represent infection, the challenge to the clinician is to localize the anatomic level of infection. Localization is critical in the management of candiduria. No useful test to differentiate *Candida* invasion of kidneys from the frequent lower tract *Candida* infection exists, other than the rare detection of *Candida* hyphae or pseudohyphae within casts (see Fig. 55.5). Quantitative cultures, fungal morphology on microscopy, and pyuria also have little value in localizing infection (Fig. 55.6). Nonspecific evidence of upper UTI is suggested by declining renal function, constitutional features, and radiographic findings on CT scanning and ultrasonography. Serologic tests for *Candida* enolase as a marker for parenchymal invasion remain insensitive. A 5 day bladder irrigation with

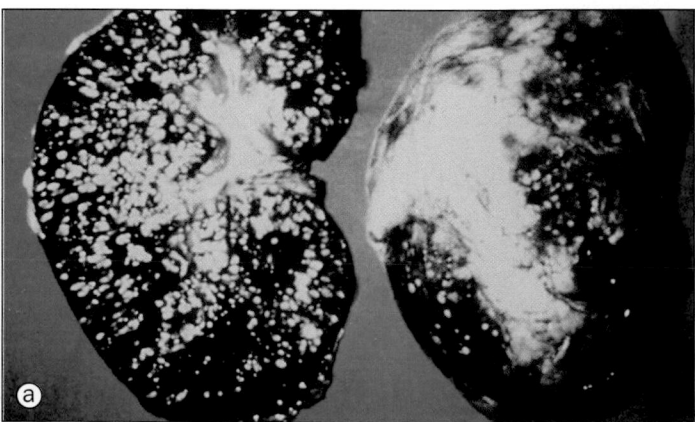
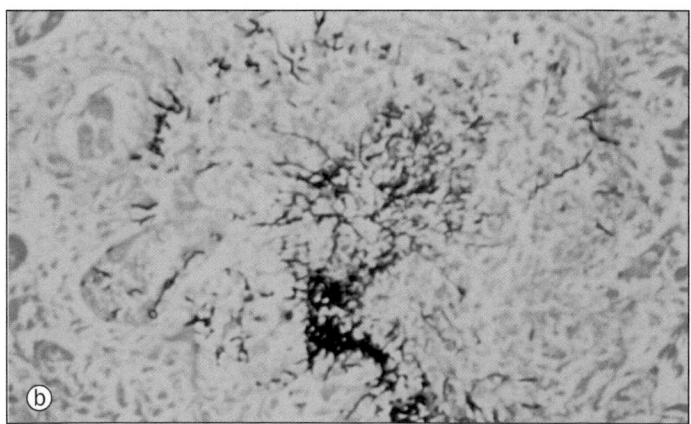

Figure 55.4 Hematogenous renal candidiasis. (a) Autopsy shows macroscopic seeding of the kidneys. (b) On microscopic examination, multiple small abscesses caused by *Candida* are evident.

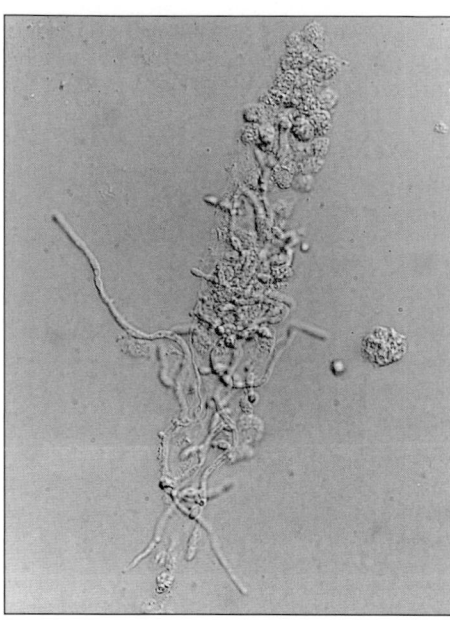

Figure 55.5 Photomicrograph of renal tubular cast containing *Candida* organisms forming hyphae, indicating renal involvement.

amphotericin B solution (50–100 mg/L 5% dextrose in water) may be effective in establishing the source of candiduria, in that persistent postirrigation candiduria is indicative of fungal infection originating above the bladder. This implies the need for further investigation and raises the suspicion of renal candidiasis. Unfortunately the lengthy nature of the conventional amphotericin B irrigation test excludes its utility in febrile, critically ill patients with candiduria. A 3-h rapid bladder irrigation test using amphotericin B at 200 mg/mL has been recommended based upon in vitro studies but has yet to be shown reliable in patients[12].

Treatment of candiduria
Asymptomatic candiduria
Asymptomatic colonization with *Candida* is the most common syndrome associated with candiduria and requires no

therapy. The candiduria is often transient and, even if persistent, uncommonly results in serious morbidity. The risk of invasive complications is small[4,10].

In a prospective, multicenter placebo-controlled study, Sobel et al[13]. found that asymptomatic candiduria resolved with urinary catheter elimination in ~ 41% of hospitalized, catheterized patients. After changing a catheter, untreated candiduria resolved in 20% of patients. Storfer et al.[14] found a similar rate of resolution of untreated candiduria.

While antifungal therapy, either with systemic amphotericin B or fluconazole or with local amphotericin B irrigation, can eliminate candiduria in catheterized patients[5,15,16] there is no evidence that patients benefit from therapy. Furthermore, relapse is frequent. For example, Sobel et al.[15] reported that fluconazole treatment resulted in high short-term rates of eradication of *Candida* from the urine, but two weeks after therapy was discontinued the frequency of candiduria was similar in the fluconazole and placebo groups. Interestingly, *C. glabrata* responded equally well to fluconazole as *C. albicans* despite having higher MICs to fluconazole. This may be due to the high concentrations (10-fold that of serum) that fluconazole achieves in the urine.

Persistent asymptomatic candiduria in patients without catheters should be investigated for upper tract disease since the likelihood of obstruction or stasis is relatively high. Persistent asymptomatic candiduria in catheterized low birth weight infants, in the renal transplant patient and in the afebrile neutropenic patient may also require antifungal therapy and investigation to exclude the possibility of renal or systemic involvement. Candiduria in these patients should be considered a complicated UTI; hence when treatment is indicated as described below, therapy should generally be for at least 14 days (Table 55.3).

The management of asymptomatic candiduria in the renal transplant patient is particularly perplexing. Many of the patients are diabetic, are receiving perioperative antibiotics and immunosuppressive agents, and/or have Foley catheters

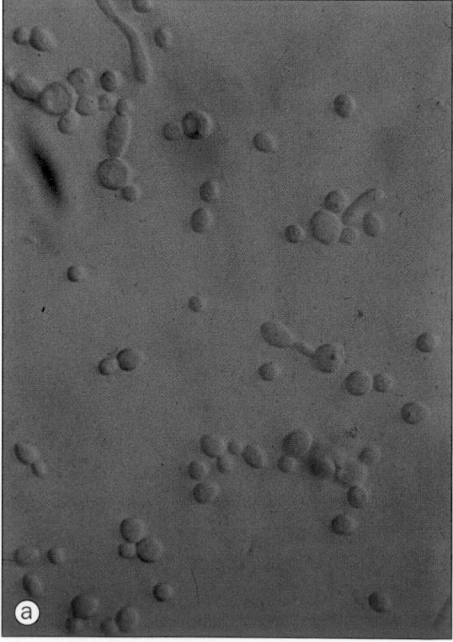

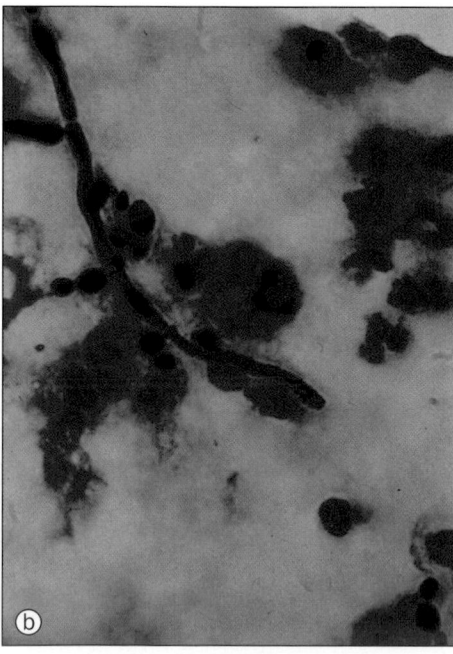

Figure 55.6 Photomicrograph of urine specimens containing *Candida*. (a) A high-power (×100) examination of urine demonstrates singlets and yeast (blastospores), budding yeast, and pseudohyphae in a patient with *C. albicans* infection. (b) A Gram stain of urine obtained from the same patient, showing pseudohyphae.

Table 55.3 Treatment recommendations for urinary tract infections with *Candida*. (LBW. low birth weight).

Treatment recommendations for urinary tract infections with *Candida*		
1. Asymptomatic candiduria	No treatment indicated (especially in catheterized patients)	
	Exceptions	
	(1) afebrile neutropenia	Systemic amphotericin B 0.6 mg/kg per d or fluconazole 6 mg/kg per d × 14 d (i.v./p.o.)
	(2) Post renal transplant	Systemic fluconazole 6 mg/kg per d × 14 d (i.v./p.o.)
	(3) Prior to elective urologic surgery	Systemic antifungal or amphotericin B bladder irrigation (50 mg/L) for 7 d if catheterized
	(4) Catheterized LBW infant	Systemic antifungal (see text)
2. *Candida* cystitis	**Options**	
	(1) Systemic fluconazole 6 mg/kg per d × 14 d	
	(2) Systemic amphotericin B (a) Single dose 0.3 mg/kg (b) Multi dose 0.6 mg/kg per d × 10–14 d	
	(3) Flucytosine for non-albicans *Candida* (e.g. *C. glabrata*) 150 mg/kg per d for 14 d	
	(4) If catheterized – amphotericin B irrigation (50 mg/L) for 5–7 d	
3. Ascending pyelonephritis	(1) Amphotericin B 0.6 mg/kg per d for at least 14 days	
	(2) Fluconazole 6–12 mg/kg per d (based on species)	
4. Disseminated/renal candidiasis	(1) Amphotericin B 0.6 mg/kg per d for 4–6 weeks (based on species)	

and intraoperative ureterocystic stent placement. The risk of ascending infection is high given the stent, glycosuria, short ureter and frequent reflux. Nevertheless, parenchymal invasion of the graft and candidemia is rare in the absence of obstruction. It is reasonable in the presence of asymptomatic infection to attempt eradication of candiduria, but many experts prefer to observe these candiduric patients until all foreign bodies are removed. When fever and sepsis due to invasive candidiasis supervenes, antifungal therapy is justified.

Patients with asymptomatic candiduria in whom urologic instrumentation or surgery is planned should have the candiduria eliminated or suppressed prior to and during the procedure in order to avoid the risk of invasive candidiasis and candidemia. Successful elimination can be achieved through amphotericin B bladder irrigation, or with systemic therapy utilizing amphotericin B, flucytosine, or fluconazole.

Candida *cystitis*

Symptomatic cystitis requires treatment with either amphotericin B bladder instillation (50 mg/L) or systemic therapy, utilizing intravenous amphotericin B, flucytosine, or fluconazole[5–13,15,17]. In contrast to fluconazole in which 80% of the drug is excreted unchanged in the urine, both ketoconazole and itraconazole are poorly excreted in the urine and should not be used. Single-dose intravenous amphotericin B 0.3 mg/kg has also been shown to be highly efficacious in the treatment of lower urinary tract candidiasis, with therapeutic urine concentrations continuing for a considerable time after the administration of the single dose of amphotericin B. This regimen may be preferable for resistant fungal species. Most patients without indwelling catheters are conveniently managed with oral fluconazole (Table 55.3).

Ascending pyelonephritis and *Candida* urosepsis

Invasive upper tract infections require systemic antifungal therapy as well as immediate investigation and visualization of the urinary drainage system to exclude urinary obstruction, papillary necrosis, and fungus ball formation[18]. The most widely accepted therapy is intravenous amphotericin B, 0.6 mg/kg daily. Duration of therapy is generally 14 days unless the infection is severe or there is evidence of candidemia. As an alternative to treatment with amphotericin B, systemic therapy with fluconazole 6–12 mg/kg daily (intravenous or oral) offers an effective and less toxic therapy, although less experience is available with its use. Since fluconazole is excreted unchanged into the urine, coexistent severe renal failure may frequently result in sub-therapeutic urinary concentrations of fluconazole. Accordingly, systemic doses of fluconazole should not be reduced in renal failure or candiduria associated with obstruction[15]. Many patients have renal insufficiency, accordingly it is tempting to use the less nephrotoxic lipid formulations of amphotericin B that are currently available. However, in spite of their clinical record of at least equivalent efficacy compared to amphotericin B, desoxycholate, the very structure that protects the kidney from the toxic effects of amphotericin B, may also impair its urinary excretion[19].

Infection refractory to medical management should be treated surgically with drainage, or in cases of a nonviable kidney, nephrectomy. An obstructed kidney with hydronephrosis requires a percutaneous nephrostomy. The management of ureteral fungal balls depends upon the extent, site, and severity of infection. In some patients, bezoars spontaneously lyse or become dislodged during placement of ureteral stents[18]. In many patients, upper tract external drainage via a nephrostomy tube must be combined with local amphotericin B or fluconazole irrigation. Occasionally, the fungal bezoars must be removed surgically.

Renal and disseminated candidiasis

Management of renal candidiasis secondary to hematogenous spread is essentially that of systemic candidiasis, including intravenous amphotericin B 0.6 mg/kg daily or intravenous fluconazole 400 mg daily (6 mg/kg)[20]. Dosage modifications may be necessary in the presence of severe azotemia. Prognosis depends upon correction of the underlying factors i.e., resolution of neutropenia or removal of the intravascular catheters implicated. Systemic candidiasis requires prolonged therapy over 4–6 weeks. Lipid formulations of amphotericin B, although less nephrotoxic than the standard desoxycholate form, have not been shown to be superior and are not currently regarded as first-line therapy for disseminated candidiasis.

CRYPTOCOCCAL URINARY TRACT INFECTIONS

Both symptomatic and asymptomatic UTI secondary to *Cryptococcus neoformans* infection can occur in AIDS patients as well as in patients with other immunocompromising conditions. In systemic cryptococcosis, cryptococcuria may occur as an early event preceding meningitis[21]. It may coexist with meningitis (30–40%) and, in this case, is a poor prognostic factor indicative of widely disseminated disease. It may occur after apparent successful antifungal therapy and may be a source of systemic infection relapse. Finally, isolated cryptococcal UTI can exist in the absence of systemic infection. However, the fact that systemic recurrence, meningitis, and death have occurred after relapse from a urinary source indicates that even in the absence of pulmonary or meningeal cryptococcosis, cryptococcuria is not benign. Hence, patients presenting with cryptococcuria should be evaluated for systemic and meningeal infection and their genitourinary tracts should also be investigated.

Clinical infection of the genitourinary tract may take three forms. Pyelonephritis is usually asymptomatic or may rarely present as a clinical pyelonephritis, particularly in immunosuppressed or diabetic patients. These patients are often found at autopsy to have disseminated infection; cryptococcal prostatitis is the most common presentation (see below); and occult cryptococcal UTI can occur, in which no localizing signs are observed. Most occult involvement occurs without an increase in serum cryptococcal antigen titer. Nevertheless, occult infection with isolated cryptococcuria and no localizing signs may represent disseminated disease, as autopsy studies have shown that disseminated cryptococcal infection is associated with renal foci of infection in 26–57% of patients. Treatment of symptomatic or asymptomatic cryptococcuria requires systemic antifungal agents, including intravenous amphotericin B 0.7 mg/kg daily or fluconazole 5–10 mg/kg daily. Duration of antifungal therapy is controversial and depends upon whether associated immunosuppression or immunodeficiency exists. In the absence of defective cell-mediated immunity, all therapy should continue for 6 weeks.

In the presence of impaired cell-mediated immunity, lifetime therapy may be indicated. The serum cryptococcal antigen can be used as a guide to therapy.

FUNGAL PROSTATITIS

Fungal prostatitis may result from local inoculation (*Candida* and *Trichosporon* species) by contaminated or infected urine, or from hematogenous spread (blastomycosis, histoplasmosis, coccidioidomycosis, aspergillosis, cryptococcosis, candidiasis, and zygomycosis). Frequently, prostatic involvement by fungi is chronic and asymptomatic, and is discovered at autopsy[1,21,22].

Candida species are the most common fungi that infect the urinary tract and hence the commonest cause of prostatitis, followed by blastomycosis and cryptococcosis. Risk factors for candidal prostatitis are similar to those for UTI, especially diabetes mellitus, antibiotic administration, indwelling catheters, and anatomic abnormalities. Considering the high prevalence of candiduria, especially in catheterized patients, *Candida* abscesses of the prostate gland are rare.

Acute prostatitis caused by *Candida* species presents with fever, constitutional findings, perineal pain, discomfort, urinary bladder irritative symptoms, and, possibly, urinary obstruction. The last is more likely in the presence of a *Candida* prostatic abscess. In most patients, urine cultures for *Candida* are positive, although rare instances of sterile urine have been reported. The presence of an abscess is confirmed by transrectal ultrasonography or CT scan. In addition to systemic antifungal therapy, focal suppuration requires drainage, either by the percutaneous route or, occasionally, by performing a transurethral prostatectomy.

Most prostatic fungal infections other than those due to *Candida* result from hematogenous dissemination, especially *Blastomyces dermatitidis*. Clinical features are identical for all the invasive mycoses. The diagnosis of chronic fungal prostatitis is usually considered when symptomatic patients have laboratory signs of urinary inflammation (pyuria) but negative bacterial cultures. A negative fungal culture of urine or secretions should, not exclude the diagnosis of chronic fungal prostatitis.

Cryptococcal infection of the prostate occurs secondary to hematogenous seeding in immunocompromised patients (especially patients with AIDS) and may accompany pulmonary infection or meningitis. Most cases of prostatic infection are asymptomatic and are only diagnosed at autopsy. Patients with AIDS are more likely to develop prostatic abscess, which may be symptomatic and present with dysuria, frequency, nausea and fever. Physical examination may only reveal variable prostatic enlargement. Although the mainstay of treatment remains intravenous amphotericin B, often in combination with flucytosine, fluconazole by virtue of its oral convenience, relative lack of toxicity, penetration, and efficacy in UTI has become the long-term treatment of choice. Nevertheless treatment failures with fluconazole have been reported. Importantly, prostatic infection is an important site of relapse of cryptococcosis after seemingly successful treatment in patients with AIDS.

REFERENCES

1. Wise GJ, Silver DA. Fungal infections of the genitourinary system. J Urol. 1993;149:1377–88.
2. Platt R, Polk BT, Murdock B, et al. Risk factors for nosocomial urinary tract infection. Am J Epidemiol. 1986;124:977.
3. Rivett AG, Perry JA, Cohen J. Urinary candidiasis: a prospective study in hospitalized patients. Urol Res. 1986;14:183–6.
4. Kauffman CA, Vazquez JA, Sobel JD, et al. Prospective multicenter surveillance study of funguria in hospitalized patients. Clin Infect Dis. 2000;30:14–18.
5. Jacobs LG, Skidmore EA, Freeman K, et al. Oral fluconazole compared with amphotericin B bladder irrigation for fungal urinary tract infections in the elderly. Clin Infect Dis. 1996;22:30–5.
6. Phillips JR, Karlowicz MG. Prevalence of Candida species in hospital-acquired urinary tract infections in a neonatal intensive care unit. Pediatr Infect Dis J. 1997;16:190–4.
7. Febre N, Silva V, Medeiros EA, et al. Microbiological characteristics of yeasts isolated from urinary tracts of intensive care unit patients undergoing urinary catheterization. J Clin Microbiol. 1999;37:1584–86.
8. Kozinn PJ, Taschdjian CL, Goldberg PK, et al. Advances in the diagnosis of renal candidiasis. J Urol. 1978;119:184–7.
9. Lehner T. Systemic candidiasis and renal involvement. Lancet. 1964;1:1414–16.
10. Ang BSP, Telenti A, King B, et al. Candidemia from a urinary tract source: microbiological aspects and clinical significance. Clin Infect Dis. 1993;17:622–6.
11. Nassoura Z, Ivatury RR, Simon RJ, et al. Candiduria as an early marker of disseminated infection in critically ill surgical patients: the role of fluconazole therapy. J Trauma. 1995;35:290–5.
12. Fong LW, Cheng PC, Hinton NA. Fungicidal effects of amphotericin B in urine: in vitro study to assess feasibility of bladder washout for localization of site of candiduria. Antimicrob Agents Chemother. 1991;35:1856–9.
13. Sobel JD, Kauffman CA, McKinsey D, et al. Candiduria – a randomized double-blind study of treatment with fluconazole and placebo. Clin Infect Dis. 2000;30:19–24.
14. Storfer SP, Medoff G, Fraser VJ, et al. Candiduria: Retrospective review in hospitalized patients. Infect Dis Clin Pr. 1994;3:23–9.
15. Fan-Havard P, O'Donovan C, Smith SM, et al. Oral fluconazole versus amphotericin B bladder irrigation for treatment of candidal funguria. Clin Infect Dis. 1995;21:960–5.
16. Leu HS, Huancy CT. Clearance of funguria with short course antifungal regimens: a prospective randomized controlled study. Clin Infect Dis. 1995;20:1152–7.
17. Wong-Beringer A, Jacobs RA, Guglielma BJ. Treatment of funguria. A critical review. J Am Med Assoc. 1992;267:2780–5.
18. Irby PB, Stoller MI, McAninch JW. Fungal bezoars of the upper urinary tract. J Urol. 1990;143:447–51.
19. Agustin J, Lacson S, Raffalli J, et al. Failure of a lipid amphotericin B preparation to eradicate candiduria: preliminary findings based on three cases. Clin Infect Dis. 1999;29:686–7.
20. Rex JH, Walsh TJ, Sobel JD, et al. Practice guidelines for the treatment of candidiasis. Infectious Diseases Society of America. Clin Infect Dis. 2000;30:662–78.
21. Byrne R, Hammil RJ, Rodriguez-Barradas MC. Cryptococcuria: case reports and literature review. Infect Dis Clin Pr. 1997;6:573–6.
22. Bailly MP, Boibieux A, Biron F, et al. Persistence of cryptococcus neoformans in the prostate, failure of fluconazole despite high doses. J Infect Dis. 1991;164:435–8.

Urinary Schistosomiasis

Rashad S Barsoum

INTRODUCTION

Schistosomiasis is a parasitic disease usually acquired by teenagers, often leading to complications that may extend throughout their fourth or fifth decades of life. It has existed since prehistoric times. Ancient Egyptians referred to schistosomiasis in medical papyri in the 16th century BC where it was referred to as 'the bloody urine disease'. It was rightly assumed to be acquired through contact with contaminated waters of the River Nile. Under the impression that the causative agent found its way into the body via the urethra, royal servants exposed to Nile water, such as those collecting the sacred papyrus leaves, were made to wear special condoms for protection[1].

Egyptian philosophers correctly assumed that schistosomiasis is caused by a worm, as proven in 1852 by Theodore Bilharz, the German physician practicing at Kasr-El-Aini Medical School in Cairo, after whom the disease has the alternative name 'bilharziasis'. However, Bilharz's observations disproved the notion that the urethra is the portal of entry. He and subsequent observers showed that any part of the skin or mucous membranes could be the portal of entry of the cercaria, the infective stage of the parasite's life cycle (Fig. 56.1). Cercariae soon mature into sexually differentiated adult worms that live, in almost continuous copulation, in the portal venous system or the perivesical venous plexus. Females leave the males only to lay eggs, traveling against the blood flow to the rectal or bladder mucosa. The ova are driven out in the respective excreta. Contact with fresh water within a couple of days allows the eggs to hatch, releasing miracidia, which infect specific snails. In this 'intermediate' host, they mature asexually into cercariae, which are eventually released and search for their 'definitive' host, usually humans, occasionally apes and cattle. The snail demography, which is altered by changes in temperature, defines the endemicity and intensity of schistosomiasis in different geographic regions[2].

Approximately 200 million inhabitants of 76 tropical countries are infected, and an additional 400 million are at risk. Seven species of schistosomiasis are significantly pathogenic to humans, of which only three are responsible for almost all of the relevant morbidity. These are *Schistosoma haematobium*, present throughout Africa, adjacent regions and an ill-defined area in India; *Schistosoma mansoni*, in Africa, South America and the Caribbean islands; and *Schistosoma japonicum* in China and the Far East (Fig. 56.2). Insignificant disease occurs when humans are accidentally exposed to other species of schistosomes such as those responsible for bird Schistosomiasis[3].

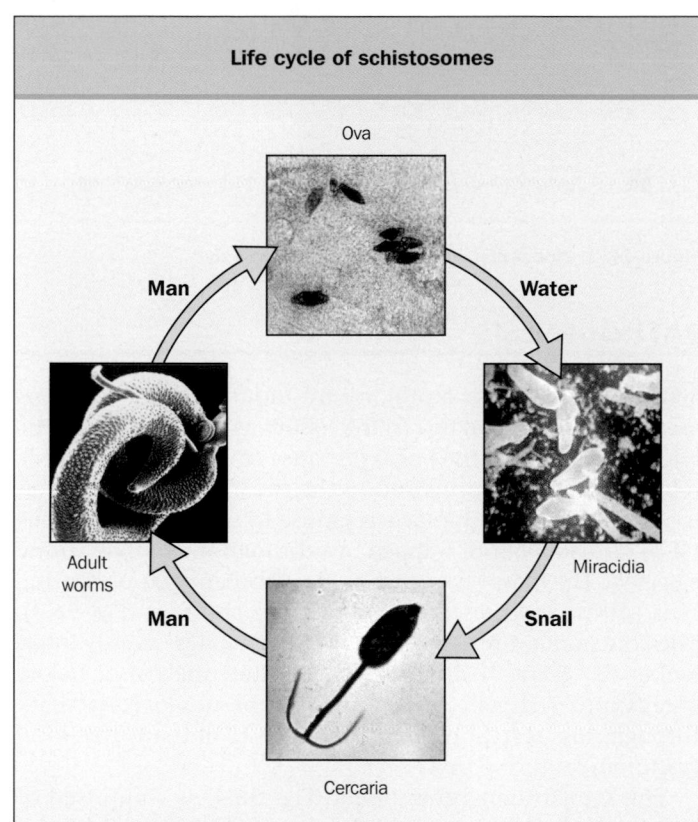

Life cycle of schistosomes

Ova

Man

Water

Miracidia

Snail

Cercaria

Man

Adult worms

Man

Figure 56.1 Life cycle of schistosomes.

S. haematobium affects the genito-urinary organs, while *S. mansoni* and *S. japonicum* affect the colon and rectum, ultimately reaching the liver and inducing periportal fibrosis. Sporadically, all three species, and particularly *S. japonicum*, can cause 'metastatic lesions' when ova are driven by the bloodstream to the lungs, brain, spinal cord, heart muscle, eyes, skin and other sites[4]. Approximately 120 million of infected subjects are symptomatic, while 20 million suffer from serious sequelae of the disease, with an estimated annual global mortality of 20 000, directly attributed to schistosomiasis[5]. Morbidity from infection is variable[6], and depends on the virulence of the infective strains, host resistance, environmental factors and standards of primary medical care. Natural and man-made ecological changes resulting from the construction of dams and artificial lakes have a major impact on the prevalence and intensity of infection and, consequently, the morbidity induced by schistosomiasis in endemic areas[5,7].

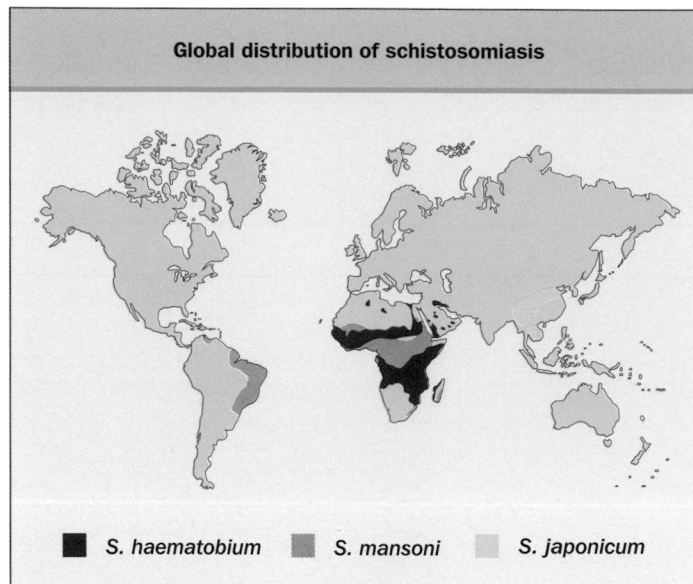

Figure 56.2 Global distribution of schistosomiasis.

PATHOGENESIS

Schistosomes induce morbidity by inducing local reactions around the deposited ova in the tissues as well as by systemic effects attributed to the host's response to circulating antigens released from the worms and/or the ova[8,9]. The local reaction is a T cell-mediated immune response to soluble egg antigens (SEA) diffusing out of trapped ova through micropores in the eggshell. These are processed by the local antigen-presenting cells (APCs) and presented to the T lymphocytes (Fig. 56.3). The concomitant release of 'classical' cytokines, mainly interleukin (IL)-1 and IL-6, leads to the differentiation of helper T cells into Th1 cells, which amplify the monocyte activity through the secretion of interferon-γ to initiate the local granulomatous response.

The schistosomal granuloma (Fig. 56.4) is comprised of mononuclear cells, eosinophils, neutrophils, basophils and fibroblasts, which are recruited and activated by a variety of Th1 pro-inflammatory lymphokines, as well as by specific chemoattractants of parasitic origin. These cells are involved in the elimination of the parasite by direct phagocytosis (monocytes), lymphocytotoxicity (T cells), antibody-dependent cytotoxicity (eosinophils) and complement-dependent and antibody-and-complement-dependent cytotoxicity (neutrophils)[8]. At a later phase, the granuloma tends to be altered through gradual switching from Th1 to Th2 activation. This is mediated by a change in the APC's phenotype and secretory function ('alternative activation')[10], thereby producing a cytokine profile that favors the release of suppressor molecules. The intensity of the inflammatory reaction is thereby reduced and progressive fibrosis is induced, largely through the integrated effects of IL-4, IL-5, IL-9, IL-10, IL-13, transforming growth factor β and somatostatin[11]. Fibrotic granulomata in the urinary bladder, lower ureters and seminal vesicles tend to become dystrophically calcified.

A humoral response also occurs to antigens from the worm's tegument, ova, and gut. Two gut antigens (termed the

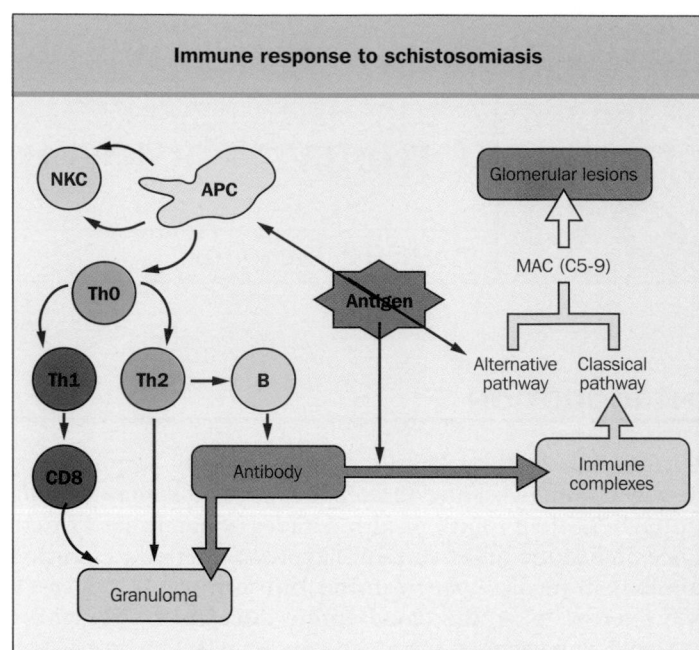

Figure 56.3 Broad lines of the immune response to Schistosomiasis. APC, Antigen presenting cell; NKC, natural killer cell; Th0, resting T-helper lymphocyte, which may be transformed into Th1 or Th2 according to prevailing cytokine profile; CD8, suppressor-killer lymphocyte; MAC, membrane attack complex.

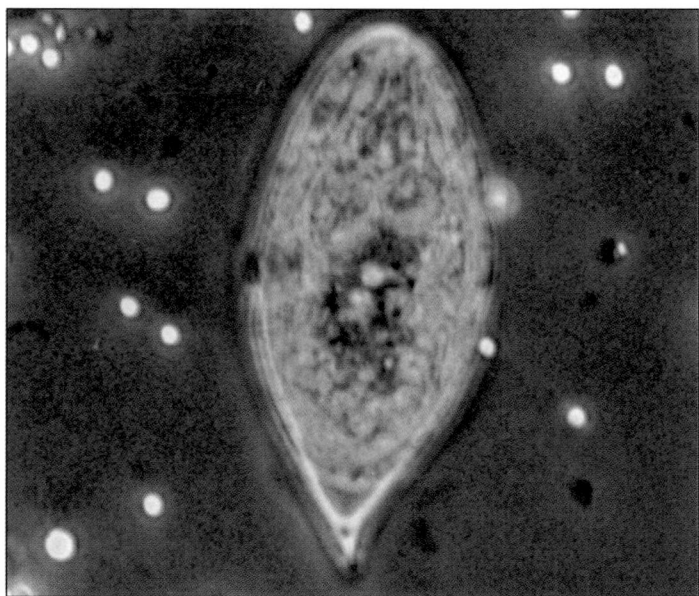

Figure 56.4 *Schistosoma haematobium* granuloma. Note the egg's terminal spike, which identifies *S. haematobium*, and the distortion of the shell under the impact of proteolytic enzymes and oxygen free radicals released by different granulocytes. In addition, note the invasion of the ovum by mononuclear cells. (Hematoxylin and eosin stain ×500.)

'circulating cathodal' and 'circulating anodal' antigen)[12] have been identified in immune complexes in glomeruli. The antibody response is biphasic, reflecting the successive Th1 and

Th2 stages of lymphocyte activation. In the Th1 phase, B cells tend to synthesize IgM, IgG_2 and IgG_3 under the influence of IL-2. During the Th2 phase, IgG_1, IgG_4 and IgA predominate. The latter immunoglobulins have a limited ability to fix complement and may even block complement deposition, hence their importance in modulating the granulomata. However, IgA predominance may be of major significance in the renal lesions of patients with significant hepatic pathology[13].

In addition to modulating the egg granuloma and modifying the systemic antibody profile in schistosomiasis, the late Th2 predominance is blamed for a number of disease associations and complications, including bacterial infection (e.g., salmonella[14], mycobacteria[15], staphylococci[16]), viral infection (HBV[17], HCV[18], human papilloma virus[19]), amyloidosis[20] and certain malignancies (urinary bladder[21], rectum[22], lymphomas[23]).

CLINICAL MANIFESTATIONS

The renal lesions in schistosomiasis reflect the two major pathogenetic mechanisms outlined above. First, there are local lesions mostly affecting the lower urinary tract and caused by the local granulomatous response to *S. haematobium* ova[24]. Second, there are lesions caused by immune-complex deposition in the glomeruli, usually associated with *S. mansoni* infections of the intestine (see Chapter 28) and less commonly with *S. haematobium* infections[8].

Schistosomiasis of the urinary tract (bilharziasis)

The lower urinary tract is the target of *S. haematobium* (and rarely *S. mansoni*) infection. Overt morbidity is extremely variable even within the same continent ranging, for example, from 2% in Nigeria to 52% in Tanzania[14].

Clinical disease starts by the coalescence of granulomata into 'pseudotubercles' in the bladder mucosa. These consolidate to form sessile, occasionally pedunculated, masses or they may ulcerate, leading to painful terminal hematuria, the typical presenting symptom of the disease. Ulcers heal by fibrosis, with calcified granulomata lying underneath the atrophic and dirty mucosa. This leads to the characteristic cystoscopic appearance of 'sandy patches' (Fig. 56.5), and to the radiological appearance of linear bladder calcifications (Fig. 56.6). Lesions may also occur in the lower ureters, bladder neck, seminal vesicles, and other organs in the vicinity.

The bladder lesions predispose to secondary bacterial infection, particularly following diagnostic or therapeutic instrumentation. This tends to persist for many decades, with little response to conventional antibiotics. *Proteus* sp. infections are notorious for favoring stone formation, which further complicates the scenario. The often relentless chronic cystitis can make the patient's life a real misery. The fibrotic process ultimately involves the bladder neck, leading to outflow obstruction, or the ureterovesical junction, leading to ureteral obstruction or vesicoureteral reflux. Involvement of the detrusor is a late event that may interfere with bladder motor function, leading to an

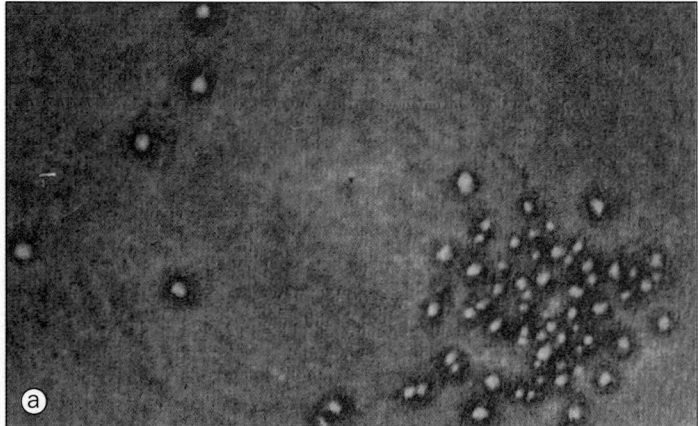
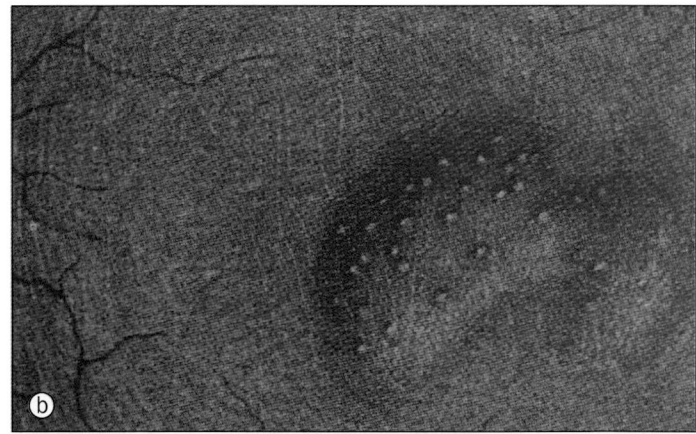
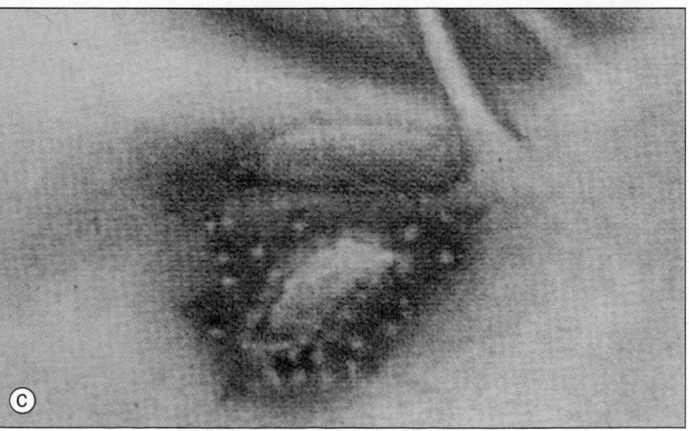
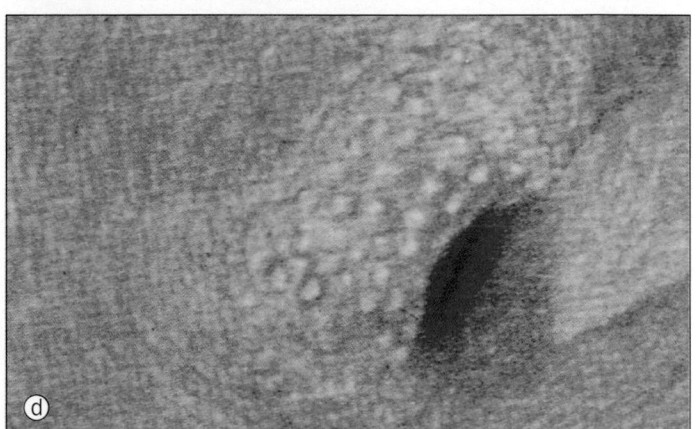

Figure 56.5 Cystoscopic appearances in urinary schistosomiasis. (a) Pseudotubercles. (b) Sessile mass covered by pseudotubercles. (c) Ulcer surrounded by pseudotubercles. (d) Sandy patches. (Courtesy of Professor Naguib Makar.)

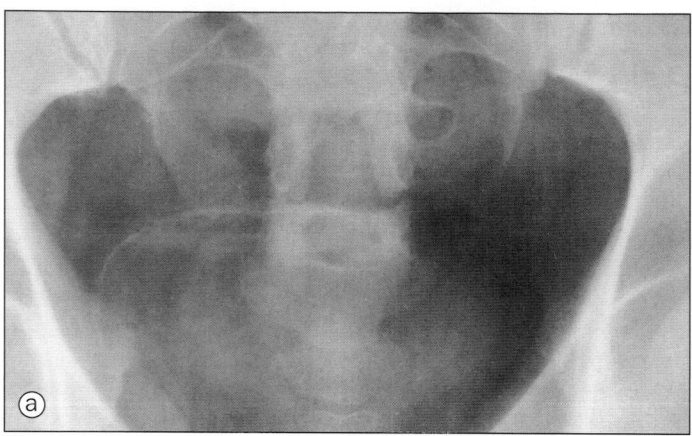
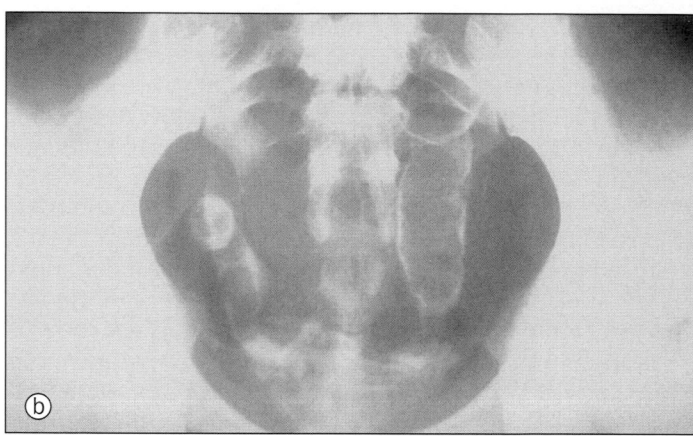

Figure 56.6 Plain radiologic appearances in urinary schistosomiasis. (a) Linear bladder calcifications. (b) Bladder calcifications with calcified left megaureter.

atonic or a hyperirritable viscus. Eventually, the bladder becomes a deformed, contracted, and calcified organ that can accommodate only a small amount of urine which it can hardly void.

Bladder cancer

Chronic schistosomal cystitis is precancerous. Instead of the conventional transitional cell type of bladder cancer, 'bilharzial cancer' is a squamous cell tumor. It is more common in males (almost 10 : 1). It is a slowly growing neoplasm that leads to extensive local infiltration before any distant (usually pulmonary) metastases are detected, owing to the obliteration of local lymphatics by extensive fibrosis. Development of malignancy is suspected when the symptoms of chronic cystitis exacerbate (along with recurrence of hematuria many years after the initial presentation) and small pieces of necrotic tissue are passed with urine (necroturia). A characteristic radiological sign is the irregular eating up of the bladder calcification in a plain radiogram. Cystography shows the tumor mass as an irregular filling defect or bladder ulcer (Fig. 56.7). Cystoscopy displays the tumor and provides the means for a histological diagnosis.

The mechanism of carcinogenesis remains uncertain. Many carcinogens of parasitic or bacterial origin (or resulting from their effects on certain urinary constituents) have been blamed, including reactive oxygen radicals that alter apoptosis genes[8], or coinfection with human papilloma virus[21].

Hydronephrosis

While ureteral strictures and calcifications are common, the hypertrophied upper ureteral musculature usually overcomes the lower obstruction, thereby limiting the upstream consequences. Nevertheless, hydronephrosis and progressive renal failure may develop when there is extensive ureteral scarring, in the presence of stones or secondary bacterial infection, or when the ureterovesical junction is incompetent. The incidence of upper urinary tract involvement varies from less than 10% in Niger to 48% in Cameroon[14].

Interstitial nephritis

Chronic pyelonephritis may result from *S. haematobium* infection complicated by obstruction, reflux and bacterial infection. Granulomata have been occasionally seen in the renal interstitium (Fig. 56.8), but are usually without functional

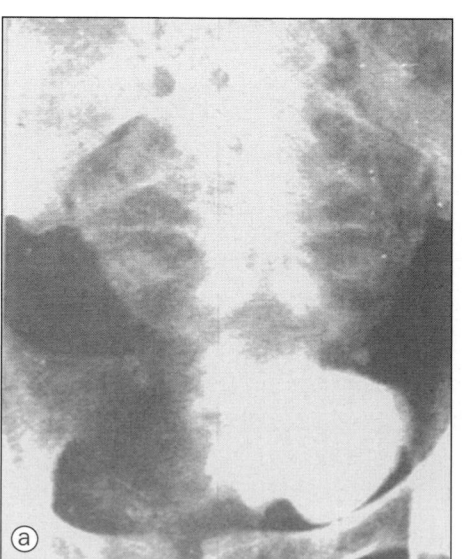
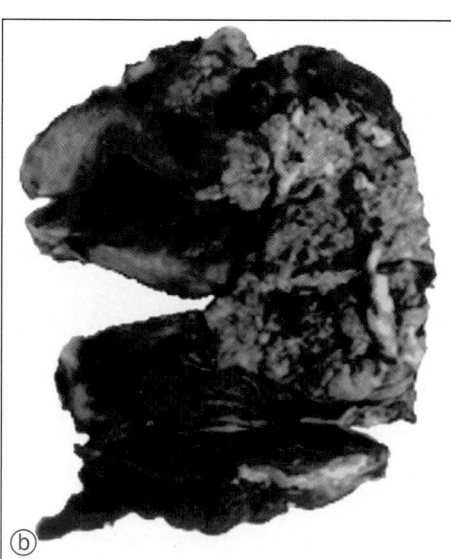

Figure 56.7 Bilharzial cancer of the urinary bladder. (a) Intravenous urogram showing the typical bladder filling defect. The left ureter is dilated and tortuous due to high-grade reflux. No dye refluxes on the right (courtesy of Professor Sameh Hannah). (b) Surgically excised urinary bladder showing a squamous cell carcinoma occupying the vault and posterior wall. Note the remarkable thickening of the bladder wall and dirty mucosa due to bilharzial chronic cystitis (Courtesy of Professor Magdy Morad).

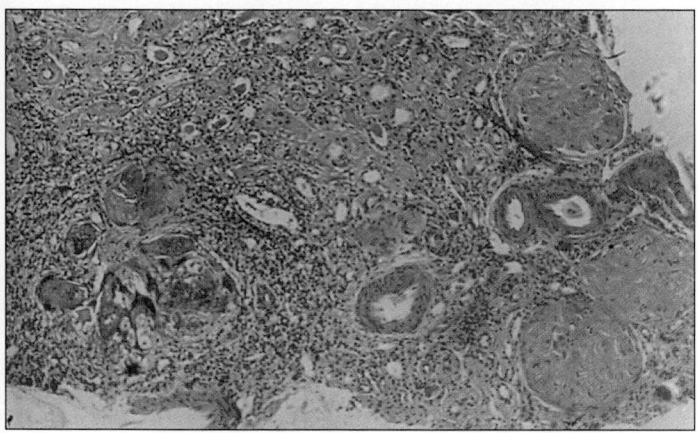

Figure 56.8 Schistosomal chronic interstitial nephritis. Note the dense cellular infiltration and fibrosis, atrophic dilated tubules, and thickened vessels. Three glomeruli heavily infiltrated with amyloid are seen on the right side and a schistosomal granuloma in the lower left corner. (Hematoxylin and eosin ×75.)

or clinical sequelae. Immune-mediated tubulointerstitial nephritis has been described with infections of *S. mansoni* in humans, but the role of immune mechanisms remains questionable in *S. haematobium* pyelonephritis.

The typical picture is that of a scarred kidney with calyceal dilatation, distortion and atrophic parenchyma. There is dense interstitial infiltration, fibrosis and periglomerular scarring. The glomeruli may show ischemic collapse or, rarely, other schistosoma-associated lesions, such as proliferative glomerulonephritis or amyloidosis[20].

The clinical picture is that of chronic tubulointerstitial nephritis (see Chapter 62), often with residual manifestations of lower urinary involvement. Hypertension is a late feature, being overcome by tubular salt wasting, particularly during the early phases of the disease. Anemia and osteodystrophy may be disproportionately severe, owing to the associated nutritional deficiency in endemic areas.

Acute pyelonephritis may be encountered with the introduction of a new ascending infection following cystoscopic or surgical manipulations especially in the setting of obstruction; this may lead to pyonephrosis, renal abscess or septicemia.

Patients with *S. haematobium* infection are prone to urinary co-infection with *Salmonella*. This association has been attributed to Th2 predominance in the late stages of the disease[25], as well as to a peculiar synergism between the two organisms that allows them to evade the host's immune defense[8]. Patients with combined infection may develop severe cystitis or acute pyelonephritis, although many become asymptomatic chronic urinary carriers of salmonellosis.

Immune-complex-mediated lesions

Glomerulonephritis

Most immune complex mediated glomerular diseases caused by schistosomiasis occur in patients with *S. mansoni*[14] (see Chapter 28). However, subclinical glomerular involvement secondary to *S. haematobium* was described in several small clinical series. Transient proteinuria, hematuria, and even the nephrotic syndrome, have been reported in an Egyptian village where the infection was introduced as a result of change in the agricultural irrigation system[26].

Most patients with glomerular disease from *S. haematobium* have mesangial proliferative glomerulonephritis (Fig. 56.9); less often, it is a mesangiocapillary pattern. Schistosomal antigens are detected in the glomerular deposits, usually along with IgM, C3 and, less frequently, IgG and IgA. These lesions tend to regress under treatment or to remain stationary even with persistence of infection. In most patients where progression was reported, there was either an associated *S. mansoni* infection or evidence of significant hepatic fibrosis.

Amyloidosis

Persistent monocyte activation by immune complexes over many years has been blamed in the pathogenesis of schistosoma-associated amyloidosis (Fig. 56.8). This lesion can be induced in animals by infection with any of the three major human pathogenic schistosomal species. Amyloid deposits of the AA type have been detected by special stains in up to 15% of histopathological specimens obtained from patients with schistosomal glomerulopathy, irrespective of the infective

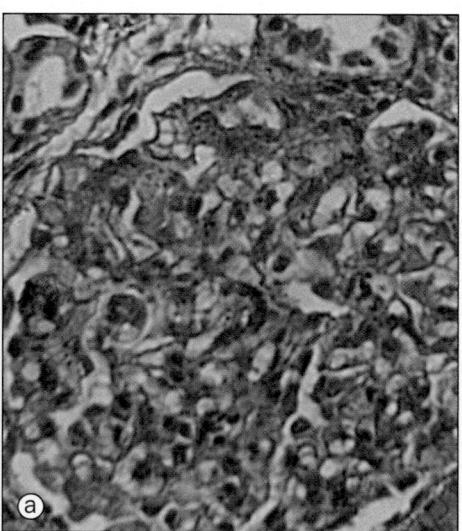

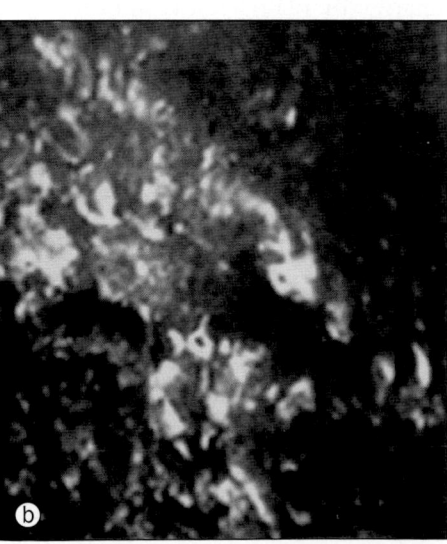

Figure 56.9 Schistosoma haematobium-associated mesangial proliferative glomerulonephritis. (a) Glomerulus showing mesangial proliferation with minimal matrix expansion. (Hematoxylin and eosin ×200). (b) Schistosomal cathodal antigen deposits in the mesangium, detected by immunofluorescence (×200).

species[20]. In a few patients, amyloid deposits have entirely replaced the background proliferative lesion. Amyloid deposits may also be found in the liver, spleen, rectal submucosa and abdominal adipose tissue.

Patients with schistosoma-associated amyloidosis usually present with proteinuria that may reach nephrotic range. The urinary sediment is benign. Hypertension is unusual, and renal function often progresses to end-stage renal disease (ESRD) within 2–3 years.

DIAGNOSIS

The diagnosis of urinary schistosomiasis is suggested in a patient presenting with painful terminal hematuria after being exposed to fresh river waters in an endemic area. It may be more difficult when the history of exposure is less convincing (e.g., swimming pools), or when the clinical presentation is atypical (e.g., bacterial pyelonephritis, typhoid or amyloidosis).

Diagnosis is confirmed by finding schistosomal ova in a fresh urine sample, with the greatest sensitivity occurring in mid-morning samples. Live ova, containing mobile miracidia, indicate active infection, while dead, calcified ova may continue to be shed from fibrotic lesions for many months or even years. A variety of serologic tests are also available for the detection of antischistosomal antibodies or schistosomal antigens[27], which provide useful tools for specific diagnosis even in 'closed infection'. They also provide quantitative appraisal of the intensity of infection and mucosal inflammation[28], and are useful in follow-up after treatment; often turning negative 3–6 months after complete eradication of infection.

Cystoscopic examination is seldom required for the diagnosis of early infection, since live ova, amidst plenty of red and pus cells, are readily detected by simple examination of the urinary sediment. Cystoscopy would show the typical 'pseudotubercles', which are easily distinguished from those of mycobacterial infection by their size and the surrounding mucosal pathology. Nodules, polyps and ulcers may be seen, as well as 'sandy patches' in late stages (Fig. 56.5).

The radiologic appearances of the bladder and seminal vesicle calcification (Fig. 56.6) are so typical that, once detected, no further confirmatory tests are required. Similarly, the plain radiographic appearances of bilharzial cancer (Fig. 56.7a) are pathognomonic.

Other imaging techniques (such as ultrasonography, intravenous or retrograde urography, computed tomography and magnetic resonance imaging scans) are useful in the diagnosis of upstream complications. Renal biopsy is essential for the diagnosis of schistosomal glomerulonephritis or amyloidosis.

NATURAL HISTORY

Early treatment of lower urinary schistosomiasis results in complete cure in almost all patients. Even early back pressure changes have been shown to resolve. On the other hand, if the disease is untreated, it tends to progress leading to bladder fibrosis, calcification, contraction and motor abnormalities. Chronic cystitis may ultimately lead to bladder cancer, the precise incidence of which among infected subjects is undetermined, though accounting for almost one-third of all

malignancies presenting to the National Cancer Institute in Egypt[21]. The 5-year survival following radical cystectomy for bladder cancer is approximately 50%.

As mentioned earlier, upstream consequences occur only in an average of 25% of cases, with a wide geographical variation. In Egypt, they are held directly responsible for 6.7% of ESRD and potentially contributing in an additional 15%[29].

Progressive glomerulonephritis is rare in *S. haematobium* infection. Early glomerular lesions have been reported to regress under treatment[14], although there have not been any controlled trials.

Although amyloid deposits may be seen in about 15% of those with glomerulonephritis, they are seldom responsible for any clinically significant disease. Response of amyloid to antischistosomal treatment is controversial[14].

TREATMENT

S. haematobium responds to treatment with old-fashioned antimony compounds, as well as the newer organophosphates (metrifonate: not available in the UK), niridazole, praziquantel, artemether and others. The current drugs of choice are metrifonate (three doses of 10 mg/kg body weight at 2-week intervals) and Praziquantel (single dose of 40 mg/kg body weight). In a recent metanalysis of five controlled trials in Africa[30], both drugs were similar in terms of cessation of hematuria and proteinuria, improvement of the nutritional state and physical fitness. Praziquantel was superior in inducing parasitiological cure; yet the reinfection rate was equally high with both drugs.

Despite being inexpensive, highly effective and virtually devoid of any side effects, Praziquantel cannot be used for chemoprophylaxis because it is active only against mature worms. Artemether, a derivative of the Chinese antimalarial Quyinghaosu alkaloid, is a promising new agent in this respect, since it can effectively kill the invading cercariae, maturing schistosomulae as well as the mature adult worms by interfering with the parasite's glycolytic pathways[31].

Antibacterial agents usually control acute episodes of secondary bacterial cystitis and pyelonephritis. However, cure requires simultaneous eradication of the parasitic infection if it is still active. This is particularly important when the concomitant bacterial infection is typhoid.

Chronic fibrotic lesions are difficult to treat. Surgical or instrumental treatment is necessary for the relief of an obstructive lesion. However, caution is required while dealing with the ureterovesical junction to avoid induction of reflux. Several plastic surgical procedures are available to restore the distorted ureteric, bladder, or urethral anatomy. Associated bacterial infections may require long-term, low-dose antibiotic therapy.

The management of ESRD in such patients can be difficult, owing to the negative effects of chronic infection; associated schistosomal lesions in the liver, lungs and other organs; and the frequent coexistence of undernutrition, viral infection, or even malignancy. Furthermore, in patients undergoing transplantation[32], the incidence of urinary leaks is manyfold higher than usual owing to the presence of fibrotic granulomata and anatomic distortion in the bladder wall. Hepatic disease may also alter the metabolism of immunosuppressive agents. Recurrence or reinfection may be encountered as a late complication.

REFERENCES

1. Ghalioungui P. Magic and medical science in ancient Egypt. London: Hodder and Stoughton; 1963.
2. Malone JB, Yilma JM, McCarroll JC, et al. Satellite climatology and the environmental risk of Schistosoma mansoni in Ethiopia and east Africa. Acta Trop. 2001;79:59–72.
3. Horak P, Kolarova L. Bird schistosomes: do they die in mammalian skin? Trends Parasitol. 2001;17:66–9.
4. Abdel-Wahab MF. Schistosomiasis in Egypt. Boca Raton, Florida: CRC Press; 1982.
5. World Health Organization Annual Report (2001): http://www.who.int/ctd/schisto/dates.htm.
6. Barsoum RS. Schistosomal glomerulopathy: selection factors. Nephrol Dialysis Transplant. 1987;2:488–97.
7. Patz JA, Graczyk TK, Geller N, Vittor AY. Effects of environmental change on emerging parasitic diseases. Int J Parasitol. 2000;30:1395–405.
8. Barsoum RS. Schistosomiasis. In: Davison AM, Cameron JS, Grunfeld JP, et al., eds. Oxford textbook of clinical nephrology, 2nd edn. Oxford: Oxford University Press; 1997:1287–302.
9. Wahl SM, Frazier-Jessen M, Jin WW, et al. Cytokine regulation of schistosome-induced granuloma and fibrosis. Kidney Int. 1997; 51:1370–5.
10. Stadecker MJ. The regulatory role of the antigen-presenting cell in the development of hepatic immunopathology during infection with Schistosoma mansoni. Pathobiology. 1999;67:269–72.
11. Chatterjee S, Van Marck E. The role of somatostatin in schistosomiasis: a basis for immunomodulation in host-parasite interactions? Trop Med Int Health. 2001;6:578–81.
12. Deelder AM. Quantitative diagnosis of Schistosoma infections by measurement of circulating antigens in serum and urine. Trop Geograph Med. 1994;46:233–8.
13. Barsoum RS, Nabil M, Saady G, et al. Immunoglobulin A and the pathogenesis of schistosomal glomerulopathy. Kidney Int. 1996;50:920–8.
14. Barsoum RS. Schistosomal glomerulopathies. Kidney Int. 1993;44:1–12.
15. Stienstra Y, van der Graaf WT, te Meerman GJ, et al. Susceptibility to development of Mycobacterium ulcerans disease: review of possible risk factors. Trop Med Int Health. 2001;6:554–62.
16. Lambertucci JR, Serufo JC, Gerspacher-Lara R, et al. Schistosoma mansoni: assessment of morbidity before and after control. Acta Trop. 2000;77:101–9.
17. Zeid AM, Hassan MM, Attia WM, et al. Hepatitis-B virus and schistosomiasis infections in childhood proteinuria. Egypt Soc Parasitol. 1994;24:371–82.
18. Abdel-Wahab MF, Zakaria S, Kamel M, et al. High seroprevalence of hepatitis C infection among risk groups in Egypt. Am J Trop Med Hygiene. 1994;51:563–7.
19. Poggensee G, Feldmeier H. Female genital schistosomiasis: facts and hypotheses. Acta Trop. 2001;79:193–210.
20. Barsoum RS, Bassily S, Soliman MM, et al. Renal amyloidosis and schistosomiasis. Trans R Soc Trop Med Hygiene. 1979;73:367–74.
21. el-Mawla NG, el-Bolkainy MN, Khaled HM. Bladder cancer in Africa: update. Semin Oncol. 2001;28:174–8.
22. Matsuda K, Masaki T, Ishii S. Possible associations of rectal carcinoma with Schistosoma japonicum infection and membranous nephropathy: a case report with a review. Jpn J Clin Oncol. 1999;29:576–81.
23. Chirimwami B, Okonda L, Nelson AM. Lymphoma and Schistosoma mansoni schistosomiasis. Report of 1 case. Arch Anat Cytol Pathol. 1991;39:59–61.
24. Badr MM. Surgical management of urinary bilharziasis. In: Dudley H, Pories WJ, Carter DC, McDougal WS, eds. Rob Smith's operative surgery. London: Butterworth; 1986.
25. Infante-Duarte C, Kamradt T. TH1/TH2 balance in infection. Springer Semin Immunopathol. 1999;21:317–38.
26. Ezzat E, Osman R, Ahmed KY, Soothill, JF. The association between Schistosoma haematobium infection and heavy proteinuria. Trans R Soc Trop Med Hyg. 1974;68:315–17.
27. Hamilton JV, Klinkert M, Doenhoff MJ. Diagnosis of schistosomiasis: antibody detection, with notes on parasitological and antigen detection methods. Parasitology. 1998;117(Suppl.):S41–57.
28. Bichler KH, Feil G, Zumbragel A, et al. Schistosomiasis: a critical review. Curr Opin Urol. 2001;11:97–101.
29. Egyptian Society of Nephrology Registry Annual Report (2000): http://www.idsc.gov.eg/health/esn/esn.htm.
30. Squires N. Interventions for treating schistosomiasis haematobium. Cochrane Database Syst Rev. 2000;2:CD000053.
31. Shuhua X, Hotez PJ, Tanner M. Artemether, an effective new agent for chemoprophylaxis against shistosomiasis in China: its in vivo effect on the biochemical metabolism of the Asian schistosome. Southeast Asian J Trop Med Public Health. 2000;31:724–32.
32. Sobh MA, El Agroudy AE, Mostaffa F, et al. Impact of schistosomiasis on patient and graft outcome after kidney transplantation. Nephrol Dial Transplant. 1992;7:858–63.

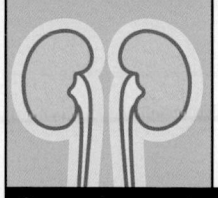

Section 11 Urological Disorders

Chapter 57
Nephrolithiasis and Nephrocalcinosis

Rebeca D Monk and David A Bushinsky

INTRODUCTION

Nephrolithiasis refers to stone formation within the renal tubules or collecting system, although the calculi are often found within the ureters or in the bladder. The principal types of renal calculi are calcium oxalate, calcium phosphate, struvite, urate and cystine. Kidney stones vary in clinical presentation from asymptomatic to large, obstructing staghorn calculi that can severely impair renal function and lead to chronic renal disease. The severity of stone disease depends on the pathogenetic factors contributing to the rate of stone formation, in addition to the stone type, size and location. In its most classic form, nephrolithiasis presents as renal colic, but may also commonly present with hematuria or urinary tract infection. Certain disorders can lead to small but diffuse renal parenchymal calcifications termed nephrocalcinosis. The calcifications, usually calcium phosphate or calcium oxalate, may deposit in the cortex or medulla, depending on etiology. Among the most common causes of stone-related nephrocalcinosis are primary hyperoxaluria and medullary sponge kidney.

NEPHROLITHIASIS

A discussion of the general features of nephrolithiasis is followed by specific features of the pathogenesis and management of the common types of renal stones.

Epidemiology

Kidney stones are common in industrialized nations with an annual incidence of over 1 per 1000 persons and a peak age of onset in the third decade of life[1]. The prevalence increases with age until approximately 70 years. Factors that determine renal stone prevalence include age, sex, race and geographic distribution. In the USA, Caucasians are much more likely to develop renal stones than African Americans, Hispanics or Asian-Americans. Men are more prone to stone formation than women, at a ratio of 2–4:1. In the USA, tendency to stone formation also depends on geographic location, with an increasing prevalence from north to south and, to a lesser degree, from west to east. It is postulated that the increase in nephrolithiasis rates in the American southeast may be linked to the greater sunlight exposure in that area. This may lead to an increase in insensible losses through sweating, which can result in more concentrated urine. The sun exposure may also enhance vitamin D production, with a subsequent increase in intestinal calcium absorption and renal calcium excretion[2].

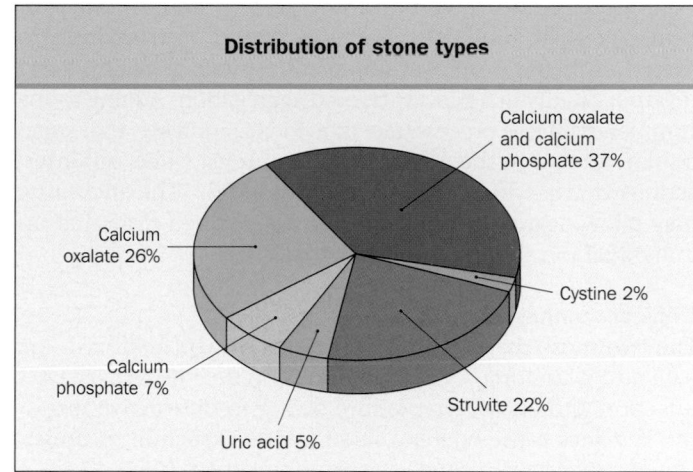

Figure 57.1 Proportion of stone types in a typical US population.

Stone type also varies with worldwide geography. In the Mediterranean and Middle Eastern countries, the percentage of stones composed of uric acid may be as high as 75%, whereas in the USA, the majority of stones are composed primarily of calcium (> 70%) with less than 10% formed purely of uric acid. Magnesium ammonium phosphate (struvite) stones account for roughly 10–25% of stones formed (with a higher incidence in the UK), and cystine stones comprise approximately 2% of stones formed (Fig. 57.1)[1,3,4].

Pathogenesis

Stone formation is a complex event that can only occur in urine that is supersaturated with respect to the constituents of the specific stone. Supersaturation is dependent on the product of the free ion activities of stone components rather than on their concentrations. While an increasing concentration of crystal constituents increases their free ion activity, other factors may serve to diminish it. If one were to dissolve calcium and oxalate in pure water, for example, the solution would become saturated when the addition of any more calcium or oxalate would not result in further dissolution. However, urine, unlike pure water, contains numerous other ions and molecules that can form soluble complexes with the ionic constituents of a stone. The interactions with these other solutes (e.g., citrate) may result in a decrease in free-ion activity, which allows the stone constituents to increase in solution to levels that would normally cause stone formation. Urinary pH can also influence free ion activity. The level of chemical free ion activity in which stones will neither grow nor dissolve is referred to as the equilibrium solubility product, or the upper limit of metastability. Above this level, the urine will be supersaturated and any stone present will grow in size.

When the solution becomes supersaturated, ions can join together in a more stable, solid phase. This so-called nucleation can be homogeneous or heterogeneous. Homogeneous nucleation refers to the joining of similar ions into crystals. The more common heterogeneous nucleation results when crystals grow around dissimilar crystals or other substances in the urine such as sloughed epithelial cells. Calcium oxalate crystals, for example, can nucleate around uric acid crystals. In order for stones to grow sufficiently large in size to obstruct prior to excretion in the urine, several small crystals generally bond together rapidly in a process termed aggregation. Adding to the complexity of this process, recent evidence indicates that small crystals anchor to the urinary epithelium via stone–cell interactions that are incompletely understood[3,5,6]. The anchoring may allow aggregation to occur in the limited time that an individual ion passes through a renal tubule.

Clinical manifestations

The two most characteristic symptoms of nephrolithiasis are pain and hematuria. Other presentations include urinary tract infection and acute renal failure owing to obstructive uropathy if stones cause bilateral renal tract obstruction or unilateral obstruction in a single functioning kidney (Table 57.1).

Pain

The classic pain of nephrolithiasis is ureteral colic. This discomfort of abrupt onset intensifies over time into an excruciating, severe flank pain that only resolves with stone passage or removal. The pain may migrate anteriorly along the abdomen and inferiorly to the groin, testicles, or labia majora as the stone moves toward the ureterovesical junction. Gross hematuria, urinary urgency, frequency, nausea, and vomiting may be present. Stones smaller than 5 mm are likely to pass spontaneously with hydration, whereas larger stones often require urological intervention (Fig. 57.2)[5]. Ureteral colic is not exclusive to stone disease and may also occur with the passage of clots from hematuria of many causes ('clot colic'), or

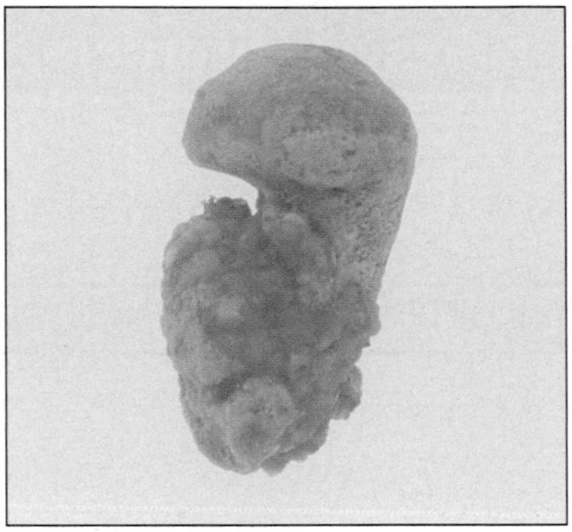

Figure 57.2 Ureteral calculus. A 1-cm wide calcium oxalate stone that provoked ureteral colic and required surgical removal.

with papillary necrosis. As well as colic, nephrolithiasis may provoke less-specific loin pain that may be poorly localized to the kidney and, therefore, has a wide differential diagnosis, particularly if not associated with other urinary symptoms.

Hematuria

Stone disease is a common cause of hematuria, both microscopic and macroscopic. Macroscopic hematuria occurs most commonly with large calculi and during urinary infection and colic. Although typically associated with loin pain or ureteric colic, the hematuria of nephrolithiasis may also be painless. The clinical differential of hematuria is therefore wide and includes tumor, infection and stones, as well as glomerular and interstitial renal parenchymal disease (Table 57.2). Painless microscopic hematuria in children may occur with hypercalciuria in the absence of demonstrable stones.

Clinical presentations of nephrolithiasis	
Presentation	**Characteristics**
Pain	Ureteral colic, loin pain, dysuria
Hematuria	–
Urinary tract infection	Recurrent, chronic infection, pyonephrosis
Asymptomatic urine abnormality	Microscopic hematuria, proteinuria, sterile pyuria
Interruption of urinary stream	–
Calculus anuria	–

Table 57.1 Clinical presentations of nephrolithiasis.

Causes of hematuria
Nephrolithiasis
Infection:
cystitis, prostatitis, urethritis, acute pyelonephritis, tuberculosis, schistosomiasis
Malignancy:
renal cell carcinoma, transitional cell carcinoma, prostatic carcinoma, Wilms' tumor
Trauma
Glomerular disease
Interstitial nephritis
Polycystic kidney disease
Papillary necrosis
Medullary sponge kidney
Coagulopathy
bleeding disorders, anticoagulation therapy
Miscellaneous
loin pain hematuria syndrome, arteriovenous malformation, chemical cystitis, caruncle, factitious

Table 57.2 Causes of hematuria.

Loin pain hematuria syndrome

Loin pain hematuria syndrome is a poorly understood condition that must always be considered in the differential diagnosis of nephrolithiasis. It is diagnosed by exclusion when patients (most typically young and middle-aged females) present with loin pain and persistent microscopic or intermittent macroscopic hematuria[7]. A most careful evaluation is required to exclude small stones, tumor, urinary infection, and glomerular disease. Angiographic abnormalities implying intrarenal vasospasm or occlusion have been reported, as have renal biopsy abnormalities typified by deposition of complement C3 in arteriolar walls. However, these findings are not consistent, nor do they provide a coherent framework to explain the pathogenesis of this condition. Loin pain hematuria syndrome is a chronic condition requiring reassurance, careful management of analgesia, and ongoing psychologic support. The condition usually remits after several years. Denervation of the kidney by autotransplantation is rarely successful[8]. Nephrectomy has been used but pain often recurs promptly in the contralateral kidney. Bilateral nephrectomy and renal replacement therapy has been reported as an approach of very last resort.

Asymptomatic stone disease

Even large staghorn calculi that have been present for a number of years may remain entirely asymptomatic, being a coincidental finding during the investigation of unrelated abdominal or musculoskeletal disease. Obstructive uropathy caused by calculi may be painless; therefore, nephrolithiasis should always be considered in the differential diagnosis of unexplained renal failure. Ultrasound is a poor imaging technique for ureteral stones and may not identify such stones in a patient with hydronephrosis (see Chapter 58, and the section on Radiologic Evaluation, below).

Clinical evaluation of stone formers

All patients with recurrent nephrolithiasis merit evaluation with the goal of determining the cause of their kidney stones. However, evaluation of patients with a single stone is somewhat controversial because of the undetermined cost–benefit ratio of stone evaluation and therapy. In the late 1980s, a National Institutes of Health Consensus Development Conference on the Prevention and Treatment of Kidney Stones determined that all patients, even those with a single stone, should undergo a basic evaluation. Those with metabolically active stones (stones growing in size or number within 1 year), all children, non-calcium stone formers, and patients in demographic groups not typically prone to stone formation, warrant a more complete evaluation[9].

The basic evaluation

The clinic evaluation of stone formers includes the general history and physical examination and requires specific data gathering on stone formation as well as specific laboratory studies (Table 57.3). In addition to the basic medical history, family history, and medications, a stone history, as well as a review of diet, fluid intake, occupation, and lifestyle, should be included.

The basic evaluation of nephrolithiasis

Stone history
- Number of stones formed
- Frequency of stone formation
- Age at first onset
- Size of stones passed or still present
- Kidney involved (left, right or both)
- Stone type, if known
- Need for urologic intervention: extracorporeal shock wave lythotripsy, percutaneous nephrolithotomy, etc.
- Response to surgical procedure
- Are stones associated with urinary tract infections?

Medical history

Medications

Family history

Occupation/lifestyle

Fluid intake/diet

Physical examination
- Evidence of systemic causes of stones, e.g., tophi

Laboratory data:
- Urinalysis
- Urine culture
- Stone analysis
- Blood chemistry:
  - —Sodium, potassium, chloride, bicarbonate,
  - —Creatinine, calcium, phosphorus, uric acid
  - —Intact parathyroid hormone level if calcium elevated

Radiologic evaluation:
- KUB
- IVU
- CT IVU
- Ultrasound

Table 57.3 The basic evaluation of nephrolithiasis.

History

The medical history serves to explore a systemic etiology for the nephrolithiasis. Any disease that can lead to hypercalcemia (including malignancy, hyperparathyroidism and sarcoidosis) can result in hypercalciuria and calcium stone formation. A number of malabsorptive gastrointestinal disorders [including Crohn's disease and sprue (celiac disease)] can result in calcium oxalate stone formation as a result of volume depletion and hyperoxaluria. Uric acid stones often occur in patients with a history of gout.

The stone history (Table 57.3) includes the number and frequency of stones formed, patient age at incidence of first stone, size of stones, stone type (if known), and whether the patient required surgical removal of the calculi. This information indicates the severity of the stone disease as well as providing clues to the possible etiology of the stone formation. For example, large staghorn calculi that do not pass spontaneously and recur despite frequent surgical intervention are more consistent with struvite than calcium oxalate stones. Stones that develop at a young age may be caused by cystinuria or primary hyperoxaluria. Stone response to surgical intervention is also significant. Cystine stones, for example, do not fragment well with lithotripsy. If stones recur frequently in a single kidney, a congenital abnormality in that kidney, such as megacalyx or medullary sponge kidney, should be explored.

Family history is important because a number of stone types have a genetic basis. Idiopathic hypercalciuria is clearly inherited apparently through a number of genes; cystinuria is an autosomal recessive disorder; and, in some patients, hyperuricosuria has been associated with rare inherited metabolic disorders. There are also rare X-linked causes of calcium stones and nephrocalcinosis[11].

Review of all medications is essential. A number of medications are known to potentiate calcium stone formation (e.g., loop diuretics promote calcium excretion) and several have been implicated in uric acid lithiasis (salicylates, probenecid) (Table 57.4). Certain drugs can precipitate into stones themselves, such as rapidly infused intravenous acyclovir, triamterene and the antiretroviral agent, indinavir.

The social history in these patients should include details regarding their occupation and lifestyle. Cardiothoracic surgeons and real-estate agents, for example, may minimize fluid intake to avoid bathroom breaks during the workday. People who engage in vigorous outdoor activities, such as running, may not rehydrate adequately to keep up with insensible losses. In patients already prone to nephrolithiasis, this may lead to production of excessively concentrated urine and precipitation of stone crystals.

A complete dietary history and review of fluid intake is essential in determining potential causes or contributors to stone formation. It is important to have the patient cite commonly consumed foods with each meal, with particular attention paid to sodium-containing foods, as well as quantities of calcium, animal protein, purine and oxalate (Table 57.5). It is particularly important to review dietary calcium as many patients with nephrolithiasis are erroneously instructed to eliminate all calcium from their diet, a suggestion that can result not only in bone demineralization, particularly in women, but also in an increase in stone formation[6].

Foods high in oxalate and purine
High oxalate foods
(avoid in setting of hyperoxaluria) Green beans Beets Celery Green onions Leeks Leafy greens: collard greens, dandelion greens, swiss chard, spinach, escarole, mustard greens, sorrel, kale, rhubarb Cocoa Chocolate Black tea Berries: blackberries, blueberries, strawberries, raspberries, currants, gooseberries Orange peel Lemon peel Dried figs Summer squash Nuts, peanut butter Tofu (bean curd)
High purine foods
(avoid in setting of hyperuricosuria) Organ meats: sweetbreads, liver, kidney, brains, heart Shellfish Meat: beef, pork, lamb, poultry Fish: anchovies, sardines (canned), herring, mackerel, cod, halibut, tuna, carp Meat extracts: bouillon, broth, consomme, stock Gravies Certain vegetables: asparagus, cauliflower, peas, spinach, mushrooms, lima and kidney beans, lentils

Table 57.5 Foods high in oxalate and purine.

Physical examination

The physical examination may be helpful in uncovering systemic disorders that predispose patients to nephrolithiasis. While most patients with idiopathic hypercalciuria are healthy and have a normal physical examination, the presence of tophi in others may provide evidence for hyperuricosuria and uric acid stone formation. Similarly, a patient with paraplegia and a chronic indwelling bladder catheter may be predisposed to chronic urinary tract infections and struvite stone production.

Laboratory findings

The basic evaluation includes several urine and blood tests that help to determine metabolic factors that may lead to stone formation. The urinalysis is particularly useful: the urine pH is generally high in patients with struvite and calcium phosphate stones but low in patients with uric acid and calcium oxalate stones. The specific gravity, if high, will confirm inadequate fluid intake in many patients. Hematuria may imply active stone disease with crystal or stone passage. Examination of the urine may reveal red blood cells along with characteristic crystals (Fig. 57.3). The presence of bacteria in urine with a pH greater than 6–6.5 may be indicative of struvite stone disease. In this case, a urine culture should be obtained. Since many bacteria can produce urease even when urine bacterial colony counts are low, the microbiology laboratory should be instructed to type the organism even if there are fewer than 100 000 colony-forming units/mL.

Medications associated with nephrolithiasis and nephrocalcinosis
Calcium stone formation:
Loop diuretics Vitamin D Glucocorticoids Antacids (calcium and noncalcium antacids) Theophylline Acetazolamide* Amphotericin B*
Uric acid stone formation:
Salicylates Probenecid Allopurinol (usually associated with xanthine stones)
Medications that may precipitate into stones:
Triamterene Acyclovir (if infused rapidly intravenously) Indinavir
* Associated with nephrocalcinosis

Table 57.4 Medications associated with nephrolithiasis and nephrocalcinosis.

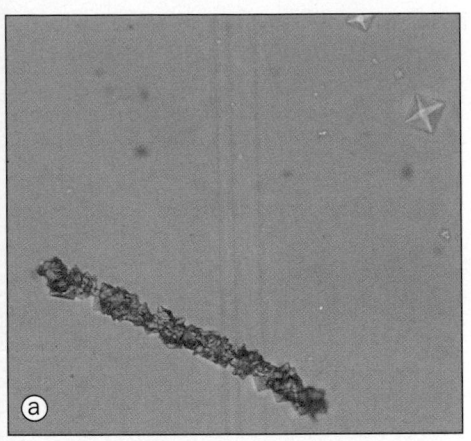
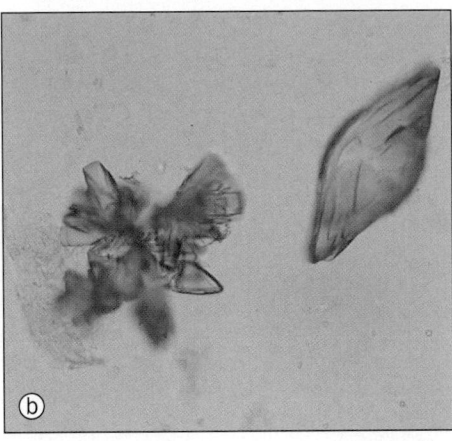
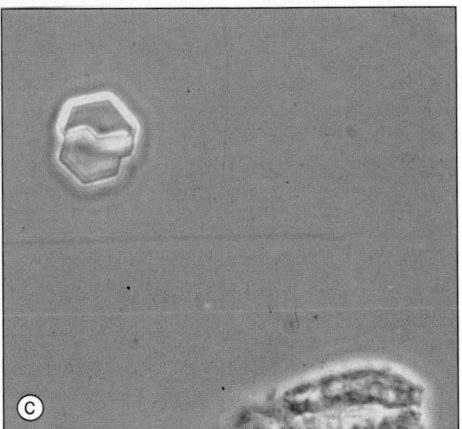
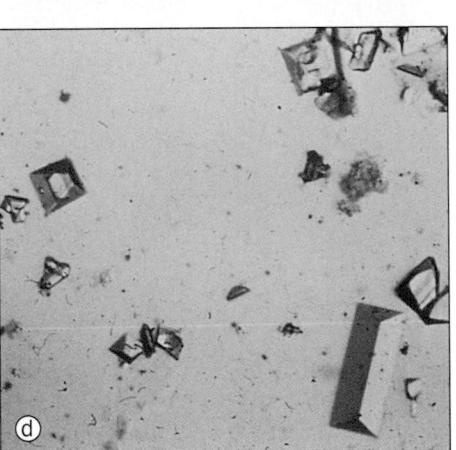

Figure 57.3 Urine crystals. (a) Oxalate crystals: a pseudocast of calcium oxalate crystals accompanied by crystals of calcium oxalate dihydrate. (b) Uric acid crystals: complex crystals suggestive of acute uric acid nephropathy or uric acid nephrolithiasis. (c) A typical hexagonal cystine crystal; a single crystal provides a definitive diagnosis of cystinuria. (d) Coffin lid crystals of magnesium ammonium phosphate (struvite). (Courtesy of Dr Patrick Fleet.)

Blood tests required in the basic evaluation are electrolytes (sodium, potassium, chloride and bicarbonate), creatinine, calcium, uric acid and phosphorus. If the serum calcium is elevated or at the upper limit of normal, especially if the serum phosphorus is low, a parathyroid hormone level should also be obtained. A low potassium or bicarbonate level may indicate a cause for hypocitraturia, such as occurs in distal renal tubular acidosis.

Stone analysis

Patients should be encouraged, whenever possible, to retrieve any stone they pass for chemical analysis. This stone analysis may be most helpful in defining an underlying metabolic abnormality and indicating a direction for treatment.

Radiologic evaluation

Patients with no contraindication to radiographic evaluation should have a plain film of the abdomen performed that includes views of the kidneys, ureters and bladder. This will reveal any opacifications in the areas of the kidneys and ureters that could be attributed to calcium, cystine, or struvite stones (Fig. 57.4). Uric acid and xanthine calculi are radiolucent, however, and will not be visible on plain films. An intravenous urogram (IVU) is also an excellent initial screening test, as all stones are readily visible (as filling defects); however, an IVU should be avoided in patients with renal insufficiency or other contraindications to the use of contrast.

The IVU may demonstrate urinary tract obstruction caused by calculi (Fig. 57.5). Another advantage of the IVU is that it can also demonstrate any abnormality in the genitourinary tract that may predispose the patient to stone formation, such as medullary sponge kidney (see Chapter 47) or calyceal anomalies (see Chapter 52). During acute episodes of colic, the IVU, by creating a strong osmotic diuresis, may assist in flushing out the stone.

The unenhanced helical computed tomography (CT) scan, also known as spiral CT, or CT-IVU, has increasingly become the diagnostic test of choice for the diagnosis of acute renal colic. This test has a high sensitivity and specificity for detecting ureteral stones and ureteral obstruction. An advantage of a CT-IVU over the standard IVU is that it can be performed without radiographic contrast or bowel preparation. It is also a more rapid test with results being available in minutes rather than hours, making it a more practical test in the emergency room setting, although an experienced radiologist, generally required for optimal interpretation of the images, may not be available at all times in urgent care facilities. Another disadvantage of the CT-IVU is the radiation dose, which is approximately three times that of a conventional IVU[10]. Renal ultrasound is also very useful in evaluating the presence of renal stones. All kidney stones (radiolucent and radio-opaque) should be visible on ultrasound, but ureteral stones may be missed. This is an excellent screening test in certain patients, such as pregnant women, who should avoid radiation exposure.

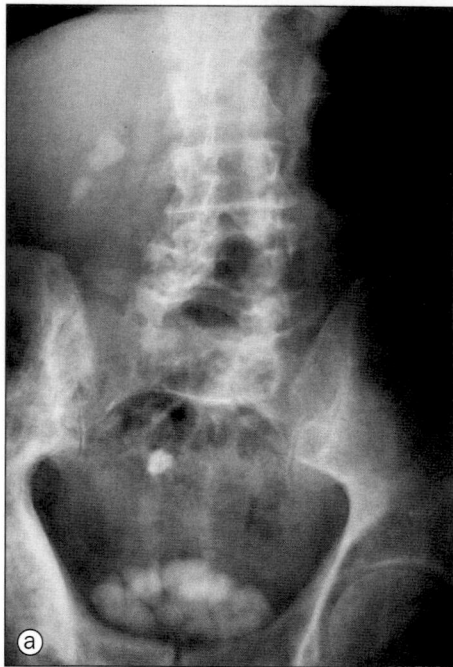
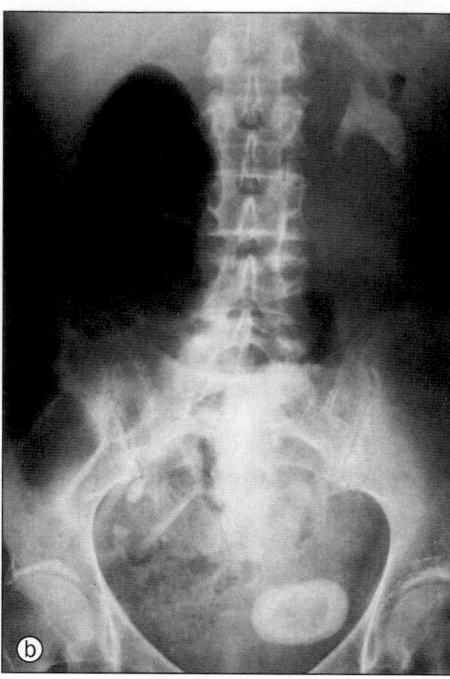

Figure 57.4 Radio-opaque renal calculi. X-ray examination showing multiple cystine stones in the right kidney, right ureter, and bladder. (b) Struvite stones: left staghorn calculus and a single bladder stone.

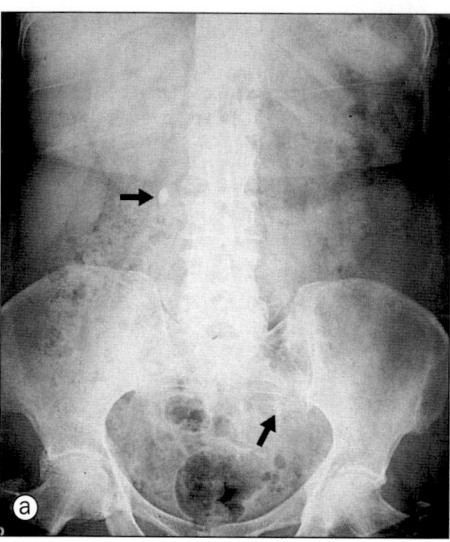
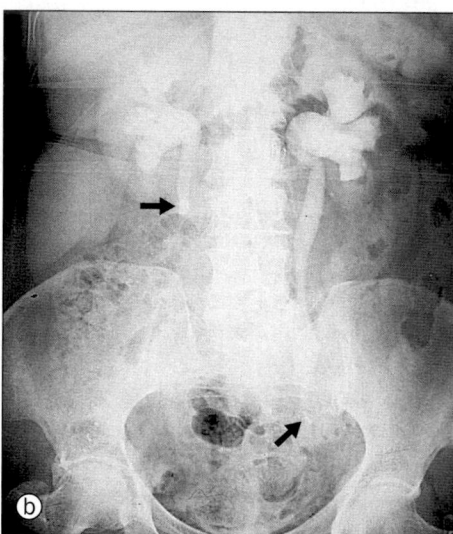

Figure 57.5 Obstructive uropathy resulting from nephrolithiasis in a patient with acute renal impairment. (a) X-ray examination showing a stone in the right upper ureter and a very small stone in the lower left ureter (arrows). (b) Intravenous urography at the same time showing bilateral hydronephrosis caused by ureteral obstruction.

The complete evaluation

A complete evaluation should be undertaken in patients with multiple or metabolically active stones (i.e., stones that grow in size or increase in number within a year). All children, non-Caucasians (demographic groups not typically prone to stone formation), and patients who form stones other than calcium-containing calculi should also undergo a complete evaluation. In addition to the basic evaluation, the complete evaluation includes a 24-h quantification of urinary supersaturation for calcium oxalate, brushite (calcium phosphate) and uric acid (Table 57.6). Urine for supersaturation analysis has been shown to correlate well with stone composition. Patients can bring their specimens to a local laboratory or may directly mail them to specialized laboratories that measure calcium, oxalate, citrate, uric acid, creatinine, sodium, potassium, magnesium, sulfate, phosphorus, chloride, urine

urea nitrogen and pH. The levels are entered into a software program that calculates supersaturation for calcium oxalate, calcium phosphate and uric acid. Desirable levels of supersaturation are noted in the results, as well as dietary and pharmacologic recommendations that may assist in achieving them[12].

In the absence of urine for supersaturation analysis, most laboratories assess urine volume and the quantity of calcium, oxalate, phosphorus, uric acid, sodium, citrate and creatinine excreted in a 24-h urine collection (Table 57.6). Urine creatinine is useful in assessing adequacy of the collection. In an adequate collection, men should excrete at least 15 µmg/kg (132 µmol/kg) creatinine daily, and women 10 µmg/kg (88 µmol/kg) daily. A disadvantage of the standard 24-h urine collection is that laboratories vary in the preservatives required to process the various constituents. Many require more than

Optimal 24-h urine values in recurrent nephrolithiasis	
24-h urine values	
Volume	> 2–2.5 L
Calcium	< 4 mg/kg (0.1 mmol/kg), ~300 mg (7.5 mmol) in men, ~250 mg (6.3 mmol) in women
Oxalate	<40 mg (0.36 mmol)
Uric acid	<750 mg (4.5 mmol) in women and < 800 mg (4.7 mmol) in men (can be pH-dependent)
Citrate	>320 mg (17 mmol)
Sodium	< 3000 mg (< 130 mmol)
Phosphorus	<1100 mg (35 mmol)
Creatinine> 10 mg/kg (88 μmol/kg) in women and > 15 mg/kg (132 μmol/kg) in men, if specimen is a complete collection	
Urine supersaturation values	
Calcium oxalate supersaturation	<5
Calcium phosphate supersaturation	0.5–2
Uric acid supersaturation	0–1

Table 57.6 Evaluation of nephrolithiasis: optimal 24-h urine values.

one collection to measure all the urinary constituents, limiting compliance with the collection and therefore, the accuracy of the results.

Patients should be encouraged to perform the collection on a typical day while eating a typical diet, though many patients prefer to collect the urine on weekends when their diet and habits may differ from usual workdays. Specialized testing, such as the use of high or low calcium diets, is not recommended[9]. When collecting the 24-h urine, the first morning urine should be discarded; then all urine should be collected for the next 24 h, including the next morning's urine. This procedure must be explicitly reviewed with the patient or an over- or under-collection may result.

General treatment

Intervention for stone removal may be required when pain, obstruction and infection due to nephrolithiasis do not respond to conservative management. These aspects of stone management are discussed in Chapter 59. The risk for developing renal insufficiency varies with different types of stone, and this must also be taken into account in planning the management of nephrolithiasis[13]. Here, we discuss medical management strategies to minimize stone recurrence.

Patients who are seen by stone 'specialists' often have a decrease in stone recurrence even without pharmacologic intervention[14]. This phenomenon, termed the 'stone clinic effect', has been ascribed to modifications in diet and fluid intake. These nonpharmacologic measures include an increase in fluid intake, which will concomitantly increase urine volume, and restriction of sodium, which reduces urine calcium excretion, and animal protein. Though dietary calcium restriction continues to be prescribed by many physicians,

increasing evidence indicates that this is not beneficial and can actually increase the rate of stone formation (see section below on Calcium Stones)[6].

Fluid intake
An increase in urine volume to greater than 2–2.5 L daily is of proven efficacy in reducing the incidence of stone formation. Larger volumes are known to reduce calcium oxalate supersaturation, as well as precipitation of other crystals[14,15]. Increased fluid intake to augment urine volume has also been the mainstay of therapy for patients with uric acid and cystine stones. The period of maximum risk for stone formation is at night, when urine concentration is physiologically increased. Patients should be encouraged to drink enough fluid in the evening to provoke nocturia and then drink further fluid before returning to bed.

Salt intake
Sodium excretion by the renal tubules augments urine calcium excretion. Conversely, dietary salt restriction, which diminishes sodium excretion, is associated with a decrease in calcium excretion[16]. Patients should be instructed to limit daily sodium intake to 2 g (approximately 87 mmol sodium).

Dietary protein
Animal protein ingestion can increase the frequency of renal stone formation by a number of mechanisms. Metabolism of certain amino acids leads to generation of sulfate ions, which render urinary calcium ions less soluble. In addition, the metabolic acidosis that results from protein ingestion leads to calcium release from bone and a consequent increase in the filtered load of calcium. Acidosis also decreases renal tubule calcium reabsorption, which leads to hypercalciuria. Urinary citrate excretion is also pH dependent, with acidosis leading to a decrease in citrate excretion. The result of increased animal protein intake is an increase in urinary calcium ions that are rendered less soluble because of concomitant sulfate excretion and hypocitraturia. The low urine pH during acidosis, coupled with increased uric acid excretion from the metabolism of animal protein, can result in uric acid lithiasis. For these reasons stone formers should consume a moderate protein diet (0.8–1.0 g/kg daily)[1].

Dietary calcium
Despite conventional wisdom, recent studies have demonstrated a decrease in stone incidence when people consume high calcium diets. The beneficial effect of dietary calcium on reducing stone formation has been attributed to the binding of ingested oxalate by the additional calcium. Given the high lithogenic potential of oxalate, a decrease in absorbed and excreted oxalate would diminish calcium oxalate crystal formation. Women also appear to have reduced stone formation on a higher calcium diet, but may be prone to forming more stones when taking calcium supplements. It has been postulated that this increase may be due to timing the supplement calcium ingestion apart from meals, which would enhance calcium absorption without reducing oxalate absorption[17-19].

The benefit of a gender and age appropriate calcium diet in decreasing stone formation in addition to the risk of bone demineralization with calcium restriction have rendered the low calcium diet obsolete in treating patients with calcium nephrolithiasis[20, 21].

SPECIFIC FORMS OF STONE DISEASE

Calcium stones

Calcium-containing kidney stones are most common, comprising around 70% of all stones formed. Most calcium stones are composed of calcium oxalate, either alone or in combination with calcium phosphate or urate. A small percentage of stones are composed entirely of calcium phosphate[1]. Most calcium stones do not exceed 1–2 cm in width, although surgical intervention is often required when they grow to be greater than 5 mm.

Calcium stones may develop as a result of excessive excretion of calcium (hypercalciuria), oxalate (hyperoxaluria), and uric acid (hyperuricosuria), insufficient citrate excretion (hypocitraturia), renal tubular acidosis, certain medications, and congenital abnormalities of the genitourinary tract (Fig. 57.6). Specific therapy for patients with calcium stones depends on any underlying metabolic abnormality. Nonspecific therapy (see above) should always be instituted; however, more definitive treatment is often required.

Hypercalciuria
Etiology

The most common pattern of hypercalciuria is an isolated excessive excretion of urine calcium with no other demonstrable abnormality of calcium metabolism, known as idiopathic hypercalciuria. These patients generally exhibit excessive intestinal calcium absorption and may also have decreased renal tubular calcium reabsorption and decreased bone mineralization. The etiology of this systemic disorder in calcium transport has, at least in hypercalciuric stone forming rats, been linked to an excessive number of receptors for vitamin D[22]. Metabolic disorders leading to an elevation in serum calcium, parathyroid hormone or $1,25(OH)_2D_3$ may result in hypercalciuria.

Treatment

For hypercalciuria, the usual first-line therapy is a thiazide diuretic. Chlorthalidone 25–50 mg is the drug of choice, as it requires only once daily administration. Indapamide (1.25–2.5 mg daily) does not tend to raise serum lipids as much as other thiazides and is often preferred for patients with cardiac risk factors or elevated serum lipids. On commencing these medications, patients should be instructed to increase their dietary potassium intake, and a serum potassium level should be checked 7–10 days later. If the level is low, oral potassium supplementation should be initiated. Potassium citrate is preferred over potassium chloride as citrate complexes urinary calcium further lowering supersaturation. However, most patients find potassium citrate liquid preparations unpalatable. Urocit-K is a wax matrix tablet that is well tolerated and is available in 5- and 10-mmol preparations. Generally, patients are able to maintain a normal serum potassium level with Urocit-K 20–40 mmol daily in single or divided doses. The serum potassium and bicarbonate levels should be rechecked 7–10 days later for further dose adjustment. As citrate is a base, potassium citrate may excessively raise the serum bicarbonate level and a change to potassium

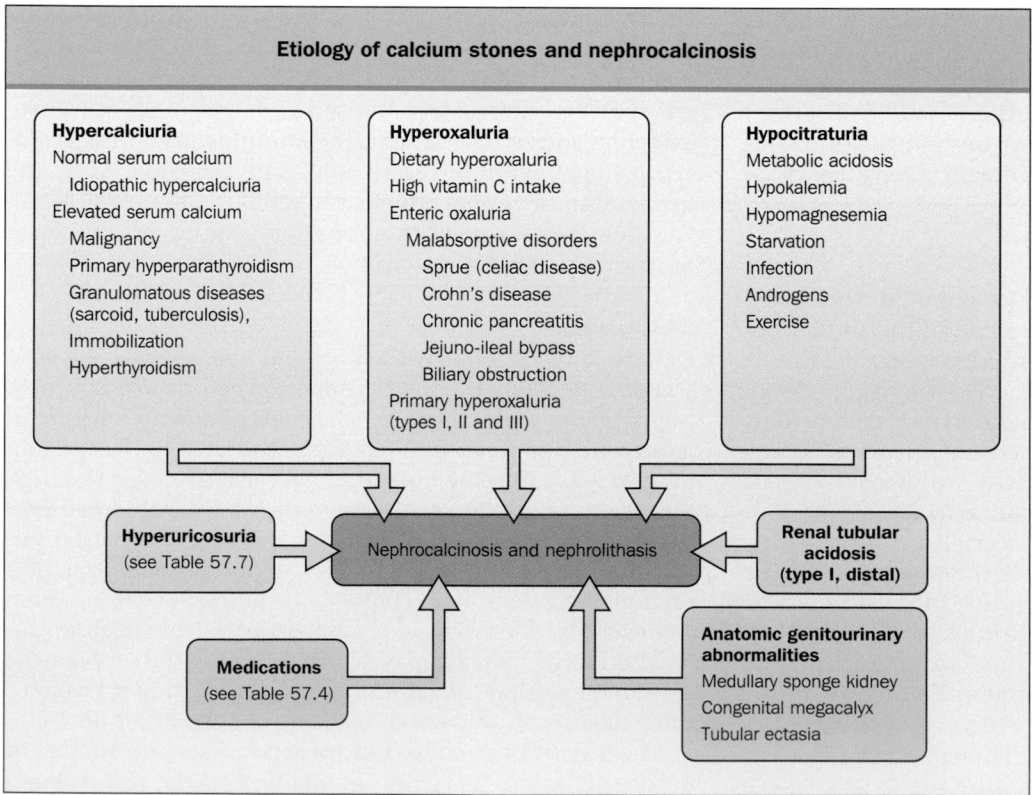

Figure 57.6 Etiology of calcium stones and nephrocalcinosis.

chloride may be required. The 24-h urine calcium, sodium and citrate should be rechecked after several weeks. If the calcium excretion remains elevated, the thiazide dose should be increased. If the sodium excretion also remains high, patients should be encouraged to limit their sodium intake further as they will not have adequate response to the diuretic on a high-sodium diet. If the potassium remains low despite supplementation or the calcium excretion remains high despite increased thiazide dosing, addition of a potassium-sparing diuretic may be advantageous. Triamterene can precipitate into stones; therefore, amiloride (starting dose 5 mg daily) should be used, or a combination tablet that includes both a thiazide and amiloride[1,5,23].

Dietary calcium

Previously there were attempts to divide hypercalciuric patients into distinct pathophysiological groups: those with excessive renal calcium excretion ('renal leak') and those who absorbed excessive amounts of calcium via the gastrointestinal tract ('absorptive hypercalciuria'). For the latter group, a low-calcium diet was suggested. However, studies have shown that hypercalciuric patients generally do not have a transport defect limited to a single site. In both hypercalciuric rats and in humans placed on a low-calcium diet, there is a continuous, wide spectrum of calcium excretion, with many subjects excreting more calcium than they consume. This negative calcium balance must be derived from demineralization of bone, the largest repository of calcium in the body[22,24].

Clinical support for the use of an ample calcium diet to prevent recurrent calcium oxalate stone formation in hypercalciuric men was recently provided by a randomized prospective study comparing the rate of stone formation in men assigned to a low calcium diet with those assigned to a normal calcium, low sodium and low animal protein diet[20]. The 60 men assigned to the low calcium diet were twice as likely to have recurrent stones at 5 years compared to those on the normal calcium, low sodium, low animal protein diet. Urinary calcium oxalate supersaturation also diminished more rapidly in those on the higher calcium diet and remained lower than that of men on the low calcium diet for most of the 5-year study. This reduction in supersaturation was due to a greater fall in urinary oxalate in the men eating the normal calcium, low sodium and low animal protein diet[20,21].

Hyperoxaluria

Etiology

Elevated urinary oxalate levels can result from excessive dietary intake (dietary oxaluria), gastrointestinal disorders that can lead to malabsorption (enteric oxaluria), or an inherited enzyme deficiency that results in excessive metabolism of oxalate (primary hyperoxaluria(PH)) (Fig. 57.6).

Dietary excess of oxalate generally does not raise urinary oxalate values to levels exceeding 60 mg/24 h (0.54 mmol/24 h). Enteric oxaluria may occur in a number of disorders in which malabsorption results in excessive colonic absorption of oxalate. These include sprue (celiac disease), Crohn's disease, chronic pancreatitis, and short bowel syndrome. Urinary oxalate values are generally greater than 60 and can exceed 100 mg/24 h (0.54 and 0.9 mmol/24 h). In PH, the tremendous oxalate production generated results in widespread calcium oxalate deposition throughout the body at an early age. This infiltration of calcium oxalate into organs can result in cardiomyopathy, bone marrow suppression, and renal failure. Urinary oxalate values may range from 80 to 300 mg/24 h (0.72–2.70 mmol/24 h). There are three types of PH[25]. In types I and II, the enzyme defect is in the liver glyoxalate pathway. In type I, the defective enzyme is alanine–glyoxalate aminotransferase; in type II, there is a failure of glyoxalate reduction to glycolate. In type III, there is absorptive hyperoxaluria without detectable small intestinal disease.

Treatment of dietary and enteric hyperoxaluria

Treatment of dietary oxaluria consists of dietary oxalate restriction. Patients should be given a list of foods that have a high oxalate content and told to either avoid them or eat them in moderation (Table 57.5). In addition, calcium carbonate (500–650 mg/tablet, two to three tablets with each meal) may be added at meals and snacks to bind any intestinal oxalate and prevent absorption.

Specific therapy of the malabsorptive disorder, such as a gluten-free diet for patients with sprue, is the first line of treatment for enteric oxaluria. In certain diseases, such as short bowel syndrome resulting from surgical bowel removal, specific therapy may not be feasible. More generalized therapy of steatorrhea, such as a low-fat diet, cholestyramine, and administration of medium-chain triglycerides, may reduce fat malabsorption as well as oxalate absorption and subsequent excretion. The low-oxalate diet and mealtime calcium carbonate prescribed for patients with dietary oxaluria is also helpful for these patients. The diarrhea associated with these disorders may result in low urine volumes, hypokalemia, hypocitraturia and hypomagnesuria. Patients should therefore be advised to increase their fluid intake and to take potassium citrate (in this case, the liquid, although unpalatable, is better absorbed than the wax matrix Urocit-K tablets) as well as a magnesium supplement. Magnesium also serves as a urinary stone inhibitor and can be given as magnesium gluconate 0.5–1 g every 8 h or magnesium oxide 400 mg every 12 h.

Treatment of primary hyperoxaluria

PH is a severe disorder that currently can only be cured with liver transplantation to replace the defective hepatic enzyme. Pyridoxine (vitamin B_6) may reduce oxalate production in patients with type I. Efforts should be made to render the calcium and oxalate more soluble in the urine by raising the urinary pH (to at least 6.5) and giving supplemental citrate and magnesium. Potassium citrate and magnesium supplementation can be prescribed as above. Orthophosphate is also an effective inhibitor of urinary calcium oxalate precipitation and can be safely administered in patients with a creatinine clearance greater than 50 mL/min. As oxalate is poorly excreted in the setting of renal insufficiency and is not removed well by dialysis, renal transplantation serves not only to improve renal function, but also to improve oxalate excretion and diminish systemic oxalosis[26,27].

Hypocitraturia

Citrate inhibits stone formation. A number of conditions can inhibit urinary citrate excretion, predisposing patients to stone formation. Excessive protein intake, hypokalemia, metabolic acidosis, exercise, hypomagnesemia, infections, androgens, starvation and acetazolamide have all been implicated in decreased urinary citrate excretion. Therapy of hypocitraturia involves treatment of the underlying condition and commencing potassium citrate supplementation. The potassium salt is preferred over sodium citrate as sodium promotes renal calcium excretion. Again, tablets such as Urocit-K at 15–25 mmol, two or three times daily, are considered by most patients to be more palatable than the liquid. In patients with renal insufficiency, potassium levels should be monitored carefully, as the dosage may need to be decreased in the setting of hyperkalemia[1,5,28].

Distal renal tubular acidosis

Patients with distal (type I) renal tubular acidosis have impaired distal tubular excretion of hydrogen ions. This results in a non-anion gap metabolic acidosis and an alkaline urine. The acidosis causes calcium and phosphate to be released from bone with an ensuing increase in renal excretion of these ions. The acidosis also leads to an increase in citrate reabsorption by the proximal tubule. The end result is a high urinary pH, hypocitraturia (with urinary citrate levels generally <100 mg/24 h (0.53 mmol/24 h)), and increased renal excretion of calcium and phosphate, all of which increase the propensity for calcium phosphate precipitation. Nephrocalcinosis in this setting is not uncommon. The metabolic acidosis and hypocitraturia should be treated with a combination of sodium citrate (or bicarbonate) and potassium citrate (or bicarbonate). Often large amounts of base, 1–2 mmol/kg daily in two to three divided doses, are required to correct the acidosis[1]. Distal renal tubular acidosis is discussed further in Chapter 11.

Hyperuricosuria

Calcium oxalate crystals often nucleate around other crystal types such as uric acid. Hyperuricosuria contributes to calcium oxalate nephrolithiasis in approximately 10–15% of calcium stones. Patients with hyperuricosuric calcium oxalate nephrolithiasis have hyperuricosuria in the setting of normal urinary calcium and oxalate levels. In contrast to patients with pure uric acid stones, however, they tend to have a higher urinary pH (> 5.5). Therapy of hyperuricosuria consists of increased fluid intake and changing to a low-purine diet. If uric acid excretion remains elevated, allopurinol may be initiated at 100–300 mg daily[29,30].

Uric acid stones
Epidemiology

The prevalence of uric acid stones depends greatly on geographic location. In the USA, uric acid stones comprise 5–10% of all stones formed, whereas in Germany and Mediterranean countries such as Israel, the percentage of uric acid stones is much greater. The stones are radiolucent and, therefore, poorly visible on plain films. They are detectable on ultrasound and computed tomography, and as filling defects on pyelography (Fig. 57.7).

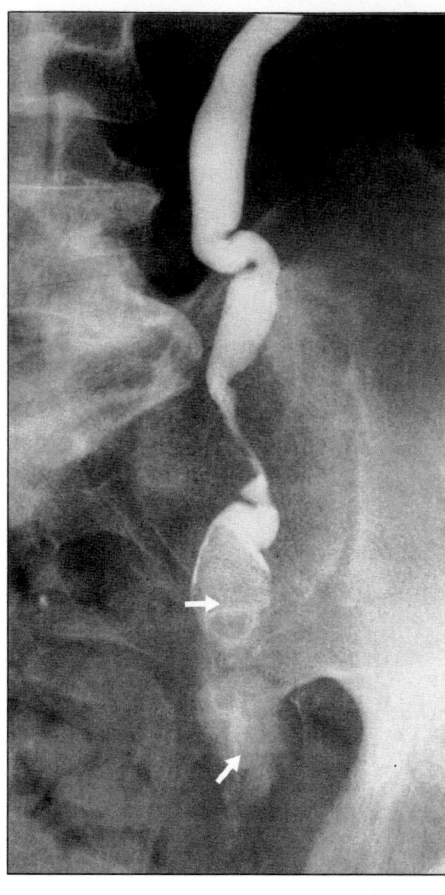

Figure 57.7 Radiolucent urate calculi. Antegrade pyelogram showing multiple radiolucent urate stones (arrows) obstructing the lower ureter.

Etiology and pathogenesis

Causes of hyperuricosuria include excessive dietary purine or protein intake, disorders associated with cellular breakdown (tumor lysis syndrome, myeloproliferative disorders, hemolytic anemia), gout, uricosuric medications, and certain inborn errors of metabolism.

Three major factors influence uric acid stone formation: a low urine pH, low urine volume, and elevated urinary uric acid levels (Table 57.8). Uric acid is poorly soluble at pH < 5.5. Solubility increases with increasing urine alkalinity such that urine at a pH of 6.5 can contain over six times the quantity of uric acid present at a pH of 5.3, without exceeding supersaturation. Metabolic acidosis associated with chronic diarrheal disorders and diets high in animal protein predisposes to formation of an acidic urine. Insufficient fluid intake and excessive extrarenal fluid losses such as from sweating and diarrhea contribute to formation of concentrated urine[31].

Treatment

Treatment of uric acid stones involves increasing urine volumes and pH as well as decreasing uric acid excretion. Increasing fluid intake to at least 3 L daily is suggested in order to achieve a urine volume of greater than 2.5 L. Greater intake may be required with excessive insensible or gastrointestinal losses. Alkaline urine not only can prevent uric acid stone formation, but may also result in stone dissolution. In order to raise the urine pH, potassium salts such as potassium citrate are advocated. While sodium salts such as sodium bicarbonate alkalinize the urine and enhance uric acid solubility, the added sodium increases sodium urate formation, which serves

Uric acid stones
Low urine pH (≤ 5.5)
High animal protein diet
Diarrhea
Low urine volume
Inadequate fluid intake
Excessive extrarenal fluid losses
Diarrhea
Insensible losses (perspiration, etc.)
Hyperuricosuria
Excessive dietary purine intake
Hyperuricemia
Gout
Intracellular to extracellular uric acid shift
Myeloproliferative disorders
Tumor lysis syndrome
Inborn errors of metabolism
Lesch–Nyhan syndrome
Glucose-6-phosphatase deficiency
Medications (see Table 57.4)

Table 57.7 Uric acid stones.

as a nidus for calcium oxalate precipitation at a higher pH. Potassium citrate (preparations discussed above) at a starting dose of 40–50 mmol/day in divided doses is recommended, increasing the dose as necessary to achieve a urine pH of approximately 6.5–7. Patients should be prescribed pH-sensitive dipsticks so that they can monitor their urine pH at various times of the day and adjust their dosing accordingly. If urine pH remains low despite high doses of potassium citrate (e.g., >100 mmol daily) or if the dose results in hyperkalemia, acetazolamide may be initiated. This carbonic anhydrase inhibitor produces an alkaline urine similar to that seen in renal tubular acidosis. Patients should be cautioned not to exceed a urine pH of approximately 7 because this may result in calcium phosphate precipitation.

A low-purine and low-animal-protein diet is also useful in both raising urinary pH and decreasing uric acid excretion. Purine-rich foods include organ meats (liver, kidney, sweetbreads, etc.), shellfish, meats, certain fish (salmon, tuna, mackerel, herring) and gravies. Most vegetables are low in purine, except asparagus, cauliflower, beans, lentils, peas, spinach, and mushrooms (Table 57.5)[32]. In situations in which uric acid excretion remains high despite dietary intervention, as in patients with disorders of cellular catabolism, allopurinol should be prescribed. Low doses should be used initially (100 mg), increasing to 300 mg as needed to keep urinary uric acid excretion below 750 mg/24 h (4.5 mmol/24 h).

Struvite stones

Struvite stones are also referred to as 'infection stones' or 'triple phosphate stones'. The stones grow rapidly to a large size, can reduce renal function in the affected kidney, and are difficult to eradicate. Because of the significant morbidity in patients with struvite stones, they have also been termed 'stone cancer'[33]. Most staghorn calculi, large stones that penetrate more than one renal calyx, are composed of struvite. Their formation requires the presence of urease-producing bacteria in the urine (Table 57.8).

Factors associated with struvite stone formation
Urease-producing bacteria
Proteus
Haemophilus
Yersinia species
Staphylococcus epidermidis
Pseudomonas
Klebsiella
Serratia
Citrobacter
Ureaplasma
[*Escherischia coli* is **not** a urease producer]
Elevated urinary pH

Table 57.8 Factors associated with struvite stone formation.

Etiology and pathogenesis

Struvite stones form when urease production by urinary bacteria results in the formation of ammonium ions as well as alkaline urine. In this setting, phosphate is present in its trivalent form and combines with three cations, ammonium, magnesium, and calcium, the latter as a component of carbonate apatite. Women are more prone to struvite nephrolithiasis than men because of an increased propensity to urinary tract infections. Other groups predisposed to developing struvite stones through infections or urinary stasis are patients with indwelling urinary catheters, neurogenic bladders, genitourinary tract anomalies and spinal cord lesions. The presence of an alkaline urine (pH 7), urease-producing bacteria in the urine, and large stones should alert one to the diagnosis of struvite nephrolithiasis[33].

A number of Gram-negative and Gram-positive bacteria have been implicated in urease production and consequent struvite formation, with the most common being *Proteus* sp. (Table 57.8). *Escherichia coli*, which is frequently present in urine cultures, is not a urease producer. Bacterial urease production occurs even with low colony counts; as a result, bacterial identification should specifically be requested from the microbiology laboratory even when the colony count is less than 100 000 colony-forming units/mL. If there is a strong suspicion for struvite stones but no organism is detected in the urine, a repeat culture for *Ureaplasma urealyticum* should be considered. As this urease-producing mycoplasma species does not grow on ordinary culture medium, a specific request to culture it may be required.

Treatment

Struvite stones require aggressive medical and surgical management. Therapy with an appropriate, culture-specific antibiotic is important to reduce further stone growth and for stone prevention. Bacteria will remain in the stone interstices, however, and stones will continue to grow unless chronic antibiotic suppression is maintained or the calculi are completely eradicated. Given the need for complete stone removal in order to effect a cure, early urological intervention is advised. Stones < 2 cm may respond well to extracorporeal shock-wave lithotripsy (ESWL); however, larger stones will likely require percutaneous nephrolithotomy (PCNL) or a combination of both ESWL and PCNL (see Chapter 59). Any stone fragments retrieved should be cultured and culture-specific antibiotics continued. Once the urine is sterile, usually around 2 weeks after initiation of therapy, the dose is halved. Monthly urine cultures should be obtained and if they remain sterile for 3 consecutive months, antibiotics may be discontinued, although surveillance urine cultures should continue monthly for a full year[34].

Adjunct medical therapies have included urease inhibitors and chemolysis. The most commonly used urease inhibitor is acetohydroxamic acid. By inhibiting urease, these agents retard stone growth and prevent new stone formation. Unfortunately, they have numerous side effects that limit their use, although adverse effects resolve on discontinuation of the drug. In addition, they require adequate renal clearance in order to be effective and therefore are not useful in patients with renal insufficiency [creatinine > 2 mg/dL (180 μmol/l)][33]. Chemolysis refers to irrigation of the kidney via a nephrostomy tube or the ureter with a solution designed to dissolve the stones. The most common solution is 10% hemiacidrin, which contains carbonic acid, citric acid, D-gluconic acid, and magnesium at pH 3.9. Use of lavage chemolysis is controversial as it has been associated with a high mortality rate in the past. However, it is felt to be relatively safe with appropriate precautions to monitor for urinary tract infections, obstruction to flow, intrapelvic pressures and magnesium levels. While it is not felt to be a treatment of choice for large stones, it may be useful in certain cases where surgical techniques have been effective but have left residual stone fragments.

Cystine stones

Cystinuria is a rare hereditary disorder in which there is a tubular defect in dibasic amino acid transport, resulting in increased cystine, ornithine, lysine and arginine excretion. The stone disease is usually clinically manifest by the fourth decade of life. Because of the high sulfur content of the cystine molecule, the stones are apparent on plain radiographs (Fig. 57.4a) and will often present as staghorn calculi or multiple bilateral stones. Cystinuria, in which cystine accumulates only in the lumen of the renal tubules, is distinct from cystinosis, in which there is widespread intracellular cystine accumulation. Cystinosis and cystinuria are discussed further in Chapter 50. There are at least three distinct types of cystinuria that can be classified by intestinal transport studies.

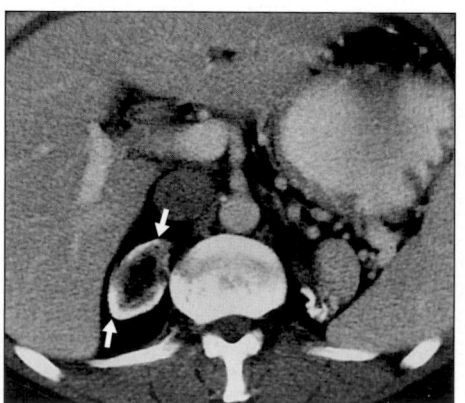

Figure 57.8 Cortical nephrocalcinosis. Non-contrast computed tomography (CT) showing cortical nephrocalcinosis (arrows) in the right kidney following cortical necrosis.

Cystine is poorly soluble with a solubility of only approximately 300 mg/L (1.25 mmol/L) at a neutral pH. Normal cystine excretion of approximately 30–50 mg (0.12–0.21 mmol) per day is readily soluble in the usual daily urine output of approximately 1 L. However, homozygote cystinurics often excrete 250–1000 mg (1.04–4.20 mmol) cystine per day, with heterozygotes excreting an intermediate amount. Treatment must be directed at decreasing the urinary cystine concentration below the limits of solubility. The dietary precursor of cystine, methionine, is an essential amino acid; therefore, it is impractical to reduce intake. Increasing urine volume so that cystine remains below the limits of solubility is often practical; however, sometimes 4 L of urine per day is necessary. Increasing urine pH above 7.5 will increase cystine excretion but this is often difficult to achieve on a chronic basis. D-Penicillamine (starting dose 250 mg daily, maximum dose 2 g daily) or tiopronin will both bind cystine and reduce urinary supersaturation; however, side effects may limit their use.

NEPHROCALCINOSIS

Introduction

Nephrocalcinosis refers to calcification within the renal parenchyma[11,35]. The disorder may be symmetric, or in anatomic disorders such as medullary sponge kidney, may involve only a single kidney.

Etiology and pathogenesis
Cortical nephrocalcinosis
Cortical nephrocalcinosis is usually the result of dystrophic calcification, which follows parenchymal tissue destruction rather than the precipitation of excessive urinary constituents. It is secondary to infarction, neoplasm and infection. It is typically asymmetric and is usually localized to the renal cortex (Fig. 57.8). Causes of cortical nephrocalcinosis include transplant rejection, cortical necrosis, tuberculosis, ethylene glycol toxicity, and chronic glomerulonephritis.

Medullary nephrocalcinosis
Medullary nephrocalcinosis is typically associated with elevated urinary levels of constituents that can precipitate, usually calcium, phosphate and oxalate, or occurs with alkaline urine (Table 57.9). Any disorder that can lead to hypercalcemia and/or hypercalciuria may be implicated. Instead of stone formation, smaller parenchymal calcifications deposit in the medulla, which are usually bilateral and relatively symmetrical (Fig. 57.9). Some metabolic disorders, particularly oxalosis due to primary hyperoxaluria, can result in both medullary and cortical nephrocalcinosis (Fig. 57.10)[35].

The common etiologies for nephrocalcinosis vary considerably with age. In adults, the most common causes of medullary nephrocalcinosis are primary hyperparathyroidism, renal tubular acidosis and medullary sponge kidney, as well as medications such as acetazolamide, amphotericin B and triamterene (Table 57.4).

While a similar range of disorders can be seen in children, the most common associations are with furosemide [frusemide] therapy and the hereditary disorders associated

Causes of nephrocalcinosis

Medullary

   Disturbed calcium metabolism
     Hyperparathyroidism
     Sarcoidosis
     Milk-alkali syndrome
     Rapidly progressive osteoporosis
     Idiopathic hypercalciuria

   Other tubular disease
     Distal (type I) renal tubular acidosis
     Oxalosis*
     Dent's disease
     X-linked hypophosphatemic rickets
     Bartter syndrome
     Hypomagnesemia–hypercalciuria syndrome

   Anatomic disease
     Medullary sponge kidney
     Papillary necrosis

   Medications
     Acetolazomide
     Amphotericin B
     Triamterene

Cortical
   Cortical necrosis
   Transplant rejection
   Chronic glomerulonephritis
   Trauma
   Tuberculosis
   Oxalosis*

* Oxalosis typically causes both cortical and medullary nephrocalcinosis

Table 57.9 Causes of nephrocalcinosis.

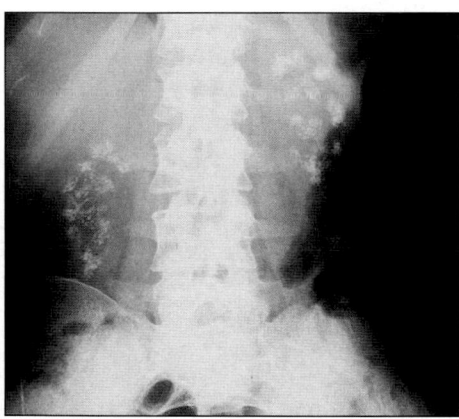

Figure 57.9 Medullary nephrocalcinosis. Plain radiograph showing bilateral metastatic medullary nephrocalcinosis in a patient with distal renal tubular acidosis.

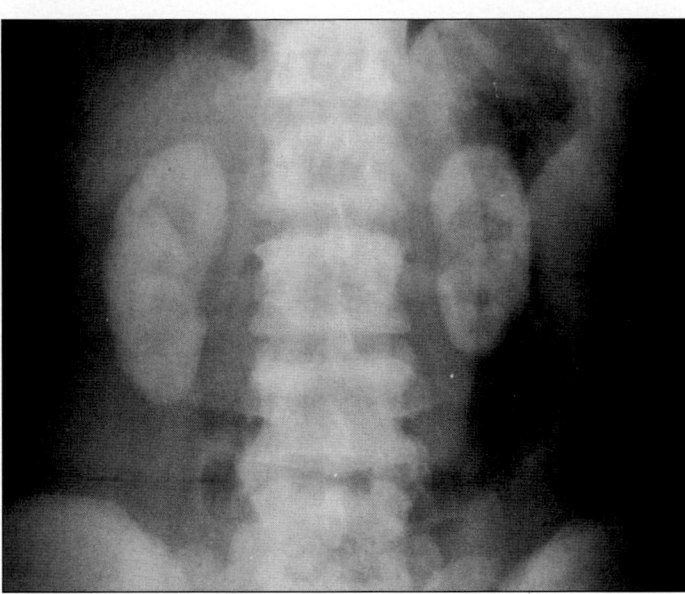

Figure 57.10 Nephrocalcinosis. Dense cortical and medullary calcification in the shrunken kidneys of a patient with oxalosis and long standing renal failure.

with hypercalciuria[36]. Furosemide, when used in premature neonates and older infants with congestive heart failure, can result in nephrocalcinosis with or without hypercalciuria. The lesions often resolve with discontinuation of therapy. A normal calcium : creatinine ratio at the time of diagnosis of nephrocalcinosis [approximately 0.40 (mg : mg) in premature infants] appears to be a good predictor of resolution.

Hereditary disorders associated with nephrocalcinosis include Dent's disease, X-linked hypophosphatemic rickets, and hypomagnesemia–hypercalciuria syndrome. Dent's disease is a rare form of hereditary hypophosphatemic rickets. Numerous mutations have been identified that lead to inactivation of CLC-5 voltage-gated chloride channels. The result is a clinical syndrome typically affecting young boys, and usually including hypercalciuria, nephrocalcinosis, nephrolithiasis, and hematuria, as well as low molecular weight proteinuria, glycosuria, aminoaciduria, hypophosphatemia, renal failure and rickets[37].

In X-linked hypophosphatemic rickets, the recommended treatment, with phosphate repletion and vitamin D, may itself result in hypercalcemia, hypercalciuria and nephrocalcinosis.

Another cause of medullary nephrocalcinosis in children is primary hypomagnesemia–hypercalciuria syndrome. In this rare autosomal recessive condition, children typically present with symptoms of urinary tract infection (most likely due to nephrolithiasis), polyuria, tetanic seizures (due to hypomagnesemia) and muscle cramps and weakness. Hypercalciuria and hypermagnesuria and a urinary concentrating defect also occur. Patients often have renal insufficiency and may require renal replacement therapy by the third decade of life. Sensorineural hearing disorders and ocular impairment may accompany the renal manifestations in a subset of patients[38].

Clinical manifestations
Patients who do not have nephrolithiasis associated with nephrocalcinosis are often asymptomatic. Ultrasonography and CT scanning are sensitive diagnostic tests for both cortical and medullary nephrocalcinosis, demonstrating the parenchymal calcifications before they can be visualized on plain radiographs. The extent of calcification correlates poorly with renal function. Patients with extensive calcification may have minimal renal impairment.

Treatment
Similarly to nephrolithiasis, treatment of nephrocalcinosis relies on therapy of the underlying disease, as well as measures to reduce hypercalcemia, hyperphosphatemia and oxalosis, if possible. The goal of treatment is usually to prevent further deposits, as therapy cannot eradicate existing calcium deposits[36].

REFERENCES

1. Monk RD. Clinical approach to adults with nephrolithiasis. Semin Nephrol. 1996;16:375–88.
2. Soucie JM, Thun MJ, Coates RJ, et al. Demographic and geographic variability of kidney stones in the United States. Kidney Int. 1994;46:893–9.
3. Mandel N. Mechanism of stone formation. Semin Nephrol. 1996;16:364–74.
4. Rodman JS, Sosa RE, Lopez MA. Diagnosis and treatment of uric acid calculi. In: Coe FL, Favus MJ, Pak CYC, et al., eds. Kidney stones: medical and surgical management. Philadelphia, PA: Lippincott Raven; 1996:973–89.
5. Coe FL, Parks JH, Asplin JR. The pathogenesis and treatment of kidney stones. N Engl J Med. 1992;327:1141–52.
6. Bushinsky DA. Renal lithiasis. In: Kelley WN, ed. Kelley's textbook of internal medicine. Philadelphia, PA: Lippincott, Williams and Wilkins; 2000:1243–8.
7. Weisberg LS, Bloom PB, Simmons RL, Viner ED. Loin pain hematuria syndrome. Am J Nephrol. 1993;229–37.
8. Sheil AGR, Chui AKK, Verran DJ, et al. Evaluation of the loin/pain hematuria syndrome treated by renal autotransplantation or radical neural neurectomy. Am J Kidney Dis. 1998;32:215–20.
9. Consensus Conference. Prevention and treatment of kidney stones. JAMA. 1988;260:977–81.
10. Greenwell TJ, Woodhams S, Denton ER, et al. One year's clinical experience with unenhanced spiral computed tomography for the assessment of acute loin pain suggestive of renal colic. BJU Int. 2000;85:632–6.
11. Wrong OM. Nephrocalcinosis. In: Davison A, Cameron JS, Grunfeld JP, et al. Oxford textbook of clinical nephrology, 2nd edn. Oxford: Oxford University Press; 1998:1375–96.
12. Asplin J, Parks J, Lingeman J, et al. Supersaturation and stone composition in a network of dispersed treatment sites. J Urol. 1998; 159:1821–5.
13. Gambaro G, Favaro S, D'Angelo A. Risk for renal failure in nephrolithiasis. Am J Kidney Dis. 2001;37:233–43.
14. Hosking DH, Erickson SB, van den Berg CJ, et al. The stone clinic effect in patients with idiopathic calcium urolithiasis. J Urol. 1983;130:1115–18.
15. Pak CYC. Prevention of recurrent nephrolithiasis. In: Pak CYC, ed. Renal stone disease: pathogenesis, prevention, and treatment. Boston, MA: Martinus Nijhoff; 1987:165–99.
16. Muldowney FP, Freaney R, Moloney MF. Importance of dietary sodium in the hypercalciuria syndrome. Kidney Int. 1972;22:292–6.
17. Lemann J Jr, Pleuss JA, Worcester EM, et al. Urinary oxalate excretion increases with body size and decreases with increasing dietary calcium intake among healthy adults. Kidney Int. 1996; 49:200–8.
18. Curhan G, Willett WC, Rimm EB, Stampfer MJ. A prospective study of dietary calcium and other nutrients and the risk of symptomatic kidney stones. N Engl J Med. 1993;328:833–8.
19. Curhan GC, Willett WC, Speizer FE, et al. Comparison of dietary calcium with supplemental calcium and other nutrients as factors affecting the risk for kidney stones in women. Ann Intern Med. 1997;126:497–504.
20. Borghi L, Schianchi T, Meschi T, et al. Comparison of two diets for the prevention of recurrent stones in idiopathic hypercalciuria. N Engl J Med. 2002;346:77–84.
21. Bushinsky DA. Recurrent hypercalciuric nephrolithiasis – does diet help? N Engl J Med. 2002;346:124–5.
22. Monk RD, Bushinsky DA. Pathogenesis of idiopathic hypercalciuria. In: Coe FL, Favus MJ, Pak CYC, et al., eds. Kidney stones: medical and surgical management. Philadelphia, PA: Lippincott Raven; 1996:759–72.
23. Coe FL, Parks JH, Bushinsky DA, et al. Chlorthalidone promotes mineral retention in patients with idiopathic hypercalciuria. Kidney Int. 1988;33:1140–6.
24. Coe FL, Favus MJ, Crockett T, et al. Effects of low calcium diet on urine calcium excretion, parathyroid function and serum $1,25(OH)_2D_3$ levels in patients with idiopathic hypercalciuria and in normal subjects. Am J Med. 1982;72:25–32.
25. Leumann E, Hoppe B. The primary hyperoxalurias. J Am Soc Nephrol. 2001;12:1986–93.
26. Smith LH. Hyperoxaluric states. In: Coe FL, Favus MJ, eds. Disorders of bone and mineral metabolism. New York: Raven; 1992:707–27.
27. Worcester EM. Stones due to bowel disease. In: Coe FL, Favus MJ, Pak CYC, et al., eds. Kidney stones: medical and surgical management. Philadelphia, PA: Lippincott Raven; 1996:883–3.
28. Pak CYC, Fuller C. Idiopathic hypocitraturic calcium oxalate nephrolithiasis successfully treated with potassium citrate. Ann Intern Med. 1986;104:33–7.
29. Millman S, Strauss AL, Parks JH, Coe FL. Pathogenesis and clinical course of fixed calcium oxalate and uric acid nephrolithiasis. Kidney Int. 1982;22:366–70.
30. Ettinger B, Tang A, Citron JT, et al. Randomized trial of allopurinol in the prevention of calcium oxalate calculi. N Engl J Med. 1986;315:1386–9.
31. Asplin JR. Uric acid stones. Semin Nephrol. 1996;16:412–24.
32. Wainer L, Resnick VA, Resnick MI. Nutritional aspects of stone disease. In: Pak CYC, ed. Renal stone disease: pathogenesis, prevention, and treatment. Boston, MA: Martinus Nijhoff; 1987:85–120.
33. Rodman JS. Struvite stones. In: Pak CYC, ed. Renal stone disease: pathogenesis, prevention, and treatment. Boston, MA: Martinus Nijhoff; 1987:225–51.
34. Wong HY, Riedl CR, Griffith DP. Medical management and prevention of struvite stones. In: Coe FL, Favus MJ, Pak CYC, et al., eds. Kidney stones: medical and surgical management. Philadelphia, PA: Lippincott Raven; 1996:941–50.
35. Ramchandani P, Pollack HM. Radiologic evaluation of patients with urolithiasis. In: Coe FL, Favus MJ, Pak CYC, et al., eds. Kidney stones: medical and surgical management. Philadelphia, PA: Lippincott Raven; 1996:369–435.
36. Alon US. Nephrocalcinosis. Curr Opin Pediatr. 1997;9:160–5.
37. Scheinman SJ, Guay-Woodford LM, Thakker RV, Warnock DG. Mechanisms of disease: genetic disorders of renal electrolyte transport. N Engl J Med. 1999;340:1177–87.
38. Benigno V, Canonica CS, Bettinelli A, et al. Hypomagnesemia-hypercalciuria-nephrocalcinosis: a report of nine cases and a review. Nephrol Dialysis Transplant. 2000;15:605–10.

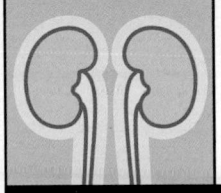

Chapter 58 — Urinary Tract Obstruction

Kevin P G Harris

INTRODUCTION AND DEFINITIONS

The complex functional and structural changes that result from obstruction of the urinary tract are relevant to the practice of both surgeons (urologists) and internists (nephrologists). Obstructive uropathy refers to the structural or functional changes in the urinary tract that impede the normal flow of urine, whereas obstructive nephropathy refers to the renal disease caused by impaired flow of urine or tubular fluid. Frequently the two coexist and their treatment requires close collaboration between nephrologists and urologists. The surgical aspects of obstruction to the urinary tract are discussed in Chapter 59. Hydronephrosis is used to describe dilatation of the urinary tract and is not necessarily synonymous with urinary tract obstruction.

Obstructive uropathy is classified according to the site, the degree, and the duration of the obstruction. Obstruction can occur anywhere in the urinary tract from the renal tubules (casts, crystals) to the urethral meatus. Causes of obstructive uropathy originating within the renal parenchyma are referred to as intrarenal and those that arise in the urinary tract as extrarenal. Extrarenal obstruction can, in turn, be divided into upper urinary tract obstruction (obstruction occurring above the vesicoureteral junction (VUJ)) and lower urinary tract obstruction (obstruction located below the VUJ). Upper tract obstruction is usually unilateral, whereas lower tract obstruction, by definition, is bilateral. Complete obstruction of the urinary tract is said to be high grade, whereas partial or incomplete obstruction is termed low grade. When the obstruction is of short duration, it is said to be acute; obstruction that develops slowly and is long-lasting is said to be chronic. Calculus, blood clot, or a sloughed papilla usually causes the former, whereas the latter occurs in congenital pelviureteral (PUJ) or VUJ abnormalities and retroperitoneal fibrosis.

As a result of obstructive uropathy, there may be marked alterations in both glomerular and tubular function (obstructive nephropathy). Unilateral obstruction in a patient with two normal kidneys will not result in significant renal impairment as the contralateral kidney is able to compensate. However, if the obstruction is bilateral (or unilateral in a single functioning kidney), renal failure will result. In acute urinary tract obstruction, changes are mainly functional, whereas with more chronic obstruction, structural damage to the kidney commonly results. The acute functional changes may recover following the effective release of the obstruction, but any structural changes will be permanent, leading to a chronic loss of functioning renal tissue and, thus, chronic impairment of renal function. Indeed, obstruction of the urinary tract remains a major cause of renal impairment worldwide.

ETIOLOGY AND PATHOGENESIS

The causes of obstructive uropathy affecting the upper and lower urinary tracts are summarized in Tables 58.1 & 58.2.

Congenital urinary tract obstruction

This occurs most frequently in males most commonly as a result of either posterior urethral valves or PUJ obstruction. PUJ obstruction usually results from deranged ureteral smooth muscle function and abnormal ureteric peristalsis.

Causes of upper urinary tract obstruction	
Intrinsic causes	**Extrinsic causes**
Intraluminal	Originating in the reproductive system
Intratubular deposition of crystals (uric acid, drugs)	Cervix: *carcinoma*
Stones	Uterus: *pregnancy, tumors,* prolapse, endometriosis, pelvic inflammatory disease
Papillary tissue	Ovary: abscess, tumor, cysts
Blood clots	Prostate: *carcinoma*
Intramural	Originating in the vascular system
Functional: *pelviureteric* or vesicoureteral junction dysfunction	Aneurysms: aorta, iliac vessels
Anatomic: tumors (benign or malignant), infections, granuloma, strictures	Aberrant arteries: pelviureteric junction
	Venous: ovarian veins, retrocaval ureter
	Originating in the gastrointestinal tract
	Crohn's disease
	Pancreatitis
	Appendicitis
	Tumors
	Originating in the retroperitoneal space
	Lymph nodes
	Fibrosis: idiopathic, drugs, or inflammatory
	Tumors: primary or metastatic
	Hematomas
	Radiation therapy

The most common causes are in bold italics.

Table 58.1 Causes of upper urinary tract obstruction.

Causes of lower urinary tract obstruction
Urethral anatomic causes
Urethral strictures: trauma, ***postinstrumentation***, infections such as gonococcal urethritis, nongonococcal urethritis, tuberculosis
Posterior urethral valves
Stones
Blood clots
Periurethral abscess
Phimosis
Paraphimosis
Meatal stenosis
Urethral functional causes
Anticholinergic drugs, levodopa
Prostate
Benign prostatic hypertrophy
Prostatic carcinoma
Prostatic calculi
Prostatic infection
Bladder anatomic causes
Bladder cancer
Schistosomiasis (*Schistosoma haematobium* infection)
Bladder calculi
Bladder trauma/pelvic fracture
Bladder functional causes
Neurogenic bladder spinal cord defects or trauma, diabetes, multiple sclerosis. Parkinson's disease, cerebrovascular accidents
The most common causes are in bold italics.

Table 58.2 Causes of lower urinary tract obstruction.

Histologically, the ureter at the point of narrowing has a preponderance of longitudinal smooth muscle fibers and a reduction in or absence of circular muscle fibers. Less commonly, PUJ obstruction is attributed to extrinsic compression by either blood vessels or fibrous bands.

If obstruction occurs early during development, the kidney fails to develop and becomes dysplastic. If the obstruction is bilateral (as with urethral valves and 30% of congenital PUJ diseases), severe renal failure results which carries a high mortality. If the obstruction occurs later in gestation and is low grade or unilateral, hydronephrosis and nephron loss will still occur, but renal function may be sufficient to allow survival. Such patients may not present until later in childhood, with an abdominal mass (either kidney- or bladder-located depending on the site of obstruction), abdominal pain, urinary tract sepsis, failure to thrive, and variable degree of renal failure. PUJ obstruction, if mild, may not present until adulthood and in some patients may be an incidental finding (Fig. 58.1). However, with increased use and improved sensitivity of antenatal scanning, congenital abnormalities of the urinary tract

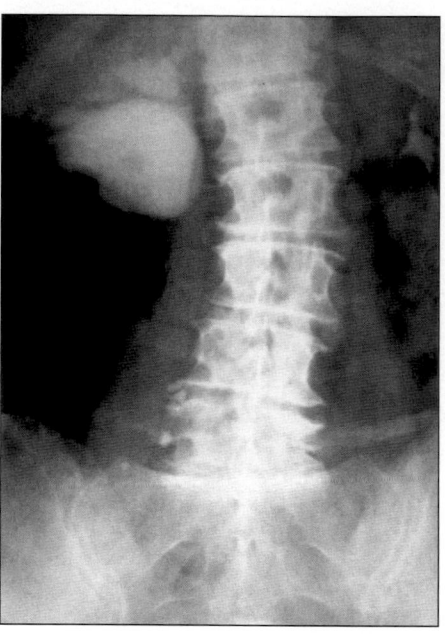

Figure 58.1
Intravenous urogram (IVU) demonstrating pelviureteric junction obstruction. The IVU was performed in a previously asymptomatic adult to investigate nonspecific right-sided loin pain. There is unilateral (right-sided) dilatation of the pelvicalyceal system with abrupt tapering to a normal sized ureter.

are now frequently identified early, allowing prompt postnatal (and in some cases antenatal) intervention to relieve the obstruction and hence preserve renal function.

Acquired urinary tract obstruction

Acquired urinary tract obstruction may affect either the upper or lower urinary tract and can result from either intrinsic or extrinsic causes. Intrinsic causes of obstruction may be intraluminal or intramural.

Intraluminal obstruction

Intraluminal obstruction may result from tubular intrarenal obstruction, of which a common cause is the deposition of uric acid crystals in the tubular lumen following treatment of hematologic malignancies (tumor lysis syndrome). It may also occur with the precipitation of Bence–Jones protein in myeloma and with the precipitation or crystal formation of a number of drugs including sulfonamides, acyclovir, methotrexate, and indinavir.

Extrarenal intraluminal obstruction in young adults is most commonly caused by renal calculi (see Chapter 57). Calcium oxalate stones are the most common. These cause intermittent acute unilateral urinary tract obstruction but marked renal impairment long term is unusual. Less common causes of urinary lithiasis such as 'struvite' stones, uric acid stones, and cystinuria are often bilateral and hence more likely to cause long term renal impairment. Renal calculi lodge more commonly in the calyx, the PUJ or VUJ junction, and at the level of the pelvic brim. Intraluminal obstruction can also result from a sloughed papilla following papillary necrosis, or blood clots following macroscopic hematuria (clot colic). Papillary necrosis occurs in diabetes mellitus, sickle cell trait or disease, analgesic nephropathy, renal amyloidosis, and acute pyelonephritis. Clot colic can occur with bleeding from renal tumors or arteriovenous malformations, following renal trauma, and in patients with polycystic kidney disease. Obstruction from blood clot has also been reported in patients with heavy glomerular bleeding, for example in IgA nephropathy.

Intramural obstruction

Intramural obstruction can result from either functional or anatomic changes. Functional disorders include vesicoureteral reflux (VUR), adynamic ureteral segments (usually at the junction of the ureter with the pelvis or bladder) and neurologic disorders. The latter cause the development of a contracted (spastic) bladder or a flaccid (atonic) bladder depending on whether the lesion affects upper or lower motor neurons and lead to impaired bladder emptying with VUR. Bladder dysfunction is very common in patients with multiple sclerosis and following trauma to the spinal cord. It is also seen in diabetes mellitus, Parkinson's disease, and following cerebrovascular accidents. Some drugs (anticholinergics, levodopa) can alter neuromuscular activity of the bladder and result in functional obstruction, especially if there is pre-existing bladder outflow obstruction (e.g., prostatic hypertrophy).

Anatomic causes of intramural obstruction of the upper urinary tract include transitional cell carcinomas of the renal pelvis and ureter and ureteral strictures secondary to radiotherapy or retroperitoneal surgery. Rarely, obstruction may result from ureteral valve malfunction, polyps, or strictures following therapy for tuberculosis. Intramural obstruction of the lower urinary tract can result from urethral strictures, which are usually secondary to chronic instrumentation or gonococcal infection, or malignant and benign tumors of the bladder. Infection with *Schistosoma haematobium* when the ova lodge in the distal ureter and bladder is a common cause of obstructive uropathy worldwide, with up to 50% of chronically infected patients developing ureteral strictures and fibrosis, with contraction of the bladder.

Extrinsic obstruction

The most common cause of extrinsic compression in women is pressure from a gravid uterus on the pelvic rim; the right ureter is more commonly affected than the left. It is usually asymptomatic and the changes resolve rapidly following delivery, although rarely, bilateral obstruction and acute renal failure (ARF) may occur. Ureteral dilatation may frequently be seen in pregnancy as a result of hormonal effects (especially progesterone) on smooth muscle, but this does not indicate functional obstruction. Carcinoma of the cervix may also cause extrinsic obstruction, as direct extension of the tumor to involve the urinary tract occurs in up to 30% of patients. Other pelvic pathologies that can cause compression of the ureter include benign and malignant uterine and ovarian masses, abscesses, endometriosis, and pelvic inflammatory disease. Compression of the ureters outside the bladder may also occur with uterine prolapse. Although rare (< 0.5%), inadvertent ligation of the ureter may occur during surgical procedures, particularly those related to obstetrics and gynecology. If unilateral, this may go undetected; if ligation is bilateral, ARF will result.

In males, the commonest cause of extrinsic obstruction of the lower urinary tract is benign prostatic hyperplasia. Carcinoma of the prostate can also result in obstruction either from direct extension of the tumor to the bladder outlet or ureters or from metastases to the ureter or lymph nodes.

Retroperitoneal pathology may also result in extrinsic obstruction of the ureters as can metastases or extension of

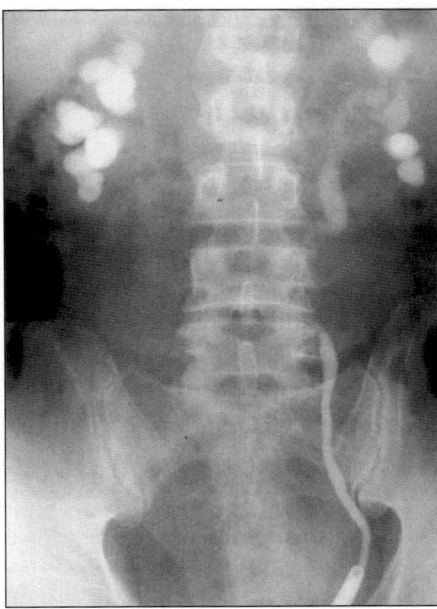

tumors from the cervix, prostate, bladder, colon, ovary, and uterus. Primary tumors of the retroperitoneum such as lymphomas and sarcomas can commonly cause obstruction. Obstruction can also result from inflammatory conditions affecting the retroperitoneum, such as Crohn's disease, inflammatory disease of the appendix, and large bowel diverticulitis. In Crohn's disease, the obstruction is usually right sided as a result of ileocecal disease. Less-common pathologies include retroperitoneal fibrosis, where thick fibrous tissue extends out from the aorta to encase the ureters and draw them medially (Fig. 58.2). Retroperitoneal fibrosis may be idiopathic but can result from inflammatory aortic aneurysms; the use of certain drugs, including β-blockers, bromocriptine, and methysergide; previous radiation, trauma, or surgery; and granulomatous disease (tuberculosis or sarcoidosis). Compression of the ureters may also occur as a result of vascular abnormalities, including aneurysmal dilatation of the aorta or iliac vessels, aberrant vessels, or anatomic variations in the location of the ureter (retrocaval ureter).

Pathophysiology

Our understanding of the consequences of urinary tract obstruction stem mainly from the study of animal models[1], with most studies focusing on the effects of short term (< 36 h) and complete ureteral obstruction in the adult rat. However, available experimental data show little species-to-species variation in the response to acute obstruction, suggesting similar changes are likely to occur in humans. The effects of long-term or partial urinary tract obstruction have been less well studied.

The effects of urinary tract obstruction on the kidney result from a variety of factors and complex interactions, with interdependent alterations in both glomerular hemodynamics and tubular function[2].

Changes in glomerular function

Glomerular filtration rate (GFR) declines progressively following the onset of complete ureteral obstruction (Fig. 58.3).

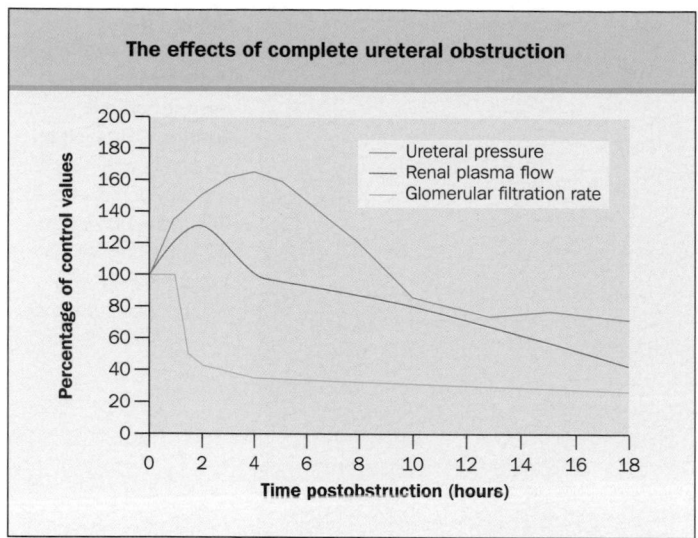

The effects of complete ureteral obstruction

Figure 58.3 The effects of complete ureteral obstruction. The relative changes in ureteral pressure, renal plasma flow, and glomerular filtration rate are shown using data from experimental studies of unilateral ureteral obstruction in rats.

Glomerular filtration is determined by the mean hydraulic pressure gradient between the glomerular capillary lumen and Bowman's space, the renal plasma flow, the ultrafiltration coefficient of the glomerular capillary wall, and the mean oncotic pressure difference across the glomerular wall. Obstruction can affect all of these, the effects varying with the duration of the obstruction, the hydration state and whether there is a contralateral functioning kidney.

Following complete ureteral obstruction, there is an initial rise in proximal tubular pressure. At the same time, afferent arteriolar dilatation occurs as a result of the generation of vasodilatory prostaglandins such as prostacyclin and prostaglandin E_2. Glomerular capillary hydraulic pressure increases but this does not offset the rise in tubular pressure and there is a net decrease in the hydraulic pressure gradient across glomerular capillaries, resulting in a decline in GFR to 80% of preobstruction values.

Approximately 2–5 h after obstruction, renal blood flow begins to decline, while intratubular pressure continues to increase. Within 5 h, proximal tubular pressure begins to decline towards control values. From this time, the main determinant of the decrease in GFR is the fall in intraglomerular capillary pressure as a result of an increase in resistance of afferent arterioles. This results in a progressive fall in renal plasma flow, which reaches 30–50% of control values by 24 h. Preferential constriction of the preglomerular blood vessels lowers both plasma flow and glomerular capillary pressure, thus resulting in a greater decrement in GFR than in plasma flow and a fall in filtration fraction. A falling filtration fraction also occurs as a result of diversion of blood to nonfiltering areas of the kidney and/or a reduction in the ultrafiltration coefficient. The relative changes in ureteral pressure, renal plasma flow, and GFR are summarized in Figure 58.3.

The intrarenal vasoconstriction results from the generation of angiotensin II and thromboxane A_2, the release of vasopressin (antidiuretic hormone) and a decrease in the production of nitric oxide. Angiotensin II and thromboxane A_2 may also reduce the ultrafiltration coefficient[2,3]. The central role of these two vasoconstrictors has been demonstrated by studies in rats in which pretreatment with angiotensin-converting enzyme (ACE) inhibitors and thromboxane synthase inhibitors virtually normalize renal function following the relief of short-term ureteral obstruction[4].

Intrarenal angiotensin II generation occurs secondary to an increase in renin release either through reduced delivery of sodium and chloride to the distal nephron (macula densa mechanism) or through a reduction in transmural pressure at the baroreceptor as a consequence of the prostaglandin-dependent dilatation of the afferent arteriole. Generation of thromboxane A_2 following ureteral obstruction occurs both in glomeruli and in interstitial infiltrating cells[5]. An interstitial infiltrate, predominantly macrophages, develops in response to chemoattractants such as monocyte chemoattractant protein 1 and osteopontin, which are presumably released in response to the increase in tubular pressure. This infiltrate has been shown to play a key role in the acute functional changes following ureteral obstruction[6].

The extent to which glomerular function recovers following the release of ureteral obstruction depends on the duration of the obstruction. Whole kidney GFR may return to normal after short term obstruction (days); however, recovery may be incomplete following prolonged obstruction. Evidence from studies in rats now suggests that even with shorter periods of obstruction (72 h) there may be a permanent loss of nephrons, and whole kidney GFR returns to normal only at the expense of hyperfiltration (increase in single nephron GFR) in the remaining functional nephrons[7].

Changes in tubular function

Abnormalities in tubular function are common in urinary tract obstruction and are manifested as altered renal handling of electrolytes as well as changes in the regulation of water excretion[2]. The degree and nature of the tubular defects following obstruction depend in part on whether the obstruction is bilateral or unilateral. These differences could result from the dissimilar hemodynamic responses, different intrinsic changes within the nephron, or differences in extrinsic factors (for example volume expansion and accumulation of natriuretic substances in bilateral obstruction) between the two states, or a combination of all three.

Following ureteral obstruction, the ability to concentrate the urine is markedly impaired, with maximum values of 350–400 mmol/kg reported in the rat. This is a consequence of multiple factors, including a loss of medullary tonicity and an overall decrease in GFR in deep nephrons. The collecting duct is also unresponsive to vasopressin, possibly as a result of decreased expression of aquaporins[8]. It is possible that the interstitial macrophage infiltrate contributes to both functional and structural tubular changes[9].

Patients with urinary tract obstruction often have urinary acidification defects. In many, this may only be detected by exogenous acid loading, but hyperchloremic acidosis caused by impaired distal acid secretion, hyporeninemic hypoaldosteronism (type IV renal tubular acidosis), or a combination of these findings have been described. This acidifying defect results from a marked increase in bicarbonate excretion and/or from a distal acidification defect, possibly as a result of abnormalities of the H^+ ATPase activity of intercalated cells of the collecting duct following ureteral obstruction.

Obstruction alters renal potassium handling. In the presence of a normal functioning contralateral kidney, potassium excretion is reduced following relief of obstruction, either in proportion to or perhaps even greater than the fall in GFR (i.e., fractional excretion of potassium is unaltered or slightly reduced). There is a defect in the distal potassium secretory mechanism following unilateral obstruction that may possibly be secondary to an unresponsiveness of that segment of the nephron to aldosterone. In contrast, following release of bilateral ureteral obstruction there is a marked increase in the net and fractional excretion of potassium. The major mechanism by which potassium losses occur in this setting is an increased delivery of sodium to the distal tubule, resulting in an accelerated sodium–potassium exchange.

Recovery of tubular function following release of obstruction is slow and it may remain abnormal even after whole kidney GFR has returned to normal. In rats, acidification and potassium-handling abnormalities persist for at least 14 d and urinary concentrating ability is abnormal for up to 60 d following the release of 24 h of unilateral ureteral obstruction. These observations are consistent with persistent alterations in distal tubular/collecting duct function and/or a loss in functioning juxtaglomerular nephrons following the release of the obstruction.

EPIDEMIOLOGY

Obstructive uropathy is a common entity and can occur at all ages. The prevalence of hydronephrosis at autopsy is 3.5–3.8%, with approximately equal distribution between males and females[10]. This is an underestimate of the true incidence since these figures exclude temporary obstruction (i.e., from renal calculi). The frequency and etiology of obstruction varies in both sexes with age. Antenatal ultrasonography more commonly identifies urinary tract anomalies as an incidental finding in the fetus, although the exact long-term significance of many of such observations remains to be determined. In children less than 10 years of age, obstruction is more common in males, with congenital anomalies of the urinary tract (urethral valves, PUJ obstruction) accounting for most cases. The overall prevalence of hydronephrosis found at autopsy in this age group is about 2%[11]. In North America, obstructive uropathy is the most common cause of end-stage renal disease (ESRD) in pediatric patients registered for renal transplantation[12]. In young adults (less than 20 years of age), the frequency of urinary tract obstruction is similar in males and females. Beyond 20 years of age, obstruction becomes more common in females, mainly as a result of pregnancy and gynecologic malignancies. The peak incidence of renal calculi occurs in the second and third decades of life, with three times more males than females being affected. After the age of 60, obstructive uropathy occurs more frequently in males than in females because of the increased incidence of benign prostatic hyperplasia and carcinoma of the prostate. Approximately 80% of men over 60 years of age have some symptoms of bladder outflow obstruction, and up to 10% have hydronephrosis. In Europe, acquired urinary tract obstruction accounts for 3–5% of the cases of ESRD in patients over the age of 65, most as a result of prostatic disease[13].

CLINICAL MANIFESTATIONS

Obstruction of the urinary tract can present with a wide range of clinical symptoms, depending on the site, degree, and duration of obstruction[2]. The clinical manifestations of upper and lower urinary tract obstruction differ. Symptoms can be caused by mechanical obstruction of the urinary tract (usually pain) or can result from the complex alterations in glomerular and tubular function that occur subsequent to obstruction (obstructive nephropathy). The latter commonly present as alterations in urine volume and as renal failure, which can be acute or chronic. For example, patients with complete obstruction may present with anuria and ARF whereas individuals with partial obstruction may present with polyuria and polydipsia as a result of acquired vasopressin resistance in the distal nephron. Alternatively, there may be a fluctuating urine output, alternating from oliguria to polyuria. Pain is a common presenting symptom of urinary tract obstruction resulting from distention of the bladder, the collecting system, or the renal capsule. Pain tends to be more common in acute than in chronic obstruction. However, it is important to note that obstructive uropathy and hence obstructive nephropathy can occur without symptoms and with minimal clinical manifestations. It may, therefore, present as unexpected acute or chronic renal failure. Thus obstruction of the urinary tract should always be considered in the differential diagnosis of any patient with renal impairment.

Pain

Pain is a frequent complaint in patients with obstructive uropathy, particularly in those with ureteral calculi. The pain is thought to be caused by stretching of the collecting system or the renal capsule. Its severity correlates with the degree of distention and not with the degree of dilatation of the urinary tract. Occasionally, the location of the pain helps to determine the site of obstruction. With upper ureteral or pelvic obstruction, flank pain and tenderness typically occur, whereas lower ureteral obstruction causes pain that radiates to the groin, the ipsilateral testicle, or the labia. Acute high-grade ureteral obstruction may be manifested by a steady and severe crescendo flank pain radiating to the labia, the testicles, or the groin ('classical' renal colic). The acute attack may last less than half an hour, or as long as a day. Pain radiating into the flank during micturition is said to be pathognomonic of VUR. By comparison, patients with chronic slowly progressive obstruction, such as those with retroperitoneal fibrosis, may have no pain or minimal pain during the course of their disease. In such patients any pain that does occur is rarely colicky in nature. In PUJ obstruction, pain may only be present following fluid loading to promote a high urine flow rate.

Lower urinary tract symptoms

Obstructive lesions of the bladder neck or bladder pathology may cause difficulties in micturition: decrease in the force and/or caliber of the urine stream, intermittency, postvoid dribbling, hesitancy, or nocturia. Urgency, frequency, and urinary incontinence can result from an inability to empty the bladder completely. Such symptoms commonly result from prostatic hypertrophy and are frequently referred to as 'prostatism', but they are not pathognomonic of this condition.

Urinary tract infections

Urinary stasis as a result of obstruction predisposes to the development of urinary tract infection. As a result, the patient may develop cystitis with dysuria and frequency or pyelonephritis with loin pain and systemic symptoms. Infection occurs more often in patients with lower urinary tract obstruction than in those with upper urinary tract obstruction.

Urinary tract infections are common in clinical practice even in the absence of urinary tract abnormalities. However, any urinary tract infection in men or young children of either sex, recurrent or persistent infections in women, infections with unusual organisms such as *Pseudomonas* spp., and a single attack of ascending infection (acute pyelonephritis) are absolute indications for further investigation. When obstruction is present, eradication of the infection is usually difficult. Infections of the urinary tract with a urease-producing organism such as *Proteus mirabilis*, predisposes to stone formation. These organisms generate ammonia, which results in urine alkalinization and favors the development of magnesium ammonium phosphate (struvite) stones. This calculus can expand to fill the entire renal pelvis, forming a staghorn calculus that can eventually lead to loss of the kidney if untreated. Thus, stone formation and papillary necrosis can also be a consequence of urinary tract obstruction as well as a cause of obstruction.

Hematuria

Trauma to the uroepithelium of the urinary tract from calculi may result in either macro- or microscopic hematuria. Any neoplastic lesion that obstructs the urinary tract and, in particular, uroepithelial malignancies may bleed, resulting in macroscopic hematuria. In addition, bleeding into the urinary tract, *per se*, may result in obstruction, giving rise to clot colic when in the ureter or clot retention if in the bladder.

Changes in urine output

Complete bilateral obstruction or unilateral obstruction in patients with a single functioning kidney (such as a renal transplant) will result in anuria. However, when the obstructive lesion is partial, urine output may be normal or increased (polyuria). A pattern of alternating oliguria and polyuria or the presence of anuria strongly suggest obstructive uropathy.

Abnormal physical findings

It is important to appreciate that physical examination can be normal. Some patients with upper urinary tract obstruction may have flank tenderness; long-standing obstructive uropathy may result in an enlarged kidney, resulting in an increased abdominal girth or a palpable flank mass. Hydronephrosis is a common cause of a palpable abdominal mass in children. Lower urinary tract obstruction will cause a distended, palpable, and occasionally painful bladder. A rectal examination and, in women, a pelvic examination should be performed since they may reveal a local malignancy or the presence of prostatic enlargement.

Acute or chronic hydronephrosis, either unilateral or bilateral, may cause hypertension as a result of impaired sodium excretion with expansion of extracellular fluid volume or from abnormal release of renin (renin-dependent hypertension). Occasionally, in patients with partial urinary tract obstruction, hypotension occurs as a result of polyuria and volume depletion.

Abnormal laboratory findings

Urinalysis may show hematuria, bacteriuria, pyuria, crystal deposition, and low-grade proteinuria, depending on the cause of obstruction. However, urinalysis may be completely negative despite advanced obstructive nephropathy.

In the acute phase of obstruction, urinary electrolytes are similar to those seen in a 'prerenal' state, with a low urinary sodium (< 20 mmol/L), a low fractional excretion of sodium (< 1%), and a high urinary osmolality (> 500 mmol/kg). However, with more prolonged obstruction, there is a decreased ability to concentrate the urine and an inability to reabsorb sodium and other solutes. These changes are particularly marked following the release of chronic obstruction and give rise to the syndrome commonly referred to as 'postobstructive diuresis'.

Polycythemia, which may subside after relief of the obstruction, has been described in obstructive uropathy. It probably results from increased erythropoietin production by the obstructed kidney.

Increases in serum urea and creatinine are the most significant laboratory abnormalities in patients with obstructive uropathy. Electrolyte abnormalities may also occur, including a hyperchloremic hyperkalemic metabolic acidosis as a result of impaired excretion of acid and potassium (type IV renal tubular acidosis), and hypernatremia as a result of acquired nephrogenic diabetes insipidus.

If obstruction develops in patients with underlying chronic renal disease, it may cause an acceleration in the rate of progression of the renal insufficiency. Occasionally, ESRD may be caused by chronic obstructive uropathy that had been asymptomatic.

Symptoms of obstruction in neonates or infants

Although it is possible to make the diagnosis of hydronephrosis and genitourinary abnormalities antenatally, obstructive uropathy may not be suspected until failure to thrive, voiding difficulties, fever, hematuria, or symptoms of renal failure appear. Oligohydramnios at the time of delivery should raise the suspicion of obstructive uropathy, as should the presence of congenital anomalies of the external genitalia. Non-urological anomalies such as ear deformities, a single umbilical artery, imperforate anus, or a rectourethral or rectovaginal fistula should prompt investigation for urinary tract obstruction. Any infant with neurologic abnormalities may have a neurogenic bladder with associated obstructive uropathy.

PATHOLOGY

The morphologic alterations in renal architecture are similar irrespective of the cause of the obstruction. Initially there is renal enlargement and edema with pelvicalyceal dilatation (Fig. 58.4). Microscopically the cortex may initially appear normal. Subsequently, there is tubular dilatation, predominantly of the collecting duct and distal tubular segments; cellular flattening and atrophy of the cells lining the proximal tubule can also occur. In most instances, glomerular structures are initially preserved, although Bowman's space may be dilated and contain Tamm–Horsfall protein; ultimately, some periglomerular fibrosis may develop. Long-standing hydronephrotic kidneys have a widely dilated renal pelvis with the renal papillae either flattened or hollowed out. Eventually, there is marked thinning of the cortex and medulla and the kidney becomes a thin rim of renal tissue surrounding a large saccular pelvis (Fig. 58.5). There is then marked atrophy of tubular structures and progressive sclerosis and fibrosis with obliteration of the nephrons.

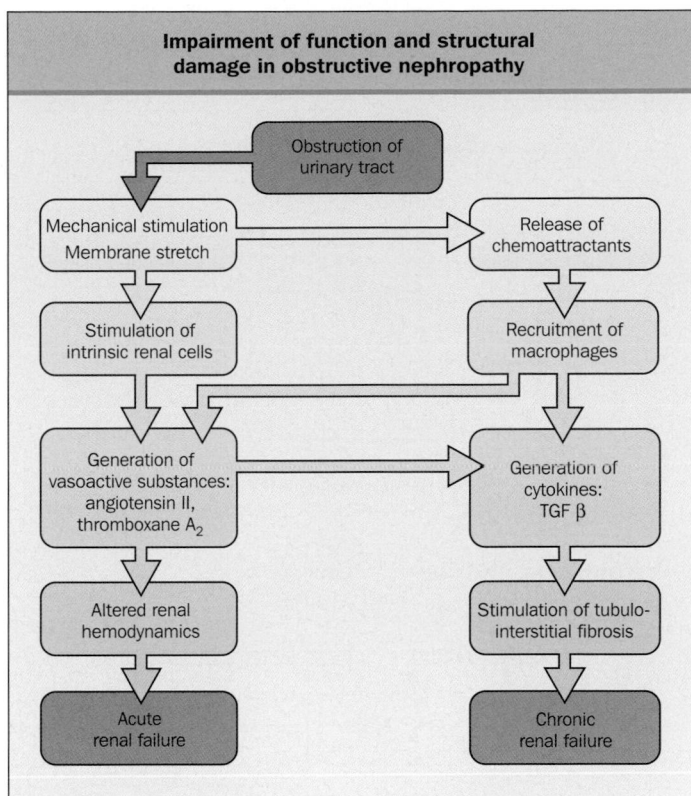

Figure 58.6 Events leading to acute impairment of renal function and chronic structural damage in obstructive nephropathy.

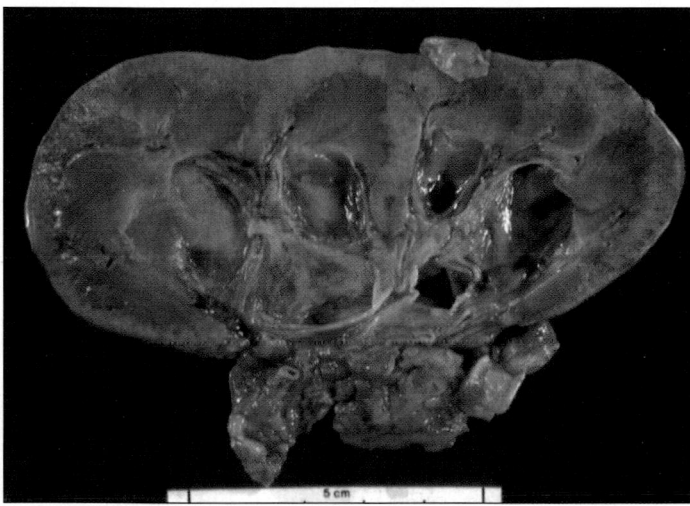

Figure 58.4 Autopsy specimen of a kidney showing the early effects of ureteral obstruction. The kidney is enlarged and edematous with pelvicalyceal dilatation. There is good preservation of the renal parenchyma.

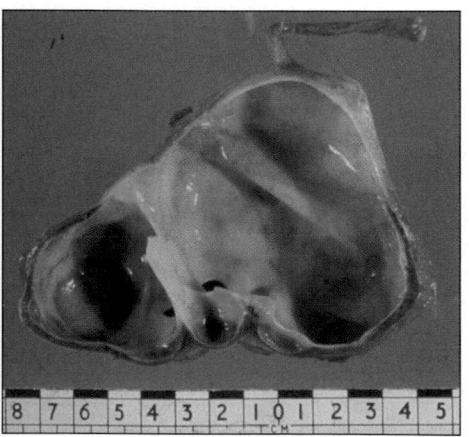

Figure 58.5 Chronic ureteral obstruction. Surgical specimen of a kidney showing gross dilatation of the pelvicalyceal system and the reduction of the renal cortex to a thin fibrotic rim of tissue. There would have been no prospect for any significant functional recovery in this kidney following the relief of the obstruction.

Ischemia as a result of the decreased renal blood flow is one of the major causes of parenchymal damage following obstruction. More recently, it has been recognized that infiltrating macrophages and T cells play a pivotal role not only in the acute functional changes that occur following obstruction but also in the chronic structural damage that results (Fig. 58.6). These biologically active cells release a number of profibrogenic cytokines, such as transforming growth factor β (TGFβ), that promote the progressive fibrosis which is characteristic of prolonged ureteral obstruction. Local angiotensin II generation may also stimulate the production of TGFβ by tubular cells, and angiotensin II receptor antagonists have been shown to decrease the degree of tubulointerstitial fibrosis in experimental obstructive uropathy[14].

Obstruction to venous drainage and the occurrence of bacterial infection (pyelonephritis) may also play a role in the development of parenchymal fibrosis.

DIAGNOSIS

The presentation of urinary tract obstruction is highly variable, from 'renal colic' to anuria with ARF and occasionally polyuria. The diagnostic approach has to be tailored accordingly (see Fig. 58.7) but a careful history and thorough physical examination are mandatory in all patients (see Clinical manifestations).

Urinalysis may provide valuable diagnostic information. Hematuria suggests that the obstructing lesion is a calculus, sloughed papilla, or tumor. Bacteriuria suggests urinary stasis,

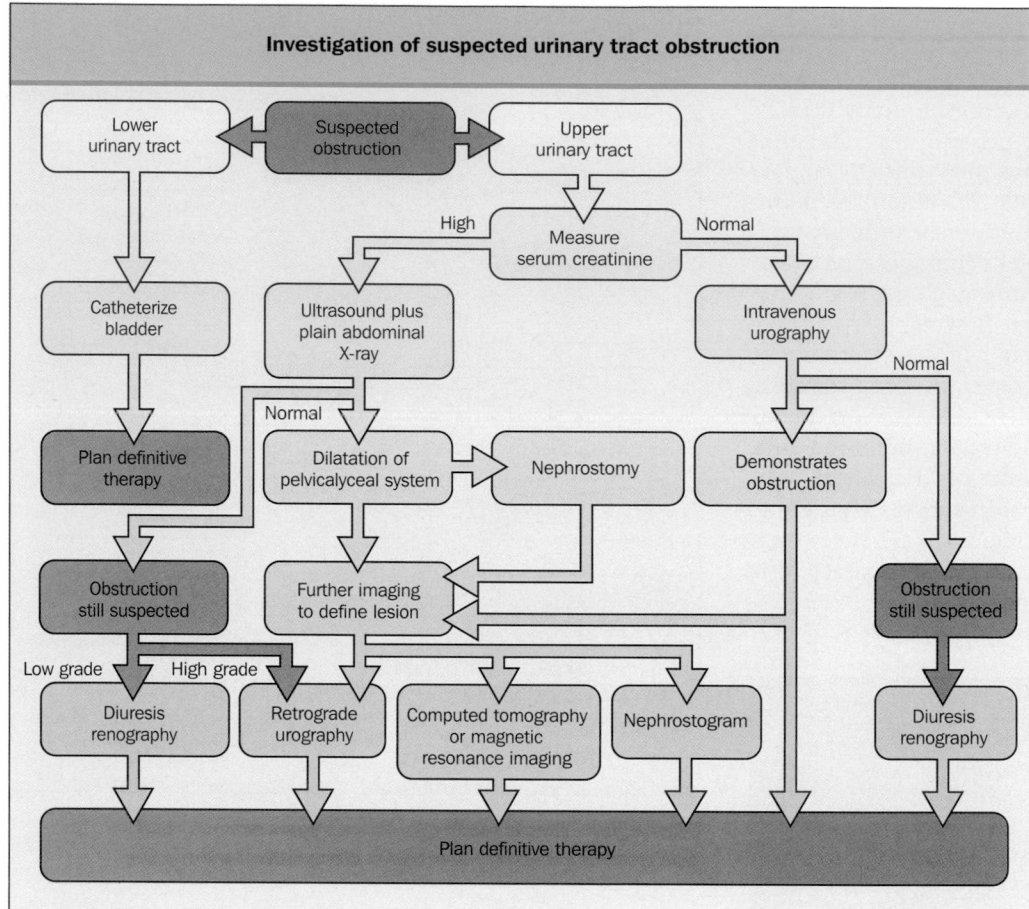

Figure 58.7 Investigation of suspected urinary tract obstruction. A full history and examination should be performed. Urine should be sent for microscopy and culture, and renal function and serum electrolytes should be measured. Increasingly, ultrasound scanning is being used as a first-line investigation for all suspected urinary tract obstruction. Insertion of a nephrostomy allows the effective relief of the obstruction and time to plan definitive therapy.

especially in males or in pregnant females; it may also be a complication of chronic obstruction caused by calculi or papillary necrosis. The presence of crystals in the urine sediment (cystine, or uric acid) may be the first indication as to the type of stone causing the ureteral obstruction or the intrarenal obstruction resulting in ARF. Laboratory studies should include an assessment of renal function (serum creatinine and urea) and the measurement of serum and urinary electrolytes.

Imaging investigations

Plain abdominal X-ray

A plain abdominal X-ray (or KUB: kidney–ureter–bladder) will allow an assessment of kidney size and contour and frequently will demonstrate renal calculi, about 90% of which are radio-opaque.

Intravenous urogram

Historically, the intravenous urogram (IVU) was the first-line investigation for suspected upper urinary tract obstruction. In patients with normal renal function it can usually define both the site and the cause of the obstruction. However, the excretion of contrast may be poor and/or delayed in patients with low GFR because of a decreased filtered load of the dye. In addition, contrast is potentially nephrotoxic. Alternative techniques, in particular ultrasound, have now become the first-line investigation to diagnose urinary tract obstruction, especially in patients with impaired renal function.

Ultrasonography

Ultrasonography can define renal size and demonstrate calyceal dilatation (see Fig. 58.8)[15]. Although sensitive for detection of dilatation of the urinary tract, it often will not detect the cause of the dilatation. Pathology within the ureter is difficult to demonstrate even in expert hands, and tiny stones will not produce an acoustic shadow. However, the presence of unilateral hydronephrosis suggests obstruction of the upper urinary tract by stones, blood clots, or tumors. When there is bilateral hydronephrosis, obstruction is more likely to be secondary to a pelvic problem obstructing both ureters or obstruction to the bladder outlet, in which case the bladder will also be enlarged. Ultrasonography should be combined with a KUB X-ray to be sure that ureteral stones or small renal stones are not overlooked.

By definition, ultrasonography produces false-negative results with nondilated obstructive uropathy (Table 58.3)[16]. Immediately following acute obstruction (< 24 h), the collecting system, which is relatively noncompliant, may not have dilated, and hence an ultrasound examination may be normal. Furthermore, if urine flow is low, as in severe dehydration or renal failure, there may be little dilatation of the urinary tract. It may also fail to dilate in slowly progressive obstruction, especially where the ureters are encased by fibrous tissue (as occurs in retroperitoneal fibrosis) or by tumor. A staghorn calculus can also hide dilatation of the upper urinary tract within its acoustic shadow. Some studies have suggested that the

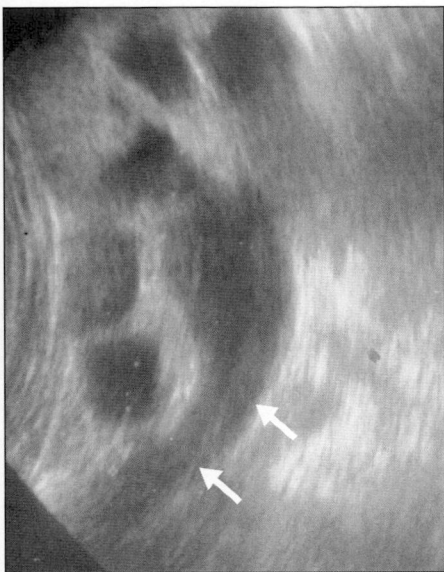

Figure 58.8 Renal ultrasound scan of a patient with obstruction of the urinary tract causing hydronephrosis. The kidney is hydronephrotic with dilatation of the pelvicalyceal system; dilatation of the upper ureter is also clearly seen (arrows).

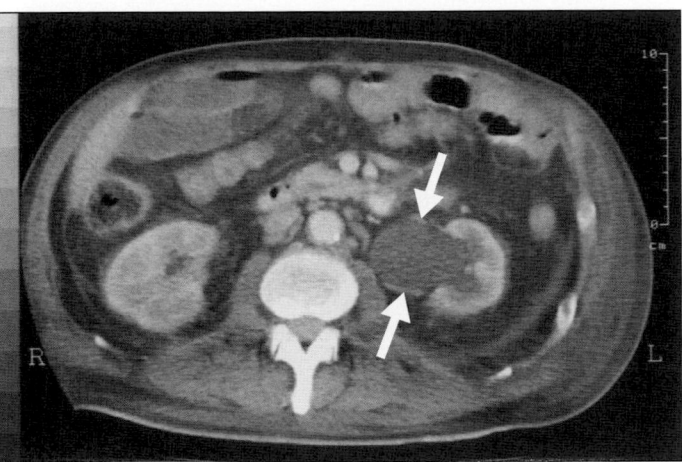

Figure 58.9 CT scan of the abdomen showing a grossly hydronephrotic kidney on the left (arrows mark dilated renal pelvis). Dilated loops of small bowel are seen in the right hypochondrium. Sequential sections demonstrated that the ureter was dilated along its length and that there was a pelvic mass, which was responsible for both bowel and left ureteric obstruction. The mass was subsequently shown to be arising from a carcinoma of the colon.

false-negative results can be decreased by using duplex Doppler ultrasound to detect a high resistive index (> 70%), which is indicative of the increased vascular resistance found in obstructed kidneys[17]. However, the use of resistive index measurements is still in a developmental phase and additional studies are needed before this technique may be used reliably for the diagnosis of obstructive uropathy.

Even in experienced hands, ultrasonography may have a significant false-positive rate, especially if minimal criteria are adopted to diagnose obstruction[15]. In addition, the echogenicity produced by multiple renal cysts may be mistaken for hydronephrosis on ultrasonography, but the former are separate structures not connected to each other and not accompanied by a large renal pelvis separating the renal sinus echoes.

Computed tomography and magnetic resonance imaging

The relative sensitivity and specificity of computed tomography (CT) and magnetic resonance imaging (MRI) and ultrasonography in detecting dilatation of the urinary tract remain to be determined. However, noncontrast-enhanced helical CT is used increasingly as the primary imaging modality for the evaluation of patients with acute flank pain. Stones

are easily detected because of their high density and hence CT can provide a highly accurate and timely diagnosis of an obstructing ureteral calculus[18]. In addition, it can provide additional useful information regarding the site and nature of the obstructing lesion, especially when this is extrinsic to the urinary tract (see Fig. 58.9). Both CT and MRI are good for demonstrating retroperitoneal pathology such as para-aortic and paracaval lymphadenopathy; retroperitoneal fibrosis can be detected by finding increased attenuation within the retroperitoneal fat resulting in encasement of one or both ureters. Hematomas can also be detected, as can primary ureteral tumors and polyps. The diagnostic potential of CT is enhanced by contrast, but this may limit its use in patients with renal impairment. In addition, it involves considerable exposure to ionizing radiation. MRI is able to provide multiplanar imaging without exposures to contrast medium or ionizing radiation. MR pyelography can rapidly and accurately depict the morphological features of dilated urinary tracts and provide information regarding the degree and level of obstruction[19]. For these reasons, MRI is an attractive technique for the evaluation of hydronephrosis in children, where in a single study without exposure to contrast or ionizing radiation, it can combine the information provided by functional and anatomic nuclear scans, voiding cystourethrography and ultrasonography[20].

Retrograde pyelography

Retrograde pyelography (see Figs 58.2 & 58.10) may be particularly useful to identify both the site and the cause of the obstruction. It is also helpful when nondilated urinary tract obstruction is suspected or when there is a history of allergic reactions to contrast material. Urinary tract infection that may become overwhelming if obstruction is present is a contraindication to retrograde pyelography.

Misdiagnosis of obstruction by ultrasonography	
False negative	**False positive**
Ultrasound performed too early following onset of obstruction	Inexperienced ultrasonographer
Decreased urine flow: dehydrated patient, renal failure	Multiple renal cysts
Encasement of ureters	
Staghorn calculus	
Ultrasound is subjective but in the hands of an expert, the diagnosis of a dilated calyceal system can be made in nearly 100% of patients.	

Table 58.3 Misdiagnosis of obstruction by ultrasonography.

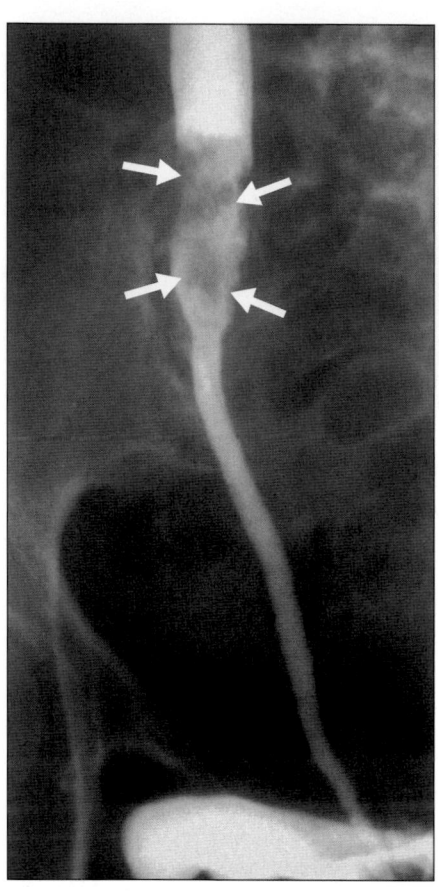

Figure 58.10 Ureteral obstruction by a tumor. A retrograde pyelogram shows the tumor is within and obstructing the ureter (arrows). Above the tumor there is dilatation of the ureter, but below it the ureter is of a normal caliber.

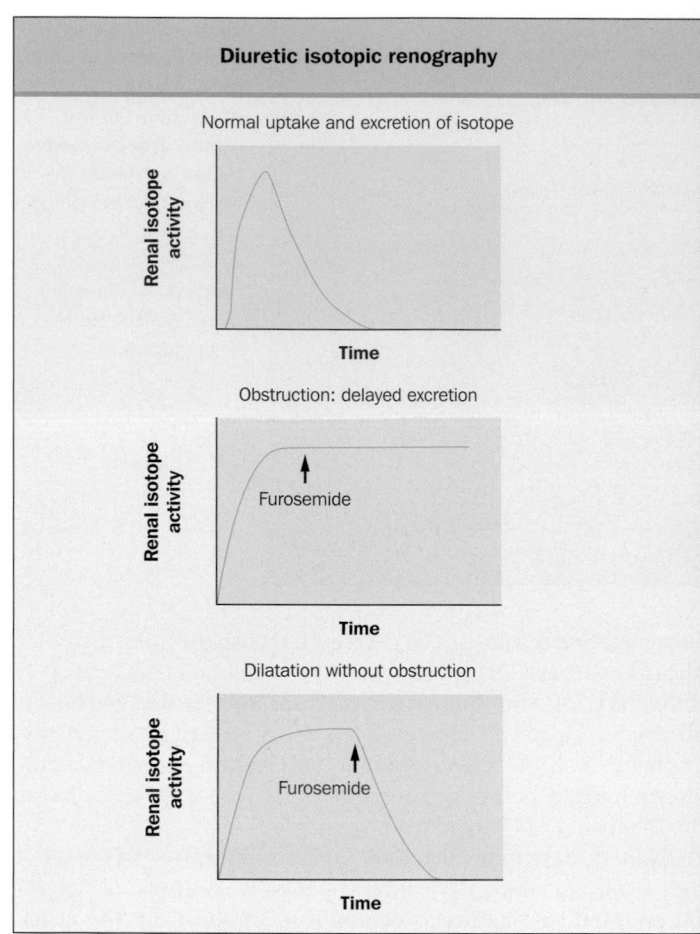

Figure 58.11 Diuretic isotopic renography. Idealized tracings for normal, obstructed, and dilatation without obstruction of the upper urinary tract. In obstruction, there is delayed excretion of the isotope despite administration of furosemide. When there is dilatation of the upper urinary tract without obstruction, the isotope is retained but is rapidly excreted following the administration of furosemide.

Isotopic renography

Isotopic renography combined with intravenous furosemide (frusemide) administered 20–30 min after injection of the isotope (diuretic renogram) may be helpful in the diagnosis of obstruction[21]. Normally there should be a rapid washout of the isotope from the kidney, and persistence of the isotope suggests that the system is obstructed (Fig. 58.11; see also Fig. 52.17). Poor renal function significantly limits the usefulness of this technique because the diuretic response to furosemide may be absent.

Pressure flow studies

Pressure flow studies (Whitaker test) are now rarely used for the diagnosis of obstruction[22]. The collecting system is punctured with a fine gauge needle and, after catheterization of the bladder, fluid is perfused at a rate of l0 mL/min. The differential pressure between the bladder and the collecting system should not exceed l5 cmH_2O; pressure greater than 20 cmH_2O indicates obstruction. Antegrade pyeloureterograms can be obtained at the same time, which may help to define the site of the obstruction.

Other evaluations

Lower urinary tract obstruction may be evaluated by cystoscopy, which allows a visual inspection of the entire urethra and the bladder. Urodynamic studies (see Fig. 52.15) may be useful in assessing bladder outlet obstruction, allows the measurement of residual urine volume after voiding, and can detect functional abnormalities of the bladder. An IVU with oblique films of the bladder and urethra during voiding (excretory cystogram) and postvoiding are also useful in evaluating the site of lower urinary tract obstruction and the amount of residual urine. A retrograde cystourethrogram will give better definition of the bladder and urethra, but bladder catheterization is required, which may be difficult if the infravesical obstruction is caused by urethral stricture or prostatic cancer.

DIFFERENTIAL DIAGNOSIS

Diagnostic uncertainty arises with nonobstructive dilatation of the upper urinary tract. This condition may be seen with VUR, diuretic administration, diabetes insipidus, congenital megacalyces, chronic pyelonephritis, and postobstructive atrophy. Although the dilatation from nonobstructive causes may not be as marked as that with obstruction, diuresis renography and/or retrograde pyelography are often required to exclude obstruction. A voiding cystogram may demonstrate the presence of VUR as a cause of the dilatation of the urinary tract.

NATURAL HISTORY

Obstructive uropathy is one of the few potentially curable renal diseases and, therefore, it should be considered in all patients with renal failure. Untreated, it will result in the progressive irreversible loss of nephrons with renal parenchyma being replaced by extracellular matrix (Fig. 58.12). If both kidneys are affected or if there is only a solitary kidney, ESRD will result. The exact prognosis will depend on the pathology responsible for the obstruction, the duration of the obstruction, and the presence or absence of urosepsis. Relief of short-term obstruction (< 1–2 weeks) usually results in an adequate return of renal function (both glomerular and tubular). With chronic progressive obstruction (> 12 weeks) there is often irreversible destruction of renal parenchyma, and renal functional recovery may be minimal even following relief of the obstruction. However, the degree of functional recovery following relief of obstruction is difficult to predict and some patients will recover meaningful renal function (i.e., have chronic renal impairment but be independent of dialysis treatment) following relief of months of chronic obstruction. In general, however, the earlier obstruction is diagnosed and hence relieved, the better the prognosis for renal functional recovery.

TREATMENT

General considerations

The treatment of obstructive uropathy is dictated by the location of the obstruction, the underlying cause, and the degree (if any) of renal impairment. If renal impairment is present, the treatment of obstruction requires close collaboration between nephrologists and urologists in order to reduce the risks associated with the metabolic and electrolyte consequences of renal failure and to optimize the chances for long term recovery of renal function. For example, complete bilateral ureteral obstruction presenting as ARF is a medical emergency and requires rapid intervention to salvage renal function. Prompt intervention to relieve the obstruction should result in a rapid improvement in renal function. With modern techniques dialysis should rarely be required in patients with ARF secondary to obstruction except to get the patient fit for intervention for example where there is life threatening hyperkalemia or fluid overload. Urological aspects of the management of obstructive uropathy are discussed further in Chapter 59.

The site of obstruction will frequently determine the approach. If the obstruction is distal to the bladder, a urethral catheter or, if this cannot be passed, a suprapubic cystostomy will effectively decompress the kidneys. Placement of nephrostomy tubes or cystoscopy and passage of a retrograde ureteral catheter will relieve upper urinary tract obstruction. Insertion of nephrostomy tubes is generally the appropriate emergency treatment for upper urinary tract obstruction, especially in the setting of ARF. They can be inserted under local anesthetic and should allow rapid recovery of renal function in most patients (> 70%), hence avoiding the need for dialysis. The rapid relief of obstruction in this way also reduces the chances of long-term permanent renal damage by reducing the stimulus for

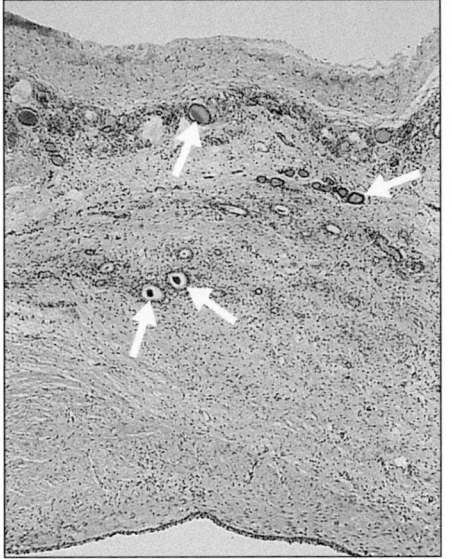

**Figure 58.12
Pathology of chronic ureteral obstruction.** This is a section of the rim of renal tissue from the kidney shown in Figure 58.5. The renal capsule is at the top, the urinary space at the bottom. The cortex is considerably thinned and only a few atrophic tubules remain (arrows) within an interstitium comprising dense fibrous tissue and a mononuclear cell infiltrate (blue staining nuclei). No glomeruli can be seen. This demonstrates why there would be no prospect for any significant functional recovery in this kidney even following the relief of the obstruction.

renal atrophy and fibrosis. However, if acute tubular necrosis has occurred as a result of obstruction, renal function may not recover immediately.

Once the obstruction is relieved by a nephrostomy, the specific site and nature of the obstructing lesion can be determined by infusing X-ray contrast media down the nephrostomy tube (nephrostogram, Fig. 58.13), and time can be taken to plan definitive therapy. Major complications (abscess, infection, and hematoma) occur in less than 5% of patients. If both kidneys are obstructed, the nephrostomy should initially be placed in the kidney with the best-preserved parenchyma, but in time bilateral nephrostomies may be required to maximize the potential for the recovery of renal function.

Infection may occur above a ureteral obstruction (pyonephrosis). In such patients, drainage of the kidney with nephrostomy tubes can play an important therapeutic role with appropriate antibiotics and supportive therapy.

A nephrostomy can be used to gauge the potential for functional recovery in patients with chronic obstruction. Failure of the kidney to recover after long-term (weeks) drainage via a nephrostomy suggests it has sustained irreversible structural damage and that there will be no benefit from performing a more definitive surgical correction of the obstructing lesion.

Specific therapies

Calculi are the most common cause of ureteral obstruction and their treatment includes relief of pain, elimination of obstruction, and treatment of infection. Ureteral obstruction by papillary tissue, blood clots, or a fungus ball is treated by procedures similar to those used for calculi. When obstruction is caused by neoplastic, inflammatory, or neurologic disease,

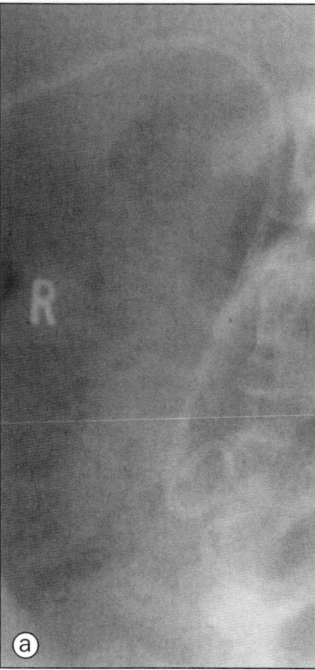
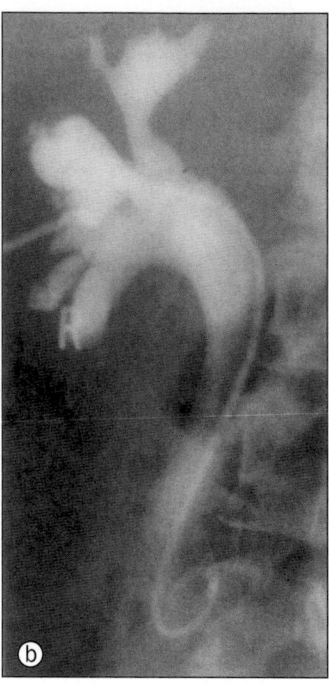
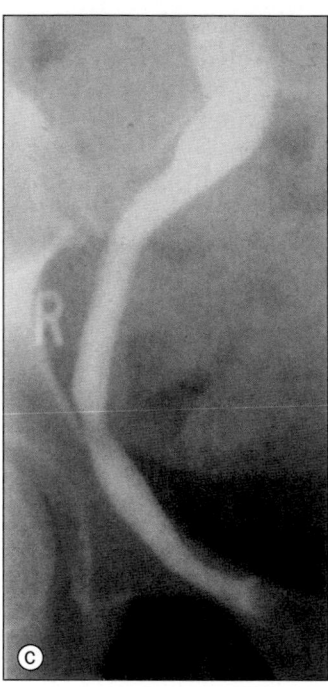

Figure 58.13 Nephrostogram. (a) A nephrostomy has been placed percutaneously into the dilated collecting system of the kidney under ultrasound control. Following infusion of contrast down the nephrostomy the pelvicalyceal system and upper ureter (b) and the lower ureter (c) are outlined. The ureter is dilated along its length but tapers abruptly at the vesicoureteral junction. In this case the obstruction was caused by a radiolucent stone.

there is unlikely to be spontaneous remission of the obstruction and some form of urinary diversion such as an ileal conduit should be considered. Some obstructing neoplastic lesions, such as lymphadenopathy from lymphoma, may respond to appropriate aggressive chemotherapy. However, when the lower urinary tract has been irreparably damaged by malignancy (bladder, cervix, or prostate), the decision whether to undertake urine diversion must be made on an individual basis and should be taken in conjunction with a multidisciplinary team involving urologists, nephrologists, oncologists and palliative care physicians. Long-term percutaneous nephrostomy may provide the best option in such patients since it has been shown to increase survival significantly (> 6 months in 50%) and decrease the number of days in hospital. This approach may also be appropriate in patients with a short life expectancy or who are unfit for major surgery. Calculus formation and pyelonephritis are long-term complications of nephrostomies.

In idiopathic retroperitoneal fibrosis, ureterolysis (in which the ureters are surgically freed from their fibrous encasement) may be beneficial, especially if combined with steroid therapy to prevent recurrence.

Functionally significant PUJ obstruction may be corrected surgically (Anderson–Hynes pyeloplasty) or by balloon dilatation of the abnormal segment of ureter, usually with good long-term results.

Benign prostatic hyperplasia is the most common cause of lower urinary tract obstruction in men. It may be mild and does not always progress. A patient with minimal symptoms, no infection, and a normal upper urinary tract can continue with assessment until he and his physician agree that further treatment is desirable. Medical therapy with either α-adrenergic blockers or 5α-reductase inhibitors may be used in patients with moderate symptoms. α-Blockers relax the smooth muscle of the bladder neck and prostate and, thus, decrease urethral

pressure and outflow obstruction. 5α-Reductase inhibitors inhibit the conversion of testosterone to the active metabolite dihydrotestosterone and, thus, reduce prostatic hypertrophy. These agents may act synergistically when given in combination. If prostatic hypertrophy results in debilitating symptoms and urinary retention or if there is recurrent infection or evidence of renal parenchymal damage, surgical intervention with transurethral resection of the prostate (TURP) is generally required.

Urethral strictures in men can be treated by dilatation or direct vision internal urethrotomy. The incidence of bladder neck and urethral obstruction in women is low, and urethral dilatation, internal urethrotomy, meatotomy, and revision of the bladder neck in females are seldom indicated. Suprapubic cystostomy may be necessary for bladder drainage in patients who cannot void after injury to the urethra or in those who have an impassable urethral stricture.

When obstruction is the result of neuropathic bladder function, dynamic studies are essential to determine therapy. The goals of therapy should be to establish the bladder as a urine storage organ without causing renal parenchymal injury and to provide a mechanism for bladder emptying that is acceptable to the patient. Patients may either have an atonic bladder secondary to lower motor neuron injury or unstable bladder function resulting from upper motor neuron dysfunction. In both cases, ureteral reflux and parenchymal damage may develop, although this is more common in patients with a hypertonic bladder. Asking the patient to void at regular intervals may be sufficient to achieve satisfactory emptying of the bladder. The best treatment for patients with an atonic bladder and significant residual urine retention associated with recurrent bouts of urosepsis is the establishment of clean intermittent self-catheterization. The aim should be to catheterize four or five times per day to ensure that the amount of urine drained from the bladder on each occasion is less than 400 mL. External sphincterotomy has also been used in men with an atonic bladder and may relieve outlet obstruction and promote bladder emptying, but it may cause urinary incontinence and the need to wear an external collection device. In patients with a hypertonic bladder, improvement in the storage function of the bladder may be obtained with anticholinergic agents. Occasionally, chronic clean intermittent self-catheterization is necessary.

Whenever possible, chronic indwelling catheters should be avoided in patients with a neurogenic bladder since they may lead to the formation of bladder stones, urosepsis, urethral erosion, and the occurrence of squamous cell carcinoma of the bladder. Patients who have chronic indwelling catheters for more than 5 years should have yearly cystoscopic examinations.

If deterioration in renal function occurs despite conservative measures, or there is intractable incontinence or a small contracted bladder, then an upper urinary tract diversion procedure such as an ileal conduit may be used to treat lower urinary tract obstruction.

Management of postobstructive diuresis

Marked polyuria (postobstructive diuresis) is frequently seen following the release of bilateral obstruction or obstruction in a single functioning kidney. Release of unilateral obstruction rarely results in a postobstructive diuresis[23], despite the presence of tubular dysfunction and a concentrating defect. This may result from intrinsic differences in the tubular response to unilateral and bilateral obstruction. Probably more importantly, in bilateral obstruction salt and water retention and renal impairment will have occurred (this is not seen in unilateral obstruction because of the presence of a contralateral normal kidney). As a result, there is an increase in natriuretic factors (including atrial natriuretic peptide) and substances able to promote an osmotic diuresis such as urea[24]. Thus the postobstructive diuresis may be in part appropriate and result from the excretion of water and electrolytes that were retained during the period of obstruction and in part inappropriate as a result of tubular dysfunction. If the latter

condition is not managed correctly, there is potential for severe volume depletion (suggested by orthostatic hypotension and tachycardia) and electrolyte imbalance, and renal function may fail to recover. Intravenous fluid as well as oral fluid replacement is usually required. Once the patient is euvolemic, urine losses plus an allowance for insensible losses should be replaced. Urine volume should be measured regularly (hourly) to determine the rate of fluid administration and serum electrolytes should be measured at least daily and as frequently as every 6 h when there is a massive diuresis. Weighing the patient daily is also helpful. Measurement of urinary electrolytes, which are typically approximately half iso-osmolar, can be used to determine the appropriate replacement intravenous fluid. Commercially available intravenous fluid preparations vary from country to country, but replacement regimens should include sodium chloride, a source of bicarbonate, and potassium. Calcium, phosphate, and magnesium replacement may also be necessary.

If fluid is administration is overzealous, the kidney will not recover its concentrating ability and a continued 'driven' diuresis will result[25]. On occasions, it may be necessary to decrease fluid replacement to levels below those of the urine output and observe the patient carefully for signs of volume depletion.

Future prospects

An understanding of the pathophysiologic changes following ureteral obstruction does hold the potential for developing effective therapies for both hastening the recovery of renal function following the relief of obstruction and limiting any permanent damage to renal tissue. Examples of potential therapies include thromboxane synthetase inhibitors/receptor blockers, ACE inhibitors, Angiotensin II receptor antagonists, antagonists of cytokines, and inhibitors of macrophage infiltration. To date, however, the value of such therapies to human disease must remain speculative and the best treatment option remains the prompt and effective relief of the obstruction.

REFERENCES

1. Harris KPG. Models of obstructive nephropathy. In: Gretz N, Strauch M, eds. Experimental and Genetic Rat Models of Chronic Renal Failure. Basel, Switzerland: Karger; 1993:156–68.

2. Klahr S, Harris KPG. Obstructive uropathy. In: Seldin D, Giebisch G, eds. The Kidney: Physiology and Pathophysiology, 2nd edn. New York, NY: Raven Press; 1992:3327–69.

3. Klahr S, Harris K, Purkerson ML. Effects of obstruction on renal function. Pediatr Nephrol. 1988;2:34–42.

4. Purkerson ML, Klahr S. Prior inhibition of vasoconstrictors normalizes GFR in postobstructed kidneys. Kidney Int. 1989;35:1305–14.

5. Harris KPG, Yanagisawa H, Schreiner G, Klahr S. Evidence for two distinct and functionally important sites of enhanced thromboxane production following bilateral ureteral obstruction. Clin Sci. 1991;81:209–13.

6. Harris KPG, Schreiner GF, Klahr S. Effect of leukocyte depletion on the function of the postobstructed kidney in the rat. Kidney Int. 1989;36:210–1.

7. Bander SJ, Buerkert JE, Martin D, Klahr S. Long-term effects of 24-hour unilateral ureteral obstruction on renal function in the rat. Kidney Int. 1985;28:614–20.

8. Kim SW, Cho SH, Oh BS, et al. Diminished renal expression of aquaphorin water channels in rats with experimental bilateral ureteral obstruction. J Am Soc Nephrol. 2001;12:2019–28.

9. Schreiner GF, Kohan DE. Regulation of renal transport processes and hemodynamics by macrophages and lymphocytes. Am J Physiol. 1990;258:F761–7.

10. Bell ET. Renal Diseases. Philadelphia, PA: Lea & Febiger; 1946:113–39.

11. Campbell MF. Urinary obstruction. In: Campbell MF, Harrison JH, eds. Urology, 3rd edn. Philadelphia, PA: Saunders; 1970:1772–93.

12. Warady BA, Hebert D, Sullivan EK, et al. Renal transplantation, chronic dialysis, and chronic renal insufficiency in children and adolescents. The 1995 Annual Report of the North American Pediatric Renal Transplant Cooperative Study. Pediatr Nephrol. 1997;11:49–64.

13. Sacks SH, Aparicio SA, Bevan A, et al. Late renal failure due to prostatic outflow obstruction: a preventable disease. Br Med J. 1989;298:156–9.

14. Ishidoya S, Morrisey J, McCracken R, et al. Angiotensin II receptor antagonist ameliorates renal tubulointerstitial fibrosis caused by unilateral ureteral obstruction. Kidney Int. 1995;47:1285–94.

15. Webb JA. Ultrasonography in the diagnosis of urinary tract obstruction. Br Med J. 1990;301:944–6.

16. Rascoff JH, Golden RA, Spinowitz BS, Charytan C. Nondilated obstructive nephropathy. Arch Intern Med. 1983;143:696–8.

17. Platt JF, Rubin JM, Ellis JH. Acute renal obstruction: evaluation with intrarenal duplex Doppler and conventional US. Radiology. 1993;186:685–8.

18. Dorio PJ, Pozniak MA, Lee FT Jr, Kuhlman JE. Non-contrast-enhanced helical computed tomography for the evaluation of patients with acute flank pain. Wis Med J. 1999,98.30–4.

19. Blandino A, Gaeta M, Minutoli F, et al. MR pyelography in 115 patients with a dilated renal collecting system. Acta Radiol. 2001;42:532–6.

20. Rodriguez LV, Spielman D, Herfkens RJ, Shortliffe LD. Magnetic resonance imaging for the evaluation of hydronephrosis, reflux and renal scarring in children. J Urol. 2001;166:1023–7.

21. O'Reilly P. Diuresis renography 8 years later: an update. J Urol. 1986;136:993–9.

22. Whitaker RH, Buxton-Thomas MS. A comparison of pressure flow studies and renography in equivocal upper urinary tract obstruction. J Urol. 1984;131:446–9.

23. Gillenwater JY, Westervelt FB Jr, Vaughan ED Jr, Howards SS. Renal function after release of chronic unilateral hydronephrosis in man. Kidney Int. 1975;7:179–86.

24. Harris RH, Yarger WE. The pathogenesis of postobstructive diuresis: The role of circulating natriuretic and diuretic factors including urea. J Clin Invest. 1975;56:880–7.

25. Bishop MC. Diuresis and renal functional recovery in chronic retention. Br J Urol. 1985;57:1–5.

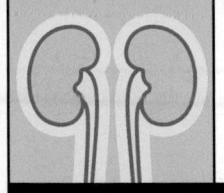

Section 11 Urological Disorders

Chapter 59

Urological Issues for the Nephrologist

J Kilian Mellon

INTRODUCTION

Close working between nephrologists and urologists is crucial to the optimal management of a number of common clinical problems. A proper understanding of urological strategies helps the nephrologist to ensure that patients presenting with these problems are given clear information and are optimally managed.

Areas where such coordinated work is most important are discussed in this chapter. They include the management of stone disease, the surgical approach to urinary tract obstruction, the investigation of hematuria and the management of renal tract malignancy.

SURGICAL MANAGEMENT OF STONE DISEASE

Introduction

In the last 20 years the management of urinary tract stones has been irrevocably changed by the introduction of extracorporeal shockwave lithotripsy (ESWL), percutaneous nephrolithotomy (PCNL) and ureteroscopy. Because of the effectiveness of ESWL, many endoscopic procedures for stones are nowadays more complex than previously. Open stone surgical techniques are a second or third line treatment in most cases. Table 59.1[1] indicates the changing use of different modalities of stone treatment since the introduction of the newer techniques.

Changing use of techniques for stone removal			
Location	1984	1990	1999
Incidence (%)			
Calyceal stones	35	43	46
Pelvic stones	42	20	13
Staghorn stones	8	3	1
Ureteral stones	15	34	40
Treatment modality			
ESWL	64	79	78
PCNL	20	5	2
Ureteroscopy	11	15	20
Open surgery	9	1	0.1

Table 59.1 Changing use of techniques for stone removal. The changes in the application of surgical techniques for stone removal since the introduction of ESWL and PCNL[1].

Indications for surgical intervention

Spontaneous stone passage can be expected in up to 80% of patients with a stone size < 4 mm. Conversely, for stones with a diameter of > 7 mm, the chance of spontaneous stone passage is very low. Stone size should be routinely measured from a plain abdominal radiograph (KUB). As well as size, other factors influencing the decision for active stone removal relate to stone size and shape, stone composition (if known), presence of infection, and stone position. Some 70% of distal ureteral stones will pass spontaneously, but only 45% of mid-ureteral stones and 25% of proximal ureteral stones. Active stone removal is strongly recommended when there is persistent pain (> 72 h) despite adequate analgesia, persistent obstruction with risk of impaired renal function (for example with pre-existing renal impairment or in a single kidney), when there is bilateral obstruction, and when there is proven associated urinary tract sepsis.

Acute surgical intervention

The goal of acute surgical intervention is to relieve obstruction. The main therapeutic options are insertion of a percutaneous nephrostomy (PCN) or a double-J ureteral stent (Fig. 59.1). Double-J stent is preferable, since it is more convenient for patient and clinical staff. PCN has the advantage that an

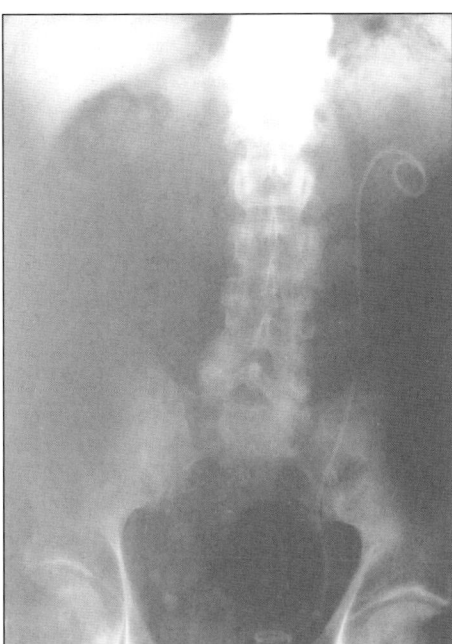

Figure 59.1 Ureteral stenting. Plain radiograph showing a double J ureteral stent in the left ureter. Note the curled ends of the stent remain in the pelvis and the bladder despite ureteral peristalsis.

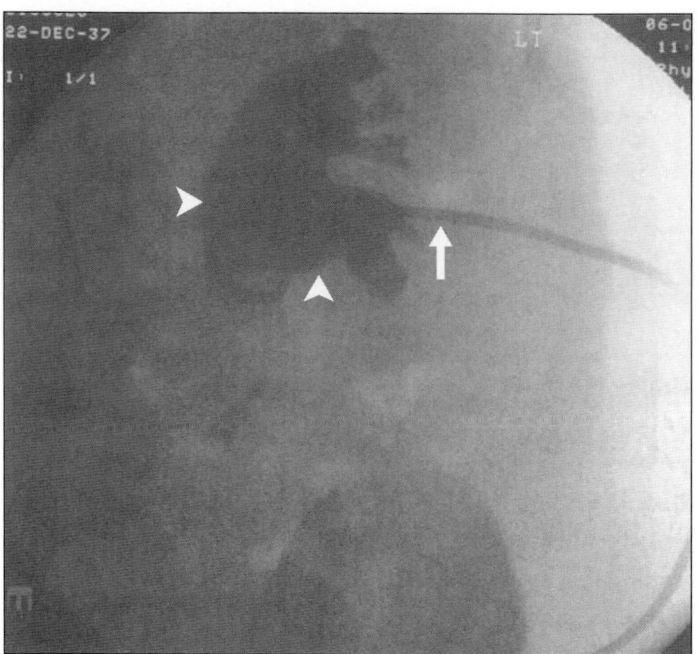

Figure 59.2 Nephrostogram in ureteral obstruction due to a stone.
Contrast is injected through a percutaneous nephrostomy tube placed in
the lower pole calyx (arrow). The contrast outlines a single large calculus
(arrowheads) producing complete obstruction at the pelvi-ureteral junction.

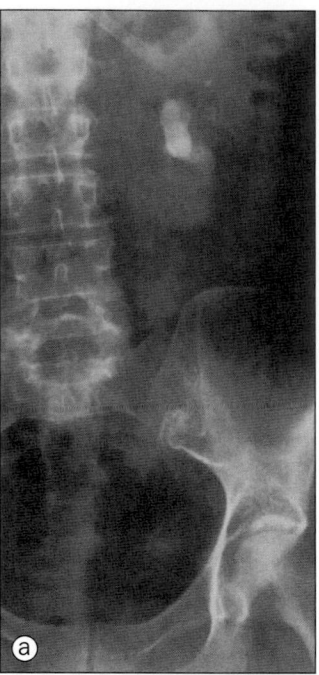
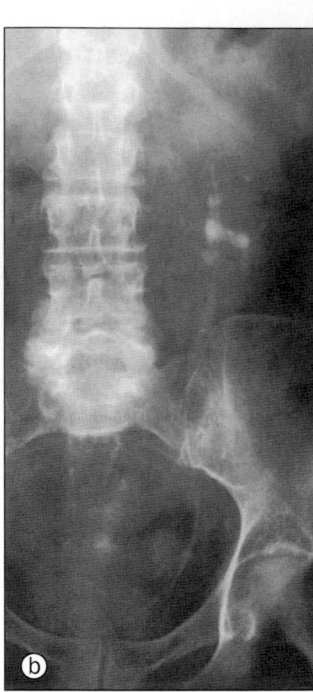

**Figure 59.3 Extracorporeal shock wave lithotripsy complicated by
'steinstrasse'.** (a) Preoperative plain radiograph showing stones in the left
renal pelvis. (b) Following ESWL, note the disappearance of the pelvic
stone and the string of stone fragments throughout the length of the
ureter. These were complicated by infection and a JJ ureteral stent was
subsequently placed to facilitate their passage. Figure 42.23a & b from
COMPREHENSIVE UROLOGY 1st Edition, Mosby.

antegrade nephrostogram can be performed to localize the
site of obstruction and define stone shape and size more
precisely (Fig. 59.2). Rarely, when neither of these options
is feasible will it be necessary to perform an urgent open
surgical procedure to remove a stone.

Elective surgical intervention
Extracorporeal shockwave lithotripsy (ESWL)
ESWL achieves stone destruction by targeting on the stone
(using ultrasound or fluoroscopy) acoustic shock wave energy
which is generated by the lithotripter using electrohydraulic,
electromagnetic or piezoelectric energy[2]. Stone fragments
may collect in the distal ureter following ESWL giving rise to
a condition referred to as 'steinstrasse' (literally *stone
street*) (Fig. 59.3). Sometimes a double-J ureteral stent is placed
endoscopically before ESWL treatment if the risk of obstruction by stone fragments is high.

The majority of patients have lithotripsy on an outpatient
basis under i.v. sedation and analgesia. Treatment sessions
are usually of the order of 30 min during which typically
1500–2500 shockwaves are delivered. The number of treatments
required depends on stone number, size and composition.

Acute complications of ESWL include hemorrhage or
hematoma, infection, injury to adjacent organs and arrhythmias. The major late complication is stone recurrence; the risks
of hypertension or renal impairment late after ESWL remain
controversial.

ESWL is the first line treatment for > 75% of stone patients.
Table 59.2 shows circumstances when ESWL is less effective
and PCNL becomes the preferred surgical approach, or a
combination of the two modalities is used.

Percutaneous nephrolithotomy (PCNL)
Preoperatively, an IVU is used to plan access, and an ultrasound scan helps determine the optimal site of puncture and
the position of the stone in the kidney (ventral or dorsal) and
to ensure neighboring organs (e.g., spleen, liver, large bowel,
pleura or lungs) are not in the planned access path. 3-D CT
scan stone reconstruction to improve localization has recently
been used in morbidly obese patients or those with malrota-
tion and renal hypermobility where ultrasound and fluoroscopy are compromised[3]. The percutaneous puncture may be
facilitated by the preliminary placement of a retrograde
ureteral catheter to dilate and opacify the collecting system
which is then punctured using fluoroscopy. The most frequently used access site is the dorsal calyx of the lower pole.
Following tract dilatation, the nephroscope is then inserted
and stone fragmentation is undertaken by ultrasonic, electrohydraulic or laser lithotripsy using a probe passed through the
nephroscope and placed on the surface of the stone. After completion of PCNL, a self-retaining balloon nephrostomy tube is
used to tamponade the tract and provide further access if
needed. Complications of PCNL include hemorrhage (from
renal or, rarely, intercostal arteries) which is treated by selective
angio-embolization. Other complications include sepsis; injury
to spleen, pleura, colon; extravasation; retained fragments; and
stone granuloma due to migration of stone fragments into the
ureteral wall. Perinephric scarring after PCNL may also make
subsequent open surgery more difficult. PCNL usually results
in minimal parenchymal injury, the amount of renal damage

Indications for PCNL		
Stone characteristics*	Large stones, > 3 cm or staghorn	
	Struvite stones	Complete removal necessary to eliminate infection and minimize stone recurrence
	Calcium oxalate stones	Difficult to pulverize by ESWL
	Cystine stones	Difficult to pulverize by ESWL
Stone position	Lower pole stones	Fragments less easily evacuated from dependent lower pole calyces, especially if collecting system dilated
Anatomic abnormalities	PUJ obstruction Calyceal diverticula Ureteral obstruction	Prevent passage of fragments after ESWL
Patient characteristics	Large patient bulk	Stone cannot be placed in focal point of ESWL machine

*Stone composition can only be defined with certainty by direct stone analysis, but advances in imaging may ultimately provide a means of accurate assessment of stone composition *in situ* before treatment, thus allowing the urologist to select the treatment most likely to succeed.

Table 59.2 Indications for PCNL. ESWL is the first choice treatment for stone intervention except in these circumstances which may favour PCNL.

averages only 0.15% of the total renal cortex[4]. 'Mini-perc', establishing a smaller than normal tract during the nephrostomy, has recently been advocated to reduce parenchymal damage even further; high stone-free rates are reported and the procedure can be converted to a bigger tract if necessary[5].

The PCNL technique is modified for special circumstances usually by altering the site of puncture – for example directly into a calyceal diverticulum or if there are ureteral stones using a higher placed puncture to permit antegrade ureteroscopy. In a transplant kidney ureteral catheterization may be difficult and ultrasound guided puncture is an alternative approach.

Indications for PCNL are shown in Table 59.2; these continue to evolve and are being challenged by developments in ureteroscopic techniques which are allowing more upper ureteral and renal pelvis stones to be dealt with using a retrograde approach.

Ureteroscopy

Recent advances in the design of endoscopes for ureteronephroscopy have rendered the entire urinary tract accessible to endoscopic examination and manipulation. Ureteroscopes may be rigid, semi-rigid or flexible. Rigid instrument channels vary in size and in number and in whether the channel is straight or curved. Ultrasound probes require straight channels but the lithoclast will pass through a gentle curvature. Flexible instruments are the only true ureteronephroscopes. They have poorer resolution and smaller working channels than rigid instruments. As well as stone fragmentation, ureteroscopy allows ureteral dilatation by bougie or balloon techniques. Calculi < 6 mm can be retrieved directly by basket, snare or wire graspers. Stone can be fragmented by ultrasonic, electrohydraulic or laser lithotripsy

using a probe passed through the ureteroscope and placed on the surface of the stone. Success rates for fragmentation of ureteral stones with one of these techniques are high, 70–80% overall.

Complications of ureteroscopic techniques include perforation, extravasation, mucosal damage, hematuria, infection, and stricture.

Management of staghorn calculus

Staghorn calculus should usually be managed by intervention since reports of conservative therapy show a high rate of nephrectomy (up to 50%) and an increase in associated morbidity (mainly renal failure) and mortality (up to 28%)[6]. Surgical options are ESWL monotherapy, complete endoscopic stone removal, or a combined approach using PCNL for debulking followed by ESWL. The advantage of the combined approach is the reduced need for additional renal access and secondary endourologic procedures. The choice of treatment depends on many factors including the age and renal function of the patient. ESWL will not usually render the patient entirely stone free (the ideal goal of treatment) especially when treating large staghorns; nevertheless achieving < 40% of a staghorn persisting as fragments can still be considered successful.

SURGICAL MANAGEMENT OF URINARY TRACT OBSTRUCTION

Upper tract obstruction

The causes of upper tract obstruction are listed in Table 58.1 and a summary of the treatment of urinary tract obstruction is found towards the end of Chapter 58. Common surgical problems are the correction of pelvi-ureteral junction (PUJ) obstruction and the management of patients with upper tract malignancy due to an underlying malignancy.

Pelvi-ureteral junction obstruction

Until recently, the standard approach to PUJ obstruction was the open surgical pyeloplasty. In recent years, minimally invasive surgery has offered alternatives including percutaneous antegrade endopyelotomy, ureteroscopic endopyelotomy and laparoscopic pyeloplasty. The role of these newer procedures is still being defined.

Upper tract obstruction due to malignancy

Upper tract obstruction due to malignancy can be as a result of direct tumor invasion, external compression due to metastatic lymph node involvement or, rarely, due to true metastasis to the ureter. Some 70% of tumours causing ureteral obstruction are genitourinary (cervical, bladder, prostate) in origin, with breast and gastrointestinal carcinomas and lymphoma comprising the majority of the remainder[7]. Ureteral obstruction may also be secondary to retroperitoneal fibrosis following combinations of surgery, systemic chemotherapy and pelvic irradiation. Upper tract obstruction due to malignancy rarely presents with classical acute ureteral colic as is typically seen with ureteral obstruction due to a benign cause such as a stone. When obstruction is due to malignancy, progressive upper tract obstruction develops, often insidiously. Progressive obstruction of one upper tract remains unrecognized until the patient presents with anuria and uremia due to subsequent compromise of the contralateral ureter.

Techniques for ureteral decompression

Where possible, a satisfactorily functioning double-J ureteral stent is preferable. The most straightforward approach is to place the stent retrogradely through a cystoscope. Bilateral stents should be placed if technically possible. However, trigonal anatomy can be distorted due to tumor infiltration making identification of ureteral orifices for double-J stent insertion impossible at the time of cystoscopy. Complications of ureteral stents include migration, obstruction with proteinaceous material, infection, and fragmentation. They may cause uncomfortable vesicoureteral reflux, and erode through the urinary tract[8]. Patients may also experience bladder spasm from irritation of the trigone, which generally subsides within several weeks of stent placement.

If stents cannot be inserted percutaneous nephrostomy (PCN) is required. PCN may also be a safer initial approach in the acute situation, particularly if a uremic patient is hyperkalemia or septic. PCN can then be followed after an interval with antegrade ureteral stenting. In patients with bilateral ureteral obstruction, it is not always necessary to insert bilateral PCN tubes. Significant palliation and return to near normal renal function can be accomplished by the insertion of a single stent, targeted at the side with the better preserved renal parenchyma as determined by CT scan or ultrasound.

Once placed PCN tubes or double-J stents need to be replaced every 4–6 months. If left longer, they become increasingly brittle and encrusted, and are liable to crack or break when manipulated.

While PCN is an accepted technique of palliative treatment when conventional ureteral stenting has failed, nephrostomy drainage has important complications including urinary tract infection, pain, intermittent hematuria and effects on the patients' psychological well-being[9]. The external bag for urinary drainage makes management at home more difficult and may interfere with activities of daily living.

Extra-anatomic stents are an alternative for patients in whom conventional stent insertion has failed or for whom permanent nephrostomy drainage is unacceptable. An extra-anatomic stent is placed by an initial percutaneous puncture and insertion of the upper end of a long (50 cm double-J stent) into the kidney. A subcutaneous tunnel is then created to bring the stent to the level of the iliac crest. A further tunnel is fashioned to bring the lower end of the stent out suprapubically, followed, finally, by suprapubic puncture of a full bladder and insertion of the lower end[10] (Fig. 59.4). Extra-anatomic stents are usually changed at intervals of 6 months.

Preliminary experience with metallic, self-expanding stents, used alone or in conjunction with double-J stents for malignant ureteral obstruction confirms their value in maintaining ureteral patency and avoiding PCN[11].

Open surgical techniques

Today, open nephrostomy, cutaneous ureterostomy, or formal urinary diversion are rarely performed and would only be considered when endourologic procedures are unsuccessful.

Major operative reconstruction (revision of ileal ureteral anastomoses, ureteral reimplantation, ileal ureter interposition) is only considered when the patient is free of disease and has a relatively good prognosis.

When is ureteral decompression justified?

The diagnosis of upper tract obstruction due to cancer can pose significant ethical issues for those involved in the patient's care. The decision to offer ureteral decompression is not straightforward and requires input not only from the urologist, but also from colleagues in radiation and medical oncology, and the palliative care team as well as careful discussion of the options with the patient and his/her family. In addition, to reach an accurate diagnosis the assistance of colleagues in radiology and pathology is often required, emphasizing the multidisciplinary approach that is mandatory in the management of this group of patients.

Ureteral decompression is justified when radiotherapy or systemic chemotherapy remain therapeutic options following improvement in renal function (*vide infra*) but may also be justified for palliation of pain or symptoms related to ongoing renal tract sepsis.

A review of patients undergoing PCN for obstructive uropathy secondary to pelvic malignant disease identified a group of patients with very poor survival in whom ureteral decompression is usually not justified (Table 59.3)[12]. Patients with gastric or pancreatic cancer survive a median of only 1.4 months following ureteral decompression, questioning the benefit of such a procedure in this setting[9]. In another report, the average survival of patients with advanced malignancies undergoing endo-urologic diversion was only 5 months, 50% of which was spent in hospital[13].

Lower tract obstruction

A list of causes of lower tract obstruction is given in Chapter 58, Table 58.2. The commonest causes relate to either benign or malignant disease of the prostate. Obstructive uropathy due

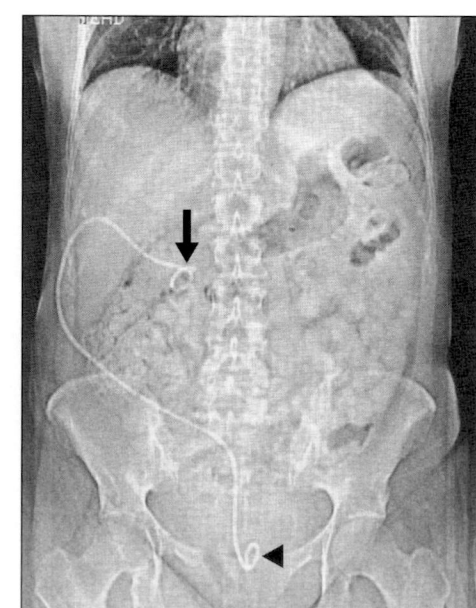

Figure 59.4 Extra-anatomic stenting for malignant ureteral obstruction. MRI scan showing placement of an extra-anatomic stent for malignant obstruction of the right ureter. The upper end of the double J stent has been placed in the right renal pelvis (arrow). The stent then runs through a subcutaneous tunnel before the lower end enters the bladder (arrowhead).

Percutaneous nephrostomy for malignant obstructive uropathy		
	Median survival	5-year survival
Group I Primary untreated malignancy	27 weeks	10%
Group II Recurrent malignancy with further treatment	20 weeks	20%
Group III Recurrent malignancy with no further treatment	6.5 weeks	None survived > 1 year
Group IV Benign disease as a result of previous treatment	Not stated	64%
Overall	26 weeks	22%

Table 59.3 Percutaneous nephrostomy for malignant obstructive uropathy. Outcome in 77 patients undergoing percutaneous nephrostomy for obstructive uropathy secondary to pelvic malignant disease[12].

to prostatic disease can be on the basis of bladder outlet obstruction (in benign prostatic hyperplasia or prostate cancer) or can be due to obstruction at the level of the vesicoureteral junctions (in prostate cancer). This distinction is easily made by the volume of residual urine in the bladder after urethral catheterization. The immediate management of bladder outlet obstruction, regardless of the prostatic pathology, is usually by the passage of a urethral catheter although suprapubic catheterization may be required if the urethral anatomy is distorted. Whereas obstructive uropathy due to tumor invasion of the vesicoureteral junctions requires insertion of either a PCN or double-J stents.

INVESTIGATION OF HEMATURIA

Macroscopic (visible) hematuria is perhaps the most important symptom in urological practice and, quite apart from being alarming to the patient, can be the first presenting sign of an underlying malignant condition of the urinary tract (often a transitional cell tumor of the bladder). Studies show that 15–22% of patients with visible hematuria have an underlying genitourinary tract malignancy.

Patients with *macroscopic* hematuria must be distinguished from those who have been found to have *dipstick* hematuria or *microscopic* hematuria in whom the risk of malignancy is significantly lower (malignancy rate: 2–11%).

The outcome of full evaluation of a large group of patients (with both macroscopic and microscopic hematuria) attending a hematuria clinic is shown in Table 59.4)[14]. As well as the small, but important group of patients in whom malignancy was identified, there is a significant pickup rate of parenchymal renal disease (~10%) in both macroscopic and microscopic hematuria. It is also important to note the sizable proportion of patients in whom a definitive diagnosis could not be reached.

Evaluation of macroscopic hematuria
All adults with a single episode of macroscopic hematuria require full urologic evaluation including renal imaging and

Outcome of evaluation in a Hematuria Clinic			
(a) Diagnoses found	All (%)	Micro (%)	Macro (%)
No diagnosis	1168 (60.5)	670 (68.2)	498 (52.5)
Renal cancer	12 (0.6)	3 (0.3)	9 (0.9)
Upper tract transitional cell carcinoma	2 (0.1)	1 (0.1)	1 (0.1)
Bladder cancer	230 (11.9)	47 (4.8)	183 (19.3)
Prostate cancer	8 (0.4)	2 (0.2)	6 (0.6)
Stone disease	69 (3.6)	39 (4.0)	30 (3.2)
UTI	251 (13.0)	128 (13.0)	123 (13.0)
Renal parenchymal disease	190 (9.8)	92 (9.4)	98 (10.3)

(b) Likelihood of finding malignancy (percentage of cases investigated) according to age		
	Macroscopic hematuria	Microscopic hematuria
Male age > 40 years	24	8
Male age < 40 years	6.5	1.7 (1 case)
Female age > 40 years	19	5.2
Female age < 40 years	none	none

Table 59.4 Outcome of evaluation in a Hematuria Clinic[14].

cystoscopy. The only exception to this rule occurs when an adult aged < 40 years gives a history characteristic of glomerular hematuria such as is typically seen in IgA nephropathy, in which dark brown hematuria lasting 24–48 h coincides with intercurrent mucosal infection, usually of the upper respiratory tract. This hematuria may be painless or there may be bilateral loin ache. These young adults should be referred first for nephrological assessment.

Evaluation of asymptomatic microscopic hematuria
Microscopic hematuria is very common, the prevalence is at least 2% of the population. It is more common in women and with increasing age (Fig. 19.6). There is no evidence to justify screening for microscopic hematuria except in specific high risk groups, for example those with occupational exposure to oncogenic chemicals or dyes (including benzene and aromatic amines).

The precise definition of microscopic hematuria remains contentious, and it has also been controversial whether these patients should be investigated by a urologist or nephrologist, and how patients should be followed up if investigations are negative[15].

In 2001, the recommendations of the American Urological Association (AUA) Best Practice Policy Panel on the management of asymptomatic microscopic hematuria in adults were published providing an evidence-based set of guidelines for family physicians, urologists and nephrologists in dealing with this condition[16]. Interpretation of the evidence continues to produce contentious results in the likelihood of identifying a cause for hematuria.

The recommended definition of microscopic hematuria is three or more red blood cells per high-power field on microscopic evaluation of urinary sediment from two of three properly collected urinalysis specimens. It is important to appreciate that dipstick positive hematuria may still herald significant disease in the absence of red cells on microscopy since red cells may lyse in alkaline or hypotonic urine before reaching the laboratory for analysis. If a careful history suggests a benign cause for the hematuria (Fig. 59.5), the patient should undergo repeat urinalysis 48 h after cessation of the implicated activity (i.e., menstruation, vigorous exercise, sexual activity or trauma). No additional evaluation is warranted if the hematuria has resolved.

Two of three positive tests is sufficient to justify evaluation, since intermittent hematuria still carries a significant risk of malignancy. Full evaluation should still be considered if there is only a single positive test or if there are only one or two red blood cells per high-power field, if there are risk factors for significant disease (Table 59.5).

Complete evaluation of microscopic hematuria includes a history and physical examination, laboratory analysis, and radiological imaging of the upper urinary tract, followed by cystoscopic examination of the bladder (Fig. 59.5). In women, urethral and vaginal examinations should be performed to exclude local causes of microscopic hematuria. In uncircumcised men, the foreskin should be retracted to expose the glans penis, if possible. If a phimosis is present, a catheter specimen of urine may be required. Patients with urinary tract infection should be treated appropriately, and urinalysis should be repeated 6 weeks after treatment. If the hematuria resolves with treatment, no additional evaluation is necessary. Serum creatinine should be measured. The remaining laboratory investigations are guided by specific findings of the history, physical examination and urinalysis. In some instances, cytological evaluation of exfoliated cells in the voided urine may also be performed. These AUA guidelines are likely to undergo continuing review. Voided urine cytology is becoming controversial as part of the urologic evaluation of hematuria, since the great majority of urothelial tumors are detected by other modalities. The role of cystoscopy in the evaluation of low risk patients is also increasingly debated. There is now evidence to justify avoiding cystoscopy in females < 40 years. However, many authorities still recommend cystoscopy in males < 40 years, since the risk of bladder cancer though very small, is higher than in young women.

The presence of significant proteinuria (> 0.3 g/24 h), red cell casts, renal insufficiency, or a predominance of dysmorphic red blood cells in the urine should prompt referral to a nephrologist and evaluation for parenchymal renal disease. When present, red cell casts are virtually pathognomonic of glomerular bleeding, but they are often absent in low-grade glomerular disease. Accurate determination of red blood cell morphology requires inverted phase contrast microscopy. In general, glomerular bleeding is associated with more than 80% dysmorphic red blood cells, and lower urinary tract bleeding is associated with more than 80% normal red blood cells[17]. This assessment is operator-dependent. An alternative is to assess urinary red cell size by Coulter counter analysis[15], since dysmorphic red cells are smaller than normal red cells, but this method is not useful when red cell numbers in the urine are

Risk factors for significant disease with microscopic hematuria	
High risk	Low risk
Age > 40 years	Age < 40 years
History of smoking	No smoking history
Occupational exposure to chemicals or dyes (benzene or aromatic amines)	No chemical exposure
History of macroscopic hematuria	No macroscopic hematuria
History of urological disease	No other urological symptoms
History of irritative voiding symptoms	
History of UTI	
Analgesic abuse	
History of pelvic irradiation	

Table 59.5 Risk factors for significant disease with microscopic hematuria.

small. Even in the absence of features of glomerular bleeding, many patients with isolated microscopic hematuria have glomerular disease, most commonly IgA nephropathy or thin membrane nephropathy[18]. Since they have a low risk for progressive renal disease, renal biopsy in this setting is not usually recommended. Nevertheless, because follow-up data are limited, these patients should be followed for the development of hypertension, renal insufficiency or proteinuria.

INVESTIGATION OF A RENAL MASS

The widespread use of abdominal ultrasound and CT scanning has resulted in the increased detection of incidental renal masses. The primary goal in investigating a renal mass is to exclude an underlying malignancy. Ultrasound has been reported to be 79% sensitive for the detection of renal parenchymal masses but does not detect lesions < 5 mm. Until recently the gold standard method of assessing renal masses was CT scanning with contrast using no more than 5 mm slices. MRI scanning, especially with T_2-weighted turbo-spin echo images, may be superior to CT in the correct characterization of benign lesions[19].

The management of a solid mass is straightforward. Any solid mass > 3 cm should be regarded as malignant and unless there are exceptional circumstances (such as high operative risk because of comorbid conditions) require surgical resection. Preoperative CT-guided biopsy is required if there is any suspicion that the histopathological diagnosis is not renal cell carcinoma, since this may alter first line treatment.

The management of mixed cystic and solid masses is more problematic. Table 59.6 shows the Bosniak classification[20] of cystic renal masses discovered on CT scanning which uses Hounsfield units to categorize these lesions in increasing probability of malignancy. This classification provides the basis for correct management according to risk of malignancy (Table 59.6)

The evaluation of multiple cystic lesions in the kidney is discussed further in Chapter 47.

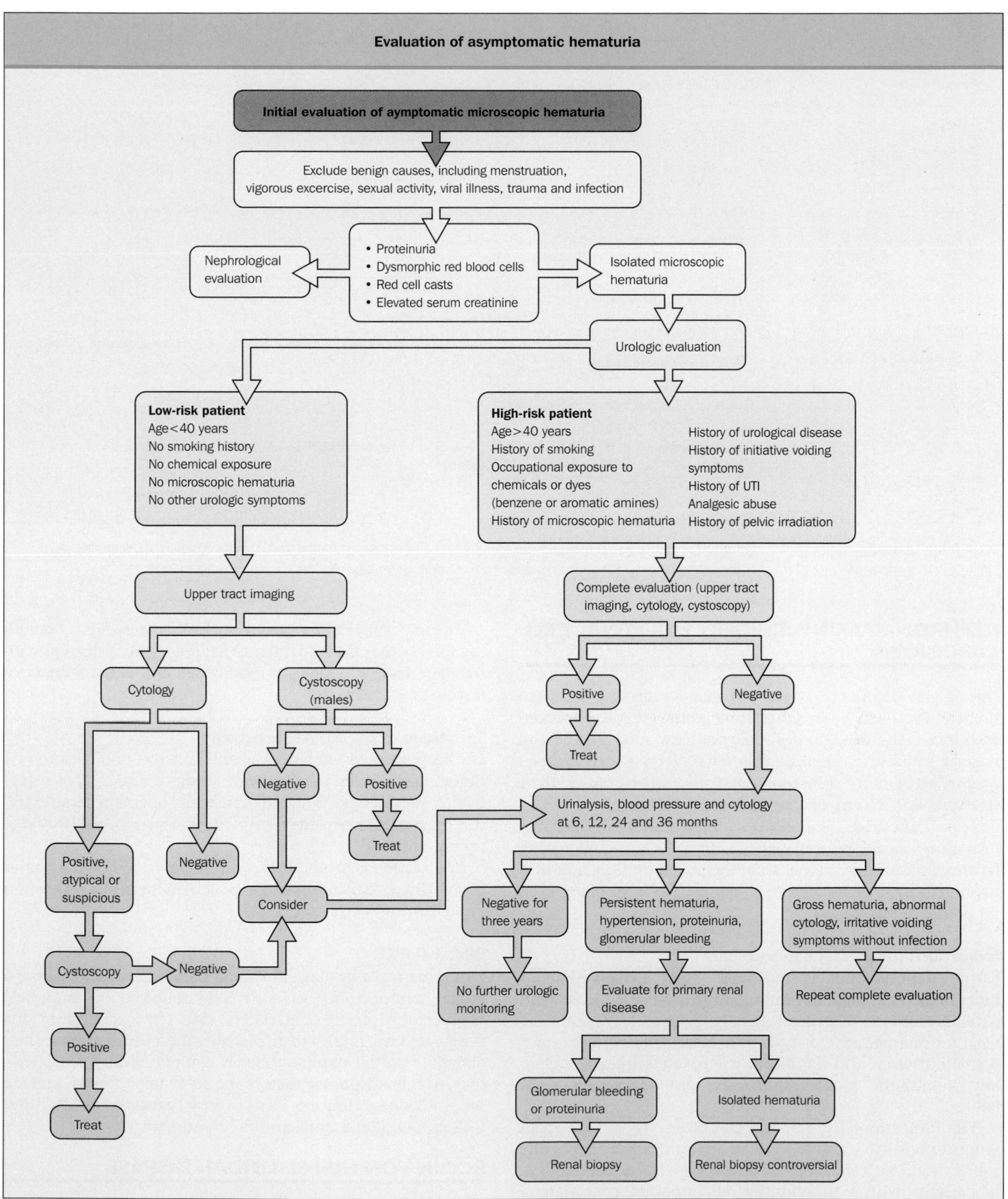

Figure 59.5 Evaluation of asymptomatic microscopic hematuria.

Urological Disorders

Classification and management of cystic renal masses			
Bosniak class	Features on imaging	Comment	Management
Class I Simple benign cysts	• Round/oval • Uniform density < 20 H • Unilocular • No perceptible wall • No contrast enhancement	Majority of asymptomatic cystic lesions	No further intervention required Repeat CT if symptoms develop
Class II Probable benign cysts	• One or two nonenhancing septa • Calcifications in the wall or septum • Hyperdense contents (50–90 H) resulting from the presence of blood, protein or colloid • < 3 cm • No contrast enhancement	Small risk that renal cell carcinoma will develop	Surveillance with 6–12-monthly CT
Class III Indeterminate cystic lesions	One or more of: • Thick, irregular borders • Irregular calcifications • Thickened or enhancing septa • Multilocular form • Uniform wall thickening • Small nonenhancing nodules	~ 40% are neoplastic MRI may improve characterization	Surgical exploration
Class IV Presumed malignant cystic masses	• Appear malignant • Heterogeneous cysts • Shaggy, thickened walls or enhancing nodules	Appearances result from necrosis and liquefaction of a solid tumor or a tumor growing in the wall	Surgical exploration

Table 59.6 Classification and management of cystic renal masses. Approach to renal mass found incidentally by ultrasound or CT scanning. All patients with symptomatic renal masses should be referred for urologic assessment. Classification after Bosniak[20]. (H-Hounsfield Units.)

NEPHRON-SPARING SURGERY FOR RENAL CELL CARCINOMA

Extrafascial nephrectomy was for many years the standard surgical approach for renal cell carcinoma (RCC). However, with increasing detection of incidental low-stage RCC, there is great interest in nephron-sparing surgery, which appears to give satisfactory long-term survival, with careful patient selection and recent advances in renal imaging, as well as improved methods of preventing ischemia. Most recently, increasing numbers of patients with RCC are undergoing laparoscopic surgery, rather than the traditional open radical nephrectomy. The laparoscopic approach is also being used for partial nephrectomy.

Indications for partial nephrectomy
Partial nephrectomy is indicated when preservation of functional renal mass has important benefits for the patient. A renal remnant of at least 20% is required to obviate the need for maintenance dialysis. When the residual renal mass is small, there is also significant risk of late sequelae, including proteinuria, glomerulosclerosis, and progressive renal failure.

The indications for partial nephrectomy include bilateral synchronous RCC, and RCC in an anatomically/functionally solitary kidney. It may also be appropriate for unilateral RCC in patients with a functioning but impaired contralateral kidney, or any concomitant condition with the potential for adversely affecting future renal function.

The role of partial nephrectomy for RCC in von Hippel-Lindau disease is controversial (see below).

The role of partial nephrectomy for unilateral RCC (including RCC which is an incidental finding) with a normal contralateral kidney is not yet established and is the subject of ongoing clinical trials.

Technique of partial nephrectomy
The technique of excision depends on size and location of tumor. Techniques used include wedge excision, polar segmental nephrectomy, major transverse resection, and extracorporeal partial nephrectomy/autotransplantation (for large central tumors).

Enucleation is problematic and should be reserved for cases of von Hippel-Lindau disease in which multiple RCCs are often located within cysts.

Bilateral RCC
This is managed by staged bilateral partial nephrectomies or a partial nephrectomy on one side followed by a radical nephrectomy on the contralateral side. The less involved side is operated on first, which obviates the need for temporary dialysis if partial nephrectomy is complicated by postoperative ATN. Predisposing factors for acute renal failure include solitary kidney, tumor > 7 cm, > 50% parenchymal excision, > 60 min ischemia time, and *ex vivo* surgery.

RCC IN VON HIPPEL-LINDAU DISEASE

VHL is a rare autosomal dominant condition with a predisposition to the development of RCC as well as retinal angiomas, hemangioblastomas of the brain and spinal cord, pheochromocytomas, cystadenomas of the pancreas and epididymis, and islet cell carcinomas of the pancreas. Individuals who inherit the disease gene may remain free of such manifestations or may develop tumors in one or more systems. There is further discussion of the genetics, clinical manifestations and general management of VHL in Chapter 47.

VHL and RCC

RCC occurs in approximately 45% of patients with VHL. Histologically, the tumors are of the clear cell type and are often multifocal and bilateral. The mean age at diagnosis is 39 years and there is a 30–35% risk of tumor progression and death.

A serial CT study identified 228 renal lesions (average 8 per patient) in patients with VHL[21]. On CT appearance, 74% were classified as cysts, 8% as cysts with solid components, and 18% as solid masses. The solid components of cysts and the solid lesions almost always contained RCC. Over a mean 2.4-year follow up (range 1–12 years), the majority of cysts remained the same size (71%) or enlarged (20%); 9% became smaller. Although it is generally thought that cysts are precursors of cancers, the transformation of a simple cyst to a solid lesion was observed in only two patients. 95% of solid lesions enlarged. Surgery is recommended when the renal tumors approach 3 cm in size, since below that size the chance of metastasis is low.

Surgical management

The results of nephron-sparing surgery for VHL appear less satisfactory than for sporadic RCC, with a high risk of local tumour recurrence. It is still unclear whether renal tumors in VHL are best managed by partial nephrectomy to preserve renal function or by immediate bilateral nephrectomy with subsequent renal replacement therapy. Bilateral nephrectomy is certainly favored in patients with multiple fast growing tumors. In one report of surgery in 65 patients with VHL, 54 patients had bilateral and 11 unilateral surgery[22]. Sixteen underwent radical and 49 partial nephrectomy. Of the latter, 51% developed recurrent tumor but only two developed metastases at a mean follow-up of 68 months. Five- and 10-year survival rates for the group undergoing partial nephrectomy were 100% and 81%. ESRD occurred in 23%. The evolving role of laparoscopic partial nephrectomy may impact on the surgical management of these patients in the near future.

REFERENCES

1. Rassweiler JJ, Renner C, Eisenberger F. The management of complex renal stones. Brit J Urol Int. 2000;86:919–28.
2. Rassweiler JJ, Renner C, Chaussy C, Thuroff S. Treatment of renal stones by extracorporeal shockwave lithotripsy: an update. Eur Urol. 2001;39:187–99.
3. Buchholz NP. Three-dimensional CT scan stone reconstruction for the planning of percutaneous surgery in a morbidly obese patient. Urol Int. 2000;65:46–8.
4. Webb DR, Fitzpatrick JM. Percutaneous nephrolithotripsy: a functional and morphological study. J Urol. 1985;134:587–91.
5. Chan DY, Jarrett TW. Techniques in endourology: mini-percutaneous nephrolithotomy. J Endourol. 2000;14:269–72.
6. Blandy JP, Singh M. The case for a more aggressive approach to staghorn calculi. J Urol. 1976;115:505–6.
7. Zadra JA, Jewett MA, Keresteci AG, et al. Nonoperative urinary diversion for malignant ureteral obstruction. Cancer. 1987;60:1353–7.
8. Saltzman B. Ureteral stents: Indications, variations, and complications. Urol Clin North Am. 1988;15:481–91.
9. Donat SM, Russo P. Ureteral decompression in advanced non-urologic malignancies. Ann Surg Oncol. 1996;3:393–9.
10. Minhas S, Irving HC, Lloyd SN, et al. Extra-anatomic stents in ureteric obstruction: experience and complications. Brit J Urol Int. 1999;84:762–4.
11. Sonnenberg E van, D'Agostino HB, O'Laoide R, et al. Malignant ureteral obstruction: Treatment with metal stents – technique, results, and observations with percutaneous intraluminal ureteral stents. Radiology. 1994;191:765–8.
12. Lau MW, Temperley DE, Mehta S, et al. Urinary tract obstruction and nephrostomy drainage in pelvic malignant disease. Brit J Urol. 1995;76:565–9.
13. Shekarriz B, Shekarriz H, Upadhyay J, et al. Outcome of palliative urinary diversion in the treatment of advanced malignancies. Cancer. 1999;85:998–1003.
14. Khadra MH, Pickard RS, Charlton M, et al. A prospective analysis of 1,930 patients with haematuria to evaluate current diagnostic practice. J Urol. 2000;163:524–7.
15. Tomson C, Porter T. Asymptomatic microscopic or dipstick haematuria in adults: Which investigations for which patients? A review of the evidence. BJU Int. 2002;90:185–98.
16. Grossfeld GD, Wolf JS Jr, Litwin MS, et al. Asymptomatic microscopic hematuria in adults: summary of the AUA best practice policy recommendations. Am Fam Physician. 2001;63:1145–54.
17. Santo NG De, Nuzzi F, Capodicasa G, et al. Phase contrast microscopy of the urine sediment for the diagnosis of glomerular and non-glomerular bleeding-data in children and adults with normal creatinine clearance. Nephron. 1987;45:35–9.
18. Topham PS, Harper SJ, Harris KPG, et al. Glomerular disease as a cause of isolated microscopic haematuria. Quart J Med. 1994;87:329–36.
19. Curry NS, Bissada NK. Radiologic evaluation of small and indeterminant renal masses. Urol Clin North Am. 1997; 24:493–505.
20. Bosniak MA. The current radiological approach to renal cysts. Radiology. 1986;158:1–10.
21. Choyke PL, Glenn GM, Walther MM, et al. The natural history of renal lesions in von Hippel-Lindau Disease: a serial CT study in 28 patients. AJR. 1992;159:1229–34.
22. Steinbach F, Novick AC, Zincke H, et al. Treatment of renal cell carcinoma in von Hippel-Lindau disease: a multicenter study. J Urol. 1995;15:1812–6.

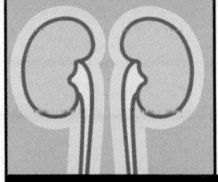

Section 12 Tubulointerstitial Disease

Chapter 60

Acute Interstitial Nephritis

Jérôme A Rossert and Evelyne A Fischer

DEFINITION

Acute interstitial nephritis (AIN) is an acute, often reversible disease characterized by the presence of inflammatory infiltrates within the interstitium. It is only a rare cause of acute renal failure, but this nephropathy should not be overlooked since it usually requires specific therapeutic interventions.

PATHOGENESIS

Most studies suggest AIN is an immunologically-induced hypersensitivity reaction to an antigen that is classically a drug or an infectious agent. There are several lines of evidence for a hypersensitivity reaction in drug-induced AIN: (1) it only occurs in a small percentage of individuals; (2) it is not dose-dependent; (3) it is often associated with extrarenal manifestations of hypersensitivity; and (4) it recurs after accidental re-exposure to the same drug or to a closely related one. Similarly, AIN secondary to infections can be differentiated from pyelonephritis by the relative absence of neutrophils in the interstitial infiltrates and the failure to isolate the infective agent from the renal parenchyma, again suggesting an immunologic basis to the disease.

Studies of experimental models of AIN have shown that three major categories of antigens can induce AIN[1-2]. Antigens may be (1) tubular basement membrane (TBM) components (such as the glycoproteins 3M-1 or TIN-Ag/TIN1); (2) secreted tubular proteins (such as Tamm–Horsfall protein); or (3) non-renal proteins (such as from immune complexes).

Although some types of human AIN may be secondary to an immune reaction directed against a renal antigen, the majority of cases of AIN are probably induced by extrarenal antigens, being produced in particular by drugs or infectious agents. These antigens may be able to induce AIN by a variety of mechanisms, including (1) binding to kidney structures ('planted antigen'); (2) acting as haptens that modify the immunogenicity of native renal proteins; (3) mimicking renal antigens, resulting in a crossreactive immune reaction; or (4) precipitating within the interstitium as circulating immune complexes.

Studies of experimental models of AIN show that their pathogenesis involves either cell-mediated immunity or antibody-mediated immunity (Fig. 60.1)[1,2]. In humans, most forms of AIN are not associated with antibody deposition, which suggests that cell-mediated immunity plays a major role. This hypothesis is reinforced by the fact that interstitial infiltrates usually contain numerous T cells, and that these infiltrates sometimes form granulomas. Nevertheless, deposition of anti-TBM antibodies or of immune complexes can be observed occasionally in renal biopsies and, in these cases, antibody-mediated immunity may play a role in the pathogenesis of the disease.

Formation of immune complexes within the interstitium, or interstitial infiltration with T cells, will result in an inflammatory reaction. This reaction is triggered by many events, including activation of the complement cascade by antibodies, and release of inflammatory cytokines by T lymphocytes and phagocytes (see Fig. 60.1)[2,3]. While the interstitial inflammatory reaction may resolve without sequelae, it sometimes induces interstitial fibroblast proliferation and extracellular matrix synthesis, leading to interstitial fibrosis and chronic renal failure[4]. Cytokines such as transforming growth factor-β appear to play a key role in this latter process.

EPIDEMIOLOGY

AIN is an uncommon cause of acute renal failure and is identified in only approximately 2–3% of all renal biopsies[5,6]. However, it may account for up to 25% of patients undergoing renal biopsy for drug-induced acute renal failure[7]. Although AIN can occur at any age, it appears to be rare in children.

Before antibiotics were available, AIN was most commonly associated with infections, such as scarlet fever or diphtheria. Nowadays, AIN is most often induced by drugs, particularly antimicrobial agents or nonsteroidal anti-inflammatory drugs (NSAIDs).

DRUG-INDUCED ACUTE INTERSTITIAL NEPHRITIS

Clinical manifestations

In the 1960s and 1970s, most cases of drug-induced AIN were caused by methicillin, and the clinical manifestations of methicillin-induced AIN were considered as the prototypical presentation of AIN. Subsequently, many other drugs have been implicated in the induction of AIN (Table 60.1), of which antimicrobial agents (in particular, β-lactam antibiotics, sulfonamides and rifampin (rifampicin)) and NSAIDs (in particular, fenoprofen) have been most commonly involved. Antiulcer agents, diuretics, phenindione, phenytoin, and allopurinol have also been reported to cause AIN. Most other drugs have only rarely been reported linked with AIN (Table 60.1). The clinical characteristics of drug-induced AIN are now recognized as much more varied than the spectrum seen in classic methicillin-induced AIN[4] (Table 60.2)[4].

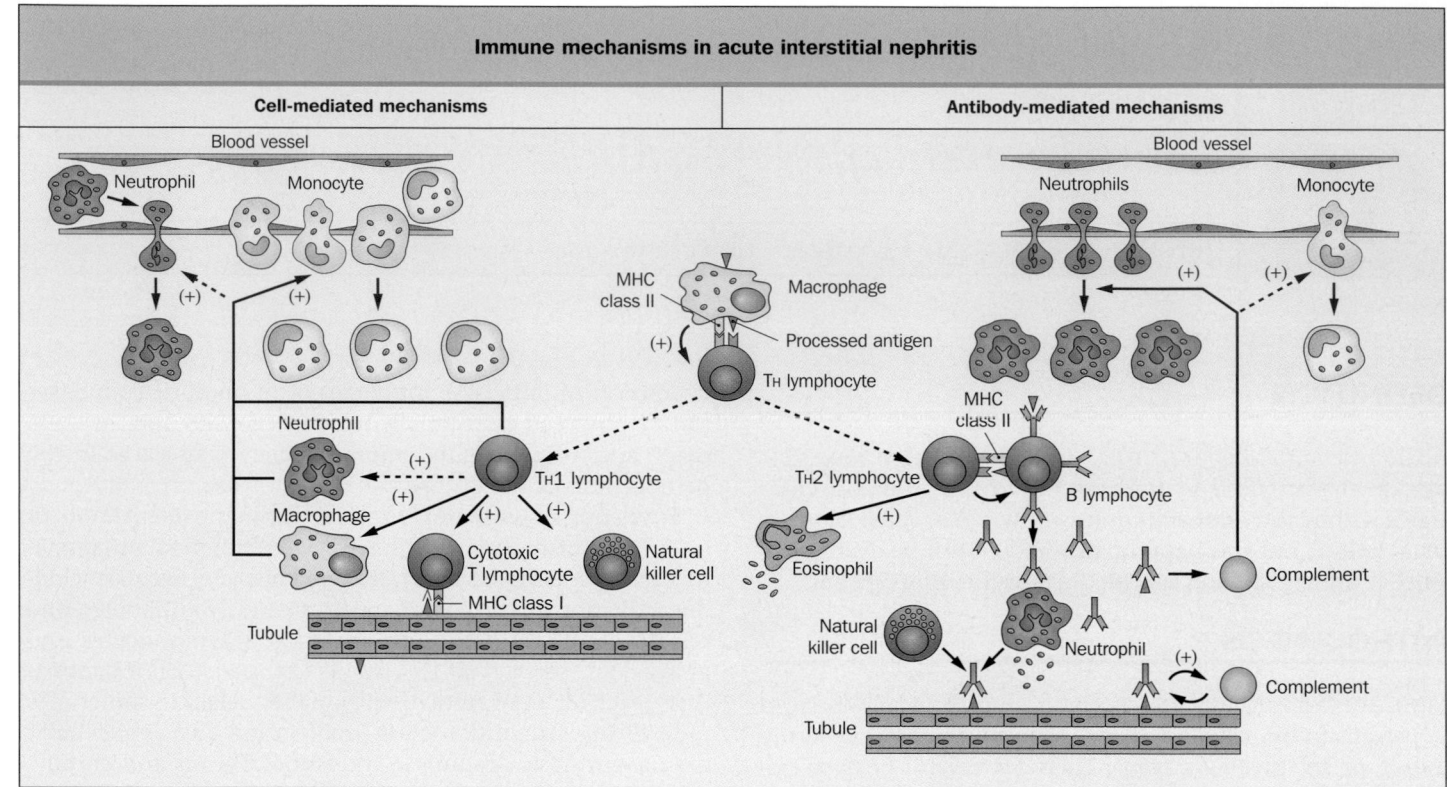

Figure 60.1 Immune mechanisms in acute interstitial nephritis[1–3]. Both cell-mediated and antibody-mediated mechanisms occur. The cell-mediated mechanism is primarily associated with macrophages and T cells; the antibody-mediated mechanism is frequently associated with neutrophil or eosinophil infiltration, as well as local complement activation.

Renal manifestations

Symptoms of AIN develop within 3 weeks after starting the inciting drug in about 80% of patients, although this can range from 1 day to more than 2 months after the beginning of the treatment. The typical presentation is that of a sudden impairment in renal function, associated with mild proteinuria (<1 g/day) and abnormal urinalysis, in a patient with flank pain, normal blood pressure and no edema. In patients with AIN not caused by methicillin, the clinical presentation is often incomplete (Table 60.2), and AIN should be considered in any patient with unexplained acute renal failure[4]. The renal dysfunction may be mild or severe, with dialysis being required in approximately one-third of patients. Hematuria and pyuria are present in approximately one-half of patients, and while leukocyte casts are common, hematuria is almost never associated with red blood cell casts. Flank pain, reflecting distension of the renal capsule, is frequent, observed in approximately one-half of patients, and can be the main complaint upon hospital admission. Occasionally, patients have a low fractional excretion of sodium.

Standard imaging procedures show kidneys normal in size or slightly enlarged, and ultrasonography usually discloses an increased cortical echogenicity (comparable to or higher than that of the liver).

Extrarenal manifestations

Extrarenal symptoms consistent with a hypersensitivity reaction are occasionally observed, including low-grade fever, maculopapular rash (Fig. 60.2), mild arthralgias and eosinophilia. If patients with methicillin-induced AIN are not considered, each of these symptoms is present in less than one-half of patients (Table 60.2), and all these symptoms are present together in less than 5% of the patients[4]. With some drugs, other manifestations of hypersensitivity such as hemolysis or hepatitis can be present. Serum IgE levels may also be elevated.

The association of acute renal failure either with a clinical sign suggestive of hypersensitivity or with an eosinophilia should lead to consideration of a diagnosis of AIN, but signs of hypersensitivity can also be observed in patients with acute renal failure not related to AIN. In a study of 81 patients with acute renal failure who had a renal biopsy, signs of hypersensitivity were found in 14% of patients with drug-induced acute tubular necrosis[7].

Other specific drug associations

The clinical and biological manifestations of AIN may have some specificity, depending on the drug involved.

As outlined above, methicillin-induced AIN was characterized by a high frequency of abnormal urinalysis and extrarenal symptoms, and by a good preservation of renal function: renal failure has been reported in only approximately 50% of patients[8–10] (Table 60.2).

More than 100 cases of rifampin-induced AIN have been reported[11,12]. The vast majority have been observed either after readministration of rifampin or several months after

Table 60.1 Drugs responsible for acute interstitial nephritis.

Drugs responsible for acute interstitial nephritis

Antimicrobial agents

Penicillin G* (benzylpenicillin)*
Ampicillin*
Amoxicillin (amoxycillin)
Methicillin*
Oxacillin*
Cloxacillin
Carbenicillin
Mezlocillin
Piperacillin
Nafcillin
Aztreonam
Cefaclor
Cefamandole
Cefazolin
Cephalexin
Cephaloridine
Cephalothin
Cephapirin
Cephradine
Cefixim
Cefoxitin
Cefotetan
Cefotaxime
Ciprofloxacin*
Norfloxacin
Piromidic acid
Erythromycin*
Flurithromycin
Lincomycin
Tetracycline
Minocycline
Spiramycine*
Gentamicin
Colistin
Polymixin B* (polymyxin B)*
Vancomycin

Teicoplamin
Rifampin* (rifampicin)*
Ethambutol
Isoniazid
Nitrofurantoin*
Sulfonamides*
Cotrimoxazole*
Acyclovir (aciclovir)
Foscarnet
Indinavir
Interferon
Quinine

NSAIDs including salicylates

Aspirin (acetylsalicylic acid)
Mesalamine (mesalazine, 5-ASA)
Sulfasalazine
Diflunisal*
Fenoprofen*
Ibuprofen*
Naproxen
Benoxaprofen
Fenbufen
Flurbiprofen
Ketoprofen
Naproxen
Pirprofen
Suprofen
Indomethacin*
Tolmetin
Zomepirac
Sulindac
Alclofenac
Diclofenac

Fenclofenac
Mefenamic acid
Niflumic acid
Piroxicam*
Azapropazone
Phenylbutazone
Phenazone
Rofecoxib

Antalgics

Aminopyrine
Antipyrine
Dipyrone (noramidopyrine metamizol)
Clometacin* (clometazin)*
Antrafenin
Floctafenin*
Glafenin*

Anticonvulsants

Carbamazepine
Diazepam
Phenobarbital (phenobarbitone)
Phenytoin*
Valproic acid (valproate sodium)

Diuretics

Chlortalidone
Etacrynic acid (ethacrynic acid)
Furosemide* (frusemide)*
Hydrochlorothiazide*
Indapamide
Tienilic acid*
Triamterene*

Antiulcer agents

Cimetidine*
Famotidine
Ranitidine
Omeprazole

Others

Allopurinol*
Alpha Methyl dopa
Amlodipine
Azathioprine
Betanidine*
Bismuth salts
Captopril*
Carbimazole
Chlorpropamide*
Cyclosporine
Clofibrate
Clozapine
Cyamemazine*
Cytosine Arabinoside
Diltiazem
D-penicillamine
Fenofibrate*
Gold salts
Griseofluvin
Interleukin 2
Lamotrigine*
Phenindione*
Phenothiazine
Phentermine/ Phendimetrazine
Phenylpropanolamine
Probenecid
Propanolol
Propylthiouracil
Streptokinase
Sulfinpyrazone

Drugs most commonly involved given in bold; * indicates a drug that can induce a granulomatous form.

Clinical manifestations of drug-induced acute interstitial nephritis (AIN)

Symptom	Methicillin	Other drugs
Flank pain	–	45%
Hypertension	–	20%
Edema	–	15%
Oliguria	25%	40%
Hematuria	90%	53%
Macroscopic hematuria	70%	17%
Pyuria	95%	50%
Mild proteinuria	80%	58%
Fever	85%	45%
Rash	25%	42%
Arthralgias	10%	12%
Eosinophilia	80%	40%

Data were pooled from different case reports, including 95 patients with methicillin-induced AIN and 175 patients with other drug-induced AIN. Patients with AIN associated with a nephrotic syndrome were not considered.

Table 60.2 Clinical manifestations of drug-induced acute interstitial nephritis (AIN).

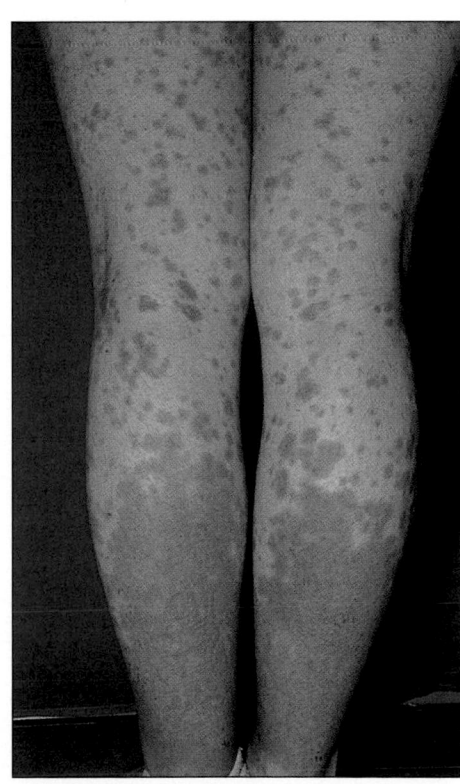

Figure 60.2 **Maculopapular rash in a patient with drug-induced acute interstitial nephritis (AIN).** Such cutaneous lesions occur in about 40% of patients with drug-induced AIN, but they can also be seen in patients with drug-induced acute tubular necrosis.

intermittent administration of the drug. Renal failure is usually associated with the sudden onset of fever, gastrointestinal symptoms (nausea, vomiting, diarrhea, abdominal pain), and myalgias. It may also be associated with hepatitis, hemolysis, and thrombocytopenia. Renal biopsy typically discloses tubular lesions, in addition to interstitial inflammatory infiltrates. Although circulating anti-rifampin antibodies are usually found in these patients, immunofluorescence staining of renal biopsies has been negative in most cases, suggesting that cell-mediated immunity plays a key role in the induction of the nephropathy. In few cases, AIN developed after continuous treatment with rifampin for 1–10 weeks. It was almost never asociated with extrarenal symptoms or with anti-rifampin antibodies, and renal biopsies disclosed severe interstitial infiltrates but few tubular lesions.

Phenindione-induced AIN is generally associated with the development of hepatitis, which can be fatal.

Allopurinol-induced AIN seems to occur more often in patients with chronic reduction in renal function and is usually seen in association with rash and liver dysfunction. It has been suggested that the decreased excretion of oxypurinol, a metabolite of allopurinol, might favor the occurrence of AIN.

AIN occurring secondary to NSAIDs is associated with nephrotic syndrome in approximately three-quarters of cases[13,14]. This nephropathy usually occurs in patients aged over 50 years and, although it has been observed with all NSAIDs, including COX-2 selective inhibitors, half of the incidents have been reported with fenoprofen. Most occurrences develop after the patient has taken NSAIDs for a few months (mean 6 months), but AIN can occur within days or after more than 1 year. With the exception of the heavy proteinuria and associated edema, the presentation of these patients is quite similar to that of patients with other drug-induced AIN (Table 60.3). The main difference is that extrarenal symptoms are present in only approximately 10% of patients. Renal disease caused by NSAIDs must be differentiated from other NSAID-induced nephropathies, including hemodynamically-mediated acute renal failure, papillary necrosis, and NSAID-induced membranous nephropathy[14].

Drugs other than NSAIDs can, rarely, induce an AIN associated with a nephrotic syndrome; a few cases have been reported after administration of ampicillin, rifampin, lithium, interferon, phenytoin, and D-penicillamine.

Pathology

The hallmark of AIN is the presence of inflammatory infiltrates within the interstitium (Fig. 60.3). These infiltrative lesions are often patchy and are most common in the deep cortex and in the outer medulla, but they can be diffuse in severe forms of AIN. They are comprised mostly of T cells and monocytes/macrophages, but plasma cells, eosinophils, and a few neutrophilic granulocytes may also be present. The relative number of $CD4^+$ T cells and $CD8^+$ T cells appears to be quite variable from one patient to another, and to be influenced by various factors including the drug. In some cases, T lymphocytes infiltrate across the TBM and between tubular cells, mainly in distal tubules, and the resulting lesion is referred to as tubulitis.

In some cases of drug-induced AIN, renal biopsy discloses interstitial granulomas (Table 60.1 and Fig. 60.4). These granulomas are usually sparse, non-necrotic, with few giant cells, and associated with nongranulomatous interstitial infiltrates. Granulomas are also found in AIN related to infection, sarcoidosis, Sjögren's syndrome, or Wegener's granulomatosis.

Interstitial infiltrates are always associated with an interstitial edema, which is responsible for separating the tubules (Fig. 60.3). They can also be associated with focal tubular lesions, which range from mild cellular alterations to extensive necrosis of epithelial cells, and which are sometimes associated with a disruption of the TBM. These tubular lesions usually predominate where the inflammatory infiltrates are most extensive.

Tubulointerstitial lesions are not associated with vascular or glomerular lesions. Even in AIN associated with a nephrotic syndrome, glomeruli appear normal on light microscopy, glomerular lesions being similar to those seen in minimal change disease (see Chapter 20).

In the vast majority of patients with AIN, renal biopsies do not show immune deposits, and both immunofluorescence

Clinical presentation of acute interstitial nephritis and nephrotic syndrome associated with NSAID use	
Symptom	Frequency
Hypertension	17%
Edema	75%
Hematuria	38%
Macroscopic hematuria	7%
Pyuria	40%
Extrarenal symptoms	10%
Eosinophilia	40%
Data were pooled from different case reports from 57 patients.	

Table 60.3 Clinical presentation of acute interstitial nephritis and nephrotic syndrome associated with NSAID use.

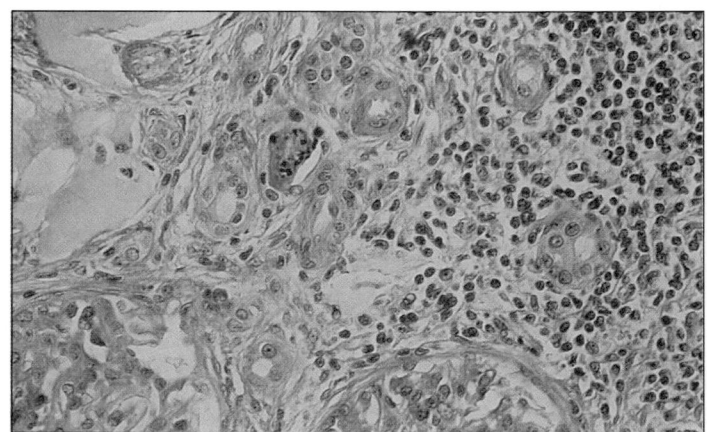

Figure 60.3 Drug-induced acute interstitial nephritis. On light microscopy, the characteristic feature is of an interstitial infiltration with mononuclear cells, with normal glomeruli. It is usually associated with interstitial edema, and with tubular lesions. (Courtesy of Dr B Mougenot.).

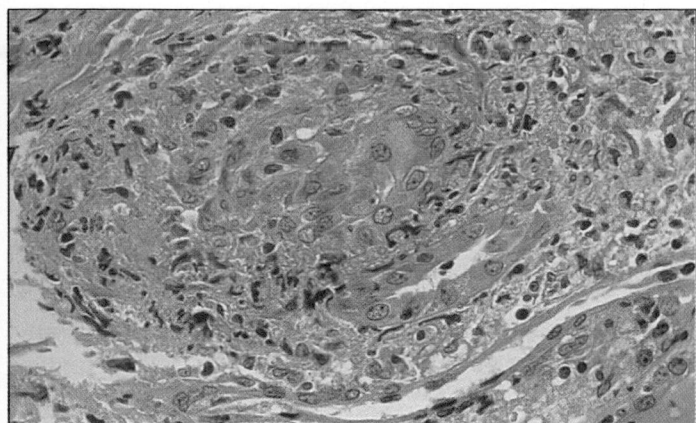

Figure 60.4 Drug-induced granulomatous acute interstitial nephritis. Some drugs can induce the formation of interstitial granulomas, which reflect a delayed-type hypersensitivity reaction. (Courtesy of Dr B Mougenot.)

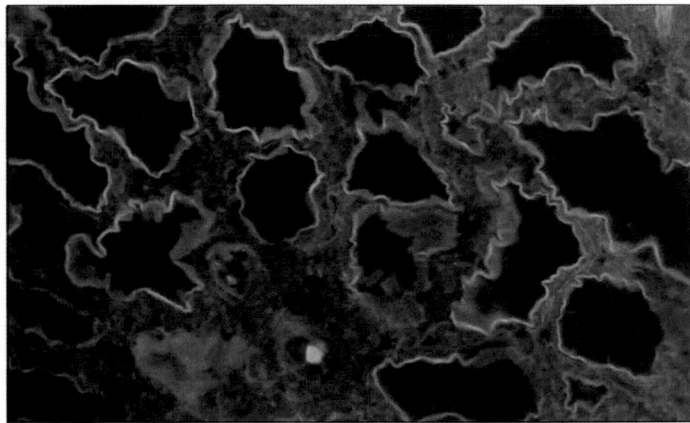

Figure 60.5 Linear deposits of immunoglobin G in methicillin-induced acute interstitial nephritis. Deposits along the tubular basement membrane (TBM) are shown on immunofluorescence microscopy. These antibodies recognize either a component of the TBM or a methicillin metabolite (dimethoxyphenylpenicilloyl) bound to the TBM. (Courtesy of Dr B Mougenot.)

and electron microscopy are negative. Nevertheless, staining of the tubular or capsular basement membrane for IgG or complement may occasionally be seen by immunofluorescence, the staining pattern being either granular or linear (Fig. 60.5). Linear fixation of IgG along the TBM indicates the presence of antibodies directed against membrane antigens, or against drug metabolites bound to the TBM and, in some cases, circulating anti-TBM antibodies have been detected. These linear deposits are seen mostly in patients taking methicillin, NSAIDs, phenytoin, or allopurinol.

Diagnosis of AIN

The most accurate way to diagnose AIN is by renal biopsy. However, both eosinophiluria and gallium scanning have been suggested as helpful in making the diagnosis.

Eosinophils can be detected in urine using either Wright's stain or Hansel's stain, which are both eosine-methylene blue combinations, but the latter appears to be much more sensitive[15,16]. This test is usually considered as positive if more

than 1% of urinary white blood cells are eosinophils. However, although eosinophiluria is frequently used to corroborate the diagnosis of drug-induced AIN, a review of four large series[15–18] shows that this test has rather low sensitivity (67%) and also a low positive predictive value, even if only patients with acute renal failure are considered (50%) (Table 60.4). In these series, the specificity of the test was 87%, and eosinophiluria was also observed in patients with acute tubular necrosis, postinfectious or crescentic glomerulonephritis, atheroembolic renal disease, urinary tract infection, urinary schistosomiasis, or even prerenal azotemia. In particular, 28% of patients with urinary tract infection had eosinophiluria.

An increased renal uptake of gallium (^{67}Ga) has been reported in AIN[19]. Analysis of available series shows that, in 45 patients with AIN, 88% had a positive renal scan (maximum after 48 h), whereas it was negative in 17 of 18 patients with

Table 60.4 Value of eosinophiluria for the diagnosis of acute interstitial nephritis.

Value of eosinophiluria for the diagnosis of acute interstitial nephritis					
	Corwin et al.	Nolan et al.	Corwin et al.	Ruffin et al.	All series
Number of patients	65	92	183	199	539
Patients with AIN					
Eosinophiluria	8	10	5	6	29
No eosinophiluria	1	1	3	9	14
Patients without AIN					
Eosinophiluria	27	12	15	10	64
No eosinophiluria	29	69	160	174	432
Number of patients	23	57	92	38	210
Patients with AIN					
Eosinophiluria	8	10	5	6	29
No eosinophiluria	1	1	3	9	14
Patients without AIN					
Eosinophiluria	6	5	2	6	19
No eosinophiluria	8	41	82	17	148

The four large available series were analysed to assess the value of eosinophiluria (defined by the presence of >1% of eosinophils in urine white blood cells) for the diagnosis of drug-induced acute interstitial nephritis[15–18].

acute tubular necrosis. However, it should be noted that these studies were small and retrospective and also that ^{67}Ga renal scanning is not specific for AIN and may be positive in patients with pyelonephritis, cancer or with glomerular diseases.

Because the clinical presentation of AIN may be polymorphic and because noninvasive diagnostic procedures have important limitations, renal biopsy is often essential for the diagnosis of AIN. Several studies have shown that prebiopsy diagnosis may be incorrect in a substantial number of patients[6].

Identification of the causative drug

Identification of the causative drug is relatively easy when AIN occurs in a patient taking only one drug, but quite often patients are taking more than one drug capable of inducing AIN. Two biologic tests have been used, primarily in research laboratories, to help identify the causative drug: the lymphocyte stimulation test, and the identification of circulating antidrug antibodies.

Identification of circulating antidrug antibodies has been used mostly for patients thought to have an AIN induced by rifampin. Antirifampin antibodies are present in most patients with rifampin-induced AIN, but unfortunately they have also been detected in patients taking rifampin and having no adverse reaction to the drug, suggesting that this test has a limited diagnostic value.

The lymphocyte stimulation test has been used since the 1960s to identify a sensitizing drug. It is based on the measurement of lymphocyte proliferation in the presence of different drugs, a high proliferative index reflecting a sensitization of T lymphocytes against the drug. It may be useful in identifying the specific drug in patients with AIN. However, it should be remembered that a positive test indicates that a patient has a hypersensitivity to the drug but does not directly prove that that drug is responsible for the renal disease.

Natural history

Drug-induced AIN was long considered benign, with complete recovery of renal function if the inciting agent was removed. For example, with methicillin-induced AIN, a complete normalization of serum creatinine has been observed in approximately 90% of azotemic patients[8–10]. Nevertheless, while hematuria, leukocyturia, and extrarenal symptoms usually disappeared within 2 weeks, complete recovery of renal function was often delayed, with an average recovery time of approximately 1.5 months.

More recent studies show that, with drugs other than methicillin, the course of AIN is not always benign and that serum creatinine remains elevated in approximately 40% of patients[4]. Moreover, as for methicillin, recovery of renal function can be delayed, and an increase in serum creatinine can persist for several weeks. Unfortunately, few prognostic factors are available. The severity of renal failure does not appear to be linked with the prognosis[4]. It has been suggested that the presence on renal biopsy of diffuse, neutrophil- or macrophage-rich infiltrates, of interstitial granulomas, or of tubular atrophy, was associated with a poor prognosis but this has not been consistently found in all series[20–24]. The best prognostic factors may actually be the duration of acute renal failure or the degree of interstitial fibrosis[22–24].

Effect of corticosteroids on the course of drug-induced acute interstitial nephritis				
	Number of patients	Mean creatinine peak value	Serum creatinine at the end of follow-up (% of patients)	
			< 1.25 mg/dL	> 2.3 mg/dL
Steroids	52	9.3 mg/dL	58%	17%
No steroids	48	6.5 mg/dL	52%	19%
Data were pooled from seven series, each with 10–23 patients[6,10,21,25–28].				

Table 60.5 Effect of corticosteroids on the course of drug-induced acute interstitial nephritis.

Treatment

In addition to removing the inciting agent, some groups have treated AIN with corticosteroids. Most commonly, patients received an initial daily dose of 1 mg/kg prednis(ol)one, which was then tapered over approximately 1 month. Analysis of series comparing patients who did or did not receive corticosteroids does not indicate that corticosteroids decrease the risk of chronic renal failure (Table 60.5), but it should be stressed that patients receiving corticosteroids tended to have a more severe alteration of renal function and that all the series were small, uncontrolled, and retrospective[6,10,21,25–28]. In contrast, analysis of available data suggests that a brief course of corticosteroids hastens the recovery of renal function. In different series, corticosteroids rapidly induced a decline in serum creatinine values in patients whose renal function did not improve within 1 week after stopping the inciting agent[5,6,28]. Interestingly, in patients with NSAID-induced AIN, corticosteroids do not seem to modify the course of the nephrotic syndrome.

We therefore recommend administering a short course of prednis(ol)one in patients whose renal function fails to improve within 1 week after stopping the inciting drug, provided that the diagnosis of AIN has been confirmed by a renal biopsy. We also treat patients with AIN who are dialysis dependent, whose nephropathy has evolved for more than 2–3 weeks, or whose renal biopsy shows severe interstitial lesions.

ACUTE INTERSTITIAL NEPHRITIS SECONDARY TO INFECTIOUS DISEASES

Infections were once the most common cause of AIN, but the frequency of AIN induced by an infection has dramatically decreased with the widespread use of antibiotics. Nevertheless, the diagnosis of infectious AIN should not be overlooked, and AIN occurring in patients treated with antibiotics should not always be attributed to the drug.

Infectious agents can cause renal parenchymal inflammation by direct infection, resulting in acute pyelonephritis (see Chapter 53). However, many infectious agents may also induce an immunologically-mediated AIN in the absence of direct invasion (Table 60.6). In this case, the clinical presentation depends mostly on the underlying infection. Histologically, lesions are identical to those described for drug-induced AIN, and they can also occasionally result in granulomas (Table 60.6). Infection-associated AIN usually resolves with the

Infections that can be associated with an acute interstitial nephritis		
Bacteria	Viruses	Parasites
Brucella	Cytomegalovirus	Toxoplasma*
Campylobacter jejuni	Epstein Barr virus*	Leishmania donovani
C. diphtheria	Hanta virus	**Others**
E. coli	Hepatitis B virus	Chlamydia
Legionella	Herpex simplex virus	Mycoplasma
Leptospira	HIV	
Mycobacterium tuberculosis*	Measles virus	
Salmonella*	Polyomavirus	
Staphylococcus	Rickettsia	
Streptococcus		
Yersinia pseudotuberculosis		
* Indicates an infection that can induce a granulomatous form.		

Table 60.6 Infections that can be associated with an acute interstitial nephritis.

treatment of the underlying infection, and corticosteroid therapy is not recommended.

An important cause of infection-associated AIN is hantavirus[29]. Hantavirus infections occur worldwide and are responsible for a disease that has been known as hemorrhagic fever with renal syndrome, epidemic hemorrhagic fever, or nephropathia epidemica. Rodents are the main reservoir of the virus, and humans are most probably infected by the airborne route. Extrarenal symptoms usually include fever, headache, lightheadedness, abdominal pain, nausea and vomiting, and thrombocytopenia; the last can be responsible for hemorrhagic complications. Acute renal failure is almost always associated with proteinuria, sometimes in the nephrotic range, and with hematuria. When a kidney biopsy is performed,

it discloses not only interstitial inflammatory infiltrates, which predominate in the medulla, but also vascular congestion and interstitial bleeding (Fig. 60.6). In approximately 50% of patients, immunofluorescence studies show granular immune deposits along the TBM and within glomeruli. Serum creatinine usually starts to decrease after a few days, and a complete recovery of renal function is the rule. Nevertheless, in the most severe incidents, recovery can be complicated by the occurrence of hemorrhagic complications or severe shock. The diagnosis is based on serologic tests, which become positive early in the course of the disease.

Tubulointerstitial lesions are common in HIV-positive patients who undergo a renal biopsy for acute renal failure[30]. Interstitial infiltrates are often associated with glomerular lesions, but they can also be isolated. These forms of AIN have been observed in both Caucasian and African American patients, and they might be related not only to drugs, to opportunistic infections but also to the HIV infection itself[30].

ACUTE INTERSTITIAL NEPHRITIS ASSOCIATED WITH SYSTEMIC DISEASES

Sarcoidosis

In sarcoidosis, renal impairment usually occurs as a complication of hypercalciuria and hypercalcemia, but granulomatous AIN associated with sarcoidosis has also been reported (Fig. 60.7)[31,32]. Presentation is usually that of acute renal failure, which can be isolated or associated with mild proteinuria and sterile leukocyturia. It is associated with extrarenal symptoms of sarcoidosis in approximately 90% of patients, the organs most frequently involved being the lymph nodes, lung, eye and liver. Nevertheless, only slightly more than half of the patients have hilar lymph nodes and/or pulmonary interstitial fibrosis at the time of diagnosis[32]. Treatment with high-dose corticosteroids quickly improves renal function, but most patients do not recover completely. Starting dose should be 1 mg/kg prednis(ol)one daily, and steroid therapy should be tapered slowly and not withdrawn before 9–12 months, in order to prevent relapses.

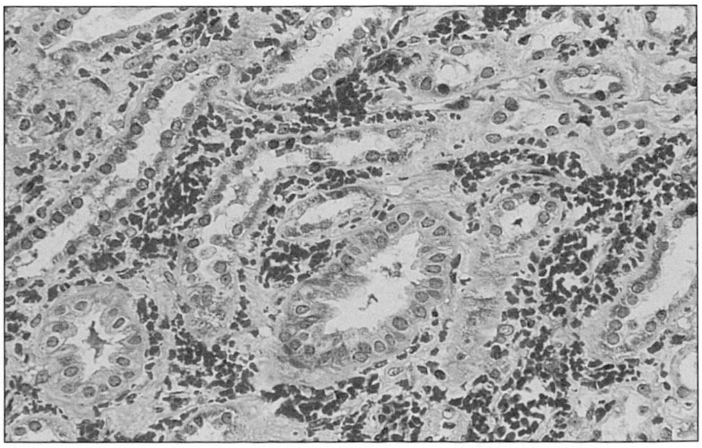

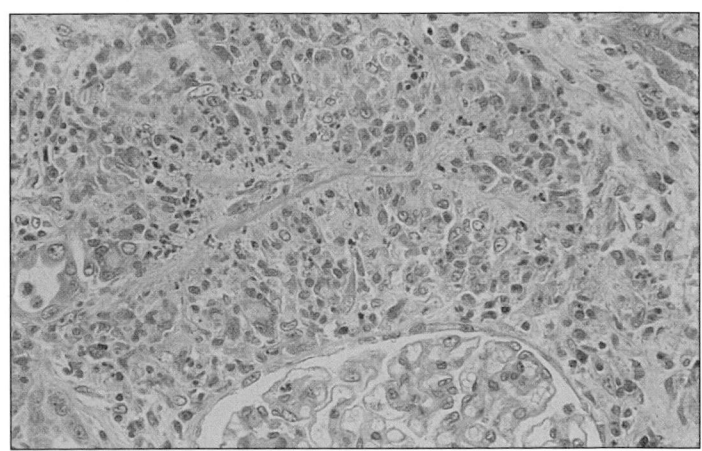

Figure 60.6 Acute interstitial nephritis secondary to hantavirus infection. Vascular congestion and foci of medullary hemorrhage are suggestive of the diagnosis. (Courtesy of Dr B Mougenot.)

Figure 60.7 Granulomatous acute interstitial nephritis in a patient with sarcoidosis. (Courtesy of Dr B Mougenot.)

Tubulointerstitial Disease

Sjögren's syndrome

Clinically significant interstitial nephritis is rare in Sjögren's syndrome and usually results in chronic tubular dysfunction[33]. Nevertheless, a few patients with Sjögren's syndrome and AIN have been reported. In these patients, treatment with high-dose corticosteroids may dramatically improve renal function.

Systemic lupus erythematosus

About two-thirds of renal biopsies performed in patients with systemic lupus erythematosus (SLE) show some tubulointerstitial involvement, but the presence of important tubulointerstitial changes in the setting of minimal glomerular abnormalities is relatively rare[34]. In these cases, renal biopsy shows typical features of AIN on light microscopy, and immunofluorescence staining always discloses immune deposits along the TBM, usually with a granular pattern. Renal function improves after high-dose corticosteroids, suggesting that SLE-associated AIN is not an indication for additional immunosuppressive drugs.

Other systemic diseases

Among patients with cryoglobulinemia and acute renal failure, a few exhibit important interstitial inflammatory infiltrates associated with granular immune deposits in the interstitium and along the TBM. This AIN is usually associated with characteristic glomerular lesions, and the treatment is that of cryoglobulinemia-induced glomerulonephritis (see Chapter 23).

Most renal lesions associated with Wegener's granulomatosis and other vasculitides consist of both an extracapillary glomerulonephritis and a tubulointerstitial nephritis. Nevertheless, a few patients with AIN and minimal glomerular lesions have been reported.

IDIOPATHIC ACUTE INTERSTITIAL NEPHRITIS

More than 50 cases of idiopathic AIN with anterior uveitis have been reported (TINU syndrome)[35,36]. This syndrome is found most commonly in girls of pubertal age, but can also occur in pubertal boys and in adults. Initial symptoms may be ocular, with ocular pain and visual impairment, or pseudoviral with fever, myalgia and asthenia. AIN is responsible for an acute renal failure, ranging from mild to severe, which may or may not be associated with abnormal urinalysis. Renal biopsy shows diffuse interstitial inflammatory infiltrates, almost always without granulomas, and without immune deposits. In children, renal prognosis is excellent, and serum creatinine usually returns to baseline values within a few weeks, with or without steroid therapy. In adults, the renal prognosis seems to be less favorable, and steroid therapy might be useful in preventing evolution to chronic renal failure. Uveitis, which can occur at any time in respect to AIN, is usually responsive to topical steroids, but it may relapse.

A few cases of idiopathic AIN have been reported. Immunofluorescence studies of renal biopsies can show linear deposits of IgG along the TBM, granular deposits of IgG along the TBM, or no immune deposits, suggesting that this entity is quite heterogenous. The treatment of patients with idiopathic AIN is still controversial. A review of available data shows that patients who received corticosteroids usually showed a dramatic improvement of renal function, but that others recovered normal renal function without any treatment[37].

ACUTE INTERSTITIAL NEPHRITIS AND RENAL ALLOGRAFTS

Acute rejection is by far the most common cause of AIN, in renal allograft recipients (see Chapter 88). Nevertheless, AIN can also be induced by drugs or infections. Cases of drug-induced AIN have been reported even in the first weeks after transplantation, when immunosuppression is maximum[38]. Among infectious AIN, the frequency of BK polyomavirus-induced AIN appears to be increasing, and it should be suspected in patients with acute deterioration of renal function and so-called 'decoy cells' in urine[39].

INFILTRATION OF KIDNEYS BY LYMPHOMA AND LEUKEMIA

Infiltration of renal parenchyma by malignant cells is common in patients with leukemia or lymphoma and may mimic AIN (Figure 15.10). Most of the time, this infiltration is totally asymptomatic or it only causes enlarged kidneys, but a few patients with acute renal failure have been reported[40]. Chemotherapy or radiotherapy may rapidly improve renal function in these patients, but before starting these treatments it is important to exclude more common causes of acute renal failure associated with neoplastic diseases.

REFERENCES

1. Wilson CB. Study of the immunopathogenesis of tubulointerstitial nephritis using models system. Kidney Int. 1989;35:938–53.
2. Neilson EG. Pathogenesis and therapy of interstitial nephritis. Kidney Int. 1989;35:1257–70.
3. Michel DM, Kelly CJ. Acute interstitial nephritis. J Am Soc Nephrol. 1998;9:506–15.
4. Rossert J. Drug-induced acute interstitial nephritis. Kidney Int. 2001;60:804–17.
5. Cameron JS. Allergic interstitial nephritis: clinical features and pathogenesis. QJ Med. 1988;66:97–115.
6. Buysen JGM, Houtlhoff HJ, Krediet RT, Arisz L. Acute interstitial nephritis: a clinical and morphological study in 27 patients. Nephrol Dial Transplant. 1990;5:94–9.
7. Landais P, Goldfarb B, Kleinknecht D. Eosinophiluria and drug-induced acute interstitial nephritis. N Engl J Med. 1987;316:1664.
8. Ditlove J, Weidmann P, Bernstein M, Massry SG. Methicillin nephritis. Medicine 1997;56:483–90.
9. Nolan CM, Abernathy RS. Nephropathy associated with methicillin therapy. Arch Intern Med. 1977;137:997–1000.
10. Galpin JE, Shinaberger JH, Stanley TM, et al. Acute interstitial nephritis due to methicillin. Am J Med. 1978;65:756–64.

11. De Vriese AS, Robbrecht DL, Vanholder RC, et al. Rifampicin-associated acute renal failure: pathophysiologic, immunologic, and clinical features. Am J Kidney Dis. 1998;31:108–15.
12. Covic A, Goldsmith DJ, Segall L, et al. Rifampicin-induced acute renal failure: a series of 60 patients. Nephrol Dial Transplant. 1998;13: 924–9.
13. Porile JL, Bakris GL, Garella S. Acute interstitial nephritis with glomerulopathy due to nonsteroidal anti-inflammatory agents: a review of its clinical spectrum and effects of steroid therapy. J Clin Pharmacol. 1990;30:468–75.
14. Kleinknecht D. Interstitial nephritis, the nephrotic syndrome, and chronic renal failure secondary to nonsteroidal anti-inflammatory drugs. Semin Nephrol. 1995;15:228–35.
15. Corwin HL, Bray RA, Haber MH. The detection and interpretation of urinary eosinophils. Arch Pathol Lab Med. 1989;113: 1256–8.
16. Nolan CR, Anger MS, Kelleher SP. Eosinophiluria: a new detection and definition of the clinical spectrum. N Engl J Med. 1986;315: 1516–19.
17. Corwin HL, Korbet SM, Schwartz MM. Clinical correlates of eosinophiluria. Arch Intern Med. 1985;145:1097–9.
18. Ruffing KA, Hoppes P, Blend D, et al. Eosinophils in urine revisited. Clin Nephrol. 1994;41:163–6.
19. Linton AL, Richmond JM, Clark WF, et al. Gallium scintigraphy in the diagnosis of acute renal disease. Clin Nephrol. 1985;24: 84–7.
20. Schwartz A, Krause PH, Kunzendorf U, et al. The outcome of acute interstitial nephritis: risk factors for the transition from acute to chronic interstitial nephritis. Clin Nephrol. 2000;54: 179–90.
21. Bhaumik SK, Kher V, Arora P, et al. Evaluation of clinical and histological prognostic markers in drug-induced acute interstitial nephritis. Ren Fail. 1996;18:97–104.
22. Ivanyi B, Hamilton-Dutoit SJ, Hansen HE, Olsen S. Acute tubulointerstitial nephritis: phenotype of infiltrating cells and prognostic impact of tubulitis. Virchows Arch. 1996;428:5–12.
23. Kida H, Abe T, Tomosugi N, et al. Prediction of the long-term outcome in acute interstitial nephritis. Clin Nephrol. 1984;22: 55–60.
24. Laberke HG, Bohle A. Acute interstitial nephritis: correlation between clinical and morphological findings. Clin Nephrol. 1980;14: 263–73.
25. Koselj M, Kveder R, Bren AF, Rott T. Acute renal failure in patients with drug-induced acute interstitial nephritis. Ren Fail. 1993;15:69–72.
26. Handa SP. Drug-induced acute interstitial nephritis : report of 10 cases. CMAJ. 1986;135:1278–81.
27. Joh K, Aizawa S, Yamaguchi Y, et al. Drug-induced hypersensitivity nephritis: lymphocyte stimulation testing and renal biopsy in 10 cases. Am J Nephrol. 1990;10:222–30.
28. Shibasaki T, Ishimoto F, Sakai O, et al. Clinical characterization of drug-induced allergic nephritis. Am J Nephrol. 1991;11:174–80.
29. Settergren B, Ahlm C, Alexeyev O, et al. Pathogenetic and clinical aspects of the renal involvement in hemorrhagic fever with renal syndrome. Ren Fail. 1997;19:1–14.
30. Nochy D, Glotz D, Dosquet P, et al. Renal disease associated with HIV infection: a multicentric study of 60 patients from Paris hospitals. Nephrol Dial Transplant. 1993;8:11–19.
31. Gobel U, Kettritz R, Schneider W, Luft F. The protean face of renal sarcoidosis. J Am Soc Nephrol. 2001;12:616–23.
32. Hannedouche T, Grateau G, Noël LH. Renal granulomatous sarcoidosis: report of six cases. Nephrol Dial Transplant. 1990;5:18–24.
33. Goules A, Masouridi S, Tzioufas AG, et al. Clinically significant and biopsy-documented renal involvement in primary Sjogren syndrome. Medicine 2000;79:241–9.
34. Singh AK, Ucci A, Madias NE. Predominant tubulointerstitial lupus nephritis. Am J Kidney Dis. 1996;27:273–8.
35. Brouland JP, Meeus F, Rossert J, et al. Primary bilateral B-cell renal lymphoma: a case report and review of the literature. Am J Kidney Dis. 1994;24:586–9.
36. Vohra S, Eddy A, Levin AV, et al. Tubulointerstitial nephritis and uveitis in children and adolescents. Four new cases and a review of the literature. Pediatr Nephrol. 1999;13:426–32.
37. Takemura T, Okada M, Hino S, et al. Course and outcome of tubulointerstitial nephritis and uveitis syndrome. Am J Kidney Dis. 1999;34:1016–21.
38. Spital A, Panner BJ, Sterns RH. Acute idiopathic tubulointerstitial nephritis: report of two cases and review of the literature. Am J Kidney Dis. 1987;9:71–8.
39. Josephson MA, Chiu MY, Woodle ES, et al. Drug-induced acute interstitial nephritis in renal allografts: histopathologic features and clinical course in six patients. Am J Kidney Dis. 1999;34:540-8.
40. Randhawa PS, Demetris AJ. Nephropathy due to polyomavirus type BK. N Engl J Med. 2000;342:1361–3.

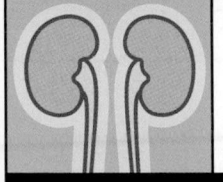

Section 12 Tubulointerstitial Disease

Chapter 61

Vesicoureteral Reflux and Reflux Nephropathy

Kelvin Lynn

DEFINITION

Primary vesicoureteral reflux (VUR) is a common congenital abnormality of the urinary tract that may be inherited. The most common presentations are fetal hydronephrosis or a urinary tract infection in early childhood. Repeated infections in infants and children with congenital or hereditary VUR may lead to renal scarring. The small, contracted, irregularly scarred kidney that occurs in association with VUR is termed reflux nephropathy (Fig. 61.1)[1]. Reflux nephropathy may present with urinary tract infections, hypertension, proteinuria or renal failure; and its presentation may not occur until adulthood[2]. While reflux nephropathy usually refers to a tubulointerstitial lesion with grossly scarred kidneys, some cases may also be associated with a glomerular lesion (focal and segmental glomerulosclerosis and hyalinosis), proteinuria and progressive deterioration of renal function[3].

Chronic interstitial inflammation associated with leukocytes (lymphocytes and polymorphonuclear cells) and macroscopic scars has often been called chronic pyelonephritis. It was previously thought that chronic pyelonephritis was almost exclusively caused by chronic bacterial infections of the kidney. Most cases of chronic tubulointerstitial inflammation with macroscopic renal scars are caused by reflux nephropathy, although similar histologic lesions (previously referred to as chronic pyelonephritis) may occur with obstructive uropathy or analgesic nephropathy (see Chapter 62)[4].

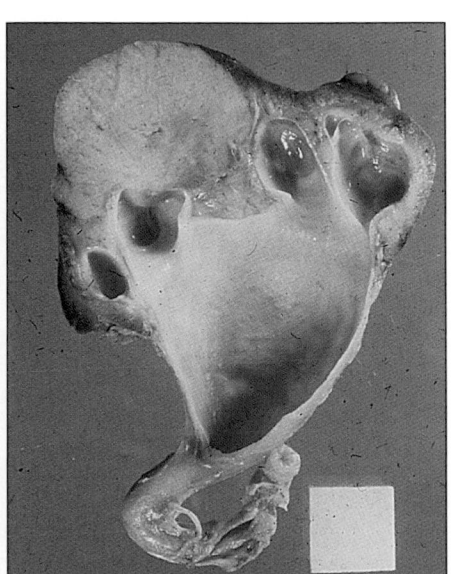

Figure 61.1 Renal pathology in reflux nephropathy. Small kidney damaged by gross vesicoureteral reflux (VUR) shows focal cortical scarring and a preserved renal lobe. (Reproduced with permission[2].)

There is scanty evidence in humans that urinary tract infection, without VUR, leads to the development or progression of renal scarring. Urinary tract infection in adults with VUR is also only rarely associated with the formation of new renal scars or progressive renal disease.

EPIDEMIOLOGY

VUR is the most common anatomic disorder affecting the urinary tract, with a prevalence of 0.4–1.8%[5]. VUR may be able to be detected *in utero* by fetal ultrasound beginning at 17 to 20 weeks' gestation. A dilated renal pelvis (> 10 mm anterioposterior diameter) suggests the diagnosis. VUR, in varying degrees of severity, has been detected by ultrasonography in up to 1.0% of healthy neonates, mostly boys. Premature infants have an increased incidence of VUR that disappears spontaneously by the time of expected maturity[6]. In babies born at term, VUR demonstrated in the first few days of life may also disappear by 4 weeks of age and will resolve spontaneously in 40% of patients by 2 years of age. Only a small number of children with VUR progress to reflux nephropathy.

Hydronephrosis is also a common fetal urinary tract abnormality. VUR is subsequently demonstrated during the neonatal period in 10–38% of such cases, depending on the fetal renal pelvic diameter chosen to initiate postnatal investigation[7,8]. Most studies of fetal hydronephrosis report a marked male preponderance and usually gross VUR.

Severe VUR and renal damage occurring in early life is more commonly observed in boys. Urinary tract infections in neonates are also associated with equal frequency of VUR in both males and females. However, after the first year of life, urinary tract infections are rare in boys, even if they have VUR[9,10].

As a consequence, reflux nephropathy is more common in girls than in boys[2,9].

Reflux nephropathy is responsible for approximately 10% of all cases of treated end-stage renal disease (ESRD) and is the commonest cause of ESRD in children[2]. ESRD from reflux nephropathy in children aged under 16 years at the time of starting renal replacement therapy is approximately equal for both sexes and, for older patients, there is only a small female preponderance[11].

ETIOLOGY AND PATHOGENESIS

Primary VUR is the regurgitation of urine through a congenitally incompetent vesicoureteral junction that starts *in utero* (Fig. 61.2). VUR may be inherited as an autosomal dominant

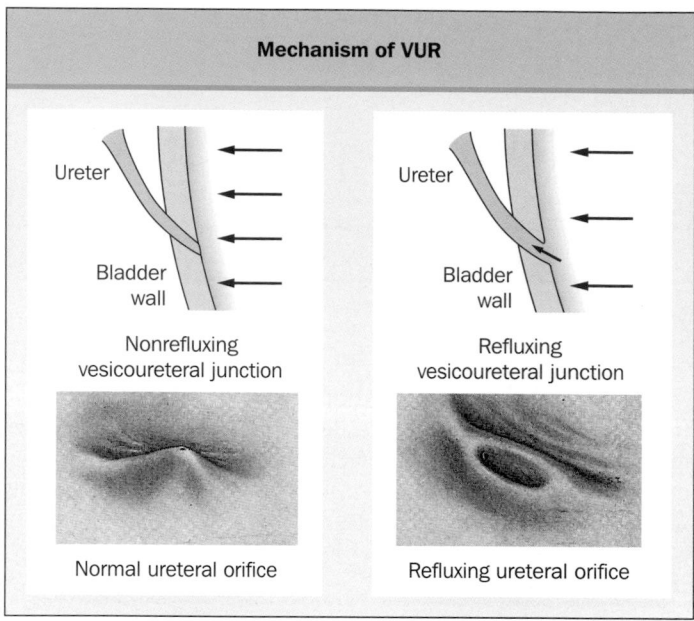

Mechanism of VUR

Ureter

Bladder wall

Nonrefluxing vesicoureteral junction

Normal ureteral orifice

Ureter

Bladder wall

Refluxing vesicoureteral junction

Refluxing ureteral orifice

Figure 61.2 Pathogenesis of VUR. (a) Competent and (b) incompetent vesicoureteral junctions and ureteral orifices.

trait[12] (Fig. 61.3). There is a 30–50-fold increase in VUR in first-degree relatives of patients with VUR or reflux nephropathy compared to the normal population, and there is preliminary evidence of linkage to chromosome 1[13]. There is a suggested linkage of some cases with the *PAX2* gene[12]. The renin–angiotensin system is also important in renal development and there was some suggestive evidence that abnormalities in the AT2 receptor might be associated with urinary tract obstruction or reflux, although these studies have not been confirmed. However, there is some evidence suggesting that the angiotensin converting enzyme (ACE) DD genotype (which is associated with higher ACE levels) may be a susceptibility factor contributing to renal scarring and more rapid deterioration in renal function in patients with reflux nephropathy[14,15].

Finally, high grade VUR is also associated with hyperreflexia of the detrusor muscle in the bladder wall which may or may not have a genetic basis[16,17].

In health, when the pressure in the bladder exceeds that in the ureter, VUR is prevented by the presence of a valve mechanism at the vesicoureteral junction (Fig. 61.2). The submucosal segment of the ureter is critical for competence. Important factors are the length of the intramural portion of the ureter, the nature of the ureteric orifice, and the integrity of the bladder wall musculature[2]. Incompetence of the vesicoureteral junction results from shortness of the submucosal segment caused by congenital lateral ectopia of the ureteric orifice. Further shortening of this segment of ureter may occur when the bladder is full. In such cases, VUR may occur only when the bladder is full or during voiding. The configuration and position of the ureteric orifice seen at cystoscopy (more lateral and wider than normal) can be correlated with the presence of VUR. The intravesical ureter lengthens with age, with the consequence that reflux often resolves.

VUR can also occur secondary to bladder disease. Lower urinary tract dysfunction resulting from detrusor instability or detrusor-sphincter dyssynergia may cause, or worsen, existing VUR[18]. Bladder inflammation, caused by tuberculosis or bilharziasis, bladder neck obstruction, surgery to the ureteric orifice, or the neurogenic bladder resulting from spina bifida or spinal cord injury may cause VUR.

Intrarenal VUR, usually at the polar regions of the kidney where focal scarring mostly occurs, may be seen in some children during micturating (voiding) cystourography (VCUG)[19] (Fig. 61.4). There is a high correlation between the areas where intrarenal reflux occurs and the associated cortical atrophy and calyceal clubbing. Intrarenal reflux usually occurs into extensively fused or compound papillae, while the simple or cone-shaped papillae do not appear to permit intrarenal reflux. Two-thirds of children's kidneys contain at least one refluxing papilla, most commonly found at the upper pole of the kidney[20].

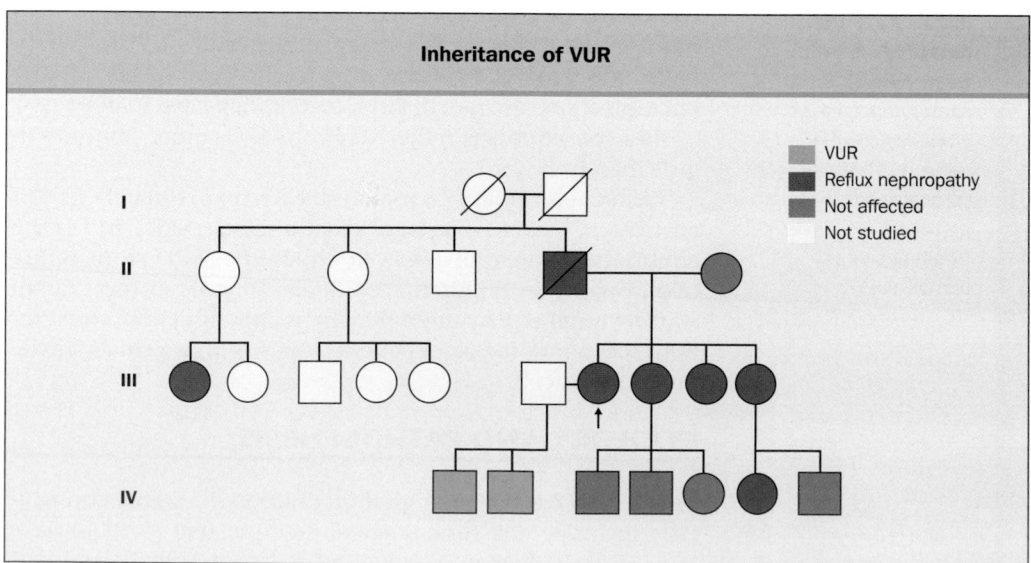

Inheritance of VUR

- VUR
- Reflux nephropathy
- Not affected
- Not studied

I

II

III

IV

Figure 61.3 Inheritance of VUR. A pedigree showing evidence of autosomal dominant inheritance of VUR. The female proband in generation III (arrow) was found to have a urinary tract infection at 4 years of age. Investigations revealed bilateral VUR and reflux nephropathy. Her father, was found to have bilateral reflux nephropathy, hypertension and proteinuria. He reached ESRD at the age of 71 years. The proband's first child was born at 36 weeks' gestation and found to have bilateral gross VUR. Repeat studies at age 6 weeks showed resolution of the VUR.

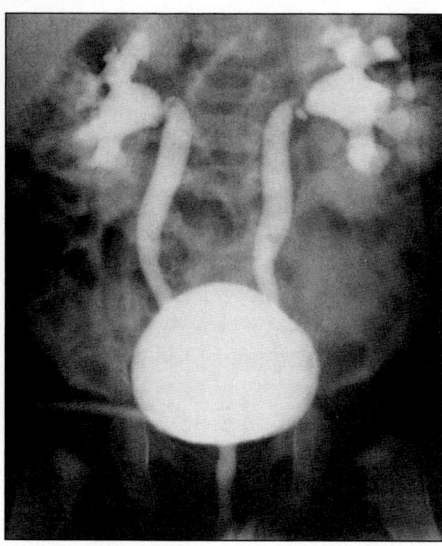

Figure 61.4 Gross VUR and intrarenal reflux. A voiding cystourethrogram showing bilateral grade V VUR and intrarenal reflux into several renal lobes in an infant presenting with urinary tract infection.

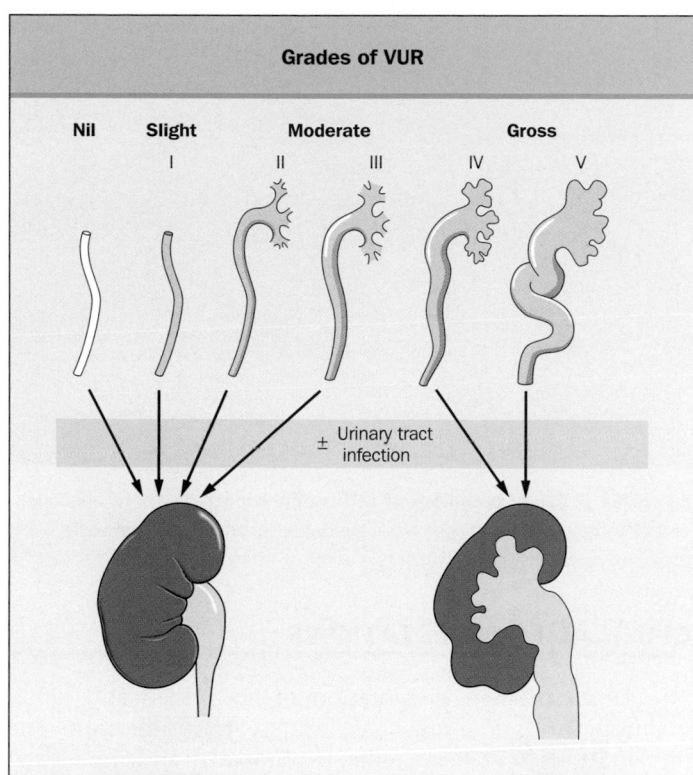

Figure 61.5 Classification of VUR and renal scarring. The relation between the grade of VUR (International Reflux Study)[21], urinary tract infection and renal scarring.

Renal scarring

There appear to be two distinct forms of renal damage associated with VUR, namely focal scars usually associated with urinary tract infection and a less specific global form resulting in a generalized reduction in kidney size[9].

Acquired renal scarring

The focal renal scars that characterize reflux nephropathy develop in infancy or early childhood. Two factors appear to be necessary for scar formation: VUR severe enough to result in intrarenal reflux and urinary infection[2,3]. The risk of renal scarring is proportional to the severity of reflux (Fig. 61.5)[21,22]. Focal renal scarring may be present at birth, with gross VUR having occurred *in utero*, but it is most commonly found after the investigation of a urinary tract infection in young girls.

Prospective studies in children suggest that the usual initiating event leading to renal scarring is a urinary tract infection. Intrarenal reflux facilitates renal parenchymal infection with subsequent scarring and contracture of the affected renal pyramids. The rest of the kidney grows normally or even becomes hypertrophic. These two processes cause the depth of the renal scar to increase with age and growth.

Primary, congenital renal scarring

Risdon[4] reported a less common, but more severe form, of reflux nephropathy that is observed primarily in boys with congenital renal maldevelopment and gross VUR in the absence of urinary infection. The kidneys in such children are small and smooth without gross focal scarring and have histologic evidence of dysplasia. This form of reflux nephropathy is often associated with fetal pelvic dilatation and renal impairment. As with other forms of reflux nephropathy, the degree of VUR is the most important determinant of renal damage[7]. In one-third of cases, there is renal impairment without a previous history of urinary tract infection. Half of the boys with gross VUR have a hypercontractile, small volume bladder[17].

Progression to ESRD

Progression to ESRD occurs in patients with gross VUR whose kidneys have sustained severe, bilateral renal scarring

Factors contributing to progression of renal impairment in reflux nephropathy
Extensive renal damage in childhood
Hypertension
Secondary focal and segmental glomerulosclerosis
Altered intrarenal and glomerular hemodynamics
? Angiotensin-converting enzyme DD genotype
Immunologic injury (e.g., immunologic response to intrarenal Tamm–Horsfall glycoprotein)

Table 61.1 Factors contributing to progression of renal impairment in reflux nephropathy.

(Table 61.1). Most of the initiating injury occurs during the first 5 years of life[2]. Less often, patients with lesser degrees of renal scarring, and sometimes only one kidney apparently involved, progress to ESRD. These patients often have proteinuria and focal segmental glomerulosclerosis in the unscarred areas of a reflux-damaged kidney or in the contralateral, macroscopically normal kidney (Fig. 61.6). It is suggested that the renal progression occurring in these patients is independent of VUR and urinary tract infection but rather is due to loss of renal mass that leads to maladaptive hemodynamic changes in the remaining glomeruli, resulting in progressive segmental focal and global glomerulosclerosis.

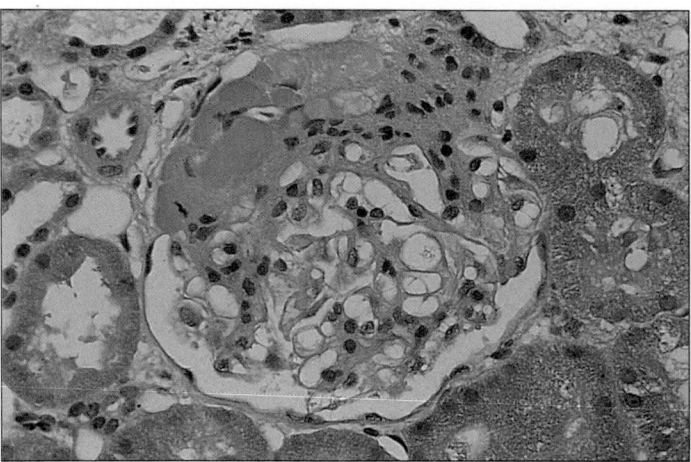

Figure 61.6 Renal pathology of reflux nephropathy. Light microscopy of a glomerulus showing segmental glomerulosclerosis and hyalinosis (hematoxylin and eosin ×400).

CLINICAL MANIFESTATIONS

The most common presentation of both VUR and reflux nephropathy is a complicated urinary tract infection. The presentations of VUR and reflux nephropathy are summarized in Tables 61.2 and 61.3.

Urinary tract infections

It is not fully understood why patients with VUR are prone to urinary infections. With severe VUR, stasis owing to the large volumes of refluxing urine probably plays a role. In 15–60%

Clinical presentations of VUR
Complicated urinary infection
Loin pain
Asymptomatic
Detected in the workup of members of an affected family
Detected by fetal ultrasonography
Detected during assessment of other urologic congenital abnormalities

Table 61.2 Clinical presentations of VUR.

Clinical presentations of reflux nephropathy
Complicated urinary infection
Hypertension benign or accelerated
During pregnancy: urine infection, hypertension, pre-eclampsia
Proteinuria
Renal failure
Urinary calculi
Asymptomatic
Detected in the workup of members of an affected family
Detected by fetal ultrasonography
Detected during assessment of other urologic congenital abnormalities

Table 61.3 Clinical presentations of reflux nephropathy.

of infants and children with urinary tract infection, there will be some form of VUR[5] and 8–13% of these will have radiologic evidence of reflux nephropathy (Table 61.4)[1].

In neonates, urinary infection usually presents as fever, jaundice, or failure to thrive. Therefore, the diagnosis of urinary tract infection may be difficult. Suprapubic aspiration of urine is a safe and effective method for obtaining uncontaminated urine.

Approximately 1% of all neonates, usually boys, have bacteriuria and approximately half have VUR of varying severity. Bacteriuria can be found on suprapubic aspiration of urine in 10% of sick infants, again mostly males. Bourchier et al. investigated 100 infants, 68 boys and 32 girls, who presented consecutively with urinary tract infection[6]. Of these, 36 infants had VUR, mostly grades III or IV. These studies show that, in neonates and infants, urinary infections are more common in boys and that with both sexes there is a high incidence of associated VUR. Studies of infants and young children with acute pyelonephritis, as defined by an abnormal scintigram using (^{99m}Tc)labeled dimercaptosuccinic acid (DMSA) as the tracer, have shown that from 30–60% have VUR. Panaretto et al.[23] found that, in preschool children, the risk factors for recurrent urinary tract infections were age less than 6 months and VUR of grades III to V.

After the first year of life, the prevalence of asymptomatic bacteriuria is very low in boys but is approximately 1% in girls. VUR is seen in one-third of preschool children with urinary infection[1,24].

Most authorities recommend that every infant or child should undergo urinary tract investigation after the first bacteriologically proven urinary tract infection[2]. There are a number of options for the appropriate investigation in such children[10,25]. A logical application of currently available techniques should take into account: (1) renal scarring is unusual after the age of 5 years; (2) VUR tends to resolve spontaneously with time; and (3) VCUG is an invasive and unpleasant procedure. In children under the age of 2 years, the first investigation remains the VCUG, together with imaging of the upper

Age, and prevalence of VUR in patients with urinary tract infection	
Age	Percentage with VUR
2–3 days	57
3–6 days	51
2–6 months	60
7–12 months	35
1–4 years	50
5–9 years	35
10–14 years	14
>14 years	10
Adult	5

Table 61.4 Age, and prevalence of VUR in patients with urinary tract infection[1].

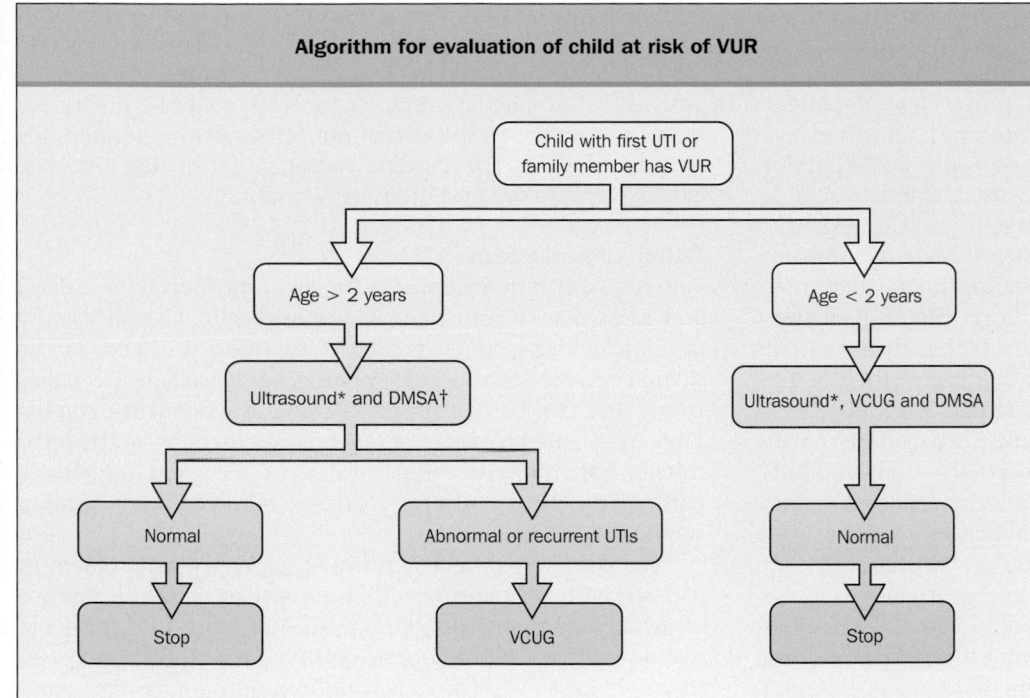

Algorithm for evaluation of child at risk of VUR

Figure 61.7 Algorithm for the evaluation of the child at risk of VUR.
*MAG3 renogram if evidence of obstruction. †> 5 years only with acute pyelonephritis.

urinary tract (Fig. 61.7). If gross VUR has been present from birth, renal scarring should be apparent by this age. If VUR is demonstrated, then further renal imaging with a DMSA scan is indicated (see Chapter 5). A VCUG can be reliably carried out as soon as any symptomatic urinary tract infection has been controlled. Delaying this investigation because of concerns of false-positive findings is unfounded.

With increasing age, other presentations of VUR become more common. Young women with urinary tract infections associated with onset of sexual activity may be shown to have reflux nephropathy not detected in infancy or early childhood. These patients may present with bacterial cystitis or acute pyelonephritis, often recurrent. Approximately 5% of sexually active women with urinary tract infection have reflux nephropathy. The diagnosis of VUR or reflux nephropathy may also be made after detection of asymptomatic bacteriuria in pregnancy.

Hypertension

Reflux nephropathy often causes hypertension, and 60% of adults with reflux nephropathy are hypertensive at presentation. Approximately 15% of adults with reflux nephropathy will present with hypertension or its complications and no history of urinary tract infection. Hypertension affects 10% of children with reflux nephropathy and is the most common cause of severe hypertension in children[25]. In adults, the hypertension is usually benign but may follow an accelerated course with deteriorating renal function. Hypertension may become apparent in women if they take the combined oral contraceptive or become pregnant. The risk of hypertension appears to be greater in males and increases with the degree of VUR, and the extent of renal damage[26,27]. Any role of the renin–angiotensin system remains unproven. The role of nephrectomy of a small contracted kidney, when the contralateral

kidney is normal or hypertrophied, in hypertensive patients for cure, or in normotensive patients for prevention of hypertension, is unclear. Hypertension accelerates the progression of reflux nephropathy and thus meticulous control of blood pressure is one of the most important aspects of its management.

Proteinuria

Proteinuria is a poor prognostic feature, indicating that the patient is likely to have focal and segmental glomerulosclerosis with hyalinosis (Fig. 61.6)[4]. Proteinuria may not be detected for many years after the renal scarring has occurred, although it may be present in childhood in patients with bilateral renal scarring. Proteinuria is more common in patients with renal impairment and severe bilateral reflux nephropathy and is one of the most serious complications of reflux nephropathy[27]. It is uncommon for the nephrotic syndrome to complicate reflux nephropathy.

Presentation during pregnancy

A pregnant woman with previously unrecognized reflux nephropathy may present during pregnancy with asymptomatic or symptomatic urinary tract infection, hypertension in early pregnancy, or severe pre-eclampsia.

Approximately 5% of women have asymptomatic bacteriuria in the first trimester of pregnancy and 5–33% of these women will have a urinary tract abnormality, most commonly reflux nephropathy. Approximately 4% of women with severe or atypical pre-eclampsia have reflux nephropathy[28]. The dilatation of the ureter seen with normal pregnancy can be distinguished from that seen with VUR. In pregnancy, the midportion of the ureter, more commonly the right, is dilated and the renal parenchymal morphology is normal.

Tubulointerstitial Disease

Renal failure

Reflux nephropathy is an important cause of chronic renal failure usually presenting with renal impairment, proteinuria, and/or hypertension. Only a small proportion of patients with renal failure have a history of urinary tract infection[11]. The urinary sediment findings are nonspecific. Older patients may have an accompanying type IV renal tubular acidosis and hyperkalemia. Reflux nephropathy should be excluded in any patient presenting with renal insufficiency and proteinuria, with or without hypertension or urinary tract infections. Approximately 10% of patients entering dialysis/transplant programs have reflux nephropathy. These patients develop ESRD at a mean age of 30 years (Table 61.5). The incidence of renal failure caused by reflux nephropathy is approximately equal between the sexes, in contrast to the female preponderance of reflux nephropathy itself in adults. This discrepancy is probably explained by the higher incidence of symptomatic urinary tract infection in girls leading to the discovery of underlying reflux nephropathy. In patients aged less than 16 years, reflux nephropathy is probably the most common cause of treated ESRD. Pretransplant bilateral nephrectomy may occasionally be necessary when there is ongoing VUR with infection that cannot be eradicated. Craig et al.[29] analyzed the incidence of ESRD in patients aged 5–44 years who were reported to the Australian and New Zealand Dialysis and Transplantation Registry (ANZDATA) between 1971 and 1998. They concluded that the treatment of VUR with ureteric reimplantation or prophylactic antibiotic therapy had not achieved a significant reduction in the incidence of renal failure due to reflux nephropathy. ESRD from reflux nephropathy is relatively rare in Swedish children. Swedish practice guidelines for the management of urinary tract infection and VUR emphasize the importance of early recognition and treatment of symptomatic urinary tract infections[10].

Familial VUR

Primary VUR is inherited in many patients (Fig. 61.3). In some patients, it may be accompanied by renal dysplasia[20]. There is a high degree of concordance in identical twins and support for autosomal dominant inheritance from fraternal twin and family studies. It is estimated that the gene frequency is 1 in 600, making VUR amongst the commonest autosomal dominant defects in humans. VUR will be found in approximately 50% of asymptomatic siblings and offspring of affected patients[13,26]. If a genetic marker for VUR could be identified, it would provide an excellent tool for screening populations at risk for VUR. The current radiologic screening tests are expensive, invasive and often unpleasant.

Other clinical features

Patients with reflux nephropathy may develop renal calculi and present with loin pain or ureteric colic. Calculi usually develop in the medullary cavities or clubbed calyces of the scarred regions of the kidney. Most renal calculi are radiopaque and can be demonstrated on intravenous urography. There is usually no evidence of a metabolic cause for the renal calculi. Patients with uncontrolled or recurrent infections, particularly those caused by *Proteus mirabilis*, may develop staghorn calculi.

Loin pain may pose a significant management problem in patients with VUR and/or reflux nephropathy. In the absence of urinary tract obstruction, continuing gross VUR, or acute pyelonephritis, reflux nephropathy does not cause pain. However, gross VUR in older children and adults may cause loin pain, particularly when the bladder is full or on the initiation of voiding. These patients may benefit from antireflux surgery.

Nocturnal enuresis and lower urinary tract dysfunction are common in children with VUR. A number of urologic abnormalities, including hypospadias, undescended testes, a bifid collecting system, and pelviureteric junction obstruction may be associated with primary VUR.

PATHOLOGY

Chronic pyelonephritis is only one of several causes of chronic tubulointerstitial nephritis and the histologic features of chronic pyelonephritis itself are nonspecific. The presence of urinary infection is insufficient to confirm the diagnosis. Most of the observations on human pathology have been made on kidneys removed because of hypertension or uncontrolled urinary tract infection, or prior to renal transplantation. The recognition of the pivotal role that VUR

Patient group	1971–80		1981–90		1991–2000	
	Male	Female	Male	Female	Male	Female
Number of patients entering renal replacement programs	2651	2147	4689	3844	9700	7202
Number of patients with reflux nephropathy (%)	173 (6.5)	203 (9.5)	293 (6.2)	368 (9.6)	360 (3.7)	492 (6.8)
Number of patients <16 years of age	110	87	162	133	202	152
Number <16 years old with reflux nephropathy (%)	27 (24.5)	29 (33.3)	31 (19.1)	28 (21.1)	35 (17.3)	18 (11.8)

Incidence of end-stage reflux nephropathy in Australia and New Zealand 1971–2000

Table 61.5 Incidence of end-stage reflux nephropathy in Australia and New Zealand 1971–2000.

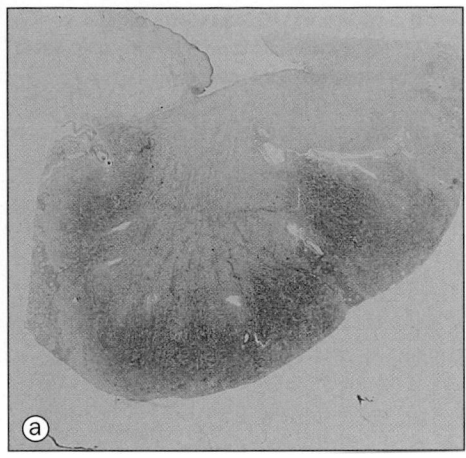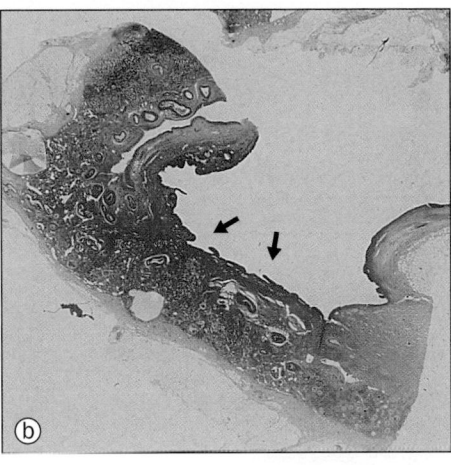

Figure 61.8 Renal pathology of reflux nephropathy. Light microscopy of a small kidney removed from an adult with advanced reflux nephropathy. (a) Preserved renal lobe; (b) full-thickness scar (arrows) (hematoxylin and eosin).

plays in the pathogenesis of reflux nephropathy has improved the understanding of chronic pyelonephritis[2]. The pathologic diagnosis of reflux nephropathy requires, in addition to the demonstration of a chronic tubulointerstitial nephritis, assessment of clinical features, particularly by radiology, and macroscopic examination of the kidney[3].

The gross changes and cardinal features of reflux nephropathy are coarse, segmental scars, most commonly at the renal poles, involving the medulla and cortex and overlying a clubbed calyx (Figs 61.1 and 61.8). Depending on the degree of scarring, the kidneys may be reduced in size. One or both kidneys may be involved. The degree of atrophy varies from lobe to lobe. Commonly, there is at least one normal or hypertrophied renal lobe. If gross VUR has persisted, the ureter will be tortuous, dilated, and hypertrophied. There may be generalized dilatation of the pelvicalyceal system with atrophy of pyramids and hypertrophy of the pelvicalyceal smooth muscle. The capsule may be thickened and adherent, particularly when urinary infections have been frequent and severe. The relationship of the full-thickness scar to the underlying dilated calyx is the critical feature that differentiates reflux nephropathy from other causes of renal scarring or small kidneys (Fig. 61.1)[18].

In the scarred areas of the kidney, the major microscopic changes are tubular atrophy or complete loss. There are variable degrees of interstitial fibrosis and chronic inflammation, with a cellular infiltrate composed mostly of lymphocytes and plasma cells (Fig. 61.9). The severity of interstitial nephritis is usually correlated with the presence of urinary infection. Lymphoid follicles may be present. Collections of dilated atrophic tubules lined by atrophic epithelium and filled with homogeneous eosinophilic casts may give a thyroid-like appearance. These changes are not specific for reflux nephropathy. Rounded masses of pale-staining material that include Tamm–Horsfall glycoprotein, which has apparently extravasated from ruptured tubules, can be seen in the outer medullary and cortical interstitium. Glomeruli within scarred areas are crowded together and may appear normal, collapsed, or completely hyalinized. Collagenous thickening of Bowman's capsule may lead to periglomerular fibrosis. Vascular changes are frequent within scars, with medial hypertrophy and concentric fibroelastic intimal hyperplasia with luminal narrowing.

In patients without severe bilateral renal scarring, ongoing VUR, hypertension, or recurrent urinary infection, renal failure

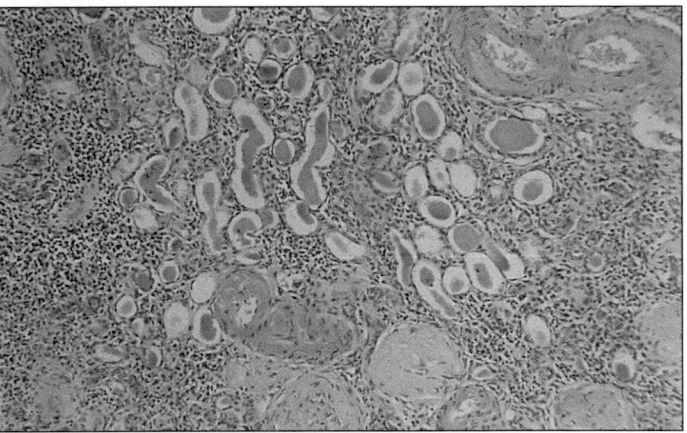

Figure 61.9 Microscopic changes in reflux nephropathy. Low-power view of renal cortex showing sclerosed glomeruli, chronic cellular infiltrate, and dilated, atrophic tubules, with eosinophilic casts and thick-walled blood vessels (hematoxylin and eosin ×40).

may develop. Clinically, these patients are characterized by the development of hypertension and, histologically, by the presence of focal and segmental glomerulosclerosis and hyalinosis affecting the unscarred regions of the kidney (Fig. 61.6)[4].

DIAGNOSIS

Algorithms describing the investigation of a child after the first urinary tract infection or the finding of fetal renal pelvic dilatation are shown in Figures 61.7 and 61.10. Screening of individuals without urinary tract infection or clinical renal disease is only warranted in the siblings and offspring of those with VUR or reflux nephropathy.

Diagnosis of VUR
Voiding cystourethrography
Voiding cystourethrography (VCUG) remains the most accurate method for detecting VUR (Figs 61.4, 61.11c and 61.12c). Radiographs are taken after bladder filling and during voiding. Bladder pressures and flow rates may also be measured. VUR is classified according to the extent and degree of ureteric filling and dilatation and the degree of dilatation of the collecting system, particularly the minor calyces. The

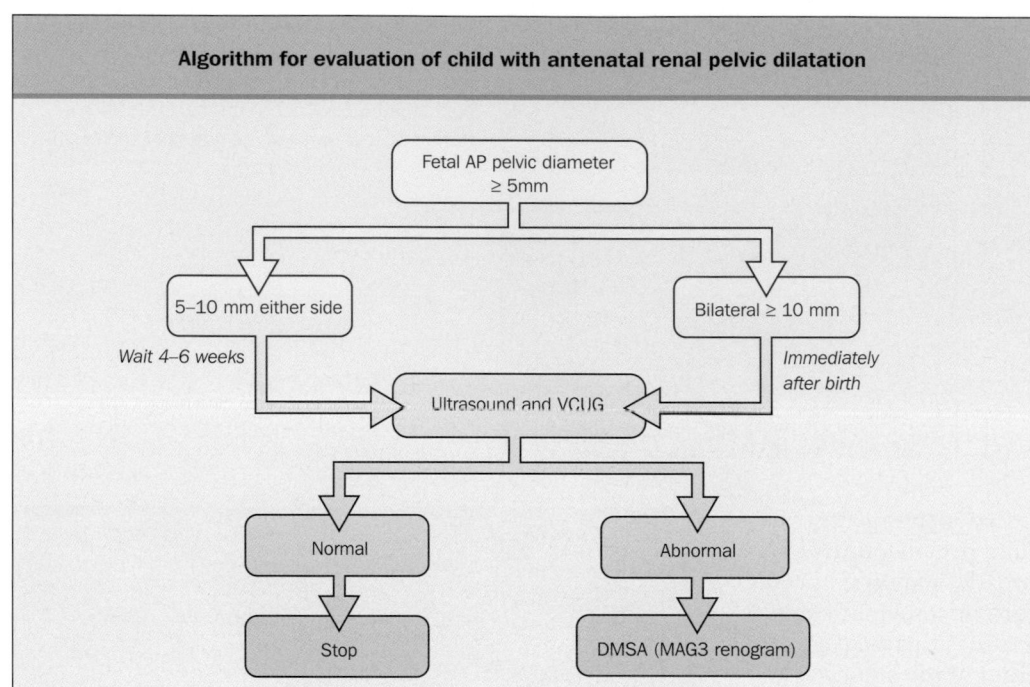

Figure 61.10 Algorithm for the evaluation of the child with antenatal renal pelvic dilatation.

bladder volume at which reflux is first seen and any intrarenal reflux should be recorded. The most widely used classification is that developed by the International Reflux Study in Children, which utilizes five grades, with three grades to describe gross VUR (Fig. 61.5 and Table 61.6)[21].

Voiding cystourethrography is not usually indicated in adults but may rarely be considered where surgical correction of VUR is warranted to manage recurrent acute pyelonephritis or flank pain with voiding.

Radionuclide micturating cystography
Substituting a radionuclide for contrast medium is an effective and sensitive means of demonstrating VUR. The estimated dose of gonadal radiation of 40–50 µGy is similar to that of a conventional VCUG. Radionuclide micturating cystography is a useful technique for follow-up of patients whose VUR is managed conservatively.

Ultrasonography
Ultrasonography, utilizing color Doppler or contrast enhancement, may demonstrate dilatation and other abnormalities of the pelvicalyceal system and ureter; in expert hands, this technique provides dynamic information on ureteric function and the position of the ureteric orifices.

Diagnosis of reflux nephropathy
Radionuclide scanning
Radionuclide scanning with DMSA is now the preferred technique for imaging reflux nephropathy. Focal defects seen with radionuclide scanning represent areas of underperfusion that are shown by reduced proximal tubular uptake of radionuclide (Figs 61.11d, 61.12b and 61.13). DMSA scanning is particularly useful for imaging the upper poles of the kidney, an area where intravenous urography (IVU) may fail to demonstrate scarring (Fig. 61.12a,b). In addition, the DMSA

	International classification of VVR
Grade	**Degree of VUR**
I	Ureter only
II	Ureter, pelvis, and calyces with no dilatation and with normal calyceal fornices
III	Mild or moderate dilatation and/or tortuosity of the ureter and mild or moderate dilatation of the pelvis; no or slight blunting of the fornices
IV	Moderate dilatation and/or tortuosity of the ureter, and moderate dilatation of the pelvis and calyces. Complete obliteration of the pelvis and calyces. Complete obliteration of the sharp angles of the fornices but maintenance of the papillary impressions in the majority of the calyces (Fig. 61.12c)
V	Gross dilatation and tortuosity of the ureter, pelvis, and calyces. The papillary impressions are no longer visible in the majority of calyces (Fig. 61.11c)

Table 61.6 International Reflux Study in Children classification of VUR (Figure 61.5)[12].

scan provides information on individual kidney function. There is excellent concordance between the findings on IVU and DMSA scanning in children with primary VUR. The DMSA scan is capable of detecting scars not apparent on IVU, suggesting that abnormalities demonstrated with radionuclide scanning precede those detected with IVU[30]. DMSA scanning is the preferred imaging technique for adults with suspected reflux nephropathy.

Ultrasonography
Ultrasonography can demonstrate many of the features of reflux nephropathy and is now being used as the first renal

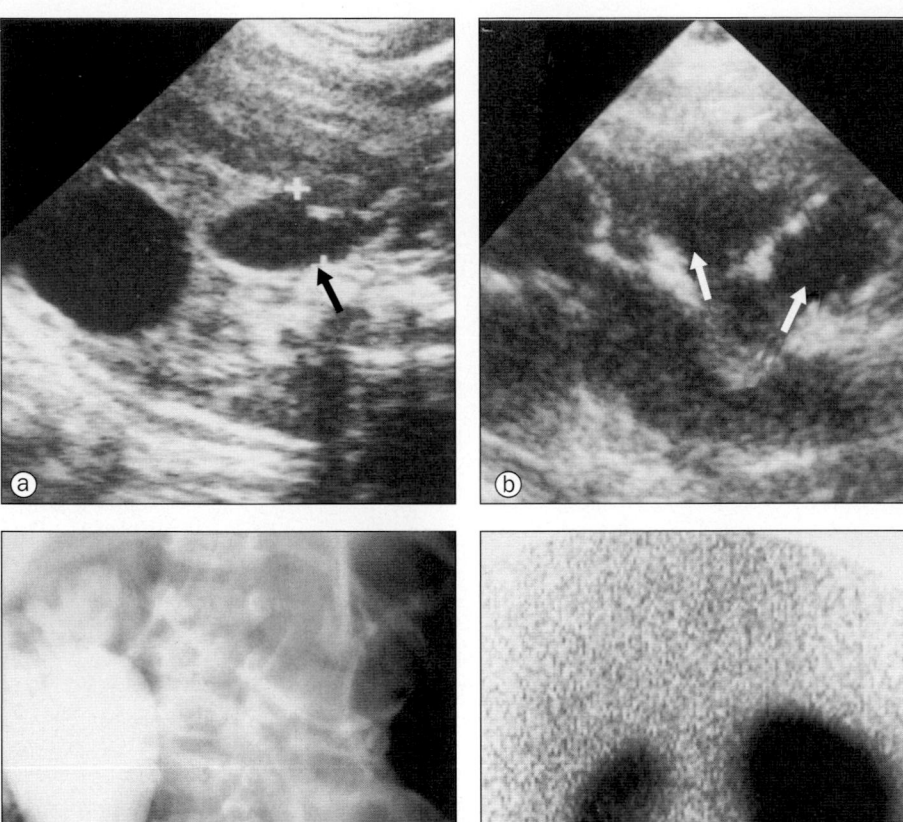

Figure 61.11 Infant with moderate antenatal renal dilatation, abnormal postnatal sonogram and grade V VUR. (a) Antenatal sonogram at 25 weeks' gestation showing longitudinal view of markedly dilated right upper urinary tract (anteroposterior diameter of renal pelvis 17 mm) (arrow). (b) Postnatal sonogram of right kidney showing pelvicalyceal dilatation and thinning of renal parenchyma (arrows). (c) VCUG showing grade V VUR on the right and grade II VUR on the left. (d) DMSA scan (anterior view) showing globally scarred right kidney with 12% uptake. (Reproduced with permission[39].)

imaging technique in many centers in the work-up of children with a urinary tract infection (Figs 61.7 and 61.11b). Ultrasonography is noninvasive, does not use ionizing radiation and gives a rapid overview of renal anatomy and the dimensions of the pelvicalyceal collecting system.

Other techniques
IVU with nephrotomography, performed in a well-prepared patient given an adequate amount of contrast medium, enables measurement of renal lengths and cortical thickness. The morphology of the papillae can be inferred from the calyceal appearances (Fig. 61.13).

[99mTc]labeled mercaptoacetyl triglycine (MAG3) renography is a dynamic study that provides information on both the renal parenchymal uptake and the pelvic and ureteric outflow. It is particularly useful in the presence of renal impairment and for the detection of urinary tract obstruction.

Computed tomography will readily demonstrate focal renal scarring but is not used routinely because of the need for intravenous contrast medium, the radiation dose and cost.

Antenatal detection of VUR
VUR is found in 10–38% of neonates or infants with antenatally detected hydronephrosis or other renal abnormalities depending on the cut-off level of renal pelvic dilatation used. The two largest studies[7,8], involving a total of 22 800 pregnancies, used a cut-off of 5 mm anteroposterior fetal renal pelvic diameter and found VUR in 22% and 10%, respectively. Postnatal urinary tract investigations should include urinary tract ultrasonography and VCUG (Fig. 61.10). The degree of fetal renal pelvic dilatation does not predict the presence of postnatal dilatation, nor the severity of VUR demonstrated by VCUG. When renal damage is present at birth, it is usually global and associated with dilating VUR in boys (Fig 61.11).

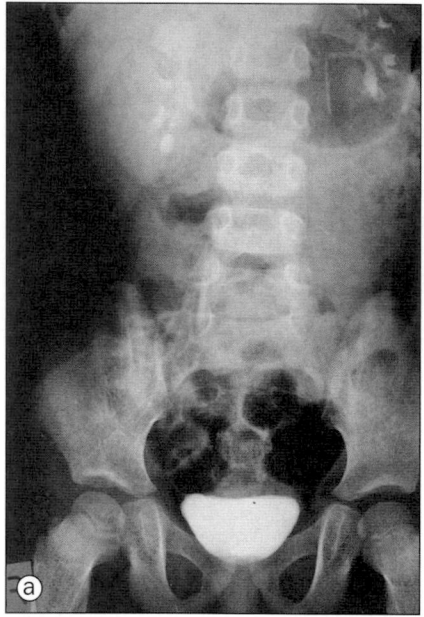 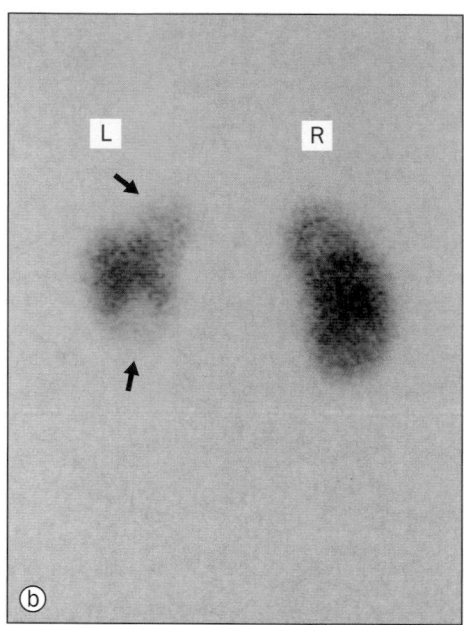 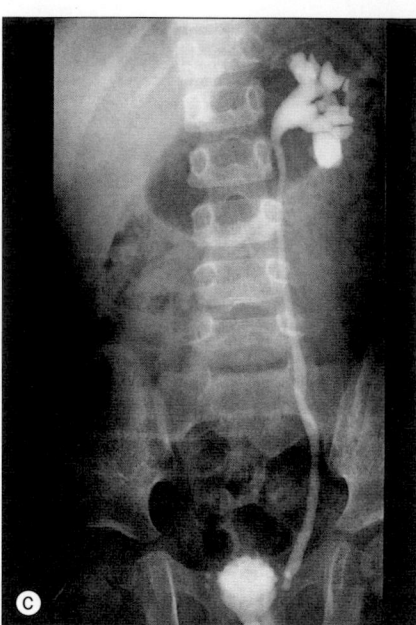

Figure 61.12 Investigation of reflux nephropathy. Investigation of a 3-year-old child with urinary tract infection. (a) Intravenous urogram showing calyceal diverticulum in the upper pole of the right kidney and renal scarring in upper pole and, probably, the lower pole of the left kidney. (b) DMSA scintigram (posterior view), demonstrating upper and lower pole scarring (arrows) in the left kidney. (c) Voiding cystourethrogram showing grade IV vesicoureteral reflux on the left.

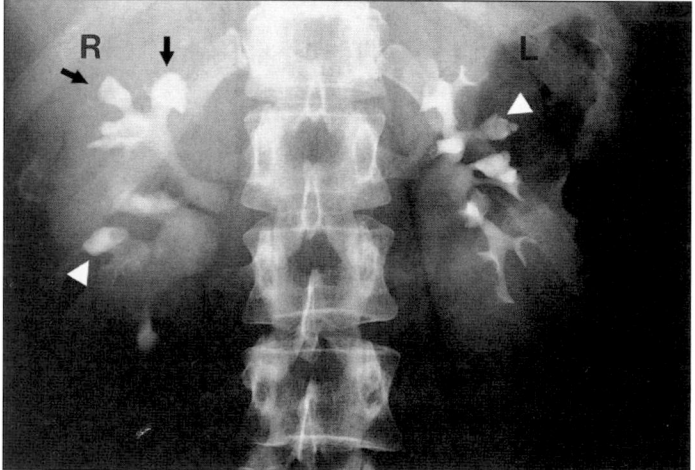

Figure 61.13 Reflux nephropathy in an adult. Intravenous urogram in a 30-year-old woman showing scarring in the upper poles of both kidneys (black arrows) and the lower pole of the right kidney (arrowhead).

DIFFERENTIAL DIAGNOSIS

Reflux nephropathy should be considered in any patient, particularly a child, with unexplained renal impairment or hypertension. The absence of a history of urinary tract infection does not exclude the diagnosis. The urinary sediment findings are unremarkable but most patients have low-grade pyuria. Nephrotic-range proteinuria is rare. In children, the differential diagnosis of a small kidney will include obstructive uropathy from a pelviureteric junction obstruction or achalasia of the ureter and congenital renal dysplasia.

Appropriate radiologic investigations should enable confident differentiation in most cases. In the adult, the differential diagnoses include obstructive uropathy, analgesic nephropathy and ischemic nephropathy. The radiologic changes in these conditions are usually distinct from reflux nephropathy. Patients with analgesic nephropathy have a lengthy history of consumption of combinational analgesics, or nonsteroidal anti-inflammatory agents, and of papillary necrosis. Obstructive uropathy results in global not focal changes to the kidney. Patients with ischemic nephropathy usually have evidence of atheromatous vascular disease affecting heart, brain or limbs; although focal scars may occur, the usual morphologic change is a global regular reduction in renal size.

NATURAL HISTORY

It is well recognized that some kidneys subjected to VUR become progressively damaged while others remain unaffected. Observations by Rolleston et al. demonstrated that the severity of VUR was the single most important factor predicting renal scarring[22]. Bailey reported on the long-term follow-up of 31 infants (16 boys) with gross VUR identified during the first year of life between 1952 and 1970[31]. These infants presented at a mean age of 15 weeks and 24 of the 31 had a urinary tract infection. None of the children underwent ureteric reimplantation. Twelve of the twenty-six children who developed reflux nephropathy had renal scarring at the time of diagnosis of VUR. The remaining 14 patients who subsequently developed reflux nephropathy did so by the age of 5 years and mostly by the age of 3 years. A group of 20 patients have remained under follow-up for up to 34 years after presentation. Four have normal kidneys, 11 have unilateral reflux nephropathy and five (two with renal impairment) have bilateral reflux nephropathy.

Smellie[32] has described the natural history of VUR in 226 children, 85 of whom had renal scarring, who presented at a median age of 5 years and were followed for up to 41 years. One hundred and ninety-three were managed conservatively and 33 were treated surgically. VUR resolved in 69% and no renal scars developed after puberty. The development of hypertension and/or renal impairment in 17 adults (7.5%) was considered predictable because of the degree of renal scarring, blood pressure and renal function in childhood.

Kidneys subjected to gross reflux usually undergo a steady decline in function, probably mediated by hemodynamic and nonimmunologic mechanisms (Table 61.1)[26]. Kidneys with lesser degrees of VUR, or no continuing reflux, are less likely to suffer a decline in individual function. Assessment of individual kidney glomerular filtration rate by radionuclide techniques has shown that only the kidneys suffering gross VUR have reduced function.

TREATMENT

The most important aim in the treatment of the patient with VUR is the prevention of renal scarring and subsequent renal failure. There is no place for antireflux surgery to prevent renal scarring in adults with ongoing VUR. The question of the best treatment for children is much more contentious. To date, there is no evidence to confirm whether medical treatment with continuous antimicrobial therapy or surgical repair is the best treatment for VUR. Few surgeons now operate on grades I–III VUR (Fig 61.5), which tend to resolve spontaneously.

Surgical versus medical treatment

There have been four controlled trials comparing medical and surgical therapy for grades II–IV VUR[18] and one for grade V VUR[33]. Unfortunately, they have not resolved the controversy regarding the best treatment for VUR, nor have they provided reassurance that either form of therapy reduces the incidence of ESRD from reflux nephropathy[29]. It should be noted that there have been no placebo controlled trials of medical or surgical treatment. Some studies have had insufficient numbers of infants, many of the children enrolled had already developed renal scars by the time of enrollment, and children with grade V VUR were excluded from all but one of the studies[33]. The complications of medical and surgical treatments were poorly reported. Surgery corrects VUR in over 95% of cases but does not decrease the incidence of urinary infections, with the possible exception of recurrent acute pyelonephritis. Antireflux surgery may be indicated in a few adults with VUR and recurrent acute pyelonephritis or flank pain with voiding.

In general, even the best designed studies have been unable to show a difference for the development of new scars or renal growth between medical and surgical treatment over follow up periods of up to 10 years. Surgery is of no benefit if proteinuria, renal impairment, or hypertension is present[34]. Prospective studies in girls over 4 years of age have shown that reflux nephropathy rarely develops in kidneys that are normal even when there is ongoing VUR and urinary infections[35]. Moreover, in careful prospective studies carried out in the UK in girls aged over 4 years with VUR, ongoing asymptomatic bacteriuria was not associated with worsening of renal function, and there

was no benefit from intermittent antimicrobial therapy, regardless of whether reflux nephropathy was present[36].

Surgery and medical treatment can be seen as equally effective, or ineffective. Each treatment has its advantages and disadvantages. Consideration of the best treatment for any child should be determined by the preferences of the parents, expected compliance with long-term medical therapy, and the knowledge that spontaneous resolution of the severe grades of VUR is uncommon. Infancy and early childhood are the critical times for the formation of scars in children with gross VUR. With this in mind, it is imperative that those at most risk of VUR and reflux nephropathy (siblings and the offspring of those with VUR) undergo screening, including renal imaging with ultrasonography and/or DMSA scintigraphy and VCUG, early in life (Fig. 61.7).

Urinary tract infections

The management of urinary tract infections in patients with VUR is the same as for any complicated urinary infection (see Chapter 53). The aim of therapy is to alleviate symptoms and to prevent bacterial invasion of the kidney. Bacteriologically confirmed urinary infections should be treated with a curative course of antibiotic therapy, usually over 5 days[2]. Combined or single-dose therapy is not indicated for infants and children with VUR and cystitis or acute pyelonephritis.

There is no evidence from randomized studies to guide the choice or duration of therapy. Some authorities recommend that infants with VUR of grade II or more should be given prophylactic antibiotics until puberty or the spontaneous or surgical correction of VUR but the benefit of this is unproven. Antibiotics that have proved effective and safe are nitrofurantoin, trimethoprim, and cotrimoxazole.

Children and adults may experience recurrent urinary infections. In addition to the treatment of symptomatic episodes, management includes maintenance of an adequate fluid intake postcoital voiding for sexually active women, and consideration for prophylactic antimicrobrial therapy (see Chapter 53). Antimicrobrial prophylaxis should be for 3–6 months initially, and then according to patient and physician choice. If there is no urinary obstruction or calculus, there is no risk of further renal scarring in adults with VUR and asymptomatic or symptomatic urinary tract infection.

Blood pressure

Hypertension in patients with reflux nephropathy, whether benign or accelerated, is usually easily controlled with standard drug therapy. Excellent control of blood pressure is the most important aspect of the long-term management of the patient with reflux nephropathy. Patients with reflux nephropathy who are hypertensive are approximately four times more likely to develop renal failure than normotensive patients[36]. Many physicians prefer to use an ACE inhibitor, particularly in patients with proteinuria and renal impairment. Currently, there are no data to indicate that any group of antihypertensive drugs is to be preferred for patients with reflux nephropathy. There is a small amount of evidence that removal of a small scarred kidney in hypertensive patients with unilateral reflux nephropathy may improve or cure hypertension[2].

Tubulointerstitial Disease

Pregnancy

During pregnancy, women with reflux nephropathy should be screened for bacteriuria at the time of diagnosis and then in each trimester. If bacteriuria is detected, it should be eradicated to reduce the risk of acute pyelonephritis. If bacteriuria recurs, antimicrobial prophylaxis (e.g., nitrofurantoin 50 mg at night) should given throughout the remainder of the pregnancy. (Chapter 44 discusses antibiotics and antihypertensives that are safe in pregnancy.) Pregnant women with reflux nephropathy, normal blood pressure, no proteinuria and normal renal function should be carefully supervised but are at low risk of developing problems during pregnancy. Urinary tract infection in the mother does not usually affect fetal outcome. There is increased risk of fetal death in pregnant women with hypertension, proteinuria and renal impairment, although long-term observations have shown recent improvement in fetal outcomes. Women with reflux nephropathy and a plasma creatinine concentration > 1.8 mg/dL (200 μmol/L) may experience an irreversible deterioration in renal function during pregnancy[37]. A prospective study of 54 pregnancies in 46 women with reflux nephropathy found pre-eclampsia in 24% with an increased risk associated with pre-existing hypertension. A deterioration in renal function occurred in 18% of pregnancies with women with mild or moderate renal impairment at greatest risk[38]. The offspring of patients with known VUR or who have a first-degree relative with VUR should be investigated as soon after birth as possible (Fig. 61.3).

REFERENCES

1. Bailey RR. The relationship of vesicoureteral reflux to urinary tract infection and chronic pyelonephritis – reflux nephropathy. Clin Nephrol. 1973;1:132–41.
2. Bailey RR. Vesicoureteric reflux and reflux nephropathy. In Schrier RW, Gottschalk GW, eds. Diseases of the kidney, 4th edn. Boston: Little, Brown; 1988:747–83.
3. Becker GJ, Kincaid-Smith P. Reflux nephropathy: the glomerular lesion and progression of renal failure. Pediatr Nephrol. 1993;7:365–9.
4. Risdon RA. Pyelonephritis and reflux nephropathy. In Tisher CG, Brenner BM, eds. Renal pathology with clinical and functional correlations, 2nd edn. Philadelphia: JB Lippincott Company; 1994:832–62.
5. Sargent MA. What is the normal prevalence of vesicoureteral reflux? Pediatr Radiol. 2000;30:587–93.
6. Bourchier D, Abbott GD, Maling TMJ. Radiological abnormalities in infants with urinary tract infections. Arch Dis Child. 1984;59:620–4.
7. McIlroy PJ, Abbott GD, Anderson NG, et al. Outcome of primary vesicoureteric reflux detected following fetal renal pelvic dilatation. J Paediatr Child Health. 2000;36:569–73.
8. Jaswon MS, Dibble L, Puri S, et al. Prospective study of outcome in antenatally diagnosed renal pelvis dilatation. Arch Dis Child Fetal Neonatal Ed. 1999;80:F135–8.
9. Wennerstrom M, Hansson S, Jodal U, Stokland E. Primary and acquired renal scarring in boys and girls with urinary tract infection. J Pediatr. 2000;136:30–4.
10. Jodal U, Lindberg U. Guidelines for management of children with urinary tract infection and vesicoureteral reflux. Recommendations from a Swedish state-of-the-art conference. Acta Paediatr. 1999;431(Suppl.):87–9.
11. Bailey RR, Lynn KL, Robson RA. End-stage reflux nephropathy. Renal Fail. 1994;16:27–35.
12. Woolf AS. A molecular and genetic view of human renal and urinary tract malformations. Kidney Int. 2000;58:500–12.
13. Feather SA, Malcolm S, Woolf AS, et al. Primary, nonsyndromic vesicoureteric reflux and its nephropathy is genetically heterogeneous, with a locus on chromosome 1. Am J Hum Genet. 2000;66:1420–5.
14. Ozen S, Alikasifoglu M, Saatci U, et al. Implications of certain genetic polymorphisms in scarring in vesicoureteric reflux: importance of ACE polymorphism. Am J Kidney Dis. 1999;34:140–5.
15. Hohenfellner K, Wingen AM, Nauroth O, et al. Impact of ACE I/D gene polymorphism on congenital renal malformations. Pediatr. Nephrol. 2001;16:356–61.
16. Greenfield SP, Wan J. The relationship between dysfunctional voiding and congenital vesicoureteral reflux. Curr Opin Urol. 2000;10:607–10.
17. Sillen U. Vesicoureteral reflux in infants. Pediatr Nephrol. 1999;13:355–61.
18. Bailey RR. Vesicoureteric reflux and reflux nephropathy. In Cameron S, Davison AM, Grunfeld J-P, et al., eds. Oxford textbook of clinical nephrology. Oxford: Oxford University Press; 1992:1983–2002.
19. Maling TMJ, Rolleston GL. Intra-renal reflux in children demonstrated by micturating cystography. Clin Radiol. 1974;25:81–5.
20. Ransley PG, Risdon RA. Renal papillary morphology in infants and young children. Urol Res 1975;3:111–13.
21. International Reflux Study Committee. Medical versus surgical treatment of primary vesicoureteral reflux : a prospective international reflux study in children. J Urol. 1981;125:277–83.
22. Rolleston GL, Shannon FT, Utley WLF. Relationship of infantile vesicoureteric reflux to renal damage. Br Med J. 1970;1:460–3.
23. Panaretto KS, Craig JC, Knight JF, et al. Risk factors for recurrent urinary tract infection in preschool children. J Paediatr Child Health. 1999;35:454–9.
24. Craig JC, Irwig LM, Knight JF, et al. Symptomatic urinary tract infection in preschool Australian children. J Paediatr Child Health. 1998;34:154–9.
25. Agarwal S. Vesicoureteral reflux and urinary tract infections. Curr Opin Urol. 2000;10:587–92.
26. Dillon MJ, Goonasekera CD. Reflux nephropathy. J Am Soc Nephrol. 1998;9:2377–83.
27. Zhang Y, Bailey RR. A long term follow up of adults with reflux nephropathy. NZ Med J. 1995;108:142–4.
28. Bailey RR. Reflux nephropathy and hypertension. In Hodson CJ, Kincaid-Smith P, eds. Reflux nephropathy. New York: Masson; 1979:263.
29. Craig JC, Irwig LM, Knight JF, Roy LP. Does treatment of vesicoureteric reflux in childhood prevent end-stage renal disease attributable to reflux nephropathy? Pediatrics. 2000;105:1236–41.
30. Stokland E, Hellstrom M, Jakobsson B, Sixt R. Imaging of renal scarring. Acta Paediatr. 1999;431(Suppl.):13–21.
31. Bailey RR. Long-term follow-up of infants with gross vesicoureteric reflux. In Hodson CJ, Heptinstall RH, Winberg J, eds. Reflux nephropathy update. Basel: Karger; 1983:146–51.
32. Smellie JM, Prescod NP, Shaw PJ, et al. Childhood reflux and urinary infection: a follow-up of 10–41 years in 226 adults. Pediatr Nephrol. 1998;12:727–36.

33. Smellie JM, Barratt TM, Chantler C, et al. Medical versus surgical treatment in children with severe bilateral vesicoureteric reflux and bilateral nephropathy: a randomised trial. Lancet. 2001;357:1329–33.

34. Kohler J, Thysell H, Tencer J, et al. Long-term follow-up of reflux nephropathy in adults with vesicoureteral reflux – radiological and pathoanatomical analysis. Acta Radiol. 2001;42:355–64.

35. Cardiff-Oxford Bacteriuria Study Group. Long-term effects of bacteriuria on the urinary tract on schoolgirls. Radiology. 1979; 130:343–50.

36. El-Khatib MT, Becker GJ, Kincaid-Smith PS. Reflux nephropathy and primary vesicoureteric reflux in adults. QJ Med. 1990;77: 1241–53.

37. El-Khatib M, Packham DK, Becker GJ, Kincaid-Smith P. Pregnancy-related complications in women with reflux nephropathy. Clin Nephrol. 1994;41:50–5.

38. North RA, Taylor RS, Gunn TR. Pregnancy outcome in women with reflux nephropathy and the inheritance of vesicoureteral reflux. Aust NZ J Obstet. Gynaecol. 2000;40:280–5.

39. Anderson NG, Abbott GD, Mogridge N, et al. Vesicoureteric reflux in the newborn: relationship to fetal renal pelvic diameter. Pediatr Nephrol. 1997;11:610–16.

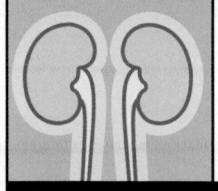

Chapter 62

Chronic Interstitial Nephritis

Rowan G Walker

DEFINITIONS

Chronic tubulointerstitial nephritis (TIN, often referred to as chronic 'interstitial' nephritis) is a histologic lesion characterized by progressive scarring of the tubulointerstitium, with tubular atrophy, macrophage and lymphocytic infiltration and interstitial fibrosis. There are many primary as well as secondary causes of chronic TIN (Table 62.1) and, indeed, all progressive renal diseases will be associated with tubulointerstitial scarring (often with glomerulosclerosis) (see Chapter 66). The importance of tubulointerstitial fibrosis is emphasized by the recognition that the degree of tubulointerstitial change not only correlates with the current renal function, but also strongly predicts outcome in almost all diseases (Fig. 62.1)[1].

In this chapter, we will discuss primary chronic tubulointerstitial diseases; the reader is referred to other chapters for discussions on the tubulointerstitial disease accompanying glomerulonephritis (see Chapter 18), diabetes (see Chapter 32), hypertension (see Chapter 36), polycystic kidney disease (see Chapter 46), and with aging or obesity (see Chapter 65). It is also useful clinically to subdivide the primary causes of chronic interstitial disease into those diseases in which the kidney shrinks but remains smooth and evenly contoured ('macroscopically' normal) and those where focal scarring leads to an irregular, abnormal, and often shrunken kidney ('macroscopically' abnormal) (Table 62.2).

PATHOGENESIS

The normal renal interstitium

The renal interstitium is made up essentially of a loose matrix of collagens (especially types I and Ill), proteoglycans, and fluid, in which both resident cells and nonresident cells are distributed. These cells include matrix-producing fibroblasts, macrophages, and dendritic cells. The interstitial matrix, situated as it is between the tubules and vessels, is obviously important for both the structural and the functional integrity

Correlation of renal function with interstitial disease

Legend:
- Acute glomerulonephritis
- Chronic glomerulonephritis
- Interstitial nephritis
- Nephrosclerosis
- Miscellaneous causes

Y-axis: Glomerular filtration rate as inulin clearance (mL/min) — 0, 20, 40, 60, 80, 100, 120, 140, 160

X-axis: Interstitial disease (semi-quantitative injury scores at biopsy) — 0 1 2 3 4 5 6 7 8 9 10 11 12

Figure 62.1 Renal function closely correlates with tubulointerstitial disease. (Adapted with permission.)

Major etiologies of chronic tubulointerstitial disease	
Primary	**Secondary**
Analgesic nephropathy	Glomerulonephritis
Vesicoureteral reflux and reflux nephropathy	Diabetes
Chronic obstruction	Hypertension
Sickle cell nephropathy	Polycystic kidneys
Metabolic ($\downarrow$ K$^+$. $\uparrow$ Ca^{2+})	Aging
Chronic urate nephropathy	Obesity
Heavy metals (lead, cadmium, arsenic)	Progressive renal disease of all etiologies
Immune mediated: lupus, Sjögren's disease	
Sarcoidosis	
Chinese herbal nephropathy	
Balkan nephropathy	
Radiation	
Transplant: chronic rejection, cyclosporine, tacrolimus	
Idiopathic	
Common causes are in italic.	

Table 62.1 Major etiologies of chronic tubulointerstitial disease.

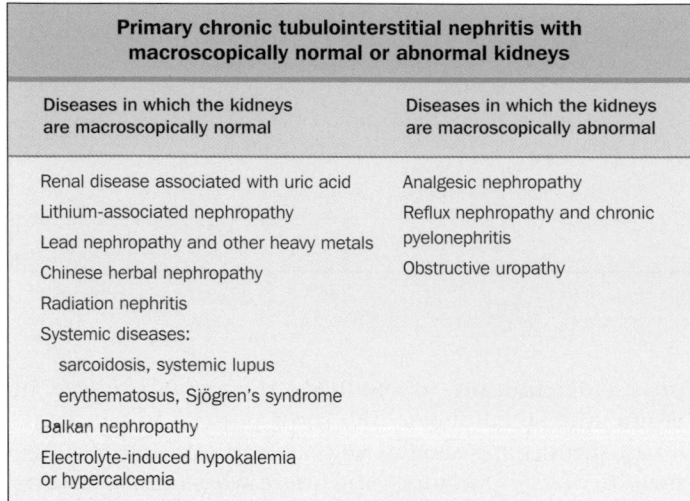

Primary chronic tubulointerstitial nephritis with macroscopically normal or abnormal kidneys

Diseases in which the kidneys are macroscopically normal	Diseases in which the kidneys are macroscopically abnormal
Renal disease associated with uric acid	Analgesic nephropathy
Lithium-associated nephropathy	Reflux nephropathy and chronic pyelonephritis
Lead nephropathy and other heavy metals	Obstructive uropathy
Chinese herbal nephropathy	
Radiation nephritis	
Systemic diseases:	
sarcoidosis, systemic lupus	
erythematosus, Sjögren's syndrome	
Balkan nephropathy	
Electrolyte-induced hypokalemia or hypercalcemia	

Table 62.2 Primary chronic tubulointerstitial nephritis with macroscopically normal or abnormal kidneys.

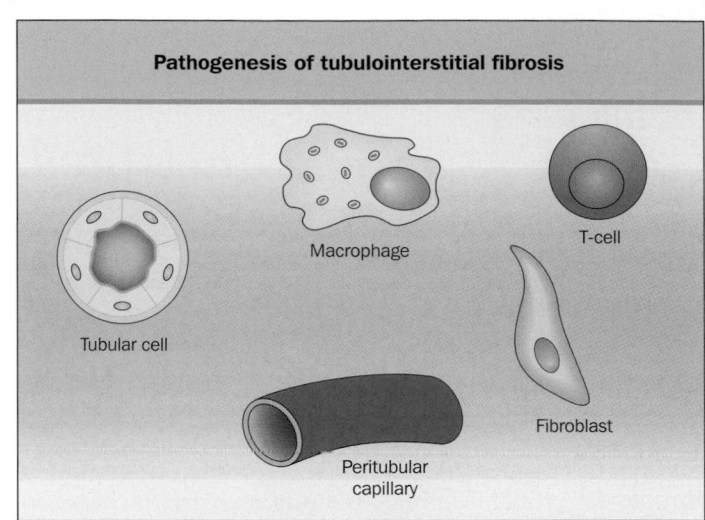

Figure 62.2 Pathogenesis of tubulointerstitial fibrosis. Injury to the tubule and peritubular capillary leads to the generation of chemotactic and adhesive factors that result in macrophage and T-cell accumulation. Local macrophage and fibroblast activation ensues, driven by growth factors such as platelet-derived growth factor and transforming growth factor-β, which results in collagen production by tubular cells and fibroblasts, eventually culminating in the fibrotic lesion.

of the kidney. Diffusion of oxygen from the peritubular capillaries to the tubules and the transfer of solute and water will largely be influenced by the width and the constituents within the interstitium. Any alteration to the interstitial matrix could therefore have profound effects on fluid and electrolyte balance and on renal function.

Mechanisms of tubulointerstitial injury

The tubulointerstitium can be injured in a variety of ways, including by toxins (e.g., heavy metals), drugs (e.g., analgesics), crystals (e.g., calcium phosphate, uric acid), infections, obstruction, lipid deposition, immunologic mechanisms, acute elevations in capillary pressure and by ischemia. Glomerular disease can also injure the tubulointerstitium through mechanisms that may involve glomerular cytokine release, effects of proteinuria, ischemia, or crossreactive immunity.

Regardless of the initiating mechanism, the tubulointerstitial response is quite similar (Fig. 62.2)[1–3]. This includes an early tubular cell proliferation in association with tubular dilatation and cast formation, and later tubular atrophy and apoptosis. There is proliferation of the interstitial fibroblast, with expression of contractile proteins such as α-actin. This suggests a change to a 'myofibroblast' phenotype, such as seen in healing wounds. There is also a focal loss of peritubular capillaries, which occurs in association with expansion of the interstitium with collagens I, III and VI. The tubular basement membrane (TBM) is thickened with increased matrix, especially collagen type IV. There is also an accompanying infiltration with inflammatory cells including macrophages and lymphocytes, especially T cells. Eventually, there is progressive apoptosis of all cell populations, resulting in a densely fibrotic and hypocellular lesion.

The processes responsible for these changes have been examined primarily in experimental models of renal disease. Proteinuria has been found to be a major mechanism for initiating tubular injury; this may be due to cytokines and pro-oxidant molecules present in the proteinuric urine, as well as complement components that are then activated to form the

complement membrane attack complex (C5b-9) which can directly activate the tubular cells. Ischemia induced by intrarenal vasoconstriction and/or loss of peritubular capillaries also leads to tubular injury and fibrosis, which is often most severe in the outer medulla and juxtamedullary regions where the kidney is normally borderline hypoxic. The injury to the tubules and peritubular capillaries are often primary events and result in the release of chemotactic substances (chemokines and lipid factors) and expression of leukocyte adhesion molecules (such as interstitial cell adhesion molecule-1 and osteopontin). These attract macrophages and lymphocytes into the interstitium. Tubular cells also express human leukocyte antigens (HLA) and secrete complement components and vasoactive mediators, which may further stimulate or attract macrophages and T cells. Growth factors released by tubular cells and macrophages, such as platelet-derived growth factors (PDGF) and transforming growth factor (TGF)-β, may stimulate the fibroblast proliferation and activation. The local fibroblast and tubular cell activation results in increased collagen synthesis which, coupled with the local expression of collagenase inhibitors, results in increased matrix deposition and accumulation. The source of fibroblasts and myofibroblasts in renal interstitial fibrosis remains controversial. Historically, it was assumed that these cells had their origin in an intrinsic fibroblast population, but alternative explanations include migration from perivascular areas and 'transdifferentiation' of tubular cells into fibroblasts.

The role of the immune system in various tubulointerstitial injuries is also being explored. Rarely, humoral (antibody)-mediated injury to the tubulointerstitium can occur, such as in some patients with lupus nephritis with TBM deposits, occasional patients with antiglomerular basement membrane (GBM) nephritis with cross-reactive antibody to TBM, and in patients with acute methicillin-induced nephritis with IgG staining of the TBM. Other tubulointerstitial diseases may be cell mediated. In these diseases, which have been primarily characterized in mice, Nielson has suggested that there may be three phases: an afferent phase characterized by recognition of antigen and expression of antigen; a regulatory phase during which the host modifies its response to the immune stimulus; and an effector phase during which tissue damage occurs under the influence of antigen (tissue)-specific T cells[4].

The tubulointerstitial injury may lead to nephron loss as a consequence of disruption of the tubular segments or indirectly by leading to periglomerular fibrosis that constricts the outflow of the urine from Bowman's space into the proximal tubule, leading to the development of 'atubular glomeruli'. The interstitial infiltration of inflammatory cells (macrophages and lymphocytes) may also release oxidants and angiotensin II that can lead to local vasoconstriction, modulating glomerular hemodynamics, and impairing sodium excretion; indeed, there is evidence that they may contribute to the pathogenesis of some forms of salt-sensitive hypertension[5].

EPIDEMIOLOGY

Whilst chronic TIN characterizes progressive renal disease of all etiologies, primary forms of chronic TIN account for relatively few patients reaching end-stage renal disease (ESRD). For example, of the new cases recorded in 1996 in the Australia and New Zealand Dialysis and Transplant Registry[6], very few (< 3%) had chronic TIN in which the kidneys are macroscopically normal (Table 62.3). For certain conditions where the kidneys are macroscopically abnormal, such as reflux nephropathy, analgesic nephropathy, obstructive uropathy and cystic renal disease, the major histologic lesions are also 'tubulointerstitial' and this certainly expands the proportion of TIN causes of ESRD toward 20% (Table 62.3). Reports from other areas of the world have also indicated quite a variable incidence of chronic tubulointerstitial disease in patients with ESRD, with a range from 42% in Scotland to 3% in the USA[7]. The marked variability in incidence may relate to differences in how diagnoses are made, differences in

Etiology of end-stage renal disease in Australia and New Zealand, 1996		
	(%)	n
Glomerulonephritiis	30	518
Analgesic nephropathy	5	79
Polycystic kidneys	6	109
Reflux nephropathy	5	89
Hypertension	14	239
Diabetic nephropathy	22	381
Miscellaneous	11	190
Uncertain diagnosis	7	118
	100	1723

Table 62.3 Etiology of end-stage renal disease in Australia and New Zealand, 1996

etiologies and toxin/drug exposure, and better measures to prevent or treat the various conditions.

In this regard, epidemiologic studies looking for risk factors in patients with idiopathic chronic tubulointerstitial disease have identified a number of risk factors, including occupational exposure to industrial toxins (such as lead), exposure to aristolochic acids (from herbal remedies), hypertension, hyperuricemia, a history of analgesic abuse, and exposure to grain in granaries as opposed to silos.

CLINICAL MANIFESTATIONS

Most patients with primary chronic tubulointerstitial disease will have non-nephrotic proteinuria and a relatively inactive urinary sediment, usually with white blood cells and, rarely, white blood cell casts. A concentrating defect is often apparent (with polyuria and nocturia) and may occasionally be severe enough to result in a nephrogenic diabetes insipidus. Other tubular defects may relate to the main site of injury, resulting in either proximal tubule defects (with amino-aciduria, phosphaturia, proximal renal tubular acidosis (RTA) or, rarely, Fanconi's syndrome) or distal tubular defects (especially type IV RTA). Many diseases are also associated with the inability to conserve salt on a low-salt diet (resulting in salt-wasting syndromes). However, there is evidence that certain tubulointerstitial diseases, particularly if they are associated with microvascular disease, may also be associated with a relative inability to excrete salt, especially when the patient is placed on a high-salt diet[8]. Thus, some tubulointerstitial diseases, such as lead nephropathy, gouty nephropathy, cyclosporine nephropathy and analgesic nephropathy, are frequently associated with salt-sensitive hypertension. Consequently, primary and acquired tubulointerstitial disease may present problems of either salt excretion or salt conservation[8].

PATHOLOGY

Since progressive interstitial disease (particularly interstitial fibrosis) is part of a common final pathway for all causes of renal disease[1], the identification of any specific histologic features in chronic TIN is problematical. Virtually all of the major histologic features are 'nonspecific' and it is rather the absence of specific glomerular features that points to the tubulointerstitium as the primary area of insult in the pathologic process. However, as progressive tubulointerstitial damage occurs, the glomeruli may become secondarily involved, with glomerulosclerosis occurring as a consequence of glomerular hypertension and hyperfiltration.

Interstitial fibrosis

Interstitial fibrosis is an essential histologic feature of chronic TIN and is characterized by expansion of the interstitial space with increased interstitial collagens. The pattern (focal or diffuse) will vary with the nature of the original insult (Fig. 62.3).

Tubular atrophy

Tubular atrophy is a nonspecific lesion seen frequently in areas of developing interstitial fibrosis. The TBM is often thickened, tubules may be dilated or atrophic and are often

Tubulointerstitial Disease

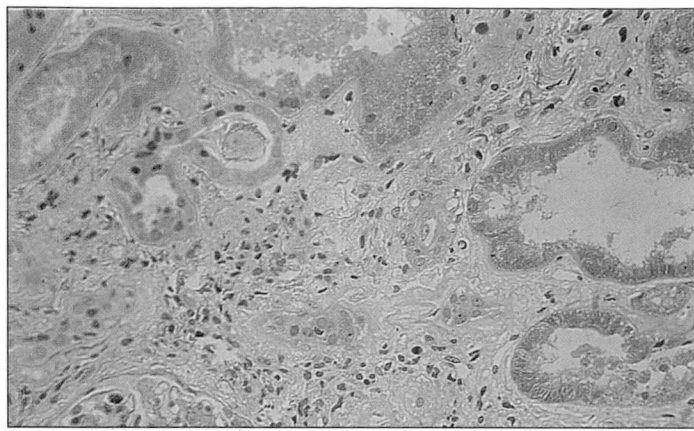

Figure 62.3 Interstitial fibrosis. The normal tubulointerstitium has been replaced by fibrotic tissue (green), which is composed largely of collagen (Trichrome ×400).

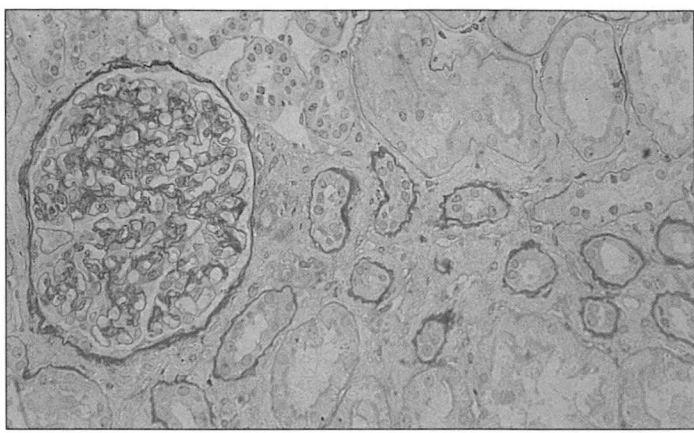

Figure 62.4 Tubular atrophy. Atrophic tubules, with thickened basement membranes, are separated from each other by interstitial fibrosis. (Periodic acid–Schiff stain ×400).

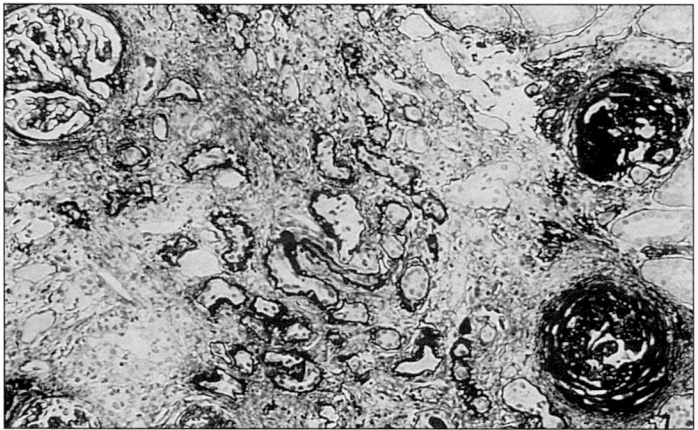

Figure 62.5 Secondary glomerulosclerosis. Obliteration of the capillary loops with capillary collapse and scarring, resulting in globally sclerosed glomeruli. (Silver stain ×200).

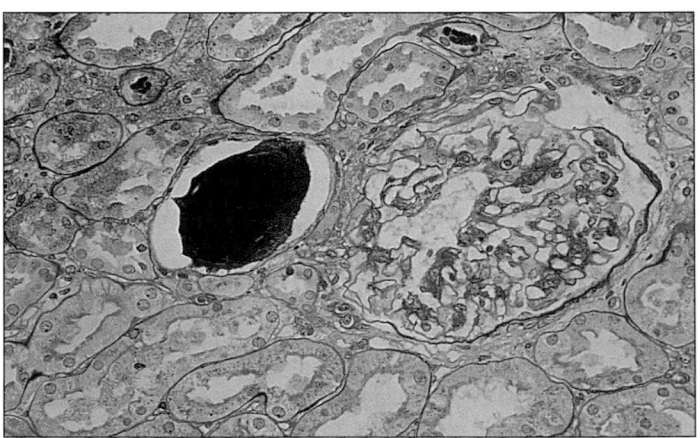

Figure 62.6 Tubular casts. Casts are periodic acid–Schiff stain (PAS) positive and usually contain Tamm–Horsfall protein. Some may contain desquamated tubular cells and macrophages. (Periodic acid–Schiff ×400).

separated from each other by dense interstitial fibrosis (Fig. 62.4). In some conditions (e.g., lithium-associated nephropathy), the degree of tubular atrophy correlates with a functional abnormality such as impairment of urine-concentrating ability (Fig. 62.13).

Glomerulosclerosis

Glomerulosclerosis occurs secondary to the tubulointerstitial insult. The normal glomerular structure is replaced by global fibrosis. In progressive renal impairment (hyperfiltration), surviving glomeruli may be normal or show focal and segmental hyalinosis lesions, as would be the case in any renal disease under such conditions (Fig. 62.5). Occasionally, glomeruli are structurally preserved with normal appearing capillaries but are nonfunctional due to periglomerular fibrosis that prevents outflow of the urine into the proximal tubules ('atubular glomeruli').

Cast formation

The presence of casts within tubular lumina is a highly nonspecific finding. The casts may contain desquamated tubuloepithelial cells embedded in Tamm–Horsfall protein (Fig 62.6). Occasionally the casts take on a homogenous waxy appearance in dilated tubules suggesting a chronic obstructive element to the tubulointerstitial damage.

Interstitial cell infiltrate

Interstitial cell infiltrate is not an invariable finding. Cells in the infiltrate include lymphocytes and monocyte–macrophages (Fig. 62.7). Depending on the etiology of the tubulointerstitial disease, there may be other cells such as neutrophils, eosinophils, or plasma cells. Infiltrating cells are usually in patches (focal) but may be more diffuse.

ETIOLOGIES

Tables 62.1 and 62.2 list the major causes of primary chronic TIN and give subdivisions into conditions where the kidneys are macroscopically normal and those where the kidneys are structurally abnormal. Certain diseases are discussed elsewhere, including sickle cell nephropathy (see Chapter 51), urinary tract obstruction (see Chapter 58), vesicoureteral

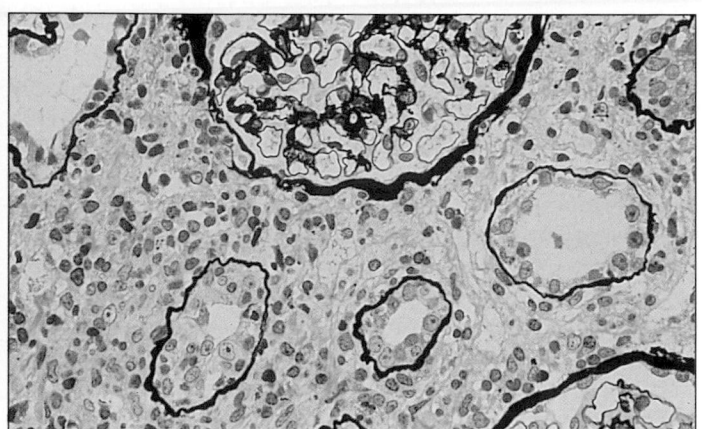

Figure 62.7 Interstitial infiltrates. A variable feature of tubulointerstitial nephritis is the presence of inflammatory cells, which primarily consist of macrophages and lymphocytes. (Trichrome ×400).

reflux and chronic pyelonephritis (see Chapter 61), cyclosporine nephropathy (see Chapter 88) and chronic rejection (see Chapter 90).

Diseases resulting in macroscopically abnormal kidneys
Analgesic nephropathy
Definition and epidemiology

Analgesic nephropathy was first recognized as an entity in the early 1950s in Swiss watch factory workers, who were habitually taking large amounts of over-the-counter analgesics, particularly combination analgesics containing phenacetin. Shortly thereafter, it was recognized as a major cause of ESRD, especially in certain areas of Europe and Australia. In two Australian States, Queensland and New South Wales, as many as 25% of patients with ESRD in the 1970s were diagnosed with analgesic nephropathy. In contrast, analgesic nephropathy was less frequently diagnosed in the USA, which likely related to less clinical awareness of the entity as well as the lower availability of phenacetin-containing analgesic mixtures. Importantly, the recognition of analgesic mixtures containing phenacetin as a risk factor for renal disease led to the banning of such compounds in a number of countries. Whereas the restriction of compound analgesic sales in Scandinavian countries, and also in Finland, Canada and the UK, led to variable effects on the incidence of ESRD, a significant decline in the incidence of ESRD was observed in Australia[9]. Following the introduction of the legislation, the number of new patients commencing dialysis fell from 7.69 per million population (p.m.p.) in 1980 to 5.85 p.m.p. in 1990 ($P < 0.003$), with the decline in patients requiring dialysis being most pronounced for those between the ages of 40 and 49 years ($P < 0.00001$). By the early 1990s, the percentage of hemodialysis patients diagnosed with analgesic nephropathy was 9% in Australia, 3% in Europe, and 0.9% in the USA[10]. The incidence of analgesic nephropathy for new cases of ESRD in Australia is currently 5%[10].

Etiologic agents

The clinical syndrome of analgesic nephropathy results from abuse of compound analgesics containing aspirin or antipyrine, combined with phenacetin, acetaminophen (paracetamol) or salicylamide, and caffeine or codeine. Recently, it has been suggested that a similar lesion can be induced with chronic nonsteroidal anti-inflammatory agent (NSAID) use. NSAIDs reported to induce analgesic nephropathy include alclofenac, antipyrine, benoxeprofen, fenoprofen, ibuprofen, indomethacin, mefenamic acid and naproxen; there are also reports suggesting aspirin and acetaminophen may have contributory roles. While the role of non-phenacetin compounds in causing analgesic nephropathy remains controversial[11], there is some evidence that the chronic use of aspirin or acetaminophen may accelerate renal progression of any etiology[12]. In this regard, it is important to recognize that agents that block intrarenal prostaglandin synthesis, such as NSAIDs, can be acutely nephrotoxic, and can cause an acute reversible decline in glomerular filtration rate (GFR) or an acute tubular necrosis, especially in the setting of volume depletion (see Chapter 15); acute papillary necrosis may also occur particularly if large doses are ingested. NSAIDs may also be idiosyncratically associated with a minimal change-like lesion with acute TIN (see Chapter 60).

Because of the uncertainties surrounding toxicologic data and pathogenesis, it is difficult to establish the critical amounts and periods of intakes of the various analgesic agents required to produce analgesic nephropathy. Epidemiologic studies generally show a dose-dependent risk for developing analgesic nephropathy with compound analgesics, especially with those containing phenacetin, and it has been estimated that there is a 15- to 20-fold increased relative risk for the development of chronic renal disease when the total consumption of phenacetin exceeds 1.0 kg.

Pathogenesis

The principal site of renal injury with chronic analgesic abuse is the medulla, a site that is vulnerable because of the concentration of toxic metabolites built up by the counter-current mechanism and because of the low oxygen tension present in this region. The injury may relate to the net effects of several metabolites. For example, phenacetin is converted to acetaminophen, which can deplete cells of glutathione and result in the generation of oxidative and alkylating metabolites. Aspirin and NSAIDs can result in the reduction of vasodilatory prostaglandins; caffeine may be metabolized to adenosine, with vasoconstrictive effects within the kidney. Collectively, these substances may lead to oxidant and ischemic injury to the medulla, an effect that is exacerbated in the setting of volume depletion. Renal papillary necrosis with features of an ischemic infarct may develop, with atrophy of the overlying cortex leading to chronic interstitial changes.

Pathology

The major pathologic change of analgesic nephropathy is renal papillary necrosis, a coagulative necrosis induced by thrombosis and infarction that involves the medulla and includes the loops of Henle, the vasa recta, the medullary interstitial cells, and the collecting ducts (Fig. 62.8). The cortical changes of chronic interstitial nephritis overlying the

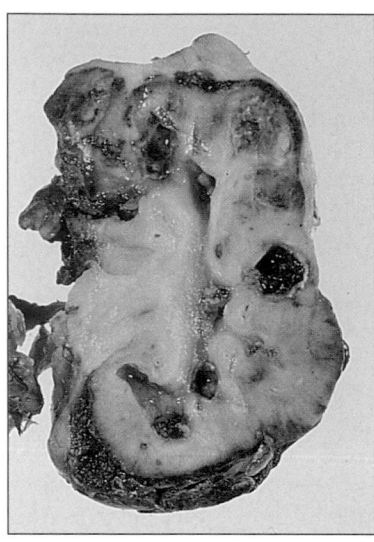

Figure 62.8 Papillary necrosis. Autopsy macroscopic appearance of papillary necrosis in a patient with long-standing analgesic nephropathy.

necrotic papilla are secondary and comprise tubular atrophy, interstitial fibrosis, and a mononuclear cellular infiltrate. The presence of a golden-brown lipofuchsin-like pigment in tubular cells, and the characteristic analgesic microangiopathy or capillary sclerosis, is highly indicative of an analgesic etiology. Glomerular changes of focal glomerular sclerosis and hyalinosis are similar to those described in reflux-associated nephropathy and tend to be late features.

Clinical features

Most patients are female and have a history of chronic pain syndromes and other symptoms suggestive of a broader analgesic syndrome. An addictive and dependent personality trait characterized by introversion or psychoneurosis may be present in some patients. Peptic ulcer disease and gastrointestinal symptoms are also present in many patients.

The renal function abnormalities of analgesic nephropathy include impaired urine-concentrating ability, urinary acidification defects and impaired sodium conservation. The urinalysis often shows pyuria with or without urinary tract infection, micro- or macrohematuria, and non-nephrotic proteinuria. Proteinuria occurs in at least half of the patients and increases

progressively as GFR decreases with advanced disease. The proteinuria is of both tubular and glomerular origin, the latter as a consequence of secondary glomerulosclerosis that develops as renal function deteriorates. A progressive increase in urinary β_2-microglobulin (a marker of tubulointerstitial disease) is indicative of a poor prognosis. Hypertension is a frequent clinical feature.

Patients with analgesic nephropathy are also at risk for premature atherosclerosis, with a nearly three-fold increased risk for cardiovascular mortality and a two-fold increased relative risk for cardiovascular disease, fatal or nonfatal myocardial infarction, heart failure or stroke. Atheromatous renal artery stenosis is also much more common in analgesic abusers. The increased atherogenic tendency relates to multiple factors including hyperlipidemia, hypertension, smoking, and probably the formation of atherogenic oxidized low-density lipoproteins under the oxidative influence of phenacetin.

An important association of analgesic nephropathy is the increased risk of transitional cell carcinoma of the uroepithelium (renal pelvis, ureter, bladder and proximal urethra). This should be especially considered in patients with gross hematuria.

Diagnosis

The disease is suggested by a history of analgesic abuse coupled with radiologic findings showing either papillary necrosis (by intravenous urography; Fig. 62.9) or bilateral atrophic but often asymmetric kidneys; the radiologic findings are not always easily distinguished from those of reflux nephropathy (Fig. 62.10). Papillary calcification is a very helpful diagnostic feature and may be best documented by a noncontrast computed tomography scan[10]. The differential diagnosis of papillary necrosis includes diabetic nephropathy, sickle cell nephropathy, and, very rarely, obstructive uropathy and reflux nephropathy.

Treatment

Management consists of avoiding phenacetin analgesic mixtures and reducing (ideally stopping) ingestion of analgesic medications. No specific treatments are available, and management is similar to that for all patients with chronic renal

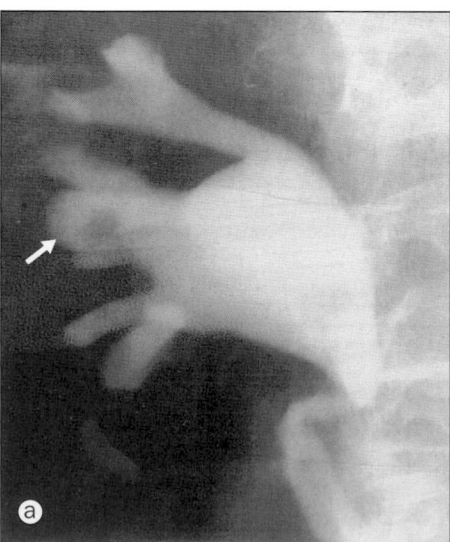

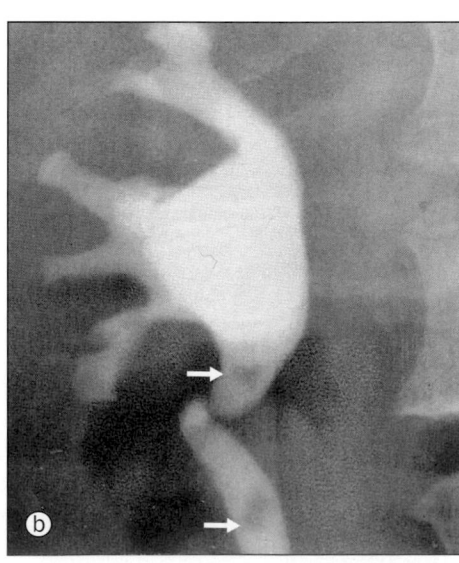

Figure 62.9 An intravenous urogram of a patient with analgesic nephropathy. (a) The pyelogram shows evidence of a necrotic papilla in the lateral minor calyx producing a 'ring' sign (arrow). (b) Two radiolucencies can be seen (arrows), one in the pelvis of the ureter and one in the proximal end of the right ureter, caused by sloughed papillae.

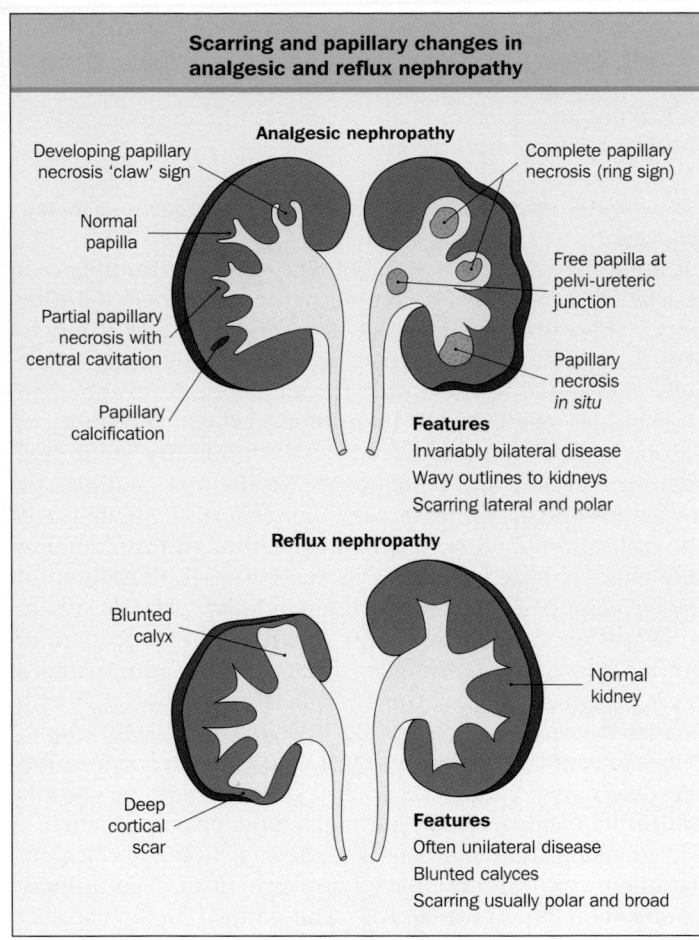

Scarring and papillary changes in
analgesic and reflux nephropathy

Analgesic nephropathy

Developing papillary
necrosis 'claw' sign

Normal
papilla

Partial papillary
necrosis with
central cavitation

Papillary
calcification

Complete papillary
necrosis (ring sign)

Free papilla at
pelvi-ureteric
junction

Papillary
necrosis
in situ

Features

Invariably bilateral disease
Wavy outlines to kidneys
Scarring lateral and polar

Reflux nephropathy

Blunted
calyx

Normal
kidney

Deep
cortical
scar

Features

Often unilateral disease
Blunted calyces
Scarring usually polar and broad

Figure 62.10 Pattern of scarring and range of papillary changes in analgesic nephropathy compared with reflux nephropathy.

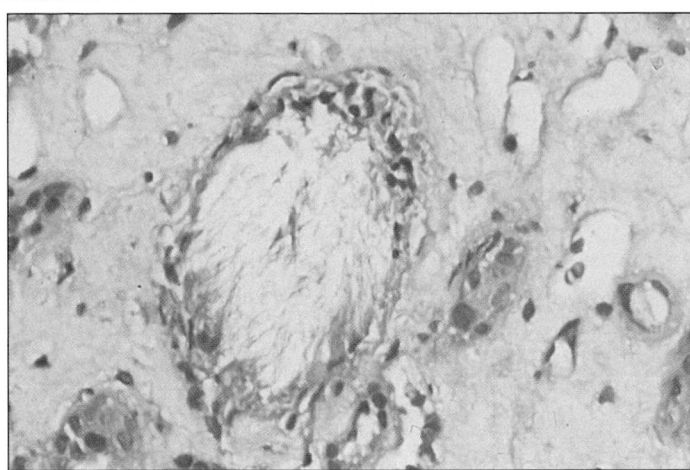

Figure 62.11 Urate crystal in the interstitium of a patient with gout. (Adapted with permission.)

insufficiency, including careful monitoring of blood pressure. Because of the increased incidence of uroepithelial tumors, close follow-up is necessary. Further work-up is indicated if patients develop new symptoms (such as hematuria or flank pain) suggestive of cancer.

Diseases with macroscopically normal kidneys

Chronic urate nephropathy

Renal disease is frequently associated with chronically elevated uric acid levels (hyperuricemia), especially in patients who have had gout for many years. Renal functional abnormalities are observed in 30–50% of subjects, and histologic changes are observed in over 90%[13]. The histologic lesion, which is often called chronic urate or chronic gouty nephropathy, is characterized by tubulointerstitial fibrosis, often with arteriolosclerosis and glomerulosclerosis. Within the kidney, one can often find precipitated uric acid crystals in the tubules and in the interstitium (particularly in the medulla) (Fig. 62.11)[13].

It is important to distinguish chronic urate nephropathy from acute urate nephropathy. The latter is a type of acute renal failure usually observed in patients with rapid cell turnover (such as may occur in patients undergoing chemotherapy for malignancy) in which there is a marked increase in uric acid generation. This leads to supersaturation

in the urine, with intratubular precipitation and obstruction (see Chapter 15). Similarly, both entities are distinct from the patient with occasional kidney stones formed from uric acid (uric acid nephrolithiasis, see Chapter 57).

Although many patients with long-standing gout have some degree of renal impairment in association with chronic tubulointerstitial disease with urate deposition, it remains controversial whether the renal disease is secondary to chronic hyperuricemia or whether it is due to coexistent hypertensive renal disease or the renal changes associated with aging[14]. It has been suggested that chronic hyperuricemia and uricosuria result in intratubular crystal deposition, with local obstruction and rupture into the interstitium where they enlist a chronic granulomatous response and interstitial fibrosis; however, it is difficult to ascribe the diffuse renal disease to the presence of focal crystalline deposits[14]. More recently, there have been a few experimental studies that suggest that hyperuricemia may induce chronic renal injury independent of crystal formation[15,16]. Specifically, the induction of mild hyperuricemia in rats (by administering an inhibitor of uricase) was associated with the development of hypertension, microvascular disease (a preglomerular arteriolopathy), interstitial fibrosis, and mild glomerulosclerosis; features identical to chronic gouty nephropathy[15,16]. Experimentally induced hyperuricemia was also shown to accelerate progression of renal disease in rats with cyclosporine nephropathy or with remnant kidneys[17,18]. The mechanism was shown to be mediated by activation of the renin angiotensin system, by stimulation of COX2, and by inhibition of local nitric oxide synthases[15–18].

Clinically, patients present with hypertension with mild azotemia, mild proteinuria, an unremarkable urinary sediment, and minimal tubular dysfunction (usually impairment of urine-concentrating ability manifest as isosthenuria). While the diagnosis of uric acid nephropathy primarily depends on histologic findings, it should be particularly considered if there is a disproportionate elevation of serum uric acid in relation to the degree of renal insufficiency (Table 62.4)[19].

The most important diagnosis to exclude in a patient considered to have gouty nephropathy is primary lead intoxication. Several studies have found that chronic lead exposure

Expected relationship of serum creatinine and uric acid levels			
Serum creatinine		Corresponding serum uric acid level	
mg/dL	µmol/L	mg/dL	µmol/L
< 1.5	132	9	536
1.5–2.0	132–176	10	595
>2.0	176	12	714
(Adopted from Murray and Goldberg.)			

Table 62.4 Expected relationship of serum creatinine and uric acid levels. Serum uric acid disproportionately elevated above the expected values for the serum creatinine suggests a diagnosis of chronic uric acid nephropathy.

can result in similar clinical features, with hypertension, hyperuricemia, glomerular and tubular dysfunction, and interstitial fibrosis[20]. Diagnosis is best made by the ethylenediaminetetracetic acid (EDTA) lead chelation test (see below). In addition, the diagnosis of hereditary hyperuricemia and renal disease should be considered for patients presenting in adolescence or during early adulthood (see below).

Treatment consists of lowering uric acid with xanthine oxidase inhibitors (allopurinol) with a target serum uric acid of 5.5 mg/dL [325 µmol] or lower. As allopurinol is excreted by the kidneys, it is prudent to initiate treatment at 100 mg per day, with increasing the dose to 200 or 300 mg/day if tolerated. Occasional patients develop a hypersensitivity syndrome (0.1%) that can be fatal, and this risk is increased in patients with renal dysfunction. Alternative agents (uricosurics) are generally less effective in the setting of reduced renal function, although benziodarone or benzbromarone may provide benefit if the GFR is > 30 mL/min.

Hereditary hyperuricemia and renal disease

A hereditary form of hyperuricemia with renal impairment and hypertension has been described in several families. The disorder is autosomal dominant[21]. The condition is characterized by hyperuricemia (usually without gout) from severe impairment of uric acid excretion. Renal vasoconstriction is prominent. The renal lesion shows tubulointerstitial fibrosis, glomerulosclerosis and preglomerular microvascular disease; interestingly, urate crystal deposits are often absent. Although the condition has only a variable response to therapy with allopurinol, the timing of administration appears critical. Some degree of prevention of progression may be achievable if the drug is administered early but therapy may be near ineffective once tubulointerstitial injury and renal insufficiency are established.

Lithium nephropathy

In the mid-1970s it was recognized that long-term administration of lithium salts to patients with severe unipolar and bipolar affective illness may be associated with the development of chronic renal disease. Several different forms of renal injury were identified[22,23]. However, it should be remembered that, because the therapeutic index of the lithium ion is

low, the most important complication of long-term lithium therapy remains the development of acute lithium intoxication. The kidneys are exclusively responsible for the excretion of lithium and, therefore, are pivotal to the development of this important complication.

Lithium-associated polyuria, polydipsia, and nephrogenic diabetes insipidus

Lithium ingestion is associated with the development of resistance to vasopressin (antidiuretic hormone), resulting in polyuria (urine volume > 3 L/24 h) and polydipsia in up to 40% of patients. Lithium accumulates in the collecting tubule cells after entering these cells through sodium channels in the luminal membrane. It then interferes with the ability of vasopressin to increase water reabsorption by inhibiting adenylate cyclase and hence cAMP production; and also by decreasing the apical membrane expression of aquaporin 2, the collecting tubule water channel. Although this common side effect is widely regarded as reversible, lithium-induced impairment of urine-concentrating ability was shown in some patients to persist many months after cessation of lithium therapy. Interestingly, lithium is also (unusually) a cause of hypercalcemia. This complication is associated with increased release of parathyroid hormone. Persistent hypercalcemia could potentially exaggerate the tubular concentrating defect and contribute to the development of chronic interstitial nephritis in lithium-treated patients (see below).

Paralleling the nephrogenic diabetes insipidus in lithium treatment is a lithium-induced impairment in distal urinary acidification (type 1 (distal) RTA) This partial functional defect is virtually never of clinical importance. A lithium-induced decrease in the activity of the H^+ ATPase pump in the distal nephron (collecting ducts) may be at least partly responsible for this defect.

Acute lithium toxicity

Acute impairment of GFR and tubular injury (acute tubular necrosis) associated with episodes of acute lithium intoxication has for many years been a recognized potential complication of lithium therapy.

Histologically, the most distinctive changes are seen in the distal convoluted tubules, in which there is ballooning, swelling and vacuolation of the cell cytoplasm, accompanied by strands and granules of periodic acid–Schiff positive staining material (glycogen). This lesion is both acute and reversible (Fig. 62.12).

Chronic lithium nephropathy

A striking new observation in the 1970s was the recognition that, in lithium-treated patients, the polyuria (and polydipsia) was not always reversible. A large number of studies subsequently showed a correlation between the duration of lithium therapy and persistent impairment of urine-concentrating ability (Fig. 62.13)[22,23]. Biopsies in these patients subsequently revealed a focal chronic interstitial nephropathy with interstitial fibrosis, tubular atrophy, and glomerular sclerosis. A characteristic finding is the presence of microcystic changes in the distal tubule. Patients at particular risk seemed to be those with severely impaired urine-concentrating defects and those with a history of repeated episodes of acute lithium intoxication.

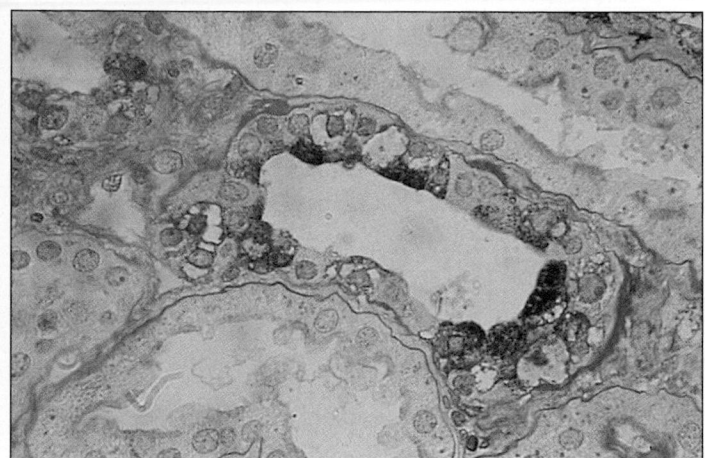

Figure 62.12 Renal histologic change in acute lithium toxicity. Glycogen granules in the distal tubular cells, with variable degrees of vacuolation of the cytoplasm. (Periodic acid–Schiff ×600).

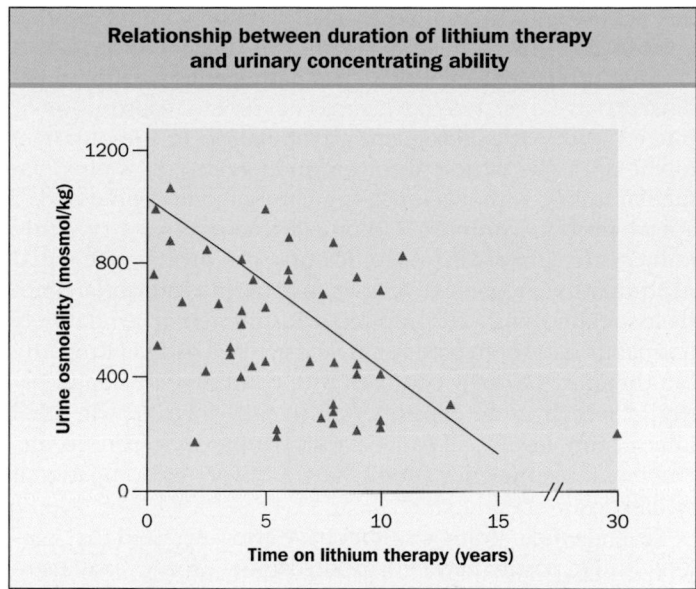

Figure 62.13 Inverse relationship between duration of lithium therapy and urinary concentrating ability (fluid deprivation test) in 46 patients on maintenance lithium therapy.

Interestingly, most patients with chronic lithium nephropathy have a relatively preserved GFR in relation to the distal tubular defect(s). Although a small number of patients have renal impairment, there is no correlation between GFR and the duration of lithium therapy (unlike with the concentrating defect). Furthermore, in patients taking lithium who do not have repeated episodes of acute lithium intoxication, the role of lithium in chronic interstitial disease remains controversial because similar degrees of chronic interstitial change, including interstitial fibrosis, have been noted in patients with affective disorders not being treated with lithium, although the characteristic microcystic dilatation of the distal tubules is generally absent[21]. The role of other psychotropic medication in this setting is unknown. If chronic TIN does occur in association with long-term stable maintenance therapy with lithium, it probably requires many years of therapy, and the consequent degree of renal insufficiency, as indicated above, is relatively mild. Perhaps the most important factor in preservation of renal function and histology is prevention of episodes of acute intoxication.

Management of lithium-associated renal disease

After ruling out other causes of polyuria and polydipsia, especially psychogenic polydipsia (or potomania), a reduction of the dose of lithium should first be considered, aiming for therapeutic concentrations (12-h serum lithium concentrations) of 0.4–0.6 mmol/L or converting to a single daily dose aiming for a lower minimum serum lithium concentration. The potassium-sparing diuretic amiloride can also reduce the urine output by up to 50% and has the added advantage of blocking lithium uptake through the sodium channels in the collecting duct[24]. Amiloride is most effective when the concentrating defect is mild and potentially reversible and has generally been disappointing in patients with severe defects in urine-concentrating ability. Although thiazide diuretics are effective in treating lithium-induced polyuria, they should be avoided as they pose risks for the induction of acute lithium intoxication because the resultant volume contraction causes

an increase in sodium and lithium reabsorption in the proximal tubule. The use of NSAIDs is also not recommended.

A practical approach to the patient on long-term lithium treatment should include a regular (at least yearly) estimation of renal function measured as serum creatinine, creatinine clearance and 24-h urine volume. Because progressive renal injury with a reduced GFR (or raised serum creatinine) in a patient without prior acute lithium intoxication is relatively unusual, a raised serum creatinine should initially be treated with dose reduction. For persistently elevated serum creatinine estimations, a renal biopsy should be considered, although the result would not often lead to a recommendation to cease lithium entirely. At all times, the risk of discontinuation of lithium in a patient with a severe unipolar or bipolar affective disorder needs to be considered against the minimal risk of progressive renal injury.

Lead nephropathy

Lead intoxication may occur in a variety of ways, particularly in children exposed to lead-based paints, in adults drinking 'moonshine', and in residents living close to smelting factories and other industries expelling lead into the environment[25]. Acute intoxication is rare but may present with abdominal pain, encephalopathy, hemolytic anemia, peripheral neuropathy, and proximal tubular dysfunction (as manifested by either a proximal RTA or Fanconi's syndrome). In contrast, chronic lead intoxication may be subtle and may manifest primarily with impaired renal function, gout ('saturnine') and hypertension. Occasionally, patients may manifest other signs of chronic lead intoxication including peripheral motor neuropathies, anemia with 'basophilic' stippling and perivascular cerebellar calcifications.

The earliest renal manifestations of chronic lead nephropathy are primarily limited to impaired proximal tubular function, giving rise to hyperuricemia, (resulting from diminished uric acid secretion) and, occasionally, aminoaciduria or renal glycosuria. Chronic lead exposure can ultimately lead to a chronic interstitial nephritis. The pathogenesis of the renal disease may be related to the proximal tubule reabsorption of filtered lead, with subsequent accumulation in the proximal tubule cells. The earliest histologic findings also show proximal tubular injury, with intranuclear inclusion bodies composed of a lead–protein complex. Prolonged lead exposure typically induces the major histologic features of chronic interstitial nephropathy: progressive tubular atrophy and interstitial fibrosis associated with chronic renal insufficiency, a relatively normal urinalysis, hypertension, and gout[25]. Lead nephropathy can therefore be easily confused with chronic urate nephropathy in which urate deposits (tophi) may form in the renal interstitium. Ideally, all patients with significant hyperuricemia and renal insufficiency should have a history of occupational lead exposure excluded[20,25].

Several epidemiologic studies have also suggested that low-level lead exposure may be associated with chronic renal insufficiency and/or hypertension in the general population. In these studies, an increase in lead burden has been shown, but whether or not the association has a causal significance has yet to be established[26].

Diagnosis of chronic lead intoxication is made by the calcium disodium edetate ($CaNa_2$ EDTA) lead chelation test. $CaNa_2$ EDTA is administered (two doses of 0.5 g in 250 mL 5% dextrose given 12 h apart) and urine is collected for 3 days, as urinary excretion is slowed in the setting of renal failure. Normal urinary lead levels are less than 650 mg per 3 days. Treatment involves the use of infusions of $CaNa_2$ EDTA together with removal of the source of lead. The likelihood of a satisfactory response to $CaNa_2$ EDTA will be influenced by the degree of interstitial fibrosis that has already occurred. In the industrial and occupational settings, such as foundry workers and individuals working with lead-based paints and glazes, preventative measures to minimize exposure and low-level absorption are essential.

Other heavy metals

Cadmium

Cadmium can also cause renal disease. It is a metal used in a variety of industries, especially in the manufacturing of alloys and electrical equipment. A major outbreak of cadmium toxicity occurred in Japan as a result of industrial contamination of the Jinzu river in the Toyama prefecture, leading to contamination of rice crops. The disease, named itai-itai or 'ouch-ouch', primarily affected older women and was characterized by proximal tubular dysfunction, anemia, severe osteomalacia and, rarely, progressive chronic interstitial disease. Cadmium workers also have a higher incidence of hypertension and renal stones (the latter caused by hypercalciuria). Prevention is the only effective treatment.

Arsenic

Arsenic is present in insecticides, weed killers, wallpaper and paints. It may rarely cause renal disease. Chronic arsenic toxicity most commonly manifests as sensory and motor neuropathies, distal extremity hyperkeratosis, palmar desquamation, diarrhea and nausea, Aldrich–Mees lines (linear white bands on the nails) and anemia. However, both proximal tubular dysfunction (RTA) and chronic interstitial fibrosis may occur. Diagnosis is made by demonstrating an elevated urinary arsenic level.

Gold and mercury

Exposure to gold (such as from therapy in rheumatoid arthritis) and mercury may be associated with the development of membranous nephropathy that may or may not be accompanied by tubulointerstitial injury (see Chapter 22).

Radiation nephritis

The clinical manifestations of radiation nephritis or nephropathy encompass two main classifications. In 'acute' radiation nephritis, the patient gradually develops symptoms and signs such as edema, hypertension (including occasionally accelerated hypertension), dyspnea, headache, and nocturia. Proteinuria may be marked, whereas the urine sediment is relatively unchanged. Anemia (normochromic, normocytic, or microangiopathic) is likely to be present as is mild-to-moderate renal impairment. Progression to a 'chronic' form of radiation nephritis may follow the acute phase or chronic radiation nephritis may present as a more indolent process, with proteinuria and progressive azotemia and eventually the development of ESRD.

The precise pathogenetic mechanism of radiation nephritis remains obscure. The progression of histologic features include early degenerative, inflammatory and thrombotic changes that lead ultimately to severe glomerular sclerosis, tubular atrophy with associated thickening of the TBM and interstitial fibrosis. Glomerular lesions vary from relatively modest mesangial cell changes (increased cells, increased matrix and mesangiolysis) to frank glomerular capillary and arteriolar necrosis, which may include evidence of thrombosis. Typically the capillary walls are thickened and show 'splitting'. Larger vessels may show patchy intimal proliferation and thickening, intimal fibrosis and fibrinoid necrosis. Interstitial changes, particularly tubular atrophy, may occur even in the absence of glomerular lesions. Severe disease is characterized by progressive interstitial fibrosis and the presence of interstitial inflammatory cells.

The similarities in certain pathologic characteristics of radiation nephritis with those of hemolytic uremic syndrome (HUS) and thrombotic thrombocytopenic purpura, particularly the interposition of amorphous material (deposits) between split layers of the GBM, have raised speculation as to the possible pathogenetic process. Endothelial cell injury, possibly leading to local intravascular coagulation, is one such postulated mechanism. Certainly, the lesions of HUS and associated deterioration in renal function are more prevalent in bone marrow transplant recipients treated with combined radiotherapy and chemotherapy than in those treated with chemotherapy alone. Radiation nephritis has also been seen in bone marrow transplant recipients following total body irradiation and particularly in patients receiving cyclosporine[27]. Cyclosporine is certainly implicated in the development of thrombotic microangiopathy, but whether it enhances the development of radiation nephropathy is not established.

Prevention is the major therapeutic approach to radiation nephritis. Preliminary studies suggest that the risk of developing this condition may be minimized by proper shielding of the kidneys and/or by fractionating the total body irradiation into several small doses over several days. Minimizing the total dose of irradiation to the kidney to less than 20–30 Gy (1 Gy = 100 rad) is recommended. No specific treatment is available for established radiation nephritis; consequently, control of hypertension and supportive treatment for renal insufficiency is the general approach. It seems appropriate to use an angiotensin converting enzyme (ACE) inhibitor in patients who become hypertensive[28].

Balkan nephropathy
Etiology and pathogenesis
Balkan nephropathy is a form of chronic TIN almost exclusively found in some well-defined areas in former Yugoslavia, Bulgaria and Romania (Fig. 62.14)[29]. Balkan nephropathy is geographically localized to a few areas along the Danube's tributaries in regions characterized by plains and low hills that generally have a high humidity and high rainfall. The precise etiology of Balkan nephropathy has never been established, but a variety of factors have been implicated, including genetic factors, environmental agents (such as trace elements and fungal and plant toxins), and immune disturbances.

It has been argued that the inheritance of Balkan nephropathy, the familial nature of which has been recognized for many years, may be polygenic and that manifestations of the genotype might be influenced by the environment. In endemic areas, likely affected individuals are villagers, but several members of one family (household) across one or more generations may be affected with many unaffected households being present in the same area. Bulgarian genetic studies favor an autosomal dominant form of inheritance with linkage to 3q25 on chromosome 3[30]. A partial deficiency of lecithin–cholesterol acyltransferase (LCAT) has been demonstrated in the healthy relatives of patients with Balkan nephropathy. Although familial LCAT deficiency is a rare cause of progressive renal disease, a possible association with the abnormalities of Balkan nephropathy remains unestablished. A search for potential viral etiologies has also been unrewarding. The disease also appears to not be mediated by any primary immune-mediated disease process. Despite significant parenchymal damage, interstitial inflammatory cells are not prominent and immune reactants (such as C3, IgG, and IgM) are only focally present in the mesangium, along the TBM, and in the walls of blood vessels. Various trace elements (lead, cadmium, manganese and silica) and/or fungal and plant toxins have been investigated as possible pathogens. Ochratoxin A, which is a product of the fungus *Penicillium*, has in particular been implicated, although the evidence for this remains unconvincing[30].

The most exciting association has been with contamination of wheat flour with aristolochic acids, which were derived from seeds of *Aristolochia clematis*[30]. Aristolochic acids present in Chinese herbal preparations have been linked to chronic tubulointerstitial disease in Belgium (from *Aristolochia fangchi*)[31] and to a Fanconi's syndrome in Japan (from *Aristolochia manshuriensis*)[32]. The clinical and histologic features of the interstitial disease in the Belgian cases (termed Chinese herbs nephropathy) are remarkably similar to Balkan nephropathy (see below).

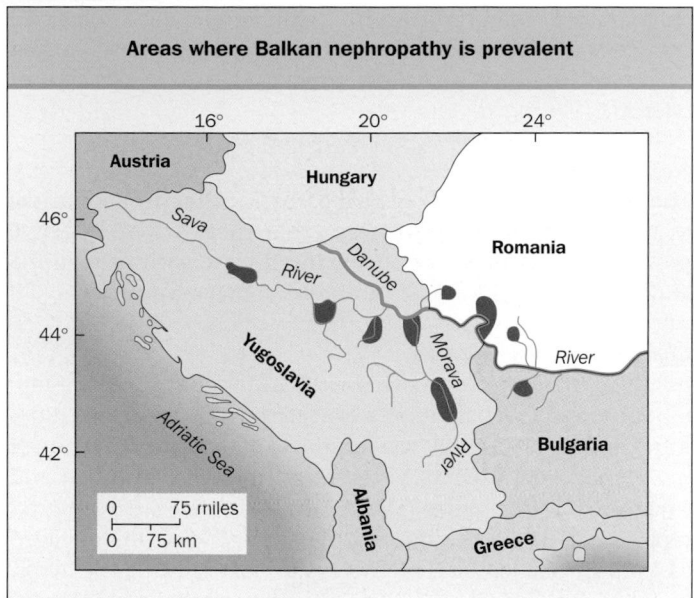

Areas where Balkan nephropathy is prevalent

Figure 62.14 Geographic regions where Balkan nephropathy is prevalent. (Adapted with permission.)

Clinical presentation and diagnosis
Apart from the epidemiologic features described above, the diagnosis of Balkan nephropathy is based on clinical, functional, and histologic characteristics. Balkan nephropathy is a tubulointerstitial kidney disease progressing slowly to ESRD, usually in the fifth or sixth decade of life. Normochromic normocytic anemia disproportionate to the degree of renal impairment is an early feature, whereas salt retention and/or hypertension occurs in the late stages[30].

Proteinuria is usually mild or intermittent but may increase in advanced stages of the disease. An unremarkable urinary sediment is characteristic of Balkan nephropathy, with mild increases in urinary leukocytes and erythrocytes. Macroscopic hematuria suggests the presence of a uroepithelial carcinoma which may involve the bladder, ureter or renal pelvis. The increased incidence of tumors of this type is similar to that observed in both analgesic nephropathy and Chinese herbs nephropathy.

Abnormal renal tubular function, such as impaired acidification, decreased ammonia and increased uric acid excretion, and urine-concentrating defects with renal salt wasting, may precede the decrease in GFR. A symmetric, smooth reduction of the kidney size is characteristic.

Pathology
Proximal tubular lesions characterize the renal biopsy findings in the early stage of disease, with predominantly focal tubular atrophy, interstitial edema and sclerosis, and sometimes mononuclear cell infiltrates. Progression of disease is associated with marked tubular atrophy and interstitial fibrosis. Major changes in the interstitial vasculature (capillaries), such as endothelial cell edema with consequent narrowing of the capillary lumen, have been found in the postglomerular vascular network. These changes correlate with the development of interstitial edema and fibrosis. Early glomerular

changes are mild and focal, with moderately increased numbers of mesangial and endothelial cells. In the advanced stages of the disease, most glomeruli are hyalinized or sclerotic.

Treatment

The treatment of Balkan nephropathy is primarily supportive as the unknown etiology means that there are no effective preventive measures. For advancing disease with proteinuria and/or hypertension, ACE inhibitors are recommended.

Chinese herbs nephropathy

In 1992, an outbreak occurred, primarily in Belgium, of a rapidly progressive renal failure associated with progressive tubulointerstitial fibrosis. It was found to be caused by Chinese herbs that were used as a part of a 'slimming' regimen and that one of the herbs (*Stephania*) had been inadvertently replaced with *A. fangchi*. Most patients were middle-aged women with at least a 6-month history of ingesting the herbs. In these patients, renal failure was often discovered incidentally and was characterized by progressive loss of renal function over several months. The histologic lesion is almost identical to that observed in Balkan nephropathy and, similar to Balkan nephropathy, it is also associated with a marked increased incidence of uroepithelial tumors (Figs 62.15 and 62.16).

There is excellent evidence that the aristolochic acids are responsible for the tubulointerstitial injury. First, there is a direct relationship between the dose of aristolochic herbs ingested and the degree of renal failure in these patients[33]. Second, the administration of aristolochic acid to rats and rabbits has also resulted in tubulointerstitial disease and uroepithelial atypia[34].

Although most patients are managed conservatively, one study suggests that progression of renal failure could be slowed by prednisone therapy (1 mg/kg for 1 month followed by a slow tapering of the dosage) (Fig. 62.17)[31].

Hypokalemic nephropathy

Functional abnormalities

Impaired urine-concentrating ability characterized symptomatically by nocturia, polyuria, and polydipsia may be a feature of chronic hypokalemia [usually when the plasma potassium concentration is consistently < 3.0 mmol/L]. The renal defect, which develops gradually over several weeks, is associated with decreased collecting tubule responsiveness to vasopressin, possibly occurring in part through decreased expression of aquaporin 2, the water channel that fuses with the luminal membrane under the influence of vasopressin. Hypokalemia also increases the tubular production of ammonia and ammonium ions and enhances bicarbonate reabsorption. Mild-to-moderate hypokalemia can impair the ability to excrete a sodium load. An opposite effect may be seen with severe hypokalemia (plasma potassium concentration usually 2 mmol/L). In this setting, maximum sodium chloride reabsorption may be impaired; the exact mechanism is unclear.

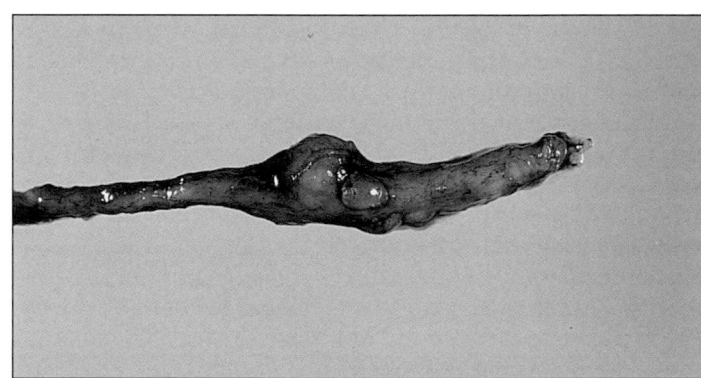

Figure 62.16 Urothelial carcinoma involving the right ureter of a patient with Chinese herbs nephropathy. (Courtesy of M Depierreux MD.)

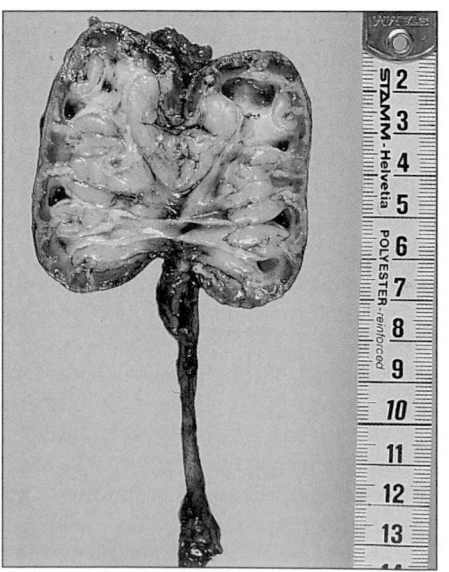

Figure 62.15 Severe atrophy of a kidney in a patient with Chinese herbs nephropathy. Microscopic examination revealed multifocal urothelial lesions ranging from moderate dysplasia to *in situ* carcinoma. (Courtesy of M Depierreux MD.)

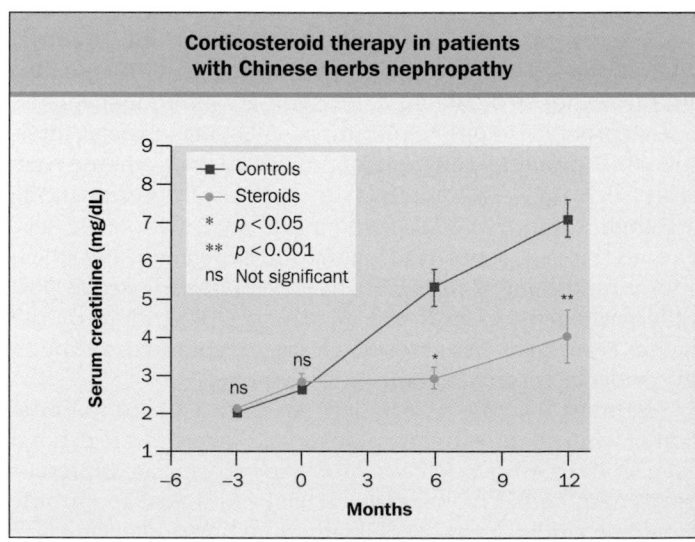

Figure 62.17 Effect of corticosteroid therapy on renal function in patients with Chinese herbs nephropathy. Values are means ± SEM for a control group ($n = 23$) and a group treated with steroids ($n = 12$). Results were compared by Student's t-test for unpaired data. (Adapted with permission.)

Pathology

Hypokalemic nephropathy may result from chronic potassium depletion. Characteristic vacuolated lesions in the cytoplasm of epithelial cells of the proximal tubule and occasionally the distal tubule are observed. This abnormality generally requires at least 1 month to develop and is readily reversible with potassium repletion. More prolonged hypokalemia can lead to more severe changes, predominantly in the renal medulla, including interstitial fibrosis, tubular atrophy, and cyst formation. There is experimental evidence that this may relate to intrarenal vasoconstriction induced by the hypokalemia; indeed both angiotensin receptor antagonists and endothelin receptor antagonists can partially ameliorate the injury[36]. Local ammonia production stimulated by the hypokalemia can also lead to intrarenal complement activation that may contribute to the renal injury; furthermore, the associated intracellular acidosis can stimulate cell proliferation which may account for the occasional development of cysts in hypokalemic subjects[35]. Correction of the hypokalemia can lead to a decrease in the number and size of cysts, although the tubulointerstitial lesions and associated renal insufficiency may be irreversible. There is some experimental evidence that these chronic lesions may lead to the development of sodium-sensitivity[37]. Patients with surreptitious diuretic use, laxative abuse, or primary hyperaldosteronism are at risk of developing chronic lesions.

Hypercalcemic nephropathy

Functional abnormalities

Irrespective of the cause of the hypercalcemia, patients with an elevated serum calcium concentration frequently develop renal functional abnormalities. Impaired urine-concentrating ability is seen most commonly; this manifests as polyuria and polydipsia. The mechanism is incompletely understood but the impairment relates both to reduction in medullary solute content and to interference with the cellular response to vasopressin. Much less commonly, hypercalcemia can also cause an episode of acute renal insufficiency; this defect is usually reversible with correction of the hypercalcemia. Irreversible renal failure is a rare consequence of long-standing hypercalcemia and is almost invariably associated with calcium crystal deposition in the interstitium of the kidney.

Pathology

The most distinctive histologic feature of long-standing hypercalcemia is the occurrence of calcific deposits in the interstitium ('nephrocalcinosis'). Depending on the cause of the metabolic defect, these deposits can be microscopic or macroscopic and most commonly occur in the renal medulla. Macroscopic nephrocalcinosis is often detected on X-ray and/or ultrasound, with the latter being more sensitive but less specific. Ultimately, the demonstration of microscopic nephrocalcinosis may require a renal biopsy, where the other features of chronic interstitial nephritis, such as interstitial fibrosis, tubular atrophy and secondary glomerular sclerosis are often present.

Acute oliguric renal insufficiency can be caused by tubular obstruction with calcium phosphate crystalline casts, but this syndrome most commonly occurs in the context of malignant disease where severe hyperphosphatemia is present.

Renal interstitial disease in sarcoidosis

One of the more common renal presentations of sarcoidosis results from the hypercalcemia that these patients often develop as a consequence of enhanced 1,25–dihydroxyvitamin D_3 production by activated macrophages in the lymph nodes and lungs[38]. The hypercalcemia may result in nephrogenic diabetes insipidus, nephrolithiasis, nephrocalcinosis or, rarely, renal insufficiency. Even more rare is the development of an acute interstitial nephritis with mononuclear cells and noncaseating granulomas (see Chapter 60). This lesion, which is generally steroid responsive, may progress to chronic tubular atrophy and interstitial fibrosis. Glomerular disease (including membranous nephropathy, a proliferative/crescentic glomerulonephritis, and focal glomerulosclerosis) may also rarely occur and is associated with microhematuria and heavy proteinuria.

Renal interstitial disease in systemic lupus erythematosus

Tubulointerstitial disease may occasionally be the only manifestation of lupus nephritis[39]. However, the presence of an interstitial infiltrate and associated tubular injury with or without immune deposits along the TBM is not an uncommon finding in lupus nephritis and is usually seen with concurrent glomerular disease. The severity of the tubulointerstitial involvement has important prognostic significance, correlating positively with the presence of hypertension, elevated plasma creatinine and a progressive clinical course. This possibility of interstitial involvement (without glomerular disease) is suggested by a rising plasma creatinine concentration and a urinalysis that shows a relatively benign or normal urine sediment. Interstitial involvement may be accompanied by signs of tubular dysfunction such as type I or type IV RTA, by isolated hyperkalemia resulting from impaired distal potassium secretion, or by hypokalemia resulting from salt-wasting and secondary hyperaldosteronism. Corticosteroid therapy is usually very effective in preserving renal function in this disorder[39].

Sjögren's syndrome

Sjögren's syndrome may be associated with chronic interstitial disease. The clinical and biochemical manifestations of the interstitial nephritis may be the presenting or only features of Sjögren's syndrome and include a variable, but generally mild, elevation in the plasma creatinine concentration, a relatively benign urinalysis, and abnormalities in tubular function, including Fanconi's syndrome, type 1 (distal) RTA (25% of patients), hypokalemia, and nephrogenic diabetes insipidus (impaired tubular responsiveness to vasopressin). The metabolic acidosis is usually mild, but some patients present with quite a low plasma bicarbonate concentration (< 10 mmol/L) and a low plasma potassium concentration (< 1.5–2.0 mmol/L) resulting from concurrent urinary potassium wasting. Muscle paralysis and respiratory arrest have been reported as the presenting symptoms of Sjögren's syndrome and are the consequences of the severe hypokalemia. The mechanism responsible for type I RTA is incompletely understood but may be related to loss of the H^+ ATPase pump in the intercalated cells of the collecting tubules[29]. Notably, hypokalemia may occur in the absence of RTA[40]. The primary defect is thought to be sodium wasting, which has two potentiating effects on potassium secretion: it increases sodium delivery to the potassium secretory site in the collecting tubules and, because of the associated volume depletion, increases the secretion of aldosterone.

The histologic lesion is characterized by a lymphocytic and plasmacytic interstitial cell infiltrate, tubular cell injury and, rarely, granuloma formation. This progresses over time to tubular atrophy and interstitial fibrosis. Treatment with corticosteroids at the stage of cellular infiltration is frequently beneficial but is not effective if irreversible tubulointerstitial injury has occurred. Regardless, progression to ESRD is a rare event. The glomeruli are typically normal, although rare cases of membranoproliferative glomerulonephritis and membranous nephropathy have been reported. There are no clear treatment guidelines for the glomerular involvement; corticosteroids are most often used but spontaneous remission of glomerular lesions can occur.

Epstein–Barr virus associated chronic interstitial nephritis
There is also recent evidence that some cases of idiopathic chronic interstitial nephritis may be associated with chronic intrarenal infection with Epstein–Barr virus (EBV)[41]. Specifically, there have been a number of cases of interstitial nephritis of unknown etiology in which EBV DNA was localized to proximal tubular cells by *in situ* hybridization; the proximal tubular cells were also shown to express CD21, which is the receptor for EBV on B lymphocytes. These patients had presented with slowly progressive renal failure of unknown etiology. Further studies are necessary to determine if the EBV infection was responsible for the chronic renal scarring.

NATURAL HISTORY AND TREATMENT

The importance of chronic tubulointerstitial injury in progressive renal disease is indicated by the observations that it is the degree of tubulointerstitial injury and not glomerular injury that best correlates not only with current renal function but also with prognosis (Fig. 62.1).

For the most part, therapy applied in the chronic interstitial nephritides will be directed at preventing progressive renal injury and particularly interstitial fibrosis. These are discussed in more detail in Chapter 66. In some conditions where there is evidence of relatively acute inflammation in the tubulointerstitium, or where the renal lesion is secondary to a systemic illness such as systemic lupus or sarcoidosis, there is a role for corticosteroids. Careful monitoring for the development of uroepithelial tumors is also necessary in those diseases in which these tumors occur at increased frequency, most notably analgesic nephropathy, Balkan nephropathy, and Chinese herbs nephropathy. Medullary renal cancers are also increased in sickle cell patients with renal disease (see Chapter 51).

The most acceptable therapies in chronic progressive impairment have some potential to influence the development of interstitial fibrosis directly[3]. For example, control of hypertension and hyperlipidemia have the potential to reduce vascular injury and therefore reduce ischemia in the tubulointerstitium. In addition, reducing glomerular hyperfiltration (e.g., with a low-protein diet) reduces the work load on tubular epithelial cells, leading to less ammoniogenesis, reduced complement activation, and a lower production of various oxygen radicals. All of these changes have the potential to stimulate interstitial inflammation and injury. Most clinicians also favor the use of ACE inhibitors, which reduce glomerular and systemic pressures, decrease proteinuria, and increase renal blood flow. These drugs have shown promise in slowing progression in both experimental and human renal diseases. Other agents, such as drugs aimed at blocking other vasoactive mediators (such as endothelin) or cytokines (PDGF and TGF-β antagonists) are on the horizon but are still not available clinically.

REFERENCES

1. Schainuck LI, Striker GE, Cutler RE, Benditt EP. Structural–functional correlations in renal disease. Hum Pathol. 1970;1:631–41.
2. Eddy AA. Molecular basis of renal fibrosis. Pediatr Nephrol. 2000;15:290–301.
3. Becker GJ, Hewitson TD. The interstitium in renal disease. J Intern Med. 1997;242:93–7.
4. Nielson EG. Pathogenesis and therapy of interstitial nephritis. Kidney Int. 1989;35:1257–70.
5. Rodriguez-Iturbe B, Pons H, Herrera-Acosta J, Johnson RJ. Role of immunocompetent cells in nonimmune renal diseases. Kidney Int. 2001;59:1626–40.
6. Disney APS (ed.). Twentieth Report of the Australian and New Zealand Dialysis and Transplant Registry (ANZDATA). Adelaide, South Australia: Queen Elizabeth Hospital; 1997:28.
7. Rastegar A, Kashgarian M. The clinical spectrum of tubulointerstitial nephritis. Kidney Int. 1998;54:313–27.
8. Johnson RJ, Herrera-Acosta J, Schreiner GF, Rodriguez-Iturbe B. Subtle acquired renal injury as a mechanism of salt-sensitive hypertension. N Engl J Med. 2002;346:913–23.
9. Nanra RS. Analgesic nephropathy in the 1990s – an Australian perspective. Kidney Int. 1993;42:S86–92.
10. Russ GR (ed.). Twenty Fourth Report of the Australian and New Zealand Dialysis and Transplant Registry (ANZDATA). Adelaide, South Australia: Queen Elizabeth Hospital; 2001:13.
11. DeBroe ME, Elseveirs MM. Analgesic nephropathy. N Engl J Med 1998;338:446–51.
12. Ad Hoc Committee of the International Study Group on Analgesics and Nephropathy. Relationship between nonphenacetin combined analgesics and nephropathy: a review. Kidney Int. 2000;58:2259–64
13. Fored CM, Ejerblad E, Lindblad P, et al. Acetaminophen, aspirin, and chronic renal failure. N Engl J Med. 2001;345:1801–8.
14. Johnson RJ, Kivlighn S, Kim Y-K, et al. A reappraisal of the pathogenesis and consequences of hyperuricemia in hypertension, and renal disease. Am J Kidney Dis. 1999;33:224–34.
15. Nickeleit V, Mihatsch MJ. Uric acid nephropathy and end stage renal disease – review of a non-disease. Nephrol Dial Transplant. 1997;12:1832–8.
16. Mazzali M, Hughes J, Kim YG, et al. Elevated uric acid increases blood pressure in the rat by a novel crystal-independent mechanism. Hypertension. 2001;38:1101–6.
17. Mazzali M, Kanellis J, Han L, et al. Hyperuricemia induces a primary renal arteriolopathy in rats by a blood pressure-independent mechanism. Am J Physiol Renal Physiol. 2002;282:F991–7.

18. Mazzali M, Kim YG, Suga S, et al. Hyperuricemia exacerbates chronic cyclosporine nephropathy. Transplantation. 2001;71:900–5.
19. Kang DH, Nakagawa T, Feng L, et al. A role for uric acid in the progression of renal disease. J Am Soc Nephrol. 2002;13:2888–97.
20. Murray T, Goldberg M. Chronic interstitial nephritis: etiologic factors. Ann Intern Med. 1975;82:453–9.
21. Loghman-Adham M. Renal effects of environmental and occupational lead exposure. Environ Health Persp. 1997;105:928–39.
22. Puig JG, Miranda ME, Mateos FA, et al. Hereditary nephropathy associated with hyperuricemia and gout. Arch Intern Med. 1993;153: 357–65.
23. Walker, RG. Lithium nephrotoxicity. Kidney Int. 1993;42:S93–8.
24. Timmer RT, Sands JM. Lithium intoxication. J Am Soc Nephrol. 1999;10:666–674
25. Batlle DC, von Riotte AB, Gaviria M, Grupp M. Amelioration of polyuria by amiloride in patients receiving long-term lithium therapy. N Engl J Med. 1985;312:408–14.
26. Bennett WM. Lead nephropathy. Kidney Int. 1985;28:212–20.
27. Sanchez-Fructuoso AI, Torralbo A, Arroyo M, et al. Occult lead intoxication as a cause of hypertension and renal failure. Nephrol Dial Transplant. 1996;11:1775–80.
28. Cohen EP, Lawton CA, Moulder JE, et al. Clinical course of late-onset bone marrow transplant nephropathy. Nephron. 1993;64:626–35.
29. Cohen EP, Lawton CA, Moulder JE. Treatment of radiation nephropathy with captopril. Radiat Res. 1992;132:346–50.
30. Feder GL, Radovanovic Z, Finkelman RG. Relationship between weathered coal deposits and the etiology of Balkan endemic nephropathy. Kidney Int. 1991;40:S9–11.
31. Stefanovíc V. Balkan endemic nephropathy: a need for novel aetiological approaches. QJ Med. 1998;91:457–63.
32. Vanherweghem J-L, Abramowicz D, Tielemans C, Depierreux M. Effects of steroids on the progression of renal failure in chronic interstitial renal fibrosis: a pilot study in Chinese herbs nephropathy. Am J Kidney Dis. 1996;27:209–15.
33. Tanaka A, Nishida R, Maeda K, et al. Chinese herb nephropathy in Japan presents adult-onset Fanconi syndrome; could different components of aristolochic acids cause a different type of Chinese herb nephropathy? Clin Nephrol. 2000;53:301–6.
34. Martinez MM, Nortier J, Vereerstraeten P, Vanherweghem J-L. Progression rate of Chinese herb nephropathy: impact of *Aristolochia fangchi* ingested dose. Nephrol Dial Transplant. 2002;17:408–12.
35. Debelle FD, Nortier JL, De Prez EG, et al. Aristolochic acids induce chronic renal failure with interstitial fibrosis in salt-depleted rats. J Am Soc Nephrol. 2002;13:431–6.
36. Alpern RJ, Toto RD. Hypokalemic nephropathy – a clue to cystogenesis. N Engl J Med. 1990;322:398–9.
37. Suga S, Mazzali M, Ray PE, et al. Angiotensin II type 1 receptor blockade ameliorates tubulointerstitial injury induced by chronic potassium deficiency. Kidney Int. 2002;61:951–8.
38. Suga S, Phillips MI, Ray PE, et al. Hypokalemia induces renal injury and alterations in vasoactive mediators that favor salt sensitivity. Am J Physiol Renal Physiol. 2001;281:F620–9.
39. Göbel U, Kettritz R, Schneider W, Luft FC. The protean face of renal sarcoidosis. J Am Soc Nephrol. 2001;12:616–23.
40. Berden JH. Lupus nephritis. Kidney Int. 1997;52:538–58.
41. Cohen EP, Bastani B, Cohen MR, et al. Absence of H^+-ATPase in cortical collecting tubules of a patient with Sjögren's syndrome and distal renal tubular acidosis. J Am Soc Nephrol. 1992;3:264–71.
42. Becker JL, Miller F, Nuovo GJ, et al. Epstein-Barr virus infection of renal proximal tubule cells: possible role in chronic interstitial nephritis. J Clin Invest. 1999;104:1673–81.

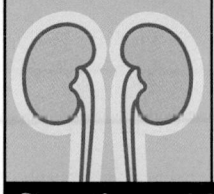

Chapter 63

Atheromatous Renovascular Disease

Julia Lewis and Barbara Greco

INTRODUCTION

Atheromatous renal artery disease is common and has varied clinical manifestations. Improved sensitivity of screening tests allow easy identification of renal artery stenosis. Advances in pharmacologic management of hypertension as well as technical advances in endovascular and surgical revascularization have led to more frequent referrals for intervention. Yet, the optimal approach to atheromatous renovascular disease remains controversial and a challenge to clinicians.

CLINICAL SYNDROMES SECONDARY TO ATHEROMATOUS RENAL DISEASE

Atheromatous renal disease may present clinically as one of several clinical syndromes, with some overlap (Table 63.1).

Nonhemodynamically significant atheromatous renal artery disease (stenosis < 50%) may be present with no clinical sequelae. Because these lesions may progress to clinically significant stenosis with hypertension and/or renal ischemia, close follow-up is necessary. For borderline lesions (50–70%), there is no accurate diagnostic maneuver to determine hemodynamic significance making optimal management of these lesions controversial.

Second, hemodynamically significant renal artery stenosis can present predominantly as renovascular hypertension (RVH) without significant detectable renal insufficiency. This subject is covered extensively in Chapter 39.

Third, significant renovascular stenosis can present as renal insufficiency usually, but not always, associated with some degree of hypertension. This clinical entity has been termed ischemic renal disease (IRD), ischemic nephropathy or renovascular renal insufficiency.

Fourth, atheroembolism (cholesterol embolization) may result from proximal aortorenal atherosclerosis and has a clinical course quite distinct from the other clinical syndromes.

Transplant renal artery stenosis (TRAS) is another clinical setting in which atheromatous disease along with mechanical, hemodynamic, and immunologic processes diminish perfusion to the allograft, resulting in hypertension and renal insufficiency. Because the course of TRAS is different from that of native kidney IRD and classic RVH, it will be considered separately in this chapter.

Finally, acute renal infarction is another clinical manifestation of atheromatous reno-occlusive disease; it is usually associated with renal artery thrombosis secondary to embolism, dissection or aneurysm of the renal vessel. This is discussed in Chapter 64.

ISCHEMIC RENAL DISEASE

Definition

Critical reduction in renal blood flow to the functioning renal parenchyma as a result of atheromatous stenotic narrowing of the renal artery can result in a state of diminished glomerular filtration rate (GFR) known as IRD. IRD occurs when renal perfusion pressure drops below the limits of autoregulatory compensation, equivalent to 60–70 mmHg. This generally corresponds to a renal artery luminal diameter narrowing of 70% or greater. Over time, progressive renal injury and atrophy develop and this can lead to permanent loss of renal structural and functional integrity. Generally, the term IRD refers to the hemodynamic and, therefore, potentially reversible component of this chronic ischemic state, though it is important for the clinician to recognize the irreversible consequences of untreated chronic renal ischemia.

IRD is associated with three anatomic variations: unilateral stenosis or occlusion in a single kidney, bilateral critical renal artery stenosis or occlusion, or unilateral critical renal artery stenosis or occlusion with contralateral renal nonfunction (Fig. 63.1). When critical atheromatous renovascular disease compromises function unilaterally, there is generally ipsilateral atrophy and a compensatory increase in function and sometimes

Clinical syndromes associated with atheromatous renovascular disease

Ischemic renal disease (IRD)
    ACE Inhibitor induced acute renal failure
    Azotemia in a patient with renovascular hypertension
    Flash pulmonary edema
    Unexplained azotemia in the elderly

Atheroembolic renal disease
Transplant renal artery stenosis (TRAS)
Renovascular hypertension (RVH; see Chapter 39)

Acute renal infarction (see Chapter 64)
    Dissection of the aorta and/or renal artery
    Aneurysm of the renal artery
    Thrombosis of the renal artery

Hemodynamically in significant atheromatous involvement of the renal vessels in a patient with extrarenal atherosclerosis: requires close follow-up to detect progression to significant disease

Table 63.1 Clinical syndromes associated with atheromatous renovascular disease.

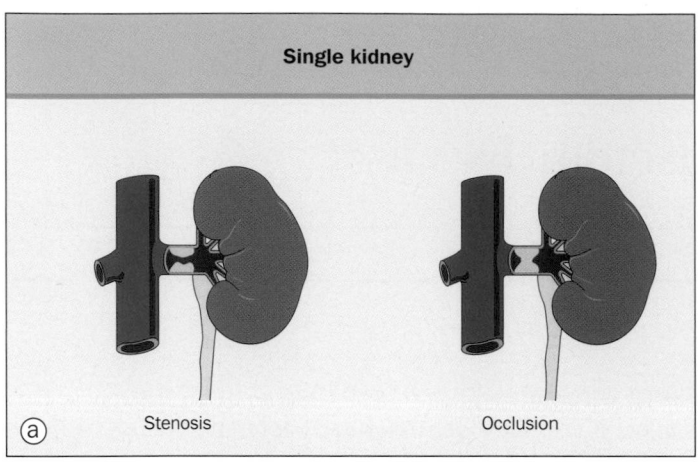

Single kidney

Stenosis   Occlusion

(a)

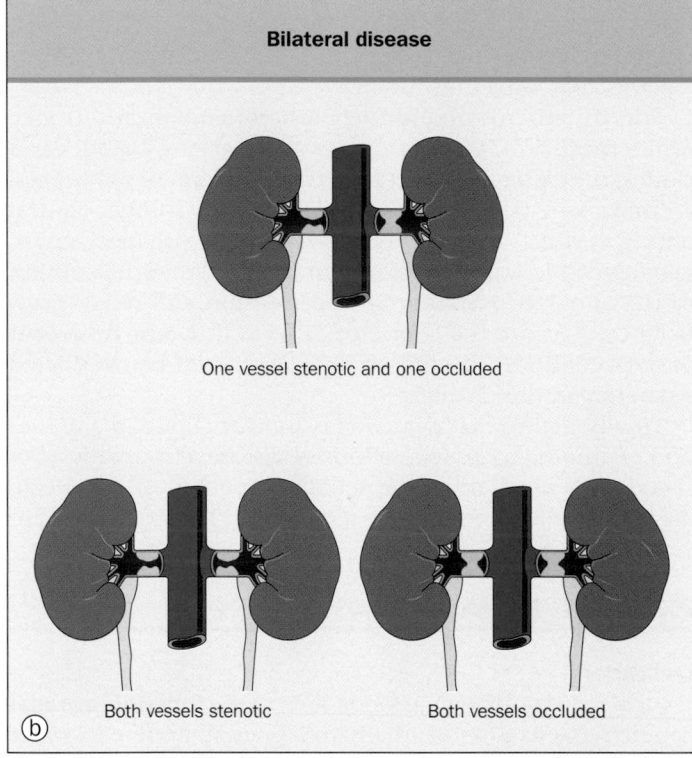

Bilateral disease

One vessel stenotic and one occluded

Both vessels stenotic   Both vessels occluded

(b)

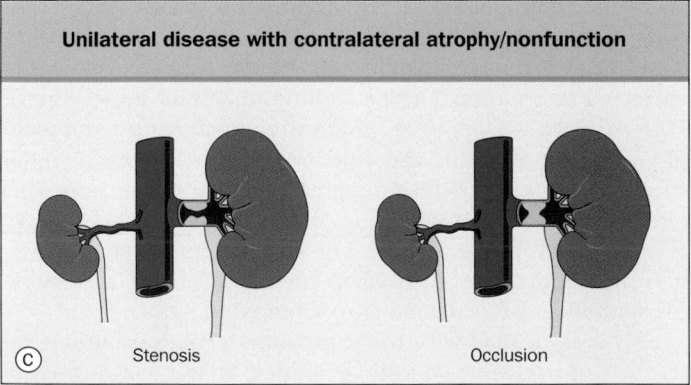

Unilateral disease with contralateral atrophy/nonfunction

Stenosis   Occlusion

(c)

Figure 63.1 Anatomic variations of ischemic renal disease. The renal artery can be partially or totally occluded in situations of (a) single functioning kidney, (b) bilateral disease or (c) unilateral disease with contralateral nonfunction.

size of the contralateral normal kidney. Although total renal function may be normal in this setting, more commonly, the contralateral kidney has developed hypertensive injury damage or injury from long-standing compensatory hyperfiltration. The presence of parenchymal renal disease in the hypertensive, nonstenosed kidney may make it difficult to ascertain the role of the ischemic kidney with unilateral renal arterial disease in the overall decrement in GFR.

Etiology and pathogenesis

IRD develops when atheromatous disease compromises blood flow to the functioning renal parenchyma. This usually requires a stenosis of 70% or higher that results in a reduction in renal perfusion pressure which prevents the kidney from effectively autoregulating its renal blood flow and GFR. As a consequence, there is decreased delivery of oxygen and nutrients to the renal parenchyma, resulting is ischemia. Ischemia is most severe in the outer medulla and medullary rays, as the tubules in this region are most susceptible to injury because, in the normal state, they are already borderline hypoxic due to the metabolic demands of the tubules and the countercurrent circulation.

Chronic ischemia leads to renal scarring and atrophy, as well as to the production of vasoactive mediators (such as renin) that can increase blood pressure. The kidney decreases in size. The renal atrophy represents an adaptive response to renal ischemia, with histologic correlates of tubular atrophy and glomerular involution with wrinkling of the glomerular capillary wall (Fig. 63.2). Occasionally, renal atrophy may be reversed by restoration of renal perfusion, with recovery of renal function and an increase in renal size following revascularization. More commonly, renal atrophy is associated with irreversible patchy areas of cortical scarring, sclerotic glomeruli and interstitial fibrosis (Fig. 63.3). These considerations complicate decisions regarding the optimal approach to a poststenotic or post-occlusion atrophic kidney, even when distal vessel reconstitution is visible angiographicallly. The ultimate renal functional response to aggressive intervention depends on the relative contributions of the hemodynamic and structural effects of diminished perfusion to the overall reduction in GFR.

While renal arterial disease may lead to ischemia and renal atrophy, in some patients, the suprarenal, the lumbar, and the ureteric vessel complexes may provide an accessory vascular

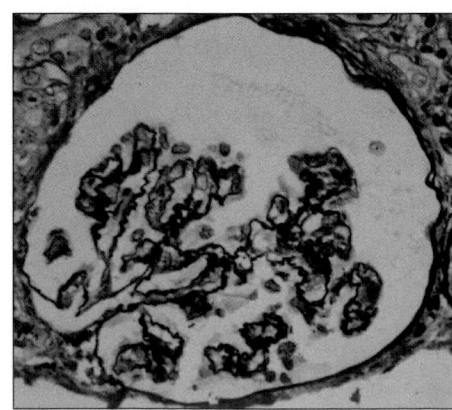

Figure 63.2 Ischemic glomerular changes. This Jones silver stain of a glomerulus demonstrates the glomerular collapse associated with wrinkling of the basement membrane characteristic of ischemia. (Courtesy of Dr R. Horn.)

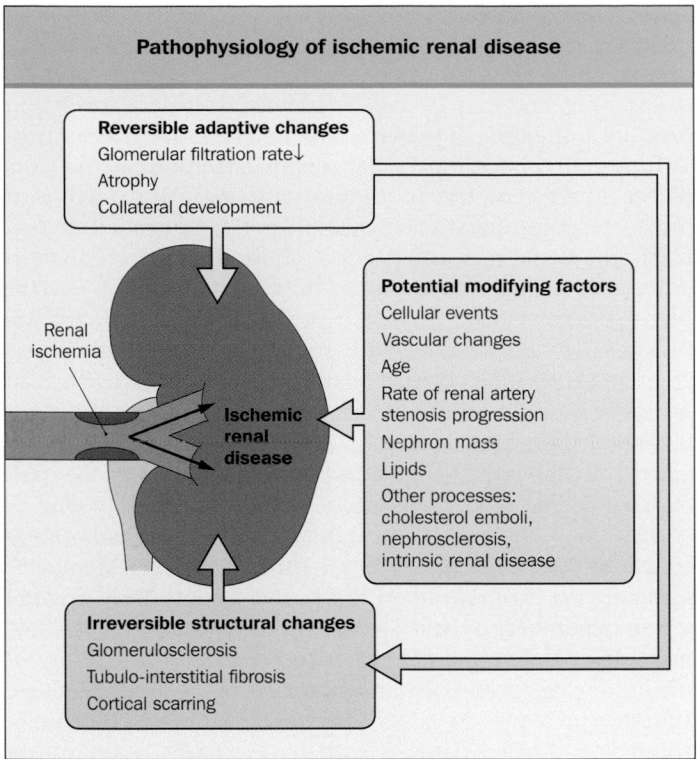

Figure 63.3 Pathophysiology of ischemic renal disease. Chronic ischemia of the kidney is associated with reversible functional involution and atrophy as well as irreversible structural changes. A number of external factors influence the renal response to chronic ischemia. (Adapted with permission[20].)

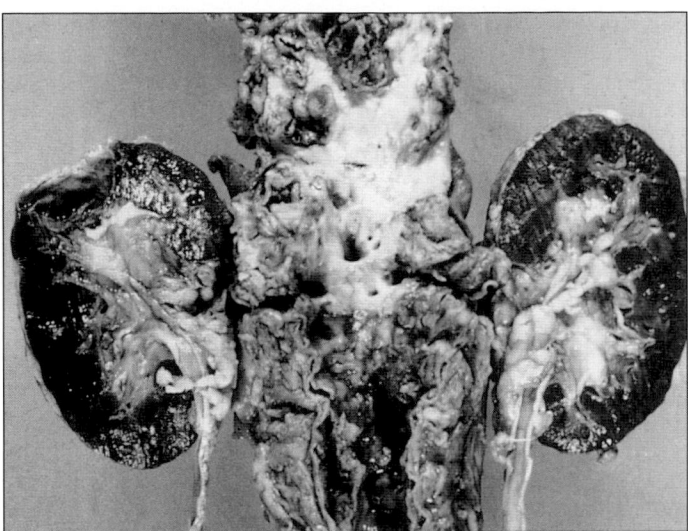

Figure 63.4 Atherosclerosis of the aorta exending into the renal artery. Section taken at autopsy of a 62-year-old man, Note the nodular scarred appearance of the kidneys caused by arterionephrosclerosis. (Adapted with permission from Dr R. Collins).

supply to the kidneys. These collaterals can maintain parenchymal viability in states of critical reduction in proximal renal blood flow. The factors determining the development and caliber of these vessels are poorly understood but likely relate to the state of the aorta, the rate of progression of main renal artery narrowing, and the condition of the intrarenal perforating arteries.

Epidemiology

Atherosclerotic renovascular disease affects older patients (generally > 50 years) with risk factors for generalized atherosclerosis. Most series report a predominance of Caucasians among their populations with significant renovascular disease. Whether this is a true racial predilection or reflects differences in screening patterns is unclear, and the answer will require prospective studies that include larger numbers of minority groups.

The prevalence of renal artery atherosclerosis is unknown because of the lack of population-based epidemiologic studies. However, autopsy studies report an overall prevalence of 4–20% with higher rates for those older than 60 years (25–30%) and 75 years (40–60%). Predictors of significant renal artery stenosis include a history of hypertension, renal insufficiency, coexisting coronary artery, carotid or peripheral vascular disease[1-3].

Angiographic studies have confirmed that, in the atherosclerotic age group, the prevalence of renovascular disease ranges between 11–42%. In patients undergoing arteriography to evaluate extrarenal atherosclerosis, unsuspected renal artery stenosis is common[4,5]. Conversely, when atheromatous renovascular disease exists, it is associated with extrarenal atherosclerosis more than 85% of the time.

Atheromatous renovascular disease frequently results from extension from diffuse aortic atherosclerosis (Fig. 63.4). Therefore, renal artery ostial disease limiting inflow to the vessel is common and present in up to 85% of cases; mid-vessel and distal renal artery stenosis account for less than 5% of cases. Bilateral renovascular disease is present in 30–80% of patients. An atrophic kidney has a 70% chance of being associated with ipsilateral significant renal artery stenosis.

The incidence of IRD as a cause of renal failure has been estimated from data derived from end-stage renal disease (ESRD) programs. The ESRD population worldwide is aging and, in the USA, the median age of patients entering renal replacement therapy is between 60–65 years. Several centers have screened their populations entering ESRD therapy for the existence of significant renal artery stenosis, either by clinical criteria or using angiography or renal duplex sonography. These data suggest IRD may have a contributory role in between 11–22% of all patients with ESRD on dialysis[6].

Clinical presentation

IRD should be considered in several clinical settings.

Acute renal failure precipitated by treatment of hypertension

Acute renal failure (ARF) may be precipitated in IRD by the treatment of hypertension, particularly with angiotensin converting enzyme (ACE) inhibitors. The sudden reduction in systemic blood pressure, in the setting of critical renal arterial stenosis, may lead to hypoperfusion of the kidney. With ACE inhibitors, there may also be alterations in glomerular hemodynamics independent of any effect on systemic blood pressure, which can lead to ARF. ACE inhibitors decrease efferent arteriolar resistance and, hence, decrease glomerular capillary filtration pressure. In the setting of renal arterial disease, the GFR may be critically dependent on angiotensin-mediated increased efferent arteriolar resistance. ARF in this setting typically occurs 1–14 days after the start of antihypertensive therapy[7] and is usually, but not always, reversible.

Most patients with renal vascular disease who are treated with ACE inhibitors will not develop acute renal failure[8]; this is likely because those with unilateral stenosis often have preserved function in the nonstenosed kidney, and because those with bilateral renovascular disease often have sodium retention and the GFR is no longer angiotensin II-dependent. However, ACE inhibitors are more likely to precipitate renal failure in patients with bilateral renal vascular disease if the patients are on diuretics that will reduce the blood volume and unmask the angiotensin II dependence of the GFR.

Because the majority of patients with renovascular disease treated with ACE inhibitors do not develop acute renal failure, it cannot be assumed that these patients do not have IRD. Conversely, acute renal failure can occur with the use of ACE inhibitors in hypertensive patients in the absence of IRD. This most commonly occurs in patients with intravascular volume depletion as, in this setting, GFR is also angiotensin II-dependent[9].

Despite widespread awareness of the potential for ACE inhibitor induced acute renal failure, surveys in England of primary care physicians have revealed that only approximately one-third of physicians routinely monitor renal function after initiating ACE inhibitor therapy[10]. However, in a prospective study, the criterion of a 20% increase in serum creatinine was 100% sensitive and 70% specific for bilateral severe renal artery stenosis. No case of acute renal failure was encountered in that study[11]. After the resolution of acute renal failure, patients should undergo evaluation for the presence of IRD. ARF can also be precipitated in a patient with IRD in the setting of hypovolemia, intrarenal cholesterol emboli or sudden renal arterial occlusion.

Patients with established RVH who develop azotemia
Patients with RVH should also be suspected of having IRD if they develop azotemia or are found to have a decrease in kidney size (by ultrasound). The vast majority of patients who present with hypertensive azotemia will have either primary renal disease or hypertensive nephrosclerosis. However, the possibility of undetected RVH and associated IRD should always be considered. Clinical factors that help distinguish RVH from essential hypertension were identified in the Cooperative Study of Renovascular Hypertension and include older age, a shorter duration of hypertension, difficult to control blood pressure, recent worsening of blood pressure, or accelerated hypertension[12]. In addition, histories of peripheral vascular disease, coronary artery disease, or cerebral vascular disease were more common in patients with RVH. Patients with RVH also have an increased prevalence of grade III or IV hypertensive retinopathy and abdominal or flank bruits. A decrease in renal function or small or asymmetric kidneys by ultrasound in the presence of these clinical clues suggests the presence of RVH and IRD.

Patients with 'flash' pulmonary edema
IRD may present as recurrent episodes of 'flash' pulmonary edema. These episodes can be unpredictable, sudden, and life threatening, and may be associated with normal or low blood pressure at the time of presentation. In a retrospective study of 191 patients undergoing renal revascularization, 17 patients (8.9%) underwent the procedure with a clinical picture of recurrent pulmonary edema and poorly controlled hypertension[13]. Renal revascularization aborted the cyclical flash pulmonary edema and improved pulmonary function even in those patients with a very poor preoperative pulmonary status. In ninety consecutive patients with renovascular disease, 23 of 56 (41%) subjects with bilateral renal artery stenosis had a history of pulmonary edema compared to 34 (12%) with unilateral renovascular disease. Seventy-seven percent of the patients with bilateral renal artery stenosis had no further pulmonary edema after renal artery stent placement in one or both arteries. The patients who did have recurrent pulmonary edema all had evidence of stent thrombosis or restenosis[14]. Although the mechanism for this is unclear, it is likely that the severe hypertension associated with IRD leads to hypertensive heart disease. As renal insufficiency progresses, the ability of the kidney to excrete salt and water becomes limited. Severe episodic increases in blood pressure in these chronically volume-overloaded patients with hypertensive heart disease may explain the flash pulmonary edema episodes. Therefore, patients who present with recurrent episodes of acute pulmonary edema associated with severe hypertension and renal insufficiency should be evaluated for the presence of IRD.

Unexplained azotemia in elderly patients
Diagnosis of IRD should also be considered in unexplained azotemia in elderly patients, particularly in those with diffuse atherosclerotic disease. As mentioned above, renal artery stenosis is prevalent in patients with atherosclerotic disease. Therefore, elderly patients who have documented peripheral vascular, cerebral vascular, or coronary artery atherosclerosis are at higher risk for occult IRD. The diagnosis of IRD should also be considered in elderly patients with unexplained azotemia who have either the recent onset of hypertension or in whom there is a recent difficulty controlling hypertension. It is important to remember that essential hypertension typically presents between the ages of 25 and 45 years. Therefore, IRD should be considered if the patient has new-onset hypertension after age 60 years, particularly if the patient is also azotemic.

Diagnosis of ischemic renal disease
Screening tests
The diagnosis of IRD involves both the identification of critical renovascular disease in patients with renal insufficiency and an assessment of the role that diminished renal perfusion is playing in the decrement in GFR.

The three best screening tests for renal artery stenosis are magnetic resonance angiography (MRA), renal duplex sonography (RDS) and spiral computed tomography (CT) (Table 63.2). A recent meta-analysis evaluated studies using CT, MRA, RDS, captopril renal scintigraphy and the captopril test for identifying renal artery stenosis in patients suspected of having

Noninvasive testing for ischemic renal disease	
Test	**Comment**
Intravenous urogram and/or renal ultrasound	Not directly helpful: can define renal anatomy (kidney size, one or two kidneys) and rule out obstruction
Plasma renin activity and captopril-stimulated plasma renin activity	Reduced specificity with renal insufficiency
Renal vein renins	Not directly helpful since bilateral disease is present
Isotopic renal blood flow and functional scans	Not directly helpful because of bilateral renal artery disease and because it is difficult to differentiate from intrinsic disease
Captopril renography	Excellent for renovascular hypertension but not accurate in severe renal insufficiency and requires great care for accuracy with moderate renal insufficiency
Doppler ultrasonography	Can be technically difficult if bowel gas or obesity interfere
Magnetic resonance angiography	Blood flow turbulence can exaggerate measured stenosis
(Adapted with permission[20].)	

Table 63.2 Noninvasive testing for ischemic renal disease.

RVH. MRA and CT proved to have much better diagnostic accuracy than ultrasonography in this population[15].

If the clinician has a moderate index of suspicion for the presence of renovascular disease and there are no contraindications, MRA is probably the best screen for the presence of significant renal artery stenosis in patients with renal insufficiency. It is noninvasive and requires no radiocontrast or nephrotoxic agents. The test requires the patient to hold his breath and to lie motionless during imaging. Studies have shown gadolinium-enhanced three-dimensional MRA to be highly sensitive (92–100%) and specific (83–95%) for accurately identifying high-grade renal artery stenosis with negative predictive values as high as 100%. The MRA may slightly overestimate the degree of stenosis, particularly in the mid to distal renal vessels, and segmental renal branches are not reliably seen. Accessory renal arteries may also be missed by MRA and there is some interobserver variability. Subtle forms of fibromuscular dysplasia may be missed by MRA[16]. CT has similar sensitivity and specificity as MRA but has the disadvantage of requiring intravenous radiocontrast administration (usually 100–150 mL) with its attendant risk of contrast induced acute renal failure. It may prove useful in following stented renal arteries for restenosis.

An in depth discussion of RDS is provided in Chapter 5. Direct interrogation of the main renal artery as well as indirect duplex evaluation of the distal arterial tree can detect lesions with > 59% renal artery stenosis. A peak systolic velocity in the main renal artery of more than 180 cm/s is the accepted threshold of detection of stenosis > 50%. This technique has been reported to be highly sensitive and specific, but caveats to technical success include operator dependency, and patient factors including habitus, echogenicity of fascia, depth or angle

of arteries and bowel gas interference. Hence, not all centers have been able to reproduce the high accuracy rates of RDS. Indeed, one prospective study comparing RDS to MRA found MRA to have greater sensitivity and negative predictive value in predicting renal artery stenoses[16]. However, RDS may be useful for following renal vessels with stents for the development of in-stent stenosis, although more studies are needed to determine its accuracy in this regard. Finally, determination of resistive-index values using RDS has been shown to predict the renal function outcome of renal revascularization[17].

There are no good tests to determine the functional significance of renal artery stenosis. Potential tests include measurement of pressure gradients across the stenosis with a ΔP of 20 mmHg considered significant. Isotopic renal blood flow and functional scan studies are not directly helpful in diagnosing IRD because they depend on a comparison of an involved and an uninvolved side whereas IRD often involves both kidneys. Captopril renography, an accurate, noninvasive screen for RVH, can be helpful in assessing the significance of renovascular disease, but its specificity is diminished with advancing renal insufficiency. Both plasma renin activity and renal vein renin measurements also have reduced specificity in the setting of renal insufficiency[18].

Diagnostic tests

MRA has become so sensitive and specific that it is considered both a screening test and a diagnostic test. The use of the MRA allows the clinician to proceed with angiography under special circumstances, such as when endovascular intervention is planned, if pressure gradient measurements are desired to determine whether the stenosis is sufficient to warrant nonmedical intervention, or if more accurate measurements of the stenosis are required. Since MRA will miss some accessory vessels, in situations of high clinical suspicion, renal angiography remains the gold standard for the identification of renal artery stenosis in IRD. Renal arteriography can be performed by conventional aortography, intravenous subtraction angiography, intra-arterial subtraction angiography or carbon dioxide angiography (Table 63.3).

Angiography in the diagnosis of ischemic renal disease				
Test	**Volume of contrast**	**Arterial puncture**	**Risk of emboli (catheterization)**	**Quality of images**
Conventional aortography	++	Yes	+++	+++
Intravenous subtraction angiography	+++	No	No	+
Intra-arterial subtraction angiography	+	Yes	++	++
Carbon dioxide angiography	None	Yes	+++	+
+ to +++ indicates increasing effect (Adapted with permission[20].)				

Table 63.3 Angiography in the diagnosis of ischemic renal disease.
Comparitive features of available angiographic techniques.

Conventional aortography produces excellent radiographic images of the renal artery and can demonstrate retrograde filling of distal renal arteries and collateral flow to the kidneys. Conventional aortography also can assess the aorta and the splenic, hepatic, celiac and iliac arteries, which might be used for extra-aortic surgical revascularization. The collateral circulation is well visualized, along with distal filling of an occluded vessel and an associated delayed nephrogram. Figure 63.5a shows an aortogram of a patient with bilateral atherosclerotic reno-occlusive disease with total occlusion of the right renal artery. Initially, the right kidney was not visualized, but the delayed view (Fig. 63.5b) demonstrates a right renal blush and distal reconstitution of the ipsilateral artery. The disadvantage of conventional aortography is that it requires an arterial puncture, the use of a reasonably large catheter (with a risk of cholesterol emboli) and the use of a moderate amount of potentially nephrotoxic radiocontrast material. Therefore, in some situations, alternate approaches should be selected.

Intravenous subtraction angiography is sensitive for identifying stenosis of the main renal artery, but does not sufficiently demonstrate accessory or branch renal arteries and uses a high volume of contrast. Intra-arterial digital subtraction angiography has a high diagnostic accuracy compared to conventional angiography. Although requiring arterial puncture, the volume of contrast is markedly reduced and the smaller catheter width decreases the risk of cholesterol embolization. Finally, carbon dioxide digital subtraction angiography has been shown to provide images that are comparable with those achieved with traditional radiocontrast angiography. This technique avoids the risk of conventional nephrotoxic agents but requires an experienced radiologist and a dedicated carbon dioxide injector. Proximal vessels are seen well, but visualization of the distal main and branch renal arteries requires the use of supplemental radiocontrast, usually less than 20 mL.

Differential diagnosis

The differential diagnosis includes hypertensive nephrosclerosis, atheroembolic renal disease, diabetic nephropathy and other unsuspected interstitial processes, such as drug-induced interstitial nephritis, urate nephropathy, autoimmune processes, and even occult glomerular diseases (e.g., focal segmental glomerulosclerosis). In patients with coexistent congestive heart failure, renal artery stenosis is often present but the predominant insult to renal function is the poor cardiac output owing to myocardial failure rather than the hemodynamic influence of the main renovascular disease. These factors make it difficult for the clinician to predict *a priori* those patients who will benefit from renal revascularization. Several investigators have commented that the only proof of the diagnosis of IRD is in the renal functional response to reperfusion. Even this is unreliable in cases where chronic ischemia has resulted in severe irreversible renal injury, often accompanied by significant atrophy. Renal biopsy has not been helpful in terms of predicting reversibility, as pathologic ischemic changes are often patchy. Thus, the clinician must carefully weigh all the factors in their individual patient before assigning the diagnosis of clinically significant IRD.

Proteinuria > 2 g/day is rare and should lead to consideration of other diagnoses. While the majority of patients (52% in

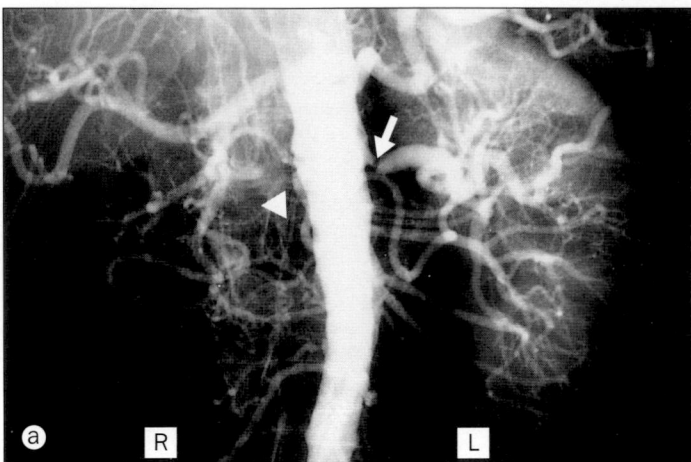

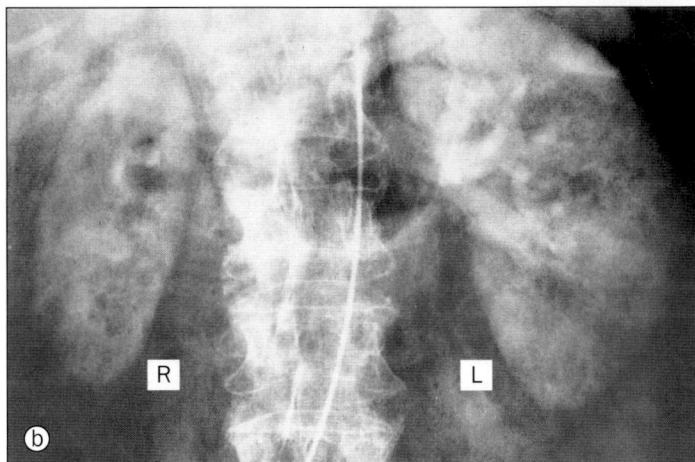

Figure 63.5 Aortogram demonstrating bilateral reno-occlusive disease. (a) This aortogram demonstrates one of the anatomic variations of ischemic renal disease (RD): the left renal artery has a tight proximal stenosis (arrow) and the right renal artery is totally occluded (arrowhead). Collateral vessels are visualized on the right. A contrast blush clearly shows the left kidney but the right kidney is not visible on this early film. (b) Delayed nephrogram, at a later time during the same aortogram, shows a viable right kidney, which appears as a delayed contrast blush. The right kidney is viable because of the collateral blood supply but, in the setting of chronic proximal renovascular disease, the kidney has atrophied.

one study) demonstrate proteinuria (< 0.5 g/24 h), proteinuria does increase with worsening renal function in patients with IRD and this suggests that the proteinuria may be a marker for worse parenchymal disease due to atherosclerotic or hypertensive parenchymal disease (including cholesterol emboli, glomerulosclerosis with ischemic changes)[19].

Natural history

Both serial angiographic studies and evaluations using renal duplex sonography have documented progression of renal artery stenosis in 40–50% of patients with atherosclerotic renovascular disease over a 1–2-year period[20] (Table 63.4). Progression is usually defined as a greater than 25% luminal diameter narrowing or progression from severe stenosis to occlusion of the vessel. In addition to progression of the arterial lesions, progression is likely if there is a 1 cm or more

Table 63.4 Natural history of renal artery stenosis.

Authors	Modality	Year	No. of patients	Length of follow-up (months)	Progression (%)	Occlusion (%)
Meaney et al.	Angiography	1968	39	6–120	36	8
Wollenweber et al.	Angiography	1968	30	12–88	63	–
Dean et al.	Angiography	1981	35	6–102	29	11
Schreiber et al.	Angiography	1984	85	12–60	44	16
Tollefson and Ernst	Angiography	1991	48	15–180	71	15
Zierler et al.	Renal duplex sonography	1994	80	6–24	42	11

Natural history of renal artery stenosis

(Adapted with permission[20].)

decrease in renal size. In 204 kidneys in 122 subjects followed for 33 months, renal atrophy was present in 16.2% of all patients and in 20.8% of patients with a > 60% renal artery stenosis[21].

The factors predicting progression have been somewhat elusive, but one consistent finding has been the close correlation between the degree of initial stenosis and progression on follow-up examination. Interestingly, progression of renovascular disease often occurs without significant change in blood pressure control, reflecting the effectiveness of current antihypertensive agents. Similarly, hyperlipidemia, a known risk factor for atherosclerosis, has not been shown to be an independent predictor of progression.

Treatment
The five major treatment options for IRD include: percutaneous transluminal renal angioplasty (PTRA), PTRA with endovascular stenting, primary renal artery stent placement, surgical revascularization and 'medical' therapy (Table 63.5).

Percutaneous transluminal renal angioplasty
Since its introduction in 1978, PTRA has proven successful in treating renal artery fibromuscular dysplasia as well as atherosclerotic renovascular disease. Immediate technical success rates of 75–80% with complication rates of 3–10% are reported and reviewed in a recent meta-analysis[22]. The application of PTRA alone to renal artery stenosis is limited by high early restenosis rates (up to 30% at 6–12 months) and inferior results in the common setting when ostial disease is present. PTRA also has a lower technical success rate when the lesions are longer or more diffuse or when the vessel is totally occluded.

Successful dilatation of the vessel can be associated with good renal functional outcomes. However, most PTRA data derive from studies with short follow-up periods. In a study undertaken in the era prior to the application of endovascular stents to the renal vasculature, 56% of patients who underwent PTRA eventually required surgical revascularization with actuarial renal artery patency: 81% in the surgical group and only 17% in the PTRA group[23].

Although PTRA can be repeated, this approach is undesirable in IRD because repeated contrast studies and endovascular

Table 63.5 Therapeutic strategies in ischemic renal disease.

Therapeutic strategies in ischemic renal disease

Surgical renal artery revascularization
  Aortorenal bypass: vein, Dacron or polytetrafluoroethylene
  Extra-anatomic repair: splenorenal, hepatorenal, ileorenal, superior mesenterorenal arteries
  Autotransplantation
  Ex vivo branch vessel repair
  Transaortic transrenal endarterectomy
  Concomitant aortic replacement and renal revascularization
Percutaneous transluminal renal angioplasty
Endovascular renal artery stenting
Medical or supportive therapy

procedures in patients with renal insufficiency pose significant risks to renal function and may offset the benefit gained by improving proximal renal blood flow.

As discussed in Chapter 39, PTRA alone offers little benefit over current antihypertensive medical therapy alone in control of blood pressure[24]. However, angioplasty has been shown to improve split renal function abnormalities associated with renal artery stenosis and to increase total GFR in patients with unilateral disease[25]. PTRA may be helpful as a bridge to more extensive vascular surgery or endovascular intervention. Renal complications of PTRA include hematoma, hemorrhage, pseudoaneurysm or dissection of the access vessel; rupture, dissection or thrombosis of the renal artery; cholesterol embolization; and ARF. In addition, cardiac morbidity and mortality have been reported. PTRA should not be undertaken lightly in this patient population.

Endovascular stents
Because of the high incidence of ostial renal artery disease, studies have failed to document long-term benefit of PTRA alone for purpose of renal preservation or salvage. Endovascular renal artery stent placement has largely supplanted PTRA alone as the preferred renal artery revascularization procedure in most centers and comparisons of PTRA

Renal function outcomes after endovascular stenting							
				Renal function outcome %			
Year	Author	n (patients)	Follow-up	Improved	Stable	Worse	Restenosis
1991	Rees	100*	7 months	36	36	28	25%
1994	Hannequin	100*	32 months	17	50	33	20%
1995	van de Ven	92*	6 months	36	64	0	13%
1996	Iannone	86*	10 months	36	45	19	14%
1997	Boisclair	100*	13 months	41	35	24	NP
1997	Harden	100*	6 months	34	34	32	13%
1998	Shannon	100*	9 months	43	29	28	NP
1998	Dorros	163*	6 months to 4 years	66–75[b]		25–33	
2000	Baumgartner	107**	12 months	35	45	27	21%
2000	Watson	25/76**[a]	8 months	25	0	0	NP
2000	Burket	37**/127*	15 months	16	9	12	NP
2001	Bush	50**	12–19 months	15	20	12	NP
2001	Beutier	63	23 months	8	41	13	17% to 19%

Table 63.6 Renal function outcomes after endovascular stenting. *Includes patients with and without renal insuficiency. **Patients with renal insufficiency. [a]Only 25 patients with 8 months follow-up. [b]Includes those with stable or improved renal function at last follow-up; the 75% and 25% values represent those stented for bilateral RAS. NP, not performed. (Adapted with permission from Leertower et al. [22].)

versus percutaneous angioplasty with stent placement show superior immediate and long-term results with stents. Initially applied to coronary and peripheral vascular circulations, a number of stents have been deployed for use in renal revascularization including Wallstent, Palmaz, Strecker, Corinthian and others. Following initial studies with high complication rates, more recent reports document excellent technical success with more acceptable mortality and morbidity rates[26] and much better long-term patency rates, although there is still a significant and definite restenosis rate of between 0% and 39% depending on the duration and type of surveillance.

Table 63.6 summarizes the data from studies of over 1000 patients undergoing renal artery stent placement for either hypertension or renal function preservation. The overall rate of improvement in blood pressure control approached 50%, with 68% of patients experiencing stabilization or improvement in renal function over a mean of 17 months. Mean restenosis rates ranged from 0–25% with follow up studies between 6–48 months. However, these studies are largely single center experiences and not randomized trials.

The effects of renal artery stenting on the course of renal insufficiency in patients with renal arterial stenosis remain controversial. First, most studies are reporting data on patients with unilateral and bilateral reno-occlusive disease, suggesting two different subgroups of renal disease, one with potential IRD and one with a combination of unilateral renal artery stenosis and contralateral nephrosclerosis. Second, many of the studies report changes in renal function as changes in serum creatinine which is a poor surrogate for changes in individual kidney GFR. Finally, long-term follow-up regarding the durability of stenting for maintaining renal artery potency is only beginning to be reported.

In one prospective study of 127 consecutive procedures, 171 renal vessels were angioplastied and stented, then followed for a mean of 15 months. Of the 37 patients with preprocedure serum creatinine greater than 1.6 mg/dL, 43% showed improved renal function but 32% were worse postintervention. The investigators found no variables predictive of improvement in serum creatinine. Thirteen of the patients died in the follow-up period and 3% experienced complications[27].

A second study focused on a subgroup of patients with presumed IRD with bilateral renal artery stenosis or unilateral stenosis in the presence of a single functioning kidney. Mean serum creatinine was 2.1 mg/dL (185 μm/L) in this cohort. Stenting resulted in significant improvements in the rate of change of renal function[26]. However, other studies have failed to demonstrate a clear benefit of stenting on renal function decline. Of concern is the large percentage of patients in some studies whose renal function declined after stenting, presumably from either thrombosis, distal cholesterol embolization or contrast acute renal failure[28].

Several studies have indicated that the rate of change of renal function prior to renal artery endovascular stenting may be the best predictor of renal function response to revascularization. In a study of 63 patients treated with renal artery stenting, those with declining renal function over the year prior to stenting experienced a reversal of the slope of decline in renal function. For patients with stable renal function prior to the procedure, stenting had no effect on renal function[29]. Of note, in this study, stented renal vessels were routinely followed angiographically and instent stenoses were treated with angioplasty. Seventy percent of the patients were on statins during the study.

Surgical revascularization

Although renal artery stenting has supplanted surgical revascularization for renal artery stenosis in many centers, there have been no prospective studies comparing efficacy in preservation or reversal of renal function and long-term vessel

Renal outcomes and mortality of surgical renal revascularization in ischemic renal disease						
Source	Year	No. of patients	Renal function result (%)			Mortality (%)
			Improved	Stable	Worse	
Luft et al.	1983	12	67	17	17	17
Jamieson et al.	1984	23	65	0	35	17
Novick et al.	1987	161	58	31	11	2.1
Hallett et al.	1987	91	22	53	25	7.1
Nally	1992	55	58	31	11	2.1
Hansen	1992	70	49	36	15	2.5
Messina et al.	1992	17	77	12	11	0
Bredenberg et al.	1992	40	55	25	20	<3
Chaikof et al.	1994	50	42	54	44	2.0
Libertino et al.	1992	91	49	35	16	6
Cambria	1996	139	54	19	27	8
(Adapted with permission[20].)						

Table 63.7 Renal outcomes and mortality of surgical renal revascularization in ischemic renal disease.

patency. Certainly, in situations of occluded renal arteries, a surgical approach is optimal. Many studies report good renal function outcomes in 70–80% of patients undergoing surgical revascularization with low mortality rates despite a population with diffuse atherosclerotic disease, and excellent long-term patency rates up to 93% at 5 years (Table 63.7). In surgical series, predictors of good renal function outcome include lower preoperative serum creatinine (< 2.0 mg/dL), the presence of bilateral renovascular disease, and recent rapid decline in renal function. These predictors are consistent with the concept that improvement is most likely when the IRD is the cause of the decrement in renal function and there is minimal intrinsic parenchymal renal disease.

Diabetics form a significant subgroup of patients with IRD. Surgical revascularization in this group is associated with similar renal functional responses but an inferior rate of blood pressure responses and a higher postoperative risk of death or eventual dialysis dependence[30].

In patients with IRD who are dialysis dependent, recovery of renal function has also been reported following surgical revascularization[31]. The best predictor of successful and sustained withdrawal from dialysis is a rapid and recent preoperative decline in GFR, often associated with occlusion of a critically stenotic main renal artery and a kidney with preserved size and extensive collateral supply. The demonstration of post-occlusion reconstitution of the renal artery by angiography is also a good predictor of successful revascularization in this setting.

When renal arterial disease accompanies an abdominal aortic aneurysm, the issue arises as to whether to perform combined aortic and renal artery repair, carry out staged surgical procedures, or use endovascular stenting to address the renal lesion and simplify the surgical procedure. There are no data to define an optimal approach in this setting. Although early reports of combined surgical procedures reported high mortality rates, these have dropped to between 2% and 13%

depending on the population and the center. However, in most centers, the mortality rate of combined procedures still exceed those for aortic or renal artery repair alone, though the margin is closing[32].

In addition to mortality rates and renal functional outcomes, the long-term survival of patients undergoing renal revascularization is improving. A study from the Cleveland Clinic reported a 2.2% mortality rate in a predominantly Caucasian population with a mean age of 59 years with documented diffuse atherosclerosis. The actuarial 5- and 10-year survival data were 81% and 53%, respectively[33]. More elderly patients in whom this disease is common would likely have worse outcomes. Cardiovascular death and stroke remain the leading causes of mortality in these patients. Improved outcomes appear to result from improved screening of patients for occult cardiovascular and cerebrovascular disease, better patient selection for surgical revascularization and optimal postoperative care. Whether the results of centers with experienced, designated renovascular surgeons can be generalized to other surgical settings is unclear.

In many centers, transaortic renal endarterectomy is the preferred operative approach to ostial renovascular disease. Aortorenal bypass with autogenous or synthetic grafts can also address the totally occluded artery or vessels with smaller luminal diameter in many cases. When severe aortic atherosclerosis is present, extra-anatomic approaches, such as hepatorenal, splenorenal and iliorenal bypasses, are often used to avoid transecting a severely diseased aorta. Subdiaphragmatic supraceliac and thoracic aortorenal bypass techniques are also gaining popularity because of the relative sparing of these aortic segments by the atherosclerotic process.

The different surgical options for atheromatous renovascular disease allow for individualization in the surgical approach. Selection of the procedure should also take into account the local experience unless referral to a more experienced center is an option.

Medical therapy

Studies from the 1980's of patients (aged 40–65 years) with renal artery stenosis and IRD randomized to medical treatment documented deterioration of renal function over a 1–2 years in 35–50%, as demonstrated by decreased renal size, rise in serum creatinine and decrease in isotopically measured GFR[34]. As such, medical therapy is generally reserved for patients with IRD who are considered nonsurgical candidates and for whom there exists an absolute contraindication to endovascular approaches. For any given patient, the overall risk profile must be considered prior to embarking on an aggressive approach, including assessment of cardiovascular status, cerebrovascular and peripheral vascular disease, age, the condition of the aorta, other comorbid conditions impacting on longevity, and quality-of-life issues. In general, a reasonable approach for whom to offer conservative therapy alone should include a clinical judgment as to the likelihood that the patient will succumb to other comorbid problems before reaching ESRD. If the patient is likely to reach ESRD in his or her lifetime, and if that patient would be considered a candidate for dialysis therapy, then surgical therapy or stenting should be considered. Although this is a controversial issue, especially in elderly patients with IRD, the data demonstrating how poorly these patients do on dialysis suggests an aggressive approach to preventing ESRD is warranted. However, there have been no prospective controlled studies comparing long-term cardiovascular outcomes and renal outcomes for patients offered intervention versus medical therapy.

Conservative management involves selection of appropriate antihypertensive agents to control blood pressure and optimize renal perfusion in the setting of a generally high-renin state. Hypertension can be managed pharmacologically in most cases, although often with less than optimal control despite triple or quadruple drug regimens. Calcium channel blockers are often used as first-line agents in this setting. The use of ACE inhibitors in this setting is controversial. As mentioned above, although they are effective in controlling blood pressure, there is a high risk of precipitating acute renal insufficiency. In addition, there is some evidence that ACE inhibitors may hasten the attendant renal atrophy and fibrosis associated with chronic renal ischemia.

Patients with renovascular hypertension and stable mild renal insufficiency whose blood pressure is controlled with medical therapy should be followed carefully at 4–6-month intervals for changes in renal size and function. It is important to remember, however, that surgical success rates are lower in patients with worse renal function and these patients have higher perioperative morbidity.

Effect of therapy on long-term outcome

IRD is associated with poor long-term survival. The mortality associated with atherosclerotic renovascular disease is largely due to cardiovascular events or stroke. Five and 10-year survival rates for patients reaching ESRD due to IRD have been reported to be as low as 18% and 5% respectively[35]. In a retrospective analysis of patients with unilateral RAS followed for a mean of 31 months, the mortality rate correlated with GFR at study entry. Patients with severe renal dysfunction requiring renal replacement therapy had the greatest mortality with median survival < 1 month. In a study of 169 consecutive patients with angiographically defined renal artery stenosis and renovascular hypertension (mean age 54 years), 44 died over a 7-year period. Age, reduced renal function, bilateral renal artery stenosis, ischemic heart disease and congestive heart failure were associated with greater risk of death. Patients who underwent renal artery interventions did not have a higher survival rate[36].

However, other more encouraging results suggest intervention to improve renal function may impact survival in this group of patients with diffuse atherosclerotic disease. Watson et al. reported 2-year survival rates of 80% among patients with ischemic nephropathy who underwent endovascular stenting[37]. In another study of 67 patients with renal artery stenosis followed for an average of 48 months, the cumulative 3-year mortality rate was 13.4%, rising to 21.2% at 4 years and 38.4% at 5 years. Risk factors for death included the presence of severe carotid disease, DD ACE genotype, smoking, duration of hypertension > 12 years and uncontrolled hypertension[38]. Clearly, the presence of renal artery stenosis is a marker for more diffuse atherosclerotic vascular disease. More information is needed to determine whether renovascular interventions alter mortality in these patients and which subgroups are most likely to benefit.

Summary of management of IRD

Both the diagnosis and management of IRD can be challenging to the clinician. Renovascular disease is often associated with some degree of parenchymal renal injury due to pre-existent hypertension and/or consequences of chronic ischemia. It is often difficult to determine whether renal insufficiency is due to a reversible decrement in GFR (IRD) amenable to improvement by renal artery revascularization. When IRD is suspected based on clinical grounds, the optimal screening test seems to be MRA. All patients with renal artery stenosis and renal insufficiency should undergo a careful evaluation for other causes of renal failure, with quantitation of proteinuria (as a clue to intrinsic renal injury), measurement of total and single kidney GFR, analysis of the rate of change in renal function over the recent preceding weeks or months and critical analysis of the anatomic information provided by all the imaging studies, including renal size, status of the aorta and caliber and degree of stenosis of the renal vessels. Intervention should be considered when there is reasonable support for the diagnosis of IRD.

Before proceeding to intervention either for preservation or retrieval of renal function, the mortality data suggest that the clinician should make some assessment of a patients' risk of developing ESRD in his/her lifetime and the risk of the intervention itself. Figure 63.6 presents an algorithm for the management of IRD. The optimal therapeutic approach should take into consideration the local endovascular interventional and renal vascular surgical expertise, the patient's renal artery and aortic anatomy, and cardiovascular risk factors.

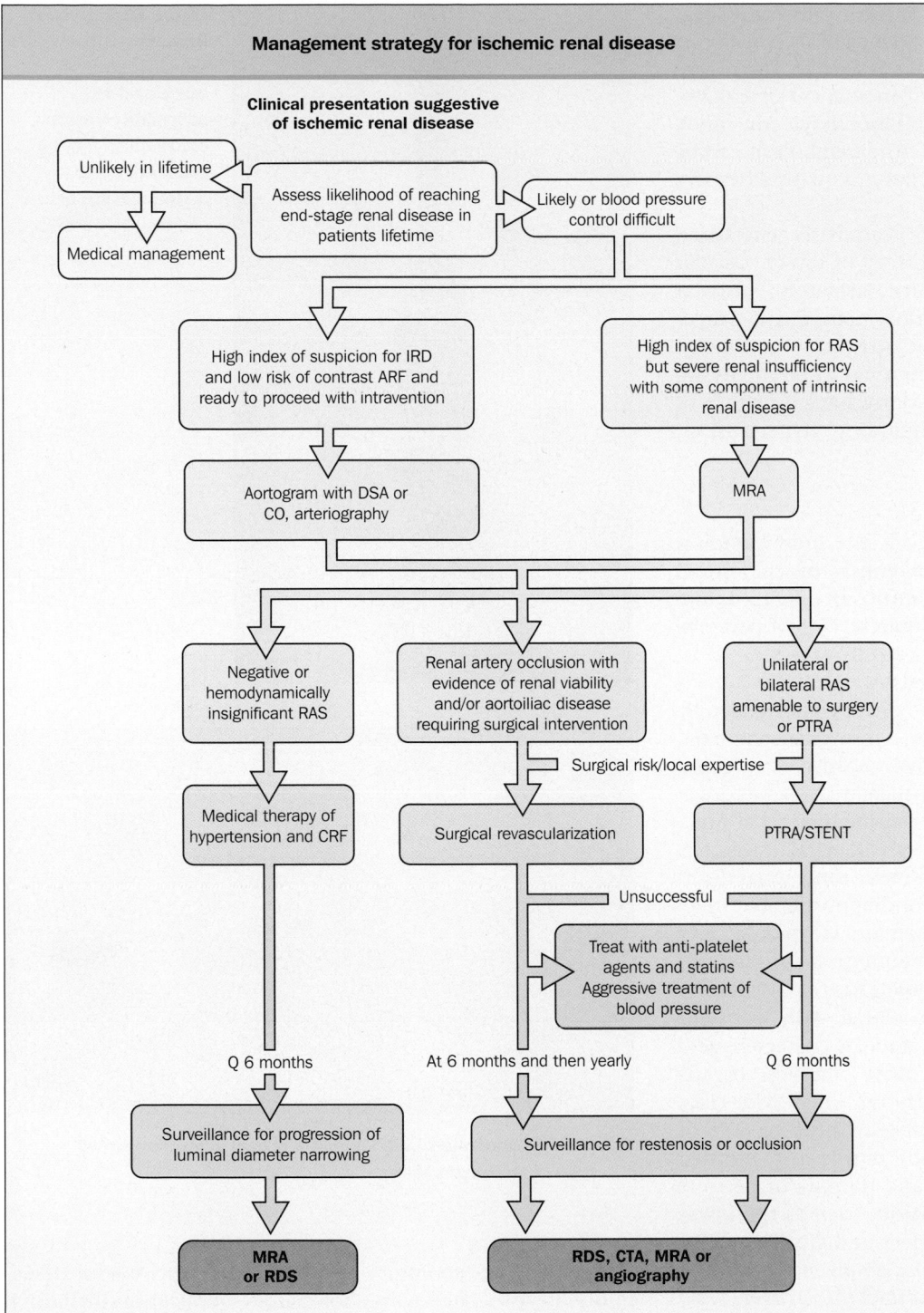

Figure 63.6 Management strategy for ischemic renal disease.

Management strategy for ischemic renal disease

Clinical presentation suggestive of ischemic renal disease

Unlikely in lifetime

Assess likelihood of reaching end-stage renal disease in patients lifetime

Likely or blood pressure control difficult

Medical management

High index of suspicion for IRD and low risk of contrast ARF and ready to proceed with intravention

High index of suspicion for RAS but severe renal insufficiency with some component of intrinsic renal disease

Aortogram with DSA or CO, arteriography

MRA

Negative or hemodynamically insignificant RAS

Renal artery occlusion with evidence of renal viability and/or aortoiliac disease requiring surgical intervention

Unilateral or bilateral RAS amenable to surgery or PTRA

Surgical risk/local expertise

Medical therapy of hypertension and CRF

Surgical revascularization

PTRA/STENT

Unsuccessful

Treat with anti-platelet agents and statins Aggressive treatment of blood pressure

Q 6 months

At 6 months and then yearly

Q 6 months

Surveillance for progression of luminal diameter narrowing

Surveillance for restenosis or occlusion

MRA or RDS

RDS, CTA, MRA or angiography

ATHEROEMBOLIC RENAL DISEASE

Definition/epidemiology

Atheroembolic cholesterol embolization renal disease is a common clinical syndrome and an important clinical presentation of atheromatous renovascular disease, accounting for up to 10% of unexplained renal failure in the elderly. Indeed, ipsilateral renal artery stenosis has been reported in up to 80% of patients with renal cholesterol embolization. These findings support the concept that cholesterol embolization may be one factor contributing to the loss of renal function in patients with atherosclerotic IRD. Autopsy studies have identified renal cholesterol embolization in 15–30% of all patients with autopsy evidence of significant atherosclerosis or abdominal aortic aneurysms.

Cholesterol embolization most commonly occurs following arterial manipulation: arteriography, vascular surgery, angioplasty and stent placement. In patients with extensive atherosclerosis with unstable plaques, this same process can occur spontaneously, independent of any vascular intervention, or following the administration of oral or intravenous anticoagulants or thrombolytic agents. The incidence of atheroembolic disease following vascular interventions is unclear. Three large series of cardiac catheterization cited incidences of < 0.2%. In selected patient groups, the incidence is clearly much higher. From the available evidence, atheroembolism can be expected to occur in up to 30% of patients with extensive aortic atherosclerosis.

Typically patients are aged 50–85 years with generalized atherosclerosis. They often have a history of recent vascular surgery or signs or symptoms of atherosclerotic vascular disease, such as claudication, abdominal pain, angina, myocardial infarction, transient ischemic attacks, retinal artery emboli, amaurosis fugax, stroke, abdominal aortic aneurysm, renovascular hypertension or IRD. Many have a history of risk factors for atherosclerosis, including hypertension, hypercholesterolemia and smoking.

Clinical presentation

Acute or subacute renal insufficiency is the most common clinical problem leading to the diagnosis of cholesterol embolization. The clinical picture is multisystemic in nature and involves the kidneys in approximately 75% of patients. At autopsy, renal involvement is observed in 92–100%.

If a large shower of atheroemboli causes significant tubular damage, the ARF may have an oliguric phase characterized by a high fractional excretion of sodium. More often, the renal failure is nonoliguric and progressive because of ongoing embolization from a nidus of unstable ulcerative plaque. Some patients develop only a moderate impairment in renal function, others progress to ESRD. Atheroembolic renal disease can also present as a more slowly progressive chronic renal insufficiency. Urinalysis findings are nondiagnostic, but may include mild proteinuria, microhematuria, pyuria and eosinophiluria. Renin release by ischemic tissue in areas of embolization can lead to labile, even malignant, hypertension early in the course, sometimes associated with transient marked proteinuria. Fever, often low-grade, is characteristic.

Although the kidneys are the most common organs involved, extarenal cholesterol embolization will provide clues for diagnosis. Cutaneous findings present in up to 60% of patients at initial presentation include purple toes, mottled skin or livedo reticularis, petechiae, and purpura or necrotic ulceration in areas of skin embolization, such as the lower back, buttocks, lower abdomen, legs, feet or digits (Fig. 63.7).

Other organs often involved include spleen (in 55% of cases), pancreas (52%), gastrointestinal tract (31%), liver (17%) and brain (14%). These can result in a number of clinical symptoms, including abdominal or muscle pain, nausea, vomiting, ileus, gastrointestinal bleeding, ischemic bowel, hepatitis, angina or neurologic deficits. When retinal cholesterol embolization occurs, refractile yellow deposits known as Hollenhorst plaques may be seen at the bifurcation of retinal vessels on fundoscopic examination (Fig. 63.8).

Diagnosis

The diagnosis of atheroembolic renal disease is strongly suspected when subacute renal failure develops following a vascular intervention in the presence of livedo reticularis.

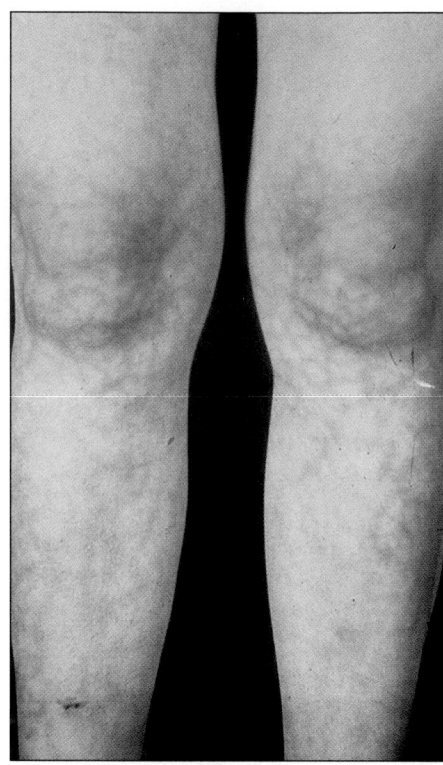

Figure 63.7 Livedo reticularis. The mottled skin changes associated with peripheral cholesterol embolization may be seen over the legs, buttocks, back, or flank and may be transient.

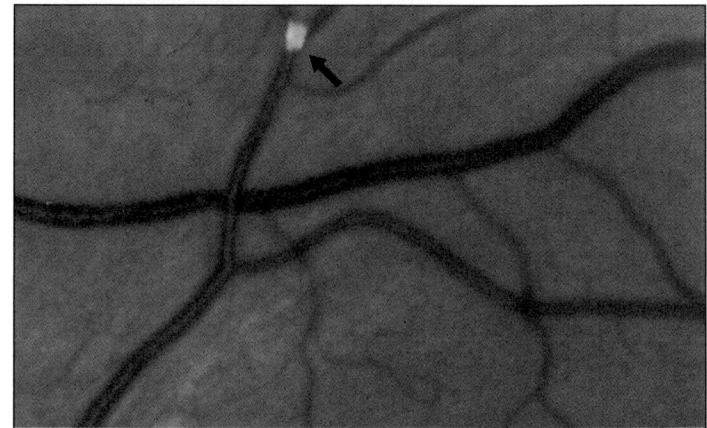

Figure 63.8 Cholesterol embolus of a retinal arteriole (arrow). (Courtesy of Mr Richard Mills.)

A myriad of laboratory abnormalities indicative of tissue injury are associated with cholesterol embolization including elevated sedimentation rate (in 97% of cases), elevated serum amylase (60%), leukocytosis (57%), anemia (46%), hypocomplementemia (25–70%) and elevated liver and muscle enzymes (38–60%). Eosinophilia, which may be transient, is seen in up to 57% of patients.

Although associated laboratory findings can be supportive, the definitive diagnosis is made by biopsy of an involved organ or system showing the cholesterol clefts within the vascular lumina, representing atherosclerotic debris that has embolized, with adjacent ischemic or infarcted segments of tissue (Fig. 63.9). A cutaneous or muscle biopsy in an involved area can preclude the need for renal biopsy.

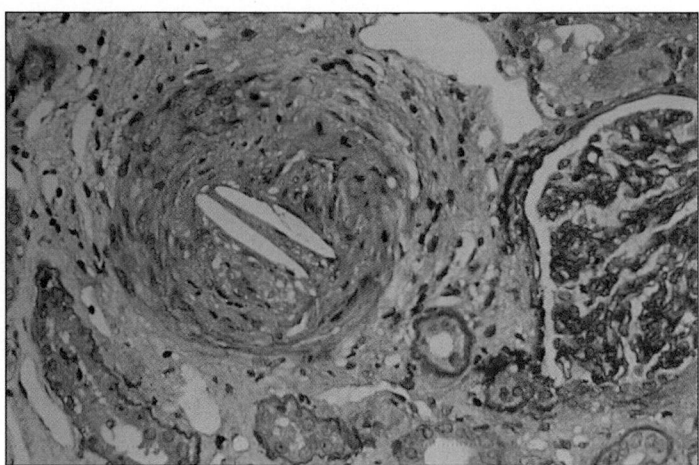

Figure 63.9 Cholesterol emboli in the kidney. Light microscopic section demonstrating cholesterol clefts with giant cell reaction and recanalization in the lumen of a medium-sized renal arteriole (periodic acid–Schiff stain) (Courtesy of Dr R Horn.)

Differential diagnosis

The systemic nature of this syndrome may mimic infection or vasculitis that may lead to delayed or missed diagnosis. Contrast nephropathy with nonoliguric acute tubular necrosis may also occur following angiography, angioplasty, or an aortic vascular surgical procedure. The frequent presence of eosinophilia and eosinophiluria, rash, fever, and renal dysfunction may also be misdiagnosed as an acute interstitial nephritis (see Chapter 60).

Pathology and pathophysiology

If clinical evidence or other pathologic evidence has not secured the diagnosis, renal biopsy may be helpful. Atheroembolic debris scatters to the smaller arteriolar branches in the involved organs, leading to ischemia and infarction. In the kidney, embolization may even extend to the level of the afferent glomerular arteriole, resulting in microinfarctions and diminished GFR.

On renal biopsy, the diagnostic finding is the presence of birefringent, biconvex, elongated cholesterol crystals or biconcave, clefts within the lumina of small vessels left behind in formalin-fixed tissue. Because of the patchy nature of this disorder, open-wedge renal biopsy guided by visualization of areas of ischemic infarction of the cortex has a higher likelihood of successfully finding diagnostic pathologic changes than does percutaneous needle biopsy. The pathologist should be alerted by the clinician that cholesterol embolization is in the differential diagnosis before the biopsy specimen is processed. In frozen sections of tissue, the cholesterol material can be identified using polarized light microscopy. Depending on the time of the biopsy with respect to the course of the illness, the pathologic findings may also include intimal thickening and concentric fibrosis of vessels as well as giant cell reaction to the cholesterol particles. Other findings include vascular recanalization and endothelial proliferation, glomerular ischemia (wrinkling of the basement membrane and glomerular collapse), and tubulointerstitial fibrosis with both an eosinophilic and mononuclear cell infiltrate. In the kidney, the most commonly affected vessels are the arcuate and interlobular arterioles, leading to patchy ischemic changes in glomeruli distal to these vessels.

Natural history

The natural history of atheroembolic renal disease is highly variable and largely determined by the extent of organ involvement and the burden of embolization. The loss of renal function caused by cholesterol embolization may result in ESRD. In a series of 24 patients with cholesterol embolization diagnosed by renal biopsy, renal function declined rapidly in 29% with a more slowly progressive course seen in 79%[39]. Among the latter group, the decline in renal function was thought to result from a combination of cholesterol embolization and IRD. There are also several reported patients with transient acute or subacute renal insufficiency followed by partial recovery of renal function that was associated with an isolated, more limited embolization event. Conversely, the outcome in diffuse cholesterol embolization can be dismal, particularly when cerebral embolization occurs or when there is a large unstable atheromatous burden. In the past, these patients have had a high mortality rate even when dialysis is offered. However, with intensive supportive therapy, recent reports suggest more favorable outcomes[40].

Management

The risk of cholesterol embolization should be considered prior to undertaking angiographic and vascular surgical procedures in patients with diffuse, extensive atherosclerotic disease. As prevention is the most effective management strategy, patients with extensive aortic atherosclerosis should be considered for alternative approaches to cardiac catherization, such as a brachial artery approach. If vascular intervention is performed, signs of embolization should be sought in both the immediate postoperative period and for several months thereafter, examining the patient's skin carefully, determining the pattern of hypertension, and ordering corroborating laboratory tests.

Once the diagnosis of cholesterol embolization is established, further endovascular interventions should be avoided to allow for stabilization of systemic and renal sequellae. Reports have documented poor outcomes in patients with cholesterol emboli that subsequently undergo coronary artery bypass surgery. When clinical factors dictate the need for aortic, renal or peripheral arterial surgery, optimal timing and surgical approach are critical. Conversely, there is a growing surgical experience with segmental aortic replacement to remove the source of emboli, particularly when atheroembolic disease occurs spontaneously. Transesophageal echocardiography is often used to identify mobile ulcerative plaque in the aorta.

ACE inhibitors are effective in managing the labile hypertension seen early in the course of cholesterol embolization. Recent reports describe some newer therapeutic approaches in the management of atheroembolic disease. First, corticosteroids have been used successfully to treat patients with systemic cholesterol embolization and associated inflammatory symptoms[41]. There have also been several reports documenting improvement or stabilization of skin signs of cholesterol embolization following administration of HMG CoA reductase inhibitors (statins)[42]. Statins should probably be part of the armamentarium treating the generalized atherosclerosis in atheroembolic disease.

Cholesterol embolization has been reported to occur in patients following treatment with anticoagulants. While direct causality between anticoagulants and cholesterol embolization has not been proven, the proposed mechanism is that anticoagulants prevent thrombus organization over the ulcerative plaques. Therefore, anticoagulation should be avoided in the acute setting of cholesterol embolization unless a strong life-threatening indication for anticoagulation is present. When dialysis support is required, consideration should be given to peritoneal dialysis or heparin-free hemodialysis until clinical stabilization occurs.

TRANSPLANT RENAL ARTERY STENOSIS

Epidemiology

TRAS is a relatively common post-transplant vascular process occurring most often in the period between 3 months and 2 years after transplantation (see Chapter 87). Its incidence is incompletely known. The highest reported incidence is 23% in a patient cohort screened angiographically versus reported incidences of between 1.3% and 12% when other screening tests are used[43]. The use of pediatric *en bloc* kidneys in adult recipients is associated with a higher rate of TRAS due to smaller donor vessel size leading to greater turbulences and mismatch between donor and recipient vessels. As the transplant population ages, there has been increasing recognition of another subset of patients with 'pseudoTRAS' in which supra-renal vascular disease results in ischemia to the allograft.

Pathogenesis

The pathophysiologic basis for TRAS is multifactorial, and may include atheromatous disease in the donor artery, intimal scarring and hyperplasia in response to trauma to the vessel during harvesting, and anastomotic stenosis which is most commonly associated with end-to-end anastomoses and may be related to suture technique. In end-to-side anastomoses, stenosis tends to develop in the postanastomotic site, suggesting that turbulence or other hemodynamic factors play a role. Immunologic causes of TRAS have also been implicated by studies correlating the incidence of TRAS with that of rejection and by comparisons of the histology of TRAS with the vascular lesions of renal allograft rejection. Localized effects of cyclosporine on vascular caliber and reactivity have been implicated in transient TRAS in some patients. Finally, CMV infection post-transplant has been associated with a higher incidence of TRAS[44].

Clinical presentation

The most common clinical presentation of TRAS is new-onset hypertension or difficult-to-control blood pressure with or without graft dysfunction occurring 3–24 months post-transplant. Patients may also present with acute renal failure or hypotension after placement on ACE inhibitors or AT1 receptor antagonists. Systolic bruits over the transplant are generally of little diagnostic value as they may represent turbulent flow in the main vessels in the absence of stenosis or biopsy-related arteriovenous fistulae. Risk factors for the development of TRAS have been identified in some series and include male gender, hyperlipidemia and elevated serum creatinine at discharge from transplantation.

Natural history

TRAS may result in poorly controlled hypertension and/or progressive loss of renal function. Spontaneous regression of TRAS may rarely occur. Most series suggest that interventional therapies may improve blood pressure and stabilize or improve renal function. One retrospective study compared the 1-, 3- and 5-year survival of 40 subjects with TRAS treated medically versus 80 subjects who underwent PTRA or surgical revascularization and could find no significant differences[45]. However, in general, some type of interventional therapy is recommended (see below).

Diagnosis

Screening tests for the presence of TRAS include plasma renin activity, captopril renography, RDS, spiral CT and MRA. The sensitivity of PRA is approximately 75% with an even lower specificity (67%). Captopril renography is not sensitive for detecting TRAS but is a good predictor of blood pressure response to intervention. RDS has great promise in transplants because it is easier to interrogate the vessel along its course. However, there is a large variability in peak systolic velocity in the renal artery. Both the ratio of velocity in the renal and iliac vessels and the resistive index in the kidney have been shown to be helpful in following the hemodynamic response to PTRA. Phase contrast MRA may have some advantages over arteriography in viewing tortuous renal arteries, and may provide additional information over doppler ultrasound regarding the aorta and iliac vessels. However, with MRA, the surgical clip artifact may obscure the proximal renal artery and often cannot resolve peripheral renal vessels. High false positive rates are associated with sharp anastomotic angles. Spiral CT has advantage over MRA from an imaging standpoint but requires a large amount of contrast.

The gold standard is selective digital subtraction angiography of the transplant artery. In situations in which the risk of contrast induced acute renal failure is high, carbon dioxide angiography can be performed safely to visualize the entire renal vessel.

Therapeutic strategies

The therapeutic options for TRAS include PTRA, with or without stents, and surgery. PTRA is the preferred initial approach in the transplant setting, with initial success rates of up to 75% and patency for follow-up periods of up to 30 months. The average complication rate for PTRA of TRAS is 10%. It is often unsuccessful when there is arterial kinking and is associated with a high complication rate in this setting. The reported rates of late restenosis are between 10% and 33%, necessitating repeated procedures. Recent reports document the safety and efficacy of endovascular stenting in treating TRAS, with fewer complications than with earlier reports for both PTRA and stenting[46].

Surgical revascularization, including resection and revision of the anastomosis, saphenous vein bypass graft and patch graft or endarterectomy, is usually reserved for patients where PTRA has been unsuccessful or complicated, or where the stenoses are distal. Although there are some data supporting the superiority of surgical repair over PTRA in TRAS in terms of long-term patency, blood pressure control and allograft function, surgical repair is fraught with difficulty and is associated with significant mortality in the transplant setting. Extensive fibrosis develops around the transplanted kidney and often involves the renal vessels, making surgical access difficult and risky. Complications include graft loss (in 15–30% of cases), ureteral injury (14%) and death (5%).

REFERENCES

1. Kuroda S, Nishida N, Uzu T, et al. Prevalence of renal artery stenosis in autopsy patients with stroke. Stroke. 2000;31:64–5.
2. Conlon PJ, O'Riordan EO, Kalra PA. New insights into the epidemiologic and clinical manifestations of atherosclerotic renovascular disease. Am J Kidney Dis. 2000;35:573–87.
3. Uzu T, Inoue T, Fujii T, et al. Prevalence and predictors of renal artery stenosis in patients with myocardial infarction. Am J Kidney Dis. 1997;29:733–8.
4. Olin JW, Melia M, Young JR, et al. Prevalence of atherosclerotic RAS in patients with atherosclerosis elsewhere. Am J Med. 1990;88(Suppl. 1):56N–61N.
5. Harding MB, Smith LR, Himmelstein SI, et al. Renal artery stenosis: prevalence and associated risk factors in patients undergoing cardiac catheterization. J Am Soc Nephrol. 1992;2:1608–14.
6. Scoble JE, Maher ER, Hamilton G, et al. Atherosclerotic renovascular disease causing renal impairment – a case for treatment. Clin Nephrol. 1989;31:119–22.
7. Hricik DE, Browning PJ, Kopelman R. Captopril induced functional renal insufficiency I patients with bilateral renal-artery stenosis or renal-artery stenosis in a solitary kidney. N Engl J Med. 1983;308:373–6.
8. Hollenberg GG, Clarkson AB, Woodroffe AJ. Medical therapy of renovascular hypertension: efficacy and safety of captopril in 269 patients. Cardiovasc Res. 1983;4:852–76.
9. Toto RD, Mitchell HC, Lee HC. Reversible renal insufficiency due to angiotensin converting enzyme inhibitions in hypertensive nephrosclerosis. Ann Intern Med. 1991;15:513–19.
10. Kulra PA, Kumwenda M, MacDowell P, Roland MO. ACE Inhibitor usage and monitoring in general practice: the need for guidelines to prevent renal failure. BMG. 1999;318:234–7.
11. van de Ven PJ, Kaatee R, Beutler JJ, et al. Arterial stenting and balloon angioplasty in ostial atherosclerotic renovascular disease: a randomized trial. Lancet. 1999;353:282–6.
12. Maxwell MH, Bleifer KH, Franklin SS. Cooperative study of renovascular hypertension: demographic analysis of the study. JAMA. 1972;220:1195–204.
13. Messina LM, Zelenock GB, Yao KA. Renal revascularization for recurrent pulmonary edema in patients with poorly controlled hypertension and renal insufficiency: a distinct subgroup of patients with arterosclerotic renal artery occlusive disease. J Vasc Surg. 1992;15:73–82.
14. Bloch MJ, Trost DW, Pickering TG, et al. Prevention of recurrent pulmonary edema in patients with bilateral renovascular disease through renal artery stent placement. Am J Hypertens. 1999;12:1–7.
15. Vasbinder GB, Nelemans PJ, Kessels AG, et al. Diagnostic tests for renal artery stenosis in patients suspected of having renovascular hypertension: a meta-analysis. Ann Intern Med. 2001;135:401–11.
16. De Cobelli F, Venturini M, Vanzulli A, et al. Renal artery stenosis: prospective comparison of color Doppler US and breath-hold, three-dimensional, dynamic, gadolinium-enhanced MR angiography. Radiology. 2000;214:373–80.
17. Radermacher J, Chavan A, Bleck J, et al. Use of Doppler ultrasonography to predict the outcome of therapy for renal artery stenosis. N Engl J Med. 2001;344:410–17.
18. Vaughn BFR Jr, Laragh JH. Renovascular hypertension: renin measurements to indicate hypersecretion and contralateral suppression, estimate renal plasma flow, and score for surgical curability. Am J Med. 1973;55:402–14.
19. Makanjuola AD, Suresh M, Laboi P, et al. Proteinuria in atherosclerotic renovascular disease. QJ Med. 1999;92:515–18.
20. Greco, BA, Breyer JB. Atherosclerotic ischemic renal disease. Am J Kidney Dis. 1997;29:167–87.
21. Caps MT, Perissinotto C, Zierler RE, et al. Prospective study of atherosclerotic disease progression in the renal artery. Circulation. 1998;98:2866–72.
22. Leertouwer TC, Gussenhoven EJ, Bosch JL. Stent placement for renal arterial stenosis: where do we stand? A meta-analysis. Radiology. 2000;216:78–85.
23. Erdoes LS, Berman SS, Hunter GC, Mills JL. Comparative analysis of percutaneous transluminal angioplasty and operation for renal revascularization. Am J Kidney Dis. 1996;27:496–503.
24. van Jaarsveld BC, Krijnen P, Pieterman H, et al. The effect of balloon angioplasty on hypertension in atherosclerotic renal artery stenosis. N Engl J Med. 2000;342:1007–14.
25. La Batide-Alanore A, Azizi M, Froissart M, et al. Split renal function outcome after renal angioplasty in patients with unilateral RAS. J Am Soc Nephrol. 2001;12:1235–41.
26. Watson PS, Hudjipetrou P, Cox SV, et al. Effect of renal artery stenting on renal function and size in patients with atherosclerotic renovascular disease. Circulation. 2000;102:1671–7.
27. Burket MW, Cooper CJ, Kennedy DJ, et al. Renal artery angioplasty and stent placement: predictors of a favorable outcome. Am Heart J. 2000;139:64–71.
28. Dejani H, Eisen TD, Finkelstein FO. Revascularization of renal artery stenosis in patients with renal insufficiency. Am J Kidney Dis. 2000;36:752–8.
29. Beutler JJ, Van Ampting JM, van de Ven PJ, et al. Long-term effects of arterial stenting on kidney function for patients with ostial atherosclerotic renal artery stenosis and renal insufficiency. J Am Soc Nephrol. 2001;12:1475–81.
30. Hansen KJ, Lundbert AH, Benjamin ME, et al. Is renal revascularization in diabetic patients worthwhile? J Vasc Surg. 1996;24:383–93.
31. Hansen KJ, Cherr GS, Craven TE, et al. Management of ischemic nephropathy: dialysis-free survival after surgical repair. J Vasc Surg. 2000;32:472–82.
32. Cambria RP, Brewster DC, L'Italien GJ, et al. Renal artery reconstruction for the preservation of renal function. J Vasc Surg. 1996;24:371–82.
33. Steinbach F, Novick AC, Campbell S, Dykstra D. Long-term survival after surgical revascularization for atherosclerotic renal artery disease. J Urol. 1997;158:388–41.
34. Dean RH, Kieffer RW, Smith BM, et al. Renovascular hypertension: anatomic and renal function changes during drug therapy, Arch Surg. 1981;116:1408–15.
35. Mailloux LU, Bellucci AG, Mossey RG, et al. Predictors of survival in patients undergoing dialysis. Am J Med. 1988,84:855–62.
36. Johannson M, Herlitz H, Jensen G, et al. Increased cardiovascular mortality in hypertensive patients with renal artery stenosis. Relation to sympathetic activation, renal function and treatment regimens. J Hypertension. 1999;17:1743–50.

37. Watson PS, Hudjipetrou P, Cox SV, et al. Effect of renal artery stenting on renal function and size in patients with atherosclerotic renovascular disease. Circulation. 2000;102:1671–7.

38. Losito A, Parente B, Cao PG, et al. ACE gene polymorphism and survival in atherosclerotic renovascular disease. Am J Kidney Dis. 2000;35:211–15.

39. Greenberg A, Bastacky SI, Iqbal A, et al. Focal segmental glomerulosclerosis associated with nephrotic syndrome in cholesterol atheroembolism: clinicopathologic correlations. Am J Kidney Dis. 1997;29:334–44.

40. Blenfant X, Meyrier A, Jacquot C. Supportive treatment improves survival in multivisceral cholesterol crystal embolism. Am J Kidney Dis. 1999;33:840–50.

41. Graziani G, Sanostasi S, Angelini C, et al. Corticosteroids in cholesterol emboli syndrome. Nephron. 2001;87:371–3.

42. Finch TM, Ryatt KS. Livedo reticularis caused by cholesterol embolization may improve with simvastatin. Br J Dermatol. 2000;143:1319–20.

43. Fervenza FC, Lafayette RA, Alfrey EJ, et al. Renal artery stenosis in kidney transplants. Am J Kidney Dis. 1998;31:142–8.

44. Pouria S, State OI, Wong W, et al. CMV infection is associated with transplant renal artery stenosis. QJ Med. 1998;91:185–9.

45. Deglise-Favre A, Hiesse C, Lantz O, et al. Long-term follow-up of 40 untreated cadaveric kidney transplant renal artery stenoses. Trans Proc. 1991;23:1342–3.

46. Bertoni E, Zanazzi M, Rosat A, et al. Efficacy and safety of palmaz stent insertion in the treatment of renal artery stenosis in kidney transplantation. Transpl Int. 2000;13:S425–30.

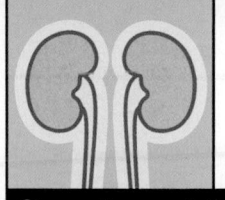

Section 13 Vascular Disease

Chapter 64 Renal Vascular Thrombosis and Occlusion

John E Scoble

INTRODUCTION

Occlusion of the renal artery or vein are both uncommon, but the prompt diagnosis and correct management of these conditions is important, since they may both be reversible causes of renal dysfunction. Although both renal artery and renal vein thrombosis may occasionally be spontaneous, more commonly they occur in the context of a hypercoaguable state or, in the case of arterial thrombosis, in the setting of pre-existing arterial disease. The major etiologies of renal artery and vein thrombosis are shown in Tables 64.1 and 64.2. A discussion of atheromatous renovascular disease is presented in Chapter 63.

RENAL ARTERY OCCLUSION

Pathophysiology

In most individuals, the kidney has a single artery, and acute occlusion may result in sudden and irreversible renal infarction, particularly if there is an inadequate collateral circulation. The potential collateral arterial vessels to the kidney are shown in Figure 64.1. Although a collateral circulation may be present even in normal kidneys, in the setting of chronic ischaemia the collateral circulation may be more extensive (see Fig. 64.2). In a study examining 301 aortograms, collateral supply to the kidney was via the adrenal arteries in 60%, the

Causes of renal artery thrombosis	
Acute	Chronic
Embolus from central source; thrombus	Atherosclerosis
Trauma	Fibromuscular dysplasia
Acute on chronic with pre-existing renal artery stenosis, e.g., with ACE inhibitors and diuretics	Takayasu's disease
	Middle aortic syndrome
Renal artery aneurysm	Renal transplant renal artery stenosis
Aortic dissection	
Aortic occlusion and retrograde thrombosis leading to renal artery occlusion	
Secondary to intervention, e.g., angioplasty	
Clotting disorder	
Antiphospholipid antibody syndrome	
Acute vascular transplant rejection	
Spontaneous	

Table 64.1 Etiology and management of renal artery occlusion.

Causes of renal vein thrombosis	
Acute	Chronic
Nephrotic syndrome	Nephrotic syndrome, especially membranous nephropathy
Clotting disorders	
Antiphospholipid antibody syndrome	Tumor
Secondary to intervention, e.g., renal venography or surgery	Retroperitoneal fibrosis
	Veno-occlusive diseases
Trauma	
Inferior vena cava occlusion	
Acute vascular transplant rejection	
Spontaneous	

Table 64.2 Etiology of renal vein occlusion.

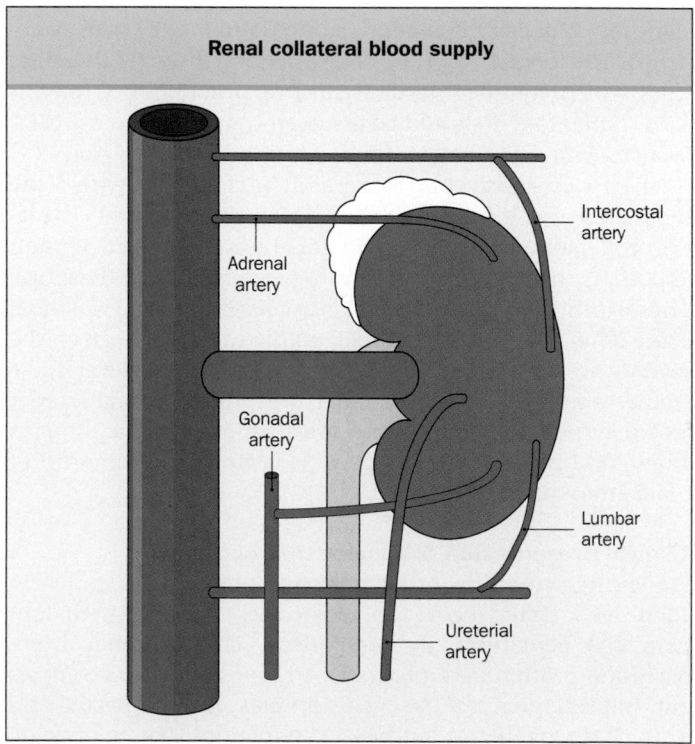

Renal collateral blood supply

Figure 64.1 A diagrammatic representation of the potential collateral arterial vessels to the kidney.

825

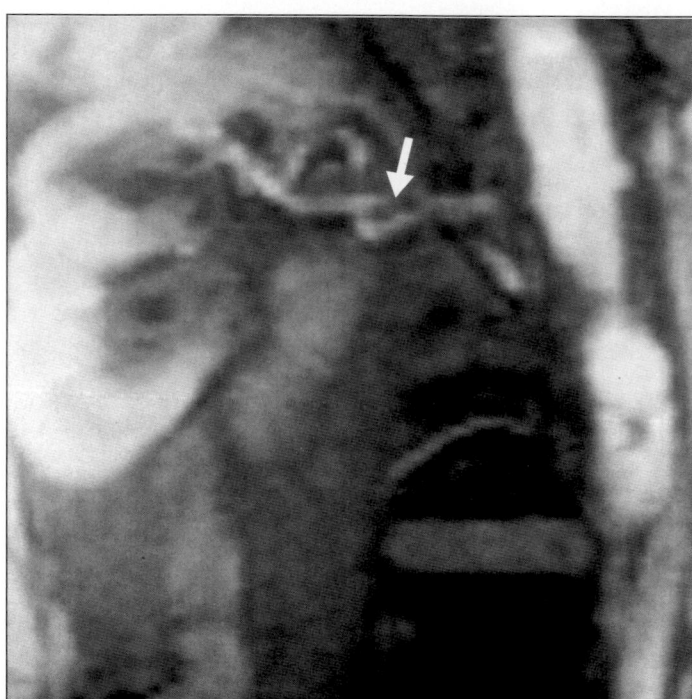

Figure 64.2 A magnetic resonance image of the aorta and right renal artery. The scan shows renal artery occlusion and a collateral artery (arrow) maintaining the renal parenchyma.

Symptoms of renal artery occlusion	
Type	**Symptoms**
Acute	Loin pain
	Hematuria
	Nausea and vomiting
	Fever
	Hypotension
	Oliguria or anuria if bilateral
	Uremic symptoms, if single kidney
Chronic	Asymptomatic
	Hypertension
	Uremic symptoms, if single kidney

Table 64.3 Symptoms of renal artery occlusion.

lumbar arteries in 55%, the ureteric arteries in 15%, and the gonadal arteries in 13%[1]. These collateral vessels may provide enough blood for the kidney to maintain its viability. Since renal arterial occlusion occurs most commonly on a background of atheromatous renovascular disease with renal artery stenosis, collateral circulation is often abnormally well established. The longest recorded renal artery occlusion with anuria from which complete resolution of renal function ensued is 42 d[2]. Therefore it should be assumed that for up to 6 weeks, kidneys with acute renal artery occlusion might be viable.

Studies by Lohse et al. in experimental animals with acute renal artery occlusion have shown that the collateral circulation will maintain renal viability for at least 3 h after occlusion and that, subsequently, severe hypertension will develop[3]. These authors suggested that revascularization of unilateral acute renal artery occlusion may not be worthwhile given the severity of the hypertension that they observed. However, these studies were performed in animals with normal renal arteries and may not be applicable to most occurrences in humans where occlusion generally develops against a background of renal artery narrowing.

Clinical presentation of renal artery occlusion

Presenting symptoms of renal artery occlusion are shown in Table 64.3. Acute occlusion most often presents with loin pain and hematuria. By comparison, chronic renal artery occlusion is often asymptomatic, and no signs may be apparent. Indeed, renal arterial occlusion may be unsuspected and only be discovered at autopsy examination. Causes of acute and chronic renal artery occlusion are shown in Table 64.1 and are discussed below.

Causes of acute renal artery occlusion

Embolus from central source

Embolus from a central source can occur with any form of central or cardiac thrombus. Because of the relatively high renal blood flow, the kidneys are frequently the target for embolism.

Trauma

Direct trauma to the kidney may, rarely, result in renal artery occlusion, usually in association with a deceleration injury. Classically, trauma to the kidney results from a fall from a great height with the patient landing on their feet. This results in the stretching of the renal arteries as the kidneys continue on their downward course after the rest of the body has stopped. The subsequent stretching and recoiling of the renal arteries results in acute thrombosis (Fig. 64.3), which is typically bilateral. Suspicion for renal vascular trauma should be increased in the emergency room if there is injury to the lumbar vertebrae. When intervention is early, there have been successful results from revascularization of traumatic renal artery occlusion. However, often the renal artery thrombosis is part of extensive and fatal injuries.

Acute renal artery thrombus resulting from 'bullet embolism' is also a rare occurrence. In one patient, a bullet had penetrated the aorta and was found at autopsy lodged in the left renal artery. The authors identified two further cases, suggesting that this may not be as uncommon as first thought would suggest[4].

Acute-on-chronic renal artery occlusion

Acute renal artery thrombosis may also occur in the setting of established renal arterial disease. For example, it may occur spontaneously or after administration of angiotensin-converting enzyme (ACE) inhibitors to patients with renal artery stenosis secondary to either fibromuscular dysplasia or atherosclerosis.

Renal artery aneurysm

Renal artery aneurysm (Fig. 64.4) may also predispose to complete occlusion or embolism to the kidney from thrombus

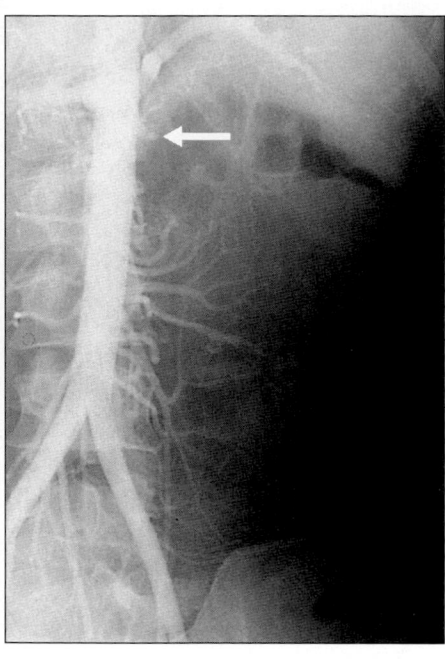

Figure 64.3 Acute renal artery occlusion caused by trauma. An aortogram showing the stump of the left renal artery (arrow) after the individual fell off his motorcycle. (Courtesy of Dr J Reidy.)

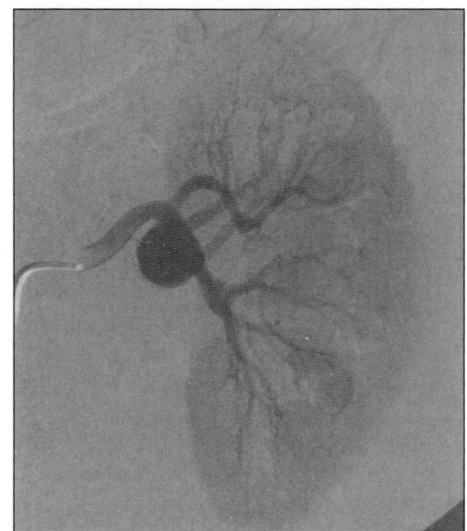

Figure 64.4 Renal artery aneurysm. Angiogram showing large renal artery aneurysm. The aneurysm is patent but is a risk factor for renal artery thrombosis.

within the aneurysmal sac. Thrombosis can occur at an early age, with one case being reported in a 6-year-old girl. Although renal artery aneurysms are rare, they may be a feature of neurofibromatosis or of fibromuscular dysplasia, both of which can also be associated with renal artery stenosis. The indications for treatment of a renal artery aneurysm are the presence of intra-aneurysmal clots, hypertension, and the potential for rupture, which is said to be high in pregnancy[5]. Treatment requires surgical repair or radiological intervention with mechanical occlusion of the aneurysmal sac.

Aortic dissection or occlusion

Aortic dissection involving the renal arteries may result in sudden impairment of renal blood flow, although in some cases blood flow is re-established via the false lumen. Aortic dissection is more likely when there is pre-existing renal artery stenosis[6]. The surgical management of aortic dissection with renal artery involvement is complex and sometimes salvage of one kidney is all that can be expected.

Aortic occlusion from atherosclerotic disease may also predispose to renal artery occlusion. In this situation, the kidneys may be vulnerable to retrograde clot propagation as the renal arteries are usually the first ostia above the occlusion. Interestingly, retrograde clot propagation is rare if the aortic occlusion results from surgical intervention[7]. It is unclear whether patients with aortic occlusion should be given anticoagulation therapy to prevent potential retrograde propagation of clot to the renal arteries.

Renal artery occlusion secondary to intervention

Renal artery occlusion may also represent a complication of angioplasty or aortic cannulation. The occlusion can result from acute thrombosis or acute dissection during or after the procedure. It is uncertain from available data whether thrombolytic therapy is indicated in acute renal artery thrombosis[8]. The treatment of renal artery dissection is usually surgical, although in theory it is possible to use an endovascular stent

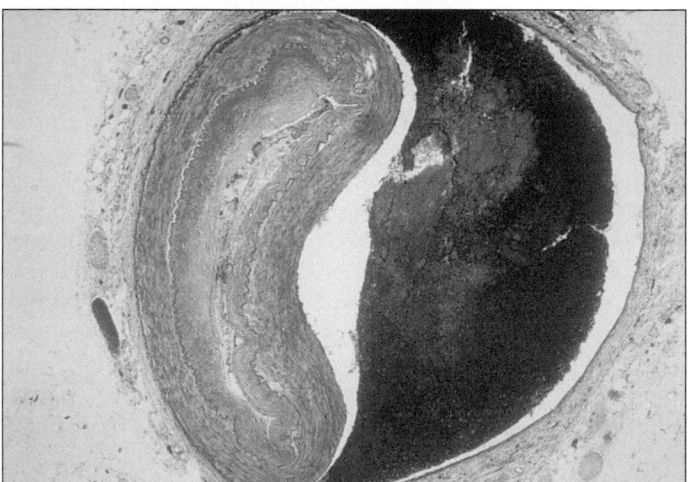

Figure 64.5 Cross-section of a renal artery with dissection following renal angioplasty. This illustrates both the dissection and the associated thrombosis. The kidney could not be salvaged at subsequent surgery.

to maintain the lumen if it can be re-established by balloon angioplasty. Figure 64.5 shows the histology of a renal artery dissection after angioplasty.

Hypercoagulable states

Several clotting disorders predispose to thrombosis of the renal artery. These include the coagulation defects associated with nephrotic syndrome, protein C deficiency, the presence of antiphospholipid antibodies, and, rarely, other coagulation defects (such as mutations in factor V and other factors). Although these lesions may cause renal artery occlusion, they are more commonly associated with renal venous occlusion. Additional predisposing causes which may provoke renal artery thrombosis in patients with a hypercoagulable state include volume depletion (for example from over-diuresis or diarrhoea) and possibly use of oral contraceptive agents[9]. These coagulation defects may require long-term anticoagulation treatment if they have presented as clinical manifestations with renal artery occlusion.

Antiphospholipid syndrome

In antiphospholipid syndrome, the presence of antiphospholipid antibodies is associated with clinical manifestations including spontaneous thromboses and spontaneous abortions. Despite the fact that the partial thromboplastin time is often prolonged, these patients are at risk for both venous and arterial thromboses. In patients under the age of 50, the antiphospholipid syndrome may account for 15–20% of all episodes of deep venous thrombosis and about a third of patients with a stroke. Nochy et al[10]. have reported on the long-term outcome of 16 patients with antiphospholipid syndrome and renal manifestations. A total of 15 of the 16 had either systemic arterial or venous thrombosis. One patient had suprarenal aortic occlusion and one renal artery occlusion. A total of 10 of the 16 patients had intrarenal arterial occlusions on biopsy. Antiphospholipid syndrome is probably the single most common cause of spontaneous renal artery occlusion. Thrombosis may not be limited to the renal arteries but may also involve the aorta, or the cerebral or mesenteric arteries[11]. Long-term anticoagulation is indicated once there has been a thrombotic event and should continue as long as antiphospholipid antibodies persist. Immunosuppressive therapy is of no proven benefit[12].

Transplant renal artery stenosis

Acute arterial thrombosis is an infrequent event leading to renal graft loss. It usually occurs in the first 24–48 h after surgery. Technical surgical factors may contribute but this is less common if a donor aortic patch is used for anastamosis. Acute thrombosis may also occur, particularly in the post surgical period, if blood volume and pressure are low subsequent to hypovolemia (over-diuresis or diarrhoea), or excessive antihypertensive therapy. Additional risk factors for transplant arterial thrombosis include unsuspected prothrombotic states, such as antiphospholipid antibodies, factor V Leiden mutation, or alterations in the plasmin/fibrinolytic system. The Factor V Leiden (R506Q) mutation has been associated with a significantly increased risk of early graft thrombosis[13]. It is important to note that none of these individuals with the FV506Q mutation had a family history of venous thrombosis and only one had a family history of arterial cardiovascular disease. It was calculated that the mutation was present in 14% of transplant venous thrombosis and 20% of all primary graft thrombosis[13].

Renal artery thrombosis may also occur later as a consequence of vascular rejection, atherosclerosis, or constriction of the renal artery at the anastamotic site. However, most documented transplant renal artery stenosis in renal allografts is not at the anastamotic site but is more distal, suggesting that surgical technique is not a prime cause of stenosis.

Another factor noted for allograft thrombosis may be the immunosuppressive regimen used. One study showed the incidence of renal vein thrombosis to be 1.2% with azathioprine-based immunosuppression and 5.6% with cyclosporine before the introduction of aspirin, which may reduce the risk of thrombosis[14]. However, other registry data have not confirmed this adverse effect of cyclosporine, nor indicated any effect of other immunosuppressive regimens on graft thrombosis.

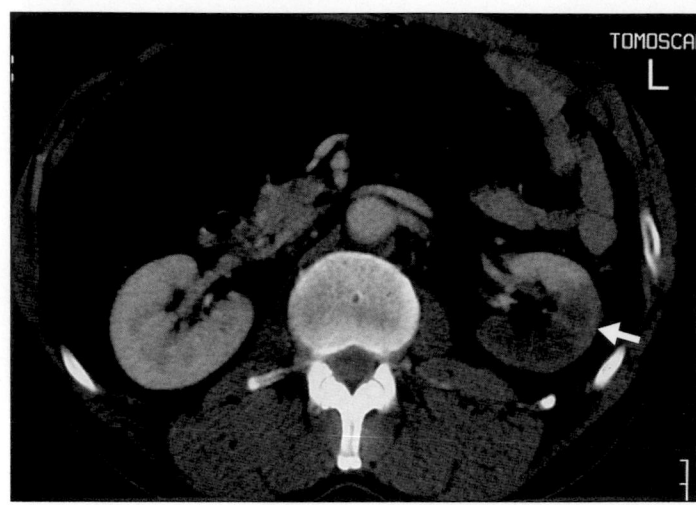

Figure 64.6 Thrombosis in a normal renal artery. Thrombosis of the left renal artery. CT scan with contrast shows hypoperfusion of most of the left kidney (dark areas, arrows) secondary to emboli or thrombosis. (From Mikhail D, et al.[23] with permission.)

Spontaneous thrombosis

Spontaneous renal artery thrombosis is a rare event, but there are a number of descriptions in the literature where no predisposing cause was found in young individuals (Fig. 64.6). Some of these cases may have been related to an undiagnosed hypercoagulable state, since they were reported before current understanding of inherited and acquired thrombophilia. Any case of renal artery thrombosis in the absence of a predisposing renal artery lesion such as atherosclerosis requires investigation for a hypercoagulable state.

Chronic renal artery occlusion

Atherosclerosis

Renal artery thrombosis occurring secondary to atherosclerotic renovascular disease is the most common cause of renal artery occlusion and is usually asymptomatic. It is often detected only when a check is made of plasma creatinine. Figure 64.7 shows the aortogram of a patient who presented with uremia and had occlusion of both renal arteries and aorta at some time prior to presentation.

Fibromuscular dysplasia

Fibromuscular dysplasia of the renal artery is an important cause of hypertension, especially in younger, female patients (see Chapter 39). It may occasionally involve other arterial vessels including the mesenteric and carotid arteries. Patients typically present with hypertension that may be malignant. Angiography shows a characteristic 'beaded' appearance of the renal arteries, which may extend into the kidney (Fig. 5.27). Although fibromuscular dysplasia is usually associated only with renal artery stenosis, renal aneurysm formation and thrombosis may occasionally occur. Patients may occasionally develop thrombotic occlusion in the setting of volume depletion or with the use of ACE inhibitors. Rare cases may occur spontaneously. These patients may present acutely (with flank pain and hematuria), or may be asymptomatic if the thrombosis develops insidiously. However, most patients

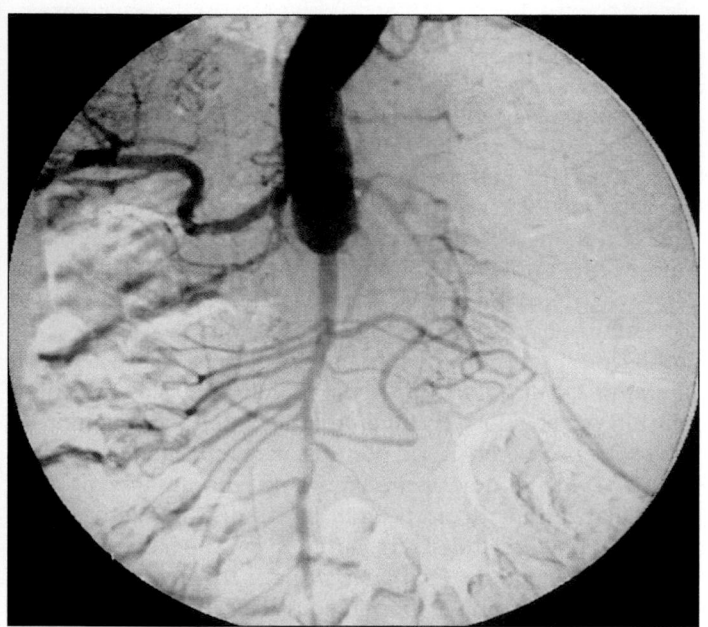

Figure 64.7 Renal artery thrombosis secondary to atherosclerosis. Aortogram of a patient with uremia who had previously had an occluded aorta. A subclavian-femoral bypass graft had been inserted and at some stage both renal arteries had become asymptomatically occluded. (From Streather[24] with permission.)

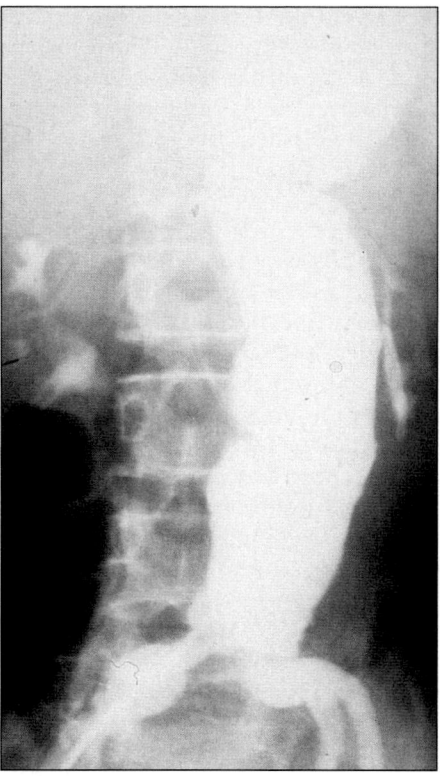

Figure 64.8 A patient with severe aortic Takayasu's disease. Note the 'ragged' appearance of the aorta (Courtesy of Dr J Reidy.)

will have a history of hypertension and will have received medical attention before occlusion occurs. It is also rare to identify an adult patient with fibromuscular dysplasia with an occluded renal artery on one side and stenosis on the other, as is commonly observed in atherosclerotic arterial disease. The incidence of renal artery occlusion in fibromuscular dysplasia is unclear from the published literature. Renal artery occlusion does not seem to follow the pattern seen in atherosclerotic disease, of significant occlusion in the setting of high-grade stenosis.

Takayasu's disease

Takayasu's disease ('pulseless disease') is a large vessel arteritis that has been primarily recognized in Japan[15]. It is uncommon in the UK, even in patients of Asian descent. It has a female to male ratio of 9:1 and has a peak onset in the 20–40 year age group. This gender ratio and age group mirror those of fibromuscular dysplasia, although the two conditions are clinically very different. Figure 64.8 shows the typical features of Takayasu's disease with a severely diseased aorta and renal artery involvement. The condition can lead to aneurysmal dilatation of the aorta as well as narrowing of the individual arteries. Unlike middle aortic syndrome (see below) there are markers of systemic inflammation such as a high erythrocyte sedimentation rate. Treatment consists of corticosteroids with revascularization by angioplasty or surgery. Because of the progressive nature of the problem, it is less amenable to treatment than fibromuscular dysplasia.

Middle aortic syndrome

Middle aortic syndrome is a rare condition that resembles an aortitis, but is not associated with any evidence of a

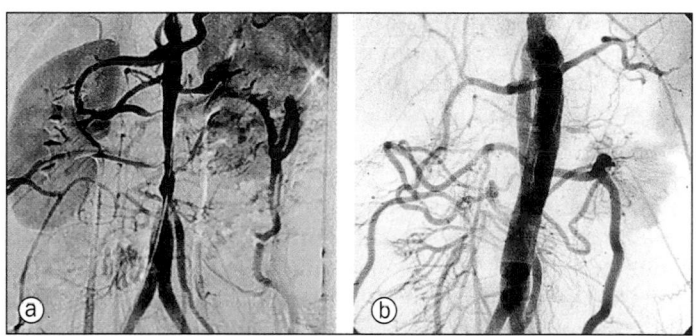

Figure 64.9 Middle aortic syndrome. (a) Angiogram showing typical smooth narrowing of the aorta. There is bilateral stenosis of paired renal arteries. (b) Angiogram after an aortic graft and reanastamosis of all four renal arteries. There is occlusion of all four renal arteries. The patient remained anuric for 60 d and became dialysis independent on day 78 without any further intervention, there had been spontaneously recanalization of one renal artery on each side (From Panayiotopoulos et al[16] with permission.)

systemic inflammatory state[16]. The characteristic angiographic appearance is shouldering and narrowing of the aorta at the level of the renal arteries (Fig. 64.9a). The smooth, constricted appearance of the aorta in middle aortic syndrome contrasts with the 'ragged' aorta characteristic of patients with atherosclerosis and Takayasu's syndrome. Middle aortic syndrome usually presents with constriction of the aorta at the level of the renal and visceral arteries. Unlike fibromuscular dysplasia, renal failure owing to progressive renal artery occlusion occurs almost inevitably in association with severe hypertension. Autologous renal transplantation is not usually an appropriate therapeutic option since the iliac vessels, the conventional site for placement of the transplanted kidney, are downstream of the usual site of narrowing unless aortic grafting is performed at the same time. The long-term prognosis must be guarded because of the progressive narrowing of the abdominal aorta.

Renal transplantation

Progressive renal artery stenosis is a particular problem in patients with renal transplants. The development of transplant artery stenosis has been associated with vascular rejection and also linked to cytomegalovirus infection. In practical terms, the stenosis resembles fibromuscular dysplasia in that it tends not to affect the ostium and can affect the vessels within the substance of the kidney. The distinction between renal artery stenosis and chronic vascular rejection, with severe narrowing of intrarenal arteries and arterioles, is not always clear cut. Results from angioplasty of these lesions appear to mirror the success seen in fibromuscular dysplasia in terms of both improved graft function and control of hypertension.

Diagnosis of renal artery occlusion

When a diagnosis of acute renal artery occlusion is considered, radiological confirmation should be obtained urgently, as early surgical or thrombolytic therapy may be necessary to salvage the kidney. The definitive examination remains contrast renal angiography; it remains the optimal technique for identifying collateral circulation, and is the only approach which allows interventional revascularization.

Recent advances in magnetic resonance (MR) angiography especially with gadolinium enhancement may in due course render renal angiography obsolete. Figure 64.2 shows the MR angiogram of a patient with occluded right renal artery with collateral blood supply maintaining kidney viability; this kidney was revascularized, restoring independent renal function. It is often difficult to image the collateral supply to the kidney, but improvements in MR scanning may make this a useful technique in the future for collateral imaging. Spiral CT scanning has also been suggested as an alternative to renal angiography. However, the required contrast load for spiral CT is considerable and greater than conventional intra-arterial digital subtraction angiography, and the post examination image analysis is often challenging. Renal arterial duplex scanning may also identify stenoses or, rarely, occlusion, but it may be difficult to demonstrate multiple renal arteries or segmental thrombosis. Nuclear medicine imaging with comparison of both renal arteries has also been advocated. Scanning using radiolabeled dimercaptosuccinic acid (DMSA) may demonstrate viable renal parenchyma even though the diethylene-triamene pentaacetic acid (DTPA) scan shows poor perfusion. Conventional CT scanning can be of use to demonstrate areas of the kidney with poor perfusion (Fig. 64.6). There is further discussion of imaging techniques in Chapter 5.

Treatment of renal artery occlusion

In principle, treatment of the underlying condition causing occlusion is paramount. In practical terms, revascularization can often be attained by anticoagulation alone if the renal artery was normal prior to occlusion. However, where the occlusion occurs in a background of chronic occlusive disease, revascularization may be necessary. The goal of imaging is not only to establish that there is an occlusion, but also to try and confirm the viability of the kidney beyond the occlusion. This may be assessed by a DMSA scan or duplex examination of the renal cortex. If there is neither DMSA uptake nor any vascular signal from the cortex then revascularization is unlikely to be successful. In extreme cases renal biopsy, either preoperative or perioperative may be required to establish viability.

It is important to note that provided there is sufficient collateral blood supply to prevent infarction successful, intervention may be delayed for a prolonged period[17]. Figure 64.9 shows the preoperative and postoperative renal angiography of a patient with middle aortic syndrome who underwent renal revascularization and aortic grafting, and postoperatively was shown to have occluded renal arteries; yet the patient became dialysis independent 78 d later without further intervention and was shown to have spontaneously recanalized both renal arteries. This illustrates the prolonged viability of a kidney with arterial occlusion and the potential for recovery even after prolonged anuria. It is likely that the pre-existing renal artery stenosis had caused the development of significant collateral renal blood supply prior to surgery.

The best course of action in an individual case is unclear[8]. Embolectomy and conservative treatment with anticoagulation have proved effective in some patients[18]. In a large series of patients[19] undergoing surgical revascularization or nephrectomy for in chronic renal artery occlusion revascularization it was shown that there was a similar outcome for blood pressure. Only revascularization in unilateral disease offered any improvement in renal function. It is important to note that the perioperative death rate in this series was 5.2% reflecting the significant comorbidity in these patients. Others suggest that, given the surgical risk of embolectomy, anticoagulation is the treatment of choice[18]. The role of systemic or intrarenal thrombolytic therapy in addition to anticoagulation is unclear[8]. Thrombolytic therapy is probably only indicated if the occlusion is very recent, for example as the result of vascular intervention. In individual cases of acute occlusion complicating antiphospholipid syndrome success has been reported with a combination of angioplasty and intra-arterial thrombolysis. There are no systematic data to support local thrombolysis over systemic thrombolysis in renal artery thrombosis. Long-term anticoagulation is required if a central source of embolization is still present.

A study from Oxford[14] has addressed preventive therapy for renal transplant thrombosis. They retrospectively analyzed the thrombosis rate before and after the introduction of aspirin as a routine treatment started immediately prior to transplantation. They found that the renal vein thrombosis rate was 5.6% prior to and 1.2% post introduction of aspirin. They reported a major bleeding complication in 2.7% of cases on aspirin, but did not provide information on bleeding risk before the introduction of aspirin. It is therefore unclear whether the introduction of aspirin to prevent allograft thrombosis is offset by an increased bleeding risk, especially in association with graft biopsy.

ACUTE AND CHRONIC RENAL VEIN OCCLUSION

Unlike renal artery occlusion, renal vein occlusion is more likely to occur without pre-existing abnormalities of the renal vein. As with renal artery occlusion, the symptoms and signs may vary, depending on whether the thrombosis is acute or chronic (see Table 64.4). A variety of aetiologies are also responsible for these conditions (see Table 64.2).

Acute renal vein occlusion

The clinical presentation of renal vein occlusion is loin pain and hematuria. These clinical signs are nonspecific and may be mistaken for renal colic or acute pyelonephritis. When renal vein thrombosis complicates the nephrotic syndrome, there may be an increment in proteinuria or deterioration in renal function. The proteinuria may diminish with systemic thrombolytic therapy for the renal vein thrombosis. The collateral veins for the kidney are different for each side. On the left there are collaterals to the ureteral, gonadal, and adrenal veins whereas on the right there is only a collateral to the ureteral vein.

Nephrotic syndrome

Renal vein thrombosis has classically been described in the nephrotic syndrome and especially in adults with membranous nephropathy. The prevalence of renal vein thrombosis in the nephrotic syndrome is difficult to determine, with estimates ranging from 5% to 62%, higher estimates occurring in reports where there had been systematic investigation to identify asymptomatic thrombosis[20]. However, a report of MRI and CT scanning in 23 patients with nephrotic syndrome without a clinical suspicion of renal vein thrombosis demonstrated only one patient with renal vein thrombosis[21]. Membranous nephropathy is the most commonly associated nephrotic syndrome seen with renal vein thrombosis; by contrast, renal vein thrombosis is uncommon in the nephrotic patient with diabetic nephropathy. There is no known explanation for these variations in risk according to underlying disease causing the nephrotic syndrome. It may just reflect the duration of the hypoalbuminemic state rather than a disease-specific effect. At one time it was considered that renal vein thrombosis could cause the nephrotic syndrome, although this is no longer considered true.

Renal vein occlusion secondary to hypercoagulable states

Renal vein thrombosis can also be seen with or without renal artery occlusion in the antiphospholipid syndrome. Renal vein thrombosis secondary to antiphospholipid antibodies may be the most common cause of spontaneous renal vein. More frequently, renal vein thrombosis will occur in the context of thrombosis in other veins or arteries. Other clotting disorders such as deficiencies in protein S, protein C, and antithrombin III may result in renal vein thrombosis. Protein C deficiency is present in approximately 1 : 16 000 to 1 : 36 000 members of the general population. Protein S deficiency is present in 1 : 20 000 of the population. Homozygous individuals with either protein C or protein S deficiency may have early-onset renal vein thrombosis as the initial presentation of their hypercoagulable state. Energetic

Symptoms of renal vein occlusion	
Type	**Symptoms**
Acute	Loin pain
	Hematuria
	Fever
	Worsening of proteinuria
	Oliguria if bilateral
	Testicular pain
	Uremic symptoms if complete occlusion and single kidney, as in renal transplantation
Chronic	Asymptomatic
	Worsening of proteinuria
	Uremic symptoms, if single kidney

Table 64.4 Symptoms of renal vein occlusion.

treatment with fresh frozen plasma and anticoagulation may help prevent further thrombotic episodes.

Renal vein occlusion secondary to intervention

Renal vein thrombosis may also occur following cannulation during renal venography. In aortic aneurysm or complicated abdominal surgery, it is not uncommon for renal veins to be ligated. Ligation of the renal vein in treatment of renal cell carcinoma usually occurs at the time of nephrectomy to prevent tumor spread.

Trauma

Renal vein occlusion appears to be rarer than acute renal artery occlusion after trauma. However, the events that cause renal artery damage are so severe that concomitant renal vein occlusion would be difficult to diagnose and less crucial for immediate management. However, cases have been described where only renal vein occlusion occurred, probably caused by hematoma around the renal vein.

Renal transplantation

Renal vein occlusion after renal transplantation often occurs in combination with acute arterial thrombosis, and the two events may be difficult to differentiate. Acute vascular rejection can cause both problems. With the increasing sophistication of Doppler ultrasound scanning, it may be possible to diagnose transplant vein thrombosis. But unfortunately, because of the absence of collateral venous drainage, these events usually result in irretrievable loss of graft function.

Spontaneous thrombosis

Cases have been reported of renal vein thrombosis in an otherwise normal individual, and are most often a consequence of severe hypovolemia.

Chronic renal vein occlusion

Chronic renal vein thrombosis is often insidious and asymptomatic, as collaterals again allow relative preservation of renal function. However, as with acute renal vein thrombosis, chronic thrombosis is associated with an increased risk of pulmonary embolism. Chronic renal vein thromboses can occur in several settings, including the nephrotic syndrome, inferior vena cava occlusion, and retroperitoneal fibrosis. It may also occur with renal cell carcinoma with spread of the tumor along the renal vein (see Table 64.2).

Diagnosis of renal vein occlusion

Previously contrast venography was the gold standard for the diagnosis of renal venous thrombosis. However, renal venography may cause thrombosis itself, as the catheter has to be advanced into the renal vein, since injection of contrast in the cava is insufficient to image the veins. It is now clear that either spiral CT scanning or MRI scanning offer the best diagnostic method and do not require venous instrumentation (Fig. 64.10). The choice between CT and MRI scanning depends on local availability. The use of gadolinium enhancement may improve the resolution of the renal vein signal and make MRI scanning more useful than CT scanning[22]. Duplex ultrasound scanning may be useful for renal vein imaging but its role is not yet established. Radionuclide scanning may be useful, renal vein thrombosis is associated with a delayed tracer clearance using DTPA. Occasionally renal biopsy undertaken for investigation of renal impairment or nephrotic syndrome suggests the presence of renal vein thrombosis, showing dilated capillaries and neutrophil infiltration. However MRI and spiral CT scanning are now superseding these other techniques.

If no aetiology for the renal venous thrombosis is apparent, studies should also be performed to look for evidence for a clotting disorder (Table 64.5).

Treatment of renal vein occlusion

As with renal artery occlusion, there are insufficient data to determine if thrombolytic therapy is superior to routine anticoagulation (with heparin followed by warfarin). There does not appear to be any advantage to intrarenal thrombolytic therapy compared with systemic administration. In the setting of a hypercoagulable state, permanent anticoagulation may be necessary, and some recommend that anticoagulation be given to all patients with nephrotic syndrome and serum albumin < 2 g/dL (20 g/L) or less even if there is no overt evidence of renal vein thrombosis (see Chapter 19).

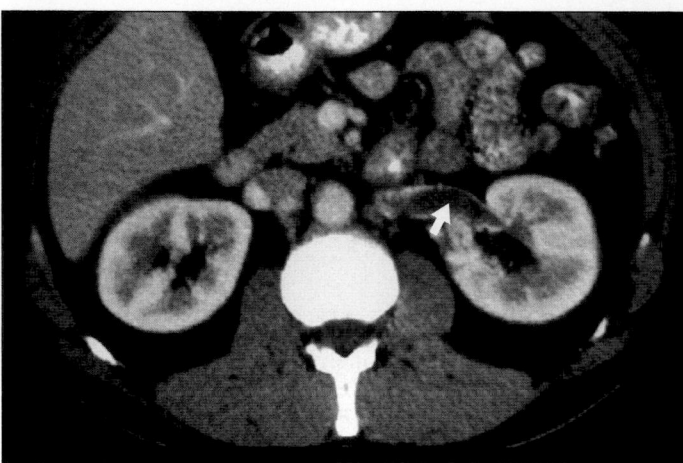

Figure 64.10 Renal vein thrombosis CT scan showing left renal vein thrombosis (arrow). (Courtesy of Dr S Rankin.)

Indications for screening for a clotting disorder
Acute renal artery thrombosis in a patient without atherosclerosis
Acute renal artery or vein thrombosis in a recent renal allograft
Documented renal vein thrombosis in the absence of the nephrotic syndrome

Table 64.5 Coagulation screening in renal vascular occlusion.

REFERENCES

1. Yune HY, Klatte EC. Collateral circulation to an ischemic kidney. Radiology. 1976;119:539–46.
2. Pontremoli R, Rampoldi V, Morbidelli A, et al. Acute renal failure due to acute bilateral renal artery thrombosis: successful surgical revascularization after prolonged anuria. Nephron. 1990;56:322–4.
3. Lohse JR, Shore RM, Belzer FO. Acute renal artery occlusion. Arch Surg. 1982;117:801–4.
4. Guileyardo JM, Cooper RE, Porter BE, McCorkle JL. Renal artery bullet embolism. Am J Forensic Med Pathol. 1992;13:288–9.
5. Abud O, Chechile GE, Sole-Balcells F. Aneurysm and arterio-venous malformation. In: Novick A, Scoble J, Hamilton G, eds. Renal Vascular Disease. London: WB Saunders; 1995.
6. Scoble JE. The epidemiology and clinical manifestations of atherosclerotic renal disease. In: Novick A, Scoble J, Hamilton G, eds. Renal Vascular Disease. London: WB Saunders; 1995:303–14.
7. Reilly LM, Sauer L, Weinstein ES, et al. Infrarenal aortic occlusion: does it threaten renal perfusion or function? J Vasc Surg. 1990; 11:216–25.
8. Wright MPJ, Persad RA, Cranston DW. Renal artery occlusion. Br J Urol. 2001;87:9–12.
9. Le Moine A, Chauveau D, Grunfeld JP. Acute renal artery thrombosis associated with factor V Leiden mutation. Nephrology Dialysis Transplant. 1996;11:2067–9.
10. Nochy D, Daugas E, Droz D, et al. The intrarenal vascular lesions associated with primary antiphospholipid syndrome. J Am Soc Nephrol. 1999;10:507–18.
11. Balligand JL, Lefebvre C, Zenagui D, Coche E. Cerebral and renal arterial thromboses in systemic lupus erythematosus with antiphospholipid antibodies: a report of two cases. Acta Clin Belg. 1990;45:372–8.
12. Joseph RE, Radhakrishnan J, Appel GB. Antiphospholipid antibody syndrome and renal disease. Curr Opin Nephrol Hypertens. 2001;10:175–81.
13. Irish AB, Green FR, Gray DWR. Morris PJ. The Factor V Leiden (R506Q) mutation and risk of thrombosis in renal transplant recipients. Transplantation. 1997;64:604–7.
14. Robertson AJ, Nargund V, Gray DWR, Morris PJ. Low dose aspirin as prophylaxis against renal-vein thrombosis in renal-transplant recipients. Nephrology Dialysis Transplant. 2000;15: 1865–8.

15. Toma H. Takayasu's arteritis. In: Novick A, Scoble J, Hamilton G, eds. Renal Vascular Disease. London: WB Saunders; 1995:47–62.

16. Panayiotopoulos YP, Tyrell MR, Koffman G, et al. Mid-aortic syndrome presenting in childhood. Br J Surg. 1996;83:235–40.

17. Masterson R, Scoble J, Taylor P, Cook G. Recovery of renal function following prolonged ischaemia in a patient with mid-aortic syndrome. Nephrology Dialysis Transplant. 2000;15:1461–3.

18. Moyer JD, Rao CN, Widrich WC, Olsson CA. Conservative management of renal artery embolus. J Urol. 1973;109:138–43.

19. Oskin TC, Hansen KJ, Deitch JS, et al. Chronic renal artery occlusion: nephrectomy versus revascularization. J Vasc Surg. 1999;29:140–9.

20. Harris RC, Ismail N. Extrarenal complications of the nephrotic syndrome. Am J Kidney Dis. 1994;23:477–97.

21. Rahmouni A, Jazaerli N, Radier CMD, et al. Evaluation of magnetic resonance imaging for the assessment of renal vein thrombosis in the nephrotic syndrome. Nephron. 1994;68:271–2.

22. Kanagasundaram NS, Bandopadhyay D, Brownjohn AM, Meaney JFM. The diagnosis of renal vein thrombosis by magnetic resonance angiography. Nephrology Dialysis Transplant. 1998; 13:200–2.

23. Mikhail A, Reidy J, Taylor PR, Scoble JE. Renal artery embolisation after back massage in a patient with aortic occlusion. Nephrology. Dialysis Transplant 1997;12:797–8.

24. Streather C, Wlodarczyk ZC, Sneddon F, et al. Progression of occlusive renal vascular disease and axillo-femoral bypass grafts. Nephrology Dialysis Transplant. 1993;8:1186–7.

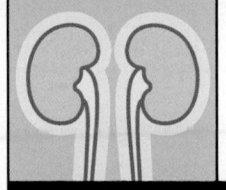

Chapter 65

Aging and the Kidney

Leon Ferder, Sharon Anderson, and Richard J Johnson

INTRODUCTION

Aging is a normal degenerative biological process that affects many organs, of which the kidney is one of the most prominently affected. Aging is associated with a decline in renal function coincident with a progressive loss of nephrons, with glomerular and tubulointerstitial scarring. These changes affect glomerular and tubular function, systemic hemodynamics and body homeostasis.

ANATOMICAL CHANGES

The human kidney reaches a maximum size of approximately 400 g (corresponding to 12 cm in length) in the fourth decade of life. Following this, there is a natural decline in renal size, amounting to an approximately 10% decrease in renal mass per decade, with a tendency for the decrease to be greater in males as opposed to females. This decline is associated with progressive cortical thinning. Renal biopsies show progressive focal and segmental glomerulosclerosis, tubulointersitital fibrosis and arteriolar hyalinosis (Fig. 65.1).

Glomerular changes

Several structural changes occur in the glomerulus with aging. Preserved glomeruli often show an increase in overall tuft cross-sectional area, strongly suggestive of glomerular hypertrophy[1]. The glomerular basement membrane also thickens with age. Most evident is the development of focal and segmental or, rarely, global, glomerulosclerosis. Whereas

the prevalence of glomerulosclerosis is < 5% of glomeruli at age 40 years, this increases to 10–30% of glomeruli by the eighth decade[2] (Fig. 65.2). In aging mice and rats, which show similar histologic changes, a strong relationship between the glomerular hypertrophy and glomerulosclerosis has been shown[3], consistent with the hypothesis that glomerular hypertrophy may predispose to the development of glomerulosclerosis[4]. The glomerulosclerosis is associated with mesangial matrix expansion and a progressive loss of capillary loops. Periglomerular fibrosis is often prominent, and there may be 'atubular glomeruli' in which the exit from Bowman's capsule to the proximal tubular lumen is blocked by fibrosis.

Tubular and Interstitial Changes

There is also tubulointerstitial injury that is greatest in the outer medulla and medullary rays. Tubules show both tubular dilation and atrophy, and are surrounded by infiltrating mononuclear cells and dense fibrosis. Studies in aging rats have more carefully characterized these changes. Many tubules have been shown to express osteopontin, which is a marker of tubular injury and a chemotactic protein. The infiltrating interstitial cells consist of both macrophages and myofibroblasts and the fibrosis is due in part to the deposition of types I and III collagen[5] which appears to be mediated by the local expression of transforming growth factor (TGF)-β[6].

Vascular Changes

Arterioles may show hyalinosis with aging. Thickening of the arterioles, or a reduction in the lumen diameter/medial

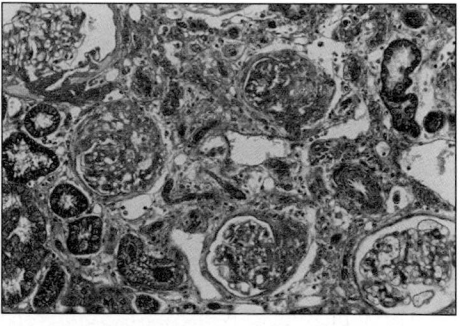

Figure 65.1 Glomerulosclerosis and tubulointerstitial fibrosis in an aging (24-month-old) Sprague-Dawley rat. Similar changes, consisting of focal segmental glomerulosclerosis, tubular atrophy, and interstitial fibrosis, occur in man (Trichrome stain ×400).

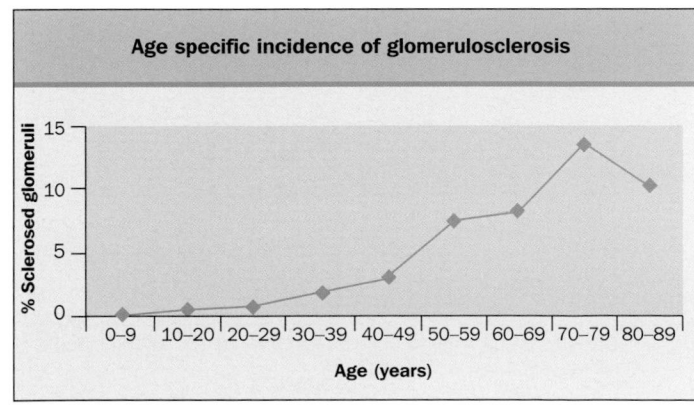

Figure 65.2 Glomerulosclerosis increases with aging in normal humans. (Adapted with permission[2].)

thickness ratio is also common with aging but is observed almost exclusively in hypertensive individuals[7]. With aging, some afferent arterioles, particularly of juxtamedullary glomeruli, develop vascular shunts to the efferent arterioles, thereby bypassing glomeruli[8]. Studies in rats have also shown focal losses of vascular endothelium in both the glomerular and peritubular capillaries[9].

FUNCTIONAL CHANGES

Glomerular filtration rate

Serum creatinine is a relatively unreliable indicator of renal function in the aging population. This is because creatinine generation reflects muscle mass, and muscle mass decreases in the aging population. Normally males excrete 20–25 mg/kg body weight of creatinine in the urine each day, and women excreted 15–20 mg/kg body weight of creatinine. However, with aging, there is a progressive decrease in urinary creatinine excretion resulting in excretion rates lower than these ranges after the age of 60 years[10] (Fig. 65.3).

When accurate creatinine clearances are performed, there is clear evidence for a reduction in renal function with age. The decrease in renal function has been corroborated by inulin clearance studies, which show a progressive fall in GFR after the age of 40 years[7] (Fig. 65.4). In one study, the mean creatinine clearance fell from 140 mL/min/1.73 m² at age 25 years to 34–97 mL/min/1.73 m² at age 75–84 years[11]. However, serum creatinine was not different between these groups due to the loss of muscle mass that occurs with aging.

Creatinine clearance values are infrequently obtained in clinical practice, and many nephrologists utilize the Cockcroft–Gault formula, which takes age into account to estimate the creatinine clearance. The creatinine clearance (in mL/min) in men is calculated: (140 – age × body weight (kg)/72 × serum creatinine (mg/dL); in women, the final value is multiplied by 0.85 (see also Fig. 3.6 in Chapter 3). While this formula is clinically helpful, it correlates only moderately with creatinine clearances in the elderly population (correlation coefficient, r, of 0.74)[12].

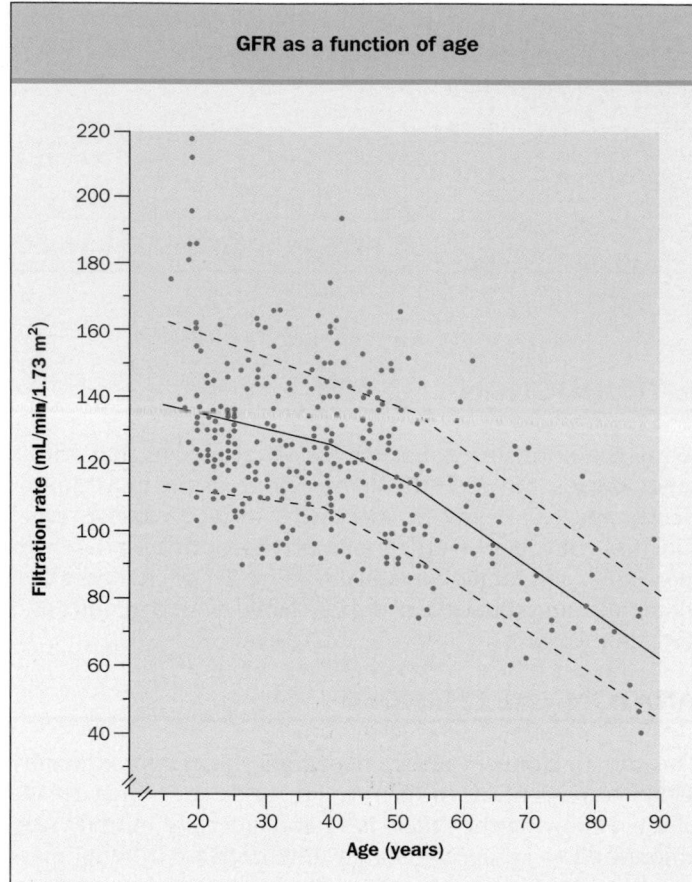

Figure 65.4 **Glomerular filtration rate (measured by inulin clearance) decreases with age in normal men.** The figure shows the sum results of 38 studies. The solid and broken lines represent one standard deviation. (Reproduced with permission[7].)

In addition to the general decrease in GFR with aging, there may be a reduction in the 'renal reserve'. Usually, GFR increases with a protein load or with feeding. Some studies suggest that aging humans show a normal increase in GFR following amino acid infusion. However, a more profound challenge was performed in aging rats; in this study aging rats showed a markedly blunted increase in GFR with feeding[13] (Fig. 65.5).

Another interesting finding is that not all individuals show a decrease in GFR with aging. In particular, in as many as one-third of subjects who remain normotensive, there is no decrease in creatinine clearance with age[7].

Renal plasma flow

There is also a normal decrease in renal plasma flow (RPF) with aging. RPF measured by PAH clearances decrease from a mean of 650 mL/min in the fourth decade to 290 mL/min by the ninth decade, and this is associated with increasing renal vascular resistance. The fall in RPF is greater in elderly subjects who are hypertensive[14]. The fact that RPF decreases relatively more than GFR explains why filtration fraction (defined as GFR/RPF) also increases with age.

The decrease in RPF does not simply reflect a decrease in renal mass. Studies by Hollenberg using a Xenon washout technique demonstrated that there is a true reduction in renal

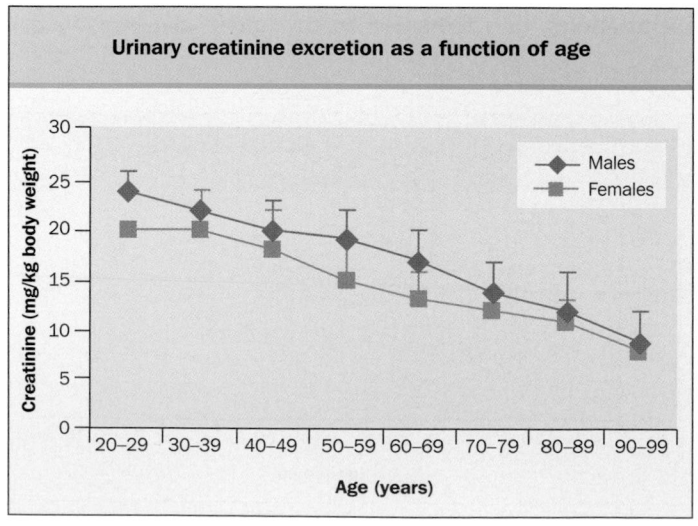

Figure 65.3 **Urinary creatinine excretion (factored for body weight) decreases with age.** (Adapted with permission[10].)

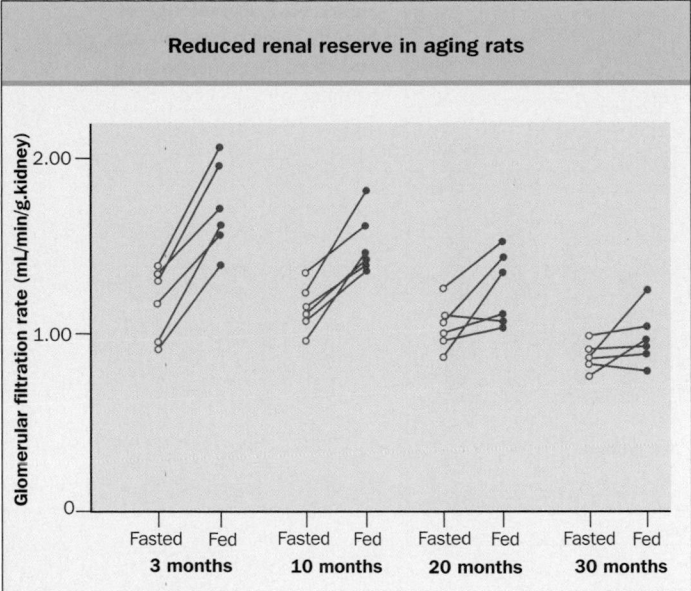

Figure 65.5 Glomerular filtration rate in starved and fed rats. Aging is associated with a fall in GFR and a blunted rise in GFR with feeding. (Reproduced with permission[13].)

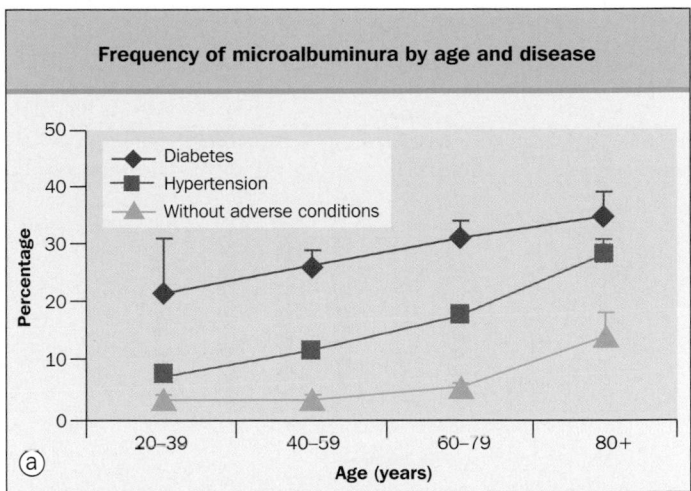

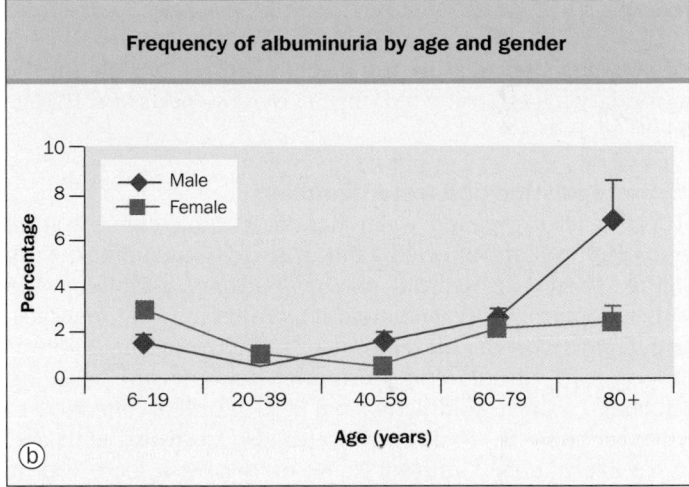

Figure 65.6 (a) Microalbuminuria increases with age. The prevalence of microalbuminuria for subjects with diabetes, hypertension, or without adverse health conditions are shown; (b) Albuminuria increases with age. (Adapted with permission[16].)

blood flow when factored for renal mass[15]. The decrease in renal blood flow especially involves the cortex, and blood flow to the medulla is relatively preserved.

Capillary permeability and proteinuria

A recent analysis of the Third National Health and Nutrition Examination Survey (NHANES) has demonstrated that both albuminuria and microalbuminuria (urinary albumin levels of 30 mg to 300 mg/day) increase progressively in the US population after the age of 40 years[16] (Fig. 65.6). The increased prevalence is most marked in diabetic and hypertensive subjects, but is also observed in the patients lacking these risk factors. The prevalence was higher in Blacks, Mexican Americans, and in those with elevated serum creatinine[16]. This is a potentially important observation, as microalbuminuria has been shown in several studies to be an independent risk factor for cardiovascular events (such as carotid disease and left ventricular hypertrophy) and cardiovascular mortality.

Sodium balance and hypertension

Sodium balance is also altered in aging. There is evidence for both impaired sodium excretion of a salt load[17] as well as defective conservation in the setting of sodium restriction[18]. Proximal sodium reabsorption (reflected by lithium clearances) is increased in aging, whereas distal sodium reabsorption may be reduced[14]. Studies in rats suggest the pressure–natriuresis is impaired in aging[19]. As the diet of most individuals in developed countries contains excess sodium (8–10 g salt/day), there is a tendency in the elderly population for total body sodium excess.

The relative defect in sodium excretion and increased total body sodium may be a predisposing factor for the development of hypertension. Blood pressure increases with age. After the age of 60 years, the majority of the population is hypertensive[20]

(Fig. 65.7). The majority (> 85%) of hypertension in the aging population is sodium-sensitive, in that restricting sodium will result in a significant fall (> 10 mmHg) in mean arterial pressure[21]. Populations that ingest low sodium diets, such as the Yanomamo Indians of Southern Venezuela, do not show the increase in blood pressure with age (see Chapter 37)[22]. Other mechanisms may also be involved in aging-associated hypertension, including loss of vascular compliance due to collagen deposition in the larger arterial vessels. Endothelial dysfunction, perhaps mediated by local oxidants, has also been shown to be increased in the aging population, and may contribute to the development of increased blood pressure.

The observation that aging associated renal and vascular changes may be responsible for the high frequency of hypertension in this population likely explains why correction of secondary forms of hypertension (such as primary aldosteronism, Cushing's syndrome, renovascular hypertension and hypothyroidism) is much more effective at curing hypertension in younger patients. In one study, diastolic blood pressure fell to < 90 mmHg in 24 of 25 subjects under the age

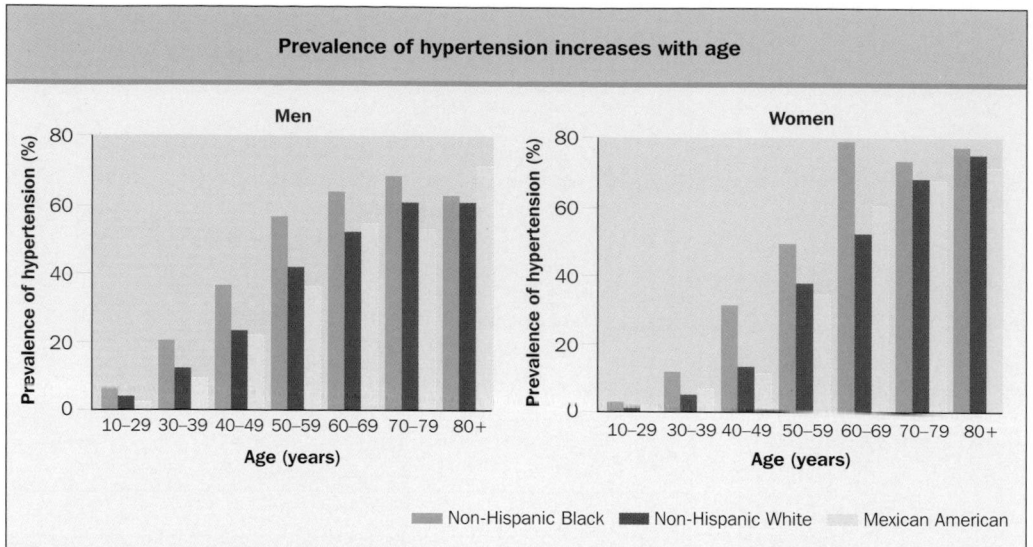

Figure 65.7 Prevalence of hypertension based on age, gender and race. (Reproduced with permission[20].)

of 40 years after treating the mechanism responsible for the secondary hypertension but only 38 of 61 subjects over the age of 40 years[23].

Osmoregulation and water handling

There is also impaired water handling. Both concentration and dilution are affected, and nocturia is common with aging. There is a reduced maximal urinary osmolarity and thirst response to hyperosmolarity, which may be predisposing factors for the development of dehydration. Subjects respond to antidiuretic hormone (vasopressin) with an increase in urine osmolality, but it is blunted compared to younger subjects. Total body water also decreases with age. Conversely, there is a slower excretion of a water load, leading to an increased predisposition to hyponatremia.

Other tubular defects and electrolyte problems

Potassium excretion is impaired and is likely due to decreased tubular mass. Hyperkalemia occurs more frequently in elderly subjects treated with drugs that interfere with potassium excretion (such as potassium-sparing diuretics) than in younger people. Hypokalemia is also common due to renal or extrarenal losses. Acid–base disturbances may result from the impaired distal tubular acidification that occurs with aging; aging subjects do not excrete an acid load as effectively as younger subjects.

Hypercalcemia is found in 2–3% of institutionalized elderly patients. Causes are multifactorial and include malignant tumors, hyperparathyroidism, immobilization, and thiazide diuretic use. Hypocalcemia is less common than hypercalcemia and is observed mainly in patients with chronic renal failure, chronic malabsorption, and severe malnutrition. Aging is associated with increased parathyroid hormone levels (which correlate inversely with GFR) and a decrease in serum calcitriol and phosphate[14]. Hypomagnesemia may be present in as many as 7–10% of elderly patients admitted to the hospital; most commonly this is the result of malnutrition, laxatives or diuretic use. Hypermagnesemia is less common and is found primarily in patients with chronic renal failure or who are taking large doses of magnesium-containing antacids.

Clinical implications

The practical implications of these limitations of glomerular and tubular function in elderly people are considerable. Fluid and electrolyte management need constant vigilance to minimize morbidity. While fluid and electrolyte homeostasis is well maintained in every day settings, older people are easily destabilized by intercurrent challenges that are well tolerated by younger patients. Moderate fluid loss (e.g., an episode of diarrhea) or moderate fluid loading (e.g., inappropriate perioperative intravenous fluids) are both poorly tolerated and may easily lead to hypovolemia and fluid overload respectively. Overzealous administration of water as 5% dextrose or 0.45% saline easily leads to hyponatremia. The acid load provoked by ischemic tissue injury or hypoxemia will be more severe in the elderly due to inadequate renal compensation. Potassium homeostasis is easily destabilized by inaccurate estimation of intravenous or oral potassium requirements.

RISK FACTORS FOR AGING RELATED RENAL DISEASE

Variability in the severity of aging related renal disease in humans and experimental animals has suggested that there may be specific risk factors for its development. For example, it is known that a percentage of normal subjects who remain normotensive will not show age-related decreases in GFR (measured as creatinine clearance)[7]. In experimental models, aging-related changes vary according to the genetic strain, gender, body mass index and diet. Specifically, disease is worse in male and obese animals, and aging changes can be retarded with protein or caloric restriction[19].

PATHOGENESIS OF PROGRESSIVE RENAL DISEASE IN AGING

A variety of mechanisms have been proposed for aging related renal changes. Senescence is associated with progressive telomere shortening of chromosomal DNA that may limit replicative capacity. In particular, a loss of mitochondrial DNA and total mitochondria occurs with aging[24,25].

A favored hypothesis is that this is due to the production of oxygen-derived free radicals that cause cumulative oxidative injury to tissues over time[26]. A loss of mitochondria would affect mitochondrial respiration and cellular energetics and may predispose to cell injury or death. Senescence is associated with accelerated apoptosis, and increased numbers of apoptotic tubular and interstitial cells have been shown in the aging rat[6].

Glomerular number has been shown to decrease from approximately one million per kidney to 600 000 or less by the eighth decade. A loss of nephrons is known to result in hyperfiltration, resulting in increased glomerular hydrostatic pressure and glomerular hypertrophy, which are known risk factors for the development of glomerular scarring[27]. Thus, it is likely that elevated glomerular pressures may contribute to glomerular scarring with aging, and this is consistent with some experimental studies[28]. However, studies in aging rats have shown that the initiation of renal damage with aging may occur independently of glomerular hypertension. Indeed, depending on the strain, glomerular hydrostatic pressures may be either elevated or normal with aging[19]. It is thus likely that glomerular hypertension, when it occurs with the decrease in nephron mass, is a contributor rather than an initiator of the renal structural changes in aging.

Recent evidence suggests a key role for angiotensin II in mediating the renal changes of aging. While aging is generally associated with extracellular volume expansion and a reduction in plasma renin activity, there is evidence in aging rats that renal angiotensin II levels are elevated. Furthermore, rats or mice treated with angiotensin converting enzyme (ACE) inhibitors or angiotensin receptor antagonists (ATRAs) from shortly after birth have less glomerulosclerosis, less glomerular hypertrophy and less tubulointerstitial fibrosis with aging[3,28]. The renoprotection may be mediated by both hemodynamic (decreasing glomerular hydrostatic pressure and increasing renal blood flow) and nonhemodynamic (direct effect to block angiotensin II-mediated cell growth or cytokine (TGF-β) generation) mechanisms[29].

One of the major mechanisms by which blockade of the renin–angiotensin system might be beneficial appears to be by preventing oxidative injury. Increased synthesis of reactive oxygen species has been demonstrated in isolated glomeruli obtained from aging rats[30]. Theoretically reactive oxygen species may be generated by infiltrating leukocytes, by tissue hypoxia or by the effects of angiotensin II to stimulate NADPH oxidases in various cells, including vascular smooth muscle cells. The administration of ACE inhibitors or ATRAs can preserve mitochondria in renal proximal tubules in association with upregulation of cellular antioxidant enzymes as rats age[31,32].

Blockade of the renin–angiotensin system in the rat also prevents or improves other age-related changes in other organs. For example, there is less left ventricular hypertrophy and myocardial fibrosis, improvement in learning capacity, increased sexual activity and decreased liver fibrosis (Fig. 65.8).

In addition to angiotensin II and reactive oxygen species, there are other potential mediators of aging-associated renal disease. In aging rats, an accumulation of TGF-β has been shown, which is an important profibrotic growth factor.

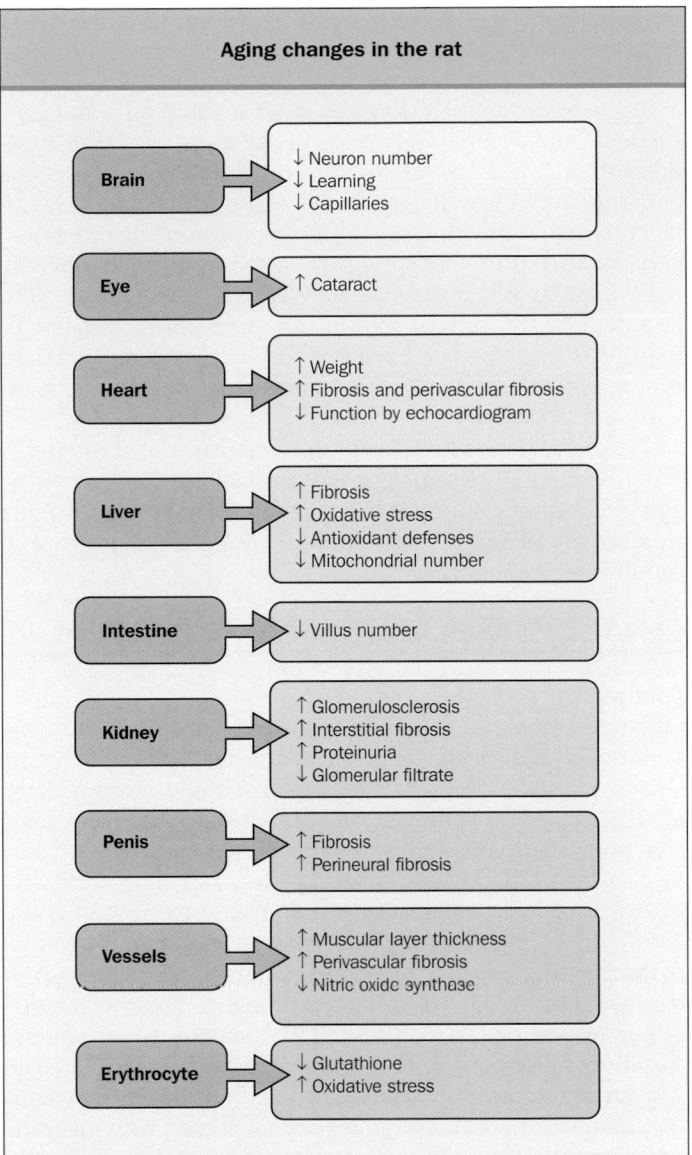

Aging changes in the rat

Brain	↓ Neuron number ↓ Learning ↓ Capillaries
Eye	↑ Cataract
Heart	↑ Weight ↑ Fibrosis and perivascular fibrosis ↓ Function by echocardiogram
Liver	↑ Fibrosis ↑ Oxidative stress ↓ Antioxidant defenses ↓ Mitochondrial number
Intestine	↓ Villus number
Kidney	↑ Glomerulosclerosis ↑ Interstitial fibrosis ↑ Proteinuria ↓ Glomerular filtrate
Penis	↑ Fibrosis ↑ Perineural fibrosis
Vessels	↑ Muscular layer thickness ↑ Perivascular fibrosis ↓ Nitric oxide synthase
Erythrocyte	↓ Glutathione ↑ Oxidative stress

Figure 65.8 Aging associated changes in the rat. The effect of aging in multiple organs is shown. These changes are reversed or ameliorated by life-long treatment of rats with agents that inhibit or block the renin–angiotensin system.

Advanced glycation endproducts (AGEs), which are observed in diabetes, also accumulate in aging, and chronic administration of aminoguanidine (an inhibitor of AGE synthesis) can reduce the incidence of glomerulosclerosis in the aging rat.

Endothelial changes also occur with aging possibly leading to more vasoconstriction that could predispose to ischemia. The vascular endothelium produces less prostacyclin and nitric oxide with aging and, in rats, this is associated with a loss of endothelial nitric oxide synthase expression in peritubular capillary endothelium. The loss of the normal endothelial vasodilatory substances may account for the increased renal vasoconstrictive response observed in aging rats to agents such as angiotensin II, endothelin-1 and nitro-L-arginine methyl ester (an inhibitor of nitric oxide synthesis)[33]. Conversely, studies in hypertensive humans have shown an impaired renal vasodilatory response to L-arginine (which stimulates NO synthesis) when older (mean age 63 years) individuals were compared to younger (mean age 23 years) subjects[34].

There is also a progressive loss of both glomerular and peritubular capillary endothelial cells in the aging rat. There is evidence that this is associated with impaired angiogenesis as a consequence of loss of constitutive angiogenic factors (vascular endothelial growth factor) and the expression of anti-angiogenic factors (thrombospondin 1)[9]. The loss of capillaries may predispose to ischemia to the tubules, whereas it may lead to loss of filtration surface area in the glomerulus. The loss of nephrons may further feedback to lead to hyperfiltration, increased glomerular pressure and the development of glomerulosclerosis.

Prolonged hyperuricemia has also been associated with renal functional and histologic changes similar to that observed in aging[35]. It is thus of interest that experimental hyperuricemia induces glomerular hypertrophy, glomerulosclerosis and tubulointerstitial fibrosis[36].

RENAL DISEASES ASSOCIATED WITH AGING

Glomerular diseases
Glomerular diseases are common in older subjects. The most common etiologies of nephrotic syndrome in the elderly are shown in Figure 65.9[37,38]. Amyloidosis should be considered in the nephrotic patient with relatively preserved renal function, a urinary sediment void of red cells or with low levels of microhematuria, normal or low blood pressure, and evidence of hepatosplenomegaly or autonomic dysfunction. Membranous nephropathy may occur and is commonly idiopathic, or may be associated with malignancies, especially of the gastrointestinal tract, lung or breast. Focal segmental glomerulosclerosis is continuing to increase in prevalence for all age groups and should be particularly considered in African American individuals. Chronic lymphocytic leukemia is common in the elderly and may be associated with membranoproliferative glomerulonephritis. Minimal change disease, although most common in young children aged 2–12 years, also has a second peak incidence in the fifth and sixth decade.

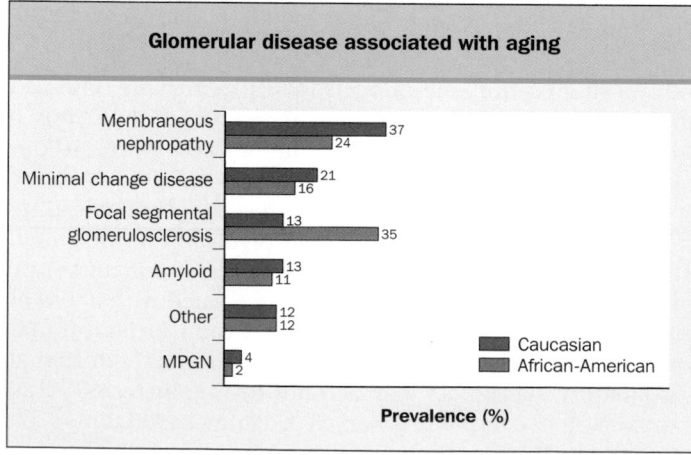

Figure 65.9 Glomerular diseases associated with aging. (Adapted with permission[36,37].)

Vasculitis, especially Wegener's granulomatosis and other forms of vasculitis associated with pauci-immune necrotizing glomerulonephritis, are common in elderly subjects and presents with a rapid onset of renal failure with red cell casts and systemic signs[39]. Other types of nephritis are also more common in the elderly (> 65 years) compared to younger adults; these include crescentic glomerulonephritis, poststreptococcal glomerulonephritis and membranoproliferative glomerulonephritis[40].

Renovascular and atheroembolic disease
There is also an increased frequency of renovascular disease and atheroembolic disease with aging (see Chapter 63). The observation of hypertension and an elevated serum creatinine, especially in an individual with a history of vascular disease, should prompt a screening test for renovascular disease, such as magnetic resonance angiography (MRA). The MRA is preferred as the study does not require contrast administration which is associated with increased nephrotoxicity in elderly subjects.

Urinary tract infections
There is an increased risk of asymptomatic bacteriuria with aging (see Chapter 53). The prevalence in women increases from 5% (less than age 50 years) to 21% (ambulatory over the age of 65 years) to 53% (institutionalized elderly women). In men the prevalence increases from 0% (less than 50 years) to 12% (ambulatory over age 65 years) to 37% (institutionalized over the age of 65 years). In men, this may relate to the increased risk for prostatic hypertrophy as well as to an increase in urinary calculi with age. Chronic instrumentation and bladder catheters in elderly subjects are also associated with increased bacterial colonization rates; treatment of these urinary tract infections should generally be based on the presence of symptoms or signs (fever, elevated white blood cell count or dysuria). Exceptions would include high risk subjects such as those scheduled to undergo urologic surgery, neutropenic patients, and patients with renal transplants (see Chapter 53).

Evaluation of hematuria
Malignancies of the urinary tract are more common in older subjects. Bladder cancer is rarely observed before the age of 40 years in men, and is even more uncommon in women under 40 years; it increases progressively after the fourth decade. Renal cell carcinomas are most commonly observed in the seventh decade, with a median age of diagnosis of 66 years and a median age of death of 70 years. As a consequence, the development of micro- or macrohematuria generally requires investigation of both the lower (cystoscopy and in men, a prostate examination) and upper tract (imaging studies) for cancerous lesions. A search for other diagnoses (including glomerular lesions, stones, idiopathic hypercalciuria, etc.) may also be indicated in the evaluation of hematuria as discussed in Chapter 19 and Chapter 59.

Nephrotoxicity and drug dosing
As mentioned, elderly subjects are prone to increased nephrotoxicity both as a consequence of their decreased renal mass

and because they are often administered medicines on the assumption that a normal or near normal serum creatinine is consistent with normal renal function. As a result, elderly subjects are prone to nephrotoxicity from nonsteroidal agents, COX-2 inhibitors, aminoglycosides, radiocontrast and chemotherapy (such as cisplatinum).

Drug dosing needs to be carefully adjusted in the aging patient. Certain common drugs frequently need adjusting for renal function; these include aminoglycosides, digoxin, procainamide, tetracycline and vancomycin. Other drugs may be commonly associated with the development of hyponatremia; these include thiazides and chlorpropamide.

END-STAGE RENAL DISEASE, DIALYSIS AND TRANSPLANTATION

It is perhaps not surprising, given the normal decrease in GFR with aging, that end-stage renal disease (ESRD) is common in the elderly. Both the incidence (number of new cases per year per million population) as well as prevalence (total number of cases per year per million population) of ESRD is higher in older subjects[41] (Fig. 65.10). Indeed, currently, the mean age for a patient to initiate renal replacement therapy is 63 years in the USA. Most cases of ESRD in older subjects are due to either diabetes or hypertension (Fig. 65.11). Glomerulonephritis and polycystic kidney disease are relatively less common. The age of an individual *per se* is no longer considered a criterion for deciding whether renal replacement therapy is appropriate. Patients often do very well with either hemodialysis or peritoneal dialysis unless there are comorbid conditions such as cardiovascular disease. Unfortunately, cardiac disease is common in elderly subjects with chronic kidney failure[41] (Fig. 65.12).

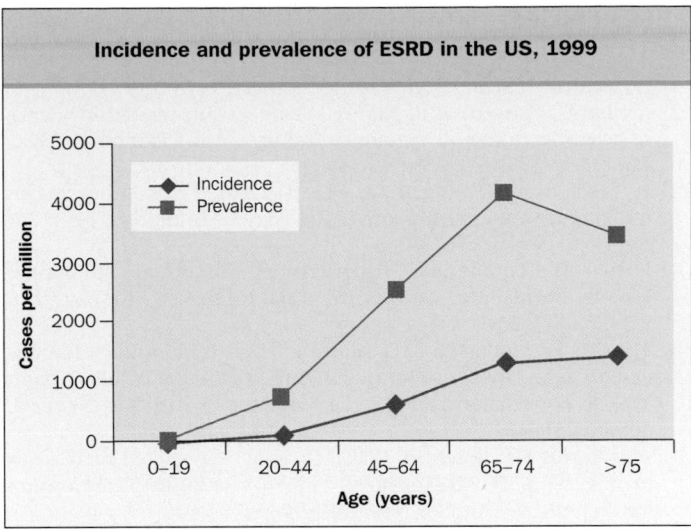

Figure 65.10 Incidence and prevalence of end-stage renal disease (ESRD) by age in the US population in 1999. (Adapted from the USRDS data base[41].)

Transplantation should be considered in the management of elderly subjects, although only a minority of elderly patients with ESRD are suitable for transplantation because of comorbid conditions, particularly cardiovascular disease and malignancy. Transplantation of subjects between the ages of 65 and 74 years is associated with superior kidney survival compared to patients at the same age who are on a transplant waiting list. Elderly subjects actually have a lower rate of graft rejection compared to younger patients. However, since they have a higher rate of death with functioning grafts, overall graft survival is similar to younger subjects[42].

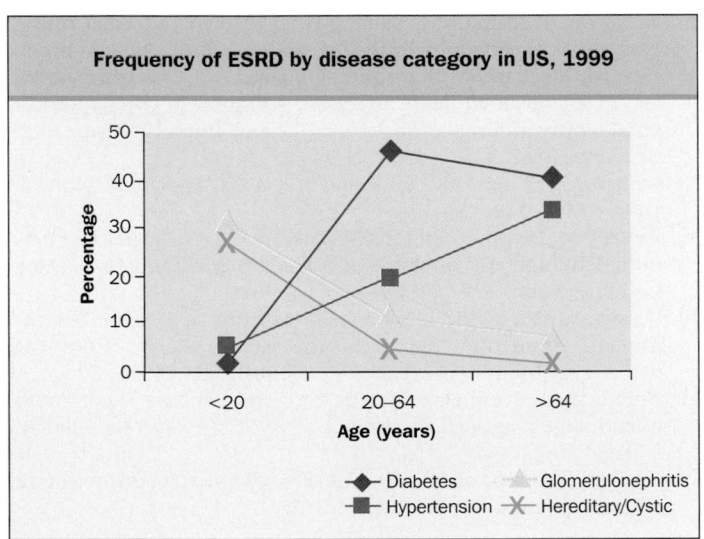

Figure 65.11 Frequency of ESRD by disease category in the US population in 1999. (Adapted from the USRDS data base[41].)

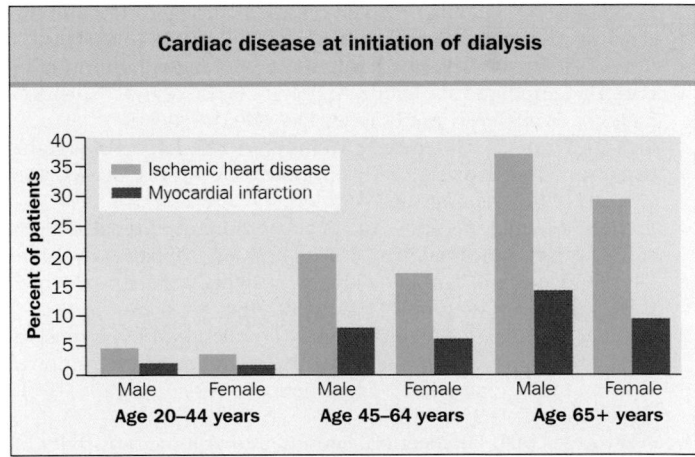

Figure 65.12 Frequency of cardiac disease in patients with ESRD being initiated on dialysis in the US. (Adapted from the USRDS data base[41].)

REFERENCES

1. McLachlan MSF. The aging kidney. Lancet. 1978;2:143–5.
2. Kaplan C, Pasternack B, Shah H, Gallo G. Age-related incidence of sclerotic glomeruli in human kidneys. Am J Pathol. 1975;80:227–34.
3. Ferder L, Inserra F, Romano L, et al. Decreased glomerulosclerosis in aging by angiotensin-converting enzyme inhibitors. J Am Soc Nephrol. 1994;5:1147–52.
4. Fogo AB. Glomerular hypertension, abnormal glomerular growth, and progression of renal diseases. Kidney Int. 2000;57:S15–21.
5. Thomas SE, Anderson S, Gordon KL, et al. Tubulointerstitial disease in aging: evidence for underlying peritubular capillary damage. A potential role for renal ischemia. J Am Soc Nephrol. 1998;9:231–42.
6. Ruiz-Torres MP, Bosch RJ, O'Valle F, et al. Age-related increase in expression of TGF-b1 in the rat kidney: relationship to morphologic changes. J Am Soc Nephrol. 1998;9:782–91.
7. Lindeman RD, Goldman R. Anatomic and physiologic age changes in the kidney. Exp Gerontol. 1986;21:379–406.
8. Takazakura E, Sawabu N, Handa A, et al. Intrarenal vascular changes with age and disease. Kidney Int. 1972;2:224–30.
9. Kang D-H, Anderson S, Kim Y-G, et al. Impaired angiogenesis in the aging kidney: vascular endothelial growth factor and thrombospondin-1 in renal disease. Am J Kidney Dis. 2001;37:601–11.
10. Epstein M. Aging and the kidney. J Am Soc Nephrol. 1996;7:1106–22.
11. Rowe JW, Andres R, Tobin J, et al. The effect of age on creatinine clearance in man: a cross-sectional and longitudinal study. J Gerontol. 1976;31:155–63.
12. Goldberg TH, Finkelstein MS. Difficulties in estimating glomerular filtration rate in the elderly. Arch Int Med. 1987;147:1430–3.
13. Corman BS, Chami-Khazraji J, Schaeverbeke J, Michel JB. Effect of feeding on glomerular filtration rate and proteinuria in conscious aging rats. Am J Physiol Renal Physiol. 1988;255:F250–6.
14. Fliser D, Franek E, Joest M, et al. Renal function in the elderly: impact of hypertension and cardiac function. Kidney Int. 1997;51:1196–204.
15. Hollenberg NK, Adams DF, Solomon HS, et al. Senescence and the renal vasculature in normal man. J Lab Clin Med. 1976;87:411–17.
16. Jones CA, Francis ME, Eberhardt MS, et al. Microalbuminuria in the US population: Third National Health and Nutrition Examination Survey. Am J Kidney Dis. 2002;39:445–9.
17. Luft FC, Grim CE, Gineberg N, Weinberger MC. Effects of volume expansion and contraction in normotensive whites, Blacks, and subjects of different ages. Circulation. 1979;59:643–50.
18. Epstein M, Hollenberg NK. Age as a determinant of renal sodium conservation in normal man. J Lab Clin Med. 1976;87:411–17.
19. Baylis C, Corma B. The aging kidney: insights from experimental studies. J Am Soc Nephrol. 1998;9:699–799.
20. Burt VL, Whelton P, Roccella EJ, et al. Prevalence of hypertension in the US adult population. Results from the Third National Health and Nutrition Examination Survey, 1988–1991. Hypertension. 1995;25:305–13.
21. Weinberger MH, Fineberg NS. Sodium and volume sensitivity of blood pressure. Age and pressure change over time. Hypertension. 1991;18:67–71.
22. Oliver WB, Cohen EL, Neel JV. Blood pressure, sodium intake, and sodium related hormones in the Yanomamo Indians, a 'no-salt' culture. Circulation. 1975;52:146–51.
23. Streeten DHP, Anderson GP, Wagner S. Effect of age on response of secondary hypertension to specific treatment. Am J Hypertens. 1990;3:360–5.
24. Murfitt RR, Sanadi DR. Evidence for increase degeneration of mitochondria in old rats. A brief note. Mech Ageing Dev. 1978;8:197–201.
25. Polson CD, Webster JC. Loss of mitochondrial DNA in mouse tissues with age. Age. 1982;5:5–133.
26. Beckman KB, Ames BN. The free radical theory of aging matures. Physiol Rev. 1998;78:547–581.
27. Anderson S, Brenner BM. Progressive renal disease: a disorder of adaptation. QJ Med. 1989;70:185–9.
28. Anderson S, Rennke HG, Zatz R. Glomerular adaptations with normal aging and with long-term converting enzyme inhibition in rats. Am J Physiol Renal Physiol. 1994;36:F35–43.
29. Inserra F, Stella I, Kurnek ML, et al. Losartan and enalapril protect against age related kidney lesions in normal rats treated from 12 to 18 months of age. J Am Soc Nephrol. 2001;12:679A.
30. Ruiz-Torres P, Gonzalezz-Rubio M, Lucio-Cazana FJ, et al. Reactive oxygen species and platelet-activating factor synthesis in age-related glomerulosclerosis. J Lab Clin Med. 1994;124:489–95.
31. Ferder LF, Inserra F, Romano L, et al. Effects of angiotensin-converting enzyme inhibition on mitochondrial number in the aging mouse. Am J Physiol Cell Physiol. 1993;34:C15–18.
32. Cavanagh EMV de, Inserra F, Ferder L, Fraga CG. Enalapril and captopril enhance glutathione-dependent antioxidant defenses in mouse tissues. Am J Physiol Regulat Integrat Comp Physiol. 2000;278:R572–7.
33. Tank JE, Vora JP, Houghton DC, Anderson S. Altered renal vascular responses in the aging kidney. Am J Physiol Renal Physiol. 1994;35:F942–8.
34. Campo C, Lahera V, Garcia-Robles R, et al. Aging abolishes the renal response to L-arginine infusion in essential hypertension. Kidney Int. 1996;49:S126–8.
35. Yu T, Berger L. Impaired renal function in gout: Its association with hypertensive vascular disease and intrinsic renal disease. Am J Med. 1982;72:95–100.
36. Nakagawa T, Mazzali M, Kang D-H, et al. Hyperuricemia causes glomerular hypertrophy in the rat. Am J Nephrol. 2002, in press.
37. Haas M, Meehan SM, Karison TG, Spargo BH. Changing etiologies of unexplained adult nephrotic syndrome: a comparison of renal biopsy findings from 1976–1979 and 1995–1997. Am J Kid Dis. 1997;30:621–31.
38. Cameron JS. Nephrotic syndrome in the elderly. Semin Nephrol. 1996;16:319–329.
39. Vassallo M, Shepherd RJ, Iqbal P, Feehally J. Age-related variations in presentation and outcome of Wegener's granulomatosis. J Roy Coll Phys Lond. 1997;31:396–400.
40. Vendemia F, Gesualdo L, Schena FP, D'Amico G. Epidemiology of primary glomerulonephritis in the elderly. Report from the Italian Registry of Renal Biopsy. J Nephrol. 2001;14:340–52.
41. United States Renal Data System. 2001 Annual Data Report: atlas of end stage renal disease in the United States. Am J Kidney Dis. 2001;38(Suppl 3):37–195.
42. Tesi RJ, Elkhammas EA, Davies EA, et al. Renal transplantation in older people. Lancet. 1994;343:461–4.

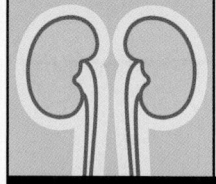

CHRONIC RENAL FAILURE: DEFINITION AND INCIDENCE

Chronic renal failure (CRF) refers to a progressive and irreversible loss of renal function. The recent Kidney Disease Outcomes Quality Initiative (K/DOQI) guidelines have classified chronic kidney diseases (CKD) into four stages using the term chronic kidney failure (CKF). Stage 1: normal or increased glomerular filtration rate (GFR) but some evidence of kidney damage reflected by microalbuminuria/proteinuria, hematuria or histological changes. Stage 2: kidney damage with a mild decrease in GFR (60–89 mL/min/1.73 m²). Stage 3: moderate decrease in GFR (30–59 mL/min). Stage 4: severe decrease in GFR (15–29 mL/min). Stage 4: kidney failure; GFR < 15 mL/min[1]. Stage 5 is when renal replacement therapy (RRT) in the form of dialysis or transplantation has to be considered to sustain life. The K/DOQI terminology has not yet been widely accepted and this chapter will use more established terms (CRF rather than CKF; chronic renal disease rather than CKD) except where information specifically relates to the K/DOQI classification.

The true incidence and prevalence of CRF within a community is difficult to ascertain as most individuals suffering from early to moderate CRF are asymptomatic. Therefore, screening for such individuals would have to rely on clinical examination (detection of systemic hypertension), biochemical measurements (serum creatinine) or urinalysis (hematuria and/or proteinuria). The point prevalence of irreversible, but not yet terminal, CRF in a community will determine whether or not population screening is feasible. In the USA, the third National Health and Nutrition Examination Survey (NHANES III: 1988 to 1994) concluded that an estimated 3% of the population (5.6 million individuals) had an elevated serum creatinine (> 1.4–1.6 mg/dL), 70% of whom were hypertensive with only a minority (27%) having blood pressure levels less than 140/90 mmHg[2]. However, a more detailed analysis by NHANES III estimated the number of individuals with different levels of GFR to be up to 114 million with stage 1 CKD, 55.3 million with stage 2 (GFR 60–89 mL/min), 7.6 million with stage 3 (GFR: 30–59 mL/min) and 0.4 million with stage 4 CKF[1,2]. The same survey found the prevalence of albuminuria estimated from the albumin–creatinine ratio to be 11.7% (20.2 million individuals)[1,2]. Such a high prevalence may reflect the increased albumin excretion rate in individuals over the age of 70 years (prevalence around 30%) and in diabetics (> 50%)[1,2]. In a single practice study in the USA of

796 subjects, proteinuria was found in 4% of the healthy and 53% of those had both hypertension and diabetes. A study in Japan found that both proteinuria and hematuria increased with age, 10% of subjects over 65 years having one or the other[3]; however, less than 2% of those reached end-stage renal disease (ESRD) in 10 years. Since whole population screening has such a low yield, one possible approach would be to screen populations at high risk such as the elderly, diabetic and hypertensive individuals, as well as high-risk communities such as African- or Native-Americans. It may also be worthwhile screening those with a family history of kidney diseases, those with autoimmune disorders, as well as those with a history of urinary tract infections. Initial screening should consist of blood pressure measurement and urinalysis (dipstix testing for albuminuria/proteinuria and hematuria). Ultrasonography has also been put forward by K/DOQI as a useful and noninvasive screening procedure[1], although this investigation is unlikely to be part of the initial screening process.

EPIDEMIOLOGY OF CHRONIC RENAL FAILURE

Since the mid-1980s, there has been a marked increase in the incidence of ESRD requiring RRT across the world. A projected analysis undertaken in the USA suggests that the incidence of ESRD will continue to rise until 2010 at a rate of 6–7% per year[4].

In the UK, the incidence of ESRD varies between 80 and 110 new patients per million of population (pmp) per year. The corresponding figure in the USA is much higher, and was around 315 pmp in 1999[5] (Table 66.1). The prevalence of patients on RRT in Europe was around 462 pmp in 1996[6] and reached 659 pmp by 1999 compared to 1217 pmp in the USA[5] (Table 66.2). In general, the incidence of ESRD increases with age, reaching around 1300 pmp per year in patients over the age of 65 years (Table 66.1). Data from Australia[7] suggest comparable incidence and prevalence of ESRD to the UK[8] and Europe (90 pmp/year and 332 respectively in 2000). On the other hand, the incidence and prevalence of ESRD in Japan is comparable to that of the USA (252 pmp/year and 1624 respectively in 2000)[9] (Table 66.2). The discrepancy between European/Australasian and American/Japanese data may reflect the higher prevalence of diabetes (in particular type 2) and hypertension in the latter. While chronic glomerulonephritis remains the most common cause of ESRD in Europe and Australia, diabetes mellitus and hypertension are the most common causes of ESRD in the USA[5–9] (Table 66.3).

Chronic Renal Failure and the Uremic Syndrome

Incidence and prevalence of ESRD in USA in 1996		
Characteristics	Incidence	Prevalence
Total population	317 pmp	1217
Age (years)		
20–44	119	745
45–64	603	2534
65–74	1317	4163
Caucasians	237	871
African Americans	953	3926
Native Americans	652	3089
Diabetes mellitus	136	411
Hypertension	83	282
Glomerulonephritis	29	194
(Data from USRDS Study 1998)		

Table 66.1 Incidence and prevalence of end-stage renal disease (ESRD) in USA in 1996.

Incidence and prevalence of ESRD					
	UK (1999)	Europe (1999)	Australia (2000)	USA (1999)	Japan (2000)
Incidence (pmp/year)	96	115	90	315	252
Prevalence (pmp)	528	659	332	1217	1624

Table 66.2 Incidence and prevalence of ESRD.

NATURAL HISTORY OF CHRONIC RENAL FAILURE

The majority of patients with CRF progress relentlessly to ESRD. A straight-line relationship is typically found between the reciprocal of serum creatinine values (1/sCr) and time. However, a significant percentage of patients do not progress in a predictable linear fashion and have breakpoints in their progression slopes suggesting an acceleration or a slowing down of the rate of progression of renal insufficiency[10]. These breakpoints could be either spontaneous or secondary to events such as infections, dehydration, or changes in the adequacy of systemic blood pressure control[10]. It is also important to appreciate that some patients with mild-to-moderate CRF have stable renal function for sustained periods of time.

The rate of progression of CRF varies according to the underlying nephropathy and between individual patients[11]. Historically, the rate of decline in GFR of patients with diabetic nephropathy (DN) has been amongst the fastest, averaging around –10 mL/min/year. Control of systemic hypertension considerably slows down the rate of decline of the GFR

Causes of ESRD				
Causes of ESRD	UK	Australia	USA	Japan
Chronic glomerulonephritis	30	30	9	47
Diabetic nephropathy	16	22	43	31
Hypertension	12	14	26	10
Chronic interstitial nephritis	8	10	2	2
Polycystic kidney disease	6	6	2	2
Miscellaneous	12	11	11	8
Uncertain	16	7	2	0

Table 66.3 Causes of ESRD.

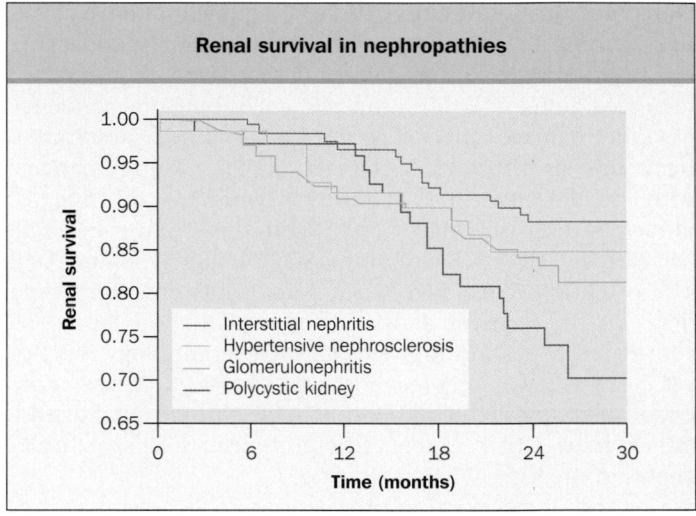

Figure 66.1 Actuarial renal survival in relation to the underlying nephropathy. (Adapted with permission[11].)

down to –5 mL/min/year with further improvement (–1 to –2 mL/min/year) expected in patients whose glycemia as well as hypertension are optimally controlled[12].

In nondiabetic nephropathy, a European study showed the rate of progression of CRF was 2.5 times faster in patients with chronic glomerulonephritis (CGN) compared to those with chronic interstitial nephritis (CIN) and 1.5 times faster than those with hypertensive nephrosclerosis (HNS) or polycystic kidney disease (PKD)[11]. In this study, the type of nephropathy was the most significant predictor of progression, with proteinuria the only continuous variable identified as an independent risk factor. The effect of proteinuria on the rate of progression of CRF was highlighted in another study where it explained the difference in the progression rates of patients with CGN, CIN and HNS, although patients with PKD with established renal insufficiency demonstrated the faster progression rate in the absence of significant proteinuria. The faster rate of progression of CRF of patients with PKD was also confirmed in other studies (Fig. 66.1)[13].

FACTORS AFFECTING THE PROGRESSION OF CHRONIC RENAL FAILURE

Factors affecting the development and progression of CRF can be divided into three categories. The first include non-modifiable susceptibility factors such as age, gender, genetics and race. The second are initiation factors necessary to initiate CRF in susceptible individuals including immune (glomerulonephritis), hemodynamic (hypertension), metabolic (diabetes mellitus and dyslipidemia) and infectious. The third group are modifiable risk factors which affect the prognosis and rate of progression of CRF, and include systemic hypertension, proteinuria, metabolic factors such as hyperglycemia and dyslipidemia, as well as smoking.

Nonmodifiable risk factors
Age
The incidence of renal disease is known to increase with age. In the UK in 1999, the incidence increased from 58 pmp per year in those under the age of 50 years to 288 pmp per year in individuals aged 65 years and over[8]. The current median age of patients with ESRD in the UK is 54 years with the highest prevalence of patients on RRT being in the 55–74 years age group (1100 pmp)[8]. In a French study, the increase was most apparent in elderly males with an annual incidence of ESRD reaching 1124 pmp per year[14]. In the USA, the annual incidence of ESRD is around 119 pmp in patients aged between 20 and 44 years, 603 pmp between 45 and 64 years, and in excess of 1300 pmp in those over the age of 65 years[5] (Table 66.1).

The etiology of CRF is also different in the elderly, with hypertension (including renovascular hypertension), diabetes and obstructive uropathy accounting for 40–60% of patients. The rate of progression of CRF is influenced by age, with elderly patients affected by glomerulonephritis having a faster rate of decline of renal function[1,14]. The faster rate of progression of glomerulonephritis in the elderly may reflect the underlying spontaneous fibrotic changes (glomerulosclerosis, interstitial fibrosis and vascular sclerosis) in the aging kidney as well as the reduced renal functional reserve. One notable exception is type 1 diabetic nephropathy where young age at diagnosis is associated with a faster rate of GFR decline.

Gender
ESRD is more common in males[5]; the incident rate in the USA in 1999 was 380 pmp/year in males compared to 266 pmp in females[5]. The majority of studies also suggest a faster rate of decline in GFR in males[1]. In nondiabetic renal disease, the rate of decline in renal function in males was found in one study to be almost twice as fast as in females, and correlated positively with mean arterial blood pressure[14]. A faster rate of progression is reported in males with membranous nephropathy, IgA nephropathy, PKD, HNS and type 1 DN[14]. Many such studies have relied on univariate analysis of risk factors; multivariate analyses have not always confirmed an independent gender-related risk factor. One study from Japan suggested that females had a faster rate of progression[1].

Race
In the USA, the incidence and prevalence of diabetic and hypertensive renal diseases are higher in African Americans and Hispanic Americans compared to Caucasians (Table 66.1)[5,15]. ESRD linked to diabetes and hypertension is three to six times more prevalent in African Americans than in Caucasians[5]. The rate of progression of diabetic and nondiabetic renal diseases is faster in African Americans than in Caucasians[15], although only one study confirmed this by multivariate analysis[1]. A faster rate of progression amongst African Americans may explain some of the findings of the Multiple Risk Factor Intervention Trial, which demonstrated a higher incidence of ESRD for all causes in African American compared with Caucasian men at all levels of blood pressure.

Among UK patients with ESRD, there is a higher incidence of diabetic and nondiabetic nephropathy in patients from the Indian subcontinent[16], while hypertensive renal disease is more common in individuals of Caribbean and African descent. Indo-Asian patients with DN may have a faster rate of decline of GFR compared to Caucasian Europeans; in one study, the proportion of patients doubling their creatinine was significantly higher in Indo-Asians compared to Caucasians or African Caribbeans despite comparable levels of blood pressure and use of angiotensin converting enzyme (ACE) inhibitors. Whether this faster rate of progression is linked to genetic predisposition remains to be determined.

Genetics
Diabetic and nondiabetic nephropathies cluster in families. Such a familial clustering appears to be stronger in the USA amongst African Americans. In diabetes mellitus, there is evidence that family histories of cardiovascular disease or hypertension are associated, respectively, with a two- or four-fold increase in the risk of developing diabetic nephropathy. Parental hypertension is also thought to be a risk factor for the progression of diabetic nephropathy and IgA nephropathy[14].

Associations have been described between certain major histocompatibility complex (MHC) antigens and susceptibility to some immune renal disease, as well as the rate of progression[14]. Patients with PKD carrying the genotype PKD1 are thought to have a worse prognosis than others[17].

New molecular genetics techniques have proved extremely powerful tools to investigate the links between genetic susceptibility and the progression of CRF. The candidate gene approach aims to detect an association between polymorphic DNA markers related to a gene coding for a factor thought to be involved in the progression of CRF. An alternative approach is based on the genome wide search for unknown genes potentially associated with progressive CRF. The candidate gene approach has focused on polymorphisms of genes coding for putative mediators of renal scarring. To date, the ACE gene has received most attention. Data have linked an insertion (I)/ deletion (D) polymorphism in the ACE gene with susceptibility and progression in diabetic and nondiabetic renal diseases[14]. In type 1 DN, a strong association has been described between disease susceptibility and the D allele which has also been linked to a faster rate of decline in renal function in IgA nephropathy, focal segmental glomerulosclerosis, reflux nephropathy and

PKD; in IgA nephropathy, this has been attributed to the higher levels of ACE and angiotensin II in DD homozygotes. Synergistic interactions between genotypes may also influence the rate of progression of CRF. A study in IgA nephropathy suggested that those with the ACE/DD genotype had a poor prognosis only in the presence of the angiotensinogen (AGT) MM genotype. Another study implied a faster rate of progression in patients with CRF who are homozygous for the ACE D allele (DD) when they were also homozygous for the cytoskeletal protein, α-adducin, G allele (ADD-G).

The response to antihypertensive treatment may also be modulated by the ACE genotype, with patients homozygous for DD having the worse response and progressive renal insufficiency, those with the II genotype having the best prognosis[14,18]. These associations remain the subject of debate.

Other candidate genes being investigated in relation to progressive renal disease, including those coding for angiotensinogen, angiotensin II receptor, nitric oxide synthase, kallikrein, and some cytokines (interleukin-1β and tumor necrosis factor-α), as well as growth factors such as transforming growth factor (TGF)-β1, known to have renal fibrogenic effects. African Americans have higher circulating TGF-β1 levels compared to Caucasians; and African Americans with progressive kidney disease have higher circulating TGF-β1 levels compared to those with stable renal function[14]. However, one study of African Americans with ESRD failed to show any association between TGF-β1 genotypes and the susceptibility to develop progressive renal failure.

The human homologue of the rat renal failure (Rf) gene has been localized on the long arm of chromosome 10. In African Americans with ESRD due a variety of nephropathies, an association between two markers (D10S1435 and D10S249) spanning 21 polymorphic regions of chromosome 10 approached significance in nondiabetic patients. The effect of this genotype on susceptibility and progression of CRF in Caucasians remains to be determined.

Modifiable risk factors

These include proteinuria, systemic hypertension, metabolic factors such as dyslipidemia, obesity and possibly hyperuricemia. In addition, recent interest has focused on the contribution of cigarette smoking, alcohol consumption and recreational drug use to the risk of development of ESRD.

Proteinuria

Many studies point to proteinuria as an important prognostic factor in the progression of kidney diseases (Fig. 66.2). Eleven studies confirmed, by multivariate analysis, that heavy proteinuria was associated with a faster rate of progression of CRF[1]. Experimental data suggest that proteinuria may also contribute directly to the progression of CRF through the initiation and progression of tubulointerstitial scarring. In a wide range of glomerulonephritis, patients with heavy and sustained proteinuria invariably have a worse prognosis compared to those with mild proteinuria or when proteinuria remits[11]. The Modification of Diet in Renal Disease (MDRD)[13] and other studies[11] have shown that baseline proteinuria is a strong predictor of subsequent decline in renal function[14]. In membranous nephropathy, the period with the highest

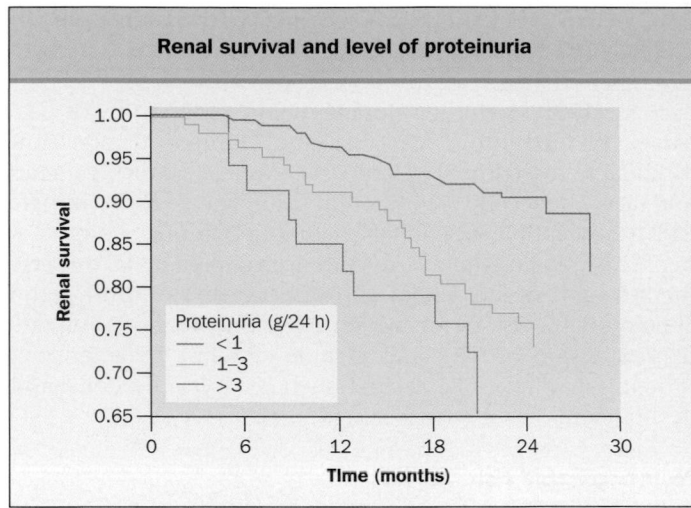

Figure 66.2 Actuarial renal survival in relation to proteinuria. (Adapted with permission[11].)

sustained proteinuria is a powerful predictor of declining renal function. The severity of proteinuria also predicts the progression of nonglomerular diseases. Furthermore, reduction of proteinuria by diet[19] or ACE inhibition[20] has been shown to predict a better outcome in diabetic as well as nondiabetic nephropathies[21].

Hypertension

Strong evidence links the progression of CRF to systemic hypertension (Fig. 66.3)[14]. The majority of clinical studies showed by either univariate or multivariate analysis that raised blood pressure is associated with a faster rate of progression of CRF[1]. It is believed that the transmission of systemic hypertension into the glomerular capillary beds, and the resulting glomerular hypertension, contribute to the initiation of glomerulosclerosis (Table 66.4 and Fig. 66.4). In one study, it was suggested that the rate of progression of CRF

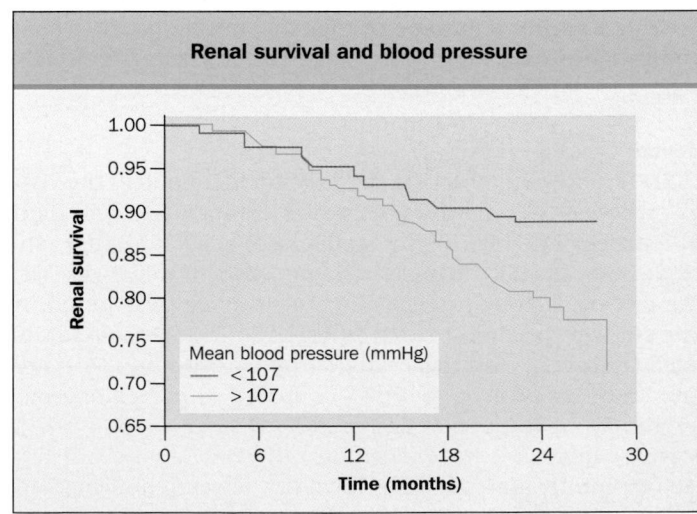

Figure 66.3 Actuarial renal survival in relation to blood pressure. (Adapted with permission[11].)

Hypotheses for the pathogenesis of glomerulosclerosis	
Hypothesis	**Author(s)**
Glomerular hyperfiltration/hyperperfusion	Hostetter and Brenner 1981
Glomerular hypertension	Anderson and Brenner 1985
Nephrotoxicity of lipids	Moorhead et al. 1982
Similarities with atherosclerosis	El Nahas 1988
	Diamond and Kamovsky 1988
Glomerular hypertrophy	Fogo and Ichikawa 1991
Nephrotoxicity of proteinuria	Remuzzi and Bertani 1990
Growth factors	
Platelet-derived growth factor	Johnson et al. 1994
Transforming growth factor β	Border et al. 1993
Mesangial/myofibroblast differentiation	Johnson et al. 1994
Podocyte injury	Kriz 1996
(Adapted with permission from El Nahas[30].)	

Table 66.4 Hypotheses for the pathogenesis of glomerulosclerosis.

is twice as fast in patients with diastolic blood pressure in excess of 90 mmHg compared to those with lower values. Intervention studies in proteinuric nondiabetic as well as diabetic nephropathies have shown that the rate of decline of GFR is almost normalized by a reduction in mean arterial pressure (MAP) by either an ACE inhibitor or an angiotensin (AT1) receptor antagonist (ATRA) to levels around 90 mmHg (125/75 mmHg). A pooled analysis of antihypertensive intervention studies in diabetic and nondiabetic nephropathies showed that the rate of decline in GFR was proportional to the level of MAP with a rate of approximately –2 mL/min/year in

those whose blood pressure levels were reduced to less than 130/85 mmHg.

The MDRD study suggested that the control of hypertension assumes more importance in proteinuric patients with CRF (> 3 g/24 h); in these patients, a lower blood pressure target (MAP 92 mmHg; 125/75 mmHg) was required to achieve the same protection of renal function as achieved in patients with less proteinuria (1–3 g/24 h) (MAP 98 mmHg; 145/85 mmHg)[22]. In the MDRD study, the rate of decline of glomerular filtration rate (GFR) was faster in hypertensive African Americans compared to Caucasians. Progression of CRF could be halted in African Americans when mean arterial pressure was reduced to less than 92 mmHg. In diabetic nephropathy, elevated blood pressure is associated with progressive proteinuria and a more rapid rate of decline in renal function.

Metabolic factors
Glycemia
While there is little doubt that poor glycemic control is a major factor in the initiation of CRF in susceptible diabetic patients, the evidence for a role for hyperglycemia in the progression of diabetic nephropathy is conflicting. Of the thirteen major studies addressing this issue, six showed an association by multivariate analysis while a similar number showed no association between hyperglycemia and the rate of progression of diabetic kidney disease[1].

Lipids
Dyslipidemia has been implicated in the pathogenesis of glomerulosclerosis and tubulointerstitial fibrosis (Table 66.5 and Fig. 66.5). A number of studies have confirmed by multivariate analysis that dyslipidemia is a risk factor for a faster rate of progression[1]. In some of these studies, patients with nondiabetic nephropathy and elevated plasma cholesterol and triglycerides appear to have a faster rate of progression of

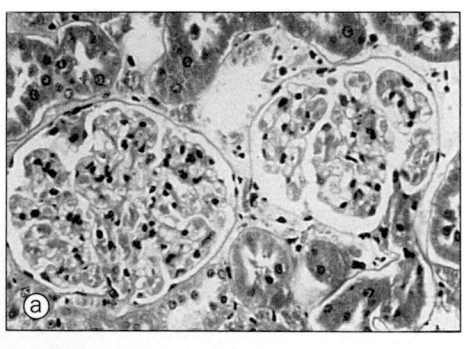
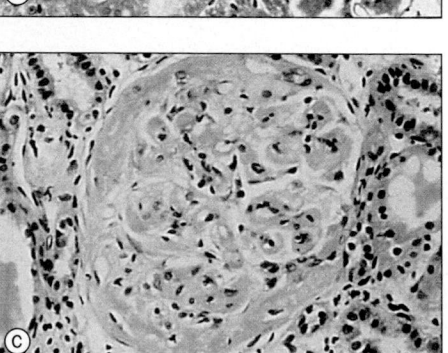
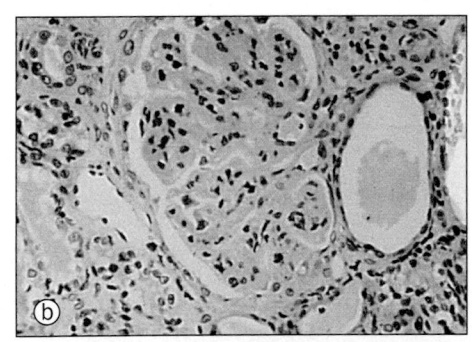
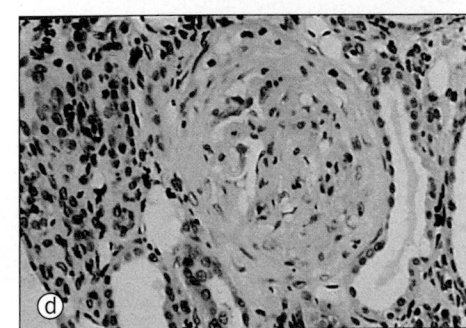

Figure 66.4 Histologic development of glomerulosclerosis. (a) Normal glomerulus; (b) mesangial hypercellularity; (c, d) glomerulosclerosis of increasing severity. Note the tubular atrophy and dilatation in (b), (c) and (d), indicating the parallel development of tubulointerstitial scarring.

Hypotheses for the pathogenesis of tubulointerstitial fibrosis

Hypothesis	Author(s)
Adaptive tubular hypermetabolism	Harris and Schrier 1988
Adaptive tubular ammoniagenesis	Nath and Hostetter 1985
Nephrotoxicity of lipids	Moorhead et al. 1982
Nephrotoxicity of proteinuria	Remuzzi and Bertani 1990
Nephrotoxicity of calcium and phosphate	Alfrey 1988
Nephrotoxicity of iron	Harris and Alfrey 1994
Nephrotoxicity of oxygen free radicals	Nath et al. 1994
Tubular cells and fibrosis	Kuncio and Neilson 1991
Tubular transdifferentiation	Okada, Strutz, and Nielson 1994

(Adapted with permission from El Nahas[30].)

Table 66.5 Hypotheses for the pathogenesis of tubulointerstitial fibrosis.

CRF compared to those without hyperlipidemia. In a prospective study baseline levels of plasma cholesterol, low-density lipoprotein cholesterol, and apolipoprotein B (apoB)-containing lipoproteins were predictors of progression along with proteinuria[23]. In this study, patients with the highest levels of circulating apoB-containing lipoproteins had the faster rate of decline of renal function. Similarly, in patients with diabetic nephropathy, elevated levels of cholesterol, triglycerides, and apoB correlated with a more rapid deterioration of kidney function[23].

Obesity

Excessive body weight and a raised body mass index have been linked to a faster rate of progression of CRF in patients with IgA nephropathy. In this study, hypertension-free survival was also considerably shorter in overweight patients compared to those with normal weight[24].

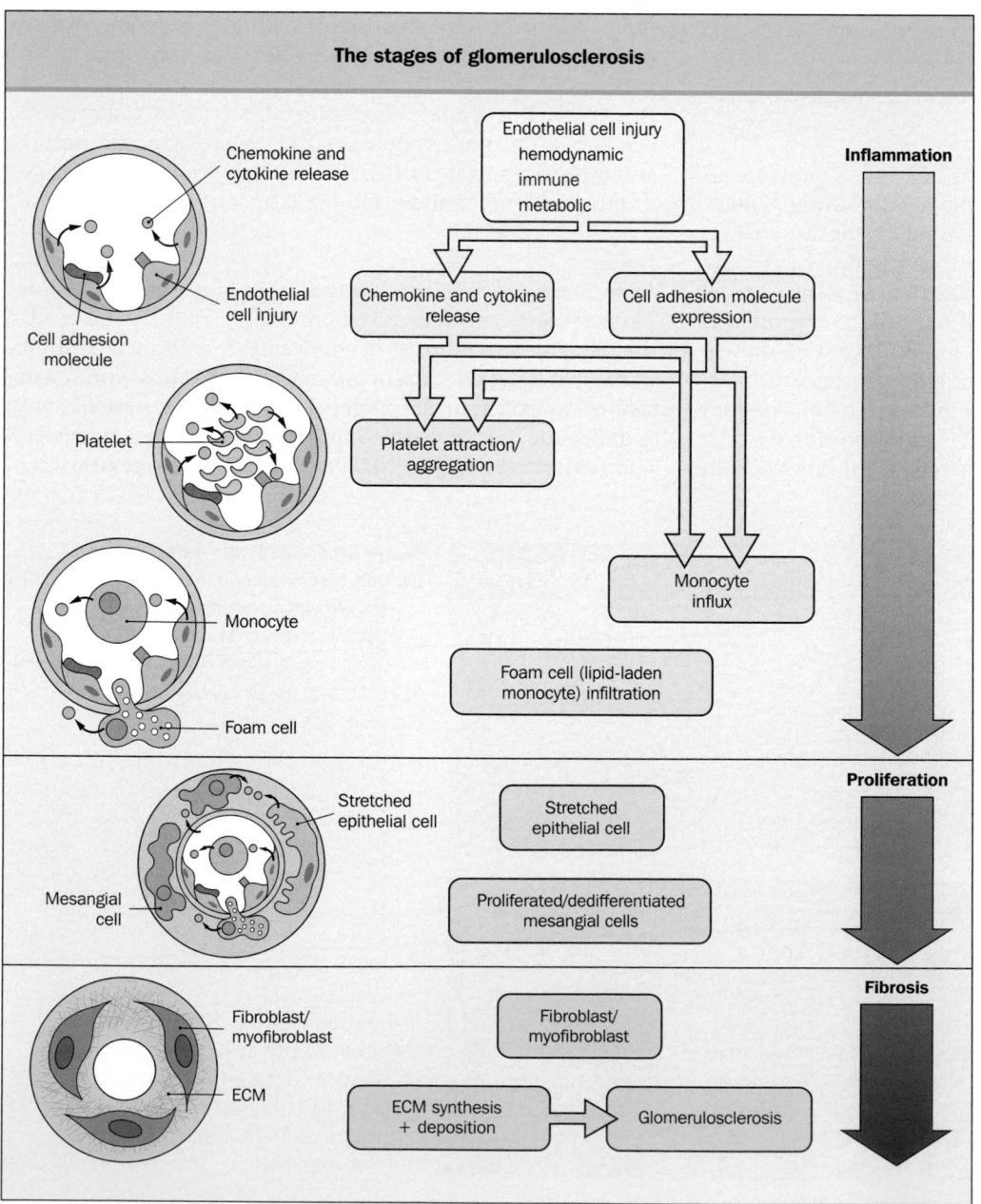

Figure 66.5 The stages of glomerulosclerosis.

Hyperuricemia

Hyperuricemia has been associated with systemic hypertension, cardiovascular and renal diseases[25]. Recent experimental data indicate that hyperuricemia may cause hypertension and renal injury through crystal-independent pathways, notably a stimulation of the renin–angiotensin system. A single Japanese study reported that hyperuricemic patients with IgA nephropathy had a worse prognosis compared to those with normal serum uric acid levels.

Miscellaneous

Smoking

Cigarette smoking causes an increase in systemic blood pressure and affects renal hemodynamics. In diabetic and nondiabetic patients, there is evidence that smoking is associated with a faster rate of decline of CRF. In one study of men with CRF, smoking increased the risk of developing ESRD threefold in patients treated with ACE inhibitors, with the odds ratio increasing to 10 in those on other antihypertensive agents[26]. The cardiovascular morbidity of diabetic patients on hemodialysis is increased in smokers compared to nonsmokers. Furthermore, the outcome of renal transplantation has also been shown to be adversely affected by smoking.

Alcohol

Some evidence links heavy alcohol consumption to progressive renal insufficiency, perhaps through the hypertensive effect of alcohol. Patients with CRF consuming more than two drinks a day had an increased odds ratio[2–4] for developing ESRD compared to those drinking less[27]. The association between alcohol consumption and hypertension is stronger in males compared to females.

Caffeine

Coffee drinking (five or more cups a day) was associated with a small increase in blood pressure in a study in US medical students[28]. Experimental data also suggest that excessive caffeine intake is associated, in a susceptible strain of obese rats, with elevated blood pressure, increased proteinuria and more severe tubulointerstitial scarring.

Recreational drugs

A case–control study in the general population conducted in the USA showed that recreational drugs are risk factors for the development of ESRD[29]. Individuals who had used heroin or opiates were at increased risk of ESRD (odds ratio 19.1). Cocaine or crack and psychedelic drugs were also associated with ESRD, although this could not be dissociated from the influence of heroin use.

MECHANISMS OF PROGRESSION OF CHRONIC RENAL FAILURE

Experimental models

Numerous experimental models have been used to study progressive kidney scarring[30]. The most commonly used model consists of a subtotal nephrectomy in the rat, leading to progressive kidney insufficiency associated with systemic hypertension, proteinuria, and progressive renal scarring.

This model progresses over weeks and is fairly representative of the late changes taking place in the remnant nephrons after a substantial loss of kidney mass and function. The study of this model led to a hypothesis implicating adaptive glomerular and tubular changes in the pathogenesis of kidney scarring (Tables 66.4 and 66.5). Models of experimental CGN have also been studied, including the nephrotoxic nephritis model (where antiglomerular basement membrane (anti-GBM) antibodies are injected into rats to reproduce an acute proliferative glomerulonephritis followed by chronic membranoproliferative and sclerotic glomerular changes). The anti-Thy1.1 model of glomerulonephritis, induced in rats by the injection of an antimesangial cell antibody, leads to mesangiolysis, followed by mesangial proliferation and sclerosis with, ultimately, healing and recovery. This gives opportunities to study the scarring as well as healing processes in injured glomeruli. Models of nephrotic syndrome and glomerulosclerosis are induced in rats by the injection of aminonucleosides (puromycin and adriamycin). In addition, a range of models of podocyte injury or dysfunction has been described including those associated with abnormalities of podocyte-associated proteins such as nephrin, podocin, α-actinin$_4$ and CD2AP. Mutations of genes coding for nephrin (NPHS1), podocin (NPHS2) and α-actinin$_4$ have been identified in patients with different types of focal segmental glomerulosclerosis resistant to steroid therapy. Experimental diabetic nephropathy can be induced in rats by the injection of the beta cell toxin, streptozotocin. However, the glomerular changes are slow to develop and are not fully representative of the changes seen in diabetic patients.

Increasingly, genetically modified rodents expressing excessive (transgenes) or absent (knockout) amounts of putative factors implicated in the progression of CRF have been studied to determine the relevance of these factors. Studies have shown that mice over-expressing certain hormones (growth hormone), autacoids (renin–angiotensin II, endothelin-1) or growth factors (TGF-β1) have a susceptibility to develop kidney scarring and fibrosis.

While these experimental models bear some similarities to progressive kidney scarring in humans and have allowed identification of mediators and pathways of scarring, they remain far from reproducing the clinical situation. Furthermore, the homogeneity of experimental animal groups often contrasts with the heterogeneity of patients studied in clinical trials. This makes the extrapolation of therapies from animals to humans difficult, as highlighted below.

Glomerulosclerosis

The progression of CRF is associated with the progressive sclerosis of glomeruli regardless of the nature of the underlying nephropathy. Since the early 1970s, numerous hypotheses have been put forward to explain the progressive sclerosis and fibrosis of the glomeruli (Table 66.4 and Fig. 66.5).

It would seem that glomerulosclerosis may evolve in stages, initially glomerular endothelial injury and inflammation, then a stage of mesangial proliferation/activation, and a final stage of glomerular sclerosis and fibrosis (Table 66.4, Figs 66.4 and 66.5). Throughout the different stages, strong similarities exist between the pathogenesis of glomerulosclerosis and that of

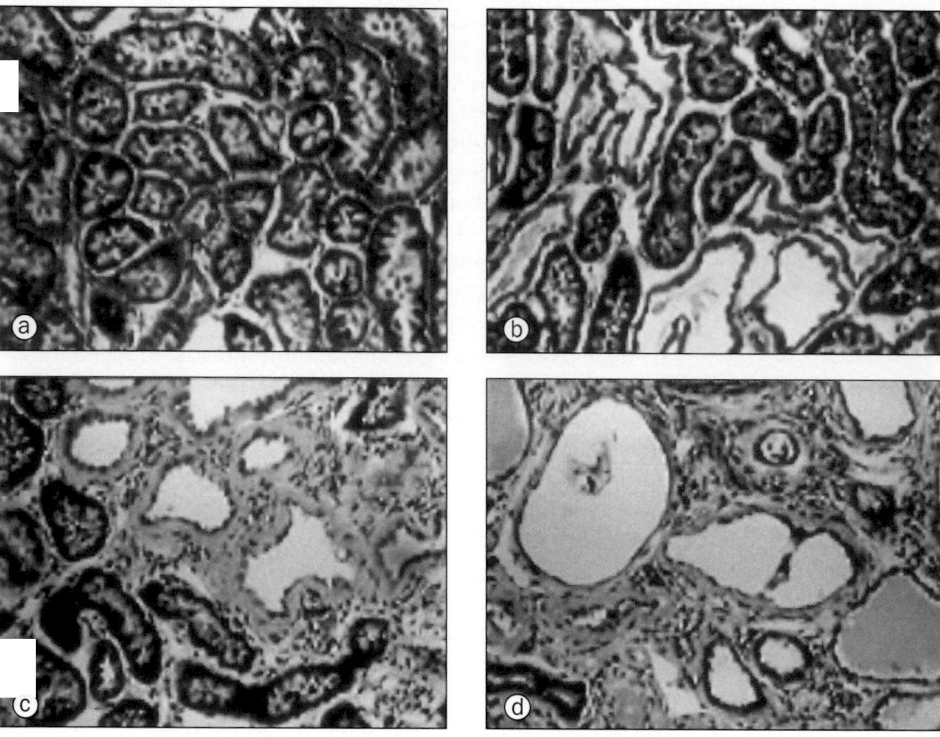

Figure 66.6 Histologic development of tubulointerstitial fibrosis. (a) Normal tubulointerstitium; (b) mild tubulointerstitial scarring with tubular atrophy and interstitial edema; (c) segmental interstitial fibrosis; (d) diffuse interstitial fibrosis with tubular atrophy and dilatation.

larger vessel atherosclerosis. The first stage of glomerulosclerosis may be initiated by damage to the endothelial cells induced by immune or nonimmune (hemodynamic or metabolic) insults. For example, raised systemic hypertension, through its unopposed transmission to poorly autoregulated remnant glomeruli, would raise glomerular capillary pressure and initiate endothelial injury. Damaged endothelium loses its anticoagulant, anti-inflammatory, and antiproliferative properties and acquires new procoagulant, proinflammatory, and mitogenic characteristics[30–32]. These are mediated through the release of procoagulant factors (such as platelet-activating factor and thromboxane amongst others) and proinflammatory and mitogenic cytokines and growth factors (interleukins, tumor necrosis factor-α and platelet-derived growth factor (PDGF)) as well as chemokines such as monocyte chemoattractant protein 1 (MCP-1) and macrophage inflammatory protein-2[30–32]. Damaged endothelium also loses its capacity to release anticoagulant as well as anti-inflammatory protective factors and expresses cell adhesion molecules. These changes lead to the attraction of platelets and inflammatory cells (neutrophils and monocytes) (Fig. 66.5) to the glomerular capillaries. Infiltrating monocytes interact with mesangial cells and stimulate their proliferation, either through direct cell–cell interactions or through the release of mitogens (such as PDGF)[30–32]. A key role has been shown for the transcription factor nuclear factor kappa B (NF-κB) in the regulation of the mesangial cell proliferative response. Proliferating and activated mesangial cells have the capacity to revert to a mesenchymal phenotype expressing markers such as α-smooth muscle actin (α-SMA) and synthesizing a range of extracellular matrix (ECM) components. Resolution of glomerular proliferation and hypercellularity may depend on apoptosis (programmed cell death) of infiltrating inflammatory cells or their efflux from the glomerular capillaries. Apoptosis of glomerular

endothelial and mesangial cells may also contribute to the resolution of injury. However, uncontrolled apoptosis may lead to glomerular cell depletion and contribute to glomerular obsolescence.

Epithelial cells may also be involved in the pathogenesis of glomerulosclerosis[33]. The inability of glomerular epithelial cells to replicate in response to injury may lead to their stretching along the GBM, exposing areas of denuded GBM that would attract and interact with parietal epithelial cells leading to the formation of adhesions[33]. The stretching of the epithelial cells along denuded areas of the GBM would also favor proteinuria and increase traffic of inflammatory, mitogenic and fibrogenic mediators. Infiltrating cells may also stimulate glomerular cells, through the release of fibrogenic growth factors (such as TGF-β1), to produce excessive ECM[33]. High circulating levels of TGF-β1 have recently been described in patients with progressive kidney disease. This growth factor is thought to play an important role in renal fibrogenesis through the stimulation of ECM synthesis together with the inhibition of its breakdown, thus contributing to irreversible glomerulosclerosis. It has also been postulated that epithelial cell injury leads to tuft-to-capsule adhesions which result, through misdirected filtration, to the accumulation of amorphous material in the paraglomerular space which sometimes extend to the neck of the tubules[33]. This leads to the disruption of glomerular–tubular junction resulting in atubular glomeruli. In addition, the misdirected filtration may contribute to tubular atrophy and interstitial fibrosis. Tuft-to-capsule adhesions may also allow the infiltration of the glomeruli by periglomerular fibroblasts thus contributing to glomerulosclerosis[33].

Tubulointerstitial scarring

The pathogenesis of tubulointerstitial fibrosis (TIF) has also received increasing attention over recent years (Table 66.5).

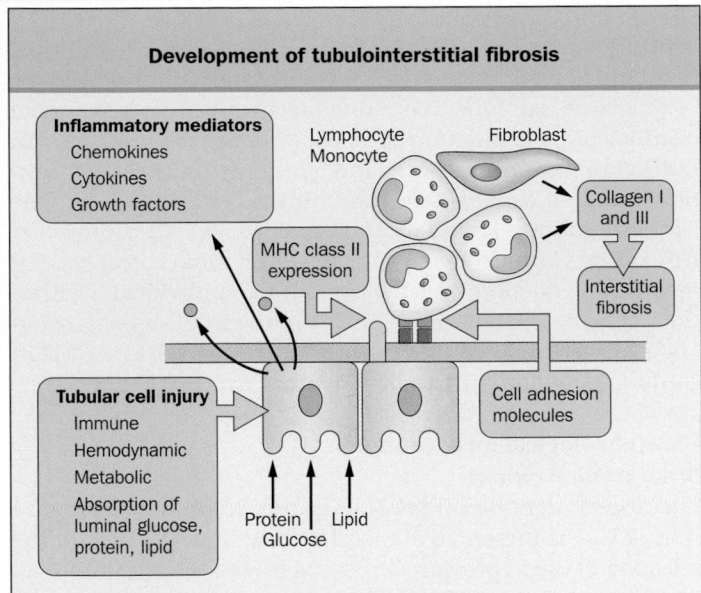

Figure 66.7 Development of tubulointerstitial fibrosis.

Severity of tubulointerstitial changes correlate better with renal function than does glomerulosclerosis. TIF is likely to evolve in stages involving inflammation, proliferation of interstitial fibroblasts, and excessive deposition of interstitial ECM, leading to fibrosis[34] (Figs. 66.6 and 66.7). Renal tubular cells play a central role in the pathogenesis of TIF. Injured tubular cells have the capacity to act as antigen-presenting cells, to express cell adhesion molecules, and to release inflammatory mediators and autacoids as well as chemokines, cytokines and growth factors[34] (Fig. 66.7). Finally, tubular cells can respond to a range of stimuli by increased synthesis of ECM. Recent evidence suggests that tubular cells respond to proteinuria by releasing many of the mediators mentioned above as well as by the synthesis of ECM[34]. In addition, the incubation of proximal tubular cells with high concentrations of albumin appears to activate NF-κB; a major transcription factor involved in the upregulation of the transcription of a wide range of chemokines and cytokines. These different pathways would establish a link between glomerular injury, proteinuria and TIF. Whether this link is solely related to the effect of proteinuria *per se* on proximal tubular cells or is associated with the lipiduria that accompanies proteinuria is currently the subject of investigation. Tubular cells might also be stimulated by the spillover of hormones such as angiotensin II and growth factors and cytokines from the injured glomeruli. Activation of tubular cells and their release of chemotactic factors (such as complement components, osteopontin and MCP-1) would attract inflammatory cells, including monocytes, to the tubules and the renal interstitium[34]. These cells would, in turn, interact with interstitial renal fibroblasts and activate them through the release of a wide range of growth factors. Activated renal fibroblasts expressing α-SMA, thus acquiring myofibroblastic characteristics, would proliferate and invade the periglomerular and peritubular spaces. These cells also synthesize ECM comprising interstitial collagens I and III, leading to its interstitial

accumulation. The resolution of deposited ECM depends on two proteolytic pathways; the first relying on the activation of matrix metalloproteinases and the second depending on the activation of the proteolytic enzyme plasmin by plasminogen activators (PA)[34]. Experimental data suggests that renal scarring is associated with the inhibition of these two collagenolytic pathways through activation of tissue inhibitors of matrix proteinases and plasminogen activator inhibitor-1 (PAI-1), disturbing the balance between ECM synthesis and breakdown to favor ECM accumulation and irreversible kidney fibrosis[34].

Vascular sclerosis
Vascular sclerosis is an integral feature of the renal scarring process. Renal arteriolar hyalinosis is present in CRF at an early stage, even in the absence of severe hypertension. Furthermore, these vascular changes are often out of proportion to the severity of systemic hypertension. Vascular sclerosis is associated with progressive kidney failure in CGN. The hyalinosis of afferent arterioles has been implicated in the pathogenesis of diabetic glomerulosclerosis. Changes in postglomerular arterioles may further exacerbate interstitial ischemia and fibrosis[35]. Recent data suggest damage to peritubular capillaries and a decrease in their numbers and function in scarred kidneys. This could also exacerbate interstitial ischemia and result in further fibrosis. A growing body of experimental evidence suggests that ischemia and the ensuing hypoxia are fibrogenic influences that stimulate tubular cells and kidney fibroblasts to produce ECM components and reduce their collagenolytic activity[36]. Loss of peritubular capillaries has been linked in experimental models of renal scarring to a fall in the renal expression of the angiogenic growth factors vascular endothelial growth factor (VEGF). Together with an overexpression by scarred kidneys of thrombospondin, an antiangiogenic factor, this would perpetuate microvascular deletion and ischemia[37]. The administration of VEGF restores the microvascular loss preserving peritubular capillaries and improving scarring and functional outcome[37]. Finally, the vascular adventitia may be a source of interstitial myofibroblasts, contributing to the development of interstitial renal fibrosis.

CLINICAL INTERVENTIONS IN CHRONIC RENAL FAILURE

Dietary interventions
Protein
A large body of experimental evidence has suggested that dietary protein restriction slows the progression of CRF and the underlying scarring process, and numerous clinical trials have evaluated the effects of a low-protein diet (LPD) on the progression of CRF. Early studies suggested that such a diet was protective. However, more scrutiny revealed the majority of the initial clinical trials on LPD in CRF to be flawed, with inadequate controls, and often relying on changes in serum creatinine to evaluate progression in spite of the fact that dietary protein restriction affects creatinine metabolism and excretion, thus rendering it an unreliable marker of progression on such a diet. More recently, better controlled,

randomized and prospective trials have been undertaken that have given conflicting and inconclusive results[38]. The largest of these trials (MDRD) involved 840 patients followed prospectively over 3 years and failed to show convincingly that LPD slows the progression of CRF[39]. However, subsequent analyses suggested that there was a positive correlation between the dietary protein intake and the rate of progression of renal insufficiency in patients with a GFR between 13 and 24 mL/min/1.73 m^2; in this group, a daily reduction of 0.2 g/kg in protein intake appeared to lead to a slowing of the decline in GFR by 1.15 mL/min/year. Four meta-analyses of the major controlled LPD trials led to conflicting results with three suggesting a beneficial effect with relative risk reduction around 35% while the largest comprising 13 randomized and 11 non-randomized clinical trials involving 2248 patients, showed a marginal benefit for LPD with treated patients having a slower decline in GFR of around 0.53 mL/min/year[40]. However, spontaneous reductions in dietary protein intake take place in patients with progressive CRF. K/DOQI Nutrition Guidelines recommend consideration of a reduction of dietary protein intake to 0.6 g/kg/day for individuals with a GFR < 25 mL/min[41] (CKD stages 4 and 5). The long-term nutritional consequences of protein deprivation cannot be excluded. For this reason, the prescription of dietary protein restriction to patients with advanced renal insufficiency warrants careful nutritional monitoring by an experienced dietitian (see Chapter 74). Clinicians must decide whether it is worthwhile to attempt to delay RRT by LPD at the risk of reaching ESRD with the patient undernourished and with the associated increased morbidity and mortality.

Phosphorus

One controlled trial of a low-phosphate diet in CRF failed to show any benefit. However, a reduction in dietary phosphorus has been advocated by some as an early and effective means of controlling hyperphosphatemia and the renal osteodystrophy associated with CRF. In addition, reduction of hyperphosphatemia may reduce the risk of cardiovascular calcifications and the associated morbidity and mortality.

Lipids

Manipulations of dietary lipids and, in particular, the supplementation of diet with fish oil (eicosapentanoic acid) have received particular attention. This is based on experimental observations of a beneficial effect attributed to the lipid-lowering effects of such a diet and its anti-inflammatory properties. In a trial of fish oil supplementation in patients with IgA nephropathy, the main endpoint, which was a 50% increase in serum creatinine, was reached in significantly fewer patients on fish oil compared to those treated with placebo[42]. However, this study was criticized for the unusually fast rate of decline of renal function of the control group. Another prospective and randomized trial in IgA nephropathy failed to show protection, and a meta-analysis of the five published studies on fish oil supplementation in failed to show a statistically significant protective effect[43]. In spite of lack of convincing evidence, both the Canadian and Australian Societies of Nephrology recommend the use of fish oil supplementation in patients with IgA nephropathy.

Salt

While dietary salt restriction has not been evaluated in CRF, it is anticipated that its antihypertensive effect would be beneficial in salt-sensitive individuals with progressive renal insufficiency. Furthermore, clinical evidence suggests that salt restriction optimizes both the antihypertensive and anti proteinuric effects of ACE inhibitors as well as ATRAs. The National Kidney Foundation Task Force on Cardiovascular Disease in Chronic Renal Disease (NKF Task Force) recommends a reduction in dietary salt to individuals within the general population with borderline hypertension (140/90 mmHg) as well as to those with stages 1 to 4 CKD in conjunction with antihypertensive agents[44] (see below).

Pharmacological interventions
Blood pressure control

The case for tight blood pressure control to minimize progression of CRF is presented above. The next consideration is the selection of blood pressure target levels. The MDRD Study suggested a lower target (MAP 92 mmHg) in patients with heavy proteinuria compared to those with mild/moderate proteinuria (98 mmHg)[22]. The same study also implied that lower targets should be sought in African Americans compared to their European counterparts. However, another study suggested no difference in the rate of decline in kidney function of patients with hypertensive nephrosclerosis with MAP 81 mmHg compared to 86.7 mmHg, and the rate of decline of these patients, with minimal proteinuria, was comparable to that of age-matched controls[14]. A pooled analysis of antihypertensive intervention studies in major studies in diabetic and nondiabetic nephropathies suggest a slowing of the rate of decline in GFR proportional to the reduction in MAP. The rate of decline of GFR reached –2 to –3 mL/min/year in patients with blood pressure levels reduced to less than 130/85 mmHg[45]. Also, intervention studies with an ACE inhibitor (REIN study) and with an ATRA (RENAAL study) suggest that a reduction in blood pressure to MAP 90 mmHg (125/75 mmHg) slows the rate of decline of GFR to near normal: approximately –2 mL/min/year.

The NKF Task Force has suggested different blood pressure targets depending on the stage of kidney disease[44]. In the general population, with normal kidney function and no proteinuria, a blood pressure goal of 140/90 mmHg is recommended. In CKD stage 1 to 4 with proteinuria < 1 g/day, the recommended target is < 135/85 mmHg. In CKD stages 1–4 with proteinuria > 1 g/day, a blood pressure goal of < 125/75 mmHg is recommended[1,44].

What antihypertensive agent should be used? A growing body of experimental data point to the nephrotoxicity of angiotensin II and, consequently, to a therapeutic advantage of ACE inhibitors compared to other antihypertensive drugs. This is often demonstrated in experimental animals and is attributed to the reduction of glomerular capillary hypertension by ACE inhibitors and their antiproteinuric effect, as well as the inhibition of angiotensin II-mediated trophic and fibrosing effects. The fibrogenic effect of angiotensin II may be mediated through its stimulation of the synthesis and release of TGF-β1, a fibrogenic growth factor, as well as that of PAI-1, a potent inhibitor of collagen proteolytic enzymes. These changes would favor the deposition and accumulation of ECM and fibrosis[30–34]. In humans, ACE inhibitors have been reported to be advantageous compared to other antihypertensive drugs in diabetic[46] as well as nondiabetic[47,48] kidney diseases. This advantage has been attributed to the antiproteinuric effect of ACE inhibitors. A recent post-hoc analysis of the REIN study suggested that renoprotection by ACE inhibitors is maximized when ACE inhibitors are started early in the course of CRF and that long-term treatment may result in GFR stabilization and the prevention of ESRD[49]. Furthermore, this analysis suggested that ACE inhibition was beneficial in patients with mild, moderate as well as advanced renal insufficiency. A meta-analysis of 11 studies suggested that ACE inhibitors reduced the relative risk of ESRD by 31%[50]. However, nondihydropyridine calcium channel blockers, such as diltiazem and verapamil, are capable of reducing proteinuria and slowing the progression of nephropathy in type 2 diabetes to the same extent as an ACE inhibitor[51]. Dihydropyridine calcium channel blockers are less protective probably because they reduce afferent arteriolar tone. β-Blockers appear less effective than ACE inhibitors in reducing proteinuria and in slowing the rate of progression of CRF. The early antiproteinuric effect of antihypertensive therapy may also predict the long-term functional improvement[20]. In type 1 diabetic nephropathy, a reversal of the decline in kidney function has been reported in up to 40–60% of patients whose MAP was maintained around 93 mmHg[12]. In this study, the beneficial effect of blood pressure normalization was independent from the type of antihypertensive agent used.

Experimental data suggest that ATRAs are as effective as ACE inhibitors in reducing proteinuria and protecting from progressive renal insufficiency. There are hypothetical considerations in comparing these two classes of drugs. ACE inhibition does not always prevent angiotensin I to II conversion because there are other proteolytic enzymes, including chymases, capable of generating angiotensin II. However, ACE inhibitors inhibit the breakdown of other autacoids, including the vasodilatory bradykinins, which accumulate and may contribute to the antihypertensive and antiproteinuric effects of such treatment. On the other hand, ATRA may divert angiotensin II to its other receptor (AT2) which mediates beneficial vasodilatory and antiproliferative pathways. Clinical trials in type 2 diabetic patients with nephropathy suggest that ATRA reduce proteinuria and slow the progression of early and advanced renal disease[52–54]. Unfortunately, these studies did not compare the efficacy of ATRA to ACE inhibitors in diabetic nephropathy. Furthermore, they compared ATRA with dihydropyridine calcium channel blockers such as amlodipine, known to be detrimental to proteinuria in diabetic patients[51]. An additive antihypertensive, and to a lesser extent antiproteinuric, effect of ACE inhibition and ATRA has been described in patients with diabetic nephropathy, although neither agent was given alone in its maximum dose to ascertain their full potential when given individually. Finally, both ACE inhibitors and ATRAs have been associated with a reduction in cardiovascular morbidity in diabetic and nondiabetic patients with CRF. With these data in mind, the NKF Task Force suggest the use of ACE inhibitors and ATRAs as first line therapies for patients with CKD (stages 1–4) in association with dietary salt restriction and diuretics[1,44]. An algorithm for the

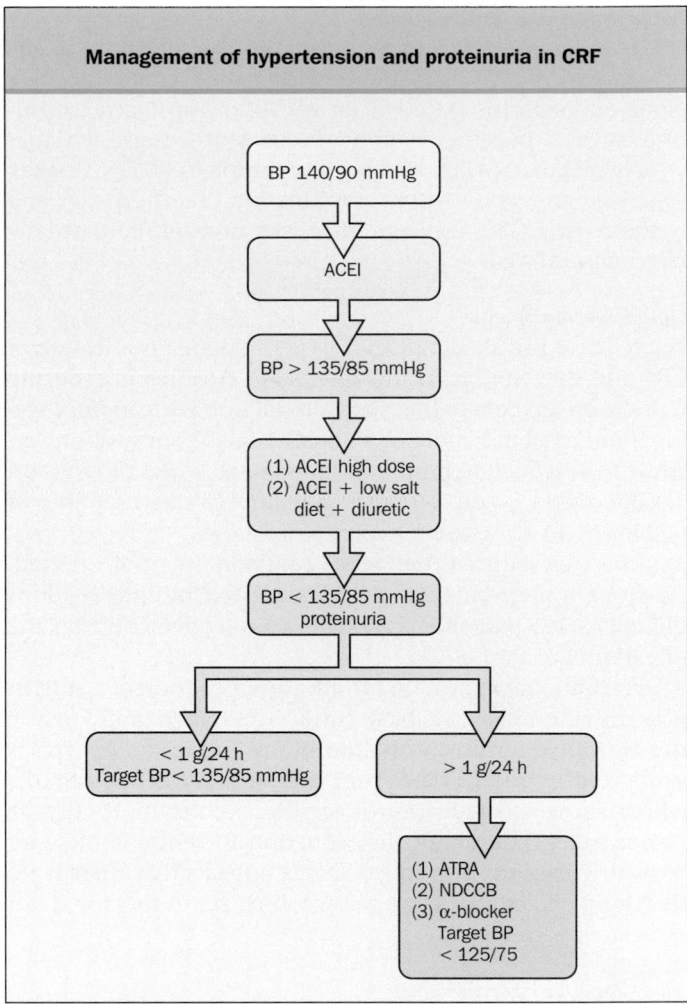

Figure 66.8 Management of hypertension and proteinuria in chronic renal failure (CRF). ACEI, Angiotensin converting enzyme inhibitor; NDCCB, nondihydropyridine calcium channel blocker; ATRA, angiotensin II receptor antagonist.

management of hypertension and proteinuria in CRF is presented in Figure 66.8.

The administration of ACE inhibitors to patients with impaired renal function warrants careful monitoring, as these agents may lead to some deterioration in renal function. A mild to moderate (10–30%) increase in serum creatinine is to be expected because these agents reduce the hyperfiltration through remnant glomeruli, but it does not justify the discontinuation of the treatment. It has been suggested that the fall in filtration fraction associated with ACE inhibition may underlie its beneficial effect. However, a further increment in serum creatinine or significant hyperkalemia would warrant the replacement of the ACE inhibitor by another antihypertensive agent. Elderly patients and those with underlying renovascular disease are particularly susceptible to the nephrotoxicity of ACE inhibitors since, in these patients, GFR may be maintained through an angiotensin II-mediated efferent arteriolar vasoconstriction. ACE inhibition in such patients can precipitate severe renal insufficiency that is not always reversible.

Antiplatelets and anticoagulants

While antiplatelet agents were initially thought to slow the progression of CRF in patients with membranoproliferative glomerulonephritis (MPGN), longer follow-up failed to confirm such a benefit. A more recent study suggested that antiplatelet therapy may reduce proteinuria in MPGN. A study suggested protection with a combination of antiplatelets and warfarin in CGN, although this was not substantiated by larger clinical trials.

Lipid-lowering agents

While there is little doubt that hyperlipidemia is a feature of CRF and that lipid-reducing agents are effective in reducing it, there are no data to link such a reduction with an improvement in renal function. A clinical trial of simvastatin, an HMG CoA reductase inhibitor, failed to slow the progression of CRF over a 2-year period in a relatively small number of patients[36]. In this study, hyperlipidemia was corrected, proteinuria was reduced, but renal function was not affected. However, a meta-analysis of 12 lipid lowering interventions including 362 patients has shown a protective effect on the rate of progression of CRF[55].

An additional indication for the administration of statins in patients with CRF would be to correct dyslipidemia and reduce the associated cardiovascular morbidity and mortality. This is supported by recent data from the Heart Protection Study, which showed a reduction of cardiovascular morbidity by statins independently of the reduction in serum cholesterol levels[56]. This study concluded that it appears that there is no threshold cholesterol value below which statin therapy is not associated with benefit.

Miscellaneous interventions

In experimental animals a range of new interventions suggest potential benefits in slowing the progression of CRF but these have not yet been investigated in clinical trials. These range from the administration of antifibrogenic growth factors such as hepatocyte growth factor and osteogenic protein-1[57], to the administration of proangiogenic factors such as VEGF[37], the administration of antifibrogenic hormones/autacoids such as relaxin, as well as the treatment with agents as diverse as aminoguanidine/advanced glycation endproduct inhibitors, heparinoids/glycosaminoglycans and miscellaneous agents such as pirfenidone.

A wide range of anecdotal interventions in patients with CRF have claimed benefit[38]. These include the administration of a dopamine analog (ibopamine), Chinese herbal extracts, oral sorbents (AST-120), and the infusion of prostaglandin E_1. The anecdotal nature of these reports precludes meaningful conclusions. More interesting are the observations of renal functional improvement in patients with moderate and even severe CRF when injected with insulin-like growth factor 1, a hormone known to have acute renal hemodynamic effects.

Interventions aimed at minimizing the complications of CRF

The interventions discussed above are primarily aimed to slow the progression of CRF. It is important to appreciate that the outcome and prognosis of patients with ESRD is often determined by associated uremic complications, such as malnutrition and hypoalbuminemia, at the initiation of RRT.

Similarly, cardiovascular complications including coronary artery disease, heart failure and left ventricular hypertrophy present at the initiation of RRT predict a poor long-term prognosis.

In order to minimize the cardiovascular complications, anemia, hypertension, hyperparathyroidism including the calcium/phosphate balance, as well as dyslipidemia, need to be corrected.

In order to minimize malnutrition, attention needs to be paid to the optimization of dietary protein and caloric intake. Metabolic acidosis has a significant catabolic effect and should be corrected.

Other complications of kidney failure need to be addressed including the early management of renal osteodystrophy. The control of hyperphosphatemia and the reduction of raised calcium phosphate product may also have an impact on the progression of cardiovascular complications and associated morbidity and mortality.

GENERAL RECOMMENDATIONS

The following general recommendations can be made for the management of patients with progressive CRF (Table 66.6).
- Frequent clinic follow-up is required with particular attention to the detection, monitoring and treatment of hypertension. Emphasis should also be on a simultaneous reduction of proteinuria (evidence-based statement).

Slowing progression of CRF	
Parameters	Interventions/target
Diet	Moderate protein restriction: 0.6–0.75 g/kg/day
	Low salt: 60–80 mmol/day (~4–6 g NaCl intake)
	Low phosphate: 600–800 mmol/day
Blood pressure control	BP < 130–135/80–85 mmHg (MAP ~ 92 mmHg)
	If proteinuria < 1 g/24 h
	BP < 125/75 mmHg (MAP ~ 90 mmHg)
	If proteinuria > 1 g/24 h
	Use an ACE inhibitor
	Add salt restriction/diuretic
	Add:
	(1) ATRA
	(2) non-dihydropyridine calcium channel blocker
	(3) α-blocker
Proteinuria	**Reduce to < 1 g/24 h**
	Use an ACE inhibitor or ATRA
Glycemia control in DM	**HbA$_{1c}$ < 8%**
Dyslipidemia	**Total cholesterol < 200 mg/dL**
	LDL cholesterol < 120 mg/dL
	Use an HMG-CoA reductase inhibitor (statin)
Smoking	No cigarette smoking
Alcohol consumption	Restriction to less than 2 drinks per/day

Table 66.6 Slowing progression of CRF. Interventions and objectives aimed at slowing the progression of CRF. Targets shown in bold.

- It is reasonable to advise patients with progressive CRF to avoid a high-protein diet, but caution should be exerted when recommending dietary protein restriction (0.6 g/kg/day) with its inherent risk of undernutrition. It may be better to start dialysis a few months earlier and be well nourished than risk malnutrition with its associated increased morbidity and mortality on dialysis (opinion). Dietary protein restriction, if recommended, should be undertaken with regular and thorough nutritional reviews and assessments.

- It is advisable that hypertensive and proteinuric patients with CRF reduce their dietary salt intake (no added salt, sodium approximately 60–80 mmol/day, or 4–6 g NaCl/day). This is all the more relevant when these patients are treated with an ACE inhibitor or AT1RA (evidence-based statement).

- It is advisable that patients with CRF reduce their saturated fat intake and control hypercholesterolemia with a statin as indicated. This would have the added potential benefit of minimizing coronary artery disease in this high-risk population (opinion).

- It is advisable that hypertensive patients with CRF reduce their alcohol consumption to less than two drinks per day (opinion).

- Patients with CRF should stop cigarette smoking (opinion).

- Attention should be paid to the early management of the complications of CRF, including anemia, metabolic acidosis, hypocalcemia and hyperphosphatemia with the associated renal osteodystrophy (evidence-based statement). Control of hyperphosphatemia should also prevent accelerated vascular, including coronary artery, calcifications and the associated cardiovascular morbidity and mortality. Control of anemia would reduce left ventricular hypertrophy and the associated cardiovascular morbidity and mortality.

- Potential nephrotoxins should be avoided, including nonsteroidal anti-inflammatory agents, nephrotoxic antibiotics, as well as intravenous radiographic contrast media; ACE inhibitors should also be used with careful monitoring.

- Nephrologists should refrain from imposing unnecessary and unproven interventions on their patients with CRF. Such interventions should first undergo the rigors of clinical trials. Clinical trials in progressive CRF remain, however, very difficult to conduct in view of the heterogeneity of the population studied, which necessitates a very large number of patients and a lengthy follow-up to reach definitive conclusions.

REFERENCES

1. National Kidney Foundation. DOQI kidney disease outcome quality initiative. Am J Kidney Dis. 2002;39:(Suppl. 1):S1–S266.
2. Coresh J, Wei GL, McQuillan G, et al. Prevalence of high blood pressure and elevated serum creatinine level in the United States: Findings from the third National Health in the United States Survey (1988–1994). Arch Int Med. 2001;161:1207–16.
3. Iseki K, Iseki C, Ikemiya Y, Fukiyama K. Risk of developing end-stage renal disease in a cohort of mass screening. Kidney Int. 1996;49:800–5.
4. Xue JL, Ma JZ, Louis TA, Collins. Forecast of the number of patients with end-stage renal disease in the United States to the year 2010. J Am Soc Nephrol. 2001;12:2753–8.
5. US Renal Data System: USRDS 2001 Annual data report. The National Institutes of Health, National Institute of Diabetes and Digestive and Kidney Diseases, Bethesda, MD. Incidence and prevalence of ESRD. Am J Kidney Dis. 2001;38 (Suppl. 3):S17–36.
6. The Annual Report on Management of Renal Failure in Europe XXVII; 1996.
7. ANZDATA Registry. Report. ANZDAT; 2001.
8. The UK Renal Registry. The Third Annual Report; December 2000.
9. Iseki K, Tozawa M, Iseki C, et al. Demographic trends in the Okinawa Dialysis Study (OKIDS) registry (1971–2000). Kidney Int. 2002;61:668–75.
10. Shah BV, Levey AS. Spontaneous changes in the rate of decline in reciprocal serum creatinine: errors in predicting the progression of renal disease from extrapolation of the slope. J Am Soc Nephrol. 1992;2:1186–91.
11. Locatelli F, Marcelli D, Comelli M, and the Northern Italian Co-operative Study Group. Proteinuria and blood pressure as causal components of progression to end-stage renal failure. Nephrol Dial Transplant. 1996;11:461–7.
12. Hovind P, Rossing P, Tarnow L, et al. Remission and regression in the nephropathy of type 1 diabetes when blood pressure is controlled aggressively. Kidney Int. 2001;60:277–83.
13. Klahr S, Breyer JA, Beck GJ, et al. Dietary protein restriction, blood pressure control and the progression of polycystic kidney disease. Modification of Diet in Renal Disease Study Group. J Am Soc Nephrol. 1995;5:2037–47.
14. Locatelli F, Del Vecchio L. Natural history and factors affecting the progression of chronic renal failure. In: El Nahas AM, Anderson S, Harris KPG, eds. Mechanisms and management of progressive renal failure. London: Oxford University Press; 2000:20–79.
15. Klag MJ, Whelton PK, Randall BL, et al. End-stage renal disease in African-American and white men. JAMA. 1997;227:1293–8.
16. Buck K, Feehally J. Diabetes and renal failure in Indo-Asians in the UK – a paradigm for the study of disease susceptibility. Nephrol Dial Transplant. 1997;12:1555–7.
17. Johnson AM, Gabow PA. Identification of patients with autosomal dominant polycystic kidney disease at highest risk for end-stage renal disease. J Am Soc Nephrol. 1997;8:1560–7.
18. Perna A, Ruggenneti P, Testa A, et al (GISEN group). ACE genotype and ACE inhibitors induced renoprotection in chronic proteinuric nephropathies. Kidney Int. 2000;57:274–81.
19. El Nahas AM, Masters-Thomas A, Brady SA, et al. Selective effect of low protein diets in chronic renal disease. Br Med J. 1984;289:1337–41.
20. Apperloo AJ, de Zeeuw D, de Jong PE. Short-term antiproteinuric response to antihypertensive treatment predicts long-term GFR decline in patients with non-diabetic renal disease. Kidney Int. 45(Suppl. 45):S147–78.
21. Jafar TH, Stark PC, Schmid CH, et al. Proteinuria as a modifiable risk factor for the progression of non-diabetic renal disease. Kidney Int. 2001;60:1131–40.
22. Peterson JC, Sharon A, Burkart JM, for the Modification of Diet in Renal Disease (MDRD) Study Group. Blood pressure control, proteinuria and the progression of renal disease. Ann Intern Med. 1995;123:754–62.

23. Attman P-O. Progression of renal failure and lipids – is there evidence of a link in humans. Nephrol Dial Transplant. 1998;13:545–7.

24. Bonnet F, Defrele C, Sassolas A, et al. Excessive body weight as a new independent risk factor for clinical and pathological progression in primary IgA nephropathy. Am J Kidney Dis. 2001;37:720–7.

25. Johnson RJ, Kivlighn SD, Kim YG, Fogo AB. Reappraisal of the pathogenesis and consequence of hyperuricemia in hypertension, cardiovascular disease and renal disease. Am J Kidney Dis. 1999;33:225–34.

26. Orth SR, Stockmann A, Conradt C, et al. Smoking as a risk factor for end-stage renal failure in men with primary renal disease. Kidney Int. 1998;54:926–31.

27. Parekh RS, Klag MJ. Alcohol: role in the development of hypertension and end-stage renal disease. Curr Opin Nephrol Hypertens. 2001;10:385–90.

28. Klag MJ, Wang NY, Meoni LA, et al. Coffee intake and risk of hypertension: the John Hopkins precursors study. Arch Int Med. 2002;162:657–62.

29. Perneger TV, Klag MJ, Whelton PK. Recreational drug use: a neglected risk factor for end-stage renal disease. Am J Kidney Dis. 2001;38:49–56.

30. El Nahas AM. Mechanisms of experimental and clinical renal scarring. In: Davison AM, Cameron JS, Grunfeld J-P, et al., eds. Oxford textbook of clinical nephrology. London: Oxford University Press; 1998:1749–88.

31. Anderson S. Glomerulosclerosis: insights into pathogenesis and treatment. In: El Nahas AM, Anderson S, Harris KPG, eds. Mechanisms and management of progressive renal failure. London: Oxford University Press; 2000:80–103.

32. Fogo AB. Progression and potential regression of glomerulosclerosis. Kidney Int. 2001;59:804–19.

33. Endlich K, Kriz W, Witzgall R. Update in podocyte biology. Curr Opin Nephrol Hypertens. 2001;10:331–40.

34. Jernigan SM, Eddy AA. Experimental insights into the mechanisms of tubulointerstitial scarring. In: El Nahas AM, Anderson S, Harris KPG, eds. Mechanisms and management of progressive renal failure. London: Oxford University Press; 2000:104–45.

35. Bohle A. Change of paradigms in nephrology – a view back and a look forward. Nephrol Dial Transplant. 1998;13:556–63.

36. Fine LG, Orphanides C, Norman JT. Progressive renal disease: the chronic hypoxia hypothesis. Kidney Int. 1998;53(Suppl 65):S74–8.

37. Kang DH, Kanellis J, Hugo C, et al. Role of the microvascular endothelium in progressive renal disease. J Am Soc Nephrol. 2002;13:806–16.

38. Coles GA, El Nahas AM. Clinical interventions in chronic renal failure. In: El Nahas AM, Anderson S, Harris KPG, eds. Mechanisms and management of progressive renal failure. London: Oxford University Press; 2000:401–23.

39. Klahr S, Levey AS, Beck GJ, and the Modification of Diet in Renal Disease Study Group. The effects of dietary protein restriction and blood pressure control on the progression of renal disease. N Engl J Med. 1994;330:877–84.

40. Aparicio M, Chauveau P, Combe C. Low protein diets and outcome of renal patients. J Nephrol. 2001;14:433–9.

41. NKF-K/DOQI clinical practice guidelines for nutrition in chronic renal failure. Am J Kidney Dis. 2000;35(Suppl 2):S1–140.

42. Donadio JV. n-3 Fatty acids and their role in nephrologic practice. Curr Opin Nephrol Hypertens. 2001;10:639–42.

43. Dillon JJ. Fish oil therapy for IgA nephropathy: efficacy and inter-study variability. J Am Soc Nephrol. 1997;11:1739–44.

44. Levey AS, Beto JA, Coronado BE, et al. Controlling the epidemic of cardiovascular disease in chronic renal disease: What do we know? What do we need to learn? Where do we go from here? Am J Kidney Dis. 1998;32:853–905.

45. Bakris GL. Preserving renal function in adults with hypertension and diabetes: a consensus approach. National Kidney Foundation Hypertension and Diabetes Executive Committees Working Group. Am J Kidney Dis. 2000;36:646–61.

46. Lewis EJ, Hunsicker LG, Bain RP, Rohde for the collaborative study group: the effect of angiotensin-converting-enzyme inhibition in diabetic nephropathy. N Engl J Med. 1993;329:1456–62.

47. Maschio G, Alberti D, Janin G, et al. Effect of the angiotensin converting enzyme inhibitor Benazepril on the progression of chronic renal insufficiency. N Engl J Med. 1996;34:939–45.

48. The GISEN group. Randomised placebo controlled trial of effect of ramipril on decline in glomerular filtration rate and risk of terminal renal failure in proteinuric, non-diabetic nephropathy. Lancet. 1997;349:1857–63.

49. Ruggenenti P, Perna A, Remuzzi G, on behalf of GISEN. ACE inhibitors to prevent end-stage renal disease: when to start and why possibly never to stop: a post hoc analysis of the REIN trial results. J Am Soc Nephrol. 2001;12:2832–7.

50. Giatras J, Lau J, Levey AS. Effect of angiotensin-converting-enzyme inhibitors on the progression of non-diabetic renal disease: a meta-analysis of randomized trials. Ann Intern Med. 1997;127:337–45.

51. Koshy S, Bakris GL. Therapeutic approaches to achieve desired blood pressure goals: focus on calcium channel blockers. Cardiovasc Drugs Ther. 2000;14:295–301.

52. Brenner BM. Effects of losartan on renal and cardiovascular outcomes in patients with type 2 diabetes and nephropathy. N Engl J Med. 2001;345:861–9.

53. Parving H-H. The effect of Irbesartan on the development of diabetic nephropathy in patients with type 2 diabetes. N Engl J Med. 2001;345:870–8.

54. Lewis EJ. Renoprotective effect of the angiotensin receptor antagonist Irbesartan in patients with nephropathy due to type 2 diabetes. N Engl J Med. 2001;345:851–60.

55. Fried LF, Orchard TJ, Kasiske BL. Effect of lipid reduction on the progression of renal disease: a meta-analysis. Kidney Int. 2001;59:260–9.

56. Collins R, Peto R, Armitage J. The MRC/BHF Heart Protection Study: preliminary results. Int J Clin Pract. 2002;56:53–6.

57. Imai E, Isaka Y. Targeting growth factors to the kidney: myth or reality? Curr Opin Nephrol Hypertens. 2002;11:49–57.

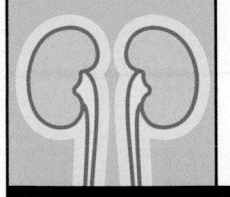

Section 14 Chronic Renal Failure and the Uremic Syndrome

Chapter 67

Clinical Evaluation and Manifestations of Chronic Renal Failure

Christopher G Winearls

INTRODUCTION

The management of chronic renal failure (CRF) is now the dominant part of the work of a clinical nephrologist. This has come about because chronic kidney disease is easily uncovered by routine blood and urine tests and treatment for end-stage renal disease (ESRD) is so successful and widely applied. This is perhaps the most important respect in which nephrology is different from other specialties that lack a simple test for organ dysfunction and a means to substitute function when the organ fails.

Although supervision of patients receiving renal replacement therapy (RRT) is the undisputed domain of the nephrologist, care of patients with progressive renal insufficiency is as important, not least because it may be possible to delay progression or halt a disease process. Moreover many of the complications and long-term problems of renal failure start well before dialysis or renal transplantation are even being discussed, and there are a number of options for preventing or ameliorating these[1].

DEFINITIONS

CRF (also known as chronic renal insufficiency) is an irreversible, usually progressive, diminution in renal function to a degree that has damaging consequences for the patient. Nomenclature and definitions have, in the past, varied but have recently been defined by an international working group, and published in the Kidney/Dialysis Outcome Quality Initiative (K/DOQI) guidelines[2], which describe the severity of renal failure in a classification of five stages of kidney disease

(Table 67.1). This classification is not yet in wide clinical use, and a traditional clinical working definition of the degree of kidney failure is shown in Table 67.2. This ranges from mild to end-stage – the degree of renal failure which would cause death if renal replacement were not instituted.

It is important to make an estimate of the severity of the CRF, which will dictate the time scale of consequences for the patient and the responses required (see Table 67.2). In practice, few nephrologists use isotopic measurements of GFR and not all will rely on the creatinine clearance, a measurement tedious for the patient, requiring a 24-h urine collection, and consequently unreliable. Quick and sufficiently reliable estimates of GFR can be obtained using the plasma creatinine, age, weight and gender of the patient using the Cockroft–Gault formula or other calculated estimates (see Chapter 3, Fig. 3.6).

EPIDEMIOLOGY

Compared with ischemic heart disease, stroke, diabetes, and cancer, renal failure is an uncommon condition, and may therefore seem a relatively minor public health problem, but because of the expense of treatment for end-stage renal disease (ESRD) it captures a disproportionate share of health care resources.

The most accurate data available are for the incidence and prevalence of ESRD, because patients would die without the provision of RRT. However there are many patients with CRF who will never require RRT, and will die *with* renal failure rather than *of* it. Examples include patients with malignant urinary tract obstruction, diabetes mellitus, or renovascular disease with widespread cerebro- and cardiovascular disease.

Stages of chronic kidney disease			
Stage	Description of kidney damage with:	GFR mL/min 1.73 m²	% US population*
1	Normal GFR but some evidence of kidney damage e.g., abnormal urinalysis or histological changes	> 90	3.3
2	Mild chronic kidney failure	60–89	3.0
3	Moderate chronic kidney failure	30–59	4.3
4	Severe chronic kidney failure	15–29	0.2
5	ESRD when RRT has to be considered	< 15 on dialysis	0.2
*Percentage of US population at each stage according to NHANES III			

Table 67.1 Stages of chronic kidney disease. Classification of chronic kidney disease according to the K/DOQI guidelines[2].

Chronic Renal Failure and the Uremic Syndrome

			Clinical classification of the severity of chronic renal failure		
K/DOQI Classification	Commonly used clinical description	GFR mL/min	Typical plasma creatinine in a 65 kg subject	Consequences	Action
3	Mild CRF	30–59	170 μmol/L 2 mg/dL	hypertension, secondary hyperparathyroidism	Treat hypertension Start phosphate restriction and phosphate binders Start Vitamin D analogue
4	Moderate CRF	15–29	350 μmol/L 4 mg/dL	*plus* anemia	Restrict dietary sodium and potassium to 60 mmol/day Advise moderate protein restriction Plan renal replacement therapy including vascular access
5	Severe CRF	< 15	700 μmol/L 8 mg/dL	*plus* sodium + water retention, anorexia vomiting, reduced higher mental function	Plan elective start of dialysis or pre-emptive renal transplant
5	ESRD	< 5	1500 μmol/L 17 mg/dL	*plus* pulmonary edema coma, fits, metabolic acidosis hyperkalemia, death	Start dialysis immediately *or* provide palliative care

Table 67.2 **Clinical classification of the severity of chronic renal failure.** The definitions and terminology of K/DOQI are not yet in wide clinical use. Many nephrologists use criteria shown in this table to describe patients with CRF and anticipate clinical problems and interventions needed as CRF progresses.

The prevalence of CRF rises steeply with age, and is higher in certain ethnic groups, including African Caribbeans, Native Americans and South Asians. It is also clear that the incidence of CRF is increasing, particularly a consequence of the sustained increase in type 2 diabetic nephropathy in many parts of the developed and developing world.

The available evidence on the incidence and prevalence of CRF is discussed further in Chapter 66.

ETIOLOGY AND PATHOGENESIS

Causes of chronic renal failure

The most reliable database of causes of renal failure is that maintained in Australia, which has a system of reporting that enjoys unparalleled loyalty from its nephrologists. The data from their registry, from a recent survey in England and Wales, and from Japan and the USA are given in Figure 66.3[3–6]. The difference in apparent prevalence of glomerulonephritis is unexplained. It may reflect the vague diagnostic criteria for the cause of renal failure used in some registries. It is likely that many patients identified as having hypertensive renal disease actually have indolent glomerulonephritis, usually IgA nephropathy. Rarer causes of ESRD not identified in substantial numbers in most registry reports are shown in Table 67.3.

Progression of chronic renal failure

Slow progression of CRF towards ESRD is the normal pattern for most chronic kidney diseases. The pathogenesis of this progression and interventions to delay the process are discussed in Chapter 66.

CLINICAL PRESENTATIONS

It is unusual for nephrologists to be the first to recognize CRF in a patient, but it is their task to confirm the diagnosis and take responsibility for the implications. The diagnosis has huge consequences for both the patients and their doctors because CRF will affect every aspect of life and health leading eventually to an odyssey of RRT when ESRD is reached. Chronic renal failure presents in three ways:

- As chronic kidney disease (K/DOQI Stages 2–4), recognized because of an abnormal plasma creatinine and blood urea, or in the context of known cause of kidney damage, e.g., diabetes, or a known familial renal disease. The patient is usually referred initially for outpatient assessment.
- Acute-on-chronic renal failure manifesting as unexpected illness; when it subsequently becomes apparent after the patient's clinical condition has stabilized that there is underlying chronic kidney disease.
- Late, as a uremic emergency, requiring urgent management for life-threatening complications of renal failure. Subsequently there is no recovery of renal function and the patient has ESRD.

Late referral of the patient with chronic renal failure

Unfortunately, a substantial proportion of patients presenting as uremic emergencies will turn out to have undiagnosed, unrecognized or neglected CRF. The problem of late referral of patients known to have renal failure is in part avoidable[7]. It is explained in part by a failure of physicians to recognize the nonlinear relation between plasma creatinine and GFR: for

Causes of chronic renal failure	
Common causes in all registries of patients with ESRD (see Fig. 66.3)	
Diabetic nephropathy	
Glomerulonephritis	
Interstitial nephritis (including pyelonephritis)	
Hypertension/vascular disease	
Hereditary/congenital disease	
Neoplasms	
Less common causes	
Group	**Causes**
Metabolic	cystinosis oxalosis nephrocalcinosis cystinuria hyperuricemia
Vascular	ischemic renal disease[a] scleroderma hemolytic uremic syndrome postpartum renal failure
Dysproteinemias	amyloid myeloma cryoglobulinemia light chain deposition disease (LCDD)
Hereditary	Alport syndrome Fabry disease tuberous sclerosis sickle cell disease
Vasculitis	Wegener's granulomatosis microscopic polyangiitis polyarteritis nodosa lupus
Malignancy	renal cell carcinoma lymphoma
Structural	cystic kidney disease other than adult-onset cystic disease; congenital and acquired abnormalities of the urinary tract, e.g., associated with spina bifida, spinal cord injury

[a]Increasingly common but not separately identified in most registries.

Table 67.3 Causes of chronic renal failure.

example a plasma creatinine of 4.5 mg/dL (400 μmol/L) is erroneously understood to imply that a patient is only 40% of the way to a need for dialysis at a creatinine of 11 mg/dL (1000 μmol/L). About 30% of patients starting RRT in the UK see a nephrologist less than 12 weeks before they start RRT. In some cases, this is unavoidable: the patients may have had a truly silent illness or an acute presentation of an irreversible renal injury, for example, myeloma, antiglomerular basement membrane (anti-GBM) disease, or cortical necrosis.

The consequences for patients of late presentation are many: they suffer a huge psychologic shock that makes coming to terms with a chronic illness difficult, they have to rely on temporary vascular access, and they often lose their jobs because of the sudden, prolonged absence from work. They will have suffered the complications of untreated renal failure, and although renal anemia can be reversed, untreated renal osteodystrophy and hypertensive damage to the heart may leave irreversible damage. They may even lose their lives from the complications of the acute uremic emergency. Those presenting late certainly have a worse prognosis although this may reflect their comorbidity[8]. The cost of initiating dialysis in patients with ESRD presenting late is very much higher than for those in whom an elective start is made[9].

THE COMPLICATIONS AND CONSEQUENCES OF CHRONIC RENAL FAILURE

Particularly at the first consultation, but also at all subsequent consultations, the nephrologist must consider the various complications and consequences of renal failure and the means to minimize immediate symptoms and reduce long-term harm. Substantial discussion of several of these aspects of CRF is provided in other chapters in this section of the book.

The clinical manifestations of mild CRF (GFR ≥ 30 mL/min) are few (Table 67.2). Most patients are asymptomatic, although biochemical evidence of secondary hyperparathyroidism may already be present. Hypertension is very common. Proteinuria or hematuria are common dependent on the cause of renal insufficiency. Isosthenuria resulting in nocturia is often the only other clinical manifestation. The following more severe manifestations then develop relentlessly as GFR declines.

Cardiovascular disease

Most patients with CRF have blood pressure that is higher than the population mean and many are frankly hypertensive (see Chapter 69). Intensive treatment and monitoring is one of the most important tasks for the nephrologist caring for these patients. Successful control has a number of benefits. First, it slows the rate of decline of renal function (see Chapter 66) and, second, it breaks the vicious circle of factors that damage both the heart and the vasculature. Most drugs act to reduce peripheral vascular resistance but equal attention must be paid to volume overload, by limiting the sodium content of the diet and administration of higher than usual doses of diuretics. Increasing evidence supports a low target blood pressure (135/85) for all patients with chronic renal disease, and a lower target for those with proteinuria > 1 g/24 h (125/75)[10,11].

Patients who smoke must be firmly warned that all patients with renal failure are more likely to die of cardiovascular disease than of renal failure and that smoking is the major multiplier of that risk. It may also contribute to progression of CRF.

Anemia contributes to cardiac dysfunction by forcing an increase in cardiac output, which is another stimulus to left ventricular hypertrophy. Reversal of anemia certainly improves cardiac function, but there is no evidence yet that it improves prognosis over the longer term. Trials are in progress.

Dyslipidemia occurs early in renal failure. At present the decision to start lipid-lowering treatment with HMG CoA reductase inhibitors is based on the same criteria that apply to the nonrenal-failure population since intervention trials have not included patients with renal failure. There is increasing opinion that the threshold for drug therapy should be lower.

Chronic Renal Failure and the Uremic Syndrome

The answer to this question is presently being sought in a randomized trial in the UK.

Anemia

Anemia probably accounts for many of the symptoms previously attributed to the general effects of uremia (see Chapter 70). Its severity is linked to the degree of renal impairment but there is considerable variation. Diabetics and those with chronic interstitial disease develop anemia earlier than those with polycystic kidney disease. A relative deficiency of erythropoietin is a sufficient if not complete explanation. Provided patients are not iron deficient and there are no other confounding factors, administration of 50–100 U/kg per week of recombinant human erythropoietin (epoetin) given subcutaneously in divided doses, will usually reverse the anemia (target hemoglobin 11.5–12.5 g/dL). A long acting erythropoietin analog, darbepoietin is now available. Because it has a prolonged half life it can be administered weekly or fortnightly. The usual dose requirement is 15–30 μg/week. The reduced dose frequency is especially convenient for those who rely on others to administer their injections. The cost is the same as recombinant erythropoietin. Treatment should be started if patients are symptomatic, have angina, or the hemoglobin falls below 11 g/dL. Whether pre-emptive treatment to maintain the hemoglobin within the normal range to prevent symptoms and protect the heart is justified remains to be established. Partial correction of anemia does not accelerate the decline of renal function but does lead to a need for more intensive treatment of blood pressure[12].

Renal bone disease

The seeds of renal bone disease are sown in the long period of CRF before RRT is begun (see Chapter 68) and there is now broad agreement that prevention of secondary hyperparathyroidism requires early treatment with vitamin D analogs (calcitriol or 1α-hydroxyvitamin D_3) and phosphate restriction[13]. There are virtually no symptoms of renal osteodystrophy in its early stages, so it takes substantial effort to motivate both patients and physicians to pay attention to calcium and phosphate balance in the predialysis period, especially when CRF is mild and the patient is otherwise asymptomatic.

Metabolic acidosis

The metabolic acidosis in CRF is caused by the failure of hydrogen ion excretion and in interstitial diseases by bicarbonate loss. The clinical consequences are subtle and are seldom sought. Patients complain of breathlessness on minor exertion, which is often incorrectly attributed to anemia or pulmonary edema. The acidosis aggravates hyperkalemia, inhibits protein anabolism, and accelerates calcium loss from bone where the hydrogen ions are buffered[14]. An uncompensated metabolic acidosis in renal failure is an indication to start dialysis. One can temporize with oral sodium bicarbonate; a dose up to 1.2 g four times daily may be tolerated, but the sodium load will aggravate hypertension. Sodium bicarbonate therapy should be restricted to normotensive patients with plasma bicarbonate concentration < 20 mmol/L. Typically, these are patients with renal failure caused by interstitial diseases such as obstructive nephropathy or reflux nephropathy.

Malnutrition

Malnutrition is common in renal failure (see Chapter 74) and is believed to increase the risk of death in patients on dialysis. It is caused by anorexia, acidosis, and insulin resistance. It is aggravated if renal insufficiency is superimposed on nephrotic syndrome. Clues to its presence are loss of weight and muscle bulk (often hidden by edema) and a low serum albumin, transferrin, and cholesterol. The creatinine will fall, which may be misinterpreted as an improvement in renal function. If patients do not respond to dietary supplements and correction of metabolic acidosis, dialysis should be instituted. It cannot be denied that balancing the need for calories and high-quality protein with limitation of phosphate, sodium, potassium, and fats is a challenge for even the most imaginative renal dietician.

Sodium and water

Patients with CRF, but otherwise in good health generally maintain sodium and water balance until the GFR is reduced very severely (below approximately 10 mL/min). This is achieved by a corresponding large increase in the proportion of the filtered sodium and water that is excreted. Similarly, to produce a given change in excretion of sodium and water at low GFR requires a magnification of the tubular response: for instance, a response that is effected by kidneys with a GFR of 120 mL/min by a change in fractional excretion of sodium from 0.5 to 3% will require a change from 5 to 30% if the filtration rate is only 12 mL/min. It is not surprising that one of the earliest effects of chronic renal disease is a limitation in the power of the kidney to compensate for changes in sodium and water intake. Patients are, therefore, advised to eschew excessively salty food, not to add it at table, and to try to adhere to a diet containing approximately 60 mmol/d sodium chloride. Salt substitutes contain potassium and should be avoided.

In healthy individuals with a normal solute intake, water excretion can be varied from approximately 20 to 1500 mL/h; in renal disease, this range is reduced in both directions. Excessive water intake will, therefore, lead to dilutional hyponatremia and inadequate intake to hypernatremia.

Potassium

Hyperkalemia (see Chapter 9) usually only becomes a problem when the GFR is <10 mL/min, and can be compensated by a diet restricted to 60 mmol potassium daily. Unlike patients with ARF, those with established CRF may tolerate plasma potassium concentrations up to 7.5 mmol/L without ECG changes or arrhythmia. To be safe, plans for dialysis are advisable if the concentration is consistently above 6.5 mmol/L. Disproportionate hyperkalemia is seen in patients with hyporeninemic hypoaldosteronism (particularly in older diabetics) and in hypercatabolic or acidotic patients. The drug therapy must be reviewed for inappropriate prescriptions, such as potassium-sparing diuretics, ACE inhibitors, and NSAIDs. The hyperkalemia of patients on ACE inhibitors is not usually clinically significant and does not necessarily mandate withdrawal of the drug. Ion-exchange resins are unpleasant to take and cause constipation and should not be used for potassium control except in emergencies.

Bleeding diathesis

Patients with renal failure have a bleeding diathesis (see Chapter 71), which is, in part, a consequence of abnormal platelet function. The silent manifestation of this is occult gastrointestinal blood loss, but patients are liable to ooze blood from incisions and particularly careful attention to surgical hemostasis is required. Epistaxes may be prolonged and menstrual periods heavy. Dentists should be warned before performing difficult tooth extractions. Medically, the problem can be limited by ensuring that the patients have undergone effective dialysis and have transfusions to hemoglobin levels of 10–12 g/dL preoperatively, and that any heparin used during dialysis has been cleared or reversed. The administration of platelets is not effective. Cryoprecipitate produces a temporary improvement in bleeding time. The synthetic vasopression analog desmopressin (DDAVP: l-deamino-8-D-arginine vasopressin) (0.3 mg/kg intravenous) is effective for about 48 h, but should not be used in patients with ischemic heart disease. The effect on water clearance may lead to hyponatremia. Conjugated estrogens provide an improvement in bleeding time that lasts up to 14 d.

Dermatologic manifestations

The dermatologic manifestations of CRF are common and frequently a source of considerable discomfort and trouble for the patient.

Pigmentation

Diffuse brown pigmentation is a common but not universal consequence of prolonged renal failure (Fig. 67.1a).

Nails

Typically the proximal part of the nail is white and the distal part is discolored brown: the so-called half and half nail. The pathogenesis of this change is not understood.

Xerosis

Dry xerotic skin is extremely common and there may be frank scaling, ichthyosis, and lichenification. The pathogenesis is not well understood. Pruritus is the usual consequence. Treatment is aimed at moisturizing the skin with emollients and oily soap substitutes.

Pruritus

Itching is a variable and unpredictable symptom of CRF[15] and can be extremely disruptive for the patient. It is usually a late manifestation, is more common in dialysis recipients, and is aggravated by heat and stress. The skin of the arms and back are usually cited as the worst-affected areas. There is often little to see except the xerosis and scratch marks in any area that the patient can reach. Sores follow where the skin has been breached. Sometimes there are keratotic papules or a nodular prurigo (Fig. 67.1b). Its pathogenesis is poorly understood but may be related to histamine release. A high calcium phosphate product (> 6.25 $(mmol^2)$, $> 77 (mg^2)$) is one cause; this can be improved by trimming the dose of vitamin D analogs and calcium-containing phosphate binders. If hypercalcemia limits the use of calcium-containing phosphate binders, sevelamer hydrochloride (2.4–4.8 g) given three times a day in divided doses before meals is an alternative. Patients will be motivated to stick to dietary phosphate restriction if their itch improves. Short-term use of aluminum-containing phosphate binders can also be justified for pruritus, which makes patients feel wretched and exhausted. Ultraviolet phototherapy is effective but not widely available and has to be limited to short courses. Naltrexone, an opioid antagonist, has been shown to be an effective short-term treatment[16]. A few patients get relief from antihistamines, such as chlorphenamine (chlorpheniramine) 4 mg three times a day, but the sedative effects may be unacceptable. They should be advised to keep cool, wear light clothes, and keep the skin

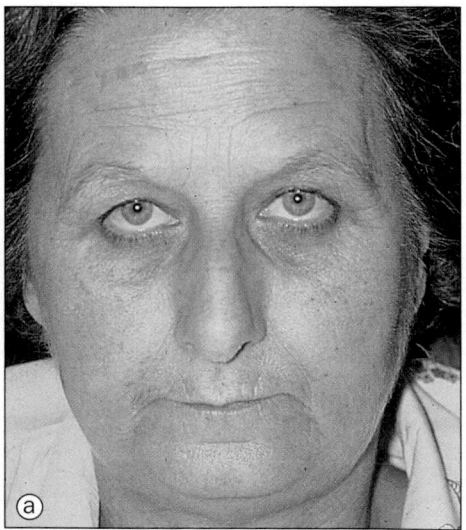
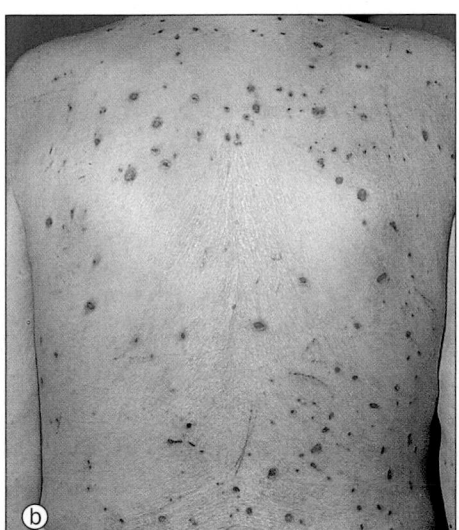
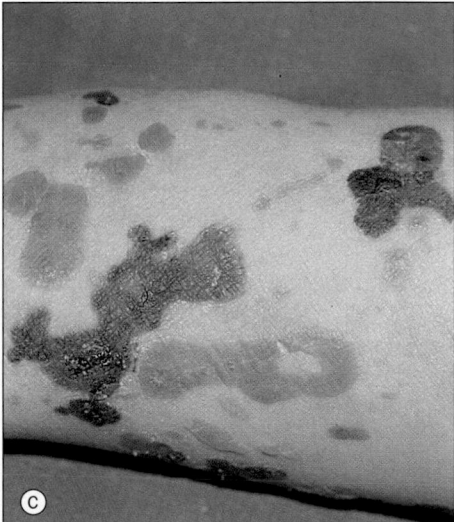

Figure 67.1 Dermatologic manifestations in chronic renal failure. (a) Pigmentation: a diffuse brown pigmentation is typical of longstanding renal failure; it may be caused by retention of b-melanocyte-stimulating hormone. (b) Nodular prurigo: extensive nodular prurigo associated with severe pruritus (note the scratch marks) in a man with advanced renal failure shortly before the initiation of renal replacement therapy. (c) Pseudoporphyria: bullous eruption in a patient on regular dialysis; the bullae are hemorrhagic in this individual because of a coincidental thrombocytopenia[14].

Chronic Renal Failure and the Uremic Syndrome

moist by adding oils to the bath or applying simple creams. Unfortunately, many patients are not helped by any of these measures. In the author's experience, well-dialyzed patients itch less, so intractable pruritus is probably an indication to start dialysis.

Bullous eruptions

Bullous skin disease in CRF is much less common than pruritus.

Pseudoporphyria

A bullous eruption that is clinically indistinguishable from porphyria cutanea tarda is occasionally seen in patients on dialysis and may also occur in patients with CRF who have not undergone dialysis (Fig. 67.1c). It appears on light exposed skin, especially in the summer, and is thought to be a consequence of retained uroporphyrins, which photosensitize the skin. An entity known as 'bullous disease of HD' has also been described; it is controversial whether this is distinct from porphyria. Iron overload may also be implicated in the pathogenesis. Epoetin treatment has been reported to ameliorate pseudoporphyria, allowing venesection to be used to reduce circulating porphyrins and iron stores[17]. The bullous lesions may take months to resolve.

Bullous drug eruptions

Fixed drug eruptions are also occasionally seen. These are also seen on light exposed skin, usually the hands, in the summer. The commonest provoking agent is high-dose furosemide (frusemide) in advanced renal failure. Resolution occurs when furosemide is withdrawn but may take several months.

Neurologic manifestations

Central nervous system

The extreme manifestation of uremic encephalopathy is coma and seizures, but this is now rare because it is a very late event in neglected renal failure. A computed tomography (CT) scan is usually normal but MRI shows diffuse changes in the white matter; lumbar puncture reveals normal CSF. More common clinical features are cognitive impairment and myoclonus, initially manifest as 'restless legs' but increasing to uncontrollable day time twitching accompanied by a demonstrable uremic flap. These features are indications to start dialysis. The electroencephalograph (EEG) is abnormal, showing widespread slow wave activity, but the EEG features do not differ substantially from those seen in other metabolic abnormalities nor does the extent of abnormality correlate well with the severity of the clinical picture. The EEG is, therefore, seldom used in diagnosis or to monitor response to treatment.

The differential diagnosis is wide, but a common problem is the additive effect of opiate toxicity owing to retention of active metabolites, which can aggravate or mimic uremic encephalopathy.

True dementia, not reversed by adequate control of uremia, may be a consequence of multiple cerebral infarction, coincidental Alzheimer's disease, or, in patients on dialysis, aluminum accumulation. In the author's opinion, uremia *per se* does not lead to dementia.

Peripheral nervous system

Asymmetric distal mixed sensorimotor polyneuropathy is common in ESRD but unusual in patients not yet requiring dialysis. Sensory symptoms usually predominate, particularly dysesthesiae with prickling or burning sensations. Motor symptoms, including foot drop, are much less common. The physical signs do not distinguish this from other causes of sensorimotor peripheral neuropathy. Nerve conduction studies show significant abnormality in up to 90% of uremic patients but clinical symptoms and disability are now rare.

The 'neurotoxin' has not been identified but it is likely to be a retained 'middle molecule', an inference that is drawn from the observation that clinically obvious neuropathy has become uncommon since dialysis is begun earlier in uremic patients.

The clinical picture may be complicated by other diseases causing peripheral neuropathy, particularly diabetes, or by a coincidental uremic mononeuropathy, most commonly median nerve compression in the carpal tunnel, caused by β_2M-amyloid (see Chapter 72).

Autonomic neuropathy

Uremic autonomic neuropathy is very variable in its clinical effects – the most substantial effect is usually sluggish cardiovascular reflexes during HD, provoking hypotension particularly during fluid removal[18]. It may be manifest as sexual dysfunction in males.

Treatment

There is no effective treatment of neuropathy in renal failure apart from adequate dialysis or successful transplantation, so management is directed towards minimizing symptoms. 'Restless legs', especially at night, are a nuisance. Clonazepam (500–2000 mg) is effective in suppressing this symptom in some but not all patients.

Endocrine abnormalities

The most obvious examples of endocrine abnormality in uremia are alterations in the vitamin D/parathyroid hormone (PTH) axis and in erythropoietin caused by damage to the endocrine function of the kidney. But there are diverse abnormalities in hormone production, control, protein-binding, catabolism, and tissue effects in uremia. Hormone concentrations may be elevated as a result of reduced degradation (insulin) or increased secretion in appropriate response to metabolic alterations (PTH). Hormone concentrations may be reduced owing to impaired renal (calcitriol, erythropoietin) or extrarenal production (estrogen, testosterone). There may also be disturbances of activation through altered prohormones. Finally, reductions in hormone-binding proteins are most commonly a consequence of protein loss in nephrotic patients or in those on CAPD.

Thyroid hormones

Total thyroxine (T_4) may be low with increased reverse triiodothyronine (T_3) as a result of impaired conversion of T_3 to T_4. Loss of thyroid-binding globulin (TBG) may further lower total circulating T_4 concentrations. However, patients are not clinically hypothyroid and measurements of thyroid-stimulating hormone remains a reliable diagnostic test for hypothyroidism in patients with renal failure.

Growth hormone

Plasma growth hormone levels are abnormally high in renal failure because of delayed clearance and alterations in hypothalamic–pituitary control of growth hormone release. In adults, the clinical implications of these changes are not clear. In children with renal failure and growth retardation, production of insulin-like growth factor 1 (IGF-1) in response to growth hormone is impaired; this can be overcome by treatment with exogenous recombinant growth hormone in supraphysiologic dosage.

Insulin

Decreased clearance of insulin seems to be balanced by increased peripheral resistance to the effects of insulin. Consequently, there are usually no clinical effects and patients are prone to neither hypoglycemia nor diabetes. However, these effects do lead to a reduced requirement for insulin in diabetics as renal function declines.

Sex hormones

Males

Prolactin levels are high in renal failure and may contribute to gynecomastia and sexual dysfunction in men. Testosterone levels are often low–normal in males and gonadotropins are raised, implying testicular failure as the cause. This is accompanied by poor spermatogenesis, leading to low sperm counts and subfertility. It is appropriate to prescribe androgen-replacement treatment if testosterone is unequivocally low, not least because this should help to prevent osteoporosis. The most important and usually neglected sexual problem in males is erectile dysfunction, which is not simply a manifestation of sex hormone deficiency. Neurologic, psychologic, and vascular abnormalities are far more important. Sildenafil (Viagra) can be effective and is safe in renal failure[19]. Reversal of anemia by epoetin improves sexual function in some patients.

Females

Raised prolactin levels contribute to infertility. In severe renal failure, the pituitary–ovary axis is disturbed. Although luteinizing hormone is raised, the normal pulsatile release and the preovulation surge are absent. Cycles are, therefore, often anovulatory, and in advanced renal failure there is usually an irregular cycle or amenorrhea. Before amenorrhea supervenes, there is often menorrhagia because of the uremic bleeding diathesis.

The common reduction in female libido is multifactorial, including psychologic influences as well as alterations in sex hormones. Occasionally, women on dialysis conceive, but they seldom carry the pregnancy to term. The special problems of pregnancy in women with renal failure are discussed in Chapter 45. The concept that this disturbance is a consequence of uremia is proved by the rapid return of menses and fertility in women who receive a well-functioning transplant.

Immunity

Infections are the second most common cause of death, after cardiovascular disease, in advanced renal failure. Although this is explained in part by the regular breaching of physical defenses – needling of vascular access, central lines, and peritoneal dialysis – uremia is also a state of chronic immunosuppression[20]. Both cellular and humoral aspects of the immune system are defective.

T-cell responses to antigen are deficient, perhaps because antigen presentation by monocytes is defective. Neutrophil activation is also deficient. Although serum immunoglobulin levels are normal, antibody responses to immunization are poor: peak antibody levels are lower and decline more quickly. Whereas over 90% of a normal population will have an effective response to hepatitis B immunization, only 50–60% of an uremic population respond and this directly relates to the severity of renal failure. This deficiency is particularly evident in immunization with T-cell-dependent antigens – for example, hepatitis B, pneumococcus, and hemophilus. The immune deficiency is not corrected by dialysis, despite the paradoxical activation of neutrophils during HD.

The practical effects of this immune depression for patients with CRF include increased susceptibility to bacterial, especially staphylococcal, infection; increased risk of reactivating tuberculosis, typically with a negative tuberculin skin test; a failure to clear hepatitis B and C infections and impaired response to hepatitis B immunization.

Although the incidence of hepatitis B is now very low in most UK and US dialysis units, it remains high (> 15% of patients) in other parts of the world, e.g., Croatia, Poland and Brazil. Containment of spread is by vigilant infection control measures and active immunization programs. Patients with CRF should be immunized against hepatitis B in the normal way as early in the course of their renal impairment as possible once they have been identified as HBs antigen and antibody negative[21]. If the patient presents with ESRD, immunization is still worthwhile but an intensified regimen is recommended – 40 μg of vaccine should be administered intramuscularly at 0, 1 and 6 months. Some 40–80% of patients will respond. Intradermal injection may be more effective – 5 μg of vaccine is injected every 2 weeks until a response is obtained.

Malignancy

Impaired immunity may be an important factor in the susceptibility of patients with renal failure to malignancy. This susceptibility is not restricted to the renal transplant recipient (see Chapter 89) or to the specific problem of malignancy developing within acquired cystic disease (see Chapter 73). In patients with ESRD who are on dialysis, increased incidences of a range of malignancies are documented including primary liver cancer, renal cancer, thyroid cancer, myeloma, and non-Hodgkin's lymphoma[22].

Psychologic manifestations

The psychologic problems of patients with CRF, usually anxiety and depression, are the predictable and understandable consequences of loss of health, control, and pleasure. They are greatest in those with the most to lose – the young and ambitious – and may be relatively minor in the elderly who are grateful that they have a treatable illness and not an immediately lethal one.

The best treatment is good empathetic symptomatic care from physicians, nurses, and other staff, with whom they can build a relationship. In particular, one should try to eliminate fear of the unknown (caused by ignorance and often by gossip in the clinic waiting room) and encourage an optimistic approach.

Psychiatrists usually have little to offer unless there is formal mental illness, but psychotherapists may be able to help with phobias, guilt, and anger. Antidepressants should be used sparingly, but gentle night sedation is frequently helpful.

MANAGEMENT OF CHRONIC RENAL FAILURE

The overall approach to the patient presenting with uremia is shown in Figure 67.2. Once any emergency treatment is over, it is necessary to establish that there is chronic rather than acute renal failure, and the cause of CRF should be identified where possible. Thereafter many centers follow patients with CRF in a dedicated 'low-clearance' clinic. This allows the most productive interaction of the patient with the members of the multidisciplinary team who manage their renal disease: nephrologist, surgeon, nurse, social worker, dietitian, and psychologist. The purposes of follow-up in a 'low-clearance' clinic are (1) to attempt to halt or delay progression of renal failure, (2) to treat or minimize the consequences of CRF, and (3) to prepare the patient for RRT (this is discussed further in Chapter 75).

Treating the uremic emergency

For patients presenting with severe renal failure, the first issue is to deal with life-threatening problems: hyperkalemia, pulmonary edema, severe metabolic acidosis, encephalopathy (uremic or hypertensive), and pericarditis/pericardial effusion. This is the so-called uremic emergency and can be the first presentation of either acute renal failure (ARF) or CRF. Whether it proves to be ARF or CRF, most of the life-threatening features of the uremic emergency and their immediate management are the same. They are summarized in Figure 67.3 and discussed further in Chapter 14.

A 'full house' uremic emergency comprising all the problems shown in Figure 67.3 is a formidable clinical challenge. Ideally it should be managed in an intensive-care unit but practical considerations, for example the institution of hemodialysis (HD), means that it is commonly dealt with in a renal ward high-dependency area. It needs an experienced nephrologist to set the priorities, and vigilant monitoring of blood pressure, oxygen saturation, level of consciousness, pH, and potassium. Medical staff should be immediately available throughout the dialysis treatment and for a few hours after, as deterioration can be sudden.

Acute or chronic renal failure?

When the crisis has been resolved, the second task is making the distinction between ARF and CRF, after which the diagnostic and management paths will diverge.

Distinguishing ARF from CRF is usually straightforward. The key evidence will come from the history. Does the patient suffer from an illness that is frequently complicated by renal failure, for example diabetes, adult polycystic kidney disease, or widespread vascular disease? Has the patient been aware of vague ill health or has nocturia been a symptom for more than 6 months? In the summer, one asks about symptoms in the

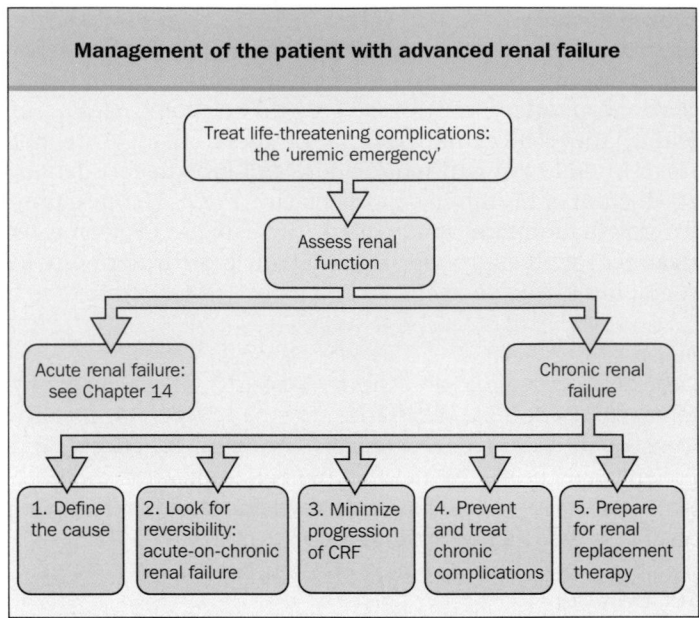

Figure 67.2 Management of the patient with advanced renal failure. Key steps in the evaluation and treatment of patients presenting with uremia.

winter and in the winter about the enjoyment of the previous summer. Are there hints from the past medical history of renal problems: for example, hypertension and/or proteinuria found during routine medical examinations or during pregnancy? Has the patient undergone any urologic procedures or suffered episodes of gout?

The examination is not usually very helpful unless the patient is pigmented and covered with scratch marks and has left ventricular hypertrophy with fundal changes of long-standing hypertension.

Of the investigations, the renal ultrasound is the most important. If small kidneys are seen with a reduction of their cortical thickness, increased echo density, scarring, or multiple cysts, this points unequivocally to a chronic process. Blood tests are less helpful unless they clinch the diagnosis of an acute illness, such as systemic vasculitis or myeloma. A normochromic anemia is usual in CRF but will also be a feature of systemic illnesses presenting with ARF. The findings of a low serum calcium and raised phosphate have no discriminatory value. Radiologic changes of renal osteodystrophy (erosion of the radial edge of the second phalanx or the lateral end of the clavicle) are late and seldom help in practice. Patients with grossly abnormal biochemical values (for example urea > 300 mg/dL (> 50 mmol/L); blood urea nitrogen (BUN) > 140 mg/dL; creatinine > 13.5 mg/dL (> 1200 mmol/L)), who appear relatively well (i.e., are still conversational and ambulant), and are still passing normal volumes of urine are more likely to have CRF. This anomaly is explained by the gradual onset of, and adaptation to, uremia.

If the urea is disproportionately high for the creatinine level measured, then dehydration, gastrointestinal blood loss, infection, and other causes of hypercatabolism should be sought. In moderate-to-severe renal failure the urea : creatinine ratio (mmol : mmol) is typically about 60 : 1; that is urea 20 mmol/L

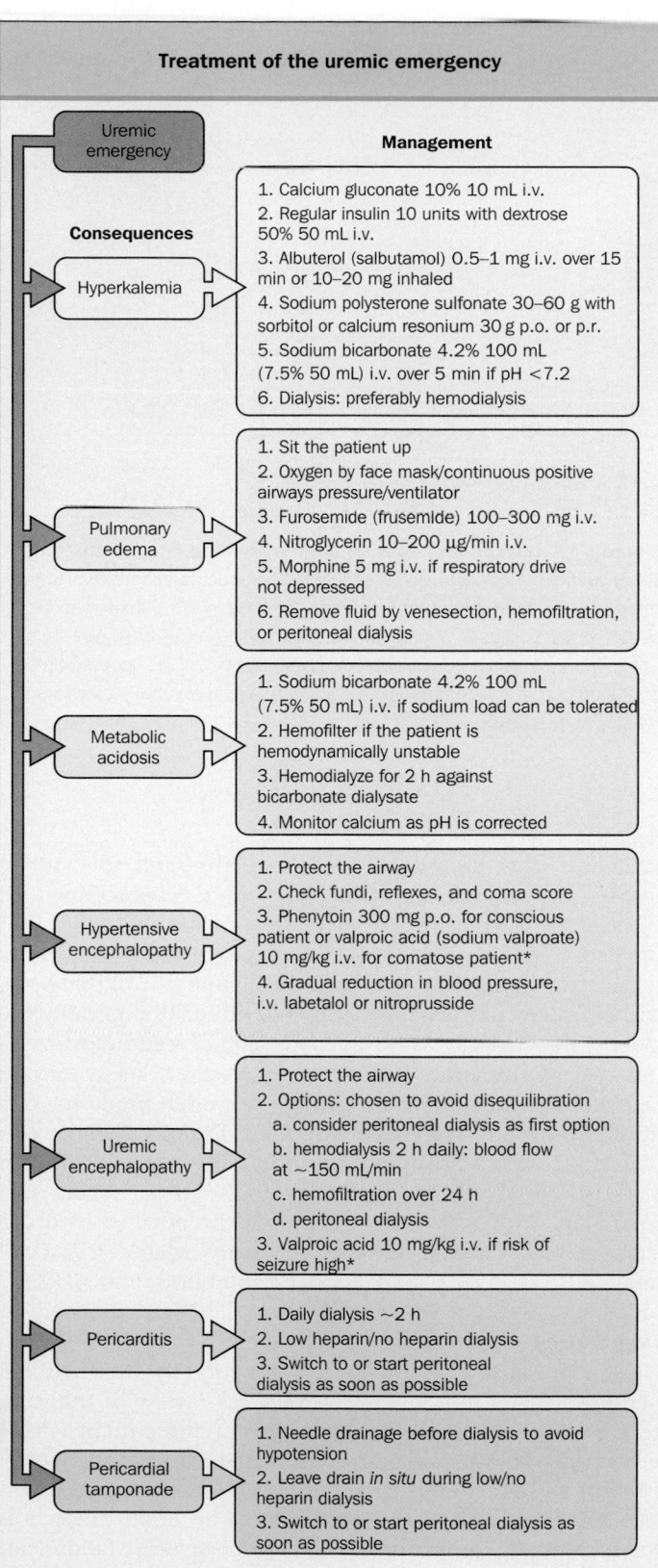

Treatment of the uremic emergency

Uremic emergency Consequences	Management
Hyperkalemia	1. Calcium gluconate 10% 10 mL i.v. 2. Regular insulin 10 units with dextrose 50% 50 mL i.v. 3. Albuterol (salbutamol) 0.5–1 mg i.v. over 15 min or 10–20 mg inhaled 4. Sodium polysterone sulfonate 30–60 g with sorbitol or calcium resonium 30 g p.o. or p.r. 5. Sodium bicarbonate 4.2% 100 mL (7.5% 50 mL) i.v. over 5 min if pH <7.2 6. Dialysis: preferably hemodialysis
Pulmonary edema	1. Sit the patient up 2. Oxygen by face mask/continuous positive airways pressure/ventilator 3. Furosemide (frusemide) 100–300 mg i.v. 4. Nitroglycerin 10–200 µg/min i.v. 5. Morphine 5 mg i.v. if respiratory drive not depressed 6. Remove fluid by venesection, hemofiltration, or peritoneal dialysis
Metabolic acidosis	1. Sodium bicarbonate 4.2% 100 mL (7.5% 50 mL) i.v. if sodium load can be tolerated 2. Hemofilter if the patient is hemodynamically unstable 3. Hemodialyze for 2 h against bicarbonate dialysate 4. Monitor calcium as pH is corrected
Hypertensive encephalopathy	1. Protect the airway 2. Check fundi, reflexes, and coma score 3. Phenytoin 300 mg p.o. for conscious patient or valproic acid (sodium valproate) 10 mg/kg i.v. for comatose patient* 4. Gradual reduction in blood pressure, i.v. labetalol or nitroprusside

Uremic encephalopathy	1. Protect the airway
	 2. Options: chosen to avoid disequilibration
	   a. consider peritoneal dialysis as first option
	   b. hemodialysis 2 h daily: blood flow at ~150 mL/min
	   c. hemofiltration over 24 h
	   d. peritoneal dialysis
	 3. Valproic acid 10 mg/kg i.v. if risk of seizure high*

Pericarditis	1. Daily dialysis ~2 h 2. Low heparin/no heparin dialysis 3. Switch to or start peritoneal dialysis as soon as possible
Pericardial tamponade	1. Needle drainage before dialysis to avoid hypotension 2. Leave drain *in situ* during low/no heparin dialysis 3. Switch to or start peritoneal dialysis as soon as possible

Figure 67.3 Treatment of the uremic emergency. *The use of anticonvulsants as prophylaxis is not 'evidence based' but the risks are small and the possible benefits considerable.

coincides with creatinine 300 µmol/L. This corresponds to a BUN:creatinine ratio (mg:mg) of 15:1.

Establishing the cause of chronic renal failure

There are five good reasons for establishing the cause of CRF whenever this can reasonably be achieved:

- where possible, to arrest the process and prevent further loss of renal function
- to inform the patient to pacify their concerns, anxieties, and sometimes anger and guilt
- to give genetic counseling if appropriate, for example in polycystic kidney disease, reflux nephropathy, and Alport syndrome
- to provide the best advice on prognosis
- to inform the decision on eligibility for renal transplantation: diagnoses such as focal segmental glomerulosclerosis, anti-GBM disease, myeloma, amyloid, and MPGN type II may influence a decision about whether or when to proceed to renal transplantation.

For most patients with CRF, establishing the cause is simple and will usually be revealed by the history. There will, for example, be no difficulty in attributing the cause of renal failure to diabetes, adult polycystic kidney disease, radiologically proven reflux nephropathy and obstruction, biopsy-proven glomerulonephritis, or systemic diseases such as systemic lupus, amyloidosis, or myeloma. The problem arises in patients with little past medical history, contracted kidneys on ultrasound, and a bland urine deposit. Renovascular disease, chronic cholesterol embolism to the kidney, chronic interstitial nephritis caused by drugs, and silent glomerulonephritis probably account for most of these. If the cause cannot be established by standard clinical methods, it should not be pursued relentlessly, for the implications for treatment are minimal. Biopsy of small kidneys is dangerous and rarely reveals a specific diagnosis. However, if interstitial tuberculosis is suspected, a biopsy for a single core of tissue for histology and culture is justifiable.

Minimizing progression of chronic renal failure

Delaying or preventing progression of established renal failure is the intent of every nephrologist and is, of course, important to the patient (see Chapter 66). Furthermore, it is welcomed by those who fund treatment of ESRD, since every year of dialysis avoided saves approximately UK£20 000 (US$33 000).

First, one concentrates on the underlying pathology and whether it can be modified or arrested (see Table 67.4). Second, one should ensure that there are no factors operating that will, independent of the underlying pathology, be harming renal function (see Table 67.5). Third, one will have to make a judgement about which interventions retard progressive glomerulosclerosis. The mechanisms involved are discussed in Chapter 66. The most fundamental factor is control of blood pressure, for which ACE inhibitors or AT1 receptor antagonists (ATRA) are preferred[23]. The recommended target blood pressure in patients with low proteinuria is < 130/80, and in proteinuric disease < 125/75. It usually takes two or more drugs to achieve (see Fig. 66.13). The controversy over dietary protection restriction is also reviewed in Chapter 66. When advising patients of the likelihood of progression, one emphasizes that

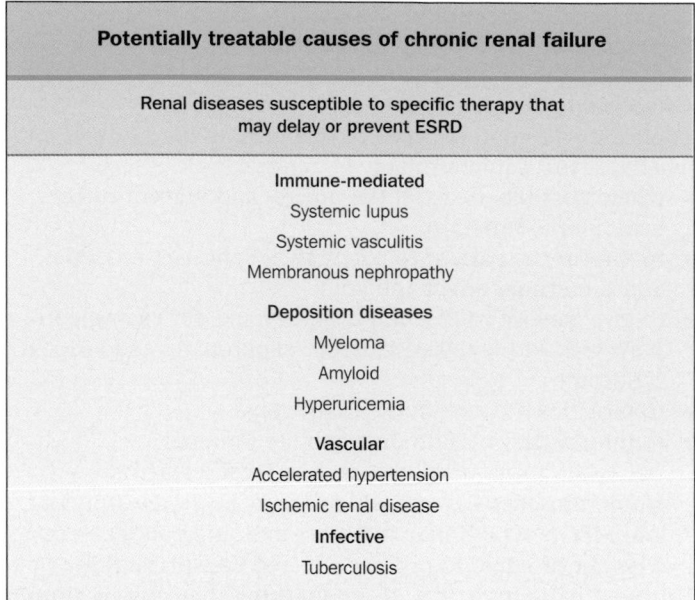

Table 67.4 Potentially treatable causes of chronic renal failure. Renal diseases susceptible to specific therapy that may delay or prevent ESRD.

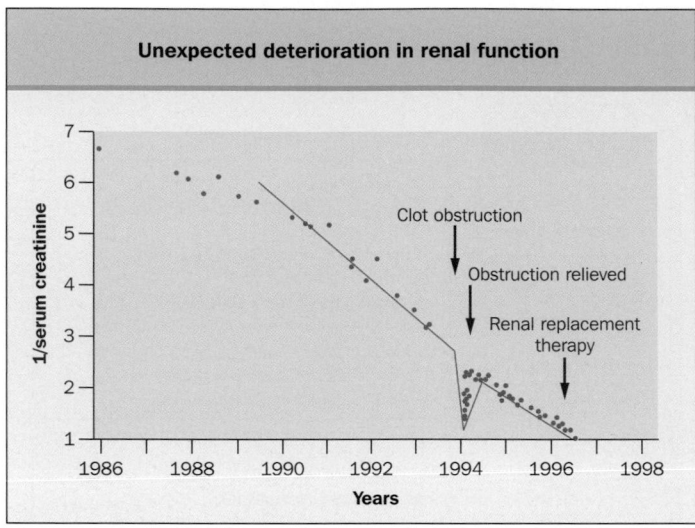

Figure 67.4 Unexpected deterioration in renal function in chronic renal failure. Reciprocal plot of sequential serum creatinine values shows the expected linear deterioration of renal function in this patient with a single polycystic kidney until an intercurrent event (in this case clot obstruction) causes an unexpected change in slope. With successful relief of obstruction, the predicted linear decline to eventual renal replacement therapy is resumed.

Causes of acute-on-chronic renal failure	
Dehydration	Obstruction
Drugs	Hypercalcemia
Disease relapse	Hypertension
Disease acceleration	Heart failure
Infection	Interstitial nephritis

Table 67.5 Causes of acute-on-chronic renal failure.

the underlying renal disease affects risk of progression – for example diabetes and polycystic kidney disease progress inexorably but relieved obstruction and treated accelerated hypertension may not. The presence of heavy proteinuria and difficult to control blood pressure are adverse prognostic signs.

Watching for unexpected deterioration in chronic renal failure

Vigilance is required for intercurrent factors which may aggravate the degree of renal failure, usually referred to as acute-on-chronic renal failure (Table 67.5). In a patient under follow-up, an unexpected deterioration can readily be identified from sequential reciprocal serum creatinine values (Fig. 67.4). The causes are, in effect, those of acute renal failure but lesser insults have greater consequences in those with pre-existing renal impairment. Although the causes can be divided conventionally into 'pre-renal', 'renal' and 'post-renal', it makes sense to run the search for the cause(s) in the order of their frequency.

Reduced renal perfusion

Whatever the underlying cause of the chronic kidney disease, any reduction in renal perfusion may reduce the GFR sufficiently to cause a rise in plasma creatinine above that predicted for the observed rate of progression and, more important, change the severity of renal failure and, therefore, the well-being of the patient. Patients with CRF, especially the elderly, may be oblivious to dehydration caused by overzealous use of diuretics, hot weather, diarrhea, or vomiting. Dehydration substantial enough to cause a rise in plasma creatinine is usually associated with a fall in body weight of at least 3 kg, with a postural drop in blood pressure. Perfusion can also be adversely affected by heart failure, myocardial infarction, and tachyarrhythmias; it is also affected by drugs such as nonsteroidal anti-inflammatory agents (NSAIDs), angiotensin-converting enzyme ACE inhibitors, and ATRAS.

Drug toxicity

Drugs may cause a decline in renal function by altering renal perfusion or by direct nephrotoxicity. A review of the drug regimen is essential in the evaluation of any patient whose renal function has taken an unexpected turn for the worse. Patients will often have been prescribed orthodox drugs such as NSAIDS, diuretics, or ACE inhibitors by other physicians for appropriate indications such as gout or heart failure. An inspection of the patient's collection of pill bottles and packs is the only way to be sure of what they are taking. The problems of iatrogenic drug nephrotoxicity is discussed further in Chapter 95.

There is a constant anxiety that deterioration in renal function may be occurring through the use of drugs causing an interstitial nephritis. If the suspicion is high, one has to choose between a renal biopsy (which has a high risk of complications because the kidneys are usually small and fibrotic), stopping the suspected drug, or prescribing a trial of steroids (prednisolone 30 mg/d for 2 weeks). In practice, few nephrologists risk performing a renal biopsy in this setting. A short course of steroids is safe and is the appropriate action if the deterioration coincides with the administration of a new drug (e.g., an antibiotic, NSAID, or allopurinol) and there are other 'allergic' manifestations such as skin rash, eosinophilia, or eosinophiluria.

Infection

Systemic infection causes a deterioration in renal function in a number of ways: the patient becomes dehydrated, renal perfusion falls, and the switch to a catabolic state causes the urea to rise. Infection of the kidneys themselves destroys nephrons and usually occurs in association with obstruction, stones, or cystic disease.

Obstruction

Minor degrees of obstruction to already damaged kidneys or obstruction of a single kidney has a marked effect on overall renal function (Fig. 67.4). The diagnosis can be difficult, especially if the anatomy of the renal tract has been distorted by chronic obstruction or surgery. The ultrasound will usually show dilated calyces, but the pictures should always be compared with previous scans when these are available. A diethylenetriamine pentaacetic acid (DTPA) renogram is not helpful when renal function is poor, and often the best policy is to relieve any potential site of obstruction by either antegrade nephrostomy and drainage or retrograde stent placement; and to review whether renal function improves.

Hypercalcemia

Hypercalcemia is most often caused by excessively high doses of vitamin D analogs and calcium-containing phosphate binders. It causes dehydration by its effect on the collecting duct inducing water loss. Rarely, the hypercalcemia will be a manifestation of malignancy, myeloma, or sarcoidosis.

Hypertension

The hypertension of CRF, especially that associated with glomerulonephritis (for example IgA nephropathy, membranoproliferative glomerulonephritis (MPGN), and membranous nephropathy), can be quite capricious and can enter an accelerated phase without an obvious explanation. The superimposed arterial and glomerular injury will aggravate rapidly the degree of renal impairment. Treatment may arrest the acceleration in decline but function is usually lost permanently.

Renal vein thrombosis

Renal vein thrombosis should be excluded by angiography or magnetic resonance imaging (MRI) in nephrotic patients whose renal function deteriorates unexpectedly.

Relapse of underlying disease

Finally, one has to consider the possibility that the underlying disease (e.g., myeloma, systemic lupus or a systemic vasculitis) has relapsed. Attempts to confirm such a suspicion will rely on clinical signs, laboratory tests, and tissue examination. A trial of immunosuppressive treatment may be justified when there is uncertainty. Although many of the diseases that cause progressive renal insufficiency behave in a predictable manner, acceleration is sometimes seen for no apparent reason. This phenomenon is most often seen in chronic glomerular disease, in particular IgA nephropathy, MPGN, and membranous nephropathy.

Staging the chronic renal failure and preparation renal replacement therapy

Despite all attempts to optimize the management of CRF, a substantial majority of patients with CRF will progress relentlessly towards ESRD. Certain milestones can be identified for the patient on the basis of the degree of renal impairment (Table 67.2).

At a clearance of < 50 mL/min, prophylaxis against secondary hyperparathyroidism should be started: dietary phosphate restriction and prescription of oral phosphate binders and 1α-hydroxyvitamin D_3 or 1,25-dihydroxyvitamin D. Immunization against hepatitis B should be arranged.

At < 20 mL/min, description and counseling on the choice of RRT should be provided and, if HD is to be the first option, natural vascular access should be fashioned. The workup for renal transplantation either for the cadaveric donor waiting list or from a living related donor should be arranged. It is important to activate transplant plans when the clearance is < 10 mL/min (so-called pre-emptive transplantation) since there is increasing evidence of improved outcome with this approach[24].

Symptomatic patients and those with refractory hypertension, hyperphosphatemia, and hyperkalemia should be started on dialysis. Diabetics often need an even earlier start to dialysis (see Chapter 34) but others may be well enough to wait until the clearance falls to below 5 mL/min. The case for starting dialysis early i.e., when GFR is ~15 mL/min is not strong[25].

Continuous clinical assessment is required in the 'low clearance' clinic to ensure management of CRF is optimal and RRT is instituted at the right time. To ensure this, a number of routine questions should be addressed at each clinic assessment (Table 67.6).

SURGERY IN THE PATIENT WITH CHRONIC RENAL FAILURE

Surgery, often complex, is being undertaken in a greater number of patients with pre-existing chronic renal impairment for conditions unrelated to renal failure. These patients also require procedures related to the complications of renal failure and the provision of RRT, for example vascular access operations, parathyroid surgery, and renal transplantation.

The perioperative period is particularly hazardous for the patient with CRF, and close liaison between nephrologist, surgeon, and anesthetist is required to optimize care.

Preoperative assessment

Modification of pre- and postoperative management will depend on the severity of renal failure. A decline in GFR of

Chronic Renal Failure and the Uremic Syndrome

Continuing assessment of the patient with advanced renal failure
Renal function
Is it worse?
If so is it at the predicted level? - use the 1/creatinine plot (see Fig. 67.4)
If not are there exacerbating factors (see Table 67.5)
Should dialysis be started?
Are there uremic symptoms?
Pericarditis
Fluid overload
Resistant hypertension
Hyperkalemia
Uncompensated metabolic acidosis
Declining intellectual function
Should access be created or transplantation planned?
Supportive treatment
Can salt, potassium, and fluid balance be improved by diet or diuretics?
Is the phosphate controlled?
Is the dose of vitamin D analog appropriate?
Should epoetin be prescribed?
Are nutritional supplements needed?
Does the patient need counseling?

Table 67.6 Continuing assessment of the patient with chronic renal failure. Questions to be posed in the clinic when reviewing the patient.

5–10 mL/min, which might easily arise during apparently uncomplicated surgery, will have different consequences in patients with mild or severe renal failure.

Volume status

The aim is for the patient to go to the operating room 'euvolemic' to avoid, on the one hand, the risk of pulmonary edema and, on the other hand, major falls in blood pressure during induction of anesthesia or after brisk intraoperative bleeding (particularly common as a result of uremic autonomic neuropathy). Because patients with renal disease have a limited capacity to regulate their salt and water excretion, they are particularly liable to imbalances in either direction.

Cardiovascular disease

Attention should be directed to the detection and assessment of coronary and hypertensive heart disease, which are so common in patients with renal disease, and to occult valvular disease, which may decompensate under anesthesia. Silent coronary disease must always be considered, especially in young diabetics.

Hypertension

Antihypertensive drugs should be maintained during surgery unless intercurrent illness has produced severe hypotension. This is particularly important with β-blockers because their abrupt withdrawal may cause rebound phenomena, and because they reduce the incidence of arrhythmias and myocardial ischemia under anesthesia.

Anemia

Anemia is usually well tolerated, except in patients with coexisting ischemic heart disease. It is important to recall that in the era before the availability of epoetin major surgery was performed in patients with hemoglobin levels as low as 6 g/dL. A preoperative hemoglobin in the range 8–10 g/dL will provide a greater safety margin in the event of hemorrhage and itself improves hemostasis. Blood should always be cross-matched for any procedure during which a brisk hemorrhage is possible and, if the surgical indication is not immediate, patients should have transfusion to a hemoglobin of over 10 g/dL. In the presence of severe coronary artery disease, it may be appropriate to attain a higher target hemoglobin before elective surgery.

Potassium

The risk of cardiotoxicity is very high when serum potassium rises above 7 mmol/L. Minor surgery in patients with moderate CRF can proceed if the serum potassium is < 6 mmol/L whereas in dialysis recipients undergoing major surgery a preoperative serum potassium of < 4.5 mmol/L should be the aim. Patients should undergo dialysis prior to surgery, but because of arrhythmias and hemodynamic instability immediately after dialysis, an interval of a few hours should be allowed before induction of anesthesia. Avoidance of hyperkalemia is vital and can sometimes be difficult, even in patients with only mild renal disease. In dialysis recipients, serum potassium must be measured before the dialysis session ends and should be reduced below 4.5 mmol/L. In dialysis patients known to have difficulty in maintaining potassium balance, dialysis on two consecutive days before surgery is a wise precaution.

Coagulopathy

Uremic coagulopathy is usually corrected by adequate dialysis preoperatively; it is generally minimized when urea is below 20 mmol/L (BUN < 56 mg/dL). If urgent surgery prevents adequate preoperative dialysis or the bleeding risk is especially high, the bleeding time should be checked and corrected with cryoprecipitate and desmopressin (see Chapter 71).

Anesthetic management

Modifications of anesthetic technique and drug prescription will depend on the severity of renal failure, the presence or absence of disease in other organs, and the type of surgery. If the patient has a functioning arteriovenous fistula, it should be covered or clearly marked to ensure it is never inadvertently cannulated. Anesthesia colleagues should also be reminded never to use forearm veins, particularly the cephalic vein, for intravenous infusions, because of the risk of damage by cannulation to these potential sites for subsequent vascular access.

Premedication and analgesia

The choice of premedication should take account of the delayed gastric emptying that is common in patients with renal failure, particularly those with diabetes mellitus with autonomic neuropathy. Premedication with agents such as metoclopramide may be helpful in reducing the risk of gastric aspiration. Opiate analgesia should be used with care as pharmacologically active metabolites are retained in renal failure and cause coma, respiratory depression, hypotension, and myoclonus. In particular, dosing schedules for patient-administered postoperative analgesia must be adjusted down to minimize the risk of opiate toxicity.

Monitoring

If substantial fluid or blood loss is expected, particularly in patients with known cardiovascular instability, the central venous pressure should be monitored. The blood pressure is best monitored using an automated sphygmomanometer; intra-arterial monitoring is rarely required, but if it is considered essential, the dorsalis pedis artery should be used to avoid damage to the radial artery, which may be required later for creation of vascular access. Where anemia and cardiorespiratory disease coexist, the use of pulse oximetry should be routine.

Induction of general anesthesia

Anesthesia may result in sudden hypotension requiring resuscitation with intravenous fluid or even pressor agents. Care must be taken to avoid overhydration, particularly in patients who have been on HD and in whom preservation of renal function is not an issue; excess fluid will require dialysis or hemofiltration for its removal. The risk of hypotension is also present during spinal and epidural analgesia, and in these circumstances it may be even more difficult to counter. Even in patients without renal disease, renal blood flow is usually reduced and autoregulation is impaired under surgical anesthesia. A variety of renal vasoconstrictor mechanisms contribute to this, including activation of the sympathetic nervous system and the renin–angiotensin system. An important defence is provided by the vasodilatory action of renal prostaglandins (PGI_2 and PGE_2). In patients with significant renal disease, this mechanism assumes greater importance and prostaglandin synthetase inhibitors should not be used in the perioperative period.

Postoperative care

The most serious, and potentially fatal, immediate postoperative complication is respiratory depression. With the use of modern muscle relaxants such as atracurium, which are rapidly cleared by mechanisms independent of renal function, the problem of recurarization because the action of muscle relaxants outlasts their antagonist should not occur. However, prolonged and excessive action of sedative and analgesic drugs and impaired gas exchange arising from undiagnosed pulmonary edema may lead to respiratory depression.

The action of most opiate analgesics is prolonged in renal failure. This is particularly striking for morphine and probably arises from retention of active metabolites such as morphine 6-glucuronide. Meperidine (pethidine) must also be avoided since its metabolite normeperidine may produce seizures and myoclonus. Fentanyl is usually the preferred opiate analgesic.

Fluid and electrolyte balance

The capacity to excrete a water load is already impaired and is aggravated during surgery when other factors such as

nonosmotic vasopressin release operate. Many patients with severe renal disease will be at risk of water intoxication from commonly prescribed postoperative regimens, which include 2–3 L of 5% dextrose/d. Since the precise limitations of renal compensation are difficult to predict, the problem can only be avoided by strict attention to fluid balance, corroborated by daily weighing of the patient and monitoring of the plasma sodium.

DRUG PRESCRIBING IN CHRONIC RENAL FAILURE

Special care must be taken with the use of all drugs, not only because their elimination may be slowed and their bioavailability altered in patients with renal failure but also because they may directly or indirectly reduce residual renal function. Before prescribing, it is prudent to ask whether these considerations apply and, if they do, whether prescription is essential, whether there is an alternative drug, and whether the dose needs to be modified.

Because the elimination of many drugs is dependent on renal function, the dose and frequency of administration must be changed in patients with renal failure. In a patient receiving maintenance dialysis, the mode of dialysis also has an important effect.

The principles of prescribing in renal failure are provided in Chapters 95 and 96. Drugs commonly used in patients with renal disease and which should be prescribed with special care are listed in Table 67.7. A more extensive list of information on dose modifications for drugs in renal failure is given in the Appendix to Chapter 96.

Pain relief in patients with chronic renal failure

The safest simple analgesic in chronic renal failure is acetaminophen (paracetamol). Unlike NSAIDs, (both COX1 and COX2 inhibitors) which can aggravate renal failure in people who rely on prostaglandin overdrive to maintain their GFR, acetaminophen does not cause renal failure. The recent epidemiological evidence suggesting that acetaminophen can also cause renal failure[26] is confounded by the fact that the high risk patients all took acetaminophen to avoid NSAIDs.

If acetaminophen does not provide enough analgesia the next stage is either acetaminophen-opioid combinations or NSAIDs. The risks of NSAIDs are that they may worsen pre-existing renal failure, hypertension and salt retention in those with cardiac failure. The risk is the same with COX1 and COX2 NSAIDs. There is no good evidence that any one NSAID is safer in renal failure than another. The first choice in chronic renal failure is an acetaminophen-opioid combination rather than NSAID, although in patients on ESRD both are valuable.

The opioid component may be excreted through the kidney, and if the metabolites are active, as they are for instance with codeine, then a given dose will give greater than expected analgesia. This will cause no problem if dose is titrated to clinical effect, rather than by the clock to a predetermined dosing schedule, when the result can be a comatose patient. NSAIDs can of course be used safely in patients already established on dialysis in whom considerations of renal effects are irrelevant. If the acetaminophen-opioid combinations do not provide

Prescribing in chronic renal failure		
Drug group or indication	Precaution	Side effect
Antimicrobials		
	Reduce dose and frequency	Ototoxic/nephrotoxic
Aminoglycosides	Reduce dose	Ototoxic/nephrotoxic
Glycopeptides (teicoplanin, vancomycin)		
β-lactams Cephalosporins,	Reduce dose	Neurotoxic at very high
Penicillins, carbapenems		concentrations
Fluoroquinolones (e.g., Ciprofloxacin)	Reduce dose	
Tetracyclines		
Cotrimoxazole	Avoid except doxycycline	
	Reduce dose	
Ethambutol		
erythromycin	Reduce dose	Optic nerve damage
	Reduce dose	Deafness, particularly in elderly
Nitrofurantoin	Reduce dose	patients
	Avoid	Peripheral neuropathy
Antivirals	Reduce dose	
Acyclovir	Reduce dose	Neurotoxic (fits)
Antifungals	Reduce dose	
Amphotericin B		Hypokalemia, tubular
Fluconazole	Reduce dose	dysfunction
Antimalarials		
Chloroquine	Reduce dose	
Quinine	Reduce dose	
Proguanil	Reduce dose	Megaloblastic anemia
Antihypertensives/cardiac		
ACEI	Reduce dose	Hyperkalemia
β-blockers	Reduce dose or frequency	Excess beta blockade
Digoxin		Digoxin toxicity
Analgesics		
Opioids	Reduce dose frequency	CNS depression
	Avoid pethidine	
Diabetes		
Sulphonylureas	Reduce dose	Hypoglycemia
Biguanides (metformin)	Avoid	Lactic acidosis
Gout and arthritis		
Allopurinol	Reduce dose	Unnecessary
Colchicine	Avoid prolonged use	Leukopenia
NSAIDs	Avoid	Reduce GFR
Anesthetics		
Pancuronium and gallamine	Do not use	Delayed excretion prolongs
		muscle paralysis
Psychotropics		
Lithium	Monitor plasma concentrations	Toxicity
Diuretics		
Frusemide	Increase dose as GFR falls	
	Slow i.v. administration of high doses	Ototoxicity
	Avoid	Hyperkalemia
Potassium sparing		Acidosis
(spironolactone and amiloride)		
Acetazolamide		
Cytotoxics/immunosuppressives		
Melphelan	Reduce dose in severe CRF	Excess effect
Cyclosporine	Avoid	Nephrotoxic/aggravates
		hypertension
Cations		
Bismuth	Avoid	Accumulates
Magnesium	Avoid	Accumulates
Sodium (Sodium bicarbonate)	Avoid	Hypertension
Anticonvulsants		
Carbemazepine	Reduce dose	Sedation

Table 67.7 Prescribing in chronic renal failure. Drugs in common use in patients with renal disease that should be used with caution and may require dose adjustment.

enough analgesia then stronger opioids may be needed. There is no advantage to meperidine (pethidine) compared with other strong opioids and there is this the specific disadvantage that the metabolite normeperidine (norpethidine) can accumulate and is a CNS toxin. The higher the cumulative dose the higher the risk of problems. Buprenorphine (sublingual or by injection) does not have these problems, and is a safer alternative for long-term use in chronic renal failure. Morphine, diamorphine, codeine and the other morphine derivatives also have an active metabolite, morphine-6-glucuronide, which will accumulate if renal function is impaired, and care should be taken to dose by effect rather than by the clock.

Greater analgesia can be achieved if acetaminophen and opioid are used together, and adding in a NSAID will further increase analgesic power. The strategy is to move up the analgesic ladder progressively by adding rather than replacing drugs, to minimize total doses of each component.

If the pains are neuropathic, then antidepressants such as amitryptiline, anticonvulsants such as carbamazepine, or gabapentin may be needed, since neuropathic pain will rarely respond well to conventional analgesia. If the patient has severe pain which is primarily provoked by movement, then conventional pain killers may not be sufficient, and antidepressants, anticonvulsants or anesthetic injections may be needed.

The treatment of acute arthritis, for example gout, is a real challenge in patients with chronic renal failure. If NSAIDs cannot be risked then a short course of colchicine 500 µg, 3-hourly (up to 6 mg) should be prescribed. Diarrhea is a predictable side effect. If this is intolerable a 5-day course of 20 mg daily prednisolone is an alternative.

MANAGEMENT OF TERMINAL UREMIA

There will be patients for whom dialysis is inappropriate or who either choose not to start or to discontinue treatment. Because, intuitively, one would predict that instituting dialysis in a patient with renal failure and other comorbid conditions should result in some improvement by ameliorating at least one element of their clinical condition, it is very hard not to start. There are those who argue that there is no harm done by starting because treatment can always be stopped or the patient will die despite dialysis. However, withdrawing dialysis or dying while on treatment are traumatic for both the patient's family and staff. If possible, one should discuss the option of not starting before treatment is actually needed. The patient will need to know what the treatment can achieve and at what cost – access, travel to dialysis, restrictions and complications. If one takes the view that dialysis is a treatment offered to allow the patient to continue living with a reasonable quality of life as opposed to delaying death in the short term, dialysis will not be offered to patients with other life limiting conditions. Certainly one could argue that it should not be started when survival beyond 3 months outside of hospital is unlikely. Indeed, at least 10% of deaths in dialysis programs follow withdrawal of treatment. The ethical and legal issues are complex and require that the patient makes the decision not to start or to discontinue when fully informed and able to do so. Withdrawal of dialysis is discussed further in Chapter 75.

Properly managed death from uremia is peaceful and free of suffering. It is important to ensure that the patient has peace of mind, i.e., they are comfortable with the decision and that their family members are understanding and supportive. They will be comforted to know that their doctor respects their decision. There are several distressing symptoms which need to be controlled. The first is breathlessness from pulmonary edema and acidosis. This is best controlled with a morphine infusion. The second is nausea and anorexia. These can be helped with regular chlorpromazine 25 mg q.i.d.; ondansetron is also effective. Food and fluid should be offered in small palatable helpings and no pressure to eat exerted on the patient. The mouth can become dry and crusted from mouth breathing and will smell foul from the uremic saliva. Regular mouth washes and gum care will help. Pruritus is managed by keeping the skin cool, and soft with emollients. The patient may not be aware of myoclonic jerks, but these may distress the family so benzodiazepines, such as clonazepam, can be prescribed.

REFERENCES

1. Walker R. General management of end-stage renal disease. BMJ. 1997;315:1429–32.
2. National Kidney Foundation. DOQI kidney disease outcome quality initiative. Am J Kidney Dis. 2002;39:S1–S266.
3. U.S. Renal Data System. *USRDS 2001 Annual Data Report: Atlas of End-Stage Renal Disease in the United States.* Bethesda, MD: National Institutes of Diabetes and Digestive and Kidney Diseases; 2001.
4. UK Renal Registry. UK Renal Registry Report. In: Ansell D., Feest TG, eds. *UK Renal Registry*. Bristol, UK: UK Renal Registry; 2001.
5. ANZDATA Registry. Australia and New Zealand Dialysis and Transplant Registry Report. In: Russ G R, ed. *ANZDATA Registry.* Adelaide, South Australia: ANZDATA; 2001.
6. Iseki K, Tozawa M, Iseki C, et al. Demographic trends in the Okinawa Dialysis Study (OKIDS) registry (1971–2000). Kidney Int. 2002;61:668–75.
7. Roderick P, Jones C, Tomson C, Mason J. Late referral for dialysis: improving the management of chronic renal disease. QJM. 2002; 95:363–70.
8. Innes A, Rowe PA, Burden RP, Morgan AG. Early deaths on renal replacement therapy: the need for early nephrological referral. Nephrol Dial Transplant. 1992;7:467–71.
9. Jungers P, Zingraff J, Albouze G, et al. Late referral to maintenance dialysis: detrimental consequences. Nephrol Dial Transplant. 1993;8:1089–93.
10. Klahr S, Levey AS, Beck GJ, et al. The effects of dietary protein restriction and blood pressure control on the progression of chronic renal disease. N Engl J Med. 1994;330:877–84.
11. National Health and Nutritional Examination Survey. The Sixth Report of the Joint National Committee on prevention, detection, evaluation and treatment of high blood pressure. Arch Intern Med. 1997;157:2413–15.
12. Roth D, Smith RD, Schulman G, et al. Effect of recombinant human erythropoietin on renal function in and chronic renal failure predialysis patients. Am J Kidney Dis. 1994;24:777–84.
13. Kanis JA. The use of alfacalcidol in the prevention of bone disease in early renal failure. Nephrol Dial Transplant. 1995;10(Suppl 4):23–8.

14. Alpern RJ, Sakhaee K. Clinical spectrum of chronic metabolic acidosis. Homeostatic mechanisms produce significant morbidity. Am J Kidney Dis. 1997;29:291–302.

15. Ponticelli C, Bencini PL. Pruritus in dialysis patients: a neglected problem. Nephrol Dial Transplant. 1995;10:2174–6.

16. Peer G, Kivity S, Agami O, et al. Randomised crossover trial of naltrexone in uraemic pruritus. Lancet. 1996;348:1552–4.

17. Peces R, Enriquez-de Salamanca R, Fontanellas A, et al. Successful treatment of haemodialysis-related porphyria cutanea tarda with erythropoietin. Nephrol Dial Transplant. 1994;9:433–5.

18. Armangol NE, Amenós AC, Illa MB, et al. Autonomic nervous system and adrenergic receptors in chronic hypotensive haemodialysis patients. Nephrol Dial Transplant. 1997;12:939–44.

19. Rosas SE, Wasserstein A, Kobrin S, Feldman HI. Preliminary observations of sildenafil treatment for erectile dysfunction in dialysis patients. Am J Kidney Dis. 2001;37(1):134–7.

20. Descamps-Latscha B, Herbelin A, Nguyen A, et al. The immune system in end-stage renal disease. Semin Nephrol. 1994; 14:253–60.

21. Rangel MC, Coronado VG, Euler GL, Strikas RA. Vaccine recommendations for patients on chronic dialysis. The Advisory Committee on Immunization Practices and the American Academy of Pediatrics. Semin Dial. 2000;13:101–7.

22. Buccianti G, Ravasi B, Cresseri D, et al. Cancer in patients on renal replacement therapy in Lombardy, Italy. Lancet. 1996; 347:59–60.

23. Ruggenenti P, Perna A, Gherardi G, et al. Renal function and requirement for dialysis in chronic nephropathy patients on long-term ramipril: REIN follow-up trial. Gruppo Italiano di Studi Epidemiologici in Nefrologia (GISEN). Ramipril Efficacy in Nephropathy. Lancet. 1998; 352:1252–56.

24. Wolfe RA, Ashby VB, Milford EL, et al. Comparison of mortality in all patients on dialysis, patients on dialysis awaiting transplantation, and recipients of a first cadaveric transplant. N Engl J Med. 1999;341:1725–30.

25. Korevaar TC, Jansen MAM, Dekker FW, et al. Bossuyt PMM, from the Netherlands Co-operative Study on the Adequacy of Dialysis Study Group. When to initiate dialysis: effect of proposed US guidelines on survival. Lancet. 2001;358:1046 50.

26. Fored CM, Ejerblad E, Lindblad P, et al. Acetaminophen, aspirin, and chronic renal failure. N Engl J Med. 2001;345:1801–8.

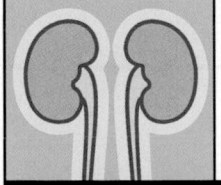

Chapter 68

Bone and Mineral Metabolism in Chronic Renal Failure

Esther A González and Kevin J Martin

DEFINITION

Disturbances of mineral metabolism are common if not ubiquitous during the course of chronic renal disease and lead to serious and debilitating complications unless these abnormalities are addressed and treated. The spectrum of disorders includes abnormal concentrations of mineral ions in serum (calcium, phosphorus and magnesium) and disorders of parathyroid hormone (parathormone (PTH)) and vitamin D metabolism. These abnormalities, as well as the presence of other factors related to the uremic state, affect the skeleton and result in the complex disorders of bone known as renal osteodystrophy. The spectrum of skeletal abnormalities seen in renal osteodystrophy (Fig. 68.1) ranges from abnormally high to abnormally low bone turnover states and includes:

- osteitis fibrosa, a manifestation of hyperparathyroidism characterized by increased osteoclast and osteoblast activity and peritrabecular fibrosis;
- osteomalacia, a manifestation of defective mineralization of newly formed osteoid most often caused by aluminum deposition;
- adynamic bone disease, a condition characterized by abnormally low bone turnover;
- osteopenia or osteoporosis;
- combinations of these abnormalities termed mixed renal osteodystrophy;

- other abnormalities with skeletal manifestations; for example, chronic acidosis and β_2-microglobulin (β_2-M) amyloidosis (see Chapter 72).

EPIDEMIOLOGY

The prevalence of the various types of renal bone disease in patients with endstage renal failure (ESRD) is illustrated in Figure 68.2[1]. In patients on hemodialysis, osteitis fibrosa and the adynamic bone lesion occur with almost equal frequency. In contrast, in patients on peritoneal dialysis, the adynamic bone lesion clearly predominates. Osteomalacia represents only a small fraction of cases in either group but is more common in certain ethnic groups, particularly Indo-Asians. This distribution of bony abnormalities represents considerable change from that identified in the late 1970s, reflecting our increased knowledge of their pathogenesis and changes in therapeutic approaches. It is important to emphasize that the abnormalities of the skeleton are not restricted to patients with ESRD, and abnormal bone histology occurs in patients with chronic renal failure (CRF) relatively early in the course

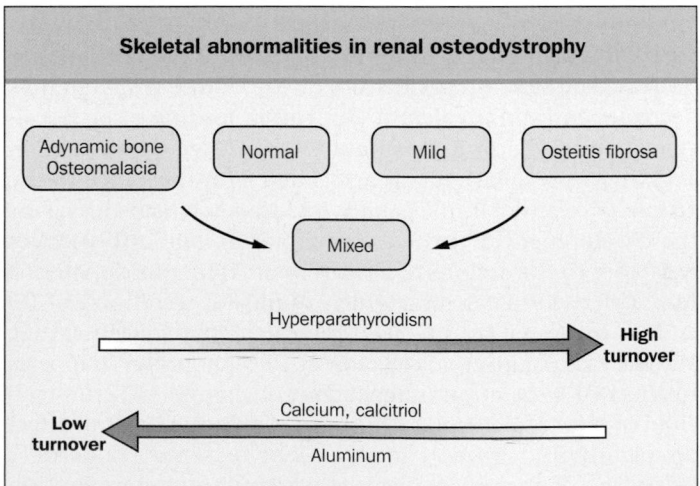

Figure 68.1 The spectrum of renal osteodystrophy. The range of skeletal abnormalities in renal bone disease encompasses syndromes with both high and low bone turnover.

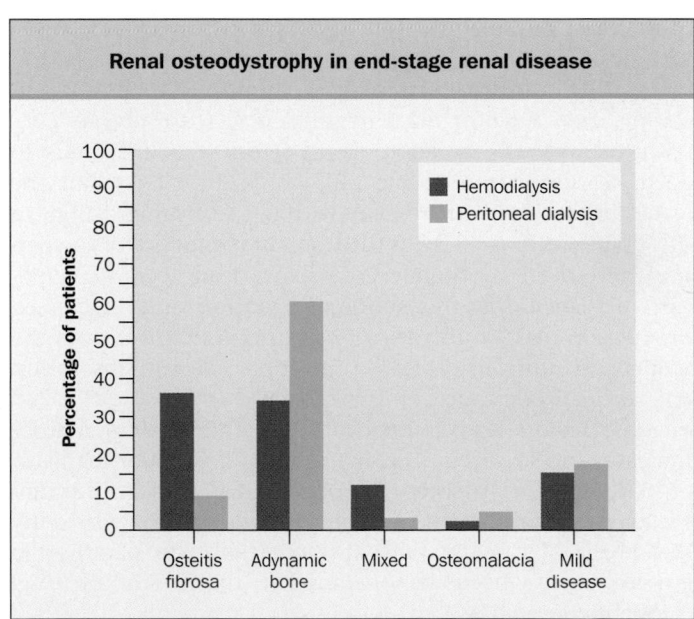

Figure 68.2 Prevalence of renal osteodystrophy in patients with end-stage renal disease. The pattern of renal osteodystrophy varied with the dialysis modality in a group of patients on hemodialysis ($n = 117$) or peritoneal dialysis ($n = 142$).

of renal insufficiency, and while manifestations of hyperparathyroidism have been clearly demonstrated, the adynamic lesion has also been found in patients before dialysis.

PATHOGENESIS

Several biochemical and hormonal abnormalities that are encountered during the course of renal insufficiency have been identified as important pathogenetic factors in the development of renal bone disease. Attention to these abnormalities forms the basis for prevention and therapy. The major factors that are operative early in the course of renal failure may change as renal disease progresses and other factors assume a predominant role. Similarly, the predominance of one particular pathogenetic mechanism over another may contribute to the heterogeneity of bone disorders that have been identified.

Osteitis fibrosa: hyperparathyroidism

Elevated levels of PTH in blood and hyperplasia of the parathyroid glands are seen early in the course of renal insufficiency. While, under normal circumstances, the level of free calcium in blood is the principal determinant of PTH secretion, during the course of renal disease, several metabolic disturbances contribute to alter the regulation of the secretion of PTH.

Abnormalities of calcium metabolism

There are three main body pools of calcium: the bony skeleton (mineral component), the intracellular pool (mostly protein bound) and the extracellular pool. The calcium in the extracellular pool is in continuous exchange with that of bone and cells and is altered by diet and excretion. Approximately half of it is protein bound; the remainder is free calcium ions in solution (free Ca^{2+}) and it is this portion that is biologically active. Calcium metabolism depends upon the close interaction of two hormonal systems: PTH and vitamin D. Perturbations of both of these systems occur during the course of renal insufficiency, with adverse consequences on the skeleton. Total serum calcium tends to decrease during the course of renal insufficiency but the levels of free calcium remain within the normal range in most patients (Fig. 68.3)[2] as the result of compensatory hyperparathyroidism. A number of factors lead towards hypocalcemia including phosphorus retention and decreased production of 1,25-dihydroxyvitamin D (calcitriol) from the kidney, resulting in decreased intestinal calcium absorption and skeletal resistance to the calcemic action of PTH. All of these factors lead to hypocalcemia unless compensatory increases in PTH occur. Because calcium is a major regulator of PTH secretion, persistent hypocalcemia is a powerful stimulus for the development of hyperparathyroidism. Persistently low levels of calcium may also contribute to parathyroid growth, as has been demonstrated in recent studies using calcimimetic agents.

Abnormalities of phosphate metabolism

With progressive renal insufficiency, there is increased phosphorus retention by the failing kidney. However,

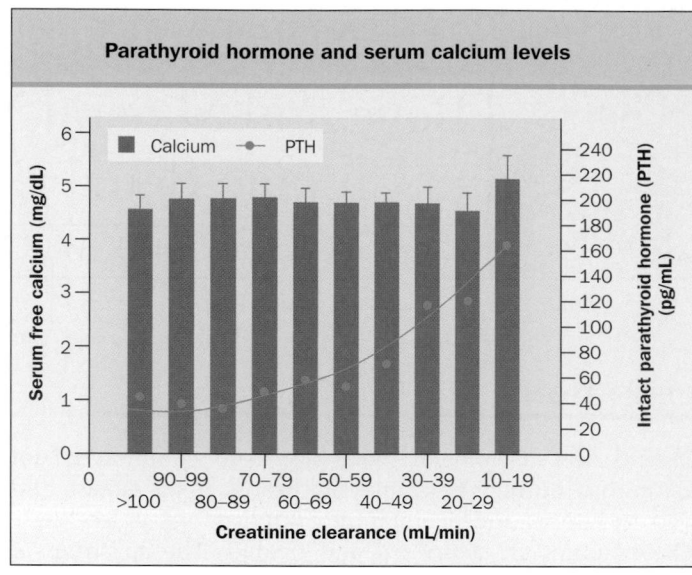

Figure 68.3 Ionized calcium and parathyroid hormone (PTH) levels in chronic renal failure. Levels of ionized calcium are maintained in advancing renal failure by progressive increases in PTH.

hyperphosphatemia does not become evident until the glomerular filtration rate (GFR) has decreased to < 20% of normal. Until that late stage in the course of CRF, compensatory hyperparathyroidism results in increased phosphaturia, maintaining serum phosphorus levels in the normal range.

It was originally proposed that the retention of phosphorus as a result of the decreased ability of the kidney to excrete the filtered phosphate load led to a decrease in serum free calcium, which in turn stimulated the secretion of PTH. Thus a new steady state was achieved in which serum phosphate was restored to normal at the expense of a sustained high level of PTH. This cycle was repeated as renal function declined until sustained and severe hyperparathyroidism was present[3]. Phosphate restriction in proportion to the decrement in GFR could effectively prevent the development of hyperparathyroidism, providing support for the role of phosphorus retention in its pathogenesis. It now appears that this is but one mechanism by which phosphate retention may lead to hyperparathyroidism (Fig. 68.4). Phosphate retention also leads to decreased production of calcitriol by the kidney, which in turn decreases intestinal calcium absorption leading to hypocalcemia, thus providing the stimulus for PTH secretion. In addition, hyperphosphatemia is associated with resistance to the actions of calcitriol in the parathyroid glands, which also favors the development of hyperparathyroidism, and also induces resistance to the actions of PTH in bone. Hyperphosphatemia may lower serum calcium, which stimulates secretion of PTH and, as suggested by studies using calcimimetic agents, may also increase parathyroid cell growth. Phosphorus *per se* appears to affect PTH secretion independent of changes in serum calcium or serum calcitriol[4,5]. Phosphorus may also have an effect on parathyroid growth independent of serum calcium[6,7]. Regardless of the mechanism by which phosphate retention causes hyperparathyroidism, it has been clearly demonstrated that restricting dietary phosphate in proportion to the decrease in GFR can prevent the development of hyperparathyroidism.

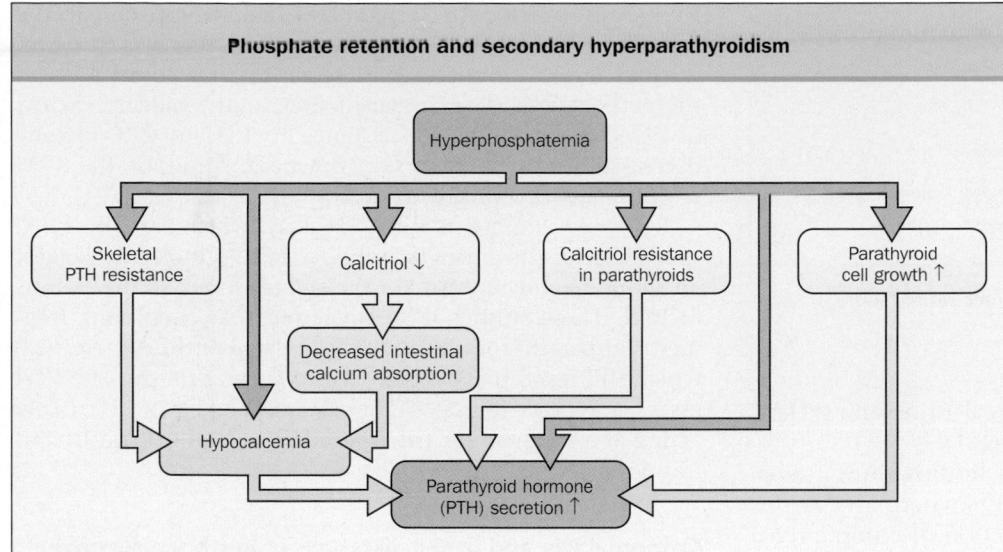

Figure 68.4 Role of phosphorus retention in the pathogenesis of secondary hyperparathyroidism. Hyperphosphatemia stimulates parathyroid hormone (PTH) secretion indirectly by inducing hypocalcemia, skeletal resistance to PTH, low levels of calcitriol and calcitriol resistance. Hyperphosphatemia also has direct effects on the parathyroid gland to increase PTH secretion and parathyroid cell growth.

Abnormalities of vitamin D metabolism

The conversion of 25-hydroxyvitamin D to its active metabolite 1,25-dihydroxyvitamin D occurs in the kidney by the enzyme 1α-hydroxylase. The kidney is the major site for calcitriol production and as functional renal mass decreases during the course of renal disease, calcitriol production falls. Plasma calcitriol concentrations may be normal in patients with mild-to-moderate renal failure; however, PTH levels are often elevated and, because PTH is a major stimulator of calcitriol production, normal levels of calcitriol may therefore be inappropriately low. Decreased production of calcitriol contributes to the pathogenesis of hyperparathyroidism by both direct and indirect mechanisms (Fig. 68.5). Calcitriol has several direct effects on the parathyroid gland. Low levels of calcitriol directly affect the transcription of the pre-pro-PTH gene[8,9] releasing the gene for PTH from suppression by the vitamin D receptor and allowing increased PTH secretion. In many tissues, vitamin D regulates its own receptor by positive feedback; the vitamin D receptor content is decreased in parathyroid tissue in CRF, which is consistent with the idea that low levels of calcitriol may be associated with decreased levels of vitamin D receptor. Conversely, administration of calcitriol might be expected to increase the vitamin D receptor content in the parathyroid glands coincident with the suppression of PTH secretion. Studies *in vitro* have shown that calcitriol is a negative growth regulator of parathyroid cells; therefore, calcitriol deficiency in CRF may facilitate parathyroid cell proliferation. Other direct consequences of low levels of calcitriol on parathyroid gland function that contribute to the pathogenesis of secondary hyperparathyroidism include increasing the setpoint for calcium-regulated PTH secretion and, possibly, decreasing levels of calcium receptors.

Low levels of calcitriol may also promote the development of hyperparathyroidism indirectly by two mechanisms. First, since calcitriol is a major regulator of intestinal calcium absorption, decreases in calcitriol production as renal function decreases can lead to progressive reductions in intestinal absorption of calcium, leading to hypocalcemia and stimulation of PTH release. Second, low levels of calcitriol have been implicated in skeletal resistance to the calcemic actions of PTH, which may also contribute to the development of hyperparathyroidism.

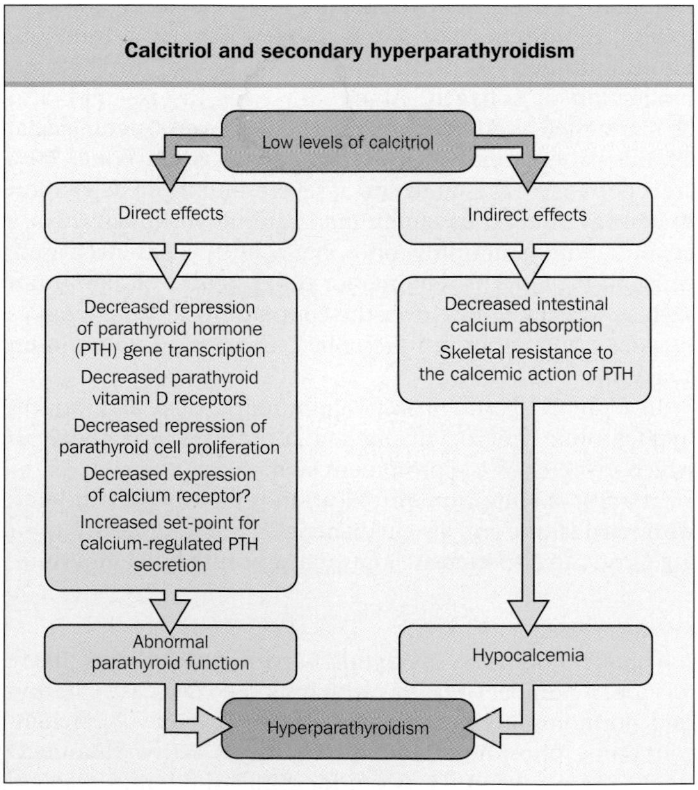

Figure 68.5 Role of low levels of calcitriol in the pathogenesis of secondary hyperparathyroidism.

Abnormalities of parathyroid gland function

There are intrinsic abnormalities in parathyroid gland function in the course of renal insufficiency in addition to those

Chronic Renal Failure and the Uremic Syndrome

Parathyroid abnormalities in chronic renal failure

Parathyroid gland hyperplasia: diffuse, nodular

Decreased expression of vitamin D receptors

Decreased expression of calcium receptors

Increased set-point of calcium-regulated PTH secretion

Table 68.1 Parathyroid abnormalities in chronic renal failure.

---

caused by hypocalcemia, low levels of calcitriol, and skeletal resistance to the actions of PTH (Table 68.1).

Parathyroid hyperplasia is an early finding during renal insufficiency. In experimental models, hyperplasia begins within a few days following the induction of chronic renal disease. The factors responsible are unclear, but parathyroid gland hyperplasia can be prevented by dietary phosphate restriction or by the use of calcimimetic agents[7,10]. Resected parathyroids from patients with severe hyperparathyroidism have nodular areas throughout the gland, which have been shown to represent monoclonal expansions of parathyroid cells[11]. The factors involved in the genesis of these monoclonal nodules are unclear, but the biologic implications are profound. Within these nodules, there is decreased expression of vitamin D receptors as well as calcium receptors[12–14]. It is not certain whether the decreased expression of these receptors is a cause or a consequence of the monoclonal transformation. However, it is clear that, in the absence of receptors for vitamin D or for calcium, efforts to regulate the secretion of these enlarged hyperplastic glands may be difficult.

Considerable advances in our understanding of the regulation of PTH secretion by calcium have followed the cloning of the parathyroid calcium receptor[15]. This receptor is involved in the mechanism for calcium-regulated PTH secretion. Parathyroid glands from hyperparathyroid subjects showed decreased expression of the calcium receptor at the mRNA and at the protein level[12,13]. Consequently, with decreased expression of the calcium receptor, altered calcium-regulated PTH secretion might be expected. Increased concentrations of calcium are required *in vitro* to suppress PTH release from the parathyroid cells of uremic patients compared to those of normal controls. Thus, the setpoint for the concentration of calcium required to decrease PTH release by 50% appears to be increased. Controversy remains whether this altered set-point is only a late finding in the abnormally functioning parathyroid glands associated with severe CRF. Decreased levels of calcitriol may play a role in this alteration of the setpoint in that administration of calcitriol to patients with ESRD has been shown to change the setpoint for PTH secretion towards normal.

Abnormal skeletal response to parathyroid hormone

Many studies have shown that in patients with renal insufficiency there is an impaired response of serum calcium to the administration of PTH and a delay in the recovery from induced hypocalcemia in the presence of larger increments in PTH levels. In CRF, the skeleton is somehow resistant to the calcemic actions of PTH, and the resultant decrease in serum calcium levels stimulates PTH secretion and contributes to the pathogenesis of secondary hyperparathyroidism. Factors involved in the skeletal resistance to PTH in CRF include decreased levels of calcitriol, downregulation of the PTH receptor and phosphorus retention.

Recent developments with PTH assays which have increased specificity for the entire 84 amino acid PTH molecule suggest an additional mechanism for skeletal resistance to the actions of PTH. These studies have suggested that circulating fragments of parathyroid hormone, truncated at the N-terminus, which still react in the older, second generation two-site PTH assays, may serve to oppose the calcemic actions of PTH, likely acting at a receptor for the C-terminal region of parathyroid hormone[16].

Osteomalacia and other disorders of low bone turnover

Because decreased levels of calcitriol are uniformly present in patients with advanced CRF, and yet osteomalacia is a relatively infrequent finding, defective mineralization of bone cannot be attributed solely to calcitriol deficiency.

Aluminum

Severe osteomalacia in patients with renal insufficiency has often been attributed to the accumulation of aluminum, which occurs mainly through the use of aluminum-containing phosphate binders. In recent years, the use of these binders has decreased markedly as the toxicity of aluminum has become recognized and, concomitantly, osteomalacia is now seen much less frequently[17]. In addition to impairing mineralization, aluminum toxicity can decrease osteoblast function, resulting in decreased cell proliferation as well as decreased production of collagen. Aluminum bone disease may also be manifested as adynamic bone without overt osteomalacia. Of the patients classified as having adynamic bone, 60% are reported to have moderate or severe aluminum deposition in bone as assessed by aluminum staining[1]. Although the use of aluminum-containing phosphate binders has decreased, constant vigilance is required for other sources of aluminum such as water supplies, over-the-counter medications such as sucralfate and other self-prescribed antacids and aluminum cookware.

In addition to osteomalacia, aluminum toxicity also induces hypochromic, microcytic anemia and causes a dementia in which myoclonus is a prominent sign.

The risk of aluminum intoxication is increased in children with renal failure and also in diabetics. Citrate administration/ ingestion can also increase intestinal absorption of aluminum.

Adynamic bone

Adynamic bone has a complex pathogenesis and likely includes a number of factors which serve to decrease parathyroid hormone levels in serum, such as the use of calcium-containing phosphate binders, the use of active vitamin D sterols, high calcium dialysate for CAPD fluid, and diabetes (Fig. 68.6)[18]. In addition, there are a number of factors in uremia which probably act directly on bone to decrease bone

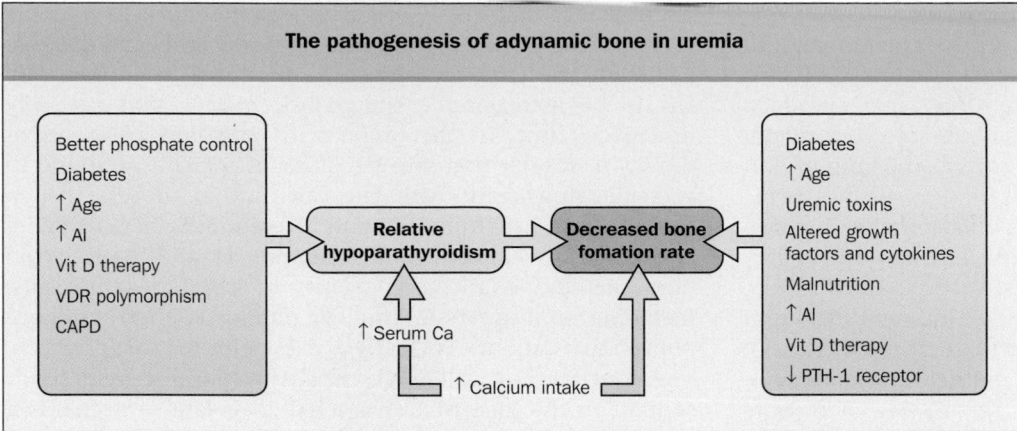

Figure 68.6 Pathogenesis of adynamic bone disease. (Adapted with permission[18].)

formation rate, such as diabetes, circulating uremic toxins, altered levels of growth factors and cytokines, malnutrition, vitamin D metabolites, and downregulation of PTH-1 receptor, and possibly direct effects of C-terminal PTH fragments on bone acting at the C-terminal PTH receptor. The clinical consequences of adynamic bone are somewhat uncertain, but appear to be associated with increased fracture risk and increased mortality. In addition, it is possible that the consequences of adynamic bone are extraskeletal. Thus, Figure 68.7 indicates a hypothetical scheme showing the possibility that when bone turnover is abnormally low, calcium and phosphate cannot be deposited in bone. Therefore, this may facilitate deposition in extraskeletal sites, and potentially contribute to vascular calcification.

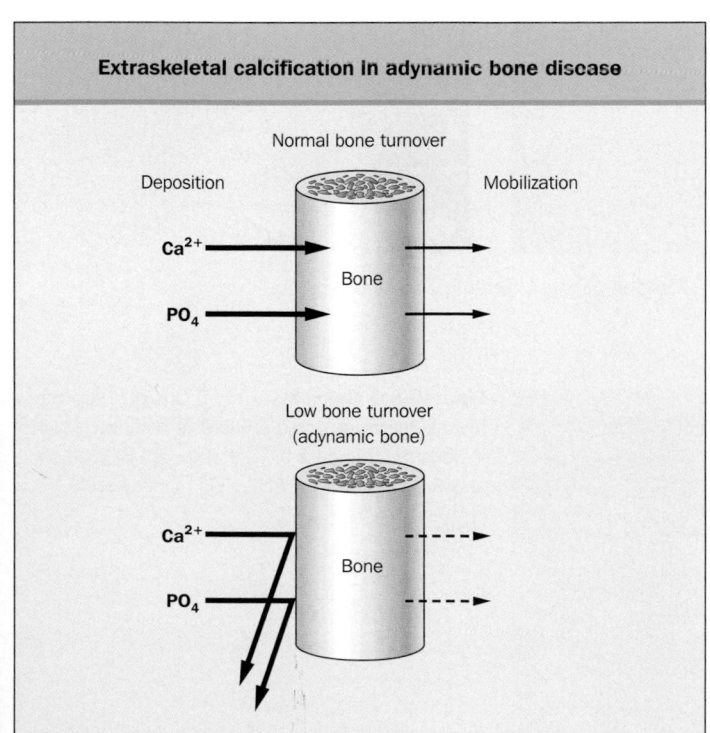

Figure 68.7 Bone turnover in adynamic bone disease. Reduced bone turnover leads to increased extraskeletal calcification.

CLINICAL MANIFESTATIONS OF RENAL OSTEODYSTROPHY

Musculoskeletal symptoms

Clinical manifestations of hyperparathyroidism and other forms of bone disease are usually nonspecific and are often preceded by biochemical or imaging abnormalities. In patients with advanced renal insufficiency who have severe bone disease, bone pain is a common manifestation. This is often nonspecific in nature and occurs in the lower back, hips and legs and is aggravated by weight-bearing. Acute, localized bone pain can also become manifest and may be suggestive of acute arthritis. Pain around joints may be caused by acute periarthritis, which is associated with periarticular deposition of calcium phosphate crystals, especially in patients who suffer from marked hyperphosphatemia. The symptoms may be confused clinically with gout or pseudo-gout and often respond to nonsteroidal anti-inflammatory agents (NSAIDs). The gradual onset of muscle weakness is also common in patients with ESRD. Many factors are probably involved in its pathogenesis, including hyperparathyroidism and abnormalities of vitamin D. An important differential diagnosis is the arthropathy associated with β_2-M amyloidosis (see Chapter 72).

Bone deformities are common in patients with severe hyperparathyroidism, particularly in children. In adults, deformities arise as a consequence of fractures, with the axial skeleton being most commonly affected. This can lead to kyphoscoliosis or chest wall deformities. Slipped epiphysis may occur in children and occasionally frank rachitic features are evident. Growth retardation is also common in children and, although some improvement has been shown with calcitriol, this has not been the universal finding. The use of growth hormone may have a role in maintaining normal growth in children.

Pruritus

Another troublesome symptom in patients with advanced renal failure is pruritus. This is especially common in patients on dialysis. Substantial or total improvement can follow parathyroidectomy. The mechanisms responsible for pruritus are not clear, but it is possibly related to calcium phosphate deposition in the skin. Parathyroidectomy should never be undertaken for pruritus alone, but only if there is also firm evidence of severe secondary hyperparathyroidism.

Chronic Renal Failure and the Uremic Syndrome

Metastatic calcification and calciphylaxis

Extraskeletal calcifications are frequently encountered in patients with advanced renal insufficiency and are aggravated by persistent elevation of the calcium-phosphate product. Most commonly, vascular calcifications are seen, but calcifications may also occur in other sites, such as the lung, and in periarticular areas (Fig. 68.8). Calciphylaxis, or calcific uremic arteriolopathy, is a severe form of vascular calcification and is found far less commonly in patients with chronic kidney disease than either arterial or cardiac valvular calcification. The syndrome is characterized by the development of painful nodules located in the lower extremities, trunk, buttocks, or other areas that then become mottled or violaceous, indurated and ultimately ulcerate (Fig. 68.9a). The more proximal lesions involving the upper thighs, buttocks and abdomen appear to be somewhat more common in recent times, and appear to be less likely associated with severe hyperparathyroidism compared to the peripheral lesions seen formerly, which were often associated with very high levels of parathyroid hormone. Biopsy of such lesions reveal calcification of the arteriolar walls of skin and muscle, with some fat necrosis, and an inflammatory infiltrate (Fig. 68.9b). While calciphylaxis most commonly occurs in patients on maintenance dialysis, it has also been described in patients with chronic kidney disease who have not yet begun dialysis. Although the true prevalence is unknown, it is generally felt to be increasing[19]. The pathogenesis is not precisely understood but, in the original investigation of this syndrome, it was felt that sensitized tissues appear to respond to a challenging agent with the calcification process, which then leads to inflammation and ulceration. Such sensitizing agents were believed to be vitamin D and parathyroid hormone and challenging agents included metallic salts, including iron dextran and egg white. A high calcium-phosphorus product is clearly a risk factor for calciphylaxis. The association of calciphylaxis with warfarin therapy lends support to the idea that an altered coagulation mechanism is present in these patients and, consistent with this, deficiencies of protein S and protein C have also been described. Therapy for this disorder is somewhat unsatisfactory, and the syndrome carries a high mortality. The principles of therapy are to reduce plasma concentration of phosphate, the avoidance of calcium-containing phosphate binders, the use of low calcium dialysate, and parathyroidectomy if PTH levels are high. In some cases, local benefit may be achieved with hyperbaric oxygen.

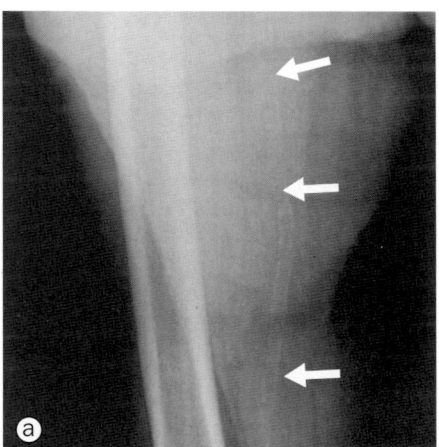
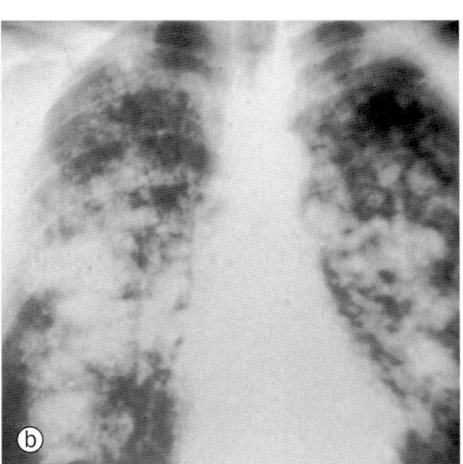
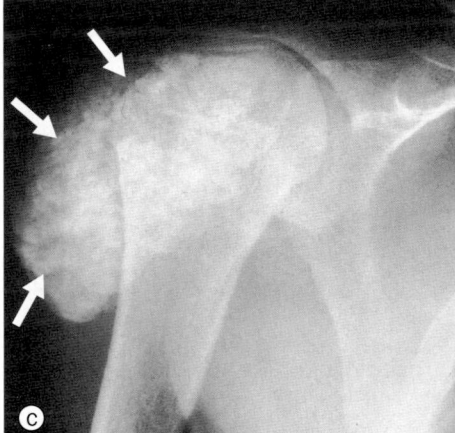

Figure 68.8 Extraskeletal calcification in chronic renal failure. (a) Arterial calcification (arrows). (b) Pulmonary calcification. (c) Periarticular calcification (arrows).

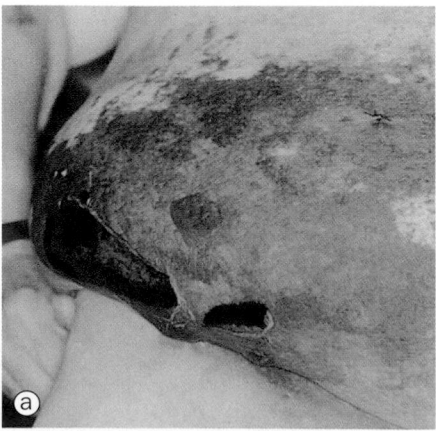
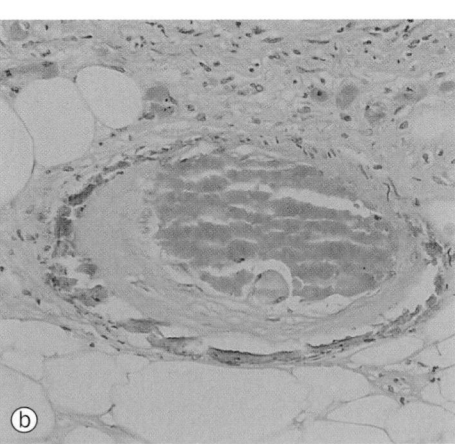

Figure 68.9 Calciphylaxis. (a) Calciphylaxis may involve the trunk or extremities as violaceous skin lesions that progress to ulceration. (b) Skin biopsy showing thrombosis of calcified blood vessel.

DIAGNOSIS AND DIFFERENTIAL DIAGNOSIS

In addition to the clinical manifestations of renal osteodystrophy, a variety of biochemical and radiographic techniques are helpful not only to establish the specific diagnosis, but also to serve as a guide for the initiation and adjustment of therapeutic interventions. Although bone biopsy is not widely utilized in clinical practice, it remains the gold standard for the diagnosis of renal osteodystrophy.

Serum biochemistry

The levels of free calcium and phosphate in serum are usually normal in patients with mild-to-moderate renal insufficiency. With advanced renal failure, the levels of serum calcium tend to fall; likewise, hyperphosphatemia does not become manifest until renal function has declined to < 20% of normal. The maintenance of serum free calcium and phosphate within the normal range during the course of CRF is largely a result of the development of compensatory hyperparathyroidism, as discussed above. Hypercalcemia may occur as a result of the administration of large doses of calcium-containing antacids or the administration of vitamin D metabolites. In addition, patients with severe hyperparathyroid bone disease, as well as those with low bone turnover syndromes, have a tendency to develop hypercalcemia. It is important to differentiate between the different causes of hypercalcemia in the setting of CRF since the management will vary greatly depending on the cause. Because the abnormalities reflect overall derangements in calcium and phosphate metabolism in CRF, the levels of serum calcium and phosphorus, when used alone, are not very useful in predicting the specific type of bone disease.

Metabolic acidosis is commonly associated with renal insufficiency and contributes to osteopenia as hydrogen ions are buffered by bone carbonate, resulting in demineralization of bone.

Parathyroid hormone

Measurements of PTH are important not only for diagnostic purposes, but also for therapeutic guidance in the management of renal osteodystrophy. With renal insufficiency, there is accumulation of circulating PTH fragments in the circulation, which complicates the interpretation of PTH assays based on assessment of the mid-region or the C-terminal portions of the molecule. Consequently, the preferred methods for measuring PTH have been the two-site immunoradiometric assay and immunochemiluminescence assay, which measure intact PTH. The levels of PTH in serum have been shown to correlate with the predominant histologic abnormality present in bone, such that elevated PTH levels are characteristic of patients with osteitis fibrosa, whereas low levels are found in patients with low bone turnover syndromes. It is well accepted that there is an element of skeletal resistance to PTH in patients with CRF; therefore, supranormal levels of PTH are required in order to maintain normal bone turnover. PTH levels two to three times normal may be appropriate for patients with advanced renal impairment. Serial measurements of PTH are useful in the initial evaluation of patients with renal bone disease and are essential during the management of these disorders in order to assess response to therapy and to avoid over- or undertreatment as either can have detrimental effects on bone histology. Recent refinements in PTH assays have led to the realization that these types of assays also measure some large fragments of PTH, which are truncated at the N-terminus. More specific assays have been developed which exclude these fragments from measurement, and work is in progress to define the clinical utility of such more specific assays[20]. As discussed above, these circulating fragments of PTH, which are truncated at the N-terminus, may have important biologic activity and their role is actively under investigation.

Vitamin D metabolites

Calcitriol levels remain within the normal range in patients with mild-to-moderate renal insufficiency because of the stimulation of 1α-hydroxylase by the high levels of PTH. With progressive decreases in renal mass, there is impaired production of calcitriol by the failing kidney, and calcitriol levels in serum fall in spite of the presence of hyperparathyroidism. Although low levels of calcitriol play a very important role in the pathogenesis of secondary hyperparathyroidism, and the adynamic bone lesion has been partially attributed to overtreatment with vitamin D metabolites, the levels of calcitriol in patients with CRF are not helpful in differentiating the histologic lesions of renal osteodystrophy. Measurements of calcitriol are not used routinely for diagnostic purposes unless extrarenal production of this metabolite is suspected, as in granulomatous disorders such as sarcoidosis.

Vitamin D deficiency is a relatively rare cause of osteomalacia in the USA and Europe but, if suspected, low circulating levels of 25-hydroxyvitamin D are diagnostic. In CRF with heavy proteinuria, there is loss of vitamin D binding protein in the urine, which may result in decreased levels of 25-hydroxyvitamin D. Vitamin D deficiency may be encountered in patients with limited sun exposure, in those with intestinal malabsorption or malnutrition, and in susceptible racial groups, particularly Indo-Asians. Therefore, measurements of 25-hydroxyvitamin D are of diagnostic value only in a very small proportion of patients with CRF who may have osteomalacia as the predominant bone lesion.

Markers of bone formation and bone resorption

Levels of circulating alkaline phosphatase offer an approximate index of osteoblast activity in patients with CRF. High levels are commonly present in hyperparathyroid bone disease, whereas low values are usually present in patients with low turnover osteodystrophy. The discriminatory power of alkaline phosphatase measurements is low. Although measurement of bone alkaline phosphatase isoenzyme is superior to that of total alkaline phosphatase, the discrimination between normal and abnormally low bone turnover remains problematic. Serial measurements of alkaline phosphatase may be useful in assessing the progression of bone disease. Osteocalcin is another marker of osteoblastic activity, but it is not superior to alkaline phosphatase for the evaluation of renal osteodystrophy. Tartrate-resistant acid phosphatase and collagen degradation products are both markers of osteoclastic activity but are not widely used in the evaluation of renal bone disease and are considered investigational at present.

Chronic Renal Failure and the Uremic Syndrome

Aluminum

Bone histology is the gold standard for the diagnosis of aluminum-related bone disease, demonstrating with specific stains the presence of aluminum at the mineralization front of bone. A noninvasive means of assessment of aluminum-related bone disease is being sought. Serum aluminum levels are useful: a random serum aluminum > 100 ng/mL usually indicates severe aluminum overload. However, serum aluminum levels usually reflect recent exposure, and iron status should be considered in their interpretation: in circumstances where aluminum therapy has recently been withdrawn or when iron overload is present, serum aluminum may be low in spite of significant tissue accumulation of aluminum. In these circumstances, liberation of aluminum from body stores by the chelator desferoxamine (desferrioxamine, DFO) may be useful. Many protocols and schedules have been described, but current recommendations state that an increase in serum aluminum of 50 mg/L (50 ng/mL) at 48 h following the administration of DFO 5 mg/kg, together with intact PTH < 150pg/mL, provides high sensitivity and specificity for aluminum overload[21].

Radiology of the skeleton

Routine X-ray examination of the skeleton is relatively insensitive for the diagnosis of renal osteodystrophy and radiographs can appear virtually normal in patients with severe histologic evidence of renal bone disease. However, subperiosteal erosions are often present in severe secondary hyperparathyroidism, detected in the hands (Fig. 68.10), clavicles and pelvis. Skull radiograph may show focal radiolucencies and a ground glass appearance, known as 'pepper pot' skull. Osteosclerosis of the vertebrae is responsible for the 'ruggerjersey' appearance of the spine (Fig. 68.11). 'Brown tumors' are focal collections of giant cells that are typical of severe hyperparathyroidism and are usually seen as well-demarcated radiolucent zones in long bones, clavicles, and digits (Fig. 68.10). Looser zones or pseudofractures are characteristic of osteomalacia. The presence of β_2-M amyloidosis is suggested by the presence of bone cysts and spondyloarthropathy[22].

Measurements of bone density

Dual-energy X-ray absorptiometry is widely used to assess bone density. However, the utility of this technique in the assessment of renal bone disease is unclear, perhaps because of the heterogeneous and complex nature of the bone histology. Other variables that may contribute to the erratic correlations of bone density measurements and bone histology in renal bone diseases include vascular and soft-tissue calcifications, age, prior therapy with corticosteroids, and limited activity secondary to chronic illness.

Bone biopsy

Biopsy of bone and the microscopic analysis of undecalcified sections following double tetracycline labeling provide definitive and quantitative diagnosis of renal bone disease[23]. Tetracycline is administered on two occasions separated by a defined interval; the quantitation of bone mineralization rate is achieved by measuring the distance between the two fluorescent tetracycline bands. Bone biopsy is not routinely performed in clinical practice because of the invasive nature

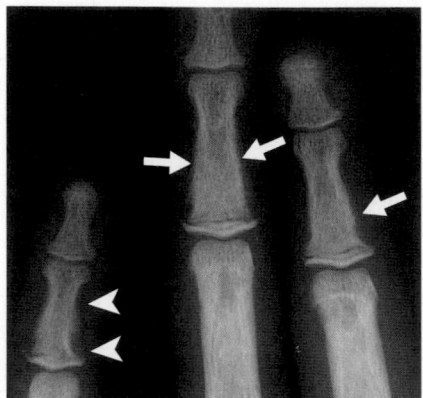

Figure 68.10 Subperiosteal erosions in hyperparathyroidism. Severe subperiosteal erosions as a manifestation of hyperparathyroidism (arrows). The extensive scalloped appearance of the middle phalanx on the left (arrow heads) represents a small brown tumor.

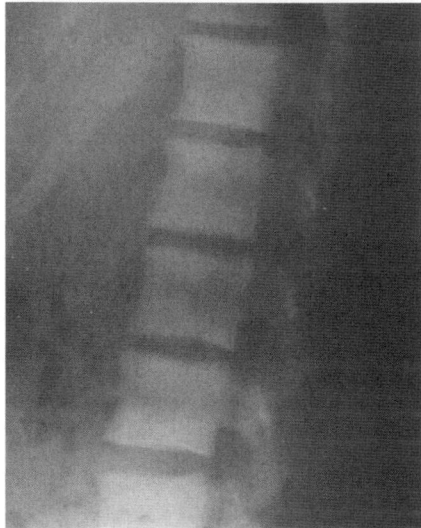

Figure 68.11 'Rugger-jersey spine' in hyperparathyroidism. Vertebral bodies show the increased density of the ground plates and central radiolucency, which gives the appearance of a 'rugger-jersey'.

of the procedure, but it is required for precise diagnosis in selected patients.

Osteitis fibrosa (hyperparathyroid bone disease) is characterized by increased bone turnover, increased number and activity of osteoblasts and osteoclasts, and variable amounts of peritrabecular fibrosis (Fig. 68.12a). Osteoid may be increased but usually has a woven pattern distinct from the normal lamellar appearance. Osteomalacia is characterized by the presence of increased osteoid seam width, increase in the trabecular surface covered with osteoid, and decreased bone mineralization as assessed by tetracycline labeling (Fig. 68.12b). The presence of aluminum can be detected on the mineralization front by specific staining (Fig. 68.12c). Aluminum-related bone disease is defined by aluminum staining exceeding 15% of the trabecular surface and a bone formation rate of < 220 mm²/mm² per day. The adynamic bone lesion is characterized by normal or decreased osteoid volume and a reduced bone formation rate. Features of osteitis fibrosa may occur together with features of osteomalacia: the combination is termed mixed renal osteodystrophy.

TREATMENT

Prevention is the primary goal in the management of renal osteodystrophy. Therapy should be initiated early in the

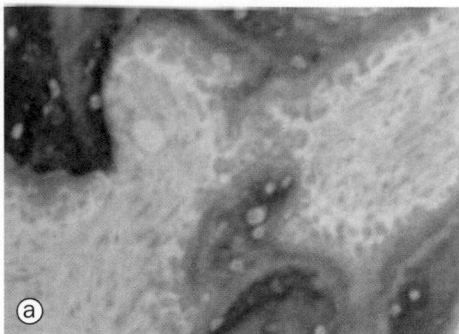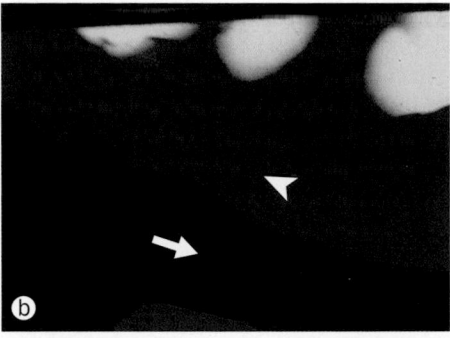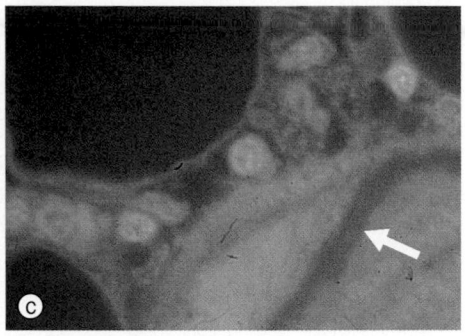

Figure 68.12 Bone histology in renal osteodystrophy. (a) Osteitis fibrosa: characteristic manifestations of severe hyperparathyroidism with increased osteoclast and osteoblast activity and peritrabecular fibrosis. (b) Osteomalacia: marked excess of unmineralized osteoid stained red (arrowhead) surrounding the mineralized bone stained black (arrow). (c) Aluminum bone disease: specific red staining shows the deposition of aluminum at the mineralization front (arrow).

course of renal insufficiency (GFR 50–80 mL/min) so that parathyroid gland hyperplasia can be prevented. Because renal osteodystrophy is usually asymptomatic early in the course of renal failure, attention is often not paid to secondary hyperparathyroidism. By the time renal failure is advanced, patients may have already developed significant skeletal abnormalities and more aggressive therapy is required in order to prevent the long-term consequences of renal bone disease.

Hyperparathyroid bone disease
Since the development of secondary hyperparathyroidism occurs during the early stages of CRF, preventative therapy should be initiated at that time to prevent further hyperplasia of the parathyroid glands, avoiding the development of nodular parathyroid hyperplasia. Based on the multiplicity of factors involved in the pathogenesis of secondary hyperparathyroidism in CRF, the successful approach to the prevention and management of this disorder involves the integration of a variety of measures directed towards the suppression of PTH secretion and the prevention of parathyroid hyperplasia.

Prevention of hypocalcemia
Hypocalcemia, if present, should be corrected since hypocalcemia is a potent stimulus for PTH secretion. Furthermore, recent studies with calcimimetic agents have shown that these agents prevent increased parathyroid cell growth[10]. In patients with hypoalbuminemia, free calcium should be measured. The initial approach to the therapy of hypocalcemia in mild-to-moderate renal insufficiency is the administration of calcium supplements such as calcium carbonate, taken between meals with increasing doses as required. Assessment of efficacy of therapy is by follow-up determinations of serum calcium and PTH. Adjunctive therapy with calcitriol should also be considered. In patients with ESRD, vitamin D metabolites are often required. The goal is to achieve levels of intact PTH of 150–250 pg/mL in patients on dialysis.

Control of phosphorus
Control of phosphorus is the cornerstone of effective management of secondary hyperparathyroidism. In mild-to-moderate renal insufficiency, a normal serum phosphorus does not necessarily indicate normal parathyroid status and, except for the late stages of CRF, normophosphatemia may be maintained at the expense of elevated serum PTH. Therefore, efforts to control phosphorus, including dietary phosphate restriction and the use of phosphate binders, should not be delayed until frank hyperphosphatemia develops.

Dietary phosphate restriction
The first step in the prevention and management of hyperparathyroidism is the restriction of dietary phosphorus intake. In experimental animals with mild CRF, dietary phosphate restriction can prevent excessive PTH synthesis and secretion, as well as parathyroid cell proliferation, independent of changes in serum calcium and calcitriol concentrations. The input of a dietitian is essential for counseling and education regarding the phosphorus content of various foods. Protein restriction and avoidance of dairy products are the mainstays of the regimen. In addition to reducing the rate of progression of renal failure, phosphate–protein restriction has been shown to increase the serum levels of calcitriol in patients with mild-to-moderate renal insufficiency. Restriction of phosphorus by severe dietary protein restriction should be avoided since it may lead to protein–calorie malnutrition. Restriction of the daily dietary protein intake to 0.8 g/kg should be sufficient to provide phosphorus restriction without the risk of malnutrition.

Phosphate binders
Restriction of dietary phosphate may be sufficient to prevent the development of hyperparathyroidism in early renal failure. As renal function deteriorates, the control of phosphorus by dietary means alone becomes difficult and it is necessary to use agents that bind ingested phosphate in the intestinal lumen in order to limit its absorption. A variety of compounds have been used for this purpose, including aluminum hydroxide, calcium-containing antacids and magnesium salts.

Aluminum-containing antacids are very effective phosphate binders but, in patients with CRF, their use can no longer be recommended because of the risk of aluminum toxicity. There are certain circumstances that limit the use of calcium-containing phosphate binders, such as hypercalcemia. In such

Chronic Renal Failure and the Uremic Syndrome

cases, aluminum-containing antacids may be used but the dose should be restricted to no more than 40–45 mg/kg per day, and frequent reassessments should be made in order to institute alternative therapy as soon as possible. Coingestion of aluminum-containing antacids together with foods containing citric acid (such as fruit juices or with sodium, calcium, or potassium citrate) may significantly increase aluminum absorption and, therefore, should be avoided.

Calcium salts taken with meals effectively bind phosphates and limit their absorption and have become the preferred agents for this purpose as the toxic effects of aluminum are recognized. Calcium carbonate has been shown to be an effective phosphate binder in 60–70% of patients on hemodialysis. The doses required to prevent hyperphosphatemia may vary according to the patient's compliance with dietary phosphate restriction as well as the degree of renal insufficiency, and generally range from 3–12 g daily. Hypercalcemia is the major potentially serious side effect related to the use of calcium carbonate. Although calcium acetate is intrinsically more effective than calcium carbonate as a phosphate binder, and lower doses of 1.5–9 g per day are usually sufficient to prevent hyperphosphatemia, the incidence of hypercalcemia during therapy with calcium acetate is similar to that associated with the use of calcium carbonate. Because calcium acetate appears to be less well tolerated, there seems to be no practical advantage over calcium carbonate. Calcium citrate is also an effective phosphate binder; however, it may potentiate aluminum intoxication by increasing the solubility of aluminum; therefore, the use of this agent should be avoided in CRF.

Magnesium salts are also effective phosphate binders for patients who become hypercalcemic on calcium-containing phosphate binders, but should be administered with caution in patients with renal dysfunction predialysis because hypermagnesemia may have serious adverse effects. In patients with ESRD on dialysis, magnesium carbonate (200–500 mg elemental magnesium per day) has been used successfully, with prevention of hypermagnesemia through a reduction in dialysate magnesium concentration. The use of magnesium carbonate also allows reduction of the dose of calcium carbonate required by approximately 50%, but its use is frequently complicated by diarrhea.

Because of the risks of hypercalcemia and the high calcium load of calcium-containing phosphate binders, alternative therapeutic approaches based upon the use of non-absorbable polymers have recently been investigated. Poly:sevelamer hydrochloride (RenaGel®) in a dose range of 2.4–4.8 g daily provides effective phosphate control without hypercalcemia[24] and also produces a significant reduction in total cholesterol. Agents such as sevelamer may offer great advantage over calcium-containing phosphate binders, although they are significantly more expensive. At present, sevelamer should be used in those patients who become hypercalcemic on calcium-containing phosphate binders, and in those in whom it is desirable to limit the calcium load, until further evidence from clinical studies is available. Sevelamer may be combined with both calcium and magnesium containing phosphate binders if necessary.

Use of vitamin D metabolites

Calcitriol deficiency contributes to the development of hyperparathyroidism by several mechanisms, and therefore there is strong rationale for the inclusion of calcitriol in the treatment regimen. Low levels of calcitriol can lead to impaired calcium absorption and hypocalcemia, increased production and secretion of PTH, altered parathyroid cell growth, and decreased levels of parathyroid vitamin D receptors. In addition, low levels of calcitriol contribute to skeletal resistance to the actions of PTH.

Calcitriol and other 1α-hydroxylated vitamin D sterols, such as 1α-hydroxyvitamin D_3, and 1α-hydroxyvitamin D_2, are effective in the control of secondary hyperparathyroidism. Calcitriol lowers PTH levels and improves bone histology. In patients with very high levels of PTH and very enlarged glands that may have severe nodular hyperplasia, the effectiveness of vitamin D metabolites may be limited since the levels of vitamin D receptor are low in such tissue. Accordingly, it would appear rational to initiate treatment of secondary hyperparathyroidism with vitamin D metabolites early in the course of the disease process when the parathyroid glands are more sensitive to such therapy, and thereby prevent the progression to a refractory stage. A beneficial effect of vitamin D metabolite therapy in the treatment of secondary hyperparathyroidism in patients with mild-to-moderate renal failure has been shown, but the concern with initiation of vitamin D therapy at this stage of renal failure is acceleration of the progression of renal disease should hypercalcemia occur. Because of the effect of calcitriol to increase intestinal phosphate absorption, hyperphosphatemia and elevations in calcium phosphate product may predispose patients to the development of metastatic calcification; however, it appears that doses of calcitriol or 1α-hydroxyvitamin D_3 up to 0.5 µg/day are not commonly associated with hypercalcemia, hyperphosphatemia, or worsening renal insufficiency. Calcitriol and 1α-hydroxyvitamin D_3 have equivalent efficacy. Another concern with the use of vitamin D metabolites predialysis is that oversuppression of hyperparathyroidism may increase the risk of adynamic bone. Accordingly, vitamin D therapy should be monitored carefully and should not be instituted without documentation of hyperparathyroidism and concomitant control of serum phosphate.

In patients with ESRD, indications for therapy with vitamin D metabolites are better defined; however, hypercalcemia and aggravation of hyperphosphatemia are frequent complications of therapy. Vitamin D metabolites are increasingly used as oral or intravenous 'pulses' given intermittently (e.g., three times weekly) rather than as continuous oral therapy. There is a growing view that pulse therapy is superior to continuous therapy in the suppression of established hyperparathyroidism, although the evidence is not yet conclusive.

In recent years, there has been considerable interest in the development of analogs of calcitriol that have less calcemic activity than the parent compound and yet retain the ability to suppress PTH release *in vivo*. Such analogs of vitamin D studied in patients with ESRD are 22-oxacalcitriol (OCT), 1α-hydroxyvitamin D_2, and 19-nor-1α,25-dihydroxyvitamin D_2 (paricalcitol)[25–27]. This last compound has been shown to

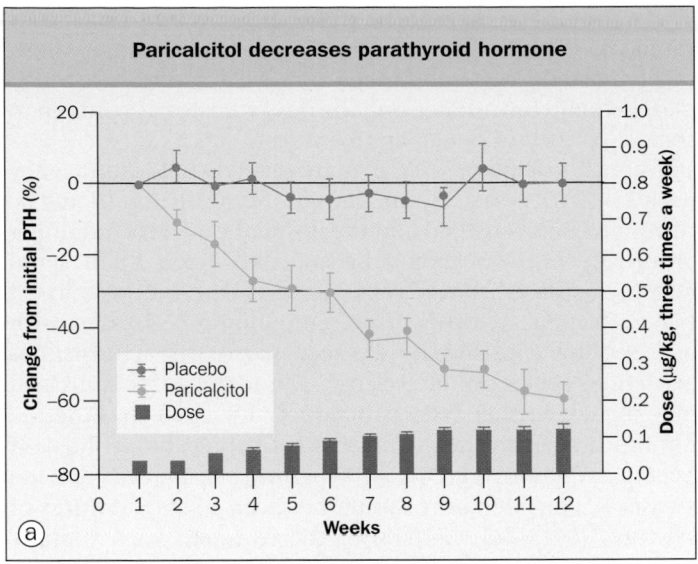

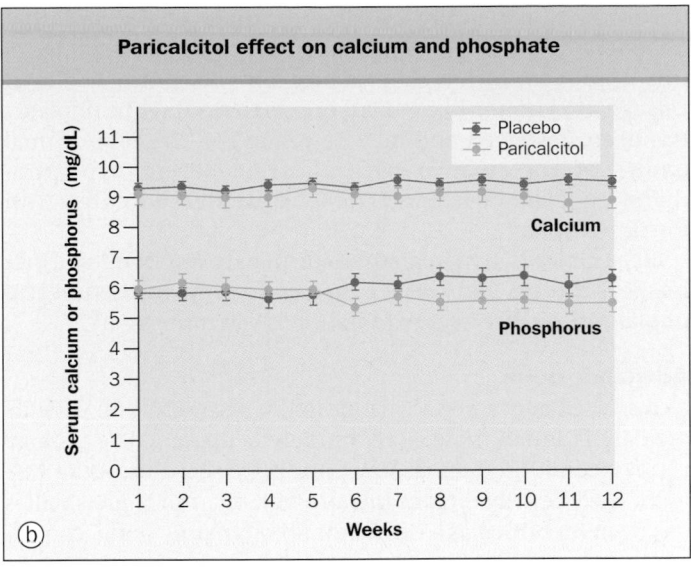

Figure 68.13 Paricalcitol as therapy of hyperparathyroidism. Paricalcitol (19-nor-1 α,25-dihydroxyvitamin D_2) (a) decreases parathyroid hormone (PTH), (b) without aggravating hypercalcemia or hyperphosphatemia.

decrease the levels of PTH in patients with ESRD without aggravating hypercalcemia or hyperphosphatemia (Fig. 68.13). The other analogs also appear to be effective, but direct comparisons between these compounds are not available at the present time. Paricalcitol is now widely used in the USA in patients in hemodialysis. It is likely that a wider therapeutic window may be offered by these analogs, which will make them the preferred treatment for hyperparathyroidism in CRF.

Role of parathyroidectomy

While the strategies discussed above are effective for the control of hyperparathryoidism in many patients, there are occasions where these steps fail or are contraindicated and surgical removal of the parathyroids should be considered (Table 68.2). Parathyroidectomy is indicated for patients with severe hyperparathyroidism who are noncompliant with diet and phosphate binders. The presence of severe hyperphosphatemia in these patients precludes the use of vitamin D metabolites because of the risk of metastatic calcification and, therefore, surgery becomes necessary for the control of hyperparathyroidism. Parathyroidectomy is also indicated in advanced hyperparathyroidism that is no longer responsive to medical therapy. Some patients with severe hyperparathyroidism may become hypercalcemic in the absence of calcitriol therapy; consequently, calcitriol and calcium-containing phosphate binders cannot be administered. In this circumstance, short-term therapy with aluminum-based phosphate binders may allow vitamin D analogs to be initiated. It is important to be certain that hypercalcemia represents severe hyperparathyroidism and is not caused by adynamic bone or osteomalacia. For hypercalcemia to occur because of hyperparathyroidism in renal failure, the levels of intact PTH generally exceeds 1000 pg/mL. Surgical parathyroidectomy might also be considered in patients with very severe hyperparathyroidism who are candidates for living related renal transplantation in the near future, particularly if they are female and have significant osteopenia. The aim of parathyroidectomy is to avoid post-transplant hypercalcemia and hypophosphatemia (owing to PTH-induced phosphaturia), as well as osteopenia. Firm guidelines have not been established for this clinical situation. Parathyroidectomy might also be considered in patients with severe hyperparathyroidism who have evidence of metastatic calcification. The development of calciphylaxis is an urgent indication for parathyroidectomy if PTH levels are elevated. Prior to parathyroidectomy, consideration should also be given to the possibility of coexisting aluminum accumulation, using DFO testing and bone biopsy if necessary, since this might predispose to osteomalacia post-parathyroidectomy.

The choice of surgical procedure for parathyroidectomy has been controversial. The most commonly used procedures are subtotal removal of the parathyroids or total removal of the parathyroids with reimplantation of parathyroid tissue in the forearm. Recurrence of hyperparathyroidism occurs in approximately 10% of patients. Total parathyroidectomy alone is less commonly performed; while this is an appropriate procedure

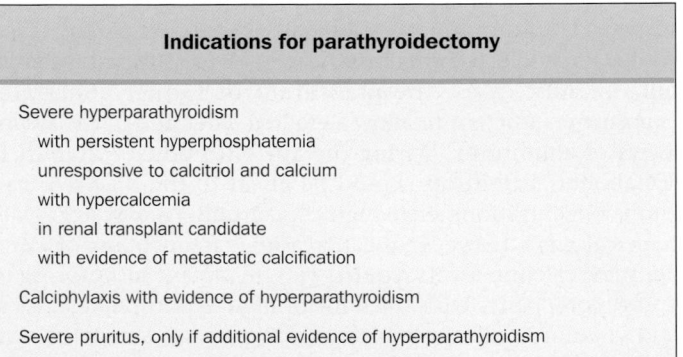

Indications for parathyroidectomy

Severe hyperparathyroidism
  with persistent hyperphosphatemia
  unresponsive to calcitriol and calcium
  with hypercalcemia
  in renal transplant candidate
  with evidence of metastatic calcification

Calciphylaxis with evidence of hyperparathyroidism

Severe pruritus, only if additional evidence of hyperparathyroidism

Table 68.2 Indications for parathyroidectomy.

Chronic Renal Failure and the Uremic Syndrome

for patients remaining on dialysis there is concern that hypoparathyroidism post-transplant may be a disadvantage of this approach, although evidence on this point is slight. Unregulated tumor-like growth of parathyroid tissue implants has been described and may be related to the monoclonal nature of the nodular hyperplasia of severe hyperparathyroidism. Our preference is for total parathyroidectomy with forearm implant.

Recurrence of hyperparathyroidism may respond to further medical therapy but further surgery to remove the forearm implant or further neck exploration is often necessary.

Adynamic bone

As discussed above, the adynamic lesion occurs both in patients predialysis and in those receiving dialytic therapy. The etiology is not clear at the present time, nor is the significance of this lesion well described. Since therapy with vitamin D metabolites has been identified as a risk factor for adynamic bone, consideration should be given to the possibility that it represents a physiologic decrease in bone turnover as a consequence of oversuppression of PTH secretion. Other possibilities should also be considered, such as defective osteoblast development or activity as a result of the uremic environment. Aluminum should be avoided in these patients and efforts should be made to decrease dialysate calcium in order to avoid oversuppression of PTH secretion. The use of calcium-containing phosphate binders is often problematic because of the increased frequency of hypercalcemia as a result of the altered calcium kinetics in these patients[28]. The novel phosphate binders that do not contain calcium discussed above may potentially be beneficial in patients with the adynamic bone lesion.

Synthesis of therapeutic strategies

The general recommendations for the prevention and therapy of renal osteodystrophy are summarized in Figure 68.14, in which therapeutic maneuvers are stratified according to the degree of renal insufficiency.

Therapy should be initiated if possible when renal insufficiency is mild (GFR 50–80 mL/min) and dietary phosphorus

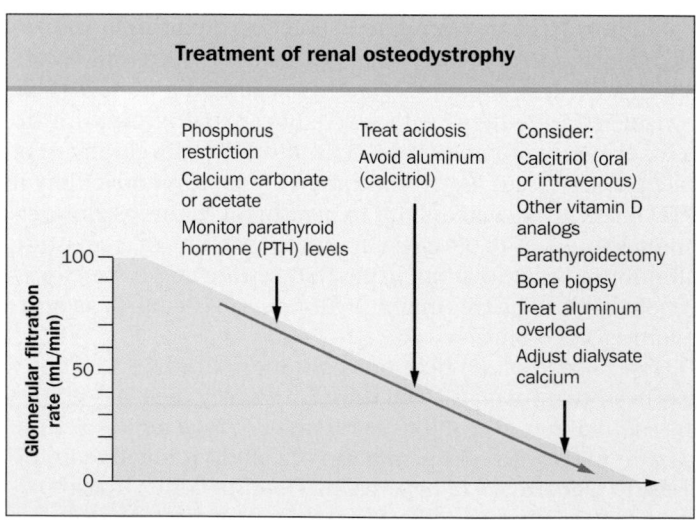

Figure 68.14 Treatment of renal osteodystrophy at various stages of renal insufficiency.

intake should be restricted at this stage. Levels of intact PTH should be measured, and if elevated above the normal range, calcium-based phosphate binders, 1–3 g/day administered with meals, should be initiated and the dose adjusted as required to achieve control of hyperparathyroidism.

As renal disease progresses to moderate renal insufficiency (GFR 25–50 mL/min), dietary phosphorus restriction should be continued or intensified and the doses of calcium-containing phosphate binders should be adjusted based upon serial measurements of intact PTH, with careful attention to avoid hypercalcemia. Acidosis, if present, should be treated with oral sodium bicarbonate because persistent acidosis has deleterious effects on the skeleton. The additional sodium load may require further salt restriction or increases in diuretics. Aluminum-based phosphate binders should be avoided. If hyperparathyroidism (PTH > 100 pg/mL) persists despite these measures, consideration should be given to the addition of calcitriol (0.25–0.5 mg/day) to the regimen. Such therapy should be monitored carefully to avoid hypercalcemia and acceleration of progression of renal failure.

When renal failure becomes advanced (GFR < 25 mL/min) or end stage, the above therapies may need to be intensified and larger amounts of phosphate binders may be required to avoid hyperphosphatemia. The use of aluminum-containing phosphate binders is particularly undesirable at this stage in view of the increased risk of aluminum accumulation with worsening renal function. With patients on dialysis, calcitriol therapy can be intensified, with attention to the serum levels of calcium and phosphate and monitoring of PTH levels. At this stage of advanced renal insufficiency, PTH levels should be maintained between 150 and 300 pg/mL in order to maintain normal bone turnover. Calcitriol may be administered orally either daily or intermittently (pulse therapy) or administered intravenously to patients on hemodialysis. During therapy with calcitriol, it is imperative to ensure that serum phosphate remains controlled and elevations of serum calcium do not occur such that the calcium phosphate product is elevated into a range at which metastatic calcification is likely. The recent introduction of vitamin D analogs into clinical practice, which are less calcemic and phosphatemic than calcitriol and yet retain the ability to suppress the levels of PTH, may be a significant advance in our therapeutic armamentarium. Parathyroidectomy needs to be considered in selected circumstances. Bone biopsy may be indicated in selected patients, particularly if aluminum overload is suspected. Aluminum overload may require chelation therapy with DFO in selected circumstances, especially if symptomatic, but, in most cases, the prevention of further aluminum exposure is sufficient to allow a gradual reduction in the serum levels of aluminum. During therapy with potent vitamin D metabolites, attention should be given to the dialysate calcium concentrations since high concentrations may aggravate hypercalcemia. However, the increasingly frequent use of lower dialysate calcium levels requires careful patient monitoring to ensure compliance with calcium-containing phosphate binders and vitamin D metabolites to avoid progressive negative calcium balance. Dialysate calcium should not be taken outside the range 1.25–1.75 mmol/L and, where possible, should be individually prescribed.

REFERENCES

1. Sherrard DJ, Hercz G, Pei Y, et al. The spectrum of bone disease in end-stage renal failure – an evolving disorder. Kidney Int. 1993;43:436–42.
2. Martinez I, Saracho R, Montenegro J, Llach F. The importance of dietary calcium and phosphorus in the secondary hyperparathyroidism of patients with early renal failure. Am J Kidney Dis. 1997;29:496–502.
3. Slatopolsky E, Caglar S, Pennell JP, et al. On the pathogenesis of hyperparathyroidism in chronic experimental renal insufficiency in the dog. J Clin Invest. 1971;50:492–9.
4. Slatopolsky E, Finch J, Denda M, et al. Phosphorus restriction prevents parathyroid gland growth. High phosphorus directly stimulates PTH secretion in vitro. J Clin Invest. 1996;97:2534–40.
5. Almaden Y, Canalejo A, Hernandez A, et al. Direct effect of phosphorus on PTH secretion from whole rat parathyroid glands in vitro. J Bone Miner Res. 1996;11:970–6.
6. Denda M, Finch J, Slatopolsky E. Phosphorus accelerates the development of parathyroid hyperplasia and secondary hyperparathyroidism in rats with renal failure. Am J Kidney Dis. 1996;28:596–602.
7. Naveh-Many T, Rahamimov R, Livni N, Silver J. Parathyroid cell proliferation in normal and CRF rats. The effects of calcium, phosphate, and vitamin D. J Clin Invest. 1995;96:1786–93.
8. Silver J, Naveh-Many T, Mayer H, et al. Regulation by vitamin D metabolites of parathyroid hormone gene transcription in vivo in the rat. J Clin Invest. 1986;78:1296–301.
9. Russell J, Lettieri D, Sherwood LM. Suppression by $1,25(OH)_2D_3$ of transcription of the pre-proparathyroid hormone gene. Endocrinology. 1986;119:2864–6.
10. Wada M, Furuya Y, Sakiyama J, et al. The calcimimetic compound NPS R-568 suppresses parathyroid cell proliferation in rats with renal insufficiency. Control of parathyroid cell growth via a calcium receptor. J Clin Invest. 1997;100:2977–83.
11. Arnold A, Brown MF, Urena P, et al. Monoclonality of parathyroid tumors in CRF and in primary parathyroid hyperplasia. J Clin Invest. 1995;95:2047–53.
12. Kifor O, Moore FD Jr, Wang P, et al. Reduced immunostaining for the extracellular Ca^{2+}-sensing receptor in primary and uremic secondary hyperparathyroidism. J Clin Endocrinol Metab. 1996;81:1598–606.
13. Gogusev J, Duchambon P, Hory B, et al. Depressed expression of calcium receptor in parathyroid gland tissue of patients with hyperparathyroidism. Kidney Int. 1997;51:328–36.
14. Fukuda N, Tanaka H, Tominaga Y, et al. Decreased 1,25-dihydroxy-vitamin D_3 receptor density is associated with a more severe form of parathyroid hyperplasia in chronic uremic patients. J Clin Invest. 1993;92:1436–43.
15. Brown EM, Gamba G, Riccardi D, et al. Cloning and characterization of an extracellular $Ca^{(2+)}$-sensing receptor from bovine parathyroid. Nature. 1993;366:575–80.
16. Slatopolsky E, Finch J, Clay P, et al. A novel mechanism for skeletal resistance in uremia. Kidney Int. 2000;58:753–61.
17. González E, Martin K. Aluminum and renal osteodystrophy: a diminishing clinical problem. Trend Endocrinol Metab. 1992;3:371–5.
18. Couttenye MM, D'Haese PC, Verschoren WJ, et al. Low bone turnover in patients with renal failure. Kidney Int. 1999;56:S70–6.
19. Mazhar AR, Johnson RJ, Gillen D, et al. Risk factors and mortality associated with calciphylaxis in end-stage renal disease. Kidney Int. 2001;60:324–32.
20. Monier-Faugere MC, Geng Z, Mawad H, et al. Improved assessment of bone turnover by the PTH-(1-84)/large C-PTH fragments ratio in ESRD patients. Kidney Int. 2001;60:1460–8.
21. D'Haese PC, Couttenye MM, de Broe ME. Diagnosis and treatment of aluminium bone disease. Nephrol Dial Transplant. 1996;11:74–9.
22. Farrell J, Bastani B. Beta 2-microglobulin amyloidosis in chronic dialysis patients: a case report and review of the literature. J Am Soc Nephrol. 1997;8:509–14.
23. Malluche H, Monier-Faugere M. The role of bone biopsy in the management of patients with renal osteodystrophy. J Am Soc Nephrol. 1994;4:1631–42.
24. Chertow GM, Burke SK, Lazarus JM, et al. Poly(allylamine hydrochloride) (RenaGel): a noncalcemic phosphate binder for the treatment of hyperphosphatemia in CRF. Am J Kidney Dis. 1997;29:66–71.
25. Martin K, González E, Gellens M, et al. 19-Nor-1a-25-dihydroxy-vitamin D_2 (paricalcitol) safely and effectively reduces the levels of intact PTH in patients on hemodialysis. J Am Soc Nephrol. 1998;9:1427–32.
26. Tan AU Jr, Levine BS, Mazess RB, et al. Effective suppression of parathyroid hormone by 1 alpha-hydroxy-vitamin D_2 in hemodialysis patients with moderate to severe secondary hyperparathyroidism. Kidney Int. 1997;51:317–23.
27. Kurokawa K, Akizawa T, Suzuki M, et al. Effect of 22-oxacalcitriol on hyperparathyroidism of dialysis patients: results of a preliminary study. Nephrol Dial Transplant. 1996;11:121–4.
28. Kurz P, Monier-Faugere MC, Bognar B, et al. Evidence for abnormal calcium homeostasis in patients with adynamic bone disease. Kidney Int. 1994;46:855–61.

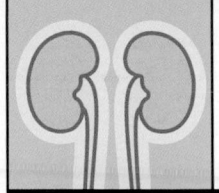

Section 14 Chronic Renal Failure and the Uremic Syndrome

Chapter 69

Cardiovascular Disease in Chronic Renal Failure

Charles R V Tomson

INTRODUCTION

Life expectancy with end-stage renal disease (ESRD) is poor despite modern renal replacement treatment (RRT). The average life expectancy of a 49-year-old with ESRD is 7.1 years, compared to 8.6 years for colon cancer, 12.8 years for prostate cancer and 29.8 years for the general population[1]. Much of the premature death of these patients, particularly in the first few years of dialysis, is attributable to cardiovascular disease, including stroke, myocardial infarction and heart failure. The increased relative risk of death from cardiovascular disease is greatest in younger patients, whose risk approaches that of the elderly without renal failure (Fig. 69.1)[2]. This increased risk has often been attributed to 'accelerated atherosclerosis' in ESRD; however, the risk markers that predict cardiovascular death in patients with renal disease differ from those in the general population[3,4], and only a quarter of cardiovascular

deaths in dialysis patients are due to myocardial infarction[5]. Much evidence points to alternative causes of cardiovascular mortality, including anemia, arteriosclerosis, vascular calcification, left ventricular hypertrophy (LVH) and remodeling, and altered energy metabolism.

EPIDEMIOLOGY

Precise epidemiologic information is difficult to obtain in chronic renal failure (CRF). The definition of myocardial infarction may be complicated by a history of angina despite normal coronary arteries and by nonspecific electrocardiogram (ECG) alterations. Sudden cardiac death may be caused by hyperkalemia rather than a primary cardiac arrhythmia. Cardiac failure may be confused with circulatory congestion in the absence of structural cardiac disease. Furthermore, it is often difficult to ascribe death to a single cause in patients with multiple pathology. Because many patients with ESRD already have clinically evident vascular disease, it is also difficult to determine from clinical or epidemiologic studies whether uremia and RRT are themselves responsible for the high risk of cardiovascular death.

Proteinuria and the nephrotic syndrome
The increased cardiovascular risk conferred by renal disease appears early in its course. Proteinuria, and even micro-albuminuria, is associated with increased cardiovascular risk not just in patients with known renal disease or diabetes but also in the general population. The risk of myocardial infarction in patients with persistent nephrotic syndrome is increased five-fold, although it is impossible to be certain that this association is causal rather than the result of the operation of confounding factors such as vascular damage caused by the underlying disease (e.g., lupus) or its treatment (e.g., corticosteroids). Possible causative factors include marked hypercholesterolemia and hypercoagulability.

Chronic renal failure
Cardiovascular disease
There is a high cardiovascular death rate among patients with CRF and a high prevalence of coronary artery disease among patients starting RRT[5]. Cardiovascular causes of death are most prominent in the first few years of dialysis and are rare in patients who have been on long-term dialysis – the reverse of what would be expected if dialysis itself caused 'accelerated' atherosclerosis[6]. Risk factors for cardiovascular disease in patients on dialysis are shown in Table 69.1.

Cardiovascular mortality in ESRD

Annual mortality (%)

100, 10, 1, 0.1, 0.01

Age (years): 25–34, 35–44, 45–54, 55–64, 65–74, 75–84, >85

Legend:
- GP male
- GP female
- GP black
- GP white
- dialysis male
- dialysis female
- dialysis black
- dialysis white

Figure 69.1 Cardiovascular mortality in renal disease. Cardiovascular mortality defined by death due to arrhythmias, cardiomyopathy, cardiac arrest, myocardial infarction, atherosclerotic heart disease, and pulmonary edema in the general population (GP) compared to end-stage renal disease (ESRD) treated by dialysis. Data stratified by age, race and gender. (Adapted with permission[2].)

Risk factors for cardiovascular disease in renal failure
Classical risk factors for atherosclerosis found in renal disease

Dyslipidemia:
    hypercholesterolemia, decreased high-density lipoprotein cholesterol,
    hypertriglyceridemia, increased very-low-density, lipoprotein remnants,
    increased lipoprotein (a), increased lipid peroxidation

Hyperinsulinemia   Smoking
Hypercoagulability   Sedentary lifestyle
Hypertension   Obesity
Other causes specific to uremia
Hyperparathyroidism
Phosphate retention
Iatrogenic iron overload
Inadequate dialysis (mechanisms uncertain)
Hyperhomocysteinemia: folate deficiency, pyridoxine deficiency

Endothelial dysfunction:
    increased plasma endothelin, impaired nitric oxide production,
    asymmetric dimethylarginine accumulation, increased oxidant stress,
    hyperhomocysteinemia

Carbamylation of matrix proteins
Carbamylation of lipoproteins (possibly resulting in increased susceptibility to peroxidation)
Decreased antioxidant defense, causing lipid peroxidation and autoantibodies to oxidized low-density lipoprotein
Hyperoxalemia

Table 69.1 Risk factors for cardiovascular disease in renal failure.

Cerebrovascular disease

Stroke accounts for approximately 10% of deaths among patients on RRT. There is an increased incidence of carotid plaques in patients with ESRD, mostly due to an excess of 'hard' calcified plaques in patients, with very few 'soft' atherosclerotic plaques, suggesting that the pathogenesis and evolution of carotid disease may be different in uremic patients from that in 'classical' atherosclerosis[7].

Peripheral vascular disease

Much of the increased risk of peripheral vascular disease in dialysis patients is amongst patients with diabetes and those with pre-existing atherosclerosis but, in hemodialysis patients, there are also associations with duration of dialysis, hypoalbuminemia, low parathyroid hormone levels and low predialysis diastolic blood pressure, but no association with hyperlipidemia or hypertension. Striking vascular calcification of peripheral arteries is often present but may not indicate the presence of endoluminal obstruction. Peripheral gangrene is often caused by small vessel disease or calcific uremic arteriolopathy rather than by proximal atheroma.

Accelerated hypertension

Accelerated hypertension as a cause of ESRD is associated with high cardiovascular mortality, presumably a result of widespread extrarenal vascular disease as a consequence of severe hypertension.

Renal transplantation

Following renal transplantation, cardiovascular disease remains the most common cause of death[8]. Among patients whose transplants have functioned for 15 years, 23% developed ischemic heart disease, 15% cerebrovascular disease and 15% peripheral vascular disease. Risk factors include diabetes, hypertension, acute rejection episodes, low levels of high-density lipoprotein (HDL), high cholesterol, age, cigarette smoking, hypoalbuminemia and male sex[9]. However, once the increased risk of early death from complications has passed, renal transplantation is associated with a reduced relative risk of death, including that from cardiovascular disease, compared to that of patients remaining on the transplant waiting list. This difference is most clearly seen in older patients and those with diabetes. As in many interventions, the greatest benefit is seen in those at highest baseline risk. However, this does not mean that transplantation would improve the prognosis of patients currently judged too 'high risk' to be entered onto the transplant list.

ETIOLOGY AND PATHOGENESIS

Several studies have shown that 'traditional' risk factors derived from the Framingham study and others underestimate cardiovascular risk amongst patients with CRF[3,4].

Hypertension in chronic renal disease

High systemic arterial BP is frequently (nearly universally) found in patients with primary renal disease, and its development commonly predates, often by years, any deterioration of renal excretory function. Both in primary renal diseases such as glomerulonephritis, reflux nephropathy and diabetic nephropathy, and in less well-defined disorders including systemic atherosclerosis, hypertension increases risk of progressive renal injury. The frequency with which 'essential' hypertension is a sole cause of renal failure ('hypertensive nephrosclerosis') in the absence of an accelerated phase is discussed in Chapter 36.

Amongst patients with chronic renal impairment, data from the Modification of Diet in Renal Disease study shows that 83% of 1795 patients screened for inclusion were hypertensive; hypertension was associated with higher body weight, male gender, lower GFR, higher age and black race, and was frequently poorly controlled[10]. Amongst dialysis patients, the prevalence of hypertension is high, apart from patients treated with long-hour dialysis and dietary sodium restriction and in those undergoing daily or nocturnal dialysis. Hypertension is common after renal transplantation[8].

Pathogenesis of hypertension in chronic renal disease

For many years there was a simplistic division of hypertension in ESRD into 'volume-dependent' and 'renin-dependent'. The extremes of this division were relatively easy to define clinically, but the majority of patients lay somewhere between the two extremes. Neither was this simple paradigm useful for treatment of hypertension in predialysis chronic renal failure. Logically, 'volume-dependent' hypertension would be expected to respond to dietary sodium restriction and/or natriuretic treatment (e.g., loop diuretics) and renin-dependent hypertension to β-blockade, angiotensin converting enzyme (ACE) inhibition or angiotensin receptor blockade. Whether patients with hypertension secondary to renal disease can be classified according to their response to different classes of antihypertensives, however, remains uncertain; many patients with renal disease and hypertension appear to require multiple antihypertensive drugs from different classes to obtain adequate BP control, suggesting a multifactorial etiology.

Several important mechanisms are involved in the hypertension of chronic renal disease. First, most patients, and particularly those on dialysis, have a component of volume expansion. Second, sympathetic overactivity is an important contributor to hypertension in polycystic kidney disease (even with normal excretory function) and in ESRD. The absence of

sympathetic overactivity amongst patients who had undergone bilateral nephrectomy suggests that this overactivity is caused by an afferent signal to the sympathetic centre arising in diseased kidneys. Several lines of evidence suggest that this afferent signal is angiotensin II; in particular, there is evidence that ACE inhibition reverses efferent sympathetic nerve activity in patients with hypertension secondary to renal disease. Third, patients with chronic renal failure have elevated serum levels of a natural inhibitor of nitric oxide (NO) synthesis, asymmetric dimethylarginine (ADMA). NO is a potent vasodilator and inhibition of NO synthesis in animals can cause hypertension. Persistent renin secretion from the diseased kidneys may also contribute to hypertension. These and other disturbances in renal disease which contribute to the pathogenesis of hypertension are shown in Figure 69.2.

Correction of anemia by epoietin can result in exacerbation of hypertension, with a syndrome of encephalopathy with cortical blindness and seizures. This complication appears more likely if anemia is corrected rapidly. The mechanism remains uncertain[12]; a failure of cardiac output to fall in response to increasing peripheral vascular resistance (as a result

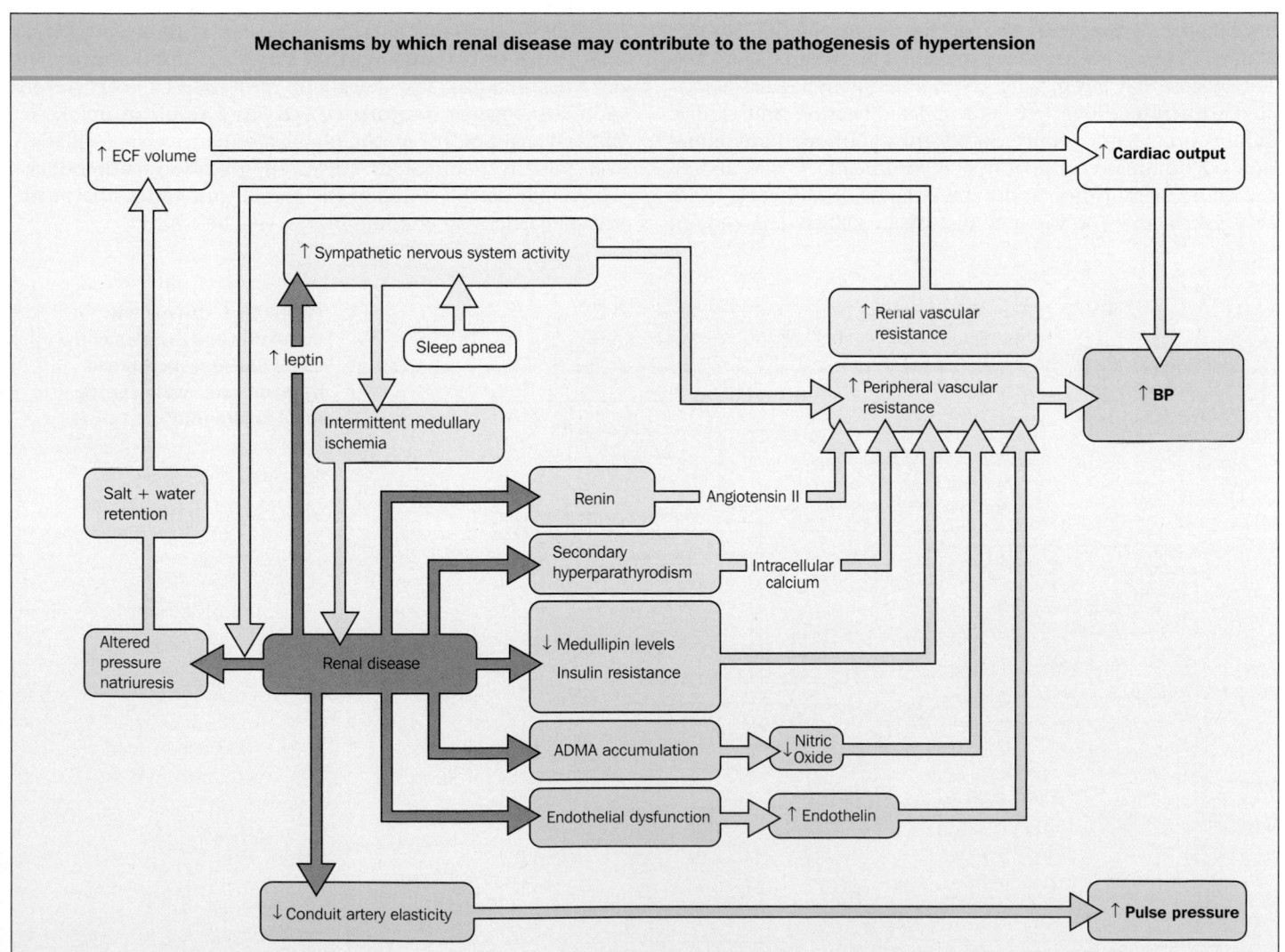

Figure 69.2 Mechanisms by which renal disease may contribute to the pathogenesis of hypertension.

of decreased hypoxic vasodilatation) is often seen. Direct pressor effects of epoietin have been described *in vitro* but the clinical relevance of these findings is uncertain.

Proteinuria

Even minor degrees of proteinuria are frequently associated with other cardiovascular risk factors, including decreased HDL cholesterol, hypertriglyceridemia, increased factor VIII von Willebrand levels, hyperfibrinogenemia and LVH. In diabetes and essential hypertension, microalbuminuria is associated with increased transcapillary escape of albumin, suggesting at least in these two situations that the appearance of albumin in the urine is simply a marker for generalized vascular endothelial dysfunction.

Chronic inflammation

Two of the strongest independent predictors of outcome in hemodialysis patients are elevated C-reactive protein and hypoalbuminemia. The two are closely correlated, as albumin is a negative acute phase reactant. Both are associated with elevated levels of proinflammatory cytokines, fibrinogen, and soluble adhesion molecules, which also predict a poor outcome. These abnormalities are associated with evidence of endothelial dysfunction. The primary cause of this chronic activation of the acute phase response is uncertain (Fig 69.3)[13]. The process may be episodic. Hypoalbuminemia is also associated with progressive left ventricular dilatation and cardiac failure and of cardiac valve calcification. Although inflammation is a dominant cause of hypoalbuminemia, it may also be caused by malnutrition and hypervolemia. Whether these are also risk factors for vascular disease in CRF is less certain,

although malnutrition might contribute via decreased intake of vitamins B_6, B_{12} and folate, causing hyperhomocysteinemia, and of arginase, impairing nitric oxide generation.

Hypervolemia

Recurrent volume overload is also a cause of premature mortality by contributing to LVH and left ventricular dilatation, although the relationship between interdialytic weight gain and mortality is U-shaped, possibly as a result of low weight gains among patients with comorbidity and advanced age[16].

Uremia and inadequate dialysis

Underdialysis, assessed either by urea clearance (Kt/V) or urea reduction ratio, is associated with increased morbidity and mortality in patients on dialysis. Cardiovascular disease accounts for a significant proportion of the increased morbidity and mortality. The exact mechanisms by which poor solute removal leads to increased cardiovascular morbidity are uncertain. Urea itself causes nonenzymatic carbamylation of proteins, including hemoglobin and lipoproteins: this might render lipoproteins more susceptible to oxidation, in a manner analogous to the increased susceptibility of glycated lipoproteins to oxidation in patients with diabetes. There is evidence available *in vitro* that urea is directly toxic to endothelial cells. Carbamylation may also inhibit antioxidant enzymes. Oxidized low-density lipoprotein (LDL) particles are more atherogenic than native LDL, as a result of uptake by the scavenger pathway. Uremia also enhances the formation and impairs removal of advanced glycation endproducts, which may partly be responsible for abnormalities such as the loss of elasticity in conduit arteries (see below).

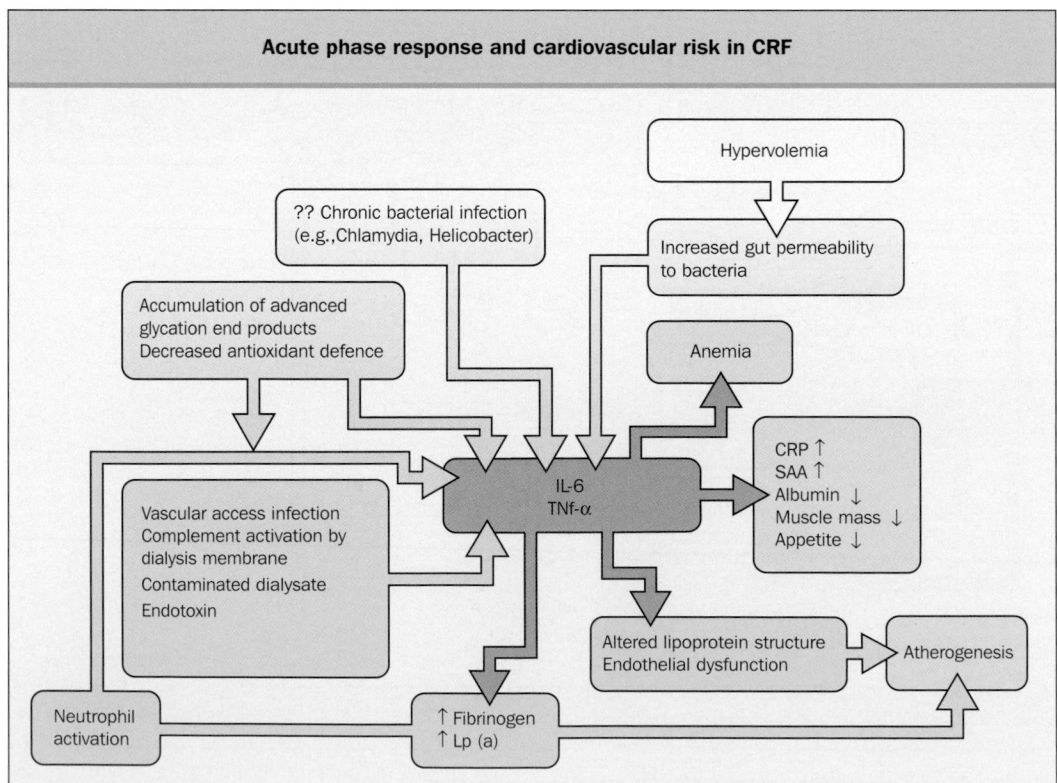

Figure 69.3 Causes and correlates of activation of the acute phase response and hypoalbuminemia in chronic renal failure (CRF).

Hyperhomocysteinemia

As in the general population, mild hyperhomocysteinemia is associated with increased cardiovascular event rates in chronic renal failure[15]. Vascular access thrombosis rates are also increased. In renal impairment only a fraction of the elevation of plasma homocysteine over normal is accounted for by deficiency of folate or the other vitamins involved in pathways of homocysteine metabolism; the remainder appears unrelated to decreased renal clearance but may be due to accumulation of inhibitors of remethylation of homocysteine. Even minor degrees of renal impairment are associated with increased plasma homocysteine. *In vitro*, high levels of homocysteine cause endothelial dysfunction, oxidative damage and thrombosis. Studies are underway to assess the effect of normalizing homocysteine levels in patients with functioning renal transplants (in whom folate supplementation is generally effective). It remains to be seen whether normalization of homocysteine levels in dialysis patients will reduce endothelial activation or cardiovascular event rates.

Insulin resistance

In nonuremic subjects, impaired insulin-stimulated glucose disposal in muscle is often part of a metabolic syndrome that also includes dyslipidemia, hypertension, endothelial dysfunction, sympathetic overactivity and, according to some investigators, microvascular angina. Many of these abnormalities, including insulin resistance, are also found in CRF and even in incipient renal disease. Whether insulin resistance is the primary defect, either in nonuremic subjects or in CRF, remains uncertain. Correction of both acidosis and hyperparathyroidism may improve insulin sensitivity in CRF, but neither has been shown to improve cardiovascular outcome.

Dyslipidemia

Numerous abnormalities of lipid and lipoprotein metabolism are described in renal disease and as a consequence of drug therapy commonly used in renal patients (Table 69.2). These abnormalities are caused by complex alterations in several pathways of lipoprotein metabolism. In addition, nonenzymatic modification of lipoprotein particles enhances their atherogenicity without affecting the measured levels of cholesterol, triglycerides, or the HDL, LDL and very-low-density lipoprotein (VLDL) fractions.

The lipid abnormalities in nephrotic syndrome and in renal transplant recipients are discussed elsewhere, see chapters 19 and 89.

Renal impairment, including hemodialysis

Two major pathways involved in lipoprotein metabolism are abnormal in CRF. Impaired action of lipoprotein lipase results in high levels of triglyceride-rich VLDL, partially metabolized remnant particles (intermediate density lipoproteins, IDL) and small dense LDL. Possible causes for the decreased lipoprotein lipase (LPL) activity include decreased synthesis of the enzyme, insulin resistance, accumulation of an inhibitor of LPL, or altered lipoprotein composition (increased ratio of apolipoprotein (apo) C-III to apoC-II). Hyperparathyroidism and chronic inflammation are both potential inhibitors of LPL activity. In hemodialysis patients, heparin may further

suppress LPL activity. Furthermore, impaired lecithin-cholesterol acyltransferase activity reduces reverse cholesterol transport, resulting in decreased HDL2 levels. Conversion from cuprophan to more biocompatible dialysis membranes improves lipid profile, with lower VLDL cholesterol levels and higher HDL2 levels, but the mechanism is unclear.

Peritoneal dialysis

Peritoneal dialysis is associated with similar abnormalities to those found in CRF combined with those found in nephrotic syndrome, with hypertriglyceridemia in 50% and hypercholesterolemia in 30% of patients. Plasma lipoproteins are lost in peritoneal effluent, HDL being lost to a much greater extent than LDL or VLDL because of its smaller size. Whether glucose absorption from dialysate contributes significantly to increased VLDL levels is unclear but this is certainly not the only explanation.

Other contributors to abnormal lipoprotein metabolism

Activation of the acute inflammatory response, discussed above, is associated with increased levels of Lp(a), a highly atherogenic particle with homology to fibrinogen. Correction of hypoalbuminemia with intravenous albumin in continuous ambulatory peritoneal dialysis patients reduces Lp(a) levels, which suggests that hypoalbuminemia contributes to increased Lp(a) synthesis independently of acute inflammation. LDL in patients with CRF is frequently modified by nonenzymatic oxidation, accumulation of advanced glycation endproducts, carbamylation, and modification by reactive carbonyl compounds. All of these alterations reduce LDL clearance and increase uptake of these particles by the macrophage scavenger receptor.

Arteriovenous fistula

A functioning arteriovenous fistula results in an increase in stroke volume, ejection fraction and cardiac output, and a fall in total peripheral resistance. This is associated with a rise in atrial natriuretic peptide, reflecting atrial stretch as a result of the increase in venous return. High-output cardiac failure

Lipid abnormalities in renal disease				
Stage of renal disease	Cholesterol levels			Triglycerides
	Total	High-density lipoproteins	Low-density lipoproteins	
Nephrotic syndrome	↑↑↑	↓	↑↑	↑
Chronic renal failure	→	↓	→*	↑↑
Hemodialysis	→	↓	→*	↑↑
Continuous ambulatory peritoneal dialysis	↑	↓	↑	↑
Transplantation	↑↑	→	↑	↑
*Composition altered				

Table 69.2 Lipid abnormalities in renal disease. Common patterns of hyperlipidemia in different stages of renal disease.

Chronic Renal Failure and the Uremic Syndrome

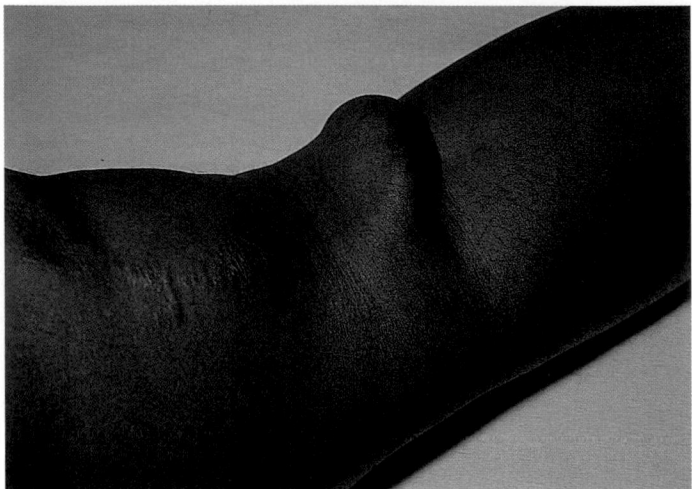

Figure 69.4 A high-flow arteriovenous fistula associated with cardiac failure.

may be precipitated by the construction of high-flow fistulae (Fig. 69.4) (e.g., brachial or femoral) in patients with pre-existing heart disease, causing impaired systolic function; however, this has not been reported with radiocephalic fistulae. A fistula blood flow of > 1500 mL/min, measured either directly or by the alteration in cardiac output during temporary occlusion, in a patient with cardiac failure and pre-existing heart disease should prompt consideration of banding the fistula to reduce flow or even of fistula ligation.

Anemia

Anemia is a major cause of LVH and left ventricular dilatation in ESRD. Partial correction of anemia with epoetin results in regression of LVH, although it has yet to be proven that this reduces cardiovascular mortality. It would be more rational to prevent the development of LVH by treatment of anemia early in the course of CRF, and trials to assess the effectiveness of this strategy are underway. Anemia also increases the chance that angina will occur at any given degree of coronary stenosis, and correction of anemia is often the best anti-anginal treatment in CRF.

Iron overload

Some studies in patients other than those with renal disease have shown an association between higher serum ferritin levels and increased cardiovascular mortality, perhaps through iron-catalyzed lipid peroxidation, which would enhance the atherogenicity of LDL. No direct association between serum ferritin and cardiovascular disease has been confirmed in patients with renal disease, although there is evidence that lipid peroxidation increases after parenteral iron administration.

Abnormalities of coagulation

In the normal population, increased activity of procoagulant proteins including factor VII and fibrinogen is associated with coronary risk. Factor VII coagulant activity and markers of thrombin activation are elevated in patients with CRF (dependent on factor VII genotype) and correlate positively with serum triglycerides and the acute phase reactants interleukin (IL)-6 and fibrinogen and negatively with serum albumin.

Endothelial function and activation

Chronic renal failure is associated with endothelial dysfunction and decreased endothelium-dependent vasodilatation. Increased serum levels of von Willebrand factor and of adhesion molecules are closely associated with increases in inflammatory cytokines and in C-reactive protein. Total body nitric oxide production is reduced in chronic renal failure. Endothelium-dependent vasodilatation is improved by hemodialysis, suggesting that a dialyzable toxin may partly be responsible. One candidate is the endogenous inhibitor of NO synthase, ADMA, the concentration of which is increased in dialysis patients, CRF patients, and even in patients with renal disease whose GFR is normal. ADMA concentration has recently been reported to be a powerful predictor of cardiovascular system event rates in hemodialysis patients. Other possible contributors to endothelial activation are hyperhomocysteinemia, hyperoxalemia, activation of the acute inflammatory response, and atherogenic lipoprotein particles.

Arterial elasticity

Decreased elasticity of conduit arteries results in increased pulse wave velocity and increased arterial wave reflection, leading to increased pulse pressure, increased central arterial systolic pressure and decreased diastolic myocardial perfusion. These changes are almost universal in dialysis patients. Increased pulse wave velocity is a powerful independent predictor of mortality in hemodialysis patients, as is increased pulse pressure. Endothelial dysfunction, damage to elastin, and medial calcification may all contribute.

Myocardial interstitial fibrosis and capillary rarefaction

Both in experimental and human uremia, there is striking diffuse interstitial fibrosis in the myocardium, combined with capillary rarefaction. In clinical (autopsy) studies, the severity of interstitial fibrosis is related to the duration of dialysis and is still present years after successful renal transplantation. The functional correlate of interstitial fibrosis is likely to be reduced diastolic compliance and increased susceptibility to arrhythmias; decreased capillary density must result in increased susceptibility to hypoxia[18].

Energy metabolism in uremia

Deficiency of L-carnitine (and reduced free carnitine : acylcarnitine ratio) is common in patients on hemodialysis. L-carnitine facilitates the entry of long-chain fatty acids into mitochondria, and deficiency would therefore be expected to impair fatty acid oxidation. There is limited evidence that carnitine supplementation may improve cardiac function and exercise capacity, and decrease the incidence of arrhythmias, in patients on dialysis.

Hyperparathyroidism, phosphate retention and vascular calcification

Patients with chronic renal disease are at markedly increased risk of vascular calcification. Serum phosphate is a powerful predictor of the development of calcification, as well as being an independent predictor of mortality in hemodialysis patients. However, in clinical studies, it is difficult to dissociate the influences of phosphate retention, duration of CRF and dialysis, and hyperparathyroidism on cardiac function, myocardial calcium content and vascular calcification. Recently, low serum levels of Ahsg/fetuin, an inhibitor of vascular calcification, have also been associated with an increased risk for vascular calcification and mortality in dialysis patients[17]. Cumulative dose of calcium-containing phosphate binders is associated with coronary artery calcification (detected by electron beam CT scanning). Early evidence suggests the use of non-calcium containing phosphate binders may reduce the rate at which coronary artery calcification develops. Warfarin (coumadin) may promote vascular calcification since it decreases synthesis of matrix GLA protein (deletion of which in transgenic animals causes striking vascular calcification). Low bone turnover, associated with over-suppression of parathyroid activity, is also associated with vascular calcification, possibly due to decreased ability of bone to 'buffer' excess calcium and phosphate. Low PTH levels are associated with poorer survival in dialysis patients, possibly because of an association with malnutrition and low phosphate intake.

Calcific uremic arteriolopathy, 'calciphylaxis', is becoming more common, perhaps due to widespread use of calcium-based phosphate binders. Other risk factors include female gender, hyperphosphatemia, and hypoalbuminemia. An association with decreased protein C and protein S activity has also been reported.

Primary hyperoxaluria
Primary hyperoxaluria complicated by ESRD results in continuous supersaturation of plasma with calcium oxalate. Unless prevented by intensive dialysis or early transplantation, the resulting systemic oxalosis results in deposition of calcium oxalate crystals in the retina, the media of blood vessels, the myocardium and resulting in peripheral gangrene, cardiomyopathy and heart block (Fig. 69.5).

Is there a specific uremic cardiomyopathy?
It has been proposed that uremia *per se* leads to impaired myocardial contractile function. Improvement after institution of dialysis or after successful transplantation suggests a dialyzable uremic toxin rather than structural alterations or ischemic damage, although chronic volume overload may be responsible by causing a reversible dilated cardiomyopathy. Contractile function improves acutely during hemodialysis, suggesting that a dialyzable uremic toxin has a direct and readily reversible cardiodepressant action. However, most studies have failed to control separately for the effects of ultrafiltration, electrolyte and acid–base changes, and changes in the plasma levels of other metabolites. One study that did control adequately for these variables showed an increase in contractility during isovolemic dialysis only if serum calcium increased as a result of using a high calcium dialysate.

CLINICAL MANIFESTATIONS

Effect of hypertension on natural history
As discussed above, hypertension is very common in chronic renal disease, especially in patients with dialysis. As well as being associated with increased cardiovascular risk, hypertension also increases the risk of progression of renal disease (see Chapter 66). The exception may be polycystic kidney disease, in which there is no evidence that reduction of blood pressure (BP) has any effect on the rate of progression. Similarly the effectiveness of BP reduction in slowing the rate of progression of other non-proteinuric renal diseases is uncertain. However these observations do not detract from the importance of aggressive antihypertensive treatment in these patients, aiming to reduce the high cardiovascular risk.

Cardiac function
Left ventricular hypertrophy
LVH (Fig. 69.6) is a potent predictor of premature mortality in patients on RRT[218]. It occurs early in the course of progressive renal failure and is frequently found in patients with renal disease, even if excretory function remains normal, perhaps

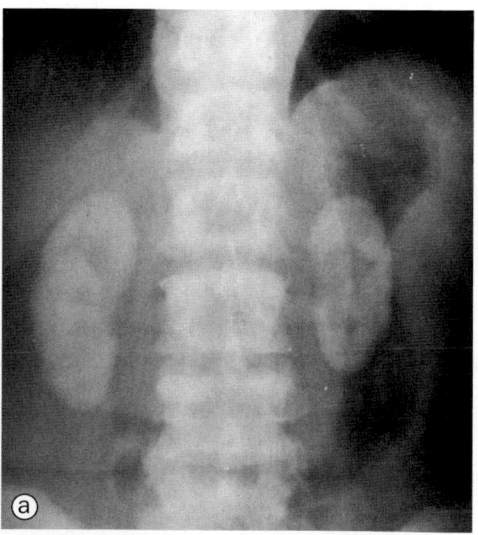

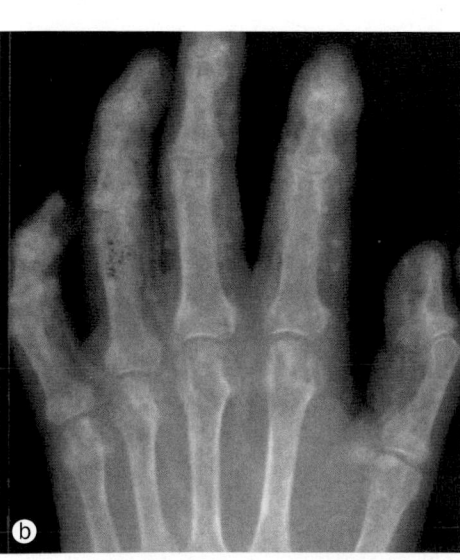

Figure 69.5 Oxalosis in ESRD. (a) Dense calcification in the shrunken kidneys of a patient with oxalosis and longstanding ESRD. (b) Vascular and subcutaneous calcification in the hand of the same patient.

Chronic Renal Failure and the Uremic Syndrome

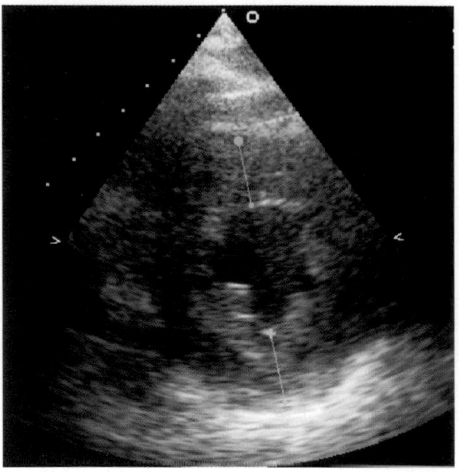

Figure 69.6 Transthoracic echocardiogram showing left ventricular hypertrophy. Markers indicate left ventricular wall thickness = 2 cm.

because of the high prevalence of hypertension and the frequent absence of a nocturnal dip in BP. However, the finding of LVH among normotensive patients with polycystic disease suggests that neuroendocrine factors may also be important, in particular the renin–angiotensin–aldosterone system, the endothelin system, and sympathetic overactivity. With progressive loss of renal function, anemia, volume overload and hyperparathyroidism all act as additional risk factors for LVH.

LVH is primarily an adaptive response, serving to normalize wall tension. Wall tension, the signal for hypertrophy, is directly proportional to wall radius and to pressure and is inversely proportional to wall thickness. Therefore, an increase in wall thickness in a patient with hypertension or with left ventricular dilatation due to hypervolemia results in normalization of wall tension. Differing stimuli to LVH cause different patterns of hypertrophy (Fig. 69.7). Pressure overload, as caused by hypertension and decreased large vessel compliance, results in concentric hypertrophy. Volume overload without any hypertrophy would normally stretch the left ventricular wall causing it to appear thinner than normal; the adaptive response to volume overload is a form of LVH in which left ventricular thickness is restored to normal (so-called 'eccentric hypertrophy'). A third variant, asymmetric hypertrophy, causes thickening of the septal wall but not the free left ventricular wall, and is thought to be caused by sympathetic overactivity. The distinction is important because the different patterns of hypertrophy involve expression of different myosin isoforms, and may have a different natural history.

Left ventricular dilatation

Left ventricular dilatation (Fig. 69.7) is also a potent predictor of poor outcome, particularly in those patients without LVH: so-called inadequate LVH. A progressive increase in the radius : wall thickness ratio may be a result of hyperparathyroidism (possibly a consequence of capillary rarefaction and interstitial fibrosis) or may simply be an end result of LVH[19]. Other potential causes include diffuse ischemic damage, recurrent volume overload or high-output arteriovenous fistulae.

Diastolic dysfunction

Abnormal diastolic relaxation is most reliably detected by pulsed Doppler measurement of the velocity of the 'e' (early, passive) and 'a' (atrial, active) components of diastolic flow across the mitral valve. Decreased left ventricular compliance caused by impaired relaxation results in an decreased e : a ratio

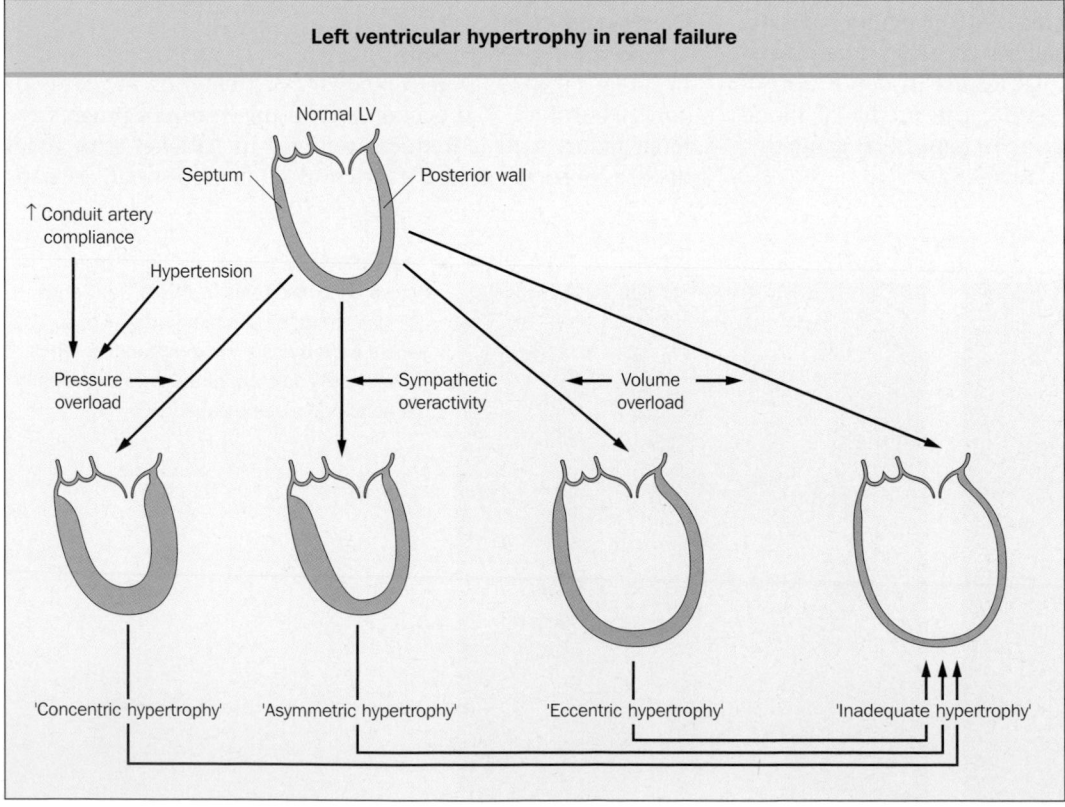

Figure 69.7 Causes of left ventricular (LV) hypertrophy in renal failure. Caution is necessary in the assessment of left ventricular mass, as echocardiographic formulae include left ventricular diameter, which may change rapidly through changes in fluid balance.

Left ventricular hypertrophy in renal failure

↑ Conduit artery compliance
Hypertension
Pressure overload
Sympathetic overactivity
Volume overload
Normal LV
Septum
Posterior wall
'Concentric hypertrophy'
'Asymmetric hypertrophy'
'Eccentric hypertrophy'
'Inadequate hypertrophy'

and is frequently found in uremic patients as a result of LVH. Diastolic dysfunction is associated with an increased risk of intradialytic hypotension, as relatively small reductions in left atrial filling have marked effects on cardiac output. Hypercalcemia, as occurs during standard hemodialysis, causes acute impairment of diastolic filling. There is no evidence that uremia *per se* causes diastolic dysfunction in the absence of LVH.

Blood vessel abnormalities

In patients with ESRD but no prior history of atherosclerosis, the dominant histologic findings in the arterial vasculature are fibrous intimal thickening, fragmentation of the internal elastic membrane and medial calcification, with a striking absence of lipid deposition. These lesions are very similar to the abnormalities associated with aging, and occur in animals even if hypertension is prevented. Increased intima-media thickness in uremic patients demonstrable by B-mode ultrasound, is related to age, smoking and serum phosphate or PTH; it is associated with increased left ventricular wall thickness, and is an independent predictor of increased mortality. The extent to which these anatomic changes are responsible for decreased conduit artery compliance remains uncertain[20].

Arterial calcification in uremia is common, often detectable on plain radiographs (Fig. 69.8) and increases with time on dialysis with increasing age and with increasing plasma phosphate and 1,25 vitamin D concentration. The calcification is often confined to the arterial media, with no endoluminal obstruction and therefore carries a different prognosis to calcification complicating atherosclerosis. Recent studies have utilized electron beam CT scanning to demonstrate a high prevalence of coronary artery calcification amongst patients with ESRD, with an association between current prescribed doses of calcium-containing phosphate binders and the extent of calcification[21]. However, the prognostic significance of coronary artery calcification in uremia is uncertain.

Calcific uremic arteriolopathy ('calciphylaxis') is a syndrome of calcification of small arterioles and venules with severe intimal hyperplasia, often complicated by thrombosis and recanalization, which results in painful skin necrosis (see Figs 68.9, 71.4 and 71.5) and peripheral gangrene. Its pathogenesis and management are discussed further in Chapters 68 and 71.

Reduced venous compliance and histologic thickening of the venous media have been reported in hypertensive but not normotensive patients on dialysis. Reduced venous compliance can be induced in sodium-sensitive patients with essential hypertension by a high salt diet, but the effect of sodium balance on venous compliance in patients on dialysis has not been studied. Failure of venoconstriction during hemodialysis is one contributor to dialysis-associated hypotension.

Autonomic dysfunction

There is decreased baroreflex sensitivity in ESRD, which may be caused by volume overload, hypertension and aging (and possibly by decreased conduit vessel elasticity); it is not clear whether a true neuropathy is also present. No relationship between altered autonomic function and cardiovascular mortality has been reported in CRF or ESRD.

Increased sympathetic nerve discharge, measured by microneurography, has been reported in patients with ESRD, although not in patients who had previously undergone bilateral nephrectomy, suggesting that the afferent signal leading to increased sympathetic nerve discharge comes from the diseased kidneys. Circulating catecholamines are increased but with reduced pressor responsiveness to α- and β-stimulation and reduced adrenoceptor numbers. Downregulation of pressor responsiveness to sympathetic stimulation may contribute to hypotension during volume removal and, in a small subset of patients on long-term dialysis, to a syndrome of chronic volume-unresponsive hypotension despite normal cardiac function.

Valvular disease

Calcification of the mitral valve annulus and the aortic valve cusps is common in CRF (Fig. 69.9). Risk factors for the presence of annular calcification include a history of hyperparathyroidism, raised calcium phosphate product, length of time on dialysis, hypoalbuminemia and advanced age.

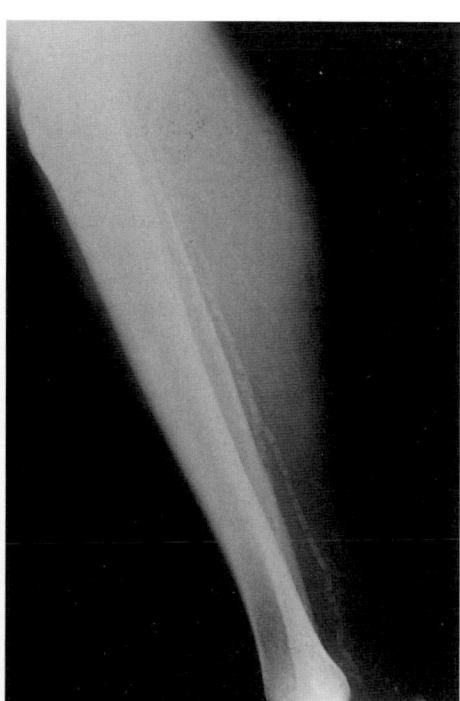

Figure 69.8 Arterial calcification in ESRD. Severe pipestem calcification in a patient on hemodialysis who had developed severe hyperparathyroidism requiring parathyroidectomy. Note calcification of subcutaneous vessels; this patient subsequently developed calciphylaxis.

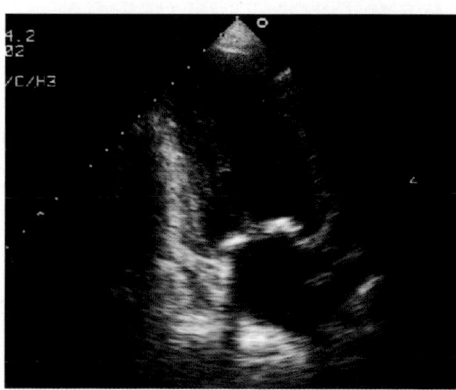

Figure 69.9 Transthoracic echocardiogram showing annular mitral ring calcification.

Chronic Renal Failure and the Uremic Syndrome

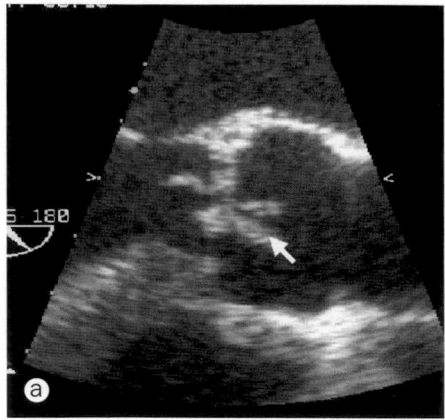
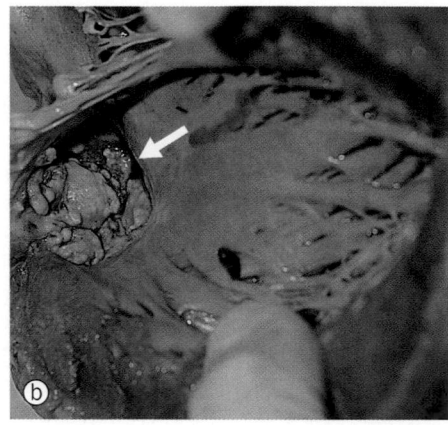
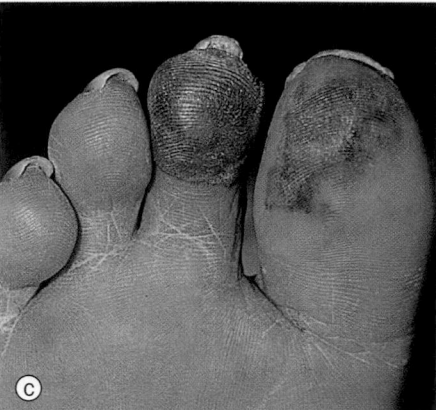

Figure 69.10 Infective endocarditis in ESRD. (a) Transesophageal echocardiogram showing vegetation on the aortic valve (arrow). (b) Vegetation on the aortic valve found at biopsy. (c) Septic embolization of the toes.

Calcification may be associated with valvular regurgitation or, occasionally, with hemodynamically significant stenosis (particularly in the aortic valve) and with the development of conduction disturbances, including complete heart block, due of involvement of the bundle of His.

Functional regurgitation of mitral and aortic valves is a frequent finding in ESRD and results from valve ring dilatation as a result of hypervolemia. Correction of volume overload by ultrafiltration leads to resolution of regurgitation, and this may be the only way of determining whether the regurgitation is functional or structural in origin.

Infective endocarditis

Infective endocarditis (Fig. 69.10) has an incidence of 2–4% in patients with ESRD, particularly in those receiving HD, in whom infection introduced via vascular access is the most important cause. Semipermanent central venous catheters are the major source: these catheters are nearly always colonized within weeks of insertion and their use is often associated with peripheral bacteremia. Dental treatment is much less commonly implicated. Whether calcified valves are more prone to infection is uncertain. The aortic valve is infected more commonly than the mitral, and right-sided lesions are uncommon. As in patients who are not receiving dialysis, the development of heart failure mandates valve replacement: without early surgery, mortality is high.

MANAGEMENT OF COMMON CARDIOVASCULAR SYNDROMES IN UREMIA

Arrhythmias

Arrhythmias are a common clinical problem in uremia particularly during hemodialysis. Sudden death is an important cause of mortality in patients with ESRD. In one study, all in-center sudden deaths were shown to be of cardiac origin, 80% caused by ventricular fibrillation and the remainder being asystolic. Hyperkalemia is the most important metabolic abnormality in ESRD associated with arrhythmias (Fig. 69.11) but serum concentrations of calcium and magnesium should also be reviewed. Asystolic cardiac arrest may be the result of hyperkalemia. Numerous ECG abnormalities have been

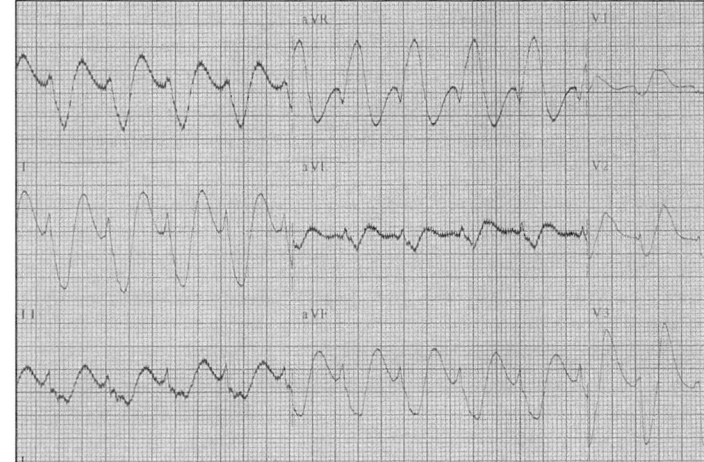

Figure 69.11 Hyperkalemia. Typical electrocardiogram changes in hyperkalemia with broad complex tachycardia and absent P waves.

reported in patients on dialysis. These abnormalities may be caused by structural heart disease, electrolyte abnormalities, or alterations in cardiac filling and may or may not be corrected by hemodialysis. For these reasons, interpretation of ECGs requires caution in ESRD (Table 69.3).

Pulmonary congestion and the assessment of left ventricular function

Breathlessness is a very common presenting symptom in uremia and is most commonly caused by pulmonary congestion, although the full range of infective, vascular and inflammatory causes of dyspnea must always be considered in the differential diagnosis. Pulmonary congestion may occur as a result of poor patient compliance with salt and water restriction or because occult loss of flesh weight results in overestimation of dry weight. The crucial distinction to be made is between hypervolemia as the sole cause of pulmonary congestion and the additional presence of left ventricular dysfunction, since this will determine whether fluid removal alone will be adequate or whether additional therapy such as ACE inhibitors and venodilators may be necessary. The additional clinical signs of raised jugular vein pulse, gallop rhythm, hepatomegaly,

Electrocardiographic abnormalities in renal failure	
Function	**Abnormality seen in renal failure**
P–R interval	Usually normal: prolongation in long-term hemodialysis
	Calcification of mitral valve annulus may involve His bundle, giving complete heart block
QRS interval	
Amplitude	Increases during ultrafiltration (correlates with reduction in left ventricular (LV) dimensions)
	LV hypertrophy (LVH) on voltage criteria found in up to 50%
Duration	Prolonged (within normal range) by hemodialysis
	Late potentials increased only in patients with pre-existing ischemic heart disease
	Prolonged in hyperkalemia
ST segment	Depression during hemodialysis does not predict coronary artery disease
	Depression or elevation may occur in hyperkalemia
	Depression during ambulatory monitoring poorly predictive of coronary heart disease (CHD)
$Q–T_c$ interval	Increases during hemodialysis (correlates with reduction in (K^+) and (Mg^{2+}))
	Increased Q–T dispersion reported in patients on dialysis
T wave	Peaking or inversion may occur in hyperkalemia
	Inversion in anterolateral leads in LVH with strain pattern
Rhythm	High incidence of atrial and ventricular arrhythmias during hemodialysis
	Risk factors: LV dysfunction, wall motion abnormalities, known coronary artery disease, positive thallium redistribution tests (even without CHD), use of cardiac glycosides, low dialysate (K^+)

Table 69.3 Electrocardiographic abnormalities in renal failure.

and peripheral edema do not help to make this distinction. Whatever the cause, these signs carry a poor prognosis.

Echocardiography

The echocardiogram is widely available but difficult to interpret in ESRD. Assessment of contractile function must be made with caution, as all of the commonly used indices (ejection fraction, fractional shortening, velocity of circumferential fiber shortening, left ventricular ejection time) may be altered by abnormal loading conditions as well as by intrinsic alterations in contractility. For example, in the isolated ventricle, ejection fraction is increased if preload is increased (because increasing preload increases end-diastolic volume) and decreased if afterload is increased (because the completeness with which the ventricle empties depends on the resistance against which it is emptying)[22]. Echocardiographic estimates of left ventricular mass are unreliable when compared to magnetic resonance imaging (MRI), particularly in the presence of left ventricular dilatation. Despite these problems in interpretation, echocardiography gives powerful prognostic information and is valuable in distinguishing between pulmonary edema due to volume overload and hypertension from that due to impaired left ventricular systolic or diastolic function. Echocardiography is usually performed when the

patient is at their prescribed 'dry weight', i.e., within 12 h of completion of hemodialysis, and allows diagnosis of valvular disease (including annular calcification), left ventricular hypertrophy, and assessment of diastolic and systolic function. Transesophageal echocardiography is far superior to transthoracic in the diagnosis of valvular vegetations complicating endocarditis.

Chest pain

The full differential diagnosis familiar to the internist must be considered in assessing the uremic patient with chest pain. However, two additional factors must be considered: (1) the high incidence of pericarditis and (2) the unusual clinical features of coronary heart disease in these patients.

Pericarditis

Two types of pericarditis are recognized in uremia. Uremic pericarditis occurs in the terminal phases of untreated uremia and is now rare, mostly being seen following withdrawal of dialysis. 'Dialysis-associated pericarditis' remains relatively common and contributes to death in up to 10% of patients, although its frequency may be decreasing.

Dialysis-associated pericarditis appears to be more frequent in patients who are under-dialyzed and is frequently precipitated by an intercurrent illness, but the exact pathogenesis remains unclear. The possibility that pericarditis is caused by the underlying disease (e.g., systemic lupus erythematosus) or drug treatment (e.g., minoxidil) should be considered. Pericardial pain and fever are the most common presenting symptoms. A pericardial rub may be present, but this may be transient. 'Classic' ECG changes are seen in a minority of patients only; echocardiography is the most useful diagnostic tool and reveals an effusion in over 90% of patients.

Because of the risk of tamponade, patients with pericarditis should be admitted to hospital. Many cases resolve within weeks, probably as a result of the resolution of the precipitating illness; it is customary to prescribe intensified dialysis, but this is of no proven benefit. Anticoagulation during dialysis should be minimized, and tamponade as a result of pericardial hemorrhage has rarely been reported. Nonsteroidal anti-inflammatory drugs reduce fever but have no effect on other complications. Decreased venous return during dialysis may precipitate tamponade; target weight may be increased temporarily to avoid this.

Fever, signs of heart failure, hemodynamic instability, neutrophilia and large effusions (Fig. 69.12) are all predictive that the pericarditis will fail to resolve. Patients with clinical or echocardiographic evidence of incipient tamponade (pulsus paradoxus, hypotension at previous target weight, diastolic collapse on echocardiography) should be referred for further intervention. This usually comprises a trial of pericardiocentesis with local instillation of steroids, followed by endoscopic or open surgical pericardiectomy if tamponade recurs.

Angina and coronary heart disease

Angina occurs as a result of typical atheromatous coronary disease and may be provoked by additional clinical events that require correction before invasive coronary management is indicated. Angina on hemodialysis is frequently provoked

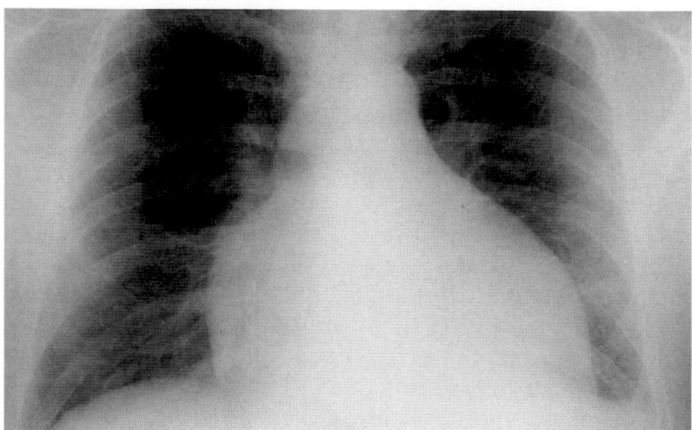

Figure 69.12 Pericardial effusion. Chest radiograph showing large pericardial effusion.

by arrhythmias or hypotension. It may also become apparent if myocardial oxygen delivery is impaired as a result of inadequately treated anemia[23].

If there is sustained ischemic pain, the diagnosis of myocardial infarction is made less straightforward by the difficulties in assessing the ECG in ESRD (Table 69.3) and also by problems in interpretation of cardiac enzymes. Borderline increases in creatine kinase have low specificity in CRF and ESRD (because of the elevated myocardial-bound creatine kinase levels that occur even in the absence of cardiac disease). Minor elevations of Troponin I (TnI) and Troponin T (TnT) are common in CRF. Both are difficult to measure reliably, and assays may be unreliable in CRF, particularly for TnT. However, moderate elevation of TnT has been repeatedly reported as a risk marker for cardiovascular events in CRF patients. This is most likely due to increases in TnI concentration in CRF patients with LVH, although the possibility that these minor elevations occur in patients with subclinical unstable coronary disease cannot easily be excluded. These minor elevations do not detract from the usefulness of these markers in the diagnosis of acute coronary syndromes, when there is a sequential rise, often to at least four times the upper limit of normal, followed by a fall towards baseline; as in patients without renal disease, a typical history and ECG changes are also crucial in establishing a diagnosis. If myocardial infarction occurs, thrombolysis should be given according to conventional criteria, although its value has not been assessed specifically in uremia.

Myocardial infarction in hemodialysis carries an extremely poor prognosis, with a 62% 1-year and 74% 2-year mortality reported in the era since the routine use of thrombolytics. Use of thrombolysis amongst hemodialysis patients is low, possibly because the presentation of myocardial infarction is frequently atypical and delayed[24]. The prognosis is equally poor in non-dialysis-dependent CRF. Renal transplant patients with acute myocardial infarction have a better prognosis than those on dialysis, although this may partly reflect selection of patients for transplantation.

Coronary angiography

Angiography is performed for conventional clinical indications, such as symptomatic angina, documented myocardial infarction, wall motion abnormalities on echocardiography, or abnormal [201]thallium distribution after exercise or dipyridamole. There is a high incidence of angina with normal coronary arteries: possible causes include severe anemia, LVH, small vessel disease (including calcific uremic arteriolopathy), endothelial dysfunction, decreased capillary density, and decreased large vessel compliance, resulting in higher pulse pressure and decreased diastolic perfusion. However, severe coronary artery disease without angina is also surprisingly common in ESRD[23]. When present, coronary disease is often diffuse and calcific, making successful revascularization difficult.

It is still not certain whether ESRD is itself a risk factor for progressive coronary atherosclerosis. Many long-term dialysis patients remain free of coronary disease, and the highest risk of coronary events is in the first year after starting dialysis[6], suggesting that the risk may be highest in the predialysis phase of CRF. Early studies reported no progression of coronary artery disease in highly selected dialysis patients undergoing repeat angiography, but a more recent study showed rapid progression in some dialysis patients, whose cardiovascular risk factors were similar to those with no progression.

Coronary revascularization

As in the general population, revascularization can be offered either to relieve symptoms or to improve prognosis. However, the evidence guiding decisions in this area is poor. There is evidence that three- and four-vessel disease carries a poor prognosis in patients being considered for transplantation, but no direct evidence on the extent to which any form of revascularization improves prognosis amongst patients with CRF. Several reports have drawn attention to a very high rate of early restenosis after percutaneous balloon angioplasty in patients with ESRD, although this might be improved by rotational atherectomy for highly calcified lesions, stenting, or placement of stents coated with heparin or rapamycin. Coronary calcification increases the risk of dissection as a complication of angioplasty.

Coronary artery bypass grafting (CABG) is safe and effective in patients with ESRD, although postoperative morbidity (including duration of mechanical ventilation, duration of inotropic support, length of stay on the intensive care unit, and length of hospital stay) is increased compared to patients with a similar severity of cardiac disease but without renal failure. These risks are further increased amongst patients with poor left ventricular function. It is still uncertain whether asymptomatic dialysis patients with prognostically important (e.g., triple vessel) coronary disease on angiography should be offered CABG or listed for transplantation without CABG; it is not clear whether either strategy would improve the outcome compared to continuing maintenance dialysis with medical management of cardiovascular risk factors.

Moderate renal impairment (serum creatinine > 1.4 mg/dL (150 μmol/L)) increases the risk of death after CABG seven-fold relative to those patients with a normal serum creatinine. For patients with CRF not yet on dialysis, there is a significant risk that coronary bypass grafting will be complicated by an irreversible loss of renal function. In these patients, angioplasty combined with intensive medical treatment may be appropriate, even if the benefit is temporary, with a view to definitive treatment when the patient has been established on dialysis. The risk of contrast nephrotoxicity should also be considered. If renal function is stable but markedly impaired, the risks of precipitating the need for dialysis have to be weighed against the possible symptomatic and prognostic benefits of surgical revascularization.

The only controlled trial comparing medical treatment with bypass grafting in ESRD enrolled 26 patients with type 1 diabetes. A significant advantage for bypass grafting was shown, but the fact that the 'medical' treatment arm consisted of aspirin and dihydropyridine calcium channel blockade, with no lipid-lowering treatment and no β-blockade makes this trial of limited relevance to modern practice[25].

EFFECTS OF HEMODIALYSIS AND ULTRAFILTRATION ON CARDIOVASCULAR FUNCTION

Acute symptomatic hypotension is the most frequent complication of hemodialysis[26]; the pathogenesis is complex but includes alterations in circulating volume, peripheral vascular resistance, venous tone, myocardial compliance and contractility, autonomic function, food consumption, and the effects of vasoactive drugs (Fig. 79.2).

Circulating volume
Circulating volume during dialysis is governed by the balance between the ultrafiltration rate and refilling from the interstitial compartment. Refilling depends first on the amount of excess extracellular fluid available for removal (i.e., the amount by which the patient is above their 'dry weight'). Second, rapid reduction in serum osmolality, seen particularly towards the start of dialysis, results in a flux of water from the extracellular to the intracellular compartment. This can be opposed by use of high initial dialysate sodium concentration, followed by a progressive reduction over the remainder of the dialysis session to avoid net sodium gain ('sodium profiling'). Third, protein flux between interstitial and vascular compartments occurs during ultrafiltration, helping to maintain circulating volume.

Peripheral vascular resistance and venous tone
Peripheral vascular resistance and venous tone both fall during dialysis (but much less during isolated ultrafiltration), possibly because of the combined effects of removal of an endogenous vasoconstrictor and warming (dialysate is conventionally used at 38°C). Acetate-based dialysis also causes vasodilatation, particularly in patients whose metabolism of acetate is slow (e.g., the elderly and those with reduced muscle bulk). Reduction in venous tone (increased venous capacitance) contributes to hypotension by causing a decrease in cardiac filling. Increased secretion of calcitonin gene-related peptide, a powerful endogenous vasodilator, in response to overhydration may allow tolerance of fluid overload between dialyses but may actually contribute to hemodynamic instability during fluid removal.

Myocardial compliance and contractility
Myocardial compliance is reduced by high calcium dialysate, resulting in impairment of left ventricular filling, particularly in patients with diastolic dysfunction caused by LVH. Myocardial contractility is increased by high calcium dialysate but may be reduced by acetate in patients with pre-existing contractile dysfunction.

Sympathetic tone
Sympathetic tone, assessed by spectral analysis of heart rate variability, increases during fluid removal (resulting in tachycardia and decreased pulse pressure) until a critical point is reached, at which sympathetic tone is withdrawn and vagal tone increased. This can best be understood as a protective reflex, preventing structural damage that might otherwise be caused by forceful contraction of an empty heart and allowing prolonged diastolic filling.

Consumption of food
Consumption of food during hemodialysis increases the risk of intradialytic hypotension, probably as a result of increased splanchnic blood flow (or preventing the reflex shutdown of splanchnic blood flow that normally accompanies ultrafiltration).

Antihypertensive drugs
Any drug that acts on vascular tone would be expected to reduce the capability of maintaining adequate venous return to the heart. Continued use of antihypertensive drugs results in setting a 'dry weight' higher than that which could be achieved with careful ultrafiltration without drugs. In particular, drugs that relax precapillary arterioles allow increased filtration from the vascular space to the interstitial space, opposing refilling and worsening intravascular hypovolemia.

Definition of 'dry weight' in dialysis patients
An important part of the dialysis prescription is the definition of a 'dry weight' for an individual patient, at which there will be signs neither of hypervolemia (e.g., peripheral or pulmonary edema, raised jugular vein pulse, third heart sound) nor of hypovolemia (decreased skin turgor, postural hypotension) (Fig. 69.13). This is often defined operationally as the weight 1 kg above that at which the patient regularly develops cramps or intradialytic hypotension during dialytic fluid removal. Given that the development of edema usually indicates an increase in extracellular fluid volume of at least 3 L in a man weighing 70 kg, the absence of edema is no guarantee that the patient is in fact 'euvolemic'. In practice, nephrologists vary considerably in how 'aggressively' they aim to correct subclinical fluid overload. At one end of the spectrum, Charra and coworkers[27] define hypertension as a feature of hypervolemia, defining dry weight as 'that body weight at the end of dialysis at which the patient can remain normotensive until the next dialysis despite retention of saline'. The success of their unit, in which 95% of hemodialysis patients are maintained normotensive without antihypertensive drugs, is attributed to long slow dialysis (typically 5–6 h, and often longer), a strict low salt diet, cessation of antihypertensives, and tolerance of a transition phase in which hypotension and cramps are relatively common before BP is normalized. At the other end of the spectrum are dialysis units that employ short, high-flux dialysis, often requiring

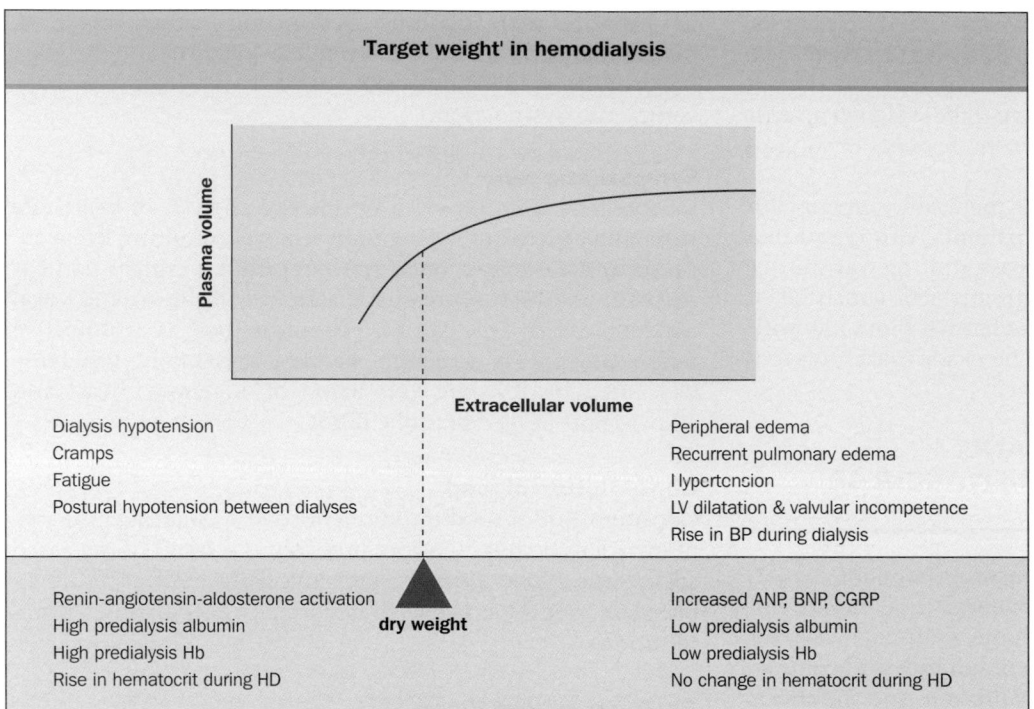

Figure 69.13 'Target weight' in hemodialysis. Many liters of excess extracellular fluid can be accommodated before obvious clinical signs (e.g., peripheral edema) are present. In contrast, a relatively small reduction in plasma volume below normal results in hypovolemic collapse. How close a patient can be brought to their ideal weight depends largely on how rapidly the correction of fluid overload is achieved. ANP: atrial nutriuretic peptide, BNP: brain nutriuretic peptide, CGRP: calcitonin gene-related peptide.

high sodium dialysate to prevent hemodynamic instability, in which well over 50% of patients are maintained on anti-hypertensives. Shorter dialysis, without a 'transition phase', is likely to be more popular with patients but may be associated with poorer survival, although it cannot be proved that this is directly a consequence of poorer attainment of true dry weight.

There are a number of techniques to assist evaluation of dry weight in individual patients. Continuous monitoring of hematocrit allows identification of patients in whom refilling balances ultrafiltration throughout dialysis ('flat-liners') as a result of being over their ideal dry weight. It also allows prediction of symptomatic hypotension from the rate of rise of hematocrit as refilling is outstripped by ultrafiltration. Measurement of inferior vena cava collapsibility during deep respiration allows direct assessment of venous return, but this can be affected by alterations in venous tone and refilling from the interstitial space: inferior vena cava diameter tends to increase rapidly in the 1–2 h after dialysis as a result of refilling, particularly after short dialysis. Multifrequency bio-impedance measurement allows assessment of extracellular and intracellular fluid volumes and changes in these volumes, but due to interindividual differences it is impossible to define a 'normal range' sufficiently accurately to allow prescription of dry weight in individual patients on dialysis. Raised plasma atrial natriuretic peptide, brain natriuretic peptide, cyclic GMP and calcitonin gene-related peptide are all sensitive markers of hypervolemia in dialysis patients. However, these measurements do not allow discrimination between normal hydration and hypovolemia.

'Online' monitoring of changes in relative blood volume in response to changes in ultrafiltration rate may be used to provide 'biofeedback' control of dialysate sodium and ultra-filtration rate, reducing the incidence of dialysis-related

hypotension and increasing dialysis efficiency, without necessarily compromising achievement of 'euvolemia'[28]. Other commonly used maneuvers to reduce dialysis-related hypotension include 'profiling' of dialysate sodium and ultrafiltration rate, use of cool dialysate, and the use of midodrine, an α-adrenergic agonist. Methylene blue, which inhibits the vasodilator action of nitric oxide, has also been reported to be useful in this situation.

Will the patient tolerate hemodialysis?

A common clinical decision is the suitability of older patients for hemodialysis rather than continuous ambulatory peritoneal dialysis if they have cardiovascular disease likely to cause intolerance of fluctuations in extracellular volume. This question is often unanswerable in the individual patient without a trial of hemodialysis. Although peritoneal dialysis offers 'gentler' steady state control of volume status, sodium sieving often makes it more difficult to achieve euvolemia with peritoneal dialysis than with hemodialysis. Apparently severe heart failure, whether judged by clinical or echocardiographic criteria, may improve substantially with the correction of hypervolemia that occurs through reversal of the valvular incompetence provoked by cardiac dilatation as well as through the improvement of volume–pressure relationships to a more favorable part of the Starling curve. Correction of anemia has also been shown to be of marked benefit to patients with cardiac failure and renal impairment.

MANAGEMENT OF CARDIOVASCULAR RISK FACTORS

'Conventional' risk factors

Unfortunately, patients with renal disease have been excluded from many of the relevant randomized trials of cardiovascular risks. Management of the renal patient with cardiovascular disease, therefore, requires careful extrapolation from these trials together with specific treatment of risk factors peculiar to the uremic state. In the general population, decisions on which patients to treat depend on the likelihood of benefit, which is highest in those patients with the most risk factors. Given the very high cardiovascular event rate in patients with renal disease, they should be included in the 'highest risk' stratum when deciding upon treatment[29].

Blood pressure reduction

Chronic renal failure

Antihypertensive treatment in patients with established renal disease has two aims: reducing the risk of cardiovascular disease (e.g., myocardial infarction, stroke, heart failure), and reducing the risk of progressive loss of GFR. The role of antihypertensive agents in slowing renal progression is discussed in Chapter 66.

Left ventricular hypertrophy is an important marker of end organ damage in hypertension, and an independent predictor of prognosis. Both in the general population and, recently, in patients with renal disease, treatment-induced regression of LVH has been associated with an improvement in prognosis. Prevention of LVH, and induction of regression of LVH when present, is therefore an important goal of antihypertensive treatment. These aims can largely be achieved by BP reduction. However, ACE inhibitors, ATRA, and calcium channel blockers may be more effective in inducing regression than other classes of antihypertensive drug. Minoxidil may even exacerbate LVH when used alone. It is also important to remember that echocardiographic measurements of left ventricular mass may be subject to artefact in the presence of anemia or hypervolemia compared to the 'gold standard' of cardiac magnetic resonance imaging.

Dialysis

Treatment of hypertension in dialysis patients should ideally be based on measurements of BP taken throughout the interdialytic period, and not only on measurements taken just prior to commencement and just after completion of hemodialysis. Ambulatory monitoring shows that BP typically rises in the 3–4 h preceding a dialysis session, and that mean interdialytic BP is better predicted by BP measurements taken at completion of hemodialysis than by those taken at the start. The rise in BP in the hours preceding dialysis is probably due to a combination of the accumulation of pressor substances and sympathetic overactivity caused by traveling and anticipation of dialysis. While there is no agreement on target BP, it seems reasonable to aim for postdialysis or interdialytic pressures of systolic BP < 130 mmHg and a diastolic BP of < 80 mmHg, as these are BP levels which are associated with the best outcomes in the general population. As in the general population, systolic hypertension is predictive of poor outcome in dialysis patients, and should also be treated. However, the proportion of patients that can achieve these targets while being treated with conventional thrice weekly dialysis remains uncertain.

The first step in BP control on dialysis is always to assess volume status, and make stepwise reductions with salt restriction to achieve dry weight. Patients may continue to be hypertensive for some days after achieving dry weight, a 'lag phase' suggesting that pressor mechanisms, though often triggered by volume, may remain active for several days after volume correction. In anephric patients BP control can always be achieved by control of extracellular volume.

The choice of drug treatment in dialysis patients is empirical. ACE inhibitors are most likely to cause regression of LVH[14]. ACE inhibitors and β-blockers are appropriate for patients with cardiac failure or ischemic heart disease. Supervised atenolol post-dialysis has been shown to be an effective strategy for improving BP control. Vasodilators are likely to increase the risk of dialysis-related hypotension.

The management of hypertension and hypotension in dialysis patients is summarized in Figures 69.14 and 69.15.

Renal transplantation

Renal transplant recipients remain at high risk of cardiovascular events. Hypertension early post-transplant is associated with an increased risk of rejection, although it is uncertain whether this is cause or effect. The aims of treatment are similar to those in CRF, as progressive deterioration in graft function may be slowed by effective antihypertensive therapy; as in CRF, patients with proteinuria should be treated with an ACE inhibitor or ATRA. Dihydropyridine calcium channel blockers ameliorate calcineurin inhibitor nephrotoxicity by counteracting their vasoconstrictor action on the afferent glomerular arteriole, and therefore have a definite role in this situation.

Hyperlipidemia

As discussed earlier, the pattern of dyslipidemia seen in CRF differs from that seen in the general population; many patients with renal disease have normal total cholesterol but raised triglycerides and abnormal lipoprotein composition. Whether the choice of treatment should be determined by the pattern of lipid abnormality, however, remains controversial. In non-renal patients at risk of cardiovascular events, HMG CoA reductase inhibitors (statins) reduce risk irrespective of initial total cholesterol level. As these agents show the greatest effectiveness in reducing cardiovascular events in patients without renal disease, they should be the agents of choice in treating patients with renal disease and hyperlipidemia, together with exercise, dietary restriction for obesity and glycemic control in diabetes. Patients with established cardiovascular disease may benefit from cholesterol-lowering therapy irrespective of serum cholesterol concentration; use as primary prevention may reasonably be confined to patients with a high total or LDL cholesterol. Both in the general population and in renal disease, there is less certainty that correction of hypertriglyceridemia is of additional benefit. Fibric acid derivatives are the drugs of choice in correcting hypertriglyceridemia, but some of these drugs may be nephrotoxic[30].

Care must be taken in the use of lipid-lowering drugs in patients taking cyclosporine, in whom there is an increased risk of myopathy, particularly with lipid-soluble agents and those which are metabolized by the cytochrome 3A4 system, which is inhibited by cyclosporine.

Chronic Renal Failure and the Uremic Syndrome

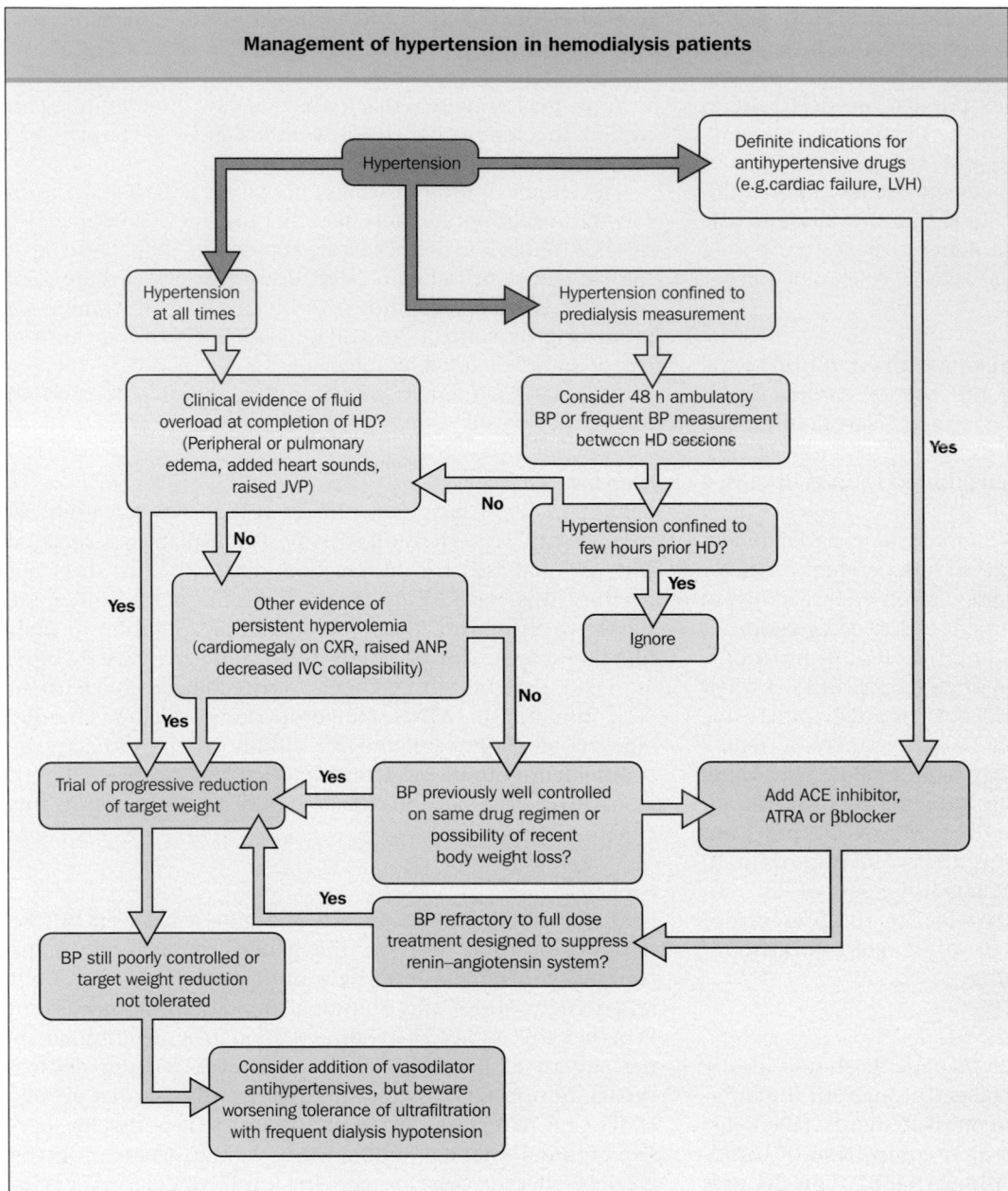

Figure 69.14 Management of hypertension in hemodialysis patients.

Figure content (flow chart): Management of hypertension in hemodialysis patients

Hypertension → Definite indications for antihypertensive drugs (e.g. cardiac failure, LVH)

Hypertension → Hypertension at all times → Clinical evidence of fluid overload at completion of HD? (Peripheral or pulmonary edema, added heart sounds, raised JVP)

Hypertension → Hypertension confined to predialysis measurement → Consider 48 h ambulatory BP or frequent BP measurement between HD sessions → Hypertension confined to few hours prior HD? — Yes → Ignore; No →

Other evidence of persistent hypervolemia (cardiomegaly on CXR, raised ANP, decreased IVC collapsibility)

Trial of progressive reduction of target weight

BP previously well controlled on same drug regimen or possibility of recent body weight loss?

Add ACE inhibitor, ATRA or βblocker

BP refractory to full dose treatment designed to suppress renin–angiotensin system?

BP still poorly controlled or target weight reduction not tolerated

Consider addition of vasodilator antihypertensives, but beware worsening tolerance of ultrafiltration with frequent dialysis hypotension

Aspirin

In the absence of direct evidence, low-dose aspirin (75–150 mg daily) should be prescribed for patients with any form of renal disease and established cardiovascular disease unless there are contraindications. Use of low-dose aspirin as primary prevention is more questionable, given the increased risk of gastrointestinal bleeding in patients with CRF.

ACE inhibitors

In addition to their use in hypertension, particularly with proteinuria, ACE inhibitors should also be prescribed to patients with impaired left ventricular function, whether ischemic or hypertensive in origin; and should also be considered for all patients with moderate or severe LVH, as they are effective at inducing regression of LVH.

β-adrenoceptor blockers

β-blockers reduce mortality after myocardial infarction, an effect that may be additive to the effects of thrombolysis, aspirin, and ACE inhibitors. They should be prescribed as secondary prevention after myocardial infarction in the absence of contraindications. They also reduce perioperative mortality in high-risk patients undergoing elective surgery, and should therefore be considered in high-risk dialysis patients likely to require surgery (e.g., transplantation).

Thrombolytic drugs

Thrombolysis should be offered to all patients with renal disease and acute myocardial infarction according to accepted indications and contraindications in the non-renal population.

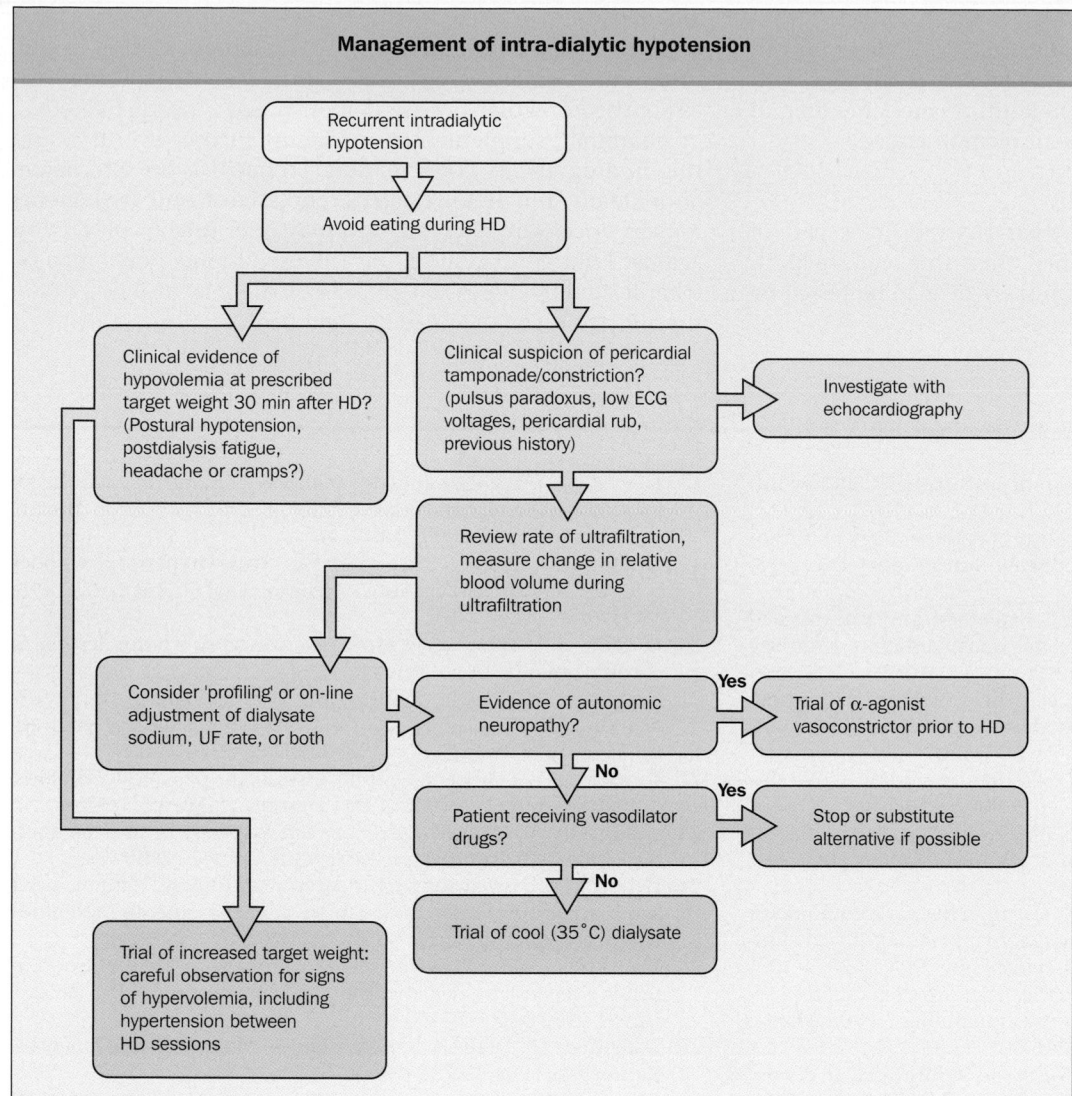

Management of intra-dialytic hypotension

Figure 69.15 Management of recurrent intra-dialytic hypotension in hemodialysis (HD) patients. (UF) Ultrafiltration.

Exercise

Exercise training is of demonstrable benefit in reducing cardiovascular risk factors and increasing quality of life in CRF and should ideally be offered to all suitable patients.

Risk factors specific for patients with renal failure

Control of hypervolemia and long-hours dialysis

The proposition that prevention of recurrent hypervolemia will reduce cardiovascular morbidity and mortality remains unproven. The debate about the overall cardiovascular benefits of long dialysis continues. The remarkable results achieved in Tassin by long-hours dialysis[12] may reflect the selection of patients for that program or some other undefined benefit of long dialysis rather than the obvious benefit of sustained normovolemia and normotension without antihypertensive therapy. Without a 'gold standard' for the assessment of dry weight by which the management of individual patients can be compared, this question is likely to remain controversial.

Sudden reductions in BP caused by rapid ultrafiltration, particularly in patients with diastolic dysfunction, may further exacerbate cardiac ischemia. This is particularly true in the presence of decreased arterial compliance, which results in systolic hypertension and decreased coronary perfusion during diastole. For these reasons, short dialysis is an inappropriate therapy for many patients for whom continuous ambulatory peritoneal dialysis or conventional hemodialysis are preferred.

Anemia

The appropriate target hematocrit to minimize LVH or other cardiac disease has not been defined. Partial correction of anemia undoubtedly allows regression of LVH, and several large studies have shown an inverse correlation between hematocrit and mortality. However, a recent study showed a trend to increased incidence of nonfatal myocardial infarction in patients with ESRD and pre-existing cardiac disease randomized to a target hematocrit of 42% compared to a target of 30%[31]. The explanation for this unexpected finding is unclear; an increased requirement for intravenous iron supplements, with resulting lipid peroxidation, is one possible contributor. Partial correction of anemia should remain the standard for high-risk patients until this issue has been resolved. In patients without established cardiac disease, the benefits of fuller correction of anemia on exercise capacity and quality of life are increasingly recognized.

Chronic Renal Failure and the Uremic Syndrome

Hyperhomocysteinemia
Neither pyridoxine nor folate supplementation are of proven benefit in reducing the cardiovascular risk associated with hyperhomocysteinemia in ESRD. Routine measurement of homocysteine levels is not at present recommended.

Hyperparathyroidism
Prevention or treatment of hyperparathyroidism is part of good practice, but the possibility that this will help to reduce cardiovascular disease is unlikely ever to be tested by a controlled trial.

Antioxidants
Vitamin E supplementation reduces lipid peroxidation in CRF to a limited extent. One small trial in dialysis patients with established vascular disease demonstrated a protective effect of vitamin E supplementation against further events[32], and this finding awaits confirmation. Probucol is an alternative antioxidant, but it lowers HDL cholesterol and its benefits remain uncertain. Ascorbic acid may offer further protection against lipid peroxidation, but the use of large doses may be complicated by hyperoxalemia; ascorbate may also potentiate the effects of iron overload on lipid peroxidation.

REFERENCES

1. Port FK. Morbidity and mortality in dialysis patients. Kidney Int. 1994;46:1728–37.
2. Foley RN, Parfrey PS, Sarnak MJ. Clinical epidemiology of cardiovascular disease in chronic renal disease. Am J Kidney Dis. 1998;32:S112–19.
3. Kasiske BL, Chakkera HA, Roel J. Explained and unexplained ischemic heart disease risk after renal transplantation. J Am Soc Nephrol. 2000;11:1735–43.
4. Cheung AK, Sarnak MJ, Yan G, et al. Atherosclerotic cardiovascular disease risks in chronic hemodialysis patients. Kidney Int. 2000;58:353–62.
5. Baigent C, Burbury K, Wheeler D. Premature cardiovascular disease in chronic renal failure. Lancet. 2000;356:147–52.
6. Mailloux LU, Bellucci AG, Wilkes BM, et al. Mortality in dialysis patients: analysis of the causes of death. Am J Kidney Dis. 1991;18:326–35.
7. Savage T, Clarke AL, Giles M, et al. Calcified plaque is common in the carotid and femoral arteries of dialysis patients without clinical vascular disease. Nephrol Dial Transplant. 1998;13:2004–12.
8. Tomson CRV. Cardiovascular complications after renal transplantation. In: Morris PJ, ed. Kidney transplantation. Philadelphia: WB Saunders Company; 2001:445–67.
9. Kasiske BL, Guijarro C, Massy ZA, et al. Cardiovascular disease after renal transplantation. J Am Soc Nephrol. 1996;7:158–65.
10. Buckalew VM Jr, Berg RL, Wang SR, et al. Prevalence of hypertension in 1,795 subjects with chronic renal disease: the modification of diet in renal disease study baseline cohort. Modification of Diet in Renal Disease Study Group. Am J Kidney Dis. 1996;28:811–21.
11. Charra B, Calemard E, Cuche M, Laurent G. Control of hypertension and prolonged survival on maintenance hemodialysis. Nephron. 1983;33:96–9.
12. Horl MP, Horl WH. Hemodialysis-associated hypertension: pathophysiology and therapy. Am J Kidney Dis. 2002;39:227–44.
13. Kaysen GA. The microinflammatory state in uremia: causes and potential consequences. J Am Soc Nephrol. 2001;12:1549–57.
14. Abuelo JG. Large interdialytic weight gains: causes, consequences, and corrective measures. Semin Dial. 1998;11:25–32.
15. Welch GN, Loscalzo J. Homocysteine and atherothrombosis. N Engl J Med. 1988;338:1042–50.
16. Amann K, Ritz E. Microvascular disease–the cinderella of uraemic heart disease. Nephrol Dial Transplant. 2000;15:1493–503.
17. Ketteler M, Bongartz P, Westenfield R, et al. Cardiovascular mortality in dialysis patients: low Ahsg/fetuin serum levels may be a crtical factor. Lancet. 2003;361 (in press).
18. Foley RN, Parfrey PS, Kent GM, et al. Serial change in echocardiographic parameters and cardiac failure in end-stage renal disease. J Am Soc Nephrol. 2000;11:912–16.
19. London GM. Heterogeneity of left ventricular hypertrophy – does it have clinical implications? Nephrol Dial Transplant. 1998;13:17–19.
20. London GM, Druecke T. Atherosclerosis and arteriosclerosis in chronic renal failure. Kidney Int. 1997;51:1678–95.
21. Goodman WG, Goldin J, Kuizon BD, et al. Coronary-artery calcification in young adults with end-stage renal disease who are undergoing dialysis. N Engl J Med. 2000;342:1478–83.
22. Tomson CRV. Echocardiographic assessment of systolic function in dialysis patients. Nephrol Dial Transplant. 1990;5:325–31.
23. Goldsmith DJ, Covic A. Coronary artery disease in uremia: etiology, diagnosis, and therapy. Kidney Int. 2001;60:2059–78.
24. Herzog CA. Dismal long-term survival of dialysis patients after acute myocardial infarction: can we alter the outcome? Nephrol Dial Transplant. 2002;17:7–10.
25. Manske CL, Wang Y, Rector T, et al. Coronary revascularisation in insulin-dependent diabetic patients with chronic renal failure. Lancet 1992;340:998–1002.
26. Daugirdas JT. Dialysis hypotension: a hemodynamic analysis. Kidney Int. 1991;39:233–46.
27. Charra B, Bergstrom J, Scribner BH. Blood pressure control in dialysis patients: importance of the lag phenomenon. Am J Kidney Dis. 1998;32:720–4.
28. Ronco C, Brendolan A, Milan M, et al. Impact of biofeedback-induced cardiovascular stability on hemodialysis tolerance and efficiency. Kidney Int. 2000;58:800–8.
29. Levey AS, Beto JA, Coronado BE, et al. Controlling the epidemic of cardiovascular disease in chronic renal disease: what do we know? What do we need to learn? Where do we go from here? National Kidney Foundation Task Force on Cardiovascular Disease. Am J Kidney Dis. 1998;32:853–906.
30. Massy ZA, Ma JZ, Louis TA, Kasiske BL. Lipid-lowering therapy in patients with renal disease. Kidney Int. 1995;48:188–98.
31. Besarab A, Bolton WK, Browne JK, et al. The effects of normal as compared to low hematocrit values in patients with cardiac disease who are receiving hemodialysis and epoetin. N Engl J Med. 1998;339:584–90.
32. Boaz M, Smetana S, Weinstein T, et al. Secondary prevention with antioxidants of cardiovascular disease in endstage renal disease (SPACE): randomised placebo-controlled trial. Lancet. 2000;356:1213–18.

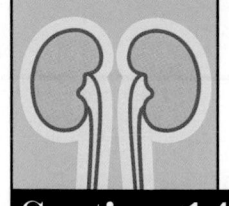

Section 14 Chronic Renal Failure and the Uremic Syndrome

Chapter 70

Anemia in Chronic Renal Failure

Joseph W Eschbach

INTRODUCTION

Anemia has been related to renal failure for over 160 years, but its etiology and management have been better elucidated during the past 20 years. Several historical observations were important in advancing our knowledge to the present era.

Kurt Reissman in 1950 was the first to demonstrate conclusively that there was a hormonal factor stimulating erythropoiesis by noting that if one partner of a parabiotic rat pair became hypoxic, both partners responded with an accelerated rate of red cell production[1]. Allan Erslev in 1953 observed that reticulocytosis developed several days after infusion into normal rabbits of large amounts of severely anemic rabbit serum, proving that there was an erythropoietic stimulating factor (ESF) in anemic sera[2]. The role of the kidney in producing ESF, later called erythropoietin, was clarified by Leon Jacobson and colleagues at the University of Chicago in 1957, who noted that hypoxia-induced erythropoiesis in rats diminished following bilateral nephrectomy[3].

In 1960, Belding Scribner at the University of Washington, Seattle, initiated chronic, maintenance hemodialysis. While other parameters of renal failure improved, the anemia did not. Patients were living longer due to dialysis therapy and the anemia became a more important complication, since multiple red blood cell (RBC) transfusions led to iron overload as patients survived for years, instead of months. This new appreciation of the importance of the anemia of chronic renal failure (CRF) resulted in a renewed interest in the pathophysiology of the anemia and its therapy.

The isolation of the human erythropoietin gene in 1983, followed by its cloning and the expression of the mature human glycoprotein hormone from the Chinese hamster ovarian cell[4], resulted in the production of sufficient quantities of recombinant human erythropoietin (epoetin) to be available for clinical trials and subsequently as a regular therapeutic agent. This is one of the major advances in the management of CRF in the past 15 years.

PATHOPHYSIOLOGY

The anemia of CRF is normochromic and normocytic and similar to that observed in acute renal failure with several exceptions. Both conditions are associated with erythropoietin deficiency and shortening of red cell survival. However, erythroid suppression is greater in acute renal failure, probably from more marked decrease in renal erythropoietin secretion because of the acute renal injury, and/or from infection/inflammation activation of cytokines, which is more common in acute renal failure. The role of uremic suppression on erythropoiesis remains controversial, although it is not as important as previously thought. *In vitro*, human uremic serum suppresses canine or murine erythroid progenitor growth, as well as myeloid and megakaryocyte growth, leading many investigators in the past to conclude that uremia directly suppressed erythroid marrow function. However, the very low incidence of leukopenia or thrombocytopenia in most patients with uncomplicated acute or chronic renal diseases, suggests that *in-vitro* erythroid inhibition by uremic serum is a nonspecific effect. This was supported by other studies indicating that sheep and human erythroid progenitor cells, regardless of whether they were from an uremic or nonuremic environment, were not suppressed by autologous uremic sera[5,6]. *In-vivo* studies indicate that epoetin is as effective in stable hemodialysis patients as in normal subjects[7], and epoetin has been extremely effective in correcting the anemia of CRF[8,9]. There are some rare patients who are refractory to epoetin, but underdialysis is usually not the cause[10].

The erythropoietin gene is located on chromosome 7[11], and encodes for a 193 aminoacid glycopeptide. Erythropoietin is predominantly synthesized by fibroblast-like interstitial cells in the kidney[12] and to a lesser extent in the liver, and secreted as a glycoprotein containing 165 aminoacids, and four carbohydrate side chains, with a molecular weight of 30 400 Da[13]. Erythropoietin production is markedly decreased in CRF, and RBC production, as quantitated by ferrokinetics, is subnormal. However, serum erythropoietin levels remain within the 'normal' range (6–30 mU/mL). Such levels are not normal since the diseased kidney is unable to respond to the anemic, hypoxemic stimulus to secrete erythropoietin to levels observed in other severe anemias not associated with renal disease ($\geq$ 100–200 mU/mL).

CLINICAL MANIFESTATIONS

Prior to the advent of epoetin and the ability to correct the anemia of CRF, most symptoms experienced by patients were thought to be related to uremia. As the result of increasing the RBC mass, independent of any change in renal function, a number of physiological improvements have occurred in CRF patients. These were first observed when the hemoglobin was increased to 10–12 g/dL, but more recently even further improvement in several parameters have occurred with normalization of hemoglobin. These changes are summarized in

Chronic Renal Failure and the Uremic Syndrome

Symptoms and signs in chronic renal failure improved with epoetin therapy	
Partial correction of anemia (hemoglobin 10–12 g/dL)	Further improvement with complete correction (hemoglobin 12–14 g/dL)
Quality of life	Quality of life
Reduction in cardiac output	Reduction in cardiac output
Reduction in LVH	Reduction in LVH
Maximal exercise capacity	Maximal exercise capacity
Cognitive function	Cognitive function
Sleep patterns	Sleep patterns
Nutrition	Nutrition
Reduction in angina, If present*	
Sexual function: nocturnal penile tumescence*	
Resumption of menses*	
Immune responsiveness*	
Platelet function improvement*	
*Not specifically studied at a normal hemoglobin.	

Table 70.1 Symptoms and signs in chronic renal failure improved with epoetin therapy.

Additional causes of anemia in chronic renal failure	
Relatively common causes	Less common causes of anemia
Iron deficiency	Hemolysis
Hypothyroidism	Aluminum excess
Active blood loss	Hyperparathyroid osteitis fibrosa
Hemoglobinopathies	Folic acid or B_{12} deficiency

Table 70.2 Possible additional causes of anemia in chronic renal failure. Causes of anemia other than erythropoietin deficiency.

Investigations for anemia of chronic renal failure
Red blood cell indices
Reticulocyte count
Serum iron and total iron-binding capacity
Serum ferritin
Test for stool occult blood
Percent of hypochromic red blood cells (if available) (serum erythropoietin level usually not indicated)

Table 70.3 Investigations for anemia of chronic renal failure.

Table 70.1. While the improvement in quality of life is the most immediate impressive change, the reduction in cardiac output (due to the decrease in anemia-induced peripheral vasodilatation) can reduce left ventricular dilatation/hypertrophy (LVH) resulting in long term benefits. Since LVH is associated with a 2.9-fold increase in mortality in end-stage renal disease (ESRD)[14], the management, and even prevention of anemia and its associated complications, represents a major therapeutic challenge which with the availability of epoetin should be met. Therefore, it is essential to optimize tissue oxygenation in CRF in order to maximize the physiological improvements noted in Table 70.1. However, prior to treating the anemia of CRF with epoetin, diagnostic work-up of anemia is essential, since other factors may be present, that if not addressed, will either result in a poor response from epoetin, and/or excessive requirement of epoetin.

DIAGNOSIS AND DIFFERENTIAL DIAGNOSIS

Anemia is almost universal in CRF once renal insufficiency ensues. However, there is no absolute level of renal failure at which anemia develops. In general, anemia is present when the glomerular filtration rate decreases to 35 mL/min, and worsens as the GFR decreases. A recent study noted that while 50% of patients with serum creatinine values of 2.1 to 3.0 mg/dL had hematocrit values < 36%, 22% of patients with serum creatinine < 2 mg/dL had hematocrit < 33%[15]. When the hematocrit/hemoglobin decreases to less than 80% of the mean values observed in normal subjects, the cause of the anemia should be investigated. This corresponds to a hematocrit of < 37%, or hemoglobin of < 12 g/dL, measured by an automated cell counter, in adult males and postmenopausal females, and a hematocrit of < 33%, or

hemoglobin of < 11 g/dL, in premenopausal females and prepubertal patients. Anemia is important to recognize since the adverse effects of anemia on the cardiovascular system (increased cardiac output, and left ventricular dilatation and hypertrophy) may occur prior to the development of overt symptoms.

While erythropoietin deficiency is the most likely cause of a normochromic, normocytic anemia in a patient with serum creatinine > 2 mg/dL, potential aggravating causes of anemia, such as iron deficiency, hypothyroidism, hemolysis and hemoglobinopathies should be excluded (Table 70.2). The minimum work up (Table 70.3) should consist of RBC indices (looking for macrocytosis or microcytosis), reticulocyte count (usually not increased in renal failure, if adjusted for the anemia), tests of iron status, and a test for occult blood in a fecal specimen. Iron status is evaluated by measurement of serum iron, total iron binding capacity (as a surrogate for transferrin) and serum ferritin levels. Transferrin saturation (%) is calculated as serum iron ×100/ total iron binding capacity. A serum erythropoietin level is not necessary if the serum creatinine is ≥ 2 mg/dL, or if a lower serum creatinine is associated with a creatinine clearance of < 35 mL/min, as is common in many elderly patients, unless the reticulocyte count is markedly increased. If there is significant reticulocytosis, this may be secondary to microangiopathic hemolytic anemia, which will transiently increase serum erythropoietin levels. Macrocytosis may suggest folate or B_{12} deficiency, but may also be observed in epoetin-induced erythropoiesis in which younger (larger) reticulocytes are released into circulation. Macrocytosis may also be due to medication being given to treat the cause of CRF, for example azathioprine. Microcytosis is present in advanced iron deficiency, aluminum excess and some hemoglobinopathies.

TREATMENT

Iron status

Iron stores should be optimized before beginning epoetin treatment. Iron deficiency may be present in 25–33% of patients presenting with anemia in CRF[16]. This can be diagnosed by a low serum iron, a transferrin saturation < 16–20%, and a serum ferritin of less than 50–100 ng/mL. The mean corpuscular volume (MCV) may be low, and the percent of hypochromic red blood cells (measured by a special adapter to the automated RBC counter) may be greater than 10%. Iron replacement therapy should be initiated, and generally oral iron will be beneficial, assuming that iron (blood) losses are not continuous. In the patient with CRF not yet requiring dialysis, 100 mg of elemental iron daily may be sufficient to replete and maintain iron stores. However, once hemodialysis and erythropoietin replacement therapy is initiated, iron requirements increase, and up to 200 mg of oral, elemental iron is needed daily. If absolute iron deficiency is present and epoetin therapy is also needed, intravenous iron replacement is necessary to replete iron stores for adequate epoetin effectiveness.

Iron preparations

The oral iron salts, iron sulfate, iron gluconate and iron fumarate, are well absorbed when given 1 h before or 2 h after a meal and not in conjunction with phosphate binders. However, for the epoetin-treated patient, at least 200 mg of elemental iron is needed daily. If oral iron does not maintain serum ferritin above 100 ng/mL (preferably above 200 ng/mL) and a transferrin saturation above 20%, then intravenous iron will be needed.

Intravenous preparations consist of iron dextran, sodium ferric gluconate and sodium ferric saccharate (sucrose). All three preparations are now available in the USA, but the rare incidence of anaphylaxis with iron dextran[17] should preclude its use[18] since the dextran sensitivity is not present with sodium ferric gluconate or iron sucrose, making these other two compounds the i.v. iron of choice. However, only iron dextran can be given in amounts greater than 300 mg at one infusion, since non-anaphylactic side effects (hypotension, nausea, or itching) occur with both iron sucrose[19] and ferric gluconate[20] at doses > 250–300 mg. Intravenous iron gluconate is available as 62.5 mg/5 mL vial, whereas iron sucrose and iron dextran are available as 50 mg/5 mL vials.

Precautions are required if iron dextran is administered. Patients sensitive to iron dextran should be identified by administering a test dose of 25 mg intravenously and observing for 15–60 min before administering the full dose. Anaphylaxis can develop in 0.7% of patients[17] and may occur after several uneventful doses. If anaphylaxis occurs it should be treated with intravenous epinephrine, diphenhydramine, and/or corticosteroids. For the hemodialysis patient iron dextran can be given as 25, 50 or 100 mg by a 1–2 min intravenous push during dialysis weekly. For CAPD or patients not requiring dialysis, it is more practical to give a larger dose, such as 500–1000 mg in 5% dextrose solution over 1 h. Iron gluconate and iron sucrose can be given i.v. without a test dose[21,22]. Iron gluconate can be given at a rate of 12.5 mg/min, not to exceed 250 mg; iron sucrose can be given at a similar rate, but not to exceed 300 mg infused over 2 h.

Epoetin

Epoetin is the primary therapeutic agent for correcting the anemia of CRF. When using epoetin several principles are important to consider: (1) there is a dose-related response between a range of 25–500 U/kg, some patients requiring a higher dose than others[8]; (2) subcutaneous injections result in approximately one third (15–50%) reduction in weekly dosing requirements compared to intravenous injections[23]; (3) iron is essential for the optimal effectiveness of epoetin; and, (4) adverse effects, such as hypertension and access clotting, are not linked to the dose or frequency of epoetin administration[23,24].

Epoetin should be used to treat the normochromic, normocytic anemia in any patient with CRF. Ideally this should begin before dialysis is required. This includes the renal transplant patient with CRF. Epoetin therapy in the USA has been suboptimal in that the mean hematocrit of CRF patients at the time that maintenance dialysis is initiated was 29.3%[25]. Epoetin should be initiated in the iron-replete patient with CRF when the hemoglobin decreases to 11.5 g/dL in premenopausal women and 13.5 g/dL in men and postmenopausal women, in order to prevent or minimize the development of increasing cardiac output which leads to LVH[26]. Unfortunately, reimbursement mechanisms in the USA at this time, prevent this optimal use of epoetin in that the hemoglobin must drop below 10 g/dL before Medicare and most private insurance companies reimburse for epoetin. Such an unphysiologic policy, based on the declaration of the FDA in 1989 that the target hemoglobin for patients with CRF should be 10–11 g/dL, allows CRF patients to develop cardiac and other anemic complications that are not easily reversed once epoetin therapy begins.

Epoetin should continue to be given s.c. once the patient begins dialysis.

Initial studies with epoetin in anemic patients with ESRD used a subnormal target hematocrit/hemoglobin. Marked improvements in many physiological parameters were noted when the hematocrit/hemoglobin increased from 21%/7 g per dL to 30%/10 g per dL, and these latter values became the target levels for many patients around the world. However, subsequent studies have shown that these levels are suboptimal in that mortality and morbidity are less when the target level is > 36%/12 g per dL, respectively. At or above these higher hemoglobin/hematocrit levels hospitalization rates due to infections are lower[27], survival improves[24,27], exercise tolerance improves[28], brain function is better[29], sleep patterns improve[30], quality of life is better[31], LVH decreases toward normal or normalizes[32], and amino acid metabolism becomes more anabolic[33]. These positive benefits from normalizing hemoglobin/hematocrit are possibly tempered by the results of a normal hematocrit study in hemodialysis patients with advance heart disease. In this study 1200 patients with a history of congestive heart failure, angina, and/or prior myocardial infarction were randomized into two groups: a hematocrit of 42% vs. 30%[24]. The study was prematurely terminated when it appeared that the incidence of non-fatal myocardial infarction or death (the primary end points of the study) was increasing in those patients randomized to the normal hematocrit. This was not a statistically significant difference but to prevent the possibility of further harm, the study was terminated. There was no relationship between the incidence of death and non-fatal myocardial infarction to the hematocrit or dose of epoetin. Paradoxically, those 200 patients that attained and maintained a normal hematocrit for 6 months, had a yearly mortality rate of 15% vs. 40% for those at 30% hematocrit, had improvement in quality of life, and for all patients there was a 30% decrease in the risk of death or myocardial infarction per 10-point increase in hematocrit, even though there were more primary events in the normal hematocrit group than in the anemic control group. These patients were older and had more comorbid factors than the average hemodialysis patient.

Initial studies with epoetin were based on its use as units/kg, but common practice has been to give it based on total units per dose, rounded to 100 units. It is available as 1000, 2000, 3000, 4000, or 10 000 U/mL vials and as a 20 000 U/2 mL multiple dose vial. Titration of dosage to maintain a stable hematocrit/hemoglobin can occur by either increasing or decreasing the dose i.v. or if administered s.c., by also reducing or increasing the frequency of hormone administration. However, administering epoetin more than three times per week, by either route, is not cost-effective. Most patients can maintain stable hematocrit/hemoglobin levels with twice weekly S.C. dosing, while many may require only weekly, and even occasionally every other week injections. On the other hand, for intravenous therapy, epoetin, because of its relatively short half-life (4–9 h)[34], is needed thrice weekly for optimal effectiveness. Most patients with optimal iron stores will require approximately 6000 units weekly for maintenance therapy, although there is much individual variation in both total dose required per week, and the most efficient frequency schedule. In the USA, because many patients with CRI must receive epoetin through the physician's office (as required for Medicare reimbursement), the logistics of travel may dictate the frequency of administration, rather than optimal clinical response.

Darbepoetin alfa

There is now another recombinant erythropoietin available for clinical use: darbepoetin or novel erythropoietic stimulating protein (NESP). While its erythropoietic action is identical to epoetin, it is a larger molecule with a three times longer half-life, due to the addition of two extra N-linked carbohydrate side chains. There are also five additional amino acids in the primary sequence. The pharmacokinetics of i.v. NESP/darbepoetin gives a mean $t\frac{1}{2}$ of 25.3 h, which contrasts to the mean $t\frac{1}{2}$ of i.v. epoetin, which is 8.5 h[35]. The $t\frac{1}{2}$ for s.c. NESP/darbepoetin is approximately 49 h[35]. This molecular change allows NESP/darbepoetin to be administered i.v. once a week, or s.c. every week or every other week. The other difference is the dosing units. NESP/darbepoetin should be initiated at a dose of 0.45–0.75 µg/kg per week and adjusted over time to achieve and maintain the target hemoglobin[36]. The initial dosing for epoetin is 150–225 U/kg per week, or approximately 6000 U/wk, in 2–3 divided doses. The clinical trials with NESP/darbepoetin indicate that it is as effective as epoetin with a similar safety profile.

Iron supplementation during epoetin or NESP/darbepoetin therapy

Once epoetin or NESP/darbepoetin therapy begins, the demand for iron increases in order to produce more hemoglobin. Iron stores are relatively small, and often the demand for iron by the epoetin-stimulated erythroid progenitor cell exceeds the rate at which the reticuloendothelial cell can release storage iron to transferrin for delivery to the erythroid marrow. As a result, functional iron deficiency often develops, which can best be corrected by the administration of intravenous iron[8]. In the normal subject, absolute iron deficiency is defined as serum ferritin < 15 ng/mL and transferrin saturation < 16% (Table 70.4). By convention, iron deficiency in the dialysis patient has been defined as serum ferritin < 100 ng/mL, transferrin saturation of < 20%, and the percentage of hypochromic RBCs > 10%. Functional iron deficiency is defined as transferrin saturation < 25% with serum ferritin > 100 ng/mL in which serial values indicate that both parameters have been decreasing during epoetin therapy. In this setting epoetin is not as effective. Some clinicians may misinterpret these values as indicating the presence of an inflammatory disorder. But once a total of 0.5–1.0 g of intravenous iron has been given in divided doses, either the hematocrit/hemoglobin rises and/or the epoetin dose decreases. An elevated serum ferritin associated with a decreased serum iron and transferrin saturation (and usually a decreased total iron binding capacity) is commonly observed in inflammatory disorders, and serial testing would show that earlier serum ferritin levels were lower, and transferrin saturation values higher than the most recent values. In functional iron deficiency there is a parallel decline in both transferrin saturation and serum ferritin levels.

It is important to understand how much iron a patient requires, since both iron deficiency and iron overload are to be avoided. Iron loss is minimal (1 mg/d) in the normal, non-menstruating subject, and absorption of food iron usually replaces such losses. However, for the patient with CRF, iron losses are usually increased, and iron available for absorption is usually decreased. For instance, in the hemodialysis patient, blood losses (1 mL of RBCs contains 1 mg of iron) related to the

Definitions of iron status			
Iron deficiency	Transferrin saturation (%) $\frac{\text{Serum iron} \times 100}{\text{Total iron binding capacity}}$	Ferritin (ng/mL)	Hypochromic RBCs (%)
In normal population	< 16	< 15	> 10
In chronic kidney disease	< 20	< 100	> 5
Functional iron deficiency	< 25 (and declining)	> 100 (but declining)	> 2.5
In inflammatory disorders	< 20 (declining)	> 100 (but rising)	

Table 70.4 Definitions of iron status.

hemodialyzer and procedure, coupled with blood losses related to surgical procedures, may amount to 3–9 mg/d, or up to 3–4 g/year. On the other hand, iron absorption, while physiologic in CRF[37], is often unable to meet the iron needs of the epoetin-stimulated erythroid marrow even if supplemental oral iron is provided. Phosphate binders and food also decrease iron absorption. Whereas iron overload was common in the era prior to epoetin therapy (because the iron infused via the cumulative effect of RBC transfusions often exceeded the dialyzer-related blood losses) iron deficiency is now very common, related to epoetin therapy. Therefore, i.v. iron must be given on a regular basis to replace the iron (blood) losses and to prevent functional iron deficiency[23].

Intravenous iron requirements will vary depending on the iron status at initiation of iron therapy, amount of blood loss related to the hemodialysis procedure, and the amount of epoetin required to achieve and maintain a stable hematocrit/hemoglobin, which is dependent upon how well the patient responds to epoetin. Correction of iron deficiency may require up to 1 g iron (iron stores are approximately 800–1200 mg)[38]; 0.5 to 1 g may be needed for new RBC formation in order to increase the hemoglobin/hematocrit up to the target range; and iron losses from blood loss may vary from 0.5–3 g/year. The National Kidney Foundation of the USA recommended through its Dialysis Outcomes Quality Initiative (DOQI) Clinical Practice Guidelines for anemia management that i.v. iron be given weekly or biweekly and that the iron status be monitored no less frequently than every 3 months with the goal of maintaining transferrin saturation of 25–35% (there is no benefit in maintaining saturation > 50%), and serum ferritin levels of 200–500 ng/mL[23], recognizing that some patients may do well within the range of 100–800 ng/mL. There is no evidence that functional iron deficiency has occurred with higher serum ferritin levels[23]. If the percentage of hypochromic RBCs is monitored, ideal i.v. iron therapy should achieve a value of < 2.5%[39]. It is best to wait 2 weeks following an i.v. iron infusion to obtain reliable serum ferritin and iron determinations.

Other possible erythropoietic stimulants

Iron and erythropoietin are the major factors needed for erythropoiesis. However, there is also the need for adequate amounts of folic acid. This may be a limiting factor, since it is water-soluble, and dialysis can result in a reduction in circulating folate levels. Most patients who eat reasonably well will ingest adequate amounts of folate to remain in folate balance, but in the epoetin stimulated patient, folic acid supplementation is essential to optimize heme synthesis.

There is controversy about whether other factors act on an adjunctive basis with iron, folic acid and erythropoietin in RBC production. Carnitine, anabolic steroids, vitamin C, and 'better' dialysis have been observed by some, but not all investigators, to improve erythropoiesis. More studies are needed to better support these contentions.

The management of anemia in CRF is summarized in Figure 70.1.

'Resistance' to epoetin

True resistance to the action of epoetin rarely occurs (Table 70.5). When defined as an inability to respond to

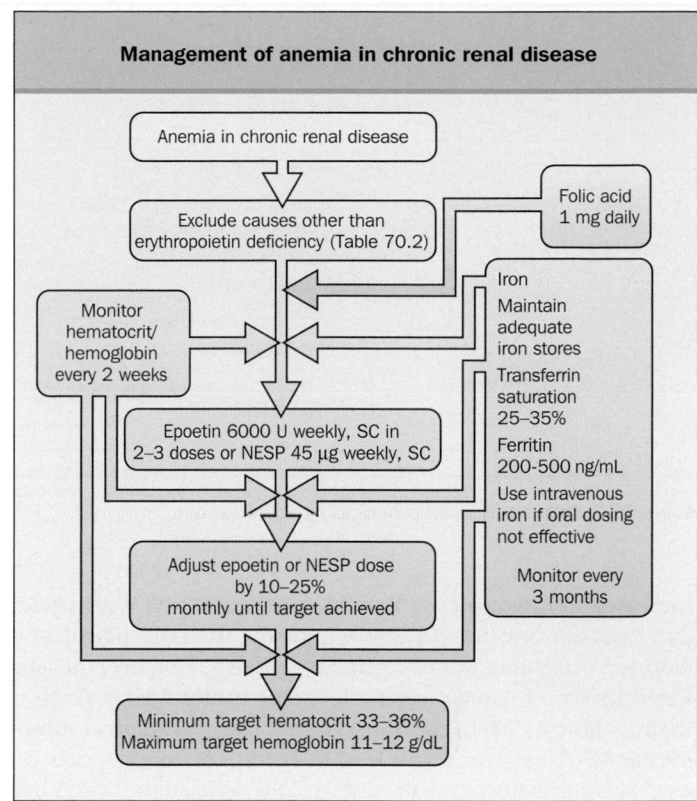

Figure 70.1 Management of anemia in chronic renal disease.

150–300 U/kg, i.v. three times a week, only 4% of over 300 iron-replete hemodialysis patients met this criteria[40]. Since the early epoetin trials, we now know that relative resistance or hyporesponsiveness is rather common. The failure to respond may be due to *insufficient epoetin*, since responsiveness is dose dependent. Assuming that enough epoetin is administered, then the majority of hyporesponsiveness in the recent past have been due to *absolute or functional iron deficiency*. Administration of up to 1000 mg of intravenous iron over 1–3 months should correct this deficiency. Now that iron stores are being better maintained, hyporesponsiveness occurs now most likely in the setting of *infection or inflammation*. Responsiveness to epoetin generally does not return, even with higher doses, until the inflammation/infection has cleared. Giving larger doses of epoetin does not overcome the inflammatory-cytokine inhibition of erythroid function in CRF, in contrast to rheumatoid arthritis, a form of chronic inflammation, when there will be a response to increasing doses of epoetin[41].

Less common causes of epoetin hyporesponsiveness include aluminum excess, hyperparathyroid osteitis fibrosa, folate deficiency, angiotensin-converting enzyme (ACE) inhibitor therapy, hemoglobinopathies and antibody production against recombinant human erythropoietin. Microcytosis in the presence of normal iron stores is suggestive of either aluminum excess or a hemoglobinopathy. Hyperparathyroidism is very common in CRF, but does not interfere with epoetin stimulation unless there is bone marrow fibrosis, which probably reduces the capacity of the marrow cavity to expand with

Causes of 'resistance' to epoetin therapy	
Common causes	**Uncommon causes**
Inadequate epoetin dosing	Aluminum excess
Absolute/functional iron deficiency	Hyperparathyroid osteitis fibrosa
Infection/inflammation	Folate deficiency
	ACE inhibitors and AT receptor antagonists
	Hemoglobinopathies
	Other primary marrow disorders, e.g., myelodysplasia
	Antibodies to epoetin

Table 70.5 Causes of 'resistance' to epoetin therapy.

increased erythropoiesis. This may be associated with intact parathyroid hormone (PTH) levels greater than 600 pg/mL and elevated bone alkaline phosphatase levels[42]. However, an elevated intact PTH level *per se* does not indicate that there is marrow fibrosis. Medical suppression therapy or surgical subtotal parathyroidectomy will lead to better epoetin responsiveness, if osteitis fibrosa is present. Folate deficiency should not occur if a folic acid supplement of 1 mg is provided orally, daily. (ACE) inhibitor and angiotensin receptor antagonist drugs are used to suppress post-transplant erythrocytosis; patients with CRF may have a blunted response to epoetin if receiving these drugs, however, this has not been an universal experience[23]. The mechanism for this phenomenon has recently been shown to be increased accumulation of a physiological inhibitor of hematopoeisis, n-acetyl-seryl-aspartyl-lysyl-proline (AcSDKP)[43] following administration of these drugs. Angiotensin II (AII) and insulin-like growth factor-1 (IGF-1) both have growth-promoting effects on erythroid progenitor cells, and ACE inhibitors can reduce IGF-1 and AII levels in transplant erythrocytosis[44]. Hemoglobin electrophoresis is necessary if none of the above causes of epoetin hyporesponsiveness can be identified. Of the hemoglobinopathies, anemia in sickle cell disease is difficult to improve with epoetin because hemolysis may be quite marked. Alpha thalassemia is more common in those of Asian descent, and often requires larger doses of epoetin to elicit an erythroid response. A bone marrow aspirate may be necessary to define rarer causes of hyporesponsiveness such as primary marrow abnormalities (i.e., myelodysplasia). There is no evidence that epoetin doses of greater than 40 000 units i.v. three times a week will overcome any of the above causes of hyporesponsiveness.

Recently, there has been a report of 13 patients treated with epoetin (12 who received epoetin alfa and one epoetin beta), who developed anti-erythropoietin neutralizing antibodies leading to absent serum erythropoietin levels and pure red cell aplasia[45]. Some, but not all, recovered erythropoietic function after discontinuing epoetin, and receiving immunosuppressive therapy or a renal transplant. The others have continued to be red cell transfusion dependent.

Epoetin therapy in the hospital

The commonest reasons for hospitalization in CRF patients are infection or the need for surgery. Both infection and the inflammatory effect of surgery will decrease the responsiveness to epoetin. In this setting, there are no data indicating whether epoetin doses should be withheld until the infection/inflammation subsides, or whether epoetin doses should be increased, in hopes of overcoming the inflammatory blockade. Since the duration of this hyporesponsiveness is difficult to predict, maintaining the prehospitalization epoetin dosage may allow for erythroid precursor receptors to remain saturated so that response will occur sooner once the inflammatory inhibition ceases. Following renal transplant surgery there is often a drop in the hematocrit/hemoglobin. There is no data to indicate whether epoetin therapy will be more effective than endogenous erythropoietin secreted from the newly engrafted organ.

Red blood cell transfusions

One of the goals of epoetin therapy is to eliminate the need for routine RBC transfusions in the CRF patient. This goal has yet to be met, although the number of transfusions is much less than in the pre-epoetin era. There are several reasons why this goal has not been achieved. In the pre-epoetin era, patients could stabilize their hematocrit/hemoglobin levels in the range of 20–28%/7–9 g per dL by avoiding the erythroid suppression from RBC transfusions. Many nephrologists unfamiliar with that era do not realize that many patients can tolerate lower hematocrit/hemoglobin levels and transfusions are now ordered for levels of RBC mass higher than observed in the pre-epoetin era. Another reason is that the target hematocrit/hemoglobin is too low at 33–36%/11–12 g per dL to tolerate acute blood loss. Blood loss that a non-anemic patient might easily tolerate, such as a drop in hematocrit from 42 to 32%, or a similar decline related to infection, would not be treated by transfusion, whereas a similar percent drop from a hematocrit of 33% in the patient on epoetin therapy, would result in a hematocrit of 25% and transfusion of several units of RBCs. The American College of Physicians state that the clinician should 'determine which, if any, symptoms or signs are likely to be reversed by giving red blood cell transfusions. If none can be identified, do not transfuse'[34].

Hypertension

An increase in blood pressure following the use of epoetin has been described in approximately 23% of patients with CRF[23]. The mechanism(s) for this action remain debated. No such hypertensive response occurs in anemic patients without renal disease treated with epoetin. Since there are erythropoietin receptors on the endothelial cell, it is intriguing to suspect that endothelial cell reactivity is increased and in selected patients a vasoactive response occurs. However, extracellular volume excess may also contribute, since optimal ultrafiltration can minimize this hypertensive response. Blood pressure can usually be controlled with either an increase in existing anti-hypertensive medication and/or adequate ultrafiltration. Rarely is it necessary to discontinue epoetin therapy, unless hypertensive encephalopathy occurs, which is unusual.

Vascular access thrombosis

Since the introduction of epoetin therapy, there has been concern that vascular access thrombosis is more likely to occur, particularly in the non-native arteriovenous graft. The preponderance of data fail to implicate the rise in hematocrit/hemoglobin or the use of epoetin in an increased incidence of vascular access thromboses[23], yet one study showed a statistically significant increase in native fistula and arteriovenous graft thromboses in hemodialysis patients with advanced cardiovascular disease when the hematocrit was increased to normal[24]. However, there was no correlation in this study of vascular access thrombosis with the epoetin dose or the actual hematocrit. Many studies have failed to note an increase in any clotting factors following the epoetin-induced rise in hematocrit/hemoglobin, even though platelet function does improve toward normal. In general, there is no need to use anticoagulant therapy when treating with epoetin.

SUMMARY

The use of epoetin has been one of the most important advances in the management of the patient with CRF, yet its use is still not optimal. Not enough patients with progressive renal insufficiency are receiving epoetin for even partial correction of their anemia and the National Kidney Foundation-DOQI evidenced-based recommendation that the target hematocrit/hemoglobin should be 33–36%/11–12 g per dL[23] has yet to be achieved for many patients. More recent studies suggest that the target hematocrit/hemoglobin should be higher, if not normal, to minimize the long-term morbidity of anemia, to more completely eliminate RBC transfusions with their associated potential complications, and to improve rehabilitation and survival.

REFERENCES

1. Reissmann KR. Studies on the mechanism of erythropoietic stimulation in parabiotic rats during hypoxia. Blood. 1950;5:372–80.
2. Erslev AJ. Humoral regulation of red cell production. Blood. 1953;8:349–57.
3. Jacobson LO, Goldwasser E, Fried W, Pizak L. Role of the kidney in erythropoiesis. Nature. 1957;179:633–4.
4. Lin F-K, Suggs S, Lin C-H, et al. Cloning and expression of the human erythropoietin gene. Proc Natl Acad Sci USA. 1985;82:7580–4.
5. Segal GM, Eschbach JW, Egrie JC, et al. The anemia of end-stage renal disease: Hematopoietic progenitor cell response. Kidney Int. 1988;33:983–8.
6. Mladenovic J, Eschbach JW, Garcia JF, Adamson JW. The anaemia of chronic renal failure in sheep: Studies in vitro. Br J Hematol. 1984;58:491–500.
7. Eschbach JW, Haley NR, Egrie JC, Adamson JW. A comparison of the responses to recombinant human erythropoietin in normal and uremic subjects. Kidney Int. 1992;43:407–16.
8. Eschbach JW, Egrie JC, Downing MR, et al. Correction of the anemia of end-stage renal disease with recombinant human erythropoietin: Results of a combined phase I and II clinical trial. N Engl J Med. 1987;316:73–8.
9. Winnearls CG, Oliver DL, Pippard MJ, et al. Effect of human erythropoietin derived from recombinant DNA on the anaemia of patients maintained by chronic haemodialysis. Lancet. 1986;2:1175–8.
10. Jacobs AA, Lada P, Zurada JM, et al. Predictors of hematocrit in hemodialysis patients as determined by artificial neural networks. J Am Soc Nephrol. 2001;12:387A.
11. Powell JS, Berkner KL, Lebo RV, Adamson JW. Human erythropoietin gene: high level expression in stably transfected mammalian cells and chromosome localization. Proc Natl Acad Sci USA. 1986;83:6465–9.
12. Maxwell PH, Osmond MK, Pugh CW, et al. Identification of the renal erythropoietin-producing cells using transgenic mice. Kidney Int. 1993;44:1149–62.
13. Egrie JC, Strickland TW, Lane J, et al. Characterization and biological effects of recombinant human erythropoietin. Immunobiology. 1986;172:213–24.
14. Silberberg JS, Barre PE, Pritchard SS, Sniderman AD. Impact of left ventricular hypertrophy on survival in end-stage renal disease. Kidney Int. 1989;36:286–90.
15. Kazmi WH, Kausz AT, Khan S, Pereira BJG. Anemia: an early complication of chronic renal insufficiency. Am J Kidney Dis. 2001;38:803–12.
16. Hutchinson F, Jones WJ. A cost-effectiveness analysis of anemia screening before erythropoietin in patients with end-stage renal disease. Am J Kidney Dis. 1997;29:651–7.
17. Fletes R, Lazarus M, Gage J, Chertow BM. Suspected iron dextran-related adverse drug events in hemodialysis patients. Am J Kidney Dis. 2001;37:743–9.
18. Hörl WH. Should we still use iron dextran in hemodialysis patients? (editorial) Am J Kidney Dis. 2001;37:859–61.
19. Chandler G, Harchowal J, Macdougall IC. Intravenous iron sucrose: establishing a safe dose. Am J Kidney Dis. 2002;38:988–91.
20. Folkert VW, Michael B. Ferrlecit Publication Committee. Safety of sodium ferric gluconate complex (SFGC) in higher individual doses. J Am Soc Nephrol. 2001;12:379A.
21. Eschbach JW, Strobos J, and The Ferrlecit Safety Study Group. Sodium Ferric Gluconate Complex (Ferrlecit®): Prospective Experience in 1122 Hemodialysis Patients. J Am Soc Nephrol. 2000; 11:249A.
22. Wyck DB Van, Cavallo G, Spinowitz BS, et al. Safety and efficacy of iron sucrose in patients sensitive to iron dextran: North American Clinical Trial. Am J Kidney Dis 2000;36:88–97.
23. Eschbach J, DeOreo P, Adamson J, et al. NKF-DOQI Clinical Practice Guidelines for the Treatment of Anemia of Chronic Renal Failure. Am J Kidney Dis. 2001;37 (suppl 1): S182–S238.
24. Besarab A, Bolton WK, Browne JK, et al. The effects of normal versus low treated hematocrit values in hemodialysis patients with cardiac disease with erythropoietin. N Engl J Med. 1998;339:584–590.
25. Obrador GT, Roberts T, St Peter WL, et al. Trends in anemia at initiation of dialysis in the United States. Kidney Int. 2001;60:1875–84.
26. Levin A, Singer J, Thompson CR, et al. Prevalent left ventricular hypertrophy and systolic dysfunction in chronic renal failure. Am J Kidney Dis. 1996;27:337–54.
27. Collins AJ, Li S, St Peter W, et al. Death, hospitalization, and economic associations among incident hemodialysis patients with hematocrit values of 36 to 39%. J Am Soc Nephrol. 2001; 12:2465–2473.

28. McMahon LP, McKenna MJ, Sangkabutra T, et al. Physical performance and associated electrolyte changes after haemoglobin normalization: a comparative study in haemodialysis patients. Nephrol Dial Transplant. 1999;14:1182–7.

29. Pickett JL, Theberge DC, Brown WS, et al. Normalizing hematocrit in dialysis patients improves brain function. Am J Kidney Dis. 1999;33:112–30.

30. Benz RL, Pressman MR, Hovick ET, Peterson DD. A preliminary study on the effects of correction of anemia with recombinant human erythropoietin therapy on sleep, sleep disorders, and daytime sleepiness in hemodialysis patients (the SLEEPO study). Am J Kidney Dis. 1999;34:1089–95.

31. Foley RN, Parfrey PS, Morgan J, et al. Effect of hemoglobin levels in hemodialysis patients with asymptomatic cardiomyopathy. Kidney Int. 2000;58:1325–35.PS.

32. Hayashi T, Suzuki A, Shoji T, et al. Cardiovascular effect of normalizing the hematocrit level during erythropoietin therapy in predialysis patients with chronic renal failure. Am J Kidney Dis. 2000;35:250–6.

33. Riedel E, Nundel M, Wendel G, Hampl H. Amino acid and α-keto acid metabolism depends on oxygen availability in chronic hemodialysis patients. Clin Nephrol. 2000;53:S56–S60.

34. Kindler J, Eckardt KU, Ehmer B, et al. Single-dose pharmacokinetics of recombinant human erythropoietin in patients with various degrees of renal failure. Nephrol Dial Transplant. 1989;4:345–9.

35. MacDougall IC, Gray SJ, Elston O, et al. Pharmacokinetics of novel erythropoietic stimulating protein compared with epoetin alfa in dialysis patients. J Am Soc Nephrol. 1999;10:2392–5.

36. Nissenson AR. Novel erythropoietic stimulating protein for managing the anemia of chronic kidney disease. Am J Kidney Dis. 2001;38:1390–7.

37. Eschbach JW, Cook JD, Scribner BH, Finch CA. Iron balance in hemodialysis patients. Ann Intern Med. 1977;87:710–13.

38. Council on Food and Nutrition, Committee on Iron Deficiency. Iron deficiency in the United States. JAMA. 1968;203:119–24.

39. Richardson D, Bartlett C, Will EJ. Optimizing erythropoietin therapy in hemodialysis patients. Am J Kidney Dis. 2001;38:109–17.

40. Eschbach JW, Abdulhadi MH, Browne JK, et al. Recombinant human erythropoietin in anemic patients with end-stage renal disease. Ann Intern Med. 1989;111:992–1000.

41. Means RT, Olsen NJ, Krantz SB, et al. Treatment of the anemia of rheumatoid arthritis with recombinant human erythropoietin: clinical and in vitro results. Arthritis Rheum. 1989;32:638–42.

42. Rao DS, Shih M-S, Mohini R. Effect of serum parathyroid hormone and bone marrow fibrosis on the response to erythropoietin in uremia. N Engl J Med. 1993;328:171–5.

43. Le Meur Y, Lorgeot V, Comte L, et al. Plasma levels and metabolism of AcSDKP in patients with chronic renal failure: Relationship with erythropoietin requirements. Am J Kidney Dis. 2001;38:510–517.

44. Glicklich D, Burris L, Urban A, et al. Angiotensin-converting enzyme inhibition induces apoptosis in erythroid precursors and affects insulin-like growth factor-1 in posttransplantation erythrocytosis. J Am Soc Nephrol. 2001;12:1958–64.

45. Casadavell N, Nataf J, Viron B, et al. Pure red cell aplasia and antierythropoietin antibodies in patients treated with recombinant erythropoietin. New Engl J Med. 2002;346:469–75.

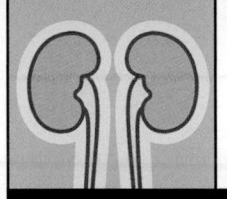

Chapter
71

Platelet Dysfunction and Coagulation Defects

James A Sloand

INTRODUCTION

A plethora of platelet and coagulation disorders exist in patients with renal insufficiency. While the balance between anticoagulation and hemostasis in a healthy population favors the latter, hemorrhagic diatheses had been a more frequent occurrence in patients with chronic renal failure (CRF) until the past decade. Patients with CRF are precariously perched, at risk for both abnormal bleeding and thrombosis, and these problems present everyday challenges to the clinician.

Uremic bleeding

Although bleeding is generally thought of as being a condition related to severe, prolonged uremia and corrected by dialysis, hemodialysis (HD) itself has actually been shown to contribute to hemostatic defects. Hemorrhagic problems have diminished in recent years. The use of recombinant human erythropoietin (epoetin), more biocompatible dialyzers, and other advances in the treatment of end-stage renal disease (ESRD) have brought about a closer return to a normal physiologic milieu. Conversely, these advances are also responsible for increased thrombotic complications in this population.

Thrombosis

The effects of epoetin on platelet–blood vessel interaction have uncovered the potential for hypercoagulability in patients with chronic renal failure. Hyperfibrinogenemia, enhanced levels of plasminogen activator inhibitor (PAI-1), deficient release or reserves of tissue plasminogen activator (t-PA), increased prevalence of antiphospholipid (APL) antibodies, diminished functional activity of protein C, and a vascular tree exposed to the damaging effects of hyperhomocystinemia and excessive oxidative stress have been well described. Fistula thrombosis and calciphylaxis are commonly recognized sequelae of these abnormalities. Atherosclerotic disease, a major cause of morbidity and mortality in ESRD, appears to be aggravated by some combination of these disorders.

Normal hemostasis

Normal hemostasis depends upon both platelets and the coagulation systems[1]. The cascade of events begins with platelet adhesion to the vessel wall (Fig. 71.1). Initial platelet adhesion requires participation of a relatively vasoconstricted vessel wall, integrity of glycoprotein Ib, the platelet receptor for von Willebrand factor (vWF), and a normal quantity of

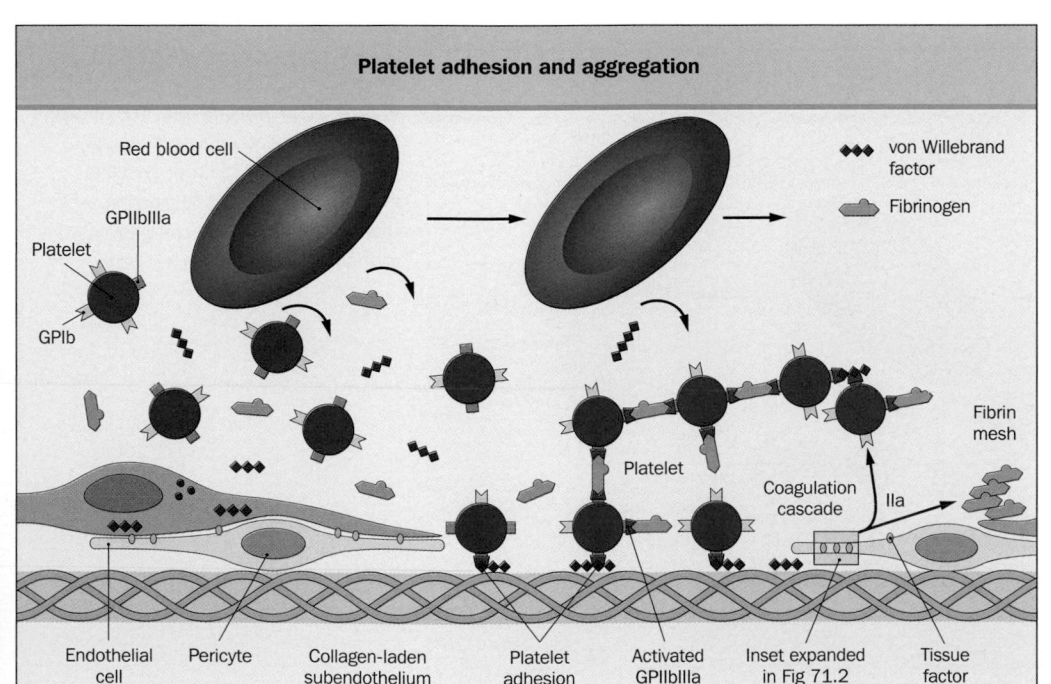

Figure 71.1 Platelet adhesion and aggregation. Platelets are pushed peripherally toward the vascular wall by red blood cells traversing centrally through the blood stream. Damage to the vessel wall results in a rent in the nonthrombogenic endothelial cell lining and exposure of subendothelial structures. While collagen supports initial platelet adhesion (and subsequent aggregation), von Willebrand factor (vWF) deposition on the subendothelium serves as the main anchor for platelet adhesion via platelet GPIb receptor. Postadhesion conformational change in platelet GPIIbIIIa receptor (fibrinogen/vWF receptor) results in interlinking platelet aggregation.

large-molecular-weight, multimeric vWF, the platelet vessel 'glue'. Endothelium-stimulated, bound platelets activate platelet fibrinogen receptors (GPIIbIIIa), allowing recruitment of circulating platelets and fibrinogen into an intricate web (aggregation). This aggregated fibrinogen–platelet mesh serves as a trap for binding and activation of other plasma clotting factors.

One of the key factors in the coagulation cascade is thrombin (factor IIa), which converts fibrinogen to fibrin. Conversion of prothrombin to thrombin is catalyzed by exposure of preceding clotting factors to tissue factor, present on damaged endothelial cells or exposed subendothelial pericytes and fibroblasts (see Figs 71.1 and 71.2). Subsequent cross-linking of insoluble fibrin results in a stable hemostatic plug.

Antithrombin III, protein C, and protein S are parts of an anticoagulant system that functions, along with plasmin generated by the fibrinolytic system, to prevent and dissolve unwanted clot (Fig. 71.3).

HEMORRHAGIC COMPLICATIONS

Pathogenesis

Primary conditions contributing to bleeding in chronic renal failure include anemia, vascular wall and platelet abnormalities[2,3]. Reduced red blood cell mass or increased vessel luminal diameter (mediated by vasodilating effects of prostacyclin and nitric oxide) decreases peripheral dispersion of platelets and their contact with the vessel wall.

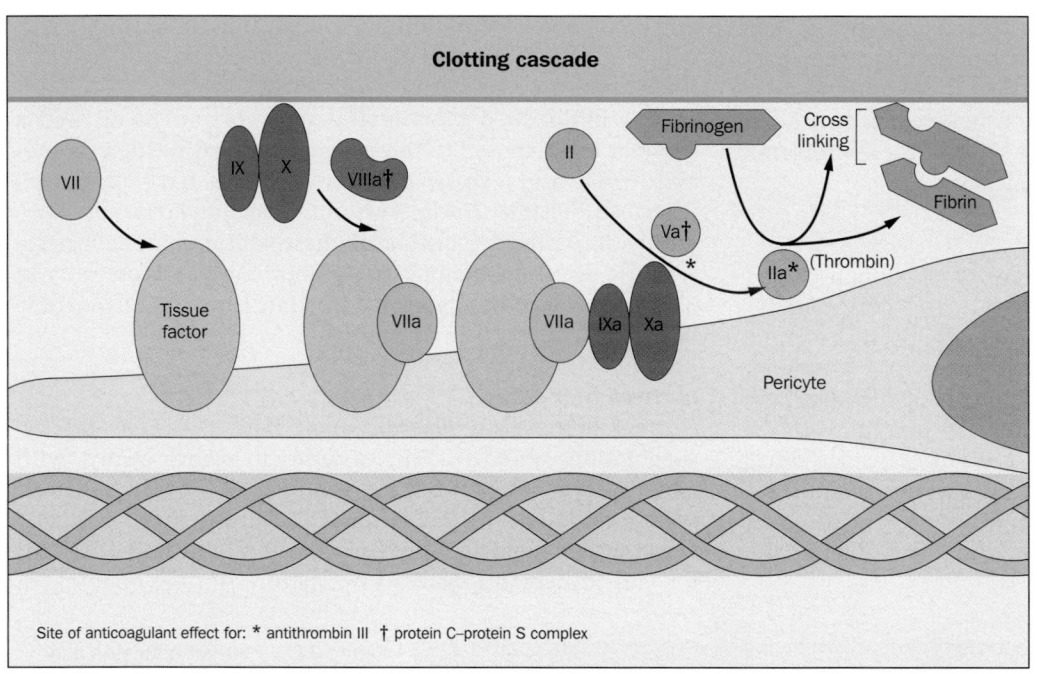

Site of anticoagulant effect for: * antithrombin III † protein C–protein S complex

Figure 71.2 Clotting cascade. Expansion of the inset in Figure 71.1 shows the clotting cascade that takes place at the damaged vessel wall. Exposure of subendothelial tissue factor, present on pericytes and fibroblasts, allows for eventual activation of prothrombin (factor II) to thrombin. Thrombin converts fibrinogen to fibrin, activates fibrin cross-linking, stimulates further platelet aggregation, and activates anticoagulant protein C. Naturally occurring anticoagulants antithrombin III, protein C, and protein S help maintain control and counterbalance on coagulation.

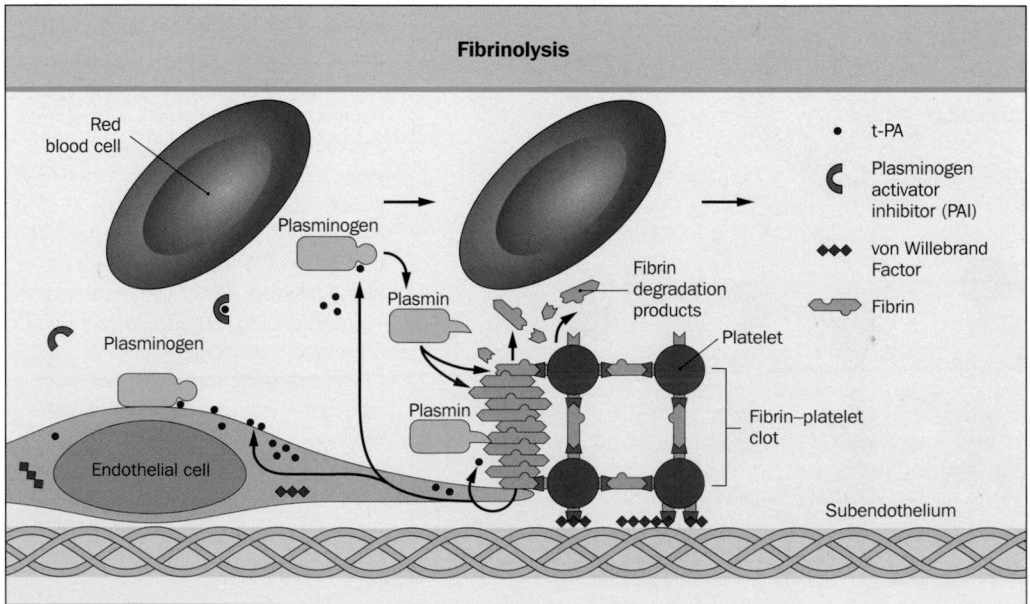

Figure 71.3 Fibrinolysis. The binding of fibrin to endothelial cells results in release of t-PA. The latter converts inactive plasminogen to plasmin, which then cleaves the fibrin clot in synchrony with blood vessel healing.

In uremia, plasma factors prevent normal platelet adhesion and aggregation by inhibiting platelet membrane receptor–ligand interplay. Increased nitric oxide synthesis, perhaps mediated by accumulation of guanidinosuccinic acid, appears to play a central causative role in disrupting normal platelet function[4]. Other uremic substances have also been reported to contribute to platelet biochemical defects and abnormal platelet aggregation. Dialysis removes many of these putative interfering uremic plasma factors, enhancing intrinsic platelet aggregatory function and leaving vWF and fibrinogen unimpeded in their interaction with platelet membrane receptors (GPIb and GPIIbIIIa). However, hemodialysis has been shown to create defects in platelet membrane receptors for vWF and fibrinogen, thus preventing normal platelet–vessel wall and platelet–platelet interaction[5,6]. This effect occurs through platelet membrane receptor modification and destruction by the hemodialysis membranes, and dissipates in the 24 h following dialysis. HD has also been associated with t-PA release from vessel walls, probably caused by vascular perturbation during extracorporeal circulation[6].

Clinical manifestations

Classically, uremic bleeding can develop in the subepidermal, submucosal, or serosal surface of any organ. Bleeding problems that occur in ESRD are usually minor, manifesting as ecchymoses or petechiae in the skin, epistaxis, gastrointestinal (GI) or gingival oozing, or prolonged hemorrhage from needle puncture or postoperative sites. Retroperitoneal hemorrhage (particularly associated with acquired cystic disease), ocular subconjunctival hemorrhage, or subcapsular hepatic hematomas are all less frequent manifestations of uremic bleeding.

While uncommon, life-threatening hemorrhagic complications can occur, in particular, from the GI tract. Platelet and vascular defects in ESRD make bleeding from any anatomic GI lesion more frequent and severe. Angiodysplasia in the mucosa and submucosa of the GI tract occurs with increased frequency in ESRD and can cause overt or occult bleeding, most often in the duodenum or stomach. These lesions may develop as a result of increased levels of prostacyclin and nitric oxide, inducing microvascular vasodilatation.

Uremic pericarditis can occur either before initiation of dialysis or during maintenance HD. Hemorrhage from the inflamed pericardium can occur in either setting, but is seen more often in HD-related pericarditis, possibly because of the combined effects of HD-related platelet defects and associated use of heparin. Hemorrhage pleuritis can occur by similar mechanisms.

Intracranial hemorrhage is a rare but potentially fatal complication occurring more often in patients with polycystic kidney disease due to an increased prevalence of arteriovenous malformations.

Renal biopsy carries an increased risk of hemorrhage in uremic patients and care must be taken to ensure bleeding time is optimized before biopsy (see Chapter 6).

Diagnosis

Abnormal bleeding associated with uremia occurs in patients with severe renal impairment, usually on or nearing the need for dialysis. There is, however, a poor correlation between uremic bleeding and the absolute level of serum urea or creatinine. Although platelet aggregation to standard agonists, clot retraction, and procoagulant activity are all abnormal in uremic patients, the only clinical test that is a marker of hemorrhagic risk is the bleeding time (BT), though it has a poor predictive value[7]. It is measured as the time to cessation of bleeding after placement of a 1 cm long by 1 mm deep incision on the volar aspect of the forearm under 40 mmHg pressure applied by a sphygmomanometer on the upper arm. As BT measures primary platelet adhesion to the vessel wall, it is not surprising that it correlates with the abnormal platelet–vessel wall interaction that characterizes uremic bleeding[4].

A reduced red blood cell mass (anemia) diminishes centrifugal dispersion of platelets, and there is a strong inverse relationship between BT and plasma hemoglobin level. Paradoxically, low t-PA levels also seem to correlate with an elevated BT. Plasma vWF levels are normal or elevated in CRI. Activated partial thromboplastin time (APTT) and prothrombin time/international normalized ratio (INR) are normal.

Treatment – Correction of bleeding

Both HD and peritoneal dialysis (PD) correct or ameliorate prolonged BT and clinical bleeding in nondialyzed or under-dialyzed patients, probably by removal of uremic plasma factors[1-3]. Hemorrhagic problems are fewer with PD than with HD. Platelet membrane receptor fragmentation by HD membranes, augmented fibrinolysis and t-PA release from HD-induced vascular perturbation, heparin exposure, and other modality-related factors[8] all contribute to this difference. Use of biocompatible dialysis membranes may reduce nitric oxide production and post-HD bleeding[4].

Correction of anemia to a hematocrit >30%, either with packed red blood cell transfusion or epoetin, results in enhanced platelet–vessel wall interaction, shortened BT, and improved hemostasis.

Estradiol (oestradiol) reduces bleeding and BT by antagonizing synthesis of nitric oxide, thereby improving platelet function and adhesion to a more vasoconstricted vessel[9,10]. Peak onset of action is 5–7 d, with efficacy continuing 5–7 d after cessation of drug administration. Estrogen can be given intravenously, orally, or transdermally. Long-term therapy is mostly limited by development of breast tenderness.

Cryoprecipitate or DDAVP are given for immediate hemorrhagic problems[9]. Both serve to increase levels of vWF, helping to overcome any adhesive deficiencies between platelets and subendothelium. Both agents can significantly improve BT. DDAVP stimulates release of vWF from endothelial cells and increases platelet adhesion receptor (GPIb) expression[11]. DDAVP is given intravenously, but can be given intranasally or subcutaneously (Table 71.1). Tachyphylaxis, related to depletion of endothelial vWF stores, limits the usefulness of this agent. The use of cryoprecipitate, a rich source of concentrated vWF and fibrinogen, is limited by the risk of transfusion-related infection (Table 71.1).

Deep-tissue biopsy or invasive surgical procedures that require improved hemostasis should ideally be scheduled the day after dialysis in patients undergoing HD[5,6] for reasons

Treatment and prevention of uremic bleeding						
Treatment	Mechanism	Prescription	Dose	Onset of action	Maximum effect	Duration of effect after cessation
Dialysis	Removes uremic platelet receptor Allows re-expression of platelet von Willebrand factor (vWF) and fibrinogen receptors	–	Per KT/V	BT may not improve immediately	Unknown	>48 h
HD	–	Avoid surgery or biopsy immediate after HD	Per KT/V	Progressive improvement in BT >4 h after HD	BT returns to baseline >16 h after HD	Until next HD
CAPD (preferred method)	Avoids platelet–dialyzer membrane interactions		Per KT/V	24 h	4–7 days	Unknown
Correct anemia (to a hematocrit >30%)	Enhances platelet-level interaction	Transfusion of packed red blood cells		Immediate	To hematocrit >30%	NA
		Intravenous or subcutaneous epoetin	See Chapter 70			
Estrogen	Vasoconstriction; enhances platelet–vessel and platelet–platelet interaction	Intravenous, conjugated	0.6 mg/kg per day (3 mg total)	6 h	6 days	14 days
		Oral conjugated	50 mg per day	3–5 days	7 days	4 days
		Topical (patch) estradiol	50–100 mg patch q3.5/day	24–48 h	5–7 days	Unknown
DDAVP (arginine vasopressin)	Enhanced platelet adhesion by increasing vWF serum levels and vWF platelet receptors (GbIb).	Intravenous	0.3 µ/kg in 50 mL normal saline over 30 min	1 h		4–8 h
		Intranasal	3 µg/kg	2 h	Unknown	Unknown
		Subcutaneous	0.3 µg/kg			
Cryoprecipitate	Enhances platelet adhesion by increasing vWF levels	Intravenous	10 U/30 min	1 h	4–8 h	24 h

Table 71.1 Treatment and prevention of uremic bleeding.

alluded to above. When there is clinical urgency or there is a high risk of postoperative bleeding, heparin use should be minimized, eliminated (using predilutional saline), or substituted with epoprostenol during HD or hemofiltration. Protamine sulfate administration, to reverse post-HD heparin effect, should be considered if there is marked, dialysis-induced prolongation of the partial thromboplastin time (PTT) and severe bleeding. A full neutralizing dose is 1 mg protamine per 100 U of heparin infused over 10 min. Reduction in protamine dosing is required in relation to the half-life of heparin (~ 60 min) and the time interval since last exposure (i.e., 10 mg protamine needed to neutralize 4000 U heparin given 2 h previously). There are few published clinical data on the use of protamine in this context, but risks of both hypercoagulability and increased bleeding in association with protamine use have been reported[12,13].

A combination of therapies may be needed to correct the hemorrhagic diathesis in some patients.

THROMBOTIC PROBLEMS

Pathogenesis
Functional protein C and protein S deficiency
Protein C is a vitamin K-dependent protease that, with the help of protein S, serves as a natural anticoagulant[14]. The activated protein C/S complex inactivates Factor VIII and Factor V, preventing unmitigated conversion of prothrombin to thrombin (see Fig. 71.2). While plasma levels of anticoagulant protein C are normal, functional activity of the protein is depressed in some patients with ESRD[14,15]. The mechanism of this functional deficit has been ascribed to a 'uremic inhibitor'. Malnutrition or sepsis can also lead to an acquired deficiency of protein C, but reduction of both measured plasma and functional levels would be expected in these conditions. The exact incidence of a protein C deficit in CRF is unknown, but it is associated with the syndrome of thrombotic vascular occlusion known as calciphylaxis or calcific uremic arteriopathy[16,17] (see below).

Deficiency of protein S has also been described in patients with CRF. As both protein C and S are phospholipid-containing proteins, antiphospholipid antibodies can also interfere with their function. The relationship between APL syndrome, functional protein C deficiency, and calciphylaxis has not been examined.

Factor V Leiden mutation
Thrombin (factor IIa) plays a pivotal role in the hemostatic process, providing the catalyst for development of the fibrin web (see Fig. 71.2) and contributing to further platelet aggregation. Activated factor V (factor Va) serves as a cofactor

necessary in the conversion of prothrombin to thrombin. Inactivation of factor V depends upon its cleavage by activated Protein C. The factor V Leiden (gene) mutation alters this cleavage site on the factor V molecule by a single amino acid substitution, rendering it resistant to degradation by activated protein C[18]. Heterozygosity for this mutation occurs in 2–5% of Western population, making it the most common cause of inherited hypercoagnability, and conferring a near seven-fold increase in risk of spontaneous venous thrombosis. The prevalence of Factor V Leiden deficiency is not increased in renal failure, but the risk of thrombotic complications is increased. This may be particularly devastating in renal transplant patients where it predisposes to renal transplant thrombosis, pulmonary embolism, and acute vascular rejection.

Antiphospholipid syndrome and antithrombin III deficiency

A significantly higher prevalence of APL antibodies is found in patients with ESRD compared with the general population, exceeding 30% in some studies[19]. Generation of these autoantibodies may be linked to accelerated apoptosis, with subsequent presentation of cellular phospholipid neoantigens to the immune system. APL antibodies may also enhance thrombin generation from prothrombin (abnormally bound by APL antibody to endothelial cells) or result in tissue factor expression by endothelial cells. Both can trigger activation of the coagulation cascade at the endothelial surface. These antibodies cross-react with phospholipid-containing proteins, including proteins C and S, rendering them functionally deficient. High circulating titers of APL antibodies have been associated with cutaneous necrosis resembling calciphylaxis and warfarin necrosis[20].

Reduced antithrombin III (AT III) activity related to uremic factors has also been described. AT III reduces conversion of prothrombin to thrombin and inactivates thrombin[21].

Fibrinolytic disorders

Inadequate release of t-PA in uremia (see Fig. 71.3) can prevent lysis of formed clot[22]. Infusion of 1-deamino-8-D-arginine vasopressin (DDAVP) not only causes vWF release from endothelial cells, augmenting platelet adhesion to the vascular wall, but is a standard fibrinolytic stimulus. Endothelial release of t-PA has been shown to be deficient in uremic patients after DDAVP infusion.

As protein C inactivates t-PA inhibitor (PAI), deficiencies in protein C activity, described above, can exacerbate defective fibrinolysis.

Hyperhomocystinemia

Homocysteine is an intermediary amino acid formed in the conversion of methionine to cysteine. There are abnormally high levels of homocysteine in ESRD, resulting from defects in homocysteine metabolism[23]. These defects may be due to low serum levels of the vitamin cofactors (folate and B_{12}) required for its metabolism. Homocysteine contributes to oxidative stress, a process that has a direct toxic effect on vascular endothelial cells. This not only enhances thrombogenesis, but plays a role in atherosclerosis. Homocysteine also inhibits protein C activation.

Heparin-induced thrombocytopenia

Heparin-induced thrombocytopenia (HIT) is a result of platelet activation by antibodies generated against complexes of heparin and platelet factor 4[24]. Despite the decrease in platelet count, HIT can cause paradoxical venous or arterial thrombosis. The incidence of this disorder in the ESRD population appears to be similar to that in the general population (~ 4%)[25] irrespective of the frequent and prolonged exposure to heparin in patients receiving hemodialysis.

Accelerated atherosclerosis

Oxidative stress, so key to development of atherosclerosis and thrombosis in the general population, appears to play an even larger role in development of vascular disease in patients with impaired renal function[26]. Diabetes, hypertension, lipid abnormalities, hyperhomocystinemia, dialyzer incompatibility, and abnormal glycation and lipoxidation of proteins in the setting of renal impairment contribute to the oxidative process. The relative contributions of exogenous calcium administration, clotting factor and fibrinolytic disorders to this process have yet to be fully defined and resolved.

Clinical manifestations

Prothrombotic abnormalities of coagulation factors and the fibrinolytic system, clinically masked by the rheologic effects of anemia, have now been exposed by routine use of epoetin. Vascular access occlusion is the most frequently recognized manifestation. The presence of APL antibodies is associated with risk of access thrombosis. The frequency of the isolated protein C functional deficit and its contribution to vascular access occlusion has not been defined.

A rare but devastating disorder associated with depressed protein C activity is calciphylaxis (see below).

Accelerated atherosclerosis is well documented in ESRD. Even after correction for age, gender, and presence of diabetes, it is manifested in a cardiovascular mortality rate 10–20 times that of the general population[27]. Peripheral vascular disease is about five times as prevalent, with patient and limb survival rates after bypass surgery about one-third those of patients without ESRD.

Diagnosis

Recurrent thrombotic events (i.e., two events over a 3-month span), including vascular access thrombosis, should prompt measurement of protein C and protein S activity, factor V Leiden status, AT III, and APL antibodies. Functional protein C activity can be measured by a protein C chromogenic or anticoagulant assay. The specific activity of protein C, calculated as its functional activity divided by its antigenic activity, is also depressed. Factor V Leiden mutation is determined by polymerase chain reaction analysis. HIT is diagnosed in a setting of thrombocytopenia (platelet count < 150 000/m² or 50% reduction) developing in a patient on heparin for HD with a positive test for heparin-induced Platelet Aggregation Test and/or ELISA for heparin-PF4 antibodies.

The presence of APL syndrome in this setting is suggested by evidence for presence of lupus anticoagulant antibodies (an elevated APTT that does not correct upon mixing with normal plasma, an elevated tissue thromboplastin inhibition assay, a

Chronic Renal Failure and the Uremic Syndrome

prolonged (diluted) Russell's viper venom time, an increased kaolin clotting time), or anticardiolipin antibodies (an increased level of IgG antibody directed at β_2-glycoprotein I)[28]. As APL antibodies are heterogeneous, no one assay will itself be more than 95% sensitive. Therefore, multiple antibody tests should be used. Conversely, the presence of antibody by any of these assays does not itself establish a diagnosis of APL syndrome. Causal relationships should be suspected in the setting of recurrent thrombosis.

Baseline plasma homocysteine levels in ESRD are 18–40 μmol/L (2.4–5.4 mg/L). The range in the normal population is 5–15 μmol/L (0.68–2.0 mg/L).

Treatment and prevention of thrombosis

If APL antibodies or abnormalities in protein C or protein S are confirmed in assays separated by one month in a setting of recurrent thrombosis, long term warfarin therapy is recommended[14,19,28], although clinical efficacy in ESRD has not been proven. A diagnosis of HIT mandates immediate discontinuation of all forms of heparin, including low molecular weight heparin to which HIT-related antibodies have strong cross-reactivity[28]. Warfarin is also indicated for recurrent thrombosis related to HIT. However, warfarin should be considered in HIT only after complete resolution of thrombocytopenia with abstinence from all forms of heparin for at least one month. This allows for recovery of Protein C levels consumed in HIT-related thrombosis. If low protein C levels persist, these patients are at high risk for development of warfarin-induced thrombosis and venous limb gangrene. Therefore, HIT should invariably be treated with a direct-acting thrombin inhibitor, such as lepirudin or argatroban[24]. The latter has the advantage of hepatic metabolism in patients with renal impairment. Cost considerations and convenience may influence decisions regarding modality change to peritoneal dialysis.

Warfarin is indicated for recurrent thrombosis related to factor V Leiden mutation[18].

The recognition of hyperhomocystinemia as a risk factor for arterial and venous thrombosis in CRF has prompted several small therapeutic trials of folate and vitamins B_6 and B_{12} supplementation. High-dose supplementation with these cofactors has been shown to reduce homocysteine levels by about 25%. There is so far no evidence that thrombotic risk is attenuated, but present evidence would at least suggest that the recommended daily (RDA) level of these vitamins should be provided (folic acid 1 mg; vitamin B_6 10 mg; vitamin B_{12} 0.006 mg). Daily doses of folic acid of 5–15 mg have been advocated for some high-risk patients.

CALCIPHYLAXIS (CALCIFIC UREMIC ARTERIOPATHY)

Pathogenesis

The skin and soft tissue necrosis seen with this disorder is characterized by extensive calcification, thrombosis and occlusion of cutaneous and subcutaneous arteries and arterioles. While the pathophysiology of this condition is unknown, the lesion may be an extreme variant of Monckeberg's or medial vascular sclerosis[29,30]. Histology shows extensive stromal and arterial calcification (see Fig. 71.4).

Venules occluded with fibrin thrombi are frequently seen. The vascular calcifications within the tunica media have enhanced expression of the bone matrix protein, osteopontin and other osteogenic markers, raising the possibility of dedifferentiation of involved vascular smooth muscle cells into osteoblast-like cells. Long-standing and poorly-controlled hyperphosphatemia may be the primary trigger to this transformation[31,32]. Low transcutaneous oxygen tension that is poorly responsive to increasing oxygen concentration suggests a fixed vascular defect. Other factors including serum calcium, parathyroid hormone, and exogenous administration of calcium and vitamin D may also play a role in the pathogenesis of this disorder. Neither vascular calcification nor histologic expression of bone-related proteins has been shown to be specific to or pathognomonic of calciphylaxis, however.

Calciphylaxis is associated with multiple coagulation abnormalities, in particular, functional protein C deficiency. Whether these deficiencies are pathogenic or an epiphenomenon is not

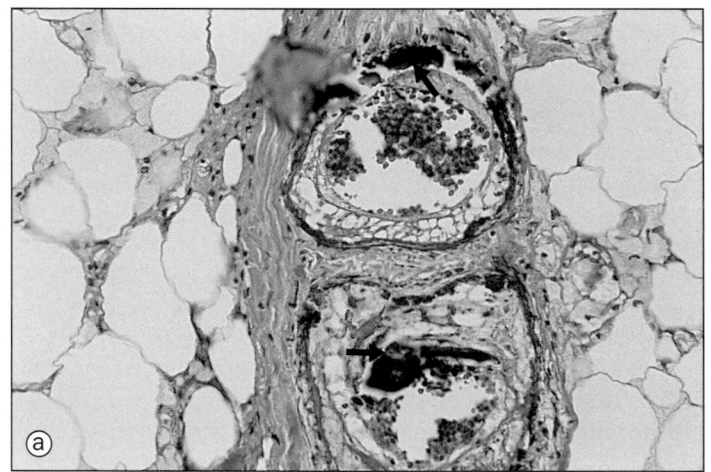

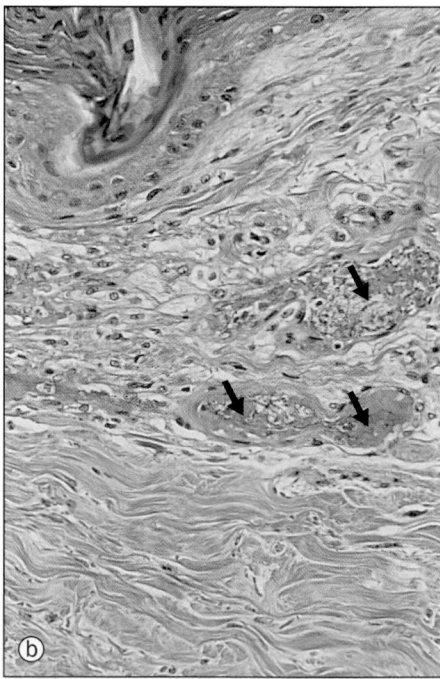

Figure 71.4 Dermatopathology of calciphylaxis. (a) Arterial calcification (arrows) seen in an area of skin necrosis associated with calciphylaxis. (b) Section of involved skin showing fibrin thrombi (arrows) in dermal venules (light microscopy, hematoxylin–eosin, 3300). (Courtesy of Drs G Scott and J Fiscella.)

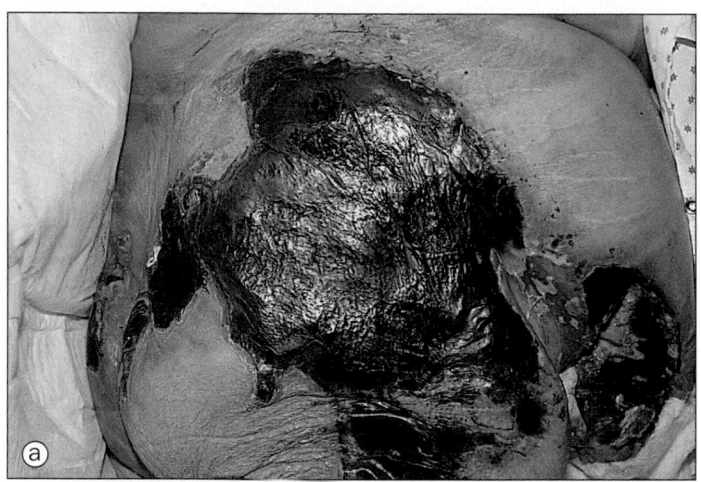
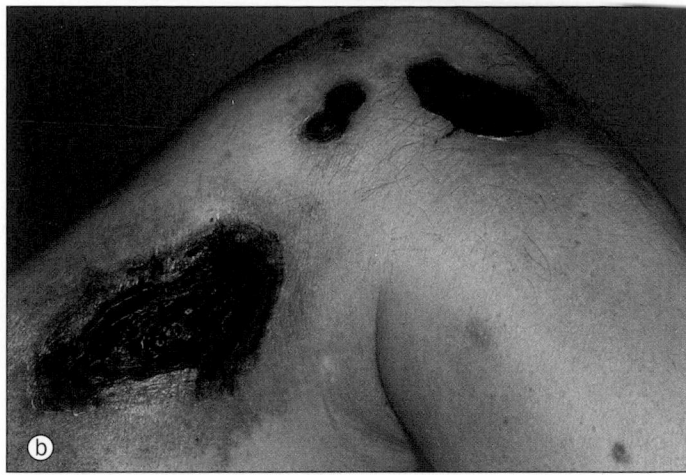

Figure 71.5 Calciphylaxis-associated skin necrosis. Initially heralded by causalgia and hemorrhagic discoloration in the affected area, calciphylaxis usually proceeds to frank necrosis. (a) Trunkal skin necrosis in the abdomen of a diabetic woman. (b) Necrotic lesions about the knee and inner thigh in a diabetic man who also developed penile gangrene from calciphylaxis. (Courtesy of Dr M Shelly.)

defined. Large-scale confirmatory studies have not been performed largely due to the sporadic nature of calciphylaxis. Even if there are no demonstrable procoagulant abnormalities, vascular patency may be further compromised by inhibition or inadequate concentrations of functional matrix Gla protein (MGP), a vitamin K-dependent inhibitor of tissue calcification[30].

Clinical Manifestations

Burning pain precedes development of hemorrhagic discoloration of affected digits, limbs, or trunkal skin. Progression to frank necrosis ensues (see Fig. 71.5), frequently requiring skin grafting and/or amputation.

Treatment

Optimal therapy for calciphylaxis may never be defined given its rarity. Aggressive wound care and normalization of serum calcium and phosphate levels are imperative, however. Avoidance of calcium-containing phosphate binders, use of low-calcium dialysate and hyperbaric oxygen are pathophysiologically promising options. Parathyroidectomy should be considered for medically uncontrollable, severe hyperparthyroidism. There are no controlled studies in the use of antiplatelet agents or systemic anticoagulants, even in the face of identified coagulation defects. While use of warfarin may seem intuitive with discovery of specific procoagulant abnormalities, inhibition of MGP may have long-term detrimental effects on vascular integrity.

REFERENCES

1. Rabelink TJ, Zwaginga JJ, Koomans HA, Sixma JJ. Thombosis and hemostasis in renal disease. Kidney Int. 1994;46:287–96.
2. Carvalho AC. Acquired platelet dysfunction in patients with uremia. Hematol Oncol Clin N Am. 1990;4:129–43.
3. Eberst ME, Berkowitz LR. Hemostasis in renal disease: pathophysiology and management. Am J Med. 1994;96:168–79.
4. Noris M, Remuzzi G. Uremic bleeding: Closing the circle after 30 years of controversies? Blood. 1999;94:2569–74.
5. Sreedhara R, Itagaki I, Lynn B, Hakim RM. Defective platelet aggregation in uremia is transiently worsened by hemodialysis. Am J Kidney Dis. 1995;25:555–63.
6. Sloand JA, Sloand EM. Studies on platelet membrane glycoproteins and platelet function during hemodialysis. J Am Soc Nephrol. 1997;8:799–803.
7. Steiner RW, Coggins C, Carvalho ACA. Bleeding time in uremia: a useful test to assess clinical bleeding. Am J Hematol 1979;7:107–17.
8. Malyszko J, Malyszko JS, Mysliwiec M. Comparison of hemostatic disturbances between patients on CAPD and patients on hemodialysis. Perit Dial Int. 2001;21:158–65.
9. Lohr JW, Schwab SJ. Minimizing hemorrhagic complications in dialysis patients. J Am Soc Nephrol. 1991;2:961–75.
10. Livio M, Mannucci PM, Vigano G, et al. Conjugated estrogens for the management of bleeding associated with renal failure. N Engl J Med. 1986;315:731.
11. Sloand EM, Kessler CM, Sloand J, Prodouz K. DDAVP corrects platelet dysfunction produced by cardiopulmonary bypass, hemodialysis, and prolonged storage: re-expression of GPIb on the platelet membrane. In: Mariana G, ed. Desmopressin in Bleeding Disorders. New York, NY: Plenum Press; 1993:147–54.
12. Mochizuki T, Olson PJ, Szlam F, et al. Protamine reversal of heparin affects platelet aggregation and activated clotting time after cardiopulmonary bypass. Anesth Analg. 1998; 87:781–5.
13. Fearn SJ, Parry AD, Picton AJ, Mortimer AJ, et al. Should heparin be reversed after carotid endarterectomy? A randomized prospective trial. Eur J Vasc Endovasc Surg. 1997; 13:394–7.
14. Nizzi FA, Kaplan HS. Protein C and S deficiency. Semin Thromb Hemost. 1999;25:265–72.
15. Faioni EM, Franchi F, Krachmalnicoff A, et al. Low levels of the anticoagulant activity of protein C in patients with chronic renal insufficiency: an inhibitor of protein C is present in uremic plasma. Thromb Haemost 1991;66:420–25.
16. Mehta RL, Scott G, Sloand JA, Francis CW. Skin necrosis associated with acquired protein C deficiency in patients with renal failure and calciphylaxis. Am J Med. 1990;88:252–57.
17. Budisavljevic MN, Cheek D, Ploth DW. Calciphylaxis in chronic renal failure. J Am Soc Nephrol. 1996;7:978–82.
18. Wuthrich RP. Factor V Leiden mutation: potential thrombogenic role in renal vein, dialysis graft and transplant vascular thrombosis. Curr Opin Nephrol Hypertens. 2001;10:409–14.

19. Brunet P, Aillaud MF, San Marco M, et al. Antiphospholipids in hemodialysis patients: relationship between lupus anticoagulant and thrombosis. Kidney Int. 1995;48:794–800.
20. Creamer D, Hunt BJ, Black MM. Widespread cutaneous necrosis occurring in association with the antiphospholipid syndrome: a report of two cases. Br J Derm. 2000;142:1199–203.
21. Vaziri ND, Gonzales EC, Wang J, Said S. Blood coagulation, fibrinolytic, and inhibitory proteins in end-stage renal disease: effect of hemodialysis. Am J Kidney Dis. 1994;23:828–35.
22. Opatrny K. Hemostasis disorders in chronic renal failure. Kidney Int. 1997;52(Suppl 62)(62):87–9.
23. Dennis VW, Robinson K. Homocysteinemia and vascular disease in end-stage renal disease. Kidney Int. 1996;50:S11–S17.
24. Deitcher SR, Carman TL. Heparin-induced thrombocytopenia: natural history, diagnosis, and management. Vasc Med. 2001; 6:113–19.
25. Yamamoto S, Koide M, Matsuo M, et al. Heparin-induced thrombocytopenia in hemodialysis patients. Am J Kidney Dis. 1996; 28:82–5.
26. Kaysen GA. The microinflammatory state in uremia: cause and potential consequences. J Am Soc Nephrol. 2001;12:1549–57.
27. Reddan DN, Marcus RJ, Owen WF, et al. Long-term outcomes of revascularization for peripheral vascular disease in end-stage renal disease patients. Am J Kidney Dis 2001;38:57–63.
28. Levin JS, Branch W, Rauch J. The antiphospholipid syndrome. N Eng. J Med. 2002;346:752–63.
29. Shanahan CM, Cary NRB, Salisbury JR. et al. Medial location of mineralization-regulating proteins in association with Monckeberg's sclerosis: evidence for smooth muscle cell-mediated vascular calcification. Circulation 1999;100:2168–76.
30. Davies MR, Hruska KA. Pathophysiological mechanisms of vascular calcification in end-stage renal disease. Kidney Int. 2001; 60:472–9.
31. Mazhar AR, Johnson RJ, Gillen D, et al. Risk factors and mortality associated with calciphylaxis in end-stage renal disease. Kidney Int. 2001;60:324–32.
32. Ahmed S, O'Neill KD, Hood AF, et al. Calciphylaxis is associated with hyperphosphatemia and increased osteopontin expression by vascular smooth muscle cells. Am J Kidney Dis 2001; 37:1267–76.

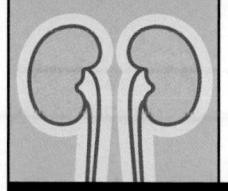

Section 14 Chronic Renal Failure and the Uremic Syndrome

Chapter 72

β₂-Microglobulin-derived Amyloid

Jürgen Floege

INTRODUCTION AND DEFINITIONS

It was first reported in 1980 that material excised from the carpal tunnel of patients undergoing chronic hemodialysis may contain amyloid. While the amyloid exhibited typical histologic features (Fig. 72.1), it could not be classified using antibodies directed against any of the known amyloidoses at that time. By identifying β₂-microglobulin as the specific amyloid precursor protein, Gejyo and colleagues established in 1985 that a novel type of amyloidosis was present in patients undergoing hemodialysis[1]. It is exclusively seen in patients with chronic uremia. Initially believed to occur only in patients on chronic hemodialysis, it was called 'dialysis amyloid' or 'dialysis-associated amyloidosis'. It soon became clear that the amyloidosis can develop in patients on any type of renal replacement therapy (patients with functioning renal transplants are exceptions) and even in uremic, predialysis patients. Therefore, it appears more appropriate to refer to it as β₂-microglobulin-derived amyloid or, in line with general amyloid terminology (see Chapter 29), as Aβ₂M-amyloid. It is a systemic type of amyloidosis but clinical manifestations of the disease are largely confined to the musculoskeletal system.

EPIDEMIOLOGY

It is important to distinguish between the prevalence of histologic amyloid deposits and clinical amyloid manifestations. In rare cases Aβ₂M-amyloid deposits may be detected histologically only a few months after the initiation of hemodialysis or even in predialysis patients[2,3]. Deposition may precede clinical manifestations by several years. Most amyloid deposits never appear to cause clinically relevant problems, which suggests that clinical assessment markedly underestimates the true prevalence of Aβ₂M-amyloidosis. Thus, the largest postmortem study available to date noted a considerable discrepancy between clinical and radiologic amyloid signs (i.e., carpal tunnel syndrome and bone radiolucencies) which were present in 2% and 4% of the patients respectively, while Aβ₂M-amyloid was demonstrated histologically in joint samples from 48% of the patients[4]. The study found that prevalence of the amyloid was already high after two years of chronic hemodialysis and increased to 100% in patients treated for more than 13 years (see Table 72.1)[4]. The joint distribution of Aβ₂M-amyloid is uneven, with the sternoclavicular joint and hips showing the highest proportion of positive samples[2].

Both clinically and radiologically, Aβ₂M-amyloid related symptoms are rarely present until therapy has continued for 5 years. After this time, there is an almost linear increase in the incidence, which in past evaluations reached nearly 100% after 15 years of treatment (see Table 72.1)[2,3]. When chronic hemodialysis patients were investigated with the more specific and sensitive diagnostic method, β₂-microglobulin scintigraphy, a more rapid increase in the prevalence of Aβ₂M-amyloidosis was detected (see Table 72.1)[5].

The occurrence of Aβ₂M-amyloidosis is not confined to patients on chronic hemodialysis with regenerated cellulosic membranes (Cuprophane®). Cases have also been described with virtually every other type of nontransplant, renal replacement therapy, including patients treated exclusively by hemodialysis or hemofiltration using synthetic high-flux membranes or peritoneal dialysis[2,3].

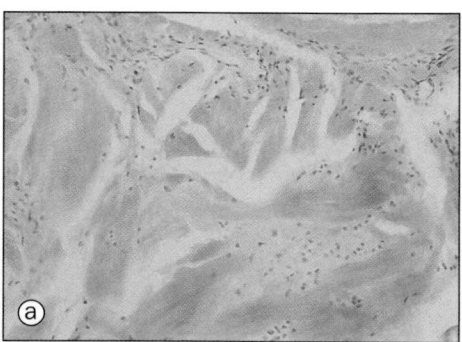 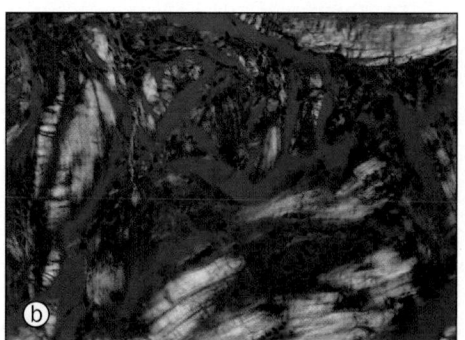 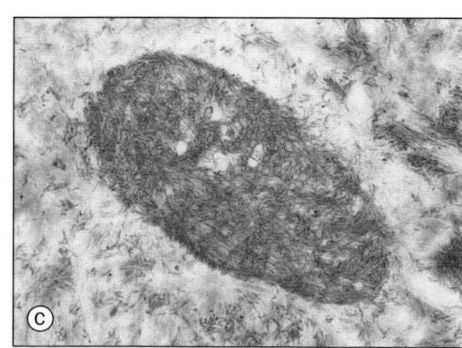

Figure 72.1 Diagnostic findings in Aβ₂M-amyloidosis. Synovial specimen of a patient on long-term hemodialysis. (a) Congo-red positive material is present in the interstitial tissue of the synovium. (b) Under polarized light, typical green birefringence can be seen. (c) Electron microscopy shows the material is composed of 8–10 nm wide, nonbranching fibrils. (Courtesy of Dr. G Ehlerding)

Epidemiology of Aβ₂M-amyloidosis				
Method of detection	Chronic dialysis treatment (years)			
	0–5	5–10	10–15	>15
Positive postmortem histology in joint samples[4] (Percentage of patients)	28	71	88	n.a.
Positive clinical and radiological signs[2,3] (Percentage of patients; range reported)	0–10	15–30	55–70	100
Positive radionuclide imaging with radiolabeled β₂-microglobulin[5] (Percentage of patients)	8	65	90	100
n.a. – not available				

Table 72.1 Epidemiology of Aβ₂M-amyloidosis. Survey of currently available histologic and clinical studies on the prevalence of Aβ₂M-amyloidosis in chronic hemodialysis patients.

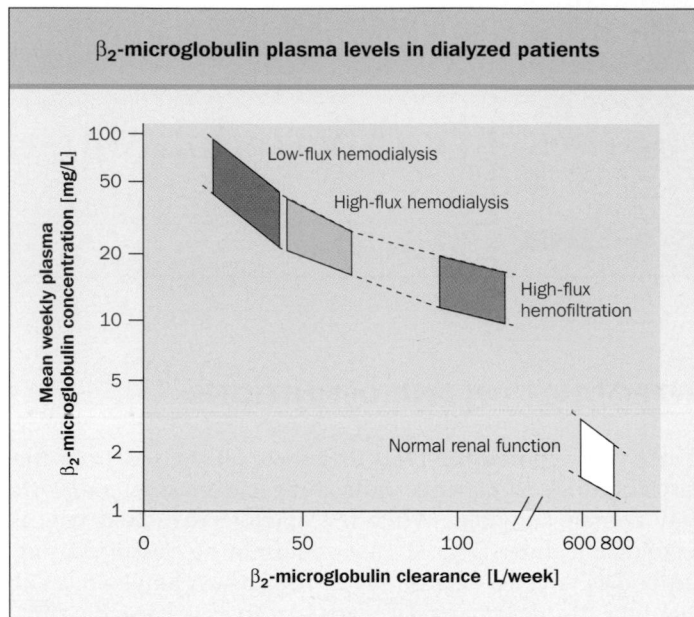

Figure 72.2 β₂-microglobulin plasma levels in dialyzed patients. Expected ranges of mean weekly β₂-microglobulin plasma levels in normal persons (or patients with good graft function) and in patients on either chronic hemodialysis or hemofiltration with β₂-microglobulin permeable or impermeable membranes.

Risk factors

Clinically, two risk factors for Aβ₂M-amyloid deposition have been identified: age at onset of renal replacement therapy and the duration of (nontransplant) renal replacement therapy[4–6]. No cases of Aβ₂M-amyloidosis have yet been described in the pediatric dialysis population. Other factors, such as hyperparathyroidism and extraosseous calcifications, as well as aluminum or iron overload, have also been suggested as risk factors for Aβ₂M-amyloid deposition. However, these may be independent events also related to the duration of renal replacement therapy.

PATHOGENESIS

The constituents of Aβ₂M-amyloid fibrils

Fibrils of Aβ₂M-amyloid are derived to a large extent from the circulating precursor protein β₂-microglobulin. The β₂-microglobulin molecule exhibits significant stretches of β-pleated tertiary conformation, which is regarded as a prerequisite for amyloidogenesis. Other molecules that are constituents of the Aβ₂M-amyloid fibrils or are bound to the fibrils include amyloid-P component, and several types of proteoglycan and antiprotease as well as immunoglobulin light chains[2].

β₂-microglobulin

The β₂-microglobulin molecule is a nonglycosylated, 11.8 kDa, single-chain protein. It forms the nonvariable light chain of the HLA class I complex and is necessary for the expression of HLA class I on the surface of nearly all nucleated cells. The β₂-microglobulin synthesis rate in healthy individuals ranges from 2–4 mg/kg per day, with a half-life of 2.5 h, and plasma concentrations vary between 1 and 3 mg/mL. Given that 95% of β₂-microglobulin elimination is achieved via glomerular filtration (with subsequent tubular reabsorption and intracellular proteolysis), it is not surprising that plasma levels are inversely related to the glomerular filtration rate. Levels in end-stage renal disease (ESRD) depend on the degree of residual renal function and can be elevated as much as 60-fold in anuric individuals owing to the prolonged plasma half-life of the protein (Fig. 72.2).

While there is no doubt that the increased burden of β₂-microglobulin in ESRD is mainly related to decreased renal excretion, it is less clear whether the rate of β₂-microglobulin synthesis is also altered in uremia. Synthesis and release of β₂-microglobulin can be stimulated in vitro by exposing cells to an acidic environment, endotoxin, and inflammatory cytokines such as interleukin-1 (IL-1), tumor necrosis factor-α (TNF-α) and interferons, many of which are present or induced during uremia or dialysis therapy[2]. However, in-vivo evidence of altered synthesis of β₂-microglobulin in dialysis patients is limited. Acutely, β₂-microglobulin plasma levels increase by about 20% during Cuprophane hemodialysis, but this has been shown to result mainly from complex water shifts. The daily synthesis rate of β₂-microglobulin is usually unchanged in dialysis patients[2]. Compared with the marked renal retention of β₂-microglobulin, any changes in its rate of synthesis are likely to be of minor importance in vivo.

Amyloid-P component

Amyloid-P component, derived from serum amyloid-P component (SAP), is a ubiquitous constituent of nearly all types of amyloid. The amyloid-P component does not form an intrinsic part of the fibrils but, rather, binds to them. It has been proposed that amyloid-P component renders the amyloid fibrils resistant to proteolytic degradation in vivo.

Proteoglycans

Proteoglycans, in particular heparan sulfate proteoglycans, chondroitin sulfate proteoglycans, and hyaluran, have been detected in or around Aβ₂M-amyloid fibrils. Experimental evidence suggests that the presence of matrix compounds, such as highly sulfated glycosaminoglycans, in particular heparan sulfate proteoglycans, are related to the onset of amyloidosis.

Antiproteases and other molecules

Antiproteases including β₂-macroglobulin, α₁-proteinase inhibitor, α₁-antichymotrypsin, antithrombin III, and tissue inhibitors of metalloproteinase, have all been identified in Aβ₂M-amyloid deposits. In every case, however, the surrounding tissues also contained these antiproteases and, consequently, it is unclear whether they play a specific role in the persistence of amyloid fibrils.

Pathogenetic concepts in Aβ₂M-amyloidosis

Given that Aβ₂M-amyloidosis is restricted to uremic patients, the increased body burden of β₂-microglobulin appears to be the basic precondition for amyloidogenesis in these patients. However, a pure 'precipitation theory' is unlikely, for the following reasons[2]:

- β₂-Microglobulin serum levels do not correlate with extent of clinical amyloid deposits.
- Local β₂-microglobulin concentrations, (e.g., in synovial fluid), are not increased above the serum concentration.
- *In vitro* formation of amyloid fibrils from purified β₂-microglobulin under physiological conditions is controversial. In most studies a nonphysiologic ambient salt concentration or prolonged incubation of synovial cells in the presence of uremic serum and endothelial cell culture supernatants was necessary to generate fibrils[2]. Copper, derived either from dialysate or dialysis membranes such as Cuprophane, may promote fiber formation at physiological conditions[7]. Of potential interest for diagnostic purposes, conformational intermediates with partial folding of β₂-microglobulin can be detected[8].

These observations have led to a search for biochemical modifications of the β₂-microglobulin molecule, which might facilitate its deposition in amyloid fibrils.

- Limited proteolysis. Partial breakdown of native β₂-microglobulin, resulting in early folding events, may occur, and would be similar to the mechanisms involved in the pathogenesis of other types of amyloid[9,10]. However, not all investigators have been able to confirm the presence of cleaved β₂-microglobulin molecules within Aβ₂M-amyloid[2].
- Advanced glycation end-products (AGE): Different sugar–protein cross-links have been detected within Aβ₂M-amyloid fibrils, including pentosidine, N-epsilon-carboxymethyllysine, and imidazolone[3]. In one study, circulating AGE-modified hemoglobin levels correlated with the progression of presumed amyloid-related bone lesions[11]. AGE-modified β₂-microglobulin species are presumably the result of oxidative or 'carbonyl stress' in chronic dialysis patients[3,12]. *In vitro*, AGE-modified β₂-microglobulin activates monocytes through the AGE receptor (RAGE) and delays monocyte apoptosis[3,12,13]. It may thereby contribute to inflammatory changes surrounding the amyloid. Possibly AGE modifications also render β₂-microglobulin more amyloidogenic or enhance the persistence of established fibrils in tissue. An unexplained finding is that radiologic signs of Aβ₂M-amyloid occur with similar frequency in both diabetic and non-diabetic dialysis patients, while diabetics have markedly higher circulating AGE levels[2].

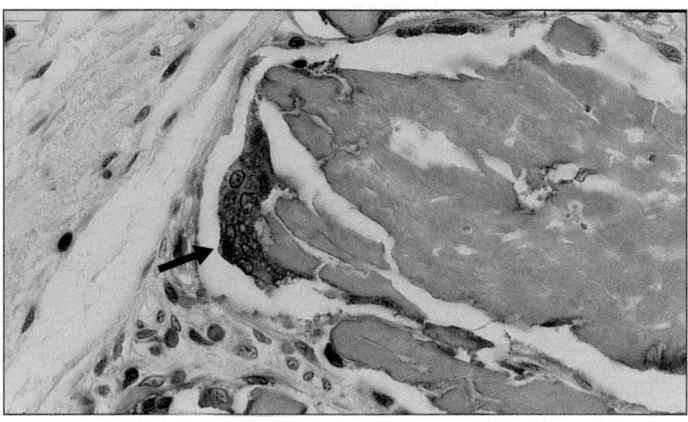

Figure 72.3 Foreign body reaction to advanced Aβ₂M-amyloid. Congo-red positive amyloid is shown in the synovium of a long-term hemodialysis patient. A multinucleated giant cell (derived from macrophages as shown by the brown immunostaining product; arrow) is noted in close proximity to the amyloid deposit. (Courtesy of Dr. G Ehlerding.)

Neither of these alterations can explain the distribution pattern of Aβ₂M-amyloidosis and additional local factors, perhaps proteoglycans, may facilitate amyloid formation at specific sites. Local inflammatory reactions, for example within synovial tissue (Fig. 72.3), appear to be the consequence of Aβ₂M-amyloid deposition rather than its cause since they exhibit characteristics of a foreign body reaction[2,14,15]. These surrounding inflammatory reactions likely contribute to the clinical manifestation of the amyloidosis, since symptoms quickly disappear after renal transplantation or the initiation of steroid therapy despite persistence of the amyloid deposits.

CLINICAL MANIFESTATIONS AND DIAGNOSIS

Clinical manifestations of Aβ₂M-amyloid deposition are largely confined to osteoarticular sites, in particular synovial membranes, while visceral manifestations are rare[2,3]. As in other types of amyloidosis, some suggestive findings but no pathognomonic clinical, or radiologic findings exist in Aβ₂M-amyloidosis.

Histology

At present, the definitive diagnosis of Aβ₂M-amyloidosis depends on histologic findings: Congo-red staining showing green dichroism under polarized light, immunohistochemical demonstration of the precursor molecule within deposits, and the electron microscopical demonstration of typical (8–10 nm wide, nonbranching, curvilinear) fibrils (see Fig. 72.1). Fat aspiration and rectal biopsy are not helpful in Aβ₂M-amyloidosis, and diagnostic material usually has to be obtained from synovial membranes or bone lesions[2]. Alternatively, detritus in synovial fluid may be used for diagnosis. Histologically, Aβ₂M-amyloid deposits may vary from pericollagenous traces to massive amyloid deposition which occupies most of the tissue. In joints, amyloid deposits can be detected in articular cartilage, the synovial membrane and villi, and in tendons as well as in subchondral bone[15].

Carpal tunnel syndrome

Carpal tunnel syndrome with dysesthesia and pain in the region of the distal median nerve, decreased motor nerve conduction velocity, and prolongation or absence of distal motor nerve latency, is a characteristic, although not pathognomonic, clinical sign of $A\beta_2M$-amyloidosis. The pain typically worsens at night and during hemodialysis. Especially when it manifests itself within the first 5 years of dialysis, other reasons for the carpal tunnel syndrome, in particular its association with diabetes, heart disease or multiple myeloma, should be considered.

Carpal tunnel syndrome induced by $A\beta_2M$-amyloid is often bilateral and usually requires surgical release of the transverse ligament and/or synovectomy of the tendon sheaths. Surgery typically reveals a hypertrophic and amyloid-laden synovial membrane or perineural connective tissue. Postoperative recurrence of the carpal tunnel syndrome may be observed within the next 2–3 years.

Osteoarthropathy of peripheral joints

Osteoarthropathy of peripheral joints is another frequent manifestation of $A\beta_2M$-amyloidosis and results from local amyloid deposition in periarticular bone and the synovial capsule (Fig. 72.4). It is characterized by recurrent or persistent arthralgias, stiffness of large and medium-sized joints and swelling of capsules and adjacent tendons. Further symptoms include recurrent joint effusions and synovitis, often in the shoulders and knees, but also in the hips, wrists, elbows, acromioclavicular joints, and feet, in which case synovial fluid should be obtained for analysis and/or a synovial biopsy should be considered. The clinical presentation may vary from frank, acute arthritis to slow, progressive destruction of the affected joints.

In the differential diagnosis, it should be remembered that as many as 95% of patients receiving long-term hemodialysis complain of shoulder pain. Apart from $A\beta_2M$-amyloid deposits this may be caused by nonamyloid-induced bursitis or tendinitis, hydroxyapatite crystal deposition, tears in the rotator cuff, cervical radiculopathy, or septic arthritis.

Ultrasonography is a noninvasive means of detecting synovial $A\beta_2M$-amyloid deposits. Thickening of the joint capsules of the hip and knee, biceps tendons, and the rotator cuffs, as well as the presence of echogenic structures between muscle groups and joint effusions have been observed in patients on long-term hemodialysis. In some cases, the ultrasound image could be correlated with the histological demonstration of $A\beta_2M$-amyloid in the respective site[3]. However, only selected joints are accessible for examination by ultrasound and the results are dependent on the observer's skill.

Radiologically, affected joints may present with single or multiple juxta-articular, cystic bone radiolucencies, which are located preferentially at the insertion sites of capsules and tendons. These cystic bone radiolucencies arise from amyloid deposition in bone and are not 'cysts' in the true sense of the word (Figs 72.4 and 72.5). Bone defects of this kind are prone to pathologic fractures, in particular if located in areas such as the femoral neck. However, bone cystic radiolucencies in patients undergoing chronic dialysis are not diagnostic of $A\beta_2M$-amyloid deposition since single, small bone cysts may be observed in

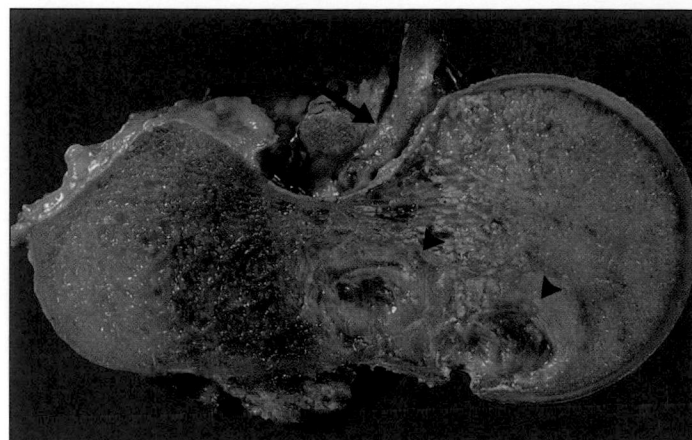

Figure 72.4 $A\beta_2M$-amyloid deposition in the femoral head. Post-mortem specimen from a long-term hemodialysis patient. Two large lesions (arrowheads), partly filled with grayish amyloid and partly cystic, are noted in the femoral head. Also note the marked thickening of the synovial capsule due to amyloid deposition (arrow).

30% of nonuremic patients. Another important differential diagnosis in uremics is the brown tumor of secondary hyperparathyroidism. Diagnostic criteria have been developed for $A\beta_2M$-amyloid-induced cystic bone radiolucencies (Table 72.2)[6].

Computed tomography (CT) and magnetic resonance imaging (MRI) also have been used to search for evidence of $A\beta_2M$-amyloidosis. However, unless very strict diagnostic criteria are fulfilled, these methods are nonspecific, as is conventional scintigraphic bone scanning[2].

Two scintigraphic methods, employing either radiolabeled SAP[2] or β_2-microglobulin[5], offer more specific detection of amyloid deposits. In long-term hemodialysis patients, intravenous injection of ^{123}I-SAP can lead to accumulation of tracer in the wrists, knees, and shoulders. Local deposition of tracer in the hip region is rare. Splenic tracer uptake in 30% of the patients was interpreted as indicating splenic amyloidosis, a conclusion not substantiated by histologic findings[2,16]. Therefore, although there is evidence that ^{123}I-SAP can accumulate in $A\beta_2M$-amyloid deposits, there are, at present, uncertainties about both the specificity and sensitivity of this scan in hemodialysis patients.

Alternatively, scintigraphy with ^{131}I-labeled β_2-microglobulin has been used[5]. Local tracer accumulations in patients on hemodialysis correlates well with clinical, radiologic, and histologic findings. The scan has a good specificity and its sensitivity exceeds markedly that of combined clinical and radiologic examination. Significant progress in improving the radiolabeled β_2-microglobulin scan recently was achieved by using human recombinant β_2-microglobulin and by substituting the radioligand iodine-131 with indium-111, reducing radiation exposure but improving optical resolution (see Fig. 72.6)[16].

Spondylarthropathy and other vertebral column involvement

Several forms of destructive spondylarthropathy are associated with long-term hemodialysis[17]. In one form, cystic bone radiolucencies dominate the picture. A second form is

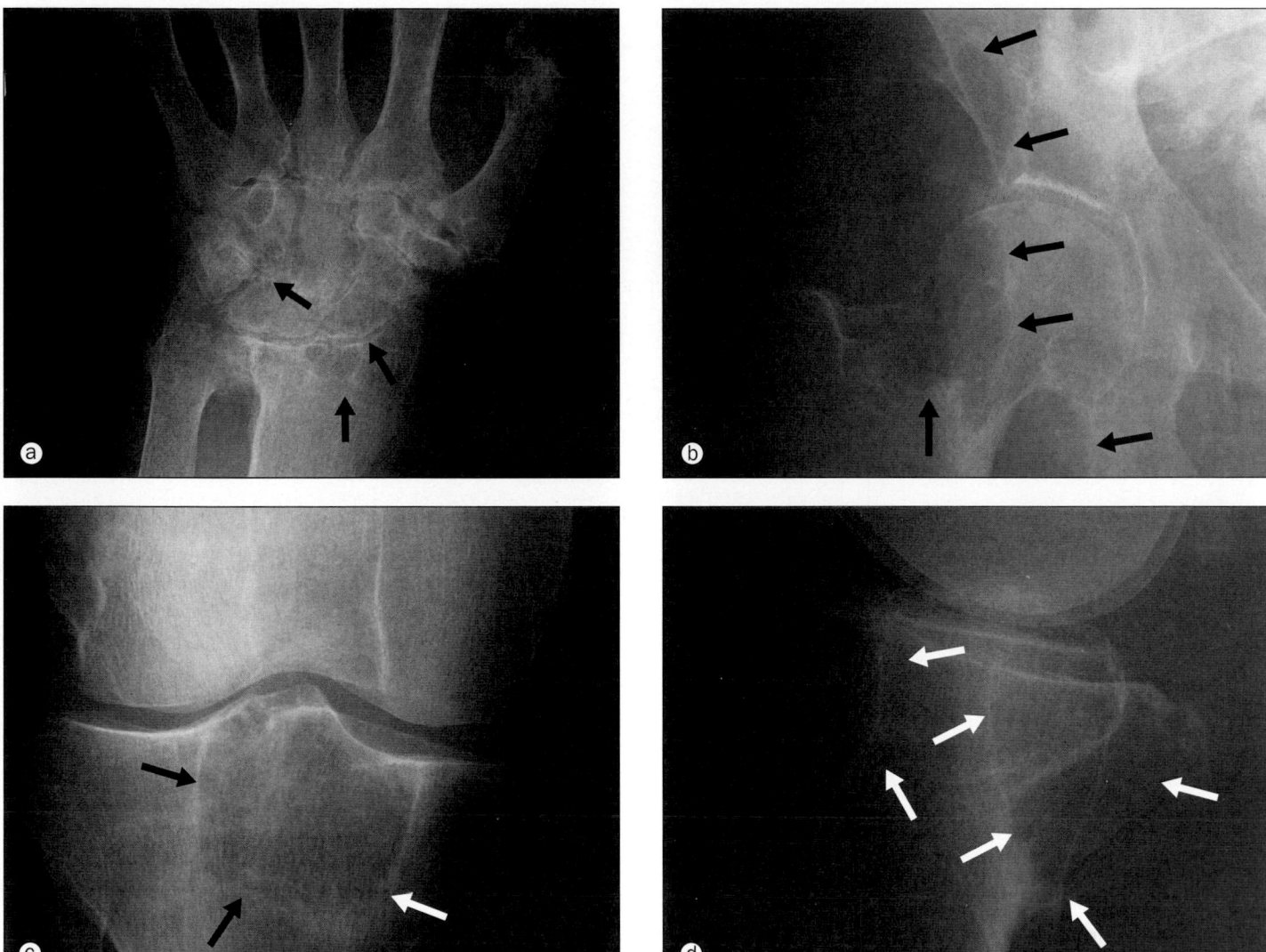

Figure 72.5 Peripheral bone 'cystic' radiolucencies in Aβ_2M-amyloidosis. Radiographic findings in a long-term hemodialysis patient. (a) Multiple 'cystic' lesions (arrows) are present in the hand bones. (b) Large cysts (arrows) in the neck of the femur and adjacent pelvic bones. (c and d) Anterior and lateral view of the head of the tibia with two very large, 'cystic' lesions (arrows) resulting in posterior bulging of the tibial plateau.

Radiologic diagnostic criteria for Aβ_2M-amyloidosis-associated cystic bone lesions
Diameter of lesions >5 mm in wrists and > 10 mm in shoulders and hips
Normal joint space adjacent to the bone defect
Exclusion of small subchondral cysts located in the immediate weight-bearing area of the joint
Exclusion of defects of the 'synovial inclusion' type
Increase of defect diameter of >30% per year
Presence of defects in at least two joints

Table 72.2 Diagnostic criteria for Aβ_2M-amyloidosis-associated cystic bone lesions[6].

more destructive, with bone fragmentation and soft tissue involvement. A third form may present with erosions and/or destructive changes of the intervertebral disk (Fig. 72.7).

Destructive spondylarthropathy has also been noted in uremic patients prior to the onset of hemodialysis as well as in patients treated with peritoneal dialysis.

Destructive spondylarthropathy in patients on long-term hemodialysis was originally attributed to the deposition of hydroxyapatite crystals, but is also associated with hyperparathyroidism, Aβ_2M-amyloid deposition, and aluminum intoxication. In present populations of dialysis patients it is very likely that Aβ_2M-amyloid plays a dominant role in the pathogenesis of spondylarthropathy. Deposits have been demonstrated in intervertebral disks, apophysial joints and ligaments. The latter may result in spinal canal stenosis requiring surgical treatment[18].

Clinical symptoms related to vertebral column involvement in the course of Aβ_2M-amyloidosis may range from asymptomatic deposits to radiculopathy, stiffness, 'mechanical ache,' and, finally, medullary compression with resulting paraplegia or cauda equina syndrome[2,3].

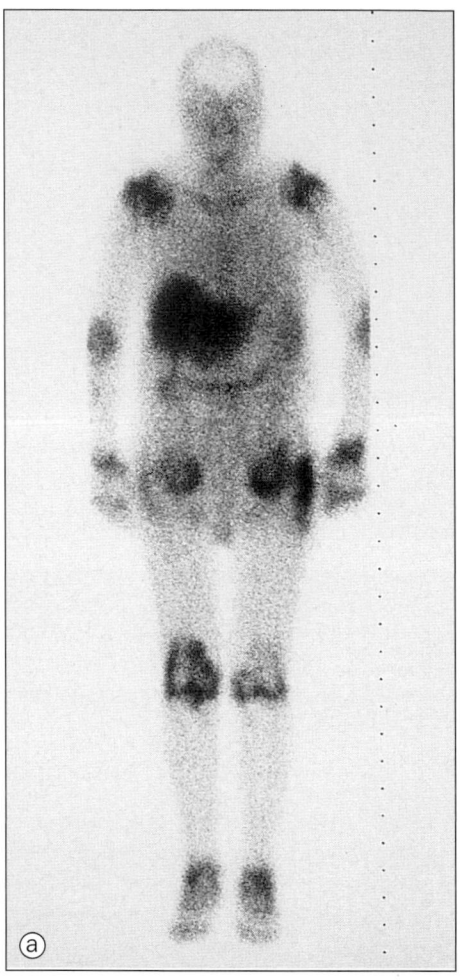 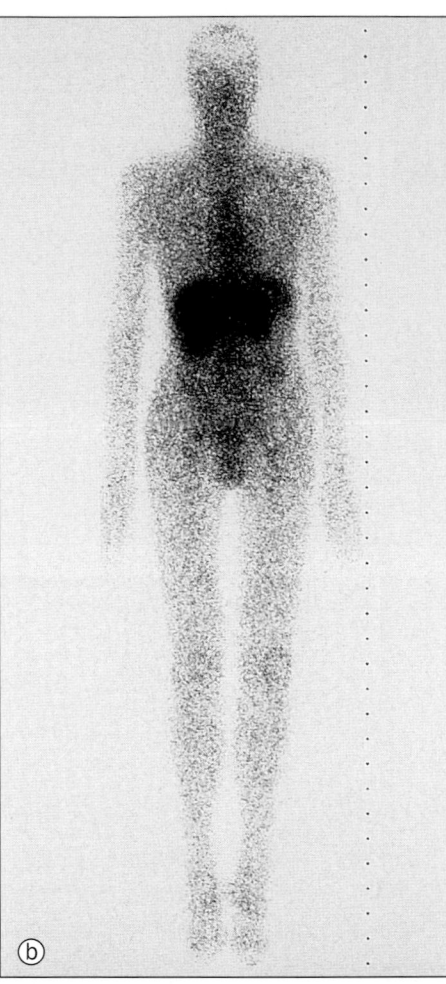

Figure 72.6 Detection of Aβ₂M-amyloidosis by ¹¹¹In-β₂-microglobulin scintigraphy. (a) Ventral image of a patient who had been on chronic hemodialysis for 16 years. Marked accumulation of the tracer is present around large joints and the sternoclavicular joint, and in the hands. Accumulation of the tracer in the liver, spleen, and gut relates to excretion of free indium. (b) Dorsal image of a patient who had been on chronic hemodialysis for 1 year only. No joint accumulation of the tracer is present. Tracer accumulation overlying the trunk relates to the blood pool (heart) and excretion of free indium as in (a). (Courtesy of Dr. J Schäffer.)

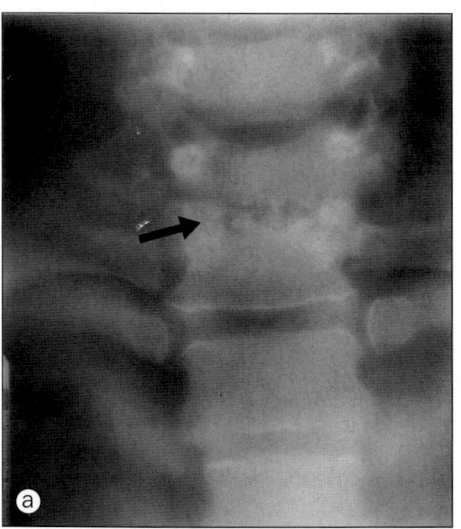 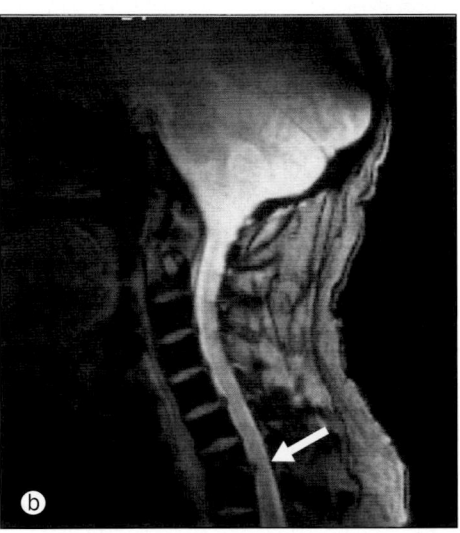

Figure 72.7 Aβ₂M-amyloidosis-associated spondylarthropathy. (a) Destruction of an intervertebral disk (arrow) in the neck vertebrae of a long-term hemodialysis patient. (b) Magnetic resonance image of the same patient as in (a). Note destruction of the intervertebral space and protrusion of material into the spinal canal (arrow).

Other musculoskeletal symptoms

As well as carpal tunnel syndrome, various other manifestations of Aβ₂M-amyloidosis may affect the hands of patients on long-term dialysis, causing severe functional deficiencies. Camptodactyly, caused by Aβ₂M-amyloid deposits along the flexor tendons of the hands, may result in prominence of the tendons upon extension ('guitar string sign') and functional contraction of the hand (Fig. 72.8). Patients undergoing dialysis can also have subcutaneous tumorous deposits of Aβ₂M-amyloid; however diffuse infiltration of the subcutaneous fat or skin has not been observed.

Systemic organ manifestations of Aβ₂M-amyloidosis

Clinically relevant involvement of other organs with Aβ₂M-amyloidosis is rare, with most organ deposits of Aβ₂M-amyloid only showing asymptomatic microscopic foci. In cases

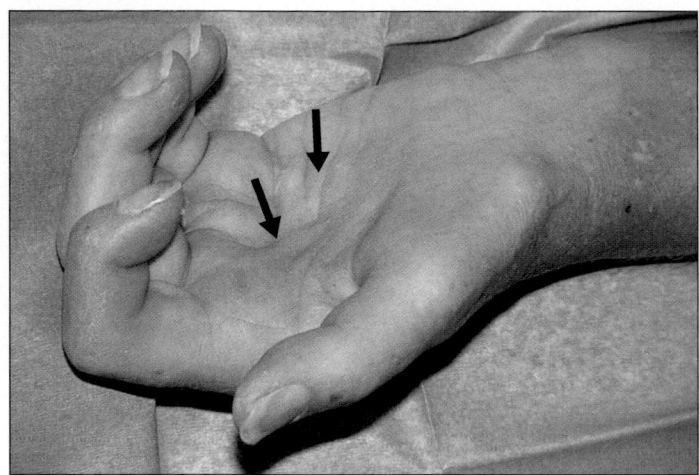

Figure 72.8 Hand involvement in Aβ_2M-amyloidosis. Hand of a long-term hemodialysis patient showing maximal extension. Note the prominence of shrunken flexor tendons (arrows). This is also known as the 'guitar string sign'.

Recommendations for the prevention and management of Aβ_2M-amyloidosis
Recommendations for prevention
• Ignore the issue of Aβ_2M-amyloidosis in all patients whose life expectancy on dialysis is below 5 years (i.e., the time when clinical manifestations first appear).
• In all other patients, attempt renal transplantation whenever possible.
• On hemodialysis, use bicarbonate-buffered dialysate and minimize microbiologic dialysate contamination.
• Use high-flux hemodialysis or hemodiafiltration in those at high risk for Aβ_2M-amyloidosis – i.e., the elderly and all patients, independent of age, who have little chance of receiving a renal transplant.
Recommendations for treatment of symptomatic Aβ_2M-amyloidosis
• Initiate symptomatic, usually orthopedic, measures depending on musculoskeletal site and symptoms of amyloid deposits.
• Attempt renal transplantation as soon as possible.
• If renal transplantation is not a short-term option, consider change to hemodialysis, or preferably hemodiafiltration, using high flux synthetic membranes and microbiologically clean dialysate (addition of adsorbent columns may also be considered, although its efficacy is less well established).
• If severe, disabling symptoms persist despite the above measures, initiate prednisone therapy at 0.1 mg/kg body weight per day.

Table 72.3 Recommendations for the prevention and management of Aβ_2M-amyloidosis.

with systemic involvement, the amyloid has been found in the walls of small blood vessels of the gastrointestinal tract, lung, heart, liver, tongue, endocrine organs, brain, and testes, as well as in the parathyroid glands[2,3]. Case reports of clinically relevant organ manifestations are almost exclusively confined to patients treated with hemodialysis for more than 15 years and have described heart failure, odynophagia, intestinal perforation of both small and large bowel, gastrointestinal bleeding and pseudo-obstruction, gastric dilatation, paralytic ileus, persistent diarrhea, macroglossia or functional tongue disturbances (abnormal taste, mobility, articulation), ureteral stenosis, and renal calculi[2,3].

NATURAL HISTORY

So long as patients are maintained on dialysis and have not yet received a renal transplant, the natural history of clinically manifest Aβ_2M-amyloidosis is usually one of slow but relentless progression. This is best illustrated by carpal tunnel syndrome induced by Aβ_2M-amyloid, which usually requires surgical intervention and thereby differs from carpal tunnel syndrome of other etiologies, which can often be managed conservatively. As shown in Table 72.1, prevalence after 15 years of chronic hemodialysis was almost 100% in past studies. No spontaneous remissions of clinical or radiologic findings have been described and at best, the inflammation accompanying, for example, synovial amyloid deposits, may vary in intensity.

TREATMENT AND PREVENTION

Present recommendations for prevention and treatment of Aβ_2M-amyloidosis are summarized in Table 72.3.

Treatment
Therapy of established Aβ_2M-amyloidosis is symptomatic. Nonsteroidal anti-inflammatory drugs, physical and surgical measures such as carpal tunnel decompression, endoscopic

coraco-acromial ligament release and bone stabilization in areas of 'cystic' destruction, are all used[2,19]. Renal transplantation can halt further progress of the disease, but it is controversial whether this can actually lead to regression of established Aβ_2M-amyloid deposits. Renal transplantation also leads to rapid symptomatic improvement, which is probably related to the use of steroids and immunosuppressive drugs.

Preliminary data suggest that prednisone (0.1 mg/kg daily) is highly efficient in relieving symptoms of Aβ_2M-amyloid-associated polyarticular arthropathy in uremic patients who have not undergone renal transplantation[20]. However, a high mortality rate was noted in treated patients although its relationship to the treatment was unclear. Therefore, at present steroids should be reserved for patients with severe, disabling symptoms.

A change of hemodialysis technique from treatment with Cuprophane membranes to 'biocompatible' hemodialyzer membranes has induced symptomatic relief in some, but not all, studies[2]. However, where studies report a symptomatic benefit, placebo effects usually have not been ruled out. Nevertheless, given the safety of such a change of technique, a trial appears appropriate in patients with a clinical suspicion of Aβ_2M-amyloid-associated symptoms. Finally, a recent prospective multicenter study described improvement of joint pain, stiffness and daily activities as well as an arrest of osteo-articular lesion progress following the start of treatment with a hemoperfusion column, that, amongst others, absorbed β_2-microglobulin[21].

Prevention
A number of strategies exist for preventing the clinical manifestations of Aβ_2M-amyloidosis[2,3,22].

Renal transplantation

Restoration of renal function by successful renal transplantation is clearly the preventive measure of choice since the amyloidosis does not occur in the presence of good renal function and because a successful kidney transplant leads within days to normalization of β_2-microglobulin plasma levels.

Increase of β_2-microglobulin removal

Given that Aβ_2M-amyloidosis is limited to patients with severe renal insufficiency, the crucial question is whether it is possible to counteract the renal retention of β_2-microglobulin in patients undergoing dialysis by an appropriate choice of renal replacement therapy. Some of the findings on nontransplant treatment modes are summarized below[2].

- Low-flux hemodialyzers with regenerated cellulosic membranes are impermeable to β_2-microglobulin.
- High-flux membranes, in particular the so-called 'synthetic' membranes, acrylonitrile, polyamide, and polysulfone, allow substantial removal of β_2-microglobulin during hemodialysis through convective mass transport as well as through adsorption. However, mass transfer is significantly lower for glycated β_2-microglobulin[23].
- Removal can be enhanced further by increasing convective transport, (i.e., by ultrafiltration), such as in hemodiafiltration and hemofiltration. However, the absolute amount of β_2-microglobulin removed decreases as plasma levels fall and currently available (nontransplant) treatment options will not achieve normal β_2-microglobulin plasma levels (Fig. 72.2). Whether a moderate, 20–30% chronic reduction of plasma β_2-microglobulin reduces the incidence of clinically manifest Aβ_2M-amyloidosis has not been tested. A higher chronic reduction in the order of 50% can be achieved by 6 nocturnal hemodialyses per week[24].
- Adsorbent columns in the hemodialysis circuit have also been used to increase β_2-microglobulin removal. Concerns about the relative nonspecificity of β_2-microglobulin adsorption and consequently the long-term safety of these devices as well as the issue of cost have so far prevented wider use of these columns.
- Continuous peritoneal dialysis allows some β_2-microglobulin removal and plasma levels in patients undergoing continuous ambulatory peritoneal dialysis (CAPD) are about 20–30% lower than those of patients on Cuprophane hemodialysis, provided that they are matched for residual renal function. However, there is no difference in the prevalence of carpal tunnel syndrome or scintigraphic evidence of Aβ_2M-amyloidosis in patients treated with Cuprophane hemodialysis and with CAPD[25]. Therefore, changing from hemodialysis to peritoneal dialysis can not be recommended for prevention of amyloid formation.

Choice of dialyzer membranes

Clinical signs of Aβ_2M-amyloid have only been compared in patients treated with either Cuprophane dialyzers or high-flux hemodialyzers. Therefore, the effects of the 'biocompatibility' of the dialyzer membrane cannot be separated from the increased β_2-microglobulin removal with the high-flux membrane, nor can it be separated from dialysate variables which are also influenced by the choice of the dialyzer membrane.

Available data on the comparison of Cuprophane and high-flux dialyzers are inconsistent[2]. Some studies demonstrated a benefit in the high-flux group and others failed to observe any difference in Aβ_2M-amyloid prevalence. In part this discrepancy may be due to the ubiquitous reliance on carpal tunnel syndrome as a sign of Aβ_2M-amyloid, which is also associated with the presence of heart disease in uremic patients[26]. Unfortunately, heart disease is an uncontrolled variable in most studies[2].

Nevertheless, three large studies suggest that high flux dialysis or (dia-)filtration may exert a beneficial effect on the signs of Aβ_2M-amyloidosis: there is a positive effect of long-term treatment with acrylonitrile hemodialyzers on some (bone cystic lesions), though not all (carpal tunnel syndrome)[6] Aβ_2M-amyloidosis associated symptoms. In a large study, the risk of carpal tunnel syndrome was reduced by 42% in the patients treated with high flux hemo(dia)filtration even after adjustment for confounding factors such as diabetes or heart disease[26]. Finally, in a Japanese registry the risk of developing signs of dialysis-related amyloidosis was 0.49 in patients using high-flux hemodialysis versus 1.0 in those using low-flux treatment and decreased further to 0.01 in patients receiving on-line hemodiafiltration[27].

Dialysate-related factors

Three studies suggest that dialysate factors may play a central role in the clinical manifestation of Aβ_2M-amyloidosis. A dramatic reduction in the prevalence of carpal tunnel syndrome occurred in patients dialyzed with ultrapure dialysate[28], perhaps suggesting that endotoxin or other bacterial products accelerate the clinical manifestation of the amyloidosis. In another study, an 80% reduction of amyloid signs in a chronic hemodialysis population did not appear to relate to an increase in the use of high flux synthetic membranes, but rather to dialysate factors such as microbiologic purity and/or the use of bicarbonate buffer[29]. Finally, in hemodialysis patients treated with a tank dialysis system, which uses essentially pyrogen free dialysate together with Cuprophane (up to 1992) or high flux synthetic membranes (from 1992 until evaluation in 1996), the prevalence of carpal tunnel syndrome in this population compared favorably to that of various other reports[30].

REFERENCES

1. Gejyo F, Yamada T, Odani S, et al. A new form of amyloid protein associated with chronic hemodialysis was identified as β_2-microglobulin. Biochem Biophys Res Commun. 1985;129:701–6.

2. Floege J, Ketteler M. Beta2-microglobulin-derived amyloidosis: an update. Kidney Int. 2001;78 (suppl):S164–71.

3. Miyata T, Jadoul M, Kurokawa K, Ypersele Strihou C de. β_2-microglobulin in renal disease. J Am Soc Nephrol. 1998;9:1723–35.

4. Jadoul M, Garbar C, Noel H, et al. Histological prevalence of β_2-microglobulin amyloidosis in hemodialysis: a prospective post-mortem study. Kidney Int. 1997;51:1928–32.

5. Floege J, Burchert W, Brandis A, et al. Imaging of dialysis-related amyloid (AB-amyloid) deposits with $^{131}I\beta_2$-microglobulin. Kidney Int. 1990;38:1169–76.

6. Ypersele Strihou C de, Jadoul M, et al. Effect of dialysis membrane and patient's age on signs of dialysis-related amyloidosis. The Working Party on Dialysis Amyloidosis. Kidney Int. 1991;39:1012–19.

7. Morgan CJ, Gelfand M, Atreya C, et al. Kidney dialysis-associated amyloidosis: a molecular role for copper in fiber formation. J Mol Biol. 2001;309:339–45.

8. Chiti F, Lorenzi E De, Grossi S, et al. A partially structured species of β_2-microglobulin is significantly populated under physiological conditions and involved in fibrillogenesis. J Biol Chem. 2001;276(46):714–21.

9. Bellotti V, Gallieni M, Giorgetti S, et al. Dynamic of β_2-microglobulin fibril formation and reabsorption: the role of proteolysis. Semin Dial. 2001;14:117–22.

10. Heegaard NH, Sen JW, Kaarsholm NC, et al. Conformational intermediate of the amyloidogenic protein β_2-microglobulin at neutral pH. J Biol Chem. 2001;31(32):657–62.

11. Motomiya Y, Iwamoto H, Uji Y, et al. Potential value of CML-Hb in predicting the progression of bone cysts in dialysis-related amyloidosis. Nephron. 2001;89:286–90.

12. Nangaku M, Miyata T, Kurokawa K. Pathogenesis and management of dialysis-related amyloid bone disease. Am J Med Sci. 1999;317:410–15.

13. Hou FF, Miyata T, Boyce J, et al. Beta2-microglobulin modified with advanced glycation end products delays monocyte apoptosis. Kidney Int. 2001;59:990–1002.

14. Garcia-Garcia M, Argiles A, Gouin-Charnet A, et al. Impaired lysosomal processing of beta2-microglobulin by infiltrating macrophages in dialysis amyloidosis. Kidney Int. 1999;55:899–906.

15. Jadoul M, Garbar C, van Ypersele de Strihou C. Pathological aspects of β_2-microglobulin amyloidosis. Semin Dial. 2001;14:86–90.

16. Ketteler M, Koch KM, Floege J. Imaging techniques in the diagnosis of dialysis-related amyloidosis. Semin Dial. 2001;14:90–3.

17. Bindi P, Chanard J. Destructive spondylarthropathy in dialysis patients: an overview. Nephron. 1990;55:104–9.

18. Nokura K, Koga H, Yamamoto H, et al. Dialysis-related spinal canal stenosis: a clinicopathological study on amyloid deposition and its AGE modification. J Neurol Sci. 2000;178:114–23.

19. Nagoshi M, Hashimzume H, Konishiike T, et al. Hemodialysis-related subacromial lesion: diagnostic imaging and minimally invasive treatment. Clin Nephrol. 2000;54:112–20.

20. Bardin T. Low-dose prednisone in dialysis-related amyloid arthropathy. Rev Rhum Engl Ed. 1994;61(suppl 9):S97–S100.

21. Kazama J, Maruyama H, Gejyo F. Reduction of β_2-microglobulin level for the treatment of dialysis-related amyloidosis. Nephrol Dial Transplant. 2001;16 (suppl)(4):31–5.

22. Zingraff J, Drueke T. Can the nephrologist prevent dialysis-related amyloidosis? Am J Kidney Dis. 1991;18:1–11.

23. Randoux C, Gillery P, Georges N, et al. Filtration of native and glycated β_2-microglobulin by charged and neutral dialysis membranes. Kidney Int. 2001;60:1571–7.

24. Raj D, Ouwendyk M, Francoeur R, et al. Beta2-microglobulin kinetics in nocturnal hemodialysis. Nephrol Dial Transplant. 2000;15:58–64.

25. Tan SY, Baillod R, Brown E, et al. Clinical, radiological and serum amyloid P component scintigraphic features of β_2-microglobulin amyloidosis associated with continuous ambulatory peritoneal dialysis. Nephrol Dial Transplant. 1999;14:1467–71.

26. Locatelli F, Marcelli D, Conte F, et al. Comparison of mortality in ESRD patients on convective and diffusive extracorporeal treatments. The Registro Lombardo Dialisi E Trapianto. Kidney Int. 1999;55:286–93.

27. Nakai S, Iseki K, Tabei K, et al. Outcomes of hemodiafiltration based on Japanese dialysis patient registry. Am J Kidney Dis. 2001;38(suppl)(1):S212–16.

28. Baz M, Durand C, Ragon A, et al. Using ultrapure water in hemodialysis delays carpal tunnel syndrome. Int J Artif Organs. 1991;14:681–5.

29. Schwalbe S, Holzhauer M, Schaeffer J, et al. β_2-microglobulin associated amyloidosis: a vanishing complication of long-term hemodialysis? Kidney Int. 1997;52:1077–83.

30. Kleophas W, Haastert B, Backus G, et al. Long-term experience with an ultrapure individual dialysis fluid with a batch type machine. Nephrol Dial Transplant. 1998;13:3118–25.

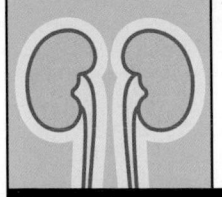

Chapter 73

Acquired Cystic Kidney Disease

Jürgen Floege

INTRODUCTION AND DEFINITION

Acquired cystic kidney disease (ACKD) was first recognized in 1847 by John Simon in patients with chronic Bright's disease. He described the development of cystic renal changes with cysts ranging from '... mustard seed to as large as cocoa nuts ...' and also noted that they '... run a slow and insidious progress during life, and often leave in the dead body no such obvious traces as would strike the superficial observer ...'. ACKD was 'rediscovered' by Dunnill et al. in 1977 in kidneys from dialysis patients[1].

EPIDEMIOLOGY

Acquired cystic kidney disease is a disease of chronic renal failure of any etiology and has to be differentiated from other types of cystic kidney disease (Chapters 46 and 47). It is usually defined as more than three to five macroscopic cysts in each kidney of a patient who does not have a hereditary cause of cystic disease. Among patients entering dialysis treatment, prevalences of ACKD ranging from 5 to 20% have been described. In both chronic hemodialysis and peritoneal dialysis patients, prevalence then increases at a similar rate and reaches 80–100% after 10 years of treatment (Fig. 73.1)[2–5]. Children are also prone to develop ACKD[5]. Several, but not all, studies have reported an increased frequency and/or faster progression in males than in females. The rate of progression appears to slow after 10–15 years of dialysis.

Following renal transplantation the course of ACKD is very variable. There may be retardation of the progressive course of the disease or regression of the cysts, in particular if good long-term graft function is maintained. However, especially in grafts with impaired or failing renal function, there may be further progression including the development of *de novo* ACKD in the graft.

PATHOGENESIS

Most cysts in ACKD develop in the proximal tubules. Although the mechanisms of proximal tubule transformation into cysts are not entirely clear, tubular epithelial cell hyperplasia is currently viewed as a central early event in ACKD pathogenesis (see Fig. 73.2)[2]. Various factors have been implicated to explain the development of tubular hyperplasia, including plasticizer, ischemia and uremic metabolites. However, the most important factor appears to be slow, progressive parenchymal loss, which could explain why the development or progression of ACKD does not appear to be influenced by the type of underlying renal disease or the choice of dialysis modality. The loss of intact nephrons is a strong stimulus for compensatory growth of the remaining, still intact nephrons, which is achieved by initial hypertrophy and later by hyperplasia. In these hyperplastic tubules a cyst will develop if transepithelial fluid secretion continues and if due to anatomic distortion or obstruction, the distal outflow is impaired. With the continuing presence of mitogenic stimuli, the epithelial layer of the cyst becomes multi-layered and atypical cells form intracystic papillary structures or mural adenomas. Activation of proto-oncogenes, chromosomal abnormalities plus additional factors such as genetic background, environmental chemicals or sex hormones, thereafter probably account for the transition of the proliferative process into malignant growth (see Fig. 73.2)[2].

CLINICAL MANIFESTATIONS

Acquired cystic kidney disease can manifest as unilateral or bilateral cysts, which are mostly cortical and variable in size and number. Rarely, severe ACKD can become macroscopically indistinguishable from adult polycystic kidney disease. In contrast to hereditary cystic diseases, the cysts of ACKD are strictly confined to the kidneys. The disease is usually

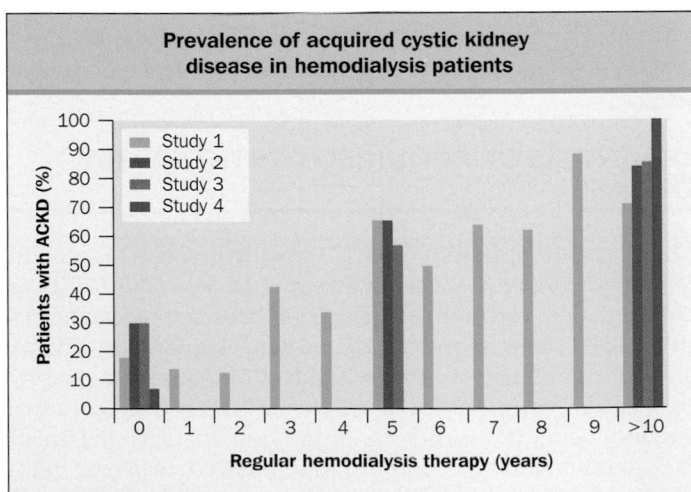

Figure 73.1 Prevalence of acquired cystic kidney disease (ACKD) in hemodialysis patients. Summary of reported ACKD prevalences in chronic hemodialysis patients in relation to the length of hemodialysis treatment. Four separate studies are shown.

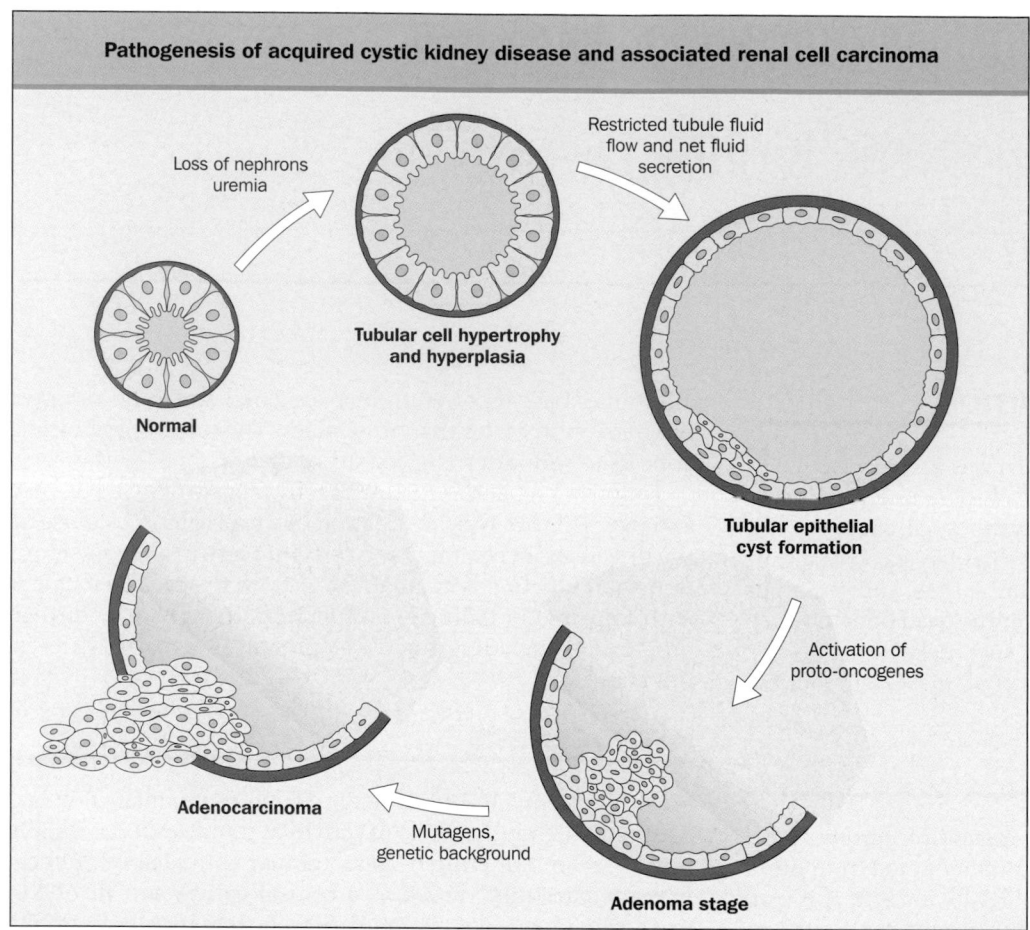

Pathogenesis of acquired cystic kidney disease and associated renal cell carcinoma

Loss of nephrons uremia

Restricted tubule fluid flow and net fluid secretion

Tubular cell hypertrophy and hyperplasia

Normal

Tubular epithelial cyst formation

Activation of proto-oncogenes

Adenocarcinoma

Mutagens, genetic background

Adenoma stage

Figure 73.2 Pathogenesis of ACKD and associated renal cell carcinoma. Diagram of events leading to the development of ACKD and subsequent malignant transformation. (Adapted from Grantham[2].)

asymptomatic and discovered accidentally during abdominal imaging procedures. Potential complications or consequences of ACKD include:

- cystic hemorrhage with or without hematuria; bleeding may evolve into cyst rupture with subsequent perinephric hemorrhage or retroperitoneal hemorrhage (Wunderlich's syndrome) which may in rare cases be severe enough to lead to hypovolemic shock
- calcifications in or around cysts and in rare cases stone formation (calcium-containing stones or β_2-microglobulin stones)
- cyst infection, abscess formation, or sepsis
- erythrocytosis in advanced cases, similar to erythrocytosis observed in polycystic kidney disease
- malignant transformation[6].

Complications of acquired cystic kidney disease

Malignant transformation, the most feared complication of ACKD, accounts for about 80% of the renal cell neoplasms observed in uremic patients. In unselected series of chronic dialysis or transplant patients, the cumulative incidence of renal cell carcinoma complicating ACKD is probably below 1%, although rates up to 7% have been reported in some small studies. These data indicate an up to 40-fold increased risk for renal cell carcinoma in ACKD patients compared with renal cell carcinoma in the general population. Risk factors include male gender (male to female ratio, 7 : 1), African American ethnicity, long duration of dialysis, and severe ACKD with

marked organ enlargement. It is unknown, whether the risk of malignant transformation differs between hemodialysis and peritoneal dialysis patients. However, cases of malignant transformation in patients treated exclusively with peritoneal dialysis have been described.

Renal cell cancers arising from ACKD are multicentric in about 50% of cases, bilateral in about 10%, and are predominantly of the papillary subtype. The large majority of ACKD-associated renal neoplasms are asymptomatic. In about 15% of cases, the tumor manifests with hemorrhage, fever, or lumbar pain.

DIAGNOSIS OF ACQUIRED CYSTIC KIDNEY DISEASE

The diagnostic approach to ACKD usually involves ultrasound (Fig. 73.3) which is a sensitive means of detecting ACKD or large renal cell carcinomas[3,7]. However, sonography can be difficult given the echogenicity of end-stage kidney parenchyma and the complexity of cysts in ACKD. Computed tomography (CT) scanning, in particular when used with early contrast-enhancement, is superior to ultrasound in detecting small malignant lesions[3,7,8]. Gadolinium-enhanced magnetic resonance imaging is also useful for detecting small carcinomas but is probably no better than CT scanning[7]. Fine-needle aspiration may be necessary to clarify equivocal findings[9]. However, even with all these imaging techniques, renal cell carcinomas (up to 8 cm) have been missed in severely distorted kidneys.

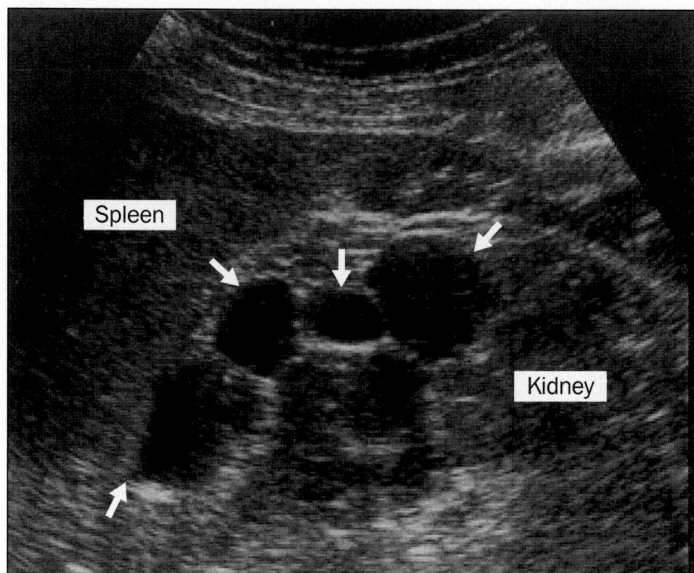

Figure 73.3 Ultrasound findings in ACKD. Ultrasound image of the left native kidney of a patient after 16 years of chronic hemodialysis. Multiple cysts are present in the renal cortex.

Because of the risk of malignant transformation, screening for ACKD on a regular basis, as well as regular follow-up imaging in cases of established ACKD, has been advocated after 3 years of renal failure. One recent proposal, modified from Truong et al.[6], is outlined in Figure 73.4. However, there is at present no consensus on screening strategies. This is because of the cost of screening as well as the risk : benefit ratio of nephrectomy in dialysis patients. A decision analysis[4] concluded that screening for ACKD (using either ultrasound or CT scanning) in young patients with a life expectancy of 25 years, offers them as much as a 1.6-year gain in life expectancy. This is similar to the gain obtained in young healthy people who stop smoking. In contrast, in ACKD patients over 60 years of age, no significant gain in life expectancy is achieved by regular screening[4]. Screening during transplant evaluation by ultrasound followed by CT in case of suspicious lesions is recommended on the basis of recent data showing a prevalence of renal cancer in up to 4% of the patients and concerns about the role of immunosuppression in accelerating tumor growth[10].

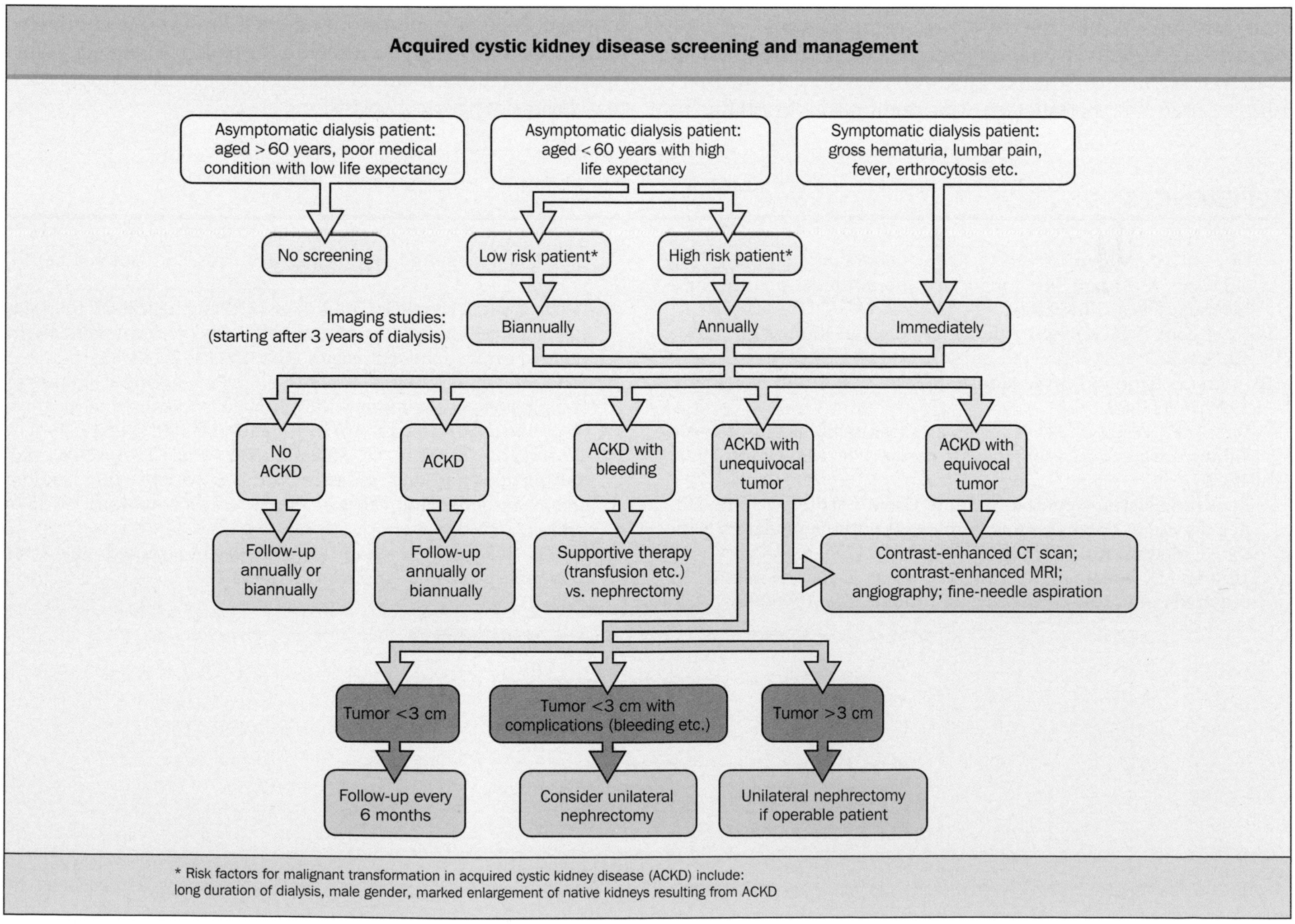

Acquired cystic kidney disease screening and management

- Asymptomatic dialysis patient: aged > 60 years, poor medical condition with low life expectancy → No screening
- Asymptomatic dialysis patient: aged < 60 years with high life expectancy → Low risk patient* / High risk patient*
- Symptomatic dialysis patient: gross hematuria, lumbar pain, fever, erthrocytosis etc. → Immediately

Imaging studies: (starting after 3 years of dialysis)
- Low risk patient* → Biannually
- High risk patient* → Annually
- Symptomatic → Immediately

- No ACKD → Follow-up annually or biannually
- ACKD → Follow-up annually or biannually
- ACKD with bleeding → Supportive therapy (transfusion etc.) vs. nephrectomy
- ACKD with unequivocal tumor → Contrast-enhanced CT scan; contrast-enhanced MRI; angiography; fine-needle aspiration
- ACKD with equivocal tumor → Contrast-enhanced CT scan; contrast-enhanced MRI; angiography; fine-needle aspiration

- Tumor < 3 cm → Follow-up every 6 months
- Tumor < 3 cm with complications (bleeding etc.) → Consider unilateral nephrectomy
- Tumor > 3 cm → Unilateral nephrectomy if operable patient

* Risk factors for malignant transformation in acquired cystic kidney disease (ACKD) include: long duration of dialysis, male gender, marked enlargement of native kidneys resulting from ACKD

Figure 73.4 Proposed approach to ACKD screening and management of suspected renal cell carcinoma. (Adapted from Truong et al.[6] and modified according to Sarasin et al.[4].)

Chronic Renal Failure and the Uremic Syndrome

NATURAL HISTORY

Microscopically, cystic dilatations of renal tubules develop once the creatinine clearance falls below 70 mL/min[11]. Macroscopic cysts start to develop when serum creatinine rises above 3 mg/dL (264 μmol/L). As discussed above, ACKD thereafter progresses and reaches a prevalence of nearly 100% after more than 10 years of dialysis (Figure 73.1). In malignant transformation, tumor growth rates are highly variable. The incidence of metastases at diagnosis (15–30% of cases) and 5-year survival rates (35%) are comparable to those observed in renal cell carcinoma in the general population. Death is usually associated with widespread metastases and accounts for about 2% of the deaths in renal transplant patients. It is not established whether renal transplantation affects the natural history of renal cell carcinoma complicating ACKD, although immunosuppression, in particular by cyclosporine, has been suggested as a risk factor for renal cell carcinoma in transplant patients with ACKD[6].

TREATMENT

Treatment for ACKD is only warranted when complications such as hemorrhage, cyst infection, or malignant transformation develop. While the first two complications may be handled conservatively and only rarely require surgery, malignant transformation should raise the question of nephrectomy. Given the perioperative morbidity and mortality of nephrectomy in dialysis or transplant patients, it is not surprising that the threshold for surgical intervention in cases of renal cell carcinoma is still controversial.

Most authors agree that tumors larger than 3 cm in diameter justify nephrectomy because above this size, renal cell carcinomas in the general population frequently metastasize (Fig. 73.4)[6]. However, it has to be stressed first that this strategy is based on an extrapolation from otherwise healthy persons, secondly that tumor size in ACKD is often difficult to establish by imaging studies (in particular given its frequent multilocular development) and last that metastases have been described even in ACKD where renal tumors were not detected by imaging studies.

In the case of tumors of less than 3 cm in diameter with no complications, the slow tumor growth may justify observation with repeated imaging studies (see Fig. 73.4). Tumor enlargement should be used as an indication for nephrectomy if permitted by the patient's status. Where complications such as back pain or persistent hematuria are present, nephrectomy has been recommended by some, but not all authors[6].

A prophylactic contralateral nephrectomy, in the case of unilateral tumors, is not routinely recommended by most investigators because of the morbidity associated with the procedure, the worsening of anemia, and the loss of residual renal function. Bilateral nephrectomy should, however, be considered in those patients likely to receive a transplant or already transplanted where there are concerns that immunosuppression may favor neoplastic growth[6].

REFERENCES

1. Dunnill MS, Millard PR, Oliver D. Acquired cystic disease of the kidneys: a hazard of long-term intermittent maintenance hemodialysis. J Clin Pathol. 1977;30:868–77.
2. Grantham JJ. Acquired cystic kidney disease. Kidney Int. 1991;40:143–52.
3. Levine E. Acquired cystic kidney disease. Radiol Clin North Am. 1996;34:947–64.
4. Sarasin FP, Wong JB. Levey AS, et al. Screening for acquired cystic kidney disease: a decision analytic perspective. Kidney Int. 1995;48:207–19.
5. Kyushu Pediatric Nephrology Study Group. Acquired cystic kidney disease in children undergoing continuous ambulatory peritoneal dialysis. Am J Kidney Dis. 1999;34:242–6.
6. Truong LD, Krishnan B, Cao JTH, et al. Renal neoplasms in acquired cystic kidney disease. Am J Kidney Dis. 1995;26:1–12.
7. Choyke PL. Acquired cystic kidney disease. Eur Radiol. 2000;10:1716–21.
8. Takebayashi S, Hidai H, Chiba T, et al. Using helical CT to evaluate renal cell carcinoma in patients undergoing hemodialysis: value of early enhanced images. AJR. 1999;172:429–33.
9. Todd TD, Dhurandhar B, Mody D, et al. Fine-needle aspiration of cystic lesions of the kidney. Morphologic spectrum and diagnostic problems in 41 cases. Am J Clin Pathol. 1999;111:317–28.
10. Gulanikar AC, Daily PP, Kilambi NK, et al. Prospective pretransplant ultrasound screening in 206 patients for acquired renal cysts and renal cell carcinoma. Transplantation. 1998;66:1669–72.
11. Liu JS, Ishikawa I, Horiguchi T. Incidence of acquired renal cysts in biopsy specimens. Nephron. 2000;84:142–7.

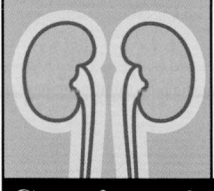

Chapter 74

Nutrition in Chronic Renal Failure

Gemma Bircher

INTRODUCTION

Diet and nutrition play an integral part in the management of individuals with renal disease. Retention of nitrogenous metabolites, a decreased ability to regulate levels of electrolytes and water, and certain vitamin deficiencies are abnormalities associated with chronic renal disease for which dietary intake can play a crucial role. Interest in the nutritional status of patients with renal failure has increased with the realization that poor nutrition predicts a poor outcome.

MALNUTRITION

Most studies that have evaluated the nutritional status of patients with end-stage renal disease (ESRD) report some degree of malnutrition in this population. The prevalence has been estimated to range from 10% to 70% in patients undergoing hemodialysis and from 18% to 50% in patients treated by continuous ambulatory peritoneal dialysis (CAPD). Advanced malnutrition not only leads to muscle wasting and general debility but also to lack of energy, nonspecific immune suppression, and poor wound healing. Malnutrition is usually chronic and slowly progressive but may accelerate rapidly with major intercurrent illness or surgery.

There is a strong relationship between the extent of malnutrition and mortality. Specifically, low serum albumin levels appear to be independently associated with an increased risk of death in patients treated with hemodialysis[1], CAPD[2], and transplantation[3] (Fig. 74.1). Malnutrition is not limited to patients receiving renal replacement therapy. There is evidence to suggest that diminished nutritional status exists even before initiation of dialysis and this has been shown to be a strong predictor of subsequent poor survival on dialysis[4-6]. This association adds weight to the argument for the earlier initiation of dialysis[7].

Why does malnutrition exist?

Several factors related to the uremic state may contribute to the high incidence of protein–energy malnutrition.

Inadequate nutrient intake

Inadequate nutrient intake is probably the most important single cause of malnutrition. Studies that have looked at the protein and calorie intakes of patients on hemodialysis have often found that they fall far short of recommendations. Reduction in nutrient intake starts in the predialysis period,

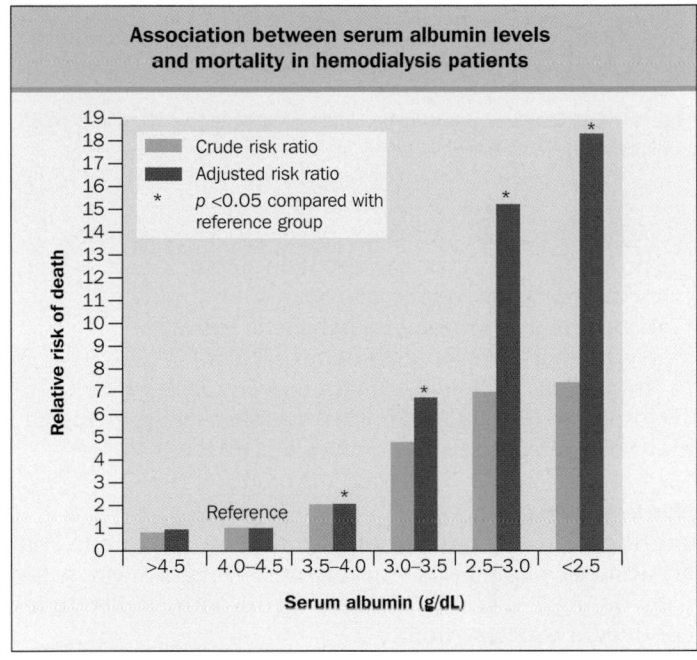

Figure 74.1 The association between serum albumin and mortality in hemodialysis patients. When serum albumin is < 25 g/L (2.5 g/dL) the relative risk of death is 20-fold compared with that in patients in the reference range (40–45 g/L (4.0–4.5 g/dL)).

with protein intake significantly reducing spontaneously as renal failure progresses[8]. The use of protein restriction to slow the progression of chronic renal failure (CRF), a controversial topic (reviewed in Chapter 66) is an imposed restriction that is of concern to many as it may increase the risk of malnutrition developing.

An important factor in the reduction of intake is anorexia, a well-known manifestation of CRF. This may exist for a number of reasons.

- Impaired taste acuity and diminished olfactory function.
- Inadequate dialysis and the use of acetate dialysate; the dialysis dose above which nutrient intake will not further improve has not been defined.
- The presence of dialysate in the peritoneal cavity may interfere with gastric emptying and intestinal motility, possibly causing discomfort or pain.
- Glucose absorbed from the dialysate may exert an inhibitory effect on food consumption.

Chronic Renal Failure and the Uremic Syndrome

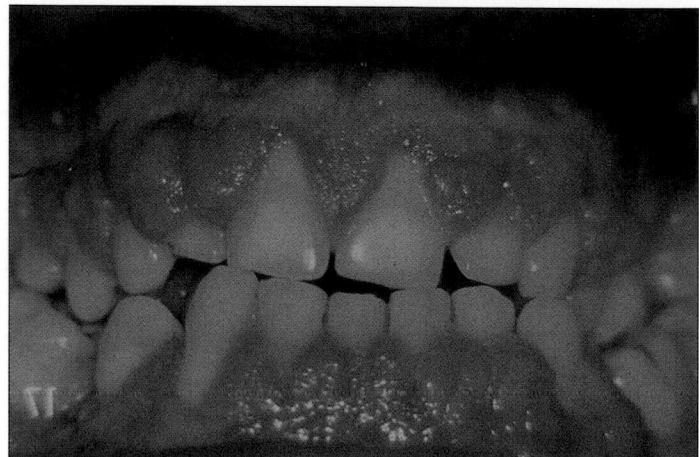

Figure 74.2 Gingival overgrowth. Gingival hyperplasia occurs in 30% of transplant recipients taking cyclosporine.

- Patients with CRF frequently have associated acute or chronic illnesses that may also reduce food intake, as can medications, autonomic gastroparesis (typically in diabetics but also seen in nondiabetic uremia), psychological and socioeconomic factors.

In transplant recipients, gingival overgrowth induced by cyclosporine (Fig. 74.2) can cause problems with eating and may have an adverse effect on nutrient intake.

Nutrient losses

Nutritional losses occur during treatment: 8–12 g amino acids are lost per hemodialysis treatment; 5–15 g protein is lost daily during CAPD, which can be significantly higher during episodes of CAPD peritonitis[9].

Protein catabolism

Metabolic acidosis, periods of acute or chronic illnesses, and the use of bioincompatible dialysis membranes may induce protein catabolism as can large doses of steroids used early in the post-transplant period, together with the stresses of surgery. Patients who present for transplantation may already have pre-existing protein malnutrition and this may be exaggerated when there is delayed graft function and continued dialysis.

Acute phase inflammatory process

There is emerging evidence that the acute phase inflammatory process not only impacts on nutritional state but also may trigger the development of atherosclerotic cardiovascular disease[10]. Malnutrition, inflammation and atherosclerosis often occur concomitantly and further studies in this area are presently underway to elucidate these relationships and possible management strategies.

Endocrine disorders

Endocrine disorders such as insulin resistance, raised parathyroid hormone concentrations (which may promote amino acid catabolism and gluconeogenesis), and vitamin D deficiency (which may contribute to proximal myopathy) may have an adverse effect on nutritional status.

Assessment of nutritional status. Common methods used to assess nutritional status are shown	
Area	**Assessments**
Physical examination	
Assessment of dietary intake	Diet history/Food diaries
Anthropometric measurements	Body weight/height/body mass index Percentage weight change Skinfold thickness Mid-arm muscle circumference
Body composition	Neutron activation Ultrasound Bioelectrical impedance Dual-energy X-ray absorptometry (DEXA)
Biochemical determinations	Serum electrolytes Serum proteins PNA/PCR Serum cholesterol Creatinine index
Subjective global assessment	
Immunological assays	Blood lymphocytes Delayed cutaneous hypersensitivity tests
Functional tests	Grip strength

Table 74.1 Assessment of nutritional status. Common methods used to assess nutritional status are shown. PNA: protein equivalent of total nitrogen appearance; PCR: protein catabolic rate.

ASSESSMENT OF NUTRITIONAL STATUS

Knowledge of the nutritional health of patients with renal disease is important for both prescription and monitoring of appropriate clinical and nutritional therapies. However, the measurement of nutritional status does not lend itself to one simple test and an optimal panel of measures for screening nutritional status is still required. Table 74.1 summarizes some of the methods used for assessing nutritional status.

Assessment begins with a careful diet history with attention to recent changes in appetite, weight, and gastrointestinal symptoms. Height/weight measures are easily obtained and can be used to determine body mass index (BMI). However, care must be taken to adjust for the presence of edema. Skinfold thickness is used to assess body fat, and muscle mass can be assessed by measurement of mid-upper arm muscle circumference (MAMC) (Fig. 74.3). The mid-point of the upper dominant arm is used as this is the arm less likely to have an arteriovenous fistula.

■ EQUATION 74.1

MAMC (cm) = mid-arm circumference (cm) – (3.14 × triceps skinfold (cm))

The measurement is taken after dialysis for patients on hemodialysis. In general, serial measurements of body composition are most useful for early detection of changes occurring over time in an individual patient, although a study of a large population of dialysis patients has been published allowing comparisons to be made[11]. Age, gender, and race all have a significant influence on the measurement. Skinfold

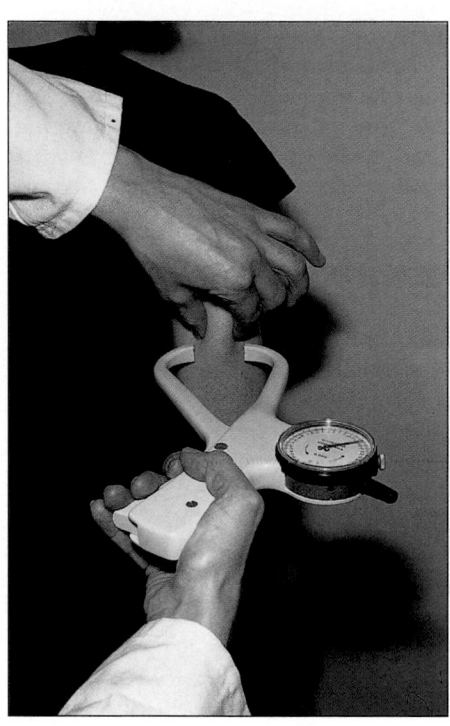

Figure 74.3 Routine measurement of skinfold thickness. The dominant arm is used in patients with renal failure.

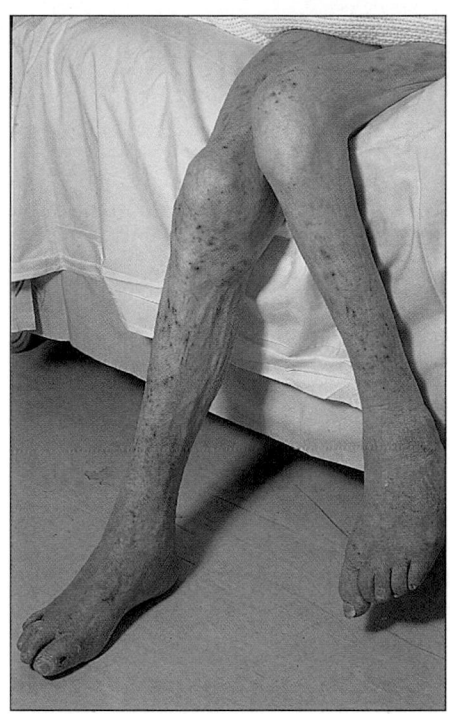

Figure 74.4 A severely malnourished hemodialysis patient. There is marked wasting of quadricep and calf muscles.

measurements are inexpensive, reproducible, relatively easy to learn and perform, and quick to carry out. However, they are observer dependent and only measure a compressible amount of subcutaneous adipose tissue thickness at a specific location.

Body composition can also be assessed by more sophisticated measurements. These include dual-energy X-ray absorptometry (DEXA), bioelectrical impedance (BEI), and neutron activation. Neutron activation is the most accurate and may be considered the 'gold standard', but it requires very expensive equipment. Both DEXA and BEI have been used to assess the body composition of patients with renal failure. DEXA is probably more accurate but again requires expensive equipment. Both techniques are affected by changes in total body water, so their use in dialysis patients is questionable.

A technique known as subjective global assessment (SGA), originally used to assess surgical patients, has been shown to be a reliable nutritional assessment tool for patients on dialysis[12,13]. A series of questions regarding recent changes in nutrient intake are used with simple observations of the patient's body weight and muscle mass to determine subjectively the nutritional status of the individual: patients are classified as well nourished, mildly malnourished/suspected malnutrition, or severely malnourished. Figures 74.4 and 74.5 show muscle wasting in a patient on hemodialysis classified by SGA as severely malnourished.

Levels of serum proteins are relatively good measures of visceral protein status in healthy individuals with normal kidney function, but unfortunately there is no single biochemical measure of somatic or visceral protein stores that is valid and reliable in patients with renal disease. Serum albumin is perhaps the most widely used and easily measured marker of nutrition. Although it remains an important index of nutritional status, its limitations must be appreciated. Fluid status, impaired liver function, age, and acute inflammatory conditions can all affect albumin levels. In addition, because of its

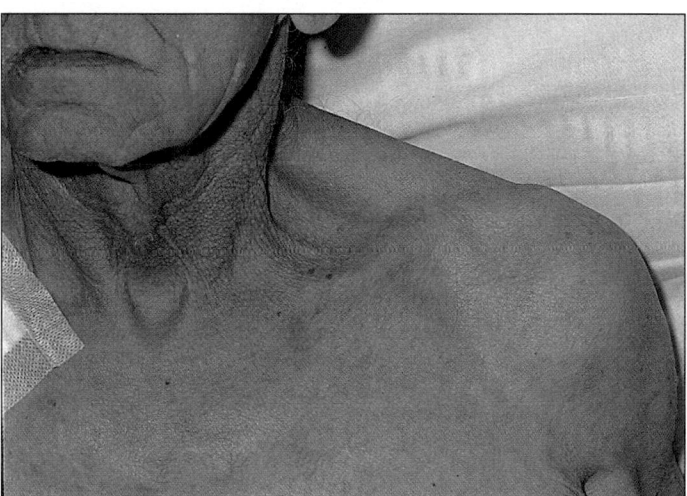

Figure 74.5 A severely malnourished hemodialysis patient. Muscle wasting around clavicle and shoulder.

relatively long half-life (20 days) and the vast capacity of the liver to synthesize albumin, a decrease in concentration may lag behind the onset of malnutrition by several months. Clinically, it may be possible to observe the growth of white nails when there has been a transient period of hypoalbuminemia (Fig. 74.6). Other serum protein markers of malnutrition have been assessed in renal failure; however all are difficult to interpret because of the influence of factors other than nutrition. Serum transferrin is linked to body iron stores and may be altered with changes in iron status. Prealbumin levels are affected by decreased renal function because the normal kidney excretes it; levels of prealbumin also decline rapidly during episodes of acute inflammation.

The excretion of the protein end product, urea, is easily measured and is often used to estimate adequacy of dialysis. The

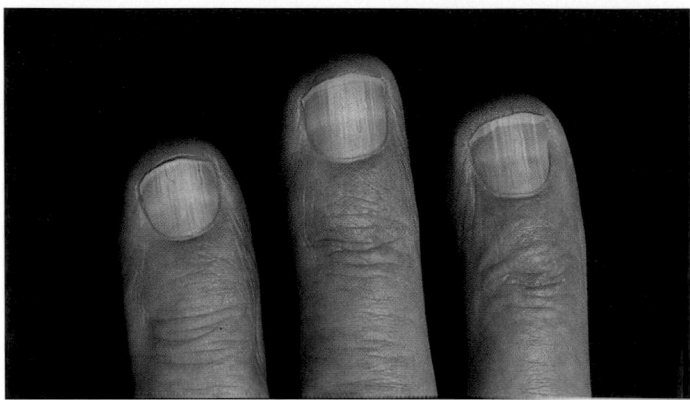

Figure 74.6 White nails in hypoalbuminemia. The white band grew during a transient period of hypoalbuminemia caused by nephrotic syndrome.

Indices of malnutrition	
Assessment	**Indices**
Biochemical parameters	Serum albumin < 40 g/L (4.0 g/dL)
	Serum transferrin < 2 g/L (200 mg/dL)
	Serum prealbumin < 300 mg/L (30 mg/dL)
	Low serum creatinine/phosphate/ potassium/urea in patients on dialysis
	Serum cholesterol < 150 mg/dL (3.8 mmol/L)
	Low creatinine index
	Low PNA/PCR
Anthropometric parameters	Continuous decline in weight
	Body mass index < 20
	Body weight < 90% of ideal
	Abnormal skinfold thickness, midarm muscle circumference and/or muscle strength

Table 74.2 Indices of malnutrition.

protein equivalent of total nitrogen appearance (PNA) can be estimated from interdialytic changes in urea nitrogen concentration in serum and the urea nitrogen content of urine and dialysate. Based on the assumption that, in steady state, nitrogen excretion equals nitrogen intake, the PNA (or protein catabolic rate (PCR)) has been used to approximate dietary protein intake in the short term. Results, however, need to be interpreted with caution (urea kinetic modeling and adequacy of dialysis are further discussed in Chapters 78 and 80). Equations used to estimate PNA can be found in K/DOQI[15].

A gradual decrease in blood urea nitrogen (BUN) and reduced phosphate and potassium levels may occur in malnourished dialysis patients because of a drop in protein intake and low serum cholesterol may indicate a poor calorie intake. A reduction in serum creatinine over time may reflect reducing muscle mass and the creatinine index (CI) can be used to assess creatinine production, and, therefore dietary skeletal muscle protein intake and muscle mass. Equations used to estimate CI can also be found in K/DOQI[15].

With the low specificity and sensitivity of many of the anthropometric and biochemical markers of malnutrition, it becomes clear that no single factor properly reflects nutritional status. Malnutrition can only be described by integrating biochemical markers and anthropometric measurements with evaluation of the subjective well-being of the patient (Table 74.2).

NUTRITIONAL GUIDELINES

Nutritional status in renal failure may be compromised by many factors, and dietary requirements can alter depending upon treatment and the current condition of the patient. Guidelines are useful, but it is important that dietary restrictions are not unnecessarily imposed and that advice is tailored to the individual and altered as circumstances dictate.

Protein/energy intake

Healthy normal subjects require a minimum of 0.6 g protein/kg body weight (BW) daily and the safe level of intake is 0.75 g/kg BW per day[14]. Protein requirements for CRF are not well defined. Benefits and safety of protein restriction remain unresolved and the level of protein intake (usually in the range 0.6–1.0 g/kg BW per day) advised during the predialysis period depends upon the personal opinion of the nephrologist involved. It is important if protein is restricted that 50% of the protein should come from high biological value sources[15] (these contain a higher percentage of essential amino acids) and patients should be monitored closely for any signs of diminishing nutritional status. Patients with nephrotic syndrome are generally advised a diet containing 1 g protein/kg BW[16].

Dialysis-dependent patients have increased protein requirements, and the consensus is that patients on hemodialysis need 1.2 g/kg BW and patients on CAPD need 1.2–1.3 g/kg BW daily[15]. The protein requirements of transplanted patients is again not clear cut but it has been recommended that a daily protein intake of 1.3–1.5 g/kg BW in the early post-transplant period is desirable, whereas 1.0 g/kg BW daily is required as a minimum for long-term intake[17]. The use of protein restriction for patients with progressive graft failure has been employed in a small number of studies but with varying results. In view of the continued increase in protein catabolism, even in patients on relatively low maintenance doses of steroids, extreme caution should be taken to ensure these patients are not further compromised.

Equally as important as protein, if not more so, is the energy intake of patients with renal failure. The few studies which have examined the caloric requirements of patients have concluded that a daily intake of 35 kcal/kg BW, for patients less than 60 years of age, and 30–35 kcal/kg BW for those over, should be used as a guide for weight maintenance[15]. In CAPD, 60–80% of the glucose in the dialysate is absorbed and may represent an additional 700 kcal/day, or a third of some patients' energy requirements. Dialysate glucose absorption depends upon the number of cycles, the dwell time, the percentage glucose concentration of the dialysate, and the peritoneal permeability to glucose. These dialysate calories should

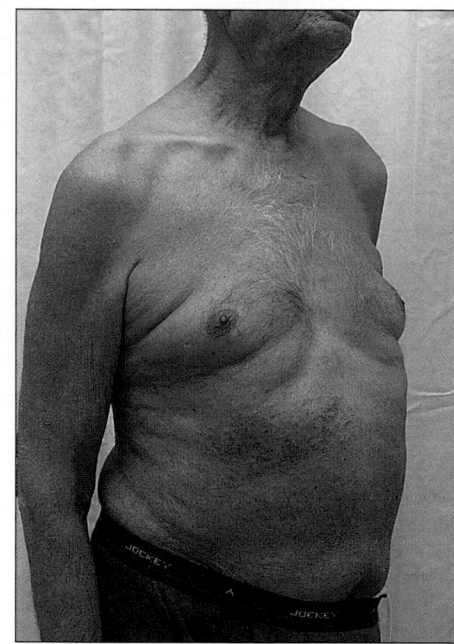

Figure 74.7 A patient on CAPD. Often there is weight gain associated with muscle loss in these patients. Note wasting of muscle around the clavicle and shoulder despite truncal obesity.

be included in the 30–35 kcal/kg BW per day guideline. It is not surprising that obesity, often with associated muscle wasting, is commonly seen in this patient group (Fig. 74.7). Patients who have received transplants may gain unwanted body fat. Average weight gains of between 8.5–14 kg have been observed over the first year[18]. Multiple factors explain this but probably the most important is the stimulation of appetite by steroids.

Fat/carbohydrate/fiber

Although disturbances of lipid metabolism are commonly seen in predialysis CRF there is a paucity of data on the effect of diet therapy in this group. A recent study indicates the difficulty for dialysis patients of complying with established lipid lowering recommendations[19]. Where possible, advice given should be in accordance with 'healthy eating guidelines' (30–35% of energy should come from fat and 50% from carbohydrate), but it must be remembered that a balance needs to be struck between healthy eating concepts and nutritional adequacy. Additional fiber, within the confines of the diet, has the benefit of helping to regulate bowel function: particularly important in CAPD patients. A high percentage of renal transplant patients have hyperlipidemia with a proatherogenic profile of increased total and LDL cholesterol and low HDL cholesterol. A few studies have looked at dietary intake and lipidemia in this group of patients and one recent study has shown the beneficial effect of a Mediterranean-style diet[20]. A diet low in fat, particularly saturated fat with an increase intake in soluble fiber, antioxidant vitamins and oily fish is recommended.

Phosphorus/calcium

Hyperphosphatemia is very commonly seen with advanced renal failure and usually becomes evident when glomerular filtration rate falls to 20–30% of normal. Foods high in protein are also high in phosphorus. It is possible to reduce daily phosphorus intake to 600–900 mg by restricting protein intake and eliminating dairy products. However, a protein intake of 1.2–1.3 g/kg BW may provide as much as 1000–1500 mg phosphorus per day, and are phosphate binders usually needed to help control serum levels, particularly when higher protein intakes are being encouraged. One session of hemodialysis eliminates approximately 500–800 mg phosphorus and CAPD permits approximately 300 mg daily to be lost.

Intestinal absorption of calcium is decreased in CRF because of the diminished production of 1,25-dihydroxycholicalciferol. In addition, phosphate restriction invariably means a reduction in dietary calcium intake. Calcium requirements in CRF are not clearly defined. Alfacalcidol or calcitriol will help to maintain normal serum calcium in predialysis and dialysis-dependent patients, although the levels need to be monitored as hypercalcemia can occur.

Serum phosphate may fall rapidly in newly transplanted patients because of the proximal tubular phosphate leak in the transplanted kidney. Restrictions can be relaxed, binders stopped, and, if necessary, supplements commenced. Clinical features of hypophosphatemia may occur when serum phosphate falls below 0.3 mmol/L; these include paresthesiae, muscle weakness and rhabdomyolysis, and leukocyte dysfunction. Transplanted patients often have reduced bone mass: contributing factors are suboptimal vitamin D levels and the action of immunosuppressive medications, which inhibit the hydroxylation of 25,hydroxy vitamin D_3. Advice to increase phosphate intake will have the additional benefit of increasing the calcium content of the diet to an adequate level.

Potassium/sodium/fluid

Depending on the treatment and the level of renal function, potassium intake may need to be reduced. Hemodialysis patients particularly if anuric, may need dietary advice bearing in mind that a protein intake of 70 g will contain a minimum of 60 mmol potassium. Potassium restriction is often not required for patients on CAPD and, indeed, some may require potassium supplementation.

The sodium content of usual diets ranges from 100 to 300 mmol per day. Mild-to-moderate sodium and fluid retention occurs in most types of renal disease and contributes to hypertension. Hemodialysis-dependent patients without residual renal function are more likely to have problems with fluid overload and hypertension. A moderately restricted diet (80–100 mmol/day) will help to prevent excessive accumulation of sodium, control thirst and aid fluid restriction. Conversely, patients who are salt wasting may require sodium supplementation. Recommendations for sodium and fluid should be individualized and based on symptoms, blood pressure, and physical examination.

Intermittent advice may be needed for hyperkalemic transplant recipients who are receiving cyclosporine or tacrolimus and moderate sodium restriction to 100 mmol/day may help with control of post-transplant hypertension.

Vitamins and minerals

Vitamin abnormalities can occur with CRF. Proposed explanations include dietary restriction, dialysate losses, and/or the necessity of an intact kidney for normal metabolism of vitamins. However, the dietary requirements for patients with

Nutritional recommendations in renal disease				
Daily intake	Predialysis CRF	Hemodialysis	Peritoneal dialysis	Transplant
Protein (g/kg ideal BW)	0.6–1.0 1.0 for nephrotic syndrome	1.2	1.2–1.3	1.3–1.5 (early post-transplant period) 1.0 long term
Energy (kcal/kg BW) 30–35% from fat 50% from carbohydrate	Age < 60 years: 35 Age > 60 years: 30–35	Age < 60 years: 35 Age > 60 years: 30–35	Age < 60 years: 35 Age > 60 years: 30–35 Includes glucose in dialysate	Age < 60 years: 35 Age > 60 years: 30–35
Sodium (mmol)	80–100 (more if salt wasting)	80–100	80–100	100
Potassium (mmol/kg ideal BW)	1.0 if hyperkalemic	1.0 if hyperkalemic	1.0 if hyperkalemic but potassium restriction is generally not required	1.0 if hyperkalemic
Phosphorus (mg)	< 1000 obligatory with protein intake	< 1200 obligatory with protein intake, use phosphate binders	< 1500 obligatory with protein intake use phosphate binders	Phosphorus restriction is normally relaxed if graft is functioning Phosphate supplements may be required
Vitamins For further details see reference 23	Vitamin B complex, folic acid, and vitamin C supplement *if* diet is protein or potassium restricted	Vitamin B complex, folic acid, and vitamin C supplement *if* diet is potassium restricted (Vitamin C *maximum* 70–100 mg daily)	Vitamin B complex, folic acid, and vitamin C supplement *if* diet is potassium restricted (Vitamin C *maximum* 70–100 mg daily)	As recommended for 'healthy eating' in general population (Vitamin C *maximum* 70–100 mg daily)

Table 74.3 Nutritional recommendations in renal disease. Recommendations are for typical patients, but should always be individualized on the basis of clinical, biochemical and anthropometric indices.

CRF are not clear cut. Dietary protein restrictions may compromise the intake of thiamine, riboflavin, pyridoxine, and vitamin B_{12}. Low-potassium diets have been shown to be deficient in thiamine, vitamin C, and folic acid. In addition, losses of water-soluble vitamins – thiamine, riboflavin, pyridoxine, and vitamin C – have been reported to occur in varying amounts during hemodialysis and CAPD.

Ideally, vitamin prescription should be based on individual monitoring but this is not always practical. In general, patients who are on diets that have restricted protein and/or potassium contents should receive a supplement of vitamin B complex, folic acid, and vitamin C. Great care should be taken with vitamin C: high-dose supplements, as frequently taken in the nonuremic population, may lead to oxalosis, and there can be extensive soft tissue calcification including blood vessels, heart, and retina (only 70–100 mg vitamin C daily is recommended).

Raised serum homocysteine is a known risk factor for cardiovascular morbidity in ESRD, and there is evidence that folic acid, B_{12} and pyridoxine supplements may lower serum homocysteine[21,22]. It is still not established whether lowering homocysteine will lead to a reduction in cardiovascular disease, and as yet there is not enough evidence to make definite recommendations for these vitamins.

Supplementation with fat-soluble vitamins is generally not recommended. Diets do not tend to be deficient, dialysis losses are minimal, and accumulation can occur. Vitamin D is generally given under close medical supervision.

Protein restriction can also lead to a reduction in intake of iron and zinc, and the use of recombinant human erythropoietin (epoetin) may increase the requirement for iron and folic acid (see Chapter 70). If a deficiency is suspected, or has been established, supplementation will be required.

Kopple has suggested recommendations for vitamin requirements in conservative treatment and in dialysis-treated patients[23]. Nutritional recommendations for typical patients are summarized in Table 74.3.

MONITORING AND TREATMENT

Monitoring of patients with CRF involves a combination of nutritional assessment, noting relevant biochemistry (potassium, phosphate, lipids), and observing fluid status. The challenge comes in giving advice that carefully balances control of electrolytes while not compromising nutritional status. Figure 74.8 summarizes the steps that may need to be taken.

Dietary intervention designed to limit dietary intake during the predialysis stage must be undertaken cautiously and the ability to achieve adequate calorie intake needs to be assessed. Patients on restricted diets should be followed very closely for signs and symptoms of malnutrition.

If potassium, phosphorus and/or cholesterol levels are low then this may, as has already been mentioned, represent a decline in nutrient intake and nutritional status. Diet restrictions should be relaxed where possible.

Strategies to treat anorexia should be considered and nutrient intake maximized by using one or more of the following methods.

Oral supplementation

If food fortification advice is not sufficient supplements in the form of high-protein/high-calorie drinks/powders and puddings are available. Prescribability depends on the country. There is, however, a need for a well-conducted controlled trial to look at the benefit of oral supplements.

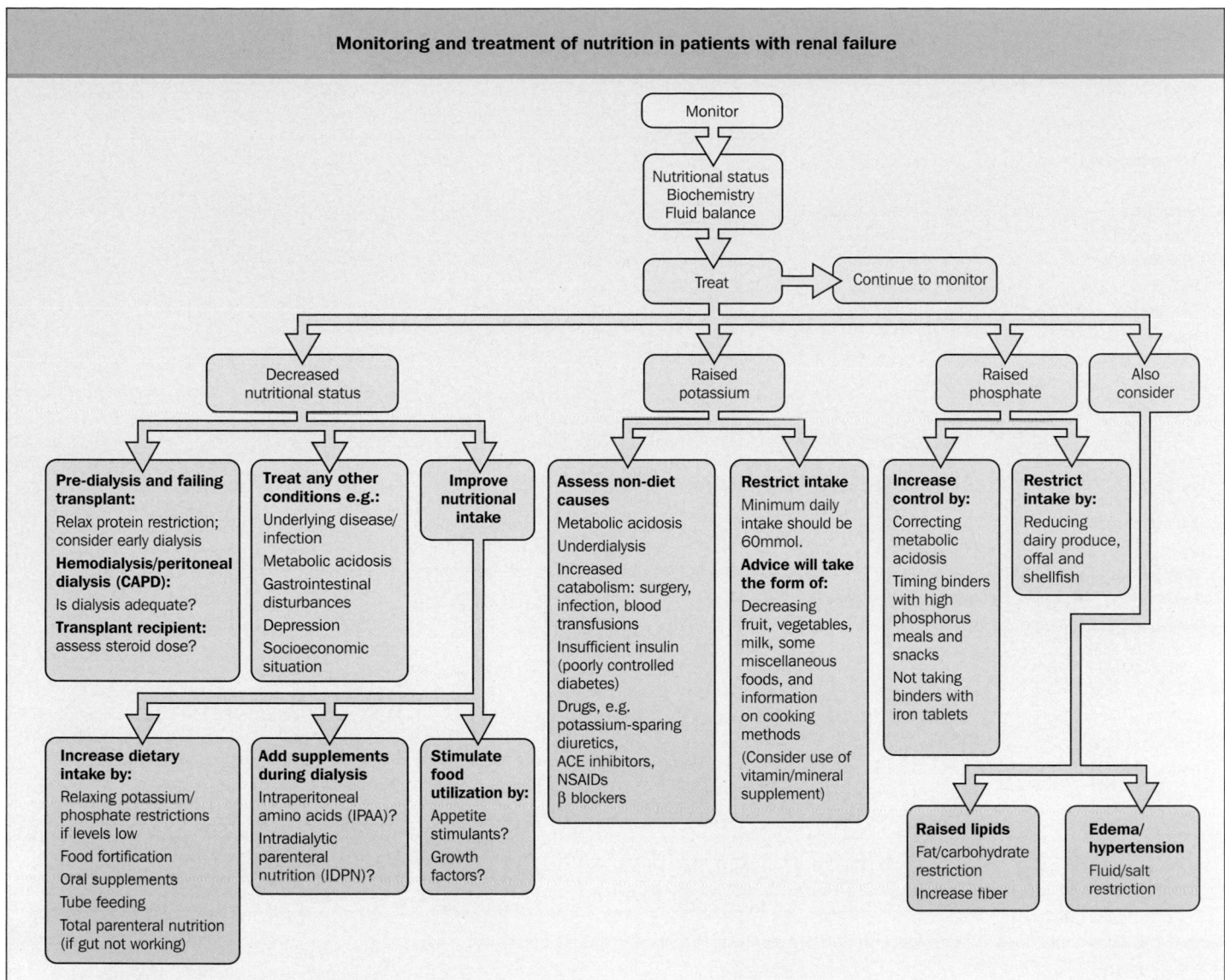

Figure 74.8 Monitoring and treatment of nutrition in patients with renal failure.

Tube feeding

There are few published reports of the use of tube feeding in adult dialysis-dependent patients, but in children there is well documented evidence of success. Use of percutaneous endoscopically placed gastrostomy (PEG) tubes is of proven value in children with CAPD, but their use in adults is not well documented. The one study, which has looked retrospectively at PEG feeding in adults on CAPD, reported frequent complications[24]. The degree of malnutrition, timing of placement of tube and rest period from peritoneal dialysis at time of PEG insertion are factors which need further study before this method of feeding can be used with confidence for adult patients on CAPD. A study of PEG feeding in hemodialysis outpatients demonstrated a benefit although the study only included eight patients studied over 3 months[25].

A selection of the enteral feeding formulae that are used most commonly in the UK and USA for patients with renal failure are listed in Table 74.4. Some of the 2-kcal/mL feeds have been designed specifically for patients with renal failure and consequently have a lower electrolyte content. If fluid and electrolyte restrictions are not necessary then standard 1-kcal/mL feeds may be used but these have not been listed.

Supplementation of dialysate fluids

Intraperitoneal amino acid (IPAA) and intradialytic parenteral nutrition (IDPN) supplementation have both been used. A 1.1% amino acid solution has been used in CAPD. The amino acids are substituted for glucose and about 80% of the amino acids are absorbed in a 4-h period. Such bags used once or twice daily may improve nutritional status, but the results are not consistent[26]. The long term effects of IPAA on nutritional status and clinical outcomes is not known. K/DOQI recommend that patients who have evidence of protein

Chronic Renal Failure and the Uremic Syndrome

Commonly used tube feeds with nutrient analysis							
Feed	Manufacturer	Country	Energy (kcal)	Protein (g)	Potassium (mmol)	Sodium (mmol)	Phosphorus (mg)
1.5 cal/mL feeds							
Comply	Mead Johnson	USA	150	6	4.7	5.2	120
Ensure plus	Abbott Nutrition (Ross)	UK/USA	150	6.3	4.7	5.2	110
Ensure plus HN	Abbott Nutrition	USA	150	6.3	4.6	6.1	100
Fresubin energy	Fresenius Kabi Ltd	UK	150	5.6	5.2	4.3	63
Fresubin energy fiber	Fresenius Kabi Ltd	UK	150	5.6	5.2	4.3	53
Fresubin HP energy	Fresenius Kabi Ltd	UK	150	7.5	6.0	5.2	63
Isosource 1.5	Novartis	USA	150	6.8	5.8	5.6	107
Isosource energy	Novartis	UK	159	5.7	3.5	3.7	75
Novosource Forte	Novartis	UK	150	6.0	3.5	3.7	75
Nutren 1.5	Nestle Clinical Nutrition	USA	150	6.0	4.8	5.1	100
Nutrison energy	Nutricia Clinical Care	UK	150	6.0	5.1	5.8	108
Nutrison energy multifiber	Nutricia Clinical Care	UK	150	6.0	5.1	5.8	108
Sondalis 1.5	Nestlé Clinical Nutrition	USA	150	5.6	4.4	3.9	80
2.0 cal/mL feeds							
Deliver 2.0	Mead Johnson	USA	200	7.5	4.3	3.5	101
Magnacal Renal	Mead Johnson	USA	200	7.5	3.3	3.5	80
Nepro	Abbott Nutrition (Ross)	UK/USA	200	7.0	2.7	3.7	70
Novasource 2.0	Novartis	USA	200	9.0	3.8	3.5	110
Novasource Renal (closed system)	Novartis	USA	200	7.4	2.8	7.0	65
Nutren	Nestlé Clinical Nutrition	USA	200	8.0	4.9	5.7	134
NutriRenal	Nestlé Clinical Nutrition	USA	200	7.0	3.2	3.2	70
Nutrison Conc LE	Nutricia Clinical Care	UK	200	7.5	3.8	4.3	75
Nutrison LP/LM	Nutricia Clinical Care	UK	200	4.0	3.8	4.3	45
Suplena	Abbott Nutrition (Ross)	UK/USA	201	3.0	2.9	3.5	79
Two Cal HN	Abbott Nutrition (Ross)	UK/USA	202	8.2	6.3	6.5	106

The information listed was correct at time of going to print but is subject to change. This is not an exhaustive list. Where a feed is available in the UK and in the USA the analysis has been quoted as per UK and there may be small differences in the micronutrient content of the feed in the USA. It is recommended that recent manufacturers nutritional data is referred to when using a feed and that this table is used as a guide only.

Table 74.4 Commonly used tube feeds with nutrient analysis. Values per 100 mL of product.

malnutrition and an inadequate dietary intake and are unable to tolerate adequate quantities of oral supplements or tube feeding may benefit from IPAA[27].

IDPN offers the advantages of providing intensive parenteral nutrient therapy with use of concentrated hypertonic solutions three times weekly during hemodialysis treatments without the need for establishing a central venous line. The nutrients, usually a mixture of amino acids, glucose, and lipid, are infused into the venous bloodline. Only about 10% of infused amino acids are lost into the dialysate. IDPN has mostly been evaluated with retrospective, small, short term studies. Data supporting the use of IDPN are weak and clear recommendations are difficult to make, but the use of IDPN in hemodialysis patients seems to be associated with decreased mortality. K/DOQI suggested that maintenance hemodialysis patients who have evidence of protein or energy malnutrition and inadequate protein or energy intake, are unable to tolerate adequate oral supplements or tube feeding may benefit from IDPN[15]. Comparison of the benefit of IDPN versus enteral nutrition is not yet available and is needed, particularly in view of the high cost of IDPN.

Appetite stimulants and growth factors

Appetite stimulants and growth factors are still in the experimental stage. However, the appetite stimulant of most interest is megestrol acetate: a progesterone derivative that has been shown to increase the appetite and nonfluid weight of cancer patients and, more recently, patients with acquired immune deficiency syndrome. A pilot study using the drug in hemodialysis patients has been published and showed an improvement in some of the nutritional parameters over a short period of time[28]. Larger and longer studies are needed.

SUMMARY

Indices of malnutrition are powerful predictors of mortality in ESRD. The high prevalence of protein–energy malnutrition in this group is clearly related to multiple factors encountered both before and after renal replacement therapy has commenced. Potentially this is a severe problem. It is the responsibility of the clinician to be aware of these risks; to implement from an early stage effective methods of assessing and monitoring nutritional status, and to act promptly if deterioration is noted.

REFERENCES

1. Lowrie EG, Lew NL. Death risk in hemodialysis patients: the predictive value of commonly measure variables and an evaluation of death rate differences between facilities. Am J Kidney Dis. 1990;15:458–82.
2. Lowrie EG, Huang WH, Lew NL. Death risk predictors among peritoneal dialysis and hemodialysis patients: a preliminary comparison. Am J Kidney Dis. 1995;26:220–8.
3. Guijarro C, Ziad MD, Massy A, et al. Serum albumin and mortality after renal transplantation. Am J Kidney Dis. 1996;27:117–23.
4. Hakim RM. Initiation of dialysis. Adv Nephrol. 1994;23:295–309.
5. Bergstom J. Nutrition and mortality in hemodialysis. J Am Soc Nephrol. 1995;6:1329–41.
6. Churchill DN, Taylor DW, Keshaviah PR. The CANUSA Peritoneal Dialysis Study Group: Adequacy of dialysis and nutrition in continuous peritoneal dialysis: association with clinical outcomes. J Am Soc Nephrol. 1996;7:198–207.
7. Churchill DN. An evidence-based approach to earlier initiation of dialysis. Am J Kidney Dis. 1997;30:899–906.
8. Ikizler TA, Greene JH, Wingard RL, et al. Spontaneous dietary protein intake during progression of chronic renal failure. J Am Soc Nephrol. 1995;6:1386–91.
9. Blumenkrantz MJ, Gahl GM, Kopple JD, et al. Protein losses during peritoneal dialysis. Kidney Int. 1981;19:593–602.
10. Stenvinkel P, Heimburger O, Paultre F, et al. Strong association between malnutrition, inflammation and atherosclerosis in chronic renal failure. Kidney Int. 1999;55:1899–1911.
11. Nelson EE, Changgi RD, Hang MD, et al. Anthropometric norms for the dialysis population. Am J Kidney Dis. 1990;6:32–7.
12. Young GA, Kopple JD, Lindholm B, et al. Nutritional assessment of continuous APD patients: an international study. Am J Kidney Dis. 1991;17:462–71.
13. Enia G, Sicuso C, Alati G, Zoccali C. Subjective global assessment of nutrition in dialysis patients. Nephrol Dial Transplant. 1993;8:1094–8.
14. FAO/WHO/UNA. Energy and protein requirements: report of a joint FAO/WHO/UNA expert consultation. Geneva: WHO; 1985:52–70.
15. K/DOQI Clinical Practice Guidelines for Nutrition in Chronic Renal Failure 2001. National Kidney Foundation.
16. Mansy H, Goodship THJG, Tapson JS, Hartley GH, Keavey P, Wilkinson R. Effect of a high protein diet in patients with nephrotic syndrome. Clin Sci. 1989; 77:445–51.
17. Pagenkemper JJ, Foulks MD. Nutritional management of the adult transplant patient. J Renal Nutr. 1991;1:119–24.
18. Pischon T, Sharma AM. Obesity as a risk factor in renal transplant patients. Nephrol Dial Transplant. 2001;16:14–17.
19. Saltissi D, Morgan C, Knight B, et al. Effect of lipid-lowering dietary recommendations on the nutritional intake and lipid profiles of chronic peritoneal dialysis and hemodialysis patients. Am J Kidney Dis. 2001;37:1209–15.
20. Barbagallo CM, Cefalu AB, Gallo S, et al. Effects of Mediterranean diet on lipid levels and cardiovascular risk in renal transplant recipients. Nephron. 1999;82:199–204.
21. Homocysteine Lowering Trialists' Collaboration. Lowering blood homocysteine with folic acid based supplements: meta-analysis of randomised trials. Br Med J. 1998;316:894–8.
22. Dierkes J, Domrose U, Basselman P, et al. Homocysteine lowering effect of different multivitamin preparations in patients with end-stage renal disease. J Renal Nutr. 2001;11:67–72.
23. Kopple JD. Nutritional therapy in kidney failure. Nutr Rev. 1981;39:193–206.
24. Fein, PA, Madane SJ, Jorden A, et al. Outcome of percutaneous endoscopic gastrostomy feeding in patients on peritoneal dialysis. Adv Perit Dial. 2001;17:148–52.
25. Sayce HA, Rowe PA, McGonigle RJS. Percutaneous endoscopic gastrostomy feeding in haemodialysis out-patients. J Hum Nutr Dietet. 2000;13:333–41.
26. Bruno M, Gabella P, Ramello A. Use of amino acids in peritoneal dialysis solutions. Perit Dial Int. 2000;20(suppl 2):s166–71.
27. Foulks CJ. An evidence-based evaluation of intradialytic parenteral nutrition. Am J Kidney Dis. 1999;33:186–92.
28. Lien YH, Ruffenach SJ. Low dose megestrol increases serum albumin in malnourished dialysis patients. Int J Artif Organs. 1996;19:147–50.

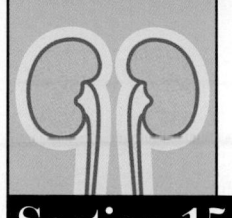

Section 15 Dialysis

Chapter 75
Selection and Preparation of Patients for Dialysis

Hugh C Rayner

HOW ARE PATIENTS SELECTED FOR DIALYSIS?

If every patient who developed end-stage renal disease (ESRD) was started on dialysis, the incidence rates of new dialysis patients in different countries would reflect the epidemiology of progressive renal disease. Incidence rates of treated ESRD patients are summarized in the annual report of the United States Renal Data System (USRDS). Data from the 2001 report show a greater than 10-fold variation across the world (Fig. 75.1) and a marked variation in the age spectrum of treated patients (Fig. 75.2). Variations of this size suggest there are marked differences between different countries in the criteria for accepting patients for dialysis.

WHAT FACTORS INFLUENCE THESE CRITERIA?

The availability of dialysis facilities
Even in relatively affluent countries such as Canada and the UK, as recently as 1995, lack of resources was given as a reason for refusing patients dialysis by 10% and 12% of nephrologists in those countries respectively[1]. The distance which the patient and primary care physician live from the nearest dialysis facility influences the local availability of treatment.

In the UK, dialysis facilities have, until recently, been concentrated in a small number of large centers and incidence rates of new dialysis patients have tended to decline the farther the population lives from one of these centers.

The availability of nephrologists
Surveys in the UK (1984 and 1996) have revealed persisting differences of opinion between general practitioners (GPs) and nephrologists about the suitability of patients for dialysis[2,3]. In regions where access to a nephrologist's opinion was not readily available, patients were often not given the opportunity of being considered for dialysis. These dialysis 'black holes' have since been targeted by UK nephrologists, who have set up outreach clinics and encouraged GPs to refer patients with renal failure for assessment. This has resulted in a dramatic increase in incidence rates in these areas.

Cultural differences
The existence of diverse attitudes to the appropriateness of starting dialysis in patients with other disabling conditions has been demonstrated in a survey of nephrologists from the USA, Canada and the UK[1]. From this survey, it was clear that severe intellectual impairment in a patient would much more

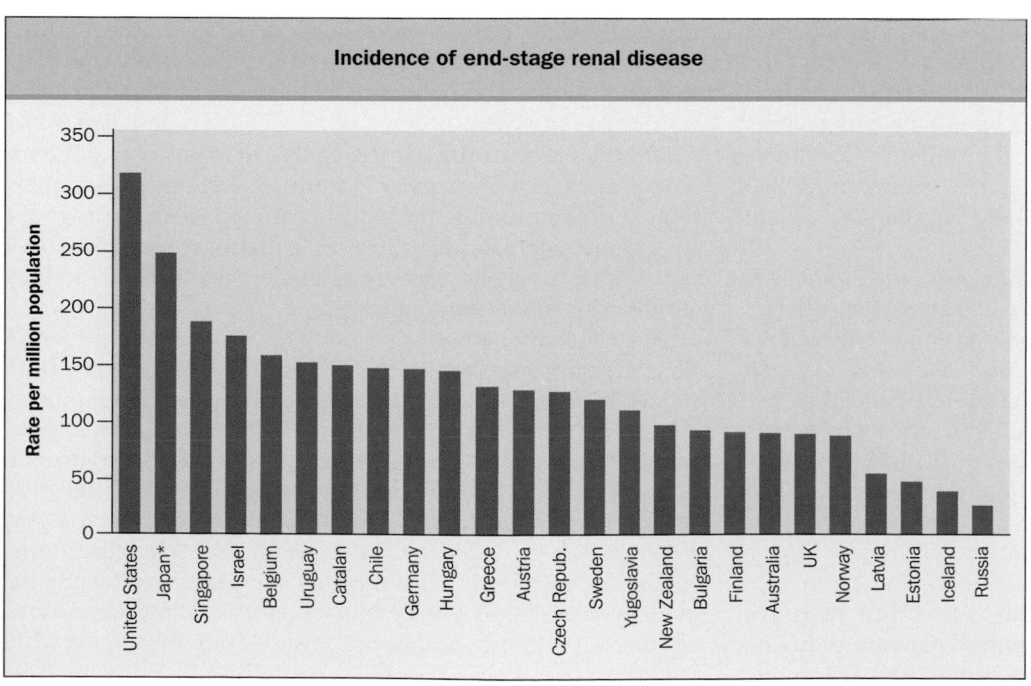

Figure 75.1 Incidence of end-stage renal disease (ESDR). Incidence rates of new ESDR patients treated in selected countries, 1999. (Data included in Figs 75.1–4 were supplied by the United States Renal Data System (USRDS). The interpretation and reporting of these data are the responsibility of the author and in no way should be seen as an official policy or interpretation of the US Government.)

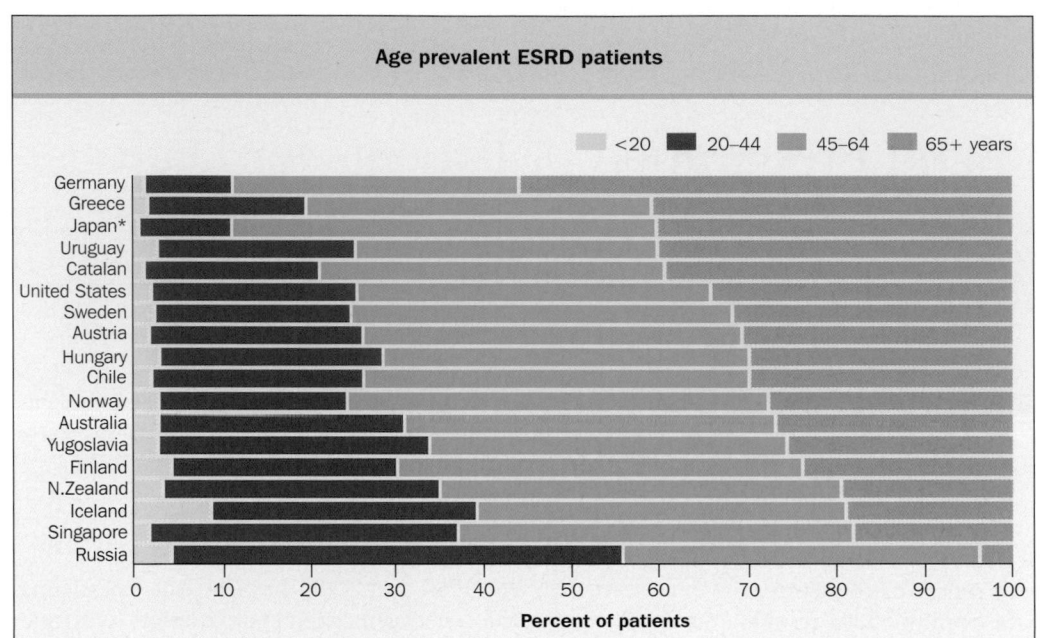

Figure 75.2 Distribution of prevalent ESRD patients by age. Distribution of prevalent ESRD patients by age treated in selected countries, 1999.

strongly influence a nephrologist in the UK not to start dialysis than in the USA. Furthermore, nephrologists in the USA were much more likely than those in the UK and Canada to start dialysis in patients with dementia or in a persistent vegetative state, if pressured to do so by family members. Fear of litigation was particularly influential in persuading US and Canadian nephrologists to offer treatment.

The RPA/ASN guidelines for the initiation of dialysis in the USA provide an approach that circumvents the issue of litigation[4].

ARE THERE OBJECTIVE CRITERIA FOR THE RATIONING OF DIALYSIS TREATMENT?

On the grounds that the greatest good should be derived from the limited resources available, it has been argued that patients who are expected to survive for only a few months should not be offered dialysis. This is supported by the view that it is preferable to avoid suffering by not starting dialysis than to withdraw treatment when the patient's condition becomes distressing[5]. Withdrawing dialysis seems more like actively causing death than withholding dialysis, where death is allowed to occur 'naturally'.

This utilitarian approach to the allocation of resources is contrary to the instincts of most doctors to act in the patient's best interest and may be unacceptable to many physicians. Furthermore, it does not take into account the value of even a short extension of life that allows the patient and his or her family to prepare for death. Nevertheless, most physicians would agree that patients who are certain to have an unacceptable quality of life on dialysis should not be offered the treatment.

The age criterion

Against this ethical background, are there any objective criteria that can be applied to identify patients who are unsuitable for dialysis? One criterion to be dismissed is age.

Although advanced age was used as a simple exclusion criterion in the early days of dialysis, the elderly are now the most rapidly growing section of the dialysis population. Their quality of life can be good; indeed their expressed satisfaction with life may be greater than that of younger dialysis patients[6].

Predictive factors

Two recent studies have attempted to identify other predictive factors. In a prospective Canadian study of patients starting dialysis[7], a comorbidity scoring system was used to quantify factors likely to predict early death and the predictive value of this scoring system was compared with the value of an estimate made by the patient's nephrologist of the probability that the patient would die within 6 months. It was not possible to predict early death accurately using either the comorbidity scoring system or the clinician's opinion. Indeed, it was impossible even to identify the small proportion of patients with a very poor prognosis. Clinicians were more accurate than the scoring system in identifying patients with less than a 50% risk of death by 6 months, but they tended to overestimate the risk of death in the worst prognostic groups. For example, 30% of patients whose predicted probability of death was considered to be ≥ 80%, in fact survived for more than 6 months.

In a UK study[8], a high-risk group of 26 patients was identified using factors associated with poor survival in a statistical model, which included poor functional status at presentation, comorbidity and underlying disease. Although these patients had a 1-year survival of only 19.2%, four patients survived at least 2 years. Furthermore, the cost incurred by this high-risk group was only 3.2% of the total cost of the chronic dialysis program. These important studies should strengthen the resolve of clinicians to resist the imposition of rationing criteria on dialysis provision. Furthermore, they warn clinicians against making self-fulfilling prophecies of early death in patients with ESRD who are denied dialysis.

HOW CAN I ADVISE MY PATIENT ABOUT PROGNOSIS ON DIALYSIS?

Despite these uncertainties, an individual patient should nonetheless be given an estimate of his or her likely future on dialysis. Factors associated with a poorer prognosis in a large number of studies include advanced age, male gender, decreased serum albumin, malnutrition, impaired functional status, diabetes mellitus and coronary heart disease. Recent data from the Dialysis Outcomes and Practice Patterns Study (DOPPS) has shown that quality of life is strongly predictive of mortality, even after statistical correction for these comorbid factors[9].

For patients whose prognosis is particularly uncertain, or where there is disagreement between the views of the patient and the dialysis team, a time-limited trial of dialysis should be offered[4]. This will give the patients and his or her family a better understanding of what life on dialysis entails and allow time for further discussion between all parties. The duration of the trial should be judged for each individual, and clinical and biochemical parameters reviewed regularly. In our experience of 31 patients over the age of 79 on hemodialysis, 10 patients who were hypoalbuminemic at the start of dialysis and whose serum albumin had fallen by more than 3 g/L to a value of < 30 g/L after 4 weeks on dialysis had all died by six months. The median survival of the other 21 patients was 1.3 years (K. Eardley, unpublished observations).

Patients with particularly poor functional status should be offered the option of nondialysis management and palliative care rather than even a trial of dialysis. Patients who are very elderly or who have significant comorbidity may have a similar life expectancy without dialysis and their quality of life may be significantly better without the burden of intensive treatment.

WHAT IF THE PATIENT DOES NOT WANT DIALYSIS?

Nephrologists may be presented with the dilemma of a mentally competent patient whom they would normally treat, but who does not wish to have dialysis[5]. From an ethical viewpoint, decisions not to start dialysis and to withdraw dialysis are justified on the principle of individual autonomy. Similarly, in the UK, they are legally based on the individual's common-law right to self-determination and, in the USA, the constitutional right of liberty. Where the patient is able to express a clear wish, the physician is obliged to respect this because to treat a patient against his will would constitute an assault. The physician must nonetheless ensure that all reversible factors have been addressed, such as unfounded fears about what dialysis will entail or a depressive illness, which is affecting the patient's judgment. It is not uncommon for patients to express a strong desire not to have dialysis, particularly if they are relatively asymptomatic, only to change their mind when they become more symptomatic. At this late stage, the basic 'will-to-survive' comes to the fore. An advance directive written by the patient should never be held as a reason against a change of heart.

WHAT IF THERE IS DISAGREEMENT ABOUT A DECISION TO DIALYSE A PATIENT?

There will inevitably be differences of opinion about the benefits of dialysis to individual patients. Dialysis nurses may disagree with the nephrologist's decision to treat a patient. If the dialysis nurses and doctors are functioning well as a team, they should feel able to express these reservations and have the issue adequately discussed. It is very demoralizing for individual staff and the team as a whole if they feel pressured into giving treatment that they feel is inappropriate.

The nephrologist may remain unwilling to offer dialysis despite the insistence of the patient, the carers or another doctor. Dialysis must never be given at the insistence of others if it is against the patient's clearly expressed wishes. However, if the patient insists on treatment against the nephrologist's advice, dialysis should usually be given while a resolution is reached. Extensive discussions and explanations of the treatment options and prognosis may be needed to gain a better understanding of the reasons behind the differing views. Helpful advice may be obtained from another physician, particularly the patient's family doctor who will have a broader understanding of the patient's circumstances. It may be appropriate to involve a psychologist, social worker or religious counselor. If the conflict persists, it may be necessary to refer the case to a formal ethics committee, if one exists locally, to clarify the issues of disagreement and enable a resolution. A physician cannot be compelled to offer treatment against his or her considered professional judgment but the patient may be transferred to another doctor or dialysis unit that is prepared to offer treatment. Only as a last resort, if no alternative dialysis unit can be found and after adequate advance notice has been given, should dialysis be withdrawn[4].

THE CHOICE BETWEEN PERITONEAL DIALYSIS AND HEMODIALYSIS

The majority of patients with ESRD are suitable for treatment with either PD or hemodialysis. It is difficult to envisage an ethically acceptable trial where patients are allocated randomly to different dialysis modalities, which would be required to compare the two treatments. A number of retrospective comparative studies have failed to indicate a consistent survival advantage for either modality when correction is made for comorbid conditions[10,11]. Recent analysis of the USRDS database has shown that patients with a serum albumin < 32 g/L who are assigned to peritoneal dialysis have a 16% higher adjusted mortality risk over the following 2 years when compared with similar hemodialysis patients ($P < 0.0005$). For those with a serum albumin > 32 g/L, survival was the same on either modality[12]. Hence, for hypoalbuminemic patients, it may be preferable to offer a period of hemodialysis during which the serum albumin may normalize, before reviewing their suitability for peritoneal dialysis.

Contraindications to peritoneal dialysis

There are a few situations where there is a consensus that peritoneal dialysis is contraindicated (Table 75.1). These have been agreed by the consensus panel of the National

Dialysis

Contraindications to dialysis modalities	
Peritoneal dialysis	
Absolute	**Relative**
Loss of peritoneal function producing inadequate clearance	Recent abdominal aortic graft
Adhesions blocking dialysate flow	Ventriculoperitoneal shunt
Surgically uncorrectable abdominal hernia	Intolerance of intra-abdominal fluid
	Large muscle mass
Abdominal wall stoma	Morbid obesity
Diaphragmatic fluid leak	Severe malnutrition
Inability to perform exchanges in absence of suitable assistant	Skin infection
	Bowel disease
Hemodialysis	
Absolute	**Relative**
No vascular access possible	Difficult vascular access
	Needle phobia
	Cardiac failure
	Coagulopathy

Table 75.1 Contraindications to dialysis modalities. Absolute and relative contraindications to hemodialysis and peritoneal dialysis. (Adapted with permission from American Journal of Kidney Disease[13].)

Kidney Foundation Dialysis Outcomes Quality Initiative (NKF-KDOQI)[13]. Relative contraindications to peritoneal dialysis include:

Fresh intra-abdominal foreign body

Patients with prosthetic aortic grafts have been successfully treated with peritoneal dialysis. Hemodialysis is usually used initially for up to 16 weeks to allow the graft to be covered with epithelium and so avoid the risk of graft infection via peritoneal dialysate. However, this risk must be balanced against that of bacterial seeding from the patient's hemodialysis access.

Body size limitations and intolerance of intra-abdominal fluid volume

Body size can be a problem at both ends of the spectrum. Small patients may be intolerant of the volume of dialysate needed to achieve adequate dialysis, particularly if they have negligible residual renal function. Alternative methods of fluid exchange such as nocturnal automated peritoneal dialysis can be used to overcome this limitation. It may also be difficult to achieve adequate clearances in large patients. The effect of increased intra-abdominal pressure can be particularly marked in patients with chronic respiratory disease, with low-back pain and with large polycystic kidneys. In general, it is hard to predict a patient's tolerance of intra-abdominal fluid and so these limitations usually appear after a patient has started peritoneal dialysis.

Bowel disease and other sources of infection

The presence of ischemic bowel disease, inflammatory bowel disease, or diverticulitis is likely to increase the incidence of

peritonitis due to organisms passing through the bowel wall into the peritoneum. Abdominal wall infection may lead to peritonitis via the exit site and catheter tunnel.

Nasal carriage of *Staphylococcus aureus* increases the risk of subsequent staphylococcal exit site infection and peritonitis. Clearance of nasal *S. aureus* with topical mupirocin cream has been shown to reduce significantly the risk of staphylococcal infection at the exit site[14]. Unfortunately, the reduction in staphylococcal peritonitis is compensated for by an increase in peritonitis due to Gram-negative organisms.

Severe malnutrition or morbid obesity

Patients should ideally commence peritoneal dialysis in an adequate nutritional state. Severe malnutrition may lead to poor wound healing and to leakage from the catheter tunnel. In addition, peritoneal protein losses during dialysis may exacerbate hypoalbuminemia. At the other end of the spectrum, it may prove difficult to satisfactorily place a peritoneal catheter through the abdominal wall in patients with morbid obesity. Thereafter, absorption of glucose from the dialysate may contribute to further weight gain.

Contraindications to dialysis modalities – hemodialysis

Contraindications to hemodialysis are few (Table 75.1). As discussed in Chapter 76, access to the circulation can usually be obtained, even in patients with extensive vascular disease or previous surgery. An aversion to needle puncture of the AV fistula is common in the early stages, but can usually be overcome by careful use of local anesthetic and nursing encouragement. Some patients with severe cardiac disease may not tolerate the shifts in volume and electrolytes that occur during hemodialysis treatment. However, there are no objective measurements that will reliably predict such patients. Where frequent episodes of intradialytic hypotension are a problem, peritoneal dialysis can be a more satisfactory treatment. Severe coagulopathy may make management of anticoagulation for the extracorporeal circuit difficult.

HOME HEMODIALYSIS

Hemodialysis patients should ideally be given the option of dialyzing at home. In the last decade, the popularity of home hemodialysis has declined, being replaced partly by peritoneal dialysis. For example, in the UK the percentage of the dialysis population on home hemodialysis fell from 35% in 1984, to 7% in 1994. Australia and New Zealand are the only other countries with a significant proportion of patients on home hemodialysis (Fig. 75.3). This has occurred for a variety of reasons. First, hemodialysis requires the presence of an assistant throughout the period of dialysis in case the patient becomes hypotensive and/or unconscious. As an increasing proportion of new dialysis patients is elderly, there may be no one available who is able or willing to take on this considerable responsibility. Second, there is the added cost of installing a dialysis machine and its associated water treatment, which is not required for peritoneal dialysis. However, the subsequent running costs are less for home than in-center hemodialysis.

Home hemodialysis can provide significant benefits for appropriate patients. It removes the inconvenience of traveling

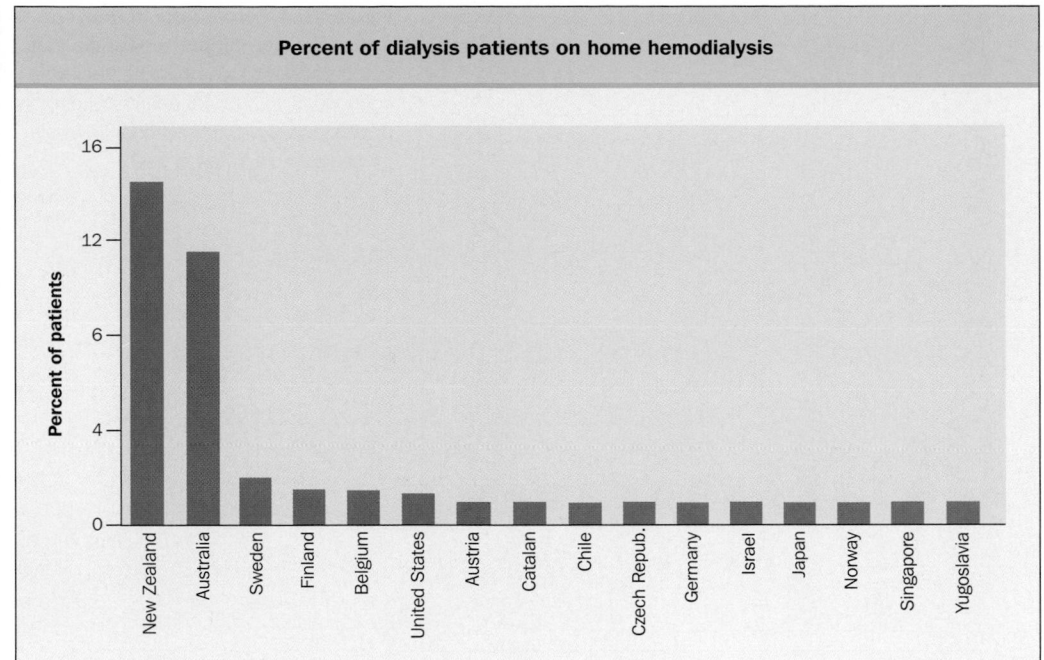

Figure 75.3 Percentage of dialysis patients on home hemodialysis. Percentage of dialysis patients on home hemodialysis in selected countries, 1999.

to and from the dialysis facility and gives patients the freedom to dialyze at a time to suit themselves. As a result they are able to perform more hours of treatment per week with less disruption to their lives. Although there is no randomized, controlled trial comparing hospital and home hemodialysis, comparative studies, where correction has been made for differences in comorbidity, do suggest that patients on home hemodialysis have a better outcome in terms of morbidity and mortality[15]. Selected patients are able to dialyze every night at home. This gives much greater clearance than is possible with thrice weekly dialysis and major improvements in anemia, blood pressure and phosphate control have been demonstrated. The inconvenience of nightly treatment is balanced by the removal of dietary restrictions and anti-hypertensive medications, and an improved quality of life[16]. With improvements in technology, this form of treatment may become much more widespread.

DO PATIENTS PREFER HEMODIALYSIS OR PERITONEAL DIALYSIS?

A number of recent studies have quantified the choices that patients would make if they were offered a free choice between hemodialysis and peritoneal dialysis. In our facility in Birmingham, UK, all patients entering the ESRD program are given 'modality-neutral' counseling and allowed to select their preferred mode of treatment[17]. Between 1992 and 1998, patient choice was restricted for medical reasons by the physician in 54 out of 333 patients (16%), peritoneal dialysis being contraindicated in 51. Of the remainder, 55% chose hemodialysis and 45% peritoneal dialysis. These relative proportions are the same as those found in a study of 5466 US patients who received a program of pre-dialysis education[18]. Independent predictors for choosing hemodialysis in our study were increasing age and male sex. Independent predictors for choosing CAPD were being married, being counseled before the start of

dialysis and increasing distance from the base unit. This last factor is a major influence in sparsely populated regions. For example in New Zealand, in 1999, 55% of patients received peritoneal dialysis (Fig. 75.4)

DO PATIENTS HAVE A FREE CHOICE OF DIALYSIS MODALITY?

Of those able to choose, almost all patients can be started on their preferred modality of dialysis[17]. However, in the US study, while 45% of patients chose peritoneal dialysis, only 33% actually started dialysis on this modality[18]. Furthermore, the major differences in dialysis modality between countries (Figs 75.3, 75.4) suggest that the type of dialysis is more often decided by physicians rather than patients. Possible factors affecting these decisions are discussed below[19,20].

Arrangements for the reimbursement of physicians and funding of dialysis facilities

The arrangements by which doctors and dialysis facilities are reimbursed for the cost of providing treatment vary widely around the world. There are also large differences between the levels of payment for hemodialysis and peritoneal dialysis in many countries. For example, in French clinics the facility is not reimbursed for peritoneal dialysis and the physicians receive no fee. In countries such as the UK and Canada, where facilities are publicly funded from taxation, the use of more expensive varieties of peritoneal and hemodialysis e.g., automated peritoneal dialysis and high-flux hemodiafiltration, is limited. Conversely, in places such as Hong Kong, where dialysis is only available in the private sector, more patients are treated by peritoneal dialysis than by hemodialysis, as the former is less expensive. In hemodialysis facilities, an arrangement whereby payment depends upon the number of patients treated creates pressure to increase patient numbers and throughput. If the patient's nephrologist has a financial interest

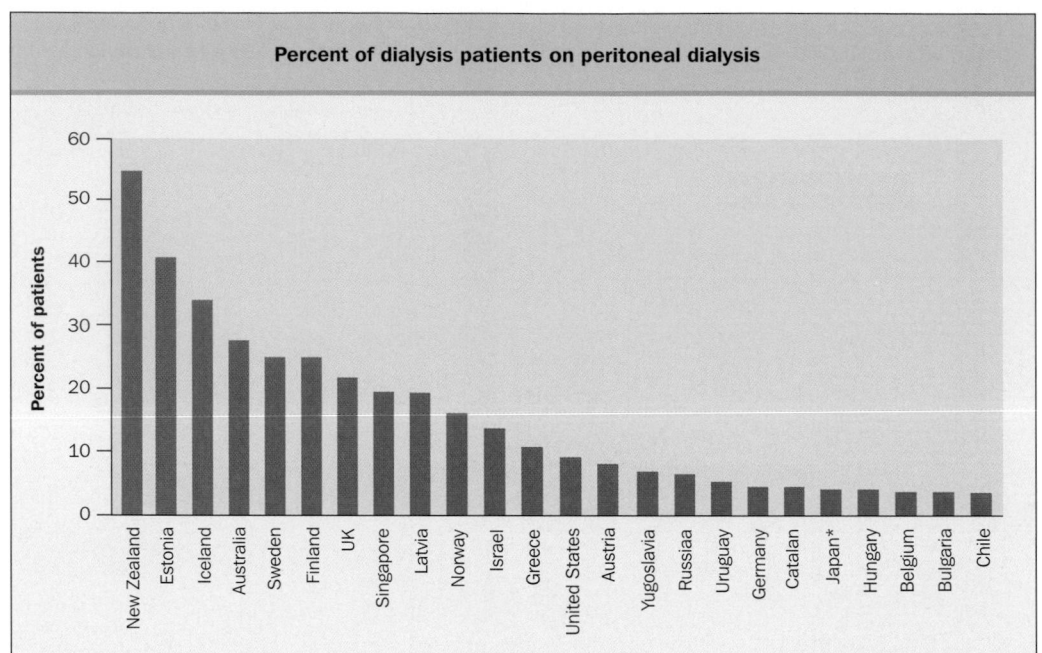

Percent of dialysis patients on peritoneal dialysis

Figure 75.4 Percentage of dialysis patients receiving peritoneal dialysis. Percentage of dialysis patients receiving continuous ambulatory peritoneal dialysis or continuous cycling peritoneal dialysis for selected countries in 1999.

in the hemodialysis facility, this may directly influence the decision on which modality of treatment to recommend.

Physician preference

There is a strong preference for hemodialysis among some influential nephrologists on both sides of the Atlantic. In a large US-based survey reported in 1997, only 25% of hemodialysis patients remembered having peritoneal dialysis discussed with them. In contrast, 68% of patients on peritoneal dialysis had had discussions about hemodialysis. Interestingly, a much greater proportion of patients on hemodialysis felt that the choice had been made by the medical team rather than by either themselves or by joint decision[21]. Since 1995, there has been a marked decline in the proportion of patients treated by CAPD in the USA (14% in 1995 to 10% in 1998) and Canada (36% in 1995 to 24% in 1999). The reasons for this are unclear[22].

THE IMPORTANCE OF DIALYSIS ACCESS

In an ideal world, every patient would make an informed choice between peritoneal and hemodialysis after a period of in-depth counseling and preparation, and dialysis access would be established in advance of starting dialysis. Ideally, access should be 3–4 months in advance for an arteriovenous fistula, and 2 weeks in advance for a PD catheter[13]. Sadly, dialysis is frequently started in less than ideal circumstances. Late presentation is a worldwide phenomenon, indicating that no system of healthcare has overcome the problems of identifying patients with chronic renal failure and bringing them to the attention of nephrologists in time (Fig. 75.5)[23,24].

Reports from both Europe and the USA clearly document the excess morbidity and mortality associated with patients presenting late in ESRD and requiring dialysis as an emergency procedure[25,26]. Patients starting dialysis as an emergency usually receive hemodialysis via a temporary vascular catheter and tend to remain on hemodialysis rather than converting to peritoneal

dialysis[17]. Compared with non-emergency patients, their length of hospital stay is significantly greater and during this time there is a higher incidence of major complications and death. A significant part of this excess mortality is related to the use of a catheter rather than a permanent arteriovenous fistula or graft. An analysis from the USRDS database shows, after adjusting for case-mix, that central venous catheters were associated with a significantly greater overall risk of death compared with arteriovenous fistulae (relative risk = 1.70 $P < 0.001$ in non-diabetic patients, 1.54 $P < 0.002$ in diabetic patients)[27].

The prevalence of catheter use within a dialysis facility is a useful composite measure of the timeliness and success of access surgery for new and existing patients, combined with the survival rate for permanent accesses. A wide variation in catheter use exists between individual dialysis units and between countries, being much greater in the USA and UK than continental Europe (Fig. 75.6). This is a serious cause for concern, since a relationship has been demonstrated between catheter use in a dialysis unit and both hospitalization and mortality[28]. The short-term convenience of tunneled hemodialysis catheters should not remove the urgency of vascular surgery in patients without a permanent access.

The detrimental effects of central venous catheters persist even after the catheter has been removed. The survival rate of subsequent arteriovenous fistulae is significantly worse in patients who have had a previous catheter in place compared with those who started directly on a fistula, even after correcting for case-mix and comorbidity[29]. Details of hemodialysis access surgery are discussed in Chapter 76 and peritoneal dialysis catheter placement is discussed in Chapter 80.

MULTI-DISCIPLINARY PREDIALYSIS PATIENT EDUCATION

Predialysis care focuses on preserving residual renal function, preventing or treating complications of chronic renal failure, ensuring that the patient has sufficient understanding of

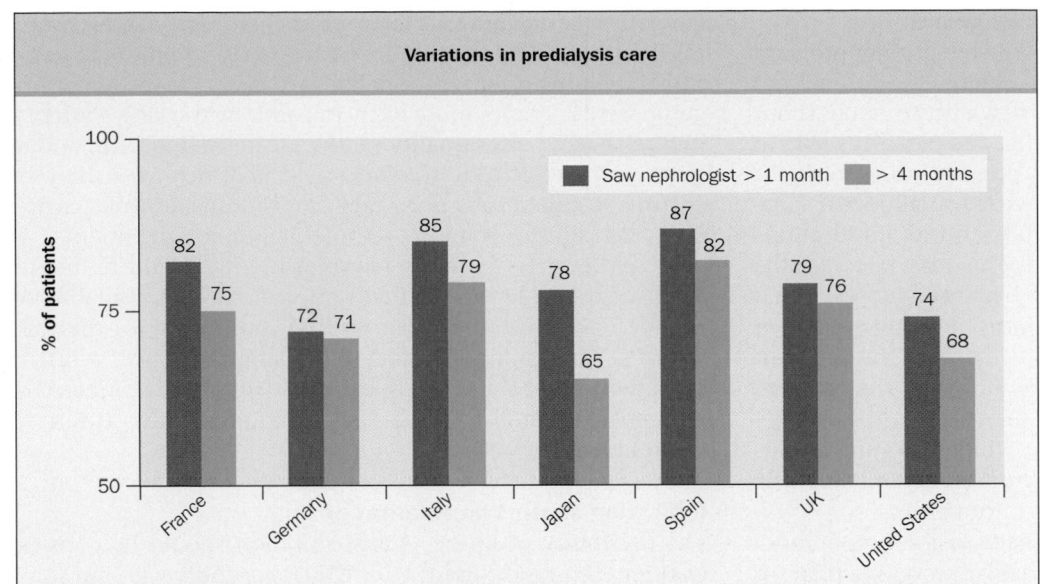

Figure 75.5 Variations in predialysis care. Percentage of patients starting hemodialysis having seen a nephrologist more than 1 month or 4 months previously by country. (Data from the Dialysis Outcomes and Practice Patterns Study.[24])

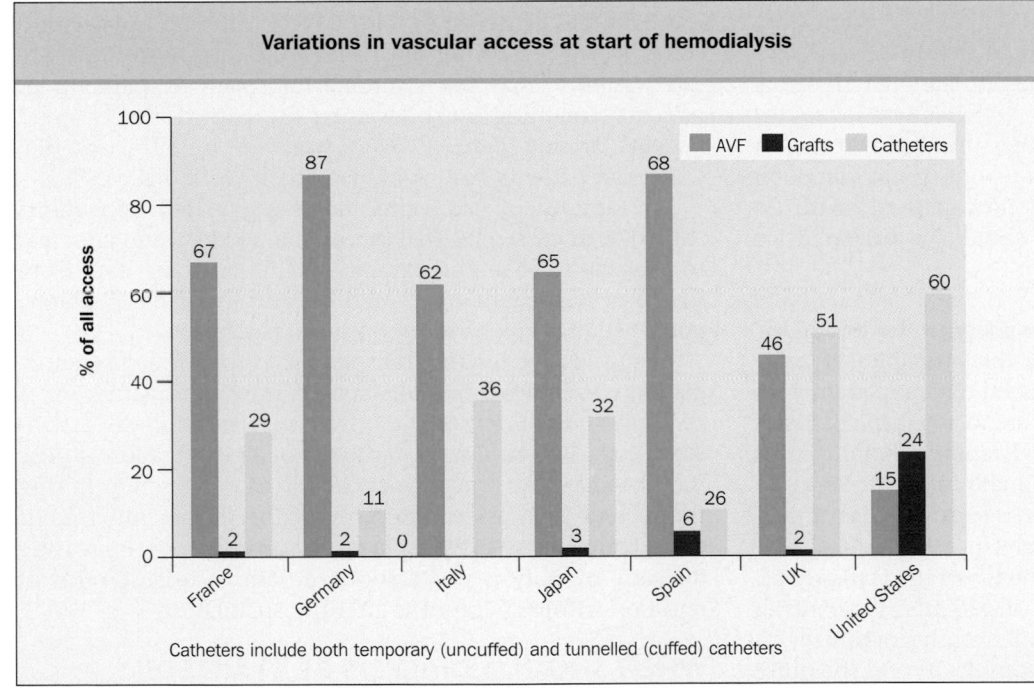

Figure 75.6 Country differences in vascular access use at start of hemodialysis. Percentage of patients starting hemodialysis using either an arteriovenous fistula, an arteriovenous graft or an intravenous catheter, by country. (Data from the Dialysis Outcomes and Practice Patterns Study.[24])

their condition to choose between peritoneal dialysis and hemodialysis, and arranging for appropriate access to be created in time for it to be functioning reliably before dialysis is required.

In addition to the nephrologist giving advice, further benefit may be gained if patients are offered a multidisciplinary educational program. This is supported by a prospective nonrandomized cohort study from Canada[30]. Conventional preparation for all patients approaching ESRD at this center consisted of a 2–3 h formal orientation session led by a nurse educator and social worker, in addition to consultations with the nephrologist totaling between 7 and 15 h per year.

This conventional preparation was compared to an intensive structured education program and a standardized follow-up regimen based in the clinic. This program was delivered by a nurse educator, social worker and dietitian as well as the patient's physician, and totaled 15–33 h per year.

Although this was a nonrandomized study, the benefits of the intensive program were impressive. They included a significant reduction in the number of patients starting dialysis urgently as inpatients on temporary vascular access (13% vs. 35%, $P < 0.05$) with only 3% of intensively educated patients requiring hospitalization for uremia compared with 11% of the conventionally prepared patients ($P < 0.05$). There were also fewer hospital admissions in the intensively prepared group, and intensively prepared patients began dialysis with better blood pressure, hemoglobin, serum calcium, and serum phosphate levels.

Estimated savings in inpatient costs from the program were considerably greater than those required to run the clinic.

When should predialysis education be given?

The aim of a predialysis educational and counseling program is to ensure that, by the time dialysis begins, the patient and his or her family know as much as they wish to know about renal failure and its treatment and that the patient is able to achieve as good a quality of life as possible on dialysis. To achieve this aim, sufficient time is needed to allow the large amount of information to be absorbed and its implications for that individual to be understood. This may take months rather than days. It is our practice to begin the process when dialysis is anticipated within 12 months. Starting education this early risks putting some patients through the program who may never actually need dialysis. However, the program should include education about the management of the pre-dialysis phase of chronic renal failure, which will still be helpful. Also, there is more harm done by not preparing a patient adequately than by giving too much information.

Predicting the start of dialysis is made easier if renal function is routinely measured by an estimate of the glomerular filtration rate (GFR) such as is derived by the Cockroft-Gault formula, rather than serum creatinine (Chapter 3). It is very easy to underestimate the severity of renal impairment from the serum creatinine alone, especially in elderly underweight patients. As a result, they frequently need to start dialysis before they have been fully prepared.

Using an estimated GFR also allows thresholds to be set which can be used to generate regular reports from a computer database, for example identifying those patients with an estimated GFR < 30 mL/min who should be prepared for dialysis by the multidisciplinary team.

How should a predialysis education program be designed?

An effective program should follow the principles of adult learning which also underlie a successful doctor–patient consultation[31,32]. The three key elements are to assess the patient's existing level of knowledge and understanding, build on this knowledge by the delivery of appropriate information in an appropriate form, and establish that the patient has understood and accepted the information given.

Education can be delivered individually or in small groups. In a group session, the wide range of patients' pre-existing understanding may make it difficult for the organizer to achieve the right level of detail and complexity. On the other hand, patients probably learn as much from fellow patients within a supportive group as they do from the group's facilitator. Furthermore, a group will help patients and their relatives appreciate that they are not alone in facing the demands of ESRD.

The predialysis program should be delivered by representatives of all members of the multidisciplinary team, both medical and non-medical. For example, a controlled trial from California has studied the value of social worker input to the predialysis program in reducing unemployment[33]. In the intervention group, patients and their relatives met regularly with a licensed social worker both before and after starting dialysis, to explore strategies for continuing the patient's current employment. The aim of the education and counseling was to change the perception among patients, relatives and employers that dialysis patients are unable to continue working.

Patients were encouraged to adapt so that dialysis fitted more easily into their lifestyle and were helped to feel more in control of their treatment. Blue-collar workers in the intervention group were 2.8 times more likely to continue working. Patients in work had a better quality of life, greater self-esteem, and a more positive attitude to work. As it is difficult for dialysis patients to regain jobs once they are lost, this result is particularly valuable for the long-term rehabilitation of patients.

In addition to formal sessions, patients should be made aware of the wide range of educational material available. A number of books have been written specifically for dialysis patients. The National Kidney Foundation produces a series of patient information leaflets and audio-visual material, and provides much useful information on the Internet (www.kidney.org).

Education about transplantation

The possibility of kidney transplantation should be considered for each new patient with ESRD. For those who are suitable, transplantation offers the prospect of improved survival and quality of life. In a US study, although the risk of death was 2.8 times higher in the first 2 weeks after transplantation compared to remaining on dialysis, the long-term mortality rate was 48 to 82% lower among transplant recipients than patients remaining on the waiting list, with relatively larger benefits among patients who were 20 to 39 years old, Caucasian patients, and younger patients with diabetes[34].

The options of cadaveric and living-related transplants should be discussed, as well as combined kidney and pancreas transplants for diabetic patients. While outcome data from the local transplanting centers should be made available, published data can be used to inform patients.

The ideal time for the transplant to be performed is before dialysis is ever begun, so-called pre-emptive transplantation. A US study showed that pre-emptive transplantation was associated with a 52% reduction in the risk of allograft failure during the first year after transplantation, an 82% reduction during the second year, and an 86% reduction during subsequent years, compared with transplantation after dialysis. Increasing duration of dialysis was associated with increasing odds of rejection within six months after transplantation[35].

WHEN SHOULD DIALYSIS BE STARTED?

In those patients under regular follow-up, where there is ready access to a dialysis program, it is usually recommended that dialysis should be started when subjective symptoms of uremia develop or when laboratory measurements indicate that ESRD has been reached. The serum levels of urea and creatinine will vary according to the patient's protein intake and muscle mass respectively and there is no single value of either that can be used as a threshold for starting dialysis. Creatinine clearance can be estimated using a formula such as that derived by Cockroft and Gault (Chapter 3), although it overestimates GFR in obese or edematous patients whose muscle mass forms a smaller proportion of their total body weight[36]. A creatinine clearance of ~ 10 mL/min is used as a threshold for nondiabetic patients. A higher threshold, 15 mL/min, should be used in diabetics, as they tend to tolerate uremia poorly and are frequently troubled by sodium retention and fluid overload. Other measurements to be taken into consideration include a rising serum phosphate, falling serum bicarbonate and protein-energy malnutrition, which develops and persists despite vigorous attempts to optimize intake. A fall in serum albumin is a late sign of reduced protein intake and debility.

Limitations of a purely clinical approach to the initiation of dialysis

Waiting for patients to develop uremic symptoms, such as anorexia, nausea, vomiting and loss of lean body weight, carries the risk that the patient will start dialysis in a malnourished state with an increased risk of mortality. Renal failure itself is a catabolic state and it is commonly difficult for patients on dialysis to regain lost weight.

Given the chronic nature of renal disease, patients frequently remain unaware of the severity of their illness. Protein intake may fall spontaneously with the result that symptoms of uremia do not develop, but this is at the expense of a loss of lean body mass. Similarly, patients may gradually reduce their activities as their exercise tolerance declines. It is only when dialysis is started that many patients appreciate how ill they have become.

Lack of awareness is a trap that can be avoided by carefully questioning the patient for insidious symptoms of uremia. For example, the patient should be asked to compare his current eating habits and lifestyle with those 6–12 months previously. Close friends and relatives provide a useful third party view of the patient's well being.

A kinetic approach to the initiation of dialysis

The current NKF-K/DOQI guidelines[13] recommend that residual renal function and protein intake should be measured formally, and a decision to start dialysis made when these values fall below the minimum recommended for patients already on dialysis; i.e., urea clearance of 7 mL/min, creatinine clearance 9–14 mL/min per 1.73 m^2 and dietary protein intake < 0.8 g/kg per day. These recommendations are based upon the rationale that, just as patients on dialysis require a minimum urea clearance and protein intake to remain healthy, patients with deteriorating native renal function should not be left for prolonged periods with inadequate renal clearance or protein intake. In other words, patients should have a 'healthy start' to dialysis. Detailed guidelines are shown in Table 75.2.

Limitations of a purely kinetic approach in the initiation of dialysis

Routine early initiation of dialysis would need to confer significant benefits to justify the added inconvenience to the patient, the additional risk of dialysis-related complications and the additional cost. As dialysis treatment has a finite life, either from loss of peritoneal function or failure of hemodialysis access, starting treatment earlier will bring forward the time when further procedures or a change of modality are necessary.

Another concern about a kinetic approach is the accuracy of measurements of residual renal function[36]. These depend upon timed collections of urine, which are notoriously inaccurate in

---

When to initiate dialysis

Unless certain conditions are met, patients should be advised to initiate some form of dialysis when the weekly renal Kt/V_{urea} (K_t/V_{urea}) falls below 2.0.

The conditions that may indicate dialysis is not yet necessary even though the weekly K_t/V_{urea} is less than 2.0 are:

1. Stable or increased edema-free body weight. Supportive objective parameters for adequate nutrition include a lean body mass >63%, subjective global assessment score indicative of adequate nutrition, a serum albumin concentration in excess of the lower limit for the laboratory and stable or rising.

2. Normalized protein nitrogen appearance (nPNA) >0.8 g/kg per day.

3. Complete absence of clinical signs or symptoms attributable to uremia.

A weekly K_t/V_{urea} of 2.0 approximates to a renal urea clearance of 7 mL/min and a renal creatinine clearance that varies between 9–14 mL/min per 1.73 m^2. Urea clearance should be normalized to total body water (V) and creatinine clearance should be expressed per 1.73 m^2 of body surface area. The glomerular filtration rate, which is estimated by the arithmetic mean of the urea and creatinine clearances, will be approximately 10.5 mL/min/ per 1.73 m^2 when the K_t/V_{urea} is about 2.0.

Table 75.2 When to initiate dialysis. NKF-DOQI Clinical Practice Guidelines for initiation of dialysis. (Adapted with permission from American Journal of Kidney Disease[13].)

---

clinical practice. This may lead to an erroneously low value for urea clearance and hence an unnecessarily early start for dialysis. Moreover, there is likely to be resistance from many patients to the suggestion that they should start dialysis when they have no symptoms of uremia. The nephrologist would need complete confidence in the laboratory values, as well as in the evidence supporting early commencement of dialysis, in order to persuade a reluctant, asymptomatic patient.

Starting dialysis is the first step in a lifelong commitment to renal replacement therapy. Patients will be asked to comply with a wide variety of inconvenient and sometimes unpleasant treatments. A high level of compliance is required for a successful outcome and, particularly in the USA, there is concern about the level of non-compliance (see Fig. 75.7). It seems reasonable to presume that the commitment to dialysis is likely to be greater if the patient feels better after it has started.

A recent prospective study in Holland provides useful data to help the patient and nephrologist agree when to commence treatment[37]. Those patients who started dialysis with less residual renal function than recommended by NKF-K/DOQI did have a poorer quality of life. However, this difference was no longer present by the end of the first 12 months of treatment. The study was too small to demonstrate a difference in mortality.

SHOULD WE DIALYSE DIFFICULT OR DISRUPTIVE PATIENTS?

Most nephrologists have had experience of treating a small number of patients who, for one reason or another, will not comply with the discipline required for maintenance dialysis and who become disruptive to the staff and other patients. This behavior can range from non-compliance with treatment, which harms the patient but is merely inconvenient to the staff, to verbal or even physical aggression towards the

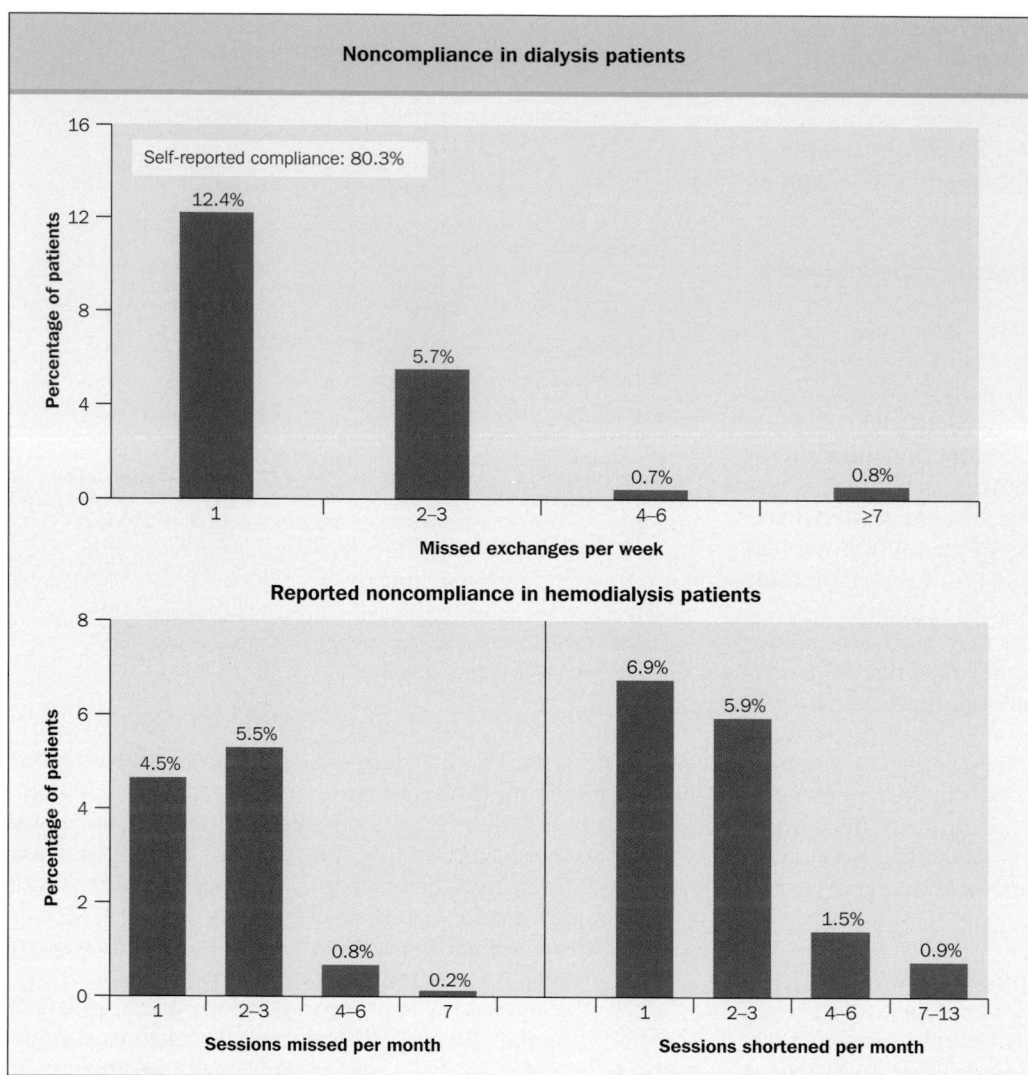

Figure 75.7 Noncompliance in dialysis patients. Admitted number of exchanges missed per week in continuous ambulatory peritoneal dialysis patients and number of hemodialysis sessions missed or shortened per month, reported by patients in the USA. (Adapted with permission from American Journal of Kidney Disease[21].)

staff and other patients in the unit. The impact of this small number of patients can be very great.

The strategy for dealing with such patients must be tailored to the individual. However, useful suggestions for resolving conflict have been provided in the RPA/ASN Clinical Practice Guideline[4] (Table 75.3) and are also available at: www.esrdnetworks.org/networks/net6/policies/po-recom.html. They emphasize the importance of understanding, information, patience and persistence. However, the bottom line for patients who are aggressive towards staff whilst on dialysis must be that they are taken off treatment and sent home (www.nhs.uk/zerotolerance/intro.htm).

RESUSCITATION AND WITHDRAWAL OF DIALYSIS

Cardiopulmonary resuscitation

If patients are to be fully involved in decision making about their treatment, two sensitive issues need to be discussed – cardiopulmonary resuscitation (CPR) and the possibility of withdrawal of dialysis. The two are not necessarily linked; patients may wish to continue with dialysis but express a desire for resuscitation not to be attempted should they suffer

a cardiac arrest. Such a decision would be supported by evidence on the outcome of CPR in dialysis patients: only six of 74 dialysis patients who received CPR survived to hospital discharge and at 6 months after CPR only two were still alive. This compares with 23 of 247 'control' patients not on dialysis being still alive at 6 months ($P = 0.044$) and this difference was not explained by age or comorbid conditions[38]. Successful CPR often resulted in a 'poor quality' death, 20 of the 27 successfully resuscitated dialysis patients dying a few days later on mechanical ventilation in an intensive care unit.

A decision not to attempt CPR must be carefully documented in the patient's medical and nursing records and all nursing staff must be made aware of it. It is important to be clear what is meant by 'cardiac arrest' and for there to be agreement on how the nursing staff should respond should the patient suffer a hypotensive 'crash' while on dialysis. These notes may form part of a complete advance directive, as discussed below.

Withdrawal of dialysis

As discussed earlier, it is not possible to predict accurately which patients will gain prolonged benefit from dialysis. Many nephrologists, therefore, operate a liberal policy of

Suggested steps for dealing with disruptive patients
Identify and document problem behaviors and discuss them with the patient
• Seek to understand the patient's perspective
• Identify the patient's goals for treatment
• Share control and responsibility for treatment with the patient
– Educate the patient so that he or she can make informed decisions
– Involve the patient in the treatment as much as possible
– Negotiate a behavioral contract with the patient
• Consult a psychiatrist, psychologist or social worker for assistance in patient management or determination of decision-making capacity
• Be patient and persistent, try not to be adversarial
• Allow the patient to ventilate concerns but do not tolerate verbal abuse or threats to staff or patients (see www.nhs.uk/zerotolerance/intro.htm)
• Contact law enforcement officials if physical abuse is threatened or occurs
• If satisfactory resolution has not occurred with the above strategies, contact the local ESRD Network to discuss the situation and ensure due process
• As a last resort, consider transferring the patient to another facility or discharging the patient
Consult with legal counsel before proceeding with plans for discharge and do not discharge without advance notice and a full explanation of future treatment options.

Table 75.3 Suggested steps for dealing with disruptive patients.
(Adapted from RPA/ASN Clinical Practice Guideline[4].)

Principles underlying withdrawal of dialysis
• The ultimate responsibility for the decision rests with the physician, not the relatives or carers.
• The patient's interests and dignity should be protected at all times.
• The process should not be rushed. If there is any doubt about the correctness of the decision, treatment should continue.
• There should be an open discussion amongst the multidisciplinary team to avoid any damaging disagreements.
• The psychological needs of the health care team should not be overlooked.
• Palliative care must be given in the most appropriate environment, e.g., a hospice or, ideally, the patient's own home.

Table 75.4 Key principles underlying the process of withdrawal of dialysis.

offering dialysis to all patients with ESRD who wish to have it. This policy ensures that no patients are denied dialysis but has the inevitable consequence that a number of patients will be started on dialysis who subsequently do not enjoy an acceptable quality of life. The possibility of withdrawing dialysis needs to be addressed if these patients are not to suffer unreasonably. Data from the USRDS[21] show that 19% of patients withdrew from dialysis prior to death. Not surprisingly, this is more common in patients over 65 years of age and in diabetics. More surprising was the marked racial variation, with African Americans having about one-third the withdrawal rate of Caucasians.

Patients may be very reticent to express a wish to withdraw from dialysis. Many see it as their duty as a patient to go along with the treatment recommended by their physician and do not wish to appear ungrateful for the efforts that are being made to keep them alive. Their physician may be the last member of the team to learn about the patient's views and it is very important that good communication exists within the multidisciplinary team so that any clues which the patient gives are passed on and acted upon.

Patients may be reluctant to discuss these issues, so staff should adopt a proactive approach and raise the issue of withdrawal of dialysis with patients who are chronically not thriving. There is good evidence that early discussion of these issues can lead to a more satisfactory outcome for patients, relatives and staff when the patient eventually dies[39]. In the USA, formal advance directives play an important part in these discussions, whilst in the UK there has been less enthusiasm for formalizing this process. Evidence from randomized trials suggests that implementing advance directives does not improve the quality of the end of patients' lives[40]. Advance directives are currently only completed by a minority of patients and even if one is in place, it does not obviate the need for staff to continue to communicate closely with the patient and his or her family in case the decision changes as death comes closer.

Where a patient is no longer competent to make a decision, an advance directive can provide a clear legal basis for the decision to stop dialysis. Indeed, in the absence of clear and convincing written evidence, some American states (e.g., Missouri and New York) insist that dialysis must be continued. In other American states and the UK, the physician is given the task of deciding on the patient's behalf. Helpful advice for dialysis staff and patients wishing to complete an advance directive is available in the RPA/ASN Clinical Practice Guideline[4] and at the website www.ageingwithdignity.org.

Once a patient has expressed a wish for dialysis to be withdrawn, or the issue has been raised by his or her relatives, the first priority must be to identify any reversible factors that may improve the patient's health sufficiently for the decision to be reversed. Once all these factors have been ruled out, the process of withdrawing dialysis should be managed according to some key principles (Table 75.4).

Withdrawing dialysis should not be seen as an admission of failure but as a final stage in the process of renal replacement therapy. This terminal phase can be uniquely rewarding, particularly if it allows a patient and his or her family and carers to prepare themselves for the patient's death. The opportunity for patients to complete unfinished emotional and financial business can make the subsequent bereavement period much less traumatic.

CONCLUSION

It behoves all nephrologists to ensure that the resources dedicated to renal failure treatment are used to best effect. As dialysis has advanced, the goal of treatment has moved from merely sustaining life to achieving as near normal a quality of life as possible. If the greatest benefit is to be gained from dialysis, the selection and preparation of patients reaching ESRD must be thoroughly addressed. Throughout this process, the patient must be an active participant whose choices are respected.

REFERENCES

1. McKenzie JK, Moss AH, Feest TG, et al. Dialysis decision making in Canada, the United Kingdom, and the United States. Am J Kidney Dis. 1998;31:12–18.
2. Challah S, Wing AJ, Bauer R, et al. Negative selection of patients for dialysis and transplantation in the United Kingdom. BMJ. 1984;288:1119–22.
3. Parry RG, Crowe A, Stevens JM, et al. Referral of elderly patients with severe renal failure: questionnaire survey of physicians. BMJ. 1996;313(466).
4. Renal Physicians Association and American Society of Nephrology. Shared Decision-Making in the Appropriate Initiation of and Withdrawal from Dialysis. Clinical Practice Guideline, Number 2. Washington, DC: Renal Physicians Association; 2000.
5. Singer PA. Nephrologists' experience with and attitudes towards decisions to forego dialysis. J Am Soc Nephrol. 1992;2:1235–40.
6. Moss AH. Dialysis decisions and the elderly. Clin Geriatr Med. 1994;10:463–73.
7. Barrett BJ, Parfrey PS, Morgan J, et al. Prediction of early death in end-stage renal disease patients starting dialysis. Am J Kidney Dis. 1997;29:214–22.
8. Chadna SM, Schulz J, Lawrence C, et al. Is there a rationale for rationing chronic dialysis? A hospital based cohort study of factors affecting survival and morbidity. Br Med J. 1999;318:217–22.
9. Mapes DL, McCullough KP, Meredith D, et al. 'Quality of Life predicts mortality and hospitalization for hemodialysis (HD) patients in the US and Europe'. American Society of Nephrology, 32nd Annual Meeting, 1999.
10. Fenton SS, Schaubel DE, Desmeules M, et al. Hemodialysis versus peritoneal dialysis: a comparison of adjusted mortality rates. Am J Kidney Dis. 1997;30:334–42.
11. Held PJ, Port FK, Turenne MN, et al. Continuous ambulatory peritoneal dialysis and hemodialysis: comparison of patient mortality with adjustment for comorbid conditions. Kidney Int. 1994;45:1163–9.
12. Stack AG, Dhingra RK, Port FK. Should patients with low serum albumin at End Stage Renal Disease (ESRD) onset be placed on peritoneal dialysis or hemodialysis Renal Association; 2001.
13. NKF-DOQI Clinical Practice Guidelines for Peritoneal Dialysis Adequacy 2000. Am J Kidney Dis. 2001;37(suppl 1):S65–S136. www.kidney.org/professionals/doqi/index.cfm.
14. Mupirocin Study Group. Nasal mupirocin prevents Staphylococcus aureus exit site infection during peritoneal dialysis. J Am Soc Nephrol. 1996;7:2403–8.
15. Woods JD, Port FK, Stannard D, et al. Comparison of mortality with home hemodialysis and center hemodialysis: a national study. Kidney Int. 1996;49:1464–70.
16. Mohr PE, Neumann PJ, Franco SJ, et al. The case for daily dialysis: its impact on costs and quality of life. Am J Kidney Dis. 2001;37:777–89.
17. Little J, Irwin A, Marshall T, et al. Predicting a patient's choice of dialysis modality: experience in a United Kingdom renal department. Am J Kidney Dis. 2001;37:981–6.
18. Golper TA, Vonesh EF, Wolfson M, et al. The impact of pre-ESRD education on dialysis modality selection. J Am Soc Nephrol. 2000;11:231A.
19. Nissenson AR, Prichard SS, Cheng IKP, et al. Non-medical factors that impact on ESRD modality selection. Kidney Int. 1993;43(suppl 40):S120–7.
20. Mendelssohn DC, Mullaney SR, Jung B, et al. What do American nephrologists think about dialysis modality selection? Am J Kidney Dis. 2001;37:22–9.
21. U.S. Renal Data System. USRDS 1997 Annual Data Report. Am J Kidney Dis. 1997;30 (suppl 1):www.usrds.org.
22. Blake PG, Finkelstein FO. Why is the proportion of patients doing peritoneal dialysis declining in North America? Perit Dial Int. 2001;21:107–14.
23. Rayner HC, Pisoni RL, Young EW, et al. Creation, cannulation and survival of arterio-venous fistulae – data from the DOPPS. Kidney Int. (submitted).
24. Young EW, Goodkin DA, Mapes DL, et al. The Dialysis Outcomes and Practice Patterns Study (DOPPS): An international hemodialysis study. Kidney Int. 2000;57(suppl 74):S74–S81.
25. Ratcliffe PJ, Phillips RE, Oliver DO. Late referral for maintenance dialysis. BMJ. 1984;288:441–3.
26. Ifudu O, Dawood M, Homel P, et al. Excess morbidity in patients starting uremia therapy without prior care by a nephrologist. Am J Kidney Dis. 1996;28:841–5.
27. Dhingra RK, Young EW, Hulbert-Shearon TE, et al. Type of vascular access and mortality in US hemodialysis patients. Kidney Int. 2001;60:1443–51.
28. Pisoni RL, Young EW, Combe C, et al. Higher catheter use within facilities is associated with increased mortality and hospitalization: results from DOPPS. J Am Soc Nephrol. 2001;12:299A (A1538).
29. Young EW, Goodkin DA, Dykstra DM, et al. Vascular access (VA) survival and prior access placement. American Society of Nephrology 32nd Annual Meeting, 1999.
30. Levin A, Lewis M, Mortiboy P, et al. Multidisciplinary predialysis programs: quantification and limitations of their impact on patient outcomes in two Canadian settings. Am J Kidney Dis. 1997; 29:533–40.
31. Tate P. The Doctor's Communication Handbook, 2nd edn. Oxford: Radcliffe Medical Press; 1997:43–54.
32. Nicholls KA. Psychological Care in Physical Illness. 2nd edn. London: Chapman & Hall; 1993:80–95.
33. Razgone S, Schwankovsky L, James-Rogers A, et al. An intervention for employment maintenance among blue-collar workers with end stage renal disease. Am J Kidney Dis. 1993;22:403–12.
34. Wolfe RA, Ashby VB, Milford EL, et al. Comparison of mortality in all patients on dialysis, patients on dialysis awaiting transplantation, and recipients of a first cadaveric transplant. New Engl J Med. 1999;341:1725–30.
35. Mange KC, Joffe MM, Feldman HI. Effect of the use or nonuse of long-term dialysis on the subsequent survival of renal transplants from living donors. New Engl J Med. 2001;344:726–31.
36. Walser M. Assessing renal function from creatinine measurements in adults with chronic renal failure. Am J Kidney Dis. 1998;32:23–31.
37. Korevaar JC, Jansen MA, Dekker FW, et al. Evaluation of DOQI guidelines: Early start of dialysis treatment is not associated with better health-related quality of life. Am J Kidney Dis. 2002;39:108–15.
38. Moss AH, Holley JL, Upton MB. Outcomes of cardiopulmonary resuscitation in dialysis patients. J Am Soc Nephrol. 1992;3:1238–43.
39. Swartz RD, Penny E. Advance directives are associated with good deaths in chronic dialysis patients. J Am Soc Nephrol. 1993;3:1623–30.
40. Anderson JP, Kaplan RM, Schneiderman LJ. Effects of offering advance directives on quality adjusted life expectancy and psychological well being among ill adults. J Clin Epidemiol. 1994;47:761–72.

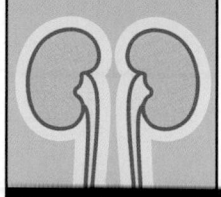

Chapter 76

Vascular Access for Hemodialysis

Peter J Conlon and Louise Giblin

INTRODUCTION

The maintenance of adequate, durable vascular access for hemodialysis is essential for the well being of the patient with end-stage renal disease (ESRD). The provision of extracorporeal hemodialytic therapy requires repetitive vascular access that can achieve a blood flow in excess of 350 mL/min. If vascular access cannot be achieved for even short periods of time the patient will die from uremia. Hemodialysis is employed in chronic maintenance hemodialysis, acute renal failure, and less commonly assisting in the elimination of poisons from the body.

For the provision of chronic maintenance hemodialysis the requirements for vascular access are very different from those for acute hemodialysis.

VASCULAR ACCESS FOR ACUTE HEMODIALYSIS

The vascular access requirements for acute hemodialysis are best served by the use of dual lumen, non-cuffed, temporary catheters. These catheters are made of a variety of materials including polyurethane, polyethylene, or polytetrafluoroethylene (PTFE). These materials have the useful property that at room temperature they are rigid, which facilitates their insertion, but when in place, they achieve body temperature and become much more flexible.

Dialysis catheters are most commonly placed in the femoral, subclavian, or jugular vein. Each of these sites has advantages and disadvantages depending on specific clinical circumstances. The femoral vein is in most patients the easiest site to insert a catheter and is associated with the lowest risk of life-threatening complications. The major disadvantages of using the femoral vein are that the patient must remain recumbent while the catheter is in place and the high rate of infection if the catheter is left in place for more than 72 h. It is preferable to use femoral catheters of 24 cm length as the recirculation in these catheters has been shown to be considerably lower than in the shorter 15 cm catheters.

For patients who require longer periods of renal replacement (> 72 h and < 3 weeks), a dialysis catheter placed in the jugular vein is preferable. The acute complications associated with both jugular and subclavian-line insertions are similar. However, subclavian-line insertions are associated with the longer-term complication of subclavian vein stenosis, thus compromising the use of the ipsilateral limb for long-term vascular access. Catheters placed under aseptic conditions in either the jugular or subclavian vein may be left in place for up to 3 weeks. Complications associated with subclavian or jugular catheters include pneumothorax and arterial or great-vein puncture with associated mediastinal, pleural, or pericardial hemorrhage. The risk of great-vein perforation is probably greatest in patients who have previously had multiple line insertions and have developed subclavian-vein stenosis. Patients with a previously documented subclavian-vein stenosis should never have a temporary catheter inserted on that side. It is imperative that a chest X-ray is taken prior to the initiation of hemodialysis after either jugular or subclavian lines are inserted. This is to exclude the development of either a pneumothorax or hemothorax and to confirm that the catheter is in a position compatible with the desired vessel. If there is any doubt that the tip of the catheter is within a great vein, a small amount of contrast should be injected into the catheter under fluoroscopic control. For patients with difficult vascular anatomy, the use of ultrasound or fluoroscopy may simplify the insertion of dialysis lines.

Acute dialysis catheter infection

All temporary catheters carry the risk of bacterial infection. Infection in these catheters is most commonly introduced by tracking along the course of the catheter from the outside or less commonly by contamination of the catheter lumen. A number of strategies have been developed to reduce the incidence of line infection such as coating these catheters with silver or antibiotics or the use of external cuffs. None of these approaches has proved particularly effective for dialysis lines.

At the first sign of systemic infection or the development of fever, the catheter should be removed and appropriate antibiotics initiated. The most common offending organisms with subclavian or jugular lines are *Staphylococcus aureus* or *S. epidermidis*. The patient should initially be treated with a loading dose of intravenous vancomycin (20 mg/kg), pending bacteriologic identification of the organism and sensitivities. Patients with femoral catheters are also highly likely to become bacteremic from Gram-negative organisms and should be empirically treated with a single intravenous dose of vancomycin (20 mg/kg) and gentamicin (2 mg/kg), pending the results of blood cultures. It is important to treat these patients for between 2 and 3 weeks and to confirm adequate antibiotic levels. Uremic patients who develop *S. aureus* bacteremia have a high incidence of metastatic complications. These patients may develop infective endocarditis, septic arthritis, or epidural abscess.

Patients who develop an exit-site infection should have a wound swab and blood sample taken for culture. If the blood cultures are positive, the catheter should be removed and appropriate antibiotics started as outlined above. If the blood cultures are negative, a course of antibiotics for 10–14 days should be given, guided by the results of the wound-swab culture.

PERMANENT VASCULAR ACCESS

There is no doubt that a pre-emptively placed forearm primary arteriovenous (AV) fistula is the most effective form of long-term vascular access for the uremic patient. Early referral to a nephrologist is necessary as it is important for physicians caring for patients with renal insufficiency to begin making plans for the provision of renal replacement therapy at an early stage and this should usually begin when creatinine clearance is < 25 mL/min or serum creatinine > 4 mg/dL (360 µmol/L)[1]. Pre-emptive planning for the provision of vascular access is certainly cost-effective; it avoids emergency placement of femoral or subclavian catheters and also reduces hospital admissions for infection and temporary access failure[2].

Types of permanent vascular access
Primary fistula
In 1962, Cimino and Brescia[2,3] described the technique of anastomosing the radial artery to the adjacent veins (Fig. 76.1). This technique allowed repeated puncturing of veins for dialysis access. The most frequent problem associated with an AV fistula is failure to mature, as manifested by early thrombosis or inadequate blood flow rates. For patients in whom it is not possible to create a primary radiocephalic AV fistula, an upper-arm brachiocephalic fistula is a second-best alternative and in our opinion much preferable to the use of a polytetrafluoroethylene (PTFE) graft (Fig. 76.2). An upper-arm brachiocephalic fistula takes many months to mature. Brachiobasilic fistulae may also be placed and although they are more likely to mature than brachiocephalic fistulae they have a higher rate of thrombosis after maturation. Recent work comparing brachiocephalic fistulae, transposed brachiobasilic fistulae and upper arm PTFE grafts show equivalent cumulative patency rates but a lower incidence of thrombosis and infectious complications with the native fistulae[4].

Up to 80% of primary AV fistulae will be functioning 3 years after creation. There are only a few exceptions when a primary AV fistula is not the preferred form of vascular access; these include patients with severe congestive heart failure or angina whom it is considered would be unable to tolerate the increased cardiac output associated with such a procedure, or patients with an estimated prognosis of less than 1 year. A primary AV fistula should be constructed in at least 50% of all new hemodialysis patients.

Polytetrafluoroethylene grafts
PTFE was introduced in 1976 as a material for vascular bypass grafts. Since that time, this material has become the mainstay for vascular access in dialysis when an autologous AV fistula is either technically impossible or has failed to mature. Using PTFE as a conduit, a fistula is created between an upper-limb

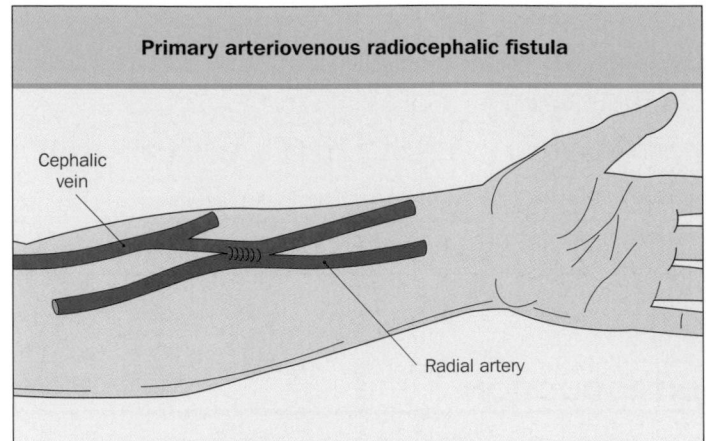

Figure 76.1 Primary arteriovenous radiocephalic fistula. Cephalic vein anastomosed to radial artery. Side-to-side anastomosis is shown, a commonly used alternative is end-to side (venous-arterial) anastomosis.

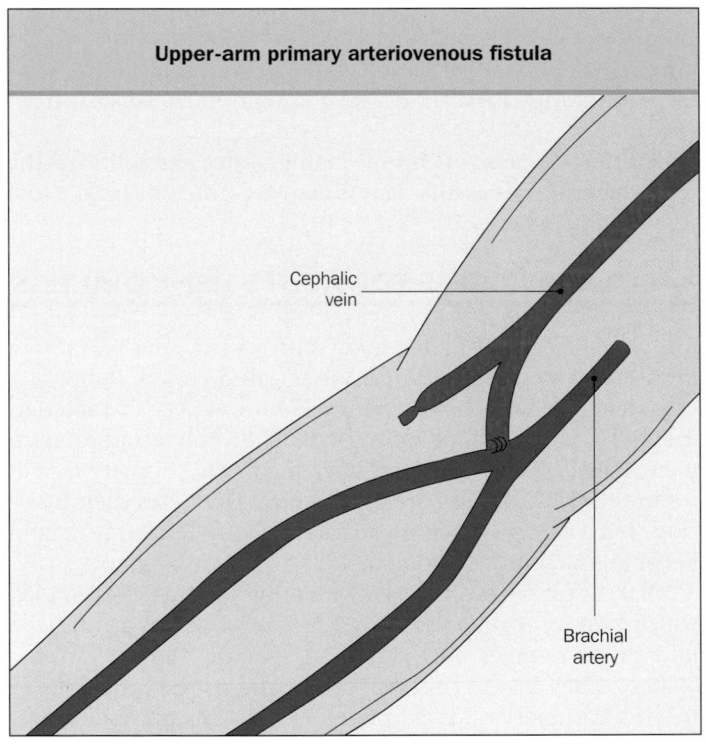

Figure 76.2 Upper-arm primary arteriovenous fistula. Cephalic vein anastomosed to brachial artery.

artery and vein (Fig. 76.3). A graft of this kind accounts for more than 80% of the vascular procedures performed in the USA[5]. In other parts of the world the reverse is the case with more than 80% of patients receiving a primary AV fistula. Recent studies have demonstrated that the use of PTFE grafts is actually increasing rather than decreasing. These discrepancies in the use of primary AV fistulae, between the USA and other parts of the world, have been attributed to the increased age of the dialysis population in the USA and the increased proportion of ESRD patients with diabetes and with poor quality vessels that provide inadequate vascular access, as

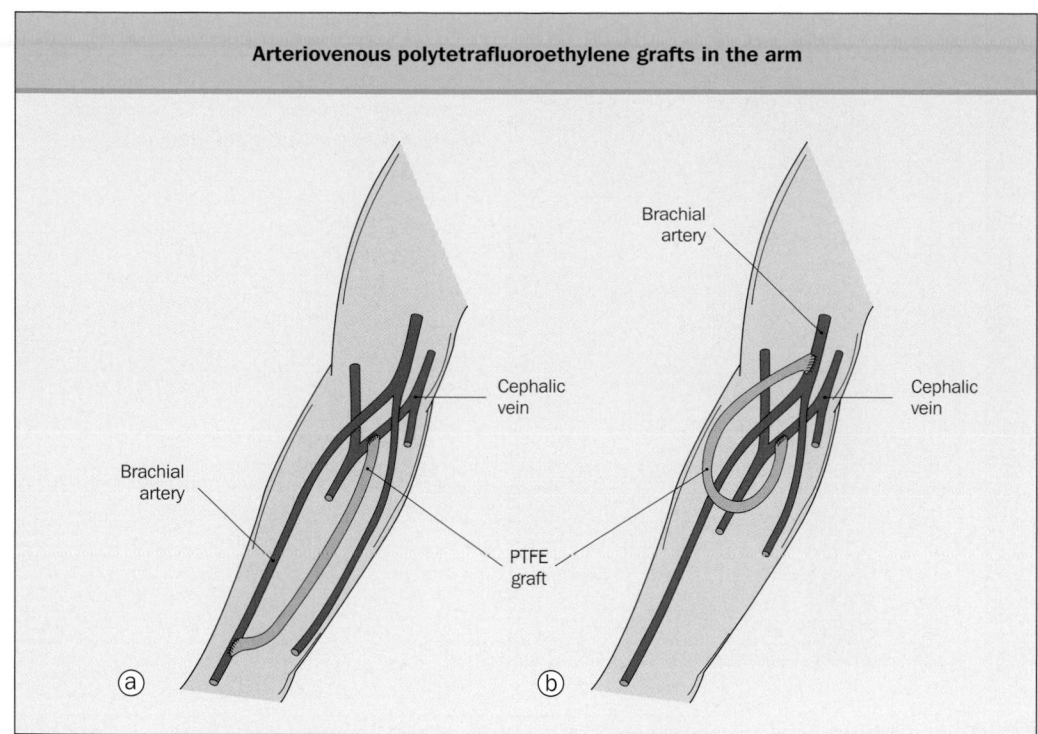

Arteriovenous polytetrafluoroethylene grafts in the arm

Brachial artery

Cephalic vein

Cephalic vein

Brachial artery

PTFE graft

(a)

(b)

Figure 76.3 Arteriovenous polytetrafluoroethylene (PTFE) grafts in the arm. (a) Straight forearm PTFE graft. (b) PTFE loop graft.

well as to the surgical practices that have evolved[6]. More than 40% of patients who present with ESRD in the USA have not had vascular access created prior to the initiation of hemodialysis.

Studies looking at the survival of PTFE grafts show cumulative patency rates for PTFE grafts between 63–90% at 1 year and 50–77% at 2 years; fewer than 50% of synthetic fistulae survive beyond the third year[7]. Most of these studies defined patency as persistent graft function, regardless of whether or not the graft had undergone revision or thrombectomy. Unassisted graft patency (i.e., graft patency without graft revision, thrombectomy, or angioplasty) has been reported to vary between 50% and 70%. The successful use of PTFE grafts for long-term vascular access requires the implementation of a rigorous, prospective intervention-plan. Nonetheless, the intervention rates to maintain this patency level for PTFE grafts are five-fold greater than for native AV fistulae[8].

Newly inserted PTFE grafts should not be cannulated for at least 14 days because adhesion of the subcutaneous tunnel and graft has not yet occurred; otherwise bleeding into the graft tunnel and hematoma formation may ruin the access site.

Prior to the creation of a new vascular access route, it is important to evaluate the patient for possible central vein stenosis. Clinical clues that should raise suspicion include edema in the extremities, collateral vein development, differential size of the extremities, and current or previous placement of a cardiac pacemaker. Complete superior vena caval obstruction may be associated with swelling of the head and neck. If any of these findings are present the patient should undergo venography (Fig. 76.4) or duplex ultrasound. Recently magnetic resonance venography has been introduced for assessment of central venous stenosis[9]. If venous stenosis is identified, it is preferable to plan access for the contralateral side, although we have had occasional success in performing angioplasty on proximal veins and then proceeding with fistula or PTFE graft insertion.

Dual-lumen cuffed tunneled catheters

Although a far inferior choice for vascular access than either a primary AV fistula or PTFE graft, dual-lumen cuffed catheters have assumed an important role in the provision of vascular access for ESRD patients[10,11]. One-year survival of this vascular access technique has been reported to vary between 49% and 75%. These catheters may be employed in a number of circumstances either as a means of initial vascular access while waiting for an AV fistula or graft to mature, or as a bridge between one access route that has failed acutely and the establishment of alternative access. There is also a group of patients in whom all alternative sites have been exhausted. These catheters are most commonly placed in the jugular vein and less commonly in the subclavian vein. They may also be placed for varying periods of time (under extreme circumstances) in the femoral vein, by a transthoracic approach into the superior vena cava, or by a translumbar route into the inferior vena cava. Dual-lumen cuffed catheters can provide adequate blood flows in order to achieve what is now the recommended dose of dialysis: Kt/V 1.3. However, blood flows are inferior to those of either a PTFE graft or primary AV fistula. The LifeSite™ Hemodialysis Access System, which has recently been developed, is a subcutaneously placed valve with an internal pinch clamp that is actuated with a standard 14-guage dialysis needle, connected to a single lumen cannula placed in the central venous circulation[12]. These devices have been demonstrated to provide increased blood flow rates when compared with other cuffed catheters but appear to have equivalent infection rates and are also expensive. The

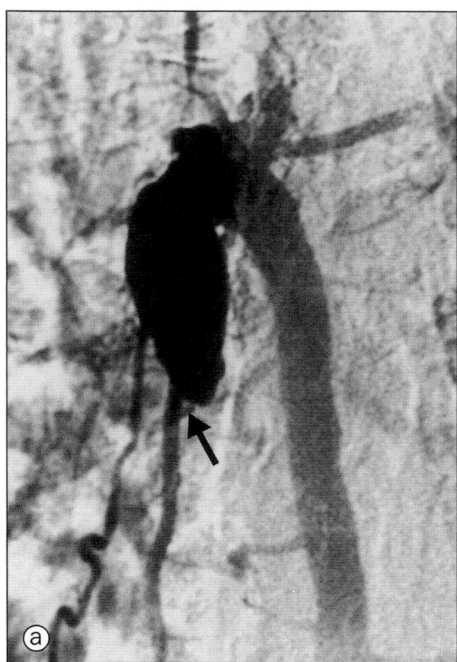

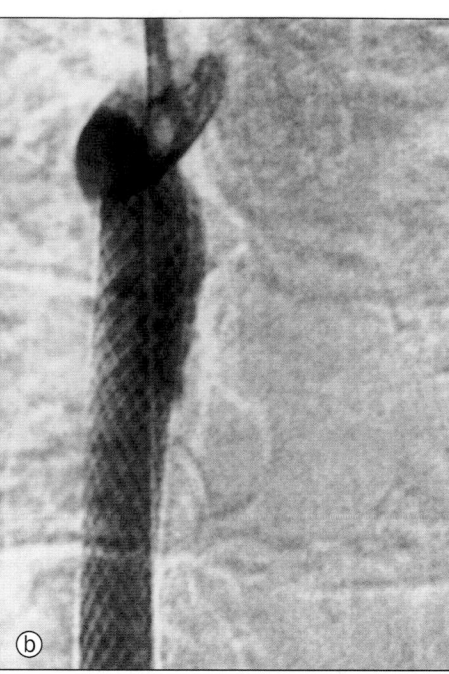

Figure 76.4 Superior vena cava stenosis. Superior vena cava stenosis following temporary subclavial dialysis catheter. (a) Venography showing tight stenosis (arrow). (b) Venography following angioplasty showing stent in situ.

techniques for placement of tunneled catheters and LifeSite devices are discussed in Chapter 77.

Whenever possible, some form of vascular access other than a cuffed catheter should be sought for a patient who has a prognosis of more than 6 months. In our opinion, the cuffed catheter is best used as a bridge between failed access and the establishment of permanent access.

THE PROBLEM OF ACCESS FAILURE

AV access failure

Thrombosis

Thrombosis is the leading cause of AV access loss. Thrombosis that occurs within 1 month of vascular access placement is the result of technical errors in fistula construction or premature use of the access. After the first month, the thrombosis rate is approximately 0.5–0.8 episodes per patient per year. The major predisposing factor to graft thrombosis is anatomic venous stenosis, being responsible for 80–90% of thromboses (see Table 76.1)[3]. The majority of venous stenoses develop within 2–3 cm of the vein graft anastomosis and are the result of progressive, fibromuscular, intimal hyperplasia and perivenous fibrosis. Previous subclavian vein cannulation, particularly if the catheter has become infected, is the major risk factor associated with subclavian vein stenosis. Arterial stenosis accounts for less than 2% of graft failures.

About 10–15% of late access thromboses occur in the absence of an identifiable anatomic lesion. Hypotension, intravascular volume depletion, and prolonged compression of the fistula during sleep or by inexperienced nursing staff may lead to markedly decreased fistula flow and subsequent thrombosis. One of the chief causes of fistula thrombosis, in the absence of identifiable anatomic stenosis, is the use of excessive and prolonged compression by patient or dialysis staff on the site of vascular access in attempting to achieve rapid homeostasis following hemodialysis.

Causes of prosthetic PTFE graft loss	
Thrombosis	
Anatomic etiology	Anastomotic stenosis
	Central venous stenosis
	Intragraft thrombosis
Non-anatomic etiology	'Low-flow' state
	Disturbed procoagulant/anticoagulant equilibrium
	Undetected anatomic lesions
	Polycythemia (relative)
Infection	
Pseudoaneurysm	
Perigraft hematoma or seroma	
'Old age' of the graft	

Table 76.1 Causes of prosthetic PTFE graft loss. Anatomic venous sterosis accounts for 80–90% of graft losses.

Arterial steal

An important complication in the creation of either a synthetic or primary AV fistula is the development of arterial steal, in which the limb distal to the AV fistula is deprived of an adequate blood supply. This complication may result in the development of severe ischemia of the hand with complete loss of function of the limb if not recognized and treated early. Until recently the standard approach was to preserve the function of the limb by ligating the fistula or, if it was apparent that the arterial anastomosis was large, to try a banding procedure to decrease flow through the fistula, although this latter strategy frequently resulted in graft thrombosis. Recently good success and preservation of the fistula access has been reported with the so called DRIL (distal revascularization-interval ligation) procedure, which involves an arterial ligation distal to the AV fistula origin (to eliminate the steal phenomenon) and an arterial bypass graft from above to below the AV fistula (to revascularize the extremity) (Fig. 76.5)[13]. However, it is not always necessary to ligate the artery and the bypass procedure alone may be sufficient. If vascular steal has developed in one limb it is usually unwise to attempt the creation of a new PTFE access in the contralateral limb.

Infection

It is unusual for primary AV fistulae to develop infection; if this does occur it will usually respond rapidly to antibiotic therapy. However, PTFE grafts frequently fail as a result of graft infection. Risk factors for infection include:

- skin pruritus with excoriation
- pseudoaneurysms
- perigraft hematomas from poor needling technique, and
- poor personal hygiene.

With prosthetic material in the vascular access channel it is uncommon to successfully salvage an infected graft with antibiotics alone. It is important that the patient is hospitalized immediately, since infected PTFE grafts are prone to sudden and torrential bleeding. Treatment will include parenteral antibiotics based on sensitivities of any isolated organisms, and surgical exploration. Despite occasional success in salvaging such a graft with local debridement and prolonged antibiotics, removal of the graft is usually required.

PTFE grafts frequently develop pseudoaneurysms from repeated needling. If these are localized, they may be repaired by surgical insertion of a patch in the graft; however, when the graft is older and has developed multiple aneurysms it will need to be replaced.

Catheter failure

The two major reasons for failure of dual-lumen cuffed catheters are thrombosis[14] and infection. In general, thrombosis is avoided by filling the lumen of the catheter (usual volume 1.3 mL) with heparin 5000 U/mL after each dialysis treatment. There are in addition a number of relatively simple strategies that will successfully prolong the life of the catheter when it presents with poor flow. The first approach should be to instil 5000 units of urokinase made up to the volume of the internal lumen of the catheter and leave it for 60 min[10] (Table 76.2). This technique should restore flow to the catheter in approximately 75% of cases. If this is unsuccessful, flow can almost always be restored by infusion of urokinase over 6 h or with the assistance of interventional radiology where contrast is injected to determine if the tip of the catheter has become misplaced or if there is a fibrin sheath enveloping the tip. A gooseneck snare[15] can then be introduced through the femoral vein, and fibrin sheaths can be stripped off the tip of the catheter with restoration of flow in about 95% of cases. Some centers have recently used recombinant tissue plasminogen activator (tPA), 2 mg inserted into each port of the central catheter, as an alternative to urokinase with similar outcomes. An infusion of tPA is also frequently effective when the urokinase or tPA 'lock' has failed[16]. If these techniques are unsuccessful, the catheter may be exchanged over a guide wire. Techniques for catheter insertion and change are discussed in Chapter 77.

The major reason for permanent catheter failure is the high infection rate. We have noted approximately four catheter-related bacteremias per 1000 catheter days. In general the guidelines for treating cuffed-catheter infection are the same as

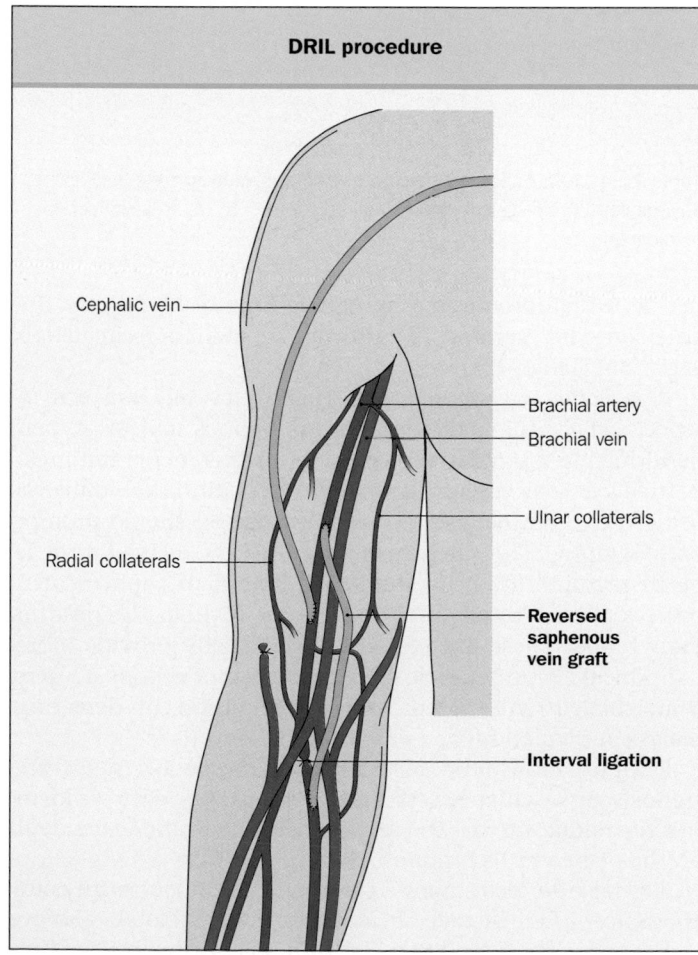

DRIL procedure

Cephalic vein

Brachial artery

Brachial vein

Ulnar collaterals

Radial collaterals

Reversed saphenous vein graft

Interval ligation

Figure 76.5 The DRIL procedure – distal revascularization-interval ligation. This arterial bypass procedure, using a reversed saphenous vein graft from above to below the fistula, corrects the steal phenomenon and allows preservation of the access.

Treatment of cuffed-catheter dysfunction

1. Attempt to aspirate occluded lumen to remove heparin.
2. Inject urokinase, 5000 units diluted in saline to completely fill the occluded lumen of the catheter.
3. Add 0.3 mL of saline and repeat in 10 min to move active urokinase to distal catheter. Leave for 60 min.
4. Aspirate catheter.
5. Repeat if necessary.
6. Urokinase infusion 5000 units over 6 hours.
7. Consider tPA 'lock' or infusion.
8. If unsuccessful, arrange contrast imaging. If imaging confirms fibrin sleeve, proceed with fibrin stripping.

Table 76.2 Treatment of cuffed catheter dysfunction. Practical approach to management of poor flow or occlusion in a cuffed-catheter.

for treating temporary catheter-mediated bacteremia (discussed above). Some authors have reported good success treating catheter-related bacteremia without catheter removal but at our institution attempts to preserve the catheter by prolonged antibiotic treatment only resulted in a 22% catheter salvage rate[17].

The catheter exit site should be inspected at each dialysis: if there is frank pus or erythema, a wound swab and blood should be taken for culture and the patient started on empiric antibiotics, pending culture results.

STRATEGIES TO PROLONG THE LIFE OF AV ACCESS

While a primary AV fistula will in general function for prolonged periods of time and require little effort to maintain function, intensive efforts are required to maintain the long-term function of PTFE grafts. Stenosis at the graft vein anastomosis and subsequent thrombosis accounts for more than 80% of PTFE graft failures. It therefore makes sense to develop strategies to predict prospectively the occurrence of graft thrombosis and arrange early intervention by surgery or endoluminal techniques such as angioplasty to dilate stenoses (discussed in Chapter 77). There are currently four techniques that have proved useful for detecting high-grade venous stenosis.

- Venous dialysis pressure measurement by dynamic and static techniques.
- Urea recirculation.
- Color Doppler scanning.
- Access flow measurement by ultrasound dilution.

Clinical features such as arm edema, pain over the access site, and prolonged bleeding after hemodialysis are relatively non-specific but may also herald impending graft thrombosis.

Pre-emptive correction of venous stenosis with angioplasty or fistula revision reduces thrombosis rates and prolongs access viability[10,18]. In a prospective study the rate of fistula thrombosis among patients, who underwent prospective monitoring for venous stenosis and its treatment once detected, was reduced from 1.4 episodes of fistula thrombosis per patient year to 0.15 episodes per patient year when compared to the rate in those patients who refused such intervention.

It is important to measure dynamic venous dialysis pressure (VDP) according to established protocols as many factors such as the rate of extracorporeal blood flow, the compliance characteristics of the tubing, and needle size can affect this value. VDP should be measured in every patient at the initiation of dialysis for 2 min, using 15- or 16-gauge needles, prior to increasing to maximum blood flow (Table 76.3). A protocol of this kind costs nothing and may be performed at every dialysis treatment. At our institution, using Cobe-Centry 3 dialysis machines, we consider three consecutive VDP values of more than 125 mmHg an indication for fistulography; the threshold for Gambro-AK 10 machines is 150 mmHg. Trends in VDP are more predictive than absolute pressure values.

Access recirculation in hemodialysis occurs when dialyzed blood returning through the venous needle re-enters the extracorporeal circuit through the arterial needle. Recirculation is usually caused by a venous stenosis proximal to the venous

---

Dynamic venous dialysis pressure monitoring

To establish a baseline and trends, initiate measurement when the access is first used.

Measure VDP from the hemodialysis machine at Qb 200 mL/min during the first 2–5 min of hemodialysis at every session.

Use 15 gauge needles (or establish own protocol for different needle size).

Pressure must exceed the threshold three times in succession to be significant.

Three consecutive VDP readings >125 mmHg is an indication for fistulography (using Cobe-Centry 3 machine).

Table 76.3 Dynamic venous dialysis pressure (VDP) monitoring. Careful adherence to protocol is needed to produce predictive data.

Urea based measurement of recirculation

Perform test after approximately 30 min of treatment and after turning off ultrafiltration:

1. Draw arterial (A) and venous (V) line samples.
2. Immediately reduce blood flow rate (BFR) to 200 mL/min.
3. Turn blood pump off exactly 10 s after reducing BFR.
4. Clamp arterial line immediately above sampling port.
5. Draw systemic arterial sample (S) from arterial line port.
6. Unclamp line and resume dialysis.
7. Measure BUN in (A), (V) and (S) samples and calculate percentage recirculation (R):

$$R = \frac{S - A}{S - V}$$

Table 76.4 Urea based measurement of recirculation. Protocol suitable for routine clinical use. R (recirculation) > 5% is an indication for fistulography.

---

needle, which produces a retrograde flow of blood into the arterial needle. A protocol for the measurement of recirculation is given in Table 76.4.

Prospective screening for abnormally elevated urea recirculation will also allow the detection of venous stenosis. When performed in a standardized fashion, urea recirculation prospectively detects venous stenosis. Recirculation exceeding 5% using the recommended two-needle method should prompt fistulography. The measurement of access recirculation is being revolutionized by the development of sophisticated devices to enable this to be carried out without the need to draw blood. These devices will undoubtedly provide more reproducible results and be more predictive of venous stenosis than the currently employed BUN-method of detecting dialysis recirculation[19].

Döppler ultrasound also may be useful for detecting stenosis in vascular access grafts. The major drawbacks of this technique are that the results are variable and dependent on the operator's technique[20].

Several new techniques have been developed to measure access flow. These include ultrasound and hemoglobin dilution techniques using a modified Fick principle. Early observations show that these techniques for determining access flow are more reproducible than assessing Doppler flow: access flows < 600 mL/min are associated with access thrombosis while access flows > 600 mL/min are unlikely to lead to thrombosis.

Indications for fistulography
Graft thrombosis
Prolonged bleeding
Fistula-arm edema
Pain in arm with dialysis
Elevated venous pressures
Increased fistula recirculation
Unexplained decrease in delivered dialysis dose
Decreased access flow
Assessment of fistulae that fail to mature

Table 76.5 Indications for contrast fistulography. Fistulography is the 'gold standard' for defining vascular access anatomy and patency.

A contrast fistulogram is the 'gold standard' for the assessment of vascular access patency as it provides detailed visualization of the fistula lumen, venous anastomosis, and proximal venous system (Table 76.5).

What to do when venous stenosis is detected

Treatment of venous stenosis with at least short-term maintenance of the vascular access channel is important clinically because it preserves other potential sites for future use. Percutaneous transluminal angioplasty, which is an outpatient procedure, corrects over 80% of stenoses in both native and synthetic fistulae and in both venous and arterial outflow tracts[3,4,20]. Pre-emptive angioplasty of a venous stenosis that narrows the lumen by more than 50% improves fistula function and prolongs access survival. Angioplasty can be performed on both anastomotic and more proximal lesions including central stenosis.

Graft function needs to be monitored closely after angioplasty, as recurrence of stenosis is frequent. If the stenosis recurs following angioplasty or shows a poor technical result with angioplasty, then surgical revision of the anastomosis should be considered.

Insertion of an endovascular stent has been widely adopted as a method of preventing recurrent stenosis after angioplasty. However, at this time controlled trials have been unable to demonstrate benefit in most patients[21]. Recent data on sirolimus (rapamycin) coated coronary artery stents have shown a reduction in the neointimal hyperplasia and restenosis. Work is currently underway to look at sirolimus coated vascular access grafts. Techniques for angioplasty and stent placement are discussed in Chapter 77.

Patients who develop recurrent graft thrombosis may be screened for hypercoagulability disorders such as antiphospholipid syndrome and protein-C or protein-S deficiency. However, in the absence of evidence of recurrent thrombosis elsewhere in the body, these tests rarely yield a positive result.

Pharmacologic strategies to prolong access survival

The effect of aspirin and dipyridamole in prolonging time to first thrombosis in PTFE grafts has previously been evaluated[22]. There was a significant reduction in the incidence of graft thrombosis in patients with newly created grafts who were treated with aspirin and dipyridamole compared to those treated with placebo. However, there was no benefit in grafts that had previously thrombosed. The NIH-sponsored Vascular Access Consortium has recently initiated a large, multi-center study to evaluate the effect of dipyridamole on vascular access outcomes[23]. Patients who repeatedly thrombose their AV access without a significant anatomic stenosis seen on fistulography have been treated with low-dose coumadin (warfarin), 1 or 2 mg/d. However, recent controlled trials using 'minidose' warfarin (1 mg/d) have not shown this approach to be effective and anticoagulation in hemodialysis patients is not without significant risk[24]. A recent randomized control trial showed that fish oil significantly decreased risk of graft thrombosis[25].

Treatment of thrombosed vascular access

Once thromboses have developed in a PTFE graft, the therapeutic options include surgical thrombectomy, thrombolytic agents and mechanical dissolution (Fig. 76.6). Interventional radiologic techniques are increasingly used and are discussed further in Chapter 77. However, available data do not yet indicate a clear-cut preference between surgical thrombectomy and revision and percutaneous mechanical or pharmacomechanical thrombolysis[10]. Thrombosis is associated with underlying venous stenosis in more than 85% of instances. It is essential that fistulography is performed rapidly and the

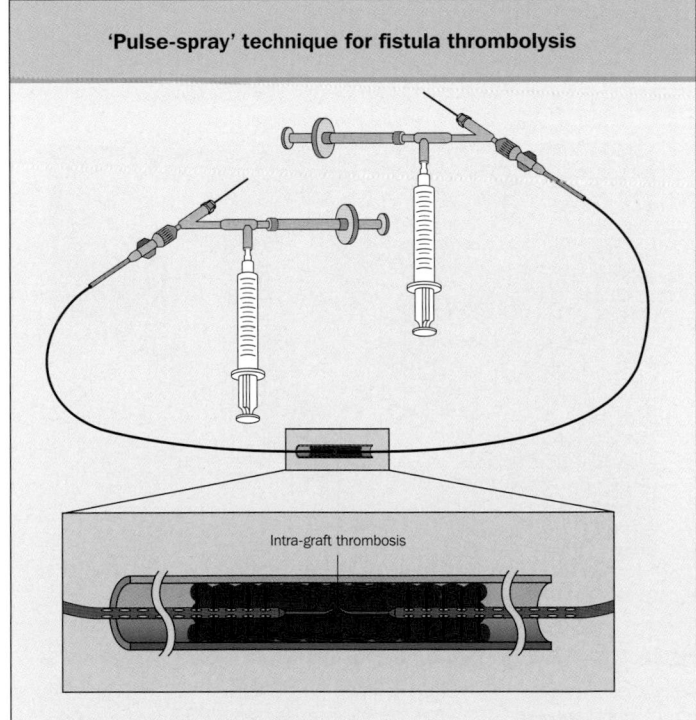

Figure 76.6 'Pulse-spray' techniques for fistula thrombolysis. Two puncture sites are made in ends of the fistula and catheters with multiple side holes are advanced and embedded in either end of the thrombus. The ends of the catheters are occluded with beaded wire. Urokinase is injected into each catheter in small volume increments at two pulses per minute. Lysis-resistant thrombus is then mechanically macerated with a balloon dilatation catheter.

Polytetrafluoroethylene vein graft

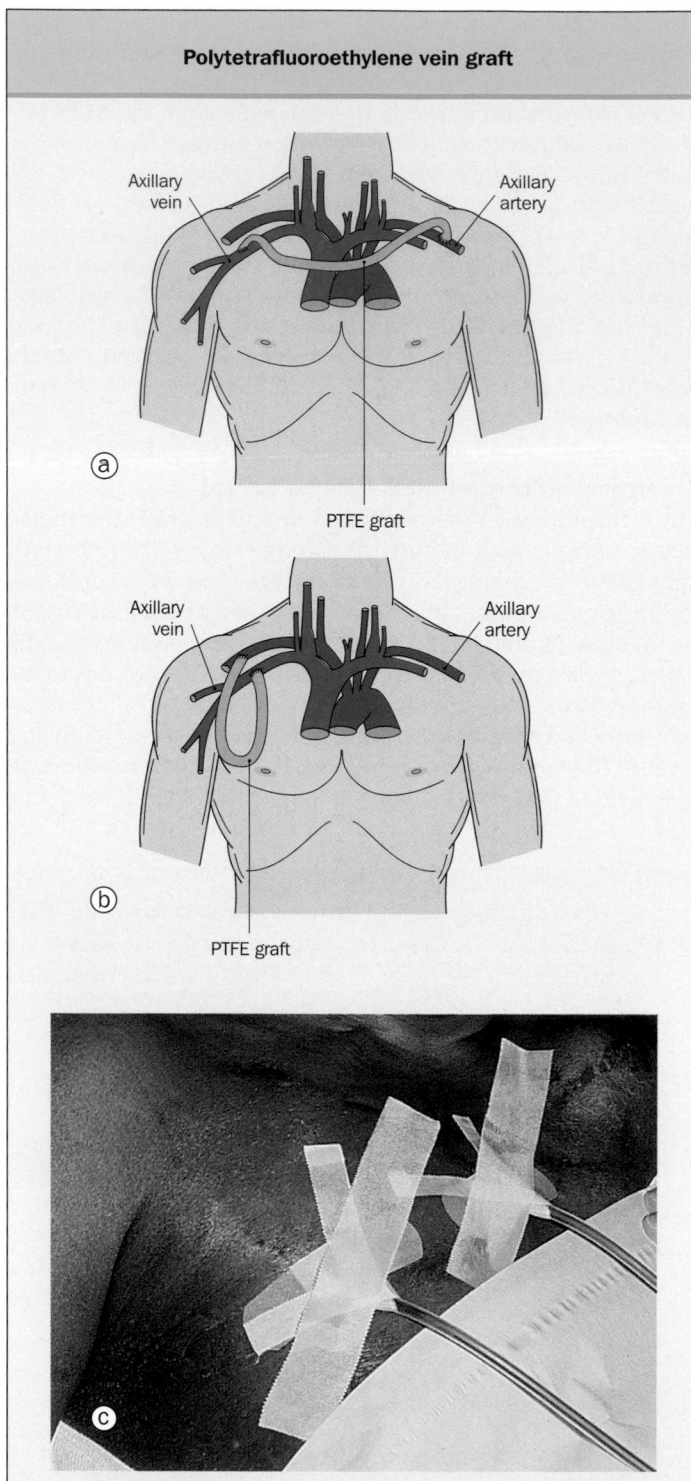

Figure 76.7 Polytetrafluoroethylene (PTFE) vein graft. (a) Ipsilateral axillary artery to contralateral axillary vein PTFE graft. (b) Ipsilateral axillary artery to axillary vein PTFE graft. (c) Axillo-axillary vein PTFE graft in use.

Polytetrafluoroethylene loop graft from femoral artery to femoral vein

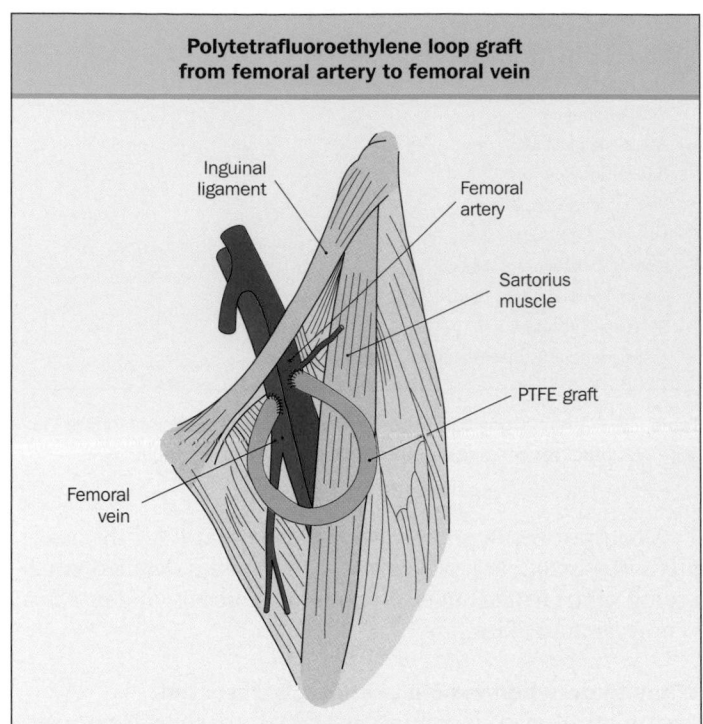

Figure 76.8 Schematic representation of polytetrafluoroethylene loop graft from femoral artery to femoral vein.

use thrombolysis or surgical thrombectomy for occluded PTFE grafts will vary between institutions depending on the relative availability of vascular, radiologic, and surgical expertise.

STRATEGIES FOR THE 'DIFFICULT' PATIENT

In general, the principle when planning vascular access should be 'as distal as possible for as long as possible'. Once sites in both lower and then upper arms have been exhausted for AV fistulae and PTFE grafts, there are a variety of more difficult options.

Our preference for the management of such patients is to create a graft from the axillary artery to the axillary vein on the opposite side. The axillo-axillary graft may also be positioned on one side of the chest (Fig. 76.7). Disadvantages of this approach include:

* difficulty in securing needles on the chest wall
* problems with hemostasis after removal of the dialysis needles
* an unwanted cosmetic result (Fig. 76.7c).

The groin is clearly not a preferred site for angio-access grafts because of increased infection as well as patient discomfort and inconvenience. However, in extreme cases of upper-extremity vascular or infectious complications, a loop thigh PTFE or saphenous vein AV graft may be constructed (Fig. 76.8) or, rarely, an axillo-femoral graft. Prior to the creation of such lower-extremity vascular access grafts, it is critically important to ensure that there is no overt vascular disease present that will place the limb in jeopardy with the shunting of blood through a graft. If all these procedures are exhausted the option of conversion to peritoneal dialysis must always be seriously considered if technically feasible.

underlying stenosis corrected. Failure to do so will result in early recurrence of thrombosis.

At our center, we have similar immediate success with surgery and thrombolysis in opening thrombosed PTFE grafts. However, grafts that have undergone surgical thrombectomy at our center have considerably superior long-term patency. The choice to

REFERENCES

1. Astor BC, Eustace JA, Coresh J, et al. Timing of nephrologist referral and arteriovenous access use in the CHOICE Study. Am J Kidney Dis. 2001;38(3):494–501.

2. Cimino JE, Brescia MJ. The early development of the arteriovenous fistula needle technique for hemodialysis. ASAIO J. 1994; 40:923–7.

3. Lazarus JM, Denker BM, Owen WF. Hemodialysis. In: Brenner BM, ed. The Kidney, 5th edn. Philadelphia, PA: Saunders; 1996: 2424–506.

4. Oliver MJ, McCann RL, Indridason OS, et al. Comparison of transposed brachiobasilic fistulas to upper arm grafts and brachiocephalic fistulas. Kidney Int. 2001;60:1532–9.

5. United States Renal Data System. 2001 Annual Data Report. United States Renal Data System: www.usrds.org.

6. Allon M, Ornt DB, Minda S, et al. Factors associated with the prevalence of arteriovenous fistulas in hemodialysis patients in the HEMO study. Hemodialysis Study Group. Kidney Int. 2000; 58(5):2178–85.

7. Ifadu O, Macey LJ, Homel P, et al. Determinants of type of initial hemodialysis vascular access. Am J Nephrol, 1997;17(5): 425–7.

8. Miller PE, Carlton D, Allon M, et al. Natural history of arteriovenous grafts in hemodialysis patients. Am J Kidney Dis. 2000; 36(1):68–74.

9. Shinde TS, Lee VS, Rofsky NM, et al. Three dimensional gadolinium enhanced MR venographic evaluation of patency of central veins in the thorax: initial report. Radiology. 1999; 213(2):556–60.

10. A report from the vascular access work group of the National Kidney Foundation. Dialysis outcomes quality initiative: clinical practice guidelines for vascular access. Am J Kidney Dis. 1997;30 (suppl 3):S150–89.

11. Schwab SJ, Buller GL, McCann RL, et al. Prospective evaluation of a dacron cuffed hemodialysis catheter for prolonged use. Am J Kidney Dis. 1988;11:166–9.

12. Beathard GA, Posen GA. Initial clinical results with the LifeSite Hemodialysis Access System. Kidney Int. 2000;58:2221–7.

13. Berman SS, Gentile AT, Stokes GK, et al. Distal revascularisation-interval ligation for limb salvage and maintenance of dialysis in ischaemic steal syndrome. J Vasc Surg. 1997;26(3):393–402.

14. Caruana RJ, Raja RM, Zeit RM, et al. Thrombotic complications of indwelling central catheters used for prolonged use. Am J Kidney Dis. 1987;9:497–501.

15. Suhocki PV, Conlon PJ, Knelson MH, et al. Silastic cuffed catheters for hemodialysis vascular access: thrombolytic and mechanical correction of malfunction. Am J Kidney Dis. 1996; 28:379–86.

16. Daeihagh P, Jordan J, Rocco M, et al. Efficacy of tissue plasminogen activator administration on patency of hemodialysis access catheters. Am J Kidney Dis. July 2000;36(1):75–9.

17. Marr KA, Schwab S, Sexton D, et al. Bacteremia in patients with central venous catheters used for hemodialysis: lack of efficacy of catheter salvage. Ann Int Med. 1997;127:275–280.

18. Windus DW, Audrain J, Vanderson R, et al. Optimization of high-efficiency hemodialysis by detection and correction of fistula dysfunction. Kidney Int. 1990;33:719–90.

19. Lindsay RM, Burbank J, Brugger J, et al. A device and a method for rapid and accurate measurement of access recirculation during hemodialysis. Kidney Int. 1996;49:1152–60.

20. Fan PY, Schwab S. Vascular access: concepts for the 1990s. J Am Soc Nephrol. 1992;3:1–11.

21. Beathard G. Gianturco self-expanding stents in the treatment of stenoses in dialysis access grafts. Kidney Int. 1993;43:872–7.

22. Sreedhara R, Himmelfarb J, Lazarus M, et al. Antiplatelet therapy in graft thrombosis; results of a prospective, randomized, double-blind study. Kidney Int. 1994;45:1477–83.

23. National Institute of Health, www.niddk.nihgov/clinical trials.

24. Mokryzycki MH, Jean-Jerome K, Rosenberg SO, et al. A randomized controlled trial of minidose warfarin for the prevention of late malfunction in tunneled cuffed hemodialysis catheters. Kidney Int. 2001;59:1935–42.

25. Schmitz PG, et al. Decreased incidence of vascular access thrombosis in patients taking fish-oil therapy versus placebo. (in press).

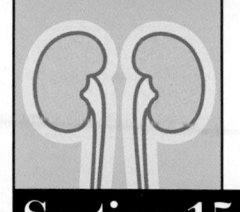

INTRODUCTION

As in other areas of medicine, the practice of nephrology is moving towards less invasive, interventional procedures. Interventional nephrology is gaining in importance and effecting significant changes in clinical management, especially in the establishment and preservation of vascular access for hemodialysis.

Numerous options are now available to provide central venous access for dialysis in patients with end-stage renal disease. While an arteriovenous (AV) fistula is the preferred access route, some patients are unable to support an AV fistula or require an interim 'bridge' access until an AV fistula or polytetrafluoroethylene (PTFE) graft can mature. For these patients, interventional nephrologists provide critical services, including placement of tunneled dialysis catheters and placement of fully-subcutaneous access devices.

Interventional radiologists also provide important services to the full spectrum of hemodialysis patients, including percutaneous management of thromboses and correction of strictures using angioplasty or stents. Percutaneous thrombectomy techniques include injection of saline, infusion of a thrombolytic agent, or mechanical removal of the thrombus. Specialized devices such as the AngioJet allow the interventional nephrologist to aspirate, fragment, and extract the thrombus. Correction of strictures in AV fistulae and grafts can be accomplished by balloon angioplasty or, occasionally, by placement of a stent graft – a thin walled polyester graft material supported by metal stents. Conventional stents are not used frequently, but may be helpful in certain situations such as an expanding aneurysm.

Indications for the appropriate use of procedures such as angioplasty, stent placement and accessory vein obliteration are not yet clearly defined. At present their application will depend on locally available expertise. Clinical studies are awaited which will identify more clearly the role of these procedures in the management of vascular access for hemodialysis.

In the USA, developments in interventional nephrology have been recognized in the recent establishment of an American Society of Diagnostic and Interventional Nephrology. A number of procedures, defined by ASDIN as *basic procedures*, are now routine procedures; these include angiography, angioplasty, placement of both short-term and long-term catheters, and flow restoration in central venous dialysis catheters. Some more complex procedures are defined by ASDIN as *advanced procedures* requiring advanced training; these include endovascular stent placement, accessory vein obliteration, and placement of central venous dialysis catheters and subcutaneous access devices. Society and certification information is available at www.asdin.org. Many of these procedures require a fully equipped endovascular X-ray suite with C-arm fluoroscopic imaging facilities.

TUNNELED DIALYSIS CATHETERS

Role of tunneled dialysis catheters

Hemodialysis requires reliable regular access to the central circulation. The long-term preferred method of vascular access is a primary AV fistula, which has the lowest rates of infection and thrombosis (see Chapter 76). However, establishment of an AV fistula is not always possible, particularly in patients with compromised vasculature and in patients who have been referred late for access creation[1]. Also, an AV fistula requires time to mature – up to several months – and the patient may require dialysis during this process. Tunneled cuffed catheters may be used as 'bridge' devices for this purpose. The tips of these large-diameter catheters are placed in the right atrium, providing faster flow with a lower risk of vessel perforation and erosion. Tunneled dialysis catheters have the advantages of universal applicability, suitability for placement in multiple sites, absence of hemodynamic consequences, immediate usability, ready removal of complicating thrombi and provision of access without venepuncture. Therefore, dialysis catheters can perform adequately as 'bridges' in many patients despite significant disadvantages including the need for fluoroscopy and a sheath for insertion, incompatibility with some drugs, moderate rates of blood flow, thrombosis, and infection[2]. Their clinical utility has led to their growing use for routine dialysis access, particularly in patients initiating hemodialysis and in patients who have exhausted all other access options. A recent US survey showed that as many as 60% of patients beginning dialysis and 30% of those who have received dialysis for longer than 60 days are dialyzed via catheters[3]. This proportion is not ideal and K/DOQI recommends that 50% of patients starting maintenance HD should be using an AV fistula. Nevertheless, tunneled dialysis catheters have a well established role in vascular access.

Site selection

The selection of a site for a tunneled catheter must take into account the risk of complications and the likely need to use a particular site for future access. The preferred location is the right internal jugular vein, which has the advantages of providing a direct route to the right atrium, while carrying a

Dialysis

lower risk of complications, including central venous stenosis, than other upper body sites[4]. Other placement options include the right external jugular vein, the left internal and external jugular veins, and translumbar access to the inferior vena cava; subclavian access should be used only when jugular access is not available[4]. The vein should be punctured under ultrasound guidance, which will demonstrate any anatomic variants and reduce the likelihood of serious complications[5–7].

Catheter selection

Dual-lumen catheters are routinely used. A wide range of dual-lumen catheters is available. One variant in catheter design which is particularly effective is the Ash Split Cath™, which is similar to a dual-lumen catheter, but has a double-D design that allows splitting of the lumens into two separate catheters at the distal tip[8]. A stepdown in the diameter of the tips slightly increases the pressure drop, ensuring flow through all the sideholes at almost any blood flow rate. The tips must be separated before the catheter is inserted.

Insertion technique

The patient is positioned on the X-ray table in a slight Trendelenburg position, and the procedure performed under local anesthesia (Fig. 77.1). A hand-held sonography transducer is used to determine the patency of the internal jugular vein and the positions of the carotid artery and sternomastoid muscle. A lateral approach to the internal jugular vein and the sternomastoid muscle or sternomastoid triangle is recommended.

An 18-gauge or a 21-gauge needle is guided into the internal jugular vein under sonographic control, and a guidewire is positioned in the superior vena cava under fluoroscopy and then passed into the right atrium and, preferably, the inferior vena cava. A subcutaneous catheter pocket is developed of sufficient size to prevent formation of kinks in the catheter as it forms a horizontal loop in the neck. A catheter of appropriate length is chosen. Typically, a 28 cm or 32 cm catheter (measured from tip to cuff) is utilized on the right side; placement in the left internal jugular vein usually requires a 32 cm or 36 cm catheter. The exit site is supraclavicular or infraclavicular, depending on previous catheter placement(s) and the patient's body habitus. A stab wound is made laterally from the exit site, and a route tunneled to the catheter pocket with a metal tunneling tool, which then engages with the catheter, and the catheter is pulled through the subcutaneous tunnel. A series of dilators is then passed over the guidewire, followed by the split sheath introducer under fluoroscopic control to avoid injury to the central blood vessels. The dilator and guidewire are then removed while exerting a tight pinch on the introducer to prevent air embolus. The patient should not breathe during this time, but may perform a Valsalva maneuver. The introducer is kept above the level of the skin as the catheter is advanced through the superior vena cava into the right atrium. Fluoroscopy is used to confirm placement, to ensure that the arterial lumen of the catheter remains in the right atrium during a deep breath, and that the venous tip does not buckle against the inferior wall of the atrium during

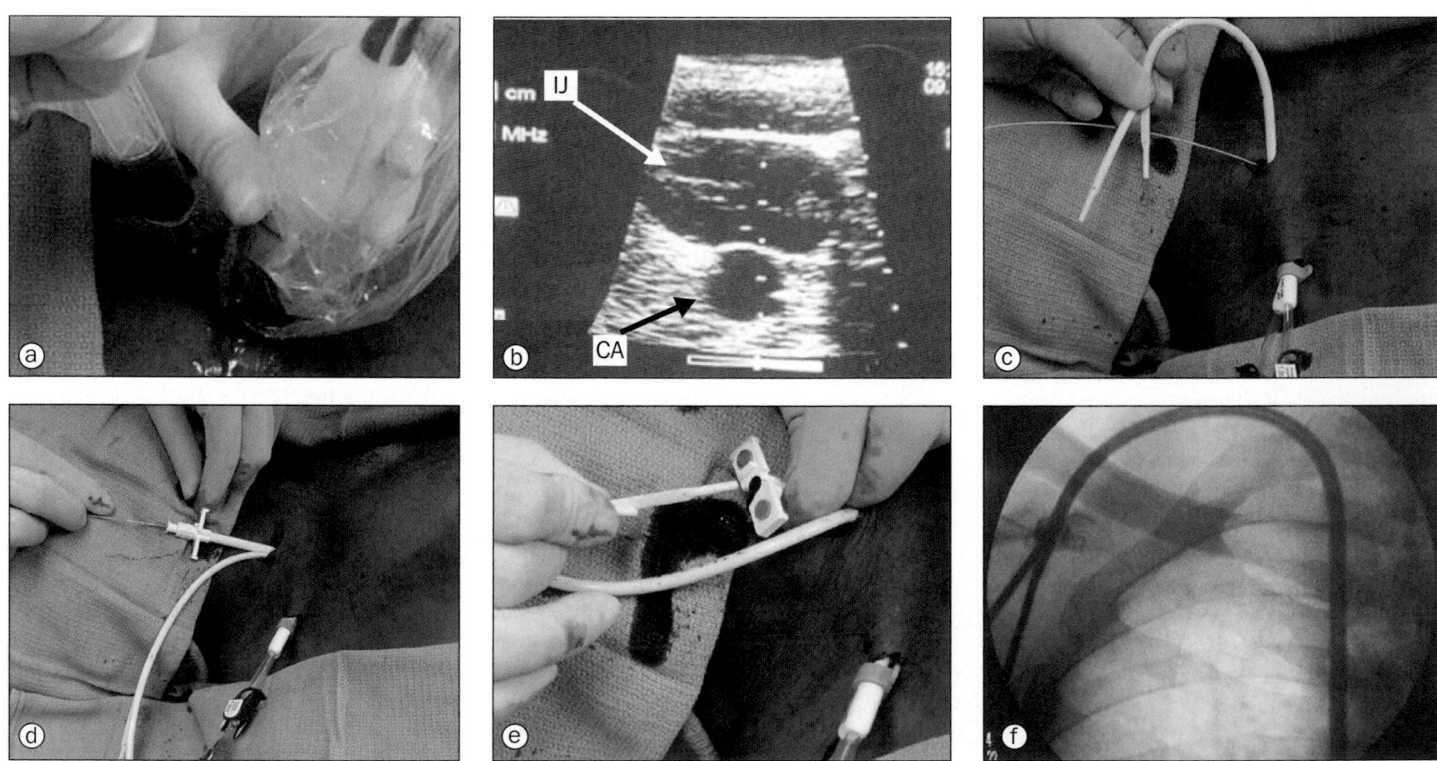

Figure 77.1 Insertion of the Ash Split Cath™. (a,b) Hand-held sonography is used to assess internal jugular vein (IJ), carotid artery (CA) and sternomastoid muscle. (c) Pulling the catheter through the subcutaneous tunnel from the pocket to the exit site. (d) Tunnel is dilated and the split sheath introducer is passed. (e) Final steps in insertion of the Ash Split Cath include pinching to prevent air embolus. (f) Fluoroscopy confirms absence of catheter kinking.

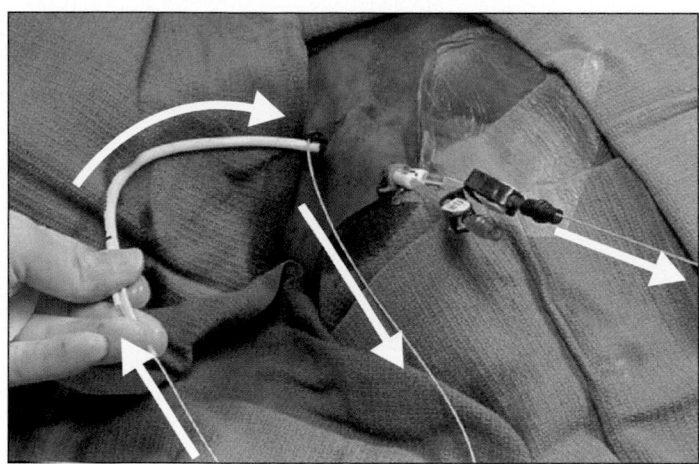

Figure 77.2 Technique of tunneled dialysis catheter exchange.
Cutdown is created proximal to the cuff and a guidewire is passed through
the cut catheter via the right atrium into the inferior vena cava. The new
catheter is exchanged over the guidewire. A new tunnel has been created
with the exit site tunneled into the established catheter pocket.

expiration. If difficulty is encountered identifying the catheter,
contrast medium may be infused. Fluoroscopy is used to
confirm that there is no kink in the catheter from the neck
incision and that the exit site position is adequate without
impingement or kinking.

Catheter exchanges

Catheter exchanges (Fig. 77.2) can be performed by a cutdown proximal to the cuff on the previous catheter. A
guidewire is passed into the cut portion of the catheter
through the right atrium to the level of the inferior vena
cava. A new exit site is tunneled to the previously created
catheter pocket. A weave technique is used, with a guidewire
being passed through the end opening of the venous limb,
out through a sidehole of the venous limb, and then through
the arterial limb end. The new catheter is then passed over
the guidewire into the right atrium, as in primary placement.
Fluoroscopy is used to confirm that there is no kinking of the
catheter in the neck and that it is positioned appropriately.

Catheter care

Care of tunneled catheters to minimize infection risk and the
prompt active treatment of suspected infection are crucial
for their optimal effectiveness and safety. These issues are
discussed further in Chapter 76.

SUBCUTANEOUS HEMODIALYSIS ACCESS DEVICES

The development of fully-implantable subcutaneous vascular
access devices is a recent innovation in vascular access[9]. The
LifeSite® Hemodialysis Access System consists of two tita-
nium-alloy subcutaneous valves with connecting silicone cannulae – one for blood draw and one for blood return – that are
placed in a central vein, preferably the right internal jugular
vein[9–12]. The cannulae are tunneled to the valves, which are
implanted side-by-side or staggered in separate subcutaneous

tissue pockets, typically below the clavicle. The subcutaneous
placement, unique internal design, and ability to perform *in
vivo* disinfection of the valve, valve pocket and buttonhole
needle tract, support higher blood flow rates and lower rates
of infection and thrombosis with the LifeSite System compared with a standard tunneled dialysis catheter[13–15]. These
properties make the LifeSite System an excellent alternative as
a 'bridge' device[16].

Insertion of the LifeSite system

Cannula insertion (Fig. 77.3) is performed using real-time
ultrasound guidance to minimize the possibility of insertion-
related complications (e.g., pneumothorax, air embolism,
hemothorax, cardiac arrhythmia) that can result from operator error. An introducer needle is inserted into the selected
vein site, and a guidewire advanced into the inferior vena
cava under fluoroscopic control. This procedure is repeated
for placement of the second guidewire into the same vein
about 0.5 cm above or below the first guidewire. The upper
guidewire should be used for the return cannula, so that the
cannulae do not cross each other. The split sheath introducer
is inserted over the guidewire, which is then removed. The
access cannula is inserted into the vein, the sheath removed,
and the placement of the cannula tip confirmed with fluoroscopy. The second cannula is placed using the same procedure.

The valve pockets (below the clavicle) are created in an area
that will not interfere with shoulder movement or clothing
straps. The valves should be placed with the upper surface
between 10 mm and 15 mm below the skin surface. If too
deep, there may be difficulties in cannulating the valves for
hemodialysis; if too shallow, insufficient tissue over the valves
may eventually lead to skin erosion.

The medial valve is connected to the cannula used for draw,
and the lateral valve is connected to the cannula used for
return. The lateral valve should be placed first, to ensure that
both valves will lie flat on the front of the chest. The valve cannulation site is 1 to 2 cm from the incision used to create the
pockets. A subcutaneous tunnel for each cannula is created
and extended to the corresponding valve pocket. Both cannula tips should be placed in the right atrium; the draw cannula tip should be placed about 2 cm above the return cannula
tip. Once the cannula tip placement has been confirmed, the
cannula can be trimmed to the appropriate length, allowing for
body movement, and connected to the valve. The valve is
secured to the fascia with nonabsorbable sutures to reduce the
risk of valve migration or rotation.

PERCUTANEOUS THROMBECTOMY

Most flow problems in established dialysis accesses are the
result of intrinsic thrombi. Several options are available to
restore flow[17]. The simplest is forceful injection of saline. If
this fails, instillation or infusion of a thrombolytic agent such
as urokinase, tissue plasminogen activator or a glycoprotein
IIb/IIIa inhibitor may be attempted. A faster treatment option
is mechanical destruction or retrieval of the thrombus with a
guidewire, Fogarty catheter, ureteral biopsy brush, or specialized device such as the AngioJet® System. A further alternative
is a combined mechanical and pharmacological approach,

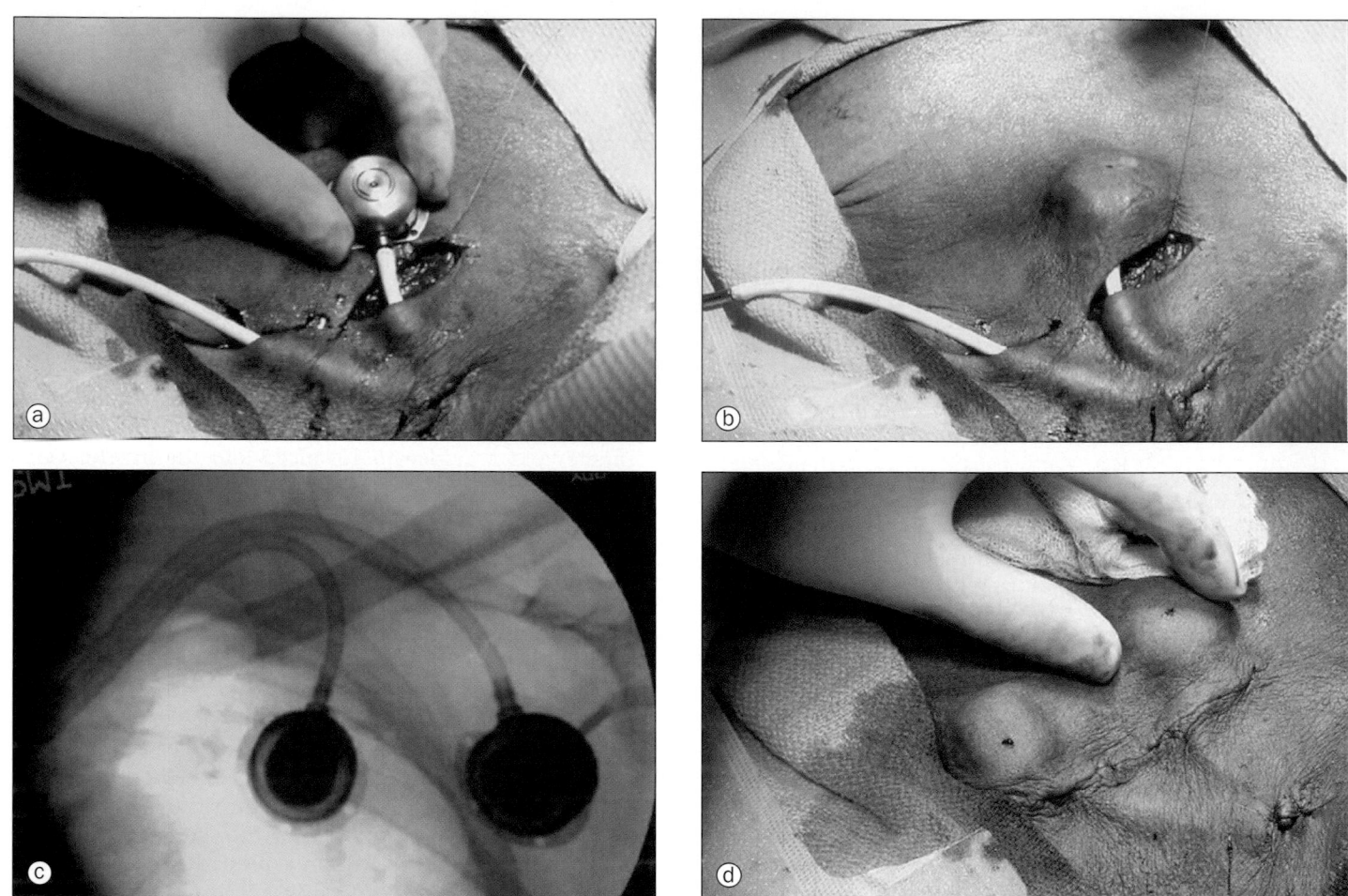

Figure 77.3 Implantation of the LifeSite® Hemodialysis Access System. Cannulae are inserted over guidewires advanced into the inferior vena cava under fluoroscopic control. (a) After cutting cannula to appropriate length, the cannula is connected to the LifeSite valve. (b) Valve is placed in tissue pocket; the flat base is secured to the underlying fascia to reduce risk of valve rotation or migration. (c) Fluoroscopy of LifeSite valves confirms proper placement. (d) Subcutaneous tissue and skin are closed. The LifeSite System is immediately ready for access by simple cannulation with a 14-gauge needle.

such as the 'pulse-spray' technique (Fig. 76.6). The advantage of a purely mechanical technique such as the AngioJet System is that risk of hemorrhage is minimized without thrombolytic agents.

Thrombectomy with the AngioJet System is accomplished using high-velocity saline jets that create localized suction at the catheter tip (Bernoulli principle), causing rapid lysis and removal of the thrombus through an exhaust lumen. The process is also known as 'rheolytic thrombectomy.' Clinical trials have demonstrated excellent results in saphenous vein grafts and coronary arteries[18]. In a prospective evaluation of rheolytic thrombectomy of thrombosed hemodialysis access grafts with the AngioJet System, recanalization was achieved in all of 18 patients without the need for adjunctive thrombolysis or surgical cutdown to complete the thrombolytic procedure, There was ≥ 50% luminal restoration in 83%; < 50% luminal restoration in 17%; following balloon angioplasty (all patients) there was no residual thrombus in 87% of patients[19].

At this time, there have been no controlled trials comparing the outcomes of different thrombectomy techniques. Choice of technique therefore depends on the local availability of expertise.

Technique for the AngioJet System

The procedure is minimally invasive, rapid, and can be performed in an outpatient setting using local anesthesia. Here it is described as applied to physical removal of thrombus from a PTFE forearm graft (Fig. 77.4a,b). Under local anesthesia the arterial side of the graft is cannulated with an 18-gauge cannula oriented toward the venous anastomosis through which is passed a guidewire followed by an introducer. If there is uncertainty whether the limb is arterial or venous, a catheter may be introduced and contrast medium injected. If the entry has been made into arterial limb, the same technique can be utilized for placement of an introducer across the venous anastomosis. The AngioJet catheter is inserted, and slow (1–2 mm/s) passes are made across the thrombosed segment until all filling defects have been removed. If the arterial thrombus cannot be removed with the AngioJet System, an embolectomy catheter may be used to pull clot into the graft for maceration with the angioplasty balloon. The absence of thrombus or stricture is confirmed by contrast radiography. If any stricture is found it must be corrected to prevent prompt recurrence of thrombosis.

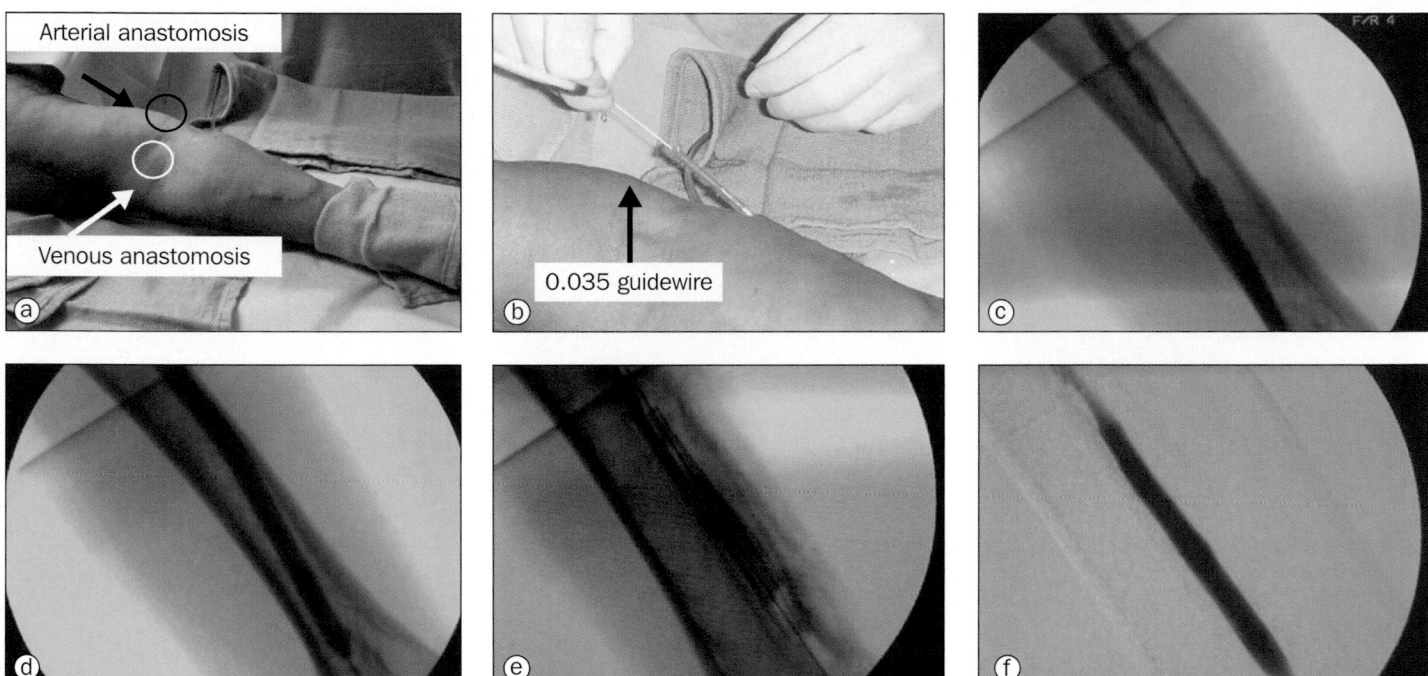

Figure 77.4 A combination of techniques used to restore flow in a PTFE forearm graft and mid upper arm basilic vein. (a) Standard aseptic technique and identification of the arterial and venous anastomoses of the graft prior to performing percutaneous rheolytic thrombectomy with the AngioJet System. (b) The arterial side of the graft is cannulated with an 18-gauge cannula oriented toward the venous anastomosis. (c) After restoring flow in the forearm graft using the AngioJet System, a high-grade stricture in the basilic vein (mid upper arm) was identified. (d) Attempt to correct the stricture with angioplasty. (e) Angioplasty resulted in rupture of the basilic vein. (f) A stent is placed to stop extravasation

At the end of the procedure, excellent thrill and bruit should be documented, the radial and ulnar should be evaluated by palpation or sonography, and good capillary refill of the hand should be noted. It is also very important to image the superior vena cava, subclavian vein, axillary vein, and upper arm veins to ensure there is no significant proximal stenosis. The graft and brachial artery should also be imaged.

CORRECTION OF STRICTURE

Angioplasty

Angioplasty is a widely used technique for relieving strictures in PTFE grafts and AV fistulae, just as in native blood vessels. However, these strictures can be resistant to dilatation.

Typical strictures in a PTFE graft extend from the venous anastomosis with endothelial hyperplasia (Fig. 77.5a). Angioplasty is achieved with an angioplasty balloon inserted over a guidewire and insufflated to a pressure of 20 to 22 atmospheres (Fig. 77.5b,c); various balloon sizes are available. Immediately after successful angioplasty, or else following arterialization of the graft, the superior vena cava, subclavian vein, and axillary vein in the upper arm should be imaged to establish patency of the venous system from the superior vena cava to the arterial anastomoses, particularly if the patient has had previous central venous catheters. Figure 77.6 shows another high-grade stricture of the basilic vein. Balloon angioplasty was performed

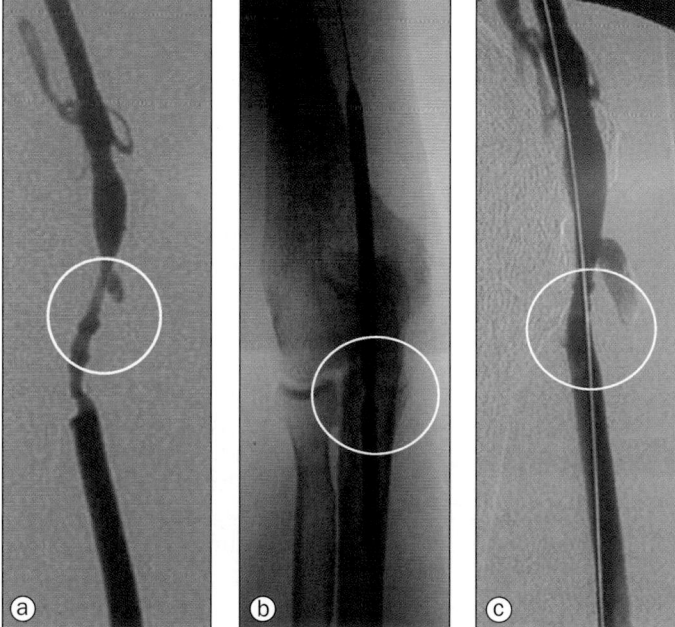

Figure 77.5 Angioplasty for relief of venous anastomotic stricture in a PTFE graft. (a) Typical stricture in a PTFE graft extending from the venous anastomosis with endothelial hyperplasia. (b) The angioplasty balloon has been inserted over a guidewire passed through the stricture. (c) Outcome of successful angioplasty (guidewire is shown remaining *in situ*).

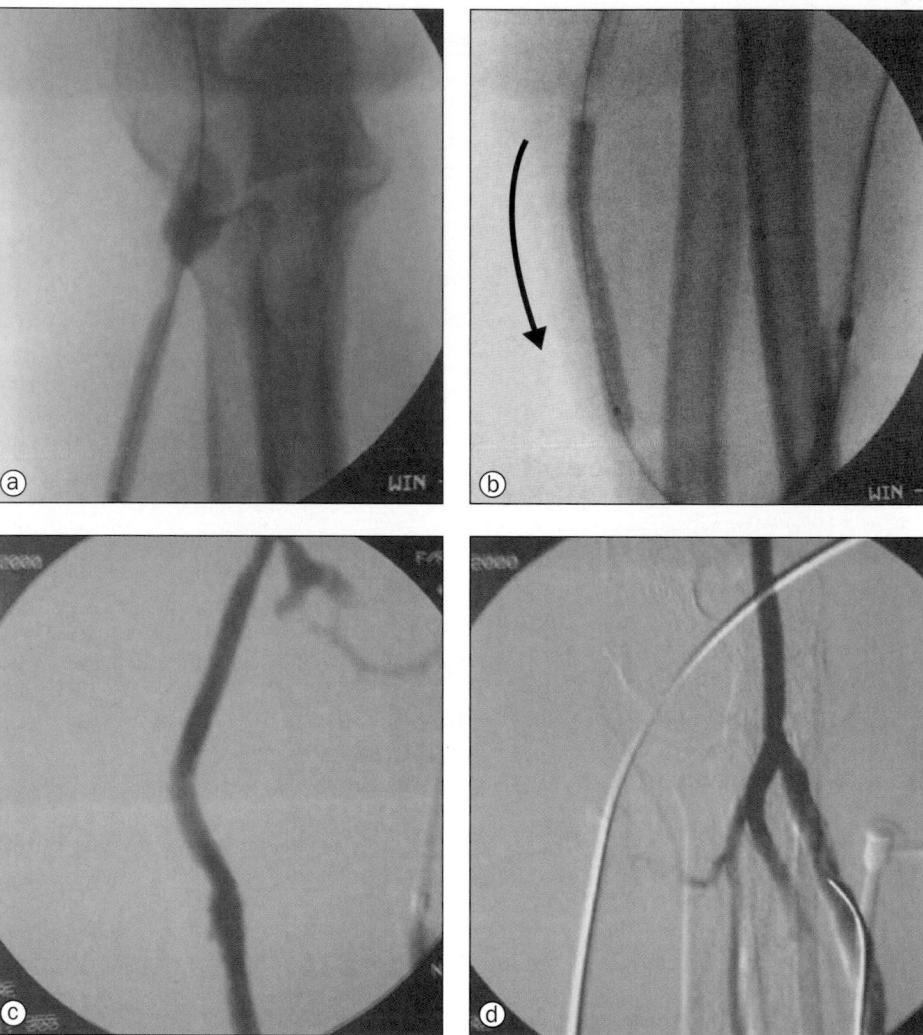

Figure 77.6 High-grade basilic vein stricture corrected with balloon angioplasty. (a) Angioplasty of venous outlet. (b) The 'pull back procedure' was performed with good effect (arrow indicates direction of balloon insertion). (c) View of the venous outflow post-thrombectomy, post-angioplasty. (d) View of post-thrombectomy inflow from the brachial artery.

with favorable results as demonstrated by unobstructed venous outflow and post-thrombectomy inflow from the brachial artery (Fig. 77.6c,d).

Stents

Endovascular stents are utilized very sparingly in AV fistulae and PTFE grafts, although there are certain situations in which they may be very helpful. At this time, controlled trials have been unable to demonstrate benefit in most patients. Recent data on sirolimus (rapamycin) coated coronary artery stents have shown a reduction in neointimal hyperplasia and restenosis; it is not yet known if such coated stents offer similar benefits in vascular access. As a rule, stents are not placed in areas that might be in an operative field at a later date. The

decision to deploy a stent will be influenced by local expertise in interventional techniques.

A stent has particular utility when there is frequent recurrence of an elastic stricture. An example of the successful use of a stent graft to correct a recurrent high-grade stricture in an upper arm PTFE graft is shown in Figure 77.7. When angioplasty alone does not lead to sustained success, other options for graft salvage include surgical revision with a patch or a jump graft, or placement of a stent.

There may also be some indications for stent graft placement in an expanding aneurysm (Fig. 77.8). Where surgical intervention for a painful aneurysm is not appropriate, a stent graft can be utilized to control its expansion. Such a procedure is somewhat controversial but may be used in urgent situations.

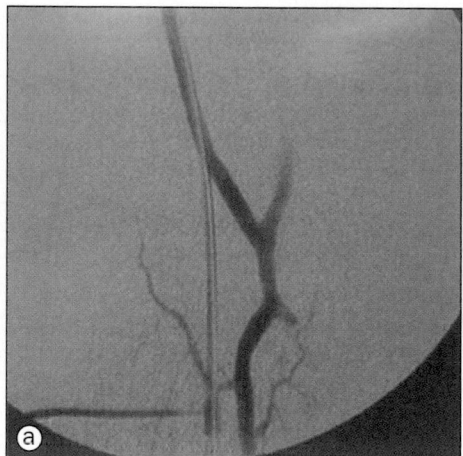

Figure 77.7 High-grade stricture in an upper arm PTFE graft, corrected with a stent graft. The patient had numerous difficulties with an elastic stricture that frequently recurred. (a) Arterial anastomosis showing needle and passage of guidewire. (b) View of a high-grade stricture associated with apparent kinking of the basilic vein into the axillary vein (arrowed). (c) Stent graft (8 mm x 4 mm) deployed over guidewire shown without contrast. (d) Stent graft in position with guidewire still in position showing correction of stricture.

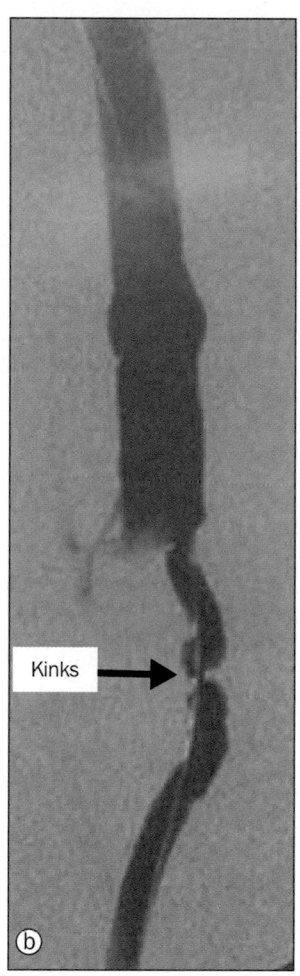

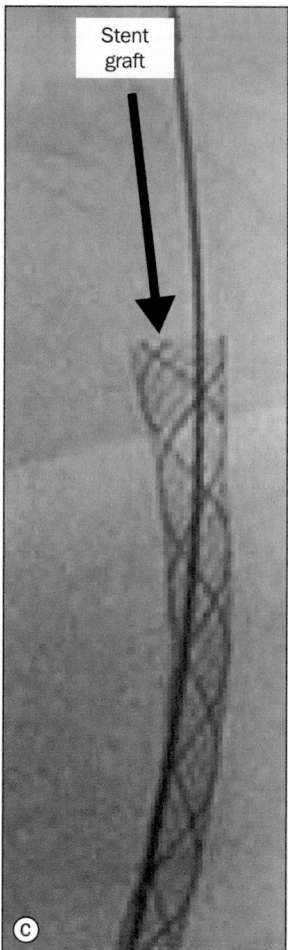

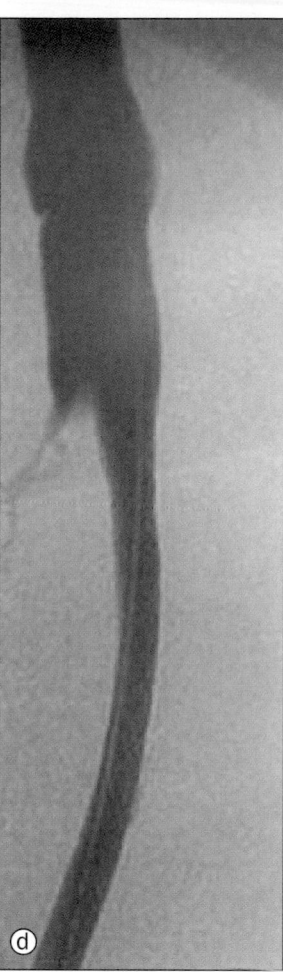

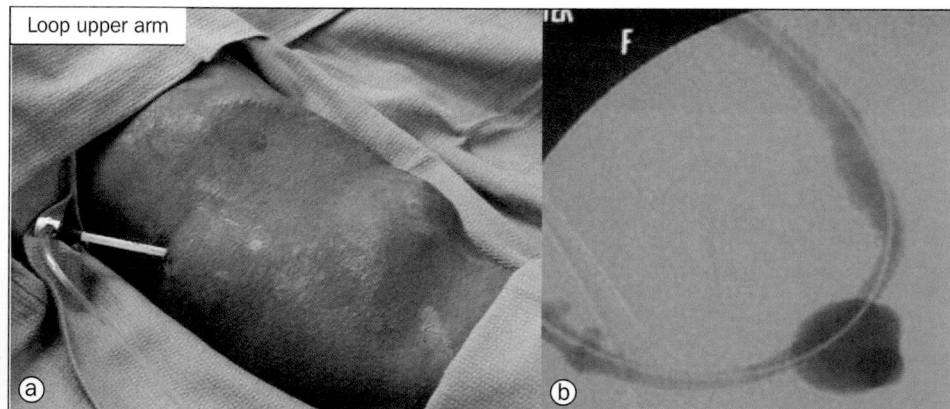

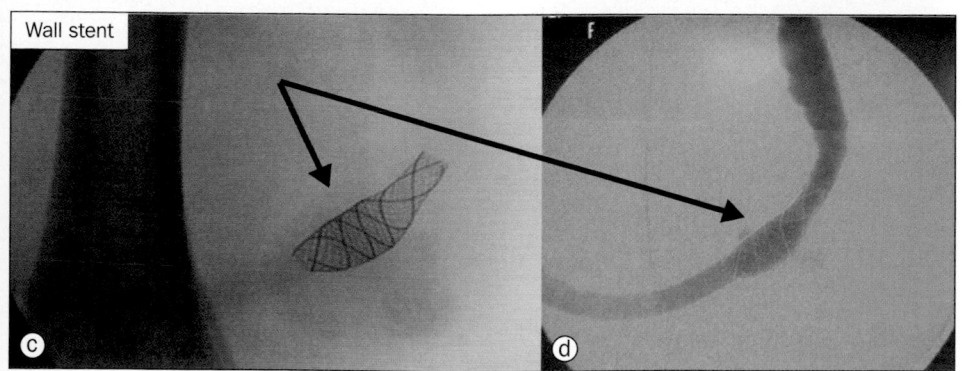

Figure 77.8 Placement of a stent graft in an expanding painful aneurysm. The patient desired to avoid surgery, so a stent graft was used to control the expansion of the aneurysm. (a) Loop graft cannulated for stent deployment. Aneurysmal area of the graft is apparent (arrowed). (b) Large aneurysm on graft. (c) Stent deployed and shown without contrast. (d) Aneurysm has been controlled by the stent.

REFERENCES

1. Butterly DW, Schwab SJ. Catheter access for hemodialysis: an overview. Semin Dial. 2001;14:411–15.
2. Ash SR. The evolution and function of central venous catheters for dialysis. Semin Dial. 2001;14:416–24.
3. Tanriover B, Carleton D, Saddekni S, et al. Bacteremia associated with tunneled dialysis catheters: comparison of two treatment strategies. Kidney Int. 2000;57:2151–5.
4. National Kidney Foundation. NKF-K/DOQI clinical practice guidelines for vascular access: Update 2000. Am J Kidney Dis. 2000;37(Suppl 11):S137–81.
5. Caridi JG, Hawkins IF, Weichmann BN, et al. Sonographic guidance when using the right internal jugular vein for central venous access. Am J Roentgenol. 1998;171:1259–63.
6. Denys BG, Uretsky BF, Reddy PS. Ultrasound-assisted cannulation of the internal jugular vein. Circulation. 1993;87:1557–62.
7. Teichgraber UKM, Benter T, Gebel M, Manns MP. A sonographically guided technique for central venous access. Am J Roentgenol. 1992;169:731–3.
8. Conz PA, Crepalki C, LaGreca G. Slow maturation of arteriovenous fistula in seven uremic patients: use of Ash Split Cath as temporary, prolonged vascular access. J Vasc Access. 2000;1:51–3.
9. Moran JE. Subcutaneous vascular access devices. Semin Dial. 2001;14:452–7.
10. Beathard GA, Posen GA. Initial clinical results with the LifeSite® Hemodialysis Access System. Kidney Int. 2000;58:2221–7.
11. Buerger T, Gebauer T, Meyer F, Halloul Z. Implantation of a new device for haemodialysis. Nephrol Dial Transplant. 2000;15:722–4.
12. Ross JR. Clinical outcomes of four hemodialysis patients implanted with the LifeSite® Hemodialysis Access System: a novel approach for vascular access. In: Henry ML, ed. Vascular Access for Hemodialysis. Vol. VII. Chicago, Illinois: WL Gore & Associates and Precept Press; 2001:109–21.
13. Schwab SJ, Weiss MA, Fushton F, et al. Multicenter clinical trial results with the LifeSite® Hemodialysis Access System. Kidney Int. 2002; in press.
14. Haynes BJ, Quarles AW, Vavrinchik J, et al. The LifeSite® Hemodialysis Access System – implications for the nephrology nurse. Nephrol Nurs J. 2002;29:27–33.
15. Rosenblatt M, Stainken B, Wesiss MA, Caridi JA. LifeSite totally implanted HD system versus Tesio Cath: Results of a comparative trial (abstract). J Vasc Interv Radiol. 2002;13(2):S39.
16. Ross J. Bridging to a high flow upper arm native fistula for hemodialysis with the LifeSite® hemodialysis access system. J Vasc Access. 2001;2:139–44.
17. Beathard G. Catheter thrombosis. Semin Dial 2001; 14:441–5.
18. Kuntz RE, Baim DS, Cohen DJ, et al. A trial comparing rheolytic thrombectomy with intracoronary urokinase for coronary and vein graft thrombus (the Vein Graft AngioJet Study (VeGAS 2)). Am J Cardiol. 2002;89:326–30.
19. Ross JR, Settum CM. Percutaneous recanalization of thrombosed hemodialysis access grafts using rheolytic thrombectomy: single-center experience. South Med J. 2000;93:S93–4.

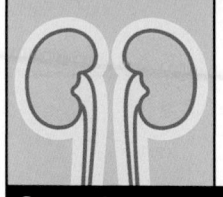

Chapter 78

Hemodialysis: Mechanisms, Outcome, and Adequacy

Ken Farrington, Roger Greenwood and Suhail Ahmad

INTRODUCTION

Successful maintenance hemodialysis was established in the 1960s. The principles of dialysis had been known for many years and its application in patients with acute renal failure had been demonstrated. Some key developments opened the door to its widespread adoption for the treatment of end-stage renal disease (ESRD). Heparin, a convenient and effective anticoagulant was already available, as was cuprophane, a membrane prepared from cellulose, which had good diffusional characteristics for urea and other small molecules. It was fortunate that its permeability to water was just enough to allow slow fluid removal from blood during dialysis (ultrafiltration) without the risk of volume depletion while using a rudimentary extracorporeal circuit. Perhaps the most important step however was the development of adequate vascular access, first the arterio-venous (AV) Scribner shunt, and then the natural AV fistula, which provided reliable, repeated access to the circulation with minimal risk of infection and thrombosis.

Even though transplantation and peritoneal dialysis subsequently appeared as successful therapies, hemodialysis (HD) remains the default therapy for all patients with ESRD and it is estimated that some one million patients worldwide are currently receiving this treatment. While there have been important technical advances, they have been relatively minor compared to the changes in dialysis schedules, the prescription and quantification of dialysis and the case-mix profile of the patients receiving the treatment.

THE DIALYSIS SYSTEM

The components of the dialysis system are illustrated in Figure 78.1. The patient's blood is circulated in a simple extracorporeal circuit and passed along one side of a semi-permeable membrane. Dialysis fluid passes along the other side of the membrane in the opposite direction (countercurrent) to optimize diffusion gradients.

The main role of the dialysis machine is to supply dialysis fluid with the intended flow rate, temperature and chemical content in a fail-safe manner. The machine mixes a pre-prepared 'concentrate' of electrolytes with treated water to produce dialysis fluid. It also removes a prescribed volume of ultrafiltrate during the dialysis session. Each machine is dedicated to a single patient but with appropriate 'disinfection' is available to treat others. Typically there are 12–30 machines in a dialysis unit, each treating three to four patients a day. Each machine receives treated water from a central water purification plant. Less commonly, machines may have their own water treatment unit.

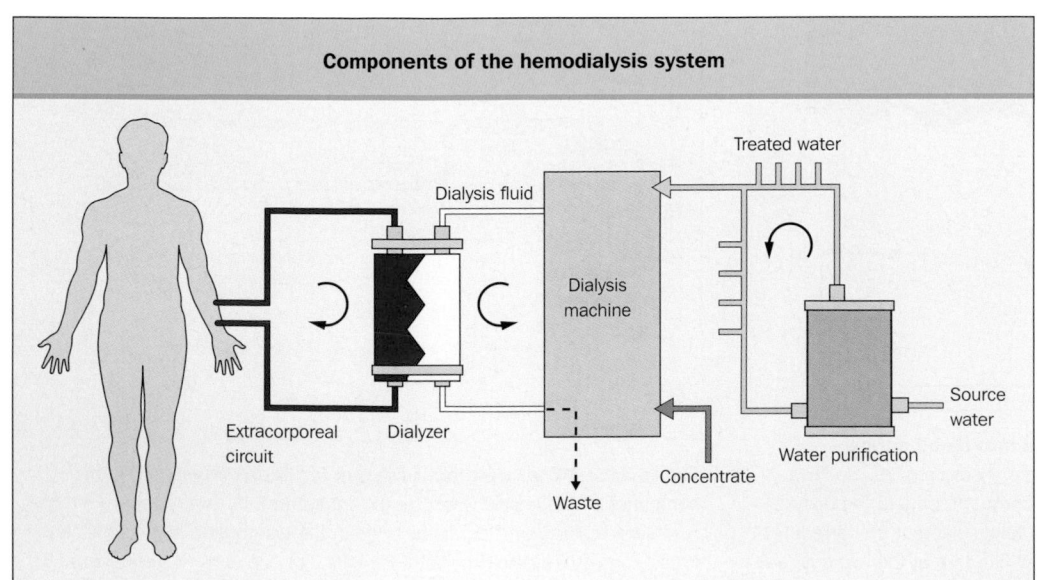

Components of the hemodialysis system

Figure 78.1 Components of the hemodialysis system.

WATER AND DIALYSIS FLUID

Background

In the 1960s, dialysis fluid, with bicarbonate as the base counteracting the acidosis of uremia, was prepared in a large mixing tank and circulated through the renal unit. The introduction of proportionating systems that mixed a concentrate of electrolytes with water at the bedside represented an improvement. The replacement of bicarbonate with acetate improved sterility, avoided precipitation of calcium salts in dialysis fluid and extended the shelf life of stored fluids.

In the early 1970s, in several units in the UK, including the unit in Newcastle upon Tyne, many patients developed rapidly progressive and fatal encephalopathy together with fracturing renal osteodystrophy. Aluminum, a deflocculating agent in local water supplies, was found to be responsible. This highlighted the serious risk of prolonged exposure of blood to large volumes of water and led to the routine use of reverse osmosis (high-pressure filtration) in water purification.

When dialysis sessions became shorter and more powerful in the 1980s, evidence of acetate intoxication emerged. Bicarbonate as the base in dialysis fluid was successfully reintroduced by mixing separate streams of electrolytes and bicarbonate immediately before delivery to the dialyzer[1].

The 'flat plate' configuration of membranes in rebuildable Kill dialyzers, almost standard during the first two decades of dialysis, and the downstream pump which created a negative pressure in the dialysis fluid, not only kept the membranes apart allowing uniform blood flow, but also prevented entry of dialysis fluid into blood. This led to complacency about microbial contamination of dialysis fluid. The 'interleukin hypothesis'[2] drew attention to the interplay between membrane type, buffer and bacteria in stimulating monocytes on the blood side of the membrane to produce cytokines. Evidence accumulated that bacteriological contamination of dialysis fluid could have serious short- and long-term consequences. It was also demonstrated that in hollow fiber (capillary) dialyzers, passage of variable amounts of dialysis fluid into blood was an inevitable accompaniment of standard dialysis[3]. So called 'backfiltration' results from the high resistance to collapse of cylindrical fibers, poor hydraulic compliance in volumetric machines and pressure gradients in blood and dialysate compartments in countercurrent mode (Fig. 78.2). The result was greater emphasis on standards of bacteriological purity in water.

Water treatment

A typical water purification plant is shown in Figure 78.3. Incoming water from the urban supply varies in quality depending on the functioning of the local grid system. The process should ensure reduced concentrations of toxic metals, chemicals and of bacteria and their breakdown products to within agreed standards. Even in the modern era, poor design, poor maintenance and failure in monitoring can have severe consequences[4]. Source water first passes through coarse filters to remove particulate matter before arriving in a holding tank. This treated water tank should be small but capable of providing an uninterrupted supply for the limited period required to take patients off dialysis, if there is a failure in the main system. Water is then pumped from the holding tank through reverse osmosis membranes into a 'ring' supplying the dialysis stations. Unused water is recirculated to avoid wastage.

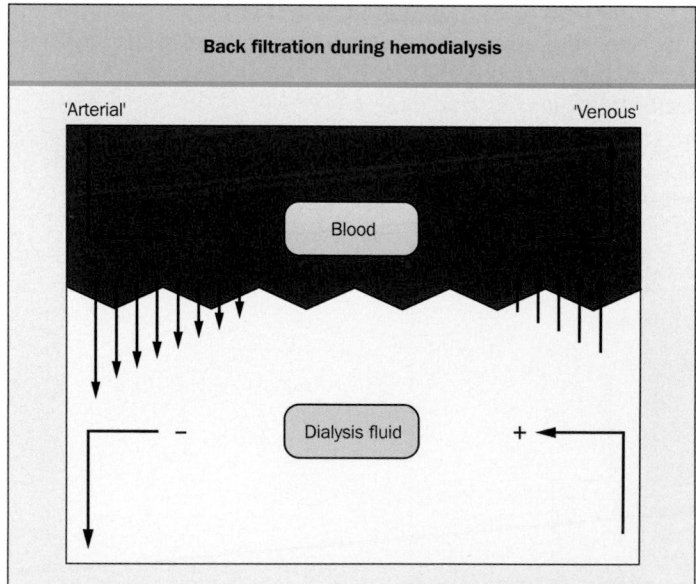

Figure 78.2 Backfiltration of dialysis fluid into blood during hemodialysis. Backfiltration results from the pressure profiles, positive (+) and negative (–), in blood and dialysate compartments of the dialyzer in countercurrent mode. Ultrafiltration, which takes place at the 'arterial' end of the dialyzer exceeds the volume of backfiltration at the 'venous' end by an amount equal to the prescribed fluid removal.

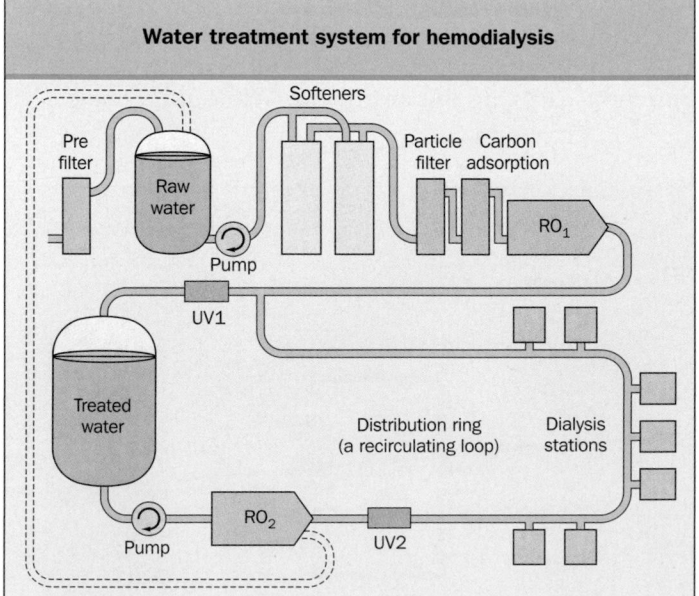

Figure 78.3 Water treatment system for hemodialysis. The main components of a typical water treatment system. In this system, a second reverse osmosis unit (RO_2) is included in the distribution ring. Ultraviolet irradiation (UV) is employed with the ROs. For economy, water rejected from RO_2 is recycled to the input raw water tank.

Softening and deionization

Softeners employ a resin coated with sodium ions, which are exchanged for calcium and magnesium ions. They are usually paired to allow one to be regenerated whilst the other is in use. Regeneration is achieved by passing brine (strong sodium chloride) across the resin. Alternatively, water may be deionized by paired cation and anion resins, which exchange these ions for water.

Carbon adsorption

Activated carbon, with high surface area, adsorbs substances such as endotoxins, chlorine and chloramines, not removed by softening. Chlorine is added to urban water for disinfection and chloramines, to reduce the odor and taste of chlorine. Several units have experienced hemolysis, anemia and epoetin resistance attributable to chloramines[5]. Common faults include carbon filters with inadequate capacity, recharging with inadequate frequency. It is important to correct these faults because chloramine removal by reverse osmosis is not very efficient.

Reverse osmosis

This process, originally designed to desalinate seawater, became essential in water treatment after the description of aluminum toxicity. The name derives from the flow direction of product water, which is the reverse of the osmotic gradient. Pumps supply water at high pressure (15–20 bar) through a tight membrane. The small pore size of these membranes (0.5–1.5 nm) provides an absolute barrier for molecules > 100–300 Da. This process rejects over 99% of all bacteria, viruses, pyrogens and organic materials. Monitoring is by comparative resistivity of inlet and outlet water.

Ultraviolet irradiation

Ultraviolet irradiation is used to damage bacteria and must be used in conjunction with reverse osmosis to ensure removal of bacterial breakdown products.

Standards for water quality

Regulatory and professional bodies such as the American Society for Medical Instrumentation (AAMI) and the UK Renal Association (RA) issue standards, but maintenance schedules and sampling methods are still in evolution. There is often a large gap between recommendations and routine practice. For water supplying the distribution ring the RA Standards reflect AAMI:

Bacterial count < 200 cfu/mL
Endotoxin count < 1 EU/mL

Where cfu = colony forming U/mL sampled water
EU/mL = Endotoxin U/mL (limulus amoebocyte lysate test, LAL)

However, using the water plant shown in Figure 78.3, ring samples taken monthly would typically yield < 1 cfu/ml and endotoxin < 0.01 EU/ml. Disinfection using citric acid is initiated if local warning limits for bacterial and endotoxin count are exceeded.

Typical concentration profile of dialysis fluid	
Component	Concentration (mmol/L)
Sodium	140
Potassium	2.0
Calcium	1.25 (5.0 mg/dL)
Magnesium	0.5 (1.2 mg/dL)
Acetate	3.0
Chloride	108
Bicarbonate	35
Glucose	5.6 (100 mg/dL)

Table 78.1 Typical concentration profile of dialysis fluid.

Dialysis fluid

A typical profile of dialysis fluid is shown in Table 78.1. The sodium concentration approximates normal plasma levels to minimize intercompartmental fluid shifts. A compromise is needed between the capacity to remove accumulated salt and water and intradialytic symptoms of cramp and hypotension. Dialysate sodium values of 135 mmol/L, have given way to higher levels, usually around 140 mmol/L. Levels higher than 140 mmol/L tend to cause thirst and to exacerbate hypertension. The potassium level is a compromise between a high removal rate and potentially dangerous intradialytic hypokalemia. The tendency to negative calcium balance is counteracted by use of dialysis fluid ionized calcium levels, which allow modest net gain. Levels of 1.75 mmol/L were generally used until calcium salts (carbonate and acetate) replaced aluminum hydroxide as the preferred phosphate binder. To avoid hypercalcemia, dialysis fluid calcium concentrations have fallen to 1.25 mmol/L in most centres. Bicarbonate is now the standard base, 35 mmol/L or more being necessary to normalize predialysis serum bicarbonate. Unlike acetate, bicarbonate solutions are not bactericidal and must be supplied separately from other constituents. Alternatively, bicarbonate in powder or granule form is used. The remaining constituents are usually provided as a liquid 'acid' concentrate with small amounts of lactate or acetate to ensure stability. There is still no consensus on whether glucose is a required component. Some argue that dialysis is more physiologic if glucose is included at approximately the plasma concentration, particularly in diabetics and in rapid high-efficiency dialysis where hypoglycemia is a theoretical risk.

THE DIALYSIS MACHINE

Standard diffusive dialysis

The principal sections and components of a dialysis machine are illustrated in Figure 78.4. Incoming water is warmed by a heater and by effluent dialysis fluid. Deaeration of the water, achieved by recirculation through a throttle valve/vacuum arrangement, renders the fluid noncompressible to allow accurate volumetric performance. Acid concentrate is mixed with water in a ratio of approximately 35:1. Similarly proportioned bicarbonate solution is then added to make the final solution. The balance chamber (electromagnetic flow cell in some machines) ensures identical flows in and out of the internal hydraulic circuit in which there is always a constant volume. The dialysate flow-rate can be set between 500–800 mL/min, fluid passing through the dialyzer and to waste via the balance chamber.

An ultrafiltration pump removes dialysis fluid at the prescribed rate from the internal hydraulic circuit. Since the volume of the internal hydraulic circuit is maintained constant, fluid must be withdrawn from the patient's blood through the dialysis membrane in a volume exactly equal to that which has been removed by the ultrafiltration pump. This is the principle of volumetric ultrafiltration.

High-flux dialysis and hemodiafiltration

Concerns about the biocompatibility of cuprophane, and its poor clearance of middle molecules, especially β_2-microglobulin, have fueled the increasing use of high-flux membranes, and investment in the use of ultrapure water for preparation of dialysis fluids. Hemofiltration is a purely convective mode, which greatly improves middle molecule clearance,

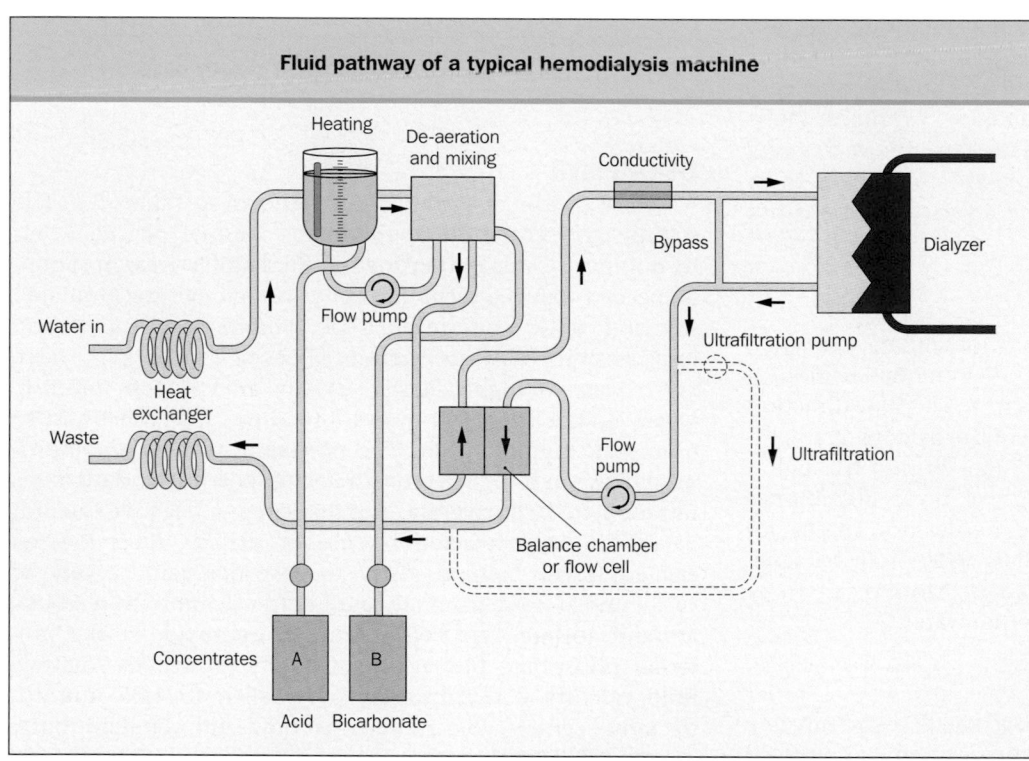

Figure 78.4 The principal components and pathway of a typical hemodialysis machine.

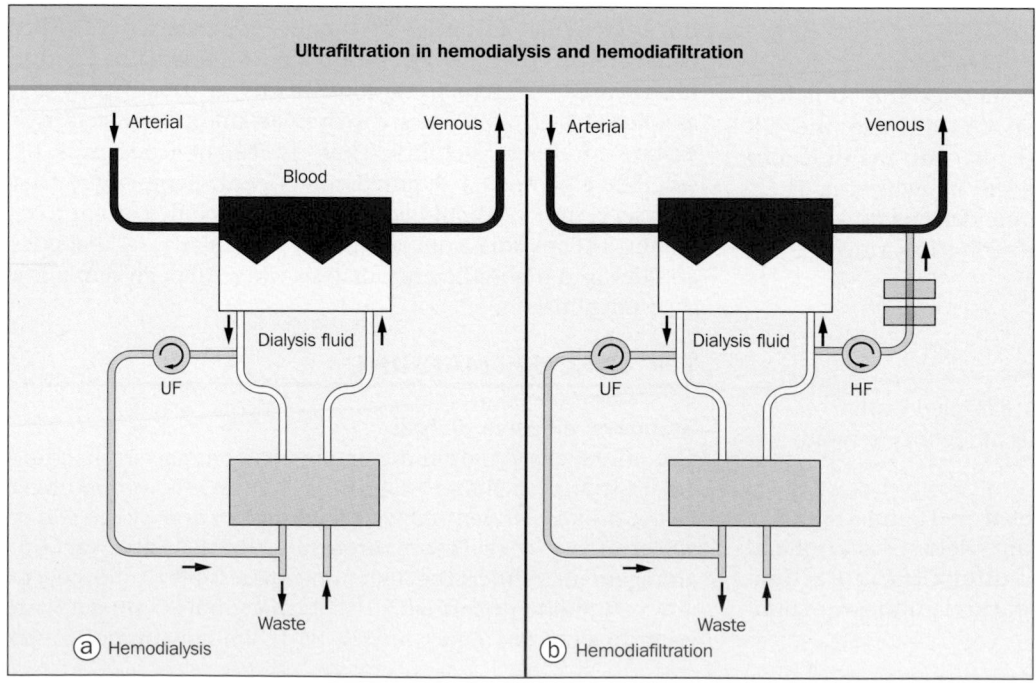

Figure 78.5 Principles of ultrafiltration in hemodialysis and hemodiafiltration. (a) Diffusive dialysis showing the ultrafiltration pump (UF) removing fluid from the internal hydraulic circuit. (b) Online hemodiafiltration showing inclusion of an extra pump (HF) and infusion of dialysis fluid into blood via two filters in series. The ultrafiltration pump (UF) is common to both systems.

but small molecule clearance is poor, and sterile pyrogen free substitution fluid is required so the technique is less suitable for maintenance treatment of ESRD patients. It has however been highly successful as a continuous treatment in patients with acute renal failure particularly in the context of multiple organ failure in the intensive care unit. Hemodiafiltration (HDF) adds a greater convective component (hemofiltration) to the diffusive and convective clearances offered by high-flux hemodialysis, and allows the benefits of both modalities to be maximized. The capacity to utilize dialysis fluid as the infusion fluid, made possible by use of ultrapure water in its preparation, or by filtering the dialysate makes the technique economically viable and HDF is gaining popularity as a routine treatment. In a typical session, 12–20 litres of water above the desired ultrafiltration (the interdialytic weight-gain) are removed and the deficit made up by infusion of an equivalent volume of physiological fluid (Fig. 78.5). If the infusion point is upstream of the dialyzer it is referred to as predilution, and if downstream, as postdilution HDF. Some would argue that HDF is the natural evolutionary end point of the dialysis process given current available technology and materials. HDF is discussed further in Chapter 82

Safety and disinfection

In standard dialysis, a conductivity meter, situated immediately before the dialyzer, monitors the integrity of the main operating system, which produces dialysis fluid. If the conductivity, which effectively measures sodium concentration, deviates by a few percent from the set point, the dialysis is stopped and dialysis fluid is directed through a bypass channel so protecting the patient. The chance of simultaneous failure of the operating system and monitor is approximately 10^{-8} per hour, which is considered an acceptable risk for any patient-connected equipment. In HDF the same monitor operates but there is additional protection from infused bacteria by filtration. Machines are usually heat disinfected between treatments, and chemically disinfected at the end of the dialysis day.

THE EXTRACORPOREAL CIRCUIT

The blood pathway and monitors

In the ideal situation, arterial blood is taken from and returned to an AV fistula via 'arterial' (A) and 'venous' (V) needles placed upstream and downstream, respectively, to prevent recirculation. Forward flow to the dialyzer is induced by a peristaltic pump, the blood returning to the patient via a collection (drip) chamber designed to detect air accumulation and to facilitate monitoring of the 'venous' return pressure (Fig. 78.6). Infrared scanning or ultrasound detects a falling blood level, due to accumulation of air in the system. The purpose is prevention of air embolism.

Monitoring of venous return pressure (P) was originally designed to detect accidental disconnection of the circuit from the V needle, an important consideration when patients often slept during long nocturnal dialyses. When transmembrane pressure control of ultrafiltration was introduced in the late 1970s, the monitor was used to reflect the pressure in the dialyzer blood compartment. The advent of volumetric machines

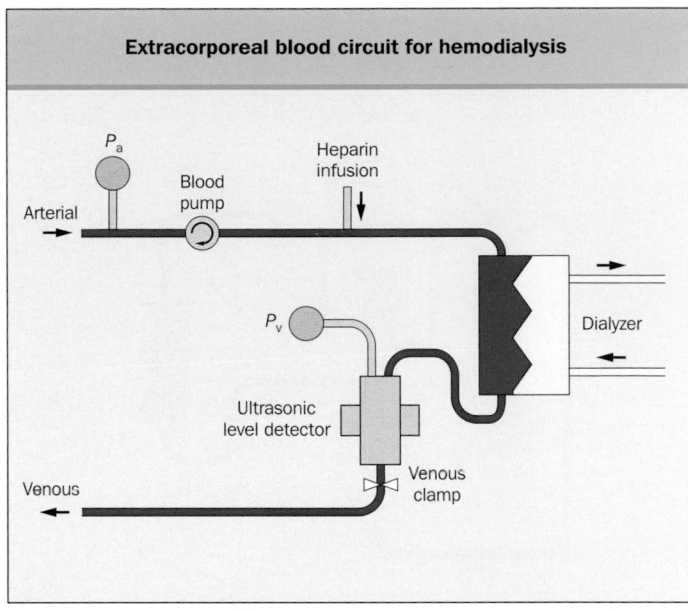

Figure 78.6 Extracorporeal circuit for hemodialysis. Blood flow is 200–500 mL/min and dialysis fluid flow is 300–800 mL/min.

rendered such monitoring of secondary importance. Monitoring arterial line pressure is a relatively new addition, serving to protect the fistula by detecting excessive negative pressure.

Tidal flow (single-needle) dialysis

Using one needle rather than two has clear attractions but less blood can be processed because of interrupted flows. Longer dialysis times are required for comparable efficiency. The flexibility to offer single-needle dialysis is important since the proportion of patients with an AV fistula is falling worldwide. Many patients now have short segments of PTFE grafts or 'permanent' tunneled catheters in the major veins of the neck or groin. A typical single-needle dialysis system is shown in Figure 78.7. 'Arterial' and 'venous' pumps work alternately; a pressure/capacitance device between the two pumps switches flow. The proportion of processed blood 'recirculating' directly from the V into the A line at the beginning of the arterial phase, can be minimized by ensuring the removal of a high 'tidal volume' usually about 40 mL each cycle.

Access recirculation

In certain situations, it is possible for processed blood to 'recirculate' within the fistula from the V needle into the A needle. Since AV fistula blood flows are usually several hundred mL/min recirculation does not occur when the needles are appropriately placed in a single vein draining directly from the anastomosis. However, recirculation can occur when a plexus of veins drain the fistula or when the fistula flow is low due to stenotic segments. Recirculation can also occur if the V needle is inadvertently placed upstream of the A needle. In the case of twin-lumen tunneled catheters, recirculation tends to be minimized by the high blood flow in the vessel in which the catheter tip is placed. Recirculation reduces the efficiency of dialysis.

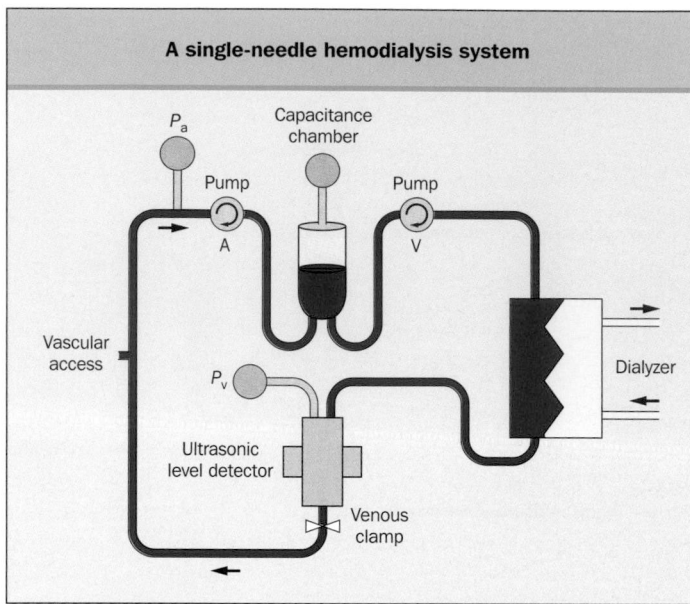

A single-needle hemodialysis system

Figure 78.7 Single-needle hemodialysis system. Flow is switched as pressure in the capacitance chamber reaches high then low limits. The venous clamp is closed during the A phase.

There are a number of physical methods, which may be employed to detect and quantitate access recirculation. Saline or dialysis fluid (via the dialyzer) can be injected into the V line and its appearance detected in the A line. The principle of thermal or optical dilution can be employed which in the former case requires cooling of the injectate. Cardiopulmonary recirculation, which is distinct from access recirculation, is an unavoidable consequence of using an AV fistula as vascular access; 5–10% of blood, which has entered the pulmonary circulation from the fistula, returns directly to the fistula without first passing through tissue capillary beds.

Blood side monitors

Blood volume monitoring
Blood volume change during dialysis contributes to symptomatic hypotension. Blood volume change is chiefly determined by water-flux, the circulating red cell volume remaining constant. Conductivity measurement, optical transmission (infrared), and ultrasound are physical techniques that can reflect blood volume change. Sophisticated algorithms have been developed to accommodate nonlinearity and differences in optical transmission of oxygenated and deoxygenated blood. Many modern machines are equipped with relative blood volume monitors, which may require a specially designed segment in the extracorporeal blood tubing. Freestanding devices are also available, which generally employ inexpensive disposable add-ons to the extracorporeal circuit.

Heat transfer
The improved blood pressure stability, which is a feature of hemofiltration and isolated ultrafiltration has been attributed to cooling of the blood during the treatment. This has led to speculation that an increase in body core temperature and

resulting heat shock might be an important factor in intradialytic hypotension. It is feasible to monitor the temperature of afferent and efferent extracorporeal blood so accurately that zero heat transfer can be prescribed (Blood temperature Module [BTM], Fresenius Medical Care).

Dialysis fluid side monitoring
Online clearance
A number of methods exist which allow dialysis quantification by real-time monitoring. Online urea monitoring involves measurement, by the urease reaction, of the urea content of blood water or spent dialysate samples at multiple points throughout the dialysis. The standard urea kinetic parameters (Kt/V and nPCR) can be derived together with a number of less well-established parameters such as 'whole body urea clearance' (see below, 'Adequacy'). The sodium ion can be used as a surrogate for urea. Sodium clearance measurements are derived from the conductivity differences between dialysate inlet and outlet at two different levels of dialysate inlet conductivity. The resulting 'ionic dialysance' approximates the 'effective' urea clearance[6] reflecting the presence of recirculation and other factors, which may reduce dialysis efficiency. Online monitoring of ionic dialysance allows assessment of the adequacy of each treatment.

Profiled dialysis
In sodium profiling the sodium content of the dialysis fluid is varied throughout the course of the session. The aim of this is to attempt to prevent osmotic disequilibrium (causing headache and other associated symptoms) and at the same time, prevent intradialytic hypotension by supporting plasma refilling. A whole range of profiles has been used: decreasing, increasing, and alternating. Decreasing profiles are by far the commonest and can be linear, stepwise or exponential[7], typically tapering from around 150 to about 130 mmol/L, and designed to maintain a mean of around 140 mmol/L over the whole session. During the initial part of the dialysis session, the rate of fall of urea concentration in the extracellular fluid (ECF) is maximal. An intercompartmental disequilibrium is established which results in an intracellular shift of water leading to cellular swelling (and headache) and ECF volume depletion (and hypotension). A higher initial dialysis fluid sodium concentration results in net gain of sodium during this period thus preventing intracellular shifts and preserving ECF volume. Interdialytic thirst and hypotension are prevented by a corresponding reduction in dialysis fluid sodium levels in the latter part of dialysis. Delivery of the required negative sodium balance by the end of the dialysis is achieved predominantly by ultrafiltration. Ultrafiltration can also be profiled to match the sodium profile (dual profiling).

DIALYZERS/FILTERS

Membrane configuration
Rebuildable with 1 m² sheets of cuprophane and reusable by disinfection and storage with formaldehyde, the Kiil dialyzer set the standard by which all future developments would be compared. It employed the principle of slow flow and a thin film across a large surface area to maximize

Types of dialyzer			
Membrane type	Hydraulic permeability	Examples	Biocompatibility profile
Regenerated cellulose	Low flux	Cuprophane	Poor
Modified cellulose	Low/high flux	Cellulose acetate Cellulose diacetate Saponified cellulose ester	Intermediate
Synthetic	High/low flux	Polyacrylonitrile Polysulphone Polyamide Polycarbonate Polymethylmethacrylate	Good

Table 78.2 Types of dialyzer. There is much overlap between the extent of biocompatibility and permeability.

diffusion while containing only a small volume of fluid (< 150 mL) during treatment. The first disposable dialyzers were multilayered flat plate construction. Capillary 'hollow fiber' dialyzers quickly replaced these. Hundreds of fibers in bundles are secured at each end of a plastic cylinder. Blood enters and leaves via manifolds, designed to create uniform flow across the capillary bundles. Dialysis fluid in countercurrent mode weaves through the fiber bundles. New membranes were rapidly introduced, some synthetically produced from basic chemical building blocks. The most dramatic change was the availability of membranes with high hydraulic permeability, so called high-flux dialyzers. They offered potential for convection as well as diffusive solute removal, explaining why the terms 'dialyzer' and 'filter' have become interchangeable.

Performance characteristics

Dialyzers are now available with a wide range of diffusive and ultrafiltration characteristics (Table 78.2). They tend to be classified according to their flux and biocompatibility profile (see below). Diffusive performance is measured as clearance of different size molecules tested *in vitro*. The flux (hydraulic permeability) is quantified *in vitro* and expressed as mL water/min per 100 mmHg.

Biocompatibility

Dialysis differs from the physiologic (biocompatible) ideal in many ways, not least because of exposure of blood to foreign materials and the appearance of micro-organisms and their breakdown products in blood via the dialysis fluid. This can activate several response systems. The alternative pathway of complement is activated by blood/membrane contact. Peridialytic elevations of plasma C3a and C5a levels have been reported. A number of physiologic events or clinical symptoms observed during dialysis can be ascribed to this activation such as anaphylaxis (rarely) and pulmonary sequestration of neutrophils leading to hypoxemia[8]. The negative charge on the surface of dialyzer membranes is responsible for the activation of the contact system of plasma, which results in the cleavage of kininogen to release

bradykinin. The inactivation of the latter depends on kininase, which is blocked by angiotensin-converting enzyme (ACE) inhibitors. Impaired removal of bradykinin from the circulation has resulted in episodes of collapse in several patients taking ACE inhibitors who were using the AN69 polyacrylonitrile membrane, one of the most negatively charged membranes (see Chapter 79).

The 'interleukin hypothesis'[2] suggested that some long-term as well as some acute complications of HD, may result from cytokine release from mononuclear cells stimulated by membrane contact and by contaminants in dialysis fluid. Cytokine induction is greater during HD with complement-activating membranes (e.g., cuprophane) and in the presence of contaminated dialysis fluid. All types of dialyzer have been shown, *in vitro*, to have some permeability to pyrogenic bacterial fragments. Paradoxically, high-flux dialyzers often have a high adsorptive capacity for pyrogens and may constitute a better barrier between activated mononuclear cells and dialysis fluid. The 'biocompatibility' of membranes can be ranked according to the degree of complement activation and cytokine release they engender. Unmodified cellulosic membranes perform poorly, synthetic perform best, with modified cellulose occupying an intermediate position (see Table 78.2). It is questionable whether it is still justifiable to use 'standard' dialysis with cuprophane membranes, especially if compliance with water quality standards is poor. Though randomized controlled trials are lacking, attaining sterile pyrogen-free dialysis fluid seems a worthwhile and achievable goal. Pressure from patients and practitioners is likely to result in the widespread adoption of the most biocompatible dialyzers. In the USA, less than 25% of patients now use cellulosic membranes. Whether transition from low to high-flux membranes will also follow may be governed by the incidence of complications related to β_2-microglobulin levels.

Reprocessing for single patient use

Reprocessing of dialyzers was necessary in the first decade of dialysis. The introduction of mass-produced disposable dialyzers reduced this need. Subsequently, the desire for the quality enhancement obtainable by use biocompatible synthetic membranes and the need to live within budgetary constraints has reversed this trend. Fortunately, newer disinfectants such as peracetic acid and automated reuse systems have rendered reprocessing safe, environmentally friendly and acceptable to staff. Rigorous procedures are necessary to ensure that reprocessed dialyzers remain dedicated to the individual patient and to ensure that disinfection procedures have been carried out correctly. Provided these systems are in place, most authorities agree that reuse is an acceptable and safe practice. Small molecule clearance is uninfluenced by reprocessing provided clotting of dialyzer capillaries is minimal. The loss of internal dialyzer volume, which results from clotting, forms the basis of quality control in automated reuse. While it has been shown that some diminution of β_2-microglobulin clearance appears after multiple-use, the effect has little influence on clinical outcomes. Predialysis β_2-microglobulin levels in patients on high-flux dialysis or hemodiafiltration with reuse are about 50% of those in patients on standard dialysis.

DIALYSIS SCHEDULES

In the early days of dialysis, patients received 24 h of dialysis a week administered in a single session or 2×12 h sessions. Further division to 3×8 h sessions was associated with a noticeable improvement in well being. Further sub-division to 6×4 h sessions pioneered in the home eventually faltered due to machine reliability problems. Thrice weekly sessions were not only compatible with improved rehabilitation but conveniently allowed a 6-day working week for renal centers. Most HD patients remain on thrice-weekly sessions, which is accepted as the minimum frequency, which can provide adequate treatment for the majority. Despite a vigorous defense of long dialysis times (6–8 h sessions), which can achieve superior volume/blood pressure control, there has been an inexorable decline in treatment times throughout the world conditioned by economic constraints, better tolerance and patient preference. The mean treatment in the UK is now 3 h 46 min. While current evidence suggests adequate dialysis can be delivered in short sessions by employing high blood flows with large dialyzers, there is little doubt that significant difficulties controlling phosphate and blood pressure levels are encountered with these modern schedules, both of which impact on the morbidity and mortality of the dialysis population.

For such reasons, there has been a resurgence of interest in home hemodialysis. It represents an 'escape' from institutional dialysis and holds the possibility that the increased quantity of dialysis it allows, will improve longevity and reduce morbidity from bone and cardiovascular complications. More dialysis can be achieved by increasing the frequency of dialysis rather than simply the duration of sessions. In the future there will likely be a cohort of motivated patients wishing to dialyze six times a week either in the center or at home for relatively short sessions, say 2 h. Alternatively, patients may wish to dialyze slowly overnight 6 nights a week. This approach has already been shown to produce excellent results[9].

ULTRAFILTRATION AND DRY WEIGHT

Most patients with ESRD are hypertensive, even in the absence of clinical signs of fluid overload. In the early days of dialysis, it was observed that slow removal of excess fluid during the first few months of dialysis results in normalization of blood pressure in most patients. The initial intense thirst gradually subsided as patients were 'dried out'. The pathophysiologic state of patients who reach and maintain their 'dry weight' is probably unique to HD. Achievement and maintenance of dry weight was considered to minimize cardiac strain, reduce progression of left ventricular hypertrophy and thereby the risk of premature death. A patient reaching dry weight will have no signs of fluid overload such as elevated jugular venous pressure or peripheral edema, will have normal predialysis blood pressure (< 140/90 mmHg) and will not be unduly susceptible to intradialytic hypotension and muscle cramps. In the modern era, the definition of 'dry weight' has become confused. Few patients ever reach the ideal described above. The mean age of patients has risen dramatically as has the extent and severity of comorbid conditions, predominantly cardiovascular. This mitigates against success in achieving dry weight as do the short and powerful dialysis sessions that are now commonplace. The advent of better-tolerated and more effective hypotensive drugs has made clinicians more ready to prescribe than subject patients to a potentially painful period of 'drying out'. Also unhelpful has been the change in the mechano-physical technique of ultrafiltration. The evaluation of dry weight in dialysis patients is discussed further in Chapter 69.

INFECTION CONTROL

Adherence to universal precautions minimizes the risk of cross-infection by blood-borne viruses. Potential transmission from contaminated external surfaces, rather than through the dialyzer membrane, is the major cross-infection risk. Screening of patients before dialysis initiation, for evidence of prior infection with Hepatitis B and C is routine, and should be repeated at least 6 monthly thereafter. Hepatitis B surface antigen negative patients should be vaccinated; hepatitis B positive patients should be segregated and use a dedicated machine. Hepatitis C and HIV positive patients should be managed similarly.

OUTCOME ON HEMODIALYSIS

Survival has been the main focus of outcome research in HD. Much less is known about treatment-associated morbidity as reflected in such parameters as hospitalization rates and quality-of-life measures. The main source of knowledge about outcomes is registry data. Only recently has information begun to emerge from randomized controlled trials. Registry data has been available since the advent of renal replacement therapy for ESRD. The European Dialysis and Transplant Association (EDTA) Registry provided comprehensive data from the 1970s until the early 1990s, when voluntary returns from some countries fell, undermining the validity of the data. By contrast, the United States Renal Data System (USRDS), which was not initiated until 1988, has obtained most of its data from the Healthcare Finance Administration, which tends to be accurate and complete as it is linked to the remuneration system for the treatment. The USRDS database is widely available to the biomedical and economic research communities and has been an effective stimulus for important outcome studies in HD. Other registries have survived through co-ordinated effort and provide complete and invaluable data e.g., Australia and New Zealand Dialysis and Transplant Registry (ANZDATA).

Changing demographics of the hemodialysis population

HD was very successful from the beginning in prolonging life. Survival in all age groups improved in Europe from the early 1970s to early 1980s. Patients who survived beyond the first 2 years spent an impressively small amount of time in hospital. Comparison of survival between different eras is hampered by a number of factors including changes in selection criteria, case-mix and technology. In the early 1980s, the mean age of HD patients in Europe was 52 years, and less than 5% were diabetic; few had diseases of other organ systems.

Subsequent liberalization of acceptance onto dialysis programs in Europe has gradually produced a dialysis population with characteristics that increasingly resemble that in the USA. Patients are older, with a mean age well over 60: more than 15% are diabetic (the figure approaches 50% in the USA) and many more are afflicted by nonrenal comorbidities, particularly degenerative vascular disease. In general they are much more dependent for support on family and social agencies. These factors all have a major impact on outcome, both in terms of survival and successful rehabilitation. The increasing shortage of donor organs has resulted in tighter selection criteria for transplantation. The proportion of dialysis patients considered suitable for transplantation is steadily decreasing. In addition the limitations of peritoneal dialysis (PD) as a long-term treatment have become apparent. Many patients require transfer from PD to HD for reasons of failing adequacy or infection. Age, nonrenal comorbidity and increased dependency are more likely to be seen as precluding transplantation and mitigating against the choice of peritoneal dialysis as the appropriate modality, rather than as a bar to renal replacement therapy. HD is thus the default mode of renal replacement therapy.

Factors affecting survival on dialysis
A range of factors reported to affect survival on dialysis are shown in Table 78.3.

Adequacy of dialysis
There is increasing emphasis on the importance of the adequacy of dialysis as a predictor of survival on dialysis. The assessment and measurement of HD adequacy are discussed in detail later in this chapter. Information about the significance of dialysis adequacy is now available both from analysis of registry data and more recently from randomized controlled trials.

Age and comorbidity
Age and nonrenal comorbidity at HD initiation are powerful predictors of outcome. HD patients can be categorized into high-, medium- and low-risk groups with profound differences in survival on the basis of factors present at HD initiation including age, severity of comorbidity and functional capacity assessed by Karnovsky performance scale[10]. While all these factors predict survival, age is heavily outweighed as a risk factor by comorbidity and functional capacity. Late referral for dialysis is also a major determinant of poor survival. Such analyses demand a reappraisal of the aims of treatment for patients in these different risk-groups. Patients in the low-risk group have the prospect of long-term survival and strategies for prevention of late complications of ESRD should be maximized, particularly in those not suitable for transplantation. For such patients increased treatment such as is offered by daily nocturnal dialysis may be an option. In the medium- and high-risk group, dialysis can be seen for many patients as a palliative therapy. Patients will often succumb to coexistent degenerative diseases, some of which may be accelerated by ESRD and its treatment. Dialysis for some patients in the high-risk group may do no more than prolong the process of dying.

Poor outcome in hemodialysis
Factors reported to be associated with poor outcome in HD patients
Hemodialysis treatment related factors
Inadequate dose: Lower URR, Kt/V, etc.
Shorter dialysis hours
Persistent metabolic acidosis
Dialyzer: bioincompatible membrane?
Associated clinical conditions
Diabetes mellitus
Poor blood pressure control
Cardiomyopathy
Peripheral vascular disease
Impaired functional capacity (e.g., Karnovsky performance scale)
Malnutrition
Protein-calorie malnutrition
Hypoalbuminemia
Hypophosphatemia
Hypocholesterolemia
Muscular wasting
Miscellaneous factors
Hyperphosphatemia: elevated calcium-phosphorus product
Anemia
β-2 microglobulin related amyloidosis

Table 78.3 Poor outcome in hemodialysis.

Comparisons with other modalities
There are major differences between modern HD and PD populations, most of which stem from differing selection criteria. Hemodialysis patients are older, have a greater comorbid load, and are more functionally impaired and dependent. Clinical imperatives around selection frustrate any hopes of valid randomized controlled comparisons of outcomes. Most available data are from registries or from observational cohort studies. When these data are corrected to take account of case-mix, and the therapies are matched with respect to delivered dialysis dose, little difference in survival can be demonstrated[11]. Technique survival is much better in HD. Similar case-mix issues dominate comparisons of survival between the dialysis and transplantation modalities.

Preservation of residual renal function
Residual renal function appears to be lost more rapidly in conventional hemodialysis than in CAPD. In hemodialysis using high-flux biocompatible membranes and ultra-pure water, residual renal function appears to decline at a rate indistinguishable from that in CAPD[12]. This may have important implications since preservation of residual renal function has major benefits and is emerging as a valid therapeutic goal.

DIALYSIS ADEQUACY

The current definition of adequate dialysis is the minimum dose below which the outcome is significantly worse, rather than the optimum dose to return the patient to full health.

To date, no study has been conducted to define 'optimum' and compare it with 'minimum' dose. There is ample evidence and general agreement that the dose of dialysis directly influences patient outcome in terms of survival and morbidity. However, there is no consensus about what constitutes an adequate dose, or the best method to measure the dose, or the best dialysis technique to deliver that dose.

Assessments of dialysis adequacy

Great attention is paid to the dose of dialysis, usually assessed by measurement of solute clearance by KT/V_{urea} or urea reduction ratio (URR), and attainment of agreed standards for these parameters (see below). However, dialysis adequacy must not be assessed by solute clearance alone. A global review of the patient including clinical and other laboratory data is necessary to make a judgment on patient well-being and treatment adequacy. There are several strong, independent predictors of patient outcome, which must be considered at least as important as solute clearance (Table 78.3). All of these may be influenced by adequate dialysis, but nevertheless are predictors of patient outcome independent of the dialysis dose.

Blood pressure

Blood pressure (BP) is a powerful predictor of survival in dialysis patients. Among the best survival in hemodialysis patients ever reported is from Tassin, France where > 95% of their patients have BP < 140/90 without any medications[13], with a further advantage in life expectancy for those with low normal BP. This strongly suggests that the target BP in dialysis patients should be lower, perhaps < 130/80 mmHg (see Chapter 69). Maintaining dry weight by ultrafiltration, and judicious control of sodium balance are very effective in normalizing the BP, and it has been suggested that adequate UF must be considered as part of the measurement of dialysis adequacy.

However the relationship between BP and survival in dialysis patients is a 'J-shaped curve'. Low pre- and postdialysis systolic blood pressures have both been associated with an increase in mortality risk[14]. This is probably accounted for in part by the association of hypotension and severe cardiac dysfunction. Difficulties in defining hypertension in HD patients may also contribute to the apparent 'J-shaped curve'[15]. Mean nocturnal blood pressure and 24-h pressure derived from ambulatory readings may be better predictors of cardiovascular mortality in this setting[16]. Notwithstanding these confusions there is concern that shortened dialysis times have increased the prevalence of hypertension and added to the increasing cardiovascular mortality of HD patients. Longer conventional sessions, short daily and daily nocturnal dialysis have all been associated with improved blood pressure control.

Nutrition, inflammation, and cardiovascular disease

Measures of nutritional status of patient are powerful independent predictors of survival on HD. Anthropometric measures as well as biochemical markers such as serum albumin, prealbumin, creatinine, BUN, phosphorus, cholesterol, have all been associated with survival. Low body mass index (BMI) strengthens the relationship between Kt/V and mortality[17]. Even very low urea reduction ratio (≤ 45%) is associated with

no increase in mortality risk in those with normal serum albumin[17]. Nutrition for patients on HD is discussed further in Chapter 74.

There are also strong correlations between malnutrition, cardiovascular disease and markers of inflammation, particularly C-reactive protein levels, in HD patients. There are many potential causes of inflammation including clinical and subclinical infections related to vascular access devices and factors related to the dialysis process itself. Use of biocompatible membranes[18] and ultrapure water[19] may reduce the inflammatory response and improve nutritional status.

Phosphate

While low serum phosphate may be associated with poor nutritional status and is associated with increased risk of death, recent reports also strongly suggest an association between high serum phosphate (and calcium–phosphate product) and increased mortality[20,21] (Fig. 78.8). Thus, aggressive prevention of elevated phosphate while maintaining good nutrition is critical in the management of dialysis patients.

Acidosis

Improved survival has been reported with normal predialysis bicarbonate concentration. Metabolic acidosis is associated with increased protein catabolism, decreased protein synthesis and poor protein nutrition. K/DOQI guidelines on nutrition recommend maintaining normal predialysis serum bicarbonate. This can usually be achieved by increasing dialysate bicarbonate to 35–40 mmol/L, but occasionally oral intake of an alkaline salt (such as sodium bicarbonate) may be necessary. Reducing catabolism will also reduce acid production and improve serum bicarbonate.

Amyloid

Beta$_2$-microglobulin (β_2M) is the major constituent of dialysis-associated amyloidosis, the prevalence of which increases with duration of dialysis, approaching 80% after 15 years on

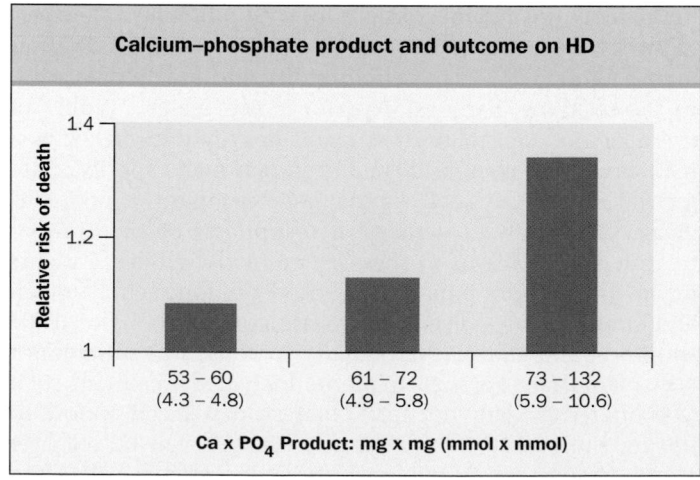

Figure 78.8 Outcome on hemodialysis in relation to calcium–phosphate product. Calcium–phosphate product > 72 ,mg × mg is associated with a significant increase in relative risk of death. (Data from Block et al.[20].)

dialysis. It is a major cause of morbidity if not mortality on HD. High-flux techniques, in contrast to both cuprophane and low-flux biocompatible dialyzers maintain relatively low β_2M levels[22], which may be sustained over periods of up to 10 years despite declining residual renal function. Membrane flux rather than biocompatibility appears to be the main determinant of β_2M levels. It remains to be clearly demonstrated that reduced β_2M levels translate into reduced amyloid load, though the relative risk of carpal tunnel surgery in patients treated with hemofiltration or hemodiafiltration appears substantially lower than in those on conventional dialysis[23]. Frequent nocturnal hemodialysis may give even lower β_2M levels[24]. β_2M-derived amyloid is discussed further in Chapter 72.

MEASUREMENT OF DIALYSIS DOSE

Uremic toxins
The size and kinetics of uremic toxin(s) are still debated. Some argue that uremic toxins are small molecules (SM) and focus on the control of urea as the surrogate marker for these toxins. Others argue that the uremic toxins are larger than urea and that dialysis should attempt to reduce these middle size molecules (MM), molecules larger than SM, but smaller than albumin.

Increasing efficiency of solute removal by improving blood flow, dialysate flow and dialyzer efficiency without increasing dialysis time will improve dialysis of all molecules to a certain point, however beyond this point further increase in dialysis efficiency will be more pertinent for SM than for MM (Fig. 78.9). For MM, total duration of dialysis becomes more important than other factors mentioned above. This point is perhaps the most important factor in the understanding of dialysis dose measurement. The MM concept focuses on duration and frequency of dialysis, longer and more frequent

treatment being more effective in controlling MM. The SM concept supports fast, more efficient dialysis (independent of treatment time) which will control urea more effectively. High-flux dialysis techniques, in contrast to both cuprophane and low-flux biocompatible techniques improve MM clearance and maintain relatively low β_2M levels, which may be sustained over periods of up to 10 years despite declining residual renal function.

Principles of solute clearance
Some basic knowledge of solute clearance is necessary in order to understand the limitations of current methods for measuring dose of dialysis. Assume that uremic toxins are dissolved in water and distributed in total body water. Figure 78.10 depicts a container representing total body water with dissolved solute (toxin) in it. Assume that this fluid is passed through the dialyzer and completely cleared of the solute (undetectable in postdialyzer fluid) and returned to a new container, and that it takes 4 h for all the fluid from container 1 to pass through the dialyzer into the container 2. Thus in 4 h, the total body water was cleared of the solute (toxin) i.e., clearance of solute (K) multiplied by 4 h (the time of dialysis, t) is equal to the volume of container 1 which is the volume of distribution of solute (V). Thus $Kt = V$ or $Kt/V = 1$. However, total body water is not distributed in one compartment but in intracellular and extracellular compartments, and the extracellular compartment is further subdivided into

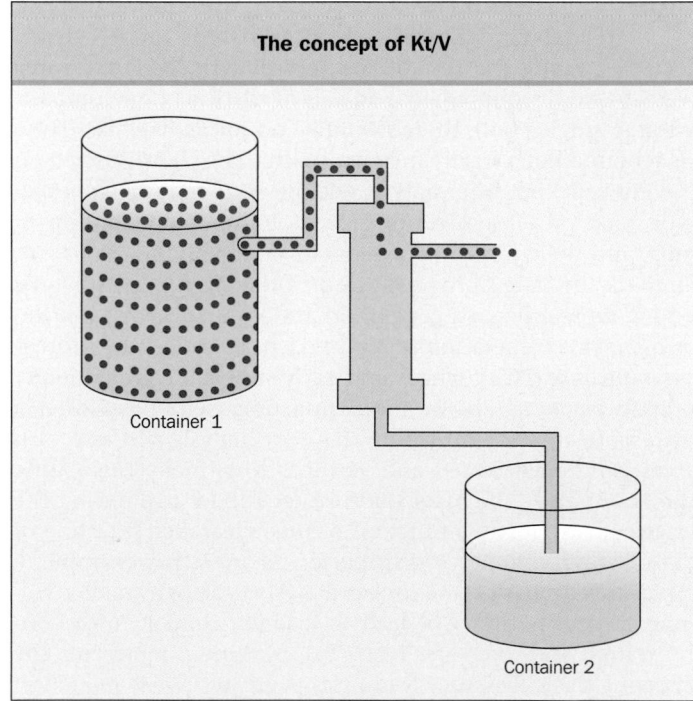

The concept of Kt/V

Container 1

Container 2

Figure 78.10 Solute removal during HD – the concept of Kt/V. The solute (red) in the total body water (Container 1) is entirely removed as all the fluid passes through the dialyzer during time (t) to Container 2. The clearance of solute (K) multiplied by t therefore equals the volume of container 1, which is the volume of distribution of solute (V). Thus Kt = V, or Kt/V = 1. This simple model assumes total body water is distributed in one compartment, which is not the case (see text).

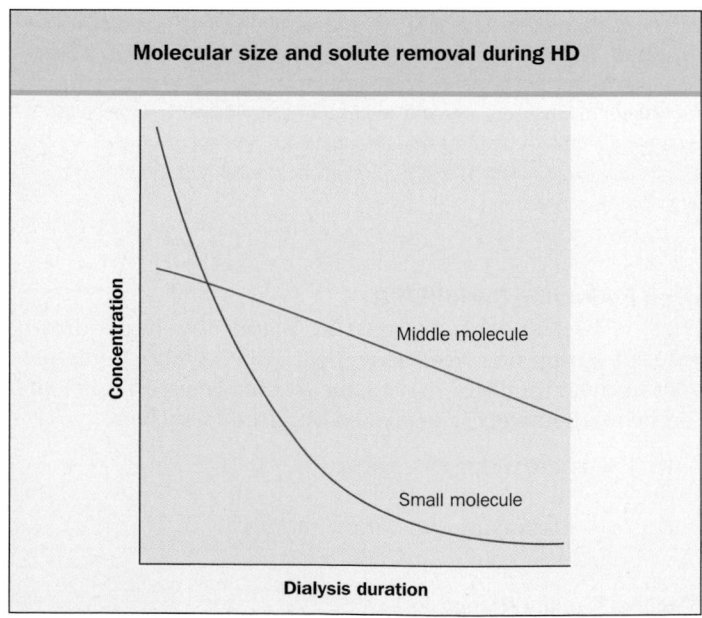

Molecular size and solute removal during HD

Concentration

Middle molecule

Small molecule

Dialysis duration

Figure 78.9 Differences in solute removal during HD according to molecular size.

a smaller plasma volume and larger interstitial volume. Solute movement from one compartment to another is controlled by the concentration gradient and characteristics of the barrier separating the two compartments; unfortunately only plasma volume, the smallest compartment, is accessible to dialysis and measurement of solute concentration.

Quantification of dose of dialysis

In 1971 the 'square meter hypothesis' was proposed which for the first time utilized the dialyzer performance (clearance) and duration of dialysis to calculate the dose of dialysis, and reported the impact of this concept on patient outcome[25], suggesting that a minimum of 21 m²-h/week dialysis was necessary to prevent uremic neuropathy. This was followed by the concept of 'liter/kilogram' (total blood flow (L)/body weight (kg)) to measure the dose[26], further refined by Kjellstrand who proposed clearance × body weight or body volume. Both these are very similar in concept to Kt/V. Later Gotch and Sargent presented urea kinetic modeling (UKM) which focused exclusively on controlling the solute concentration of urea as the means of providing adequate dialysis[27].

Measurement of Kt/V

Each of the three methods used in current practice to obtain Kt/V have advantages and disadvantages. In assessing KT/V it is also important to define the contribution of residual renal function as well as solute removal by dialysis.

Urea kinetic modeling (UKM)

Figure 78.11a depicts the (A) decrease in urea during dialysis, (B) a rapid rebound immediately after dialysis and (C) steady increase during the rest of the interdialytic period. If urea were to be distributed in and removed from one compartment (a single pool), there would be no immediate postdialysis rebound but a steady increase in urea (E). UKM is based on the concept that interdialytic decline in urea represents dialytic removal (clearance) of urea, volume of distribution of urea, and the effect of urea generation during the treatment. Similarly the rate of increase in urea during the interdialytic period represents urea generation and volume of distribution of urea. Urea generation in turn is dependent on the protein catabolic rate (PCR), which, in steady state, is equal to dietary protein intake (DPI). By measuring urea before and after a dialysis treatment and before the next dialysis all these variables can be calculated and verified thus finally calculating the Kt/V value. The magnitude of decline in urea during the treatment is mostly a function of urea clearance (K), time of dialysis and volume of distribution of urea. For example, a rapid urea clearance or a longer dialysis time or a smaller volume of distribution will lead to a larger drop in urea concentration and vice versa (Fig. 78.11b). Line A represents the effect of faster clearance leading to a greater (75%) reduction in urea, compared with the slower clearance and 63% urea reduction (line A-1). In another situation, if the clearance were the same for A and A-1 but the V were different, the line A will represent smaller V (rapid and larger urea reduction) than represented by A-1 (larger V and slower the urea decline). Similarly, E and E-1 will represent smaller and larger V, respectively with similar urea generation.

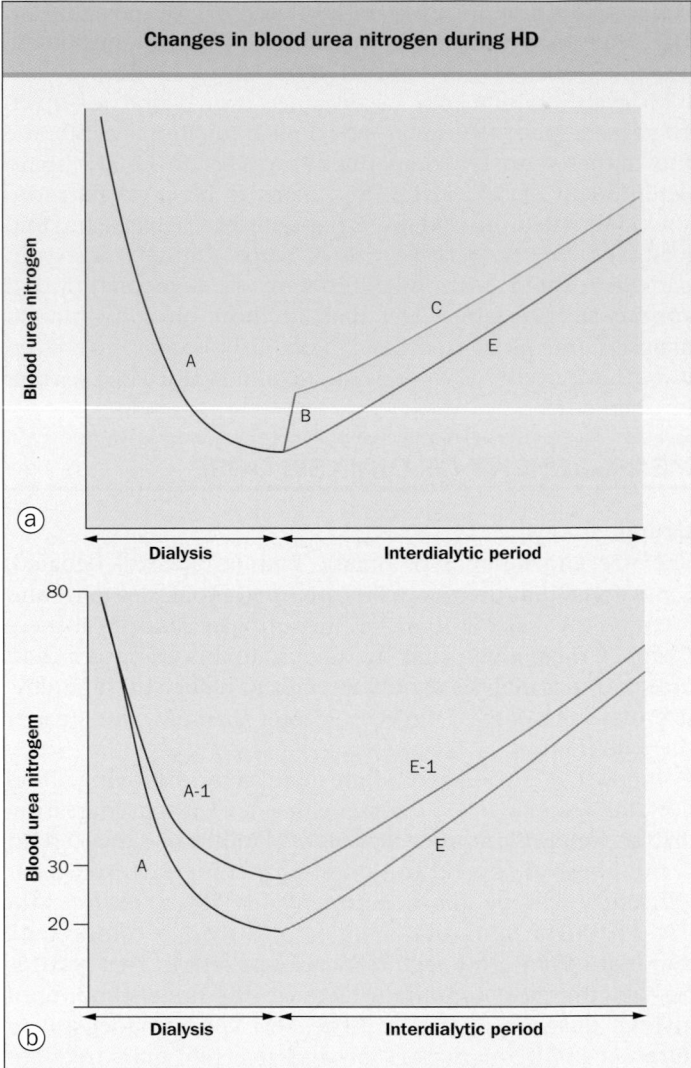

Figure 78.11 Changes in blood urea nitrogen during HD. (a) Decrease in urea during dialysis (A) is followed by a rapid rebound immediately after dialysis (B) and steady increase (C) during the interdialytic period. If urea were distributed in a single compartment there would be steady increase (E) without rebound. (b) Line A-1 represents either slower clearance of urea compared to A, or the same clearance but a larger volume of distribution (V). Similarly E and E-1 represent smaller and larger V with similar urea generation.

Urea Reduction Ratio (URR)

There is a relationship between Kt/V and how much urea is reduced during one treatment, URR (1-postdialysis urea/predialysis urea). Actually the decline in urea is exponential and can be mathematically expressed by formula:

Kt/V = – natural log (1 – URR)
or
Kt/V = – natural log (post-urea/ pre-urea)

Modified formula (Daugirdas)

Daugirdas modified this simple formula to account mathematically for the additional effects of the small amount of urea generated during the dialysis and also the effect of ultrafiltration on urea removal[28].

$$Kt/V = -LN\ (R - 0.008 \times T) + (4 - 3.5 \times R) \times UF/V\ or\ W$$

Where LN is natural log; T is duration of dialysis in hours; UF is ultrafiltration volume or interdialytic weight loss; V is postdialysis volume of distribution of urea, which can be substituted with W, postdialysis weight, assuming V is 55% of W.

Single pool vs multiple pool urea distribution

Figure 78.11a shows that urea removal is rapid in the early part of dialysis and after dialysis ends there is a rapid rebound of urea (line B) which is in excess of urea generation (lines C and E). The two major components of this rapid rebound are recirculation of dialyzed blood (access and cardiopulmonary recirculation) and sequestration of urea in pools such as muscle which are not receiving proportionally enough blood, so that effective V is reduced and there is faster interdialytic decline and rapid postdialytic rebound. Therefore single pool Kt/V would overestimate total body urea removal and thus reduction. Measurement of urea 30–60 min after the dialysis session ends enables equilibrated Kt/V (eKt/V) to be calculated, but this is not practical for routine clinical care. Alternatively, Daugirdas and Schneditz proposed the following formula to calculate eKt/V from single pool Kt/V:

For peripheral arteriovenous access:
$$eKt/V = Kt/V - 0.6 \times (Kt/V)/T + 0.03$$

For central venous access:
$$eKt/V = Kt/V - 0.47 \times (Kt/V)/T + 0.02$$

Planning the dialysis prescription

Variables influencing the delivery of the required dose of dialysis are dialyzer clearance, duration of dialysis treatment, blood flow rate and dialysate flow rate.

Dialyzer clearance is determined by the surface area and permeability of the dialyzer membrane. It is denoted as mass transfer area coefficient or KoA, which can be defined as the maximum clearance of a solute (e.g., urea) by the dialyzer when the blood and dialysate flows are not limiting factors. Nomograms are available giving the relationships between clearance and KoA for varying blood flow rates (Qb) and dialysate flow rates (Qd) (Fig. 78.12). The KoA (or clearance) reported by the manufacturer should be reduced by 20–30% before using it for further calculations. High efficiency dialyzers have KoA_{urea} > 700 mL/min and for the traditional dialyzer KoA_{urea} varies between 400 and 700 mL/min. Access recirculation will reduce the effective Qb and the K will be lower than assumed for that Qb. If Qd is slow, all the dialyzer membrane may not be penetrated thus reducing the effective surface area and both K and KoA. Time of dialysis (T) is measured in minutes and must be the actual dialysis time free of interruption and during which the actual Qb and Qd, for which K is assumed, are operational.

Most of the errors in using UKM occur because of V_{urea}. V_{urea} is equal to total body water (TBW) which in average size males and females are about 58% and 50% of body weight,

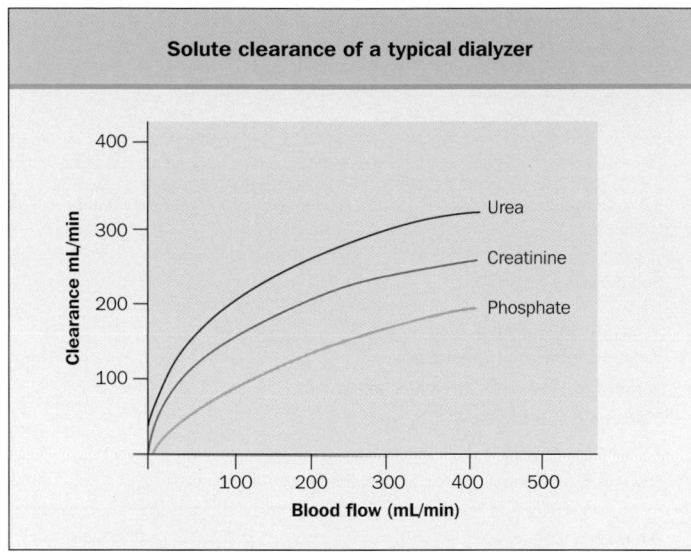

Figure 78.12 Nomogram defining dialyzer characteristics.
Diagrammatic representation of *in-vitro* clearance of different solutes over a range of blood flow rates in a typical dialyzer.

Patient samples and data for urea kinetic modeling
Predialysis and postdialysis blood urea for the first dialysis treatment of the week (sample collection as in Table 78.5)
Predialysis blood urea for the next dialysis treatment (see Table 78.5)
Predialysis and postdialysis patient weights at the first dialysis treatment of the week
Actual dialysis treatment time in minutes
Effective dialysis clearance, as measured in the hemodialysis unit (not *in vitro* clearance reported by the manufacturer); alternatively, computer programs hold dialyzer clearances that can be used for the calculation

Table 78.4 Patient samples and data required for formal urea kinetic modeling.

respectively. However major fluctuations in TBW, and in lean body mass change this relationship. V can also be calculated from body surface area by using Watson's formula[29]. The patient data required for UKM are shown in Table 78.4. Once V is determined and K is calculated, then dialysis time required for a desired value of Kt/V can be established. If using UKM, then the slopes of curves B and E (Fig. 78.12a) can be used to verify V. A major discrepancy should indicate that the source of error could be in K. However, even with this verification a major postdialysis urea rebound will potentially cause error in the estimation of V. Another common source of inaccuracy in UKM is in the collection of blood samples, which requires the utmost attention to detail (Table 78.5). A number of clinical and laboratory factors can result in real or apparent shortfall in delivery of the planned dialysis dose (Table 78.6). If a real shortfall in Kt/V is identified, there are a number of options for increasing dialysis dose (Fig. 78.13).

Blood sampling for urea kinetic modeling
Predialysis sample
Sample from fistula needle immediately after insertion (ideally insert without prefilling); if fistula needle prefilled or the patient is dialyzing via an indwelling catheter, withdraw and discard 10 mL blood to avoid contamination before sampling
Postdialysis sample
If postdialysis sample is contaminated by recirculation or saline washback, the dialysis dose will be overestimated
At end of dialysis set ultrafiltration rate to zero
Slow pump speed to 50–100 mL/min
Exactly 10 s later stop blood pump
Disconnect and draw 3 mL blood from fistula needle tubing
Analysis
Send all samples together to the laboratory for analysis consecutively in the same batch

Table 78.5 Sampling technique for urea kinetic modeling.

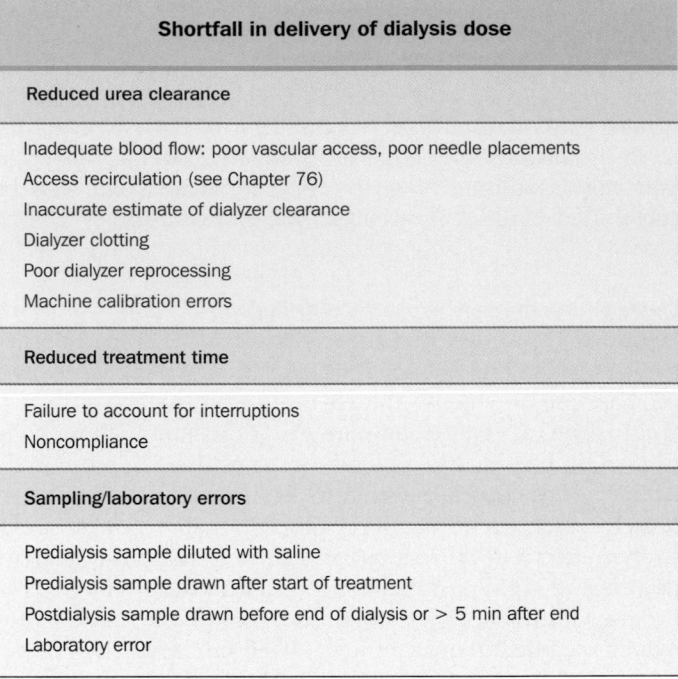

Shortfall in delivery of dialysis dose
Reduced urea clearance
Inadequate blood flow: poor vascular access, poor needle placements
Access recirculation (see Chapter 76)
Inaccurate estimate of dialyzer clearance
Dialyzer clotting
Poor dialyzer reprocessing
Machine calibration errors
Reduced treatment time
Failure to account for interruptions
Noncompliance
Sampling/laboratory errors
Predialysis sample diluted with saline
Predialysis sample drawn after start of treatment
Postdialysis sample drawn before end of dialysis or > 5 min after end
Laboratory error

Table 78.6 Causes of shortfall in delivery of dialysis dose.
Explanations to consider when delivered dialysis dose assessed by urea kinetic modeling fails to achieve the prescribed dose.

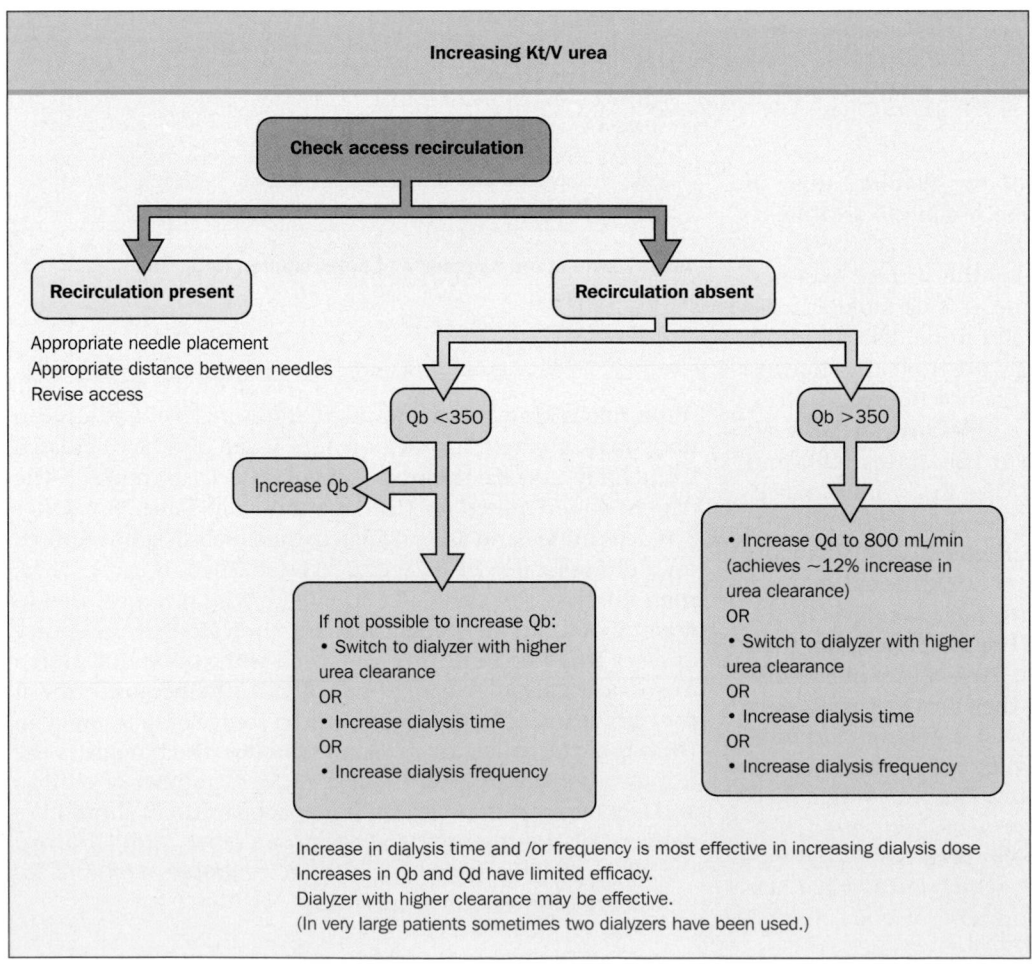

Figure 78.13 Steps to increase Kt/V urea. Adjustment of dialysis prescription to achieve required delivered dialysis dose.

STANDARDS OF DIALYSIS ADEQUACY

The National Cooperative Dialysis Study (NCDS)[30] first observed reduced morbidity in those patients who had lower time average concentration of urea (TAC$_{urea}$), whether patients were dialyzed for shorter or longer times, thus supporting the SM concept and underplaying the importance of dialysis time. However, subsequent analysis of NCDS showed that the duration of dialysis was also important in terms of patient outcome. NCDS demonstrated a relationship between medium-term morbidity and mortality and adequacy, defined by Kt/V, suggesting that a threshold Kt/V between 0.8 and 1, divided adequate from inadequate treatment[30]. This 'threshold' concept has been challenged. Some units which routinely deliver a Kt/V up to 1.6 by thrice weekly HD[13], appear to have better outcomes even adjusting for comorbidity. Retrospective analyses of quality-adjusted survival data[31], have suggested continuous improvement in outcome as Kt/V increases beyond 1, and this is supported by a recent prospective observational study, the Dialysis Outcome and Practice Patterns Study (DOPPS)[32].

Based on these data DOQI and the UK Renal Association both recommended a minimum dialysis dose of Kt/V 1.2, or URR 65%[33]. Support for these recommendations is not universal and the concept of Kt/V$_{urea}$ has been challenged If patients are segregated in racial and gender subgroups, USRDS data shows that African American men in the USA receive a lower dose of dialysis than Caucasian females, yet the adjusted mortality among African American males is better[34]. This apparent paradoxical relationship may be related to the body size, which increases V, resulting in a smaller calculated Kt/V, underscoring the limitations of calculated Kt/V. Similarly, long-term follow-up data from Tassin, France have the best ever reported patient survival on HD (60% survival over 10 years), has shown that the length of dialysis and dialysis index of MM not Kt/V$_{urea}$ predicted patient survival[13]. Analysis of the USRDS data found that a 10% increase in vitamin B$_{12}$ (MM) removal resulted in a 5% improvement in survival, which was independent of Kt/V$_{urea}$[35].

Remarkably good results from daily dialysis also support the concept of MM, since a change to daily dialysis, while maintaining the same weekly Kt/V, resulted in improved patient outcome[36]. More frequent dialysis, similar to longer dialysis, increases the removal of the slowly diffusing MM from extravascular to vascular compartment. Despite these uncertainties, minimum targets of Kt/V > 1.2 and URR > 65% are generally accepted. It is important to consider that these represent minimum standards and therefore the median Kt/V value among patients in any dialysis facility should be higher.

Findings from the HEMO Study, a large prospective study in which patients were assigned to three-times-a-week high (equilibrated Kt/V = 1.45) or standard (equilibrated Kt/V = 1.05) dialysis doses and high- or low-flux membranes in a randomized 2 × 2 factorial design, suggest that over a 3-year mean follow-up period, there were no statistically significant differences in overall mortality for the various combinations of dosage and membrane type[37]. This appears to confirm as adequate the minimum HD dose recommended by current treatment guidelines and suggest that, in general, higher doses and special membrane types provide no added benefit. However, differences were noted in subgroup analyses. Among women, the higher dialysis dose appeared to reduce the risk of death and hospitalization, and among people who had been on hemodialysis longer than 3.5 years when they joined the study, high-flux membranes appeared to reduce the risk of death. Analysis of USRDS data also shows that use of high-flux synthetic membrane dialyzers is associated with lower mortality risk[38]. These possible benefits of high-flux membranes suggest that clearance of larger molecules may have a role in defining adequacy of dialysis. It also appears that reuse, a strategy devised to allow the widespread economic use of synthetic membranes, is a safe procedure, mortality being no greater in reuse than no-reuse units. Reprocessed dialyzers may be more biocompatible than new dialyzers, producing fewer intradialytic symptoms, less complement activation, and a diminished initial fall in neutrophil count.

REFERENCES

1. Mion CM, Hegstrom RM, Boen SIM, Scribner BH. Substitution of sodium acetate for sodium bicarbonate in the bath fluid for haemodialysis. Trans Am Soc Artif Intern Organs. 1964;10:110–14.
2. Henderson LW, Koch KM, Dinarello CA, Shaldon S. Haemodialysis hypertension: the interleukin hypothesis. Blood Purif. 1983;1:3–8.
3. Stiller S, Mann H, Brunner H. Backfiltration in hemodialysis with highly permeable membranes. Contrib Nephrol. 1985;46:23–32.
4. Jochimsen EM, Carmichael WW, An JS, et al. Liver failure and death after exposure to microcystins at a haemodialysis center in Brazil. N Engl J Med. 1998;338:873–8.
5. Eaton JW, Kolpin CF, Swofford HS, et al. Chlorinated urban water: a cause of dialysis-induced hemolytic anemia. Science. 1973;181(98):463–4.
6. Katopodis KP, Hoenich NA. Accuracy and clinical utility of dialysis dose measurement using online ionic dialysance. Clin Nephrol. 2002;57(3):215–20.
7. Stiller S, Bonnie-Schorn E, Grassman A, Uhlenbusch-Korwer I, Mann H. A critical review of sodium profiling for hemodialysis. Semin Dialysis. 2001;14(5):337–47.
8. Hakim RM, Breillatt J, Lazarus JM, Port FK. Complement activation and hypersensitivity reactions to dialysis membranes. N Engl J Med. 1984;311:878–82.
9. Pierratos A. Nocturnal home haemodialysis: an update on a 5-year experience. Nephrol Dial Transplant. 1999;14(12):2835–40.
10. Chandna SM, Schultz L, Lawrence C, et al. Factors affecting survival and morbidity on chronic dialysis. Brit Med J. 1999;318:217–23.
11. Keshaviah P, Collins AJ, Ma JZ, et al. Survival comparison between hemodialysis and peritoneal dialysis based on matched doses of delivered therapy. J Am Soc Nephrol. 2002;13 (suppl)(1):S48–S52.
12. McKane W, Chandna SM, Tattersall JE, et al. Identical decline of residual renal function in high-flux biocompatible hemodialysis and CAPD. Kidney Int. 2002;61(1):256–65.
13. Charra B, Calemard E, Ruffet M, et al. Survival as an index of adequacy of dialysis. Kidney Int. 1992;41(5):1286–91.
14. Port FK, Hulbert-Shearon TE, Wolfe RA, et al. Predialysis blood pressure and mortality risk in a national sample of maintenance hemodialysis patients. Am J Kidney Dis. 1999;33(3):507–17.

Dialysis

15. Mitra S, Chandna SM, Farrington K. What is hypertension in chronic haemodialysis? The role of interdialytic blood pressure monitoring. Nephrol Dial Transplant. 1999;14(12): 2915–21.

16. Amar J, Vernier I, Rossignol E, et al. Nocturnal blood pressure and 24-hour pulse pressure are potent indicators of mortality in hemodialysis patients. Kidney Int. 2000;57(6):2485–91.

17. Owen WF, Lew NL. Liu N92, et al. The urea reduction ratio and serum albumin concentration as predictors of mortality in patients undergoing hemodialysis. N Engl J Med. 1993;329: 1001–6.

18. 3rd PTF, Wingard RL, Husni L, et al. Effect of the membrane bio-compatibility on nutritional parameters in chronic hemodialysis patients. Kidney Int. 1996;49(2):551–6.

19. Tielemans C, Husson C, Schurmans T, et al. Effects of ultrapure and non-sterile dialysate on the inflammatory response during in vitro hemodialysis. Kidney Int. 1996;49(1):236–43.

20. Block GA, Hulbert-Shearon TE, Levin NW, Port FK. Association of serum phosphorus and calcium x phosphate product with mortality risk in chronic hemodialysis patients, a national study. Am J Kid Dis. 1998;31:607–17.

21. Goodman WG, Goldin J, Kuizon BD, et al. Coronary artery calcification in young adults with end stage renal disease who are undergoing dialysis. N Engl J Med. 2000;342:1478–83.

22. Pickett TM, Cruickshank A, Greenwood RN, et al. Membrane flux not biocompatibility determines beta-2-microglobulin levels in hemodialysis patients. Blood Purif. 2002;20(2):161–6.

23. Locatelli F, Marcelli D, Conte F, et al. Comparison of mortality in ESRD patients on convective and diffusive extracorporeal treatments. Regist Lomb Dialisi E Trapianto Kidney Int. 1999;55: 286–93.

24. Raj D, Ouwendyk M, Francoeur R, Pierratos A. β_2-Microglobulin kinetics in nocturnal haemodialysis. Nephrol Dial Transplant. 2000;15:58–64.

25. Babb AL, Strand MJ, Uvelli DA, et al. Quantitative description of dialysis treatment: a dialysis index. Kidney Int. 1975;5(suppl): 23–29.

26. Milutinovic J, Babb AL, Eschbach JW, et al. Mathematical formulation of the dialysis index for middle molecules, DI (MM). Artif Organs. 1978;2:51–4.

27. Gotch FA, Sargent JA. A mechanistic analysis of the National Cooperative Dialysis Study (NCDS). Kidney Int. 1985;28(3):526–34.

28. Daugirdas JT. Second generation logarithmic estimate of single-pool variable volume Kt/V: an analysis of error. J Am Soc Nephrol. 1993; 4:1205–13.

29. Watson P, Watson I, Batt R. Total body water volumes for adult males and females estimated from simple anthropometric measurements. Am J Clin Nutr. 1980;33:27–39.

30. Lowrie E, Laird NM eds. National Cooperative Dialysis Study. Kidney Int. 1983;28 (suppl):S19–S26.

31. Hornberger JC. The hemodialysis prescription and quality-adjusted life expectancy. J Am Soc Nephrol. 1993;4:1004–20.

32. Locatelli F, Andrulli S, D'Amico M. Evaluation of dialysis outcomes: experimental versus observational evidence. J Nephrol. 2001;14 (suppl 4):S101–8.

33. Hemodialysis Adequacy Work Group. NKF-DOQI clinical practice guidelines for hemodialysis. Am J Kidney Dis. 1997;30 (suppl 2): 15–66.

34. Owen WF, Coladonato J, Szczech L, Reddan D. Explaining counter-intuitive clinical outcomes predicted by Kt/V. Semin Dialysis. 2001;14:268–70.

35. Leypoldt JK, Cheung AK, Carroll C, et al. Effect of dialysis membrane and middle molecule removal in chronic hemodialysis patient survival. Am J Kidney Dis. 1999;33:349–55.

36. Kooistra MP, Vos J, Koomans HA, Vos PF. Daily home hemodialysis in The Netherlands: Effects on metabolic control, haemodynamics and quality of life. Nephrol Dial Transplant. 1998;13:2853–60.

37. Mitka M. How to reduce mortality in dialysis patients still a puzzle. JAMA 2002;287:2643–4.

38. Port FK, Wolfe RA, Hulbert-Shearon TE, et al. Mortality risk by hemodialyzer reuse practice and dialyzer membrane characteristics: results from the USRDS dialysis morbidity and mortality study. Am J Kidney Dis 2001;37(2):276–86.

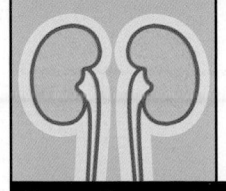

Chapter 79

Acute Complications of Hemodialysis

Bertrand L Jaber and Brian J G Pereira

DIALYSIS REACTIONS

During hemodialysis (HD), blood is exposed to surface components of the extra-corporeal circuit including the dialyzer, tubing, sterilization processes and other foreign substances related to the manufacturing and reprocessing procedures. This interaction between the patient's blood and the extracorporeal system can lead to various adverse reactions[1]. (Fig. 79.1)

Anaphylactic and anaphylactoid reactions
Clinical presentation

Anaphylaxis is the result of an IgE-mediated acute allergic reaction in a sensitized patient whereas anaphylactoid reactions result from the direct release of mediators by host cells. The onset of symptoms usually occurs within the first 5 min of initiating dialysis, although a delay of up to 20 min is possible. Symptoms vary from subtle to quite severe and

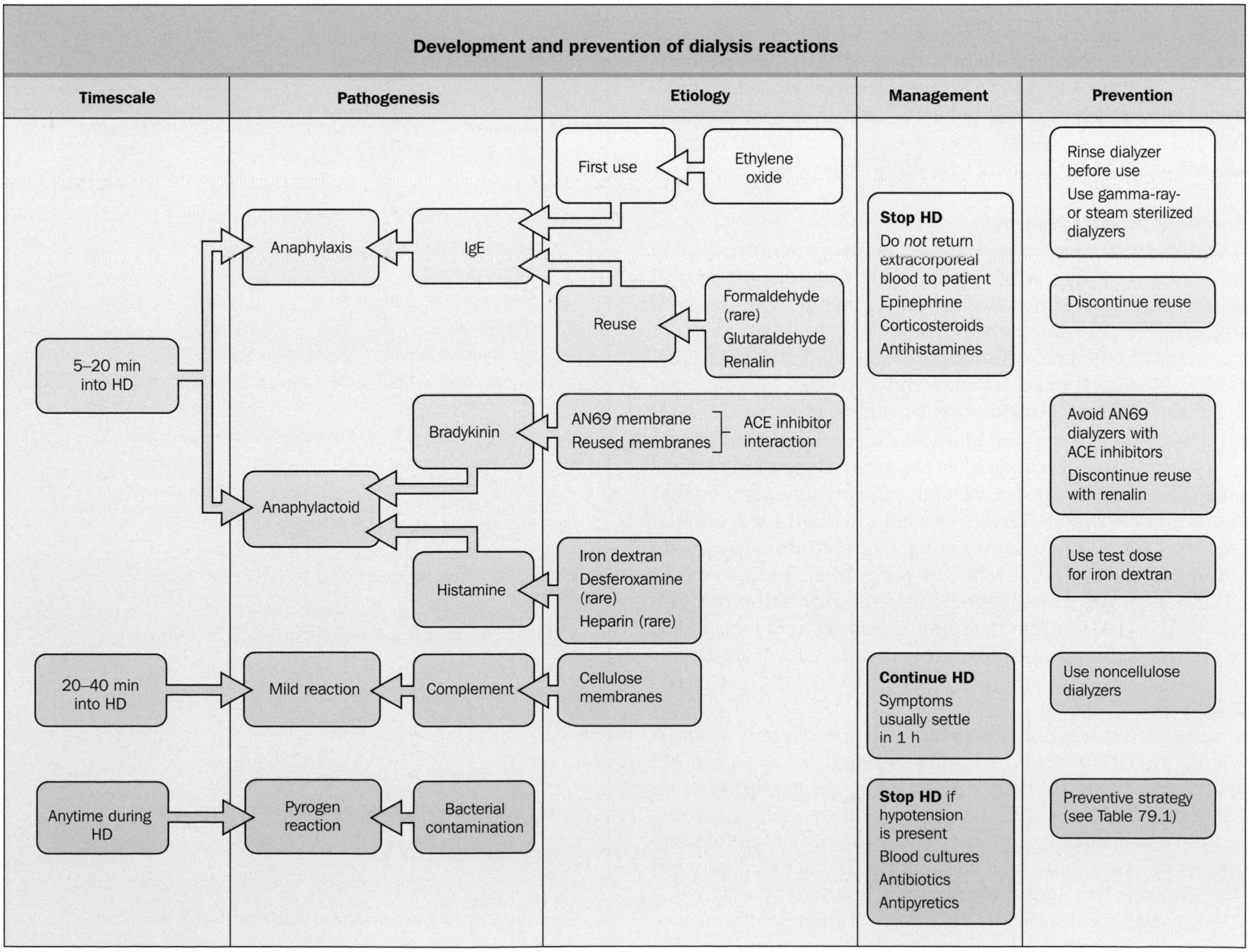

Development and prevention of dialysis reactions

Timescale	Pathogenesis	Etiology	Management	Prevention
5–20 min into HD	Anaphylaxis ← IgE	First use ← Ethylene oxide	**Stop HD** Do *not* return extracorporeal blood to patient Epinephrine Corticosteroids Antihistamines	Rinse dialyzer before use / Use gamma-ray- or steam sterilized dialyzers
		Reuse ← Formaldehyde (rare) / Glutaraldehyde / Renalin		Discontinue reuse
	Anaphylactoid ← Bradykinin	AN69 membrane / Reused membranes ⌐ ACE inhibitor interaction		Avoid AN69 dialyzers with ACE inhibitors / Discontinue reuse with renalin
	Anaphylactoid ← Histamine	Iron dextran / Desferoxamine (rare) / Heparin (rare)		Use test dose for iron dextran
20–40 min into HD	Mild reaction ← Complement	Cellulose membranes	**Continue HD** Symptoms usually settle in 1 h	Use noncellulose dialyzers
Anytime during HD	Pyrogen reaction ← Bacterial contamination		**Stop HD** if hypotension is present Blood cultures Antibiotics Antipyretics	Preventive strategy (see Table 79.1)

Figure 79.1 Development and prevention of dialysis reaction.

include burning/heat throughout the body or at the access site; dyspnea; chest tightness; angioedema/laryngeal edema; paresthesias involving the fingers, toes, lips or tongue; rhinorrhea; lacrimation; sneezing or coughing; skin flushing; pruritus; nausea/vomiting, abdominal cramps and diarrhea. Predisposing factors include a history of atopy, elevated total serum IgE, eosinophilia and the use of angiotensin converting enzyme (ACE) inhibitors. The etiology of dialysis reactions is diverse and requires a thorough investigation.

First use reactions

The majority of these reactions are ascribed to the manufacturer's dialyzer sterilant, ethylene oxide (ETO). The potting compound that anchors the hollow fibers in the dialyzer housing acts as a reservoir for ETO and may impede its washout from the dialyzer, leading to sensitization. When conjugated to human serum albumin (HSA), ETO acts as an allergen. Using a radioallergosorbent test (RAST), specific IgE antibodies against ETO-HSA are detected in two-thirds of patients with such reactions. However, 10% of patients with no prior history of dialysis reactions have a positive RAST.

Reuse reactions

As most residual ETO is washed out of the dialyzer during first use, reuse reactions are likely to be due to the disinfectants used for dialyzer reprocessing. These agents include formaldehyde, glutaraldehyde, and peracetic acid/hydrogen peroxide (renalin), and in allergic patients, specific IgE antibodies against formaldehyde are occasionally detectable.

Bradykinin-mediated reactions

Anaphylactoid reactions can occur in patients on ACE inhibitors who are dialyzed with AN69 dialyzers. Binding of factor XII to this sulfonate-containing membrane results in the formation of kallikrein and release of bradykinin which in turn, leads to the production of prostaglandin and histamine, with subsequent vasodilatation and increased vascular permeability. ACE inactivates bradykinin, and therefore, ACE inhibitors can prolong the biological activities of bradykinin.

Anaphylactoid reactions have also been observed in patients on ACE inhibitors who were dialyzed with membranes that had been reprocessed. Renalin was the sterilant used, and the reactions abated once reprocessing was discontinued, despite continued use of ACE inhibitors. It has been speculated that renalin may oxidize cysteine-containing proteins that are adsorbed on the dialyzer membrane, leading to the formation of cysteine sulfonate and contact activation of factor XII.

Drug-induced reactions

Anaphylactoid reactions to parenteral iron dextran occur in 0.6–1% of HD patients. *In vitro*, dextran produces a dose-dependent basophil histamine release. At a clinical dose > 250 mg, iron dextran is associated with hypotension and a serum sickness-like syndrome may ensue. It is therefore recommended to initiate iron dextran as a 25 mg test dose, with staff available to respond to reactions, followed by a course of 100 mg/dialysis session for 10 doses[2]. Intravenous iron gluconate or saccharate are alternatives increasingly used for patients requiring intravenous iron supplementation because

of rare anaphylactoid reactions to dextran. Patients rarely exhibit hypersensitivity to heparin formulations, which respond by substituting beef with pork heparin, or vice versa.

Treatment and prevention

Treatment of anaphylactic/anaphylactoid reaction requires the immediate cessation of HD without returning the extracorporeal blood to the patient. Epinephrine, antihistamines, corticosteroids and respiratory support should be provided, if needed. Specific preventive measures include rinsing the dialyzer immediately before first use, substituting ETO- with gamma- or steam-sterilized dialyzers, avoiding AN69 membranes in patients on ACE inhibitors, and discontinuing reprocessing procedures in selected cases.

Mild reactions

Mild reactions occur 20–40 min after initiating dialysis with unsubstituted cellulose dialyzers and consist of chest/back pain. Dialysis can be continued as symptoms usually abate after the first hour, suggesting a relation to the degree of

---

Strategies to prevent bacterial contamination

- Strict adherence to the AAMI standards

Type of fluid	Microbial count	Endotoxin
– Water products	< 200 cfu/mL	< 2 EU
– Dialysate	< 2000 cfu/mL	no standard
– Reprocessed dialyzers	No growth	–

- Use appropriate germicide
    - 4% formaldehyde*
    - 1% formaldehyde heated to 40°C*,†
    - glutaraldehyde†
    - hydrogen peroxide/peracetic acid mixture (Renalin®)*,†
    - heat sterilization (105°C for 20 h) for reprocessing of polysulfone membranes.†
- Wash and rinse the vascular access arm with soap and water
- Prior to cannulation, inspect vascular access for local signs of inflammation
- Scrub the skin with povidone iodine or chlorhexidine, and allow to dry out for 5 min prior to cannulation
- Record temperature prior to and at the end of dialysis
- When central delivery system is used:
    - clean and disinfect connecting pipes regularly
    - remove residual bacteria or endotoxin by additional filtration
- When single-patient proportioning dialysis machine is used:
    - freshly prepare bicarbonate dialysate on a daily basis
    - discard unused solutions at the end of each day
    - rinse and disinfect containers with fluids that meet AAMI standards
    - air-dry containers prior to dialysate preparation
- Follow manufacturer's guidelines for use of preservative-free medications

AAMI, Association for the Advancement of Medical Instrumentation; cfu, colony forming unit.
*A minimum of 11- or 24-h exposure to peracetic acid or formaldehyde is required, respectively.
†These germicides are all equivalent or superior to 4% formaldehyde.

Table 79.1 Strategies to prevent bacterial contamination.

complement activation. Indeed, these reactions decrease with the use of substituted and reprocessed unsubstituted cellulose membranes. Oxygen therapy and analgesics are usually sufficient. Preventive measures include automated cleansing of new dialyzers or using noncellulose dialyzers.

Microbial contamination

Several factors that are operative during dialysis place patients at risk for exposure to bacterial products, including contaminated water/bicarbonate dialysate, improperly sterilized dialyzers, and cannulation of infected grafts or fistulas[1]. Soluble bacterial products can diffuse across the dialyzer into the blood, resulting in cytokine production and consequently, pyrogen reactions. When bacterial contamination becomes excessive, pyrogen reactions with or without bacteremia can result.

Pyrogen reaction is a diagnosis of exclusion, as early septicemia should first be ruled out. Careful examination of the dialysis access is warranted and blood cultures should be obtained. Treatment includes antipyretics, broad-spectrum antibiotics, discontinuation of ultrafiltration whenever hypotension is present and selective hospitalization. An outbreak of bacteremia among several patients, involving a similar organism should prompt a thorough search for bacterial contaminants in the dialysis equipment[1]. Attention should also be paid to single-use vials that are punctured several times, such as Epoetin alfa, which was recently linked to an outbreak of bloodstream infection[3]. Strategies for the prevention of pyrogen reactions are summarized in Table 79.1.

CARDIOVASCULAR COMPLICATIONS

Hypotension

Intradialytic hypotension occurs in 10–30% of treatments, ranging from asymptomatic episodes to marked compromise of organ perfusion resulting in myocardial ischemia, cardiac arrhythmias, vascular thrombosis, loss of consciousness, seizures or death. Further, in patients with acute renal failure, intradialytic hypotension may induce further renal ischemia and retard recovery of renal function. The pathogenesis of intradialytic hypotension is complex[4] and is summarized in Figure 79.2.

The immediate treatment is to restore the circulating blood volume by placing the patient in a Trendelenburg position, reducing or stopping ultrafiltration, and infusing isotonic normal saline. With the advent of newer dialysis engineering principles, better preventive strategies have emerged. These include the use of bicarbonate dialysate, volumetric control of ultrafiltration, sodium modeling and better assessment of patient's 'dry weight'. Both midodrine, an oral selective alpha 1 agonist, and cool dialysate, which increases the release of catecholamines are also useful preventive therapies[5]. Salt poor albumin offers no advantage over normal saline and costs more. Other preventive strategies include correction of anemia and hypoalbuminemia, withdrawal of antihypertensive drugs before dialysis, avoidance of food before and during dialysis, counseling patients about weight gain and treatment of congestive heart failure or arrhythmias.

If hypotension recurs soon after the initiation of dialysis, pericardial effusion and tamponade is a life-threatening condition, which should be considered.

Hypertension

Hypertension during or immediately after dialysis constitutes an important risk factor for cardiovascular mortality. Its mechanism is primarily volume-dependent. However, in a number of patients, blood pressure remains elevated despite fluid removal, a syndrome called dialysis-refractory hypertension. These patients are usually young with pre-existing

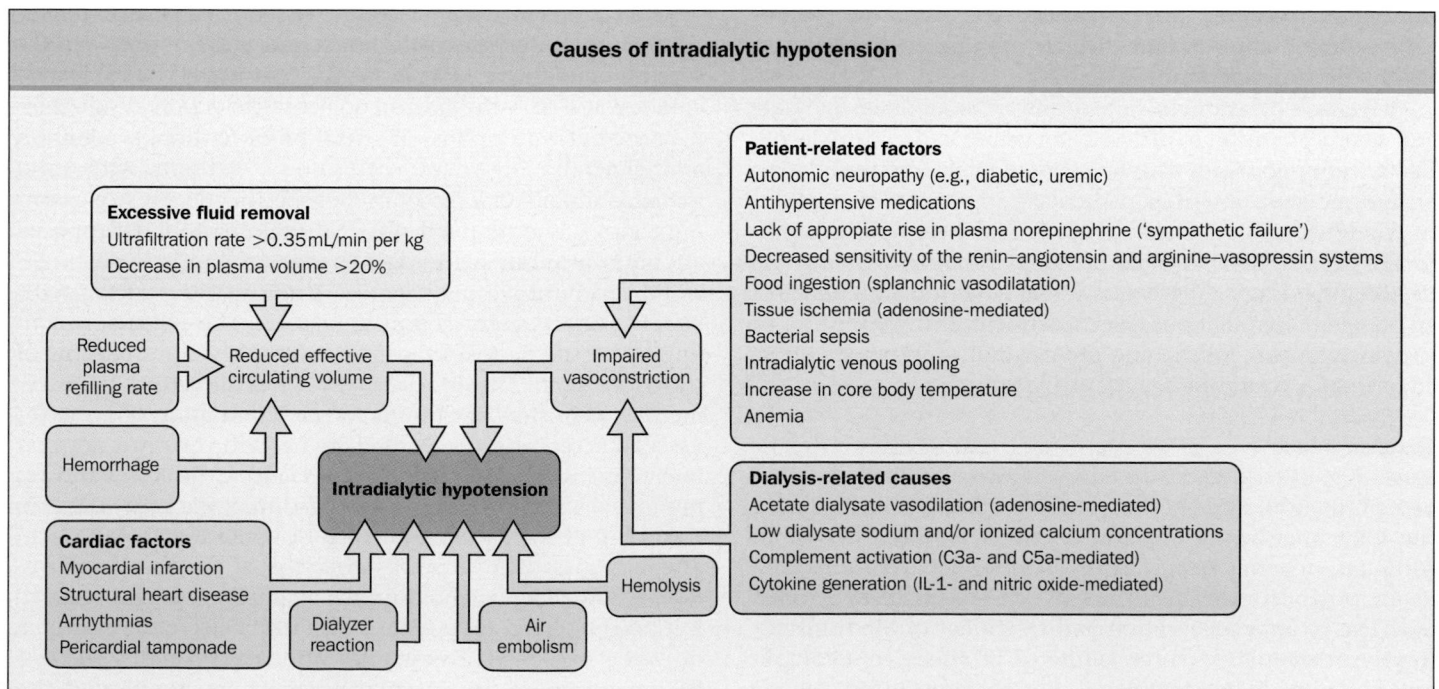

Causes of intradialytic hypotension

Excessive fluid removal
Ultrafiltration rate >0.35mL/min per kg
Decrease in plasma volume >20%

Reduced plasma refilling rate

Reduced effective circulating volume

Hemorrhage

Cardiac factors
Myocardial infarction
Structural heart disease
Arrhythmias
Pericardial tamponade

Dialyzer reaction

Air embolism

Intradialytic hypotension

Impaired vasoconstriction

Hemolysis

Patient-related factors
Autonomic neuropathy (e.g., diabetic, uremic)
Antihypertensive medications
Lack of appropiate rise in plasma norepinephrine ('sympathetic failure')
Decreased sensitivity of the renin–angiotensin and arginine–vasopressin systems
Food ingestion (splanchnic vasodilatation)
Tissue ischemia (adenosine-mediated)
Bacterial sepsis
Intradialytic venous pooling
Increase in core body temperature
Anemia

Dialysis-related causes
Acetate dialysate vasodilation (adenosine-mediated)
Low dialysate sodium and/or ionized calcium concentrations
Complement activation (C3a- and C5a-mediated)
Cytokine generation (IL-1- and nitric oxide-mediated)

Figure 79.2 Pathogenesis and causes of intradialytic hypotension.

hypertension and have excessive interdialytic weight gain and a hyperactive renin–angiotensin system in response to fluid removal[6].

Epoetin has been associated with a 20–30% incidence of new onset or exacerbation of hypertension. Further, among patients receiving intravenous (not subcutaneous) epoetin, elevated levels of endothelin-1 (a potent vasoconstrictor) have been shown to correlate with increased blood pressure. Intradialytic hypertension can be precipitated by the use of hypernatric dialysate (sodium modeling)[7]. Finally, clinicians should also be aware of possible dialytic removal of certain antihypertensive drugs (see Chapter 96).

Treatment requires an accurate determination of the patient's 'dry weight'. It is reasonable to avoid the use of sodium modeling, reduce the 'dry weight' by 0.5 kg, observe the clinical response, and re-evaluate periodically. Once 'dry weight' is achieved, optimization of antihypertensive drug therapy is warranted, including withholding antihypertensive medication before dialysis.

Cardiac arrhythmias

Intradialytic arrhythmias are common and are often multifactorial in origin[8,9]. Left ventricular hypertrophy, congestive cardiomyopathy, uremic pericarditis, silent myocardial ischemia and conduction system calcification are frequently encountered in adult dialysis patients. In addition, polypharmacy coupled with the constant alterations in fluid, electrolyte and acid/base homeostasis, may precipitate intradialytic arrhythmias. Hypocalcemia and hypomagnesemia have additive effects on hypokalemia, whereas hypercalcemia and hypokalemia can precipitate arrhythmias in patients on digoxin. Further, myocardial ischemia due to a decrease in myocardial oxygen delivery (e.g., intradialytic hypotension) or an increase in myocardial oxygen consumption (e.g., volume overload) can trigger arrhythmias in patients with underlying coronary artery disease. The range of electrocardiographic abnormalities which may be encountered in renal failure are shown in Table 69.3.

Preventive measures include the use of bicarbonate dialysate and careful attention to dialysate potassium and calcium levels. Use of zero potassium dialysate should be discouraged due to arrhythmogenic potential, particularly in patients on digoxin, its where serum potassium should not fall below 3.5 mmol/L. Serum digoxin levels should be regularly monitored and the need for the drug regularly reassessed. Finally, maintenance of an adequate hemoglobin level, treatment of hypertension or congestive heart failure and antianginal prophylaxis offers additional precautions against arrhythmias.

Sudden death

Some 80% of sudden deaths during dialysis are due to ventricular fibrillation, and they are more frequently observed after the long interdialytic interval on thrice weekly dialysis[10,11]. Although ischemic heart disease increases the risk for sudden death, other catastrophic intradialytic events need to be ruled out. The prompt recognition and treatment of life-threatening hyperkalemia, often encountered in young, noncompliant patients, is imperative. Profound generalized muscle weakness may be a warning sign of imminent life-threatening hyperkalemia. When cardiopulmonary arrest occurs during dialysis, an immediate decision must be made as to whether the collapse is due to an intrinsic disease or whether technical errors such as air embolism, unsafe dialysate composition, overheated dialysate, line disconnection or sterilant in the dialyzer have occurred. Air in the dialysate, grossly hemolyzed blood, and hemorrhage due to line disconnection can be easily detected. However, if no obvious cause is identifiable, blood should not be returned to the patient, particularly if the arrest occurred immediately upon initiation of dialysis. A patient exposed to formaldehyde may have complained earlier, of burning at the access site. If the possibility of a problem with dialysate composition is remote, blood may be returned to the patient. However, blood and dialysate samples should be immediately sent for electrolyte analysis, the dialyzer and blood lines saved for later analysis, and the dialysis machine replaced until all of its safety features have been thoroughly evaluated for possible malfunction. While the management of cardiopulmonary arrest during dialysis should follow the standard principles of cardiopulmonary resuscitation, the diagnosis and management of technical errors is discussed later.

Dialysis-associated steal syndrome

The construction of an arteriovenous fistula or graft frequently results in reduction of blood flow to the hand. Although clinically significant ischemia does not usually result, symptoms are by no means rare, particularly in diabetics or elderly patients with peripheral vascular disease. Dialysis-associated steal syndrome has been reported in 6.4% and 1% of patients with radiocephalic fistulas or grafts, respectively. The clinical presentation, differential diagnosis and evaluation of dialysis-associated steal syndrome are summarized in Table 79.2[12,13].

Treatment depends on the clinical severity of ischemia and vascular access anatomy[13]. Severe ischemia can cause irreparable injury to nerves within hours and must be considered a surgical emergency. Mild ischemia, manifested by subjective coldness and paresthesias and objective reduction in skin temperature but with no loss of sensation or motion, is common and generally improves with time[14]. Patients with mild ischemia should undergo symptom-specific therapy (e.g., wearing a glove) and frequent physical examination, with special attention to subtle neurologic changes and muscle wasting[15]. Failure to improve may require surgical intervention with banding or access correction or ligation. The simplest way to improve distal perfusion is ligation of the venous outflow of the fistula/graft. This procedure provides immediate improvement in perfusion but results in the elimination of a site for vascular access and the immediate need to construct another one. Other techniques that do not sacrifice the access and yet improve distal perfusion include ligation of the artery distal to the origin of the fistula/graft with or without establishing an arterial bypass (Fig 76.5) or narrowing of the fistula/graft to reduce flow. Percutaneous luminal angioplasty or laser recanalization is reserved for patients with inflow or outflow arterial disease. Persistence of symptoms after an apparently successful correction of the vascular access flow should alert the clinician to other unrelated causes.

Dialysis-associated vascular steal syndrome
Clinical Presentations
(symptoms often aggravated on dialysis)
Hand numbness, pain or weakness
Coolness of distal arm
Diminished pulses
Acrocyanosis, gangrene
Differential diagnosis
Consider:
Dialysis-associated cramp
Polyneuropathy – diabetes, uremia
Entrapment neuropathy – Aβ2M-amyloid
Reflex sympathetic dystrophy
Calciphylaxis
Evaluation of steal severity
Pulse oximetry
Plethysmography
Doppler flow
Angiography
Treatment options
(depending on severity)
Symptomatic (e.g. gloves)
Surgical
With preservation of vascular access – banding to reduce flow, DRIL procedure (Fig 76.5)
With loss of vascular access - ligation

Table 79.2 Dialysis-associated vascular steal syndrome.

NEUROMUSCULAR COMPLICATIONS

Muscle cramps

Muscle cramps occur in 5–20% of patients late during dialysis and frequently involve the legs. They account for 15% of premature discontinuations of dialysis or 'sign-offs'[16]. Electromyography shows increased tonic muscle electrical activity throughout dialysis, and elevated serum creatinine kinase levels may be seen.

Although the pathogenesis is unknown, dialysis-induced volume contraction and hypo-osmolality are common predisposing factors. However, hypomagnesemia and carnitine deficiency may also play a role.

The acute management is directed at increasing plasma osmolality. Parenteral infusion of 23.5% hypertonic saline (15–20 mL), 25% mannitol (50–100 mL) or 50% dextrose in water (25–50 mL) are equally effective. However, hypertonic saline may result in postdialytic thirst, and both hypertonic saline and mannitol cause transient warmth/flushing during the infusion. Furthermore, large and repetitive infusions of mannitol may lead to increased thirst, interdialytic weight gain and fluid overload. Overall, dextrose in water is preferred, particularly in nondiabetics.

Preventive measures include dietary counseling about excessive interdialytic weight gain. In patients without clinical signs of fluid overload, it is reasonable to increase the 'dry weight' by 0.5 kg, and observe the clinical response. Quinine sulfate (260–325 mg) or oxazepam (5–10 mg) given 2 h prior to dialysis may also be effective. However, in the USA, the Food and Drug Administration regards quinine sulfate as both unsafe and ineffective for the prevention of cramps. The use of sodium gradient during dialysis is effective as well. Proposed strategies include, starting with a dialysate sodium concentration of 145–155 mmol/L and a linear decrease to 135–140 mmol/L by the completion of the treatment. A comparison of sodium modeling using an exponential, linear or step program has yielded similar results[17]. In anecdotal reports, 5 mg enalapril twice weekly may be effective, presumably by inhibiting angiotensin II-mediated thirst. Finally, stretching exercises and carnitine supplementation (20 mg/kg per dialysis session) may also be beneficial.

Restless legs syndrome

Patients complain of crawling sensations in their legs that occur exclusively during sleep or inactive seated or recumbent wakefulness, such as during dialysis. Although the tendency to move can be momentarily suppressed, it is ultimately irresistible to move the legs, which yields prompt relief. Some patients also complain of pain at the same site. As a consequence, most patients have insomnia, and some suffer from anxiety or mild depression. The results of neurologic and electromyographic examinations are generally unremarkable.

Iron deficiency anemia, vascular insufficiency, chronic lung disease and abuse of caffeine have all been implicated in the pathogenesis of restless legs[18]. The differential diagnosis is peripheral neuropathy, in which paresthesias are constant and unrelieved by activity. When symptoms develop in a stable dialysis patient, anxiety, peripheral vascular disease and inadequate dialysis need to be considered.

Whereas temazepam (a short-acting benzodiazepine) is temporarily effective when administered at bedtime, opiates are remarkably efficient but have the potential for abuse and development of tolerance. Carbamazepine and levodopa have also been advocated but tolerance may develop rapidly. Hence, a reasonable approach is to alternate chemically unrelated agents on a weekly/biweekly basis. These agents should be given early enough before dialysis to allow for absorption. Transcutaneous electric nerve stimulation should be reserved for refractory cases. More recently, pramipexole, a dopamine receptor agonist, as primary therapy, has been associated with excellent outcomes in a nondialysis population[19].

Dialysis disequilibrium syndrome

Despite a decline in its incidence, dialysis-disequilibrium syndrome (DDS) is still observed sporadically in patients who are initiated on HD with large-surface area and high-flux dialyzers and shorter dialysis time. Risk factors include young age, severe azotemia, low dialysate sodium concentration and pre-existing neurological disorders.

DDS commonly presents with restlessness, headache, nausea, vomiting, blurred vision, muscle twitching, disorientation, tremor and hypertension. More severe manifestations include obtundation, seizures and coma. DDS usually develops towards the end of dialysis but may be delayed for up to 24 h. Although cerebral edema is a consistent finding on computerized tomographic (CT) scanning, DDS remains a clinical diagnosis since laboratory tests, including electroencephalography (EEG) are nonspecific. It is usually self-limited but full recovery may take several days.

The pathogenesis of DDS is still a subject to debate. The 'reverse urea effect' theory, which proposes that a transient osmotic disequilibrium occurs during dialysis as a result of a more rapid removal of urea from blood than from cerebrospinal fluid (CSF) has been disputed[20]. In animals undergoing rapid dialysis, despite the correction of systemic acidosis, a paradoxical CSF acidosis develops which is aborted by slower dialysis. Additional mechanisms include the intracerebral accumulation of idiogenic osmoles such as inositol, glutamine and glutamate.

In high-risk patients, preventive measures include the use of volumetric controlled machines, bicarbonate dialysate, sodium modeling, earlier recognition of uremic states and earlier initiation of dialysis. In addition, short and more frequent dialysis treatments are recommended using small-surface area dialyzers and reduced blood flow rates. The target reduction in plasma urea should initially be limited to 30%. The prophylactic use of mannitol or anticonvulsants is not recommended.

Seizures

Intradialytic seizures occur in < 10% of patients, and tend to be generalized but easily controlled. However, focal or refractory seizures warrant evaluation for focal neurological disease, particularly intracranial hemorrhage. Causes of seizures are summarized in Figure 79.3.

Treatment of established seizures requires cessation of dialysis, maintenance of airway patency, and investigation for metabolic abnormalities. Intravenous diazepam or clonazepam, and phenytoin may be required. Intravenous administration of 50% dextrose in water should be administered promptly if hypoglycemia is suspected.

Headache

Dialysis headache is common and consists of a bifrontal discomfort that develops during dialysis, and may become intense and throbbing, accompanied by nausea and vomiting. It is usually aggravated by the supine position, but there are no visual disturbances.

Although its etiology has not been elucidated, dialysis headache may be a subtle manifestation of DDS or may be related to the use of acetate dialysate. Furthermore, it may be a manifestation of caffeine withdrawal due to dialytic removal of caffeine.

Management consists of oral analgesics (acetaminophen), and preventive measures include slow dialysis with reduced blood flow rates, change to bicarbonate dialysate, coffee ingestion during dialysis and use of reprocessed dialyzers.

HEMATOLOGICAL COMPLICATIONS

Complement activation and dialysis-associated neutropenia

During dialysis with unsubstituted cellulose dialyzers, the free hydroxyl groups present on the membrane cause activation of the alternative pathway of complement[21]. This results in activation and increased adherence of circulating neutrophils to the endothelial capillary pulmonary vasculature, leading to transient neutropenia that reaches a nadir after 15 min dialysis, followed by a rebound leucocytosis 1h later. Although the long-term clinical relevance of this phenomenon remains speculative, its contribution to acute intradialytic morbidity is discussed later.

Intradialytic hemolysis

Acute hemolysis can be due to faulty dialysis equipment, chemicals, drugs, toxins or patient-related factors[22] (Fig. 79.4).

Figure 79.3 Causes of hemodialysis-associated seizures.

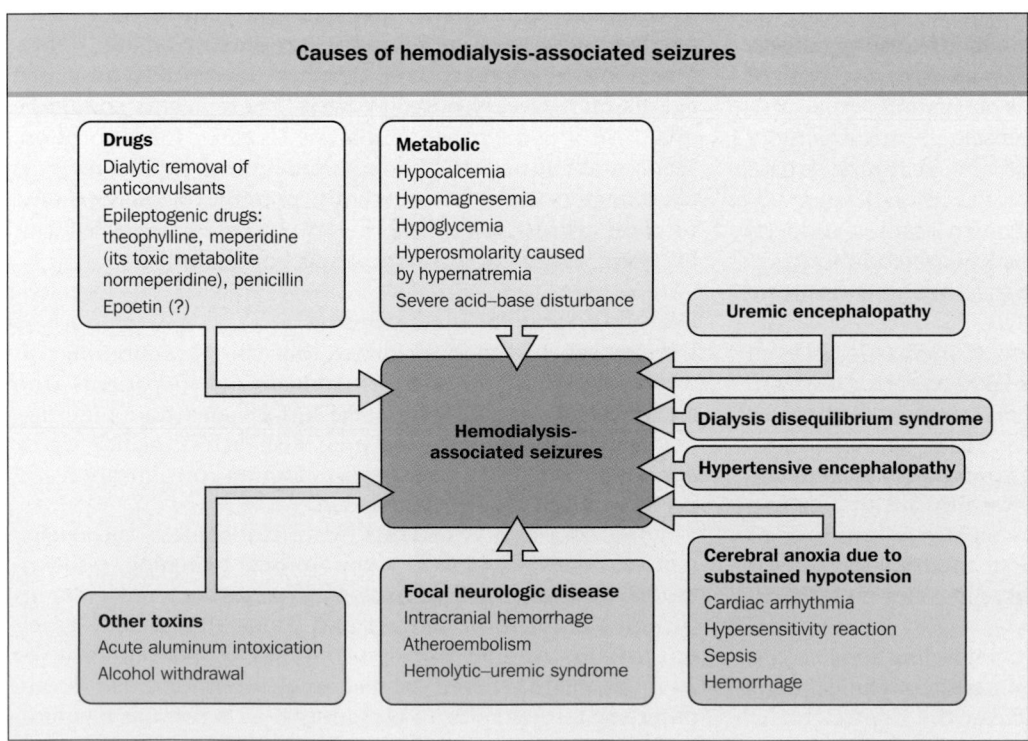

Causes of hemodialysis-associated seizures

Drugs
Dialytic removal of anticonvulsants
Epileptogenic drugs: theophylline, meperidine (its toxic metabolite normeperidine), penicillin
Epoetin (?)

Metabolic
Hypocalcemia
Hypomagnesemia
Hypoglycemia
Hyperosmolarity caused by hypernatremia
Severe acid–base disturbance

Uremic encephalopathy

Hemodialysis-associated seizures

Dialysis disequilibrium syndrome

Hypertensive encephalopathy

Other toxins
Acute aluminum intoxication
Alcohol withdrawal

Focal neurologic disease
Intracranial hemorrhage
Atheroembolism
Hemolytic–uremic syndrome

Cerebral anoxia due to substained hypotension
Cardiac arrhythmia
Hypersensitivity reaction
Sepsis
Hemorrhage

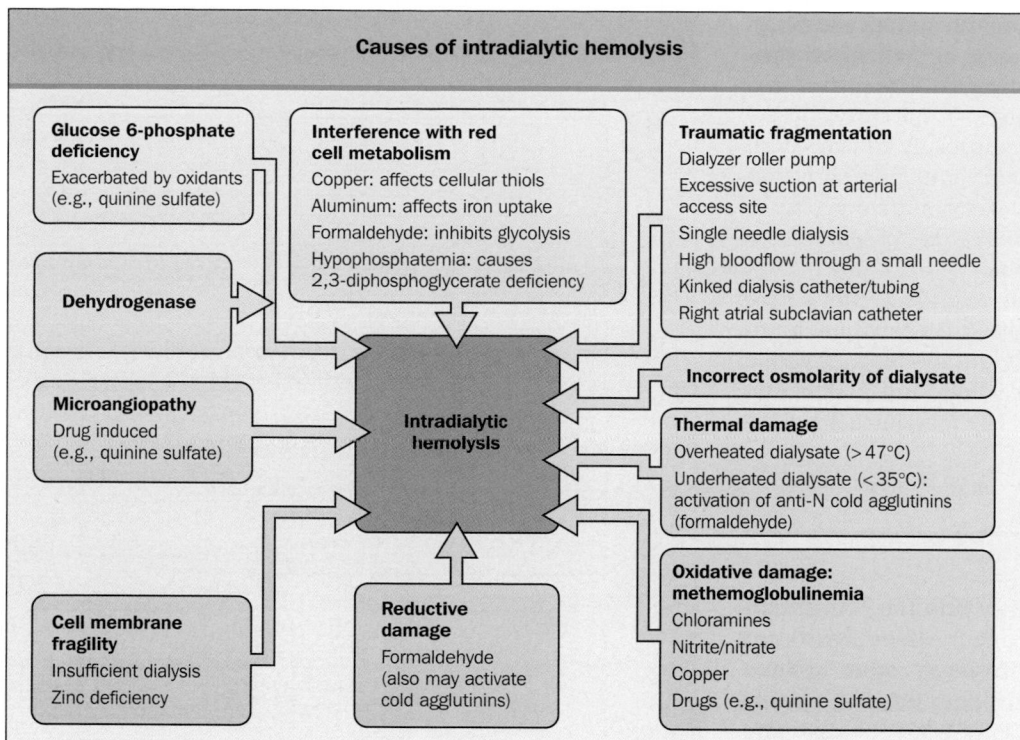

Figure 79.4 Causes of intradialytic hemolysis.

With the advent of better dialysis equipment and the widespread use of deionization systems, traumatic red blood cell (RBC) fragmentation caused by poorly designed blood pumps, and methemoglobinemia caused by water contamination with chloramine or copper are never seen today. However, nitrate/nitrite intoxication causing methemoglobinemia still occurs sporadically in patients on home HD who use well water that is contaminated with urine from domesticated animals. Further, during dialyzer reprocessing, formaldehyde retention can result in hemolysis by inducing formation of cold agglutinins or inhibiting RBC metabolism.

The diagnosis of acute hemolysis is self-evident when grossly translucent hemolyzed blood is observed in the tubing. Patients with methemoglobinemia have nausea, vomiting, hypotension and cyanosis, and oxygen therapy does not improve the black-colored blood present in the extracorporeal circuit. Copper contamination should be suspected in the presence of skin flushing and abdominal pain or diarrhea.

Evaluation should include reticulocyte count, haptoglobin, lactate dehydrogenase, blood smear, Coombs test and measurement of methemoglobin. ^{51}Cr-RBC survival and bone marrow examination may occasionally be indicated if there is recurrent hemolysis. More importantly, analysis of tap water for chloramines and metal contaminants and thorough analysis of the dialysis equipment for clues of increased blood turbulence are recommended.

Hemorrhage

Bleeding complications are commonly related to the use of intradialytic anticoagulation, which further confounds the uremic bleeding diathesis[23] (see Chapter 71). In addition, dialysis patients are prone to spontaneous bleeding at specific sites, such as gastrointestinal arteriovenous malformations, subdural, pericardial, pleural, retroperitoneal and hepatic subcapsular spaces, and ocular anterior chamber. Despite its limitations, the bleeding time remains the best indicator of hemorrhagic tendency. In addition to specific measures directed to the site of hemorrhage, reversal of uremic platelet dysfunction is imperative. Strategies include the use of epoe or RBC transfusions to achieve a hematocrit > 30% in order to improve rheological platelets–vessel wall interactions; intravenous conjugated estrogens at 0.6 mg/kg per day for 5 consecutive days; intravenous/subcutaneous 1-deamino-8-D-arginine vasopressin (DDAVP) at 0.3 µg/kg over 15–30 min; and/or intravenous infusion of cryoprecipitate. For patients experiencing severe bleeding, it is advisable to consider heparin-free dialysis, using normal saline flushes every 15–30 min with ultrafiltration adjustments, regional heparin or citrate anticoagulation, low-molecular-weight heparin, heparin modeling or prostacyclin. In patients scheduled for elective surgery or invasive procedures, aspirin should be stopped a week earlier, the dose of anticoagulant reduced to minimum and the hematocrit maintained above 30%. In some cases, DDAVP and/or estrogens may also be required.

PULMONARY COMPLICATIONS

Dialysis-associated hypoxemia

In most patients, the arterial Pao_2 drops by 5–20 mmHg (0.6–4 kPa) during dialysis, reaching a nadir at 30–60 min, and resolves within 60–120 min following discontinuation of dialysis. This drop is usually of no clinical significance to patients unless there is pre-existing chronic cardiopulmonary disease.

Hypoventilation is the main implicated factor and is primarily central in origin due to a drop in carbon dioxide production following acetate metabolism (specific to acetate dialysate), loss of carbon dioxide in the dialyzer (with both acetate and bicarbonate dialysate), and rapid alkalinization of body fluids (specific to bicarbonate dialysate, particularly with large surface-area dialyzers)[24]. In addition, acetate-induced respiratory muscle fatigue can lead to hypoventilation, especially in acutely ill patients. Further, a commonly observed ventilation/perfusion mismatch may be due to pulmonary leukoagglutination (due to complement activation) and/or impaired cardiac output (due to acetate-induced myocardial depression).

In high-risk patients with fluid overload, preventive measures consist of using intradialytic oxygen supplementation, conventional bicarbonate dialysate and biocompatible membranes. Optimizing hematocrit values and performing sequential ultrafiltration followed by HD may further reduce the likelihood of hypoxemia.

TECHNICAL MALFUNCTIONS

Air embolism

The most vulnerable source of air entry into the extracorporeal circuit is the prepump tubing segment, where significant subatmospheric pressures prevail. However, other sources need to be considered including intravenous infusion circuits especially with glass bottles, air bubbles from the dialysate and dialysis catheters. High blood flow rates may allow rapid entry of large volumes of air despite small leaks.

Clinical manifestations depend on the volume of air introduced, the site of introduction, patient's position and the speed at which air is introduced[25]. In the sitting position, air entry through a peripheral vein bypasses the heart and causes venous emboli in the cerebral circulation. The acute onset of seizures and coma in the absence of precedent symptoms such as chest pain or dyspnea is highly suggestive of air embolism. In the supine position, air introduced through a central venous line will be trapped in the right ventricle where it forms a foam, interferes with cardiac output, and if large enough, leads to obstructive shock. Dissemination of microemboli to the pulmonary vasculature results in dyspnea, dry cough, chest tightness or respiratory arrest. Further, passage of air across the pulmonary capillary bed can lead to cerebral or coronary artery embolism. In the Trendelenburg position, air emboli migrate to the lower extremity venous circulation, resulting in ischemia, due to increased outflow resistance. Foam may be visible in the extracorporeal tubing and cardiac auscultation may reveal a peculiar churning sound.

The immediate management of clinically suspected air embolism is summarized in Figure 79.5. Prevention depends primarily on dialysis machines that are equipped with venous air bubble traps and foam detectors located just distal to the dialyzer, and a venous pressure monitor at the venous end. The detector is attached to a relay switch that simultaneously activates an alarm, shuts off the blood pump and clamps the venous bloodline if air is detected. Therefore, dialysis should never be performed in the presence of an inoperative air detection alarm system. Glass bottles should be avoided since they create vacuum effects that can permit air entry into the extracorporeal system. Dialysis catheters should be aspirated and flushed with saline prior to connection. Dialyzer rinsing, prior to use, should expand all compartments to remove residual air bubbles.

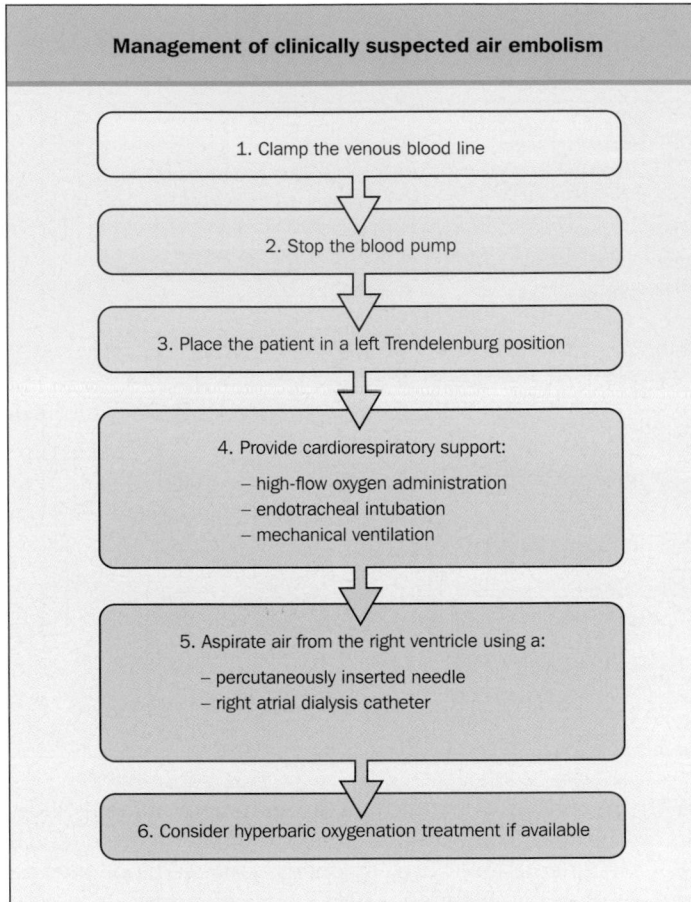

Management of clinically suspected air embolism

1. Clamp the venous blood line

2. Stop the blood pump

3. Place the patient in a left Trendelenburg position

4. Provide cardiorespiratory support:
   – high-flow oxygen administration
   – endotracheal intubation
   – mechanical ventilation

5. Aspirate air from the right ventricle using a:
   – percutaneously inserted needle
   – right atrial dialysis catheter

6. Consider hyperbaric oxygenation treatment if available

Figure 79.5 Management of clinically suspected air embolism.

Incorrect dialysate composition

Incorrect dialysate composition occurs as a result of technical or human errors. Since the primary solutes constituting the dialysate are electrolytes, the dialysate concentration will be reflected by its electrical conductivity (see Chapter 78). Therefore, proper proportioning of concentrate to water can be achieved by a meter that continuously measures the conductivity of the dialysate solution as it is being fed to the dialyzer. Life-threatening electrolyte and acid–base abnormalities are avoidable if the conductivity alarm is functioning properly and the alarm limits are set correctly. However, in dialysis machines that are equipped with conductivity-controlled mixing systems, the system automatically changes the mixing ratio of the concentrates until the dialysate solution conductivity falls within the set limits. This may inadvertently lead to dialysate without any bicarbonate, with apparently acceptable conductivity. Therefore, if conductivity-controlled systems are used, it is safer to also check the dialysate pH prior to dialysis. Conductivity monitors can fail or can be improperly adjusted due to human error. Therefore, it is important to add human monitoring of dialysate composition before every treatment, whenever a machine has been sterilized, moved about, and whenever a new concentrate is used. Furthermore, many nonstandardized solutions are available, some of which may be used with an inappropriate proportioning system. Therefore, it is also essential that the supplies match the machine-proportioning ratio for which they were prepared to obtain the appropriate final dialysate composition.

Hypernatremia

Hypernatremia occurs when concentrate or the ratio of concentrate to water is incorrect, and the conductivity monitors or the alarms are not functioning properly. Hyperosmolality results in intracellular water depletion. Clinical manifestations include thirst, headache, nausea, vomiting, seizures, coma or death. Aggressive treatment is mandatory, and includes cessation of dialysis, hospitalization, and infusion of 5% dextrose in water. Dialysis should be resumed using a different machine, and the dialysate sodium level should be 2 mmol/L lower than the plasma level and isotonic saline should be concurrently infused. Dialysis against a sodium level 3–5 mmol/L lower than the plasma level may increase the risk of disequilibrium. Ultrafiltration with equal volume replacement with normal saline is another option.

Hyponatremia

Failure to add concentrate, inadequate concentrate to water ratio, or conductivity monitor or alarm malfunction can cause hyponatremia. Hyponatremia can also occur during the course of dialysis with a proportioning system, if the concentrate container runs dry and the conductivity set limits are inappropriate. Acute hypo-osmolality causes hemolysis with hyperkalemia and hemodilution of all plasma constituents. Symptoms include restlessness, anxiety, pain in the vein injected with the hypotonic hemolyzed blood, chest pain, headache, nausea, and occasional severe abdominal/lumbar cramps. Pallor, vomiting and seizures may be observed. Treatment consists of clamping the bloodlines and discarding the hemolyzed blood in the extracorporeal circuit. High-flow oxygen and cardiac monitoring are imperative because of hyperkalemia and potential myocardial injury. Dialysis should be restarted with a new dialysate batch containing low potassium, and high transmembrane pressure should be applied to remove excess water. Correction of plasma sodium concentration should be achieved by no more than 1–2 mmol/L per h. Anticonvulsants are indicated for seizures and blood transfusions for severe anemia.

Metabolic acidosis

Although acute intradialytic metabolic acidosis can be a manifestation of improper mixing of concentrates or failure of pH monitors, other causes need to be ruled out including diabetic or alcoholic ketoacidosis, lactic acidosis, toxic ingestions, or dilutional acidosis[26]. The diagnosis is usually suggested by the acute onset of hyperventilation during HD and confirmed by laboratory evaluation. In most circumstances, correcting the underlying cause and using bicarbonate dialysate at the appropriate concentration (35 mmol/L) are adequate measures.

Metabolic alkalosis

Severe intradialytic metabolic alkalosis is rare and may be due to error in dialysate concentrates, reversed connection of bicarbonate and acid concentrate containers to the entry ports of the dialysis machine, pH monitor malfunction or the use of regional citrate anticoagulation. The most common cause however, is hydrochloric acid loss as a result of vomiting or nasogastric suction. Attention should also be directed at identifying sources of added alkali[27]. Further, the combination of sodium polystyrene sulfonate and aluminum hydroxide can lead to absorption of alkali that is normally neutralized in the small intestine.

Acute treatment is rarely necessary unless a technical error has occurred. Usually, removal of the alkali source is sufficient, and H2-antagonists or proton pump inhibitors may be successful if gastric acid loss is present. The administration of sodium chloride to anephric patients with chloride-sensitive alkalosis will not repair the alkalosis. If a more rapid reduction in plasma bicarbonate is desired, modifying the dialysate bath by replacing alkali with chloride, substituting bicarbonate with acetate dialysate, using acid dialysate or infusing hydrochloric acid are cumbersome measures. Conventional bicarbonate dialysis or dialysis using lower dialysate bicarbonate levels (25–30 mmol/L) is probably as effective.

Respiratory acidosis

REDY sorbent dialysis is a dialysate regenerating system that consists of a sorbent cartridge that has three different layers that participate in the regeneration process. During dialysate regeneration, acute hypercapnia can develop. Indeed, the breakdown of urea that occurs in the second layer generates NH_4^+ and HCO_3^-. The third layer is a cation exchanger that exchanges Na^+ and H^+ for NH_4^+, hence carbonic acid is formed when HCO_3^- combines to H^+. Fortunately, protons are partially buffered in the blood and carbon dioxide is normally eliminated by the lungs. However, the excess of carbon dioxide may be limited in critically-ill patients with underlying pulmonary disease, resulting in hypercapnia and a superimposed or worsening respiratory acidosis.

Temperature monitor malfunction

Malfunction of the thermostat in the dialysis machine can result in the production of excessively cool or hot dialysate. Whereas cool dialysate is not dangerous and may have beneficial hemodynamic effects, overheated dialysate can cause immediate hemolysis and life-threatening hyperkalemia, particularly if the dialysate temperature rises above 51°C. In such an event, dialysis must be stopped immediately and blood in the system be discarded. The patient should be monitored for hemolysis and hyperkalemia. Dialysis should be resumed to cool the patient by using a dialysate temperature of 34°C, to treat hyperkalemia and to allow blood transfusions if necessary. Visual and audible alarms are mandatory to prevent this complication.

Blood loss

Intradialytic blood loss can result from arterial or venous needle disengagement from the access, separation of the venous or arterial line connections, femoral or central line dialysis catheter perforation or dislodgment, or rupture of a dialysis membrane with or without malfunction of the blood leak detector. Clinical findings include hypotension, loss of consciousness, or cardiac arrest. In addition, following traumatic insertion of a dialysis catheter, blood loss can result in pain/mass from a rapidly expanding hematoma; chest, shoulder or neck pain from intrapericardial blood loss; back, flank, groin or lower abdominal pain/distention from retroperitoneal bleeding; or hemoptysis from blood loss in the lungs. Acute management includes the discontinuation of HD, pressure application for local hemostasis, hemodynamic support, oxygen administration and surgical intervention if needed.

MISCELLANEOUS COMPLICATIONS

Postdialysis syndrome

An ill-defined 'washed out' feeling or malaise during or after HD is a common nonspecific symptom that is observed in about one third of patients[28], and has multifactorial origins. Reduced cardiac output, peripheral vascular disease, depression, poor conditioning, postdialysis hypotension, hypokalemia or hypoglycemia, mild uremic encephalopathy, myopathy due to carnitine deficiency and membrane biocompatibility through cytokine production have all been incriminated. The use of glucose/bicarbonate dialysate and L-carnitine supplementation (20 mg/kg per d) has been shown to improve postdialysis well being. Although there are insufficient data to support the use of L-carnitine to improve quality of life in unselected dialysis patients, the most promising of the proposed applications is for the treatment of epoetin-resistant anemia[29].

Pruritus

Pruritus is common and the etiology is often multifactorial including xerosis, hyperparathyroidism and inadequate dialysis. In many cases, pruritus is more severe during or after dialysis and may be an allergic manifestation to heparin, ETO, formaldehyde or acetate. In a subgroup of patients, use of gamma-sterilized dialyzers, cessation of use of formaldehyde and switching over to bicarbonate dialysate may result in cessation of itching. Eczematous reactions to antiseptic solutions, rubber glove or puncture needle components, puncture needles, or collophane used to secure dialysis needles should also be considered[30].

Therapies include the use of emollients and antihistamines, activated charcoal, ultraviolet therapy, sunbathing, ketotifen (a mast cell stabilizer), epoetin therapy or topical capsaicin. Finally, dialysis adequacy should always be assessed.

Priapism

Priapism occurs in < 0.5% of male HD patients. It is not related to sexual activity and occurs while on dialysis. The patient is usually awakened from sleep by a painful erection. Although the majority of cases are idiopathic, secondary causes include heparin-induced hyperviscosity, high hematocrit due to androgen or epoetin therapy, dialysis-induced hypoxemia and hypovolemia due to excessive ultrafiltration, particularly in African American males with sickle cell disease, and the use of β-blockers, such as prazosin.

Urological referral is mandatory. Acute treatment consists of corporal aspiration and irrigation. Although surgical bypass provides venous egress from the corpora cavernosa, secondary impotence commonly develops but may be effectively treated by a penile prosthesis.

Hearing and visual loss

Intradialytic hearing loss may be due to bleeding in the inner ear as a consequence of anticoagulation, or cochlear hair cell injury from edema.

Intradialytic visual loss is rare, but can be caused by central retinal vein occlusion, precipitation of acute glaucoma, ischemic optic neuropathy secondary to hypotension or Purtscher's-like retinopathy secondary to leukoembolization.

Finally concomitant ocular and hearing impairment can occur following the use of outdated cellulose acetate dialyzer membranes[31].

REFERENCES

1. Jaber BL, Pereira BJG. Dialysis reactions. Semin Dial. 1997; 10:158–65.
2. National Kidney Foundation – Dialysis Outcome Quality Initiative. NKF-DOQI clinical practice guidelines for the treatment of anemia of chronic renal failure. Am J Kidney Dis. 1997; 30:192S–240S.
3. Grohskopf LA, Roth VR, Feikin DR, et al. Serratia liquefaciens bloodstream infections from contamination of epoetin alfa at a hemodialysis center. N Engl J Med. 2001;344:1491–7.
4. Daugirdas JT. Dialysis hypotension: a hemodynamic analysis. Kidney Int. 1991;39:233–46.
5. Cruz DN, Mahnensmith RL, Brickel HM, Perazella MA. Midodrine and cool dialysate are effective therapies for symptomatic intradialytic hypotension. Am J Kidney Dis. 1999;33:920–6.
6. Rahman M, Dixit A, Donley V, et al. Factors associated with inadequate blood pressure control in hypertensive hemodialysis patients. Am J Kidney Dis. 1999;33:498–506.
7. Sang GL, Kovithavongs C, Ulan R, Kjellstrand CM. Sodium ramping in hemodialysis: a study of beneficial and adverse effects. Am J Kidney Dis. 1997;29:669–77.
8. Bailey RA, Kaplan AA. Intradialytic cardiac arrhythmias: I. Semin Dial. 1994;7:57–8.
9. Kant KS. Intradialytic cardiac arrhythmias: II. Semin Dial. 1994; 7:58–60.
10. Chazan J. Sudden deaths in patients with chronic renal failure on hemodialysis. Dial Transplant. 1987;16:447–8.
11. Bleyer AJ, Russell GB, Satko SG. Sudden and cardiac death rates in hemodialysis patients. Kidney Int. 1999;55:1553–9.
12. Kwun KB, Schanzer H, Finkler BA, et al. Hemodynamic evaluation of angioaccess procedures for hemodialysis. Vasc Surg. 1979; 13:170–7.
13. Schanzer H, Skladany M, Haimov M. Treatment of angioaccess-induced ischemia by revascularization. J Vasc Surg. 1992; 16:861–6.
14. NKF-K/DOQI. Clinical Practice Guidelines for Vascular Access: Update 2000. Am J Kidney Dis. 2001;37:137S–181S.
15. Mattson WJ. Recognition and treatment of vascular steal secondary to hemodialysis prostheses. Am J Surg. 1987;154:198–201.
16. Canzanello VJ, Burkart JM. Hemodialysis-associated muscle cramps. Semin Dial. 1992;5:299–304.

17. Sadowski RH, Allred EN, Jabs K. Sodium modeling ameliorates intradialytic and interdialytic symptoms in young hemodialysis patients. J Am Soc Nephrol. 1993;4:1192–8.
18. Krueger BR. Restless legs syndrome and periodic movements of sleep. Mayo Clin Proc. 1990;65:999–1006.
19. Montplaisir J, Nicolas A, Denesle R, Gomez-Mancilla B. Restless legs syndrome improved by pramipexole: a double-blind randomized trial. Neurology. 1999;23:938–43.
20. Arieff AI. Dialysis disequilibrium syndrome: current concepts on pathogenesis and prevention. Kidney Int. 1994;45:629–35.
21. Cheung AK. Biocompatibility of hemodialysis membranes. J Am Soc Nephrol. 1990;1:150–61.
22. Eaton JW, Leida MN. Hemolysis in chronic renal failure. Semin Nephrol. 1985;5:133–9.
23. Remuzzi G. Bleeding in renal failure. Lancet. 1988;i:1205–8.
24. Cardoso M, Vinay P, Vinet B, et al. Hypoxemia during hemodialysis: a critical review of the facts. Am J Kidney Dis. 1988; 11:281–97.
25. O'Quin RJ, Lakshminarayan S. Venous air embolism. Arch Intern Med. 1982;142:2173–6.
26. Gennari FJ. Acid–base balance in dialysis patients. Semin Dial. 2000;13:235–40.
27. Gennari HJ, Rimmer JM. Acid–base disorders in end-stage renal disease: part II. Semin Dial. 1990;3:161–5.
28. Parfrey PS, Vavasour HM, Henry S, et al. Clinical features and severity of nonspecific symptoms in dialysis patients. Nephron. 1988;50:121–8.
29. NKF-K/DOQI. Clinical practice guidelines for nutrition in chronic renal failure. Am J Kidney Dis. 2000;35:S54–5.
30. Weber M, Schmutz JL. Hemodialysis and the skin. Contr Nephrol. 1988;62:75–85.
31. Hutter JC, Kuehnert MJ, Wallis RR, et al. Acute onset of decreased vision and hearing traced to hemodialysis treatment with aged dialyzers. Jama. 2000;283:2128–34.

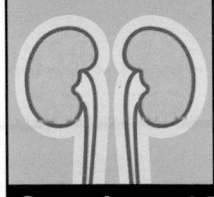

Section 15 Dialysis

Chapter 80

Peritoneal Dialysis: Principles, Techniques, and Adequacy

Simon J Davies and John D Williams

INTRODUCTION

Peritoneal dialysis (PD) is in widespread use for the treatment of end-stage renal disease (ESRD), being used by more than 120 000 patients worldwide. PD should not be thought of as a technique in competition with hemodialysis (HD) but rather as a complementary modality and part of the range of therapies that can be offered to the patient with ESRD. Peritoneal dialysis should, therefore, be part of an integrated program of renal replacement therapy that comprises HD, PD, and transplantation[1]. As a result, individuals will move from one type of treatment to another as their particular circumstances dictate (Fig. 80.1).

In current practice, PD is best used for subjects with some residual renal function. Individuals have, however, successfully used continuous ambulatory PD (CAPD) for up to 18 years. At present many patients will have to transfer to alternative modes of treatment after several years of PD if the adequacy of their regimen cannot be satisfactorily maintained. Ideally, renal replacement therapy should begin with PD (subject to patient choice) and then move as required to HD or transplantation (Fig. 80.1). Selection of dialysis modality is discussed further in Chapter 75.

PRINCIPLES OF PERITONEAL DIALYSIS

The basic principle of dialysis is the separation of substances in solution by their varying diffusion down a concentration gradient, through a semipermeable membrane. In addition, some solute is removed by convection or solvent drag. In PD, the peritoneum is used as the porous membrane. The peritoneum, unlike the HD membrane, allows some loss of proteins as well as much smaller solutes. Fluid removal is along an osmotic gradient rather than as a result of a pressure gradient. Mathematically, the dialysis function of the peritoneal membrane can best be represented by a three pore model (see Fig. 80.2a)[2]. The smallest pores, < 0.5 nm in diameter, only permit the passage of water. The small pores, about 4 nm in diameter, allow the diffusion of smaller solutes and water.

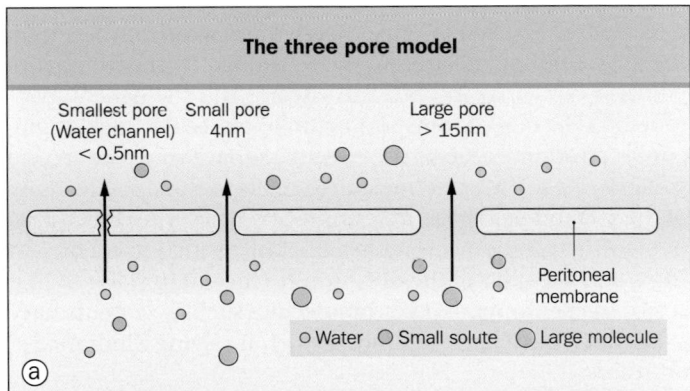

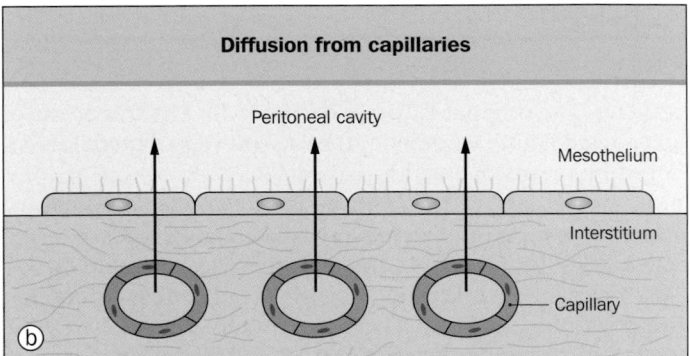

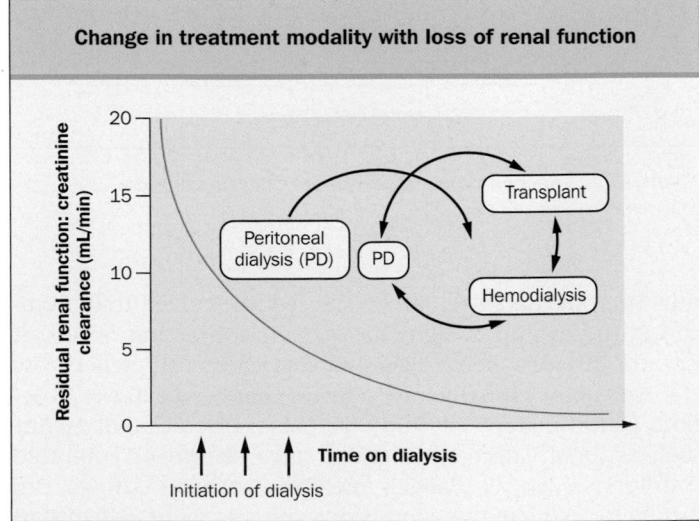

Figure 80.1 The place of peritoneal dialysis as first-line therapy for advanced uremia. Peritoneal dialysis is often the preferred therapy at the initiation of dialysis when there is significant residual renal function. As residual renal function declines, PD becomes part of an integrated renal replacement therapy with hemodialysis and transplantation.

Figure 80.2 Principles of peritoneal dialysis. In the three pore model of peritoneal transport (a), the smallest pores probably represent aquaporins. Diffusion from capillaries into the peritoneal cavity (b) depends on the intrinsic permeability of capillaries and also on the number of perfused capillaries (the effective surface area).

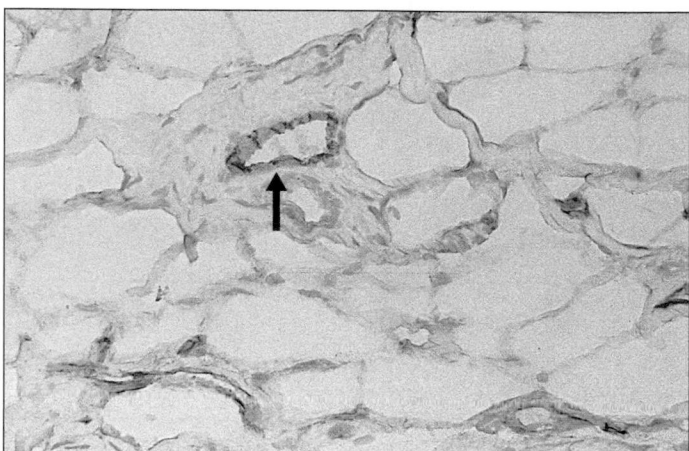

Figure 80.3 Aquaporins in the peritoneal membrane. Aquaporins stained red in peritoneal capillary endothelial cells (arrow). (Courtesy of Dr M Ho-dac Pannekeet.)

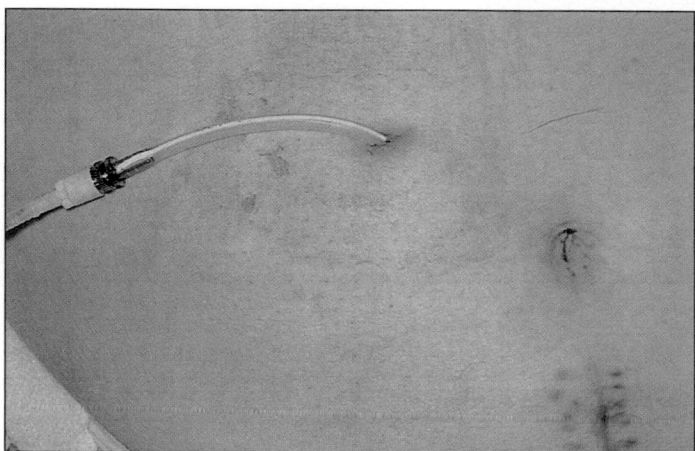

Figure 80.4 A recently implanted peritoneal dialysis catheter *in situ*.

There are also a small number of large pores, average effective radius > 15 nm, that permit macromolecules such as proteins to diffuse into the peritoneal cavity. The morphologic counterpart of these mathematically derived concepts is still unclear, but it is likely that specialized water channels, aquaporins, in peritoneal capillaries represent the smallest pores (Fig. 80.3).

Transport across the peritoneal membrane is linked to the vascular surface area and the intrinsic permeability of the peritoneum, which is determined by the permeability of the capillaries (see Fig. 80.2b). The effective surface area is less than the anatomic equivalent and is determined by the number of perfused capillaries in both the visceral and the parietal peritoneum. The rate of transport of small molecules such as glucose or creatinine reflects the effective surface area. The second variable, the intrinsic permeability, refers to the size selectivity of the membrane. This is determined by measuring the restriction coefficient for macromolecules. The restriction coefficient represents the ratio of the diffusion coefficient in water to that across the peritoneum. Macromolecules such as proteins have restriction coefficients significantly >1, implying hindrance to diffusion.

ACCESS

Access to the peritoneal cavity is obtained by the use of a catheter. The original catheter designed for the treatment of acute renal failure was made from a semi-rigid material introduced by means of a stylet. This device is no longer in common use because of the high incidence of dialysate leakage and infection. Most catheters nowadays are derivatives of the one devised by Tenckhoff and Schecter (Figs 80.4 and 80.5)[3]. This consists of a silastic tube with side holes along the intraperitoneal portion. There are usually one or two cuffs made of Dacron, allowing tissue ingrowth, which not only secures the device in place but prevents pericatheter leakage and infection. The original Tenckhoff catheter was straight, being inserted caudally, the inner cuff lying on the peritoneum and the outer close to the skin exit; the tube itself skirting the umbilicus. A number of different versions have

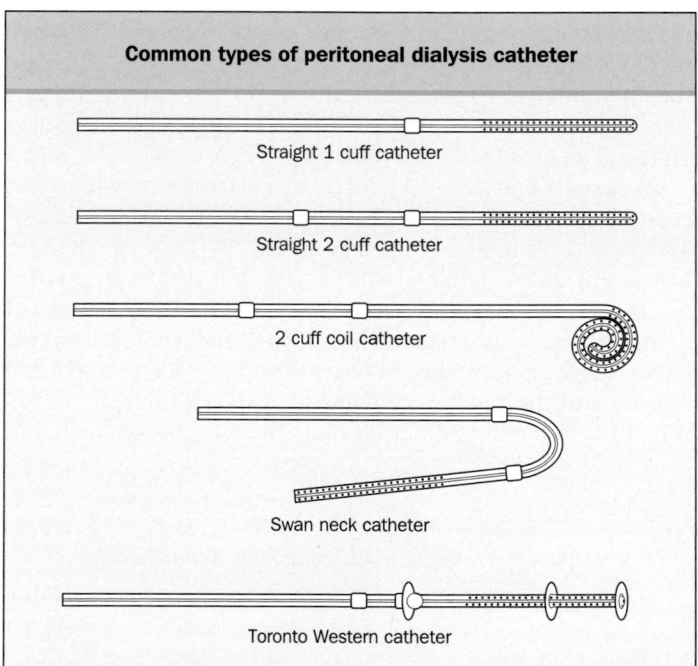

Common types of peritoneal dialysis catheter

Straight 1 cuff catheter

Straight 2 cuff catheter

2 cuff coil catheter

Swan neck catheter

Toronto Western catheter

Figure 80.5 Common types of peritoneal dialysis catheter.

now been devised (Fig. 80.5). The few controlled trials comparing the various designs have given conflicting results. It has, for instance, been suggested that those catheters whose exit sites point caudally have a lower chance of exit site infection. Unfortunately, no study has taken into account factors such as nasal carriage of *Staphylococcus aureus* or comorbid conditions such as diabetes mellitus; both are known risk factors for exit site infection. Consequently, hard evidence to determine which design is the clinically most effective is not yet available.

Silastic PD catheters can be inserted by a variety of techniques. The original method involved dissection under local anesthetic down to the linea alba and then the insertion of a metal trocar and cannula through which the catheter was placed using a metal rod as a stiffening device. Many units perform a minilaparotomy under general anesthetic and ensure pelvic placement of the catheter under direct vision. An alternative is to use a minilaparoscope (Needlescope), which allows the operator to view the peritoneal cavity, choose a position, and then insert the cannula through the sheath of the scope, again using a rod as a stiffener. A further variation is to use a Seldinger technique, the catheter being slid over a guide wire placed into the peritoneal cavity. There is some evidence that placing the catheter through the rectus sheath lateral to the linea alba may reduce the risk of subsequent hernia formation. The subcutaneous tunnel is usually constructed with a sharp-ended tunneling instrument. The aim is to ensure that the outer cuff rests in the subcutaneous tissue at least 2 cm from the actual exit site.

TECHNIQUES OF PERITONEAL DIALYSIS

Peritoneal dialysis involves filling the peritoneal cavity with dialysate, allowing this fluid to dwell for a certain period, draining it out, and then replacing it with fresh dialysate (Fig. 80.6). The dwell time to achieve full equilibration between dialysate and plasma solute concentrations is ~4–5 h, whereas maximum ultrafiltration using glucose solutions is usually between 2 to 3 h. Each time the procedure is carried out is called an exchange or cycle. If the exchange dwells are short, for example 1–2 h, then the procedure is called intermittent PD (IPD). IPD is commonly performed in hospital using a machine ('cycler'). It is also used when the patient needs dialysis but the intraperitoneal volume has to be reduced to prevent leakage. This may occur following catheter insertion, hernia repair, or an abdominal operation. IPD can also be performed when the patient needs rapid correction of fluid overload, when 60 min exchanges using a high osmolality solution (e.g., 3.86% dextrose) will result in optimal ultrafiltration. IPD can be performed manually but this is labor intensive.

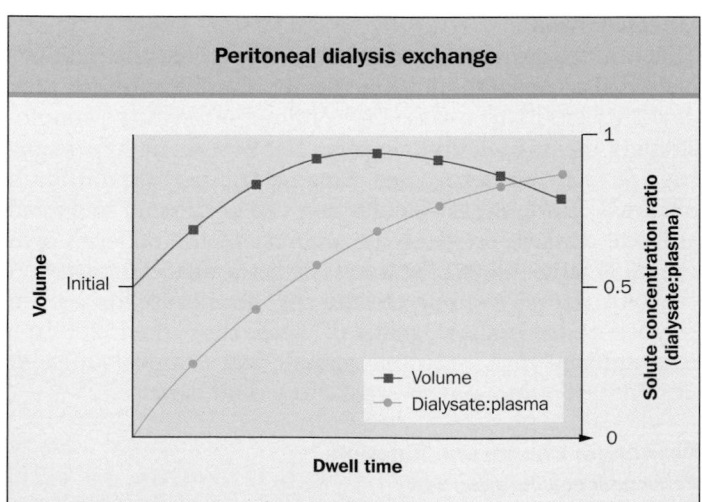

Figure 80.6 Peritoneal dialysis exchange. Changes in intra-abdominal volume and small solute concentration during a dialysis exchange.

CAPD is in widespread use for the long-term treatment of ESRD. Usually four exchanges are carried out every 24 h (although in many individuals five exchanges may be necessary to ensure adequate dialysis). The exact timing is not important and can be adjusted to suit individual patient convenience. Dialysis will remain efficient so long as the exchanges are reasonably spaced out during the waking hours. Each exchange time (if the catheter is not malfunctioning) should be about 30 min. CAPD is an entirely manual technique though there are devices to help patients with problems of manual dexterity.

CAPD must take place 7 days a week to ensure adequate solute removal. Using CAPD, the plasma levels of urea, creatinine, potassium, bicarbonate, and phosphate remain stable throughout the 24 h, unless there is some other intervention, for example a change in the dose of phosphate binder. Sometimes for reasons of efficient solute exchange or adequacy (see below) five bags per 24 h are used[4]. This can be done manually but it is also possible to have the fifth bag exchanged using an exchanger device at night. This drains out the used fluid and instils new dialysate at a predetermined time while the patient sleeps.

All other forms of chronic PD require a machine or cycler to exchange the dialysis fluid. Most cyclers can be programmed to alter inflow volume, inflow time, dwell time, and drain time. They also usually warm the fluid prior to inflow and monitor outflow volume, measuring any excess drainage as ultrafiltration. Alarm conditions include failure of inflow, overheating, and poor drainage. This form of PD is commonly referred to as automated PD (APD). APD can be confined to night-time exchanges, with the abdomen being left dry or empty during the day (nocturnal or NPD). If fluid is left intraperitoneally during the day the technique is often referred to as continuous cyclic PD (CCPD). Some cyclers have an additional function whereby after the initial inflow, not all the fluid is allowed to drain. The subsequent inflow volumes are correspondingly reduced and after a preset number of cycles complete drainage occurs. Therefore, for a period some of the dialysate remains in the abdomen. This technique is called tidal PD. It is used when improved solute clearance is needed (see Adequacy).

CAPD has the great advantage over APD of simplicity, but it does involve a bag exchange in the middle of the day. APD has the advantage of social convenience, particularly for those in occupations that render a midday exchange difficult or who require a helper. Sometimes, however, for reasons of adequacy, APD may need to be combined with extra exchanges during the day.

The exchange volume used should be appropriate to the patient's size. As a generalization, adult patients weighing < 60 kg should start with 1.5 L bags; those weighing 60–80 kg should receive 2 L exchanges; and if over 80 kg, then 2.5 L should be used. These volumes may need to be increased later to maintain total solute clearance.

PERITONEAL DIALYSIS FLUIDS

All PD fluids contain sodium, calcium, magnesium, and chloride. At present they usually include lactate as the source of bicarbonate/buffer although newer fluids are now becoming routinely available which contain either bicarbonate alone or a mixture of bicarbonate and lactate as a source of buffer.

PD fluid is also available with several different calcium concentrations, varying from 0 to 7 mg/dL (0–1.75 mmol/L). A calcium concentration of 5 mg/dL (1.25 mmol/L) is in widespread use as first-line therapy. Care must be taken when using calcium containing phosphate binders to avoid hypercalcemia.

Glucose is usually present as the osmotic agent and is available in a variety of concentrations. An alternative osmotic agent to glucose is glucose polymer (icodextrin), which has a mean molecular weight of 20 000[5]. This is available as a 7.5% solution with the same electrolyte composition as glucose-based dialysate. The osmolality of glucose polymer fluid is the same as for normal plasma (290 mosmol/L), unlike 1.36% glucose dialysate (350 mosmol/L). Glucose polymer induces fluid removal by colloid osmosis, which is the osmotic effect induced by a large molecule that either is not absorbed or diffuses very slowly. It is most valuable when used for a long dwell, for example overnight, and particularly for patients who tend to absorb glucose rapidly (see loss of ultrafiltration).

An alternative dialysis fluid, which is also commercially available, replaces glucose with a 1.1% amino acid mixture. This fluid has the same osmolality as 1.36% dextrose. There is some evidence that regular daily use of this dialysate may augment certain nutritional indices[6] but there are no data yet demonstrating if it will improve long-term patient outcome. Use of this fluid in earlier studies had a tendency to increase acidosis, which could have prevented any nutritional gain.

Conventional commercial dialysis fluid has an acid pH (~ 5.3), a high concentration of lactate and high levels of glucose degradation products (GDPs) that are toxic to a variety of cells *in vitro*. Recently dialysate fluids with neutral pH, reduced GDPs and in some cases bicarbonate buffer, have been developed to improve biocompatibility. Those using bicarbonate alone or a bicarbonate/lactate mixture result in significantly less infusion pain and are as effective as lactate at correcting acidosis when used at the same total buffer ion concentration[7]. Each of these new, more biocompatible solutions requires dual compartment bag systems to enable separate sterilization of glucose at low pH. This is followed by mixing with fresh buffer to achieve a physiologic pH and prevent precipitation of bicarbonate. Prospective, randomized studies of these fluids have been associated with improvement in dialysate effluent markers of peritoneal membrane integrity. Their effects on long-term membrane function remain unknown at this stage.

Alternative fluid compositions under evaluation include the use of pyruvate as an alternative to lactate, glycerol instead of glucose, and certain additives that might help preserve the peritoneal membrane, for example N-acetylglucosamine and hyaluronic acid.

ASSESSING PERITONEAL CLEARANCES AND FUNCTION

Unfortunately, the transport of fluid and solute across the peritoneal membrane varies considerably from patient to patient and also with time in individual patients. It is therefore necessary to assess peritoneal function at regular

Assessment of peritoneal function
Solute clearance
Total solute clearance: weekly creatinine clearance, weekly urea clearance
Rate of small solute transport: peritoneal equilibration test
Ultrafiltration
Charts
Bag weights
Number of hypertonic bags used
Calculation from peritoneal equilibration test
Sodium sieving (to test water channels)

Table 80.1 Assessment of peritoneal function.

intervals. The methods commonly used to measure solute clearance and assess peritoneal function are summarized in Table 80.1.

Peritoneal solute clearance

The only way to measure solute clearance accurately is to collect all the used dialysate for 24 h and take a plasma sample during this period. The concentrations of urea and creatinine are measured in dialysate and plasma. Together with the 24-h dialysate volume, this gives the 24-h clearance. By convention, the results are usually multiplied by seven, to give weekly clearance. In order to compare patients, some sort of normalization is performed. For creatinine clearance, this is usually related to a body standard surface area of 1.73 m^2.

Urea clearance is expressed as Kt/V (where Kt represents weekly clearance and V the volume of distribution of urea). The volume of distribution can be estimated by various techniques but each has a considerable error when compared with the gold standard, namely direct measurement of total body water. Unfortunately, measuring the latter is not practical for routine clinical use.

Ultrafiltration

This can be assessed in a number of ways. First the patient's daily dialysis record will show the net ultrafiltration for each day. This should be assessed in conjunction with the composition of the utilized fluid, in particular how many hypertonic bags per day are being used. Second, the net ultrafiltration obtained during the 24-h collection can be directly measured and will confirm or refute the accuracy of the patient's own charts. Finally, the PET indicates the peritoneal ultrafiltration capacity, the net volume of achieved ultrafiltrate for a given glucose concentration gradient: when less than 200 mL it is unlikely that an anuric patient will achieve sufficient ultrafiltration to maintain satisfactory fluid balance.

Peritoneal membrane function
Peritoneal equilibration test

The peritoneal equilibration test (PET) gives information on the rate of peritoneal transport of small solutes and ultrafiltration capacity (Table 80.2)[8]. Peritoneal solute transport reflects the effective peritoneal surface area, whereas the ultrafiltration capacity is a composite measure of peritoneal ultrafiltration efficiency. After an overnight dwell, fluid is drained out of the peritoneal cavity, the contents of a 2.27% glucose bag are infused and allowed to dwell for 4 h. At the end of this period, the dialysate is drained out and measured. The net volume represents the ultrafiltration capacity. The concentrations of glucose and creatinine in the outflow and plasma are measured, as is the concentration of glucose in the initial inflow. The results are expressed as the ratio of dialysate to plasma creatinine concentration (D/P creatinine);

and as the ratio of dialysate glucose at 4 h to dialysate glucose at time zero (D/D_0) (Table 80.2 and Fig. 80.7). When the test is properly performed, the results are usually in inverse proportion, so the higher the D/P creatinine the lower the D/D_0 glucose. Clearly, the higher the ratio for creatinine at 4 h, the faster the rate of transport for small solutes across the peritoneal membrane. Conventionally, the results obtained from the test (peritoneal transport) are used to divide patients into four transporter types: high, high-average, low-average, and low transporters (Fig. 80.7).

Table 80.2 The peritoneal equilibration test.

Peritoneal equilibration test			
Time point	Action	Technique	Data collected
Overnight	Dwell of 8–12 h	Must use 1.36 or 2.27% glucose	Dwell time(h) Glucose concentration
	Drain of overnight dwell	Drain over at least 20 min with patient vertical	Drainage volume
	Infusion	Infuse 2 L warm 2.27% glucose fluid: 200 mL/min for 10 min exactly with the patient supine and rolled from side to side every 2 min	
Completion of infusion (D_0) and end of dwell time (D_2)	Collect dialysate samples	Drain 200 mL into bag; draw off 5 mL (discard); draw 5 mL sample; reinfuse remainder	Creatinine and glucose at D_0, D_2
D_2	Collect blood samples		Creatinine, glucose, and urea in plasma (P)
D_4	Collect dialysate	Drain over 20 min with patient vertical	Ultrafiltration volume V
		Weigh bag (less weight of empty bag, liner) and add weight of samples D_0, D_2	
		Mix bag contents well; draw 5 mL (discard); draw 5 mL sample	Creatinine and glucose at D_4
	Calculation* and classification	Calculate D/P creatinine for D_2, D_4	
		Calculate D/D_0 glucose for D_2, D_4	
		Classify using graph (Fig. 80.7)	

*Glucose interferes with creatinine estimation in dialysate. The correction factor is determined by the assessing laboratory.

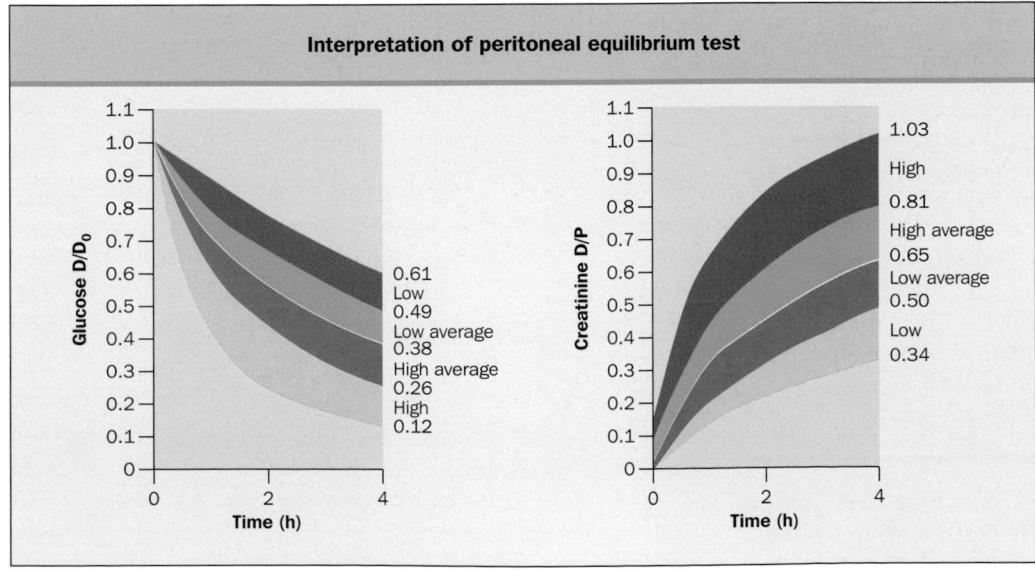

Figure 80.7 Interpretation of the peritoneal equilibration test. Changes in solute concentration during a peritoneal equilibration test allow classification into different transport types. Creatinine is corrected for glucose interference in its assay. (Adapted from Twardowski et al.[8])

Standard permeability analysis

Standard Permeability Analysis (SPA) is a test similar to the PET, in which a 3.86% dextrose bag is instilled. After a dwell of 1 h, a dialysate sample is taken and the sodium concentration is compared with that of the inflow. Although not universally accepted, this test has been proposed for the assessment of aquaporin water channel function. If the water channels are functioning normally, the sodium concentration in the dialysate should decrease by more than 13%, so-called sodium sieving[9]. If there is little or no decrease, then the peritoneal aquaporin water channels may no longer be functional. Ultrafiltration capacity < 400 mL in SPA suggests peritoneal ultrafiltration failure.

Other tests

More sophisticated tests of peritoneal function, such as mass transfer area coefficient and permeability for proteins are used as research tools but are not required for routine clinical use.

Residual renal function

When assessing peritoneal function, it is important to measure the contribution of residual renal function to total solute clearance and fluid loss. This is best done by obtaining all the urine passed during the same time as the 24-h dialysate collection and measuring urea clearance (C_u) and creatinine clearance (C_{Cr}) and urine volume. Creatinine clearance is corrected to apparent glomerular filtration rate (GFR) by the formula: $(C_u + C_{Cr})/2$.

If the daily urine volume is < 200 mL, the contribution of residual renal function will be too small to measure accurately.

OUTCOME OF PERITONEAL DIALYSIS

Several observational studies of patients commencing renal replacement therapy with CAPD were performed during the 1990s[10–12]. These defined factors predicting patient and technique survival, which include demographic factors such as age and comorbidity, but also aspects of the treatment which can potentially be modified.

The most important of these is maintenance of residual renal function. While PD is associated with relative prolongation of residual renal function when compared to HD, it is also dependent on the contribution of residual renal function for its success as a treatment modality, at least as currently practiced.

These studies have also shown that peritoneal membrane function and fluid balance are important for patient and especially technique survival. High solute transport is associated with worse outcome, probably because the high solute transport results in poor ultrafiltration, since glucose is rapidly absorbed, intraperitoneal glucose concentration is not maintained and there is loss of osmotic gradient. The importance of fluid balance is also emphasized by the observation in the NECOSAD study that high blood pressure at the commencement of PD is an independent adverse factor[11].

ADEQUACY

Assessment of the adequacy of PD should include all aspects of renal function replacement (both excretory and endocrine). Control of the consequences of endocrine dysfunction, for example anemia and renal osteodystrophy, are discussed in other chapters. In assessing the adequacy of excretory function, equal emphasis should be given to fluid balance as well as low molecular solute clearance. The various measures used to assess PD adequacy are summarized in Table 80.3.

Solute clearance

There are a few small retrospective studies of small solute clearance which suggest that for CAPD, a weekly Kt/V of < 1.5 or a weekly creatinine clearance of < 50 L/1.73 m² is associated with a worse outcome in terms of morbidity and mortality. One large prospective study has been carried out in North America, the CANUSA study[10], which recorded the outcome for a cohort of 680 patients starting CAPD, with an average follow-up of 2 years. In the CANUSA study, patients who maintained higher small solute clearance over the study period, whether assessed by urea or creatinine clearance, had better outcomes. This survival advantage, however, was entirely attributable to maintained residual renal function. Furthermore, there was no apparent upper limit beyond which further increases in clearance were not associated with improved outcome. The ADEMEX study[13], the only randomized controlled trial designed to test the value of increasing peritoneal solute clearance, did not show any survival advantage in maintaining a total creatinine clearance above 60 L/1.73 m² compared with less than 50 L/1.73 m². These studies demonstrate clearly that renal and peritoneal solute clearances cannot be equated, and every attempt should be made to maintain residual renal function for as long as possible. As residual function is lost it is appropriate to increase peritoneal clearances to maintain minimum values of urea and/or creatinine clearance, e.g., weekly Kt/V > 1.7 or creatinine clearance > 50 L/1.73 m².

Increasing peritoneal solute clearance to compensate for the loss of residual renal function is best achieved by increasing dialysate volume or modifying dwell time. Simple calculation shows that for a patient with average peritoneal transport an increase in clearance is difficult to achieve with four bags a

Criteria for peritoneal dialysis adequacy	
Criteria	**Assessment**
Solute clearance	Weekly Kt/V urea >1.7 (including residual renal function)
	Weekly creatinine clearance >50 L/1.73 m²
Fluid balance	No edema
	No postural hypotension
Electrolyte balance	Serum potassium <6.0 mmol/L
Acid–base balance	Serum bicarbonate >24 mmol/L
Nutrition	Daily protein intake: 1.2–1.5 g/kg
	Body mass index 20–30
	Stable midarm muscle circumference
	Serum albumin >3.5 g/dL
	Serum cholesterol >150 mg/dL (3.8 mmol/L)

Table 80.3 Criteria for peritoneal dialysis adequacy.

day if the patient weighs more than 65 kg[14]. However, studies have not shown that large body size is an independent risk factor predicting poor outcome with CAPD.

Higher clearances can be achieved if larger volumes or a fifth exchange are instituted, or if there is a change to APD. This inevitably increases costs and, being more complicated, may impair the patient's quality of life or reduce compliance. However, there are at present no data relating solute clearance (of urea or creatinine) achieved by APD to patient outcome. Each patient must be assessed separately and prescribed an individual PD regimen. It is important to measure renal and peritoneal clearances of urea and creatinine every 4–6 months (or more frequently if there is any suggestion that the patient could be underdialyzed as judged by an increasing plasma creatinine or clinical signs). Present evidence is good enough to recommend augmenting peritoneal clearance by whatever is the best technique for the individual if the weekly Kt/V is < 1.7 and/or the weekly creatinine clearance is < 50 L/1.73 m² surface area, bearing in mind that body composition and membrane function will have a significant impact on the ease with which these targets can be met. A patient with high solute transport will achieve peritoneal creatinine clearance targets relatively easily, whilst in an obese individual it may be impossible to reach an adequate Kt/V urea. A number of computer programs are commercially available that use data from PET and 24-h collection of dialysate and urine to offer a range of treatment options together with the predicted clearances. If, despite adjusting the PD regimen to the maximum possible, including the use of daytime bags with APD, the clearances remain persistently well below the values recommended, then serious consideration should be given to transferring the patient to HD.

Strategies for enhancing solute clearance on PD are summarized in Table 80.4.

Fluid balance

It is important to maintain normal fluid balance if survival of patients receiving PD is to be optimized. Outcome is known to be worse for patients who lose residual renal function, or have high peritoneal small solute transfer rates, or who are high transporters in the PET (which results in a more rapid absorption of glucose and the loss of osmotic gradient)[12]. Both these conditions are associated with inadequate fluid removal and, therefore, an increased tendency to fluid overload. When PD is commenced, there tends to be a fall in blood pressure during the first few months. With time the blood pressure rises again and the number of antihypertensive agents needed for treatment increases[15]. Left ventricular hypertrophy is often present at the start of dialysis and is an independent risk factor for mortality during PD. Factors influencing progression of left ventricular hypertrophy include anemia and hypertension[16]; abnormalities of ventricular function can also occur. It is likely that fluid overload contributes to these cardiac problems.

Assessment of fluid balance is not always easy during long-term PD. Individuals with no edema may still have a degree of fluid excess, particularly those who are hypertensive. Early in PD treatment, continuing urine output often helps to maintain fluid balance[17]. As urine output is progressively lost, however, some patients will tend to become fluid overloaded (especially those with increased peritoneal small-solute transfer i.e., high transporters). Regular assessment of fluid removal should be made at the same time as measuring solute clearance.

It is important to instruct patients to restrict fluid intake as urine output falls. The use of a loop diuretic (e.g., furosemide (frusemide) 250 mg daily) will maintain urine volumes, but does not maintain renal clearance[18]. Ultrafiltration is first augmented by increasing the dialysate glucose concentration to 2.27% or 3.36%. Patients with increased peritoneal small-solute transfer may, however, still tend to absorb the fluid, particularly during long dwells, and this reduces net ultrafiltration. Use of an osmotic agent with a much higher molecular weight can overcome this problem, at least for a while. The only licensed product is the glucose polymer (icodextrin). Randomized control trials using icodextrin for the long, day-time dwell in APD patients have demonstrated improved ultrafiltration[19], and this regimen should be used in patients with poor ultrafiltration associated with high solute transport. Alternatively, frequent short dwells using a cycler may prevent fluid absorption and improve removal. Strategies for maximizing fluid balance according to membrane function are summarized in Chapter 81.

Peritoneal dialysis regimens				
	Peritoneal solute transport characteristics (D/P$_{creatinine}$ at 4 h)			
Patient body surface area (m²)	Low (< 0.5)	Low-average (0.5– < 0.65)	High-average (0.65–0.82)	High (> 0.83)
< 1.7	CAPD/APD 10–12.5 L	CAPD/APD+ 10–12.5 L	APD+* 10–12.5 L	APD* 10–12.5 L
1.7–2.0	CAPD+/APD 12.5–15 L	APD+ 12.5–15 L	APD+* 12.5–15 L	APD+* 12.5–15 L
> 2.0	CAPD+, HD	APD+ 15–20 L	APD+* 15–20 L	APD+* 15–20 L

The total volume of dialysate fluid required increases with body size, using 2.5 or even 3.0 L exchanges. As solute transport increases, the use of APD using shorter overnight exchanges, is favored over CAPD. Both CAPD and APD may have to be augmented by the use of an additional exchange (denoted +); this is given by way of an additional tea-time exchange in CAPD patients or by employing an exchange device that delivers a single additional exchange at night. *The use of glucose polymer (icodextrin) solution for the long exchange will enhance both solute clearance and ultrafiltration.

Table 80.4 Peritoneal dialysis regimens. Typical PD regimens required to achieve adequate solute clearances according to patient size and membrane characteristics in anuric patients.

Electrolyte balance

Sodium balance during PD is closely associated with fluid balance since all water losses whether from the peritoneum or in urine are accompanied by some sodium. In general, problems with fluid overload are associated with sodium excess in the body. In the absence of urine output, there can be no substantial removal of sodium if there is no peritoneal ultrafiltration. Since sodium intake in food cannot be avoided, the consequence will be a progressive positive sodium balance. Therefore, measures to maintain fluid equilibrium will usually affect sodium at the same time. It is important to control dietary sodium intake if there are any problems with fluid removal.

Dialysate potassium is zero to aid control of potassium balance. In the absence of inadvertent potassium loading or catabolic events, changes in plasma potassium mainly result from variations in dietary intake. Due to the continuous nature of PD dietary potassium restriction is less severe than for HD patients. Alterations in total body potassium with time on PD reflect changes in nutrition, in particular a reduction in lean body mass.

Acid–base balance

Commonly used commercial dialysate contains lactate, which is absorbed during the dwell and converted by the body into bicarbonate (the main extracellular buffer), thus correcting uremic acidosis. Short-term studies have shown that correcting acidosis during PD decreases protein degradation. One long-term (1-year) study has suggested that nutritional indices are better if 40 mmol/L lactate is used rather than 35 mmol/L[20]. One measure of PD adequacy is therefore correction of acidosis, usually judged clinically by plasma bicarbonate. PD fluid containing bicarbonate is equipotent in maintaining plasma bicarbonate concentration. For the majority of patients to sustain a normal plasma bicarbonate, the concentration of bicarbonate in the inflow should be 38–40 mmol/L.

Nutrition

One further criterion for adequate dialysis is the preservation of good nutrition. Assessments of dietary intake and nutritional status are important. If there is evidence of poor nutrition then the possibility of underdialysis should be considered. This is discussed further in Chapter 74.

Quality of life

One factor in assessing the success or otherwise of PD or any other renal replacement therapy is the patient's quality of life. Since there are no randomly allocated prospective trials comparing PD with HD or renal transplant, the information available could well be subject to bias, particularly in relation to patient selection. At present, it would appear that the patients' perception of their own quality of life is much better if they have a working transplant than if they receive either type of dialysis[21]. Comparisons between PD and HD are difficult. It has been suggested that individuals receiving home HD have a better quality of life than those on other types of dialysis. Such people, however, are highly selected. Comparative data suggest that the illness intrusiveness of either form of dialysis is comparable to that of other chronic diseases such as rheumatoid arthritis. It is clear that patients who choose PD themselves feel they have a better quality of life than those who are obliged to receive PD because of resource limitations on HD[22]. There is some evidence that patients on PD are more likely to be employed compared with those on HD[22–24]. It is often not recognized that one of the supposed advantages of PD, namely that it is a home-based therapy, may have a negative effect on the family. Though most patients are trained to do the bag exchanges themselves, in practice a carer often becomes involved. The continuous nature of the therapy can then lead to stress and exhaustion for the carer. A further factor that is of crucial importance is the hemoglobin level of the patient. It is very clear that correction of anemia, usually by epoetin therapy, is associated with a significant improvement in quality of life.

PD is not, and never can be, associated with a normal quality of life. This can, however, be optimized by respecting patient choice, reducing complications including anemia, and encouraging patient independence.

REFERENCES

1. Coles GA, Williams JD. What is the place of peritoneal dialysis in the integrated treatment of renal failure? Kidney Int. 1998; 54:2234–40.
2. Flessner MF. Peritoneal transport physiology: insights from basic research. J Am Soc Nephrol. 1991;2:122–35.
3. Tenckhoff H, Schechter H. A bacteriologically safe peritoneal access device. Trans Am Soc Artif Intern Organs. 1973;10:363–70.
4. Blake P, Burkart JM, Churchill DN, et al. Recommended clinical practices for maximising peritoneal dialysis clearances. Perit Dial Int. 1996;16:448–56.
5. Mistry CD, Gokal R. Peers E and the MIDAS Study Group. A randomized multicentre clinical trial comparing isosmolar Icodextrin with hyperosmolar glucose solutes in CAPD. Kidney Int. 1994;46:496–503.
6. Kopple JD, Bernard D, Messana J, et al. Treatment of malnourished CAPD patients with an amino acid based dialysate. Kidney Int. 1995;47:1148–57.
7. Coles GA, Gokal R, Ogg C, et al. A randomised controlled trial of a bicarbonate and a bicarbonate/lactate containing dialysis solution in CAPD. Perit Dial Int. 1997;17:48–51.
8. Twardowski ZJ, Nolph KD, Khanna R, et al. Peritoneal equilibration test. Perit Dial Bull. 1987;7:138–47.
9. Pannekeet MMH, Krediet RT. Water channels in the peritoneum. Perit Dial Int. 1996;16:255–9.
10. CANADA-USA. (CANUSA) Peritoneal Dialysis Study Group. Adequacy of dialysis and nutrition in continuous peritoneal dialysis: association with clinical outcomes. J Am Soc Nephrol. 1996; 7:198–207.

11. Jager KJ, Merkus MP, Dekker FW, et al. Mortality and technique failure in patients starting chronic peritoneal dialysis: results of the Netherlands Cooperative Study on the Adequacy of Dialysis. NECOSAD Study Group Kidney Int. 1999;55:1476–85.

12. Davies SJ, Phillips L, Russell GI. Peritoneal solute transport predicts survival on CAPD independently of residual renal function. Nephrol Dial Transplant. 1998;13:962–8.

13. Paniagua R, Amato D, Vonesh E, et al. Effects of increased peritoneal clearances on mortality rates in peritoneal dialysis: ADE-MEX, a prospective, randomized, controlled trial. J Am Soc Nephrol. 2002;5:1307–20.

14. Nolph KD, Jensen RA, Khanna R, Twardowski ZJ. Weight limitations for weekly urea clearances using various exchange volumes in continuous ambulatory peritoneal dialysis. Perit Dial Int. 1994;14:261–4.

15. Faller B, Lameire B. Evolution of clinical parameters and peritoneal function in a cohort of CAPD patients followed over 7 years. Nephrol Dial Transplant. 1994;9:280–6.

16. Harnett JD, Kent GM, Barré PE, et al. Risk factors for the development of left ventricular hypertrophy in a prospectively followed cohort of dialysis patients. J Am Soc Nephrol. 1994;4:1486–90.

17. Lysaght M, Vonesh EF, Gotch F, et al. The influence of dialysis treatment modality on the decline of remaining renal function. Trans Am Soc Artif Intern Organs. 1991;37:598–604.

18. Medcalf JF, Harris KP, Walls J. Role of diuretics in the preservation of residual renal function in patients on continuous ambulatory peritoneal dialysis. Kidney Int. 2001;59:1128–33.

19. Posthuma N, Wee PM ter, Verbrugh HA, et al. Icodextrin instead of glucose during the daytime dwell in CCPD increases ultrafiltration and 24-h dialysate creatinine clearance. Nephrol Dial Transplant. 1997;12:550–3.

20. Stein A, Moorhouse J, Iles-Smith H, et al. Role of an improvement in acid–base status and nutrition in CAPD patients. Kidney Int. 1997;52:1089–95.

21. Khan IH, Garratt A, Kumer A, et al. Patients' perception of health on renal replacement therapy: evaluated using a new instrument. Nephrol Dial Transplant. 1995;10:684–9.

22. Szabo E, Moody H, Hamilton T, et al. Choice of treatment improves quality of life. A study on patients undergoing dialysis. Arch Intern Med. 1997;57:1352–6.

23. Manen JG van, Korevaar JC, Dekker FW, et al. R T Changes in employment status in end-stage renal disease patients during their first year of dialysis. Perit Dial Int. 2001;21:595–601.

24. Merkus MP, Jager KJ, Dekker FW, et al. Quality of life in patients on chronic dialysis: self-assessment 3 months after the start of treatment. Am J Kidney Dis. 1997;29:584–92.

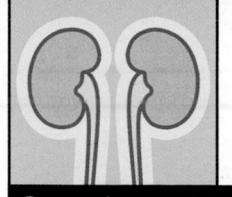
Chapter 81

Complications of Peritoneal Dialysis

Simon J Davies and John D Williams

INTRODUCTION

Changes in peritoneal structure and function on peritoneal dialysis

Loss of peritoneal function is a major factor leading to treatment failure in peritoneal dialysis (PD). Although the precise biological mechanisms responsible for these changes have not been defined, it is widely assumed that alterations in peritoneal function are related to structural changes in the peritoneal membrane. There is accumulating, albeit indirect, evidence that continuous exposure to bioincompatible dialysis solution components, as well as repeated episodes of bacterial peritonitis (Fig. 81.1), play a major role in the long term changes seen in peritoneal function (ultrafiltration loss and increased solute clearance). To date, however, the relationship between structure and function has not been fully defined. Although a number of studies have identified various mesothelial, vascular and interstitial changes in peritoneal morphology during PD neither the factors responsible for these changes nor the time scale over which they develop have been identified. The changes observed include, loss or degeneration of mesothelium, sub-mesothelial thickening (variously described as fibrosis or sclerosis), changes in the structure and number of blood vessels and vascular basement membrane reduplication.

Recent studies have quantified the changes within the sub mesothelial collagenous zone and demonstrated a progressive increase in thickness with time on PD. (Fig. 81.2). Changes within the peritoneal vascular bed have also been identified.

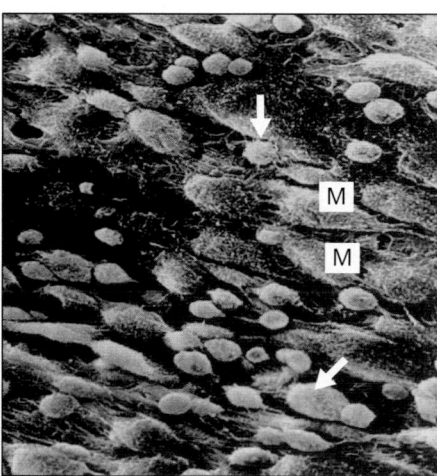

Figure 81.1 Peritonitis. Scanning electron micrograph of the peritoneum from a patient receiving peritoneal dialysis who has peritonitis. The small round cells (arrowed) are phagocytes, which are widely distributed among the mesothelial cells (M). (×1800)

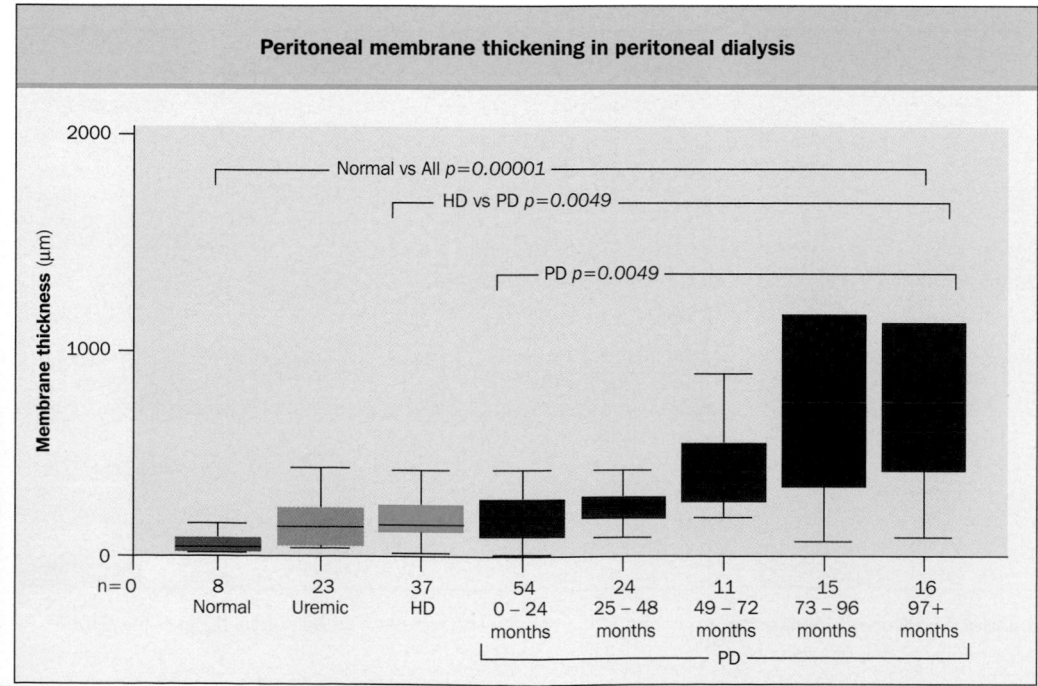

Figure 81.2 Peritoneal membrane thickening in peritoneal dialysis. The thickness of the submesothelial collagenous zone of the peritoneal membrane in normal individuals, in undialyzed uremics, in HD and those who have received PD for different periods of time. Membrane thickness is significantly increased in all uremic and dialysis patients compared to normal. Membrane thickness increases significantly with duration of PD, and is increased in PD patients as a group compared to HD.

Dialysis

These include progressive changes to the structure of small venules ranging from subtle thickening of the subendothelial matrix through to complete obliteration of vessels (Fig. 81.3)[1]. In one study, the extent of these changes in a small group of patients correlated with the loss of ultrafiltration[2]. There is thus accumulating evidence that changes occur in both the interstitial and vascular compartments of the dialyzed peritoneal membrane. Whilst it is likely that these changes are related to time on dialysis, to peritonitis and perhaps to dialysis solution components, the exact relationships are poorly understood as is the possible contribution of uremia.

In a small proportion of patients, there is extensive thickening and fibrosis of the peritoneal membrane (Fig. 81.4)[3]. This can occur after severe or recurrent peritonitis. It was originally described following exposure to acetate in the dialysate, the use of chlorhexidine as an antiseptic, and the administration of the β-blocker practolol. Clinically, it usually presents with poor ultrafiltration and reduced peritoneal transport.

Some patients develop an encapsulating, sclerotic reaction, in which the bowel is enveloped in a thick cocoon of fibrous tissue, causing obstruction (Fig. 81.5). Such individuals present with anorexia, nausea, malnutrition, and partial or complete intestinal obstruction. Whether this is a variant of extensive peritoneal fibrosis or a separate entity is unknown.

INFECTIOUS COMPLICATIONS

Peritonitis

Though the introduction of 'disconnect' delivery systems has reduced the incidence of peritonitis, it remains one of the most important complications of long-term PD and is a major cause of treatment failure.

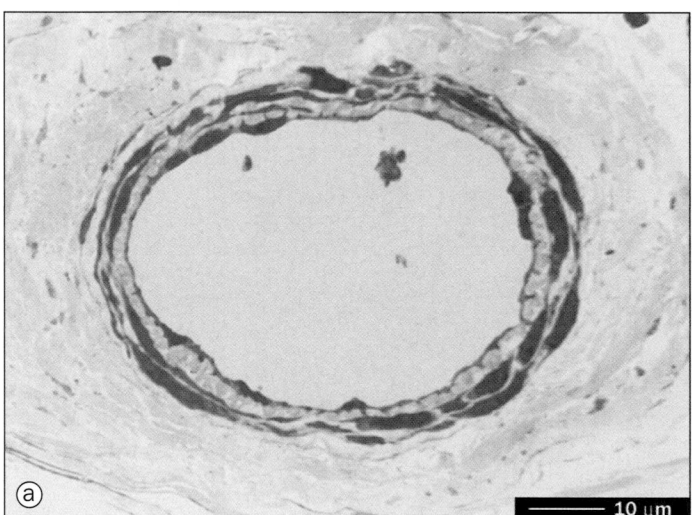
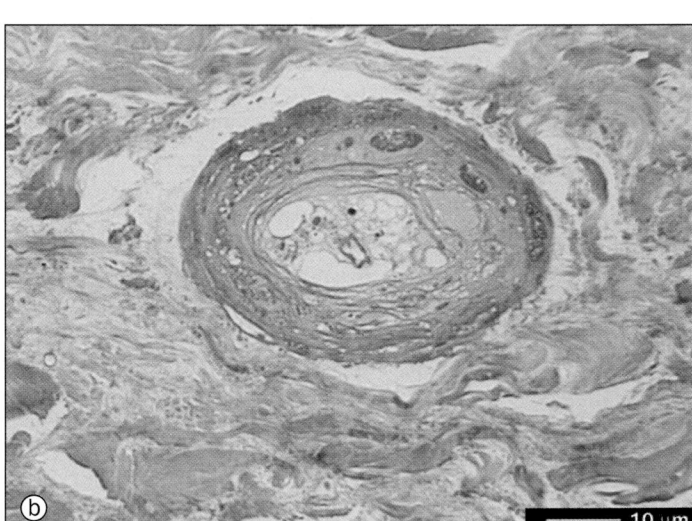

Figure 81.3 Blood vessels in the parietal peritoneum. Transverse sections of peritoneal arterioles (a) normal, (b) vasculopathy in a patient on PD; the vascular lumen is occluded by connective tissue containing fine calcific stippling (toluidine blue).

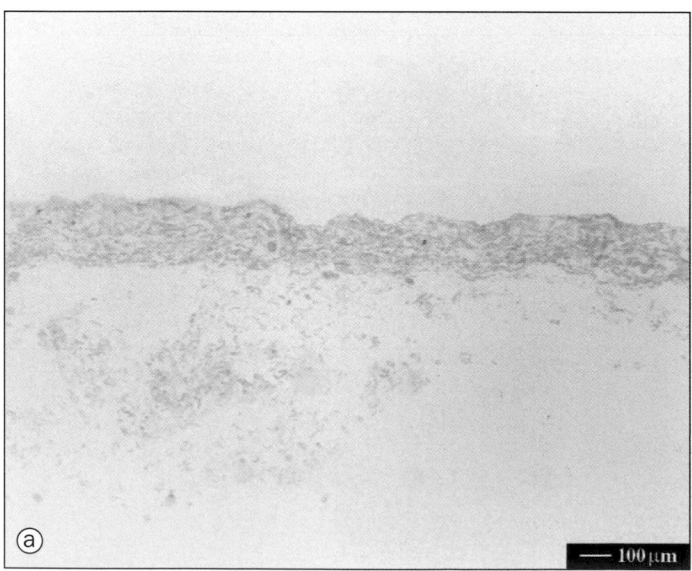
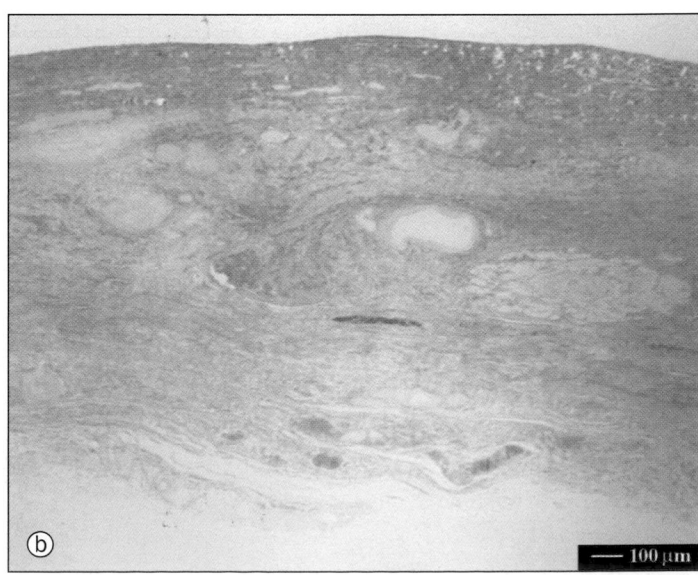

Figure 81.4 Morphological changes in the parietal peritoneal membrane. (a) normal; (b) a patient who has been on peritoneal dialysis for 10 years; note the marked thickening of the submesothelial compact zone (toluidine blue).

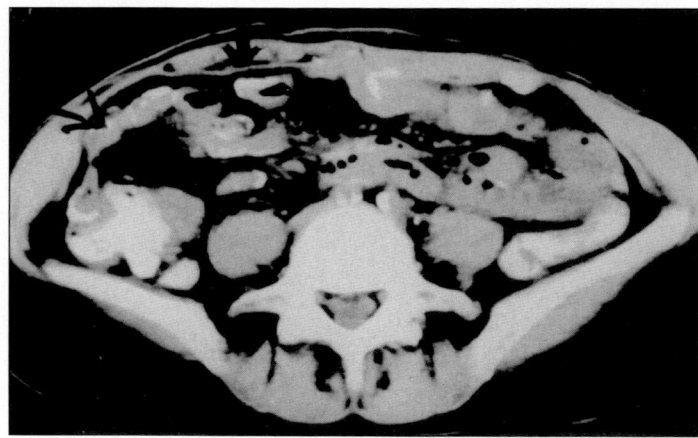

Figure 81.5 Sclerosing encapsulating peritonitis. Abdominal CT scan of a patient with sclerosing encapsulating peritonitis. The thickened peritoneum is clearly visible. (With permission from Dr S Campbell, Princess Alexandra Hospital, Brisbane, Australia.)

Diagnosis of peritonitis

The diagnosis of peritonitis should be suspected in any patient who develops a cloudy bag and/or abdominal pain. Fever may also be present but is not a universal feature of peritonitis. Patients should be advised to contact their dialysis unit immediately if they observe a cloudy bag or develop persistent abdominal pain. Samples of the dialysate should be taken for cell count and microbiologic examination. The diagnosis of peritonitis is confirmed by finding > 100 white blood cells/mm^3 (1×10^7 cells/L). A Gram stain of the spun deposit should also be performed to help to identify the type of causative organism, though initial treatment will often have to be empirical pending full culture and sensitivity results. Various culture techniques have been proposed, but white cell lysis is often helpful in increasing the yield of a positive growth.

Based largely on experience in children, it has been shown that the same diagnostic criteria can be used for patients on automated PD (APD)[4]. Occasionally, if the patient has had a dry abdomen during the day, the initial drain on connection may be cloudy. This will, however, clear within one or two cycles and the majority of the cells will be found to be mononuclear. If cloudy fluid and/or abdominal pain occur, then a dialysate sample should be examined as with continuous ambulatory PD (CAPD). Should there be any doubt, then a further exchange with at least a 1-h dwell should be performed and the fluid re-examined.

Treatment of peritonitis

There is no gold standard treatment for peritonitis in a PD recipient. Most centers use an intraperitoneal regimen for the administration of antibiotics. A number of regimens have been found reasonably effective but none give a 100% cure rate with no relapse. A further complicating factor is the recent emergence of vancomycin-resistant enterococci. There is concern that large-scale use of vancomycin selects for these organisms with the potential of transfer of the resistance, especially to methicillin-resistant *Staphylococcus aureus* (MRSA). As a consequence, alternative regimens, avoiding vancomycin have been proposed.

The Advisory Committee on Peritonitis Management of the International Society of Peritoneal Dialysis has recently published detailed guidelines and algorithms for the management of this condition[4]. The recommended initial empirical therapy is a first-generation cephalosporin, such as cefazolin (cephazolin) or cefalothin (cephalothin) (Fig. 81.6). This is administered as a loading dose in the first bag and then as a maintenance dose in subsequent bags. Once the culture result is available, the regimen should be modified accordingly (Table 81.1). Though *in vitro* tests may suggest resistance of coagulase-negative staphylococci to cephalosporins, the *in vivo* concentration of the drug is usually sufficient to overcome this potential problem. If, however, clinical improvement is slow or fails to occur, vancomycin may be given at a dose of 30 mg/kg intraperitoneally every 7 days. If the organism is MRSA, vancomycin should be given using the same regimen. Finally, for uncomplicated Gram-positive infections an oral cephalosporin can be substituted for the intraperitoneal cephalosporin during the second week of therapy.

If the culture is negative, then cephalosporin should be continued for 2 weeks, assuming there is a clinical response (Table 81.1). If a Gram-negative organism is identified, the subsequent management will depend on the sensitivity (Table 81.1). The isolation of multiple organisms including anaerobes strongly suggests major bowel pathology. Metronidazole should be added to the regimen. In this situation, an urgent laparotomy may be required. A wide variety of antibiotics other than those cited have been tried with success. In particular, a commonly used strategy is to include an oral quinolone, such as ciprofloxacin, instead of an aminoglycoside[2] (see Fig. 81.6), since ototoxicity and loss of residual renal function may occur with aminoglycosides. At present, it is recommended that for Gram-positive organisms, therapy should be for 14 days except in the case of *S. aureus*, when 21 days is suggested. For culture-negative episodes, 14 days of therapy should suffice. The same is true in the case of single organism Gram-negative peritonitis. For *Pseudomonas*, *Xanthomonas* spp. or multiple organisms, 21 days is recommended. Fungal or yeast infections require 4 to 6 weeks of therapy (or 7–10 d of therapy after catheter removal).

Many patients can be treated successfully as outpatients. It is extremely important, however, that they are followed up either in the clinic or by telephone. In most cases, clinical resolution, as judged by the clearing of the bags, starts within 48 h. If there is no improvement within 96 h, despite using the correct antibiotic, as judged by sensitivity tests, the fluid must be retested for cell count, Gram-stain, and culture. In the case of a persistent *S. aureus* infection, an underlying tunnel infection should be excluded. In all other situations where there is a failure to improve, serious consideration should be given to removing the catheter. In addition, the possibility of intra-abdominal or gynecologic pathology or the presence of unusual organisms such as mycobacteria should be considered.

For patients on APD, similar protocols to those outlined above are used, but the dialysis should be modified to a regimen lasting a full 24 h with 3- to 4-h dwells. Once there is clinical resolution, the usual APD regimen can be recommenced but with a daytime bag containing the antibiotic(s) until completion of the treatment.

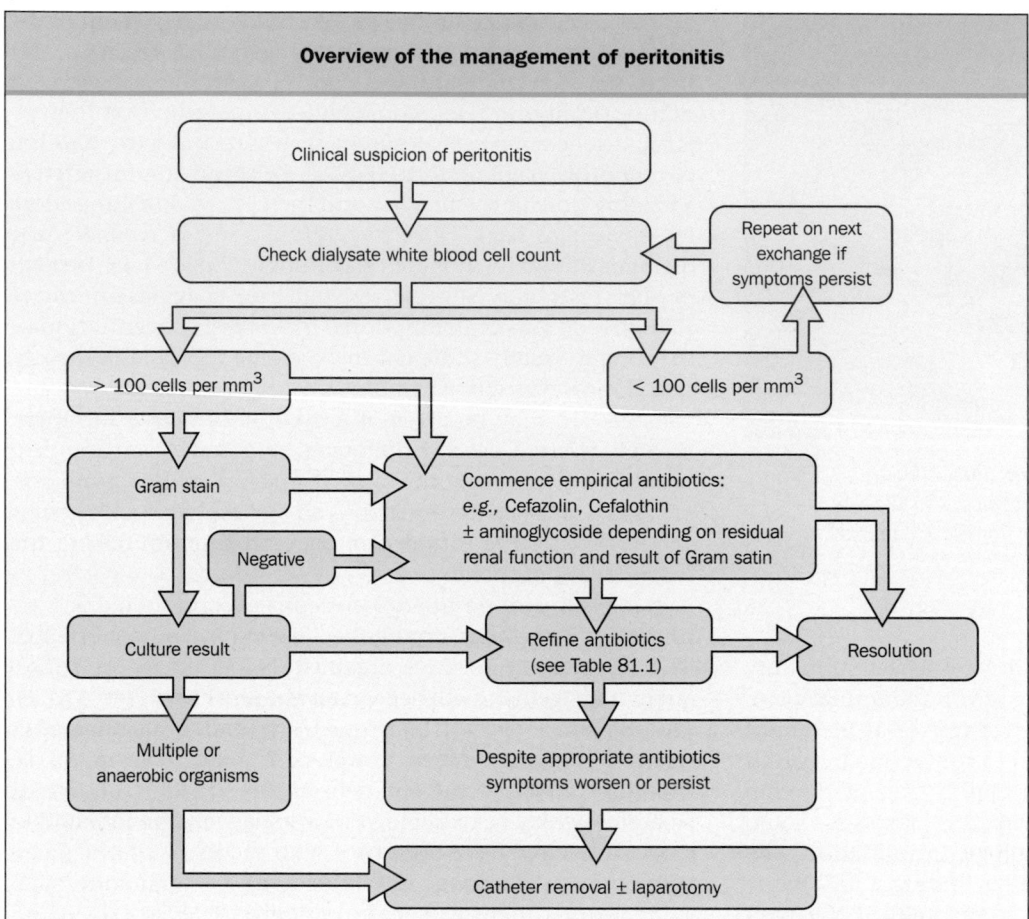

Figure 81.6 Management of PD peritonitis. See text and table 81.1 for further discussion of antisocial regimens.

Fungal peritonitis

If peritonitis is caused by yeasts or fungi, the peritoneal catheter should be removed. There is limited experience with drug treatment. The recommendation for adults is daily fluconazole at an oral or intraperitoneal dose of 200 mg and flucytosine at a loading dose of 2 g orally with a maintenance dose of 1 g daily. Amphotericin (amphotericin B) is no longer recommended. Unfortunately, oral flucytosine is not universally available.

Relapsing peritonitis

Relapsing or recurrent peritonitis is defined as a separate infective episode caused by the same organism within 4 weeks of finishing the previous course of antibiotics. In Gram-positive infections, a 4-week course of a cephalosporin together with oral rifampin (rifampicin) should be tried. The recurrence of S. aureus infection should trigger the search for a pericatheter infection. Relapsing MRSA peritonitis will require a prolonged course (4 weeks) of vancomycin or clindamycin. If enterococci or Gram-negative organisms are the cause, then the possibility of intra-abdominal pathology or an abscess should be considered, although these organisms are frequently water borne. If a patient has other gastrointestinal specific symptoms, such as change in bowel habit, then colonoscopy should be performed, but this is only essential if multiple organisms have been isolated. Again, a repeat course of antibiotics chosen by sensitivity testing

Suggested antibiotic regimens when dialysate culture result is available	
Culture	**Antibiotic**
Enterococci (including vancomycin-resistant enterococci	Ampicillin
Staphylococcus aureus ¶	Cephalosporin/Floxacillin (flucloxacilin)
Methicillin-resistant (MRSA) ¶	Vancomycin
Other Gram-positive organisms §	Cephalosporin/Floxacillin
Gram-negative organisms (including Pseudomonas species) ¶	Cefazolin, quinolone or aminoglycoside*, depending on sensitivities and residual renal function (*avoid unnecessary use if residual function present).
Multiple/anaerobic organisms ¶	Metronidazole ± laparotomy
Culture negative §	Continue empirical treatment

Notes: Except for culture negative episodes, empirical treatment is stopped once the sensitivities are known. Treatment should be for 2 weeks (§) or 3 weeks as indicated (¶). All antibiotic regimens should be developed in consultation with local microbiology practices.

Table 81.1 Antibiotic regimens for PD peritonitis. Suggested antibiotic regimens when dialysate fluid culture is available.

should last 4 weeks. Removal of the catheter should be considered if there is no improvement within 4 days, or earlier if clinically indicated. There are theoretical benefits to the withdrawal of PD as replacement renal therapy for a brief period and avoiding an intraperitoneal foreign body and altered host defenses by instilling dialysate. Some centers, however, have practiced simultaneous removal and replacement of the catheter, under antibiotic cover, with success[5].

Prevention of peritonitis

Because of the high rate of peritonitis experienced during the early years of CAPD, considerable efforts have been made to prevent this serious complication. To date, however, there is no evidence that a correctable biologic defect predisposes patients to an increased risk of peritonitis. In contrast, significant advances have been made in the design of delivery systems, resulting in the 'Y system', which significantly reduces the rate of infection. The use of such a system has now become the standard for CAPD[6].

S. aureus nasal carriage is associated with an increased chance of peritonitis caused by this organism. Regular use of mupirocin either intranasally or applied to the catheter exit site may reduce the rate of *S. aureus* peritonitis[7], though whether resistance will occur with long-term use is unclear.

Unfortunately, there is no proven method of decreasing the incidence of Gram-negative infection. This type of organism often causes problems in the elderly, possibly as a result of diverticular disease. Except for the avoidance of constipation and encouraging regular bowel movements by the judicious use of fiber, no other measure can be recommended at present.

Eosinophilic peritonitis

Eosinophilic peritonitis is diagnosed when a patient presents with a cloudy bag of effluent that is found on microscopy to contain eosinophils rather than neutrophils. The fluid is also culture negative. It is an uncommon event, but tends to occur within the first few weeks of starting PD. The cause is unknown but it is assumed to be some form of reaction to the cannula or to the dialysate. The condition is usually self-limiting and no treatment is required.

Exit site infection

Exit site infection is an important complication of long-term PD, occurring on average at a rate of 0.48 episodes per patient-year (Fig. 81.7)[8]. The most common infecting organism is *S. aureus*, either alone or in association with another species of bacteria[9]. The diagnosis is suspected on clinical grounds, usually by the presence of marked erythema and/or discharge from the exit site. Increased scab formation also makes the diagnosis likely. There is often, but not invariably, local tenderness around the exit site and over the outer cuff. Although a positive culture is not essential to diagnose exit site infection, an attempt to determine the causative microorganism should be made. It is essential to culture any exudate rather than just sample the surrounding skin.

Consensus guidelines for management of exit site infection have been published[10].

If there is any discharge and/or significant associated cellulitis, it is important to start with a systemic antibiotic. Since *S. aureus* is the most common infecting organism, an agent effective against this species should be prescribed. Unless there

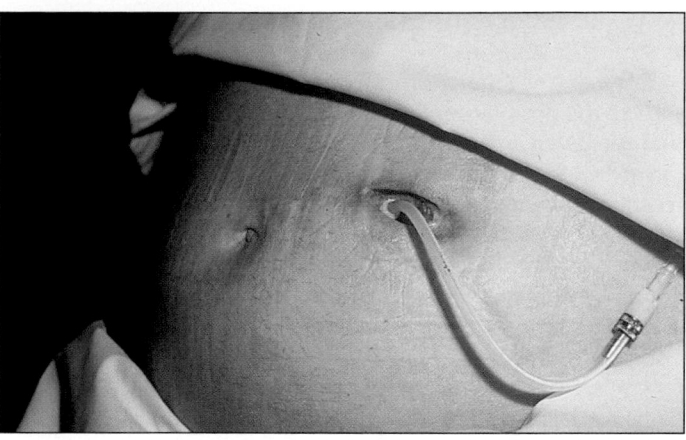

Figure 81.7 Exit site infection. A severe exit site infection that has exposed the outer cuff of the cannula.

is prior evidence that the patient carries MRSA, flucloxacillin (500 mg four times daily) is appropriate, or a cephalosporin if the patient is allergic to penicillin. In most patients, the drug can be given orally, but if the individual is systemically ill, the antibiotics should be administered intravenously until clinical improvement occurs. Hospitalization is not necessary for most patients. If the infection is MRSA, the organism may occasionally be sensitive to a cephalosporin, but most patients should be given vancomycin (1 g i.v., or i.p. if the dwell time is at least 6 h). The dose is repeated once a week for up to 4 weeks.

Should the culture grow a Gram-negative organism, ciprofloxacin in an oral dose of 500 mg twice daily will be effective in most patients. Other antibiotics should be substituted according to the *in vitro* sensitivity results. It is recommended that treatment should continue for a minimum of 2 weeks. In Gram-positive infections, if there is no improvement within 7 d, rifampin (rifampicin) 600 mg daily should be added. If complete healing does not take place after 4 weeks of therapy, further measures should be considered, such as exteriorizing and shaving of the outer cuff. Should this cuff be visible or even close to the exit site, it is likely to be involved in the infection. There is often temporary resolution of infection following this procedure but it may only prolong catheter life for 6 to 12 months. If despite this step the infection persists or relapses, catheter removal must be considered since there is a high risk of the exit site infection leading to peritonitis. It is important that the new exit site is formed in a different part of the anterior abdominal wall. If the infection is controlled and there is no evidence of sepsis along the tunnel, it is possible to insert a new catheter under antibiotic cover at the same time as the old one is removed.

Whenever exit site infection occurs, increased local measures are necessary. The site should be cleaned at least once and preferably twice daily with povidone–iodine or hydrogen peroxide. Should there only be erythema and no significant discharge, these measures may be effective on their own. Topical mupirocin has also been advocated for treatment, though experience is limited. Where there is exuberant granulation tissue formed, the application of a silver nitrate stick is advocated, taking care to avoid the surrounding skin[7,11]. Failure of initial therapy or recurrence of infection should be considered as strong indications for catheter removal and replacement.

Since exit site infection can be intractable, prophylaxis must start at the time of implantation. There are studies suggesting that the use of a single dose of parenteral antibiotic at the time of insertion reduces the early infection rate. In view of the recent emergence of vancomycin-resistant organisms, it is clear that this antibiotic must no longer be used for this purpose. A cephalosporin is probably the best alternative, although because of the association between nasal carriage of *S. aureus* and exit site infections, preoperative nasal mupirocin might also prove effective[7].

The next important preventive measure is the avoidance of dialysate leakage. This can be minimized by implanting the catheter through the rectus sheath and/or not commencing PD for at least 2 weeks after insertion. Should dialysis be necessary, small volumes (500 mL for adults) with no dwell should be used initially; slowly increasing over 10 days. In addition, catheter movement should be minimized using tape and a dressing of gauze with a nonocclusive cover. This should not be changed for several days unless there is excessive bleeding. Daily dressing should start between 2 and 8 weeks postimplantation. The regular use of povidone–iodine is associated with reduced infection compared with the use of soap and water.

Several studies have specifically addressed the prevention of *S. aureus* exit site infections. Benefits have been reported with daily topical mupirocin[7,11]. Recently, a large European randomly allocated prospective study showed that the regular use of nasal mupirocin by patients who were proven nasal carriers of *S. aureus* reduced the rate of exit site infection by this organism by two-thirds compared with that seen using a placebo nasal ointment[11]. The most cost-effective regimen has yet to be determined.

Tunnel infection

Tunnel infection is a relatively rare problem, defined as an infection occurring between the two cuffs. The diagnosis is suggested by the classical signs of inflammation appearing along the line of the catheter. Sometimes, but not always, there is an associated exit site infection. The diagnosis may be aided by the use of ultrasound (Fig. 81.8)[12]. If this shows a fluid collection around the cannula, a tunnel infection should be suspected. The treatment of tunnel infection is similar to that of exit site infection and requires the systemic administration of antibiotics. The chances of resolution, however, are much lower and catheter removal will probably be required. This is mandatory if there is an associated peritonitis.

NONINFECTIOUS COMPLICATIONS

Ultrafiltration failure

Problems with ultrafiltration may be transient or long-standing. Acute peritonitis is a common cause of ultrafiltration failure, which improves as infection is controlled. Inadequate ultrafiltration leading to fluid overload is one of the commonest problems associated with long-term PD. One study suggested that up to 31% of patients had a problem by 6 years of treatment[13]. There is no ideal definition of ultrafiltration failure, but both patient and membrane factors need to be taken into account. From the patient perspective there is concern if more than two hypertonic (3.86% anhydrous glucose) dialysis exchanges per 24 h are required to maintain fluid balance. In these circumstances peritoneal membrane function tests should be performed to establish the ultrafiltration capacity of the membrane. Low drain volumes alone do not make the diagnosis. If the patient has a good urine output it is not uncommon for some of the dialysate to be absorbed, particularly during a long dwell.

An algorithm for investigating apparent problems with ultrafiltration is shown in Figure 81.9. It is important to check the actual drainage volumes by asking the patient to bring their bags to the unit. The total volume of outflow over 24 h should be compared with previous records to see if any decrease has occurred. If there is no difference, ultrafiltration has not changed. Under such circumstances, the next step is to measure the 24-h urine volume. A decrease in residual renal function will be manifest as fluid overload unless ultrafiltration is increased or fluid intake is curtailed. The final step in assessing fluid overload is to measure fluid intake. If fluid intake is excessive, then measures must be undertaken to correct this. In the short term, restricting fluid intake may suffice but usually extra hypertonic bags are needed until fluid status improves as judged by weight, blood pressure and edema. If there has been

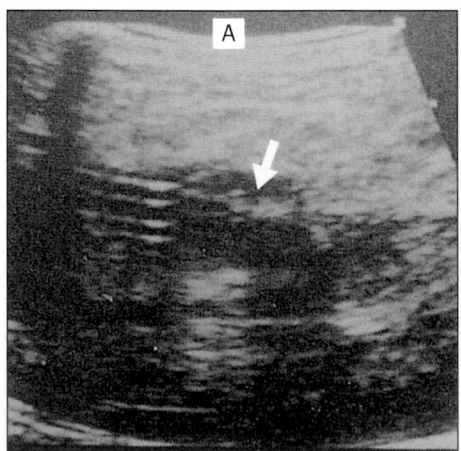
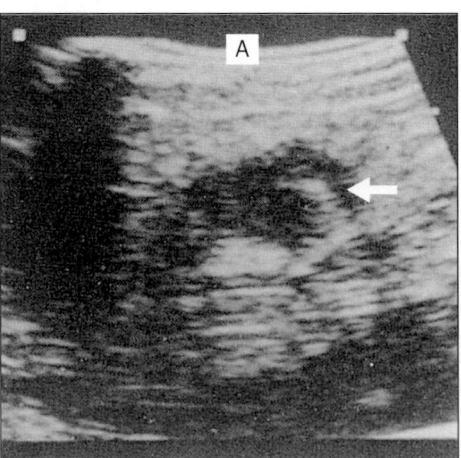

Figure 81.8 Ultrasound appearance of tunnel infection. Note the fluid collection around the catheter in two different views (arrows). A, abdominal surface. (With permission from Holley et al.[12].)

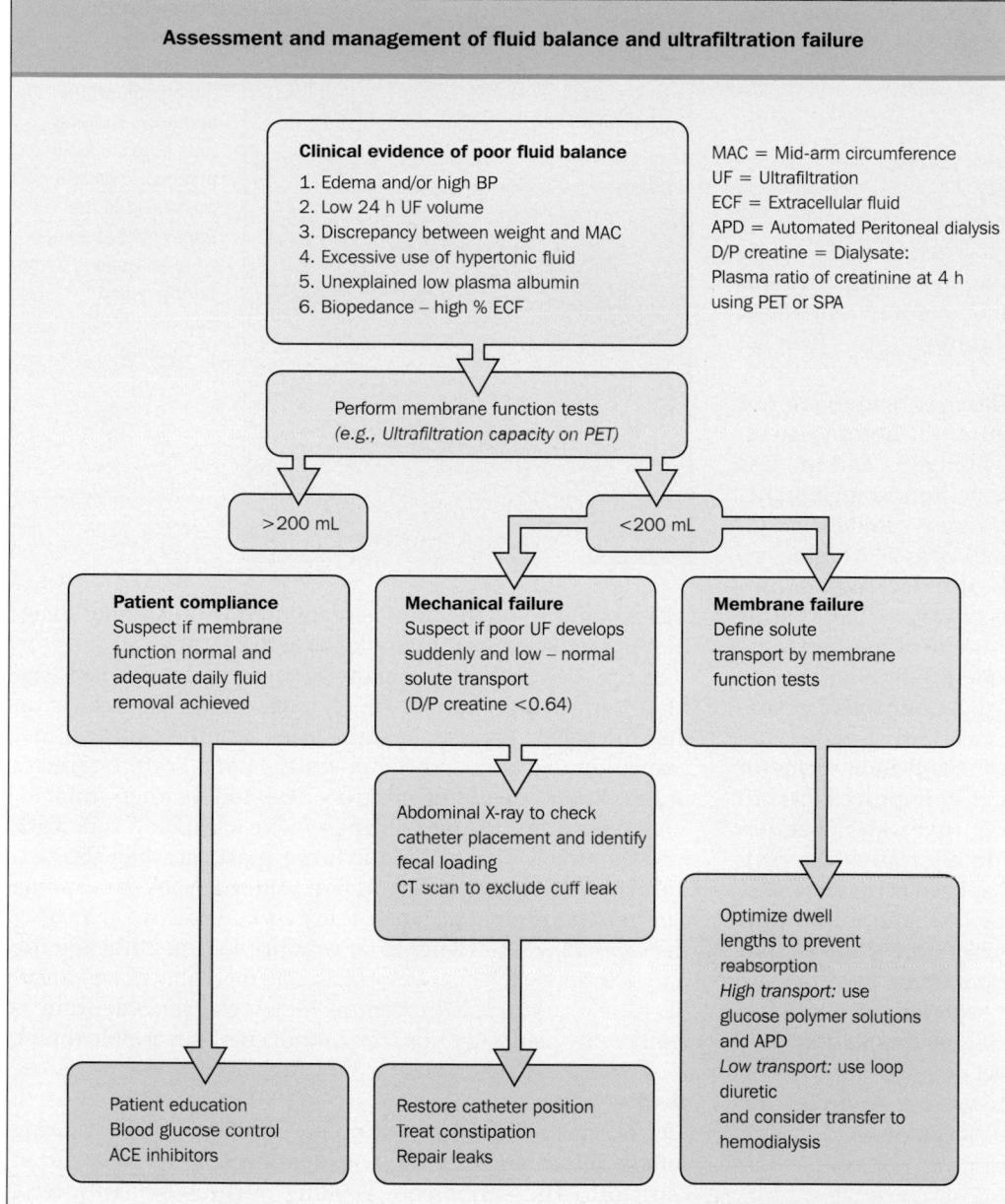

a loss of residual renal function this may expose a problem with ultrafiltration. This is best assessed using the peritoneal equilibration test (PET) (see Chapter 80). Ultrafiltration failure is likely if the ultrafiltration capacity is < 200 mL using a routine PET with 2.27% glucose, or < 400 mL using a modified standard permeability analysis (SPA) with 3.86% glucose (see Chapter 80). Ultrafiltration failure can then be categorized further according to the low molecular weight solute transport. High solute transport failure is present when the dialysate: plasma creatinine ratio at 4 h is > 0.64.

Management of high solute transport ultrafiltration failure (dialysate : plasma creatinine ratio > 0.64)

In patients with high transport failure, there is a more rapid absorption of glucose from the peritoneal cavity, which results in the early loss of the osmotic gradient. Short dwell periods reduce the degree of fluid reabsorption. One approach to improving fluid loss is to use four bags during the waking hours and remain dry overnight. Alternatively, a change to automated PD(APD) using several short overnight cycles with a dry day may improve the situation. If there is a significant urine output, a loop diuretic in high dosage (e.g., furosemide (frusemide), 250 mg daily) should be tried. It has also been claimed that a short period of temporary hemodialysis leads to improvement[14] although there are no controlled clinical trial data to support this.

An alternative approach is the use of a high-molecular-weight osmotic agent. Such a molecule is more slowly absorbed than glucose and, therefore, generates an osmotic effect for much longer. Only one agent is currently available, glucose polymer or icodextrin, which has a molecular weight of approximately 20 000. A 6-month clinical trial showed reasonable clinical efficacy with no obvious adverse effects[15]. There is also cumulative evidence from patients who have now been treated for more than 3 years. Icodextrin is of particular value when used for long dwell periods (overnight for CAPD or in the daytime as an adjunct to APD). In several countries it is licensed and available as a 7.5% solution.

Management of low transport ultrafiltration failure (dialysate : plasma creatinine ratio < 0.64)

Although less common, the management of low transport ultrafiltration failure is more difficult. It is essential to exclude any form of mechanical failure, such as an occult peritoneal cuff leak or an inguinal hernia using contrast enhanced computerized tomographic (CT) scanning, and manage appropriately (see below).

The causes of low transport ultrafiltration failure are not fully understood but may include peritoneal fibrosis, excessive fluid reabsorption, possibly via lymphatics, and the loss of water channels (aquaporins) in the peritoneal membrane, presumably in the endothelium of peritoneal capillaries[16].

Usually during the first part of a dwell with 3.86% glucose, there is a rapid dilutional increase in the dialysate sodium concentration (sodium sieving). With loss of water channels this phenomenon is not seen and its measurement has been suggested as a diagnostic test, although poor ultrafiltration of any cause will result in reduced sodium sieving. Completely removing glucose from the dialysis regimen substituting a combination of bags containing icodextrin, glycerol and amino acids for several weeks has been claimed to result in improved ultrafiltration and sodium sieving (suggesting that water channels have been restored)[17]. Alternatively simply resting the peritoneum by changing to hemodialysis has been tried. Otherwise there is no satisfactory treatment for low solute transport ultrafiltration failure. If there is a reasonable urine output (> 200 mL/24 h), the addition of a loop diuretic may increase urine volumes, but often a permanent switch to hemodialysis is necessary. In patients with sclerosing encapsulating peritonitis, laparotomy will reveal a bowel covered in a cocoon of fibrous tissue. In some cases this tissue can be peeled off, freeing the bowel and thus relieving obstruction.

Catheter malfunction

Inflow failure

A 2 L bag of dialysate should take 15 min or less to run into the peritoneal cavity. If inflow is significantly slowed or even stopped completely, mechanical causes should first be evaluated. One should first ensure the tubing and catheter are not kinked, that any clamp or roller is open for the inflow position, and that any frangible seal is fully broken. In the absence of such problems, the catheter should be flushed vigorously with 20 mL heparinized saline. If the catheter now becomes patent, it is wise to add heparin 500 u/L for the next few cycles, because the cause of the blockage is often a fibrin plug. Should the catheter remain blocked, the abdomen must be X-rayed. If the catheter is in a satisfactory position in the pelvis, an attempt to restore patency should be made using urokinase: 2 mL of saline containing 25 000 units urokinase are infused into the lumen of the catheter and left *in situ* for 2 to 4 h. The catheter is then flushed; if inflow is restored heparin should be added to the dialysate for the next few cycles. Should this procedure not be successful but fibrin is

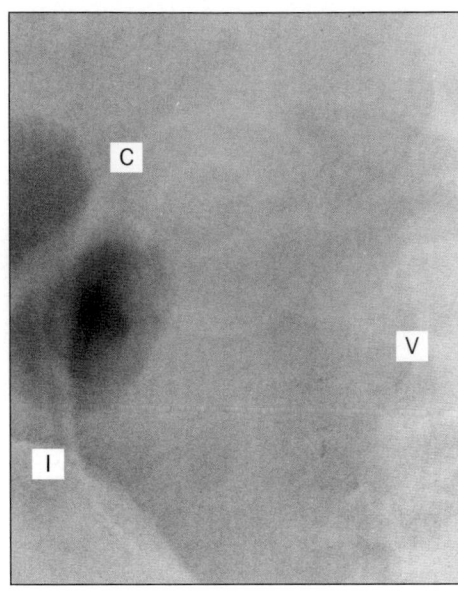

Figure 81.10 Catheter malposition. Plain radiograph of the abdomen showing marked fecal loading and curled catheter misplaced in the upper right abdomen. C: radio-opaque stripe on the curled catheter; I: ilium; V: vertebra.

still thought to be the cause, an endoscopy brush may sometimes prove successful in unblocking the catheter.

If the X-rays show the catheter to be malpositioned (Fig. 81.10), an attempt should be made to reposition the catheter tip into the pelvis. This can be done using a sterile semirigid rod, shaped into a curve and slid down the lumen of the catheter under X-ray screening control. The rod is then rotated. Sometimes the catheter will then move easily and slide back into the pelvis. This technique is not practical when the cannula has a swan-neck configuration. Alternatively, the cannula can be repositioned at laparotomy or peritoneoscopy. Often the cannula will be found to be wrapped in omentum and the only solution will be to carry out an omentectomy or an 'omental hitch', a surgical procedure in which the omentum is temporarily held away from the cannula by a dissolvable suture.

Outflow failure

The reasons for outflow failure are similar to those causing inflow failure. In addition, constipation is a well-recognized cause of outflow problems. Loading of the bowel with fecal material is often obvious on a plain X-ray of the abdomen. If constipation is the cause, it should be treated with oral laxatives or an enema. Magnesium-, phosphate-, or citrate-containing enemas should be avoided because of potential toxicity. Sometimes a strong laxative such as sodium picosulfate is necessary to ensure sufficient evacuation to permit drainage of the dialysate. Subsequently, bowel action should be kept regular by increasing the fiber in the diet and, if necessary, the addition of a mild laxative such as lactulose or senna.

Fibrin in the dialysate

During peritonitis, it is common for fibrin to be present in the dialysate. If there is any restriction of dialysate flow, heparin (500 u/L) should be added to the bags. A small number of patients have fibrin formation in the absence of peritonitis. Immediately on drainage, the bag may appear cloudy, but on standing the fibrin will aggregate. The first time this happens, a sample must be sent to the microbiology laboratory to exclude infection. If this proves negative, the patient can be reassured. If catheter plugging occurs, regular use of heparin is recommended.

Fluid leaks

External leaks

On occasion, fluid may leak from the exit site or even the incision used to insert the cannula into the peritoneal cavity. This is usually a problem that occurs early, particularly if dialysis is started soon after cannula insertion. Whenever possible, elective insertion of the catheter should be performed at least 2 weeks before dialysis is required. In addition, the use of the paramedian approach for the peritoneal entry site is thought to minimize the chances of this complication. If a leak occurs, PD should be withheld for as long as possible. If dialysis is necessary, temporary use of hemodialysis should be employed for 2 weeks. Alternatively, after at least 48 h of a 'dry' abdomen, PD can be recommenced with the aid of a cycler using a low volume (500 mL for adults) and no dwell. Volumes are then progressively increased over 10 days. Should the leak recur despite either of these regimens, surgical repair of the peritoneal entry site or replacement of the catheter at a different site will be required. Once again the abdomen should be left 'dry' for 2–4 weeks to allow full healing.

Internal leaks

Isolated abdominal wall edema

Isolated edema of the abdominal wall suggests an internal leak from the peritoneal cavity. This is particularly likely to occur from the catheter insertion site or a previous incision. It also sometimes occurs in association with an overt hernia. The site of the leak can be visualized by CT scanning following intraperitoneal instillation of contrast. It may be necessary for the patient to stand or perform other maneuvers to increase intra-abdominal pressure before the leak is demonstrated. An alternative diagnostic test is to perform scintigraphy after injecting a compound such as technetium-99m-diethylenetriamine pentaacetic acid (^{Tc99m}DTPA) (Fig. 81.11). A surgical repair will be required if a major leak is visualized. Often,

however, the patient can be managed conservatively by bed rest, using low-volume cycles with little or no dwell. Cessation of PD for 2 weeks with temporary hemodialysis may also allow the leak to seal permanently.

Isolated genital edema

Isolated genital edema can be caused by the same processes as abdominal wall edema and the management is identical. In addition, genital edema can also be caused by a patent processus vaginalis with or without an associated inguinal hernia. The leak may be visualized using CT or scintigraphy. Any hernia requires surgical repair, but once again a small leak may seal off spontaneously if PD is either suspended or continued using bed rest, low volumes, and a scrotal support for affected male patients.

Hydrothorax

A pleural effusion can occur with generalized fluid overload or local lung disease, but occasionally it is caused by a leakage of dialysate through the diaphragm (Fig. 81.12). This more commonly occurs on the right side. A leak is most simply confirmed by aspirating a sample of the effusion and finding that its glucose concentration is higher than the patient's blood glucose. Initially, conservative measures should be tried. These include stopping PD, aspirating the effusion to dryness, and leaving the abdomen dry for 2 weeks (using hemodialysis if necessary). This regimen is effective in a number of patients. If the condition recurs, then pleurodesis should be tried. Various agents have been advocated, including tetracycline, talc, autologous blood, and fibrin glue, but there are no comparative studies to indicate the best regimen.

Herniae

Herniae are relatively common in patients on PD[18]. The major risks are incarceration and strangulation of bowel. The commonest sites are inguinal, incisional, pericatheter, and periumbilical. Any patient commencing long-term PD with a hernia present should have it repaired. This can be done at the same time as catheter insertion. Pericatheter herniae are

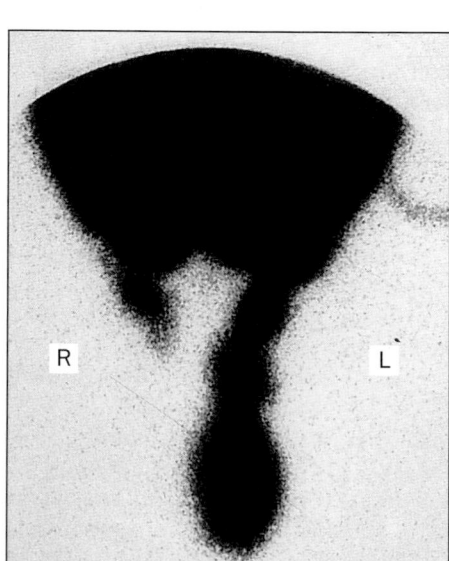

Figure 81.11 Inguinal hernia during peritoneal dialysis. Peritoneal scintigram of a male patient on peritoneal dialysis, showing bilateral inguinal hernias. The left hernia extends into the scrotum; the right hernia is less extensive.

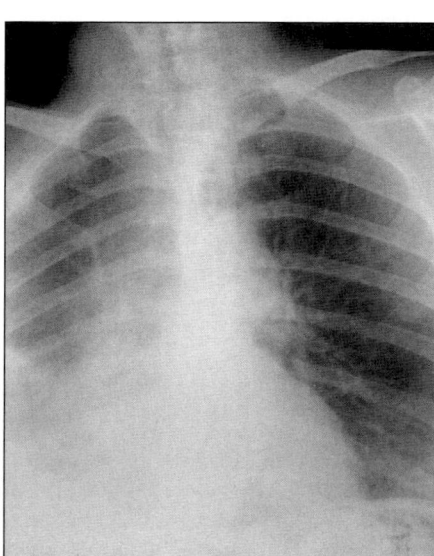

Figure 81.12 Hydrothorax in peritoneal dialysis. Chest radiograph showing a right-sided pleural effusion caused by a diaphragmatic leak.

less likely if the catheter is inserted in a paramedian position and PD is not started within 14 days of the procedure. If a hernia subsequently develops during PD treatment, it should be electively repaired. Postoperatively, the patient should be treated by low-volume (500 mL) cycles with no dwell using a cycler. The volume is progressively increased and CAPD can recommence after 10 days. Alternatively, the patient can be treated by temporary hemodialysis. Should herniae become a recurrent problem, a switch to nocturnal PD (NPD) should be seriously considered since intra-abdominal pressure is lower in the supine position. The only other option is a transfer to hemodialysis.

Pain
Inflow pain
Soon after the commencement of PD, patients may experience pain during inflow of the fluid. This is particularly likely to occur if dialysis begins immediately or within a few days of catheter insertion. It is presumably related to blunt trauma of the peritoneum. This problem usually disappears with time but may require the temporary use of simple analgesics. Slowing the rate of fluid inflow will often reduce the symptoms. Curled-tip catheters are also thought to reduce the likelihood of this type of pain. The introduction of air can produce discomfort. Care with the bag-exchange technique should eliminate this hazard. Pain often occurs during peritonitis. The treatment is the same as for any case of peritonitis together with sufficient analgesia if clinically necessary. Finally, a small number of individuals get persistent inflow pain. A randomized controlled trial has demonstrated that bicarbonate dialysis fluid at physiologic pH is associated with a dramatic improvement in infusion pain in such individuals[19].

Backache
Backache occurs in a minority of patients, particularly those undergoing CAPD or having a daytime dwell in association with APD. The presence of a large volume of fluid in the abdomen distorts the normal posture, exacerbating any tendency to lordosis of the spine. Patients with pre-existing back problems are most likely to have an exacerbation of their backache, though not all will be affected. It is important to investigate the symptom to exclude treatable or serious disease. This includes plain radiographs of the spine and, if necessary, magnetic resonance imaging. Renal osteodystrophy, if present, must be treated appropriately. If, however, the problem appears to be caused by degenerative disease of the spine (spondylolisthesis or osteoporosis) then adjusting the PD regimen can be of benefit. Reducing the volume of dialysate may help but it can adversely affect adequacy (see Chapter 80). Avoidance of fluid in the abdomen while the patient is upright will often allow considerable improvement. This means transferring those on CAPD to NPD and avoiding a daytime dwell. If this is ineffective, a switch to hemodialysis should be tried. In addition to the above measures, back exercises are sometimes of value.

Outflow pain
Some patients have discomfort or even pain when the fluid runs out. This emptying sensation is abolished when the next cycle runs in. This commonly occurs during peritonitis but may be experienced in the absence of infection during the first few weeks of treatment. In the latter situation, the symptom usually disappears with time.

Bleeding
Exit site
The exit site can be a source of blood loss at any time while a peritoneal cannula is in place. A common cause is the removal of a crust before actual separation has occurred. The bleeding almost invariably stops with local pressure, but a new raw area remains that is liable to become infected. Regular cleansing of the exit site with povidone–iodine will reduce the chances of this complication. Patients must be instructed not to pull off the crust but await its natural separation. Severe infection of the exit site may, on occasion, be accompanied by secondary hemorrhage. This will usually respond to firm pressure. The subsequent management is the same as for any exit site infection.

Blood-stained dialysate
Blood-stained dialysate is uncommon. It is rarely serious but causes considerable alarm to the patient. There is sometimes a clear history of trauma to the abdomen or of unexpected strain. A few female patients relate the episode to their menstrual cycle at the time of ovulation or menstruation. The treatment is to flush the abdomen with a few cycles of dialysate containing heparin (500 u/L) to minimize the chances of clotting in the cannula. The problem usually resolves spontaneously and often is only visible in one outflow. It is unusual for the blood-stained dialysate to be associated with infection, though it is wise to have the fluid cultured. Routine use of antibiotics is not necessary. In the rare event of significant hemorrhage, an urgent laparotomy may be required.

Nutritional problems
Malnutrition
Cross-sectional surveys of patients receiving PD show that about 40% have malnutrition and 8% having severe protein–calorie depletion[20]. Malnutrition is an adverse risk factor for morbidity and mortality of patients on PD; this poor nutrition is multifactorial. The assessment and management of malnutrition are discussed further in Chapter 74. It has been suggested that ideally patients should consume daily at least 1.2–1.3 g protein/kg body weight. In practice, many subjects take only 0.8 g/kg daily and seem to be nutritionally stable. It is likely that they have achieved a steady state but with a lower total body nitrogen or lean body mass.

Patients on CAPD have abnormal eating behavior with smaller meals and slow eating compared with normal subjects. The full peritoneal cavity may produce easy satiety, and some patients complain of feeling bloated. However, studies have shown that there is no actual difference in food consumption with or without dialysate in the abdomen.

One obvious contributing factor is protein loss via the peritoneum, which averages 8 g/d but can be as high as 20 g/d. It increases considerably during peritonitis. Patients with high solute transport also have high peritoneal protein losses, in particular albumin, in both cases a reflection of a larger effective peritoneal surface area. The ensuing hypoalbuminemia combines with less good ultrafiltration to exacerbate the extracellular fluid expansion in these patients.

Another important influence on nutrition is the acid–base status of the patient. Correction of acidosis reduces protein catabolism. One study compared the use of 35 mmol/L lactate dialysate with fluid containing 40 mmol/L lactate[21]. After 1 year, the group receiving the higher lactate concentration had increased serum bicarbonate levels and, more importantly, had gained more weight with a greater increase in mid-arm muscle circumference. This implies that protein anabolism had taken place as the result of better acid–base correction.

The serum albumin tends to be lower in patients on PD than in subjects receiving hemodialysis. Metabolic studies suggest that, despite this finding, the total albumin pool is normal in stable patients on CAPD. Low serum albumin has been suggested as a marker of malnutrition. There is certainly an inverse relationship between serum albumin concentration and mortality, but there is some evidence that this is because low albumin is a marker of other diseases rather than of malnutrition alone.

Correction of malnutrition is not easy. Clearly patients should be encouraged to increase protein and calorie intake. Food supplements are of particular value during intercurrent illness. One report suggested that the regular use of a calorie supplement was associated with increased total body nitrogen after several months, but this remains to be confirmed. Correction of acidosis is clearly important. This is best achieved by using dialysate with higher levels of potential buffer, but if necessary oral bicarbonate may be added. Avoidance of peritonitis is crucial to minimize protein losses, but currently there is no way the obligatory loss of protein during PD can be regulated.

Amino acid-based dialysate improves nitrogen balance in malnourished patients but the long-term benefits are still unclear[22]. Usually one bag a day is recommended during the daytime when calories are being consumed in order to promote anabolism and avoid the risk of the absorbed amino acids being used for energy production. Earlier reports noted a tendency to acidosis with this type of dialysate, which would negate any beneficial effect. Close observation of the plasma bicarbonate is necessary, with correction as required.

Though it seems eminently desirable to improve nutrition, currently no conclusive data confirm that this actually improves patient outcome.

Lipids

The use of glucose-based hyperosmolar solutions for PD results in a significant increase in the glucose load experienced by the patient. A number of reports have measured the daily glucose absorption, which is estimated to be 100 and 200 g/d, producing 400–800 kcal. The resultant metabolic effect is a persistent tendency for patients on CAPD to develop obesity, hyperglycemia, and hyperinsulinemia; they may even develop frank diabetes. This glucose load is also thought to contribute to be atherogenic. Serum triglycerides and cholesterol increase during the first year on CAPD, with increases in very-low-density and low-density lipoproteins (VLDL and LDL). The greater the degree of hyperlipidemia at the start of therapy, the worse will be the changes with time on CAPD. In addition, there is some evidence that lipoprotein (a) levels may increase with time on CAPD (although this has not been consistently confirmed). Proatherogenic lipid levels are more common in patients on CAPD than on hemodialysis. A number of studies have demonstrated the effectiveness of cholesterol-lowering agents in patients on CAPD. Hydroxymethylglutaryl (HMG) CoA reductase inhibitors (statins) are of proven efficacy in reducing total cholesterol and LDL cholesterol while increasing high-density lipoprotein (HDL) cholesterol. However the long-term effects of such intervention on cardiovascular morbidity and mortality in CAPD patients have yet to be established.

Other complications
Bone disease

Renal osteodystrophy probably occurs as frequently during PD as with hemodialysis. It has been suggested that adynamic bone disease is more common in patients on PD but the clinical significance of this finding is still not clear. The management of renal osteodystrophy during PD is the same as for any uremic patient (see Chapter 68). As noted in Chapter 80, dialysate with a variety of calcium concentrations is available and the most appropriate should be chosen for the individual.

Anemia

On average, patients on PD have higher hemoglobin levels than do patients on hemodialysis, although typically at least 60% of patients on CAPD will require epoetin. The treatment of renal anemia is discussed in Chapter 70.

REFERENCES

1. Williams JD, Craig KJ, Topley N, et al. Morphological changes in the peritoneal membrane of patients with renal disease. JASN. 2002;13:470–9.
2. Honda K, Nitta K, Horita S, et al. Morphological changes in the peritoneal vasculature of continuous ambulatory peritoneal dialysis patients with low ultrafiltration. Nephron. 1996;72:171–6.
3. Rubin J, Herrara GA, Collins D. An autopsy study of the peritoneal cavity from patients on continuous ambulatory PD. Am J Kidney Dis. 1991;17:97–102.
4. Keane WF, Bailie GR, Boeschoten E, et al. Adult peritoneal dialysis-related peritonitis treatment recommendations: 2000 update. Perit Dial Int. 2000;20:396–441.
5. Paterson AD, Bishop MC, Morgan AG, Burden RP. Removal and replacement of Tenchkoff catheter at a single operation. Lancet. 1986;I:1245–7.
6. MacLeod A, Grant A, Donaldson C, et al. Effectiveness and efficiency of methods of dialysis therapy for end-stage renal disease: systematic reviews. Health Technol Assess. 1998;2:111–20.
7. Bernardini J, Piraino B, Holley J, et al. A randomized trial of Staphylococcus aureus prophylaxis in peritoneal dialysis patients: mupirocin calcium ointment 2% applied to the exit site versus cyclic oral rifampin. Am J Kidney Dis. 1996;27:695–670.
8. Luzar MA. Exit site infection in continuous ambulatory peritoneal dialysis: a review. Perit Dial Int. 1991;11:333–40.

9. Gokal R, Alexander S, Ash S, et al. Peritoneal catheter and exit site practices. Towards optimum peritoneal access. 1998 update. Perit Dial Int. 1998;18:11–33.

10. Khanna R, Twardowski ZJ. Recommendations for treatment of exit-site pathology. Perit Dial Int. 1996;16 (suppl 3):S100–4.

11. The Mupirocin Study Group. A controlled trial of nasal mupirocin in the prevention of exit site infections due to S. aureus during CAPD. J Am Soc Nephrol. 1996;7:2403–8.

12. Holley JL, Foulks CJ, Moss AH, Willard D. Ultrasound as a tool in the diagnosis and management of exit site infections in patients undergoing continuous ambulatory peritoneal dialysis. Am J Kidney Dis. 1989;14:212.

13. Heimbürger O, Waniewski J, Werynski A, et al. Peritoneal transport in CAPD patients with permanent loss of ultrafiltration capacity. Kidney Int. 1990;38:495–506.

14. Alvaro F de, Castro MJ, Dapena F, et al. Peritoneal resting is beneficial in peritoneal hyperpermeability and ultrafiltration failure. Adv Perit Dial. 1993;9:56–61.

15. Gokal R, Mistry CD, Peers E, et al. A United Kingdom Multicentre study of icodextrin in continuous ambulatory PD. Perit Dial Int. 1994;14 (suppl 2):S22–7.

16. Pannekeet MMH, Krediet RT. Water channels in the peritoneum. Perit Dial Int. 1996;16:255–9.

17. Ho-dac-Pannekeet MM. Struijk DG, Krediet RT. Improvement of transcellular water transport by treatment with glucose free dialysate in patients with ultrafiltration failure. Nephrol Dial Transplant. 1996;6:A255.

18. Bargman JM. Non infectious complications of PD. In: Gokal R, Nolph KD, eds. Textbook of peritoneal dialysis. Dordrecht, Netherlands: Kluwer; 1994:555–590.

19. Mactier RA, Sprosen TS, Gokal R, et al. Bicarbonate and bicarbonate/lactate peritoneal dialysis solutions for the treatment of infusion pain. Kidney Int. 1998;53:1061–7.

20. Young GA, Kopple JD, Lindholm B, et al. Nutritional assessment of continuous ambulatory PD patients: an international study. Am J Kidney Dis. 1991;17:462–70.

21. Stein A, Moorhouse J, Iles-Smith H, et al. Role of an improvement in acid–base status and nutrition in CAPD patients. Kidney Int. 1997;52:1089–95.

22. Kopple JD, Bernard D, Messana J, et al. Treatment of malnourished CAPD patients with an amino acid based dialysate. Kidney Int. 1995;47:1148–57.

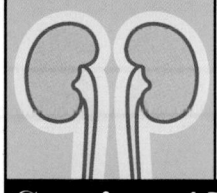

Chapter 82

Other Dialysis Modalities

Mark R Marshall and Thomas A Golper

CONTINUOUS RENAL REPLACEMENT THERAPY

Introduction

Continuous renal replacement therapy (CRRT) involves the application of lower solute clearances and ultrafiltration rates (UFR) for substantial periods of every day. Solute removal is achieved using dialysis (diffusion), filtration (convection) or a combination. Kramer initially promoted CRRT for hypotensive patients[1], and Paganini convincingly demonstrated its efficacy in 1984 in patients hemodynamically intolerant to a regimen of conventional bicarbonate buffered intermittent hemodialysis (IHD)[2].

CRRT is used to complement or supplant IHD in critically ill patients with acute renal failure (ARF). IHD is relatively inexpensive, and provides high solute clearances over brief treatment times allowing convenient access to the patient for various procedures. However, the relatively high UFR may lead to hemodynamic instability. The delivered dose of dialysis also tends to be low which may affect patient outcome. Solute control is episodic and subsequent water shifts may increase brain edema and intracranial pressure.

CRRT provides better stability due to lower UFR and better steady-state control of azotemia even in severely catabolic patients. An additional advantage may be the more effective removal of immunomodulatory substances, such as endotoxin and cytokines[3]. However, interruptions to CRRT because of circuit clotting or out-of-unit procedures lead to a reduction in dialysis dose from 'down-time', as well as expense related to blood circuitry changes. Mean operating time for CRRT has been reported at 21.9 h/d[4].

Techniques of continuous renal replacement therapy

CRRT is categorized by standardized nomenclature according to vascular access and mechanisms of solute removal.

Vascular access

Arteriovenous (AV) denotes an extracorporeal circuit in which an arterial catheter allows blood to circulate by systemic blood pressure. A venous catheter is placed for return. AV circuits are simple, but involve arterial puncture that can lead to distal embolization, hemorrhage and vessel damage. Blood flow can be erratic predisposing to clotting. VV (venovenous) denotes a dual lumen catheter placed in a central vein, achieving reliable rapid circulation of blood by a mechanical pump.

Mechanisms of solute removal

Hemodialysis

Diffusive transport favors the removal of solutes < 300 Da. During CRRT, small solute clearance can be defined by the degree to which dialysate is saturated with urea (expressed as the ratio of dialysate to blood urea nitrogen, or DUN/BUN). Blood and dialysate flow rates (Qb, Qd) during CRRT are usually relatively low (100–200 mL/min, 1–2 L/h, respectively). Under these conditions, DUN/BUN is 1.0 indicating complete saturation. Urea clearance is therefore equal to Qd, and unaffected by Qb, until it falls to below 50 mL/min[5].

With increasing Qd, there are proportionally decreasing gains in urea clearance as the DUN/BUN progressively falls. Figure 82.1 illustrates this principle, and the flattening of the curves describe the conditions where increases in Qb do not

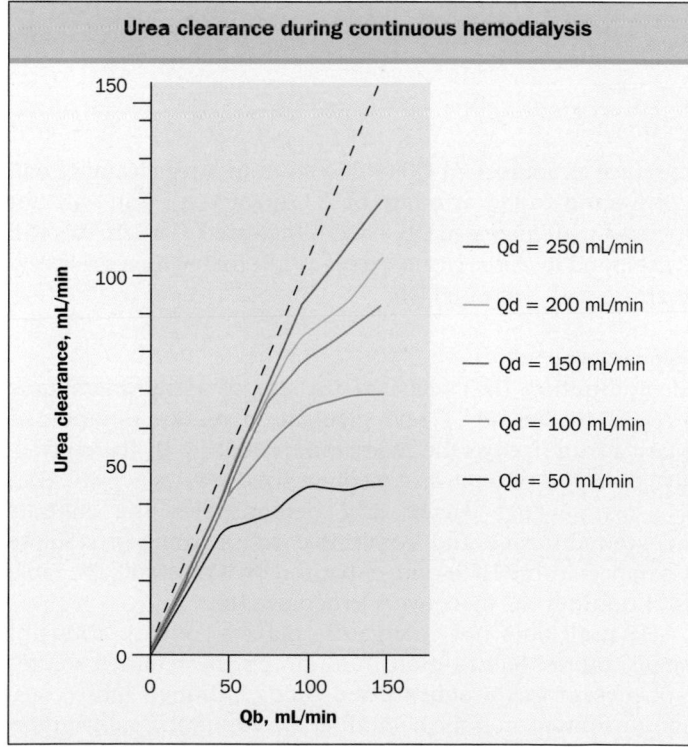

Figure 82.1 Determinants of urea clearance during continuous hemodialysis. Relationship among urea clearance, Qb, and Qd during continuous hemodialysis. The flattening of the urea clearance curves describe the conditions in which increases in Qb do not enhance clearance. (Reproduced with permission from Kudoh and Iimura[6].)

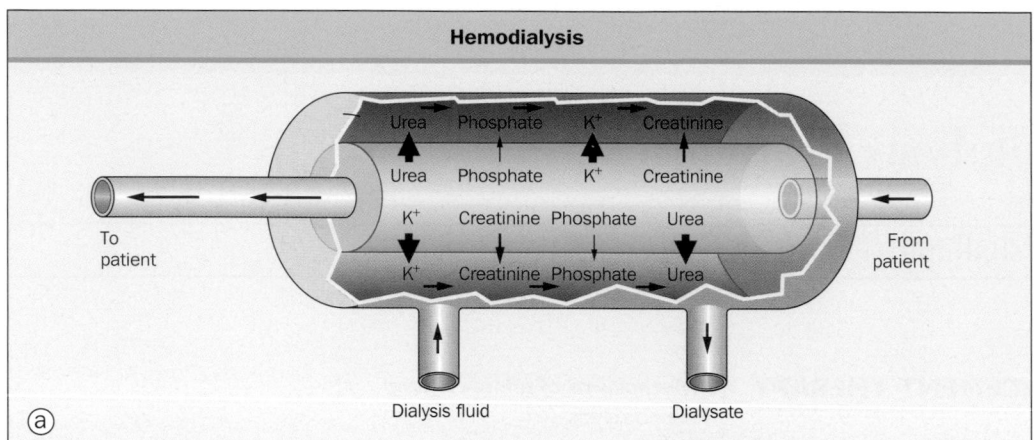

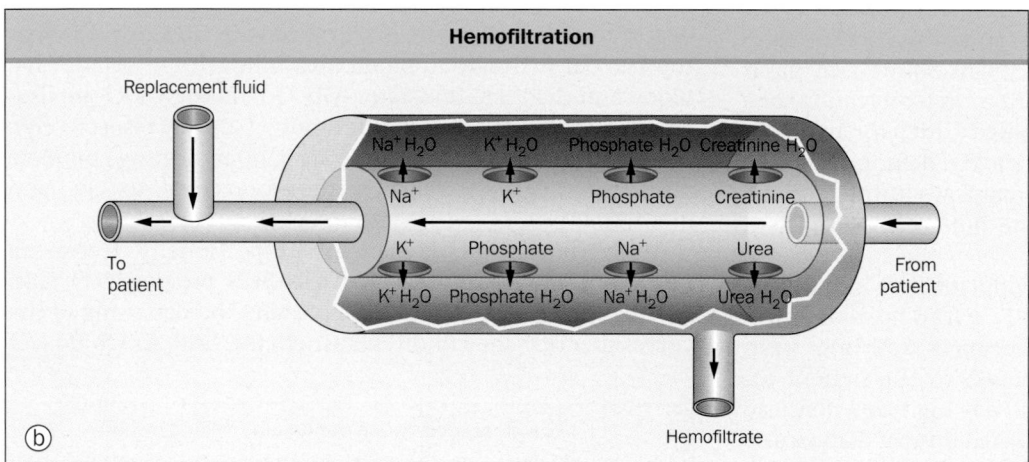

Figure 82.2 Comparison of fluid and solute movements across the membrane in hemodialysis and hemofiltration. (a) Demonstrates this movement in hemodialysis, and (b) in hemofiltration. The arrows that cross the membrane indicate the predominant direction of movement of each solute through the membrane; the relative size of the arrows indicates the net amounts of the solute transferred. Other arrows indicate the direction of flow. (Reproduced with permission from Forni and Hilton[7]).

enhance clearance[6]. At Qb of 200 mL/min, urea clearance will correspond to Qd at a rate of 2 L/h (or less), and will not increase with increased Qb. If Qd is increased to 4 L/h, this will correspond to a urea clearance of ~ 3 L/h that will progressively increase with increased Qb.

Hemofiltration

Hemofiltration (HF) refers to the use of a transmembrane hydrostatic pressure (TMP) gradient to induce filtration of plasma water across the membrane, resulting in the convective transport of small and medium sized solutes (< 5–10 kDa) by solvent drag. Figure 82.2 demonstrates the contrast between diffusive and convective solute transport. Solute clearance during HF is only enhanced by increased UFR. Table 82.1 outlines the maneuvers to achieve this.

HF itself does not change the plasma concentrations of small solutes. Substitution fluid dilutes the retained solutes not present in the substitution fluid. Although more commonly infused after the hemofilter (postdilution), substitution fluid can also be infused before the hemofilter (predilution), which increases net filtrate output by around 25% and lowers prefilter plasma concentrations of urea, hemoglobin and clotting factors. This enhances urea diffusion from within erythrocytes into the plasma increasing urea clearance by up to 15%. Filter patency may also be improved and anticoagulant

Increasing solute clearance in hemofiltration
Increase transmembrane pressure
Suction on filtrate side
Predilution fluid replacement
Increase filter hydraulic permeability
Increase filter surface area
Increase blood flow
Add diffusion dialysis to convective ultrafiltration (hemodiafiltration, HDF)

Table 82.1 Maneuvers to increase urea clearance by hemofiltration in acute renal failure.

requirements decreased. The prime disadvantage of the predilution mode is the cost of increased fluid replacement.

Hemodiafiltration

Hemodiafiltration (HDF) refers to a combination of dialysis and filtration. Solute is removed primarily by diffusion, but 25% or more may be removed by convection.

Specific techniques

The CRRT techniques described here are shown in Table 82.2 and Figure 82.3.

Comparison of continuous renal replacement modalities

Modality	Blood pump	Dialysate (D) Replacement fluid (RF)	Urea clearance (L/day)	Urea clearance (mL/min)	Middle molecular clearance	Complexity[a]
Slow continuous ultrafiltration (SCUF)	Yes/no	No	1–4	1–3	+	+
Continuous arteriovenous hemofiltration (CAVH)	No	RF	10–15	7–10	++	+
Continuous venovenous hemofiltration (CVVH)	Yes	RF	22–24	15–17	+++	++
Continuous arteriovenous hemodialysis (CAVHD)	No	D	24–30	17–21	–	+
Continuous venovenous hemodialysis (CVVHD)	Yes	D	24–30	17–21	–	++
Continuous arteriovenous hemodiafiltration (CAVHDF)	No	RF + D	36–38	25–26	+++	+++
Continuous venovenous hemodiafiltration (CVVHDF)	Yes	RF + D	36–38	25–26	+++	+++

[a]Complexity: +, most simple; +++, most complex.

Table 82.2 Comparison of different continuous renal replacement modalities. (Modified with permission from Manns et al.[8].)

Continuous renal replacement therapies

	Slow continuous ultrafiltration	Continuous hemofiltration	Continuous hemodialysis	Continuous hemodiafiltration
	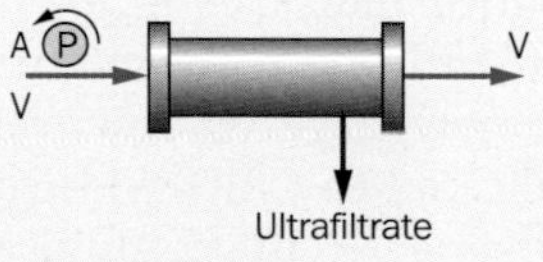	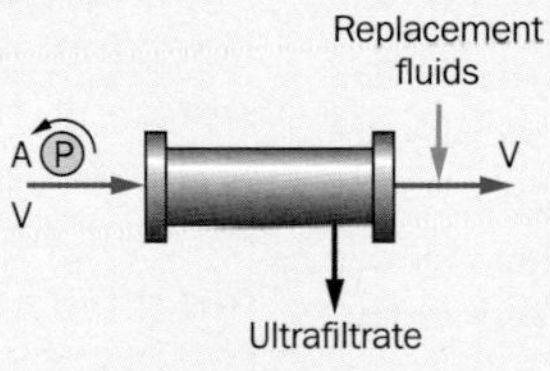	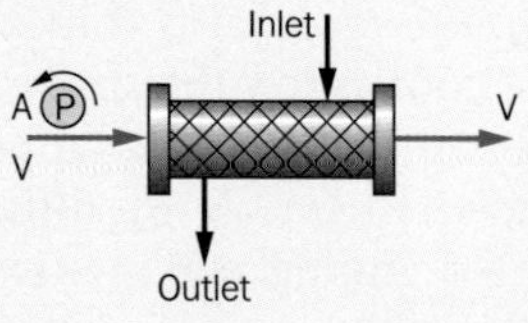	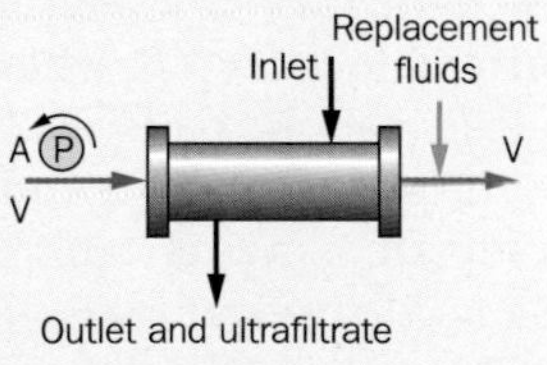
Arteriovenous (AV) or venovenous (VV)	AV or VV	AV or VV	AV or VV	AV or VV
Blood flow (mL/min)	50–100	50–200	50–200	50–200
Dialysate flow (mL/min)	–	–	10–20	10–20
Clearance (L/24 h)	–	12–36	14–36	20–40
Ultrafiltration rate (mL/min)	2–5	8–25	2–4	8–12
Blood filter	Highly permeable filter	Highly permeable filter	Low-permeability dialyzer with countercurrent flow through the dialyzer compartment	High permeability dialyzer with countercurrent flow through the dialyzer compartment
Ultrafiltrate	Corresponds exactly to the patient's weight loss	Replaced in part or completely to achieve purification and volume control	Corresponds to patient's weight loss; solute clearance by diffusion	In excess of patient's weight loss; solute clearance by both diffusion and convection
Replacement fluid	None	Yes	None	Yes, to achieve fluid balance
Efficiency	Used only for fluid control in overhydrated states	Clearance for all solutes equals ultrafiltration	Limited to small molecules	Extends from small to large molecules

Figure 82.3 Continuous renal replacement therapy modalities. The pump P is used only in venovenous modes. (Modified from Ronco[9] with permission.)

Dialysis

Slow continuous ultrafiltration

Slow continuous ultrafiltration (SCUF) is a dehydrating procedure providing slow fluid removal by filtration. Convective solute clearance is equal to the ultra filtration rate (UFR) (generally 4–5 mL/min). In patients who are uremic or hyperkalemic, this minimal solute removal must be supplemented with either intermittent or continuous hemodialysis.

Continuous arteriovenous hemofiltration

Continuous arteriovenous hemofiltration (CAVH) is similar to SCUF except that UFR is greater than required for the restoration of euvolemia, and substitution fluid is required to prevent hypovolemia. As with any HF procedure, the aim is to keep the filtration fraction at 10 to 20%. At 40% and above, sludging occurs in the hemofilter, predisposing to clotting. Solute clearance is directly related to UFR, which tends to be lower in CAVH than other CRRT techniques as a result of erratic and generally low Qb. In one series, survival of 29% vs 12% was reported for equivalent groups of patients treated with CVVH and CAVH respectively, probably as a result of differing UFR (16 L/d with CVVH vs 7 L/d with CAVH)[10]. This survival difference disappeared when UFR and urea clearance were not different on CAVH compared with CVVH[11].

Continuous venovenous hemofiltration

Continuous venovenous hemofiltration (CVVH) is similar to CAVH except that VV access requires a blood pump. This provides a relatively higher Qb (usually ~ 250 mL/min) allowing for a higher UFR and urea clearance. CVVH is therefore preferable to CAVH when solute removal is important, as in hypercatabolic patients. The contention that increased blood purification might correlate with survival is supported by a study of patients randomized to CVVH at different UFR. Reduced survival was reported among patients treated with UFR less than 35 mL/h per kg[12].

Continuous arteriovenous hemodialysis

Continuous arteriovenous hemodialysis (CAVHD) differs from CAVH in that solute removal is dependent on dialysate flowing through the hemodialyzer in a compartment separated from the blood by the dialysis membrane. Unlike CAVH, UFR is not maximized, but set as required to restore euvolemia. Thus, fluid removal with CAVHD is slower than with CAVH alone, but greater solute clearance is achieved.

Continuous venovenous hemodialysis

Continuous venovenous hemodialysis (CVVHD) is similar to CAVHD except that VV access is used. A prospective study of comparing CVVHD with CAVHD found no difference in urea clearance (37 L/d vs 33 L/d) or in survival (52% vs 43%)[11].

Continuous arteriovenous hemodiafiltration

Continuous arteriovenous hemodiafiltration (CAVHDF) is similar to CAVHD, except that UFR is greater than required for the restoration of euvolemia, and substitution fluid is infused to prevent volume depletion. CAVHDF combines diffusion, which favors small solutes removal, with convection, which removes both small and medium sized solutes.

Continuous venovenous hemodiafiltration

Continuous venovenous hemodiafiltration (CVVHDF) is similar to CAVHDF except that VV access and blood pump are utilized.

Choice of continuous renal replacement therapy technique

The choice of CRRT technique is dependent on equipment availability, clinician expertise, prospects for vascular access, and whether the primary need is for fluid and/or solute removal. This last factor is often the most important, since each technique provides different rates of solute and fluid removal (see Table 82.3). The substantially enhanced clearance capabilities of CAVHD/CAVHDF or CVVHD/CVVHDF allow these techniques to be applied to hypercatabolic or intoxicated patients. Most clinicians prefer pumped VV circuits because of reliable Qb and low vascular complications rates. CRRT is increasingly routine in the management of ARF in the intensive care unit (ICU), with suitably trained ICU nursing staff managing the therapy and dialysis staff providing back-up when required. Continuous therapies are generally well tolerated with a low rate of complications. The potential complications are listed in Table 82.4[14].

Technical considerations

Equipment

Venovenous CRRT requires a blood pump, a hemofilter or hemodialyzer, arterial and venous pressure monitors, an air detection system, a method for removing air bubbles, and a system to balance dialysate inflow/substitution fluid with dialysate outflow/filtrate. Most major manufacturers of dialysis equipment now have commercially available integrated machinery dedicated to CRRT with computerized volumetric balancing allowing accurate fluid removal (reviewed by

Choice of renal replacement technique in acute renal failure		
Primary therapeutic goal	Clinical condition	Options for renal replacement therapy
Solute removal	Stable, catabolic	IHD
	Unstable, catabolic	CAVH, CVVH, CVVHD, SCUF + IHD
	Unstable, noncatabolic	CAVH, CVVH, SCUF + IHD, CEPD
Fluid removal	Stable	IIUF
	Unstable	IIUF, SCUF
Solute and fluid removal	Stable	IHD
	Unstable	CAVHD, CVVH, CVVHD, CAVH + IHD, IIUF + IHD
Blood detoxification	Unstable	CVVH, CVVHD, ?plasma exchange

[a]CEPD, continuous equilibrium pentoneal dialysis; IIUF, intermittent isolated ultrafiltration; see text for other definition or abbreviations for modalities.

Table 82.3 Choice of renal replacement technique in acute renal failure. (With permission from Golper[3].)

Complications of continuous replacement therapy
Technical complications
Vascular access malfunction
Blood flow reduction and circuit clotting
Line disconnection
Air embolism
Fluid and electrolyte balance errors
Loss of filter efficiency
Clinical complications
Bleeding
Thrombosis
Infection and sepsis
Biocompatibility and allergic reactions
Hypothermia
Nutrient losses
Inadequate blood purification

Table 82.4 Complications of continuous renal replacement therapy. (Reproduced with permission from Ronco and Bellomo[14].)

Ronco[15]). Continuing technical innovations are aimed at simplifying treatment delivery, and improving reliability and safety of equipment.

Vascular access catheters

Temporary dialysis catheters can be inserted into the internal jugular, subclavian, or femoral veins. These catheters easily allow a Qb of 250 mL/min. CRRT provides sufficient solute removal that the 20% recirculation rate in such catheters does not compromise overall solute control.

Extracorporeal blood pumps

Many different pumps can be used for CRRT. These pumps require alarms on both the arterial and venous lines and an air detection system. An additional roller pump can be utilized to regulate UFR. This second pump can also be used for dialysate in continuous HD or infusate in continuous HF.

Hemofilters

The artificial kidneys used for CAVH or CVVH are usually referred to as hemofilters although this label is more accurately applied to specific devices with properties that maximize convective transport by a high intrinsic ultrafiltration coefficient. The sieving coefficients of small solutes are preserved throughout the life of such hemofilters. Conventional inexpensive hemodialyzers can serve as hemofilters by occluding one of the dialysate ports and connecting the other to a filtrate line drainage system. To achieve adequate UFR, the surface area must be large (~ 2 m²) for low-flux or alternatively more modest (~ 0.5 m²) for high-flux hemodialyzers. Some CRRT machines however, require the use of a specific hemofilter because of the unique cartridge module requirement of the machine (e.g., Prisma – Gambro/Hospal).

CAVH and CVVH can be undertaken using most commercially available hemodialyzers and hemofilters. For CAVHD and CVVHD, hemodialyzers comprised of polysulfone, PAN or AN69 are preferred due to the relatively poorer diffusive transport characteristics of those comprised of polyamide[16]. Biocompatible membranes are favored due to observations suggesting a survival advantage and more rapid renal recovery in patients with ARF.

Anticoagulation

Anticoagulation during CRRT ideally should prevent clotting in the extracorporeal circuit without producing significant systemic anticoagulation. A heparin–saline mixture of 5 U/mL can be infused into the most proximal port of the extracorporeal circuit. The activated partial thromboplastin time (APTT) in the venous return limb is kept at 1.5 to 2 times the control value and the systemic APTT below 50 s. This typically requires an initial bolus dose of up to 2000 units and maintenance infusion of 300–400 U/h. The heparin–saline mixture should be concentrated or diluted as necessary to keep the infusion rate between 100 and 200 mL/h, allowing thorough mixing with inflowing blood and acting as a form of predilution fluid replacement. If the extracorporeal circuit clots more frequently than every 12 h, more aggressive anticoagulation is indicated.

Low molecular weight heparin is theoretically advantageous because of increased antithrombotic activity and decreased hemorrhagic risk. However disadvantages include a prolonged half-life (approximately doubled when GFR < 5 mL/min), incomplete reversal with protamine, and limited availability of appropriate monitoring by serial anti-factor Xa determinations.

For those receiving systemic anticoagulation with heparin, the incidence of significant bleeding complications is between 25–30%, and 4% of such patients die as a result of hemorrhage[8]. A minority of patients (~10%) can successfully avoid any anticoagulation during CRRT, such as those with a coagulopathy. Alternatives to systemic anticoagulation include regional citrate calcium chelation with calcium reversal, or regional heparin anticoagulation with protamine reversal. For CVVHD, a prefilter infusion of 4% trisodium citrate (3 to 7% of Qb), with a postfilter infusion of calcium chloride may be used. This requires dialysate that is hyponatremic (117 mmol/L) and devoid of alkali[17]. For CVVH, a prefilter infusion of substitution fluid can be used that is calcium free and contains citrate (40 mmol/L) instead of lactate or bicarbonate. The lowest rates of hemorrhage and greatest prolongation of filter life are associated with regional citrate anticoagulation. Regional heparin anticoagulation results in modest prolongation of filter life, but has not yet been shown conclusively to decrease hemorrhagic complications. A further alternative is prostacyclin (epoprostenol), a potent inhibitor of platelet aggregation. Prostacyclin is vasodilatory, however, causing a variable but occasionally marked decrease in blood pressure. Regional techniques are suitable for patients with bleeding diatheses or at major risk for hemorrhage, or alternatively those with very low levels of antithrombin III and heparin cofactor II who may be prone to premature clotting with the usual heparin regimens.

Substitution fluids

One frequently employed substitution fluid regimen consists of a blended mixture of 1 L of each of four different solutions:

- isotonic saline (0.9% NaCl) plus 7.5 mL 10% calcium chloride (5.2 mmol calcium)
- isotonic saline plus 1.6 mL 50% magnesium sulfate (3.2 mmol magnesium)
- half-isotonic saline
- half-isotonic saline plus 150 mmol sodium bicarbonate.

The four solutions are kept separately until allowed to mix via a multiprong adapter just before entering the blood pathway. Alternatively, commercial substitution fluids are available (Table 82.5).

A preprinted flowsheet documents all fluids given and removed, on an hourly basis, and improves the organization of fluid balance and accounting. The rate of fluid replacement is determined by a formula comparing the net balance in the previous hour (all output, including the ultrafiltrate, minus all input) to the desired net fluid loss. The formula excludes fluids or blood products specifically given for hypotension. If, for example, output was 2000 mL, input was 500 mL, and the desired net loss was 200 mL, then 1300 mL is given as replacement fluid in the next hour. It is also important periodically to ensure the filtration fraction (UFR divided by plasma flow rate) is between 10 and 20% so as to minimize filter clotting.

Recent technical innovations

High volume hemofiltration (HVHF)

HVHF has been safely used in experimental animal models and patients with septic shock. Humoral inflammatory cytokine systems in this setting produce a variety of middle to large molecules with cardiodepressant, vasodilatory, or immunomodulatory properties. Experimental and clinical studies confirm that HVHF removes a range of cytokines by a combination of convection and adsorption[18], but it remains unclear whether this strategy improves patient outcomes. There are some data demonstrating better preservation of cardiovascular function with HVHF, but this has not been corroborated in controlled studies.

Sustained low-efficiency dialysis or extended daily dialysis

Experience is increasing with hybrid therapies that utilize standard IHD equipment and accessories, but with lower solute clearances and UFR maintained for prolonged periods of time (Table 82.6). The systems are fully monitored and have computerized volumetric ultrafiltration control. Qd and urea clearances are higher in this form of CVVHD. This compensates for the absence of additional filtration and also allows for scheduled 'down time' without compromise in dialysis dose.

Sustained low-efficiency dialysis (SLED) or extended daily dialysis (EDD) provides a high dose of dialysis with minimal urea disequilibrium, on-line bicarbonate dialysate, excellent control of electrolytes, and good tolerance to ultrafiltration. Hemodialyzer clotting is a common complication; monitoring the degree to which dialysate is saturated with urea may enable

Replacement fluid for hemofiltration	
Component	Concentration (mmol/L)
Sodium	140
Potassium	1.0
Calcium	1.6 (6.4 mg/dL)
Magnesium	0.75 (1.8 mg/dL)
Chloride	100.7
Lactate	54
Glucose	12 (216 mg/dL)
Osmolarity	300 mOsm/L

Table 82.5 A commercial replacement fluid for hemofiltration. This fluid (Gambro HF21) is commercially available and could be used instead of the author's recommended mix (see text).

Sustained low efficiency dialysis (SLED)				
Sustained low efficiency dialysis regimens at four hospitals				
	BIMC	GND	UAMS	UCD
Hemodialysis machine	Fresenius 2008H	Fresenius Genius®	Fresenius 2008H	Fresenius 2008H
Hemodialyzer	Fresenius F40	Fresenius F60S	Fresenius F8	Toray 2.0
Duration (h)	Continuous	18	12	8
Time of day	Continuous	Nocturnal (start 2 p.m.)	Nocturnal (start 7 p.m.)	Diurnal
Frequency	Continuous	Daily	Daily/5–6 days a week	Daily/6 days a week
D_B (mL/min)	150–200	70	200	150–200
D_D (mL/min)	100	70	100	300
Dialysate	Bicarbonate	Bicarbonate	Bicarbonate	Bicarbonate

SLED regimens utilized at the following academic centers; Beth Israel Medical Center New York [BIMC]; Gemeinschaftspraxis fur Nephrologie/Dialyse, Germany [GND]; University of Arkansas for Medical Sciences [UAMS]; and University of California at Davis [UCD]. (Modified from Marshall and Golper[36] with permission of UpToDate®)

Table 82.6 Sustained low efficiency dialysis (SLED)

elective blood circuit changes and optimization of anticoagulation, prior to complete clotting. Survival in the largest reported observational series did not differ from that predicted by a variety of illness severity scores[20]. Renal replacement therapies that are the easiest to administer will be the most popular if all such outcomes are equivalent, and SLED/EDD may become the therapy of choice in this setting, as it is safe, convenient, inexpensive and effective in achieving goals for solute and fluid removal.

Outcome of continuous renal replacement therapy

The prime advantage of CRRT appears to be the increased hemodynamic stability it affords in the critically ill. Observational reports have previously suggested improved survival with CRRT, but numerous confounding variables have made definitive comparison with IHD difficult. A recent randomized controlled study did not demonstrate any differences in mortality, length of hospital stay, and recovery of renal function between groups treated with CRRT and IHD[21]. Although this study is hard to interpret because of irregularities in the randomization process, a preliminary report from the Cleveland Clinic in which patients were well matched before randomization and received equivalent dialysis dosage also showed no difference in survival or duration of ARF[22]. To resolve this question will require large studies with rigorous standardization of patient care between groups[23].

Cost

Extracorporeal circuits and artificial kidneys for CRRT are more expensive than those for IHD. In the United States, the reimbursement structure inflates the price of substitution fluid that is made *de novo* in hospital pharmacies. CRRT is therefore more expensive than IHD in the US, but this is not necessarily so elsewhere. For example, a comparison at Guys Hospital, London in the late 1990s showed no substantial difference between the estimated cost of CVVHD (£744 (US$1190) weekly) and intermittent HD (£697 (US$1152) weekly)[23].

Drug dosing in continuous renal replacement therapy

For patients undergoing CRRT, 20 L of daily filtrate correspond to a glomerular filtration rate (GFR) of 14 mL/min and the dosage of drugs should be calculated as for a patient with a GFR of 14 mL/min. Although losses of dopamine, epinephrine (adrenaline), and norepinephrine (noradrenaline) do occur, these agents are usually dosed by titration. Any drug with a low therapeutic index that can be readily measured should be measured frequently early in the course of CRRT, until a stable pattern appears. One day of CRRT is in general comparable to one IHD treatment with regard to drug removal. Details of dosing for specific drugs in those patients on CRRT are given in the Appendix to Chapter 96.

ALTERNATIVE MODALITIES FOR MAINTENANCE RENAL REPLACEMENT THERAPY

Clinical outcomes in end-stage renal disease (ESRD) are determined by removal of both small and larger solutes. The most clinically apparent uremic complication attributable to larger solutes is dialysis related β_2-microglobulin derived amyloidosis.

Alternative modalities are available that provide enhanced middle molecule clearance using convective solute transport.

Hemofiltration

HVHF has been used as maintenance renal replacement therapy. When acetate buffered IHD was widely used, HVHF offered an advantage in reducing hemodynamic instability. However, no such advantage is evident from comparisons of HVHF to bicarbonate buffered IHD[24]. Figure 82.4 describes solute clearance profiles during postdilution HVHF compared with IHD when using the same high-flux membrane with a pore radius of 4 nM[25]. Although small solute clearance is generally insufficient to achieve currently recommended adequacy targets even when enhanced by predilution, the several fold higher middle molecule clearance seems to negate any detrimental clinical consequence[26]. HVHF has largely been superseded by other modalities that combine both diffusion and convection for optimal clearance of all uremic solutes.

Hemodiafiltration

Approximately 10 000 patients worldwide are now treated with hemodiafiltration (HDF). The technique consists of hemodialysis with highly permeable membranes so that UFR is greater than required for the restoration of euvolemia, and substitution fluid is infused to prevent volume depletion. Dialysate provides diffusive small solute clearance as good as in any form of HD. The UFR can provide convective medium sized solute clearance as good as that seen during HVHF. HDF offers the highest solute flux per membrane surface area for all solutes.

Infusion can be in predilution or postdilution mode. Unlike HVHF, predilution decreases small solute removal during HDF. The gains from the increased filtration fraction are outweighed by the reduced concentration gradient for diffusion and the reduction in dialysate flow due to the larger requirement for

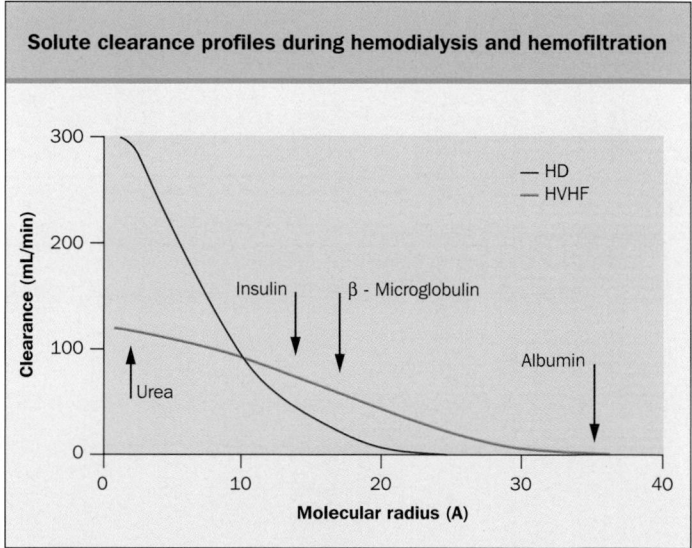

Figure 82.4 Solute clearance profiles during hemodialysis compared with postdilution HVHF. These curves were calculated as described in the text. Molecular weights of certain solutes are indicated. (Reproduced with permission from Leypoldt[25].)

substitution fluid. For these reasons, HDF is usually performed in postdilution mode, although predilution is still possible and occasionally indicated under extraordinary circumstances. Convective clearance should exceed 50 mL/min to effectively remove medium and large sized solutes. For comparison, high flux IHD clears up to 30 mL/min by internal filtration and back-transport within the hemodialyzer[27]. HDF treatments are not standardized and are prescribed to exchange anywhere between 8–60 L per treatment[28].

HDF is more expensive than IHD because of the need for hemodiafilters and substitution fluid. These increased costs are partially offset by online production of substitution fluids. Cost-per-treatment analysis has estimated this excess cost at about $US11 per session[29], although one report from a British dialysis unit showed comparable costs between online HDF and high flux IHD[30].

Online hemodiafiltration
Originally, substitution fluid for HDF was supplied in autoclaved bags, which was expensive and limiting due to the small range of fixed fluid compositions available. Online production of substitution fluids was introduced in 1985, and has made HDF convenient and affordable by using sterile dialysate as substitution fluid. Dialysate is passed through a series of ultrafilters that remove bacteria and endotoxin by virtue of a pore size of 0.22 μm and specific adsorptive properties. A fraction of this sterile dialysate is then redirected to become substitution fluid and infused directly into the blood lines. Ultrapurity of online substitution fluids prepared in this manner is at least equivalent to commercially available prepacked fluids[27].

Water quality
Online HDF requires ultrapure dialysate. This is defined by a resistivity in the range 0.1–0.5 MΩ/cm, and very low levels of bacterial and endotoxin contamination (< 100 c.f.u./L and < 0.03 EU/L of endotoxin with *Limulus* amoebocyte lysate assay). Ultrapure water, is generated by one or two stage reverse osmosis in series in addition to the usual softeners and charcoal filters. It should be distributed using a loop that is well maintained and designed to prevent stagnation and recontamination[29]. Water that meets the prevailing standard for IHD (AAMI, European Pharmacopoeia) can also be used for HDF, providing there is satisfactory dialysate purification within the machine[27].

Hemodiafiltration machines
Safety demands specifically designed HDF machines, which have a different dialysate flow path from conventional IHD machines (Fig. 82.5). Fresh dialysate is generated at

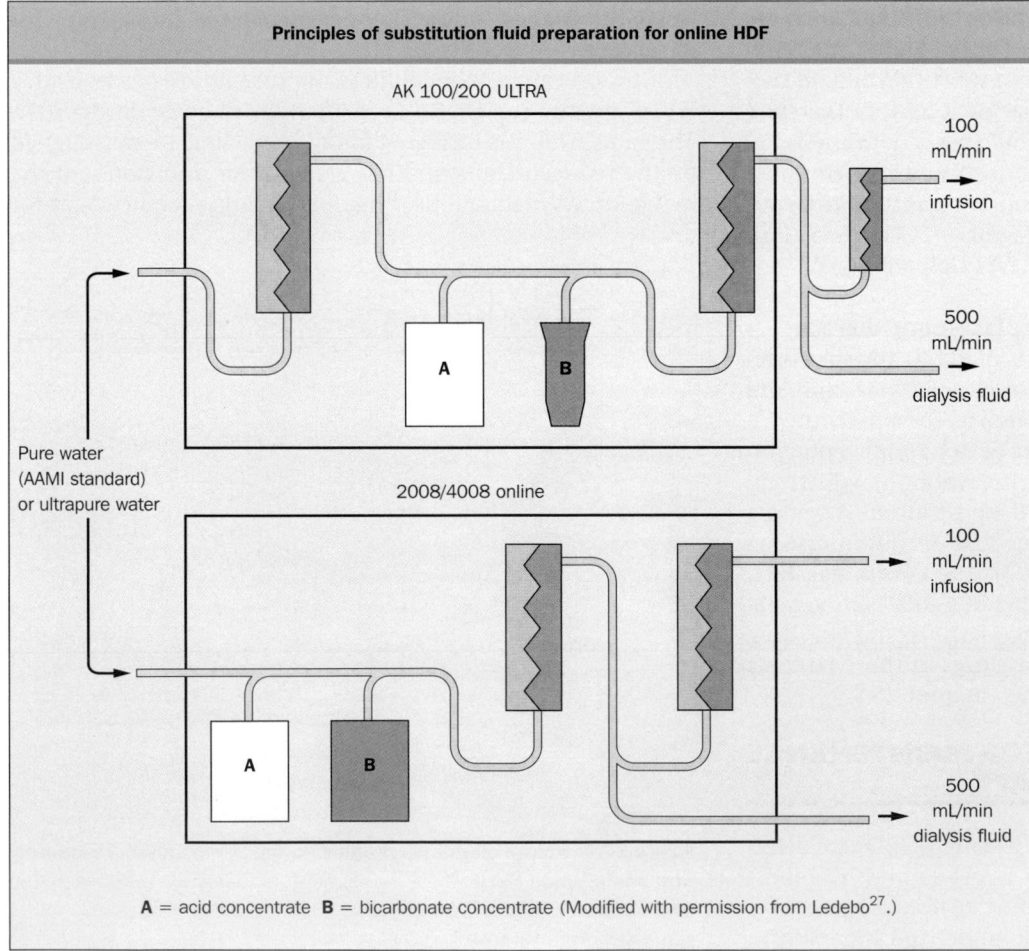

Principles of substitution fluid preparation for online HDF

AK 100/200 ULTRA

100 mL/min → infusion

500 mL/min → dialysis fluid

Pure water (AAMI standard) or ultrapure water

2008/4008 online

100 mL/min infusion

500 mL/min dialysis fluid

A = acid concentrate B = bicarbonate concentrate (Modified with permission from Ledebo[27].)

Figure 82.5 Principles of substitution fluid preparation for online HDF in two commercially available systems. A, acid concentrate; B, bicarbonate concentrate. (Modified with permission from Ledebo[27].)

600 mL/min, and 100 mL/min diverted and infused into the patient. Dialysate purification occurs by an initial ultrafilter placed immediately after the proportioning system, and a second after dialysate is diverted as substitution fluid. An additional ultrafilter is placed at the water inlet in some machines. It is recommended that the entire dialysate flow path is heat disinfected after each treatment, and filled with chemical disinfectant when not in use.

Efficacy of hemodiafiltration

HDF delivers a high dialysis dose in a short time. Reported single pool Kt/V ranges from 1.2 to 1.6. Bicarbonate-buffered infusate facilitates the correction of acidosis, and may necessitate a reduction in dialysate bicarbonate concentration to prevent postdialysis metabolic alkalosis[29]. Removal of phosphate in general is limited by the delayed intercompartmental transfer rather than dialysis efficacy, and reduction of serum phosphate is no different from that seen during conventional IHD[27]. The calcium content of the infusate contributes to the overall calcium load, although problematic hypercalcemia with HDF has not been reported. However, when calcium salts are used as phosphate binders, it may be necessary to reduce the dialysate calcium concentration.

Back-transport of bacterial derived substances into the patient's circulation from dialysate has been shown to exacerbate the systemic inflammatory response as evidenced by associated increases in levels of circulating proinflammatory cytokines and acute phase reactants, and activation of peripheral blood mononuclear cells. Ultrapure dialysate during HDF ameliorates this response. The uremic inflammatory state has been associated with excess total and cardiovascular mortality in ESRD patients, leading to speculation that the use of ultrapure dialysate might decrease the incidence of cardiovascular disease.

It has been consistently shown that serum concentrations of β_2-microglobulin ($\beta_2 M$) in patients treated by HDF are lower than in those treated with conventional IHD, and comparable to those on CAPD. This is as a result of both greater $\beta_2 M$ clearance, and reduced generation by peripheral blood mononuclear cells as a result of ultrapure dialysate.

Recently, it has also been shown that advanced glycation end-products and advanced oxidized protein products, which may be an important group of uremic toxins with molecular masses up to 15 kDa, are best cleared by HDF.

Clinical outcomes

HDF is postulated to overcome some of the short and long-term dialysis-related problems seen in patients receiving conventional IHD. HDF attributes favoring hemodynamic stability include the cooling effect of substitution fluid due to heat loss in the circuit, lower sodium removal when the substitution fluid sodium concentration is equal to the dialysate sodium concentration, the removal of endogenous vasodilatory substances, and high fluxes of calcium which may contribute to increased cardiac output and peripheral vascular resistance[29]. Hemodynamic stability is better during HDF compared to acetate buffered IHD. Although a similar advantage is reported in comparison to historical controls treated with bicarbonate buffered IHD, two prospective controlled trials have not resolved the issue arriving at diametrically opposed conclusions[31,32]. Persistent hypertension during HDF has been reported to necessitate a switch from this modality[33].

HDF allows a large dialysis dose to be achieved in a relatively short time. This is useful in achieving adequate Kt/V in larger patients. The prevalence of dialysis related amyloidosis is lower with HDF compared to conventional low flux IHD[34]. Relative protection of residual renal function is associated with increased membrane and water biocompatibility during high flux hemodialysis, and this is also postulated but not proven to be an attribute to HDF.

Clinical studies to date have not confirmed the theoretical expectation that HDF might improve cardiovascular morbidity and overall patient mortality[28,34].

Acetate-free biofiltration

Acetate-free biofiltration (AFB) is an HDF technique performed with standard IHD machinery and high-flux biocompatible hemodialyzers, base-free dialysate and a continuous postdilution infusion of a sterile isotonic bicarbonate solution. The most commonly used commercially available solution contains a bicarbonate concentration of 145 mmol/L, and is usually infused at between 8–10 L per treatment to compensate for bicarbonate lost into the dialysate. Because of the high UFR, no backfiltration occurs and risk of exposure to bacterial derived substances is low. Water quality need not be ultrapure, but should meet the prevailing standard for IHD. Other substantial technique differences between AFB and bicarbonate buffered IHD are listed in Table 82.7.

Acetate free biofiltration and bicarbonate hemodialysis		
	Acetate-free biofiltration	Bicarbonate hemodialysis
Acetate	None	Small amount of acetate (4–5 mmol) for chemical stability
Dialysate circuit	No bicarbonate	Possible precipitation of calcium salts
Sterility	Sterile bicarbonate infusion fluid and bacteriostatic dialysate concentrate	Possible bacterial and endotoxin contamination of the basic concentrate
Ultrafiltration	High ultrafiltration rate: no backfiltration; in any case dialysate is sterile	Possible backfiltration at low ultrafiltration rates
Bicarbonate balance	Personalized balance because easily predictable levels of administered and lost bicarbonate	Unpredictable because of the complex connective and diffusive bicarbonate transfer across the dialysis membrane

Table 82.7 Comparison of acetate-free biofiltration with bicarbonate hemodialysis. (Reproduced with permission from Zucchelli[35].)

Dialysis

Most studies of clinical outcomes with AFB have been uncontrolled observations over short periods. When compared to bicarbonate based IHD, AFB has been associated with less left ventricular hypertrophy[36], improved clearance of small and medium solutes, and better correction of acidosis[36]. There may be fewer undesirable intradialytic symptoms such as hypotension, muscle cramps, and vomiting, which has been attributed to the complete absence of acetate exposure during treatments[31]. Reports so far have been inconclusive with regard to the impact of AFB on patient survival, nutritional parameters, or quality of life[37].

REFERENCES

1. Kramer P, Kaufhold G, Grone HJ, et al. Management of anuric intensive-care patients with arteriovenous hemofiltration. Int J Artif Organs. 1980;3:225–30.
2. Paganini EP, O'Hara P, Nakamoto S. Slow continuous ultrafiltration in hemodialysis resistant oliguric acute renal failure patients. Trans Am Soc Artif Intern Organs. 1984;30:173–8.
3. Hoffmann JN, Hartl WH, Deppisch R, et al. Hemofiltration in human sepsis: evidence for elimination of immunomodulatory substances. Kidney Int. 1995;48:1563–70.
4. Frankenfield D, Reynolds H, Wiles C, et al. Urea removal during continuous hemodiafiltration. Crit Care Med 1993;22:407–12.
5. Sigler MH. Transport characteristics of the slow therapies: implications for achieving adequacy of dialysis in acute renal failure. Adv Ren Repl Ther. 1997;4:68–80.
6. Kudoh Y, Iimura O. Slow continuous hemodialysis – new therapy for acute renal failure in critically ill patients – Part 1. Theoretical considerations and new technique. Jpn Circ J. 1988;52:1171–82.
7. Forni LG, Hilton PJ. Continuous hemofiltration in the treatment of acute renal failure. N Eng J Med. 1997;336:1303–9.
8. Manns M, Sigler MH, Teehan BP. Continuous renal replacement therapies: an update. Am J Kidney Dis. 1998;32:185–207.
9. Ronco C. Continuous renal replacement therapies for the treatment for acute renal failure in intensive care patients. Clin Nephrol. 1993;40:187–98.
10. Storck M, Hartl WH, Zimmerer E, Inthorn D. Comparison of pump-driven and spontaneous continuous haemofiltration in postoperative acute renal failure. Lancet. 1991;337:452–5.
11. Bellomo R, Parkin G, Love J, Boyce N. A prospective comparative study of continuous arteriovenous hemodiafiltration and continuous venovenous hemodiafiltration in critically ill patients. Am J Kidney Dis. 1993;21:400–4.
12. Ronco C, Bellomo R, Homel P, et al. Effects of different doses in continuous veno-venous haemofiltration on outcomes of acute renal failure: a prospective randomised trial. Lancet. 2000; 356(9223):26–30.
13. Golper TA. Continuous renal replacement therapy in acute renal failure. In: Rose BD, ed. Up to Date, Wellesley, MA; 9.1.2001.
14. Ronco C, Bellomo R. Complications with renal replacement therapy. Am J Kidney Dis. 1996;28(suppl 3):S100–4.
15. Ronco C, Brendolan A, Dan M, et al. Machines for continuous renal replacment therapy. In: Ronco C, Bellomo R, Greca G La, eds. Blood Purification in Intensive Care. Contrib Nephrol. Basel, Switzerland: Karger; 2001:323–34.
16. Relton S, Greenberg A, Palevsky PM. Dialysate and blood flow dependence of diffusive solute clearance during CVVHD. ASAIO J. 1992;38:M691–6.
17. Mehta RL, McDonald BR, Aguilar MM, Ward DM. Regional citrate anticoagulation for continuous arteriovenous hemodialysis in critically ill patients. Kidney Int. 1990;38:976–81.
18. Vriese AS De, Colardyn FA, Philippe JJ, et al. Cytokine removal during continuous hemofiltration in septic patients. J Am Soc Nephrol. 1999;10:846–53.
19. Marshall MR, Golper TA. Sustained low efficiency or extended daily dialysis. In: Rose BD, ed. Up to date, Wellesley, MA; 9.1.2001.
20. Marshall MR, Golper TA, Shaver MJ, et al. Sustained low-efficiency dialysis for critically ill patients requiring renal replacement therapy. Kidney Int. 2001;60:777–85.
21. Mehta RL, McDonald B, Gabbai FB, et al. A randomized clinical trial of continuous versus intermittent dialysis for acute renal failure. Kidney Int. 2001;60:1154–63.
22. Sandy D, Moreno L, Lee JC, Paganini EP. A randomized, stratified, dose equivalent comparison of CVVHD and intermittent HD support in ICU acute renal failure (Abstr.). J Am Soc Nephrol. 1998; 9:225A.
23. Silvester W. Outcome studies of continuous renal replacement therapy in the intensive care unit. Kidney Int. 1998;53 (suppl 66):S138–41.
24. Maggiore Q, Pizzarelli F, Dattolo P, et al. Cardiovascular stability during haemodialysis, haemofiltration and haemodiafiltration. Nephrol Dial Transplant. 2000;15(suppl 1):68–73.
25. Leypoldt JK. Solute fluxes in different treatment modalities. Nephrol Dial Transplant. 2000;15(suppl 1):3–9.
26. Vanholder RC, Ringoir SM. Adequacy of dialysis: A critical analysis. Kidney Int. 1992;42:540–58.
27. Ledebo I. On-line hemodiafiltration: technique and therapy. Adv Ren Replace Ther. 1999;6:195–208.
28. Wizemann V, Lotz C, Techert F, Uthoff S. On-line haemodiafiltration versus low-flux haemodialysis. A prospective randomized study. Nephrol Dial Transplant. 2000;15(suppl 1):43–8.
29. Canaud B, Bosc JY, Leray H, et al. On-line haemodiafiltration: state of the art. Nephrol Dial Transplant. 1998;13(suppl 5):3–11.
30. Tattersall JE, Greenwood RN, Farrington K. Safety of on-line hemodiafiltration. Kidney Int. 1997;52:1119.28.
31. Locatelli F, Mastrangelo F, Redaelli B, et al. Effects of different membranes and dialysis technologies on patient treatment tolerance and nutritional parameters. Kidney Int. 1996;50:1293–302.
32. Movilli E, Camerini C, Zein H, et al. A prospective comparison of bicarbonate dialysis, hemodiafiltration, and acetate-free biofiltration in the elderly. Am J Kidney Dis. 1996;27:541–7.
33. Ward RA, Schmidt B, Hullin J, Hillebrand GF, Samtleben W. A comparison of on-line hemodiafiltration and high-flux hemodialysis: a prospective clinical study. J Am Soc Nephrol. 2000;11:2344–50.
34. Locatelli F, Marcelli D, Conte F, et al. Comparison of mortality in ESRD patients on convective and diffusive extracorporeal treatments. Kidney Int. 1999;55:286–93.
35. Zucchelli P. Acetate-free biofiltration. In: Maeda K, Shinato T, eds. Effective Hemodiafiltration. Basel: Karger; 1994:105–13.
36. Schrander Meer A van der, Wee PM ter, Kan G, et al. Improved cardiovascular variables during acetate free biofiltration. Clin Nephrol. 1999;51:304–9.
37. Galli G, Panzetta G. Acetate free biofiltration (AFB): from theory to clinical results. Clin Nephrol. 1998;50:28–37.

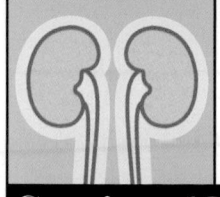

Chapter 83

Plasma Exchange

Jeremy Levy and Charles Pusey

INTRODUCTION

The place of plasma exchange (plasmapheresis) in the management of renal disease remains controversial, largely because of the paucity of controlled studies comparing plasma exchange with other treatments. The techniques for separating plasma from cells were initially developed during the 1940s and 1950s, but only put into widespread clinical use after early reports of the beneficial effects in Goodpasture's disease in the mid-1970s. More recently, plasma exchange has been used to remove many large-molecular-weight substances from plasma, including pathogenic antibodies, cryoglobulins, and lipoproteins.

TECHNIQUES

Therapeutic plasma exchange can be carried out either by centrifugal cell separators or, more commonly in renal units, with hollow fiber plasma filters and standard hemodialysis equipment (see Figs 83.1 and 83.2). Centrifugal devices allow

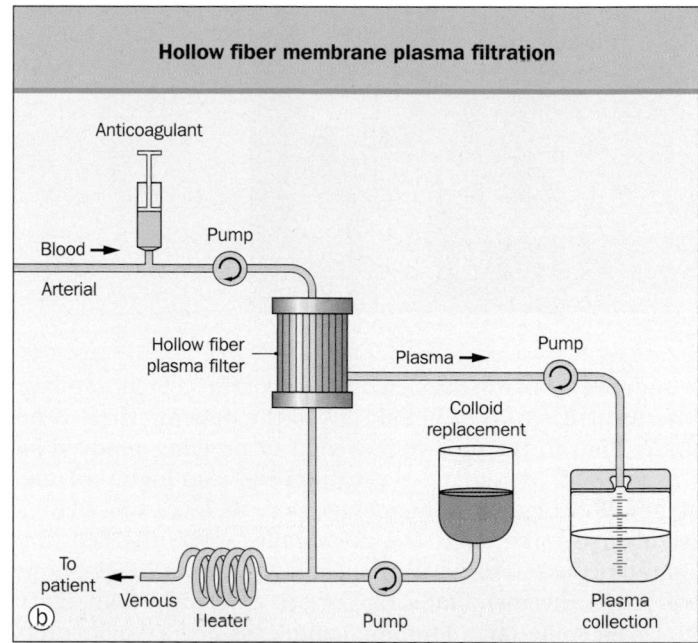

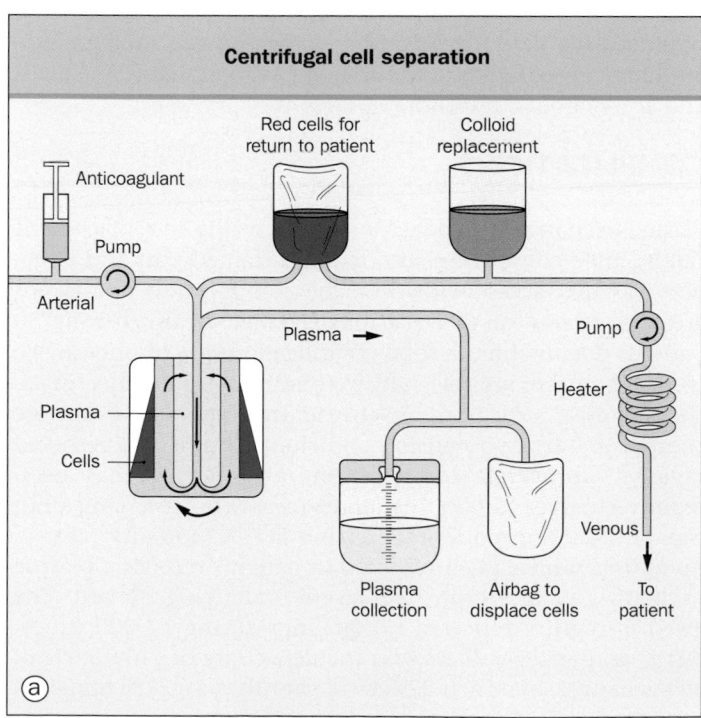

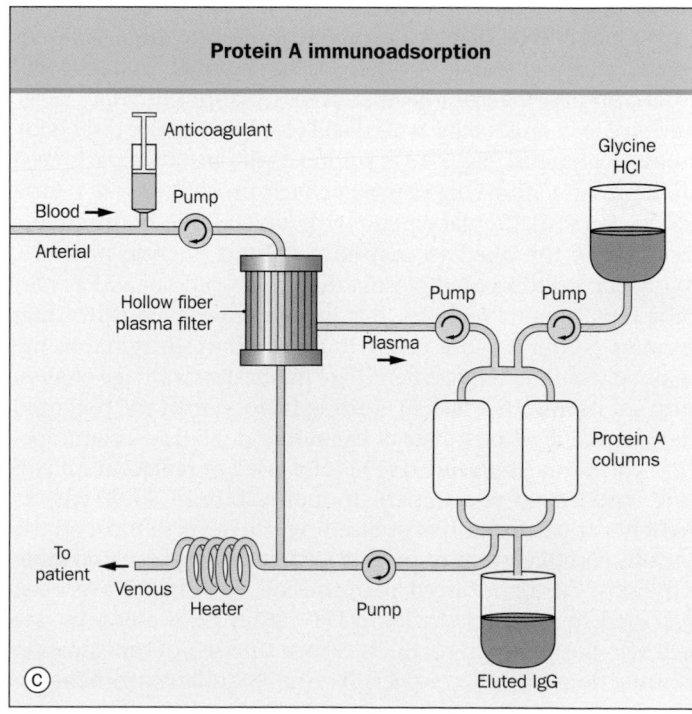

Figure 83.1 **Plasma exchange and immunoadsorption techniques.** Techniques include (a) centrifugal cell separation, (b) hollow fiber membrane plasma filtration, and (c) protein A immunoadsorption.

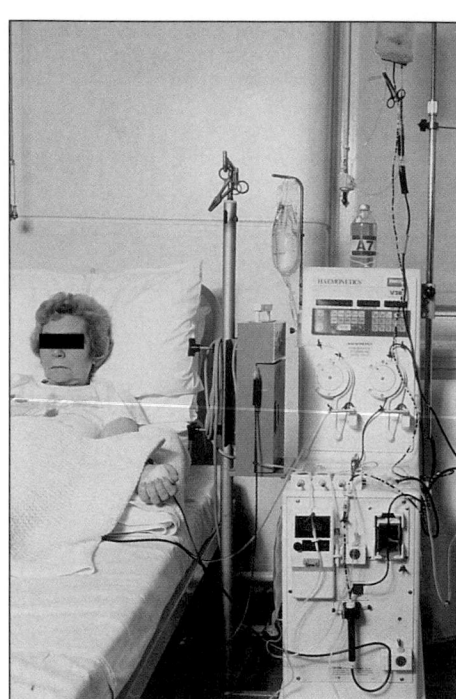

Figure 83.2 A centrifugal cell separator used for plasma exchange.

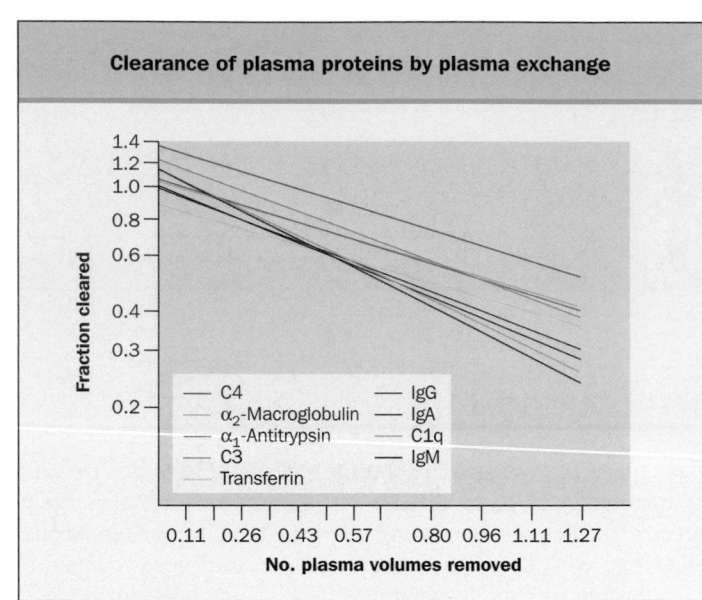

Figure 83.3 Clearance of plasma proteins by plasma exchange. Clearance from the intravascular compartment varies with the plasma volume exchanged and between individual proteins. (Adapted with permission from Derksen et al.[1].)

withdrawal of plasma from a bowl with either synchronous or intermittent return of blood cells to the patient. There is no upper limit to the molecular weight of proteins removed by this method. Membrane plasmafiltration uses highly permeable hollow fibers with membrane pores 0.2–0.5 μm. Plasma readily passes through the membrane, while the cells are simultaneously returned to the patient. All immunoglobulins will cross the membrane (IgG more efficiently than IgM); however, some large immune complexes and cryoglobulins may not be adequately cleared.

Both methods of plasma exchange require large volumes of colloid replacement. A single plasma volume exchange will lower plasma macromolecule levels by approximately 60%, and five exchanges over 5–10 d will clear 90% of the total body immunoglobulin (Fig. 83.3)[1]. For most patients, this is achieved by removing 50 mL/kg plasma at each procedure (~ 4 L for a 75 kg person). Replacement with crystalloid is untenable because of the need to maintain colloid oncotic pressure. Synthetic gelatin-based plasma expanders can be used as part of a replacement regimen but have a shorter half-life than human albumin. As a result, human albumin remains the mainstay of fluid replacement. The major disadvantage of albumin solutions is the lack of clotting factors, with the potential development of postplasma exchange depletion coagulopathy. Fresh frozen plasma (FFP) is also used as replacement colloid, usually in addition to human albumin solutions, in patients at particular risk of bleeding. However, almost all the serious complications of plasma exchange (hypotension, anaphylaxis, citrate-induced paresthesiae, urticaria) have been reported in patients receiving FFP rather than albumin (see below)[2]. Both human products carry a tiny risk of transmission of infectious diseases, especially viral. Standard regimens for plasma exchange are summarized in Table 83.1.

More recently, protein A immunoadsorption techniques have been utilized to remove immunoglobulin alone from plasma, without the need for replacement fluids and without depletion of clotting factors and complement (Fig. 83.1c). Protein A selectively binds the Fc domains of immunoglobulin molecules, and the immunoadsorption columns can be repeatedly regenerated. This technique has been used to treat Goodpasture's disease, systemic lupus, vasculitis and to remove anti-HLA antibodies in highly sensitized transplant recipients, with equal efficacy as plasma exchange. Specific ligands have also been immobilized onto columns for more specific removal of potentially pathogenic serum factors; ligands used include antihuman IgG, C1q, phenylalanine, hydrophobic amino acids and acetylcholine receptor peptides.

COMPLICATIONS

Plasma exchange is expensive (mostly owing to replacement fluids), time consuming, and requires trained staff and large-bore vascular access. However, the complication rate is not great. A review of 699 plasma-exchange treatments in 50 patients documented a total complication rate of only 9.7%, of which approximately half were minor (leg cramps, dizziness, nausea, urticaria). Seventeen treatments (7.4%) were complicated by hypotension and chest pain, which resolved rapidly. An overall complication rate of 1.4% has been reported in over 15 000 treatments in patients receiving albumin, and 20% in patients receiving FFP[2,3]. Mortality rates of up to 0.05% have been reported in patients receiving plasma exchange, all of whom had severe underlying disease. The Swedish registry reported no fatalities during 14 000 procedures, and an overall adverse incidence rate of only 5.6% of all exchanges, of which 22% were paresthesiae, 21% transient hypotension, 14% urticaria and 7% nausea[4].

Other complications directly attributable to plasma exchange include citrate-induced hypocalcemia and citrate-induced

	Antiglomerular basement membrane antibody (anti-GBM) disease	Small vessel vasculitis	Cryoglobulinemia	Recurrent focal segmental glomerulosclerosis (FSGS) after transplantation	Hemolytic uremic syndrome (adults and nondiarrheal in children) and thrombotic thrombocytopenic purpura
Indication					
Duration of treatment	Daily, at least 14 days until anti-GBM antibodies <20%	Daily, 7–10 days depending on clinical response	At least 7–10 days or until clinical response	Daily, at least 10 days initially, then continuing less frequently, often for months	Daily for 7–10 days or until platelet count > 80–100 × 10⁹/L
Exchange volume	50 mL/kg each treatment	As for anti-GBM disease	As for anti-GBM disease	As for anti-GBM disease	As for anti-GBM disease
Replacement fluid	Human albumin 5% (unless bleeding risk)	As for anti-GBM disease	As for anti-GBM disease	As for anti-GBM disease	Fresh frozen plasma (FFP) or cryo-poor FFP
Additions to replacement fluid	20 mL 10% calcium gluconate (occasionally more), 3 mL 15% KCl if not dialysis dependent, heparin 5000–10 000 units (unless citrate anticoagulation)	As for anti-GBM disease	As for anti-GBM disease	As for anti-GBM disease	As for anti-GBM disease (may need more calcium because of increased volume of FFP)
Immunosuppression	Prednisolone and cyclophosphamide	As for anti-GBM disease	Prednisolone and cyclophosphamide in type II (caution if HCV positive)	None	None
Variations	Fresh frozen plasma 5–8 mL/kg as part of exchange volume if hemorrhage risk (renal biopsy in last 48 h, lung hemorrhage, platelets < 40 × 10⁹/L (but usually withhold plasma exchange), fibrinogen < 15.5 g/L). Immunoadsorption may be as effective.	As for anti-GBM disease. Immunoadsorption may be as effective.	As for anti-GBM disease	As for anti-GBM disease. May need to include replacement immunoglobulins if continuing long term. Immunoadsorption may be as effective.	

Table 83.1 Practical regimens for plasma exchange in renal disease.

metabolic alkalosis. Citrate is usually present in the FFP or is administered in the extracorporeal circuit as an anticoagulant; it binds free calcium in plasma. Some patients experience symptomatic hypocalcemia, which can be averted by infusing 10–20 mL 10% calcium gluconate during each plasma exchange. Alkalosis is rare and is caused by metabolism of citrate to bicarbonate, and failure to excrete the latter in patients with renal impairment.

Plasma exchange predictably increases the risk of bleeding as a result of depletion of coagulation factors in patients receiving albumin as sole replacement colloid. Prothrombin time is increased by 30%, and partial thromboplastin times by 100% after a single plasma volume exchange. Patients at risk of bleeding (alveolar hemorrhage, postbiopsy, postoperative) should receive FFP (300–600 mL) with replacement fluids. Dilutional hypokalemia is avoided by adding potassium to the replacement albumin. An increased incidence of infection secondary to hypogammaglobulinemia has not been confirmed in recent series[3,4]. Sepsis related to intravenous access is the commonest infectious complication of plasma exchange.

MECHANISM OF ACTION

Plasma exchange removes large-molecular-weight substances from the plasma, including antibodies, complement components, immune complexes, endotoxin, lipoproteins and von Willebrand factor multimers. The pathogenicity of autoantibodies in anti-glomerular basement membrane (anti-GBM) disease provided the impetus for developing plasma exchange therapy but it is now clear that antibodies, although necessary, are not sufficient to cause the necrotizing glomerulonephritis in Goodpasture's disease. Therefore, plasma exchange may well have benefits in addition to simply clearance of autoantibodies. Plasma exchange has been successfully used in a number of other diseases characterized by autoantibodies, including myasthenia gravis, hemolytic anemia, Eaton–Lambert syndrome, anti-neutrophil cytoplasm antibody (ANCA)-associated systemic vasculitis, and in patients with cytotoxic anti-HLA (human leukocyte antigen) antibodies. The clearance of antibodies from patients is variable and depends on a number of factors, including the rate of equilibration of macromolecules between the intra- and extravascular compartments. IgM antibodies are cleared more effectively by centrifugal plasma exchange than other classes of immunoglobulin as they are retained in the vascular compartment almost wholly. Rebound increase in antibody production will occur unless there is concomitant immunosuppression to prevent resynthesis.

Plasma exchange has also been shown to remove immune complexes, which may have clinical significance in cryoglobulinemia and systemic lupus. Plasma exchange improves reticuloendothelial clearance of senescent red blood cells. There is no good evidence that removal of cytokines has any significance. Plasma exchange certainly reduces plasma viscosity, with consequent improved blood flow in the microvasculature.

INDICATIONS FOR PLASMA EXCHANGE

Anti-glomerular basement membrane antibody disease

Plasma exchange removes anti-GBM antibodies very effectively. Most patients can be depleted of pathogenic antibodies after seven to ten plasma volume exchanges if further antibody synthesis is inhibited by the concurrent use of cyclophosphamide and corticosteroids. Prior to the introduction of this therapy, the mortality from Goodpasture's disease was over 90%, and only 11% of patients who were not dialysis dependent at presentation survived with preserved renal function[5]. The use of plasma exchange improved the outcome considerably: 70–90% of patients now survive. However, only 50% of survivors retain independent renal function overall, and 10% (at best) of those who are dialysis dependent at presentation (see Table 83.2)[5]. There has only been one small controlled trial of plasma exchange in the treatment of Goodpasture's disease that utilized a low intensity of plasma exchange[6]. A total of 17 patients were randomized to receive steroids and cyclophosphamide, with or without plasma exchange. Only two of the eight receiving plasma exchange developed end-stage renal disease (ESRD) compared with six of the nine receiving drugs alone.

Long-term data from 71 patients with antiglomerular basement antibody disease confirmed the benefit of a treatment regimen including plasma exchange, since most patients with mild to moderate renal failure retained independent renal function over 10–25 years[7]. Patients who presented with serum creatinine less than 5.7 mg/dL (500 µmol/L) had 95% renal survival at one year and 74% at last follow-up. In patients who presented with dialysis dependent renal failure, 8% and 5% had independent renal function at one year and last follow-up. However, patients with severe renal failure (serum creatinine >5.7 mg/dL, 500 µmol/L), but not requiring immediate dialysis, had a good outcome with intensive treatment with 82% renal survival at one year and 69% at last follow-up. Combining all of the available published data for patients with Goodpasture's disease, 74% of patients presenting with serum creatinine < 5.7–6.6 mg/dL (500–600 µmol/L) will retain renal function, in contrast to 11% of those presenting dependent on dialysis (Table 83.2).

Recommendation: All patients presenting predialysis should receive intensive plasma exchange with daily 4 L exchanges initially for 14 d, using 4.5% albumin solution (supplemented with calcium) as replacement fluid. Fresh plasma (300–600 mL) is added for patients actively bleeding, or those who have had recent surgery or biopsy. We reserve aggressive treatment in dialysis-dependent patients for those with biopsy or clinical evidence of recent onset disease. Pulmonary hemorrhage is an independent indication for plasma exchange.

Small vessel vasculitis

The majority of patients with rapidly progressive glomerulonephritis (RPGN), other than anti-GBM disease, have small vessel vasculitis with ANCA detectable in their serum, and there is increasing evidence that these autoantibodies are

Summation of available observational and randomised controlled trials		
A: Anti-GBM disease	Scr<6.6 mg/dL at presentation	SCr>6.6 mg/dL at presentation
Independent renal function at 1 year	81/116	16/149
Number receiving plasma exchange	86	109
B: RPGN – nonanti-GBM disease	Successfully treated with plasma exchange	Successfully treated with oral or intravenous drugs alone
Nonrandomized studies	79/108	79/132
Randomized controlled trials	31/42	8/25

Table 83.2 Summation of available patient outcome in observational and randomized controlled trials in rapidly progressive glomerulonephritis. Studies in anti-GBM disease are summarized in reference[7].

pathogenic. Plasma exchange was initially introduced in such patients because of the similarity of the histologic changes to those seen in Goodpasture's disease, and the supposition that immune complexes may be instrumental in disease pathogenesis. Six controlled trials of plasma exchange in nonanti-GBM RPGN have been reported (Table 83.2)[8–13].

Glockner et al. could not demonstrate additional benefit of twice weekly plasma exchange in 14 patients with RPGN compared with 12 controls treated with oral steroids and cyclophosphamide, regardless of the degree of renal failure of the patients[8]. However, in this study the plasma-exchange protocol was of very low intensity and cyclophosphamide was only used for 1 week. Furthermore, the patients were a heterogeneous group including those with lupus, polyarteritis nodosa, and scleroderma as well as small vessel vasculitis; in addition, those with oliguria were excluded.

Pusey et al. conducted a randomized prospective controlled trial of plasma exchange in addition to oral immunosuppression in 48 patients with small vessel vasculitis[9]. Plasma exchange was intensive (at least five exchanges in the first 7 d), but was of no benefit in patients with moderate or severe renal disease not requiring dialysis, since almost all of these patients improved. However, 10 of 11 dialysis-dependent patients receiving plasma exchange discontinued dialysis, compared with only three of eight in the control group. Patients surviving long term maintained independent renal function.

The Canadian Apheresis Study Group[10] randomized 32 patients with nonanti-GBM RPGN to receive intravenous methylprednisolone (10 mg/kg per d for 3 d) and azathioprine with or without plasma exchange (10 exchanges in the first 16 d). Once again there was no significant benefit of additional plasma exchange in patients who were not dependent on dialysis; however, a nonsignificant trend in benefit was apparent in dialysis-dependent patients.

Guillevan et al. conducted two trials in patients with polyarteritis nodosa, microscopic polyangiitis and Churg Strauss syndrome in which patients received methylprednisolone, prednisolone and cyclophosphamide with or without plasma

Renal conditions for which plasma exchange may be indicated			
Conditions for which plasma exchange has an established role		**Conditions for which plasma exchange may be useful**	
Condition	Comment	Condition	Comment
Antiglomerular basement membrane antibody disease	Especially nonoliguric renal failure predialysis and for pulmonary hemorrhage	Nephrotic proteinuria post-transplantation caused by recurrent focal segmental glomerulosclerosis (FSGS)	Transient reduction in proteinuria in most patients. 50% achieve long-term remission.
Antineutrophil cytoplasmic antibody (ANCA) associated vasculitis	Only for patients with dialysis dependent renal failure and/or pulmonary hemorrhage	Acute vascular allograft rejection	May help in patients with resistant rejection
Hemolytic uremic syndrome (HUS) in adults or nondiarrheal HUS in children	Plasma exchange or infusion both may be beneficial although exchange allows greater volume of plasma to be infused. Full exchange for plasma rather than albumin.	Highly sensitized transplant recipients	May help remove anti-HLA antibodies and allow successful transplantation
Thrombotic thrombocytopenic purpura (TTP)	Plasma exchange or infusion both beneficial although exchange allows greater volume of plasma to be infused. Full exchange for plasma rather than albumin.	Systemic lupus	May be of use in the most severe disease or cerebral lupus; no clear benefit in moderately severe renal involvement
Type I and II cryoglobulinemia	Patients improve symptomatically, vasculitic syndrome improve, variable effect on renal function, no controlled trials.	Myeloma with cast nephropathy	Conflicting reports; probably of benefit in severe acute renal impairment
		Crescentic IgA nephropathy	Possible short-term benefit
		Focal segmental glomerulosclerosis (primary FSGS)	Up to 40% remission rate of nephrotic syndrome in steroid resistant patients

Table 83.3 Renal conditions for which plasma exchange has an established role or may be useful.

exchange (60 mL/kg, 3/week for 3 or 4 weeks)[11,12]. Very few of the patients included had rapidly progressive glomerulonephritis. There was a trend to better outcome in patients receiving plasma exchange but no statistically significant difference in outcome. Most recently, Zauner et al. prospectively randomized 39 patients with nonanti-GBM crescentic nephritis to receive plasma exchange (40 mL/kg per day, for 3–12 exchanges) in addition to pulsed methylprednisolone, oral steroids and oral cyclophosphamide[13]. Six of 11 dialysis dependent patients recovered renal function but there was no difference in outcome between the two groups.

Frasca et al. reported their uncontrolled experience with plasma exchange in ANCA-associated RPGN[14]. Ten dialysis-dependent patients with Wegener's granulomatosis or microscopic polyangiitis treated with oral steroids, cyclophosphamide, defibrotide (an antithrombotic agent) and daily plasma exchange (three to ten exchanges) all recovered renal function. Levy and Winearls retrospectively examined the outcome of all patients presenting to a single unit with pauci-immune RPGN[15]. In that study, plasma exchange was of less benefit: nine of 11 dialysis-dependent patients who received plasma exchange recovered renal function compared with five of nine without such treatment. Gaskin et al. reviewed their experience in using intensive plasma exchange in addition to prednisolone and cyclophosphamide in dialysis dependent patients with ANCA associated vasculitis, and showed that 74% recovered renal function[16]. Finally, Stegmayr et al. conducted a prospective randomized controlled trial of plasma exchange or immunoadsorption in addition to conventional immunosuppression in 38 patients with RPGN[17]. They showed excellent recovery of renal function in 70% dialysis dependent patients with nonanti-GBM disease.

Plasma exchange is therefore likely to be of significant benefit in dialysis-dependent patients with pauci-immune crescentic nephritis (Table 83.3), but not in patients with less severe renal disease. Combining the results of the controlled trials, 31 out of 42 (74%) dialysis-dependent patients treated with plasma exchange recovered renal function compared with only 8 of 25 (32%) treated with drugs alone. A prospective randomized controlled multi center trial comparing plasma exchange with intravenous methylprednisolone in patients with ANCA-associated systemic vasculitis and severe renal impairment has just been completed (MEPEX) and the results are due to be reported during 2002[18].

Recommendation: We perform plasma exchange in patients with small vessel vasculitis who present with dialysis dependent renal failure, or with pulmonary hemorrhage. Exchanges are performed with albumin replacement unless there is a bleeding risk (as for anti-GBM disease).

Other crescentic glomerulonephritis
Crescent formation is a common histologic finding in a number of other patterns of nephritis, including postinfectious glomerulonephritis, infective endocarditis, IgA nephropathy, membranoproliferative glomerulonephritis (MPGN) and membranous nephropathy. Plasma exchange has been used in the treatment of a number of these conditions, despite the lack of substantive evidence that the renal injury is caused by

circulating antibodies or immune complexes. There are no controlled trials. In crescentic IgA nephropathy there are anecdotal reports of short-term benefit in patients with severe renal impairment but longer-term follow-up has proved disappointing. Roccatello et al. reported six patients with crescentic IgA nephropathy treated using intravenous methylprednisolone, cyclophosphamide, and plasma exchange[19]. All of the patients improved in the short term; however, repeat renal biopsies revealed persistent crescents, and half of the patients subsequently lost independent renal function. Other case reports have not even shown short-term benefits.

Plasma exchange has also been used in a number of isolated cases of MPGN and postinfectious crescentic nephritis, but overall no convincing data have been published to justify the widespread use of plasma exchange in other nephritides.

Recommendation: We reserve plasma exchange in IgA nephropathy for patients with rapidly deteriorating renal function and extensive crescents in the biopsy.

Focal segmental glomerulosclerosis

Plasma exchange and protein A immunoadsorption have been used to treat patients with primary FSGS. The results have been less good than in patients with recurrent disease after transplantation, and in general less than 40% of patients achieve either partial or complete remission[20]. The place for extracorporeal therapies in this setting remain to be defined.

Hemolytic uremic syndrome/thrombotic thrombocytopenic purpura

Over the last 5 years, the pathogenesis of TTP in particular has become better understood, and clearly distinguishable from HUS[21]. In both diseases, endothelial activation leads to thrombotic microangiopathy, but through independent mechanisms. Childhood diarrheal associated HUS (D+ HUS) is usually caused by bacterial verotoxins, and has a good prognosis. Most children will recover fully with supportive care and management of fluid and electrolyte imbalance and hypertension. Two controlled trials of plasma infusion (at least 10 mL/kg daily) in childhood HUS complicated by dialysis-dependent renal failure could not demonstrate any clinical benefit (as determined by hypertension, renal dysfunction, and proteinuria) in either short- or medium-term follow-up[22].

In contrast, mortality from HUS and TTP in adults remains high despite aggressive treatment regimens. There has been much debate as to the role of plasma infusion versus plasma exchange in HUS/TTP, and whether it is the removal or replenishment of factors that is critical for treatment efficacy. A single prospective controlled trial has compared plasma infusion with plasma exchange in 102 adults presenting with TTP in Canada in 1982–1989[23]. Plasma exchange of 1–1.5 plasma volumes was performed at least seven times in the first 9 d. All patients received aspirin and dipyridamole. The outcome after the first cycle of treatment was substantially better in those patients receiving plasma exchange: 47% of patients had a platelet count greater than 150×10^9 cells/L and no new neurologic features, compared with only 25% of those receiving plasma infusion. Two of the patients in the plasma exchange group died (4%) compared with 12 (24%) of those infused. At 6 months,

survival remained substantially better in the plasma exchange group (50% vs. 78%). However, the plasma exchange patients received a mean of 21.5 L of plasma compared with only 6.7 L in those treated with plasma infusion. The benefit of plasma exchange may, therefore, simply be to allow greater replenishment of plasma rather than removal of pathogenic factors. Subsequent studies have reinforced the value of plasma exchange in patients especially with TTP[24]. Whether FFP or cryosupernatant fraction is better as replacement plasma remains unclear.

More recently, the etiopathogenesis of TTP has been clarified[21]. Patients with TTP have a defective vWF cleaving protease – an enzyme which normally degrades large vWF multimers. Accumulation leads to systemic platelet activation under conditions of high shear stress (the microcirculation) and thrombosis. The value of plasma infusion and removal in TTP is therefore both to replenish vWF cleaving protease and to remove the large vWF multimers from circulation. In contrast the cause of HUS remains unclear in most cases. Some patients have defective regulation of the complement pathway (e.g., factor H deficiency and uninhibited activation of complement), while in others infections or drugs cause platelet or leukocyte activation and complement activation and consumption. Direct activation of endothelial cells may also be a cause. Plasma exchange and infusion has not been subjected to any controlled trials in pure HUS, but uncontrolled series suggest benefit in both diarrheal and nondiarrheal adult HUS[25].

Recommendation: We use plasma exchange in all adults with HUS and perform all exchanges against FFP or cryo-poor FFP.

Systemic lupus

Plasma exchange has been used extensively in patients with lupus. Most studies have included patients with diverse patterns of disease, and often only mild renal involvement. A randomized prospective trial could show no benefit of plasma exchange over conventional immunosuppression for renal, serologic, or clinical outcomes, both in the short and long term[26]. However, patients with crescentic lupus nephritis and those with the most severe renal dysfunction (dialysis dependency) were excluded. Anecdotal evidence suggests that plasma exchange may benefit patients with crescentic nephritis, pulmonary hemorrhage, cerebral lupus, or severe lupus unresponsive to conventional drugs, or in patients for whom cytotoxic therapy has been withdrawn because of bone marrow suppression or other toxicity. The results of a multicenter trial in which plasma exchange is synchronous with intravenous cyclophosphamide are awaited, however reports from a single center including patients in the trial are not encouraging. Immunoadsorption may be more successful in the severe forms of lupus nephritis.

Cryoglobulinemia

In type I cryoglobulinemia, usually associated with myeloma or lymphoma, a monoclonal immunoglobulin causes hyperviscosity and cryoprecipitation. Such antibodies are easily removed by plasma exchange, often with immediate benefit for the patient. Cytotoxic agents are used simultaneously to inhibit further paraprotein production. There are no controlled trials of the use of plasma exchange, but symptoms are closely related to the presence of the cryoimmunoglobulin, and hence treatment with plasma exchange is efficacious.

Patients with type II (mixed essential) cryoglobulinemia develop a monoclonal antibody (usually IgM) with specificity for a second, usually polyclonal, immunoglobulin. The resulting immune complexes can be deposited in the microcirculation and are particularly associated with MPGN. Type II cryoglobulins occur most commonly with lymphomas and hepatitis C virus infection. Plasma exchange is effective at clearing the immune complexes in this condition, though in long-term follow-up the cryoglobulins often recur, and sustained benefit has not been clearly demonstrated. Despite these reservations, many of the acute features of cryoglobulinemia do resolve with plasma exchange, particularly arthralgia, skin lesions, and digital necrosis, and patients with RPGN can recover renal function. Concomitant immunosuppression with cytotoxic agents may prevent resynthesis of the cryoproteins, although many patients require long-term intermittent plasma exchange to control symptoms. Patients with hepatitis C virus associated cryoglobulinemia may respond to antiviral therapies such as interferon or ribavirin, although published reports show only a limited response. Immunosuppressive treatment should be used with caution in these patients.

Myeloma

Plasma exchange has been reported to be of benefit in patients with myeloma and either cast nephropathy or light chain renal toxicity[27], though two controlled trials have provided conflicting results[28,29]. Zuchelli et al. randomized 29 patients with acute renal failure and myeloma with Bence–Jones proteinuria to receive steroids and cyclophosphamide, with or without plasma exchange (five exchanges on 5 consecutive days) after hydration and diuretic challenge[28]. The results suggested a clear benefit for plasma exchange in this setting: 11 of 13 dialysis-dependent patients treated with plasma exchange improved after initiation of therapy, compared with only two of 11 dialysis-dependent control patients. Unfortunately, the patients receiving plasma exchange underwent dialysis thrice weekly by hemodialysis, whereas those in the control group received alternate daily intermittent peritoneal dialysis, which may have influenced the outcome.

A second prospective trial of plasma exchange in 21 patients with myeloma and renal failure showed no benefit[29]. Only five patients were oliguric, 13 required dialysis and plasma exchange was only performed three times per week for 1–4 weeks. However, of the five oliguric patients only three improved, all of whom had received plasma exchange; of 12 initially dialysis-dependent patients, the only ones to establish independent renal function (three) had all received plasma exchange.

Recommendation: We use plasma exchange in myeloma patients with acute renal failure and a measurable paraprotein, after aggressive hydration and correction of other reversible causes (such as hypercalcemia and sepsis), and after performing a renal biopsy. Patients will usually receive high dose prednisolone as part of their chemotherapy for myeloma, and we begin this early since an acute interstitial infiltrate is a common feature and may respond to steroids. We perform 5–7 exchanges for albumin (unless there is a bleeding risk).

Transplantation

Vascular rejection

Vascular rejection is associated with both anti-HLA and antiendothelial antibodies. Studies in the 1980s suggested that combining plasma exchange with cyclophosphamide could deplete circulating antibodies and improve renal function. Subsequent controlled studies have been performed in heterogeneous patient populations, with conflicting results. Gurland et al. reviewed data on 157 patients included in five trials and could not demonstrate any significant difference in the outcome of acute vascular rejection in patients treated with or without plasma exchange[30]. More recently, Frasca et al. documented reversal of acute (but not chronic) rejection in 75% of 62 patients treated with plasma exchange[31]. A number of reports have shown plasma exchange to be effective at reversing up to 50% of episodes of acute vascular rejection resistant to corticosteroids, but there are no studies comparing plasma exchange with antibody therapy in resistant rejection. Plasma exchange has also been used in the treatment of chronic rejection, but without any convincing evidence for efficacy.

Anti-HLA antibodies

Highly sensitized patients with preformed anti-HLA antibodies have been treated both pre- and post-transplantation with plasma exchange or immunoadsorption to reduce cytotoxic antibody levels[32]. Patients usually received intensive immunoadsorption or plasma exchange pretransplantation to ensure a current negative cross-match immediately prior to transplantation; some received longer-term immunoadsorption/plasma exchange in combination with steroids and cyclophosphamide in the months preceding transplantation. Reisaeter et al. treated 100 patients with high-titer cytotoxic antibodies with plasma exchange or immunoadsorption in addition to cyclophosphamide and prednisolone[32]. Renal transplants were given to 83 patients, of whom 15 had a pre-transplant positive cross-match towards the donor. Graft survival rates at 1 and 4 years were 77% and 64%, respectively, in living donor transplants, and 70% and 57%, respectively, in first cadaveric graft recipients.

Recurrent focal segmental glomerulosclerosis

Plasma exchange and protein A immunoadsorption have both been used to treat recurrence of nephrotic syndrome after transplantation in patients with recurrent focal segmental glomerulosclerosis[20]. An undefined factor causing increased permeability of glomerular capillaries can be found in most patients with recurrent disease. There are no controlled trials of plasma treatments in recurrent FSGS, and most series are small. Dantal et al. demonstrated an 82% reduction in urinary protein excretion in eight patients with recurrent nephrosis during plasma protein adsorption; however, the effect was transient and persisted for less than 2 months in seven of the eight patients[33]. Other investigators have obtained remissions in approximately 50% patients, and a significant reduction in graft loss due to recurrent disease compared with historic controls[20]. More intensive treatment regimens have led to more persistent remissions. Both plasma exchange and protein A immunoadsorption have also been used prophylactically in patients deemed to be at high risk for recurrence.

CONCLUSION

Plasma exchange has a valuable role in the management of renal disease. However, it is necessary to define its role more clearly, if possible in controlled trials, so that the treatment can be targeted at those patients who will benefit. Such clarity has not been achieved for many of the renal disorders in which plasma exchange is used. The development of more specific and targeted antibody-removal technology will reduce the incidence of complications and may allow more efficacious therapy.

REFERENCES

1. Derksen RH, Schuurman HJ, Meyling FH, et al. The efficacy of plasma exchange in the removal of plasma components. J Lab Clin Med. 1984;104:346–54.
2. Reutter JC, Sanders KF, Brecher ME, et al. Incidence of allergic reactions to FFP or cryo-supernatant in the treatment of thrombotic thrombocytopenic purpura. J Clin Apheresis 2001; 16(2):134–8.
3. Pohl MA, Lan SP, Berl T. Plasmapheresis does not increase the risk of infection in immunosuppressed patients with severe lupus nephritis. Ann Intern Med. 1991;114:924–9.
4. Norda R, Bersems O, Stegmayr B. Adverse events and problems in therapeutic apheresis. A report from the Swedish registry. Transfus Apheresis Sci. 2001;5(1):33–41.
5. Levy JB, Pusey CD. Anti-GBM antibody mediated disease. In: Wilkinson R, Jamison R, eds. Nephrology. London: Chapman and Hall;1997:599–615.
6. Johnson JP, Whitman W, Briggs WA, Wilson CB. Plasmapheresis and immunosuppressive agents in antibasement membrane antibody-induced Goodpasture's syndrome. Am J Med. 1978; 64:354–9.
7. Levy JB, Turner AN, Rees AJ, Pusey CD. Long term outcome of anti-Glomerular basement membrane antibody disease treated with plasma exchange and immunosuppression. Ann Intern Med. 2001;134:1033–42.
8. Glockner WM, Sieberth HG, Wichmann HE, et al. Plasma exchange and immunosuppression in rapidly progressive glomerulonephritis: a controlled multi-center study. Clin Nephrol. 1988;29:1–8.
9. Pusey CD, Rees AJ, Evans DJ, et al. Plasma exchange in focal necrotizing glomerulonephritis without anti-GBM antibodies. Kidney Int. 1991;40:757–63.
10. Cole E, Cattran D, Magil A, et al. A prospective randomized trial of plasma exchange as additive therapy in idiopathic crescentic glomerulonephritis. Canadian Apheresis Study Group. Am J Kidney Dis. 1992;20:261–9.
11. Guillevin L, Fain O, Lhote F, et al. Lack of superiority of steroids plus plasma exchange to steroids alone in the treatment of polyarteritis nodosa and Churg Strauss syndrome. A prospective randomised trial in 78 patients. Arthritis Rheum. 1992;35:208–15.
12. Guillevin L, Lhote F, Cohen P, et al. Lack of superiority of corticosteroids plus pulse cyclophosphamide and plasma exchanges to corticosteroids plus pulse cyclophosphamide alone in the treatment of polyarteritis nodosa and Churg Strauss syndrome patients with poor prognostic factors. A prospective randomised trial in 62 patients. Arthritis Rheum. 1995;38:1638–45.
13. Zauner I, Bach D, Kramer BK, et al. Predictive value of initial histology and effect of plasmapheresis on long term prognosis of rapidly progressive glomerulonephritis. Am J Kidney Dis. 2002; 39(1):28–35.
14. Frasca GM, Zoumparidis NG, Borgnino LC, et al. Plasma exchange treatment in rapidly progressive glomerulonephritis associated with anti-neutrophil cytoplasmic autoantibodies. Int J Artif Organs. 1992;15:181–4.
15. Levy JB, Winearls CG. Rapidly progressive glomerulonephritis: what should be first-line therapy? Nephron 1994;67:402–407.
16. Gaskin G, Pusey CD. Systemic vasculitis. In: Cameron JS, et al., eds. Oxford Textbook of Clinical Nephrology. 2nd edn. Oxford: Oxford University Press; 1997.
17. Stegmayr BG, Almroth G, Berlin G, et al. Plasma exchange or immunoadsorption in patients with rapidly progressive crescentic glomerulonephritis. A Swedish multi-center study. Int J Art Organs. 1999;22:81–7.
18. Rasmussen N, Jayne DRW, Abramowicz D, et al. European therapeutic trials in ANCA associated systemic vasculitis: disease scoring, consensus regimens and proposed clinical trials. Clin Exp Immunol. 1995;101(suppl 1):29–34.
19. Roccatello D, Ferro M, Coppo R, et al. Treatment of rapidly progressive IgA nephropathy. Contrib Nephrol. 1995;111:177–82.
20. Bosch T, Wendler T. Extracorporeal plasma exchange in primary and recurrent focal segmental glomerulosclerosis. A review. Ther Apheresis. 2001;5(3):155–60.
21. Moake JL. Thrombotic thrombocytopenic purpura. Annu Rev Med. 2002;53:75–88.
22. Rizzoni G, Claris-Appiani A, Edefonti A, et al. Plasma infusion for hemolytic uremic syndrome in children. J Pediatr. 1988; 112:284–90.
23. Rock GA, Shumak KH, Buskard NA, et al. Comparison of plasma exchange with plasma infusion in the treatment of thrombotic thrombocytopenic purpura. Canadian Apheresis Study Group. N Engl J Med. 1991;325:393–7.
24. Lara PN, Coe TL, Zhou H, et al. Improved survival in patients with thrombotic thrombocytopenic purpura-hemolytic uremic syndrome. Am J Med. 1999;107:573–9.
25. Dundas S, Murphy J, Soutar RL, et al. Effectiveness of therapeutic plasma exchange in the 1996 Lanarkshire Eschericia coli O157: H7 outbreak. Lancet. 1999;354(9187):1327–30.
26. Korbet SM, Lewis EJ, Schwartz MM, et al. Factors predictive of outcome in severe lupus nephritis. Lupus Nephritis Collaboration Group. Am J Kidney Dis. 2000;35(5):904–14.
27. Moist L, Nesrallah G, Kortas C, et al. Plasma exchange in rapidly progressive renal failure due to multiple myeloma. A retrospective case series. Am J Nephrol. 1999;19(1):45–50.
28. Zucchelli P, Pasquali S, Cagnoli L, Ferrari G. Controlled plasma exchange trial in acute renal failure due to multiple myeloma. Kidney Int. 1988;33:1175–80.
29. Johnson WJ, Kyle RA, Pineda AA, et al. Treatment of renal failure associated with multiple myeloma. Arch Intern Med. 1990;150:863–9.
30. Gurland HJ, Blumenstein M, Lysaght MJ, Samtleben W, Stoffner D. Plasmapheresis in renal transplantation. Kidney Int. 1983;23 (suppl 14):82–4.
31. Frasca GM, Martella D, Vangelista A, Bonomini V. Ten years experience with plasma exchange in renal transplantation. Int J Artif Organs. 1991;14:51–5.
32. Reisaeter AV, Leivestad T, Albrechtsen D, et al. Pretransplant plasma exchange or immunoadsorption facilitates renal transplantation in immunized patients. Transplantation. 1995;60:242–8.
33. Dantal J, Bigot E, Bogers W, et al. Effect of plasma protein adsorption on protein excretion in kidney-transplant recipients with recurrent nephrotic syndrome. N Engl J Med. 1994;330:7–14.

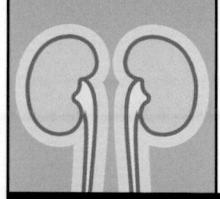

Chapter 84

Immunologic Principles of Kidney Transplantation

Luis G Hidalgo and Philip Halloran

INTRODUCTION

Kidney transplantation between nongenetically identical humans leads to the activation of a large number of alloreactive T lymphocytes that can exert effector functions leading to the destruction of the transplant. The massive response is invoked due to the large number of T cells capable of recognizing allogeneic major histocompatibility complex (MHC). Unlike most responses to cognate antigens where approximately $1/10^6$ of the T cell population may respond, up to 5% of the T cell population may respond to an allogeneic stimulus. Many arms of the immune system are activated during rejection including the generation of cytotoxic T lymphocytes (CTLs), delayed-type hypersensitivity (DTH) responses, and alloreactive antibodies. In this chapter we will discuss the mechanisms of T cell activation, polymorphism of MHC genes and the roles of the MHC in rejection, and the course of rejection.

The relationship between tissues of individuals is called syngeneic for identical twins, allogeneic for nonidentical members of the same species, and xenogeneic for members of different species. The prefixes allo- and xeno- designate components of the respective immune response e.g., alloantibody. This chapter is devoted to allotransplantation but alludes briefly to xenotransplantation. The mechanism of action, pharmacokinetics, administration, and side effects of immunosuppressives are discussed in Chapter 85.

IMMUNE CELLS THAT MEDIATE REJECTION

Alloresponses involve two groups of immune cells: lymphocytes and antigen presenting cells (APC). T and B lymphocytes mediate adaptive immune responses through their antigen-specific receptors, which permit them to express specificity, adaptation and tolerance, memory, and self/non-self recognition. NK cells are not antigen-specific, but express receptors for MHC class I and may have roles in transplantation, especially bone marrow transplantation. However, their role in allotransplantation remains unclear and is not discussed here. APC are cells required for the activation of T cells, engulfing and destruction of micro-organisms, and the generation of successful immune responses. The most effective APCs are dendritic cells (DCs) which are specialized cells in peripheral tissues and lymphoid tissues belong mainly to the monocyte lineage.

T cells

T cells arise in the thymus from bone marrow-derived precursors, somatically rearranging the genes for their antigen-specific receptors (TCRs). Thus each cell expresses a unique TCR which will then be expressed by all its daughter cells, forming a T cell clone. As T cells mature in the thymus, they undergo positive and negative selection. Positive selection identifies useful clones recognizing foreign antigens in the context of self MHC. Negative selection prevents potentially destructive autoreactive clones from maturing. Mature T cells expressing their clone-specific TCRs then leave the thymus. T cells are divided into two subpopulations: CD4 T cells (sometimes called helper cells) and CD8 T cells. CD4 T cells direct many aspects of the antigen-specific immune responses, while CD8 T cells are precursors of potent cytotoxic T cells (CTL), which are major effectors against intracellular pathogens. The TCRs of CD4 T cells are selected to interact with class II MHC molecules, and the TCRs of CD8 T cells with class I MHC molecules. The essential role of T cells in the generation of immune responses is demonstrated by the immunocompromised phenotype of nude mice that lack T cells[1].

B cells

B cells arise and mature in the bone marrow. B cells express immunoglobulin as their B cell receptors (BCRs). The precursors somatically rearrange their BCR (immunoglobulin, Ig) genes to express clone-specific Ig receptors. They are also selected negatively, deleting strong autoreactivity. When they leave the bone marrow they express BCRs on their surface. When their BCR is stimulated by antigen, B cells secrete immunoglobulins (antibodies) of the same specificity as their BCRs. The antibodies interacting with antigen activate the effector systems such as complement, NK cells, phagocytes, and mast cells. B cells can differentiate into plasma cells that are very efficient in secreting antibody. Antibody mediated responses are called 'humoral' and play an important role in some types of kidney allograft rejection.

APC

APCs are specialized cells capable of activating T cells. Antigen is endocytosed by APCs and then displayed on MHC molecules on their surface. T cells recognize and interact with antigen-MHC to become activated. Additional costimulatory molecules are expressed by APCs that allow for the optimal activation of T cells. Dendritic cells (DC), macrophages, and B cells are considered APCs with DC being the most effective

APC. Immature DCs live in the interstitial areas of the kidney, and are activated by stimuli (innate immunity, endotoxin, possibly tissue injury) to mature and move to the T cell areas of lymphoid tissues.

T CELL ACTIVATION

The activation of T cells is a crucial step in the generation of immune responses to specific antigens (Fig. 84.1) It begins with naïve T cells which have not yet encountered their cognate antigen, i.e., the MHC-peptide complex whose shape engages their TCR with sufficient affinity to trigger activation. The trafficking pattern of naïve T cells is restricted to secondary lymphoid organs such as lymph nodes, and spleen. They cannot enter organs such as kidney. They traverse from blood to lymphoid organs, where they pass through the T cell areas, enter lymph vessels and return to the blood.

Within secondary lymphoid organs naive T cells interact with DC that have migrated from the periphery in response to infection or injury. DC are the sentinels of the immune system. Immature DCs pick up material for surveillance and sense environmental disturbances in the peripheral tissues. They respond to disturbances such as endotoxin by maturing into potent APCs, and migrating to lymphoid organs[2]. DCs are highly 'intelligent' cells, interpreting the environment and determining whether the environment suggests that antigen should lead to an immune response, no response, or tolerance.

Thus the movement of DCs and the movement of naive T cells are co-ordinated to bring them into contact in the T cell areas of secondary lymphoid organs. If naive T cells encounter their cognate antigen presented on mature DC they become activated. Following activation, CD4 T cells move to the B cell region of secondary lymphoid organs to provide help to B cells, permitting them to class switch from IgM to IgG and to become antibody producing plasma cells. Activated T cells also leave the lymphoid organs and are now able to enter peripheral tissues, particularly sites of inflammation to apply their effector functions[3].

CD4 T cells can become effector cells but also are important regulatory cells in the generation of nearly all forms of immunity and the prevention of autoimmunity. They exert their effects through the production of cytokines and by direct contact between their surface molecules and other cells. CD4 T cells are required to provide help for the generation of plasma cells and CTL. One type of CD4 T cell attracting considerable interest is the CD4-CD25 T cell population discussed below.

As the host defense challenge subsides, the majority of T cells generated in an immune response will be deleted through cell death, either activation-induced cell death (AICD) triggered by antigen, or cell death secondary to antigen withdrawal, which acts by stopping growth factor production. Programmed cell death spares only sufficient antigen-specific memory cells to maintain the capacity to produce an efficient rapid response upon re-exposure to the same antigen.

Antigen presentation

Allografts (tissue transplants between members of the same species) induce alloimmune responses due to the recognition of nonself antigens from the graft by recipient T cells. Recipient T cells may encounter alloantigen through either direct or indirect pathways[4].

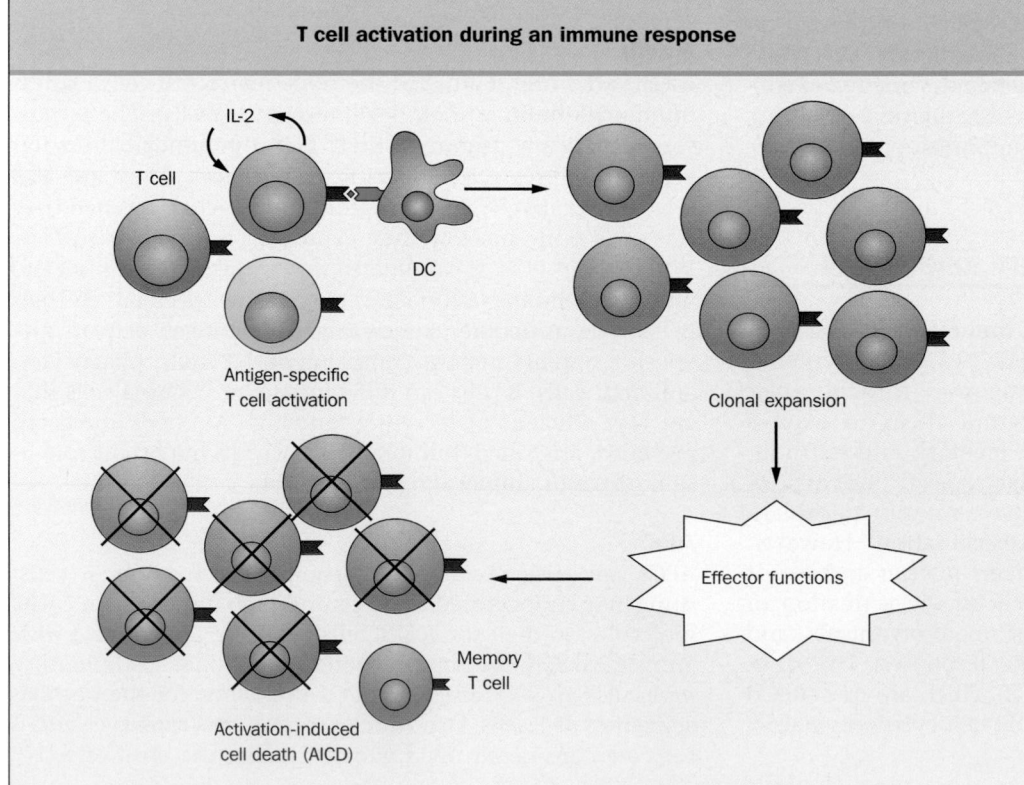

T cell activation during an immune response

IL-2

T cell

DC

Antigen-specific
T cell activation

Clonal expansion

Effector functions

Memory
T cell

Activation-induced
cell death (AICD)

Figure 84.1 T cell activation during an immune response. Only those naive T cells specific for the antigen being presented by DC (dendritic cells) are activated and begin to produce IL-2. IL-2 drives the clonal expansion of the activated clone, which go on to become effector cells. The majority of the activated clones undergo apoptosis by AICD.

Indirect antigen presentation is the way antigen is normally presented in immune responses. Antigen is taken up by APCs, processed intracellularly, and then presented as peptides on MHC molecules. In alloimmune responses graft-derived cells or released antigens can be taken up by recipient APCs. Recipient APCs process donor antigens and present donor MHC-derived peptides on recipient MHC molecules to T cells initiating the alloimmune response.

Direct antigen presentation involves the recognition of intact donor MHC on the surface of donor cells. Donor APCs may migrate from the graft to recipient lymphoid organs and activate alloreactive T cells to begin the alloresponse. Direct antigen presentation also occurs when recipient T cells encounter the allograft and recognize nonself antigens within the allograft. B cells also recognize intact donor MHC antigen by their B cell receptors leading to alloantibody production. The best evidence for direct recognition is the strong *in vitro* responses generated by cultured T cells with allogeneic APCs.

Major histocompatibility complex

MHC genes (in humans, the histocompatibility locus antigen (HLA)) encode molecules crucial to the initiation and propagation of immune responses. The HLA locus maps to a 3.5 million base pair region on chromosome 6 and is divided into three regions: the class II region, the class III region, and the class I region. Only the class I and class II regions encode proteins involved in antigen presentation. The key MHC genes are the class I genes (namely HLA-A, -B, and -C) and the class II genes (including HLA-DP, -DQ, and -DR).

The class I and II proteins share overall structural homology but are functionally different[5]. MHC class I molecules are single polypeptide chains of 45 kDa noncovalently associated with a smaller 12 kDa protein, $\beta2$-microglobulin. The class I heavy chain consists of three alpha domains ($\alpha1$, $\alpha2$, and $\alpha3$) and a short cytoplasmic tail (Fig. 84.2b). The membrane proximal $\alpha3$ domain and the $\beta2$-microglobulin are Ig domains, while the $\alpha1$ and $\alpha2$ domains are 'sheet-and-helix' domains, each constructed to form a long α-helix and an antiparallel β-sheet (Fig. 84.2a). The two sheet and helix domains assemble face-to-face to form a long β-sheet bounded by two α-helices, making up the peptide binding groove. The membrane-proximal Ig domain binds to $\beta2$-microglobulin, which is like a single Ig domain. Thus the structural elements of class I are two α-helices, a β-pleated sheet, and two membrane-proximal Ig domains, with a membrane anchor.

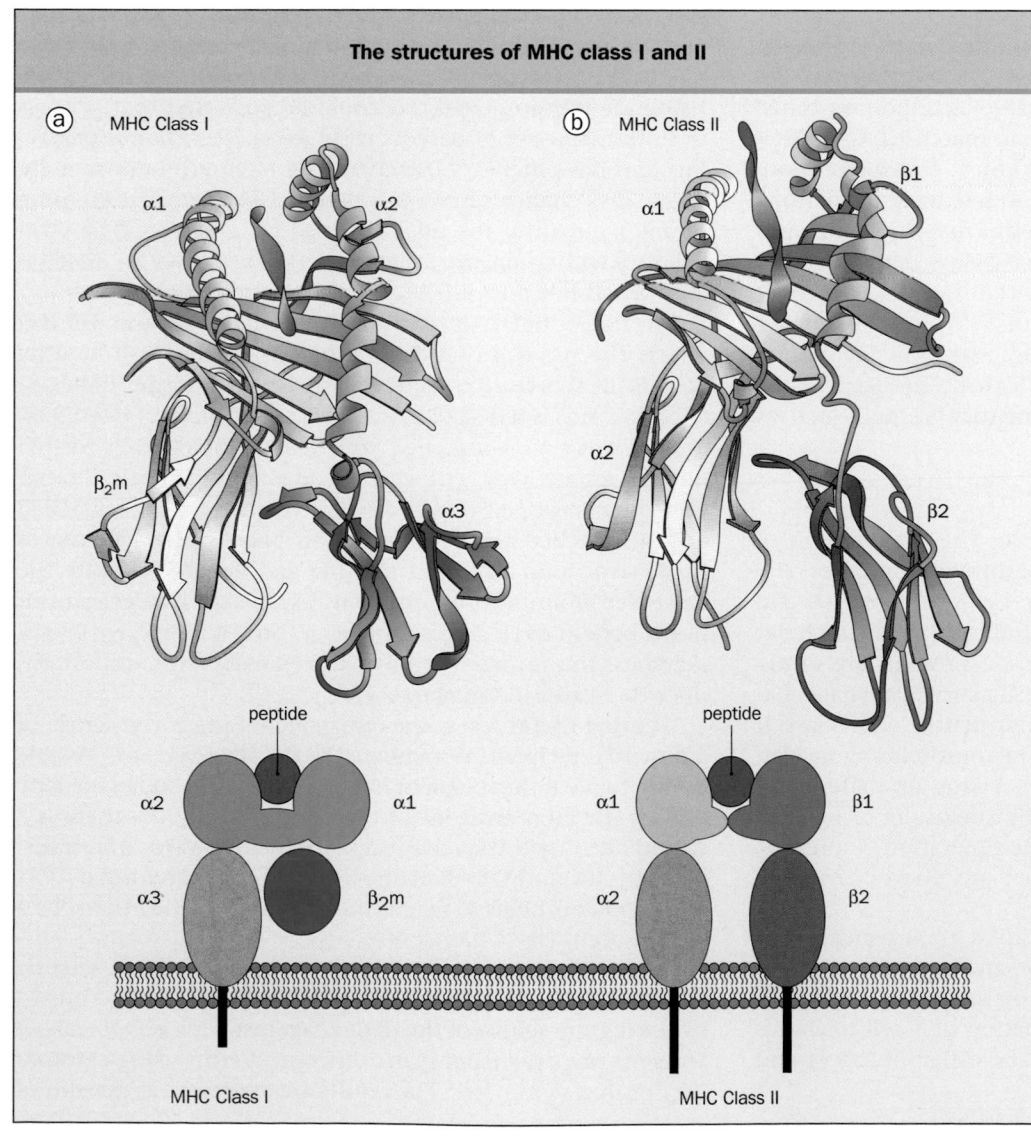

The structures of MHC class I and II

(a) MHC Class I

$\alpha1$ $\alpha2$

β_2m $\alpha3$

peptide

$\alpha2$ $\alpha1$

$\alpha3$ β_2m

MHC Class I

(b) MHC Class II

$\beta1$

$\alpha1$

$\alpha2$

$\beta2$

peptide

$\alpha1$ $\beta1$

$\alpha2$ $\beta2$

MHC Class II

Figure 84.2 The structures of MHC class I and class II. (a) MHC class I is composed of a heavy chain divided into $\alpha1$, $\alpha2$, and $\alpha3$ domains, noncovalently associated with β_2-microglobulin. The $\alpha1$ and $\alpha2$ domains make up the floor and the walls of the peptide binding groove. (b) MHC class II is a dimer composed of an α and a β chain. Each chain is divided into two domains with $\alpha1$ and $\beta1$ making up the floor and walls of the peptide binding groove.

Transplantation

Class II proteins are heterodimers of an α and a β chain each crossing the membrane. The α2 and β2 domains are adjacent to the cell membrane and are Ig domains while the peptide binding groove is composed of the α1 and β1 domains (Fig. 84.2b). The structural elements of class II are two α-helices, a β–pleated sheet, and two membrane-proximal Ig domains, with two membrane anchors (Fig. 84.2b).

Class I molecules present peptide (usually derived from endogenously synthesized proteins) to CD8 T cells. Class II proteins present peptide (usually derived from endocytosed proteins synthesized outside the cell) to CD4 T cells. Each molecule contains a groove that can hold peptides of 8 to 10 amino acids for class I or 8 to 25 amino acids for class II.

MHC class I and class II genes are highly polymorphic in the regions that encode the amino acids lining the peptide-binding groove. The polymorphism helps to ensure survival of a population by increasing the variety of peptides that can be presented to T cells. MHC polymorphism decreases the chance of encountering pathogens that may induce poor immune responses within a population leading the demise of the population due to disease. However, the polymorphism also predisposes to allograft rejection as the antigen presenting structures of one person are seen as foreign by another person.

HLA-A and HLA-B products are expressed on most somatic cells, but the amount expressed varies. DR antigens also are widely expressed or inducible, and serve as important transplantation antigens. Efforts are made to match HLA-A and -B and -DR genes and proteins in kidney transplantation. Although Class II expression is mainly restricted to marrow-derived APCs including DC, B cells, macrophages, and Langerhans cells, humans also express class II products on some endothelial cells (EC) and epithelial cells. Moreover both class I and class II antigens can be induced on many cells by interferon-γ (IFN-γ), in synergy with other cytokines. In the absence of IFN-γ little MHC can be induced in the kidney even during strong inflammatory stimuli such as allograft rejection[6,7].

Function of MHC

Class I and II systems are designed for the presentation of antigen from different sources and for different purposes. The class I system is designed to sample cytosolic proteins and detect foreign proteins that would indicate an intracellular infectious agent such as a virus. Class I proteins are recognized by CD8 T cells and thus provide a surveillance mechanism to target infected cells for destruction. The class II system is designed to sample extracellular proteins by specialized APC, which are very efficient in taking up material by phagocytosis or endocytosis. Class II proteins are recognized by CD4 T helper cells and allow for the generation of immune responses to invading pathogens that are phagocytosed by APC early on in infection.

MHC products also play important roles in the regulation of T cell function, including the positive and negative selection of developing T cells, stimulation of naive T cells that is necessary for their survival, the induction of T cell tolerance and anergy, and interaction with NK and other inhibitory and activating receptors.

HLA matching and transplantation

The class I and II HLA proteins are the most polymorphic loci in the human genome. Initially, the polymorphisms were defined by HLA serologic typing using sera from multiparous women or persons that had received multiple blood transfusions. Approximately 30 serotypes have been identified for HLA-A, 70 for HLA-B, and 10 for HLA-C. The development of molecular biology techniques (polymerase chain reaction (PCR), sequencing) has made possible the analyses of the HLA allelic sequence diversity at the DNA level. By DNA typing many more polymorphisms have been identified; over 230 for HLA-A, over 470 for HLA-B, nearly 120 for HLA-C, and over 380 for HLA-DR. The most currently updated source for HLA alleles can be found at the website www.anthonynolan.com/HIG/index.html. Currently, PCR methods allow for rapid DNA sequence-based typing of human populations although serological methods are still sometimes used for identifying HLA antigens.

HLA profiles

HLA genes are codominantly expressed meaning that both copies of each HLA gene will be expressed as antigens. Tissue typing identifies the two alleles encoded at each of the three loci (A, B, DR). One allele for each of HLA-A, -B, and -DR (i.e., one haplotype) will have been inherited from the mother and a second haplotype will have been inherited from the father. Using Mendelian genetics it could be predicted that siblings from the same set of parents will have a 25% chance of having zero mismatches, 50% chance of having one mismatch, and a 25% chance of two mismatches. The term HLA typing means to identify the alleles carried by a person. The term 'HLA matching' means assigning a donor kidney to a recipient with as few mismatches as possible, after typing both.

The degree of HLA matching at the HLA-A, -B, and -DR loci affects the survival of kidney allografts, as demonstrated by data from the United Network for Organ Sharing database (UNOS)[8]. This is reflected in the 3-year graft survival rates: 93% and 85% for HLA-matched and mismatched living related donors, respectively. The same trend is observed in cadaveric donor grafts with 82% and 76% survival rates for HLA-matched and mismatched living related donors, respectively. Differences in survival rates and graft half-life are observed despite the improved immunosuppression in use today. However, most of the benefit of HLA matching is in those who receive 0 mismatches: the number of mismatches seems less important, once there are HLA mismatches.

Another useful test is the crossmatching test: the serum of a potential recipient is incubated with cells from the possible donor, to see if the recipient has antidonor antibodies, usually against the HLA antigens of the donor. If they do, there is a strong likelihood that the recipient would destroy the transplant by antibody-mediated rejection. Crossmatching donors and recipients helps to determine whether a kidney transplant should occur (see Chapter 86).

Anti-HLA antibodies in the serum of a person can be assessed as panel reactive antibodies (PRA). This is determined by testing the serum of the patient against a 'panel' of cells or antigens prepared from many different donors using cytotoxicity or flow cytometry. The results are expressed as percent of positive donors. PRA can also be identified in ELISA-based methods, using purified HLA antigens instead of cells from each donor. Alloreactive antibodies can be generated by prior sensitization through blood transfusions, previous transplants, or by pregnancy.

Crossmatching helps to prevent a transplant from being given to a recipient who has pre-existing antibodies to the transplant. PRA helps to assess how much HLA antibody a person has, which predicts whether they will have difficulty getting a transplant.

GENERATION OF T CELL EFFECTOR FUNCTIONS

Alloreactive T cells can be found in the naive and memory T cell populations but both require recognition of nonself MHC molecules to become activated. Naive T cells may be triggered by donor or recipient APCs to proliferate and develop effector functions in secondary lymphoid organs. Memory cells may be activated in the same manner or they may also become activated by recognizing cells in the allograft directly. The difference is that naive cells are restricted to trafficking only within lymphoid organs while memory cells can enter peripheral tissues. Reactions mediated by naive T cells require longer to develop than those mediated by memory T cells, which can be generated more quickly and with higher numbers of cells (secondary response). During allograft rejection both populations are probably activated simultaneously.

T cell proliferation generally occurs in secondary lymphoid organs and is mostly driven by T cell growth factors such as IL-2 and possibly IL-15. Proliferation of alloreactive clones generates a considerable number of responding T cells including CD4 and CD8 T cells, and B cells. These can injure the allograft through the generation of alloantibody by B cells, the generation of CTL, and by mediating DTH responses. Each CD4 T helper cell can activate several B cells to produce antibody or recruit and activate a large number of macrophages for a DTH response. CTLs can destroy the cells of the allograft directly. Although CTLs can only kill one target at a time, a single CTL can kill multiple targets over a short amount of time. Exactly how T cells create the typical lesions of graft rejection is not clear.

The T cell receptor

T cells express TCRs that recognize peptide–MHC complexes on the surface of other cells. TCRs are heterodimers composed of an α and a β chain, or a γ and a δ chain. Expression of αβ and γδ TCRs are mutually exclusive. The majority of T cells (approximately 95%) have αβ TCRs and they account for all T cell functions in kidney transplantation. A minority (approximately 5%) express γδ TCRs, but are generally restricted to epithelial tissues and their role in alloimmunity is not known.

Each α and β chain contains a constant domain and a variable domain. These domains are similar to the C and V domains of Ig and are in the Ig superfamily. The diversity in the TCR repertoire is encoded in the V domains of the α and β chains. These V domains have 3 hypervariable loops or complementary determining regions (CDRs) that form the antigen binding site

at the end of the TCR, interacting with the sheet and helix domains of the MHC. Of these CDRs, CDR3 is most variable. Much of the peptide contact is made by the CDR3 loop. This interaction enhances the specificity of antigen recognition by T cells since the most variable region of the TCR interacts with the diverse peptides that are presented in MHC molecules[9].

Normally an individual's TCRs recognize a universe of MHC–peptide shapes that form the surface of MHC–peptide molecules that are viewed as self and remain nonreactive. For each individual self-reactive peptide–MHC shapes were deleted in the thymus by negative selection. Peptide–MHC shapes that are later encountered are identified as non-self, or potentially infected self, such as a peptide from a virus that creates a new peptide–MHC shape, and this triggers a response. The shapes of one person's peptide–MHC universe differs from another because of peptides they contain or because of polymorphisms in the amino acids of the MHC itself, resulting in the predisposition for alloreactivity.

CD4 and CD8 Coreceptors

TCR–MHC interaction alone is not enough to invoke T cell activation. Specific coreceptor molecules are also found on the T cell surface that enhance the affinity of TCR interaction with a peptide–MHC complex, and help recruit signaling molecules to engaged TCRs. CD4 and CD8 bind to conserved regions of MHC molecules. CD4 is a monomeric membrane glycoprotein containing four Ig-like domains. CD8 can be an αβ heterodimer or an αα homodimer consisting of a single Ig-like domain. Both CD4 and CD8 have a cytoplasmic tail that can associate with signaling proteins such as the protein tyrosine kinase (PTK) *lck*, important in T cell activation.

Expression of CD4 and CD8 divides mature T cells into two distinct subsets due to their mutually exclusive expression. T helper cells that recognize MHC class II molecules on APCs express CD4 while CTL that recognize MHC class I molecules on target cells express CD8. Both coreceptors interact with the nonpolymorphic regions of their respective MHC molecules; CD4 binds the membrane proximal β2 domain of class II and CD8 interacts mostly with the α3 and the α2 domains of class I.

T cell signaling

The antigen-specific receptor of T cells (TCR) does not have signaling properties directly associated with it, having only a short cytoplasmic tail that is unable to transduce signals. The signaling complex noncovalently associated with TCRs is known as the CD3 complex and is composed of three different chains; CD3γ, CD3δ, and CD3ε (Fig. 84.3). A homodimer of ζ chains completes the signaling complex.

Engagement of the TCR by MHC, along with the other required receptor engagements, initiates the signaling process from the CD3 complex[10]. The first event to occur following TCR engagement is the activation of *lck* associated with CD4 or CD8 molecules. Activated *lck* phosphorylates tyrosine residues on the CD3 molecules, which then serve as anchoring sites for PTK ZAP-70. ZAP-70 phosphorylates several downstream substrates including adaptor and linker molecules that lead to the activation of phospholipase C (PLC-γ1). PLC-γ1 hydrolyzes PIP_2 to the potent second messengers IP_3 and

Transplantation

The T cell receptor complex

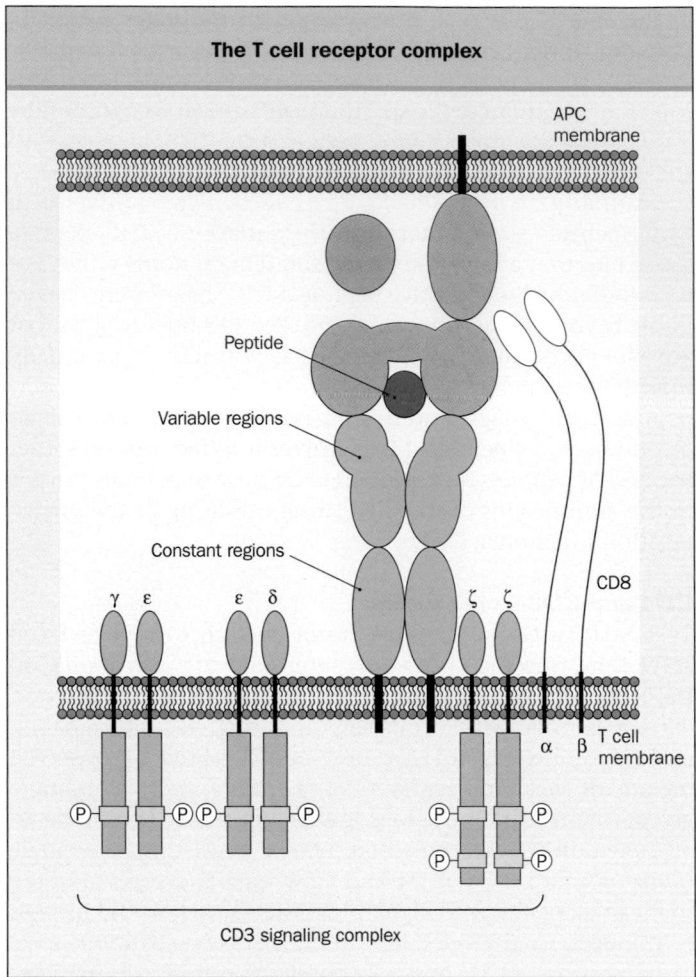

Figure 84.3 The T cell receptor (TCR) complex. Antigenic peptides are presented in the groove of an HLA molecule and are recognized by the variable regions of the TCR. Binding of CD8 (or CD4) to the HLA molecules increases the affinity of the TCR-MHC interaction. Triggering of the TCR by antigen starts a signaling cascade started by the signaling complex made up of CD3 γ, ε, and δ chains as well as the ζ chain homodimer.

diacylglycerol (DAG). DAG activates protein kinase C (PKC) leading to the activation of the NF-κB pathway while IP_3 acts on the endoplasmic reticulum to induce the release of intracellular Ca^{2+}.

The release of intracellular Ca^{2+} from the endoplasmic reticulum opens calcium channels that are linked to depletion of ER calcium stores, the so-called calcium release activated calcium (CRAC) channels. These channels generate a calcium current (I_{CRAC}). The I_{CRAC} then activates the protein serine phosphatase calcineurin. Calcineurin dephosphorylates the transcription factor NF-AT allowing it to translocate into the nucleus. The translocation of NF-AT and NF-κB, along with other transcription factors, allows for the transcription of the genes for IL-2 and other cytokines, as well as the genes for the high affinity subunit of the IL-2 receptor (CD25), and thus permit clonal expansion. Cyclosporine and tacrolimus are immunosuppressive due to their ability to prevent translocation of NF-AT through the inhibition of calcineurin (see Chapter 85).

The immune synapse

The molecular interaction between a T cell and an APC is architecturally organized into a structure known as the immune synapse (IS)[11]. The mature IS is characterized by the bull's eye arrangement of supramolecular activation clusters (SMACs) that form during T cell-APC contact. The center of the SMAC (cSMAC) contains the TCR and important cytoplasmic signaling molecules on the T cell and MHC–peptide complexes on the APC. The peripheral SMAC (pSMAC) contains the integrin LFA-1 on the T cell and its ligand ICAM-1 on the APC. IS stabilization correlates with full T cell activation and is dependent on TCR signaling.

Costimulation

Costimulation is the second signal required for the activation of T helper cell (Figure 84.4). Signal 1 is provided by the recognition of peptide–MHC by the TCR but another signal (Signal 2) is necessary for optimal IL-2 production, IL-2 receptor expression and cell-cycle progression according to the two-signal model of T cell activation. The TCR dictates the specificity of the response while costimulation amplifies and prolongs the response and allows for the generation of effector function. Costimulation is probably a checkpoint developed by the immune system to prevent the generation of autoimmune cells. The activation of a naive T helper cell in the absence of signal 2 leads to anergy, perhaps because of an inhibitory molecule called Cbl. Thus costimulation removes this inhibition, and determines whether a T cell will proceed with clonal expansion and development of effector function or become anergic (Fig. 84.4).

CD28 was the first costimulatory molecule identified on T cells and binds to B7 molecules on APCs. CD28 costimulation is mostly required by T helper cells but does not appear to be as important in the activation of CTLs[12].

The CD40-CD40L system plays an ancillary role as an amplifier of costimulation. CD40L (a member of the TNF superfamily) is expressed on T cells activated by TCR stimulation. CD40L binds to CD40 expressed on B cells, DC, macrophages, and endothelial cells (EC). When CD40L engages CD40 a differentiation signal is sent that allows the APC to perform more specialized tasks. CD40 ligation induces class switching allowing the production and secretion of specialized, higher affinity antibodies, affords the ability to prime precursor CTLs following T helper cell interaction, leads to activation associated with expression of chemokines, adhesion molecules, and other inflammatory mediators, and increases production of proinflammatory cytokines and nitric oxide in B cells, DC, EC, and macrophages, respectively. The roles of CD40-CD40L in modulating costimulation and class switching in the immune system made it a potential target for immunosuppression. However, clinical trials using anti-CD40L antibody have so far been disappointing.

The B7 superfamily and their receptors are also involved in costimulation. Of these, B7 related protein-1 (B7RP-1) and its T cell counterpart, inducible costimulator (ICOS) are important. ICOS is a member of the CD28 family that is induced on activated T cells within 24–48 h of activation. ICOS induces production of IFN-γ, IL-4, IL-10, and IL-2 independent of CD28. ICOS-B7RP-1 interactions are required for antibody production

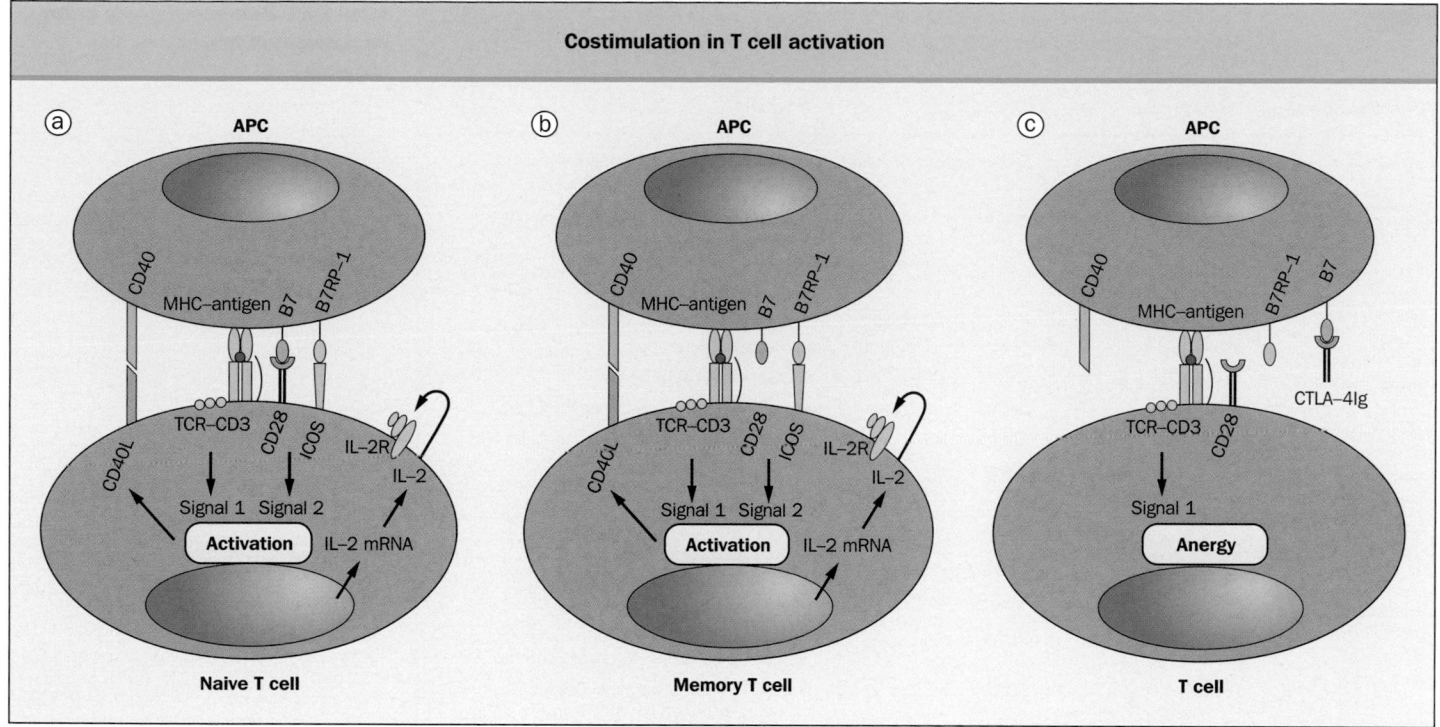

Figure 84.4 Costimulation in T cell activation. (a) Naive T cells require ligation of CD28 by B7 on the APC. Signal 1 is provided by the recognition of antigen by the TCR while signal 2 is provided by ligation of CD28 and ICOS by their respective ligands. Signal 1 and 2 leads to activation of the T cell and expression of IL-2, IL-2R, and CD40L. (b) Memory T cells do not require costimulation through CD28 to become activated. Costimulation through ICOS is sufficient for memory T cell activation. (c) Absence of B7, or blocking of B7 with CTLA-4Ig, leads to anergy of the T cell.

through their role in T cell-dependent B cell activation. Unlike CD28 or CD40L, ICOS is expressed on memory T cells suggesting an important role for ICOS in the regulation of effector and memory T cells[13].

T cell activation is terminated through a number of events, one of which is the membrane expression of the inhibitor of costimulation, CTLA-4. CTLA-4 is similar to CD28 in that it also interacts with B7 but unlike CD28, it sends an inhibitory signal and is not expressed on resting T cells. TCR engagement causes CTLA-4 expression but only following 24 h of stimulation, thus providing an effective regulatory feedback mechanism. Although CTLA-4 surface levels are not as high as CD28, it has higher affinity for B7 molecules allowing it to outcompete CD28 for B7 binding. CTLA-4 has two effects: it removes B7 from CD28, eliminating the CD28 signal, and it delivers a poorly understood negative signal itself to terminate T cell activation. The higher affinity of CTLA-4 for B7 is the reason behind the immunosuppressive effects of the soluble fusion protein CTLA-4Ig that efficiently blocks B7 expressed on APCs.

T cell differentiation

CD4 and CD8 T cells are both produced in the thymus from which they leave to enter the circulation as naive T cells. Naive T cells are restricted to recirculating between secondary lymphoid organs and blood until they encounter antigen. Naive T cells are small in size with little cytoplasmic space and condensed chromatin and reside in the paracortical region of lymph nodes. DC enter lymph nodes and migrate into the T cell region in the paracortex. After encountering a DC expressing antigenic MHC and costimulatory receptors, T cells are induced to undergo gene transcription in order to differentiate to effector T cells.

One of the first cytokines produced is IL-2 that helps to drive T cell division during clonal expansion. Activated T cells expressing IL-2R then migrate to the B cell region of the lymph node located in the cortex. T cells recruited to the cortex provide help to differentiating B cells. Other interleukins such as IL-15 also contribute to this response.

As T cells leave the lymph node they have undergone multiple rounds of division and express their respective effector molecules between 3–5 days following activation. After activation, T cells change their chemokine receptor expression to permit them to enter the peripheral tissues. Those that enter the graft promote inflammation. The activated T cells become responsive to inflammatory chemokines and home to inflamed sites (Table 84.1). The activated T cells rapidly accumulate in the interstitium of the allograft as the response mounts in the first few days.

Effector functions of T cells

CD4 and CD8 T cells play different roles during immune responses. CD4 T cells may be both effectors and regulators. CD4 T cells are important cytokine-secreting cells that help to modulate the type of immune response. They first express IL-2, and later a wide variety of cytokines. After prolonged stimulation CD4 T cells sometimes tend to express groups of several groups of cytokines, probably depending on the local environment and the nature of the antigen and the APC. The

Transplantation

Proteins involved in the recruitment of leukocytes into allografts			
Protein type	Name	Ligand	Function
Selectins	L-selectin	Sialated glycoproteins	Present on activated EC, mediates initial rolling of leukocytes on endothelium
Chemokines	MCP-1/CCL2	CCR2	Recruitment of monocytes, immature DC, T cells and NK cells
	MIP-1α/CCL3	CCR1	Recruitment of monocytes, immature DC, T cells, and neutrophils
	RANTES/CCL5	CCR1, CCR4, CCR5	Recruitment of monocytes, DC, T cells, NK cells and neutrophils
	IL-8/CXCL8	CXCR1, CXCR2	Recruitment of neutrophils
	MIG/CXCL9	CXCR3	Recruitment of activated/memory T cells
	IP-10/CXCL10	CXCR3	Recruitment of activated/memory T cells
	Lymphotactin/XCL1	XCR1	Recruitment of T cells
Ig superfamily	ICAM-1	LFA-1	Present on activated EC, mediates tight adhesion of leukocytes to endothelium
	ICAM-2, -3	LFA-1	Present on activated EC, mediates tight adhesion of leukocytes to endothelium (not as strong as ICAM-1)
	VCAM-1	VLA-4	Present on activated EC, mediates rolling and tight adhesion of leukocytes to endothelium
	CD31	CD31	Present at intercellular junctions on EC, mediates extravasation of leukocytes across endothelium

Table 84.1 Proteins involved in the recruitment of leukocytes into allografts.

T helper 1 (Th1) pattern of cytokines includes IL-2, IFN-γ, and lymphotoxin while Th2 pattern includes IL-4, IL-5, IL-10 and IL-13. These cytokine patterns are never observed as unique patterns in transplantation. Thus rejecting grafts typically have high levels of IFN-γ, TNF-α, and IL-10 mRNA, and cannot be called a pure Th1 response. Through their cytokine production (Table 84.2) CD4 T helper cells affect the allo-immune response by:

- stimulating production of nitric oxide, reactive oxygen species, and TNF-α in macrophages
- providing help to B cells to enhance their antibody production
- increasing MHC expression in the allograft through the production of IFN-γ
- CD4 T cells may sometimes be killers through expression of the apoptosis triggering molecule Fas ligand (FasL). However, whether this is important in killing graft cells is unknown. FasL is important in lymphocyte homeostasis: mice and humans with disruptions in the FasL-Fas system manifest lymphoproliferation and autoimmunity.

Many cells in the graft express and present class II MHC to alloreactive CD4 T cells. IFN-γ is strongly expressed during rejection and induces MHC class II expression in vascular endothelial cells, epithelial cells, and parenchymal cells in the graft. Ischemic injury to the graft also induces class II expression. Secretion of IFN-γ is thought to occur only while the TCR is engaged by antigenic MHC. A mild increase in MHC expression caused by ischemic injury can serve as the alloantigen for infiltrating alloreactive CD4 T cells to induce secretion of IFN-γ and other effector cytokines that further amplify class II expression and inflammation. The precise role of class II expression by donor cells in the graft remains controversial because kidney grafts lacking all class II are still rejected[14].

Alloantibody responses are generated simultaneously with T cell responses against foreign MHC antigens, particularly the class I antigens. T helper cell-dependent B cell activation is as an important component of the effector functions of graft rejection. Naive or memory B cells become activated by the cross-linking of the BCR by intact antigen (donor MHC). They also express donor peptides in their class II molecules to permit them to be recognized and helped by peptide-specific primed T cells. T helper cells stimulate B cells to become antibody producing plasma cells. T helper cells expressing CD40L engage CD40 on B cells and provide the signal required by B cells to undergo class switching (switch from producing IgM to IgG). Alloantibody produced during rejection is mainly IgG, and primarily participates in the destruction of the vascular endothelium of the graft (e.g., peritubular capillaries).

CD8 T cells can also express a number of effector functions, including cytokine production and cytotoxicity. Thus they can also participate in rejection through DTH or through cytotoxicity.

GRAFT REJECTION

Recruitment of cells into allografts

The leukocytic infiltrate observed in rejection is composed of mononuclear cells including T cells, macrophages, B cells and plasma cells. T cells serve as the main effectors and regulators of the alloimmune response. Macrophages serve as possible effectors and in the removal of apoptotic cells while B cells and plasma cells serve in the production of alloantibodies within the graft. The recruitment of these cells into the graft is a result of the combination of chemokine expression and adhesion molecule expression by the endothelium of the graft (Table 84.1). The endothelium of postcapillary venules

Table 84.2 Cytokines involved in allograft rejection.

Cytokines involved in allograft rejection		
Cytokine	Source	Biologic activity
IL-1	Macrophages, EC, NK cells	Proinflammatory, costimulates T cell and macrophage activation, enhances NK cell activity
IL-2	Activated T cells	Promotes T cell proliferation, induces NK activity, responsible for AICD of activated T cells
IL-4	Activated T cells	B and T cell growth factor, promotes allergic responses, increases MHC expression on B cells
IL-5	Activated T cells	Eosinophil growth factor and chemoattractant
IL-6	Macrophages, EC, T cells	Lymphocyte differentiation, stimulates production of acute-phase proteins
IL-10	T cells, macrophages	Anti-inflammatory, suppresses cytokine production and MHC expression on APC
IL-12	Macrophages, DC, B cells	Proinflammatory, stimulates IFN-γ production by T and NK cells, enhances NK cell activity
IL-15	Epithelial cells, stromal cells, macrophages	T cell growth factor, supports NK cell development, required for memory T cell survival
IFN-γ	Antigen-engaged T cells, NK cells	Increases MHC expression, increases cytotoxic activity of macrophages, promotes recruitment of activated T cells by EC
TGF-β	T and B cells, macrophages, platelets	Anti-inflammatory, promotes wound healing
TNF-α	Macrophages, NK cells, T and B cells	Proinflammatory, cytotoxic, activates EC and fibroblasts

in the graft serve as the entry point of recipient leukocytes from the bloodstream into the allograft. Graft endothelial cells are activated by proinflammatory cytokines and injury to express adhesion molecules and chemokines necessary for transendothelial migration.

The recruitment of leukocytes is initiated by the release of chemokines by tubular cells, interstitial cells, endothelial cells, and infiltrating recipient cells within the allograft. T cells expressing the respective chemokine receptors extravasate through the endothelium and are guided by a chemokine gradient towards the tubules of the graft where they cross the basement membrane resulting in tubulitis. The invasion of epithelial layers by CTL, including tubulitis, appears to be restricted to a specific subset of CTL. CD8 CTL expressing the integrin CD103, which binds to its ligand E-cadherin present on cells comprising epithelial layers including renal tubules, are exclusively found in tubules during acute rejection[15,16]. The ability of CD103 CTL to bind E-cadherin on tubular epithelium may be an important factor in the pathogenesis of acute renal allograft rejection.

Binding of chemokines to chemokine receptors induces a conformational change in integrins, which are normally present on circulating leukocytes in an inactive state. Tight adhesion occurs when activated integrins bind their Ig superfamily ligands such as ICAM and VCAM. The most common integrins present on lymphocytes are: LFA-1 that binds ICAM-1 and -2, and VLA-4 that binds with VCAM-1. ICAM-1, VCAM-1 and E-cadherin are expressed on the tubular epithelium of rejecting grafts where they play a role in the development of tubulitis. Unfortunately, blocking of adhesion has not been that successful at treating rejection, likely due to

redundancy among the multiple adhesion molecules and ligands that mediate leukocyte adhesion.

As a result of cytokines from infiltrating T cells the graft changes its pattern of gene expression. IFN-γ from the T cells induces a massive increase in MHC class I and class II in the epithelium and endothelium in the graft which are important for peptide loading and antigen presentation. Other genes such as adhesion molecules are also expressed.

T cell mediated rejection

Most rejection in clinical kidney transplantation is mediated by T cells and may consist of either delayed type hypersensitivity (DTH) or cytotoxic responses. Activated T helper cells secrete cytokines that induce the influx of nonspecific inflammatory cells including macrophages in the DTH response. DTH responses lead to the destruction of allograft cells through induction of the various cytotoxic mechanisms of the macrophages, including reactive oxygen species and proteolytic enzymes, plus vasomotor changes mediated by eicosanoids. The interstitial infiltrate and some of the vasospasm and edema in the rejecting kidneys can be considered an analogue of DTH.

T cell cytotoxicity results from two principal mechanisms. First, activated CTLs may kill their targets by releasing the cytotoxic molecules perforin and granzyme B from stored granules (Fig. 84.5). Granzymes bind their receptors on the target cell surface and perforin inserts into the membrane in a Ca^{2+}-dependent manner. The cytotoxic molecules are internalized into vesicles from which perforin releases granzyme into the cytosol. In the cytosol granzymes use their serine esterase activity to initiate a cascade of events that leads to apoptosis.

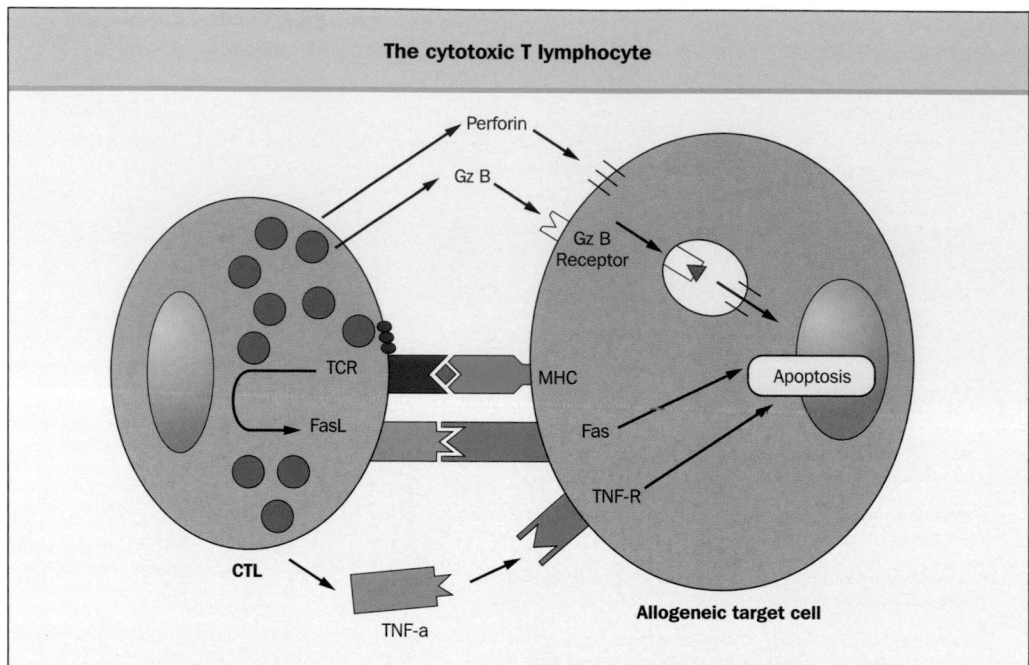

The cytotoxic T lymphocyte

Figure 84.5 Cytotoxic mechanisms of T lymphocytes. TCR of alloreactive CTL recognize allogeneic MHC on target cells. CTL mobilize cytotoxic granules containing perforin and granzyme B (GzB) towards the target cell releasing the cytotoxic molecules into the intercellular space. Perforin inserts into the target cell membrane and GzB binds to its receptor and both are internalized to induce apoptosis. TCR stimulation increases expression of FasL on the CTL surface and binds the Fas receptor triggering the apoptotic cascade. CTL can produce TNF-α which binds the TNF-R on the target cell leading to apoptosis.

Second, activated CTLs and T helper cells also use the Ca^{2+}-independent Fas/FasL pathway. Engagement of Fas on target cells by FasL from CTLs results in apoptotic death of the graft cell. While CD8 T cells are present in large numbers in renal allograft rejection, mice lacking CD8-associated cytotoxic molecules still reject grafts relatively briskly.

Most studies suggest that deterioration of renal function in T cell mediated rejection correlates with invasive lesions, where T cells invade the epithelium (tubulitis) (Fig. 84.6) and arterial endothelium (endothelialitis) (Fig. 84.7). One possibility is that T cells must express specialized molecules to interact with these structures. For example, CD103 may permit CD8 T cells to engage the renal epithelium[15,16]. Future research focusing on the pathogenesis of these lesions should ultimately be able to identify the molecular basis of tubulitis and endothelialitis.

Alloantibody mediated rejection

Alloantibody-mediated rejection is classically associated with the triad of decreased renal function, the presence of anti-donor antibody in recipient serum, and a renal biopsy showing neutrophils in peritubular capillaries with endothelial damage[17]. Alloantibodies are cytotoxic through their ability to activate complement as well as by recruiting leukocytes with receptors for attached antibodies (FcR) or complement. The

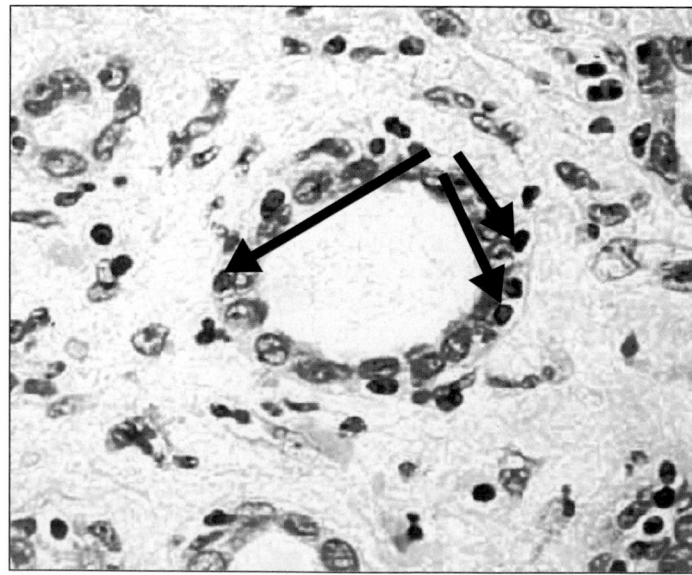

Figure 84.6 Tubulitis. Infiltration of tubular epithelium by T lymphocytes that have crossed the basement membrane (arrows).

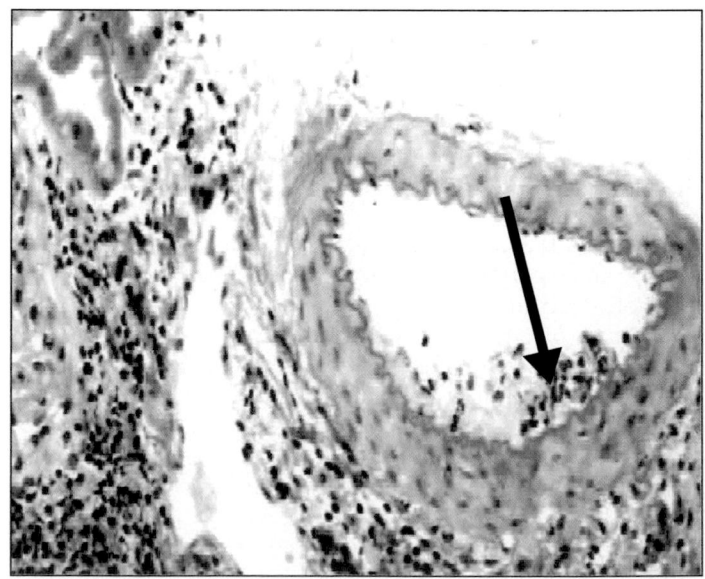

Figure 84.7 Endothelialitis. Invasion of the endothelium of a large artery by graft infiltrating T lymphocytes.

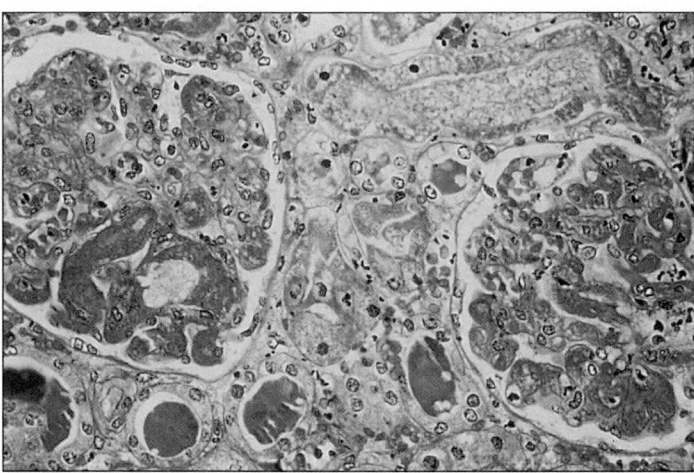

Figure 84.8 Hyperacute rejection. Hyperacute rejection of a kidney transplant showing glomerular and peritubular capillary infiltration and tubular coagulation leading to necrosis and glomerular thrombosis.

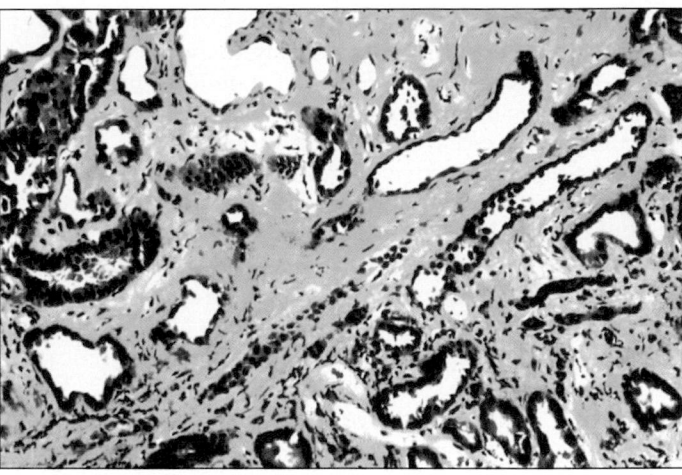

Figure 84.9 Interstitial fibrosis and tubular atrophy. Fibrosis of the interstitium is depicted in blue.

demonstration of C4d deposition in the peritubular capillaries is now the basis for the diagnosis of antibody-mediated rejection[18,19].

If recipients have been sensitized by previous transfusions, pregnancies, or transplants bearing donor MHC molecules, they may have preformed alloantibody against the donor. This can lead to disastrous *hyperacute rejection*, even on the operating table[20]. The entire endothelium of the graft is injured, and the large vessels usually fail (Fig. 84.8). This is prevented by crossmatching. For the same reason, recipients must be compatible with the donor at the ABO blood group locus. Hyperacute rejection is now very rare due to crossmatching practices.

Late deterioration of kidney transplants

Approximately 40% of late graft loss is due to nonspecific deterioration in the absence of other specific diseases, often described as 'chronic rejection'. 'Chronic rejection' of kidney transplants is commonly defined as an alloimmune response causing the slow deterioration of graft function accompanied with pathology showing tubular atrophy, interstitial fibrosis (Fig. 84.9), and fibrous intimal thickening of arteries (Fig. 84.10). Unfortunately, the term 'chronic rejection' is ambiguous as it fails to differentiate between the presence of an active alloimmune response causing tissue damage (rejection) and the state of the transplanted tissue (e.g., fibrosis and atrophy)[17]. Whereas some cases are due to true rejection (and which may be suspected in the presence of endothelialitis or tubulitis), other cases may represent the hemodynamic consequences of hypertension, accelerated senescence of the allograft, the development of an allograft glomerulopathy, or the development of chronic calcineurin toxicity or other diseases (see Chapter 90)[17,19,21–25]. A new consideration is nephropathy due to BK virus[26].

We have recently proposed that the term chronic rejection be replaced by accurate terms that convey whether rejection is active, the status of the parenchyma, and whether transplant glomerulopathy and other specific diseases are present[17]. Deterioration in a renal transplant often reflects the effects of

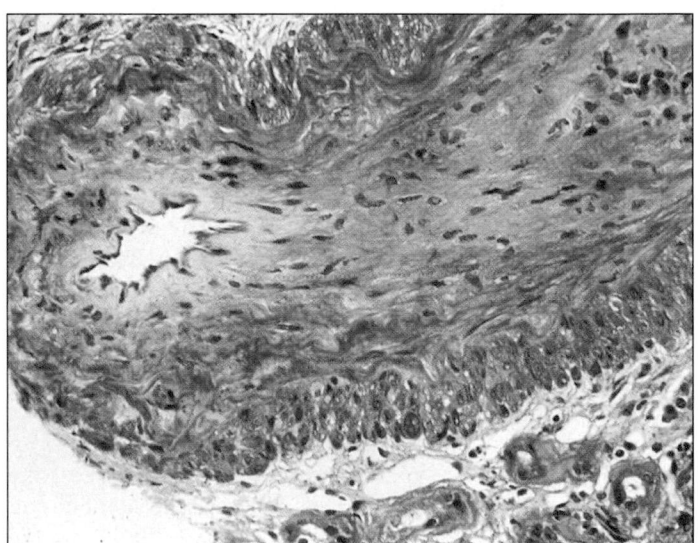

Figure 84.10 Fibrous intimal thickening. Thickening of the intima surrounding a small artery.

more than one process e.g., transplant glomerulopathy and calcineurin inhibitor nephrotoxicity.

TOLERANCE INDUCTION

Tolerance is a state of antigen-specific unresponsiveness where responses to other antigens are maintained. Normally, the immune system recognizes but does not respond to self-antigens. The education of the immune system begins in the thymus with the deletion (negative selection) of self-reactive T cells in a process known as central tolerance. Self-reactive T cells that escape negative selection in the thymus can be tolerized in the periphery through incompletely understood mechanisms. Central and peripheral tolerance use many processes including apoptosis, anergy, and suppression to neutralize self-reactive T cells.

Transplantation

Transplantation biologists have been searching for ways to induce tolerance to allografts as a way to avoid immunosuppressive treatment of the recipient. Life-long immunosuppression of recipients increases the risk of life-threatening infections and cancer. With induced tolerance the recipient's immune system selectively ignores the transplant without compromising protection against pathogens. Almost fifty years ago Billingham, Brent, and Medawar demonstrated that it was possible to induce tolerance in newborn mice by exploiting the mechanism of central tolerance[27]. Tolerance induction as a therapeutic procedure in humans has yet to be achieved but is likely to utilize the mechanism of peripheral tolerance and not central tolerance.

The mechanisms proposed for transplantation tolerance induction can be divided into deletional and nondeletional immunoregulatory states. Peripheral tolerance to allografts can be induced in experimental animals through costimulation blockade of CD28 and CD40L pathways[28] or by using sirolimus[29]. Costimulatory blockade inhibits T cell proliferation yet allows AICD to occur. AICD is necessary for tolerance induction since its inhibition prevents tolerance to allografts[29]. These studies demonstrate that apoptosis of alloreactive T cells is necessary in the induction of peripheral tolerance.

The immunoregulatory mechanisms governing peripheral tolerance involve the participation of DC and CD4CD25 regulatory T cells (Treg). Under normal steady state conditions, DC traffic from peripheral tissues to draining lymph nodes. In the periphery, DC can acquire self-antigens in the form of apoptotic bodies (generated by constant cell turnover). Phagocytosis of apoptotic cells in the absence of inflammation leads to a tolerogenic state in DCs, which could help to tolerize self-reactive T cells[30]. The tolerogenic mechanisms of DC remain largely unknown but the ability to mimic the induction and maintenance of peripheral tolerance by DC opens the possibility of a biologic therapy to graft rejection.

CD4CD25 Treg have recently been shown to suppress the expansion of conventional T cells in a contact-dependent, CD28-independent manner requiring CTLA-4[31]. Treg display an anergic phenotype with no production of IL-2 or effector cytokines such as IL-4 or IFN-γ. Studies in mice have revealed that depletion of Treg cells induces autoimmune diseases including gastritis, diabetes, and thyroiditis[32]. The reintroduction of CD4CD25 Treg inhibits disease development indicating a role for these cells in self-tolerance. The suppressive effects of these cells have also been observed in the inhibition of responses across minor histocompatibility differences[33]. Better understanding of the mechanism of suppression is necessary for the development of immunosuppressive treatments to induce tolerance.

Xenotransplantation

Transplantation is now the preferred treatment for organ failure but the short supply of human organs is a critical limiting factor. Xenotransplantation; the transplantation of cells, tissues, or organs across species barriers, could provide a solution to the organ shortages. With the application of new technologies such as transgenic animals and cloning it may be possible to overcome the immunologic problems associated with xenotransplantation. The pig is emerging as the most likely source of xenografts due to their availability and reproductive potential, physiologic and anatomic similarity to humans, as well as our ability to generate transgenic pigs. The recent generation of heterozygous gene-deficient pigs[34] allows for the possibility to generate pigs that will be more resistant to the robust immunologic attack by human recipients.

The major barrier in pig-to-primate transplantation is the presence of the saccharide galactose α-1,3 galactosyl (Galα1,3Gal) that is present on all cells of lower mammals but absent in humans. Humans develop anti-Galα1,3Gal natural antibodies that probably arise early in life as a result of stimulation by gut bacteria. Anti-Galα1,3Gal antibodies are capable of fixing complement once bound to porcine endothelium and mediate the hyperacute rejection of the xenograft. Complement regulatory proteins (such as CD55, CD59, and DAF) normally protect endothelium from complement-mediated attack but are species specific and therefore unable to prevent the complement activation that occurs with xenografts[33]. Natural killer cells may also participate by a variety of mechanisms.

Hyperacute rejection therefore may result and is mediated by complement activation with neutrophil infiltration and platelet thrombi (Fig. 84.8). Xenografts that do not undergo hyperacute rejection proceed to develop acute vascular rejection/delayed xenograft rejection (DXR). DXR destroys a xenograft over a period of days to weeks and is characterized by intravascular coagulation, focal ischemia, and endothelial swelling. Inflammatory cells such as NK cells and macrophages are observed in DXR but it is thought that although they contribute to tissue injury, they do not initiate the injury. The likely initiator is xenoreactive antibodies based on the ability of complete Ig depletion or depletion of anti-Galα1,3Gal to delay DXR. The exact mechanism of antibody-mediated DXR remains uncertain.

REFERENCES

1. Pantelouris EM. Observations on the immunobiology of 'nude' mice. Immunology. 1971;20(2):247–52.

2. Baggiolini M. Chemokines and leukocyte traffic. Nature. 1998; 392:565–8.

3. Braakman E, Tunen A van, Meager A, Lucas CJ. IL-2- and IFN gamma-enhanced natural cytotoxic activity: analysis of the role of different lymphoid subsets and implications for activation routes. Cell Immunol. 1986;99(2):476–88.

4. Gould DS, Auchincloss H. Jr. Direct and indirect recognition: the role of MHC antigens in graft rejection. Immunol Today. 1999; 20(2):77–82.

5. Jones EY. MHC class I and class II structures. Curr Opin Immunol. 1997;9(1):75–9.

6. Halloran PF, Miller LW, Urmson J, et al. IFN-γ alters the pathology of graft rejection: protection from early necrosis. J Immunol. 2001;166:7072–81.

7. Goes N, Sims T, Urmson J, et al. Disturbed MHC regulation in the interferon-γ knockout mouse. J Immunol. 1995;155:4559–66.

8. Cecka JM. The UNOS scientific renal transplant registry. In: Cecka JM, Terasaki PI, eds. Clinical Transplants. Los Angeles, CA: UCLA Tissue Typing Laboratory; 1999:1–21.

9. Reiser J-B, Darnault C, Guimezanes A, et al. Crystal structure of a T cell receptor bound to an allogeneic MHC molecule. Nat Immunol. 2000;1(4):291–7.

10. Wange RL, Samelson LE. Complex complexes: signaling at the TCR. Immunity. 1996;5:197–205.

11. Bromley SK, Burack WR, Johnson KG, et al. The immunological synapse. Annu Rev Immunol. 2001;19:375–96.

12. Coyle AJ, Gutierrez-Ramos JC. The expanding B7 superfamily: increasing complexity in costimulatory signals regulating T cell function. Nat Immunol. 2001;2(3):203–9.

13. Hutloff A, Dittrich AM, Beier KC, et al. ICOS is an inducible T-cell co-stimulator structurally and functionally related to CD28. Nature. 1999;397:263–6.

14. Sims TN, Afrouzian M, Urmson J, et al. The role of the class II transactivator (CIITA) in MHC class I and II regulation and graft rejection in kidney. Am J Transplant. 2001;1(3):211–21.

15. Hadley GA, Rostapshova EA, Gomolka DM, et al. Regulation of the epithelial cell-specific integrin, CD103, by human CD8+ cytolytic T lymphocytes. Transplant. 1999;67(11):1418–25.

16. Robertson H, Wong WK, Talbot D, Burt AD, Kirby JA. Tubulitis after renal transplantation: demonstration of an association between CD103+ T cells, transforming growth factor beta1 expression and rejection grade. Transplant. 2001;71(2):306–13.

17. Trpkov K, Campbell P, Pazderka F, et al. Pathologic features of acute renal allograft rejection associated with donor-specific antibody. Transplant. 1996;61:1586–92.

18. Feucht HE, Schneeberger H, Hillebrand G, et al. Capillary deposition of C4d complement fragment and early renal graft loss. Kidney Int 1993;43:1333–8.

19. Collins AB, Schneeberger EE, Pascual MA, et al. Complement activation in acute humoral renal allograft rejection: diagnostic significance of C4d deposits in peritubular capillaries. J Am Soc Nephrol. 1999;10:2208–14.

20. Kissmeyer-Nielsen F, Olsen S, Peterson VP, Fjeldborg O. Hyperacute rejection of kidney allografts associated with pre-existing humoral antibodies against donor cells. Lancet. 1966;2: 662–5.

21. Racusen LC, Solez K, Colvin R. Fibrosis and atrophy in the renal allograft: interim report and new directions. Am J Transplant. 2002;2(3):203–6.

22. Halloran PF. Call for revolution: A new approach to describing allograft deterioration. Am J Transplant. 2002;2(3):195–200.

23. Halloran PF, Melk A, Barth C. Rethinking chronic allograft nephropathy: the concept of accelerated senescence. J Am Soc Nephrol. 1999;10(1):167–81.

24. Bonsib SM. Acute rejection-associated tubular basement membrane defects and chronic allograft nephropathy. Kidney Int. 2000;58(5):2206–14.

25. Solez K, Vincenti F, Filo R. FK506 Kidney Transplant Study Group. Histopathologic findings from two-year protocol biopsies from a US multicenter kidney transplant trial [abstract]. Intl Cong Immunosuppression. 1997;124

26. Nickeleit V, Klimkait T, Binet IF, et al. Testing for polyomavirus type BK DNA in plasma to identify renal-allograft recipients with viral nephropathy. N Engl J Med. 2000;342(18):1309–15.

27. Billingham RE, Brent L, Medawar PB. Actively acquired tolerance of foreign cells. Nature. 1953;172:603–6.

28. Larsen CP, Elwood ET, Alexander DZ, et al. Long-term acceptance of skin and cardiac allografts after blocking CD40 and CD28 pathways. Nature. 1996;381:434–8.

29. Wells AD, Li XC, Li Y, et al. Requirement for T-cell apoptosis in the induction of peripheral transplantation tolerance. Nat Med. 1999;5(11):1303–7.

30. Toby P, Coates P, Thomson AW. Dendritic cells, tolerance induction and transplant outcome. Am J Transplant. 2002;2:299–307.

31. Takahashi T, Tagami T, Yamazaki S, et al. Immunologic self-tolerance maintained by CD25(+)CD4(+) regulatory T cells constitutively expressing cytotoxic T lymphocyte-associated antigen 4. J Exp Med. 2000;192(2):303–10.

32. Sakaguchi S, Sakaguchi N, Shimizu J, et al. Immunologic tolerance maintained by CD25+ CD4+ regulatory T cells: their common role in controlling autoimmunity, tumor immunity, and transplantation tolerance. Immunol Rev. 2001;182:18–32.

33. Taylor PA, Noelle RJ, Blazar BR. CD4(+)CD25(+) immune regulatory cells are required for induction of tolerance to alloantigen via costimulatory blockade. J Exp Med. 2001;193(11):1311–8.

34. Lai L, Kolber-Simonds D, Park KW, et al. Production of alpha-1,3-galactosyltransferase knockout pigs by nuclear transfer cloning. Science. 2002;295(5557):1089–92.

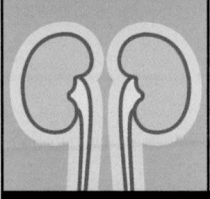

Chapter 85

Immunosuppressive Agents used in Transplantation

Anette Melk and Philip Halloran

INTRODUCTION

Ideally, a host would accept a renal transplant by induction of antigen-specific nonresponsiveness (immunologic tolerance). No current method induces specific tolerance, and transplantation requires immunosuppressive therapies. The current goal is to use immunosuppressive agents that are potent, selective, and reversible, with reliable delivery and long-term safety. Most therapies alter immune response mechanisms but are not immunologically specific, and a careful balance is required to find the dose that prevents rejection of the graft while minimizing the risks of oversuppression: the development of infection and certain types of cancer.

It is true that a few patients with organ transplants successfully can withdraw their immunosuppression without rejecting their grafts for long periods of time. Nevertheless, they are rare exceptions, and they may eventually reject, even after years.

Current immunosuppressive agents reduce acute rejection but do not induce tolerance, and few people can be withdrawn from immunosuppression without risk of rejection and graft loss. Antigen-specific T cells with reactivity to the foreign antigen persist in the host indefinitely. Nevertheless, some graft and host adaptation must occur because the level of immunosuppression required in the long-term patient is very low compared with the levels required in the first weeks. It is this adaptation that makes long-term immunosuppression possible;

Table 85.1 Classification of immunosuppressive therapies.

Classification of Immunosuppressive therapies	
Therapies	Examples
Physical therapies	
Irradiation	Total lymphoid irradiation, UV irradiation
Anatomic/physical manipulation	Thoracic duct drainage, thymectomy, splenectomy, plasma exchange, other depleting therapies
Pharmaceutical therapies: small molecule drugs	
Glucocorticoids	
Immunophilin-binding drugs	Calcineurin inhibitors: cyclosporine, tacrolimus
Inhibitors of cell division/nucleotide metabolism	TOR (target of rapamycin) inhibitors: sirolimus and everolimus
	Nonselective antiproliferative and cytotoxic drugs: azathioprine, cyclophosphamide
	Lymphocyte-selective specific drugs: mycophenolate mofetil, mizoribine (only in Japan), (potential drugs: brequinar, leflunomide)
	Deoxyspergualin
Pharmaceutical therapies: protein drugs	
Antibodies against immune proteins	Polyclonal antilymphocyte globulin (ALG): horse antithymocyte globulin (ATG), rabbit ALG or ATG
	Murine monoclonal antibodies: anti-CD3 (OKT3), anti-CD25, anti-LFA (leukocyte function-associated antigen), anti-ICAM (intercellular adhesion molecule)
	Humanized murine monoclonal antibodies: anti-IL-2R (interleukin 2 receptor)
Fusion proteins	Immunoglobulin based: CTLA4Ig
	Immunotoxins: IL-2 toxin
Cytokines and cytokine receptors	Natural immunosuppressive cytokines: IL-10, IL-4, transforming growth-factor β (TGFβ), interferon-γ (IFN-γ)
	Solubilized ligands, receptors: IFN-γ receptor
Peptides	Mimicking parts of immune molecules
Intravenous immunoglobulin (IVIg)	

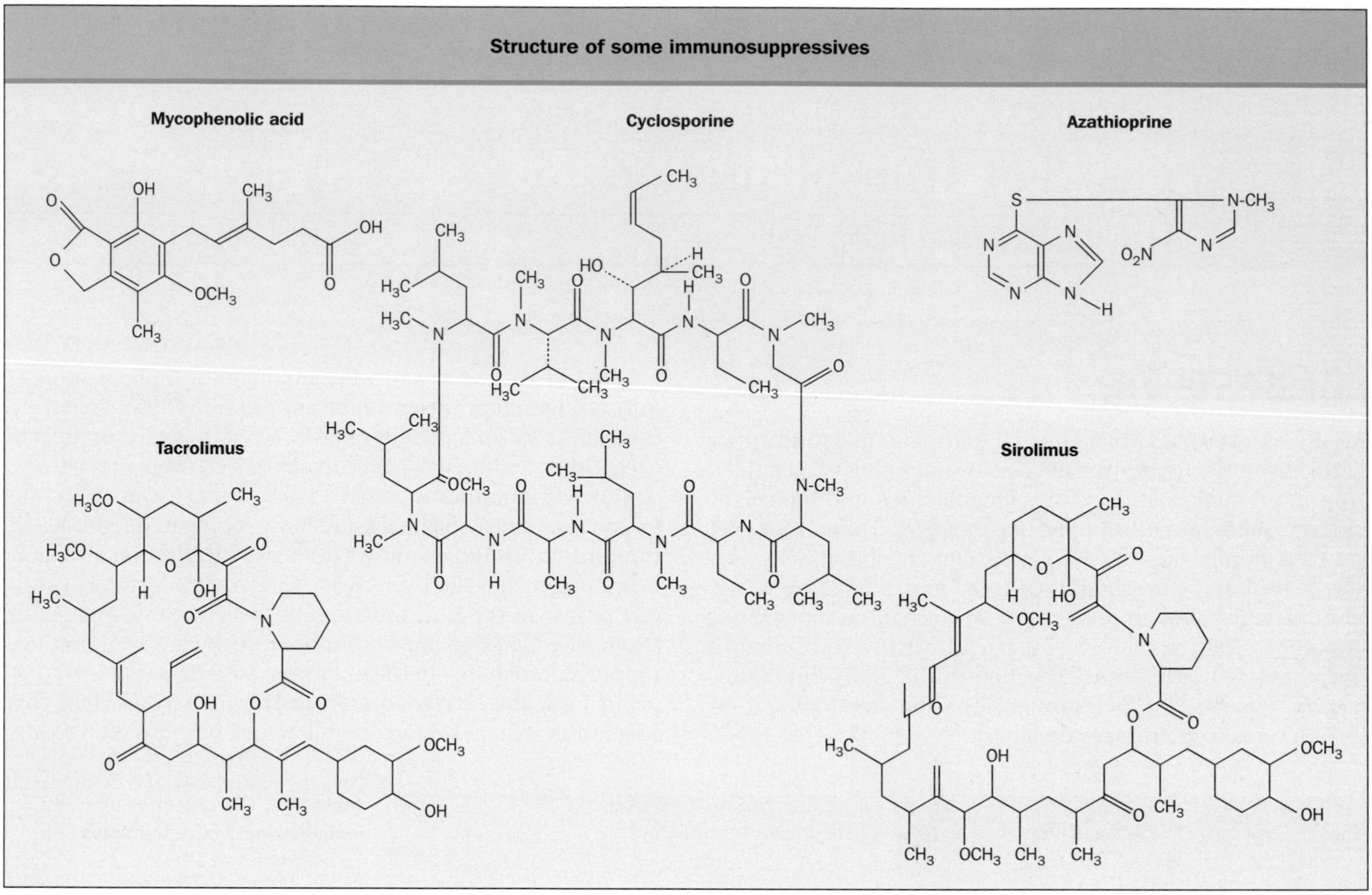

Figure 85.1 Structure of mycophenolic acid, cyclosporine, azathioprine, tacrolimus, and sirolimus. These are all small molecules with molecular weights of 320, 1203, 277, 804, and 914, respectively.

however, the long-term risk of cancer in the immunosuppressed patient remains increased. Thus the distinction between immunosuppression and induction of tolerance is partly artificial: all immunosuppression involves some apparent antigen specific adaptation, a downregulation of the host response to the graft; and many tolerance protocols involve some nonspecific immunosuppression.

The common immunosuppressive agents used in transplantation include the corticosteroids, azathioprine, mycophenolate mofetil, the calcineurin inhibitors cyclosporine and tacrolimus, and antibodies to cell surface antigens on lymphocytes (antilymphocyte globulin (ALG), monoclonal anti-CD3 (OKT3) and anti-CD25, and others) (Table 85.1). Newer agents are inhibitors of the target of sirolimus and everolimus, new monoclonal antibodies (e.g., anti-CD40L, anti-CD80, anti-CD86, anti-ICAM-1), and an antisense oligonucleotide for ICAM-1. The structures of some immunosuppressives are shown in Figure 85.1. Our discussion will focus on these agents and how they inhibit the immune response.

THE IMMUNE RESPONSE

The principles of host recognition and response to foreign antigens are discussed in Chapter 84. By the time transplantation is completed, the graft has experienced acute injury that increases the expression of major histocompatibility complex (MHC) molecules, including constitutively expressed (class I, HLA-A and HLA-B) and inducible (class II, HLA-DR) antigens by cells within the graft. Injury recruits lymphocytes and antigen-presenting cells (APCs: typically monocytes, macrophages, and dendritic cells) from the host. These injury-related events may influence the probability of rejection and may contribute to the superior outcome in transplants from live donors (with less injury) versus those from cadaveric donors.

Allorecognition of donor MHC molecules may occur either by the direct route (host T cells recognize donor MHC on donor cells) or indirectly (host T cells recognize donor MHC as peptides in the MHC groove of host APCs). T cell receptors (TCR) engaging MHC–peptide complexes provides signal 1. Costimulatory signals from the APC engaging receptors on the T cells provide signal 2 (Fig. 85.2). The major costimulatory molecules of the APC are B7-1/B7-2, which bind CD28 on the T cells. Activated T cells express CD40L, which can activate the APC by engaging CD40 on the APC, and Fas ligand (FasL), which binds Fas on other lymphocytes or other cells to induce apoptosis in the Fas-bearing cell. Activation of signals 1 and 2 is followed by T cell activation with production of many cytokines. Cytokines, such as interleukin 2 (IL-2), engage other specific receptors on the T cells to provide 'signal 3', the signal for cell division and

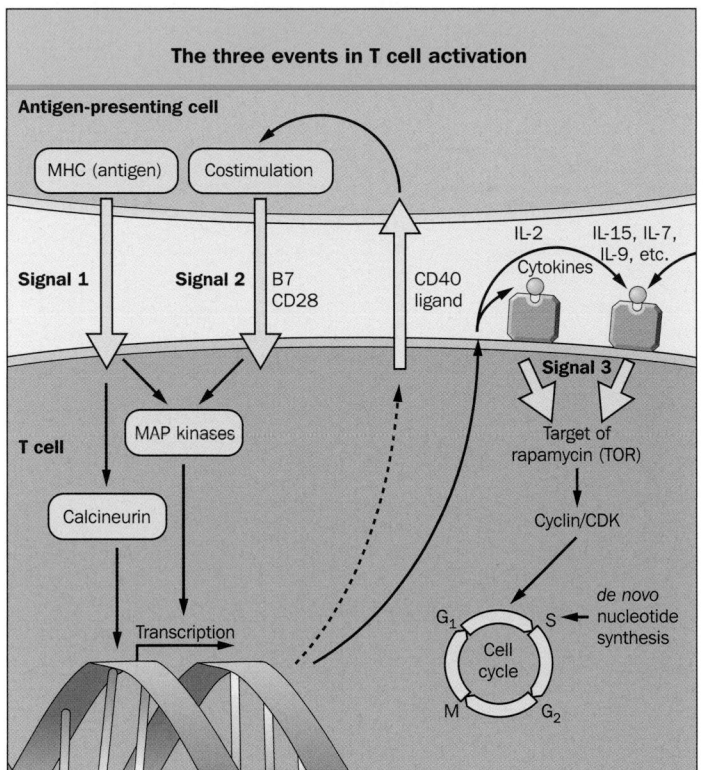

Figure 85.2 The three events in T cell activation. Engagement of the T cell receptor with the antigenic peptide in the context of self-MHC class II molecule leads to the activation of the calcineurin pathway and results in the induction of cytokine genes (e.g., IL-2) (signal 1). Signal 2, the co-stimulatory signal, involves the engagement of CD28 with members of the B7 family. This synergizes with signal 1 to induce cytokine production. Interaction between cytokine production and its corresponding receptor leads to induction of cell division, probably through the target of rapamycin (TOR) pathway. This constitutes signal 3.

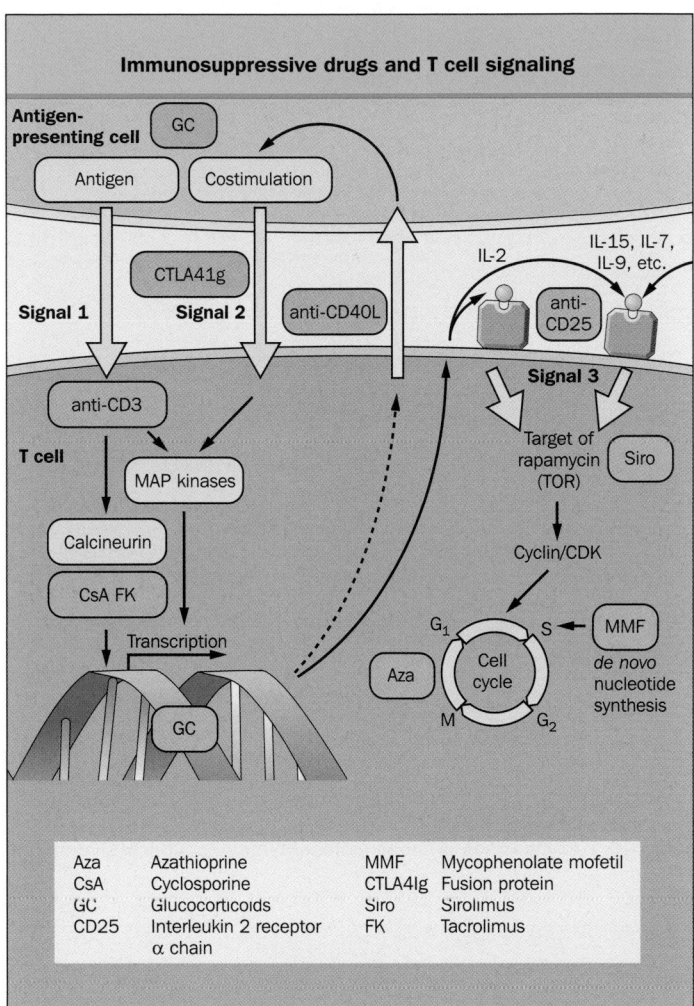

Aza	Azathioprine	MMF	Mycophenolate mofetil
CsA	Cyclosporine	CTLA4Ig	Fusion protein
GC	Glucocorticoids	Siro	Sirolimus
CD25	Interleukin 2 receptor α chain	FK	Tacrolimus

Figure 85.3 Effects of immunosuppressive drugs on T cell signaling.

CORTICOSTEROIDS

Corticosteroids, developed in the early 1950s, represent one of the principal types of agent used for both maintenance immunosuppression and treatment of acute rejection (Fig. 85.4).

Pharmacokinetics and absorption

The major corticosteroids used are prednisone or prednisolone (given orally with comparable efficacy) and methylprednisolone (given intravenously with 25% more potency). These agents are rapidly absorbed and have short plasma half-lives (60–180 min) but long biological half-lives (18–36 h). The effect of prednisone (dose/weight) is greater in the setting of renal failure or hypoalbuminemia, in women, and in the elderly, whereas less prednisone effect is observed in children. Prednisone should be dosed on body weight independent of obesity, whereas methylprednisolone should be administered based on ideal weight. In practice methylprednisolone is given in standard doses. Certain drugs can decrease steroid efficacy by increasing metabolism: rifampin (rifampicin), phenytoin, phenobarbital (phenobarbitone), and carbamazepine. In contrast, increased steroid effects may be observed in patients

clonal expansion. The engagement of CD40 by CD40L and the cytokines and growth factors from T cells regulate the T cell response, recruit and activate inflammatory cells, and alter adhesion molecules to cause mononuclear cells to accumulate in the graft. Depending on the type and degree of signaling, full activation of the T cell may occur, or T cells may undergo partial activation, apoptosis, anergy, or neglect (ignoring the antigen). T cells also bind via CD40L to CD40 on the B cell, thereby directing the switch from IgM to IgG production by the B cell and promoting the maturation of IgG-producing B cells.

Chemotactic factors (chemokines) and expression of adhesion proteins and foreign (MHC) antigens initially mediate localization (homing) of the T (CD4 and CD8) cells to the endothelium of the graft. Lymphocyte recirculation depends on being able to enter and leave lymphoid tissue.

CD8 T cells recognize peptide in the groove of class I MHC to become cytotoxic T cells (CTL). Graft rejection is associated with infiltration by cytotoxic (CD8) lymphocytes. Delayed type hypersensitivity may also be involved in T cell mediated damage. Antibody-mediated injury may also occur, and is damaging to endothelium (see Chapter 84).

Summaries of the effects of immunosuppressive drugs are presented in Figure 85.3, Tables 85.2 and 85.3.

Transplantation

Comparison of small molecule immunosuppressive drugs

Agent	Action	Toxicity	Uses in renal transplant
Corticosteroids ('steroids'): prednisone, methylprednisolone	Binds to steroid receptor to create a complex that enters the nucleus and binds to DNA and/or interacts with transcription factors and activators to alter transcription positively or negatively; acts particularly through regulation of factors AP-1 and NF-κB	'Cushingoid features', skin thinning, osteoporosis, diabetes	Prophylaxis against rejection; reversal of rejection; used in short-term high doses or long-term maintenance doses
Cyclosporine	Binds to intracellular protein called cyclophilin to create a complex that gives partial inhibition of essential phosphatase calcineurin	Nephrotoxicity, hyperlipidemia, hypertension, gum hyperplasia, skin changes; less neurotoxicity and diabetes than tacrolimus	Long-term oral maintenance therapy against rejection, usually with steroids
Tacrolimus	Binds to intracellular protein tacrolimus-binding protein to create a complex that inhibits calcineurin	Nephrotoxicity, more neurotoxicity and diabetes but less hypertension, gum hyperplasia, skin changes than with cyclosporine	Long-term maintenance therapy against rejection; 'rescue' of patients with severe or refractory rejection, usually with steroids
Sirolimus (everolimus (RAD) is an analog in development)	Binds to intracellular protein tacrolimus-binding protein to create a complex that inhibits 'target of rapamycin' (TOR), a kinase involved in signal transduction from cytokine/growth factor receptors to the nucleus to initiate cell cycling	Hyperlipidemia, thrombocytopenia leukopenia, impaired wound healing	Usually used with cyclosporine plus steroids
Mycophenolate mofetil	The ester bond is broken to release the active drug mycophenolate (MPA), which inhibits the enzyme inosine monophosphate dehydrogenase (IMPDH)	Diarrhea, occasional mild anemia, leukopenia	Usually used with cyclosporine or tacrolimus, plus steroids
Azathioprine	Incorporated as a purine into DNA; interferes with DNA synthesis; other effects on purine metabolism	Leukopenia, anemia, thrombocytopenia, megaloblastoid changes	Usually used with cyclosporine or tacrolimus, plus steroids

Table 85.2 Comparison of small molecule immunosuppressive agents

Some protein immunosuppressive drugs

Agent	Action	Toxicity	Uses in renal therapy
Mouse monoclonal anti-CD3 (OKT3)	Binds to CD3 complex associated with T cell receptor (TCR) and triggers then blocks the TCR and inactivates or kills the T cell; short half-life and eventually neutralized by antibody response	'First-dose' cytokine-release syndrome (fever, chills, 'flu-like' symptoms); plus occasional acute pulmonary edema, acute renal failure, encephalopathy	Prophylaxis against rejection; reversal of severe rejection; daily i.v. dose for 7–14 days
Polyclonal horse or rabbit antilymphocyte or antithymocyte globulin (ALG, ATG)	Contains many antibodies against proteins on lymphocytes that alter traffic, trigger, kill, and sequester the T and B lymphocytes	'First-dose' cytokine-release syndrome; thrombocytopenia, leukopenia	Prophylaxis against rejection; reversal of severe rejection
Humanized or chimeric anti-CD25 basiliximab and daclizumab	Binds to CD25 in IL-2 receptor complex; rendering all T cells resistant to IL-2; long half-life (same as human IgG, 21 days) once CD25 is saturated	Virtually none	Prophylaxis against rejection: interval dosing to saturate the CD25 for 4–16 weeks; usually used with cyclosporine plus steroids

Table 85.3 Some protein immunosuppressive agents.

receiving oral contraceptives, estrogens, ketoconazole, and erythromycin.

Mechanism of action

Corticosteroids have both anti-inflammatory and immunosuppressive actions. Lymphopenia and monocytopenia occur, with inhibition of lymphocyte proliferation, survival, activation, homing, and effector functions. Corticosteroids suppress production of numerous cytokines and vasoactive substances, including IL-1, tumor necrosis factor α (TNFα), IL-2, MHC class II, chemokines, prostaglandins (via inhibition of phospholipase A_2), and proteases. Corticosteroids also cause neutrophilia (often with a left shift), but neutrophil chemotaxis and adhesion are inhibited. They also affect nonhematopoietic cells.

Corticosteroids exert their effect by binding to corticosteroids receptors (CR), which belong to a family of ligand-regulated transcription factors called nuclear receptors. CR are normally present in the cytoplasm in an inactive complex with heat shock proteins (hsp90, hsp70, and hsp56). The binding of corticosteroids to the CR dissociates hsp from the CR and forms the active corticosteroids–CR complex, which migrates to the nucleus and dimerizes on palindromic DNA sequences

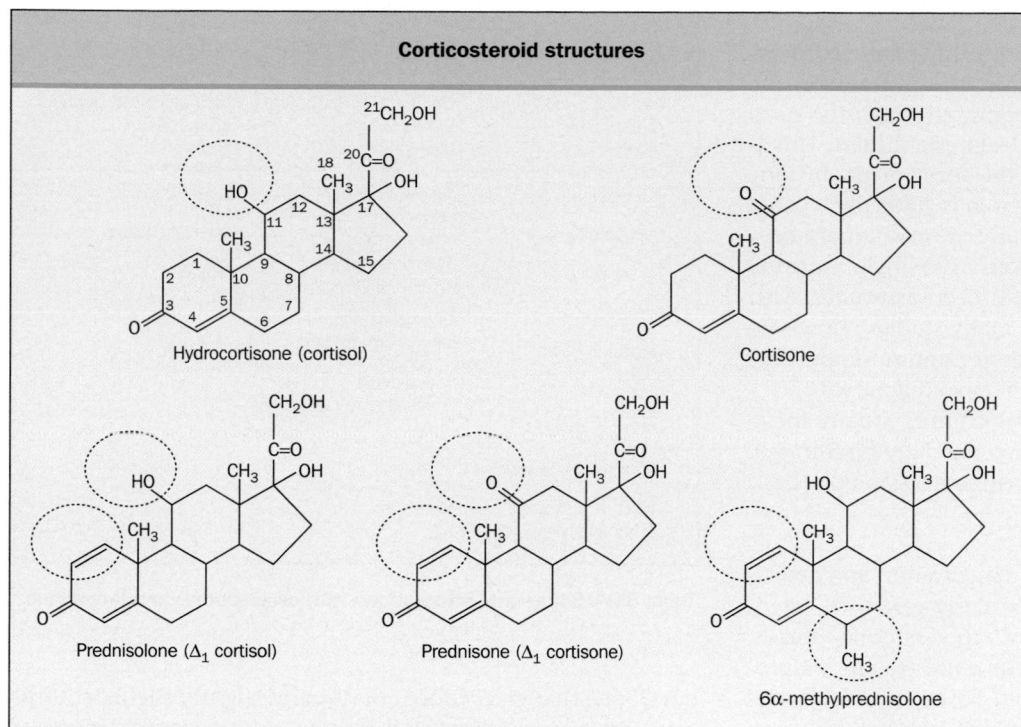

Figure 85.4 Structural formulae of the corticosteroids cortisol, cortisone, prednisolone, prednisone and 6α-methylprednisone.

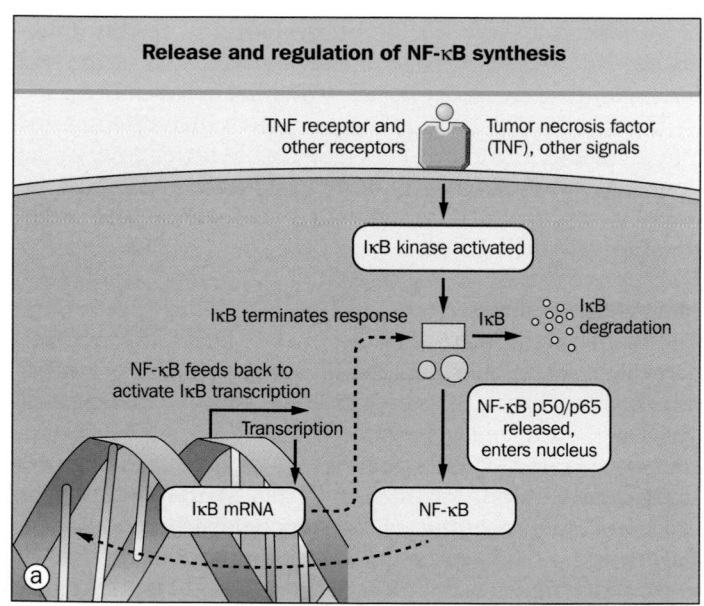

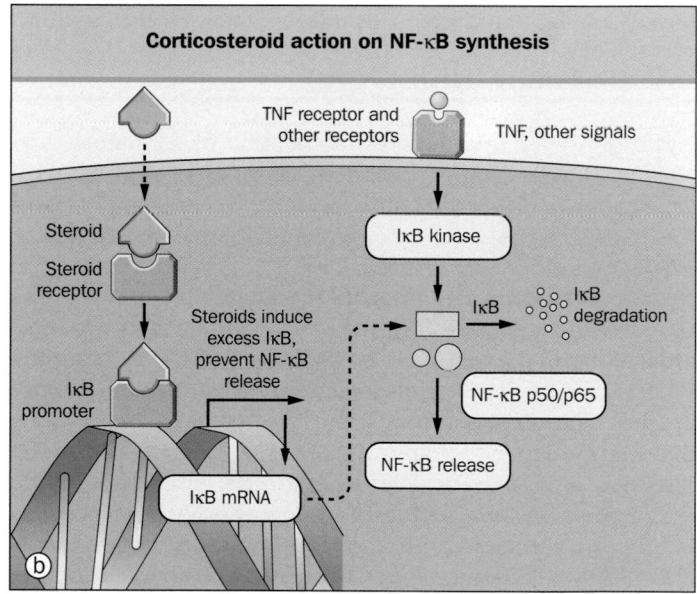

Figure 85.5 Corticosteroids and regulation of transcription factors. (a) The mechanism of NF-κB and its regulation by induction of synthesis of its inhibitor IκB. Activation of IκB kinase leads to IκB degradation; released NF-κB enters the nucleus and activates IκB transcription. Synthesis of IκB feeds back to terminate the cycle. (b) The mechanism of corticosteroid immunosuppression by inhibition of NF-κB. The corticosteroid–corticosteroid receptor complex migrates to the nucleus and interacts with the promoter of the IκB gene to induce the synthesis of excess IκB, the natural inhibitor of NF-κB. IκB in excess prevents the release of NF-κB to the nucleus upon stimulation by cytokines such as tumor necrosis factor (TNF).

in many genes, called the corticosteroid response element (CRE). The binding of CR in the promoter region of the target genes can lead to either induction or suppression of gene transcription (e.g., of cytokines). CR also exert effects by interacting directly with other transcription factors independent of DNA binding. One principal effect of corticosteroids on immune and inflammatory responses may be attributable to their ability to affect gene transcription by regulating key transcription factors involved in immune regulation: activator

protein-1 (AP-1) and nuclear factor-kappa B (NF-κB). The regulation of NF-κB by steroids may operate by induction of IkB, the inhibitor of NF-κB (Fig. 85.5). Other effects of corticosteroids are mediated through the release of a regulatory protein, lipocortin, which inhibits phospholipase A_2, thereby inhibiting the production of leukotrienes and prostaglandins. The total immunosuppressive effect of corticosteroids is complex, reflecting effects on cytokines, adhesion molecules, apoptosis, and activation of inflammatory cells.

Administration

In many transplant centers, high-dose intravenous corticosteroids (e.g., methylprednisolone 1 g) is administrated in the perioperative period as induction therapy, although the need for such high steroid pulses has not been established. This is followed by oral steroid, usually in the form of prednisone (e.g., 30 mg/d). The dose of the oral steroid is gradually tapered to a maintenance dose of 5–15 mg daily or on alternate days over a period of months, usually taken as a single morning dose. Complete steroid withdrawal has been associated with an increased incidence of rejection in many studies[1]; however, protocols using combinations with newer immunosuppressive agents show promise for this approach[2] (see Chapter 88).

The first-line treatment of acute rejection is usually intravenous methylprednisolone at 250–500 mg daily for 3 to 4 d. This regimen reverses about 75% of acute rejection episodes.

Side effects

Side effects of corticosteroid therapy are common and associated with significant morbidity, particularly cataracts, osteoporosis, and avascular necrosis of the femoral heads. Infection risk is excessive if high-dose pulse therapy is prolonged (typically > 3 g). Corticosteroid dosage should, therefore, be decreased gradually during rejection treatment even if serum creatinine fails to improve. Interestingly, corticosteroids are not associated with increased risk for malignancy.

CALCINEURIN INHIBITORS

Cyclosporine, a lipophilic cyclic peptide of 11 amino acid residues, and tacrolimus, a macrolide antibiotic, are drugs with similar mechanisms of action and have become major maintenance immunosuppressive agents used in transplantation.

Pharmacokinetics and drug interactions

Cyclosporine and tacrolimus are both variably absorbed and are metabolized extensively by the liver (via the cytochrome P450 system). Cyclosporine is excreted primarily by the biliary system. The absorption of some cyclosporine preparations may be bile dependent and, therefore, may be reduced in the presence of cholestatic liver disease. The absorption of the microemulsion formulation of cyclosporine or of tacrolimus is bile independent. Neither cyclosporine nor tacrolimus is affected by alterations in renal function. Both cyclosporine and tacrolimus bind to cells and to plasma components (primarily lipoproteins for cyclosporine and albumin for tacrolimus) in the blood; consequently, they must be assayed in whole blood. Many drugs and agents can affect cyclosporine and tacrolimus levels through effects on their absorption or metabolism (Table 85.4).

Cyclosporine is usually administered initially as 8–10 mg/kg daily in divided doses (or intravenously using one-third the oral dose over a 24-h period) during the induction phase, with target trough blood levels of 150–300 μg/L for the first 6 months. Doses are reduced after 6 months (typically 4–6 mg/kg daily); long-term target blood levels of 75–125 μg/L appear to provide comparable patient and graft survival as higher blood levels but with less risk of malignancy[3]. Recently a microemulsion form of cyclosporine (Neoral) has been

Drug interactions with cyclosporine and tacrolimus		
Increase cyclosporine or tacrolimus blood levels	Decrease cyclosporine or tacrolimus blood levels	Increase cyclosporine or tacrolimus nephrotoxicity
Ketoconazole	Anticonvulsants: phenytoin, phenobarbital (phenobarbitone), carbamazepine, others	Amphotericin B
Fluconazole		Aminoglycosides
Erythromycin		Cisplatin
Diltiazem	Antibiotics: rifampin (rifampicin), rifabutin	
Verapamil		
Nicardipine	Nonsteroidal anti-inflammatory drugs	
Metoclopramide		
Methylprednisolone		
Sirolimus (increases cyclosporin levels)		

Table 85.4 Some drug interactions with cyclosporine and tacrolimus.

developed that gives more reliable and slightly higher absorption and may require a slightly lower dose. Generic forms of cyclosporine are becoming available soon. Oral formulations of cyclosporine may not be equivalent and readily interchangeable, and knowledge of the characteristics of the oral formulations is necessary before switching between them.

Tacrolimus is 20- to 30-fold more potent than cyclosporine and, therefore, is administered at a 20-fold lower dose. Initial dosing is usually 0.2 mg/kg daily in divided doses orally (or 0.05–0.1 mg/kg daily intravenously over 24 h), and target trough levels are 5–20 μg/L.

Mechanism of action

Cyclosporine and tacrolimus act by inhibiting the calcium-dependent serine phosphatase calcineurin, which normally is rate limiting in T cell activation (Fig. 85.6). Calcineurin is activated by the engagement of the TCR, activation of tyrosine kinases and of phospholipase C-γ1, release of inositol triphosphate, release of calcium stored in the endoplasmic reticulum, and opening of membrane calcium channels. Calcineurin provides an essential step for transducing signal 1 to permit cytokine and CD40L transcription. A high cytoplasmic calcium concentration activates calcineurin, which then dephosphorylates regulatory sites in key transcription factors, the 'nuclear factors of activated T lymphocytes' ($NFAT_p$ and $NFAT_c$). This causes the NFAT proteins to translocate (with calcineurin) into the nucleus and bind to their DNA target sequences in the promoters of cytokine genes. Calcineurin has been implicated in the dephosphorylation of transcription factor Elk-1, and indirectly in the activation of Jun/AP-1 and NF-κB.

Cyclosporine and tacrolimus cross cell membranes freely and bind to immunophilins (cyclophilin and FK-binding protein 12 (FKBP12), respectively), which are ubiquitous and abundant intracellular proteins with isomerase activity. The active complex then binds to a site on calcineurin and blocks its interactions with key substrates. The inactivity of calcineurin

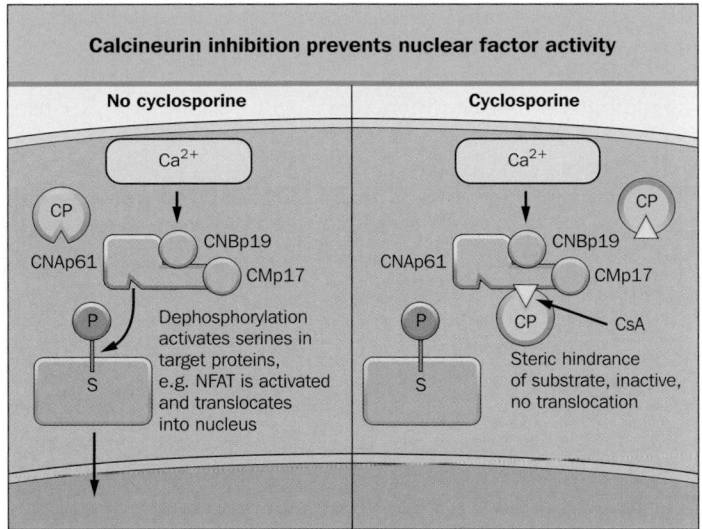

Figure 85.6 Calcineurin inhibition prevents nuclear factors (NFAT) dephosphorylation, activation, and translocation. In the absence of cyclosporine calcium activates calcineurin by exposing its phosphatase site, which, in turn, activates its target protein, for example, the transcription factor NFAT. Cyclosporine forms a complex with cyclophilin (CN), which binds to calcineurin (CN) and sterically hinders the phosphatase site.

bound to cyclosporine–cyclophilin or tacrolimus–FKBP12 is the key to the immunosuppressive effect and some of the toxic effects of these drugs. While inhibition of calcineurin has many effects on the T cell, the best studied is the blocking of the translocation (movement) of the NFAT proteins from the cytoplasm into the nucleus.

Cyclosporine and tacrolimus partially inhibit the calcineurin pathway at therapeutic blood levels (e.g., trough levels of 200 µg/L cyclosporine or 5–20 µg/L tacrolimus)[4]. However, even partial inhibition of calcineurin reduces the transcription of many genes associated with T cell activation (e.g., IL-2, interferon-γ (IFN-γ), granulocyte–macrophage colony-stimulating factor (GM-CSF), TNF-α, IL-4, CD40L). Therefore, the functional consequence of partial calcineurin inhibition is probably a quantitative limitation in cytokine production, CD40L expression, and lymphocyte proliferation. The effect of cyclosporine and tacrolimus on calcineurin *in vivo* is rapidly reversible, emphasizing the importance of patient compliance, drug monitoring, and reliable formulations for delivery. The effects on non-T cells could also be clinically significant.

Efficacy: comparison of cyclosporine and tacrolimus

To date, most studies suggest similar graft and patient survival with either cyclosporine or tacrolimus. In some clinical trials, tacrolimus was associated with fewer acute rejections. These trials are hard to interpret because it is not clear whether equivalent dosing strategies were used for the two drugs. In clinical practice, the rejection rates obtained with the drugs reflect the dose and the blood levels obtained. Conversion from cyclosporine to tacrolimus has been widely used as rescue therapy for refractory rejection in patients taking cyclosporine, with success rates as high as 75%[5]. The relative frequency of late graft deterioration in patients treated with tacrolimus versus cyclosporine has been similar.

Side effects

Cyclosporine and tacrolimus have similarities and differences in their toxicity profiles (see Table 85.2). Both can cause nephrotoxicity, hyperkalemia, hyperuricemia (with occasional gouty attacks), hypomagnesemia (secondary to urinary loss), hypertension, diabetes, and neurotoxicity (especially tremor). Certain side effects, such as gingival hyperplasia, hirsutism, hypertension, and hyperlipidemia, are more commonly observed with cyclosporine, whereas tremor and glucose intolerance are more common with tacrolimus. Cyclosporine may also be associated with coarsening of facial features, especially in children. Bone pain that is responsive to calcium channel blockers may also occur with cyclosporine use and sometimes may require changing to tacrolimus. Both cyclosporine and tacrolimus may contribute to the development of post-transplant diabetes, which regresses after dose reduction in some but not all patients. There has been concern that tacrolimus may rarely induce hypertrophic cardiomyopathy in children[6]. Some observations in mice suggest a role for calcineurin and NFAT proteins in cardiac development and heart failure, but there is no clinical evidence for this effect.

The most common serious problem with the calcineurin inhibitors is nephrotoxicity, with both a reversible vasomotor component and an irreversible component. Both cyclosporine and tacrolimus can cause acute elevations in serum creatinine that reverse with reduction of the dose, apparently caused by renal vasoconstriction which itself may be mediated by calcineurin inhibition. Chronically, cyclosporine and tacrolimus can induce a tubular atrophy and interstitial fibrosis with characteristic hyalinosis of the afferent arteriole. This lesion appears to result from long-standing renal vasoconstriction, perhaps mediated in part by an increase in local vasoconstrictors (angiotensin II, endothelin-1, thromboxane, and sympathetic nerve transmitters) and an inadequate vasodilatory response (impaired nitric oxide formation). The importance of this lesion is apparent from studies in cardiac and liver transplant recipients, in which cyclosporine or tacrolimus use is associated with progression to end-stage renal disease (ESRD) in many patients. This problem was more acute at a time when higher doses of cyclosporine were administered for longer periods. Currently, cyclosporine and tacrolimus toxicity is associated with only mild to moderate declines in renal function. However, as the number of patients with long-standing nonrenal transplants increases, there is increasing concern about future ESRD in this population. It is important to react to potential toxicity by renal biopsy to make the diagnosis and to reduce or stop the calcineurin inhibitor if possible.

Experimentally, cyclosporine nephropathy is exacerbated in the presence of sodium restriction/volume depletion and is lessened by treatment with angiotensin-converting enzyme (ACE) inhibitors, calcium channel blockers, vasodilators (hydralazine), and corticosteroids.

Cyclosporine and tacrolimus can cause hemolytic uremic syndrome, probably through endothelial dysfunction. This complication, which is usually associated with elevated drug levels, may respond to temporary withdrawal of cyclosporine or tacrolimus, plasma exchange, switching to another calcineurin inhibitor, or switching to another class of immunosuppressive drug.

Conclusions

Cyclosporine and tacrolimus are widely used for renal transplants. Tacrolimus is often considered for patients with multiple or severe rejection episodes, cardiovascular risks such as hypertension and hyperlipidemia, and other side effects such as gum hyperplasia and hirsutism. Another group that benefits from tacrolimus is children with growth retardation, because corticosteroids can be reduced or even stopped. Patients in whom cyclosporine seems to be more beneficial are those who experience or are at risk for the side effects of tacrolimus, such as the development of diabetes. Calcineurin inhibitor sparing protocols have also been attempted using newer immunosuppressive drugs such as mycophenolate and sirolimus. An increasing number of patients are being withdrawn from calcineurin inhibitors late following transplantation, but the rate of rejection and long-term safety of this practice remains to be established.

AZATHIOPRINE

Azathioprine, developed by Nobel Prize laureates Elion and Hitchings in the 1950s, has been widely used in renal transplantation for four decades. Azathioprine is a purine analog derived from 6-mercaptopurine (6-MP).

Pharmacokinetics

Azathioprine is administered orally at 2–3 mg/kg per d (when used without calcineurin inhibitors), but is often used at lower doses when it is supplementing cyclosporine or tacrolimus. It is metabolized in the liver to 6-MP and further converted to the active metabolite thioinosinic acid (TIMP) by the enzyme hypoxanthine–guanine phosphoribosyltransferase. Some but not all of the immunosuppressive activity of azathioprine is attributable to 6-MP. Because 6-MP is degraded by xanthine oxidase, allopurinol (a xanthine oxidase inhibitor) will increase the levels of TIMP. Therefore, azathioprine doses must be reduced by about two-thirds in patients taking allopurinol.

Mechanism of action

Azathioprine acts mainly as an antiproliferative agent by interfering with normal purine pathways, by inhibiting DNA synthesis, and by being incorporated itself into DNA, thereby affecting the synthesis of DNA and RNA[7]. TIMP interferes with the synthesis of guanylic and adenylic acids from inosinic acid by inhibiting several enzymes. TIMP is also converted to thioguanylic acid, a precursor for thiodeoxyguanosine triphosphate, which is incorporated into the developing strands of DNA and interferes with the DNA synthesis. TIMP also interferes with the induction of a number of coenzymes such as that produced by nicotinamide mononucleotide-adenylyl transferase. By inhibiting the synthesis of DNA and RNA, azathioprine suppresses the proliferation of activated B and T lymphocytes. In addition, azathioprine has been shown to reduce the number of circulating monocytes by arresting the cell cycle of promyelocytes in the bone marrow.

The antiproliferative action of azathioprine probably explains much of its observed effects on the immune system and its toxicity. Azathioprine shows some selectivity in its effects with certain cell types and different kinds of immune reaction[7]. For instance, it has been shown that the primary immune responses are more susceptible to azathioprine than the secondary responses despite the fact that there is a more rapid proliferation of lymphocytes during a secondary response.

Side effects

The major side effect of azathioprine is bone marrow suppression. All three hematopoietic cell lines can be affected, leading to leukopenia, thrombocytopenia, and anemia. The hematologic side effects are dose related and can occur late in the course of therapy. They are usually reversible upon dose reduction or temporary discontinuation of the drug. Other important side effects include increased susceptibility to infection, increased risk of malignancy, hepatotoxicity, and hair loss. The mean cell volume (MCV) is commonly increased in patients on full-dose azathioprine, and red cell aplasia can eventually result. Interactions between azathioprine and ACE inhibitors have been reported, causing anemia and leukopenia.

MYCOPHENOLATE MOFETIL

Dosage and pharmacokinetics

Mycophenolate mofetil, a semisynthetic ethyl ester of mycophenolic acid (MPA), is rapidly and completely absorbed and hydrolyzed by esterases to yield the active drug MPA. Doses are usually 1g orally twice daily. Mycophenolate blood levels are currently not monitored[8]. The mycophenolate dose should be reduced with active cytomegalovirus (CMV) infection. When mycophenolate is associated with diarrhea (a side effect of mycophenolate, see below), spreading the dose to 500 mg four times a day may be effective in controlling the diarrhea. A new enteric form of MPA is also being developed for use in renal transplantation.

MPA is metabolized in the liver by β-glucuronidase enzymes to the glucuronide (MPAG), which is excreted in the urine and to a lesser extent in the bile. There is an extensive enterohepatic circulation. Mycophenolate may not be absorbed well in the setting of antacids or cholestyramine use. MPAG levels are high in patients on mycophenolate, particularly in patients in renal failure, but the MPAG is itself probably inactive. The high levels of MPAG in the gut may explain the gastrointestinal toxicity, especially the diarrhea. MPA levels are lower in patients on cyclosporine than in patients on tacrolimus.

Mechanism of action

MPA acts by blocking *de novo* purine synthesis in lymphocytes. Purines can be generated either by *de novo* synthesis or by recycling (salvage pathway), and lymphocytes preferentially use *de novo* purine synthesis whereas other tissues such as brain use the salvage pathway. MPA uncompetitively inhibits inosine monophosphate dehydrogenase (IMPDH), which is the rate-limiting enzyme in the *de novo* synthesis of guanosine monophosphate (GMP) (Fig. 85.7). Inhibition of IMPDH creates a relative deficiency of GMP and a relative excess of AMP. GMP and AMP levels act as a control on *de novo* purine biosynthesis, which is essential for T and B lymphocyte proliferation but not for division in other cells. Therefore mycophenolate, by blocking IMPDH, creates a

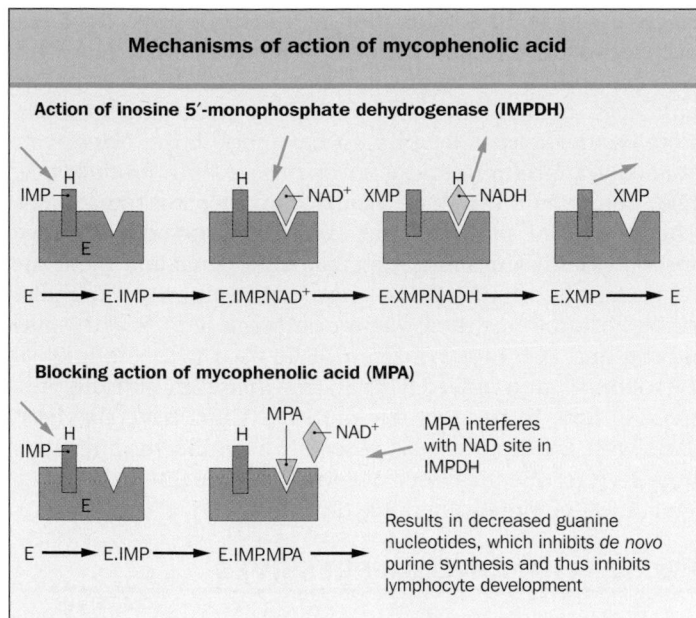

Mechanisms of action of mycophenolic acid

Action of inosine 5'-monophosphate dehydrogenase (IMPDH)

$$E \longrightarrow E.IMP \longrightarrow E.IMP.NAD^+ \longrightarrow E.XMP.NADH \longrightarrow E.XMP \longrightarrow E$$

Blocking action of mycophenolic acid (MPA)

MPA interferes with NAD site in IMPDH

Results in decreased guanine nucleotides, which inhibits *de novo* purine synthesis and thus inhibits lymphocyte development

$$E \longrightarrow E.IMP \longrightarrow E.IMP.MPA \longrightarrow$$

Figure 85.7 Mechanism of action of mycophenolic acid (MPA).
Inosine 5'-monophosphate (IMP) dehydrogenase (IMPDH) catalyzes the NAD^+-dependent oxidation of IMP to xanthosine 5'-monophosphate (XMP) (top). MPA, an uncompetitive inhibitor of IMPDH, binds to IMPDH after the release of NADH but before the production of XMP; it interferes with the NAD^+ site by mimicking the nicotinamide portion of the NAD^+ cofactor and a catalytic water molecule (bottom).

block in *de novo* purine synthesis that selectively interferes with proliferative responses of T and B lymphocytes, inhibiting clonal expansion and thus inhibiting antibody production, the generation of cytotoxic T cells, and the development of delayed type hypersensitivity.

The drug mizoribine also inhibits IMPDH but differs from mycophenolate in being a purine and a competitive inhibitor. Mizoribine is used for transplant immunosuppression in Japan.

Efficacy

Three multicenter clinical trials established the efficacy of mycophenolate in addition to cyclosporine plus corticosteroids in the primary prevention of renal allograft rejection in clinical renal transplantation compared with treatment with azathioprine or placebo. Mycophenolate reduced rejection by about 50% and also reduced the requirement for steroids or anti-CD3/antithymocyte globulin (OKT3/ATG) treatment for acute rejection and graft loss owing to rejection. As with other new immunosuppressives, this may be contributing to the improvement in long-term function and graft and patient survival. Triple therapy with mycophenolate, corticosteroids, and either cyclosporine or tacrolimus has become widespread in the management of transplant recipients. Mycophenolate can also be added to cyclosporine or tacrolimus for rescue and in reversing refractory acute rejection in renal transplant patients[9].

Side effects

The major toxicity is gastrointestinal, chiefly diarrhea, probably as a result of the high concentrations of MPAG in the

gut. Mycophenolate has no organ toxicity and does not cause lipid disorders but can cause increased CMV, leukopenia, and perhaps, mild anemia. MPA has been associated with protection from *Pneumocystis carinii* pneumonia (PCP) and may actually have some anti-PCP activity because *Pneumocystis carinii* has IMPDH activity. Mycophenolate should not be used in pregnant transplant patients since its safety in pregnancy has not yet been established.

Conclusion

Many renal transplant recipients now receive cyclosporine, mycophenolate, and corticosteroids, with or without antibody induction therapy, at least in the first year after renal transplantation. Mycophenolate is also used in transplantation for rescue from refractory rejection. The key features of mycophenolate are moderate potency with good selectivity and few major side effects and a high oral availability with no requirement for monitoring. The drawback of mycophenolate is expense and the necessity to use it with cyclosporine or tacrolimus. Trials of mycophenolate without cyclosporine or tacrolimus are in progress, but the use of monitoring will have to be reconsidered if mycophenolate becomes the main long-term immunosuppressant.

TARGET OF SIROLIMUS INHIBITORS

Sirolimus, a relative of tacrolimus, is a macrolide product of a soil organism found in Easter Island (Rapa Nui) and is related to the 'mycin' antibiotics. Like tacrolimus, sirolimus is a prodrug that must bind to FKBP12 to be active, but unlike tacrolimus–FKBP12, the sirolimus–FKBP12 complex cannot inhibit calcineurin. Everolimus (RAD) is an analog of sirolimus that is still in clinical trials but seems to have similar effectiveness and side-effect profile as sirolimus.

Mechanism of action

Sirolimus binds to FKBP but does not inhibit calcineurin or the calcium-dependent activation of cytokine genes (Fig. 85.8). Instead it inhibits signal 3 and thus cell division driven by certain cytokine receptors (e.g., IL-2). Unlike cyclosporine or tacrolimus, sirolimus blocks IL-2 mediated signal transduction and cell proliferation and blocks lymphocyte responses to IL-4, IL-7, IL-15, and other cytokines and growth factors[10]. Sirolimus–FKBP12 engages a kinase enzyme called 'target of rapamycin' or TOR[11]. TOR is critical in transducing a signal from these cytokine receptors to the mechanisms controlling cell division. TOR acts to inhibit an inhibitor, called 4E-BP1, and activate a ribosomal enzyme, p70 S6 kinase[12]. Both of these proteins are important for the translation of the mRNAs for certain proteins needed for progression from the G_1 phase to the S phase of DNA synthesis. Therefore cytokines must activate these steps to trigger G_1 to S progression and act via TOR and its effects on 4E-BP1 and p70 S6 kinase.

Sirolimus has complementary effects with cyclosporine and anti-CD25 antibodies; this relation has been referred to as the 'cytokine paradigm'[13]. Sirolimus is a potent immunosuppressive, particularly when paired with cyclosporine, but bioavailability has been problematic and monitoring is necessary.

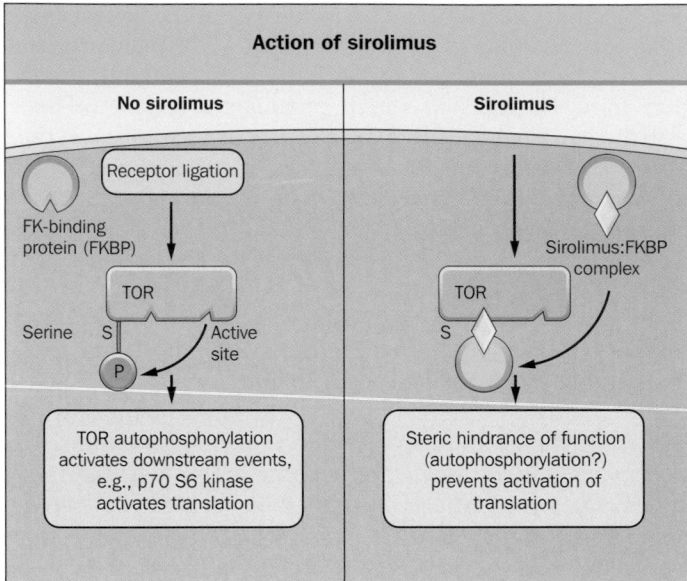

Figure 85.8 Action of sirolimus. In the absence of sirolimus, receptor ligation causes activation of a kinase enzyme called target of rapamycin (TOR). Sirolimus prevents the activation of TOR by binding to FK-binding proteins (FKBP) and preventing autophosphorylation of TOR through steric hindrance.

Pharmacokinetics

Sirolimus is available as tablet or oral solution. Maximal concentrations are reached after 1 h. The drug is mainly metabolized by the cytochrome P450 system, like tacrolimus and cyclosporine. The drug is more than 90% excreted by the biliary system, but great variations in elimination time have been found, especially prolonged times in patients with hepatic impairment. Sirolimus is widely distributed in tissues, including blood cells. Detection of drug levels uses whole blood samples. Interactions have been shown for high-fat meals and the drugs diltiazem and ketoconazole leading to increased sirolimus levels; whereas rifampin (rifampicin) and anticonvulsants decreased sirolimus levels. Sirolimus also results in an increase in mycophenolate levels. The more important interaction is with cyclosporine: sirolimus levels are increased by concomitant administration of the micro-emulsion formulation of cyclosporine and sirolimus increases cyclosporin levels about two-fold through competition for the cytochrome P450 system.

In clinical trials, sirolimus is given as a once daily dose of 2 mg or 5 mg, respectively. Whether monitoring or weight adjustment is needed is not yet clear. Because of the interaction cyclosporine levels must be adjusted accordingly.

Clinical trials

Clinical trials of sirolimus and everolimus in combination with cyclosporine and corticosteroids have been successful at reducing biopsy-proven acute rejection in renal transplant recipients compared to placebo or azathioprine. Whether sirolimus or everolimus can be used without calcineurin inhibitors is being evaluated: a study comparing sirolimus plus corticosteroids with cyclosporine plus corticosteroids suggested that sirolimus alone may be approximately equivalent

to cyclosporine. In combination with cyclosporine, sirolimus decreases acute rejection episodes by about 85–90%. However, the addition of sirolimus or everolimus to cyclosporine enhances cyclosporine nephrotoxicity and hypertension. Combinations with tacrolimus have not been extensively studied yet. Sirolimus and mycophenolate both produce anemia, and combining these agents may increase the anemia. The toxicity of sirolimus and everolimus includes impaired wound healing thrombocytopenia, leukopenia and moderate to severe hyperlipidemia, but not hypertension. In the pilot studies of sirolimus there was an outbreak of PCP, with some deaths, and PCP prophylaxis must be used with sirolimus or everolimus[14], and indeed with all transplant immunosuppressives, at least in the first few months. There have also been cases with aphthous mouth ulcers. No significant differences were seen for the incidence of CMV and Epstein–Barr virus as well as for lymphoproliferative disorders.

PROTEIN IMMUNOSUPPRESSIVES

Protein immunosuppressives have been used in renal transplantation since the introduction of antilymphocyte globulin (ALG) or antithymocyte globulin (ATG), followed by mouse monoclonal anti-CD3 (OKT3). Recently, humanized mouse monoclonal antibodies have been introduced, and many other monoclonal or fusion proteins, such as CTLA4Ig, await evaluation. Novel strategies such as use of antisense RNA, gene therapy, and various peptides are under development. However, none of the latter group shows promise of full-scale clinical trials soon. Table 85.3 gives an overview of protein or peptide-based biologic immunosuppressives. Some of these agents are very potent and have long-term consequences, including viral infections (CMV, Epstein–Barr virus) and a higher long-term rate of lymphomas.

Polyclonal antibodies

Polyclonal ALT/ATG antibodies are crude polyclonal IgG preparations that remain effective but are unselective. They are usually made in horses or rabbits and consist of IgG preparations from animals repeatedly immunized against human lymphoid cell lines, lymphocytes, or thymocytes. They are absorbed with other cell types to reduce cross-reacting antibodies against other human tissue components, but there is always some residual undesirable activity. They act in three ways: by activating or altering the function of lymphocytes, by lysing lymphoid cells, and by altering the traffic of lymphoid cells and sequestering them. They are potently immunosuppressive but often produce serious side effects. By triggering T cells, they generate significant first-dose effects, with release of TNF-α, IFN-γ, and other cytokines, causing a first-dose reaction (flu-like symptoms, fever, and chills; see below).

Monoclonal antibodies against immune proteins

The first monoclonal antibody for routine antirejection therapy in renal transplantation was murine monoclonal anti-CD3 (OKT3). The CD3 complex is the transducer associated with the TCR and is essential for T cell triggering. OKT3 binds to the ε-chain of this complex and paralyzes T cell recognition, but at the expense of triggering the T cells to release

TNF-α and other cytokines, which give fevers and other flu-like first-dose symptoms. OKT3 is highly effective in reducing CD3 counts and creates potent suppression of T cells for several days, during which there is virtually no T cell function. However, being a mouse protein, the monoclonal antibody evokes a host antibody response that neutralizes the antibody and renders it useless. The usual OKT3 dose is 5 mg intravenously every day for 7, 10, or 14 days. It can be used as prophylaxis against rejection or as treatment to reverse rejection.

OKT3 must be used with caution because of the severe first-dose effects or 'cytokine release syndrome'. It is wise to premedicate the patient with corticosteroids, antihistamine, and possibly, indomethacin. The first-dose reaction can produce acute renal failure or pulmonary edema as a result of capillary leak. Pulmonary edema is more frequent if the patient has volume expansion. Therefore, it is often necessary for a patient requiring OKT3 to undergo dialysis before the first dose to minimize the risks of pulmonary edema. First-dose reactions may include gastrointestinal upset (diarrhea), headache, and rarely, severe CNS manifestations such as cerebral edema or cortical blindness. The second and third doses may also be associated with symptoms, but the later doses may be asymptomatic.

Many other mouse monoclonal antibodies are or have been in development, but few will make it into the clinic as transplant immunosuppressives. The murine monoclonal products will probably be replaced by humanized or chimeric monoclonal antibodies (Fig. 85.9), which originate from mouse or rat monoclonal products. To humanize a mouse monoclonal, the sequences encoding the antigen-combining sites are transferred into human immunoglobulin genes, which are transfected into mouse hybridomas to secrete the new product with the specificity of the original mouse monoclonal antibody in a human immunoglobulin framework. Chimeric antibodies use the same strategy but for the entire V region.

Two new monoclonal anti-CD25 antibodies are in use: one humanized (daclizumab) and one chimeric (basiliximab). Both antibodies are directed against CD25, the IL-2 receptor 55kDa α-chain. The IL-2 receptor consists of three transmembrane protein chains: CD25, CD122, and CD132. CD25 is present on nearly all activated T cells but not on resting T cells. IL-2 induces clonal expansion of activated T cells. Although CD25 does not transduce the signal, it is responsible for the association of IL-2 with the β- and γ-chains, which triggers the activated T cell to undergo rapid proliferation. These antibodies bind to activated T cells and render them resistant to IL-2 by blocking, shedding, or internalizing the receptor; they may also deplete and sequester some activated T cells. However, IL-2 receptor functions are partially redundant; because other cytokine receptors have overlapping functions, e.g., IL-15 receptors. Therefore, saturating IL-2 receptors produces stable but relatively mild immunosuppression and is only effective when other immunosuppressives are also used (e.g., cyclosporine, corticosteroids).

The studies on the two monoclonal antibodies produced similar results[15–17]. Both compounds (plus cyclosporine and corticosteroids) reduced the frequency of acute rejection by about one-third, with virtually no side effects. These studies show no evidence of increased infections, even with CMV.

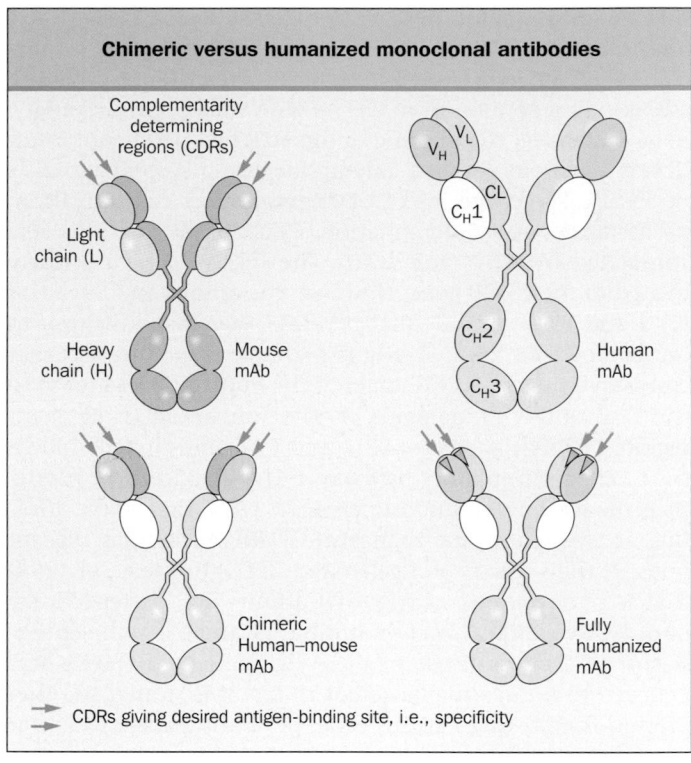

Chimeric versus humanized monoclonal antibodies

CDRs giving desired antigen-binding site, i.e., specificity

Figure 85.9 Chimeric versus humanized monoclonal antibodies. Chimeric monoclonal antibodies consist of human constant (C) regions and mouse heavy and light chain variable (V) regions. A chimeric antibody therefore, retains the binding specificity of the original mouse antibody but contains fewer amino acid sequences foreign to the human immune system. Humanized monoclonal antibodies retain only minimum necessary parts of the mouse antibody. These complementary-determining regions (CDRs) are built into a human antibody, i.e., only the antigen-binding site is combined with human V region framework and human C region sequences. These monoclonal antibodies retain the ability to recognize the target sequence.

The use of anti-CD25 antibodies did not result in increased malignancies or post-transplant lymphoproliferative disorders. Recent studies suggest a potential role of those antibodies in replacement of corticosteroids and reduction of calcineurin inhibitors. Another potential application is delayed graft function when the use of calcineurin inhibitors should be avoided. However, given the limited efficacy of anti-CD25 monoclonals, they are not generally used for prophylaxis in highly sensitized patients or for reversing rejection episodes.

Monoclonal anti-CD40 ligand

The monoclonal anti-CD40L has produced relatively long-lasting graft survival in mice, and in monkeys[18]. CD40 is expressed on antigen presenting cells and interacts with its ligand on activated T cells. The interaction is an essential signal for B cell class switching (IgM to IgG) and anti-CD40L may be useful for controlling alloantibody responses. Anti-CD40L does not produce tolerance: it produces sustained immunosuppression followed by a long period of stability, which then eventually passes off. Anti-CD40L is an immunosuppressive drug that can be used with or without CTLA4Ig. Recent phase I trials were terminated because of excessive occurrence of thromboses and acute rejections.

CTLA4 immunoglobulin and anti-CD80 and -CD86 antibodies

CTLA4Ig is a fusion protein (Fig. 85.10) created by combining a B7-binding domain from CTLA4 with the Fc portion of IgG. As noted above, the binding of the TCR by MHC is not a sufficient signal to activate T lymphocytes: a second signal is necessary. The triggering of CD28 promotes T cell activation, proliferation, and differentiation. CD28 binds to and is also stimulated by B7–1 and B7–2. The CTLA4 gene is closely related to the CD28 gene. However, the affinity of CTLA4 for B7–1 and B7–2 exceeds that of CD28 thereby allowing it to out compete CD28. CTLA4Ig is a soluble fusion protein that consists of the variable domain of the human CTLA4 fused to the C_H2 and C_H3 domains of the human IgG1 constant region. CTLA4Ig saturates B7–1 and B7–2 and thereby blocks the CD28 costimulatory pathway. CTLA4Ig in human psoriasis is moderately immunosuppressive. CTLA4Ig is more effective as a single agent than anti-CD40L antibodies. Recent phase II trials use second generation CTLA4Igs (e.g., LEA294) that were developed with greater affinity and better efficacy in order to avoid calcineurin inhibitors. There is some enthusiasm for long-term use of CTLA4Ig. Initially CTLA4Ig was believed to induce tolerance but in fact it is similar to other immunosuppressives at this time, permitting adaptation but not inducing tolerance.

Monoclonal antibodies against B7–1 and B7–2 (CD80 and CD86) have been used in nonhuman primates and have been found to delay the onset of rejection. In combination with cyclosporine or corticosteroids they were able to prolong graft survival. Clinical trials might emerge based on this data.

Intravenous immunoglobulin

There is a considerable potential for intravenous immunoglobulin (IVIg) in control of antibody responses and possibly other responses in transplantation[19]. It is used in studies together with plasma exchange, tacrolimus and mycophenolate both to desensitize highly immunized patients before transplantation and also to treat recipients suffering from humoral rejection after transplantation. The mechanism of action of IVIg is not understood. It may work by increasing immunoglobulin metabolism, by triggering inhibitory Fc receptors on immune cells, possibly through triggering of inhibitory phosphatases such as SHP-1, or by inducing apoptosis of B cells. Although IVIg has many applications in transplantation, its high cost and limited supply are serious barriers. Perhaps its action can be achieved more cheaply in other ways (e.g., by new monoclonal antibodies). IVIg can also occasionally produce acute renal failure[20].

OTHER IMMUNOSUPPRESSIVES

There are several drugs in various stages of development for which no firm plans as clinical transplant immunosuppressives are known. Leflunomide is an inhibitor of the enzyme dihydroorotic acid dehydrogenase, which is a key enzyme in pyrimidine synthesis. Leflunomide has been in phase II and III trials for rheumatoid arthritis and it has been shown to be immunosuppressive in transplant models. A recent case report[21] advocates its use in renal transplantation.

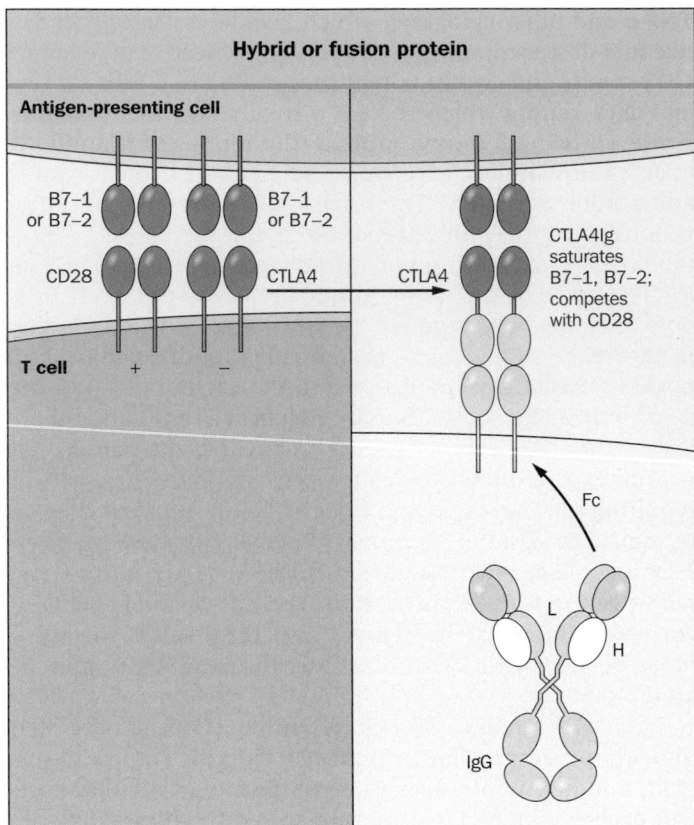

Figure 85.10 Hybrid or fusion protein. A ligand is combined with the Fc portion of the IgG H chain, e.g., CTLA4Ig. In theory, this fusion should prevent the costimulatory signal required for activation of T lymphocytes (see text).

FTY720, derived from metabolite of *Isaria sinclairii*, is an analogue of sphingosine-1-phosphate. It does not inhibit T cell proliferation but alters lymphocyte trafficking and thereby has an interesting mechanism of action. It acts by triggering sphingosine phosphate receptors. Lymphocytes enter lymphoid tissues in their normal circulation, then must re-enter the lymph vessels. If their sphingosine receptors are triggered they cannot re-enter the lymph vessels and are trapped in the lymphoid tissues[22]. This prevents them from infiltrating the graft and results in suppression of graft rejection. A phase II trial has been completed but cardiac toxicity emerged as a significant problem. This dose-dependent bradycardia is of particular concern during the 'loading phase'. At present, no new patients are enrolled in clinical trials.

An antibody against intercellular adhesion molecule 1 (ICAM-1) that blocks the interaction between ICAM-1 and leukocyte function-associated antigen-1 (LFA-1) as well as an antisense oligonucleotide based on the mRNA sequence of ICAM-1 (ISIS 2302) that prevents protein translation have been explored as possible immunosuppressives and anti-inflammatory agents with promising results. A monoclonal antibody against LFA-1 was compared to rabbit antithymocyte globulin for induction therapy. The results for incidence of acute rejection and graft survival were comparable. There is also interest in a humanized monoclonal anti-CD20 antibody (Rituximab) for depleting B cells and stopping alloantibody production in sensitized patients and those with alloantibody-mediated rejection.

REFERENCES

1. Kasiske BL, Chakkera HA, Louis TA, Ma JZ. A meta-analysis of immunosuppression withdrawal trials in renal transplantation. J Am Soc Nephrol. 2000;11(10):1910–17.
2. Landsberg DN, Cole EH, Russell D, et al. Renal transplantation without steroids – One year results of a multicentre Canadian pilot study. Transplant. 2000;69(8):S134.
3. Dantal J, Hourmant M, Cantarovich D, et al. Effect of long-term immunosuppression in kidney-graft recipients on cancer incidence: randomised comparison of two cyclosporin regimens. Lancet. 1998;351:623–8.
4. Batiuk TD, Kung L, Halloran PF. Evidence that calcineurin is rate-limiting for primary human lymphocyte activation. J Clin Invest. 1997;100:1894–901.
5. Woodle ES, Thistlethwaite JR, Gordon JH, et al. A multicenter trial of FK506 (tacrolimus) therapy in refractory acute renal allograft rejection: a report of the Tacrolimus Kidney Transplantation Rescue Study Group. Transplant. 1996;62:594–9.
6. Atkison P, Joubert G, Barron A, et al. Hypertrophic cardiomyopathy associated with tacrolimus in paediatric transplant patients. Lancet. 1995;345:894–6.
7. Elion GB. The pharmacology of azathioprine. Ann NY Acad Sci. 1993;685:400–7.
8. Mathew TH. Tricontinental Mycophenolate Mofetil Renal Transplantation Study Group. A blinded, long-term, randomized multicenter study of mycophenolate mofetil in cadaveric renal transplantation. Results at three years. Transplant. 1998;65:1450–4.
9. The Mycophenolate Mofetil Renal Refractory Rejection Study Group. Mycophenolate mofetil for the treatment of refractory, acute, cellular renal transplant rejection. Transplant. 1996;61:722–9.
10. Sehgal SN. Immunosuppressive profile of rapamycin. Ann NY Acad Sci. 1993;696:1–8.
11. Brown EJ, Schreiber SL. A signaling pathway to translational control. Cell. 1996;86:517–20.
12. Chung J, Kuo CJ, Crabtree GR, Blenis J. Rapamycin-FKBP specifically blocks growth-dependent activation of and signaling by the 70 kD S6 protein kinases. Cell. 1992;69:1227–36.
13. Kahan BD. Camardo JS. Rapamycin: clinical results and future opportunities. Transplant. 2001;72(7):1181–93.
14. Murgia MG, Jordan S, Kahan BD. The side-effect profile of sirolimus: a phase I study in quiescent cyclosporin-prednisone-treated renal transplant patients. Kidney Int. 1996;49:209–16.
15. Vincenti F, Kirkman R, Light S, et al. Interleukin-2-receptor blockade with Daclizumab to prevent acute rejection in renal transplantation. N Engl J Med. 1998;338:161–5.
16. Nashan B, Moore R, Amlot P, et al. Randomised trial of basiliximab versus placebo for control of acute cellular rejection in renal allograft recipients. Lancet. 1997;350:1193–8.
17. Bumgardner GL, Hardie I, Johnson RW, et al. Results of 3-year phase III clinical trials with daclizumab prophylaxis for prevention of acute rejection after renal transplantation. Transplant. 2001;72(5):839–45.
18. Kirk AD, Harlan DM, Armstrong NN, et al. CTLA4-Ig and anti-CD40 ligand prevent renal allograft rejection in primates. Proc Natl Acad Sci USA. 1997;94:8789–94.
19. Glotz D, Haymann JP, Sansonetti N, et al. Suppression of HLA-specific alloantibodies by high-dose intravenous immunoglobulins (IVIg). A potential tool for transplantation of immunized patients. Transplant. 1993;56:335–7.
20. Cayco AV, Perazella MA, Hayslett JP. Renal insufficiency after intravenous immune globulin therapy: A report of two cases and an analysis of the literature. J Am Soc Nephrol. 1997;8:1788–94.
21. Pascual J, Orte J, Marcen R, et al. Use of leflunomide in human renal transplantation. Transplant. 2001; 72(10):1709.
22. Mandala S, Hajdu R, Bergstrom J, et al. Alteration of lymphocyte trafficking by sphingosine-1-phosphate receptor agonists. Science. 2002;296(5566):346–9.

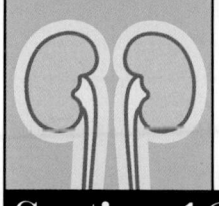

Chapter 86

Evaluation of Renal Transplant Donor and Recipient

Andries J Hoitsma and Lukas B Hilbrands

RECIPIENT

Introduction

In the early days of renal transplantation, the mortality rate of patients subjected to the procedure was high. This was caused by the combined risks of the operative procedure and the intensive immunosuppressive treatment that followed. Through substantial improvements in treatment, the risk of death in the first year after renal transplantation has decreased to below 5%. As a consequence, the selection criteria used in evaluating a potential candidate for renal transplantation no longer need to differ from those used in patients undergoing comparable operative procedures. Although renal transplantation is not a life-saving operation, it is the best treatment option for those patients with end-stage renal disease (ESRD) that are accepted to the waiting list.[1] However, not all patients can be listed for transplantation because of an unacceptable risk of complications. In aged patients, patients with complicating diseases, or those in whom prolonged immunosuppression carries particular risks, it may therefore be very difficult to weigh the advantages of renal transplantation against its risk. This has resulted in considerable variation in acceptance criteria at different centers. In a survey conducted in the USA in 147 centers, the approach appeared particularly variable with regard to the presence of viral hepatitis and cardiovascular disease (Fig. 86.1)[2]. In a more recent survey of European transplant centers also controversy was found with respect to oxalosis, gastric ulcers, and lack of compliance[3].

Careful screening of the recipient is required and this can best be done by using standardized procedures. Areas deserving particular attention are given in Table 86.1. Detailed guidelines to screen a recipient for renal transplantation have been published,[4] and a more recent overview is given by the EBPG (European Best Practice Guidelines for Renal Transplantation) expert group on renal transplantation[5]. An important aspect is that all candidates for renal transplantation should be informed about mortality, morbidity, results compared with dialysis, and also about data concerning different sources of kidneys, including marginal donors.

Exclusion policies in renal transplant programs

Conditions

Condition	Centers excluding a condition (%)
Positive for HIV antibodies	92
Inoperable multivessel coronary artery disease	74
Older than 70 years	34
Positive for hepatitis B surface antigen	22
Positive for hepatitis C antibodies	5

Figure 86.1 Exclusion policies in renal transplant programs.
Evaluation of candidates for renal transplantation in 147 transplant centers in the USA. (With permission from Ramos et al.[2].)

Assessment of the patient before transplantation

History and physical examination
- Cause of renal failure
- Infections (especially urinary tract, viral, tuberculosis)
- Previous transplantation
- Cardiovascular risk
- Previous or current malignancies
- Respiratory, gastrointestinal disease
- Pregnancies
- Dental evaluation

Special laboratory and radiologic examinations
- Screening for HIV, hepatitis B and C, cytomegalovirus, Epstein–Barr virus, tuberculosis (Purified protein derivative, PPD skin test)
- Liver function tests
- Calcium and phosphate metabolism
- Urine culture
- Electrocardiogram
- Chest radiograph
- Abdominal ultrasound
- Prostate specific antigen (PSA) for men > 60 years old

Immunologic investigations
- Blood group and HLA typing
- Screening for HLA antibodies and autoreactive antibodies
- Cross-matching

Table 86.1 Assessment of the patient before transplantation.

Routine assessment of the patient before transplantation

In Table 86.1 the most important items that should be carefully worked out before transplantation are listed. Several of these items are discussed in the section about special patient groups. Patients should preferably have a body mass index below 30, because the outcome of renal transplantation in obese patients is worse than that in nonobese patients[6].

Abdominal ultrasound gives information on the kidney size, and in patients with polycystic disease it may assist in reaching a decision regarding the need for pretransplant nephrectomy. The discovery of asymptomatic gallstones is used as a reason for laparoscopic cholecystectomy before transplantation in some centers, since there is some evidence of an increased risk for complications after surgery in renal transplant patients[7].

Immunologic investigations before transplantation

ABO blood groups

The ABO blood group antigens act as strong transplantation antigens and, therefore, there should be ABO compatibility between donor and recipient. An exception can possibly be made for the transplantation of kidneys of blood group A2 into O or B recipients, but this is only if the pretransplant titer of anti-A antibody in the recipient is low[8]. Blood group antigens other than ABO (e.g., rhesus antigen) do not behave as histocompatibility antigens.

HLA antigens

The HLA-A, HLA-B, and HLA-DR antigens are the major histocompatibility (MHC) antigens in transplantation. In animal models, graft survival shortens with increasing mismatches for MHC antigens. In clinical transplantation, such a correlation is more difficult to detect, mainly because immunosuppressive therapy dampens the rejection response. Nevertheless, in large studies of cadaveric transplants a 5–10% increased survival over 3–10 years can be demonstrated in completely matched compared with mismatched kidneys. Grafts fully matched for all HLA-A, HLA-B, and HLA-DR antigens should, therefore, be given preference in donor–recipient selection. Donor–recipient combinations fully mismatched for all four B and DR antigens should be used only after weighing the potential decrease in kidney survival with other variables such as the waiting time of the recipient and the potential of matching (ethnic diversity). As will be discussed below, this does not apply to living donor transplantation.

In cadaveric kidneys mismatched for one to three of the HLA-B and HLA-DR antigens, there is also a decreased graft survival with an increasing number of mismatches, but here the differences are relatively small. For these mismatches, the advantage of the local use of a less well matched kidney has to be weighed against the disadvantage of the prolonged ischemia time associated with transport of the kidney to another center where the better-matched recipient is located[9]. Prolonged ischemia (> 36 h) increases the risk of acute tubular necrosis. The dilemma is also illustrated in Figure 86.2, which shows that mismatched donor kidneys with immediate diuresis have a better graft survival than well-matched kidneys without immediate function[10]. These data suggest that the exchange of kidneys with more than zero mismatches should no longer be based on HLA matching's criteria. An exception should be made

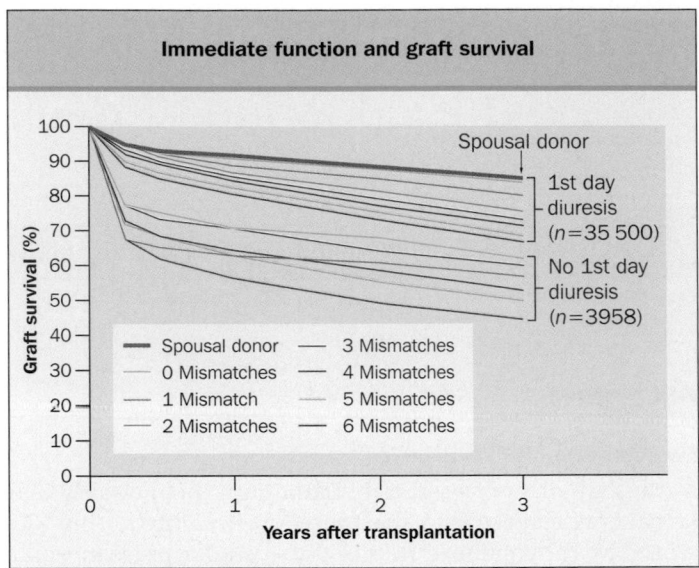

Figure 86.2 Survival of first cadaveric grafts according to urine flow on the first day. The grafts were further grouped on the basis of the number of HLA-A, HLA-B, and HLA-DR mismatches. The spousal-donor group is included for comparison. (With permission from Terasaki et al.[10].)

for a kidney offered to a highly sensitized patient with a negative cross-match.

HLA antibodies and cross-matching

Lymphocytotoxic antibodies against HLA antigens may be present in the recipient as a consequence of sensitization by blood transfusions, pregnancy, or a previous transplant. If these antibodies are specifically directed against the HLA antigens of the graft, they may cause hyperacute or accelerated rejection of the graft. Therefore, sera from potential candidates for transplantation should be screened every 3 months against a panel of representative donor lymphocytes for the presence of panel reactive antibodies (PRA). If positive responses are found, it is important to define the immunoglobulin class of the PRA and, if possible, their specificity. The principle of screening for HLA antibodies is illustrated in Figure 86.3. The class I (A and B) antibodies of the IgG class are almost always detrimental and the presence of the corresponding antigens in the donor should be avoided. Most IgM antibodies against lymphocytes are probably harmless. If they do not show a definite HLA specificity, their presence can be disregarded. In many patients, they are broadly reactive and react also with the recipient's own lymphocytes (autoantibodies). Since they can cause false-positive cross-matches (see below), they should be removed from the serum. This is most commonly achieved by testing the serum in the presence of dithiothreitol (DTT), a reducing agent that destroys IgM but leaves IgG intact. In some patients, such as those with systemic lupus, IgG autoantibodies against lymphocytes may be present, and removal of these reactive autoantibodies from the serum by prior absorption with autologous lymphocytes should also be done during the testing process.

Analogous to the common practice in blood transfusion, a cross-match of the lymphocytes of the donor with the recipient's

Screening for anti-HLA antibodies

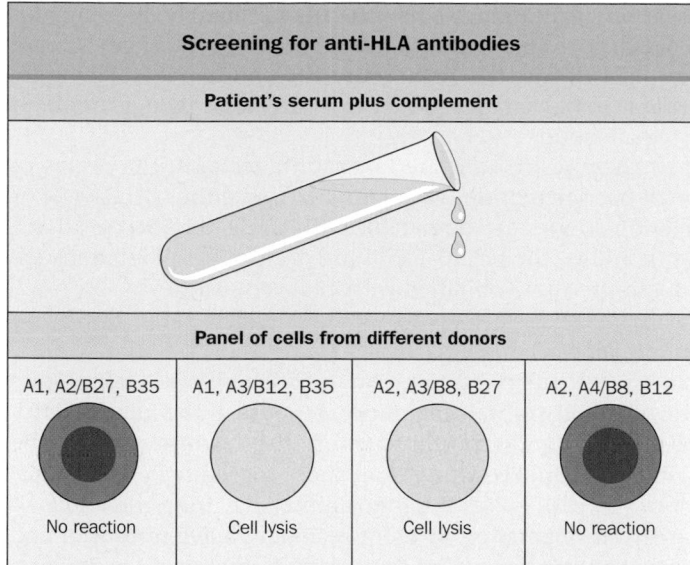

Figure 86.3 Principle of screening for anti-HLA antibodies. The patient's serum is tested with a panel of cells of known HLA types. The most common HLA antigens are represented in such panels. In this example, the A3 antigen is the only antigen present in the two lysed cell populations and absent from the nonlysed samples. Therefore, the patient's serum contains anti-HLA-A3 antibodies.

Interpretation of the cross-match test

Antibody	Cross-match normal procedure		Cross-match + dithiothreitol		Antibody-mediated graft damage
	T cells	B cells	T cells	B cells	
IgG class I	+	+	+	+	Yes
IgM class I	+	+	–	–	Yes, IgM class I antibodies may be harmless if present in old sera only but not in the current serum
IgG class II	–	+	–	+	Yes
IgM class II	–	+	–	–	Unknown
IgM autoantibodies	+	+	–	–	No

Table 86.2 Interpretation of the cross-match test.

serum should be performed before transplantation. Evidence suggests that a cross-match is not necessary for patients who never had any PRA in previous screenings, because in these cases the cross-match will always be negative[11].

In sensitized patients, more sensitive cross-matches using separated T and B cells are necessary. T cells express class I antigens (HLA-A and B) whereas B cells express both class I and class II (HLA-DR) antigens. The possible results of these tests and their interpretation are given in Table 86.2. Both a recent serum and the historical sera, in which PRA have been demonstrated earlier, should be included in the test. A positive DTT cross-match with donor T cells in one or more of these sera is generally considered to be an absolute contraindication for transplantation. Tests with isolated B cells are necessary to identify antibodies against HLA-DR with sufficient sensitivity. A positive B cell cross-match, in the presence of a negative T cell cross-match, can be caused by antibodies against HLA-DR, nonspecific antibodies, or autoantibodies. Only HLA-DR antibodies of the IgG class are potentially destructive. By performing all tests also in the presence of DTT most false-positive cross-matches can be eliminated. Flow cytometry is a more sensitive method for detecting reactive IgG antibodies. This method will detect cytotoxic antibodies of low titer and non-complement-fixing antibodies that have remained undetected in the routine cross-match procedure. The test has not found wide application because of its relatively high false-positive rate and because the role of noncomplement-fixing antibodies in the induction of graft damage is uncertain. It may be helpful in situations where the patient has a high PRA as a result of previous sensitization against HLA.

The most problematic patients are those that develop high titers of PRA antibodies (typically > 85% against a panel of class I (HLA-A and B) antigens. Most patients with high PRA have been sensitized by either a prior transplantation, by previous pregnancies, or by previous blood transfusions. Interestingly, many of these patients have only one antibody that cross-reacts with many HLA antigens by binding an antigen that serves as a 'public epitope'. Several groups are typing these public epitope antibodies as a means to determine *a priori* if they can be used to predict the subsequent cross-match.

Special patient groups

Those with absolute and relative contraindications

Although renal transplantation is a complicated procedure, there are only a few absolute contraindications, which are summarized in Table 86.3. The most important absolute

Contraindications for renal transplantation

Absolute contraindications
- High perioperative risk
- Active cancer
- Active infection, including HIV-seropositivity
- Life expectancy < 2 years
- Liver cirrhosis, unless combined liver and kidney transplantation
- Poorly controlled psychosis
- Active substance abuse
- ABO incompatibility
- Positive T cell cross-match

Relative contraindications
- Chronic active hepatitis
- Coronary heart disease
- Active peptic ulcer disease
- Cerebrovascular disease
- Medical noncompliance
- Active hepatitis B virus infection (HBV DNA+, HBeAg +)

Table 86.3 Absolute and relative contraindications for renal transplantation.

Transplantation

contraindication is transplantation in a patient who is unlikely to survive the operation. However, this is often hard to predict, and strict criteria are not available. For instance, there is no definite upper age limit for renal transplantation. Transplantation in patients older than 70 years is not frequently performed but is certainly possible when their physical condition is good. The decision is even more difficult in patients with complicating diseases that imply a shortened life expectancy. In these patients, the advantages of renal transplantation must be carefully weighed against the risks, but as a general rule transplantation should not be offered to a patient whose life expectancy is less than 2 years.

Active infection is a strong contraindication. In particular, identification of urinary tract infections is mandatory before renal transplantation, and such infections should first be treated with the appropriate antibiotics. If treatment is not successful because of anatomic abnormalities, surgical correction should be considered. Also, the presence of other infectious foci should be excluded. Renal transplantation into patients with HIV infection has generally been regarded as contraindicated because the use of immunosuppressive medication can cause an acceleration of the course of the disease. With the availability of highly active antiretroviral therapy, this policy may be reconsidered in individual cases. However, the toxicity and potential interaction of immunosuppressive and antiviral drugs hinder safe transplantation in HIV-infected patients. In several centers hepatitis B positivity is a relative contraindication against renal transplantation (see below).

Finally, the risk for noncompliance should be determined, since this is one of the major causes for graft failure after transplantation. This may be very hard to evaluate, and sometimes the help of other specialists (psychiatrists, psychologists, social workers) will be required.

In conclusion, there are few absolute contraindications to renal transplantation. The consequence of this is that the acceptance criteria will vary between transplantation centers. The cost–benefit ratio for the potential recipient should always be determined by the physician but should also be considered by the recipient.

Children

Although there are conflicting results in the literature, the success rate of renal transplantation in children younger than 2 years seems to be lower than in older children. In children, vascular thrombosis is an important cause of graft loss. In children younger than 2 years, the risk of thrombosis in a cadaveric graft may be as high as 9%, decreasing to 5.5 and 4.4% in children aged 2–5 and 6–12 years, respectively[12]. Results after transplantation of a kidney from a living donor in very young children are also worse than those in older children even though they are much better than the results obtained with a kidney from a cadaveric donor.

In addition to the age of the recipient, also the age of the donor affects the success rate in pediatric transplantation. Lower graft survival rates with transplantation of kidneys from donors under 5 years is mainly due to a higher risk of graft thrombosis. Moreover, recent data indicate that very good results in children can be achieved with adult-size kidneys, especially when there is no acute tubular necrosis[13].

At our institution, we have set the minimal body-weight for a pediatric recipient at 11 kg, which usually correlates with an age of 24–30 months. In most of these children it is technically feasible to transplant a kidney from an adult, particularly from a female donor.

If these restrictions are taken into account, the results of renal transplantation (with kidneys from either a cadaveric or a living donor) are comparable with those obtained in adults. As in adults, the results for living donor transplantations are superior to those obtained with cadaveric kidneys.

Elderly patients

Elderly patients (> 60 years) with ESRD are often not offered the possibility of transplantation because of the increased risk of mortality and morbidity. Before the cyclosporine era, the results were indeed worse than those for younger age groups. However, with newer immunosuppressive drugs the results of renal transplantation in older recipients have improved and nowadays the survival of transplant recipients 60 to 74 years of age is superior compared to waiting-list patients of the same age[1]. The loss of grafts from rejection is even less than in younger patients (Table 86.4)[14]. This is most likely explained by the decrease of immune responsiveness with aging. However, the loss of functioning grafts as a result of the death of the recipient is higher, resulting in an overall result comparable to that in other age groups. This illustrates that age by itself is not a contraindication for renal transplantation. Careful examination for the existence of comorbidity, especially cardiovascular diseases, in these patients may prevent early mortality after renal transplantation and may further improve graft survival results. However, since these patients are now also eligible for transplantation, an increase of the donor shortage can be expected. A solution for this problem might be the expansion of the donor pool by including older donors. Registry data show that kidney grafts from old donors have a shorter graft survival[15]. This may not be a problem for older recipients because they will require a functioning graft for a shorter period than younger patients.

Patients with urologic problems

Urologic examinations, including voiding cystourethrography, urodynamic studies, and cystoscopy, should only be performed in patients with a prior urologic history[16]. The presence of vesicoureteral reflux is only an indication for

Renal transplantation in older people			
	Age (years)		
Responses	<60	>60	p
Rejection episodes (%)			
None	46	56	0.02
More than 1	25	12	0.001
Immunologic graft loss at 3 years (%)	31	11	0.0009

Table 86.4 Renal transplantation in older people. Change in immunologic responsiveness with age. (With permission from Tesi et al.[14].)

nephroureterectomy if there is a hydroureter or if the reflux is the cause of recurrent infections. In patients with bladder abnormalities, every attempt should be made to correct the problem surgically. Patients with long-standing anuria during the dialysis period may have a very small bladder capacity, which may increase the risk of surgical complications. Nevertheless, the bladder quickly regains its original capacity after successful transplantation. Infravesical obstruction, for instance caused by urethral valves, should be corrected only if there is still diuresis, otherwise the correction should be delayed until after a successful transplantation. In patients with a neurogenic bladder without urinary incontinence but with an inability to void spontaneously, self-catherization is a feasible solution. If the patient's own bladder cannot be used, kidney transplantation can be performed with implantation of the ureter into a urinary diversion. Ileal or colonic conduits have been used for this purpose and excellent results have been reported. The conduit must be constructed at least 6 weeks before transplantation.

High-risk patient groups
Diabetic nephropathy
Patients with diabetic nephropathy form a special category of transplant recipients because apart from the nephropathy other complications almost invariably occur. The most important causes of death in patients with diabetic nephropathy and a renal transplant are myocardial infarction and congestive heart failure. Although the risk for atherosclerosis is greater in diabetics over the age of 45 years and in those with a history of smoking, neither clinical symptoms nor the cardiovascular risk profile are sufficiently reliable to document or exclude the presence of coronary artery disease.[17] Therefore, non-invasive screening tests (see below) should be carried out in all diabetic transplant candidates before transplantation. If abnormalities are found, coronary angiography is indicated before a renal transplantation can be performed. In addition, special attention should be directed to urinary bladder emptying and the presence of foot ulcers.

Since patient survival and quality of life are substantially better after renal transplantation than with hemodialysis, diabetic patients should already be considered for transplantation when the creatinine clearance falls below 15–20 mL/min. The availability of a living donor graft may provide the opportunity to circumvent the need for dialysis. Early renal transplantation can prevent the progression of uremic neuropathy, although the extrarenal complications of the diabetes mellitus are not halted. A discussion of kidney/pancreas transplantation (including the work-up and efficacy) in diabetes is provided in Chapter 93.

Cardiovascular disease
Cardiovascular disease is the most important cause of death after renal transplantation. Major risk factors are age > 50 years, diabetes mellitus, history of angina pectoris, congestive heart failure, and an abnormal electrocardiogram. The cardiac mortality after renal transplantation in patients with one or more risk factors was found to be as high as 17% at a mean follow-up of 2 years, whereas it was 1% in the low-risk group[18]. In the high-risk group, the cardiac prognosis is determined by the extent of coronary artery disease and by left ventricular function. Although definitive recommendations do not exist, we consider work-up by a cardiologist warranted in high-risk patients, as summarized in Table 86.5. Resting echocardiography is a valuable tool to detect valvular diseases and to evaluate (residual) left ventricular function. Noninvasive methods to screen for the presence of coronary artery disease are hampered by the fact that uremic patients (and especially those with diabetes) frequently have a poor exercise tolerance and can have non-specific basal ECG abnormalities. Combined dipyridamole and exercise thallium imaging as well as dobutamine stress echocardiography probably have the highest sensitivity and specificity in these circumstances[19,20]. We advocate to repeat the screening for coronary artery disease every two years in high risk patients who are on the waiting list. Patients with a positive screening test should undergo coronary arteriography. If there is significant narrowing of the major coronary vessels, revascularization before transplantation is recommended. Several studies suggest that in dialysis patients bypass surgery leads to a better long-term outcome as compared to percutaneous transluminal coronary angioplasty[21], although the results of the latter procedure may be improved by stenting and use of antiplatelet therapy.

Routine examination of the iliac vessels is not necessary. If there is a history of claudication or when physical examination reveals signs of arterial insufficiency, non-invasive vascular studies can help to select patients in whom angiography is indicated. If an aortoiliac reconstruction is necessary it should preferably be performed prior to transplantation as a scheduled procedure.

In patients with a history of transient ischemic attacks or cerebrovascular accident, carotid Doppler studies should be performed to screen for the presence of vascular disease requiring intervention.

Hereditary diseases with increased risk
Another special group of transplant candidates is formed by patients who have an original kidney disease, often of genetic origin, that causes increased risks after transplantation. A good example is primary hyperoxaluria type I. This disease is caused by a deficiency of the enzyme alanine glyoxalate aminotransferase and it leads to nephrolithiasis and nephrocalcinosis.

Indications for cardiological evaluation before renal transplantation
Previous myocardial infarction
Angina pectoris
Congestive heart failure
Cardiac murmur*
Abnormal ECG
Diabetic nephropathy
Age above 70, or above 45 in diabetics
Signs of peripheral vascular disease
*In many cases echocardiography will be sufficient.

Table 86.5 Indications for cardiological evaluation before renal transplantation.

ESRD usually occurs in these patients before the age of 20. As a consequence, oxalate excretion is completely interrupted and oxalate deposition throughout the body proceeds at an increased rate. After renal transplantation, there is an increased risk of graft destruction by massive deposition of oxalate, especially in patients with primary nonfunction. Strategies to reduce oxalate deposition in the kidney include aggressive preoperative dialysis, forced diuresis and administration of pyridoxine, orthophosphates, and thiazide diuretics after transplantation. Since the enzyme defect can be reconstituted by liver transplantation, combined liver and renal transplantation has become the treatment of choice[22]. It should be preferably carried out when the glomerular filtration rate drops below 25 mL/min. Isolated kidney transplantation, preferably with a living donor kidney to avoid delayed graft function, can be considered in adults with a late-onset form of the disease.

A second group of special patients are those with cystinosis. This disease is caused by an autosomal recessive defect of cystine transport and leads to cystine deposition in all tissues. In the kidney, the cystine crystals cause interstitial inflammation and progressive fibrosis, leading to ESRD. Early treatment with phosphocysteamine retards the progression of renal failure. When ESRD has occurred, renal transplantation is the treatment of choice and cystinosis does not recur in the graft. However, the nonrenal complications of cystinosis tend to progress after renal transplantation.

The third group consists of patients with Fabry's disease. This rare X-linked disorder of glycosphingolipid metabolism is most severe in hemizygous females and leads to renal failure in the fourth decade of life. Contrary to initial reports of a high mortality rate after transplantation, recent experience is much more favorable. Recurrence of the disease in the renal transplant has been reported, but it does not lead to renal failure. Furthermore, recurrence may become less of an issue once recombinant alpha-galactosidase A becomes widely available.

Other renal diseases

Certain types of glomerulonephritis may recur following renal transplantation (see Chapter 91). In many of the diseases, such as systemic lupus and vasculitis, the likelihood of recurrence may be greater if the disease was fulminant and if the period on dialysis was short (< 3 months). However, neither extrarenal manifestations nor markers of disease activity, such as titers of antineutrophil cytoplasmic antibody (ANCA) or antinuclear antibody, always correlate with disease recurrence. In contrast, the continued presence of circulating antibodies against the glomerular basement membrane (GBM) (detected by either enzyme immunoassay or indirect immunofluorescence) is generally considered a contraindication to renal transplantation because of the increased risk for disease recurrence. Focal segmental glomerulosclerosis (FSGS) is also a disease with a high recurrence in transplants. Recurrence rates are higher in living donor allografts as opposed to cadaveric donor kidneys, but overall allograft survival is not reduced due to the lower frequency of rejection in the living donor kidneys[23]. As a consequence, transplantation with a living donor allograft is acceptable, unless a prior allograft has been lost to recurrent disease. Since a remission of recurrent FSGS can be

induced with plasma exchange, it has also been proposed to start plasma exchange prior to a planned transplantation to prevent recurrence[24]. More studies will be required before this policy should be uniformly adopted.

Malignancy

It is not an uncommon occurrence that a patient proposed as a candidate for renal transplantation has previously been treated for a malignancy. There is a great variation among the rates of recurrence of different tumors. Penn has provided helpful guidelines for waiting times based on data collected in an international transplant tumor registry[25]. Of all patients with a pretransplant tumor, 22% developed a recurrence of the malignancy after transplantation. Not unexpectedly, the interval between the treatment of the patient and the transplantation played an important role. The recurrence rates were 53, 34, and 13% in patients transplanted at 0–24, 24–60, and more than 60 months, respectively, after treatment for the malignancy. There was also a substantial variability among the rates of recurrence of different tumors. Transplantation guidelines for specific tumors are given in Table 86.6. A waiting time of 2 years seems a reasonable compromise with most tumors. Patients with acquired cystic kidney disease have an increased risk for the development of renal carcinoma. For this reason, it is recommended to perform ultrasound screening every 1–2 years after transplantation.

Hepatitis B virus infection

Carriers of the hepatitis B (HBV) surface antigen (HBsAg) who have no markers for active viral replication (HBeAg or HBV-DNA) are eligible for transplantation, although reactivation of the HBV infection can occur in these patients as a result of the immunosuppressive therapy. In contrast, patients with active HBV infection, or with chronic active hepatitis or cirrhosis on liver biopsy, are usually not considered candidates for transplantation. Transplantation in these patients carries an increased risk for progression of their liver disease as well as an

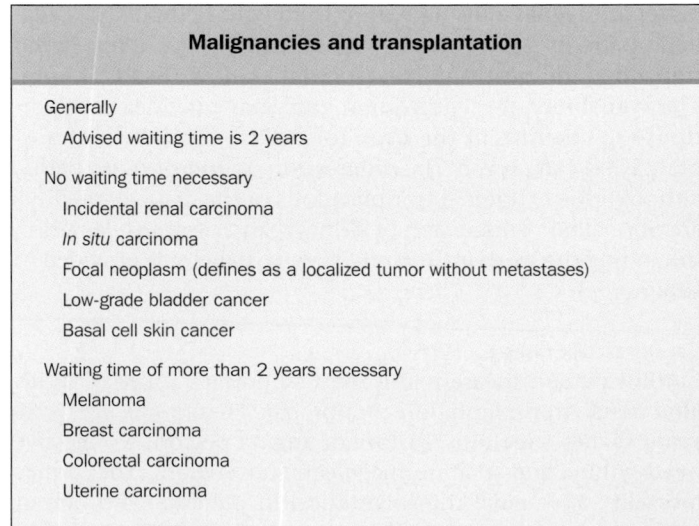

Malignancies and transplantation

Generally
    Advised waiting time is 2 years

No waiting time necessary
    Incidental renal carcinoma
    In situ carcinoma
    Focal neoplasm (defines as a localized tumor without metastases)
    Low-grade bladder cancer
    Basal cell skin cancer

Waiting time of more than 2 years necessary
    Melanoma
    Breast carcinoma
    Colorectal carcinoma
    Uterine carcinoma

Table 86.6 Guidelines for transplantation in patients with previous malignancies. (With permission from Penn.[25].)

increased risk for infections. Patients with active hepatitis should be treated with interferon-α and/or lamivudine prior to transplantation and should ideally not be placed on the waiting list unless they are no longer infectious (negative for HBeAg and HBV DNA). Treatment of hepatitis B viral infection in the transplant recipient is difficult as interferon-α may precipitate rejection and experience with lamivudine is limited. In patients with cirrhosis renal transplantation is contraindicated and continuation on dialysis or a combined liver and kidney transplantation should be discussed.

Hepatitis C viral infection

The clinical course of patients with hepatitis C (HCV) infection appears to be similar to that in nontransplant patients, but this observation is based on studies with a relatively short follow-up. The pretransplant serum level of alanine aminotransferase has no predictive value for the course of liver disease after transplantation in HCV infection, and as a consequence many centers recommend liver biopsy in these patients. In patients with signs of chronic active hepatitis or cirrhosis on biopsy, the risk for progressive liver disease after renal transplantation is increased. In patients with cirrhosis a combined kidney and liver transplantation should be considered. Patients with chronic hepatitis may be candidates for interferon-α therapy during the dialysis period, although there are no data showing that this interferon therapy improves survival after transplantation[26].

Tuberculosis

Tuberculosis reactivates more frequently in patients under immunosuppression, particularly when the tuberculin test is positive and there is radiologic evidence of inactive tuberculosis. Tuberculosis prophylaxis is indicated in patients at risk, but the difficulty lies in the identification of such patients. A negative tuberculin test, for instance, is unreliable because in patients with chronic renal failure the test can be a false negative as a consequence of a decreased cellular immune responsiveness. Moreover, the prophylactic treatment with isoniazid (drug of choice) is potentially hepatotoxic, especially if used together with azathioprine. It may also interfere with the metabolism of cyclosporine. Patients who have received adequate treatment in the past do not need prophylactic treatment. If this is not the case and radiologic evidence of an inactive tuberculosis infection exists, prophylactic treatment with isoniazid (300 mg daily) during the first 9 months after transplantation (or ideally before transplantation) is recommended.

Pre-emptive transplantation

Transplantation in patients with progressive chronic renal disease who are not yet dialysis dependent (creatinine clearance < 15 mL/min) has the potential to avoid dialysis related morbidity and is cost-saving. Especially when living donor kidneys are used, pre-emptive transplantation results in longer allograft survival than transplantation performed after the initiation of dialysis[27]. Therefore, pre-emptive transplantation should be encouraged for all patients whenever a living donor is available. Several patient categories can particularly benefit from pre-emptive transplantation, such as children, diabetics, and patients with primary hyperoxaluria type I. Transplantation with a cadaveric donor kidney before the end-stage of renal failure has been reached is not generally applicable as long as there is a waiting list of patients on dialysis.

Special therapeutic or preparatory measures
Nephrectomy

Bilateral nephrectomy before transplantation is only performed for special indications. Gross abnormalities of the urinary tract (with or without renal stones), accompanied by persistent infections, are absolute indications for removal of one or both kidneys. To avoid persistent infections after nephrectomy, abnormal ureters are also removed. Otherwise, the ureters should be left in place, because the ureter can be used after transplantation for a new anastomosis with the pelvis of the graft if urologic complications occur. Another indication for nephrectomy is a very large kidney, for instance in polycystic kidney disease, which will hinder the placement of the new graft. In the exceptional cases where hypertension does not respond to fluid removal and is drug resistant, there may be an indication for nephrectomy. Since the morbidity of the nephrectomy in patients with ESRD is relatively high, the operation should not be performed to normalize an otherwise treatable hypertension before transplantation or to prevent the occurrence of post-transplant hypertension. In retransplant patients, removal of a prior graft is only necessary when there are signs of active rejection or infection or if placement of a subsequent graft would otherwise not be possible. There is no evidence that the presence of a failed graft influences the course of a second graft.

Blood transfusion

Since blood transfusions can cause sensitization against HLA antigens, it seemed logical to avoid them as much as possible before transplantation. This probably explains why the report of Dossetor in 1967, suggesting that many blood transfusions exerted some protective effect against rejection, was initially neglected by transplant clinicians. The transfusion effect was rediscovered by Opelz and Terasaki in 1973. They showed a correlation between the number of pretransplant blood transfusions and graft survival rates. Subsequently, it has been claimed that the graft-protecting effect could be induced by a single transfusion, whereas others have maintained that graft survival rates improve further with increasing numbers of transfusions. This controversy has never been resolved. Subsequent evidence that a single blood transfusion is only protective if there is sharing of one HLA-DR antigen (or one HLA-B and one HLA-DR antigen) between donor and recipient has remained unconfirmed. However, there is general agreement that perioperative transfusions do not have a protective effect. The controversial reports on the effect of transfusion and the fact that the mechanism by which the transfusion has its effect has never been clarified have led many centers to abandon pretransplant transfusions. Moreover, with the introduction of recombinant epoetin, the need for transfusions to treat the anemia of chronic renal failure has vanished. With the current immunosuppressive possibilities the 1 year graft survival is about 90% in nontransfused patients, thus equivalent or even better than the results in transfused patients in previous studies. As transfusions still carry a small risk of allo-immunization and transmission of infectious diseases, the use of pretransplant transfusions to improve cadaveric graft survival is no longer recommended.

Donor-specific transfusion

In living donor transplantation, excellent results have been reported in recipients who received three blood transfusions from their related kidney donors with one or two haplotype mismatches. Unfortunately, this procedure also induced the production of donor-specific cytotoxic T cell antibodies in about 20% of the recipients, thus precluding transplantation of a kidney from that particular donor. Attempts to prevent the sensitization under an umbrella of immunosuppressive therapy have only been partly successful. As a consequence, this approach has not found wide acceptance in renal transplantation. Procedures such as infusion of stem cells or bone marrow cells seemed a promising procedure[28], but until now there are no new studies to support this strategy.

Highly sensitized patients

For patients who have formed antibodies against HLA antigens, it is more difficult to find a suitable organ with a negative cross-match. This is particularly a problem for patients who are highly immunized (with a high PRA) who have antibodies against most HLA antigens. Of course, transplantation of an HLA-identical kidney could circumvent the problem, but with the exception of a kidney from an HLA-identical sibling donor, these kidneys are not easily found. An effective, but laborious, approach is to test serum of the patient against all possible HLA antigens in a search for antigens that will produce a negative cross-match. Some groups are also attempting to identify the specificity of the antibodies directed against the public epitope antigens on the HLA class I molecules that are responsible for the elevated PRA. In this way, acceptable mismatches can be traced before transplantation and this increases the chances of a suitable match for a sensitized recipient. A somewhat simpler method to find suitable kidneys for highly immunized patients is to perform a cross-match against each available donor in a large donor pool. Graft survival results of patients receiving transplants in these programs have been quite satisfactory[29].

Another possible solution is the active removal of the circulating antibodies by plasma exchange or extracorporeal immunoadsorption. Resynthesis of antibodies is prevented by concomitant immunosuppression. With these methods the titer of the antibodies is reduced. When the antibody titer was decreased by immunoadsorption, these patients prove to have reactivity only against a few HLA specificities. It is then much easier to find a suitable donor with a negative cross-match. The results of this approach show an increase of negative cross-matches after immunoadsorption, but the number of patients subsequently receiving a transplant is too small to evaluate the graft survival rates. Apart from the removal of antibodies against HLA antigens, removal of natural anti-A or anti-B antibodies has also been carried out in order to perform a transplantation of ABO-incompatible kidneys from living donors. This is only possible with a pretransplant splenectomy. The whole procedure has many side effects and should only be performed in patients for whom there is no other satisfactory solution[30]. An exception to this rule can possibly be made for the transplantation of kidneys with blood group A2 into non-A recipients (see above).

Immediate preoperative dialysis

Dialysis immediately preceding transplantation should only be carried out if hyperkalemia or an unacceptable fluid overload occurs. In all other situations, dialysis should be avoided because of an increased risk of bleeding complications after transplantation. If pretransplant dialysis must be performed, it is important to keep the patient well hydrated, since this improves the chances of immediate graft function. Patients on peritoneal dialysis should continue dialysis until the time of the transplantation. The peritoneal cavity should be drained before surgery.

DONOR

Donor organs can be obtained from living donors or from cadaveric sources. Each method has its individual risks and advantages.

Living donor

Advantages and risks

The use of kidneys from living donors for transplantation finds its most important justification in the existing shortage of organs from cadaveric donors. A second consideration is that the results in terms of graft survival and quality of life of the recipient are better when organs from living donors are used (Fig. 86.4).

The acute mortality risk related to surgery is very low. Estimates vary from 1 in 1600 to 1 in 3000 kidney donations

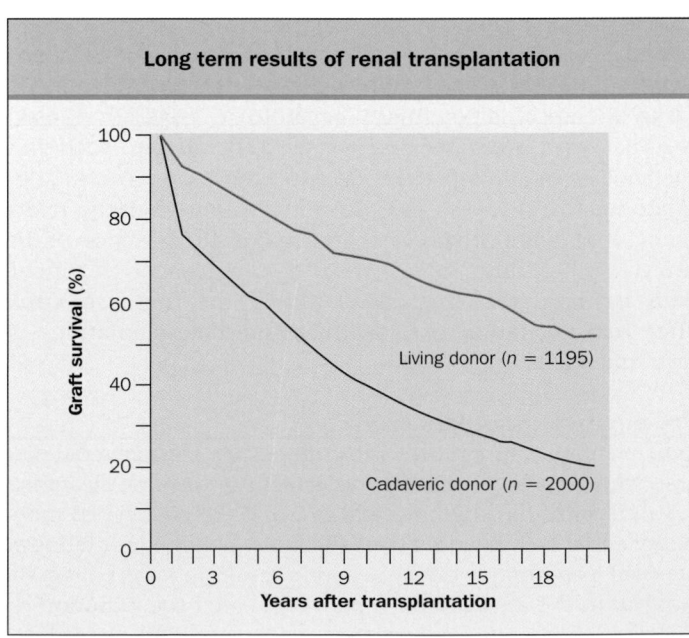

Figure 86.4 Comparison of the long term follow-up of living related transplants and cadaveric transplants in the Netherlands between 1966 and 2001.

(0.03%)[31]. Bay and Hebert compared this risk with other daily risks[32]. Using the rate of mortality from traffic accidents in Ohio, they calculated that a kidney donor incurs as much risk from the transplant procedure as the average Ohio citizen does of dying in a traffic accident for each 2–4 years of residence in Ohio. Such comparisons may be helpful in explaining the acute mortality risk of surgery to a prospective donor. Nephrectomy can be performed by open surgery or by a laparoscopic procedure. Major complications (bleeding, pneumothorax requiring a chest tube, wound infection, pneumonia) occur in 3% of the open procedures. Estimates of minor complications (asymptomatic pneumothorax, urinary retention, urinary tract infection) amount to 17%[33]. With the use of laparoscopic removal of kidneys, the number of hospitalization days and overall morbidity are reduced. In a systematic review comparing the open procedure with the laparoscopic procedure Merlin et al. concluded that the evidence base for laparoscopic live donor nephrectomy was inadequate to make safety and efficacy recommendations[34]. Although the complications from any type of donor nephrectomy are relatively low and in general treatable, the donor should be carefully informed about these potential problems.

There have been ample discussions about the long-term risks of living with a single kidney after donation. Mainly based on results obtained in experimental animals, it has been suggested that hyperfiltration in the remaining single kidney might lead to focal glomerulosclerosis and renal insufficiency. Data from life insurance companies do not show a shorter life span in otherwise healthy individuals with a single kidney. Also, follow-up studies of kidney donors demonstrate that long-term consequences of the procedure are absent or negligible (Table 86.7)[35]. A most impressive argument stems from a study in which 62 American soldiers who lost one kidney during World War II were traced 45 years later. They were compared with 620 control individuals. There were no increased mortality, no increased prevalence of hypertension, and no signs of renal dysfunction that could be related to the loss of one kidney in the past[36].

Women of childbearing age can also serve as kidney donors. The course of subsequent pregnancies is similar to that in the general population and changes in renal function have not been noted.

The advantages for the recipient of a kidney from a living donor are considerable. With good planning, the transplantation can be performed before the patient has to be treated with dialysis. A second advantage is that in almost 100% of the cases, a living donor kidney starts to function immediately after transplantation, whereas in cadaveric kidney transplantation 20–30% of the kidneys go through a period of acute renal failure. This difference is important, because ultimate graft survival rates are at least 10% higher in kidneys with immediate function after transplantation (see Fig. 86.2).

If kidneys from living related donors are used, the degree of HLA matching between the donor and recipient is also important. When donor and recipient are HLA-identical siblings, graft loss from rejection is as low as 3%. The results are somewhat less good when donor and recipient are haploidentical or completely mismatched for the HLA antigens, but they are still substantially better than those obtained with cadaveric kidneys.

Kidney donation by living unrelated donors who are emotionally related to the recipient (e.g., spouse) is also an option. The results obtained with unrelated, and most often completely mismatched living donors, are surprisingly good and virtually equal to the graft survival of haploidentical kidneys from living related donors[10]. These encouraging results can most probably be explained by the absence of delayed graft function in these kidneys and by the fact that the absence of ischemic damage makes the kidney less sensitive to the rejection process.

Routine assessment

The donor should be healthy and free from complicating diseases. A definite age limit for donation cannot be given. Also at older age, the clinical condition and renal function are the decisive criteria for acceptance as a kidney donor. The topics that deserve special attention in the assessment of a living donor are given in Table 86.8. Preoperative visualization of

---

Follow-up of living donors 20 years after uninephrectomy

Assessment	Donors (n = 57)	Sibling controls (n = 50)	p
Serum creatinine (mg/dL (μmol/L)	1.1 (98)	1.1 (98)	NS
Patients on antihypertensive drugs (%)	32	44	NS*
Patients with proteinuria (%)	23	22	NS

* Also no significant difference from age-matched general population.

Table 86.7 Follow-up studies of living donors 20 years after uninephrectomy. (With permission from Najarian et al.[35].)

Assessment of a prospective living donor

History
  Exclude hereditary renal diseases
  Exclude congenital abnormalities of the urinary tract
  Exclude recurrent urinary tract infections

Physical examination
  Careful measurement of blood pressure

Laboratory tests
  Blood group and HLA typing
  Urinalysis (protein, glucose)
  Urine culture
  Careful examination of the urinary sediment
  Serum creatinine
  Screening for HIV, hepatitis B and C, cytomegalovirus, Epstein–Barr virus
  Electrocardiogram

Radiologic examination
  Spiral computed tomographic angiography (Spiral CT)

Table 86.8 Important factors in the assessment of a prospective donor.

the renal arteries is mandatory in each living donor procedure. Spiral computerized tomography or magnetic resonance angiography are nowadays first choice, because of the potentially lower morbidity, improved donor convenience, and reduced cost. In case of ambiguity renal angiography is still the gold standard.

Evaluation and selection of cadaveric donors

Because of the shortage of donor organs, all brain dead patients should be evaluated for the suitability to become a donor. An absolute contraindication for donation is the risk of transmission of a disease from donor to recipient. Patients with sepsis, acute hepatitis, HIV-infection or behavior associated with a high risk for HIV-infection, or a history of malignancy (except non-invasive brain tumor or non-metastatic skin tumor) are therefore excluded for donation. Most centers do not accept organs from a donor who is a hepatitis B virus carrier (HbsAg positive) or who is positive for HCV antibody, although transplantation of these organs into recipients with similar positive tests does not carry a large additional risk. Preferably, the function of the donated kidney should be normal. The lack of kidney donors necessitates the acceptance of kidneys with less than optimal function, although there is no consensus on the minimal requirements for acceptance. Since renal function decreases with age and donor age is one of the major determinants of outcome after transplantation, an upper age limit of about 70 is commonly used. Serum creatinine at admission should be in the near normal range (estimated creatinine clearance > 60 mL/min), but a temporary decline in renal function with subsequent signs of improvement is acceptable. The presence of proteinuria (> 0.5 g/24 h) indicates structural renal damage and is a valid reason for nonacceptance. However, one should be aware of the fact that the use of gelatin-based plasma expanders can interfere with several urinary protein assays, leading to apparently high protein concentrations while the dipstick reaction remains negative[37]. When it is difficult to determine whether a kidney is acceptable for transplantation, the medical history of the donor (diabetes mellitus, hypertension, cardiovascular disease) and a procurement renal biopsy may help in reaching a decision.

To ameliorate the shortage of donor organs, both kidneys from an otherwise nonacceptable donor have been used for dual transplantation into one recipient[38]. The results of this strategy are quite promising, although it remains a challenge to develop accepted criteria for deciding when to perform single, dual, or no transplantation.

Cadaveric donor management prior to transplantation

In the brain-dead donor, maintenance of a stable blood pressure and a continuous diuresis is of utmost importance to prevent the ischemic damage that may lead to acute tubular necrosis and delayed graft function after transplantation. The donor should be kept well hydrated by liberal infusion of fluid and plasma substituents. One should be cautious with the infusion of large amounts of hydroxyethyl starch solutions, since these have been associated with renal dysfunction in kidney donors and patients with sepsis[39]. Diabetes insipidus can be treated by the administration of vasopressin.

Pressor agents, such as dopamine, are frequently required to maintain blood pressure.

Donors with nonbeating hearts

It has been suggested that a 20% increase in the number of available cadaveric kidneys can be achieved through using donors with nonbeating hearts. Potential donors are those who have a permanent circulatory arrest either occurring in the intensive care unit or shortly after their admission to an emergency service. The kidneys are cooled by *in situ* perfusion with a special double-balloon triple-lumen catheter (Fig. 86.5). If effective cooling can be attained within 45 min of the circulatory arrest, these kidneys can be used for transplantation[40]. With the use of machine perfusion and viability testing even longer warm ischemia times may turn out to be acceptable in selected cases.[41] Since there is an increased incidence of delayed graft function in recipients of these kidneys, one might expect that the graft survival rates would be lower than that for kidneys from brain-dead cadaveric donors. So far such a difference has not been found (Fig. 86.6)[40,42].

Mismatch in size and age

There is controversy in the literature with regard to the acceptability of very young cadaveric kidney donors. Some centers find that kidneys from children less than 5 years of age do less well when transplanted to either children or adults. In a large North American study, the risk of vascular thrombosis was 8.3% compared with 3.9% with kidneys from donors more than 5 years of age[12]. Others did not find such a difference. Most centers accept kidneys from donors older

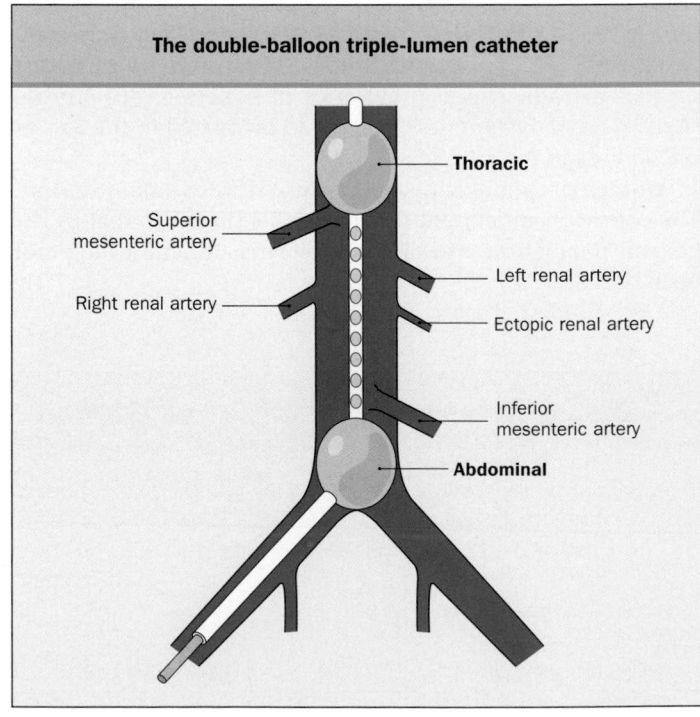

The double-balloon triple-lumen catheter

Thoracic

Superior mesenteric artery

Right renal artery

Left renal artery

Ectopic renal artery

Inferior mesenteric artery

Abdominal

Figure 86.5 The double-balloon triple-lumen catheter *in situ*. Two lumina are used for inflation of the balloons. The third lumen is used for infusion of the cooling fluid for the kidneys.

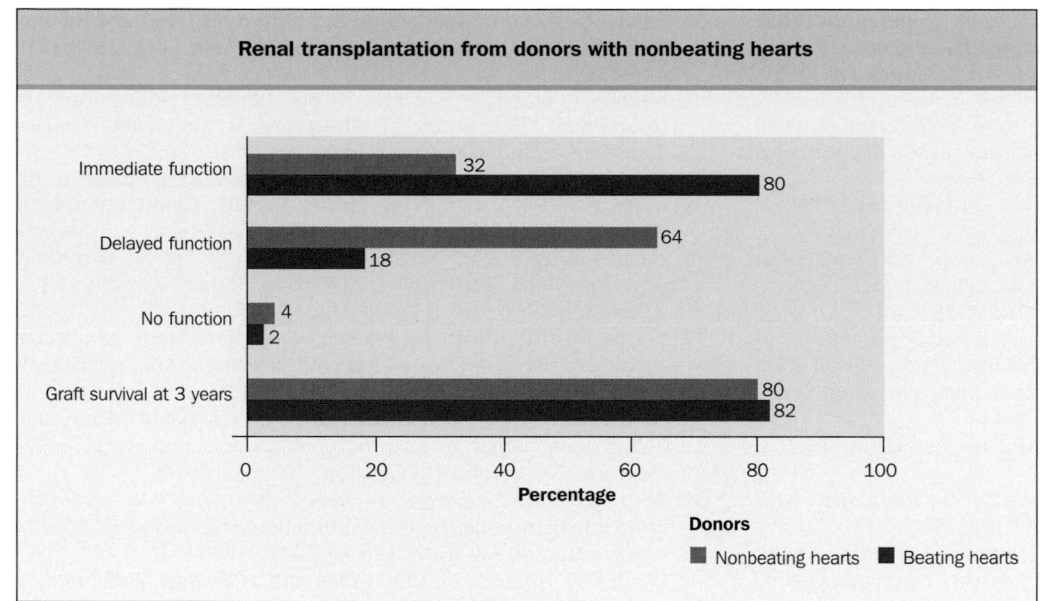

Figure 86.6 Kidney transplants from donors with nonbeating hearts. Results of a case-control study (comprising 47 cases and 94 controls) with a mean duration of follow up of 3.7 years[40].

than 2 years. Other centers do not hold a lower age limit. In the latter, both kidneys from very small children are engrafted en bloc.

It has also been suggested that kidney grafts that are small relative to recipient size may have a decreased survival, most likely as a result of progressive glomerulosclerosis as a consequence of hyperfiltration in a reduced number of nephrons[43].

The same sequence of events may explain why transplantation with kidneys from older donors, already damaged by glomerulosclerosis, is associated with a decreased graft survival. Kidneys from aged donors should, therefore, preferably not be given to children or young adults. Alternatively, a larger supply of nephrons can be achieved by transplanting two kidneys into one recipient.

REFERENCES

1. Wolfe RA, Ashby VB, Milford EL, et al. Comparison of mortality in all patients on dialysis, patients on dialysis awaiting transplantation, and recipients of a first cadaveric transplant. N Engl J Med. 1999;341:1725–30.
2. Ramos EL, Kasiske BL, Alexander SR, et al. The evaluation of candidates for renal transplantation. The current practice of U.S. transplant centers. Transplantation. 1994;57:490–7.
3. Fritsche L, Vanrenterghem Y, Nordal KP, et al. Practice variations in the evaluation of adult candidates for cadaveric kidney transplantation: a survey of the European Transplant Centers. Transplantation. 2000;70:1492–7.
4. Kasiske BL, Ramos EL, Gaston RS, et al. The evaluation of renal transplant candidates: clinical practice guidelines. Patient Care and Education Committee of the American Society of Transplant Physicians. J Am Soc Nephrol. 1995;6:1–34.
5. Berthoux F, Abramowicz D, Bradley B, et al. European best practice guidelines for renal transplantation (part 1). Nephrol Dial Transplant. 2000;15(suppl 7):1–85.
6. Halme L, Eklund B, Kyllonen L, Salmela K. Is obesity still a risk factor in renal transplantation? Transpl Int. 1997;10:284–8.
7. Graham SM, Flowers JL, Schweitzer E, et al. The utility of prophylactic laparoscopic cholecystectomy in transplant candidates. Am J Surg. 1995;169:44–8.
8. Alkhunaizi AM, Mattos AM de, Barry JM, et al. Renal transplantation across the ABO barrier using A2 kidneys. Transplantation. 1999;67:1319–24.
9. Morris PJ, Johnson RJ, Fuggle SV, et al. Analysis of factors that affect outcome of primary cadaveric renal transplantation in the UK. HLA Task Force of the Kidney Advisory Group of the United Kingdom Transplant Support Service Authority (UKTSSA). Lancet. 1999;354:1147–52.

10. Terasaki PI, Cecka JM, Gjertson DW, Takemoto S. High survival rates of kidney transplants from spousal and living unrelated donors. N Engl J Med. 1995;333:333–6.
11. Matas AJ, Sutherland DE. Kidney transplantation without a final crossmatch. Transplantation. 1998;66:1835–6.
12. Singh A, Stablein D, Tejani A. Risk factors for vascular thrombosis in pediatric renal transplantation: a special report of the North American Pediatric Renal Transplant Cooperative Study. Transplantation. 1997;63:1263–7.
13. Sarwal MM, Cecka JM, Millan MT, Salvatierra O Jr. Adult-size kidneys without acute tubular necrosis provide exceedingly superior long-term graft outcomes for infants and small children: a single center and UNOS analysis. United Network for Organ Sharing. Transplantation. 2000;70:1728–36.
14. Tesi RJ, Elkhammas EA, Davies EA, et al. Renal transplantation in older people. Lancet. 1994;343:461–4.
15. Cecka JM. The UNOS Scientific Renal Transplant Registry – 2000. Clin Transpl. 2000;14:1–18.
16. Glazier DB, Whang MI, Geffner SR, et al. Evaluation of voiding cystourethrography prior to renal transplantation. Transplantation. 1996;62:1762–5.
17. Koch M, Gradaus F, Schoebel FC, et al. Relevance of conventional cardiovascular risk factors for the prediction of coronary artery disease in diabetic patients on renal replacement therapy. Nephrol Dial Transplant. 1997;12:1187–91.
18. Le A, Wilson R, Douek K, et al. Prospective risk stratification in renal transplant candidates for cardiac death. Am J Kidney Dis. 1994;24:65–71.
19. Dahan M, Viron BM, Faraggi M, et al. Diagnostic accuracy and prognostic value of combined dipyridamole-exercise thallium imaging in hemodialysis patients. Kidney Int 1998; 54:255–62.

20. Herzog CA, Marwick TH, Pheley AM, et al. Dobutamine stress echocardiography for the detection of significant coronary artery disease in renal transplant candidates. Am J Kidney Dis. 1999; 33:1080–90.

21. Szczech LA, Reddan DN, Owen WF, et al. Differential survival after coronary revascularization procedures among patients with renal insufficiency. Kidney Int. 2001;60:292–9.

22. Cochat P. Primary hyperoxaluria type 1. Kidney Int. 1999;55: 2533–47.

23. Baum MA, Stablein DM, Panzarino VM, et al. Loss of living donor renal allograft survival advantage in children with focal segmental glomerulosclerosis. Kidney Int. 2001;59:328–33.

24. Ohta T, Kawaguchi H, Hattori M, et al. Effect of pre- and postoperative plasmapheresis on posttransplant recurrence of focal segmental glomerulosclerosis in children. Transplantation. 2001; 71:628–33.

25. Penn I. The effect of immunosuppression on pre-existing cancers. Transplantation. 1993;55:742–7.

26. Morales JM, Campistol JM. Transplantation in the patient with hepatitis C. J Am Soc Nephrol. 2000;11:1343–53.

27. Mange KC, Joffe MM, Feldman HI. Effect of the use or nonuse of long-term dialysis on the subsequent survival of renal transplants from living donors. N Engl J Med. 2001;344:726–31.

28. Pauw L De, Abramowicz D, Donckier V, et al. Isolation and infusion of donor CD34+ bone marrow cells in cadaver kidney transplantation. Nephrol Dial Transplant. 1998;13:34–6.

29. Doxiadis II, Meester J De, Smits JM, et al. The impact of special programs for kidney transplantation of highly sensitized patients in Eurotransplant. Clin Transpl. 1998;12:115–20.

30. Shishido S, Asanuma H, Tajima E, et al. ABO-incompatible living-donor kidney transplantation in children. Transplantation. 2001; 72:1037–42.

31. Johnson EM, Remucal MJ, Gillingham KJ, et al. Complications and risks of living donor nephrectomy. Transplantation. 1997; 64:1124–8.

32. Bay WH, Hebert LA. The living donor in kidney transplantation. Ann Intern Med. 1987;106:719–27.

33. Shaffer D, Sahyoun AI, Madras PN, Monaco AP. Two hundred one consecutive living-donor nephrectomies. Arch Surg. 1998;133: 426–31.

34. Merlin TL, Scott DF, Rao MM, et al. The safety and efficacy of laparoscopic live donor nephrectomy: a systematic review. Transplantation. 2000;70:1659–66.

35. Najarian JS, Chavers BM, McHugh LE, Matas AJ. 20 years or more of follow-up of living kidney donors. Lancet. 1992;340: 807–10.

36. Narkun-Burgess DM, Nolan CR, Norman JE, et al. Forty-five year follow-up after uninephrectomy. Kidney Int. 1993;43: 1110–15.

37. Keijzer MH de, Klasen IS, Branten AJ, et al. Infusion of plasma expanders may lead to unexpected results in urinary protein assays. Scand J Clin Lab Invest. 1999;59:133–7.

38. Dietl KH, Wolters H, Marschall B, et al. Cadaveric two-in-one kidney transplantation from marginal donors: experience of 26 cases after 3 years. Transplantation. 2000;70:790–4.

39. Schortgen F, Lacherade JC, Bruneel F, et al. Effects of hydroxyethyl starch and gelatin on renal function in severe sepsis: a multicentre randomised study. Lancet. 2001;357:911–16.

40. Hordijk W, Hoitsma AJ, Vliet JA van der, Hilbrands LB. Results of transplantation with kidneys from non-heart-beating donors. Transplant Proc. 2001;33:1127–8.

41. Daemen JW, Oomen AP, Janssen MA, et al. Glutathione S-transferase as predictor of functional outcome in transplantation of machine-preserved non-heart-beating donor kidneys. Transplantation. 1997;63:89–93.

42. Metcalfe MS, Butterworth PC, White SA, et al. A case-control comparison of the results of renal transplantation from heart-beating and non-heart-beating donors. Transplantation. 2001;71:1556–9.

43. Brenner BM, Milford EL. Nephron underdosing: a programmed cause of chronic renal allograft failure. Am J Kidney Dis. 1993; 21:66–72.

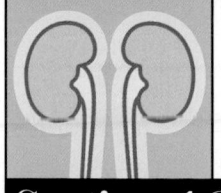

Chapter 87 Renal Transplant Surgery

Hans Sollinger and Yolanda Becker

LIVING DONOR NEPHRECTOMY

Transplants from living donation have excellent long-term function with a half-life of 12–20 years vs. 8–9 years for cadaveric donation[1]. Living donation minimizes ischemia time resulting in fewer complications and a lower incidence of delayed graft function. Siblings, parents, and 'emotionally related' individuals are routinely evaluated for donation. The evaluation of the donor is addressed in Chapter 86.

Renal arteriography, CT scanning with 3D reconstruction (Fig. 87.1) or magnetic resonance angiography (MRA) is performed preoperatively to assess renal vasculature. The left kidney is preferentially chosen because it has a longer renal vein. If the left kidney has vascular anomalies, the right kidney can be used. If both donor kidneys have multiple arteries, *ex vivo* renal artery reconstruction can be performed. Intravenous urography is also performed to exclude urologic anomalies (extrarenal pelvis, double ureter). The nephrectomy can be performed using the traditional open technique or the newer laparoscopic procedure.

Open nephrectomy

For the open technique, a 7–10 cm flank incision is made extending from the tip of the 12th rib toward the umbilicus (Fig. 87.2). Dissection of the renal artery, vein, and ureter is carried out with an extraperitoneal approach. The ureter is ligated and divided near the bladder. All efforts are made to avoid stripping the ureter to minimize damage to its blood supply. Donors should be kept well hydrated. Furosemide and mannitol are given just prior to removal of the donor kidney to ensure a brisk diuresis. The kidney is placed in a basin of ice slush and then cold heparinized normal saline with lidocaine added is flushed through the renal artery.

Laparoscopic nephrectomy

Laparoscopic donor nephrectomy was introduced in 1995 and is a popular method of nephrectomy because it allows a decreased length of hospital stay, less need for pain medication, and faster return to full activity[2]. By removing perceived disincentives to donation, some centers have experienced an increase in living donation by as much as 40%[3].

In early series, only left nephrectomies were performed because of the longer renal vein. A total of four 12 mm operating ports are required. A camera is placed in the left lower quadrant port. Using a harmonic scalpel, the surgeon mobilizes the left colon, and dissects the gonadal vessel complex carefully to preserve the periureteric vessels, and then clips and divides the adrenal and gonadal vein. After visualization of the renal vessels, the ureter is divided as distal to the kidney as possible, and the renal artery and then vein are divided. The kidney is placed in an extraction bag and removed through a Pfannenstiel incision (Fig. 87.3).

Laparoscopic right nephrectomies were initially associated with increased risk for thrombosis and delayed graft function, but can now be performed safely using a modified hand assisted technique that allows for retraction of the right renal vein and division of the vein close to the vena cava[4].

Laparoscopic vs. open nephrectomy

The open nephrectomy has a long record of safety, shorter operative time, and minimal warm ischemia time. However, the donor experiences a longer convalescence (6–8 weeks),

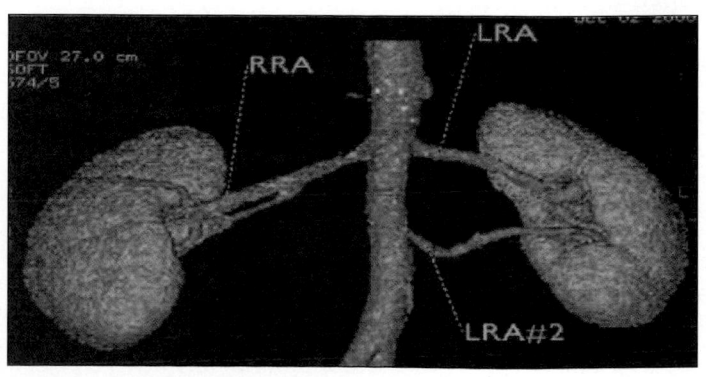

Figure 87.1 Donor preoperative CT angiogram. 3D reconstruction showing two left renal arteries.

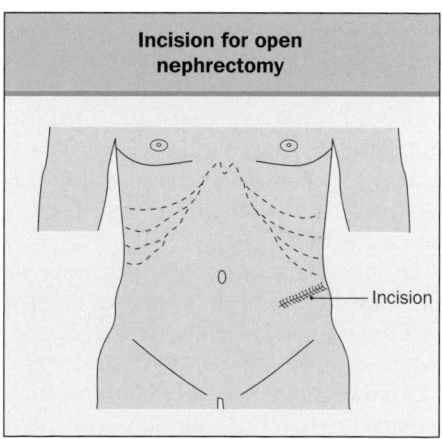

Incision for open nephrectomy

Figure 87.2 Incision for open nephrectomy. A right or left flank incision is used for initial exposure.

Transplantation

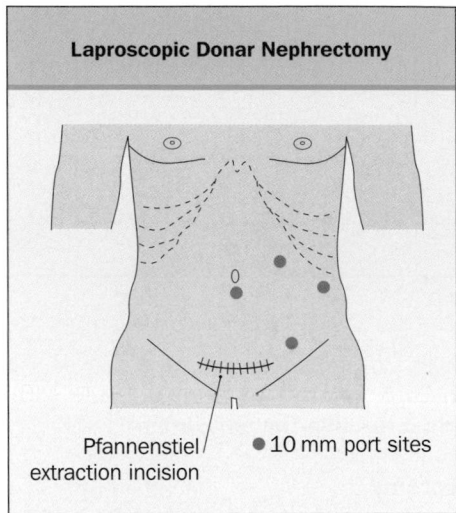

Laproscopic Donar Nephrectomy

Pfannenstiel
extraction incision ● 10 mm port sites

Figure 87.3 Port positions for laparoscopic donor nephrectomy. The kidney is retrieved through the Pfannenstiel incision.

Components of UW (University of Wisconsin) solution	
Component	Concentration
Potassium lactobionate	100 mmol/L
Raffinose	30 mmol/L
Hydroxyethylstarch	50 g/L
Potassium biphosphate	25 mmol/L
Glutathione	3 mmol/L
Adenosine	5 mmol/L
Allopurinol	1 mmol/L
Magnesium sulfate	5 mmol/L
Penicillin	200 000 U/L
Insulin	100 µg/L
Dexamethasone	16 mg/L
Sodium ions	25 mmol/L
Potassium ions	125 mmol/L

Table 87.1 Components of UW (University of Wisconsin) solution[6].

has more postoperative pain, and a longer scar. In a randomized controlled trial, laparoscopic donor nephrectomy was shown to be associated with 47% less analgesic requirements, 33% more rapid return to activity (2–4 weeks) and 73% less pain reported at 6 weeks compared to open nephrectomy[2]. Laparoscopic nephrectomy is safe, has excellent recipient outcomes, and is associated with a shorter average hospital stay (1–3 d) vs. the open technique (4–5 d)[5]. By decreasing the morbidity associated with the donor operation, more potential living donors may volunteer for evaluation.

RENAL PRESERVATION

Preservation of cadaveric organs is crucial to allow time for matching, sharing of organs, and preparation of the recipient. Damage from hypothermia and reperfusion must be minimized. The original 'Collins' solution used for cold storage was replaced in the late 1980s, when Belzer and Southard developed the UW solution (ViaSpan, Dupont Pharma, Wilmington, DE) which has extended preservation time up to 72 h for kidneys[6] (Table 87.1). Lactobionate, raffinose, and hydroxyethylstarch are added to minimize hypothermic cell swelling.

Cadaveric organs can be preserved by cold storage (used in 70% of centers) or by machine-driven pulsatile perfusion (used in 30% of centers and also by the authors). Pulsatile perfusion is associated with less delayed graft function; in one study the rate was 8.8% vs. 20.2% with routine cold storage ($P = 0.001$)[7]. Delayed graft function is associated with poorer long-term graft survival, which suggests that machine perfusion is a better method. A comparison of cold storage vs. machine perfusion in over 800 kidney transplants revealed similar graft survival rates in the two groups despite the fact that the machine perfused kidneys had been procured from higher risk donors (older age, higher serum creatinine)[7].

Pulsatile perfusion may provide extra benefit as it allows the kidney to function aerobically due to the supply of oxygen and substrate, and due to the removal of metabolic end products. Decisions about whether or not to use a kidney from a marginal donor can be based on data retrieved from machine perfusion. Both an increase in perfusate calcium[8] and high perfusion pressures on the machine are associated with poor or delayed graft function.

RENAL TRANSPLANT TECHNIQUE

Preoperative preparations
The patient with end-stage renal disease (ESRD) may require dialysis immediately prior to transplant to optimize hemodynamic status and electrolyte balance. After induction of general anesthesia, a foley catheter is inserted and an antibiotic solution is instilled to sterilize the bladder. A first-generation cephalosporin is administered within 1 h of the skin incision and for 24 h postoperatively. Peritoneal dialysis patients need to empty their peritoneum of dialysate prior to going to the operating room. Catheters for peritoneal dialysis can be removed at the time of transplant. However, we prefer to remove them 4–6 weeks after transplantation when steroid dosage is lower and transplant function is stable.

Operative technique
The right side is generally chosen for the initial transplant, as adequate exposure of the left iliac vein can be more difficult. However, some surgeons prefer to use the ipsilateral side of the donor organ. A curvilinear incision is made from above the iliac crest to the inguinal ligament lateral to the symphysis pubis. The external oblique muscle, fascia, and internal oblique and transversalis muscles are divided and the peritoneum is swept medially. The iliac artery and vein are exposed, the overlying lymphatic tissue ligated or cauterized, and the common iliac artery is isolated to the level of the hypogastric bifurcation. If there are multiple donor renal arteries, a more extensive dissection of the recipient hypogastric artery branches may be required for later reconstruction (see below).

The common iliac vein is freed from the level of the vena cava to just superior to the inguinal ligament. While some surgeons perform the venous anastomosis at the site of the common iliac vein without further mobilization, we ligate and divide the majority of the posterior branches of the common iliac vein. This allows the vein to lie more anteriorly thereby facilitating the venous anastomosis, preventing kinking of the anastomosis, and compensating for a short right renal vein. The donor kidney is then brought to the operative field. An end-to-side donor vein to recipient common iliac anastomosis is completed. An end-to-side anastomosis of the donor renal artery to the native common iliac artery is then performed. The end-to-end anastomosis of the recipient hypogastric artery to the donor renal artery is no longer performed as it is associated with an increased risk of thrombosis and subsequent stenosis[9]. The venous clamp is removed first, followed by the distal and then proximal arterial clamp. The kidney is bathed in warm saline to minimize vasospasm. In cold stored kidneys, the vasospasm may persist and can be alleviated by the infusion of 5 mg of verapamil into the iliac artery above the renal artery anastomosis. Bleeding points along the renal capsule are electrocoagulated whereas along the ureter they are ligated with fine ligatures to avoid compromise of blood supply.

The ureteral anastomosis is designed to prevent reflux or obstruction. The ureter may be implanted into the bladder or a uretero-ureteral anastomosis may be used if the donor ureter is short. A common method of ureteroneocystostomy is the Leadbetter-Politano method in which an anterior cystotomy is made and the ureter is passed through the submucosal tunnel and implanted just lateral to the ipsilateral native ureteral orifice. An alternative method is the Liche technique, in which a single cystotomy is made in the anterolateral surface of the bladder. The ureter is implanted in an end-to-side fashion and the bladder muscularis reapproximated over the ureter to create an anti-reflux tunnel. A double J ureteral stent may be placed prior to completion of the ureteral anastomosis to decrease the incidence of postoperative urine leaks and ureteral obstruction[10]. We prefer the stented Liche (extravesical) technique. The stent is removed cystoscopically 4–6 weeks after transplantation. Foley catheter drainage of the bladder is continued for 2–3 d. A diagram of the completed transplant is shown in Figure 87.4.

Implantation into the native bladder is preferred. Patients with small bladders may require routine catheterization for a period of time. However, bladder compliance and capacity improve with time. Ureters may be implanted to a pre-existing ileal conduit.

Multiple arteries

Multiple renal arteries are found in 18–30% of all potential kidney donors. Multiple arteries may be converted to a single anastomosis (see Fig. 87.5) or multiple anastomosis may be required (see Fig. 87.6). The most common vascular complication of multiple renal arteries is renal artery stenosis which usually occurs late (> 10 d post-transplant)[11]. Revascularization of the lower pole renal arteries is particularly important because these vessels supply the ureter.

Because many transplant centers only perform left nephrectomies using the laparoscopic technique, there has been a rise in kidneys procured with multiple arteries, as these centers

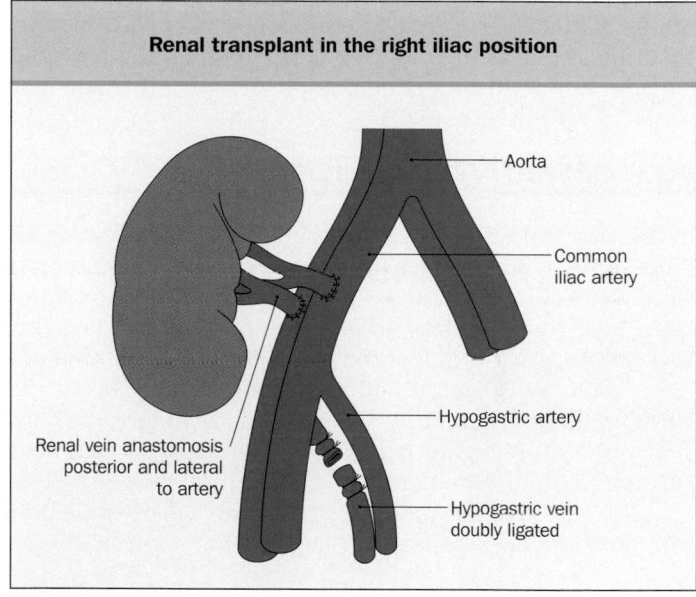

Figure 87.4 Renal transplant in the right iliac position. The completed renal transplant with a single renal artery and vein.

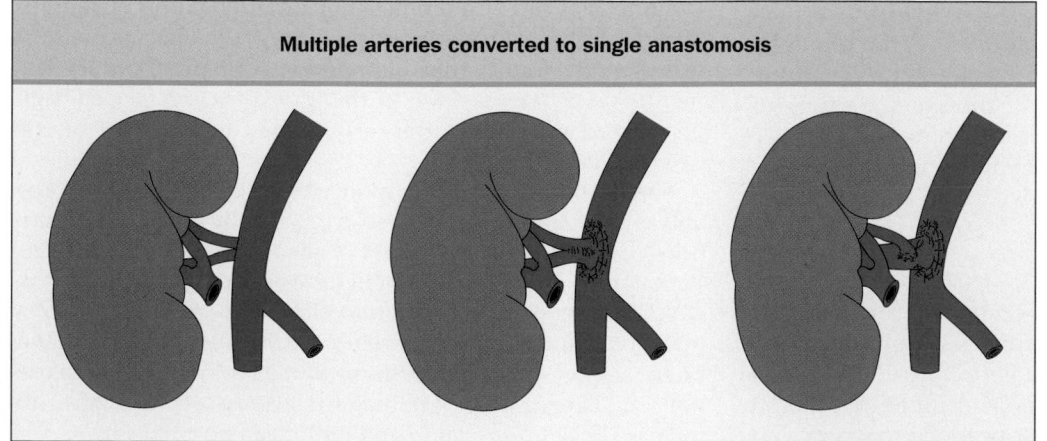

Figure 87.5 Multiple donor renal arteries. Arteries reconstructed to a single orifice for anastomosis.

Transplantation

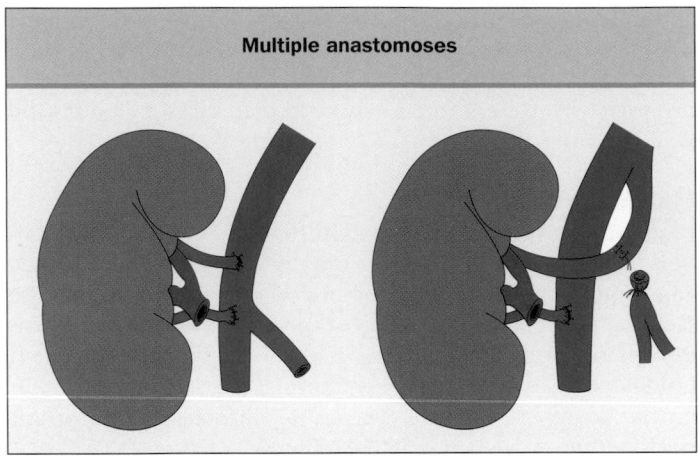

Figure 87.6 Multiple anastomoses. Multiple donor renal arteries requiring multiple reanastomoses.

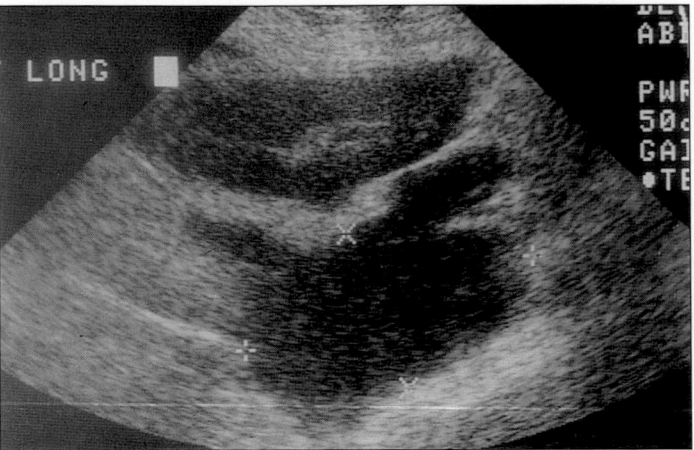

Figure 87.7 Lymphocele, ultrasound appearance. A large echolucent lymphocele can be seen inferior to the transplanted kidney.

will select a left kidney with multiple renal arteries over a right kidney with a solitary artery. There is a 15–18% incidence of multiple arteries in open live donor nephrectomies compared to an incidence as high as 27% in laparoscopically procured kidneys. At this time the complication rates for either donor or recipient are not increased[12].

POSTOPERATIVE COMPLICATIONS

In the early postoperative period, careful management of fluid status is imperative. Regular measurements of central venous pressure, especially in patients with early acute tubular necrosis, can be crucial. Intravenous fluids should be given at a rate to equal urine output plus 30 mL/h. The minimal rate should be 30 mL/h and the maximal rate 200 mL/h. Furosemide and mannitol can be used to induce diuresis. Dopamine (5–15 µg/kg per min) is employed to maintain adequate systolic blood pressure. The surgical causes of postoperative dysfunction are discussed below; whereas medical complications are discussed in Chapter 89.

Lymphocele

Presentation
Lymphoceles are collections of lymphatic fluid caused by the disruption of lymphatic vessels that lie along the course of the iliac artery and vein. On occasion, large amounts of lymph can be produced by the transplanted kidney. The incidence of lymphocele is usually less than 10%. Patients may be asymptomatic and present with an elevated serum creatinine as the lymphocele compresses part of the ureter, leading to ureteral obstruction. The lymphocele can compress the iliac vein, leading to unilateral leg swelling or deep venous thrombosis. Spontaneous lymphocele drainage also can present as a scrotal mass or swelling.

Diagnosis
Ultrasound shows a rounded echolucent mass usually located near the lower pole of the kidney that is distinct from the bladder (Fig. 87.7). Internal echoes in lymphoceles may signal infected fluid. The fluid may be aspirated under ultrasound and will have a creatinine concentration similar to serum, and

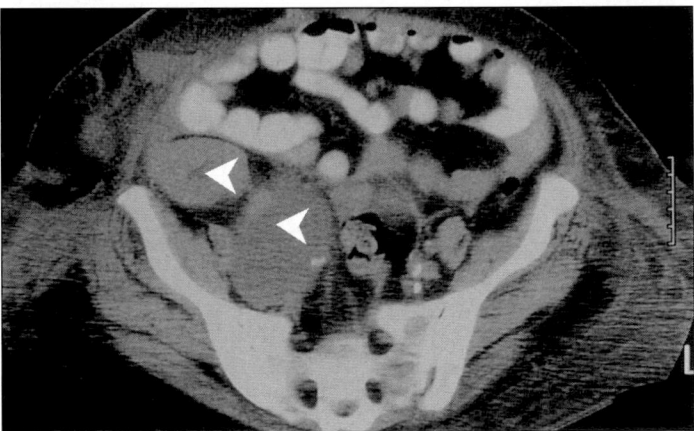

Figure 87.8 Lymphocele, computed tomography appearance. A 5 cm × 5 cm lymphocele (right arrow head) is present under the transplanted kidney (left arrow head).

an elevated protein content. Urinomas (collections of urine from urinary tract leak), are similar in ultrasound appearance but have a high creatinine level. Lymphoceles are also easily diagnosed by computed tomographic (CT) scan (Fig. 87.8).

Treatment
Lymphoceles can be minimized by careful ligation or cauterization of the lymphatics surrounding the iliac vessels. A recent study found that lymphocele formation occurs less frequently (2.1% vs. 8.5%) if the transplant was placed high on the common iliac artery as opposed to the level of the external iliac vessels[13].

Small asymptomatic lymphoceles do not require therapy and usually spontaneously resolve. Medially located lymphoceles that compress the ureter or iliac vein require drainage. Various techniques for treatment have been described. Injection of sclerosants such as talc, tetracycline, doxycycline and povidone-iodine may be successful in up to 90% in some series[14] but often require repeated treatments with a prolonged time to resolution. Percutaneous drainage is also associated with an increased risk for infection and prolonged hospital stay[15].

The most successful therapy is an open operative procedure in which a 5–7 cm × 1–2 cm segment of the peritoneum is excised to create a window. This allows the lymph to be absorbed by the peritoneal cavity and omentum. A small section of omentum may be placed within the window to prevent closure. Laparoscopic techniques have also been used to make the peritoneal window and are associated with less pain and a shorter hospital stay when compared to the open method[16].

Obese patients are at increased risk for developing lymphoceles. For this reason, we routinely create a peritoneal window at the time of the initial transplant in this population.

Graft thrombosis
Presentation
Thrombosis of the transplant renal artery or vein is heralded by the sudden onset of oliguria. Vascular thrombosis may also be the end-point of severe rejection; however, the precise cause remains obscure in the vast majority of patients. Arterial thrombosis usually occurs within the first 24–48 h. The peak incidence of venous thrombosis is 3–9 d. Risk factors for thrombosis include a history of other venous thrombosis, diabetic nephropathy, technical surgical factors, extremes of age in both donor and recipient, and hypovolemia from overdiuresis, bleeding, or diarrhea[17]. A graft with venous thrombosis may become acutely swollen and present with pain arising from compression of surrounding tissue; transplant venous thrombosis may also be associated with significant hematuria.

Diagnosis
Vascular thrombosis may be clinically difficult to distinguish from acute tubular necrosis. However, one must maintain a high index of suspicion especially in the setting of persistent graft dysfunction. Lack of function in a living donor kidney should prompt an immediate search for adequate perfusion. Isotope scanning (DTPA) is simple and accurate; isotope is quickly taken up by the transplanted kidney in a normal perfusion scan whereas no isotope is taken up during the early perfusion phase in acute arterial thrombosis. Duplex ultrasonography can also be used to demonstrate lack of flow in thrombosed vessels.

Treatment
There is no effective treatment for vascular thrombosis. This disaster is a rarity (incidence ~ 1%). There are case reports of salvaging renal transplants with venous thrombosis when operative therapy (thrombectomy, or evacuation of a hematoma causing extrinsic compression) was performed within 1 h of the event[18,19]. An urgent transplant nephrectomy is the indicated treatment for venous thrombosis to minimize the chances of graft rupture and exsanguinating hemorrhage.

A transplant with arterial thrombosis cannot be salvaged. There appears to be a higher incidence of this complication in highly sensitized patients. This suggests that antibody-mediated endothelial damage may be occurring despite the lack of evidence of rejection on biopsy[20]. Transplant nephrectomy is also required in arterial thrombosis.

Patients who have experienced graft thrombosis can be safely retransplanted[21]. However, these patients should have protein C and S, antithrombin III, factor V Leiden, and antiphospholipid antibody levels checked prior to retransplantation. If a hypercoagulable state is identified, adequate perioperative anticoagulation has been associated with a 2.6-fold decrease in the expected incidence of thrombosis[22].

Renal artery stenosis
Presentation
Transplant renal artery stenosis (TRAS) develops in 1–12% of grafts depending on the method of diagnosis and the definition of significant stenosis[23]. The stenosis usually occurs between 3 months to 2 years post-transplantation[24]. Early presentation is usually attributed to surgical technique and has been associated with end-to-end arterial anastomosis[25]. Late presentation is less well understood.

Patients classically present with worsening hypertension after a stable post-transplant course. Hypoperfusion of the transplant stimulates an increase in renin release and subsequent sodium and water retention and volume expansion. Many patients present with significant weight increases and lower extremity edema in the absence of nephrotic range proteinuria. The serum creatinine level may also rise. Angiotensin-converting enzyme (ACE) inhibitor therapy can precipitate a dramatic decrease in graft function when there is pre-existing renal artery stenosis.

While examination may reveal an abdominal bruit overlying the graft, the sensitivity and specificity of this physical sign is low. Femoral pulses should always be examined, as aorto-iliac disease may mimic renal artery stenosis. Iliac occlusive disease masquerading as TRAS occurs in up to 2.4% of patients[24]. Risk factors for the development of TRAS include extremes of donor age, recipient diabetes, and obesity.

Diagnosis
All patients with worsening graft function should undergo ultrasound examination to exclude ureteral obstruction and a biopsy to rule out other causes of hypertension including acute rejection, chronic allograft nephropathy, drug toxicity, or recurrence of renal disease. Duplex scanning with color flow Doppler may demonstrate an arterial jet or decreased flow (Fig. 87.9). Magnetic resonance angiography (MRA) is the noninvasive test of choice and does not require the administration of nephrotoxic contrast material (Fig. 87.10). Other diagnostic modalities include spiral-computed tomography, isotope renography before and after dosing with captopril, and carbon dioxide angiography[9]. Contrast angiography remains the 'gold standard'.

Treatment
Medical management
The optimal medical management of hypertension from TRAS has not been clearly delineated. Calcium channel blockers and diuretics are the mainstay of therapy. ACE inhibitors and angiotensin II receptor antagonists should be avoided as they may precipitate renal failure. Chapter 63 contains a complete review of this topic.

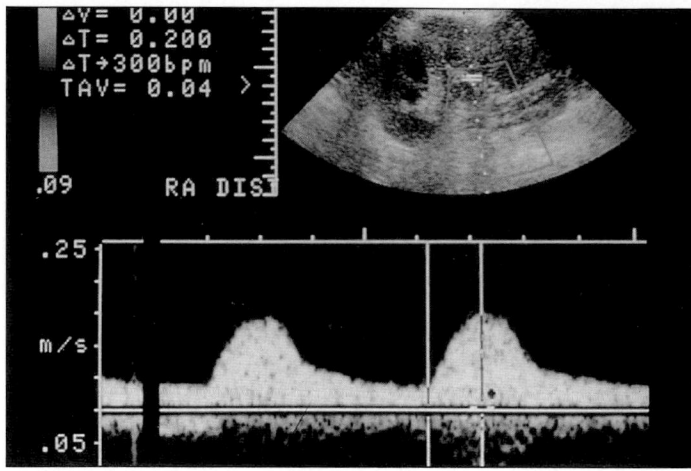

Figure 87.9 Arterial stenosis on Doppler ultrasound. Transplant arterial stenosis on ultrasound with a tardus parvus waveform.

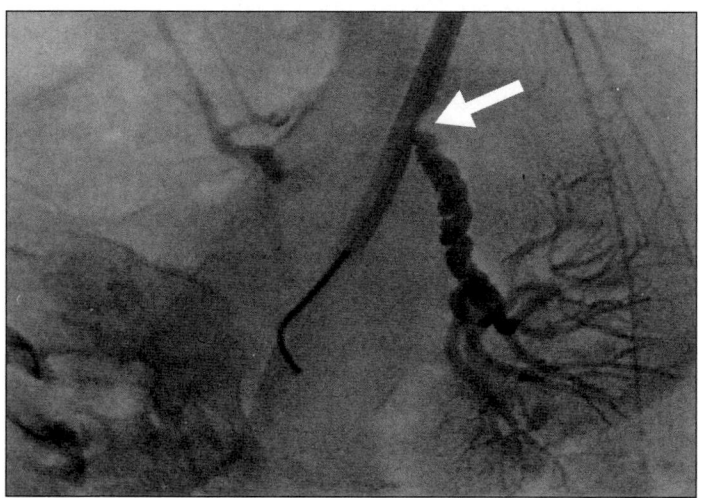

Figure 87.10 Transplant renal artery stenosis. MR angiogram (MRA). Demonstrating hemodynamically significant TRAS.

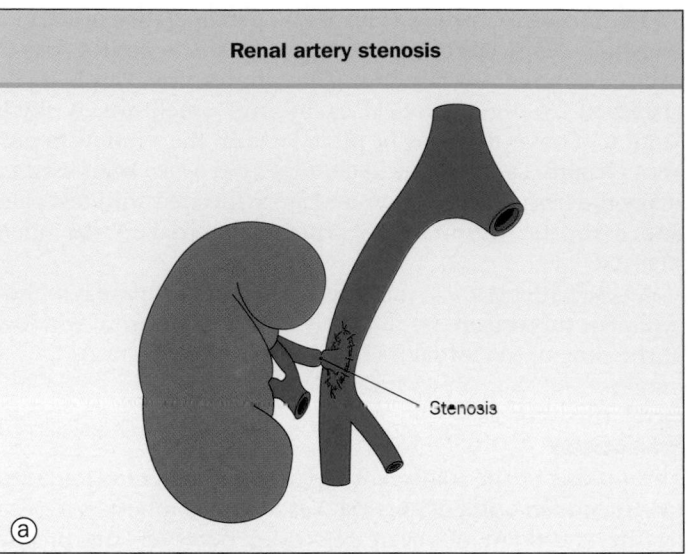

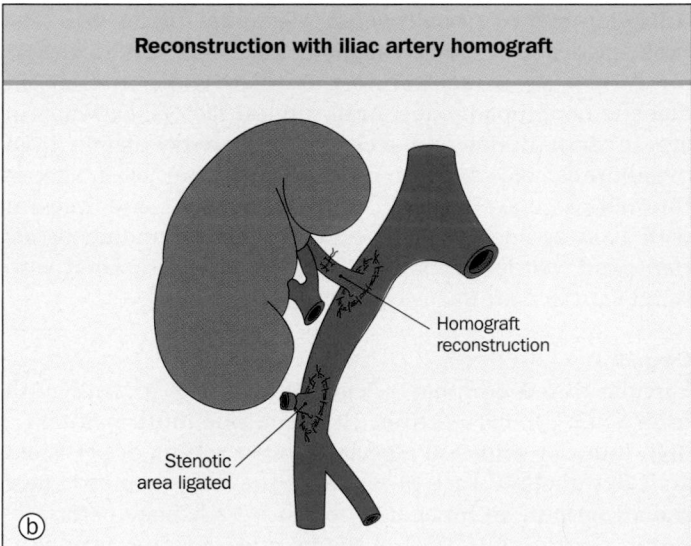

Figure 87.11 Renal artery reconstruction using an iliac artery homograft.

Percutaneous interventional management

Percutaneous transluminal angioplasty is a safe and effective therapy with a high rate of success in treating renal artery stenosis in well-selected patients. Angioplasty may alleviate stenosis and decrease the severity of hypertension in up to 80% of patients[9]. Unfortunately, restenosis occurs in up to 30% of successfully treated patients within 6 months[23]. The most suitable lesions for angioplasty are localized stenoses distal to the original anastomosis. Dilatation at the anastomosis is associated with a higher complication rate and a poorer long-term outcome. Stenting of ostial lesions after angioplasty has been used successful in the short term, but long-term results are still unknown[26].

Surgical repair

Surgical has success rates varying from 63–92%[25]. Surgical correction of TRAS can be accomplished by resection or revision of the anastomosis, patch angioplasty, localized endarterectomy or bypass with recipient saphenous vein or ipsilateral hypogastric artery. However, these techniques require extensive dissection in a scarred field that may increase the risk for complications. The authors have successfully used blood-type compatible cadaveric iliac artery as a conduit for bypass in a series of 21 patients with a 90% success rate and with only one recurrence[27]. These donor iliac arteries are routinely procured during multiorgan recoveries to reconstruct the pancreas or liver allograft. The cadaveric vessel is anastomosed to the recipient iliac artery prior to ligating and dividing the stenotic transplant renal artery to limit transplant warm ischemia (Fig. 87.11). Long-term follow up (median 42 months) resulted in only two cases of graft loss secondary to renal artery stenosis.

Comparison of treatment modalities

In the only study comparing surgical outcome (using saphenous vein graft) and percutaneous angioplasty, the authors found that while both modalities adequately treated hypertension, angioplasty was associated with a significantly higher incidence of restenosis[28]. Ruggenenti and colleagues have also shown that revascularization of the stenosis restores kidney perfusion, and normalizes blood flow and vascular shear stress[23]. With medical therapy blood pressure may be controlled but kidney perfusion is not restored. Therefore either surgery or angioplasty to restore flow is preferred.

Urine leaks

Presentation
Urine leaks present early in the postoperative period. The patient usually complains of flank pain or pain over the transplant site as urine irritates the surrounding peritoneum. The patient may have a decreased urine output, with a disproportionate rise in serum creatinine. Patients may also present with copious fluid drainage from the wound site.

Diagnosis
A renal scan with delayed images is a sensitive screening test for the detection of urinary extravasation. Cystography is also useful to exclude the bladder as the source of the leak. Ultrasound can detect a fluid collection (urinoma). If an abnormal fluid collection is noted on ultrasound, it should be aspirated in a sterile fashion and the creatinine level of the fluid should be determined to differentiate a urine leak from a lymphocele.

Treatment
Foley catheter drainage of the bladder should be instituted if a urine leak is suspected. Decompressing the bladder may reduce pressure at the site of the leak and lead to resolution without requiring further intervention. Once catheter drainage is established, efforts should be made to define the anatomy of the leak. The most common site of leakage is at the ureteroneocystostomy. Other sites of leakage include the ureter or renal calyx. Leakage from the ureter or renal pelvis may occur as a result of ischemia secondary to procurement injury.

Some leaks may be managed successfully by bladder drainage and antegrade placement of a double J ureteral stent[29]. Leaks caused by ureteral sloughing cannot be solely managed by percutaneous methods. The surgical approach to therapy depends on the amount of viable ureter. Leaks at the renal pelvis can be managed by performing a ureteropyelostomy, using the native ureter. If the ipsilateral ureter is not available, the contralateral ureter may be passed through the sigmoid mesentery and used as a conduit. Dividing the transplant ureter leads to necrosis of its distal end through compromise of the blood supply. However, if a simple anastomotic leak has occurred, it may be possible to resect the distal ureter and reimplant the ureter over a double J stent. Following repair, an indwelling stent is usually left in place for 6 weeks and removed cystoscopically.

Ureteral obstruction

Presentation
Ureteral obstruction may be asymptomatic because of the lack of innervation of the transplanted kidney and it may occur early or late. The reported incidence varies from 2–10%[30]. Causes of early obstruction are generally technical and include a twisted ureter, a badly placed suture, blood clots obstructing outflow, or edema at the anastomosis site. Causes of late obstruction are more diverse and include ureteral stricture or fibrosis, renal calculi, a mycotic mass, or a lymphocele.

Diagnosis
A rising serum creatinine is usually the first clue to diagnosis. Hydronephrosis is evident on ultrasound. Pressures within the renal pelvis are obtained (Whittaker test). Pressures >15 cm H_2O are diagnostic of obstruction. An intravenous urogram is useful to demonstrate the level of the obstruction but may be suboptimal in poorly functioning allografts. In these cases placement of a percutaneous nephrostomy tube and antegrade pyelography will allow definitive visualization of the lesion. The nephrostomy tube may also be used to place an antegrade stent for treatment. A furosemide renogram may be performed as a screening test but will not define anatomic detail.

Treatment
Early obstructions caused by postoperative edema can be managed nonoperatively. This complication can potentially be avoided by placement of a double J stent at the time of the neureterocystostomy. An evaluation of 670 patients undergoing living related renal transplant revealed a significantly lower complication rate (0.22% with stent vs. 8.5% without) when a stent was left in place[31]. Balloon dilatation in early obstruction has a 50–70% success rate. Late obstructions are more difficult to manage. Balloon dilatation followed by 4–6 weeks of stenting can be effective. The success rate is influenced by the location, length and extent of the stricture and varies from 16–100%[30]. Placement of stents via bladder cystoscopy is difficult because of the anterior position of the transplant ureteral orifice. The nephrostomy tube placed for diagnosis can be used for dilatation and placement of a stent. If percutaneous methods fail, an operative approach is necessary.

Resecting the region of obstruction and performing a new ureteroneocystostomy can treat very short distal ureteral obstructions. If the obstruction is proximal, a ureteroureterostomy to native ureter can be done. The native ureters may also be incorporated into a ureteropyelostomy to bypass a high obstruction[32]. A Boari flap may be constructed if the transplant ureter is too short and no native ureter is available (Fig. 87.12).

Wound infection
Wound infections occur in less than 1% of patients and are usually due to *Staph aureus*. The infection rate was higher (34%) in the 1960s and 1970s[33], probably because of the higher doses of steroids used. Wound infections usually occur around postoperative day 7 and occur more frequently in obese patients[34]. Patients with abdominal wall cellulitis distant to the site of the transplant should be investigated for the presence of a foreign body such as a retained peritoneal dialysis cuff. Therapy with systemic antibiotics should be initiated immediately when a wound infection is suspected. Early operative debridement may be necessary.

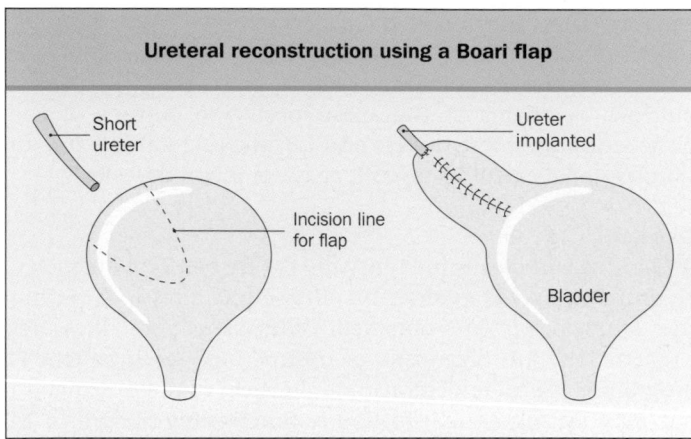

Ureteral reconstruction using a Boari flap

Short ureter

Ureter implanted

Incision line for flap

Bladder

Figure 87.12 Ureteral reconstruction using a Boari flap.

Bleeding complications

Presentation and diagnosis

The patient with ESRD and inherent platelet dysfunction is at risk for perioperative bleeding. Vasopressin (0.3 µg/kg) given immediately prior to making the incision significantly decreases bleeding in the operative field by potentiating the release of von Willebrand factor.

Bleeding from small vessels in the renal hilum may not be evident during the operation because of vasospasm. Careful monitoring of blood pressure and serial hematocrits are crucial to making the diagnosis of small vessel hemorrhage in the early postoperative period[35]. Patients may complain of pain only if a hematoma is large enough to cause peritoneal irritation. Bloody drainage from the incision and a decrease in hematocrit should prompt obtaining an ultrasound (easiest and most sensitive) or CT scan to look for a hematoma.

In rare cases, an acute rejection episode or venous thrombosis may cause rupture of the renal capsule resulting in hemorrhage with tachycardia, acute hypotension and pain due to the rapidly enlarging hematoma. The hematoma may cause sudden swelling at the incision site. If a peritoneal window was previously created, blood will drain intraperitoneally and the only sign will be sudden hemodynamic compromise.

Treatment

The best prevention for immediate postoperative bleeding is meticulous intraoperative hemostasis. Coagulation parameters (prothrombin time, partial thromboplastin time) should be checked to exclude occult intrinsic coagulopathy. Efforts should be made to correct any coagulopathy prior to transplant. Large hematomas causing compression of surrounding structures should be drained surgically. Hematomas may be a nidus for infection if left undrained. At exploration, a specific bleeding point may not be identifiable. There is usually a large coagulum and a small amount of hemorrhage from the renal capsule that is easily electrocoagulated.

If the patient's clinical condition suggests acute rupture, immediate surgical exploration is required. High dose methylprednisolone is given intraoperatively. In rare cases, the kidney can be repaired using pledgeted sutures or wrapped with a sheet of vicryl mesh similar to management of a ruptured spleen in the trauma patient. However, in most patients, the transplant will have to be removed.

TRANSPLANT NEPHRECTOMY

A nephrectomy may be required for arterial thrombosis, capsular rupture, or other technical reasons. Removal of a graft may cause a steep elevation in the percentage of preformed antibodies, making subsequent transplantation difficult. However, some patients require graft nephrectomy for persistent fever, malaise, thrombocytopenia, or graft tenderness following functional graft loss. Early graft loss within 1 year has been associated with a 90% need for transplant nephrectomy. Only 50% of grafts lost after 1 year require nephrectomy. A nonfunctional graft left in place will usually shrink and become fibrotic.

Operative procedure

Removal of a rejected graft can be a technical challenge as the renal capsule may be adherent to adjacent structures because of repeated bouts of rejection. For this reason, we prefer a subcapsular dissection. By using this method, the vascular pedicle may be identified at the base of the graft. A large vascular clamp may be placed and the kidney removed. The hilum is then suture ligated leaving a cuff of donor vessel in place[36].

Absolute hemostasis is the key to prevention of further complications. The entire raw surface of the remaining capsule should be cauterized using the argon beam coagulator or electrocautery. Closed suction drains will frequently not drain collected coagulum and can serve as a source of possible infection. Intravenous perioperative antibiotics as well as antibiotic irrigant are routinely used.

REFERENCES

1. Cecka JM. The UNOS Scientific Renal Transplant Registry. In: Cecka JM, Terasaki PI, eds. Clinical Transplants. Los Angeles: UCLA Tissue Typing Laboratory; 2000.

2. Wolf JS, Merion RM, Leichtman AB, et al. Randomized controlled trial of hand-assisted laparoscopic versus open surgical live donor nephrectomy. Transplantation. 2001;72(2):284–90.

3. Schweitzer EJ, Wilson J, Jacobs S, et al. Increased rates of donation with laparoscopic donor nephrectomy. Ann Surg. 2000; 232(3):392–400.

4. Johnson MW, Andreoni K, McCoy L, et al. Technique of right laparoscopic donor nephrectomy: A single center experience. Am J Transplant. 2001;1:293–5.

5. Jacobs SC, Cho E, Dunkin BJ, et al. Laparoscopic live donor nephrectomy: the University of Maryland 3-year experience. J Urol. 2000;164(5):1494–9.

6. Ploeg RJ, van B, Langendijk PT et al. Effect of preservation solution on results of cadaveric kidney transplantation. The European Multicentre Study Group. Lancet. 1992;340:129–37.

7. Sellers MT, Gallichio MH, Hudson SL, et al. Improved outcomes in cadaveric renal allografts with pulsatile preservation. Clin Transplant. 2000;14(6):543–9.

8. Polyak MM, Arrington BO, Stubenbord WT, et al. The influence of pulsatile preservation on renal transplantation in the 1990s. Transplantation. 2000;69(2):249–58.

9. Fervenza FC, Lafayette RA, Alfrey EJ, Petersen J. Renal artery stenosis in kidney transplants. Am J Kidney Dis. 1998;31:142–8.

10. Butterworth PC, Horsburgh T, Veitch PS, Urological complications in renal transplantation: impact of a change of technique. Br J Urol. 1997;79:499–502.

11. Benedetti E, Troppmann C, Gillingham K, et al. Short- and long-term outcomes of kidney transplants with multiple renal arteries. Ann Surg. 1995;221:406–14.

12. Troppmann C, Wiesmann K, McVicar JP, et al. Increased transplantation of kidneys with multiple renal arteries in the laparoscopic live donor nephrectomy era: surgical technique and surgical and nonsurgical donor and recipient outcomes. Arch Surg. 2001;136(8):897–907.

13. Sansalone CV, Aseni P, Minetti E, et al. Is lymphocele in renal transplantation an avoidable complication? Am J Surg. 2000; 179:182–5.

14. Caliendo MV, Lee DE, Queiroz R, Waldman DL. Sclerotherapy with use of doxycycline after percutaneous drainage of postoperative lymphoceles. J Vasc Interventional Radiol. 2001; 12(1):73–7.

15. Thurlow JP, Gelpi J, Schwaitzberg SD, Rohrer RJ. Laparoscopic peritoneal fenestration and internal drainage of lymphoceles after renal transplantation. Surgical Laparoscopy. Endosc Percutaneous Tech. 1996;6:290–5.

16. Risaliti A, Corno V, Donini A, et al. Laparoscopic treatment of symptomatic lymphoceles after kidney transplantation. Surg Endosc. 2000;14(3):293–5.

17. Bakir N, Sluiter WJ, Ploeg RJ van S, Tegzess AM. Primary renal graft thrombosis. Nephrology, Dialysis Transplantation. 1996; 11:140–7.

18. Nerstrom B, Ladefoged J, Lund F. Vascular complications in 155 consecutive kidney transplantations. Scand J Urol Nephrol. 1972; 6 (suppl 74).

19. Humar A, Sharpe J, Hollomby D. Salvage of a renal allograft with renal vein occlusion secondary to extrinsic compression. Am J Kidney Dis. 1996;28:622–3.

20. Harmer AW, Haskard D, Koffman CG, Welsh KI. Novel antibodies associated with unexplained loss of renal allografts. Transplant Int. 1990;3:66–9.

21. Humar A, Key N, Ramcharan T, et al. Kidney retransplants after initial graft loss to vascular thrombosis. Clin Transplant. 2001; 15(1):6–10.

22. Friedman GS, Meier-Kriesche H-U, Kaplan B, et al. Hypercoagulable states in renal transplant candidates: impact of anticoagulation upon incidence of renal allograft thrombosis. Transplantation. 2001;72:1073–8.

23. Ruggenenti P, Mosconi L, Bruno S, et al. Post-transplant renal artery stenosis: the hemodynamic response to revascularization. Kidney Int. 2001;60(1):309–18.

24. Becker BN, Odorico JS, Becker YT, et al. Peripheral vascular disease and renal transplant artery stenosis: a reappraisal of transplant renovascular disease. Clin Transplant. 1999;13(4):349–55.

25. Rengel M, Gomes-Da-Silva G, Inchaustegui L, et al. Renal artery stenosis after kidney transplantation: diagnostic and therapeutic approach. Kidney Int Suppl. 1998;68:S99–S106.

26. Bertoni E, Zanazzi M, Rosat A, et al. Efficacy and safety of Palmaz stent insertion in the treatment of renal artery stenosis in kidney transplantation. Transplant Int 2000.13(Suppl 1):S425–30.

27. Shames BD, Sollinger JS, D'Alessandro AM, et al. Surgical repair of transplant renal artery stenosis with preserved cadaveric iliac artery grafts. Ann Surg. 2002; (in press).

28. De M, Pirson Y, Dautrebande J, Treatment of renal graft artery stenosis. Comparison between surgical bypass and percutaneous transluminal angioplasty. Transplantation. 1989;47(5):784–8.

29. Swierzewski SJ, Konnak JW, Ellis JH. Treatment of renal transplant ureteral complications by percutaneous techniques. J Urol 1993;149:986–7.

30. Hobart MG, Streem SB, Gill IS. Renal transplant complications. Minimally invasive management. Urol Clin North Am. 2000; 27(4):787–798.

31. Kumar A, Verma BS, Srivastava A, et al. Evaluation of the urological complications of living related renal transplantation at a single center during the last 10 years: Impact of Double-J Stent. J Urol. 2000;164:657–60.

32. Nargund VH, Cranston D. Urological complications after renal transplantation. Transplant Rev. 1996;10:24–33.

33. Stephan RN, Munschauer CE, Kumar MS. Surgical wound infection in renal transplantation: outcome data in 102 consecutive patients without perioperative systemic antibiotic coverage. Arch Surg. 1997;132:1315–18.

34. Pirsch JD, Armbrust MJ, Knechtle SJ, et al. Obesity as a risk factor following renal transplantation. Transplantation. 1995; 59: 631–3.

35. Gritsch HA, Rosenthal JT. The transplant operation and its surgical complications. In: Danovitch GM, ed. Handbook of Kidney Transplantation. Philadelphia, PA: Lippincott. 2001:146–62.

36. O'Sullivan DC, Murphy DM, McLean P, Donovan MG. Transplant nephrectomy over 20 years: factors involved in associated morbidity and mortality. J Urol. 1994;151:855–8.

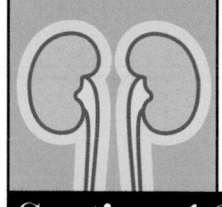

Chapter 88

Prophylaxis and Treatment of Renal Transplant Rejection

Venkataraman Ramanathan and Anthony J Langone

INTRODUCTION

Renal transplantation is the preferred modality of treatment for selected patients with end-stage renal disease. The number on the transplant waiting list continues to increase each year, but the number of available cadaver kidneys (5000–6000/year) has remained static for the past decade resulting in a growing demand vs. supply gap. The main focus has been to avoid rejection in the post-transplant period since acute rejection is a strong predictor for chronic allograft nephropathy (CAN) and chronic attrition of the graft. Preventing chronic rejection and prolonging the half-life of the graft can decrease the need for retransplants. The number of acute rejection episodes[1], late post-transplant rejection (> 60 d)[1], severity of rejection, vascular component[2,3], and failure of renal function to return to baseline after anti-rejection therapies are the strongest predictors of CAN. In recent years, an acute rejection episode is more predictive of chronic allograft failure than in the past[4].

Considering the correlation between acute rejection and CAN, there is increasing rationale to develop immunosuppressive strategies that can eliminate acute rejection entirely. A general description of the immunosuppressive agents used in renal transplantation is provided in Chapter 85. This chapter will review the prophylaxis and the diagnosis of acute rejection, the expanding treatment options available to combat rejection, and the persistent challenges that daunt physicians.

INDUCTION THERAPY

The risk of graft loss is greatest in the immediate postoperative period. Hence, many transplant centers have resorted to an aggressive periengraftment immunosuppression protocol, a strategy known as induction. African Americans, retransplanted patients, recipients of poorly matched kidneys, and patients with high panel reactive antibodies (PRA) are considered high immunologic risk patients and many transplant centers will use antilymphocyte antibodies as induction therapy. In patients with low immunologic risk, many centers induce with anti-interleukin 2 receptor (anti-IL2R) antibodies or no induction therapy is used. Currently, there is no consensus whether anti-IL2R antibodies prolong graft life or which commercially available anti-IL2R antibody or antilymphocyte antibody is most efficacious in preventing rejection.

Burgeoning knowledge from immunologic research has resulted in an explosion of new drugs to combat acute rejection. One can also individualize therapy in induction and maintenance of immunosuppression. While some centers initiate immunosuppression a few days prior to engraftment, the majority of centers start the induction therapy on the day of surgery. Three immunosuppressant classes are used in induction protocols including polyclonal antilymphocyte antibodies, monoclonal antilymphocyte antibodies and anti-IL2 receptor antibodies.

Polyclonal antilymphocyte antibodies

Poly and monoclonal antilymphocyte antibodies have been successfully used to treat acute rejection[5], improve long term allograft survival[6], prevent or delay first acute rejection episodes[7,8], and avoid calcineurin inhibitor nephrotoxicity[9] in organs with delayed graft function[10,11].

Polyclonal sera, against human lymphocytes, are obtained from rabbit (Thymoglobulin) or horse (ATGAM) sources. Polyclonal antibodies are utilized for rejection prophylaxis in high-risk patients and for the treatment of vascular or steroid-resistant cellular rejection. ATGAM and Thymoglobulin contain antibodies to a wide variety of T cell and major histocompatibility complex (MHC) antigens. With the first doses of these agents, T cell derived cytokines are released and can result in fever, nausea, vomiting, chills and rigors for the patient. Pre-medication with steroids, antihistamines and antipyretics are often necessary to mitigate these symptoms. Repeated use of Thymoglobulin or ATGAM can result in serum-sickness, commonly manifested as a rash, fever and severe arthralgias. Anti-heterologous proteins (antihorse and antirabbit antibodies) should be screened for during prolonged use of these agents as antibody formation leads to decreased efficacy of the drug and increases the risk of serum sickness. Leukocyte depletion and thrombocytopenia are common and often require dose reduction or cessation of other medications with similar side effects. The dose of ATGAM is 10–30 mg/kg per d for 7–14 d and it requires infusion via a central vein. Thymoglobulin is also infused centrally at a dose of 1–1.5 mg/kg per d. Close monitoring of CD3 cell counts are useful to ensure efficacy of the administered agent; occasionally doses can be reduced to every other day if CD3 counts are adequately suppressed. The possibility of acute rejection becomes remote with absolute CD3 counts less than 50 cells/µl. When polyclonal antibodies are utilized for induction, and absolute CD3 counts are reduced appropriately, this single agent provides enough protection against rejection that the introduction of calcineurin inhibitors can be delayed if it is feared that their use may be acutely nephrotoxic.

Early introduction of calcineurin inhibitors (cyclosporine and tacrolimus) can lead to or prolong delayed graft function

(DGF) in kidneys sensitive to the vasoconstrictive effects of these agents (e.g., cadaveric kidneys with prolonged cold ischemia time or kidneys from donors with long-standing hypertension or atherosclerosis). Withholding these agents in patients with DGF, while covering them with antilymphocyte preparations permits the delay of introduction of calcineurin inhibitors and at the same time reduces the rate of rejection and improves graft outcome[11]. Unfortunately, withholding other agents from the regimen such as steroids, may lead to worse outcomes[12]. Anti-IL2R antibodies do not appear to offer as much protection and delaying the use of calcineurin inhibitors might lead to increased rates of rejection.

Induction with antilymphocyte antibody is not universal. A recent analysis of USRDS data revealed that antilymphocyte induction was associated with significant relative risk for patient death from cardiovascular and infectious causes in the first 6 months post-transplantation[13]. These drugs were also associated with a significant risk for long-term malignancy-related death. In view of these complications, some centers avoid routine induction with antibodies.

Monoclonal antilymphocyte antibodies

OKT3, a monoclonal antibody directed against the CD3 complex on mature human T lymphocytes, is produced by the hybridization technique. OKT3 is currently used for rejection prophylaxis in induction protocols and for the treatment of severe rejection. The binding of this drug to the CD3 complex causes the T cell receptor to undergo endocytosis with eventual removal by the reticulo-endothelial system. The absolute number of CD3 T lymphocytes are measured to ensure efficacy of the delivered agent. OKT3 is delivered at a standard adult dose of 5 mg i.v. through a filter in a peripheral vein while following recommended guidelines (Table 88.1). As with polyclonal sera, the first few doses of OKT3 can result in a cytokine release syndrome. Fever, chills, capillary leak, non-cardiogenic pulmonary edema and nephrotoxicity have been described and require the coadministration of antipyretics, antihistamines and steroids to mitigate the symptoms. Chimeric OKT3 single chain variable fragment IgM antibodies have been developed that do not induce a significant T cell proliferation or cytokine release (IL-2, TNF-alpha and IFN-gamma) in *in vitro* assays, while their CD3-modulating properties were retained[14]. These compounds have not yet been approved for clinical use.

Historically, when mono and polyclonal antibodies have been compared they have shown equivalent efficacy[15,16]. As an induction agent[17], and in patients with delayed graft function, some studies found no differences in graft survival between the two agents[18]. Despite these findings, most centers that utilize antibody induction have avoided OKT3 induction and have relegated its use for severe rejection episodes. In addition OKT3 has been shown rejections resistant to polyclonal agents[19]. OKT3 appears to lead to post-transplant lymphoproliferative disorders and more frequent and severe cytomegalovirus (CMV) infections and hence there is need to limit its use.

Anti-Interleukin-2 receptor antibodies

Interleukin-2 (IL-2) is an important target for more specific immunosuppression. Genetically engineered, monoclonal IL-2

Guidelines for OKT3 administration

Confirm euvolemia: no pulmonary edema on chest radiograph

  Diuretics (for volume overload)

  Ultrafiltration (for volume overload)

Premedication: For the first two doses of OKT3

  Acetaminophen

  Antihistamines

  Methylprednisolone

    2 doses of 250 mg i.v.

    6 h and 1 h prior to OKT3

Administration:

  5 mg i.v. bolus through a filter for 7–14 d

  Can be administered via a peripheral line

Vital signs monitoring

  First hour: every 15 min

  Next 2 h: every 30 min

Monitoring

  First course: check CD3

  Second course:

    Check for antibody titers prior to the administration

  Measure CD3 at least twice weekly

Cyclosporine/Tacrolimus

  50% reduction in dose during OKT3 therapy

  Restart the original dose 3 d prior to the completion of OKT3

Table 88.1 Guidelines for OKT3 administration.

---

receptor antibodies, daclizumab and basiliximab, have been shown in several trials to be of therapeutic use in clinical transplantation[20,21]. The anti-IL-2 receptor (IL-2R) monoclonal antibody is a human IgG antibody that binds to the α-chain of the IL-2R, present only on the cell surface of activated T cells. Hence, monoclonal antibodies targeted against IL-2R α-chain can block lymphocyte activation and its effects, while the resting T lymphocytes are undisturbed. Because of their relatively benign side effect profile and apparent efficacy in reducing acute rejection rates, many centers utilize these chimeric (basiliximab) and humanized (daclizumab) monoclonal antibodies in induction therapy. Unlike the polyclonal sera, these agents do not induce immune complex reactions, bone marrow suppression or increase the incidence of opportunistic infections like CMV.

In a recent trial involving tacrolimus-mycophenolate mofetil-steroid protocol, induction with daclizumab was compared with OKT3[22]. The daclizumab arm had a lower acute rejection rate, hospitalization for infections and CMV infections. However, the patient and graft survival rates were similar at 1 year. A recent US multicenter open-labeled trial randomized patients to basiliximab and antithymocyte globulin (ATG) to evaluate economic and quality of life measures. The authors concluded that the use of ATG was significantly more expensive due to the cost of the induction agent itself in addition to increasing hospital costs. They found no difference in quality-adjusted survival between the agents[23]. Newer regimens utilizing smaller total doses of ATG, while providing the same immunosuppressive efficacy might eliminate these cost differences. In a subpopulation of sensitized recipients, anti-CD 25 drugs offer inferior protection from rejection compared to antilymphocyte globulins[24].

Other drugs

During induction, methylprednisolone (250–1000 mg) is administered intravenously as a single dose during the operation. The mechanism of action of steroids is poorly understood. Postulates include the induction or synthesis of a protein that inactivates nuclear factor kappa B, suppression of macrophage IL-1 production, and a direct cell membrane effect. Steroids also inhibit the synthesis of cytokines.

When one should deliver the first dose of calcineurin inhibitor after transplantation is controversial. While some centers start these agents in the immediate postoperative period, others tend to wait until there is graft function as shown by a brisk diuresis and a decrease in serum creatinine. Another practice is to give one-half the standard dose of the drug (2 mg/kg per dose for cyclosporine) as a 'test dose' and then change to full dose (8 mg/kg per d in two divided doses) if there is no deterioration of renal function. The goal of therapy is to prevent rejection while avoiding toxicity.

MAINTENANCE IMMUNOSUPPRESSION

Calcineurin inhibitors

There has been a substantial improvement in the short and long-term graft and patient survival rates after kidney transplantation[25] since the introduction of cyclosporine in the early 1980s. While monotherapy with calcineurin inhibitors is practiced in some transplant centers, the usual maintenance regimen consists of three drugs, if steroids are to be continued indefinitely. By binding to their respective immunophilins (cyclosporine to cyclophilin and tacrolimus to FK binding protein), the calcineurin inhibitors inhibit the enzyme responsible for activation of IL2 gene transcription.

With regards to comparing the efficacies of tacrolimus and cyclosporine, a meta-analysis of four randomized trials revealed that treatment with tacrolimus was associated with a reduction in episodes of acute rejection, a reduction in the use of antilymphocyte antibodies to treat rejection, and an increased prevalence of new onset diabetes mellitus compared with treatment with cyclosporine[26]. However a major limitation to this observation was the use of an older preparation of cyclosporine, Sandimmune (with poor bioavailability and dependance on the patient's bile production for absorption) rather than Neoral (a newer microemulsion preparation). Vincenti et al. extended their Phase III US multicenter trial to 5-years of follow up and intent-to-treat analysis revealed similar patient and graft survival rates between Sandimmune and tacrolimus arms[27]. When crossovers due to rejection from Sandimmune group were considered as graft failures, it was observed that tacrolimus group had superior graft survival. In a recent multicenter randomized European trial[28], tacrolimus was compared to microemulsified cyclosporine and the rate of biopsy confirmed acute rejection and steroid-resistant acute rejection was significantly lower in tacrolimus group compared to cyclosporine. In this study azathioprine and corticosteroid were used in addition to calcineurin inhibitors. There were no significant differences in survival of patients or grafts or in renal function. With the addition of mycophenolate mofetil and sirolimus, the division between microemulsified cyclosporine and tacrolimus may be narrower. No definitive superiority has been shown in long-term graft survival between neoral and tacrolimus so far.

Avoidance, withdrawal and reduction in the dose of calcineurin inhibitors have been an area of controversy. Improvement in graft and patient survival rates since the 1980s, are attributable to the use of cyclosporine. However, calcineurin inhibitors have had a paradoxical impact on long-term transplant outcomes even though they have reduced acute rejection episodes. Calcineurin inhibitor related vasoconstriction leads to a state of chronic ischemia. The drug also appears to increase levels of transforming growth factor-β (TGF-β) and osteopontin (a macrophage chemoattractant), which have been implicated in interstitial fibrosis. The typical pathologic features of cyclosporine toxicity include obliterative arteriopathy, interstitial fibrosis, tubular atrophy and vacuolization. Similar to steroid withdrawal, the withdrawal of cyclosporine has no impact on short-term graft survival. In fact, there may be a slight improvement in the serum creatinine. The initial improvement in serum creatinine is merely due to the expected relief of cyclosporine induced arteriolar constriction. The question remains whether calcineurin inhibitor-free regimens can maintain adequate immunosuppression without contributing to long-term graft loss.

Trough levels (c_{min}) are followed routinely and frequently in the near term after surgery. Target 12-h trough levels are center dependent and range between 200–300 µg/L for cyclosporine and 10–15 µg/L for tacrolimus the first 3–6 months after transplantation. Lower blood levels are targeted and monitoring is less frequent after the first year when the risk of acute rejection is lower. Area under the curve (AUC) is a true measure of drug exposure for efficacy and toxicity. In those patients who may possess unusual absorption rates or metabolism kinetics, an area under the curve (AUC) study can be performed. This cumbersome and expensive, yet gold standard measure is obtained by measuring serial serum levels of the respective drug at multiple time points between drug ingestion and re-dosing. Based on the AUC, the ideal dose can be calculated. Unfortunately, the ideal dose may change over time. Cyclosporine trough levels, especially with older nonemulsified preparations (i.e., Sandimmune) have been found to correlate poorly with the true AUC whereas tacrolimus trough levels are more accurate. An abbreviated pharmacokinetic study that involves measurement of c_{min} and a blood level 2 h after the administration of the drug (c2) has the ability to predict the AUC for a given cyclosporine dose with much greater accuracy than trough levels alone. Many centers are incorporating c2 measures when cyclosporine is the calcineurin inhibitor of choice. With resolution of the uremic milieu, the ability to absorb these drugs becomes greater with time prompting the astute physician to closely monitor drug levels and make frequent dose adjustments.

Although the benefit of therapeutic blood level monitoring has been accepted, there are very few studies addressing the optimal interval for monitoring. Even though the Clinical Practice Guidelines of the American Society of Transplantation[29] recommends monitoring cyclosporine levels frequently early after transplantation, after dose changes, during periods of growth in pediatric recipients and administration of drugs that interact with cyclosporine metabolic pathway, there is poor evidence to support this recommendation. Most transplant centers check the blood level of the drug during each clinic visit.

Steroids

Most transplant centers taper to an oral maintenance dose of prednisone (5–10 mg/d) by the third month after transplantation. Steroid withdrawal and steroid avoidance protocols have been attempted to eliminate the metabolic, cosmetic and osseous ill effects of steroids. The Canadian Multicenter Transplant Study Group[30] showed that chronic graft attrition rates were higher in the steroid withdrawal group, even though there were no early problems. In contrast, the European Collaborative Transplant Study group showed that the group with the least steroid exposure had a better long-term survival[31]. However, a weakness to this retrospective study was that the group with the least steroid exposure had a higher cyclosporine dosage. These studies were done with two-drug regimens or with azathioprine. Now, with the introduction of more potent drugs like tacrolimus, mycophenolate mofetil and sirolimus, these protocols are being re-evaluated. Studies with short-term follow up have shown the feasibility of steroid withdrawal in renal and kidney-pancreas transplantation. Long-term studies are needed to test if these new drugs provide adequate immunosuppression after the withdrawal of steroids.

Mycophenolate mofetil

Mycophenolate mofetil specifically inhibits the rate limiting enzyme inosine monophosphate dehydrogenase (IMPDH) in the *de-novo* synthesis of purines, a pathway crucial to T and B lymphocytes. The FDA approved mycophenolate in 1995 for rejection prophylaxis in renal transplantation based on three large randomized trials[32–34]. Mycophenolate is administered orally a few hours prior to surgery. The typical dose is 1 g twice daily with most centers recognizing an additional benefit to using a higher dose (3 g/d) for African American patients. Mycophenolate has an additional benefit toward chronic rejection by blocking the glycosylation of proteins thereby preventing the targeting of several growth factor receptors to the membrane. Analysis of the data from US Kidney Transplant Scientific Registry revealed that MMF decreased the relative risk for development of chronic allograft failure by 27% and this benefit was independent of its effect on acute rejection[4].

The side-effect profile of mycophenolate includes gastrointestinal discomfort, diarrhea, leukopenia, and thrombocytopenia. MMF might increase the risk of cytomegalovirus (CMV) disease. When a patient develops severe GI symptoms on mycophenolate mofetil, management should include endoscopic evaluation and biopsy to rule out invasive CMV gastritis and esophagitis.

Sirolimus

Sirolimus, a macrolide antibiotic isolated from *Streptomyces hydroscopicus*, is a new potent immunosuppressive agent. The drug inhibits a cytosolic enzyme called target of rapamycin (TOR), which plays a crucial role in the immune response by regulating the growth and proliferation of lymphocytes during the G_1 phase of the cell cycle. Sirolimus binds to the same cytoplasmic binding protein, FKBP, to which tacrolimus binds, but the resulting complexes have different actions. Unlike the calcineurin inhibitors, it does not affect the cytokine transcription (IL-2) and is not believed to be nephrotoxic.

The exact role for sirolimus in our current maintenance immunosuppressive strategy is unclear. Some centers have utilized sirolimus instead of mycophenolate mofetil, while some have used this drug in calcineurin inhibitor withdrawal or avoidance protocols. Early withdrawal of calcineurin inhibitors with replacement of sirolimus appears to be safe resulting in low rates of rejection and better allograft function and histology at one year[35]. Patients with biopsy-proven calcineurin inhibitor toxicity also appear to benefit from conversion to sirolimus. Newer protocols with complete avoidance of calcineurin inhibitors but incorporation of sirolimus are currently being evaluated. Cyclosporine and sirolimus appears to be a potent combination that may even safely allow withdrawal of steroids[36]. Unfortunately significant pharmacologic interactions between the agents require separation of dosing by 4 h. Tacrolimus with sirolimus protocols have been proven both safe and efficacious. Simultaneous dosing also appears to be safe as drug levels of the two agents remain unaffected and no significant toxicities have been reported.

Experimental evidence suggests that sirolimus ameliorates chronic allograft rejection by reducing the expression of growth factor mRNAs. The release of cytokines (platelet derived growth factor, basic fibroblast growth factor, insulin-like growth factor), upregulation of surface adhesion molecule expression, and generation of inflammatory mediators have been implicated in CAN and sirolimus confers protection against CAN by inhibiting these cytokines. Long-term clinical trials are needed in humans to confirm this protection against CAN.

Another intriguing role for sirolimus is in the maintenance of tolerance. The interaction between the alloantigen and CD3-T cell receptor (Signal 1) initiates a cascade of events that results in the activation of the enzyme calcineurin. Both signal 1 and the costimulatory pathway are required for T cell activation. The presence of an antigen and activation of the signal 1 pathway in the absence of the costimulation pathway results in an anergic response. Therefore, costimulatory pathways have been the targets of tolerance induction. A second method of tolerance induction in the periphery involves T cell apoptosis through IL-2. IL-2 generates both a T cell activation signal and a programmed cell death signal. Hence, blockade of IL-2 synthesis may not only prevent T cell activation but also block apoptotic signal and tolerance development. Thus, the calcineurin inhibitors may prevent tolerance as it blocks IL-2 generation. Sirolimus blocks IL-2 induced proliferation, but not the generation of IL-2, and when combined with costimulatory blockade may induce tolerance[37].

Drug combinations

With the advent of newer immunosuppressive medications, numerous combinations of maintenance immunosuppression are possible. Many protocols have been attempted with the common goal of minimizing the chance of rejection while inflicting minimal side effects on the recipient. Three-drug regimens have been developed with the hope of reducing calcineurin inhibitor toxicity. It is believed that adding more agents would allow for adequate immunosuppression with less maintenance doses of calcineurin inhibitors. A prospective, randomized trial was performed to determine if there were differences in patient and allograft outcomes in patients who received monotherapy (cyclosporine alone), dual (cyclosporine + steroids) or triple therapy (cyclosporine, steroids and azathioprine). Despite a significantly higher rate of acute rejections in the monotherapy group, graft and patient survival did not differ after nine years of follow up[38]. In addition, monotherapy was associated with fewer extra-renal complications. Furthermore, a meta-analysis of trials comparing dual versus triple therapy regimens could not find an advantage in using three agents[39].

Sirolimus can replace mycophenolate in patients who suffer gastro-intestinal intolerance. Sirolimus appears to have an anti-proliferative effect and may retard cancer progression. In transplant recipients with a prior history of cancer, this anti-proliferative benefit may make sirolimus the drug of choice. Further studies are required to confirm this hypothesis. In patients with severe delayed graft function, immunosuppression can be maintained with mycophenolate, sirolimus and prednisone, thus avoiding calcineurin inhibitors until renal recovery.

If the patient maintains a stable clinical course, a gradual dose reduction is attempted to decrease the risk of known side effects to immunosuppression (e.g., bone marrow suppression, nephrotoxicity, GI intolerance, glucose intolerance, osteoporosis, hypertension, opportunistic infections and malignancy).

DIAGNOSIS OF ACUTE REJECTION

Acute rejection is defined as an immunologic process resulting in a serum creatinine increase of ≥ 0.4 mg/dL (36 µmol/L) over baseline, and histologic confirmation that has been standardized to the Banff criteria[40]. Fever, oliguria and graft tenderness, formerly clinical signs of acute rejection, are uncommon in the era of calcineurin inhibitors. More than half of patients with acute rejection have neither fever nor decreased urine output[41]. Only a Grade III rejection is likely to be associated with the presence of clinical signs (Fig. 88.1). The allograft biopsy remains the gold standard for confirming the diagnosis of acute rejection. It is always important to rule out obstruction as the cause of an elevated creatinine with a renal ultrasound. Similarly, one should perform a good history and physical examination with emphasis on the volume status of the patient. Volume contraction, especially in the presence of calcineurin inhibitors, can worsen renal function.

The differential diagnosis for elevated serum creatinine (Table 88.2) depends on the time frame after transplantation. In the immediate post-transplant period, acute tubular necrosis from ischemia injury, hyperacute or accelerated rejection, and urologic or vascular complications should be considered.

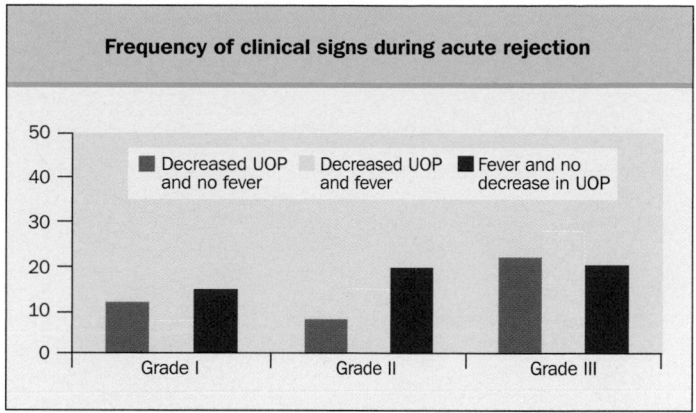

Figure 88.1 Frequency of clinical signs during acute rejection as reported in the Efficacy Endpoints database. Rejection severity is graded by the Banff Criteria. (Reproduced with permission from Schroeder and Moore[41].)

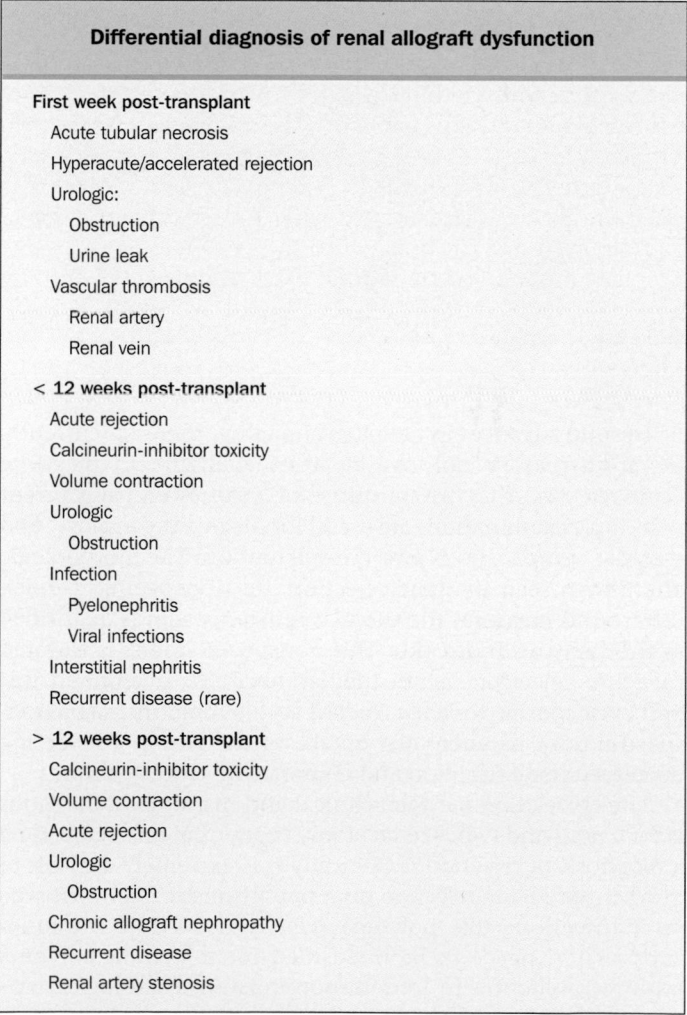

Table 88.2 Differential diagnosis of renal allograft dysfunction.

In the first few months, acute rejection, cyclosporine or tacrolimus nephrotoxicity, pyelonephritis and urinary tract obstruction are more likely.

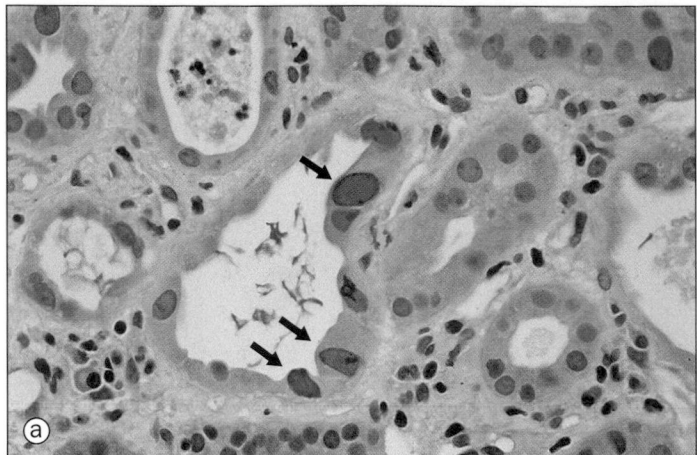

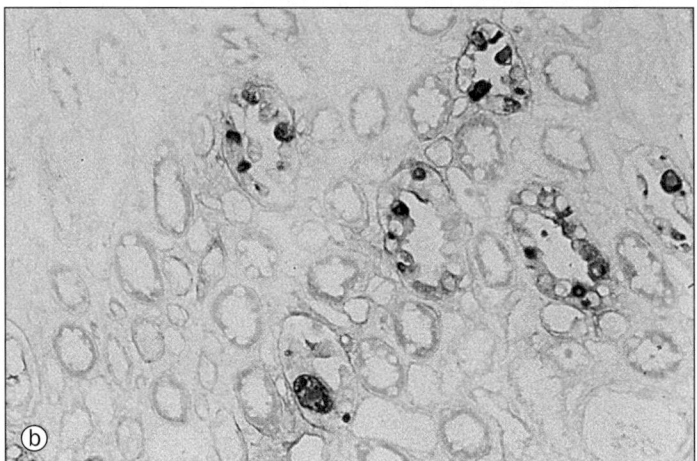

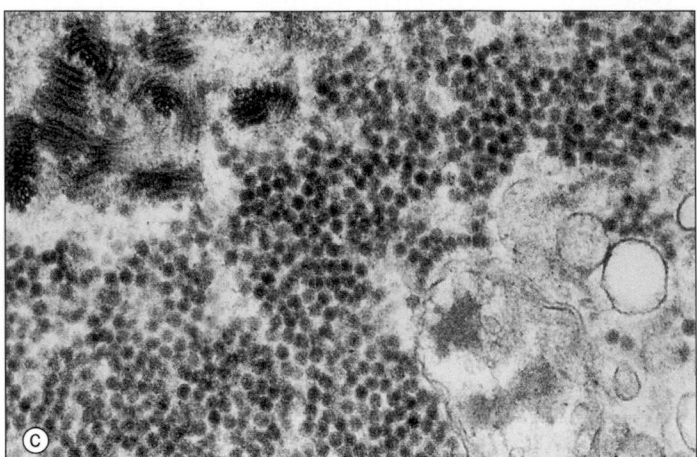

Figure 88.2 BK Polyoma virus infection. (a) BK Polyoma virus infection is suspected when there is a pleomorphic interstitial infiltrate comprised of lymphocytes, frequent plasma cells and occasional neutrophils, with inclusions typical of virus within tubular nuclei (arrows) Periodic acid-Schiff stain, ×400). (b) Definitive diagnosis is made by in situ hybridization looking for viral DNA ×200). (c) Electron microscopy shows the presence of the viral inclusions within tubular nuclei. (Courtesy of Dr Luan Truong.)

Despite advances in radiologic imaging, there are currently no confirmatory noninvasive tests available to diagnose acute rejection that can substitute for a kidney biopsy. Current radiologic examinations are useful for diagnosing urologic and vascular complications post-transplantation. The morphologic alterations seen in acute rejection are nonspecific. Duplex ultrasound measures the vascular resistance and is quantified as the Resistive Index (RI). This nonspecific index is elevated in acute rejection, acute tubular necrosis, pyelonephritis, and cyclosporine toxicity. Nuclear studies demonstrate a nonspecific poor parenchymal uptake of the isotope, reflecting decreased renal function and clearance in acute rejection.

The correlation between clinical and histological diagnosis is very poor and hence renal biopsy is essential for establishing a diagnosis of rejection[42]. Clinically it is extremely difficult to differentiate acute rejection from opportunistic nephrotrophic viral infections like polyoma (Fig. 88.2). While immunosuppression needs to be intensified for rejection, polyoma requires reduction in immunosuppression. Histological evidence of cyclosporine or tacrolimus toxicity can be evident with therapeutic or even low drug levels.

If the patient has normal clotting parameters, informed consent is obtained and the patient receives a transplant ultrasound to rule out obstruction and determine the best site to biopsy. Local anesthetic is delivered followed by a slow advancement of the biopsy needle to the capsule of the kidney.

An 18 or 16 gauge needle previously placed into a spring-loaded automatic biopsy gun is thrown between 0.5 and 1.5 centimeters into the parenchyma of the kidney. Ideally, a pathologist will be present to confirm the origin of the tissue and the adequacy of the sample. The Banff 97 classification[43] defined an 'adequate' specimen as a biopsy with 10 or more glomeruli and at least two arteries; the threshold for a minimal sample is seven glomeruli and one artery (Table 88.3). Two separate cores containing cortex should be obtained since histologic evidence of rejection may be focal (Fig. 88.3).

The messenger RNA (mRNA) encoding cytotoxic proteins, perforin and granzyme B, are higher in urinary cells from patients with biopsy–confirmed acute rejection[44]. Urinary measurement of these proteins, other soluble adhesion molecules and upregulated cytokines are not currently utilized as diagnostic tools in routine clinical practice.

An increase in serum creatinine occurs only after a significant loss of glomerular filtration rate. In other words, significant parenchymal damage may have already occurred if the clinician relies on an increase in creatinine to diagnose acute rejection. Future availability of sophisticated urinary and blood tests, that truly mirror intragraft immunologic events, may identify patients at risk earlier. Whether such noninvasive monitoring for subclinical rejection leads to improved graft survival remains to be seen.

PATHOLOGY

A formalized classification of acute rejection pathology originated in a meeting held at Banff, Canada. This classification has lead to a standardization of biopsy interpretation and has helped define objective end points for clinical trials of new immunosuppressive medications. The Banff 1997 classification is described in Table 88.4.

Adequacy of renal transplant biopsy	
Unsatisfactory	Less than 7 glomeruli and no arteries
Marginal	7 glomeruli with one artery
Adequate	10 or more glomeruli with at least two arteries
Minimum sampling	
7 slides	3 H&E, 3 PAS or silver stains, and 1 trichrome, section thickness 3–4 µm.
(Reproduced with permission from Racusen et al.[43].)	

Table 88.3 Adequacy of renal transplant biopsy.

According to the Banff schema, Type I is defined as a tubulointerstitial rejection without vascular involvement and is further subdivided into type IA with moderate tubulitis and type IB with severe tubulitis (Fig. 88.4). Type II and III have blood vessel involvement in addition to the tubulointerstitial involvement described in Type I.

Tubulitis, a cardinal feature of rejection, is expressed as the number of mononuclear cells per tubular cross section or group of 10 tubular cells. The infiltrating mononuclear cells in the tubular epithelium should have breached the basement membrane and lie beneath or between the tubular cells. Tubulitis should not be graded in atrophic tubules (i.e., tubules with > 50% reduction in caliber) or areas of scarring as this may

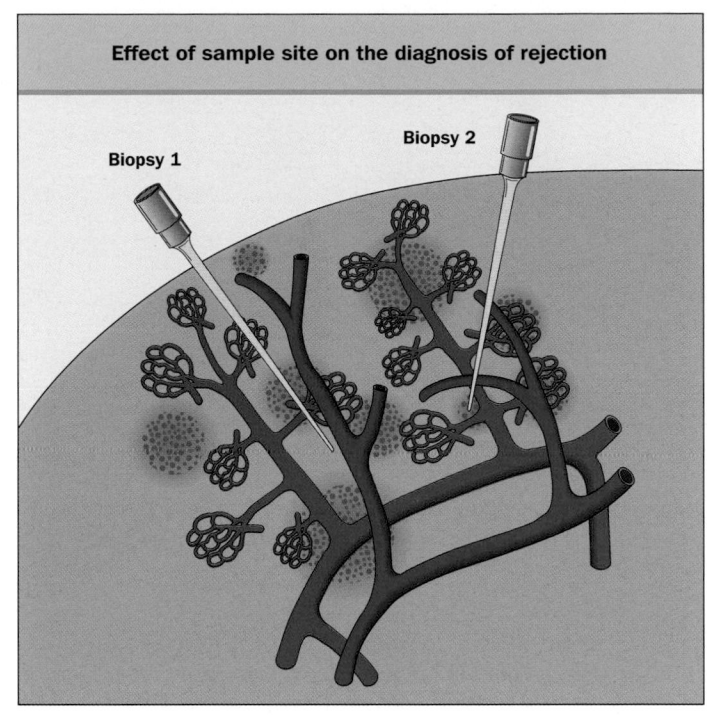

Figure 88.3 Effect of sampling error on the diagnosis of rejection. Acute rejection begins as patchy, focal infiltrates and only becomes homogenous in advanced stages. Compare the intensity of mononuclear infiltrate that would be seen in biopsy core 1 vs core 2. Routinely taking two core biopsies can help decrease the sampling errors, which can affect the histologic interpretation of rejection.

Table 88.4 Banff 1997 Classification.

Banff 1997 Classification	
Classification Type/grade	Histopathological findings
1. Normal	
2. Antibody mediated rejection-demonstrated to be due, at least in part, to antidonor antibodies	
Immediate (hyperacute)	Polymorphonuclear cell accumulation in glomerular and peritubular capillaries with subsequent endothelial damage and capillary thrombosis
Delayed (accelerated acute)	
3. Borderline changes: 'Suspicious' for acute rejection	
'Suspicious'	This category is used when no intimal arteritis is present, but there are foci of mild tubulitis (1 to 4 mononuclear cells/tubular cross section) and at least 10 to 25% of interstitium affected
4. Acute rejection	
IA	Cases with significant interstitial infiltration (> 25% of parenchyma affected) and foci of moderate tubulitis (> 4 mononuclear cells/tubular cross section or group of 10 tubular cells)
IB	Cases with significant interstitial infiltration (> 25% of parenchyma affected) and foci of severe tubulitis (> 10 mononuclear cells/tubular cross section or group of 10 tubular cells)
IIA	Cases with significant interstitial infiltration and mild to moderate intimal arteritis (v1)
IIB	Cases with severe intimal arteritis comprising > 25% of the luminal area (v2)
III	Cases with 'transmural' arteritis or fibrinoid change and necrosis of medial smooth muscle cells (v3 with lymphocytic inflammation)
(Reproduced with permission from Racusen et al.[43].)	

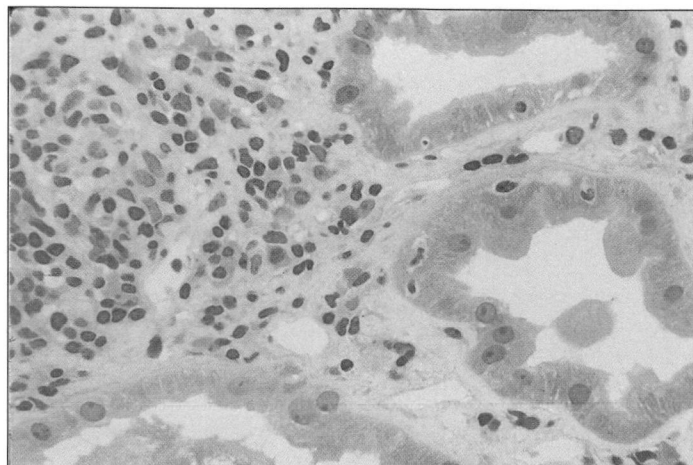

Figure 88.4 Type I acute rejection. Type I acute rejection is manifest by interstitial lymphoplasmacytic infiltrate with lymphocytes invading the tubules (Periodic acid-Schiff stain, ×200).

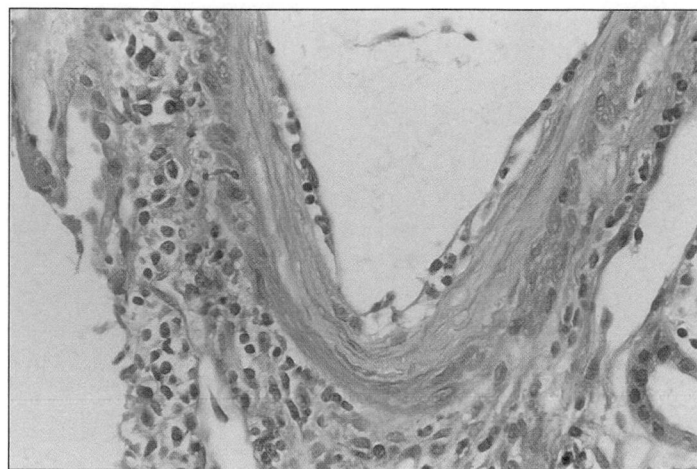

Figure 88.5 Type II acute rejection. Type II rejection, so-called acute vascular rejection, is manifest by endothelialitis with lymphocytes infiltrating beneath the arterial endothelium (Periodic acid-Schiff, ×200). (Courtesy of Dr Agnes Fogo.)

represent a nonspecific response. The threshold of > 4 mononuclear cells per tubular cross section for acute rejection, is supported by the observation that treatment of this degree of tubulitis after protocol biopsies, resulted in better allograft function after two years of follow up[45].

A significant background interstitial inflammation, with > 25% of the parenchyma involved, is required for the diagnosis of acute rejection. Areas of fibrosis and the immediate subcapsular cortex should not be assessed for the degree of interstitial inflammation. The classical cellular infiltrate of rejection is comprised of T lymphocytes. Eosinophils, neutrophils and plasma cells can occasionally be seen in the infiltrate of acute rejection. Many eosinophils may represent a hypersensitivity reaction. Their presence in acute rejection is of no prognostic significance. Plasma cells may signal infection, but when associated with acute rejection, the presence of plasma cells is a poor prognostic indicator of recovery. If the plasma cells are atypical and displace normal structures, post-transplant lymphoproliferative disorder should be considered. It is noteworthy that the severity of the interstitial inflammation and degree of tubulitis do not correlate with the response to antirejection therapy.

The presence of vasculitis on the biopsy portends a poor response to traditional antirejection therapies. Type II rejection is characterized by intimal arteritis and further subcategorized to type II A and type II B depending on the degree of involvement (Fig. 88.5). Type III rejection has evidence of 'transmural' arteritis and/or arterial fibrinoid change and necrosis of medial smooth muscle cells. Similar to the tubulitis scoring, the grading for vascular rejection should be done on the blood vessel most involved.

Since many centers perform 'protocol biopsies' in spite of unaltered renal function, the physician is faced with the dilemma of finding a 'borderline rejection'. Borderline changes are defined as mild tubulitis (1 to 4 mononuclear cells/tubular cross section) and at least 10–25% involvement of the parenchyma with inflammatory cells[43]. This category is used only when there is no evidence of intimal arteritis. These mild changes should be interpreted in a clinical context. If there is

evidence of diminished renal function, therapy may be required. Whether these changes represent an early acute rejection remains an unanswered question. In a retrospective analysis of borderline infiltrates, a rise in serum creatinine, persistently elevated creatinine after the initial kidney biopsy, or histologic findings of glomerulitis were statistically associated with progression of these infiltrates to acute rejection in the short term[46]. Since the majority of these infiltrates did not culminate in acute rejection, many centers are reluctant to perform 'protocol biopsies' if the patient has stable renal function and further burden the patients with more immunosuppression. However a prospective and long-term follow up study is needed to confirm this observation.

The prevalence of 'subclinical rejection' is approximately 30% in the first 3 months post-transplantation. A randomized study was performed by Rush et al to determine whether the treatment of subclinical rejection with corticosteroids was associated with improved outcomes in these patients[45]. The patients were randomized to biopsies at 1, 2, 3, 6, and 12 months (biopsy group), or to 6- and 12-month biopsies only (control group). Patients in the biopsy arm of the study had a significant decrease in early (months 2 and 3) and late (months 7 to 12) acute rejection episodes, a reduced chronic tubulointerstitial score at 6 months, and a lower serum creatinine at 24 months than did patients in the control arm. There were more infections, but no increase in mortality among the biopsy group. Even though this study suggested that early protocol biopsies and the treatment of subclinical rejection with corticosteroids might lead to better histologic and functional outcomes, the concept of protocol biopsies has not yet received universal acceptance.

A type III rejection strongly suggests an antibody-mediated pathology. Severe vessel involvement with fibrinoid changes, extensive endothelial damage with glomerular and small vessel thromboses, glomerulitis, and focal interstitial hemorrhage suggest antibody-mediated rejection. A repeat crossmatch should be done in such a scenario. Banff classification identifies two types of antibody-mediated rejection and they include immediate (hyperacute rejection) and delayed (accelerated

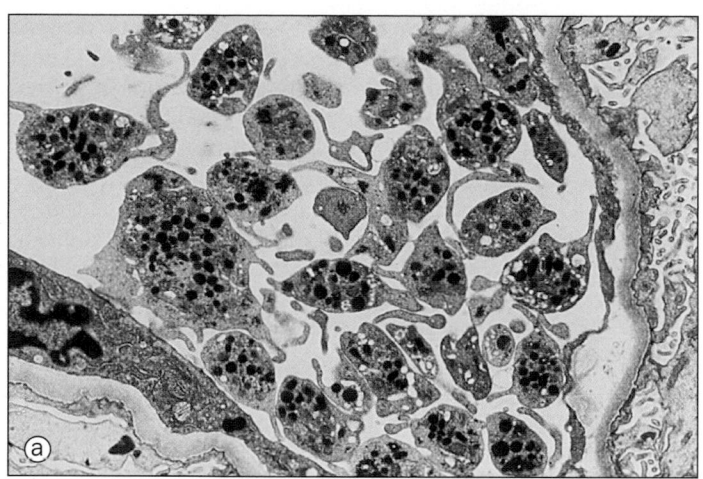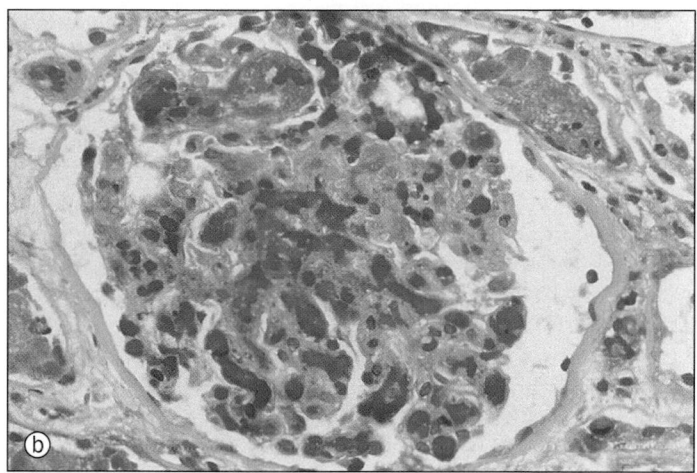

Figure 88.6 Hyperacute rejection. Hyperacute rejection refers to immediate rejection of the kidney, due to presensitization of the recipient to graft endothelial alloantigens. An early lesion is accumulation of platelets in glomerular capillaries (a), followed by further endothelial damage, resulting in capillaries filled with sludged red blood cells and fibrin, as illustrated here (a, Electron Microscopy, Courtesy of Dr Charles Alpers; b, Hematoxylin and eosin, courtesy of Dr Agnes Fogo.)

acute) forms. Hyperacute rejection (Fig. 88.6) occurs in the setting of preformed antibodies (e.g., ABO incompatibility) and is characterized by a cyanotic and flaccid kidney once the vascular anastomoses are completed. Surgical removal is usually the only treatment. Accelerated rejection occurs at between 3 and 14 days post-transplantation and presents as a severe rejection requiring treatment with antilymphocyte antibodies and possibly plasma exchange. Only 30% would be expected to recover to baseline function with treatment.

It is difficult to distinguish acute humoral rejection from acute cellular rejection pathologically. Since acute humoral rejection activates the classical complement pathway, C4d deposition into the peritubular capillaries has been shown to be a marker of acute humoral rejection[47]. As one would expect, the presence of C4d staining is correlated with increased rates of acute graft loss and decreased long-term graft survival. In addition, it has been shown that C4d staining can be used to differentiate the substantial number of patients with chronic rejection secondary to humoral mechanisms. The ability to differentiate the etiology of graft dysfunction in this population may lead to specific therapies against chronic rejection.

TREATMENT OF ACUTE REJECTION

Once the diagnosis of acute rejection is confirmed, the choice of antirejection medication depends on the histology. Pulse steroids with intravenous methylprednisolone are appropriate first line treatment for mild rejection. If there is evidence of vascular rejection on the biopsy and significant reduction in renal function, initial treatment is started with OKT3 or polyclonal antibody. While the actual dose of the pulse therapy varies between centers, most centers resort to three intravenous doses before switching to high dose oral corticosteroids. Pulse steroids reverse 70–80% of acute rejections. The patients who respond to methylprednisolone cannot be distinguished from nonresponders until at least 5 d after the initiation of therapy for acute rejection[48]. Hence most physicians do not resort to OKT3 or antilymphocyte preparations

until 5 d of steroid therapy if serum creatinine is stable. The reversal of histologic features may require as long as 10 d after methylprednisolone therapy. A corticosteroid resistant rejection is defined as a rejection episode in which 250 to 1000 mg of methylprednisolone is administered daily with failure to maintain or reduce the serum creatinine by the third day of therapy[40]. In addition, the serum creatinine will continue to rise if not treated with a different therapy. Glucose intolerance, psychiatric disturbances including mood changes, hypertension, and opportunistic infections are side effects of high dose methylprednisolone therapy. From the Efficacy Endpoints Database it is clear that the presence of Grade III rejection on kidney biopsy predicts steroid resistance[41].

OKT3 is highly effective for the treatment of rejection and can reverse almost 90% of first rejections. In view of the profound immunosuppression that follow courses of OKT3 and the risks including opportunistic infections and lymphoproliferative disorders, most centers reserve this therapy for vascular and severe steroid resistant rejections. The typical dosage of OKT3 is 5 mg/d as a peripheral intravenous bolus for 10–14 d. As described earlier, released cytokines can lead to fever and rigors with the first few doses. If fever recurs after an afebrile period, a complete fever workup should be performed (including testing for CMV). The completion of OKT3 therapy is followed by a resurgence in CD3 counts with the development of a steroid responsive acute rejection episode in half of the cases. As with induction, calcineurin inhibitors can be withhheld or halved during OKT3 therapy. This strategy avoids over immunosuppression while minimizing the nephrotoxic potential of calcineurin inhibitors while the graft is recovering from an acute rejection injury. Calcineurin inhibitors are restarted before the cessation of OKT3 therapy to achieve therapeutic concentrations of the drug prior to the withdrawal of OKT3. Recent data suggest that the production of human anti-mouse antibodies may be decreased if cyclosporine and mycophenolate mofetil are continued simultaneously. A few centers have utilized high-dose tacrolimus to treat acute rejection in lieu of antilymphocyte antibodies.

Transplantation

Approximately 15 to 20% of patients have recurrent episodes of acute rejection. Approximately half of the patients who receive OKT3 will produce antimouse antibodies. Low antibody titers (< 1:100) can be overcome with an increase in the dose, whereas higher titers (> 1:100) or recurrent rejection beyond 3 months is associated with a reversal rate of less than 25%. Late rejection, a prelude to chronic attrition of the graft, responds poorly to antirejection strategies. In such a scenario, for small increases in serum creatinine, it is prudent to withhold aggressive treatment considering the unfavorable risk-benefit ratio.

For treatment of mild rejection with intravenous steroids, hospitalization is not required. Similar to induction, when immunosuppression is intensified for rejection, antimicrobial prophylaxis is restarted. Recipients who are CMV antibody positive are at the highest risk for CMV disease and infection after treatment with antilymphocyte antibodies for acute rejection and hence should receive prophylactic ganciclovir for 3 months.

CHEMOPROPHYLAXIS

A major concern during intense immunosuppression for acute rejection is CMV infection. A CMV seronegative recipient who receives a seropositive donor kidney (CMV D+/R–) is at the highest risk for infection and disease. Acyclovir, ganciclovir, valacyclovir and CMV hyperimmune globulins have been studied as chemoprophylactic agents for CMV disease. Currently, acyclovir and hyperimmune globulins are infrequently used for prophylaxis. Even though the currently available antiviral drugs do not prevent CMV infection in the CMV (D+/R–) group, they attenuate the severity of disease. In this group, intravenous ganciclovir is administered concomitantly with antilymphocyte preparations followed by conversion to oral ganciclovir for a total of 3 months. Oral ganciclovir (1000 mg t.i.d.) is administered for patients who receive conventional immunosuppression without antilymphocyte products and the dose is adjusted for level of renal function. Even though the practice guidelines consensus[49] in the CMV (D–/R+) and CMV (D+/R+) groups vary with the administration of antilymphocyte preparations, many centers have resorted to oral ganciclovir for all patients other than the CMV (D–/R–) group. Valacyclovir, a drug that is rapidly metabolized to acyclovir, has been shown to prevent CMV disease in high-risk transplant patients. A new oral prodrug version of ganciclovir known as valganciclovir has greater bioavailability than the older version and can be substituted for i.v. ganciclovir since an oral dose of 900 mg twice daily (adjusted for renal function) achieves equivalent blood levels as 5 mg/kg twice daily dosing of the intravenous preparation.

Trimethoprim-sulfamethoxazole is given as an oral single strength preparation daily for 6 months to 1 year for the prevention of urinary tract infections, other bacterial infections, toxoplasmosis, *Pneumocystis carinii* pneumonia, and nocardia infection.

With induction therapy and high dose steroid usage, concomitant oral administration of nystatin ('swish and swallow', 5 mL p.o. t.i.d.) prevents oral candidiasis and is typically discontinued when oral steroids are tapered to their maintenance level.

REFERENCES

1. Basadonna G, Matas A, Gillingham K, et al. Early versus late acute renal allograft rejection: Impact on chronic rejection. Transplantation. 1993;55:993–5.
2. Saase J Van, Woude F Van der, et al. The relation between acute vascular and interstitial renal allograft rejection and subsequent chronic rejection. Transplantation. 1995;59:1280–5.
3. Chavers B, Mauer M, Gillinghan K. Histology of acute rejection impacts renal allograft survival in patients with a single rejection episode. J Am Soc Nephrol. 1995;6:1076.
4. Ojo AO, Meier-Kriesche HU, Hanson JA, et al. Mycophenolate mofetil reduces late renal allograft loss independent of acute rejection. Transplantation. 2000;69:2405–9.
5. Cosimi AB. Treatment of rejection: Antithymocyte globulin versus monoclonal antibodies. Transplant Proc. 1985;17:1526–9.
6. Abramowicz D, Norman DJ, Vereerstraeten P, et al. OKT3 prophylaxis in renal grafts with prolonged cold ischemia times: association with improvement in long-term survival. Kidney Int. 1996;49:768–72.
7. Khana L, Ackermann J, Lefor W, et al. Uses of Orthoclone OKT3 for prophylaxis of rejection and induction in initial nonfunction in kidney transplantation. Transplant Proc. 1990;22:1755–8.
8. Charpentier B. Induction versus noninduction protocols in anti-calcineurin based immunosuppression. Transplant Proc. 2001;33:3334–6.
9. Novick AC, Ho-Hsieh H, Steinmuller D, et al. Detrimental effects of cyclosporin on initial function of cadaver renal allografts following extended preservation. Transplantation. 1986;42:154–8.
10. Steinmuller DR, Hayes JM, Novick AC, et al. Comparison of OKT3 with ALG for prophylaxis for patients with acute renal failure after cadaveric renal transplantation. Transplantation. 1991;52:67–71.
11. Lange H, Muller TF, Ebel H, et al. Immediate and long-term results of ATG induction therapy for delayed graft function compared to conventional therapy for immediate graft function. Transpl Int. 1999;12:2–9.
12. Cantarovich D, Giral-Classe M, Hourmant M, et al. Prevention of acute rejection with antithymocyte globulin, avoiding corticosteroids, and delaying cyclosporin after renal transplantation. Nephrol Dial Transplant. 2000;15:1673–6.
13. Meier-Kriesche HU, Arndorfer JA, Kaplan B. Association of antibody induction with short and long-term cause-specific mortality in renal transplant recipients. J Am Soc Nephrol. 2002;13(3):769–72.
14. Choi I, Ines C De, Kurschner T, et al. Recombinant chimeric OKT3 scFv IgM antibodies mediate immune suppression while reducing T cell activation in vitro. Eur J Immunol. 2001;31(1):94–106.
15. Mariat C, Alamartine E, Diab N, et al. A randomized prospective study comparing low-dose OKT3 to low-dose ATG for the treatment of acute steroid-resistant rejection episodes in kidney transplant recipients. Transpl Int. 1998;11:231–6.
16. Kumar MSA, Cahill K, Kumar AMS, et al. ATGAM versus OKT3 induction therapy in cadaveric kidney transplantation: patient and graft survival, CD3 subset, infection, and cost analysis. Transplant Proc. 1998;30:1351–2.

17. Frey DJ, Matas AJ, Gillingham KJ, et al. Sequential therapy – a prospective randomized trial of MALG versus OKT for prophylactic immuno-suppression in cadaver renal allograft recipients. Transplantation. 1992;54:50–6.

18. Steinmuller DR, Hayes JM, Novick AC, et al. Comparison of OKT3 with ALG for prophylaxis for patients with acute renal failure after cadaveric renal transplantation. Transplantation. 1991;52: 67–71.

19. Norman DJ, Kahana L, Stuart FP Jr, et al. A randomized clinical trial of induction therapy with OKT3 in kidney transplantation. Transplantation. 1993;55:44–50.

20. Vincenti F, Kirkman R, Light S, et al. Interleukin-2-receptor blockade with daclizumab to prevent acute rejection in renal transplantation. Daclizumab Triple Therapy Study Group. N Engl J Med. 1998;338(3):161–5.

21. Kahan BD, Rajagopalan PR, Hall M. Reduction of the occurrence of acute cellular rejection among renal allograft recipients treated with basiliximab, a chimeric anti-interleukin-2-receptor monoclonal antibody. United States Simulect Renal Study Group. Transplant. 1999;67(2):276–84.

22. Ciancio G, Burke GW, Suzart K, et al. Daclizumab induction, tacrolimus, mycophenolate mofetil and steroids as an immuno-suppression regimen for primary kidney transplant recipients. Transplantation. 2002;73(7):1100–6.

23. Polsky D, Weinfurt KP, Kaplan B, et al. An economic and quality-of-life assessment of basiliximab vs antithymocyte globulin immunoprophylaxis in renal transplantation. Nephrol Dial Transplant. 2001;16:1028–33.

24. Mariat C, Afiani A, Alamartine E, et al. A pilot study comparing basiliximab and anti-thymocyte globulin as induction therapy in sensitized renal allograft recipients. Transplant Proc. 2001;33: 3192–3.

25. Hariharan S, Johnson CP, Bresnahan BA, et al. Improved graft survival after renal transplantation in the United States, 1988 to 1996. N Engl J Med. 2000;342:605–12.

26. Knoll GA, Bell RC. Tacrolimus versus cyclosporin for immuno-suppression in renal transplantation: meta-analysis of ran-domised trials. BMJ. 1999;318:1104–7.

27. Vincenti F, Jensik SC, Filo RS, et al. A long-term comparison of tacrolimus (FK506) and cyclosporin in kidney transplantation: evidence for improved allograft survival at five years. Transplantation. 2002;73(5):775–82.

28. Margreiter R. European tacrolimus vs ciclosporin microemulsion renal transplantation study group. Efficacy and safety of tacrolimus compared with ciclosporin microemulsion in renal transplantation: a randomized multicenter study. Lancet. 2002; 359(9308):741–6.

29. Kasiske BL, Vazquez MA, Harmon WE, et al. Recommendations for the outpatient surveillance of renal transplant recipients. J Am Soc Nephrol. 2000;11(15):S9.

30. Sinclair NRS. Low dose steroid therapy in cyclosporin treated renal transplant recipients with well functioning grafts. J Can Med Assoc. 1992;147:645–57.

31. Opelz G. Effect of the maintenance immunosuppressive drug regimen on kidney transplant outcome. Transplantation. 1994; 58:443–6.

32. Tricontinental Mycophenolate Mofetil Renal Transplantation Study Group. A blinded, randomized trial of mycophenolate mofetil for the prevention of acute rejection in cadaveric renal transplantation. Transplantation. 1996;61:1029–37.

33. Sollinger HW. Mycophenolate Mofetil for the prevention of acute rejection in primary cadaveric renal allograft recipients. Transplantation. 1995;60:225–32.

34. The European Mycophenolate Mofetil Cooperative Study Group. Placebo controlled study of mycophenolate mofetil combined with cyclosporin and corticosteroids for prevention of acute rejection. Lancet. 1995;345:1321–6.

35. Ruiz JC, Campistol JM, Mota A, et al. Early cyclosporin A with-drawal in kidney transplant recipients under a sirolimus based immunosuppressive regimen: Pathological study of graft biopsies at 1-year post transplant. Transplant Proc. 2002;34:92–3.

36. Mahalati K, Kahan BD. A pilot study of steroid withdrawal from kidney transplant recipients on sirolimus-cyclosporin A combi-nation therapy. Transplant Proc. 2001;33:3232–3.

37. Li Y, Zhen XX, Chang X, et al. Combined costimulation blockade plus rapamycin but not cyclosporin produces permanent engraft-ment. Transplantation. 1998;66:1387–8.

38. Montagnino G, Tarantino A, Segoloni G, et al. Long-term results of a randomized study comparing three immunosuppressive schedules with cyclosporin in cadaveric kidney transplantation. J Am Soc Nephrol. 2001;12:2163–9.

39. Helderman JH, Buren DH Van, Amend WJC, Pirsch JD. Chronic immunosuppression of the renal transplant patient. J Am Soc Nephrol. 1994;4:S2–S9.

40. Guttman RD, Soulillou JP, Moore LW, et al. Proposed consensus for definitions and endpoints for clinical trials of Acute Kidney Transplant Rejection. Am J Kid Dis. 1998;31:S40–S46.

41. Schroeder TJ, Moore LW. Efficacy endpoints conference on acute rejection in kidney transplantation: summary report of the data-base. Am J Kid Dis. 1998;31:S31–S39.

42. Al-Awwa IA, Hariharan S, First MR. Importance of allograft biopsy in renal transplant recipients: correlation between clinical and histologic diagnosis. Am J Kid Dis. 1998;31:S15–S18.

43. Racusen LC, Solez K, Colvin RB, et al. The Banff 97 working classi-fication of renal allograft pathology. Kidney Int. 1999;55:713–23.

44. Li B, Hartono C, Ding R, et al. Noninvasive diagnosis of renal-allo-graft rejection by measurement of messenger RNA for perforin and granzyme B in urine. N Engl J Med. 2001;344(13):947–54.

45. Rush D, Nickerson P, McKenna RM, et al. Beneficial effects of treatment of early subclinical rejection: A randomized study. J Am Soc Nephrol. 1998;7:2129–34.

46. Meehan SM, Siegel CT, Aronson AJ, et al. The relationship of untreated borderline infiltrates by the Banff criteria to acute rejection in renal allograft biopsies. J Am Soc Nephrol. 1999; 10(8):1806–14.

47. Collins AB, Schneeberger EE, Pascual MA, et al. Complement activation in acute humoral renal allograft rejection: diagnostic significance of C4d deposits in peritubular capillaries. J Am Soc Nephrol. 1999;10:2208–14.

48. Shinn C, Malhotra D, Chan L, et al. Time course of response to pulse methylprednisolone therapy in renal transplant recipients with acute allograft rejection. Am J Kid Dis. 1999;34:304–7.

49. Jassal SV, Roscoe JM, Zaltzman JS, et al. Clinical practice guide-lines: Prevention of cytomegalovirus disease after renal trans-plantation. J Am Soc Nephrol. 1998;9:1697–708.

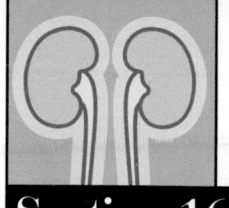

Section 16 Transplantation

Chapter 89

The Medical Management of the Renal Transplant Recipient

William E Braun

Renal transplant recipients may develop a variety of complications related to the allograft, immunosuppression, progression of pre-existing disease, and aging with the appearance of new diseases. Major causes of death for recipients with functioning renal allografts are directly related to these factors and include cardiovascular disease (CVD) that accounts for approximately 46% of patient mortality, infection 20%, malignancy 13%, and liver failure[1].

CARDIOVASCULAR DISEASE

About 23% of patients develop coronary heart disease (CHD), 15% cerebrovascular disease, and 15% peripheral arterial disease by 15 years after renal transplantation[2].

Coronary heart disease

Studies of renal transplant recipients in the late 1970s and early 1980s indicated a three-fold greater prevalence of CHD compared to a nontransplant population[3]. However, the relative risk of CHD has progressively decreased to 0.60 between 1986 and 1992, and 0.27 since 1992, along with a 50% reduction in post-myocardial infarction (MI) mortality[3]. This improvement has occurred despite the increase in renal transplant operations in older (> 60 years) and diabetic patients, who account for about 12% and 30%, respectively, of all transplant recipients.

For clinical purposes, coronary risk factors may be considered in three groups: nonmodifiable, difficult-to-modify, and modifiable (Table 89.1)[3,4]. Transplantation confers additional risks for CHD particularly because key immunosuppressive medications can cause hypertension (calcineurin inhibitors (cyclosporine more than tacrolimus) and corticosteroids), hyperlipidemia (cyclosporine, corticosteroids, and sirolimus), impaired glucose tolerance (calcineurin inhibitors (tacrolimus more than cyclosporine) and corticosteroids)[1], and allograft dysfunction (calcineurin inhibitors). Because of these and other side effects, corticosteroid-free and/or calcineurin-free immunosuppressant protocols are currently being studied in renal transplant recipients. Consequently, coronary risk factors specific for transplantation, such as prednisone dose, cyclosporine dose, and post-transplant diabetes mellitus, may be in transition to becoming modifiable risk factors in the near future.

Risk assessment for CHD in renal transplant recipients requires not only recognition of symptomatic CHD (angina pectoris, congestive heart failure, arrhythmia, and syncope) but also an evaluation every 1–2 years of asymptomatic patients who have acquired individual risk factors for CHD or

whose aggregate level of risk factors warrant further testing for CHD. Risk assessment for CHD based on the Framingham Heart Study[5] and the National Cholesterol Education Program[6] emphasize the importance of risk factors commonly found in renal transplant recipients in whom their pathologic consequences are amplified[3]. Those with the highest risks of CHD (> 20% at 10 years) have either established CHD or 'CHD risk equivalents' that include diabetes, other forms of atherosclerotic disease, and multiple risk factors – diseases found in most transplant recipients[6].

When a high-risk patient has been identified, a proactive management algorithm may be employed (Fig. 89.1). The most frequently used noninvasive tests for CHD include exercise-based cardiac stress testing utilizing $^{99m}T_c$sestamibi, with or without a second isotope, ^{201}thallium, and pharmacologic stress tests such as dobutamine echocardiography and dipyridamole thallium for patients unable to exercise. There are currently insufficient data to recommend electron beam computerized axial tomography (CT) scanning and coronary calcium scoring as a first-line means of screening for CHD. Following a positive stress test, coronary angiography is typically done (Fig. 89.1). High-grade stenosis (usually > 70%) may be treated when feasible with percutaneous transluminal angioplasty (PTCA) and coronary artery stenting, or may require coronary artery bypass grafting. However, it is well known that the culprit lesion associated with an acute MI may be located not at the site of greatest occlusion but rather at a site where only 'minor' disease was detected by angiography.

Patients with known CHD or at high risk for CHD should take an aspirin or enteric-coated aspirin in a dose of 65–325 mg daily for those without aspirin sensitivity[2]. For secondary prevention of cardiac morbidity and mortality β-adrenergic receptor blockers have also been recommended.

Cerebrovascular disease

Clinical screening for subtle symptoms and signs of carotid artery occlusive disease should be part of the annual examination. It should be noted that CHD and carotid artery occlusive disease are strongly predictive of one another. Hyperhomocysteinemia as well as traditional risk factors contribute to carotid artery stenosis and cerebrovascular disease. The benefit of carotid endarterectomy is well established in symptomatic patients with high-grade carotid artery stenosis. In asymptomatic patients, ≥ 80% occlusive disease is usually the threshold for intervention, although patients with ≥ 60% narrowing are also candidates when carotid endarterectomy can be performed with ≤ 3% perioperative morbidity and

Coronary risk factors in the general population and in renal transplant recipients									
	Not modifiable			Difficult-to-modify			Modifiable		
	A*	B	C	A	B	C	A	B	C
General population*	aging		family history of premature CHD male gender ethnic characteristics	cigarette smoking pretransplant diabetes mellitus†	elevated Lp$_{(a)}$ levels small LDL particles coagulation factors inflammatory factors (CRP, myeloperoxidase)	obesity physical inactivity insulin resistance psychosocial factors	hypertension LDL cholesterol $\geq$ 160 mg/dL (or lower depending on additional risk factors) HDL cholesterol $\leq$ 35 mg/dL	elevated triglycerides elevated plasma homocysteine levels	
		Unclassified but important: 1. Plaque burden itself, i.e., pretransplant asymptomatic CHD without myocardial dysfunction; age is a surrogate marker 2. Atherosclerosis already in other vascular beds							
	Not modifiable			Difficult-to-modify			Modifiable		
Renal transplant recipients‡	ESRD due to Type 1 diabetes ESRD due to Type 2 diabetes, especially in women diabetes not causing renal disease pretransplant nephrectomy for polycystic kidney disease pretransplant splenectomy (possibly reflecting other risk factors such as thrombocytosis and hypercholesterolemia)			current smoking 2 or more first-year rejections (possibly reflecting the need to use higher prednisone and cyclosporine doses, as well as an inflammatory state) serum albumin < 4 g/dL (possibly reflecting an inflammatory state with elevated C-reactive protein) post-transplant diabetes mellitus			cholesterol > 200 mg/dL triglycerides > 350 mg/dL proteinuria if possible, avoid pretransplant splenectomy, and nephrectomies for polycystic kidney disease develop immunosuppression protocols that can effectively prevent rejection (< 10% the first year) while reducing or avoiding prednisone and/or cyclosporine that promote hypertension, hypercholesterolemia and diabetes mellitus.		

* A = causal, B= conditional, C= predisposing (Adapted and modified with permission from Grundy SM. Primary prevention of coronary heart disease; integrating risk assessment with intervention. Circulation. 1999;100:988–98, and Kasiske and Ballantyne[1].
† Modifiable by pancreas or pancreatic islet cell transplantation.
‡ Adapted and modified with permission from: Kasiske[3]; Kasiske BL, Chakkera HA, Roel J. Explained and unexplained ischemic heart disease risk after renal transplantation. J Am Soc Nephrol. 2000;11:1735–43; and Kasiske BL, Guijarro C, Massy ZA, et al. Cardiovascular disease after renal transplantation. J Am Soc Nephrol. 1996;7:158–65.

Table 89.1 Coronary risk factors in the general population and in renal transplant recipients.

mortality in a combination with aggressive management of modifiable risk factors.

In patients with autosomal dominant polycystic kidney disease (ADPKD) the prevalence of an intracranial aneurysm (ICA) identified by magnetic resonance angiography (MRA) is 12% overall, 24% in those with a positive family history of an ICA or subarachnoid hemorrhage in conjunction with ADPKD, and 5% in those with a negative family history. An excruciating headache ('thunderclap') followed by a variable period of improvement may indicate sentinel bleeding (prerupture) from an ICA and requires urgent or emergent treatment. Cerebral angiography is usually performed in patients with acute symptoms or those with an ICA of $\geq$ 7 mm for whom surgery may be planned. Periodic screening of asymptomatic ADPKD patients with MRA about every 5 years has been suggested[7].

Peripheral arterial occlusive disease

Peripheral arterial occlusive disease (PAOD) is common after renal transplantation, particularly in the presence of diabetes mellitus (type 1 diabetes), older age recipients, smoking, and male gender. Progressive PAOD leading to limb loss has also been described in renal transplant recipients who were neither diabetic nor smokers, with the same allograft functioning for more than 20 years[4]. This development appears to be the consequence of pre-existing atherosclerosis with calcification that had been initiated during the period of pre-existing chronic renal failure. Symptoms of claudication and diminished pulses in the lower extremities are classic findings with PAOD and can normally be confirmed by measuring the ankle–brachial (A/B) index with pulse–volume recordings at rest and with exercise. The A/B index values may be falsely elevated when there is vascular calcification because such vessels tend to be incompressible. The use of toe peripheral vascular resistance may be more informative, although data are limited. In the general population more than 50% of patients with PAOD on the basis of abnormal A/B index ratios do not have typical claudication or critical leg ischemia[8]. An A/B index value more than 0.90 at rest but decreasing by 20% after exercise is diagnostic of PAOD. An initial A/B index value of 0.90 at rest indicates probable PAOD, an A/B index of

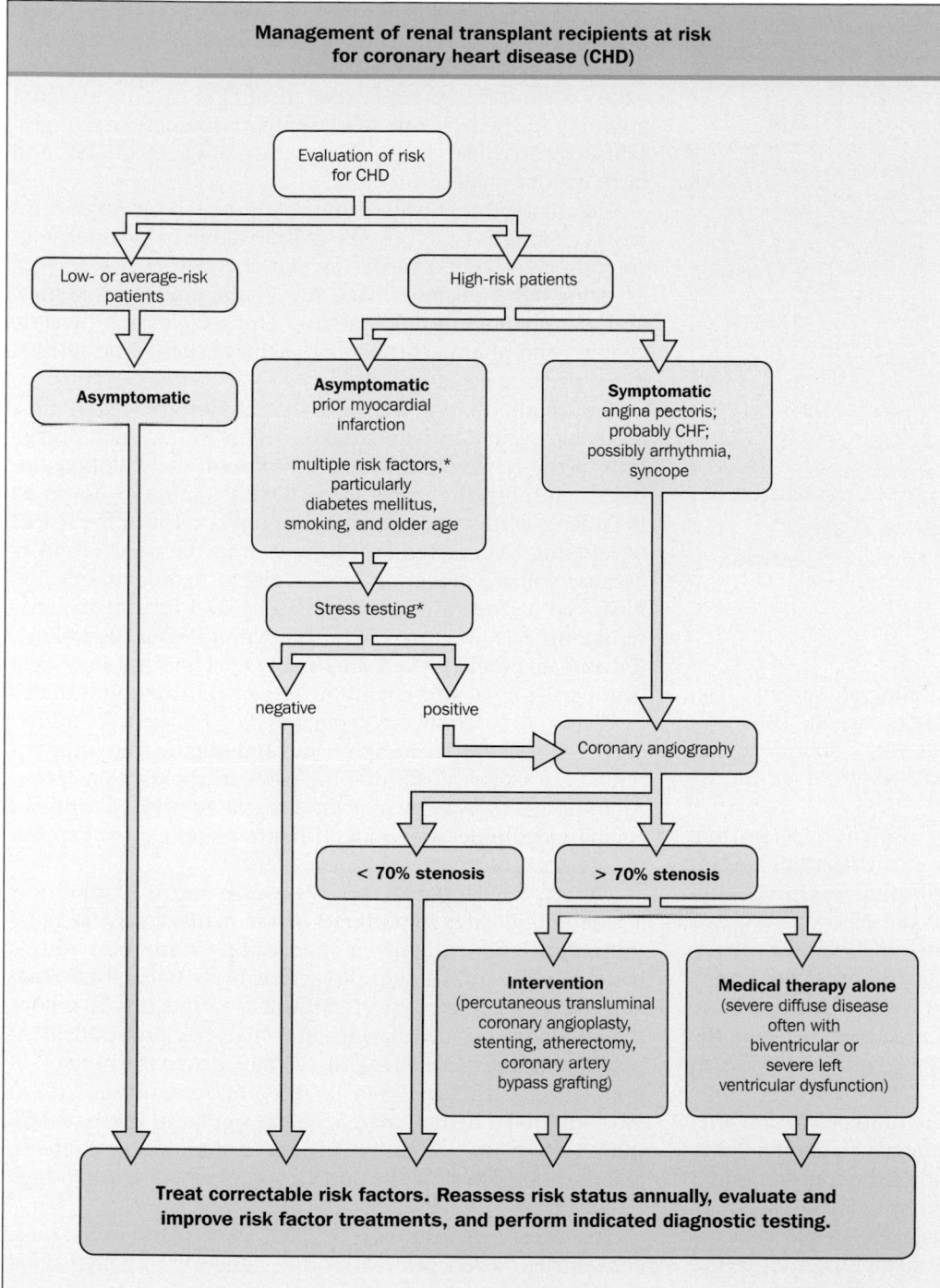

Figure 89.1 Management of renal transplant recipients at risk for CHD.

0.70–0.89 represents mild disease, 0.40–0.69 moderate disease, and < 0.40 severe disease. For the more severe degrees of PAOD angiography will usually be performed in preparation for possible endovascular or surgical intervention. Nonionic radiocontrast material, CO_2 angiography, or MRA have been employed in order to minimize the risk of ionic contrast nephrotoxicity.

Hypertension

The prevalence of hypertension after renal transplantation is influenced by several factors that include variable definitions of hypertension, donor source, immunosuppressive medications, time after transplantation, and level of allograft function. A more revealing stratification of blood pressure (BP) goals has been recently published[9]. It has been recognized that a continuum of CVD risk extends from optimal (< 120/80 mmHg) to normal (< 130/85 mmHg), to high-normal (130–139 systolic or 85–89 mmHg diastolic), and to hypertensive BP levels (≥ 140/90 mmHg) (see Chapter 36). In addition to contributing to cardiovascular and cerebrovascular mortality, systolic BP levels in increments of 10 mmHg extending from 120 to > 180 mmHg have been shown to

Transplantation

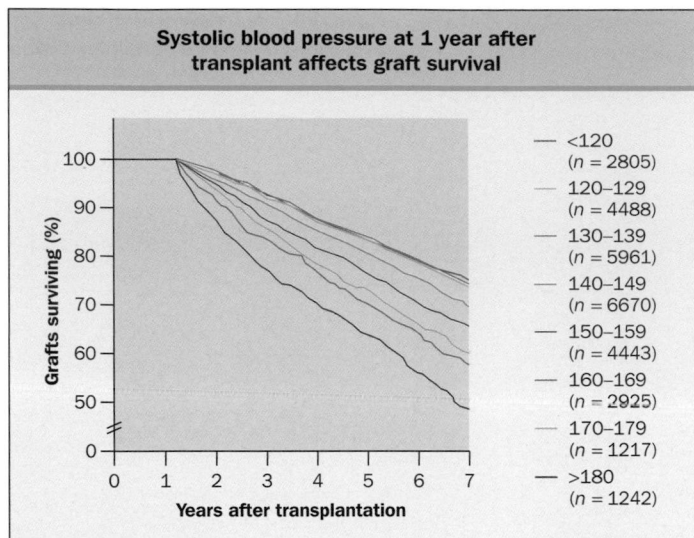

Figure 89.2 Effects of systolic blood pressure at 1 year on cadaveric kidney transplant graft survival. (Adapted with permission from Opelz et al., Kidney Int. 1998;53:217–22.)

have a striking effect on 1-year renal allograft survival (Fig. 89.2)[1]. The adverse effect of elevated systolic BPs was present even in patients with diastolic BPs < 90 mmHg and even in those who had not experienced rejection within the first year.

The most common causes of post-transplant hypertension, often combined, include the use of corticosteroids and/or calcineurin inhibitors (particularly cyclosporine), chronic allograft nephropathy, excess weight gain, acute rejection, recurrent or *de novo* glomerulonephritis, and transplant renal artery stenosis. The prevalence of hypertension in the pre-cyclosporine era ranged between 42 and 72% at 1 year, and from 46 to 71% at 5 years after transplantation, compared to ranges in the cyclosporine era of 63 to 78% at 1 year, and 70 to 85% at 5 years[2].

Cyclosporine has been a major cause of hypertension after renal transplantation, and to a greater degree than tacrolimus. Early after transplantation when cyclosporine doses are usually the highest, hypertension is caused by vasoconstriction of the afferent arterioles and to a lesser degree systemic vasoconstriction, direct effects on other vasoconstrictors, interference with vasodilators, sodium retention, and volume expansion. With prolonged cyclosporine exposure there may be the development of arteriolopathy, ischemic and focal segmental glomerulosclerosis, and interstitial fibrosis accompanied by worsening renal function that become fixed factors in sustaining hypertension. Renal artery stenosis should be suspected in the presence of a systolic and, particularly, a diastolic bruit over the renal transplant artery or in the area of the ipsilateral iliac artery (see Chapter 63). Excess renin output from the native kidneys may also contribute to hypertension for an indeterminate time after transplantation. The role of genetically influenced essential hypertension in the recipient and donor, and the observation that hypertension follows the kidney, are discussed in Chapter 36. Primary hyperaldosteronism has also been

recognized after transplantation[10]. Coconspirators in the development of hypertension include bad lifestyle habits (excess intake of calories and lack of exercise leading to obesity, excess sodium intake, and excess alcohol or cocaine use) and a variety of medications (e.g., sympathomimetic decongestants, nonsteroidal anti-inflammatory drugs (NSAIDS), and birth control medication).

The management of post-transplant hypertension encompasses treating as far as possible specific causes of hypertension, correcting associated cardiovascular risk factors (see above), assessing target organ damage (e.g., brain, eye, heart, kidney, and peripheral arterial system), and employing lifestyle changes and pharmacotherapy to achieve normal or optimal blood pressure goals.

Treatment of hypertension that is not the result of a reversible, secondary cause usually begins with sodium restriction in the range of 3000 mg (130 mmol) daily. Potassium-based salt substitutes must be used with caution or not at all in patients with impaired renal function because of the risk of developing hyperkalemia. Diuretics must be used carefully because volume depletion may augment hemodynamically-mediated cyclosporine nephrotoxicity and further increase serum uric acid and the possibility of clinical gout (see below). Calcium channel blockers are usually effective and may help counter the renal afferent arteriolar vasoconstriction induced by cyclosporine. However, verapamil and diltiazem (nondihydropyridines), and nicardipine and amlodipine (dihydropyridines) can cause substantial increases in cyclosporin levels. Amlodipine especially may be associated with peripheral edema. Nifedipine, isradipine, and nitrendipine do not appear to significantly affect cyclosporine levels.

The use of angiotensin converting-enzyme (ACE) inhibitors is assuming greater importance in the management of renal transplant recipients. Their increasingly important role is based not only on their antihypertensive but also their renal and cardiac protective effects, as well as a capability to reduce the incidence of new diabetes in a high-risk non-transplant population that bears a striking resemblance to the transplant population[11]. The angiotensin receptor antagonists (ATRA) have intrarenal hemodynamic effects similar to those of ACE inhibitors, as well as antiproteinuric and antifibrotic effects, and the ability to slow the progression of renal failure in type II diabetics.

The use of ACE inhibitors or ATRA, particularly in the presence of high levels of cyclosporine, seriously impaired renal function, or transplant renal artery stenosis may cause acute renal failure and/or significant hyperkalemia. These adverse effects may also be exacerbated by volume contraction (e.g., excessive diuresis, uncontrolled hyperglycemia, gastrointestinal losses) and the use of NSAIDs. When cyclosporine is used in high doses after renal transplantation, it may be safer to postpone ACE inhibitors or ATRA use until lower maintenance levels are achieved. The safest approach to instituting an ACE inhibitors or ATRA after transplantation would be to have ultrasonographic evidence that the transplant artery is not significantly narrowed (< 60%). If an ultrasound study were not possible, then close observation of serum creatinine after starting an ACE inhibitors or ATRA is indicated to assure stable renal function.

Hyperlipidemia

The abnormal lipid profile that occurs in 50–80% of renal transplant recipients treated with prednisone and cyclosporin is characterized by an increase in total, low-density lipoprotein (LDL), and very low-density lipoprotein (VLDL) cholesterol, and apolipoprotein B levels[1,3,4]. High-density lipoprotein (HDL) cholesterol levels may be low, normal, or slightly elevated, and lipoprotein-(a) (Lp$_a$) levels may be high or normal. Elevated LDL cholesterol and low HDL cholesterol levels have been associated with an increased risk for CHD after renal transplantation.

Although hyperlipidemia following renal transplantation is multifactorial, immunosuppressive medications play a large role[1]. Calcineurin inhibitors, particularly cyclosporine, and corticosteroids increase serum cholesterol levels. Nevertheless severe hypercholesterolemia and hypertriglyceridemia were more frequent with sirolimus than with cyclosporine (44% vs. 14%, and 51% vs. 12%, respectively) and reached maximum levels after about two months of treatment[12]. Although cholesterol and triglyceride levels are lower with tacrolimus than with cyclosporine, tacrolimus allows greater LDL oxidation[1].

The mechanisms for hyperlipidemia after renal transplantation are complex. They include alterations in cholesterol-rich lipoprotein metabolism (increased synthesis of VLDL causing increased LDL levels; glucocorticoid and cyclosporin interference with LDL receptor activity; reduced hepatic LDL receptor number or function), changes in the metabolism of triglyceride-rich lipoprotein (increased hepatic production of VLDL caused by hyperinsulinemia associated with glucocorticoid-related insulin resistance; decreased VLDL turnover possibly related to decreased activity of lipoprotein lipase and hepatic triglyceride lipase), and, in the case of sirolimus, blockade of lipoprotein lipase.

Although hyperlipidemia often improves within the first 6 months after transplantation as doses of prednisone, cyclosporine, and sometimes sirolimus are reduced, levels that are still abnormal frequently persist and require treatment. Therapeutic lifestyle changes that focus on diet and exercise, and medication are the two lines of therapy to lower LDL cholesterol[6]. Medications to treat hyperlipidemia include HMG Co-A reductase inhibitors (statins), bile acid sequestrants, nicotinic acid, and fibric acid derivatives. Statins will be the most frequently used class of medications because of the high frequency of LDL cholesterol post-transplantation. Goals for LDL levels can be judged by the recent NCEP guidelines (Table 89.2)[6]. Renal transplant recipients, just as those with chronic renal failure, should generally be treated aggressively[2,3]. When statin drugs are used in the presence of cyclosporine, doses of statins can usually be lower because cyclosporine increases statin blood levels several-fold[3]. Statins currently consist of atorvastatin, fluvastatin, lovastatin, pravastatin, and simvastatin. Approximate therapeutic equivalencies are achieved by 10 mg of atorvastatin, 20 mg of simvastatin, 40 mg of pravastatin, 40 mg of lovastatin, and 80 mg of fluvastatin. At these doses the LDL cholesterol decrease is approximately 34% with very little change in HDL levels. Impaired renal function may necessitate the use of lower doses of statins. Recent studies suggest that statins may offer protection against CHD by other mechanisms that include a decrease in the level of circulating endothelin-1, decreases in systolic and diastolic BP as well as pulse pressure, reduced levels of C-reactive protein, a decrease in acute primary coronary events, and antiproliferative effects. The major statin side effects are hepatotoxicity with increased liver enzymes, and myopathy/rhabdomyolysis with increased creatine kinase (CK) enzymes. Contraindications to the use of statins include active or chronic liver disease. Statins metabolized by the CYP3A4 system (atorvastatin, simvastatin, and lovastatin) have their levels increased by drugs also metabolized by the CYP3A4 system: e.g., cyclosporine, tacrolimus, sirolimus, macrolide antibiotics, azole antifungal agents, fibric acid derivatives, and niacin, as well as by grapefruit juice. Patients should be monitored every 3–6 months or as clinically indicated with alanine aminotransferase (ALT) levels for hepatic toxicity and CK enzymes levels for muscle toxicity.

Severe hypertriglyceridemia (> 500 mg/dL (5.6 mmol/L)) has become more frequent since the introduction of sirolimus. Although sirolimus-associated hypertriglyceridemia may decrease as sirolimus doses are reduced, levels may still be significantly elevated and require treatment. In some cases extremely high triglyceride levels in excess of 1500 mg/dL (that may cause pancreatitis and avascular necrosis) may persist and require a change in immunosuppression, often to tacrolimus.

LDL cholesterol goals and cutpoints for therapeutic lifestyle changes and drug therapy in different risk categories			
Risk category	LDL goal (mg/dL)	LDL level at which to initiate therapeutic lifestyle changes (mg/dL)	LDL level at which to consider drug therapy (mg/dL)
CHD or CHD risk equivalents (10-year risk > 20%)	< 100	≥ 100	≥ 130 (100–129: drug optional)
2+ risk factors	< 130	≥ 130	10-year risk 10–20%: ≥ 130 10-year risk < 10%: ≥ 160
0–1 risk factor	< 160	≥ 160	≥ 190 (160 to 189: LDL-lowering drug optional)
Executive Summary of The Third Report of The National Cholesterol Education Program (NCEP) Expert Panel on Detection, Evaluation, And Treatment of High Blood Cholesterol In Adults (Adult Treatment Panel III). JAMA. 2001;285:2486–97.			

Table 89.2 LDL cholesterol goals and cutpoints for therapeutic lifestyle changes and drug therapy in different risk categories.

In less extreme cases, treatment consists of a low-calorie, low-fat diet, exercise program, and typically the addition of a fibric acid derivative or nicotinic acid. Depending on dosage, both fibric acid derivatives and nicotinic acid may decrease triglycerides by as much as 20–50% while increasing HDL cholesterol 10–20% (fibric acid derivatives) or 15–35% (nicotinic acid)[6]. Side effects of nicotinic acid include flushing, hyperglycemia, hyperuricemia with the possibility of gout, upper gastrointestinal distress, and hepatotoxicity. Contraindications to the use of nicotinic acid are chronic liver disease and severe gout, with relative contraindications being diabetes mellitus, hyperuricemia, and peptic ulcer disease. Fibric acid side effects include dyspepsia, gallstones, myopathy, and unexplained nonCHD deaths in the WHO study. Contraindications to fibric acid use include severe renal disease and severe hepatic disease. Of the major fibric acid medications (bezafibrate, ciprofibrate, fenofibrate, and gemfibrozil), the first three can cause increases in serum creatinine in cyclosporine-treated patients and higher plasma homocysteine (tHcy) levels. Bile acid sequestrants for the treatment of hypercholesterolemia are difficult to use in renal transplant recipients who have multiple medications throughout the day that may have their absorption affected by these agents.

Hyperhomocysteinemia

Hyperhomocysteinemia (i.e., fasting plasma homocysteine > 10 µmol/L) occurs in about two-thirds of renal transplant recipients. In the general population mild-to-moderate elevations of homocysteine are a significant and independent risk factor for coronary, cerebrovascular, and peripheral arterial disease. Elevated levels of homocysteine cause endothelial injury, enhancement of coagulation, proliferation of vascular smooth muscle cells, and the production of other toxic products[13]. Four factors known to increase homocysteine levels are deficiencies of folate, B_6 (pyridoxine), B_{12} (cyanocobalamin), and impaired renal function. Although definitive studies are not yet available, treatment of hyperhomocysteinemia seems warranted because of the significantly increased risk of CHD in renal transplant recipients. Treating deficiencies of folate, B_6, and B_{12} as well as correctable causes of renal insufficiency may improve elevated levels of homocysteine.

Post-transplant diabetes mellitus (PTDM)

PTDM has been reported to occur in 4–20% of patients with renal transplants, about 40% of whom require insulin therapy[14]. PTDM has been described within 3 weeks to more than 20 years after transplant with the same functioning allograft but is most often detected within the first year[4,14]. Risk factors for PTDM include African American and Hispanic race, excess body weight, increasing age > 45 years, male gender, family history of diabetics, cadaver–allograft recipient, acute rejection history, cytomegalovirus (CMV) and hepatitis C virus (HCV) infection, several HLA antigens (A30, B27, and B42), and the use of corticosteroids and tacrolimus more so than cyclosporine. Azathioprine and mycophenolate mofetil (MMF), both purine antagonists, do not appear to be diabetogenic; mycophenolate may mitigate the diabetogenic effect of tacrolimus[1]. Early studies with sirolimus indicate that at blood levels about 15 ng/mL, it is not diabetogenic.

Numerous new medications for the treatment of diabetes mellitus will often require collaborative management with an endocrinologist or diabetologist. These agents need to be reviewed by the transplant nephrologist because of side effects such as edema (particularly the thiazolidinedione derivatives, pioglitazone and rosiglitazone), higher blood levels and hypoglycemia risk in the presence of impaired renal function (insulin, metformin, sulfonylurea derivatives), lactic acidosis (metformin), and metabolism by CYP3A4 for short-acting insulin secretogogues such as repaglinide and nateglinide. Intensive glucose control can reduce diabetic complications but at the risk of hypoglycemic events.

Comprehensive diabetic care should be provided to patients with PTDM and should include diabetes education, diet instruction, monitoring of glycemic control with a home glucose diary, hemoglobin A_1C levels approximately every 3 months, regular ophthalmologic exams, regular foot care, evaluation of complications from different neuropathies, and at least annual clinical evaluation of their cardiovascular system.

Although infrequent, diabetic nephropathy has been reported in at least three patients who developed *de novo* PTDM. One patient had the nephrotic syndrome and mesangial changes two years after transplantation; the second patient developed the nephrotic syndrome 11 years after the onset of steroid-induced diabetes and had diffuse mesangial changes; the third case developed diabetes mellitus 10 years after transplantation, about 1 g of proteinuria per 24 h, and in less than 6 years nodular diabetic glomerulosclerosis developed[15].

Prednisone withdrawal is usually associated with significant decreases in total cholesterol levels and the number of antihypertensive medications needed, but there is very little information concerning its effect on PTDM. Of 14 patients who developed PTDM the eight in a steroid withdrawal protocol were reduced to four, whereas the six in the prednisone continuation group were increased to eight, a 50% reduction vs. 33% increase, respectively[16].

Post-transplant erythrocytosis

Between 4% and 22% of renal transplant recipients will develop post-transplant erythrocytosis (PTE) defined as a persistently elevated hematocrit > 51%. Risk factors for PTE include: presence of native kidneys, male gender, excellent allograft function with absence of rejection episodes, smoking, hypertension, and diabetes mellitus. The mechanism of PTE appears to involve angiotensin II stimulation of early erythroid precursors that have an increased number of angiotensin type I receptors which correlate with hematocrit levels in patients with PTE. Thromboembolic complications in the legs, lungs, and brain may occur in up to 22% of PTE patients. Primary treatment for PTE is either an ACEI or ATRA. At times phlebotomy may be a helpful adjunct; native kidney nephrectomies have been used in the past.

MALIGNANCY

Recurrent malignancies

Because immunosuppression increases the risk for malignancy, patients should be carefully evaluated for cancer during the pre-transplant work-up. For many pre-existing

Post-transplant recurrence rates of malignancies	
Recurrent rate	Type of malignancy
Low (0–10%)	Incidental renal cell, testicular, cervical, and thyroid cancer, lymphoma
Medium (11–25%)	Carcinomas of the corpus uteri, colon, prostate (nonfocal), and breast, Wilms' tumor
High (> 25%)	Invasive bladder cancer, sarcomas, melanomas, symptomatic renal cell carcinoma, nonmelanomatous skin cancer, multiple myeloma
Adapted with permission from Penn[17].	

Table 89.3 Post-transplant recurrence rates of malignancies.

Relative risk for malignancies after renal transplantation	
Malignancy	Relative risk
Non-Hodgkin's lymphoma	28–49
Kaposi's sarcoma (certain ethnic groups)	400–500
Skin cancer (squamous cell is greater risk than basal cell)	4–21
Melanoma	8–9
Carcinoma of cervix	14
Carcinoma of vulva or anus	100
Hepatobiliary carcinoma	30
Renal carcinoma	10–100
Other cancers (lung, colon)	1.5
Adapted with permission from Penn[18].	

Table 89.4 Relative risk for malignancies after renal transplantation.

cancers a 2-year tumor-free interval before transplant is recommended, but greater and lesser times are appropriate for certain cancers (see Chapter 86). Despite such precautions, these malignancies may recur, and the risk of that happening largely relates to the type of underlying malignancy and subsequent immunosuppression (see Table 89.3)[17].

De novo malignancies

Renal transplant recipients are at increased risk for *de novo* malignancies (Table 89.4)[18]. In addition to cancer risks present in the general population, the new risks for renal transplant recipients are primarily related to the dose, duration, and type of immunosuppressants, and in part to the ability of these agents to promote replication of various oncogenic viruses. These viruses include human papillomaviruses (HPV) associated with cervical and vulvar carcinoma, as well as squamous-cell carcinoma of the head and neck in a nontransplant population, Epstein–Barr virus (EBV) with post-transplant lymphoproliferative disorder (PTLD) most often represented by non-Hodgkin's lymphoma (NHL) and some squamous cell carcinomas of the skin, hepatitis B virus (HBV) and HCV with hepatocellular carcinoma (HCC), and human herpesvirus (HHV) 8 with Kaposi's sarcoma[2].

Cancer surveillance guidelines are given in Table 89.5. More frequent and invasive testing may be necessary for patients with high-risk features, such as intensive immunosuppressive therapy (particularly with polyclonal antibodies, OKT3 monoclonal antibody, and high-dose mycophenolate), long duration of immunosuppressive therapy, age over 55 years, history of cancer before transplantation, and certain lifestyles.

Cancer of the skin and lips

More than one-third of *de novo* malignancies in organ transplant recipients are cancers of the skin and lip, most frequently squamous cell carcinomas[1]. Skin cancers in transplant recipients are strikingly increased in regions with high sun exposure, occur at a younger age, and tend to be multifocal, have a more aggressive course, and lead to death more often than in the general population. Avoidance of direct sun exposure, especially from 11:00 a.m. to 3:00 p.m. and the use of protective clothing and sun blockers that interfere with ultraviolet A and B rays are standard precautions. The continued use of azathioprine in patients with multiple or severe skin

cancers should be carefully evaluated because a metabolite of azathioprine, thioguanine, is believed to be a chemical carcinogen for the skin.

Periodic skin self-examinations and regular dermatologic screening examinations are recommended[2]. The primary treatment of these lesions is early surgical excision. Patients with severe recurrent lesions have been treated with 5-fluorouracil and low-dose acetretin.

Post-transplant lymphoproliferative disorder (non-Hodgkin's lymphoma)

Within the first few months after renal transplant there is a rapidly increasing risk for the development of NHL. NHL has been reported to occur between 1 and 254 months after transplantation with an average onset at 32 months[18]. The clinical presentation is varied and may include systemic symptoms such as fever, night sweats, and weight loss, or more localized symptoms of the respiratory tract (infection, mass, tonsillitis, or even gingival involvement), gastrointestinal tract (diarrhea, pain, perforation, bleeding, mass), or nervous system (headache, seizure, confusion). Special characteristics of post-transplant NHL include involvement of the central nervous system in 26% of patients with 63% of the lesions confined to the brain, extranodal involvement (often intra-abdominal or pulmonary) in 70% compared with 35% in nontransplant patients, and direct invasion of the allograft itself in 20%, a situation that may be clinically and sometimes histologically confused with rejection[18]. Factors that increase the risk of NHL include the use of polyclonal antibodies, monoclonal OKT3 antibody, cyclosporine, tacrolimus, and mycophenolate; an age of 18 years or younger; prior seronegativity for EBV; a high level of EBV replication in the oropharynx; and preceding CMV infection. About 85% of NHL cases have a B-cell origin and incorporate the EBV genome.

Complete remissions may be achieved in about 25% of patients with NHL, and approximately 25% of total remissions are induced by a decrease or elimination of non-glucocorticoid immunosuppressants. (i.e., antiproliferative agents (azathioprine

Preventive care recommendations for adult cancer surveillance			
Screening for	Starting at age	Preventive care	How often?*
Colorectal cancer	average risk: 50	colonoscopy or fecal occult blood test plus flexible sigmoidoscopy	colonoscopy: every 10 years fecal occult blood test: every year flexible sigmoidoscopy: every 5 years
	increased risk: 40		If you have a parent, brother, or sister who has had colorectal cancer at age 60 or younger, you should have a colonoscopy every 5 years beginning at age 40 or 10 years younger than the youngest family member with cancer. If the relative was > 60 years, colonoscopy every 10 years.
			Two or more first-degree relatives with colorectal cancer may indicate an inherited colon cancer syndrome. Consider referral to Medical Genetics.
Females			
Breast cancer	40	breast physical examination and screening mammography	Every year If your mother or sister has had breast cancer, you may want to begin screening before age 30
Cervical cancer	18	Pap smear and pelvic examination	Every year for 3 years. If all three smears are normal, begin having Pap smears once every 3 years if you do not have any of the following risk factors: HIV-positivity infection with certain types of human papillomavirus (HPV) cigarette smoking multiple sex partners prior abnormal Pap smear or cervical dysplasia chronic immunosuppression for organ transplantation If you have any of the above risk factors, obtain a Pap smear and pelvic exam every year.
Males			
Prostate cancer	50	1. Digital rectal exam	1. Every year 2. Discuss with your physician
		2. PSA testing	If you are African American, have a family history of prostate cancer, or are receiving chronic immunosuppression for organ transplantation, you should have a digital rectal exam every year and discuss the frequency of PSA testing with your physician beginning at age 40.

* Please review these recommendations with your physician to decide on the best course of preventive care for you based on your personal and family medical history. Adapted from the Cleveland Clinic Foundation Cancer Surveillance Task Force, December 2001.

Table 89.5 Preventive care recommendations for adult cancer surveillance.

or mycophenolate) and calcineurin inhibitors (cyclosporine and tacrolimus)). Under these circumstances, the prednisone dose is typically increased in order to afford protection for the allograft. In a recent series of 42 adult patients with PTLD, 30 treated with reduction in immunosuppression alone and 12 with additional surgical resection of all known disease, a complete remission was achieved in 31 of the 42 patients (74%)[19]. Quintuple therapy consisting of reduction of immunosuppression, acyclovir, interferon-α, high-dose intravenous gammaglobulin, and anti-CD19 monoclonal antibodies achieved complete remissions in seven transplant recipients (kidney, kidney–pancreas, liver, heart)[20]. Additional therapy may involve surgical excision, chemotherapy, radiotherapy, acyclovir, gancyclovir, immunostimulation with drugs such as interferon-α, gammaglobulin, anti-CD19 and anti-CD20 monoclonal antibodies, the latter reported to be associated with a fatal reactivation of CMV infection.

Renal carcinomas
Up to 4% of renal transplant recipients may develop renal carcinoma. The overwhelming majority of renal carcinomas occur in the native kidneys, but some have been inadvertently transplanted with the allograft, and others may develop *de novo* in the allograft many years after transplantation. Risk factors for renal carcinoma include previous analgesic abuse, prior history of renal cell carcinoma, retained polycystic kidneys, tuberous sclerosis, and acquired renal cystic disease. The course of renal cell carcinomas and urothelial cancers may be particularly aggressive in renal transplant recipients. Thorough investigation of hematuria in the transplant recipient with urine cytology, cystoscopy, and either contrast-enhanced computed tomography (CT) or magnetic resonance imaging (MRI) is important if these lesions are to be detected at an early stage.

Hepatobiliary carcinomas
Renal transplant recipients who have chronic liver disease or known cirrhosis should be monitored at regular intervals for the development of hepatocellular carcinoma (HCC). The etiology of chronic liver disease in these patients is most often chronic HBV and/or HCV infection. The risk of HCC in renal transplant recipients is approximately 30-fold higher

than that in the general population but reaches 100-fold in Taiwan[2]. For patients with chronic liver disease or cirrhosis from HCV, the time of occurrence of HCC is in the range of 25 to 30 years after the onset of the disease. Because testing for HCV was not generally available until about 1991, the time of onset for most patients is uncertain. Monitoring transplant recipients at risk for HCC (cirrhosis, HCV, seropositivity for HBsAg) involves annual monitoring of serum alphafetoprotein, and periodic imaging studies of the liver.

INFECTION

Infections are a major complication of transplantation and have been categorized according to their usual time of occurrence following transplantation (Table 89.6)[21]. Infections that occur shortly after transplantation or during the initial hospitalization are usually caused by common nosocomial bacterial and candidal infections associated with the surgical wound, lines for vascular access, the respiratory and urinary tracts. Except for HSV, other viral infections are very uncommon this early. Organisms transmitted with the donor

organ, or untreated infections in the recipient, are fortunately rare. However, recipients who have additional risk factors (see below) may have atypical infections earlier than first-time renal transplant recipients.

Because of the cumulative effects of high levels of immunosuppression, infections between 1 and 6 months are typically caused by opportunistic organisms. The most important viruses are CMV, EBV, VZV, HBV, HCV and respiratory tract viruses. Bacterial infections caused by *Legionella* sp. (Fig. 89.3), *Nocardia* sp., *Listeria* sp., and even tuberculosis may occur. The most serious fungal infections are those caused by *Cryptococcus* (Fig. 89.4), *Mucor*, and *Aspergillus*; protozoal infections include *Pneumocystis carinii*, and *Toxoplasma* sp. A rare but important infection to recognize is disseminated strongyloidiasis, which is most likely to develop in patients from regions where *Strongyloides* sp. are endemic such as the southeastern region of the USA and southeast Asia (Fig. 89.5). Urinary tract infections are frequent and have a greater likelihood of causing bacteremia than do those in non-transplant patients. Acute respiratory failure simulating opportunistic infection and subsequent pulmonary fibrosis may occur with

Table 89.6 Infections following renal transplantation.

Infections following renal transplantation		
1st month after transplantation	**Months 1–6**	**After 6 months**
Postoperative bacterial infections: urinary tract respiratory vascular access-related wound	Opportunistic or unconventional infections: Viral: CMV, HHV-6, HHV-7, EBV, VZV, influenza, RSV, adenovirus	Late opportunistic infections: *Cryptococcus*, CMV retinitis or colitis, VZV, parvovirus B-19, polyomavirus (BK, JC), *Listeria*, tuberculosis
Nosocomial: including *Legionella* sp.	Fungal: *Aspergillus* sp., *Cryptococcus*, *Mucor*	
	Bacterial: *Nocardia*, *Listeria*, *Mycobacterium* sp., *Legionella*, tuberculosis	Persistent infections: HBV, HCV
Viral: HSV, HBV, HCV, HIV		Associated with malignancy: EBV, papillomavirus, HSV, HHV-8
Fungal: candida	Parasitic: *Pneumocystis carinii*, *Toxoplasma* sp., *Strongyloides* sp, leishmaniasis	Community acquired
Organisms transmitted with donor organ		Unusual sites: e.g., paravertebral abscess
Untreated infection in recipient		

* Geographically focused infections will need to be considered in certain cases, such as malaria, leishmaniasis, trypanosomiasis, and strongyloidiasis.
Adapted from Fishman and Rubin[21].

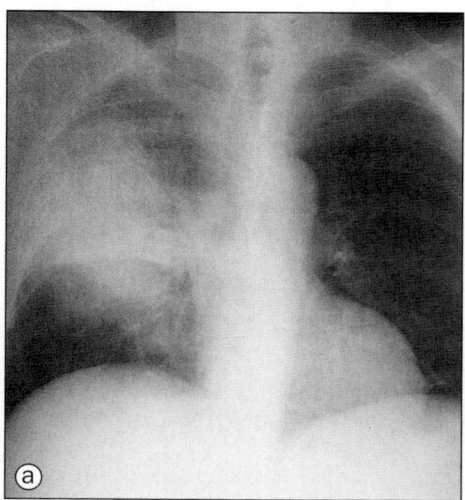
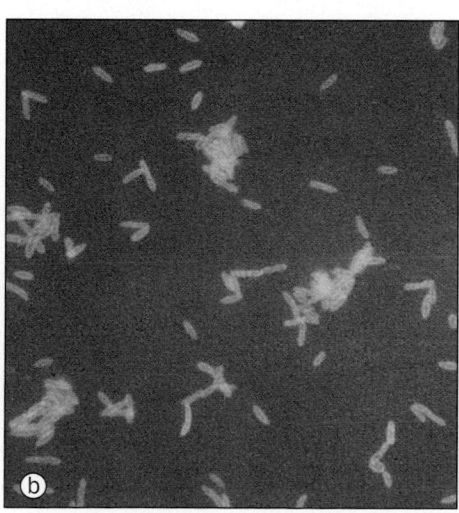

Figure 89.3 Legionnaire's disease in a renal transplant recipient. (a) Chest radiograph showing a right lower lobe pneumonia. (b) Culture of sputum showing Legionella pneumophila, as identified by immunofluorescent staining with a specific antibody. (Courtesy of R Johnson.)

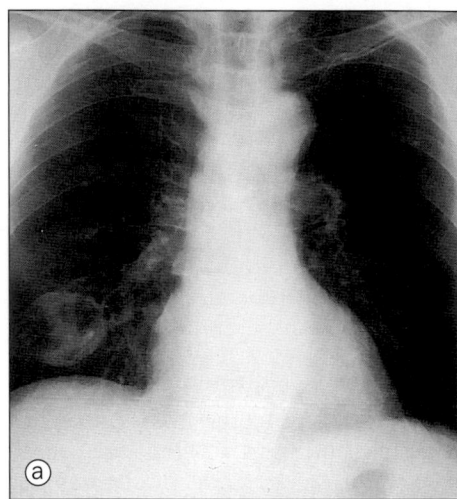

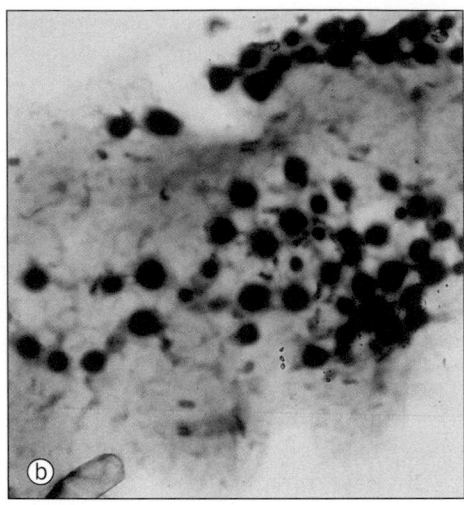

Figure 89.4 Cryptococcal lung infection in a renal transplant recipient. (a) Chest radiograph showing an irregular thick-walled cavitating mass in the right lower lobe. (b) Gram stain of of bronchoalveolar lavage shows numerous cryptococci. (Courtesy of R Johnson.)

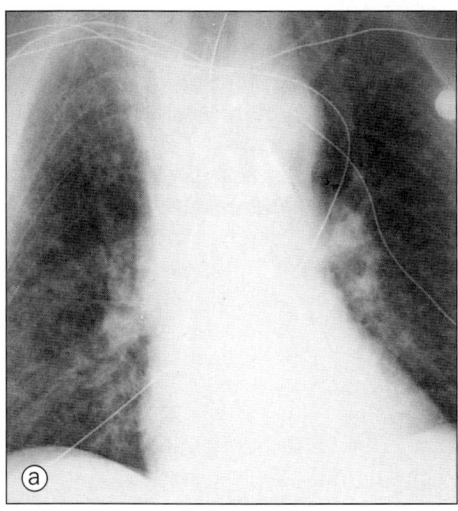

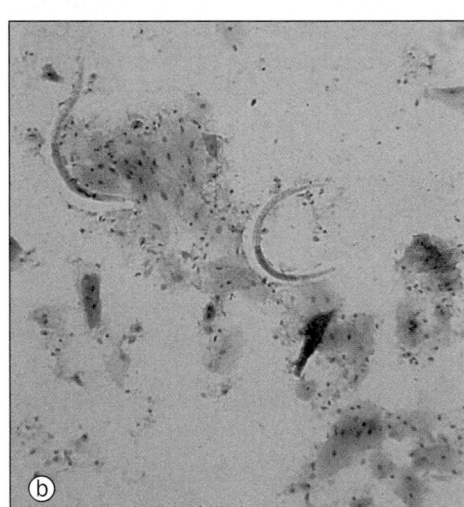

Figure 89.5 Disseminated strongyloidiasis in an immunocompromised patient. (a) Chest radiograph showing a diffuse bilateral interstitial process. (b) Gram stain of sputum from the same patient shows filariform larvae of Strongyloides stercoralis. (Courtesy of R Johnson.)

mycophenolate, and interstitial pneumonitis may develop with sirolimus, apparently in a dose-related manner. A wide variety of infections may occur beyond 6 months (Table 89.6).

Additional risk factors for severe and/or opportunistic infections include: intensive immunosuppression especially with polyclonal or monoclonal antibodies, repeated courses of intravenous methylprednisolone, and high-dose mycophenolate; chronic renal insufficiency; long duration of immunosuppressive therapy (e.g., > 20 years); repeat renal transplantation; leukopenia often related to therapy with azathioprine, mycophenolate, or CMV infection; splenectomized state; hypogammaglobulinemia which may require specific treatment; seronegativity for CMV, EBV, or HSV; diabetes mellitus; liver disease; and malnutrition.

Cytomegalovirus infection

CMV infections constitute one of the most common and potentially serious infections in renal transplant recipients. Their risk of CMV infection is based on the relationship of the donor's CMV status (D^+ or D^-) to that of the recipient (R^+ or R^-). For example, the combination of D^+/R^- (primary infection) is associated with > 60% occurrence of symptomatic CMV disease; D^+/R^+ (reactivation or superinfection) with a 20–40% occurrence; and D^-/R^+ (reactivation) with about a 15% occurrence. When polyclonal or monoclonal antibody

therapy is used together with mycophenolate, a calcineurin inhibitor, and prednisone, any R^+ recipient has a 50% risk of recurrence.

Typically CMV infections occur 3–12 weeks after transplantation with a peak around 6 weeks. However, in the cyclosporine era, CMV infections appear to have two additional features. First, occurrences may be much more delayed after renal transplant, in terms of months to years, and second, there may be one or more recurrences. The initial infection and recurrences are enhanced by the use of polyclonal antibody or monoclonal OKT3 either for induction therapy or treatment of rejections. High-dose mycophenolate (1.5 g q12 h) is also an additional risk for CMV infections, but data concerning standard dose mycophenolate are conflicting.

The clinical presentation of CMV infection may range from subtle findings of low-grade fever, malaise, and leukopenia with mild atypical lymphocytosis to life-threatening multilobar pneumonia. CMV can infect the gastrointestinal tract (particularly the esophagus, stomach, or colon where it may cause colitis and diarrhea, or mimic a neoplasm or ischemic colitis); liver, pancreas, gallbladder, retina, CNS, ureter, and myocardium. The diagnosis is confirmed by demonstration of CMV viremia usually by blood tests for CMV DNA or antigenemia, or of tissue invasion by biopsy. Involvement of the renal allograft by CMV is unusual, but has been reported to cause glomerular injury including endothelial cell swelling or necrosis, immunotactoid glomerulopathy, and typical but not specific intranuclear inclusions with a characteristic 'owl eye' appearance on light microscopy[22]. CMV hemolytic uremic syndrome/thrombotic microangiopathy has also been described and may respond to intravenous Ig infusions[23]. Although primary CMV infection (D+/R-) has received the most attention because of the severity of the infection in these individuals, the worst graft and patient survival in some studies was in the D+/R+ and not the D+/R- group[23].

Approaches to controlling CMV infection in renal transplant recipients include: avoiding CMV-positive kidneys for CMV-negative recipients, prophylaxis and pre-emptive therapy protocols, monitoring during and after intensive immunosuppressant treatment, and therapy of established disease[23]. Generally, avoidance of CMV-positive donors for CMV-negative recipients is not achievable or feasible on a large scale. Currently, oral ganciclovir in doses of 1000 mg orally three times a day for at least 3 months is being used in renal transplant recipients at risk for CMV disease. Valacyclovir in doses of 2 g four times a day (with reduced doses for impaired renal function) has been shown to reduce the occurrence of CMV disease and decrease the risk of acute allograft rejection and HSV disease[23]. Other prophylaxis for the D+/R- recipient has included use of CMV-intravenous immmunoglobulin that does not prevent primary infection but is capable of reducing the frequency of serious disease[23]. An oral form of ganciclovir, valganciclovir (not to be confused with valacyclovir) has shown promising results in that doses of 450–900 mg orally produce ganciclovir levels comparable to intravenous ganciclovir at doses of 2.5–5 mg/kg.

Standard treatment of CMV disease is intravenous ganciclovir for 2–4 weeks. Before intravenous therapy is stopped, viremia should be cleared. In patients with primary infection, typically D+/R-, the relapse rate is approximately 50–75%, compared with 10–20% in R+ recipients. CMV resistance to ganciclovir is just beginning to be reported in renal transplant recipients. One such case resolved with discontinuation of mycophenolate and a course of intravenous ganciclovir[23].

CMV infections may predispose transplant recipients to additional infections ranging from conventional bacteremias to opportunistic infections, as well as to a 7- to 10-fold increased risk for PTLD. This state of CMV-associated suppression may allow one to use lower doses of immunosuppression and still preserve allograft function under circumstances in which the patient's general ability to respond to infection would be compromised by continued high-dose immunosuppression.

HHV-6 and HHV-7 infections

In addition to CMV, other members of the betaherpesvirus subfamily include HHV-6 and HHV-7. HHV-6 infections usually occur 2 to 4 weeks after transplantation and may cause skin rash, hepatitis, myelosuppression, interstitial pneumonitis, and encephalitis. These reactivations of HHV-6 and less often primary infections frequently occur simultaneously with CMV infection and intensify its severity. A fatal primary infection due to HHV-6 (variant A), apparently transmitted by the renal allograft and appearing within 3 weeks of transplantation, caused an acute hemophagocytic syndrome with hepatitis, CNS involvement, and fulminant candidemia[24].

In a prospective study of HHV-6, HHV-7, and CMV in 52 renal transplant recipients, CMV was found in 58%, HHV-7 in 46%, and HHV-6 in 23% of recipients. HHV-7 infection was detected earlier than CMV, was associated with more episodes of rejection, and led to a significant increase in CMV disease when co-infecting the recipient[25].

Parvovirus B-19 infection

Human parvovirus B-19 is a single-stranded DNA virus known to cause erythema infectiosum in children and severe symptomatic anemia in renal allograft recipients[26]. The erythroid progenitor tropism of parvovirus B-19 in immunosuppressed individuals who fail to mount an adequate humoral immune response can produce severe anemia with low reticulocyte counts and hypoplastic bone marrow showing intranuclear inclusions consistent with parvovirus[26]. Because IgM antibody production in renal transplant recipients may be suppressed, diagnosis is usually suspected by the clinical presentation and bone marrow examination, and confirmed by parvovirus B-19 PCR testing. Treatment with intravenous Ig and decreased immunosuppression generally results in a favorable response. Thrombotic microangiopathy and a collapsing form of focal segmental glomerulonephritis (FSGS) have been associated with parvovirus B-19 infection (Chapter 21).

Polyomavirus infections

Polyomavirus (PV) is a double-stranded DNA virus with two strains associated with human disease: BK virus and JC virus[27]. About 60–80% of immunocompetent adults are serologically positive for PV, have PV residing in a latent state in the kidney, and experience no functional impairment even with viral activation denoted by PV-infected cells in the urine ('decoy cells')[27]. The PV-BK virus in renal transplant recipients may cause acute tubulointerstitial nephritis, ureteral stenosis, hemorrhagic cystitis, severe allograft dysfunction, and a systemic vasculopathy associated with extensive capillary leakage and myocardial infarction[27,28]. Tubular necrosis is the main cause of allograft dysfunction and is a direct consequence of extensive replication of the BK virus[28]. Reactivated JC virus may cause progressive multifocal leukoencephalopathy. The background for both of these PV viruses is believed to be a state of high immunosuppression often developing after treatment of recurrent rejection episodes and in some cases associated with conversion from cyclosporine to tacrolimus, and the use of mycophenolate. The diagnosis has been made by the presence of cells containing viral inclusion bodies ('decoy cells') in the urine or allograft biopsy. Detection of BK DNA by PCR has been shown to be a sensitive and specific method for identifying this agent in blood, urine and kidney tissue as a cause of viral nephropathy[27]. Treatment usually consists of judicious reduction in immunosuppression, although cidofovir, which has significant nephrotoxic potential, has also been used.

Vaccinations and prophylaxis for opportunistic infections other than CMV

Vaccines using killed, inactivated, component, and recombinant moieties are generally safe. Live virus or live organism vaccines are not recommended for immunosuppressed renal transplant recipients and include: measles–mumps–rubella, live oral polio (which is also contraindicated for household contacts who should receive inactivated polio vaccine), smallpox (vaccinia), varicella, yellow fever, adenovirus, live oral typhoid (Ty21a), and bacillus Calmette–Guérin[29]. Additionally, exposure to persons who have chickenpox or herpes zoster should be avoided until the lesions have crusted over and no new lesions are appearing. Vaccinations recommended for immunosuppressed individuals include: influenza (yearly), pneumococcal (every 2–5 years), tetanus-diphtheria toxoid (booster every 10 years), hepatitis B (three-dose series for pre-transplant patients or those at risk), hepatitis A (two-dose series for high-risk patients, travelers, and during outbreaks), and hemophilus influenza B (single-dose for patients with asplenia, human immunodeficiency virus (HIV), or Hodgkin's disease). Because the pneumococcal vaccine is a polysaccharide antigen that is T-cell independent, the antibody response to it may theoretically be better than to those vaccines that are viral protein and T-cell dependent. However, in practice, the responses to pneumococcal vaccination have been variable.

For patients who are not allergic, prophylaxis with daily trimethoprim-sulfamethoxazole (TMS) 80 mg/400 mg is routinely used as prophylaxis for approximately one year and often longer in patients at high-risk for infection with opportunistic organisms including *P. carinii*, *Listeria*, *Nocardia*, *Toxoplasma* sp., as well as common urinary tract pathogens. Prophylaxis with TMS has reduced the frequency of *P. carinii* pneumonia (PCP) from 10–12% to less than 1%, and early urinary tract infections from 30–60% to < 5%. In some centers, prophylaxis for oral and esophageal candidiasis with nystatin is used for about the first 6 weeks after transplantation.

LIVER DISEASE

Liver disease occurs frequently in renal transplant recipients and may be responsible for 8–28% of mortality beyond 7 years after transplantation (Table 89.7). It is important to distinguish acute liver dysfunction caused by medications (notably azathioprine, cyclosporine, acetaminophen (paracetamol), and antibiotics) and acute viral hepatitis (HAV, HBV, HCV, CMV, HSV, HHV-6, EBV) from those etiologies (especially HBV and HCV infections, and ethanol) that can be associated with chronic liver dysfunction resulting in cirrhosis and HCC. The mortality associated with chronic liver disease is not only a consequence of liver failure, but also results from an increased risk for infection, particularly from encapsulated bacteria such as the pneumococcus.

Hepatitis B

HBsAg positive transplant recipients should be treated with lamivudine 100 mg/day (with adjustments for impaired renal function) starting at the time of transplantation and continuing for at least 18–24 months[2]. Lamivudine, a nucleoside analogue that interferes with reverse transcriptase activity of HBV, has been shown in small studies of HBsAg-positive renal transplant recipients to have results similar to those reported for nontransplant patients, namely, reduction or clearance of HBV DNA levels and improvement in transaminase levels[2].

Liver dysfunction following renal transplantation
Occurrence
Liver disease occurs in 7–24% of patients early after transplantation
Late mortality in 8–24% of patients often beyond 7 years
Clinical picture
Acute hepatic: hepatitis A, B, C viruses, cytomegalovirus, herpes simplex virus, human herpes virus 6, Epstein–Barr virus; drugs
Chronic hepatitic: hepatitis B and C viruses
Cholestatic: usually acute (including effect of azathioprine, cyclosporine, tacrolimus), as well as other drugs
Veno-occlusive: usually chronic (associated with azathioprine and cytomegalovirus)
Infiltrative: potentially reversible (fat, iron); typically progressive (amyloid, malignancy)
Alcohol: often chronic
Morphology
Chronic persistent hepatitis
Chronic active hepatitis
Fibrosing cholestatic hepatitis
Cirrhosis
Hepatocellular carcinoma (hepatoma)
Fatty metamorphosis
Hemosiderosis
Hepatic peliosis

Table 89.7 Liver dysfunction following renal transplantation.

Lamivudine in the dose range 75 to 150 mg daily have been used in renal transplant recipients. The optimal duration of therapy is not clearly defined, but because of recurrent viremia and worsening of liver function after withdrawal, therapy may be needed for extended periods of time. The use of interferon-α is generally unacceptable because of the frequent occurrence of irreversible allograft rejection. However, the use of pegylated interferon-α before transplantation may be indicated. Some centers do not carry out transplantation in HBV carriers; liver biopsy is usually needed for that decision.

Patients vaccinated against HBV (anti-HBs+, anti-HBc−) should be tested annually for anti-HBV antibodies and should received booster vaccinations when the titer has decreased to less than 10 mIU/mL[2]. Uninfected patients who have not been vaccinated (anti-HBs−, anti-HBc−) should receive HBV vaccinations, may require increased dosing because of their immunosuppressed status, and should be monitored for an adequate antibody response[2].

Because immunosuppression favors HBV viral replication, it is not surprising that histologic evidence of worsening liver disease has been documented in as many as 85% of patients; cirrhosis develops in 28%, and HCC in 23% of those with cirrhosis[30]. Significantly worse histopathology was found in those coinfected with HBV and HCV. Serum liver enzyme changes indicate neither clear histologic distinctions nor, if normal, the absence of significant disease. Morphology of the liver is the best predictor of the clinical course. In a recent study comparing HBsAg-positive and HBsAg-negative patients, the former had significantly lower allograft survival (36% vs. 63%), and patient survival (55% vs. 80%) 10 years after transplantation[31]. Ten-year patient survival in those with HBV-related cirrhosis diagnosed pretransplantation was just $26 \pm 16\%$[31]. The major causes of death in HBsAg-positive recipients were liver disease, sepsis, and cardiovascular disease[31]. Patients with confirmed cirrhosis may be managed best with dialysis or, in the absence of viral replication, be considered for liver–kidney transplantation[30].

Hepatitis C

Between 10 and 40% of renal transplant recipients have been reported to have anti-HCV antibody, and the majority of these have HCV RNA in their serum[2,32]. There is often an increase in HCV viremia after transplantation due to immunosuppression. A very small percentage of patients who have HCV may be unable to make antibody to HCV but can be diagnosed by testing for HCV-RNA. Liver disease can be documented in 19–64% of those who are HCV-positive before transplantation compared to just 2–19% of those who are HCV-negative[32]. Elevations of liver enzymes are neither sensitive nor specific in detecting HCV infection or as a measure of severity of liver damage in renal transplant recipients[2,32].

Several glomerular lesions have been reported in association with HCV and include membranoproliferative, membranous, fibrillary, and immunotactoid glomerulonephritis, as well as thrombotic microangiopathy. HCV-positive recipients have an increased risk for vascular rejection. In addition to the well-known association of HCV with cryoglobulinemia, HCV is also associated with an increase in monoclonal gammopathies, diabetes mellitus, and death from CHD. Although HCV-positive transplant recipients have a better outcome compared to those continuing dialysis, the mortality risk after transplantation in HCV-positive recipients is 1.4- to 3.3-fold, and the risk of death from liver disease or sepsis is 2.4- to 9.9-fold that of HCV-negative recipients[32]. At 10 years following transplantation, HCV-positive patients also have a lower allograft (49%) and patient (65%) survival compared with uninfected controls (63% and 80%, respectively), although they fare better than patients who are HBsAg-positive[31].

For the same reasons as noted with HBV, the use of interferon-α is generally unacceptable for treating HCV after transplantation. However, treatment of HCV before transplantation with interferon-α (currently pegylated interferon-α) and possibly ribavirin remains an option. Alcohol can increase the viral load and worsen hepatic injury and should be avoided. Because of the tendency to chronic changes over time periods exceeding 20 years, monitoring for the development of HCC may be a lifelong necessity (see 'Hepatobiliary cancers').

GASTROINTESTINAL DISEASE

A recent review has categorized gastrointestinal (GI) complications after transplantation into seven major categories: (1) infections, (2) mucosal injury and ulceration, (3) biliary tract diseases, (4) diverticular disease, (5) perforations, (6) pancreatitis, and (7) malignancy[33]. The most common opportunistic viral infections are CMV and HSV, fungal in the form of various *Candida* species, bacterial in the form of peptic ulcer disease due to *Helicobacter pylori* and colon infections due to *Yersinia enterocolitica*, *Campylobacter*, and *Clostridium difficile*; and parasitic infections notably microsporidia, cryptosporidia, and *Strongyloides stercoralis*. The time of appearance of these infections is shown in Table 89.6. Medications are also often responsible for GI side effects, as described below.

Esophagitis

Esophagitis may be caused by *Candida* species (which often have accompanying lesions in the oropharynx) as well as by HSV-1 and CMV. CMV may cause ulcerations not only in the esophagus but also in the stomach, duodenum and colon. Esophageal symptoms or esophagitis may also be caused by medications used in transplant patients such as cyclosporine, mycophenolate, and alendronate or risedronate used for osteoporosis. Gastroesophageal reflux symptoms in a transplant recipient may warrant endoscopy not only to identify infectious causes but also to detect early malignancy.

Gastroduodenal disease

Viral infections affecting the esophagus are often present in the stomach and at times the duodenum as well. However, *H. pylori* peptic ulcer disease is also common. Treatment involves a triple-drug program for 2 weeks that involves the use of two antibiotics and a third agent such as omeprazole or lansoprazole. The fact that eradication of the infection occurred in only about half of 47 heart transplant recipients treated with this protocol raises concern that immunosuppression is supporting the infection and that a new treatment protocol for immunosuppressed patients may need to be developed[33]. Endoscopy should be performed early in the disease course in order to identify the underlying cause which in some cases may be an unsuspected malignancy. Immunosuppressive medications, particularly mycophenolate, should be reviewed for either direct or indirect effects, and the use of NSAIDs and excess alcohol ingestion corrected.

Biliary calculus disease and pancreatic lesions

The frequency of biliary calculus disease and pancreatic lesions (asymptomatic hyperamylasemia, acute pancreatitis, pseudocysts, and abscess) was modestly increased in patients receiving cyclosporine in the early years after its introduction when dosing was higher than currently. Acute pancreatitis occurs in 1.7–6.8% of renal allograft recipients and has a mortality of up to 53%[33]. Causes of pancreatitis include traditional factors (cholelithiasis, alcohol abuse, and hypercalcemia), commonly used medications (azathioprine, corticosteroids, cyclosporine, and statins), and certain viral infections such as CMV and HHV. Controversy remains as to whether asymptomatic cholelithiasis should be treated surgically before transplantation.

Diseases of the colon

Diseases of the colon may be life-threatening and difficult to diagnose after transplantation because symptoms are muted in the presence of immunosuppression, especially early after transplantation. The major disease entities include diverticulitis with abscess formation or perforation, infectious or toxin causes of diarrhea, and medication-induced diarrhea related to mycophenolate and sirolimus. mycophenolate has also been associated with colon ulceration[33]. Perforation of the colon has been reported in approximately 2% of renal transplant recipients often early after transplantation when high doses of immunosuppression (particularly corticosteroids) are being used[33]. Prompt exteriorization of the perforated colon, early and appropriate antibiotic coverage, and reduction of immunosuppressive therapy to minimal levels (such as monotherapy with prednisone 15 mg/day) have been associated with low mortality and maintenance of graft function[4,33].

MUSCULOSKELETAL DISORDERS

Persistent hyperparathyroidism

Hypercalcemia associated with persistent hyperparathyroidism is observed in about 25% of renal transplant recipients overall, but in over 40% of those who had hypercalcemia before transplantation. Spontaneous resolution of hypercalcemia occurs in about two-thirds of these cases, but in less than one-half of those patients whose hypercalcemia existed before transplantation. Although hypophosphatemia and phosphaturia are also signs of hyperparathyroidism, numerous other factors may be responsible including corticosteroids and a nonparathyroid hormone (non-PTH) circulating serum factor, possibly phosphatonin (see Chapter 10)[34]. When persistent hyperparathyroidism occurs, it is often the result of continued autonomous production from nodular hyperplastic glands, reduced density of calcitriol receptors, and lower expression of membrane calcium sensor receptors that render cells more resistant to physiologic concentrations of calcitriol and calcium. Oseteitis fibrosa, lytic lesions (Brown tumors), pathologic fractures, osteoporosis, myopathy, ectopic calcifications, and calciphylaxis are other features of hyperparathyroidism.

Patients with asymptomatic hypercalcemia should have an intact parathyroid hormone level measurement along with investigation for other causes of hypercalcemia that include excessive calcium and vitamin D ingestion, hyperthyroidism, multiple myeloma, and aluminum toxicity.

Indications for parathyroid surgery have generally been acute hypercalcemia > 12.5 mg/dL (3.2 mmol/L) without other explanation in the immediate post-transplant period, asymptomatic hypercalcemia > 12 mg/dL (3.0 mmol/L) persisting without other causation for more than 1 year after transplantation, and symptomatic hypercalcemia[35]. In one major study only 38 renal transplant recipients among 4344 renal transplant procedures (0.9%) required parathyroidectomy for tertiary hyperparathyroidism; this occurred at a mean of 2.7 years post-transplantation[35].

Osteoporosis

Progressive loss of bone mineral density (BMD) in trabecular bone such as in the lumbar vertebrae often occurs early in renal transplant recipients with a 3–7% loss within the first 6 months, followed by a loss of 1.7 ± 2.8% per year[36]. In renal transplant recipients with functioning allografts for at least 20 years and treated only with prednisone and azathioprine, as many as 40% eventually developed osteoporosis[4]. Multiple factors may contribute to the loss of BMD, including the duration of prior chronic renal failure and dialysis, aluminum exposure, persistent metabolic acidosis, hyperparathyroidism, hypogonadism, diabetes mellitus, and smoking. After transplantation, two major risk factors are cumulative corticosteroid dose and female gender (postmenopausal). Interestingly, prednisone doses below the threshold of approximately 7.5 mg/day do not appear to incur loss of BMD beyond what would be expected with age- and gender-related losses over time.

Evaluation of patients for osteoporosis relies on measurement of BMD using dual energy X-ray absorptiometry (DEXA) scan. 'T' scores obtained by the DEXA scan are based on BMD comparisons with young adults and are used to describe a 'fracture threshold' (> 2.0 standard deviations (SD) below the mean reference value of young adults) and osteoporosis itself (> 2.5 SD below).

Oral bisphosphonates such as alendronate and risedronate, calcium, and vitamin D supplements have become the major therapies for corticosteroid-induced osteoporosis. For those who cannot tolerate bisphosphonates orally, calcitonin as a nasal spray may be a useful alternative. Etidronate, a non-nitrogen-containing bisphosphonate, has been used in a cyclical fashion. Intravenous bisphosphonates such as pamidronate and ibandronate have also been used; side-effect profiles are still evolving, and long-term outcomes are not yet available. Raloxifene, a selective estrogen receptor modifier, may be useful in post menopausal women[37]. Male and female hypogonadism may require specific therapy. Other aspects of treatment include smoking cessation, avoidance of excess alcohol intake and excess caffeine, a consistent exercise program, and treatment of overt hypocalcemia and vitamin D deficiency.

Avascular necrosis

In the precyclosporine era before 1984, when corticosteroids were one of the major immunosuppressants used, the prevalence of avascular necrosis (AVN) ranged from 3 to 41%. Currently, the prevalence appears to be < 5% in major transplant centers. Most often the hip joints are involved but knees, shoulders and much less commonly ankles, elbows and wrists may be affected. Pain from AVN of the hips may occur in the inguinal area, typically when the hips are bearing weight as when walking or rising from a seated position, and sometimes may be referred to the medial aspect of the knee. Although later stages of AVN may be seen on standard radiographs, MRI can best establish the diagnosis at an early stage (Fig. 89.6). Despite controversy over the role of glucocorticoids in causing AVN, corticosteroids are still generally considered a risk factor for AVN along with frequent acute rejections, cadaver transplants, repeat transplants, alcohol consumption, and severe hypertriglyceridemia.

Nonoperative management includes the use of conservative measures, such as crutches to avoid weight-bearing on the symptomatic hip. Operative interventions include core decompression, with and without bone grafting, and reconstructive procedures that involve total hip replacement. If AVN has already occurred, a sharp decrease in corticosteroid dose or complete discontinuation does not appear to be helpful in altering the lesion and may jeopardize renal allograft function.

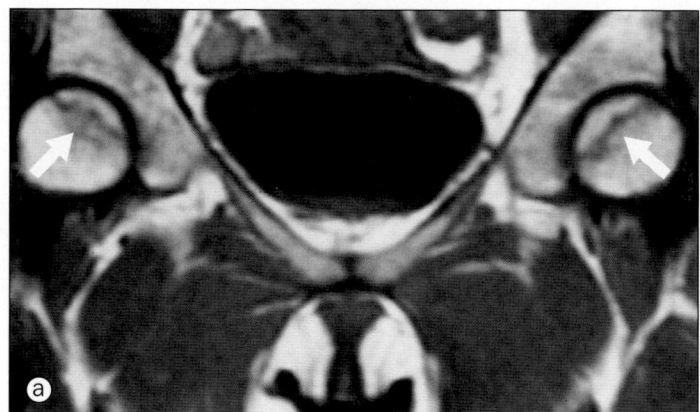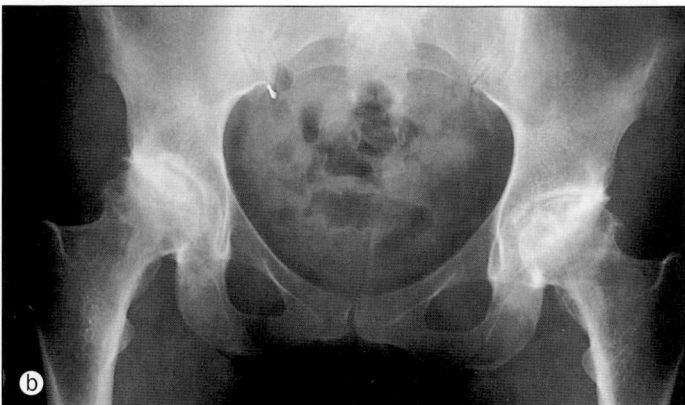

Figure 89.6 Avascular necrosis of the hip in a renal transplant recipient. (a) early changes consisting of low intensity oblique lines are noted by magnetic resonance imaging. (b) Late changes of AVN by X-ray show narrowing of the hip joint space, sclerosis of the femoral head, and flattening of the left femoral head.

Gout

In the cyclosporine era hyperuricemia has been reported in 30–84% and gout in 2–28% of renal transplant recipients[38]. In the precyclosporine era hyperuricemia ranged from 19–55%, and gout was usually absent, or at most 8%. However, gout has been reported even in the absence of cyclosporine in up to 23% of renal transplant recipients whose allograft functioned for > 20 years[4]. In addition to typical first metatarsophalangeal joint inflammation, gout after transplantation may involve more proximal joints (wrists, knees, elbows, hips, shoulders, and sacroiliac joints), have a less florid presentation because of concurrent corticosteroid use, and cause tenosynovitis of the dorsum of the foot and ankle[38].

Risk factors include cyclosporine, diuretic use, pretransplant uric acid level, obesity, and renal insufficiency. Hyperuricemia caused by cyclosporine may be due to both a decrease in the glomerular filtration rate (GFR) with decreased uric acid filtration, and an increased net reabsorption of uric acid by the proximal tubule.

Protocols for treating acute gout attacks with limited doses of colchicine, and for managing chronic tophaceous gout are shown in Tables 89.8 and 89.9. Losartan is unique among ATRA drugs by virtue of being uricosuric and having a greater effect on higher blood levels of uric acid. Other approaches to treating acute gouty attacks include an increase in corticosteroid dose or adrenocorticotrophic hormone (ACTH) given parenterally[38]. NSAIDs are best avoided. Long-term prophylaxis may include reduction or discontinuation of diuretics if possible, careful introduction and monitoring of low doses of allopurinol, and possibly a change from cyclosporine to a comparably potent immunosuppressant. If allopurinol is to be used in the presence of azathioprine, much lower doses of both medications are required (see Table 89.9), whereas, its use with mycophenolate has not been reported to require dosage reduction.

Muscle weakness

Muscle weakness following renal transplantation may have many etiologies (Table 89.10)[39]. Assuming that hereditary myopathies have not been previously overlooked, acquired forms include drug-induced/toxic, endocrine, electrolyte-related, inflammatory, and other systemic diseases[39]. Clinically, it may be useful to consider myopathies as those in which muscle enzyme tests (creatine kinase) are usually normal (e.g., associated with corticosteroids, hyperparathyroidism, diabetes, adrenal insufficiency, hyperkalemia) from those with elevated muscle enzymes (e.g., hypothyroidism, severe hypophosphatemia, severe hypokalemia, and rhabdomyolysis secondary to statins and colchicine). Neuropathies such as a sacral plexopathy, and unsuspected iliofemoral occlusive vascular disease may also be responsible for leg weakness. Neurology consultation, electromyography, muscle biopsy, and pulse volume recordings in the lower extremities may be necessary.

A protocol for the treatment of acute gout in renal transplant recipients
Objectives
Terminate the acute painful inflammatory joint symptoms while minimizing side effects*
Treatment
Day 1: colchicine 0.6 mg q1h × 2 doses maximum, but stop if diarrhea occurs
Day 2: colchicine 0.6 mg q1h × 2 doses maximum, but stop if diarrhea occurs
Days 3–10: colchicine 0.6 mg once daily; stop if diarrhea occurs
Supplementary treatment
Adjust allopurinol, azathioprine, diuretics, and diet as needed
* Potential side effects of chronic colchicine use include myelosuppression with agranulocytosis and aplastic anemia, myopathy, neuropathy, and depilation; acute toxicity includes diarrhea that may be bloody, nausea, vomiting, abdominal pain, burning of the throat and skin, shock, renal failure, ascending paralysis, and death. One should also be aware of any drug interactions. Lower doses or drug avoidance are necessary for those with GFR < 50 mL/min per 1.73 m². Adapted from Braun WE. Modification of the treatment of gout in renal transplant recipients. Transplant Proc. 2000;32:199. With permission from Elsevier Science.

Table 89.8 A protocol for the treatment of acute gout in renal transplant recipients.

Transplantation

A protocol for managing tophaceous gout in renal transplant recipients
Objective
Eliminate uric acid deposits without incurring drug toxicity* or damaging the allograft
Treatment
1. Drug regimen
a. For patients taking azathioprine (in whom allopurinol inhibits its metabolism):
—Start allopurinol 50 mg/day; reduce azathioprine by 50–75% (to about 50–75 mg/day)
—Monitor complete blood count, liver, and renal function
—Reduce or eliminate diuretic
b. For patients taking mycophenolate:
—Start allopurinol 100 mg/day
—Monitor complete blood count, liver, and renal function
—Be prepared for acute gouty attack; colchicine if needed
—Reduce or eliminate diuretics
2. Ultrasound assessment of renal allograft for obstruction or stones; treat as indicated
3. Alkalinize the urine to pH 6.5–7.0†
4. Increase hydration to 240 mL every 2 h until bedtime or as permitted by patient's cardiopulmonary and renal status
5. If GFR is > 50 mL/min/1.73 m², probenecid 250 mg *bid* may be initiated. Losartan also is uricosuric
6. If no side effects or toxicity occur, allopurinol may be cautiously increased with continued close monitoring.
* Potential side effects of allopurinol include hypersensitivity reactions involving the skin and blood, fever, malaise, myalgia, liver function changes, peripheral neuritis, myelosuppression, and gastrointestinal symptoms. Allopurinol interferes with the metabolization of azathioprine that can lead to severe agranulocytosis and myelosuppression.   Potential side effects of probenecid include gastrointestinal symptoms, hypersensitivity reactions, intrarenal precipitation of uric acid during uricosuric therapy, and the nephrotic syndrome. Probenecid can increase blood levels of sulfonamides. With impaired renal function (GFR < 50 mL/min/1.73 m²) allopurinol and probenecid need dosage reduction or avoidance.   † Approaches to alkalinize the urine (and their risks) when clinically safe include the use, preferably, of potassium citrate (hyperkalemia, alkalosis). Sodium citrate and sodium bicarbonate (hypertension, fluid retention, possibly nephrolithiasis) and acetazolamide (paresthesis, renal stone) may be more problematic.   Adapted from Braun WE. Modification of the treatment of gout in renal transplant recipients. Transplant Proc. 2000;32:199. With permission from Elsevier Science.

Table 89.9 A protocol for managing tophaceous gout in renal transplant recipients.

Etiology of muscle weakness in renal transplant recipients		
Cause	Myopathy usually with normal creatine kinase	Myopathy usually with elevated creatine kinase
Drugs	glucocorticoids*	statins (especially with cyclosporine or combinations of lipid-lowering drugs)* gemfibrozil clofibrate colchicine* cimetidine cyclosporine tacrolimus labetalol amiodarone alcohol
Endocrine	diabetes mellitus* hyperparathyroidism* adrenal insufficiency hypothyroidism*	Hyperthyroidism*
Electrolyte	hyperkalemia* hypermagnesemia hypomagnesemia*	severe hypokalemia severe hypophosphatemia
Inflammatory	most uncomplicated viral, bacterial and fungal infections	dermatomyositis polymyositis myositis in overlap inclusion body sarcoidosis viral (e.g., severe influenza, coxsackie, HIV) bacterial (e.g., clostridia, legionella) protozoal (e.g., malaria due to *Plasmodium falciparum* helminthic (e.g., trichinosis)
Other systemic diseases simulating myopathy	anemia malnutrition occult malignancy chronic hypotension, often orthostatic, or with volume depletion sleep disturbances	

*More common
Adapted and modified from Kissel JT, Amato AA, Barohn RJ, et al[39].

Table 89.10 Etiology of muscle weakness in renal transplant recipients.

Electrolyte abnormalities

Hypomagnesemia

Renal magnesium wasting is common following renal transplantation and can be caused by cyclosporine, tacrolimus, and sirolimus. Hypomagnesemia may help to explain some cyclosporine toxicity such as anorexia, nausea, vomiting, apathy, depression, tremors, and ataxia. Seizures similar to those seen with hypocalcemia and findings of nystagmus, spasticity, and positive Trousseau's and Chvostek's signs may also be present. Hypomagnesemia increases susceptibility to cardiac arrhythmias and may intensify atherogenesis in coronary vessels. Nevertheless, the great majority of renal transplant recipients with hypomagnesemia are asymptomatic. Unlike hypomagnesemia associated with cisplatin or aminoglycoside therapies, that occurring secondary to cyclosporine is generally not accompanied by hypocalcemia or hypokalemia. Oral and, if necessary, intravenous magnesium therapy is indicated.

Hypophosphatemia

Hypophosphatemia of varying degrees may be seen both early and late after transplantation. Early after transplantation, the occurrence of a massive initial diuresis (often after a living-related renal transplant in a recipient who has not required dialysis) as well as persistent autonomous hyperparathyroidism may cause hypophosphatemia. However, the presence of a non-PTH circulating serum factor (possibly phosphatonin) that increases the fractional excretion of phosphate may also be responsible for hypophosphatemia early after a successful kidney transplant[34]. Other factors tending to promote hypophosphatemia include the use of corticosteroids that inhibit proximal tubular reabsorption of phosphate, defective renal phosphate reabsorption as part of allograft injury, glycosuria, magnesium depletion, and a continued inadvertent use of phosphate-binding antacids. Severe hypophosphatemia may cause rhabdomyolysis, left ventricular dysfunction, respiratory muscle weakness, hemolysis, defects in erythrocyte metabolism, insulin resistance, osteomalacia, and renal tubular defects. The treatment of hypophosphatemia involves the treatment of any underlying conditions, and oral supplementation for most situations.

ALLOGRAFT DYSFUNCTION

The evaluation of an increase in serum creatinine carries with it a long list of differential diagnoses. The use of a more anatomically-detailed approach can be helpful in identifying the primary cause (Table 89.11). Re-evaluation of data that supported the cause of renal failure in the patient's native kidneys may be necessary because the allograft could be experiencing dysfunction from a disease not recognized in

Table 89.11 Differential diagnosis of impaired renal allograft function based on site of injury.

Differential diagnosis of impaired renal allograft function based on site of injury	
Site of impaired renal function	**Causes of impairment**
Prerenal	*Volume depletion*: excessive diuresis, hyperglycemia, vomiting/diarrhea, etc.
	Cardiac: severe congestive heart failure, acute myocardial infarction, ischemic and nonischemic cardiomyopathy, large pericardial effusions, etc.
Renovascular	*Artery stenosis*: technical, recipient atherosclerosis even in the iliac artery above the anastomosis, immunologic associated with chronic rejection; antiphospholipid antibodies especially with systemic lupus
	Venous occlusion: technical, cyclosporine and/or OKT3, occlusion with ipsilateral leg thrombophlebitis
Renal parenchymal: glomerular	*Recurrent disease*: e.g., focal segmental glomerulosclerosis, IgA nephropathy, membranoproliferative glomerulonephritis (MPGN) types I and II, diabetic nephropathy, HUS, light chain deposition, etc.
	De novo disease: membranous nephropathy, post-transplant diabetic nephropathy, etc.
	Drug/infection-induced disease: hemolytic uremic syndrome/thrombotic microangiopathy with cyclosporin or tacrolimus, cytomegalovirus, and parvovirus B-19
	Rejection: thromboses in accelerated rejection or thrombotic microangiopathy, transplant glomerulopathy/chronic rejection
	Hepatitis C: MPGN type 1, membranous nephropathy, immunotactoid and fibrillary GN, thrombotic microangiopathy
Renal parenchymal: arteriolar	*Anatomic*: thromboses with hyperacute rejection, endotheliolitis or fibrinoid necrosis with acute vascular or accelerated rejection, thrombotic microangiopathy, chronic cyclosporine arteriolopathy, nephrosclerosis, atheroemboli
	Hemodynamic: cyclosporine especially with ACE inhibitors, and/or ATRA, diuretics, nonsteroidal anti-inflammatory drugs, amphotericin B
Renal parenchymal: tubular	Acute cellular rejection with tubulitis, ischemic acute tubular necrosis worsened by cyclosporine, recurrent oxalosis, nephrotoxins, acute pyelonephritis, pigment nephropathy with high-dose statin medications + cyclosporin
Renal parenchymal: interstitial	Acute cellular rejection, acute interstitial nephritis secondary to drugs or infection, lymphoma, fibrosis associated with multiple factors including chronic rejection, cyclosporin and tacrolimus nephrotoxicity
Postrenal	*Obstruction*: any site from urethra upward, intrinsic and extrinsic ureteral occlusion, lymphocele, stone, ileal conduit problems (excess length, stone, infection)
	Extravasation: usually at the vesico-ureteral junction within 1–2 weeks after transplantation
Miscellaneous causes of a rising serum creatinine	Drugs interfering with tubular secretion of creatinine (trimethoprim-sulfamethoxazole, cimetidine), factors affecting muscle mass (weight/muscle, glucocorticoids)
Factors affecting creatinine measurement	*Alkaline picrate method*: elevated by cephalosporins (especially cefoxitin (cephoxitin)), both acetoacetic and beta-hydroxybutyric acid, possibly high vitamin C; decreased by very high bilirubin levels
	Enzymatic: elevated by flucytosine, lidocaine (lignocaine); decreased by dobutamine and dopamine
Adapted from Braun WE. In: Comprehensive Clinical Nephrology, Harcourt Publishers, 2000.	

Transplantation

Differential diagnosis of pain in the allograft area
Typically early (days to weeks); usually a surgical emergency
ruptured graft (often graft with ATN and patient still requiring hemodialysis)
acute transplant arterial or venous bleeding
acute large volume urine extravasation from ureteral dehiscence or necrosis
acute thrombosis of external iliac artery threatening leg
necrosis of graft experiencing primary non-function
rejection typically pre-cyclosporine when patient receiving only prednisone and azathioprine
Usually late
rejection in a failed allograft when immunosuppression being tapered
renal stone (rare)
Any time
acute pyelonephritis (most common)
expanding fluid collection of blood, urine, or lymph possibly causing obstruction
renal infarction (usually silent if small)
primary events occurring adjacent to or near the allograft: appendicitis, diverticulitis, strangulated hernia, bowel obstruction, iliac artery dissection or aneurysm, inflammatory bowel disease, pelvic or femoral bone pathology such as osteoporotic fractures or AVN, cellulitis of abdominal wall, broken deep sutures, pain preceding herpes zoster.

Table 89.12 Differential diagnosis of pain in the allograft area.

the native kidneys (e.g., light chain deposition disease, adult hyperoxalosis).

Proteinuria

Proteinuria occurs in approximately 10–40% of renal allograft recipients. Transient proteinuria (lasting < 6 months) may be seen with acute rejection, acute pyelonephritis, and intercurrent systemic diseases. Persistent proteinuria (lasting > 6 months) may occur with recurrent or *de novo* glomerulonephritis, chronic allograft nephropathy that may be either alloantigen-dependent or -independent, chronic rejection associated with transplant glomerulopathy, recurrent or *de novo* diabetic nephropathy, progressive cyclosporine nephrotoxicity

with ischemic and focal segmental glomerular lesions, renal vein thrombosis, reflux nephropathy, and rarely acute rejection. Proteinuria > 10 g/day is typically seen just with *de novo* membranous glomerulonephritis and focal segmental glomerulosclerosis; transplant glomerulopathy may give rise to proteinuria that approaches this range. Unusual causes of proteinuria include atheroembolic disease, and light chain deposition disease. If there is no contraindication, renal transplant biopsy should be undertaken and should include histopathologic examination by electron microscopy.

Proteinuria > 2 g/day is associated with a significant reduction in graft survival to 5.6 years compared to 16.5 years for those with proteinuria below this level[40]. Proteinuria even less than 1 g/day for over 6 months has also been associated with poorer allograft survival.

Pain in the allograft area

The differential diagnosis of pain in the renal allograft area includes very early and serious causes (e.g., ruptured allograft, necrosis of a nonfunctioning graft, acute bleeding, and/or urine extravasation), common problems such as acute pyelonephritis, other transplant-related events (expanding fluid collection of lymph, urine, or blood), acute rejection in the presence of only prednisone and azathioprine immunosuppression, very late rejection of a failed graft after tapering immunosuppression, infarction, rarely a renal stone, and a variety of other potentially serious problems in organs adjacent to the allograft (Table 89.12).

OUTPATIENT CARE

The frequency of outpatient visits and laboratory testing will vary according to the time after transplantation, the condition of the patient, and the level of allograft function. It has been noted that 'there are virtually no scientific data on which to base decisions regarding the optimal frequency or type of contact between renal transplant recipients and transplant centers'[2]. However, renal transplant recipients should have regular follow-up in a transplantation center.

REFERENCES

1. Kasiske BL, Ballantyne CM. Cardiovascular risk factors associated with immunosuppression in renal transplantation. Transplant Rev. 2002;16:1–21.
2. Kasiske BL, Vazquez MA, Harmon WE, et al. Recommendations for the outpatient surveillance of renal transplant recipients. American Society of Transplantation. J Am Soc Nephrol. 2000;11(Suppl):S1–86.
3. Kasiske BL. Ischemic heart disease after renal transplantation. Kidney Int. 2002;61:356–69.
4. Braun WE, Yadlapalli NG. The spectrum of long-term renal transplantation: Outcomes, complications, and clinical studies. Transplant Rev. 2002;16:22–50.
5. Wilson PW, D'Agostino RB, Levy D, et al. Prediction of coronary heart disease using risk factor categories. Circulation. 1998;97: 1837–47.
6. Executive Summary of The Third Report of The National Cholesterol Education Program (NCEP) Expert Panel on Detection, Evaluation, And Treatment of High Blood Cholesterol In Adults (Adult Treatment Panel III). JAMA. 2001;285:2486–97.
7. Kasiske BL, Ramos EL, Gaston RS, et al. The evaluation of renal transplant candidates: clinical practice guidelines. Patient Care and Education Committee of the American Society of Transplant Physicians. J Am Soc Nephrol. 1995;6:1–34.

8. Hiatt WR. Medical treatment of peripheral arterial disease and claudication. N Engl J Med. 2001;344:1608–21.

9. Joint National Committee. The sixth report of the committee on the Prevention, Detection, Evaluation and Treatment of High Blood Pressure (JNC-VI). Arch Intern Med. 1997;157:2413–46.

10. Fahmy HI, Melby JC, Mesler DE, et al. Primary hyperaldosteronism causing posttransplantation hypertension: localization by adrenal vein sampling. Am J Kidney Dis. 1998;31:853–5.

11. Yusuf S, Gerstein H, Hoogwerf B, et al. Ramipril and the development of diabetes. JAMA. 2001;286:1882–5.

12. Saunders RN, Metcalfe MS, Nicholson ML. Rapamycin in transplantation: a review of the evidence. Kidney Int. 2001;59:3–16.

13. Welch GN, Loscalzo J. Homocysteine and atherothrombosis. N Engl J Med. 1998;338:1042–50.

14. Jindal RM. Posttransplant diabetes mellitus – a review. Transplantation. 1994;58:1289–98.

15. Kelly JJ, Walker RG, Kincaid-Smith P. De novo diabetic nodular glomerulosclerosis in a renal allograft. Transplantation. 1992;53:688–9.

16. Hollander AA, Hene RJ, Hermans J, et al. Late prednisone withdrawal in cyclosporine-treated kidney transplant patients: a randomized study. J Am Soc Nephrol. 1997;8:294–301.

17. Penn I. The effect of immunosuppression on pre-existing cancers. Transplantation. 1993;55:742–7.

18. Penn I. Cancers in renal transplant recipients. Adv Ren Replace Ther. 2000;7:147–56.

19. Tsai DE, Hardy CL, Tomaszewski JE, et al. Reduction in immunosuppression as initial therapy for posttransplant lymphoproliferative disorder: analysis of prognostic variables and long-term follow-up of 42 adult patients. Transplantation. 2001;71:1076–88.

20. Schaar CG, van der Pijl JW, van Hoek B, et al. Successful outcome with a 'quintuple approach' of posttransplant lymphoproliferative disorder. Transplantation. 2001;71:47–52.

21. Fishman JA, Rubin RH. Infection in organ-transplant recipients. N Engl J Med. 1998;338:1741–51.

22. Birk PE, Chavers BM. Does cytomegalovirus cause glomerular injury in renal allograft recipients? J Am Soc Nephrol. 1997;8:1801–8.

23. Brennan DC. Cytomegalovirus in renal transplantation. J Am Soc Nephrol. 2001;12:848–55.

24. Rossi C, Delforge ML, Jacobs F, et al. Fatal primary infection due to human herpesvirus 6 variant A in a renal transplant recipient. Transplantation. 2001;71:288–92.

25. Kidd IM, Clark DA, Sabin CA, et al. Prospective study of human betaherpesviruses after renal transplantation: association of human herpesvirus 7 and cytomegalovirus co-infection with cytomegalovirus disease and increased rejection. Transplantation. 2000;69:2400–4.

26. Pamidi S, Friedman K, Kampalath B, et al. Human parvovirus B19 infection presenting as persistent anemia in renal transplant recipients. Transplantation. 2000;69:2666–9.

27. Nickeleit V, Hirsch HH, Binet IF, et al. Polyomavirus infection of renal allograft recipients: from latent infection to manifest disease. J Am Soc Nephrol. 1999;10:1080–9.

28. Petrogiannis-Haliotis T, Sakoulas G, Kirby J, et al. BK-related polyomavirus vasculopathy in a renal-transplant recipient. N Engl J Med. 2001;345:1250–5.

29. Avery RK. Immunizations in adult immunocompromised patients: which to use and which to avoid. Cleve Clin J Med. 2001;68: 337–48.

30. Fornairon S, Pol S, Legendre C, et al. The long-term virologic and pathologic impact of renal transplantation on chronic hepatitis-B virus infection. Transplantation. 1996;62:297–9.

31. Mathurin P, Mouquet C, Poynard T, et al. Impact of hepatitis B and C virus on kidney transplantation outcome. Hepatology. 1999;29:257–63.

32. Pereira BJ, Levey AS. Hepititis C virus infection in dialysis and transplantation. Kidney Int. 1997;51:981–99.

33. Helderman JH, Goral S. Gastrointestinal complications of transplant immunosuppression. J Am Soc Nephrol. 2002;13:277–87.

34. Green J, Debby H, Lederer E, et al. Evidence for a PTH-independent humoral mechanism in post-transplant hypophosphatemia and phosphaturia. Kidney Int. 2001;60: 1182–96.

35. Kerby JD, Rue LW, Blair H, et al. Operative treatment of tertiary hyperparathyroidism: a single-center experience. Ann Surg. 1998; 227:878–86.

36. Rodino MA, Shane E. Osteoporosis after organ transplantation. Am J Med. 1998;104:459–69.

37. Maricic MJ, Gluck OS. Osteoporosis: Therapeutic options for prevention and management. J Musculoskel Med. 2001;18:415–25.

38. Clive DM. Renal transplant-associated hyperuricemia and gout. J Am Soc Nephrol. 2000;11:974–9.

39. Kissel JT, Amato AA, Barohn RJ, et al. Muscle disease. Continuum. 2000;6(Part A of A & B):7–192.

40. Peddi VP, Dean D, Hariharan S, et al. Proteinuria following renal transplantation: Correlation with histopathology and outcome. Transplant Proc. 1997;29:101–3.

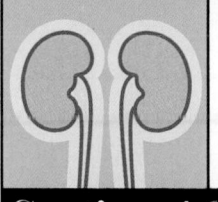
Chapter 90

Chronic Transplant Rejection

Magdalena Adeva Andany and Bertram L Kasiske

DEFINITION

There is no uniformly agreed-upon definition of chronic rejection. From a practical standpoint, it can be defined as a gradual deterioration in kidney function that occurs in the absence of other causes of allograft dysfunction. Histologically, chronic rejection is characterized by glomerular sclerosis, interstitial fibrosis, and fibrointimal proliferation in arteries (Fig. 90.1). However, biopsies often do not contain medium-size or large arteries, where the lesions of chronic rejection are most common. In addition, the intimal thickening may not be uniform and may be missed in the biopsy even if arteries are present in the sections. Glomerular sclerosis and

interstitial fibrosis are non-specific changes that can result not only from chronic rejection but also from age-related damage already present in the kidney at the time of transplantation.

Chronic rejection needs to be distinguished from other causes of graft dysfunction (Table 90.1), especially acute rejection, since the latter often responds to specific therapies. The inflammatory response seen on allograft biopsy is usually diagnostic of acute rejection, particularly when it occurs in the setting of an acute deterioration in kidney function. Recurrence of the original kidney disease can also be confused with chronic rejection (Table 90.1). It is difficult to differentiate biopsy changes of chronic rejection from those of chronic calcineurin inhibitor toxicity, e.g., toxicity from cyclosporine or

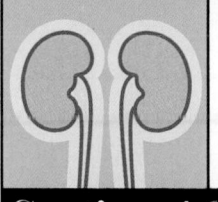

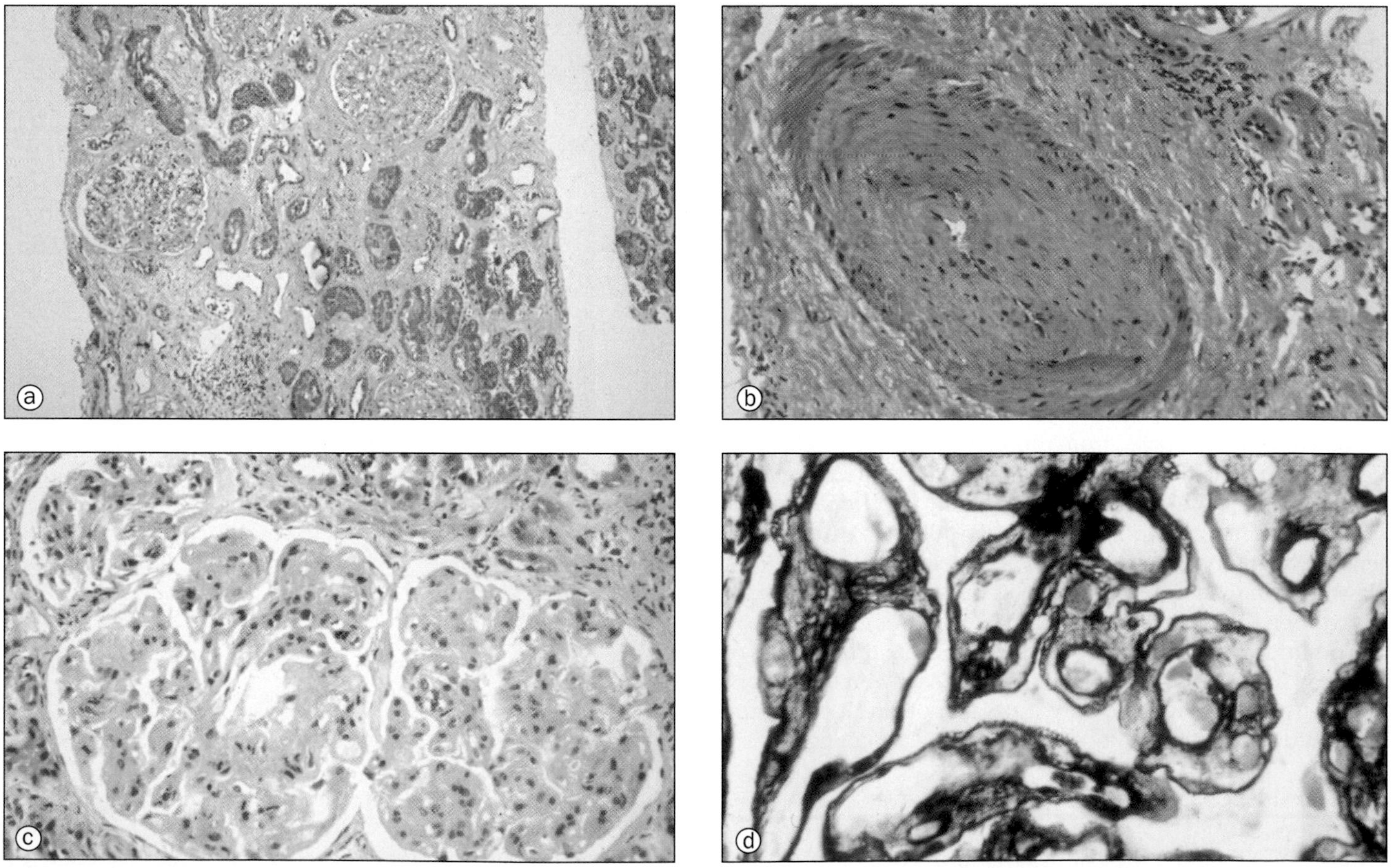

Figure 90.1 Histologic changes typical of chronic renal allograft rejection. (a) Interstitial fibrosis, glomerulosclerosis, and tubular atrophy (trichrome). (b) Fibrointimal proliferation in an intrarenal artery (hematoxylin and eosin). (c) Transplant glomerulopathy with mesangial matrix expansion and thickening of capillary loops (hematoxylin and eosin). (d) Transplant glomerulopathy showing membrane reduplication in capillary loops (silver stain).

Differential diagnosis of chronic renal allograft rejection

Acute rejection

Drug toxicity:
    Cyclosporine
    Tacrolimus
    Other drugs

De novo glomerulonephritis

Recurrence of renal disease or disease with renal sequelae:
    IgA nephropathy
    Membranoproliferative glomerulonephritis
    Systemic lupus erythematosus
    Diabetes mellitus
    Other renal diseases

Interstitial nephritis:
    Infection
    Allergic

Urinary obstruction

Renal artery stenosis (unusual)

Cholesterol emboli (rare)

Table 90.1 Differential diagnosis of chronic renal allograft rejection.

Histologic features seen in chronic rejection versus cyclosporine toxicity

Feature	Chronic rejection	Cyclosporine toxicity
Interstitial fibrosis	+++++	+++++
Glomerulosclerosis	++++	++++
Transplant glomerulopathy	+	−
Fibrointimal arterial proliferation	+++	+
Arteriolar hyalinosis	−	+

Table 90.2 Histologic features seen in chronic rejection versus cyclosporine toxicity.

tacrolimus (Table 90.2). Hyalinization of arterioles and other changes are relatively specific for acute cyclosporine toxicity, but chronic cyclosporine nephrotoxicity primarily causes interstitial fibrosis, glomerular sclerosis, and chronic arterial changes that are indistinguishable from those seen in chronic rejection.

The Banff classification of renal allograft pathology groups together under the term chronic allograft nephropathy four entities: chronic rejection, chronic cyclosporine toxicity, hypertensive vascular disease, and chronic infection or reflux. This classification scheme uses the term chronic allograft nephropathy rather than chronic rejection, even though it may be important to distinguish chronic rejection from other causes of nephropathy in managing patients. There are three grades of chronic allograft nephropathy: mild, moderate, and severe, depending on the intensity of the pathological changes[1].

EPIDEMIOLOGY

Long-term allograft survival has improved over the past decade[2] (Fig. 90.2). Much of this improvement is due to reductions in early acute rejection and improved one-year graft survival. Chronic allograft nephropathy is the leading

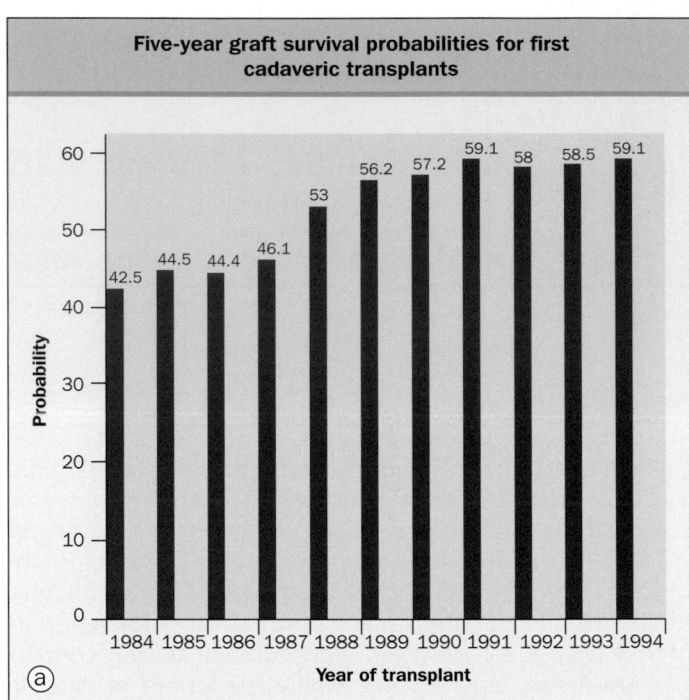

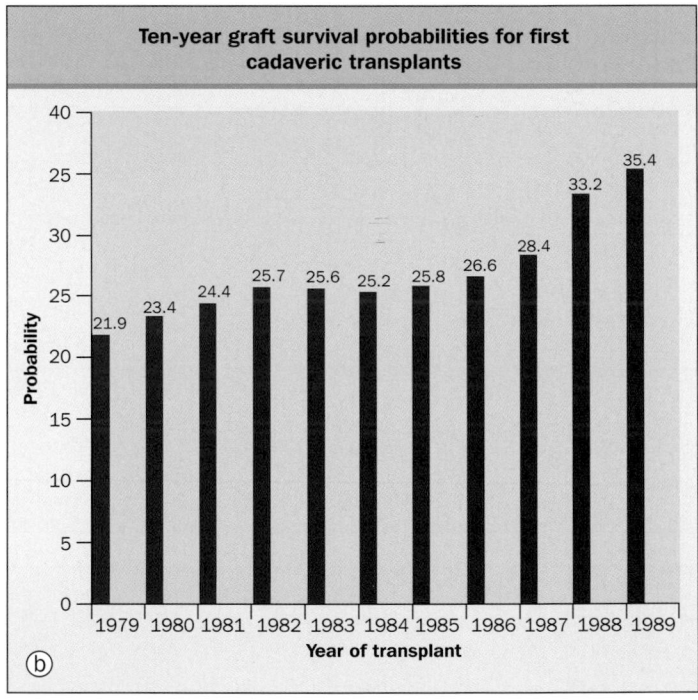

Figure 90.2 Long-term graft survival. Total graft survival probabilities for first cadaveric transplants (adjusted for age, gender, race, and primary diagnosis). (a) At 5 years. (b) At 10 years. Data from 2001 Annual Report of the USRDS[2]. Since 1988, there has been a remarkable increase in long-term kidney graft survival.

cause of death-censored late graft failure[3] (Fig. 90.3). The incidence and prevalence of chronic rejection are difficult to determine because the onset of chronic rejection is often insidious and difficult to define, especially since not every patient undergoes biopsy. However, in some studies biopsies have been obtained in all patients at defined times

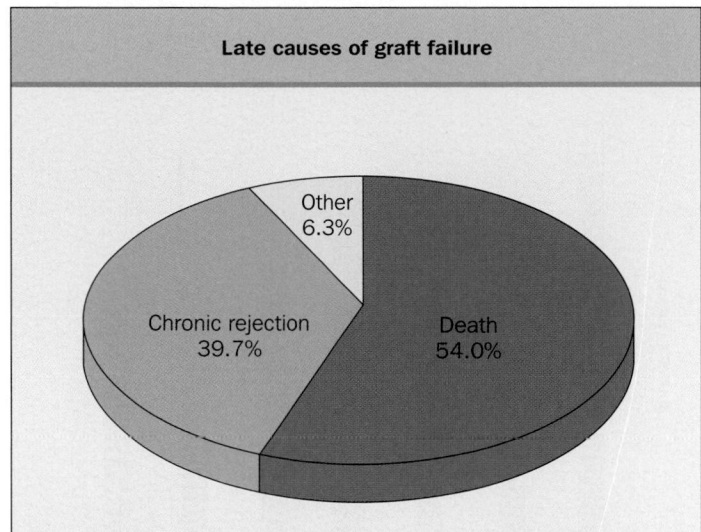

Figure 90.3 Late causes of graft failure. Assessment involved 706 patients who survived with a functioning allograft for at least 6 months after transplantation at Hennepin County Medical Center[3]. Mean follow-up to death, return to dialysis, or last clinic visit was 7.0 years. Chronic rejection was confirmed by histology in 85% of patients. The category 'other' included graft loss to acute rejection and recurrent disease.

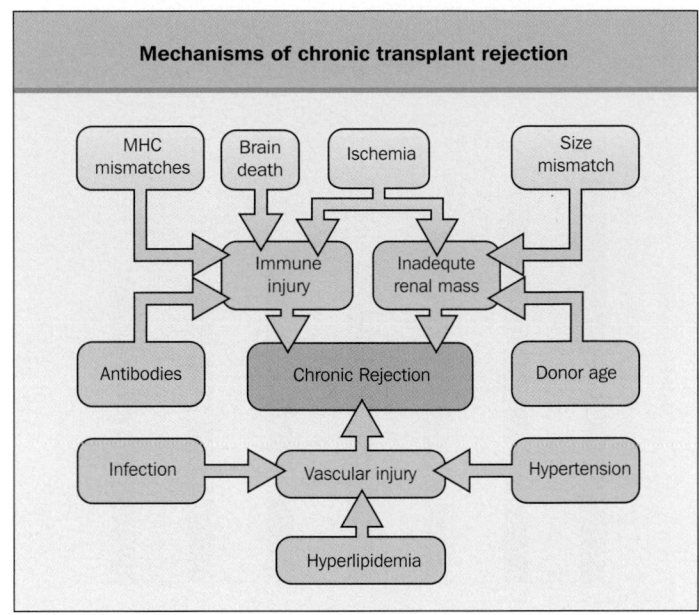

Figure 90.4 Possible mechanisms causing chronic renal allograft rejection. Antigen-dependent and antigen-independent risk factors may be involved. MHC, major histocompatibility complex.

post-transplant, i.e., protocol biopsies. Chronic allograft nephropathy was found in 24% of protocol biopsies at 3 months[4] and in 62–72% of protocol biopsies at 2 years after transplantation, in recipients treated with tacrolimus or cyclosporin, respectively[5]. A number of clinical correlates, or risk factors for late allograft failure, and presumably chronic rejection, have been identified. In single-center, multivariate analyses, independent predictors of late allograft failure include the number and severity of acute rejection episodes[3,6,7], African American race[7], older donor age[7], younger recipient age[6], proteinuria[3], serum albumin[3], and serum triglycerides[3,6].

PATHOGENESIS

The pathogenesis of chronic rejection is unknown. Both antigen-dependent (immune) and antigen-independent (non-immune) mechanisms may be important in the pathogenesis of chronic rejection (Fig. 90.4). Some antigen-independent risk factors, such as brain death and ischemia reperfusion injury, may cause an increase in expression of major histocompatibility complex (MHC) antigens and proinflammatory cytokines in the allograft. These, in turn, may lead to enhanced chemotaxis and adhesion of mononuclear cells that can cause acute and chronic rejection. Antigen-dependent damage may be mediated by cytotoxic lymphocytes and/or antibodies to the vascular endothelium. Endothelial injury from antigen-dependent or antigen-independent mechanisms may set in motion a cascade of events that leads to the chronic fibrointimal arterial changes that are often seen in chronic rejection.

Infection has been postulated to play a role in systemic atherosclerosis, and the increased incidence of viral and other infections associated with immunosuppression could also contribute to chronic rejection. A number of antigen-independent

vascular disease risk factors, such as hyperlipidemia and hypertension, could contribute to chronic allograft vasculopathy in much the same way that these risk factors play a major role in systemic atherosclerosis. It has been suggested that an inadequate amount of functioning renal mass may lead to chronic renal allograft rejection, just as an inadequate nephron mass may cause or contribute to progressive renal disease in the native kidneys, possibly as a result of glomerular hyperfiltration. Finally, senescence of the allograft, perhaps accelerated by injury response mechanisms, could play a role in the pathogenesis of chronic rejection[8].

Antigen-dependent risk factors
Major histocompatibility complex antigen mismatches
The number of mismatches in the MHC antigens (two each for the A, B, and DR loci) has a significant effect on long-term graft survival, as reflected by allograft half-life. Allograft half-life is defined as the time until one half of the grafts that were functioning at one year after transplantation have failed, due to death, return to dialysis or retransplant. Allograft half-life reflects graft failure in the late posttransplant period, when most graft failure in recipients that have not died is due to chronic rejection. In the USRDS registry data MHC mismatches had a significant effect on graft half-life among recipients of cadaveric and living donor kidneys in 1988–1998, particularly for zero-antigen mismatches (Fig. 90.5)[2]. Unfortunately, there are limitations with using registry data to draw inferences regarding chronic rejection. Registries generally do not have detailed information on acute rejection, and it is difficult to know whether the influence of MHC matching on allograft half-life is mediated by acute rejections that may then go on to cause chronic rejection.

A role for MHC matching in chronic rejection was suggested by a retrospective study of protocol biopsies at 3 months and

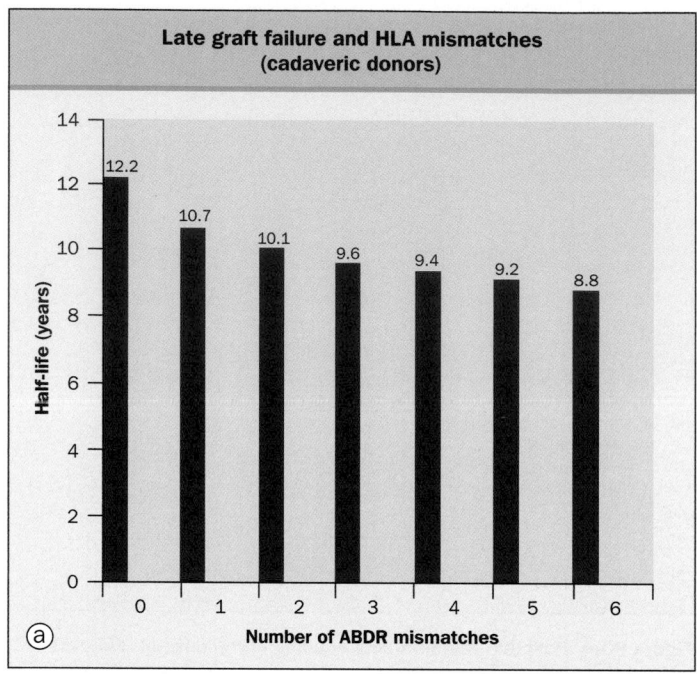

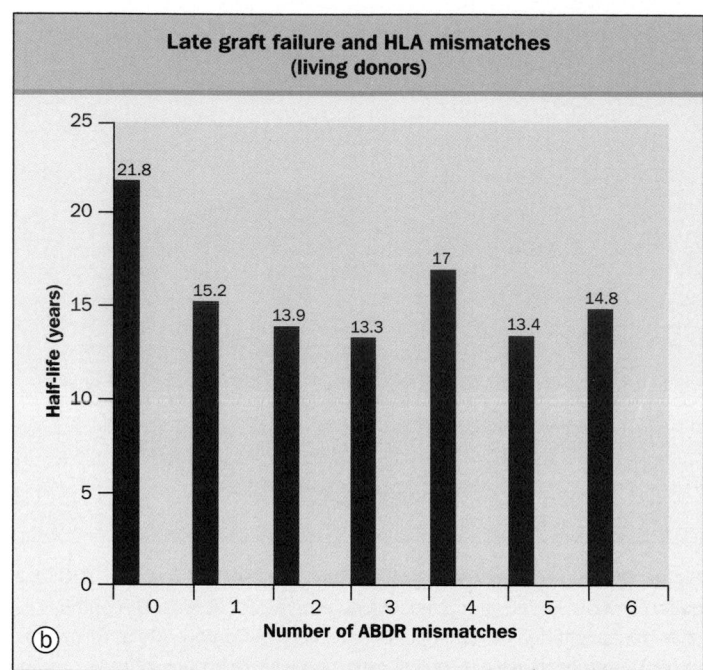

Figure 90.5 Major histocompatibility complex mismatches and late graft failure. The effect of ABDR mismatches on the rate of late graft failure as reflected by graft half-lives of kidney transplants. Patients received first kidney transplants in 1988–1998. Data are from the 2001 Annual Report of USRDS[2]. (a) Cadaveric donors. (b) Living donors. Graft survival is better for better-matched kidneys, particularly for zero-antigen mismatches.

2 years after transplantation. Biopsies were performed in kidney transplant recipients with normal renal function and who had no clinical acute rejection episodes during the 2 years of follow-up. Among recipients of cadaveric kidney transplants, histological changes of chronic allograft nephropathy were present in 25% at 3 months and 50% at 2 years, but absent in the recipients of MHC identical living-related donor kidneys. The living-related donor kidney recipients all had cold ischemia times of less than 5 h, did not have delayed graft function, and were not treated with cyclosporine[9]. Each of these factors could also explain the absence of chronic rejection in these recipients of living donor kidneys.

Antibodies

The number of preformed antibodies to MHC antigens can be estimated before transplantation. This is referred to as the degree of sensitization or cytotoxicity, and is typically measured as the percentage of lymphocytes from a random sample of individuals that react to antibodies in the recipient's serum; this value is known as the percent panel reactive antibodies (PRA). These antibodies to MHC antigens are usually the consequence of previous transplants, pregnancies, and blood transfusions. The PRA has been found to affect graft survival for first cadaver and living donor kidney transplants. Recipients with PRA ≥ 50% have a 25–30% higher risk of graft failure. Importantly, the half-life (reflecting the rate of late graft failure) is lower for recipients with a high PRA (Fig. 90.6)[2]. Peak PRA greater than 50% has been identified as a risk factor for delayed graft function[10,11], although how pretransplant antibodies reduce the long-term graft survival is not clear. Antibodies to the endothelium of the allograft may be

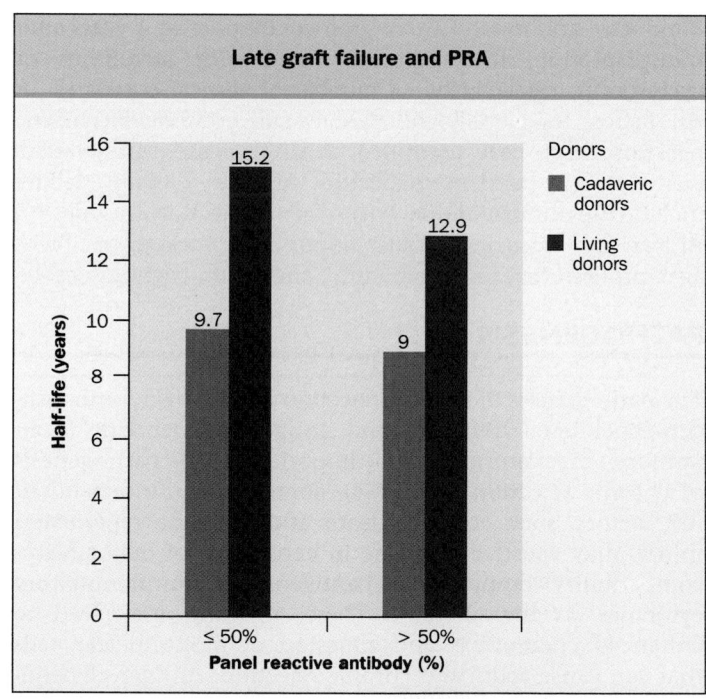

Figure 90.6 Effect of panel reactive antibody (PRA) status on long-term graft survival as reflected by graft half-lives. Data are for first cadaveric and living renal transplants with peak PRA ≤ 50% and > 50% performed from 1988 to 1998. Data obtained from 2001 Annual Report of USRDS[2]. Graft survival is lower for recipients with high PRA.

formed after transplantation as well. A number of studies have correlated the presence of antibodies to the allograft with chronic rejection, thus suggesting that antibody-mediated rejection may play a role in the pathogenesis of chronic rejection[12]. On the other hand, post-transplant antibody formation may be a result, rather than a cause, of chronic rejection.

Acute rejection

One of the best predictors of chronic rejection is acute rejection[3,6,7]. However, not all acute rejection episodes lead to chronic rejection. Although it is impossible to predict which acute rejection episodes herald chronic rejection, some studies have suggested that acute rejection episodes that are more severe, as determined by a greater decline in renal function, are more likely to be associated with chronic rejection. Similarly, acute rejection episodes that show histological evidence of vascular involvement or that occur after the first 2–3 months post-transplant are more likely to be associated with subsequent chronic rejection. Recurrent acute rejection episodes are also more likely to be followed by chronic rejection[3]. Interestingly, the effect of early acute rejections on late graft failure has been reported to be greater in recent years, even as the incidence of early acute rejections declines. This may be a result of more potent immunosuppressive agents effectively preventing mild rejections, thereby increasing the proportion of early rejections that are more severe. In other words, it is possible that 'treatable' acute rejection episodes are being prevented by more potent immunosuppressive medications, while more severe and refractory rejections remain to cause chronic rejection[13].

Subclinical rejection may also be a risk factor for late graft failure. In a prospective, observational study, 102 protocol biopsies were performed at 3 months after transplantation and recipients were followed for a median of 9.3 years. Subclinical rejection, defined as histological evidence of Banff acute rejection without acute decline on renal function, was present in 29% of protocol biopsies. Subclinical rejection at 3 months correlated both with chronic interstitial fibrosis and chronic arterial fibrointimal thickening at 12 months. Subclinical rejection was associated with increased MHC mismatch and with previous acute rejection. In this study, subclinical rejection is associated with chronic rejection, but it is not clear if this association is mediated through the presence of prior clinical acute rejection or MHC mismatch[4].

While clinical correlations are suggestive, proof that subclinical acute rejection causes chronic rejection can only come from randomized controlled trials. A small, pilot randomized trial recently reported that subclinical acute rejection occurred in 80% of 36 patients who underwent multiple, serial, protocol biopsies. Treatment of the subclinical acute rejection resulted in a lower serum creatinine at 2 years, compared with a control group of 36 patients that had fewer protocol biopsies and therefore less treatment for subclinical acute rejection[14]. Unfortunately, serum creatinine is a poor marker of kidney function, and the lower serum creatinine in the treatment group could be potentially explained by a reduction in muscle mass from the additional treatment with corticosteroids, rather than an improvement in function. The results of this trial need to be confirmed in large, adequately powered, randomized trials examining graft failure or other suitable endpoints, before we accept that treatment of subclinical acute rejection reduces the incidence of chronic rejection.

Antigen-independent risk factors

Brain death

Kidneys from living donors, regardless of their relationship with the recipients, survive longer than cadaveric donor kidneys. The half-life for cadaveric kidneys is 9.7 years, whereas the half-life for living-related and living-unrelated donor kidneys is 15.2 and 15.5 years, respectively[2]. There are a number of possible reasons why living-unrelated donor kidneys survive longer than cadaveric donor kidneys. Noncompliance is a major cause of late allograft failure and it is possible that patients with kidneys from emotionally related donors may be more likely to take immunosuppressive medications over the long term than patients with cadaveric kidneys. Transplants from living donors also have less ischemia time. Another factor could be brain death. Brain death has been shown to cause an upregulation of cytokines and growth factors in the kidney and other organs. These alterations may be related to increased levels of catecholamines associated with brain death. Experimental data suggest that the increase in tissue cytokines resulting from brain death may lead to enhanced rejection of the transplanted organ. Brain death is also associated with tissue ischemia, which is more severe in brain death related to intracerebral hemorrhage than in patients with head trauma. Retrospective analyses identify cardiovascular or cerebrovascular cause of donor death as a risk factor for worse long-term allograft survival[15].

Ischemia and reperfusion injury

Graft survival is lower for recipients with longer ischemia times. In registry data there is a 5–14% increase in graft failure for each 12 h increment of cold ischemia time, even after adjusting for the effects of transplant era, donor type, recipient age, donor age, recipient race, recipient gender, donor gender, MHC mismatches, and PRA (Fig. 90.7)[2]. This registry analysis does not take into account the presence of acute rejection, and therefore it is unclear how much of the effect of longer cold ischemia time on graft survival is mediated by acute rejection. Other analyses have found either an independent association between delayed graft function and late graft failure[16], or an association between delayed graft function and graft failure that is mediated by acute rejection[10]. Major risk factors for delayed graft function are prolonged cold ischemia time, donor age greater than 50 years, and peak PRA greater than 50%[10,11]. Ischemia and oxidative injury resulting from reperfusion of an ischemic kidney may cause an upregulation of MHC antigens and/or proinflammatory cytokines. It is possible that these changes may lead to acute rejection.

Cytomegalovirus infection

Circumstantial evidence suggests that infections may play a role in the pathogenesis of systemic atherosclerosis. One may speculate that infections that are common in kidney transplant recipients may also contribute to the allograft vasculopathy of chronic rejection. Some studies have found an association between cytomegalovirus infection and late allograft failure. However, since treatment of acute rejection can be expected to activate cytomegalovirus, it is difficult to determine whether clinical associations between cytomegalovirus

Transplantation

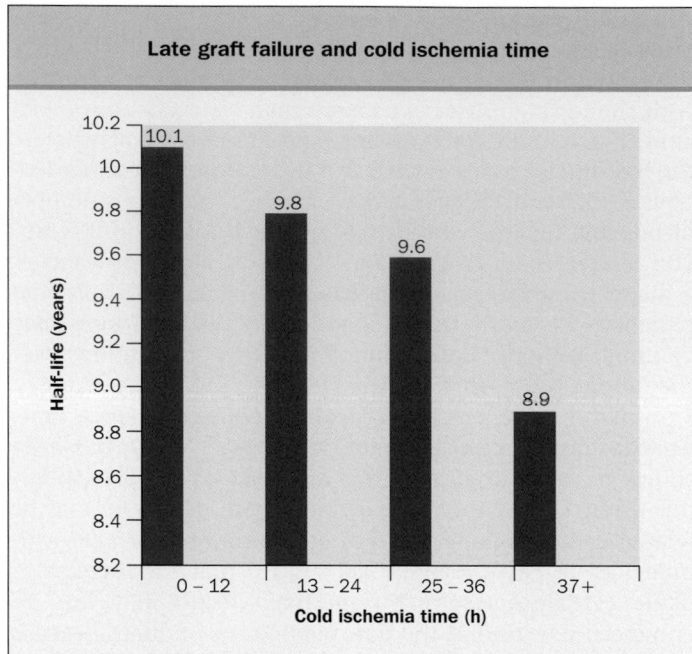

Figure 90.7 Effect of cold ischemia time on the rate of late allograft failure. Data for graft half-life, as a measure of graft survival, were collected for recipients of first cadaveric renal transplants from 1988 to 1998. Data obtained from 2001 Annual Report of USRDS[2]. Graft survival is gradually lower for recipients who have longer cold ischemia times.

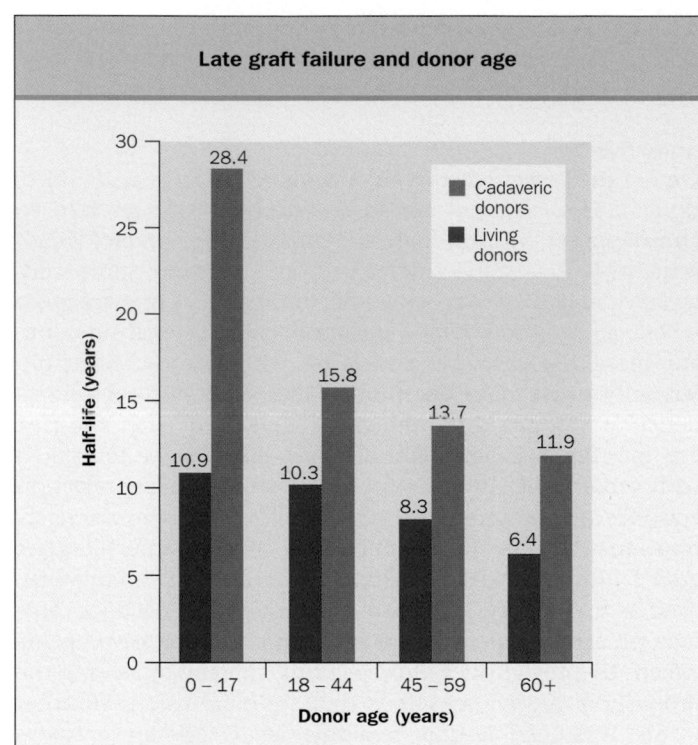

Figure 90.8 Effect of donor age on the rate of late allograft failure. Data for graft half-life, as a measure of graft survival, were collected for recipients of first cadaveric and living renal transplants in 1988–1998. Data obtained from 2001 Annual Report of USRDS[2]. Graft survival is worse for older donors, both in cadaveric and living donors recipients.

and long-term graft survival are caused by cytomegalovirus or result from the acute rejection that may be associated with both cytomegalovirus and long-term graft survival. Indeed, some have reported that cytomegalovirus disease increases the risk for chronic rejection only when acute rejection is also present[17]. However, others have failed to find an association between cytomegalovirus infection, defined by antigenemia, and allograft dysfunction at 5 years[18]. The risk for cytomegalovirus disease is highest among patients who receive kidneys from donors who have had cytomegalovirus infection. Therefore, the cytomegalovirus status of the donor does not appear to influence graft survival[19]. Altogether, it remains uncertain whether cytomegalovirus, or other infections, play a role in the pathogenesis of chronic rejection.

Kidney size mismatching

It has been postulated that an insufficient number of nephrons in the transplanted kidney may lead to compensatory increases in glomerular capillary pressures and flow rates, or to other changes that could contribute to chronic renal allograft rejection. Indeed, a number of factors that would be expected to be associated with fewer nephrons in the allograft appear to be risk factors for graft survival. These include donor age, donor kidney size, female donors, donor race, and serum creatinine at the time of discharge after transplantation[20]. However, other factors not related to the number of nephrons in the allograft could explain the associations between these risk factors and graft survival. Moreover, the effects of these factors on graft survival already appear to be fully manifest one year after transplantation, when the

incidence of graft failure owing to chronic rejection is still relatively low[20]. Therefore, the extent to which an inadequate number of functioning nephrons may contribute to chronic rejection is unknown.

Donor age

Long-term graft survival is reduced in kidneys from older donors. Older donor age is associated with higher graft failure for both cadaveric and living donor kidneys, after adjusting for transplant era, donor source (living or cadaveric), recipient age, recipient race, recipient gender, donor gender, MHC mismatches, cold ischemia time, and PRA (Fig. 90.8)[2]. There are a variety of mechanisms that could explain the effect of donor age on graft survival. However, the function of older kidneys would be expected to be proportionally reduced. Further reductions in renal function from any cause would then be expected to lead to earlier graft failure, simply because there would be less function to lose. Therefore, the higher rate of allograft failure from age need not involve other mechanisms.

Hypertension

The vasculopathy in chronic rejection resembles systemic vascular disease, raising the possibility that cardiovascular disease risk factors may play a role in chronic rejection. Hypertension occurs in over 50% of transplant recipients. In a multicenter, retrospective study of 29 751 kidney transplant recipients with 7 years of follow-up, elevated systolic and diastolic blood pressure were associated with chronic graft failure in a multivariate analysis[21]. Unfortunately, there are no intervention trials proving that aggressive blood pressure treatment reduces the incidence of graft failure from chronic rejection. Thus, the extent to which chronic rejection is a cause, or an effect, of hypertension is unclear.

Hyperlipidemia

Epidemiological studies have associated hyperlipidemia with chronic renal allograft rejection[3,6]. Foam cells and apolipoprotein deposition may also be found in the vascular lesions of chronic rejection. The results of randomized, controlled trials have suggested that 3-hydroxy-3-methylglutaryl-coenzyme A (HMG-CoA) reductase inhibitors (statins) reduce coronary artery disease and increase survival after cardiac transplantation[22]. Since the vascular abnormalities seen in chronic rejection in kidney transplant recipients is similar to recurrent coronary artery disease in heart transplant recipients, it is possible that HMG-CoA reductase inhibitors may also reduce renal allograft loss to chronic rejection. However, there are no prospective, randomized, controlled trials showing that lipid-lowering agents reduce the incidence or severity of chronic rejection.

Proteinuria

Proteinuria is a major risk factor for late renal allograft failure[3]. It is difficult to determine if proteinuria is just an early marker of chronic rejection, or if proteinuria actually causes renal injury, and thereby contributes to the pathogenesis of chronic rejection. It has been suggested that proteinuria itself might contribute to the progression of renal diseases through several mechanisms[23]. If true, nonspecific measures that reduce proteinuria, e.g., angiotensin converting enzyme (ACE) inhibitors, could theoretically retard the progression of chronic rejection. Unfortunately, large-scale clinical trials have not yet tested this hypothesis.

CLINICAL MANIFESTATIONS

Chronic rejection generally presents as a gradual increase in serum creatinine and the diagnosis is usually, but not always, made in patients who are more than 6 months post-transplantation. In addition to chronic rejection, the differential diagnosis of a rise in serum creatinine after transplantation includes acute rejection, nephrotoxicity from cyclosporine, tacrolimus, or other medications, *de novo* glomerulonephritis, recurrence of the original renal disease, infection- or drug-induced interstitial nephritis (uncommon), urinary obstruction, renal artery stenosis, and cholesterol emboli (see Table 90.1). There are no clinical signs and symptoms associated with chronic rejection, unless renal function is depressed enough that the patient has signs and symptoms of uremia. However, patients with chronic rejection often have hypertension and proteinuria.

The proteinuria in patients with chronic rejection may be in either the non-nephrotic or nephrotic range. Chronic rejection is found in about 60% of patients who undergo allograft biopsy for proteinuria. Transplant glomerulopathy has been observed in one-third of patients with chronic rejection (see

Chapter 91). The pathogenesis of transplant glomerulopathy is unknown but has been postulated to be another manifestation of chronic allograft nephropathy. Other causes of proteinuria include acute rejection, *de novo* glomerulonephritis, recurrent glomerulonephritis, and calcineurin inhibitor toxicity. Except for proteinuria, the urinalysis is usually unremarkable.

The diagnosis of chronic rejection should be confirmed with biopsy, unless contraindicated. Biopsy findings of chronic rejection are relatively nonspecific. The diagnosis can be more correctly thought of as a diagnosis of exclusion. In patients who have no evidence for acute rejection, acute cyclosporine toxicity, *de novo* glomerulonephritis, or recurrent renal disease (or other causes of renal dysfunction), the presence of glomerulosclerosis and interstitial fibrosis most probably results from chronic rejection. Fibrointimal hyperplasia of medium or large intrarenal arteries is also highly suggestive. Unfortunately, these arterial lesions may be missed in the biopsy through insufficient sampling.

TREATMENT

There is no known, effective treatment for chronic rejection (Table 90.3). Therefore, it is prudent to minimize the exposure to risk factors for chronic rejection as much as possible (Table 90.4). While often not possible, it is best to start with a low-risk, young, living-donor kidney. Avoiding prolonged cold ischemia times helps to minimize the risk for delayed graft function, and may possibly reduce the risk for early acute rejection. Optimal MHC matching may also help reduce the incidence of chronic rejection, but optimal matching is often impossible in this era of long waiting times and a growing shortage of kidney donors.

Probably the most effective preventive strategy is one that minimizes the incidence and severity of acute rejection. Early detection by frequent monitoring of serum creatinine remains the first line of defense against acute rejection. The role of protocol biopsies in detecting subclinical acute rejection, and thereby preventing chronic rejection, remains to be established. Similarly, several noninvasive techniques to detect early acute rejection are promising, but require additional study before widespread, clinical application. Frequent monitoring of serum creatinine not only facilitates the early detection of acute rejection, but may also help to identify patients who are at risk to become noncompliant with immunosuppressive

Treatment options for established chronic rejection	
Therapy	Evidence
Immunosuppression	Good
Treatment of hypertension	
Angiotensin-converting enzyme inhibitors	Good
Calcium antagonists	Good
Treatment of hyperlipidemia	
HMG-CoA reductase inhibitors	Good
Other therapies	Poor

Table 90.3 Treatment options for established chronic rejection.

Risk factor	Evidence	Relative influence
Antigen-dependent risk factors		
Clinical acute rejection	****	++++
Chronic immunological injury		
(subclinical rejection)	***	+++
Noncompliance	****	++++
MHC mismatching	***	+++
Panel reactive antibodies (PRA)	***	++
Antidonor antibodies post-transplantation	**	++
Antigen-independent risk factors		
Donor age	****	++++
Delayed graft function		
(ischemia times, donor age, PRA)	***	+++
Cadaveric (versus living) donor	****	++++
Brain death/Cause of brain death	*	++
Dyslipidemia	**	++
Hypertension	***	++
Proteinuria	****	++++
Other cardiovascular risk factors		
(smoking, fibrinogen)	*	+
Cytomegalovirus infection	*	+
Early transplant era	***	+++
Waiting list time	**	++
Female recipient gender	***	+
Younger recipient age	***	++
Female donor gender	***	+
Inadequate nephron mass	**	++
Primary renal disease	***	++

Table 90.4 Risk factors for chronic renal allograft failure.

medications. Patients who fail clinic appointments designed to monitor graft function, may be patients who are also at risk to be noncompliant with their immunosuppressive medications. Thus, follow-up regimens that require frequent monitoring of serum creatinine may help to uncover patients who need special attention to prevent noncompliance.

The optimum immunosuppression protocol to prevent chronic rejection remains to be established. There is indirect evidence to suggest that improvements in immunosuppression have led to a reduction in the incidence of late allograft failure, and presumably chronic rejection. This is reflected by the improvement in renal allograft half-life seen over the past decade. Some investigators have attempted to correlate more favorable outcomes in transplant registries with the use of specific immunosuppressive agents[24]. However, randomized controlled trials remains the only method to determine with certainty whether a particular therapy is effective. Indeed, randomized trials have established that several new immunosuppressive agents, e.g., mycophenolate mofetil, tacrolimus,

and sirolimus, are effective in reducing the incidence of acute rejection. Unfortunately, there are still no randomized trials showing that any immunosuppression effectively reduces the incidence of chronic rejection. Similarly, there are no randomized trials showing that changing in immunosuppressive medications can alter the course of chronic rejection once it has become established.

There may be other, nonimmune mechanisms that can be modified in order to ameliorate the progression of chronic rejection. Proteinuria, for example, may contribute to the chronic tubulointerstitial damage that characterizes chronic rejection. Reducing proteinuria appears to retard the rate of progression of kidney disease. In a number of studies in nontransplant kidney disease, ACE inhibitors and angiotensin II receptor antagonists (ATRA) reduced proteinuria and slowed the rate of disease progression in native kidneys. Their beneficial effects were more than could be explained by a reduction in blood pressure *per se*. The ACE inhibitors and ARTAS may cause as hyperkalemia, anemia, or worsening renal function in kidney transplant recipients, but these complications are generally reversible[25]. Unfortunately, there are no randomized controlled trials in kidney transplant recipients showing that ACE inhibitors and ARTAS slow the rate of progression of chronic rejection.

Similarly, there are no controlled trials showing that the treatment of vascular disease risk factors prevents the onset, or reduces the rate of progression, of chronic rejection. However, there are compelling reasons to treat traditional risk factors to prevent cardiovascular disease, and to hope that aggressive risk factor management may also help to preserve kidney function. In this regard, efforts should be directed at blood pressure control (goal < 140/90 mmHg), treatment of hyperlipidemia, smoking cessation, and optimal glycemic control. Although there is little direct evidence that cytomegalovirus or other infections contribute to the pathogenesis of vascular disease or chronic rejection, measures to prevent the morbidity and mortality from cytomegalovirus are warranted.

In the future, the induction of tolerance may be our best hope for preventing chronic rejection. So far, early efforts at inducing tolerance show promise, but lack strong evidence of efficacy[26]. To the extent that alloantigen-independent mechanisms are important in the pathogenesis of chronic rejection, even effective measures that induce tolerance may not be completely effective in preventing chronic rejection. In the end, a multifaceted approach to block both alloantigen-dependent and alloantigen-independent mechanisms may be the best strategy for reducing the risk of graft loss to chronic rejection.

REFERENCES

1. Racusen LC, Solez K, Colvin RB, et al. The Banff 97 working classification of renal allograft pathology. Kidney Int. 1999; 55:713–23.
2. US Renal Data System. USRDS 2001 Annual Data Report: Atlas of End-Stage Renal Disease in the United States. Bethesda, MD: National Institutes of Health, National Institute of Diabetes and Digestive and Kidney Diseases.
3. Massy ZA, Guijarro C, Wiederkehr MR, et al. Chronic renal allograft rejection: immunologic and nonimmunologic risk factors. Kidney Int. 1996;49:518–24.
4. Nankivell BJ, Fenton-Lee CA, Kuypers DRJ, et al. Effect of histological damage on long-term kidney transplant outcome. Transplantation. 2001;71:515–23.
5. Solez K, Vincenti F, Filo RS. Histopathologic findings from 2-year protocol biopsies from a U.S. multicenter kidney transplant trial comparing tacrolimus versus cyclosporin. A report of the FK506 Kidney Transplant Study Group. Transplantation. 1998; 66:1736–40.
6. McLaren AJ, Fuggle SV, Welsh KI, et al. Chronic allograft failure in human renal transplantation. A multivariate risk factor analysis. Ann Surg. 2000;232:98–103.
7. Matas AJ, Gillingham K, Humar A, et al. Immunologic and non-immunologic factors. Different risks for cadaver and living donor transplantation. Transplantation. 2000;69:54–8.
8. Halloran PF, Melk A, Barth C. Rethinking chronic allograft nephropathy: the concept of accelerated senescense. J Am Soc Nephrol. 1999;10:167–81.
9. Legendre C, Thervet E, Skhiri H, et al. Histologic features of chronic allograft nephropathy revealed by protocol biopsies in kidney transplant recipients. Transplantation. 1998;65:1506–09.
10. Boom H, Mallat MJK, Fijter JW De, Zwinderman AH. Delayed graft function influences renal function, but not survival. Kidney Int. 2000;58:859–66.
11. McLaren AJ, Jassem W, Gray DWR, et al. Delayed graft function: risk factors and the relative effects of early function and acute rejection on long-term survival in cadaveric renal transplantation. Clin Transplant. 1999;13:266–72.
12. Lederer SR, Kluth-Pepper B, Schneeberger H, et al. Impact of humoral alloreactivity early after transplantation on the long-term survival of renal allografts. Kidney Int. 2001;59:334–41.
13. Meier-Kriesche HU, Ojo AO, Hanson JA, et al. Increased impact of acute rejection on chronic allograft failure in recent era. Transplantation. 2000;70:1098–100.
14. Rush D, Nickerson P, Gough J, et al. Beneficial effects of treatment of early subclinical rejection: A randomized study. J Am Soc Nephrol. 1998;9:2129–34.
15. Matas AJ, Gillingham K, Payne WD, et al. Should I accept this kidney? Clin Transplant. 2000;14:90–5.
16. Shoskes DA, Cecka JM. Deleterious effects of delayed graft function in cadaveric renal transplant recipients independent of acute rejection. Transplantation. 1998;66:1697–701.
17. Humar A, Gillingham KJ, Payne WD, et al. Association between cytomegalovirus disease and chronic rejection in kidney transplant recipients. Transplantation. 1999;68:1879–83.
18. Dickenmann MJ, Cathomas G, Steiger J, et al. Cytomegalovirus infection and graft rejection in renal transplantation. Transplantation. 2001;71:764–7.
19. Cecka JM. The UNOS Scientific Renal Transplant Registry. In: Cecka JM, Terasaki PI, eds. Clinical Transplants 1996. Los Angeles: UCLA Tissue Typing Laboratory; 1997:1–14.
20. Terasaki PI, Koyama H, Cecka JM, Gjertson D. The hyperfiltration hypothesis in human renal transplantation. Transplantation. 1994;57:1450–4.
21. Opelz G, Wujciak T, Ritz E. Association of chronic kidney graft failure with recipient blood pressure. Kidney Int. 1998; 53:217–22.
22. Wenke K, Meiser B, Thiery J, et al. Simvastatin reduces graft vessel disease and mortality after heart transplantation: A four-year randomized trial. Circulation. 1997;96:1398–402.
23. Remuzzi G, Bertani T. Pathophysiology of Progressive Nephropathies. N Engl J Med. 1998;339:1448–56.
24. Ojo AO, Meier-Kriesche HU, Hanson JA, et al. Mycophenolate mofetil reduces late renal allograft loss independent of acute rejection. Transplantation. 2000;69:2405–9.
25. Stigant CE, Cohe J, Vivera M, Zaltzman JS. ACE inhibitors and angiotensin II antagonists in renal transplantation: an analysis of safety and efficacy. Am J Kidney Dis. 2000;35:58–63.
26. Ciancio G, Miller J, Garcia-Morales RO, et al. Six-year clinical effect of donor bone marrow infusions in renal transplant patients. Transplantation. 2001;71:827–35.

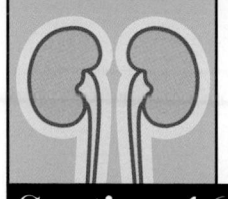

Chapter 91

Recurrent Disease in the Renal Transplant

Jeremy Hughes and Charles E Alpers

INTRODUCTION

This chapter will deal with the recurrence of the primary renal disease in the renal allograft (Table 91.1), together with the treatments currently available (see Table 91.2). The development of *de novo* glomerular disease including transplant glomerulopathy will also be briefly discussed. At the outset, it should be borne in mind that recurrence rates quoted in the literature probably underestimate the true incidence of recurrent disease for a variety of reasons. First, the primary renal diagnosis is unknown in many patients. In such cases, the development of glomerulonephritis in the transplant would be labeled as *de novo* glomerulonephritis, despite the fact that it may represent recurrent disease. It is for this reason that some studies group *de novo* disease and recurrent disease together. Second, recurrent histopathological disease that remains clinically silent will pass undetected unless transplant centers have a policy of routinely performing transplant biopsies. Third, some patients who develop deteriorating graft function may be inadequately investigated and incorrectly labeled as 'chronic rejection'. It should also be noted that recurrent disease may be an incidental histopathological finding or actively contribute to graft failure and the development of end-stage renal disease (ESRD). Overall, patients with recurrent or *de novo* disease exhibit significantly worse graft survival (40% vs. 68% for patients without recurrent or *de novo* disease at 5 years post-transplantation)[1].

Various studies indicate that recurrent disease affects between 6 and 20% of renal transplant patients overall but, not surprisingly, is more problematical in patients with ESRD secondary to glomerulonephritis or systemic diseases such as diabetes mellitus that are not cured by renal transplantation[2–4]. Risk factors affecting the incidence of recurrent disease include patient age with younger patients being more commonly affected[1]. This probably results from the fact that the incidence of renal failure secondary to diseases such as renovascular disease or hypertension is higher amongst older patients. In addition, the incidence of recurrent disease increases with the

Table 91.1 Recurrent diseases in renal transplants and effects upon graft survival.

Recurrent diseases in renal transplants		
Disease	Clinical recurrence rate (%)	Graft loss in recurrent disease (%)
Primary focal segmental glomerulosclerosis	20–50 (children), 10–15 (adults)	40–50
Membranoproliferative glomerulonephritis		
Type I	20–30	30–40
Type II	80–100	<20
Hemolytic uremic syndrome (HUS)		
Classical D+ HUS	0–13	?
Atypical D- HUS	30–50	55–100
Familial HUS	57	Approaching 100
IgA nephropathy	29–39 with increasing duration of follow-up (30–60% histologic recurrence rate)	16–33
Henoch–Schönlein purpura	Rare (despite 50% histologic recurrence rate)	Rare
Membranous nephropathy	<10 (histologic recurrence may be more common)	up to 50
Systemic vasculitis including Wegener's granulomatosis (WG) and microscopic polyangitis (MPA)	10–20 overall (WG > MPA); with extrarenal relapses occurring more commonly	Rare
Antiglomerular basement membrane antibody-mediated glomerulonephritis	<5	50
Systemic lupus erythematosus	Many studies: <1; recent study[40]: 8	Many studies: rare; recent study[40]: 44
Amyloidosis	25	Uncommon

Transplantation

Treatment and prophylaxis options for recurrent disease	
Disease	**Treatment options**
Primary focal segmental glomerulosclerosis	Consider plasma exchange or immunoadsorption for recurrent disease; other options include increasing the dosage of cyclosporine or commencing cyclophosphamide. Angiotensin-converting enzyme inhibitors and nonsteroidal anti-inflammatory agents have also been used
Membranoproliferative glomerulonephritis	
Type I	Consider aspirin and dipyridamole prophylaxis; increased immunosuppression may be of benefit in severe disease
Type II	Nil proven though anecdotal reports of aggressive disease being successfully treated with increased immunosuppression
Membranous nephropathy	Nil proven
IgA nephropathy	Nil proven
Henoch–Schönlein purpura	Consider increased immunosuppression for aggressive disease
Hemolytic uremic syndrome	Consider prophylaxis with antiplatelet agents (aspirin/dipyridamole); discontinue cyclosporine and consider plasma infusions and plasma exchange. Anecdotal reports of benefit with intravenous immunoglobulin
Systemic vasculitis and rapidly progressive glomerulonephritis	Conversion to cyclophosphamide (3 to 6 months only) and increased corticosteroid dosage
Systemic lupus erythematosus	Prophylactic anticoagulation if antiphospholipid syndrome present
Amyloidosis	Colchicine prophylaxis in familial Mediterranean fever
Antiglomerular basement membrane antibody-mediated glomerulonephritis	Conversion to cyclophosphamide, increased corticosteroids, and plasma exchange
In patients with Alport syndrome	Conversion to cyclophosphamide, increased corticosteroids, and plasma exchange, though treatment is often unsuccessful
Hepatitis C virus-associated membranoproliferative glomerulonephritis type I	Consider Interferon-α (beware of precipitation of rejection episode) and/or ribavirin
Primary hyperoxaluria	Prophylaxis with supplements of vitamin B_6, orthophosphate, citrate, and magnesium and maintenance of diuresis

Table 91.2 Treatment and prophylaxis options for diseases that may recur in renal transplants.

survival of the allograft; from 2.8% at 2 years to 9.8% and 18.5% at 5 and 8 years, respectively in one study[4]. Indeed, an increase in the incidence of recurrent disease has accompanied the overall improvement of allograft survival, resulting from a reduction in the incidence of immunological rejection[5]. This relationship was emphasized in a study of patients with renal failure secondary to glomerulonephritis who receive HLA-identical grafts. Although such patients exhibit a very low incidence of rejection, they have an increased incidence of recurrent disease (45% at 12 years) resulting in graft loss in

24% of patients at 20 years follow up[6]. In contrast, HLA-identical recipients with renal failure resulting from nonglomerular disease exhibited 100% graft survival[6]. Over recent decades we have accumulated significant information regarding the risks of recurrence of many individual diseases in renal transplant patients and these are outlined below.

DISEASE IN THE RENAL TRANSPLANT

Primary focal segmental glomerulosclerosis
Primary focal segmental glomerulosclerosis (FSGS) recurs in 20–50% of pediatric and 10–15% of adult renal transplant recipients. Patients usually present soon after transplantation with nephrotic or less commonly non-nephrotic proteinuria, and although the presentation is usually within the first two weeks, it may not occur until months after transplantation. Recurrent FSGS exerts a significant negative impact upon long-term graft survival and imparts a relative risk of 2.25 for subsequent graft failure[1]. In addition, the development of post-transplant FSGS is associated with an increased risk of developing acute renal failure and acute rejection episodes in the early post-transplant period.

Risk factors have been identified for recurrence but, since they have not been identified consistently in all studies, it is potentially hazardous to attempt to predict whether or not a recurrence will occur in individual patients. Such risk factors include young age at the onset of primary FSGS (< 6 years of age), rapid progression to ESRD (< 3 years) and diffuse mesangial proliferation in the native kidney biopsy. In addition, African American children have been reported to develop recurrent FSGS less often than Caucasian or Hispanic children which is interesting since primary FSGS is more common in African American children. Asian children appear to exhibit comparable recurrence rates[7]. In some studies, a slightly increased rate of recurrence has been noted in living related donor (LRD) grafts compared with cadaveric grafts, though graft survival is still better with LRD grafts in view of the reduced incidence of rejection[8]. More recent studies have supported the use of LRD grafts in patients with ESRD secondary to FSGS[9,10]. However, a LRD transplant should be avoided if a first transplant has succumbed to recurrent disease in view of the high risk of repeated recurrence (60–80%). Although the introduction of cyclosporine has not affected the incidence of recurrent FSGS, it is of interest that the use of antilymphocyte serum has been associated with an increased rate of recurrent disease in pediatric patients (53% vs. 11%)[11]. A recent study indicated a relatively high incidence of recurrent FSGS in adult patients (49%) and suggested that recurrence was associated with increasing age of the donor kidney[12]. Interestingly, FSGS occurs with an increased frequency in certain families and these patients with 'familial FSGS' do not seem to develop recurrent disease, although the numbers of patients involved is small. Collapsing FSGS may also recur in the renal allograft.

The treatment of recurrent FSGS is difficult and, like the primary disease, it is poorly responsive to steroids. Evidence indicates the involvement of a circulating humoral mediator in the rapid onset of proteinuria although the development of a diagnostic test to determine which patients will develop recurrent disease has been problematical[13–15]. Affected patients are usually treated with plasma exchange (PE) in an attempt to remove this factor and data strongly suggest that PE is of clinical benefit. PE can induce a dramatic remission of proteinuria and patients who relapse following cessation of PE may respond to further acute or chronic treatment. In some studies PE has also been combined with cyclophosphamide or high-dose cyclosporine treatment although it is unclear whether such combination therapy has significant added benefits[9,14]. In adult patients with recurrent FSGS PE may not be as effective as in the pediatric population[16]. In one study, the five patients who completely or partially responded to PE exhibited rapid development of recurrent disease and commenced PE within 30 days of evidence of recurrence. In contrast, seven of the eight non-responders developed disease at a later stage and did not undergo PE until at least 42 days after the development of clinical recurrence[16]. This suggests that it is important to commence PE as soon as possible after the detection of clinical relapse and certainly prior to the development of structural lesions within the kidney. Similar principles apply to the pediatric population[9]. A recent small study suggests that pre-transplant PE may be of benefit in pediatric patients[17]. However, at the present time there is no data available from controlled, randomized, prospective clinical trials regarding the effectiveness of PE and the long-term impact upon disease is still incompletely understood. Other treatments that have been used to treat recurrent FSGS include angiotensin-converting enzyme (ACE) inhibitors and nonsteroidal anti-inflammatory drugs (NSAIDs) but these treatments are very much secondary to the use of PE.

De novo focal segmental glomerulosclerosis

FSGS can develop de novo in adult recipients of pediatric donor kidneys (reduced nephron mass) as well as allografts with chronic vascular rejection (obliterative vasculopathy and glomerular ischemia). This 'secondary form' of FSGS tends to occur later, is more indolent and less commonly results in the nephrotic syndrome compared to recurrent primary FSGS. However, the presence of de novo FSGS does exert a negative impact on graft survival[18].

Membranoproliferative glomerulonephritis
Type I

Membranoproliferative glomerulonephritis (MPGN) type I recurs in 20–30% of patients[3,5], although the incidence may be overestimated since transplant glomerulopathy (see later) may exhibit a similar light microscopic appearance. In view of this, the diagnosis should be confirmed by immunofluorescence and electron microscopy, which demonstrates discrete subendothelial and mesangial immune deposits. The presence or severity of serum complement abnormalities is not predictive of recurrence. Patients can present with proteinuria or hematuria early or late following transplantation and 30–40% of affected grafts are lost[19]. Recurrence in a second transplant is common (up to 80%) if the first transplant experienced recurrence[19]. No interventional therapy is of proven benefit though there is anecdotal evidence that treatment with aspirin and dipyridamole may stabilize renal function whilst severe recurrent disease has been successfully treated with increased immunosuppression including PE and cyclophosphamide.

Hepatitis C virus (HCV)-associated MPGN may recur or occur de novo in renal transplant recipients[20,21]. HCV-associated MPGN in native kidneys is usually associated with a type II cryoglobulinemia and hypocomplementemia, but these are typically absent or less marked in recurrent disease. Interferon-α has been used to treat HCV-associated MPGN in native kidneys and, although there are some reports of the successful use of interferon-α in transplant patients, it is not without risk as it can precipitate acute rejection. Other therapeutic options include oral ribavirin[22] or possibly a combination of ribavirin and interferon-α. However, formal prospective trials need to be undertaken.

Type II

MPGN type II or dense deposit disease recurs in the majority of transplanted kidneys, affecting 80–100% of patients although electron microscopy is usually required to make a definitive diagnosis[23] (Fig. 91.1). Patients usually present with non-nephrotic proteinuria within a year of transplantation. Renal function may be adversely affected and up to 25%

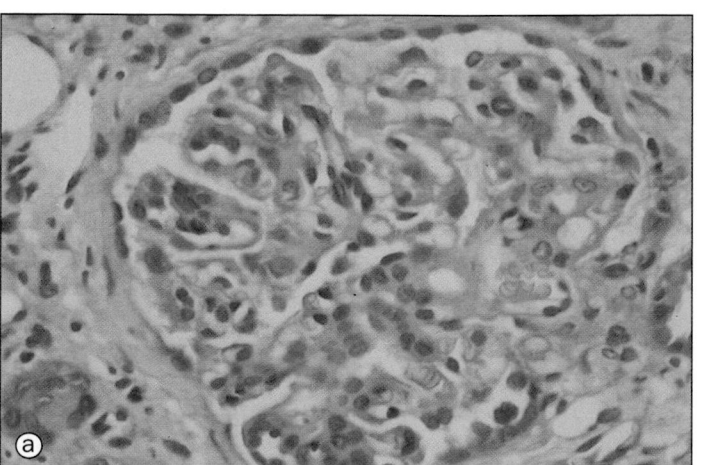
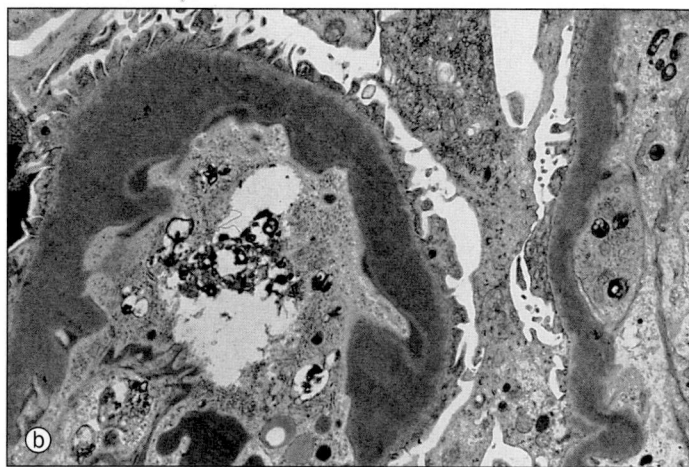

Figure 91.1 Recurrent membranoproliferative glomerulonephritis type II. (a) Light microscopy reveals irregular thickening of the glomerular basement membrane with mild mesangial hypercellularity. (b) Electron microscopy shows electron-dense material replacing and expanding much of the glomerular basement membrane. (Micrographs courtesy of DI Ansell.)

Transplantation

of grafts may be lost[23]. No correlation has been found between clinically evident recurrence and serum complement levels or the presence of circulating nephritic factor (C3Nef) activity. Lastly, MPGN type III may also recur in transplanted kidneys[24].

Recurrent hemolytic uremic syndrome

Patients with recurrent HUS can broadly be divided into classical diarrhea-associated (D+ HUS) or atypical D- HUS depending upon whether the primary disease was preceded by a diarrheal illness. In a minority of patients, the disease is familial. Most cases of D+ HUS are due to infection with verotoxin-producing E. coli.

Children whose primary disease was D+ HUS exhibit a low rate of recurrence (0–13%) with no difference evident between LRD and cadaveric grafts[25].

In contrast, patients with atypical D- HUS exhibit recurrence rates of 30–50% (Fig. 91.2) with recurrences being more common in LRD transplants[26]. Subsequent graft loss occurs in 55–100% of D- HUS patients with recurrent disease. A meta-analysis of 10 studies (159 grafts in 127 patients) performed between 1977 and 1997 indicated that most recurrences occurred within a month of transplantation and recurrent disease was associated with a significantly reduced 1-year graft survival rate (33% vs. 77% in patients without recurrence)[27]. Recurrent disease was associated with an older age at the onset of HUS (17 vs. 10 years), a more rapid progression to ESRD (0.8 vs. 2.8 years) and earlier transplantation (2.5 vs. 6 years). In addition, patients with recurrent disease had received a higher proportion of LRD transplants (52% vs. 22% in the nonrecurrence group) and had been treated more often with cyclosporine or tacrolimus (40% vs. 29% in the nonrecurrence group). However, it has been shown that cyclosporine has no detrimental effect in patients (mainly children) with D+ HUS and actually improved graft survival. It would, therefore, seem prudent to avoid cyclosporine in patients with atypical D- HUS while patients with D+ HUS may receive conventional immunosuppression.

A more recent retrospective North American study of pediatric patients indicated a recurrence rate of 8.8% (six recurrences in 68 allografts involving five patients)[28]. Five of the six affected grafts were lost despite treatment with fresh frozen plasma and PE and cyclosporine treatment was not implicated in the development of recurrent disease. In this study, 80% of affected patients had atypical D- HUS thereby reinforcing the increased tendency for recurrence in this form of HUS[28]. Less than 5% of patients have familial HUS, but unfortunately recurrence is common in these patients, affecting 57% of patients with autosomal recessive HUS in a recent study with significant graft loss[29].

Recurrent HUS does not respond particularly well to treatment. However, it is reasonable to institute plasma infusions and PE at an early stage in an attempt to prevent graft loss. General supportive measures including dialysis should be instituted. There are anecdotal reports of attempts to prevent recurrence with low-dose aspirin and dipyridamole, as well as treatment of recurrent disease with intravenous infusions of immunoglobulin but hard data regarding these treatments are lacking. Cyclosporine, if used, should be discontinued and replaced with newer agents such as mycophenolate mofetil. It should be noted that the severity of hemolysis, thrombocytopenia or renal failure is not predictive of graft loss, but outcome does seem to be worse if HUS recurs shortly after transplantation. Despite these concerns, transplantation remains the treatment of choice for patients with ESRD secondary to HUS.

De novo hemolytic uremic syndrome

HUS may be associated with cyclosporine, tacrolimus or OKT3 therapy (de novo HUS) and may be difficult to distinguish pathologically from acute vascular rejection. Recently there has also been a report of thrombotic microangiopathy occurring in HCV infected renal transplant patients who have anticardiolipin (IgG or IgM) antibodies.

IgA nephropathy

IgA nephropathy is the most common type of glomerulonephritis with a significant number of patients developing ESRD and receiving renal transplants. Recurrent glomerular IgA deposition is common in transplant recipients and affects 30–60% of allografts with higher values found in studies where all patients undergo renal biopsy. Until recently, it was believed that actual loss of graft function secondary to recurrent IgA nephropathy (see Fig. 91.3) was rare since the overall graft survival for patients with IgA nephropathy was comparable to or even better than graft survival for transplant patients with other primary diseases. However, a number of recent large, retrospective, single center studies have demonstrated that recurrent IgA nephropathy is not benign in the long term with 11–55% of patients exhibiting graft dysfunction resulting in graft loss in up to 33% of patients[30,31]. Recurrence of IgA nephropathy is unaffected by the use of cyclosporine although it is possible that immunosuppression with mycophenolate mofetil may exert a beneficial effect in the future in view of its suppressive effects upon B cells and antibody production. Recurrent disease is also unaffected by patient age or gender, ACE genotype or the clinical course

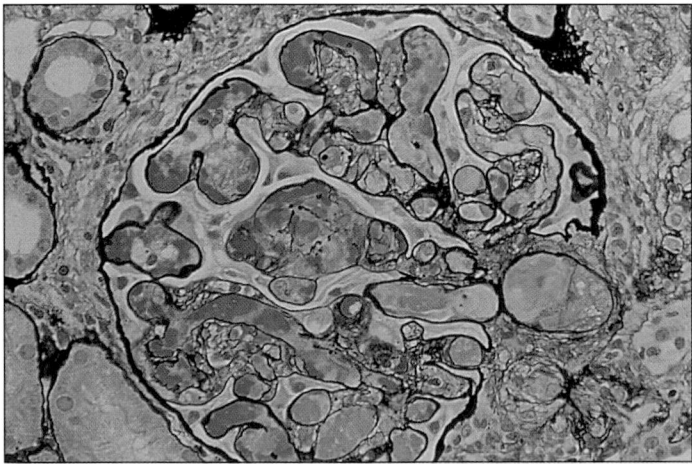

Figure 91.2 Thrombotic microangiopathy secondary to recurrent hemolytic uremic syndrome. The glomerular capillary loops and the afferent arteriole are almost completely occluded by numerous fibrin thrombi.

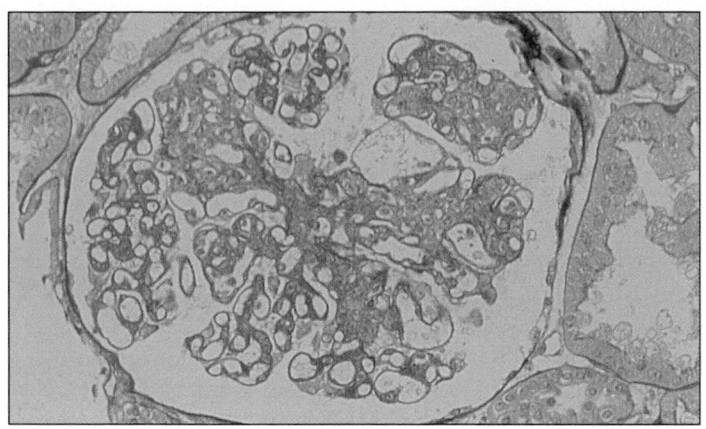

Figure 91.3 Recurrent IgA nephropathy. Light microscopy shows mild mesangial hypercellularity and increased mesangial matrix.

prior to transplantation but is directly related to the duration of follow-up[30–32]. While some studies have indicated a slightly higher rate of recurrence in patients receiving a LRD transplant others have found no difference and there is no indication to avoid LRD transplantation in these patients. However, it would be prudent to avoid a LRD transplant in patients who have lost a previous graft from recurrent IgA nephropathy since there is a high risk of recurrence in subsequent allografts. In the study by Ohmacht et al., three of five such retransplanted patients lost their grafts as a result of recurrent IgA nephropathy[30]. Affected patients exhibiting heavy proteinuria (> 1 g/d) and marked glomerulosclerosis (> 30%) are at high risk of subsequent graft loss. Therefore, it appears that recurrent IgA nephropathy behaves similarly to the primary disease, with an indolent though progressive course towards ESRD. There is no treatment of proven benefit to date for chronic recurrent disease although recurrent aggressive crescentic IgA nephropathy should, in the author's opinion, be treated with high dose prednisolone and cyclophosphamide.

Henoch–Schönlein purpura

Glomerular deposition of IgA is also common in Henoch–Schönlein purpura (HSP). Pooled data from Japan and Belgium indicated a 35% recurrence rate and a 11% graft loss rate at 5 years[33]. Recurrence is more frequent in patients who progressed to ESRD within 3 years of diagnosis. Transplantation is commonly deferred for at least a year after the purpura has resolved but recurrent disease may still occur despite this safeguard.

Membranous nephropathy

Membranous nephropathy (MN) may be a recurrent disease or arise de novo (see below), with the latter being more common. Nephrotic-range proteinuria occurs at a mean of 10 months post-transplantation, and characteristic subepithelial immune deposits have developed as rapidly as 8 d following transplantation. Recurrent MN was reported to affect < 10% of patients with MN who undergo transplantation, but this figure was derived primarily from case reports and small series of patients. Recurrent MN is not associated with pretransplant clinical course, immunosuppression regimen, recipient HLA status, degree of HLA matching or the type of transplant[34]. Recent analysis of a series of 30 patients indicated a 29% recurrence rate at 3 years post-transplantation with an increased rate of graft loss in affected patients[35] although spontaneous remission has been documented. There are no good data to support any particular therapeutic intervention in these patients.

De novo membranous nephropathy

De novo MN is the most common form of de novo glomerulonephritis and affects 1–2% of all transplant recipients, though the actual incidence may be higher since subclinical disease may be common. The incidence increases significantly over time and de novo MN is present in 15–20% of transplants of > 15 years duration[36]. After transplant glomerulopathy, it is the second most common cause of post-transplant nephrotic syndrome, accounting for 30% of cases. Patients typically develop proteinuria about 2 years following transplantation and approximately 60% are nephrotic. It has been suggested that de novo MN is more common in children and in well-matched cadaveric or LRD transplants but the data are inconsistent. It is associated with chronic rejection that often antedates the de novo MN. Indeed, it has been proposed that the pathogenesis of de novo MN is related to chronic rejection, and suggested mechanisms include alloimmune responses to major or minor histocompatibility antigens. It has also been proposed that rejection-associated damage to the glomerular capillary wall may lead to the deposition of circulating immune complexes or cause the 'unmasking' of antigens, resulting in in situ immune-complex formation. In general, the outcome of affected grafts is related to the degree and progression of chronic rejection rather than the de novo MN. There is no evidence to support any interventional treatment for this condition. Lastly, de novo MN has also been reported in patients with HCV infection[37].

ANCA-associated small vessel vasculitis

A recent pooled analysis of 127 transplanted patients with a primary diagnosis of ANCA-associated small vessel vasculitis indicated a relapse rate of 20.4% in patients with Wegener's granulomatosis (WG) and 15.7% in patients with microscopic polyangiitis (MPA) (Fig. 91.4) or pauci-immune necrotizing crescentic glomerulonephritis[38]. The relapse rate is lower than the relapse rate for patients on chronic dialysis and the relapses were 'extrarenal' in just under half of affected patients. The type of disease, pretransplantation course, use of cyclosporine and ANCA positivity at the time of transplantation did not affect relapse rate[38]. Overall, patient and graft survival is comparable to that in other nondiabetic transplant recipients of comparable age. Transplantation should be undertaken when the disease is clinically quiescent. Careful clinical monitoring is required if a previously ANCA-negative patient becomes positive or if the ANCA titer rises significantly, since this may herald a relapse. Disease relapses may be successfully treated with increased doses of corticosteroids and conversion to cyclophosphamide (for 3–6 months)[38].

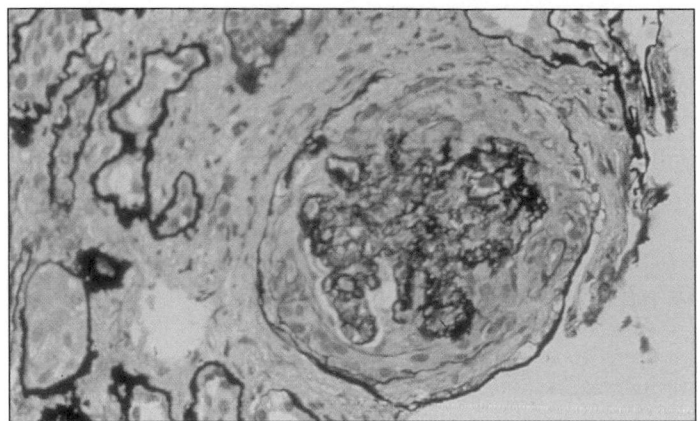

Figure 91.4 Recurrent microscopic polyangiitis. Light microscopy reveals a cellular crescent completely encircling the glomerular tuft.

Antiglomerular basement membrane antibody-mediated glomerulonephritis

The policy of delaying renal transplantation until at least 6 months after antiglomerular basement membrane (anti-GBM) antibodies have become undetectable following treatment has resulted in a reduction in the recurrence rate to < 5% in most centers, with overall graft outcome being comparable to other groups[3]. In the minority of patients who develop recurrent disease, graft loss occurs in about 50%. Recurrence of anti-GBM antibody production with associated graft injury is treated along conventional lines with conversion to cyclophosphamide (3–6 months), higher doses of corticosteroids and vigorous PE.

De novo anti-GBM disease in Alport syndrome

Although approximately 5% of patients with Alport syndrome develop de novo anti-GBM disease following renal transplantation, overall graft survival is very good. Risk factors for the development of de novo anti-GBM disease include the early onset of renal failure, deafness and large deletions in the COL4A5 gene. Affected patients develop proteinuria, hematuria and renal dysfunction, usually months following transplantation, with typical linear immunofluorescence evident on the renal biopsy. Patients are not at risk of pulmonary hemorrhage. Treatment with cytotoxic drugs and PE may be instituted but is of limited benefit and the majority of patients eventually lose their grafts. The disease typically recurs in subsequent grafts and patients should be advised of the high risk of failure. Any patient with Alport syndrome who develops hematuria, proteinuria or renal impairment should undergo a renal transplant biopsy. A recent study indicates that all patients with Alport syndrome who receive a renal transplant develop detectable autoantibodies to type IV collagen but only a minority of these patients develop clinical disease thereby indicating that other factors are important in the pathogenesis of this condition[39].

Systemic lupus erythematosus

The development of ESRD is often associated with a reduction in disease activity in systemic lupus and many reports have found that recurrent lupus nephritis is a very infrequent complication, affecting < 1–2% of patients receiving a transplant. However, a recent study of 97 transplant recipients (106 transplants) with systemic lupus, the largest single center study published to date, noted a somewhat higher recurrence rate of 8.5% (nine patients), with recurrent lupus nephritis contributing to graft failure in 44% (four patients) of the nine affected patients[40]. The mean time to recurrence was about 3 years. Recurrence can not be predicted based on the duration of pretransplant dialysis or serologic parameters (autoantibody and complement levels). There is also a slightly higher incidence of early graft loss in patients with systemic lupus that is partly related to thrombotic events secondary to associated antiphospholipid antibodies. Patients with high titers of antiphospholipid antibodies should receive anticoagulation therapy to maintain the INR > 3.0. Graft survival is superior in patients receiving LRD transplants.

Amyloidosis, monoclonal gammopathies, and mixed essential cryoglobulinemia

Recurrence of primary (AL) and secondary (AA) amyloidosis affects approximately 25% of patients. Graft loss secondary to recurrent disease is uncommon (< 10%). The documented reduction in long-term graft survival is mainly secondary to patient death as a result of extrarenal amyloid deposition, particularly in the cardiovascular system. Colchicine may reduce the recurrence of amyloidosis in the graft in familial Mediterranean fever. Light-chain deposition disease recurs in about half of patients receiving a transplant and can result in loss of the graft. Interestingly, the association of proliferative glomerulonephritis with light chain deposition in a native kidney biopsy may predispose patients to the development of recurrent disease in a renal transplant[41]. Recurrence of disease with adverse effects upon the graft has been documented in multiple myeloma and Waldenström's macroglobulinemia, but the number of patients is small. Fibrillary and immunotactoid glomerulopathies recur in over 50% of patients but the progression of disease is generally slow[42], such that the 5-year graft survival is not reduced. Mixed essential cryoglobulinemia recurs in about 50% of patients, though graft loss is uncommon[2].

Metabolic disorders

Diabetes mellitus is a common cause of ESRD. Histological recurrence of diabetic nephropathy is common following transplantation and includes arteriolar hyalinosis, thickening of the glomerular and tubular basement membranes and mesangial expansion, although nodular glomerulosclerosis is rare (Fig. 91.5). Graft loss from recurrent disease is uncommon and the main cause of graft loss is patient death as a result of associated cardiovascular disease[43].

Fabry's disease results from a deficiency of the lysosomal alpha-galactosidase A enzyme and is characterized by progressive accumulation of globotriaosylceramide and other related glycosphingolipids within the microvascular endothelial cells of critically important organs such as the kidney, heart and brain (see Chapter 48). Despite a high incidence of cardiovascular complications, renal transplantation has an excellent outcome in patients with Fabry's disease[44]. Recurrent disease in the transplant is documented but does not usually affect graft

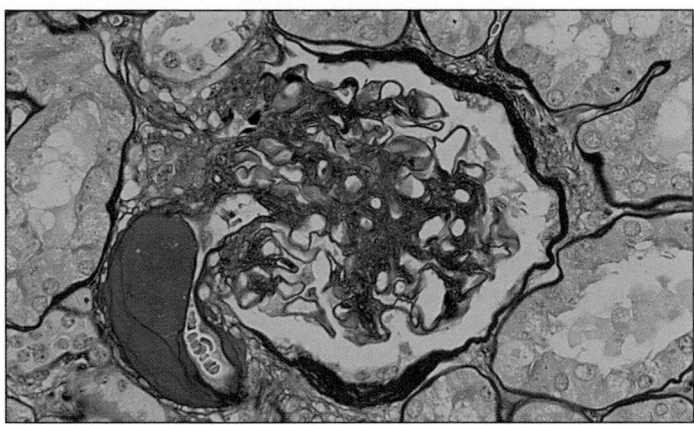

Figure 91.5 Recurrent diabetes mellitus. Light microscopy demonstrates characteristic microvascular hyalinosis, typically the first morphologic manifestation of recurrent disease, involving a hilar arteriole. Other manifestations of recurrent diabetic nephropathy that are present include diffuse mesangial sclerosis and thickened glomerular and tubular basement membranes.

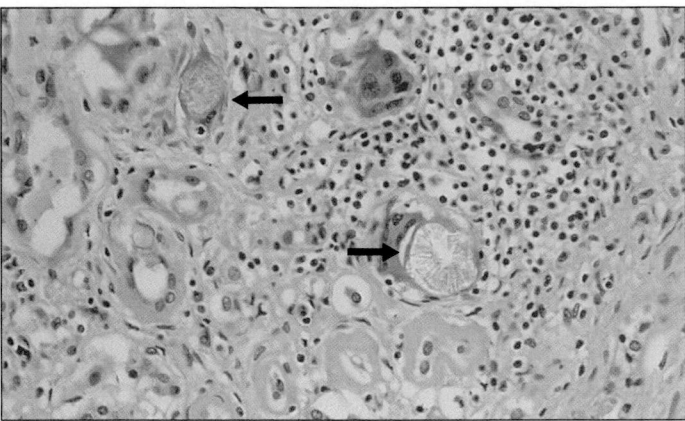

Figure 91.6 Recurrent primary hyperoxaluria. Light microscopy demonstrates oxalate crystals within the tubular lumen (arrows) with a secondary interstitial inflammatory infiltrate.

survival. In addition, the recent development of recombinant enzyme replacement therapy may well retard or reverse extrarenal manifestations of the disease in renal transplant recipients and prevent future patients developing ESRD[45].

Cystinosis is characterized by excessive intracellular accumulation of the amino acid cystine (see Chapter 50). In transplant recipients, resident cells of the renal transplant do not exhibit cystine accumulation although this may be evident in infiltrating cells from the recipient. The results of renal transplantation are good although extrarenal disease will progress if treatment with cysteamine is not maintained[46].

Primary hyperoxaluria is caused by a functional deficiency of the hepatic peroxisomal pyridoxine (B6)-dependent enzyme alanine glyoxylate aminotransferase (AGT). Renal failure with nephrocalcinosis often occurs in childhood, after which calcium oxalate is deposited systemically and particularly affects the skeleton and vasculature, resulting in systemic oxalosis. The early results of renal transplantation were disappointing (3-year survival rate < 25%) partly because the systemic oxalate pool slowly leached out causing marked hyperoxaluria with graft failure secondary to graft oxalosis (see Fig. 91.6). Children with renal failure, particularly those who do not respond to high-dose pyridoxine treatment, are best treated with a combined liver/kidney transplant, since the liver transplant cures the metabolic derangement. Patients with systemic oxalosis should receive measures to minimize deposition of calcium oxalate in the renal transplant, including aggressive pretransplant hemodialysis, the maintenance of a high urine volume, and the early commencement of dialysis if there is any significant renal insufficiency in the post-transplant period. In addition, pyridoxine (which reduces oxalate generation in up to 60% of patients) should be continued until the liver transplant is functioning well, while treatment to inhibit crystallization of urinary calcium oxalate (such as orthophosphate, citrate (if hypocitraturic), and magnesium supplements) should be continued since significant hyperoxaluria may persist for over a year.

Transplant glomerulopathy

Transplant glomerulopathy, the most common cause of nephrotic syndrome in transplant recipients, is a manifestation of chronic allograft rejection and may have a similar light microscopic appearance to MPGN, with reduplication of the GBM and mesangial cell interposition. However, subendothelial immune complexes are absent, though the subendothelial accumulation of electronlucent material is often evident. Transplant glomerulopathy is found in 4–8% of transplant biopsies in most series and is thought to be mainly secondary to immunological injury to the glomerular endothelium with both the cellular and humoral arms of the immune response implicated in its pathogenesis. There is also evidence to support a role for HCV infection[37]. For example, transplant biopsies from two patients with HCV infection demonstrated features of both MPGN type I and transplant glomerulopathy (i.e., subendothelial immune complexes and subendothelial electronlucent material)[47]. In another study, about 33% of patients with transplant glomerulopathy had positive HCV antibodies compared with only 1.9% of control patients.

Patients present with proteinuria, microhematuria, with or without renal insufficiency, and occasionally with nephrotic syndrome. The prognosis is poor, with most patients developing ESRD. No therapy is of proven benefit though ACE inhibitors may ameliorate the proteinuria and could theoretically retard the progression to ESRD.

DONOR DISEASE

Glomerular disease may be inadvertently transmitted in the donor kidney. Subclinical mesangial IgA deposits that have been identified in donor kidneys have been found to be cleared within the first year and have not been shown to cause clinically significant disease post-transplantation.

CONCLUSIONS

Clearly, recurrent and *de novo* disease is a significant problem and particularly affects certain categories of patients such as those with FSGS, HUS and MPGN. The high probability of recurrent disease in certain patients mitigates against performing a LRD transplant. However, the development of recurrent disease does allow the study of the pathogenesis of various disease processes, an example being the development of HCV-associated *de novo* and recurrent MPGN. The challenge for the future is to systematically design studies to assess the impact of various treatment strategies in these groups of transplant recipients with the aim of further prolonging graft function.

REFERENCES

1. Hariharan S, Adams MB, Brennan DC, et al. Recurrent and *de novo* glomerular disease after renal transplantation: a report from Renal Allograft Disease Registry (RADR). Transplantation. 1999; 68(5):635–41.
2. Charpentier B, Hiesse C, Marchand S, et al. *De novo* and recurrent diseases: recurrent glomerulopathies. Transplant Proc. 1999; 31(1/2):264–6.
3. Kotanko P, Pusey CD, Levy JB. Recurrent glomerulonephritis following renal transplantation. Transplantation. 1997;63(8): 1045–52.
4. Hariharan S, Peddi VR, Savin VJ, et al. Recurrent and *de novo* renal diseases after renal transplantation: a report from the renal allograft disease registry. Am J Kidney Dis. 1998;31(6): 928–31.
5. Chadban S. Glomerulonephritis recurrence in the renal graft. J Am Soc Nephrol. 2001;12(2):394–402.
6. Andresdottir MB, Hoitsma AJ, Assmann KJ, et al. The impact of recurrent glomerulonephritis on graft survival in recipients of human histocompatibility leucocyte antigen-identical living related donor grafts. Transplantation. 1999; 68(5):623–7.
7. Kim SJ, Ha J, Jung IM, et al. Recurrent focal segmental glomerulosclerosis following renal transplantation in Korean pediatric patients. Pediatr Transplant. 2001;5(2):105–11.
8. Tejani A, Stablein DH. Recurrence of focal segmental glomerulosclerosis posttransplantation: a special report of the North American Pediatric Renal Transplant Cooperative Study. J Am Soc Nephrol. 1992;2(12):S258–63.
9. Cheong HI, Han HW, Park HW, et al. Early recurrent nephrotic syndrome after renal transplantation in children with focal segmental glomerulosclerosis. Nephrol Dial Transplant. 2000; 15(1):78–81.
10. Refaie A, Sobh M, Moustafa F, et al. Living-related-donor kidney transplantation outcome in recipients with primary focal-segmental glomerulosclerosis. Am J Nephrol. 1999;19(1):55–9.
11. Raafat R, Travis LB, Kalia A, Diven S. Role of transplant induction therapy on recurrence rate of focal segmental glomerulosclerosis. Pediatr Nephrol. 2000;14(3):189–94.
12. Choi KH, Kim SI, Yoon SY, et al. Long-term outcome of kidney transplantation in adult recipients with focal segmental glomerulosclerosis. Yonsei Med J. 2001;42(2):209–14.
13. Savin V, Sharma R, Sharma M, et al. Circulating factor associated with increased glomerular permeability to albumin in recurrent focal segmental glomerulosclerosis. N Engl J Med. 1996;334(14): 878–83.
14. Dall'Amico R, Ghiggeri G, Carraro M, et al. Prediction and treatment of recurrent focal segmental glomerulosclerosis after renal transplantation in children. Am J Kidney Dis. 1999;34(6): 1048–55.
15. Godfrin Y, Dantal J, Perretto S, et al. Study of the in vitro effect on glomerular albumin permselectivity of serum before and after renal transplantation in focal segmental glomerulosclerosis. Transplantation. 1997;64(12):1711–15.
16. Matalon A, Markowitz GS, Joseph RE, et al. Plasmapheresis treatment of recurrent FSGS in adult renal transplant recipients. Clin Nephrol. 2001;56(4):271–8.
17. Ohta T, Kawaguchi H, Hattori M, et al. Effect of pre-and postoperative plasmapheresis on posttransplant recurrence of focal segmental glomerulosclerosis in children. Transplantation. 2001; 71(5):628–633.
18. Cosio FG, Frankel WL, Pelletier RP, et al. Focal segmental glomerulosclerosis in renal allografts with chronic nephropathy: implications for graft survival. Am J Kidney Dis. 1999; 34(4):731–8.
19. Andresdottir MB, Assmann KJ, Hoitsma AJ, et al. Recurrence of type I membranoproliferative glomerulonephritis after renal transplantation: analysis of the incidence, risk factors, and impact on graft survival. Transplantation. 1997; 63(11):1628–33.
20. Roth D, Cirocco R, Zucker K, et al. *De novo* membranoproliferative glomerulonephritis in hepatitis C virus-infected renal allograft recipients. Transplantation. 1995;59(12):1676–82.
21. Cruzado JM, Torras J, Gil-Vernet S, Grinyo JM. Glomerulonephritis associated with hepatitis C virus infection after renal transplantation. Nephrol Dial Transplant. 2000; 15(suppl 8):65–7.
22. Pham HP, Feray C, Samuel D, et al. Effects of ribavirin on hepatitis C-associated nephrotic syndrome in four liver transplant recipients. Kidney Int. 1998;54(4):1311–19.
23. Andresdottir MB, Assmann KJ, Hoitsma AJ, et al. Renal transplantation in patients with dense deposit disease: morphological characteristics of recurrent disease and clinical outcome. Nephrol Dial Transplant. 1999;14(7):1723–31.
24. Morales JM, Martinez MA. Munoz dBE, et al. Recurrent type III membranoproliferative glomerulonephritis after kidney transplantation. Transplantation. 1997; 63(8):1186–8.
25. Bassani CE, Ferraris J, Gianantonio CA, et al. Renal transplantation in patients with classical haemolytic-uraemic syndrome. Pediatr Nephrol. 1991;5(5):607–11.
26. Miller RB, Burke BA, Schmidt WJ, et al. Recurrence of haemolytic-uraemic syndrome in renal transplants: a single-centre report. Nephrol Dial Transplant. 1997;12(7):1425–30.
27. Ducloux D, Rebibou JM, Semhoun-Ducloux S, et al. Recurrence of hemolytic-uremic syndrome in renal transplant recipients: a meta-analysis. Transplantation. 1998;65(10):1405–7.
28. Quan A, Sullivan EK, Alexander SR. Recurrence of hemolytic uremic syndrome after renal transplantation in children: a report of the North American Pediatric Renal Transplant Cooperative Study. Transplantation. 2001;72(4):742–5.
29. Kaplan BS, Papadimitriou M, Brezin JH, et al. Renal transplantation in adults with autosomal recessive inheritance of hemolytic uremic syndrome. Am J Kidney Dis. 1997;30(6):760–5.
30. Ohmacht C, Kliem V, Burg M, et al. Recurrent immunoglobulin A nephropathy after renal transplantation: a significant contributor to graft loss. Transplantation. 1997;64(10):1493–6.
31. Bumgardner GL, Amend WC, Ascher NL, Vincenti FG. Single-center long-term results of renal transplantation for IgA nephropathy. Transplantation. 1998;65(8):1053–60.
32. Floege J, Burg M, Kliem V. Recurrent IgA nephropathy after kidney transplantation: not a benign condition. Nephrol Dial Transplant. 1998;13(8):1933–5.
33. Meulders Q, Pirson Y, Cosyns JP, et al. Course of Henoch-Schonlein nephritis after renal transplantation. Report on ten patients and review of the literature. Transplantation. 1994;58(11):1179–86.
34. Couchoud C, Pouteil-Noble C, Colon S, Touraine JL. Recurrence of membranous nephropathy after renal transplantation.

Incidence and risk factors in 1614 patients. Transplantation. 1995; 59(9):1275–9.

35. Cosyns JP, Couchoud C, Pouteil-Noble C, et al. Recurrence of membranous nephropathy after renal transplantation: probability, outcome and risk factors. Clin Nephrol. 1998; 50(3): 144–53.

36. Schwarz A, Krause PH, Offermann G, Keller F. Impact of *de novo* membranous glomerulonephritis on the clinical course after kidney transplantation. Transplantation. 1994;58(6): 650–4.

37. Morales JM, Campistol JM, Andres A, Rodicio JL. Glomerular diseases in patients with hepatitis C virus infection after renal transplantation. Curr Opin Nephrol Hypertens. 1997; 6(6):511–15.

38. Nachman PH, Segelmark M, Westman K, et al. Recurrent ANCA-associated small vessel vasculitis after transplantation: A pooled analysis. Kidney Int. 1999;56(4):1544–50.

39. Kalluri R, Torre A, Shield CF, et al. Identification of alpha3, alpha4, and alpha5 chains of type IV collagen as alloantigens for Alport posttransplant anti-glomerular basement membrane antibodies. Transplantation. 2000;69(4):679–83.

40. Stone JH, Millward CL, Olson JL, et al. Frequency of recurrent lupus nephritis among ninety-seven renal transplant patients during the cyclosporin era. Arthritis Rheum. 1998;41(4):678–86.

41. Short AK, O'Donoghue DJ, Riad HN, et al. Recurrence of light chain nephropathy in a renal allograft. A case report and review of the literature. Am J Nephrol. 2001;21(3):237–40.

42. Samaniego M, Nadasdy GM, Laszik Z, Nadasdy T. Outcome of renal transplantation in fibrillary glomerulonephritis. Clin Nephrol. 2001;55(2):159–66.

43. Kim H, Cheigh JS. Kidney transplantation in patients with type 1 diabetes mellitus: long-term prognosis for patients and grafts. Korean J Intern Med. 2001;16(2):98–104.

44. Ojo A, Meier-Kriesche HU, Friedman G, et al. Excellent outcome of renal transplantation in patients with Fabry's disease. Transplantation. 2000;69(11):2337–9.

45. Eng CM, Guffon N, Wilcox WR, et al. Safety and efficacy of recombinant human alpha-galactosidase A–replacement therapy in Fabry's disease. N Engl J Med. 2001;345(1):9–16.

46. Langlois V, Geary D, Murray L, et al. Polyuria and proteinuria in cystinosis have no impact on renal transplantation. A report of the North American Pediatric Renal Transplant Cooperative Study. Pediatr Nephrol. 2000;15(1/2):7–10.

47. Gallay BJ, Alpers CE, Davis CL, et al. Glomerulonephritis in renal allografts associated with hepatitis C infection: a possible relationship with transplant glomerulopathy in two cases. Am J Kidney Dis. 1995;26(4):662–7.

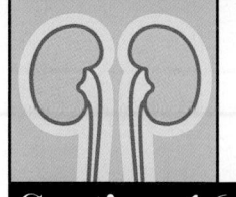

Chapter
92

Outcomes of Renal Transplantation

Colm C Magee, Glenn Chertow and Edgar L Milford

INTRODUCTION

The most convenient and widely used method of assessing renal transplantation outcomes is measurement of allograft survival. Other important measures include allograft function (typically measured by plasma creatinine), patient survival, number of rejection episodes, days of hospitalization and quality-of-life indices. Most of the data described here are derived from the United States Renal Database System (USRDS), the Collaborative Transplant Study (CTS) and the Australia and New Zealand Dialysis and Transplant Registry (ANZDATA). The USRDS reports on almost all patients transplanted in the USA; the CTS on some – but not all – patients transplanted throughout the world and the ANZDATA on all patients transplanted in Australia and New Zealand.

Actual and actuarial allograft and patient survival

Allograft survival is calculated from the day of transplantation to the day of reaching a defined end-point (either return to dialysis or retransplantation or death – whichever occurs first). In practice, survival is usually calculated by *actuarial* methods. These methods imply projection or estimation of survival as not all patients will have been followed for the same period of time. Also, as not all patients will have reached the defined end-point, censoring of such patients is required. One-year, 5-year and 10-year actuarial survival rates are frequently presented. Another actuarial measure commonly used is graft half-life (median graft survival).

Traditionally, graft survival (or its inverse, graft loss) is assessed under two distinct time phases: early and late. Early graft loss refers to loss in the first 12 months; late loss to any time thereafter. This distinction is empiric but makes clinical sense. In the first 12 months, graft loss is *relatively* common – because of technical complications such as graft thrombosis, and because of severe rejection. After 12 months, the incidence of graft loss is lower but remains quite stable over time. Usually, analysis of long-term survival is restricted to those allografts that have survived to 12 months post-transplant. The causes of late graft loss are also different and are discussed below.

Note that using the definition above, patient death is equivalent to graft loss. Graft survival can also be calculated after censoring for patient death.

Survival benefits of renal transplantation

Comparison of survival between the general dialysis population and transplanted patients is greatly affected by selection bias – only relatively healthy patients are referred for transplantation. Thus, comparisons between patients on the waiting list who do or do not receive a transplant are usually performed instead (the large increase in the number of patients on the waiting list has allowed such meaningful statistical analysis). Of course, such analyses assume that the two groups (transplanted or still on the list) can otherwise be matched – this is not necessarily true.

One study of USRDS found that during the first 106 days after transplantation the relative risk of death was greater than remaining on the waiting list (on dialysis). This mainly reflected the risks associated with the transplant procedure itself. Thereafter, however, transplantation conferred a survival benefit (Fig. 92.1). On the basis of 3–4 years of follow-up, transplantation reduced the risk of death overall by 68%[1]. Transplantation was particularly life-saving in diabetic patients.

Current short-term outcomes in renal transplantation

For recipients of a first cadaveric kidney in the USA, current unadjusted 1-year patient and graft survival probabilities are

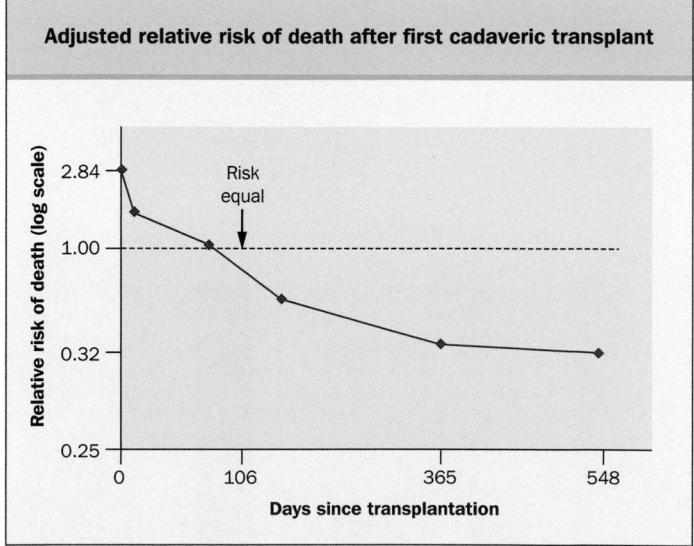

Figure 92.1 Adjusted relative risk of death among 23 275 recipients of a first cadaveric transplant. The reference group was the 46 164 patients on dialysis who were on the waiting list (relative risk, 1.0). Values were adjusted for age, sex, race, cause of end-stage renal disease (ESRD), year of placement on the waiting list, geographic region, and time from first treatment for ESRD to placement on the waiting list. (Adapted, with permission, from Wolfe et al.[1].)

approximately 95% and 89%, respectively[2]. For recipients of a first living donor kidney, current unadjusted 1-year patient and graft survival probabilities are approximately 98% and 94%, respectively. These outcomes have steadily improved over the last 25 years (Fig. 92.2). Similar outcomes have been reported from other registries[3,4]. The principal causes of graft loss in the first post-transplant year are patient death, acute rejection, graft vessel thrombosis and primary nonfunction (Fig. 92.3). The principal causes of death during this time period are cardiovascular disease (here, meaning cardiac and cerebrovascular disease) and infection[5] (Fig. 92.4).

Current long-term outcomes in renal transplantation

Although static in the 1980s, long-term renal allograft survival has steadily increased over the last 10 years[2,3]. For example, estimated graft half-lives for the USRDS 1985–1989 cohort were 7.7 years, for the 1990–1994 cohort 9.0 years and for the 1995–1999 cohort 10.9 years[5]. Figure 92.5 illustrates these changes in Caucasian American recipients. This impressive improvement has occurred even in the setting of greater use of organs from older and less optimal donors. The increasing use of elderly cadaveric donors is shown in Figure 92.6.

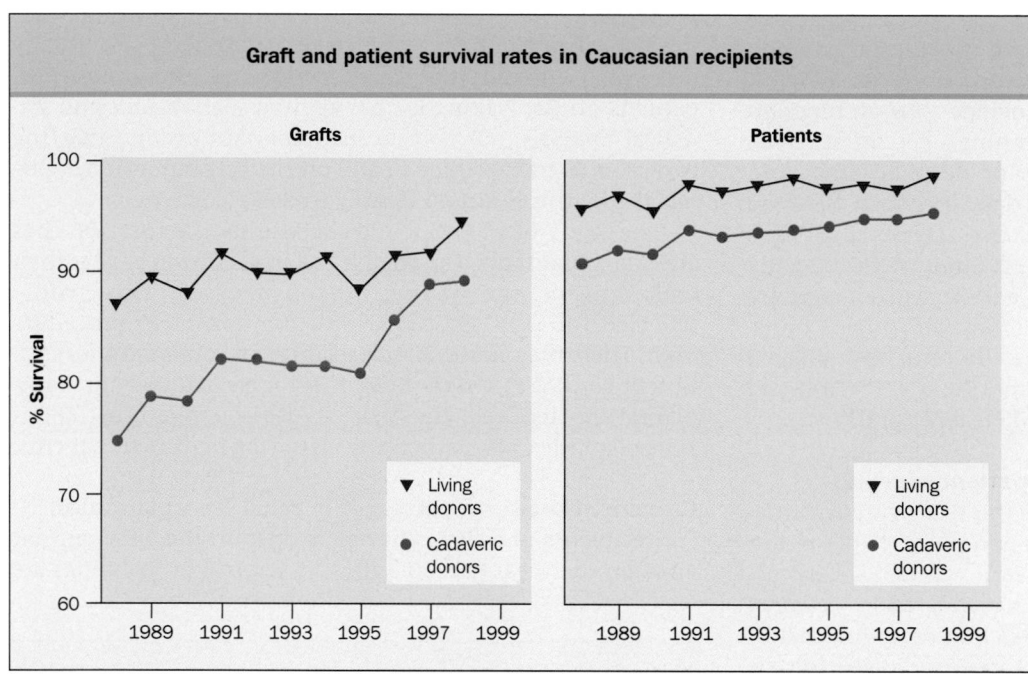

Figure 92.2 1 year graft and patient survival. Trends in 1-year graft and patient survival rates in Caucasian recipients (adjusted for age, gender, primary diagnosis; standardized to 1997). *Source*: USRDS 2001 Report.

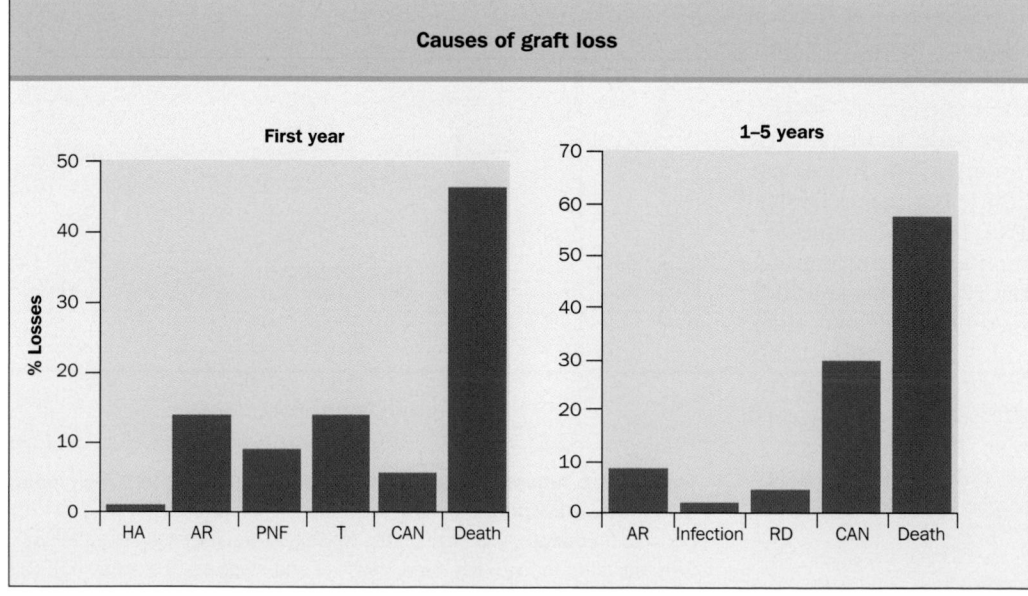

Figure 92.3 Causes of graft loss among Caucasian cadaver kidney recipients, 1995–1999. (Adapted, with permission, from Cecka[5].) HA, hyperacute rejection; AR, acute rejection; PNF, primary nonfunction; T, thrombosis; CAN, chronic allograft nephropathy; RD, recurrent disease.

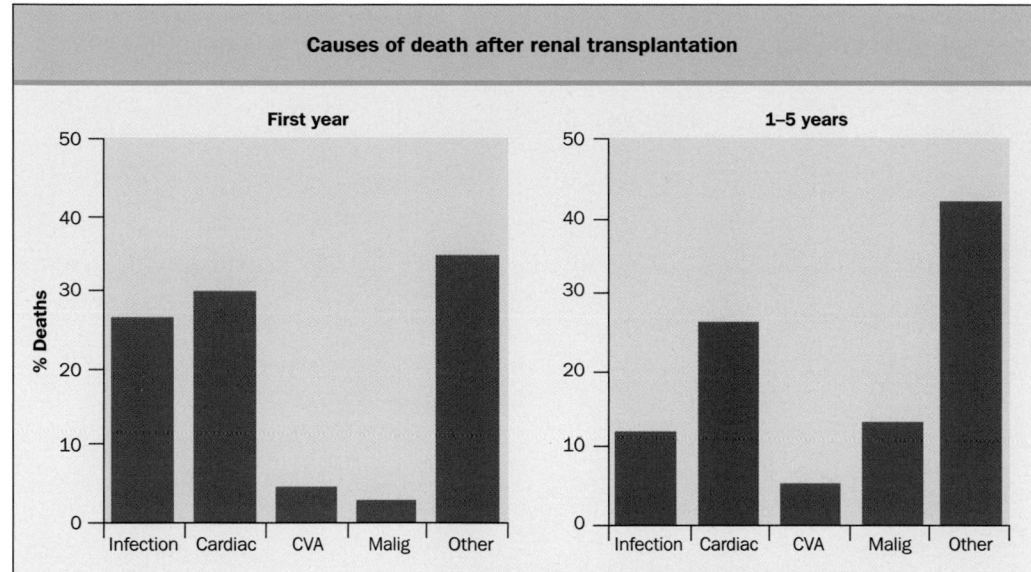

Figure 92.4 Causes of death among Caucasian cadaver kidney recipients, 1995–1999. (Adapted, with permission, from Cecka[5].). CVA, cerebrovascular accident; Malig, malignancy.

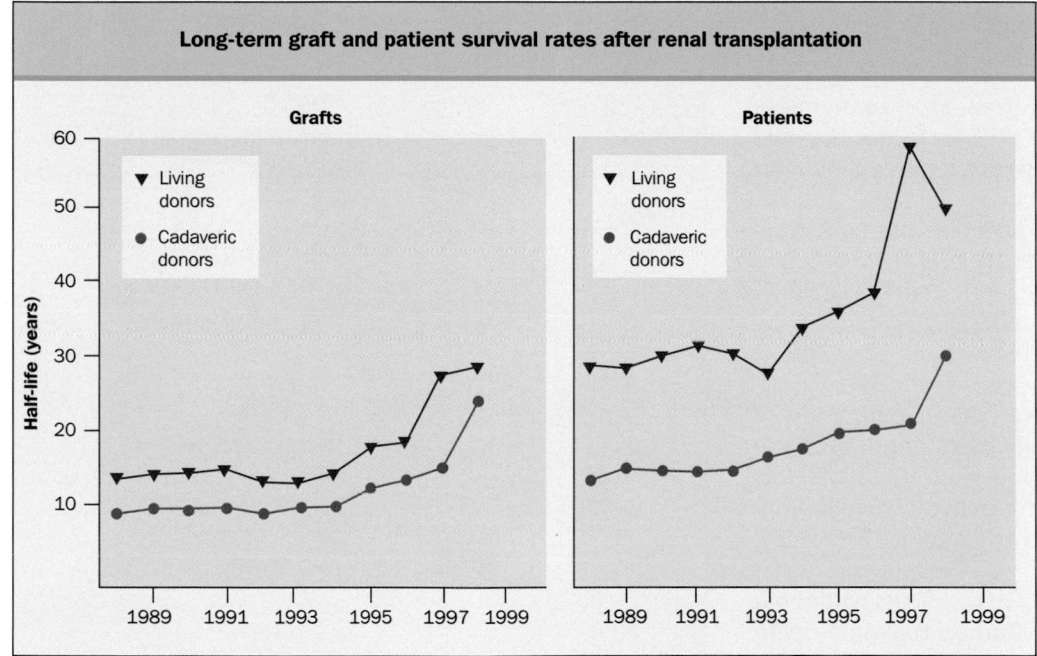

Figure 92.5 Long-term graft and patient survival after renal transplantation. Trends in long-term (as measured by half-life) graft and patient survival rates in Caucasian recipients (adjusted for age, gender, primary diagnosis; standardized to 1997). *Source*: USRDS 2001 Report.

Beyond the first post-transplant year, the principal causes of renal allograft loss are patient death and chronic allograft nephropathy (CAN); less common causes are late acute rejection and recurrent disease[5] (Fig. 92.3). The number one cause of death remains cardiovascular disease, followed by infection and malignancy (Fig. 92.4).

FACTORS AFFECTING RENAL ALLOGRAFT SURVIVAL

Prospective studies and analyses of registry data have shown that many factors are associated with renal allograft survival. These can be considered as either *donor, recipient* or *donor-recipient*. Another classification is based on factors being considered either *alloantigen dependent* or *alloantigen independent*.

Many of the factors considered below contribute to the development of CAN, which is the most common cause of nondeath graft failure.

Donor-recipient factors
Delayed graft function
Delayed graft function (DGF) is considered here because both donor and recipient factors are associated with it. DGF is usually defined as failure of the renal allograft to function immediately post-transplant, with the need for dialysis within a specified period, usually 1 week. DGF is associated with poorer graft survival, poorer graft function and greater risk of patient death[6]. This adverse impact of DGF is due in part to its association with higher rates of acute rejection. Rejection may be more common because ischemia-reperfusion injury

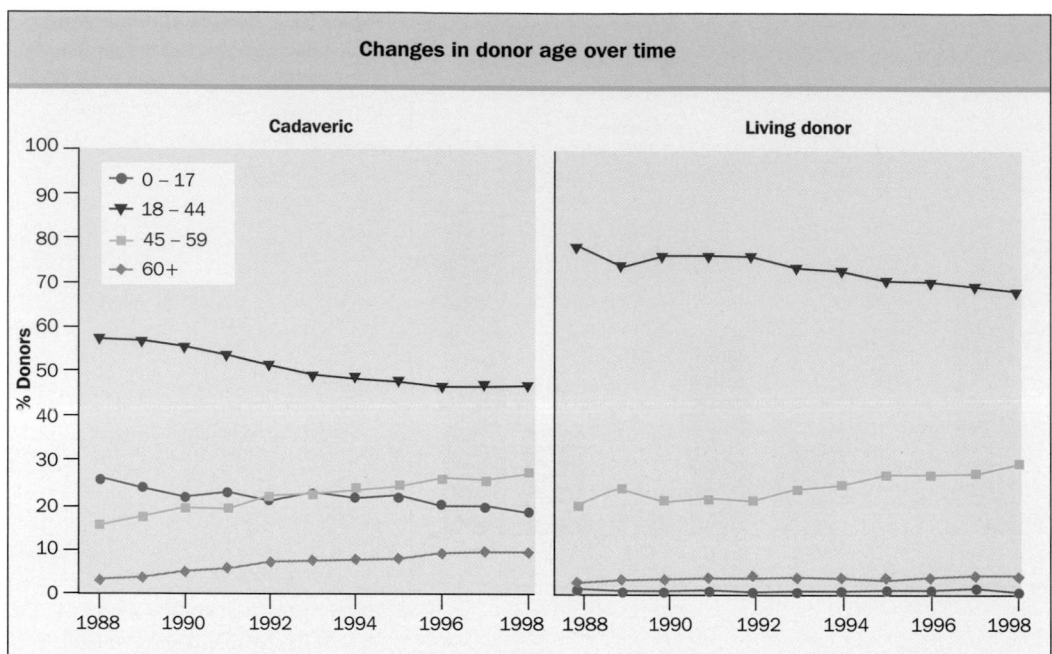

Figure 92.6 Changes in donor age over time. *Source*: USRDS 2001 Report.

increases the immunogenicity of the graft. Most studies have also demonstrated that, even in the absence of documented acute rejection, DGF is associated with poorer long-term graft function and survival.

Although the incidence of acute rejection has fallen dramatically over the last 10 years, rates of DGF have declined only slightly – to just over 20% of cadaveric grafts[6] (Fig. 92.7). Recent USRDS data show that DGF reduces graft half-life by 30% – a bigger effect than early acute rejection[7]. Thus DGF is both an outcome and a predictor.

The presence of DGF reflects a variable combination of chronic pretransplant injury (e.g., advanced donor age) and peritransplant injury (e.g., ischemia-reperfusion). Risk factors for DGF are shown in Table 92.1. Warm ischemia time is probably also a risk factor but, as it is often not accurately recorded, its impact is difficult to assess.

Slow graft function defines a group of recipients with moderate early graft dysfunction – one definition is plasma creatinine > 3.0 mg/dL (264 µmol/L) and no dialysis, at 1 week after transplant[6]. Slow graft function appears to be also associated with poorer graft function and survival. Thus, measures which simply convert grafts from delayed to slow function may be of limited benefit[6].

HLA matching

Registry data from many countries clearly demonstrate that, even with current immunosuppressive regimens and improving outcomes in the whole transplant population, better HLA matched allografts still have prolonged survival. This benefit applies both to living donor and cadaveric donor grafts and to almost all subsets of patients. Thus, the projected half-life varies from 13.0 years for first cadaveric renal allografts with zero HLA mismatches to 8.3 years for those with five or six HLA mismatches[8]. Similar results are reported by CTS (Fig. 92.8). The better outcomes are presumably related to fewer

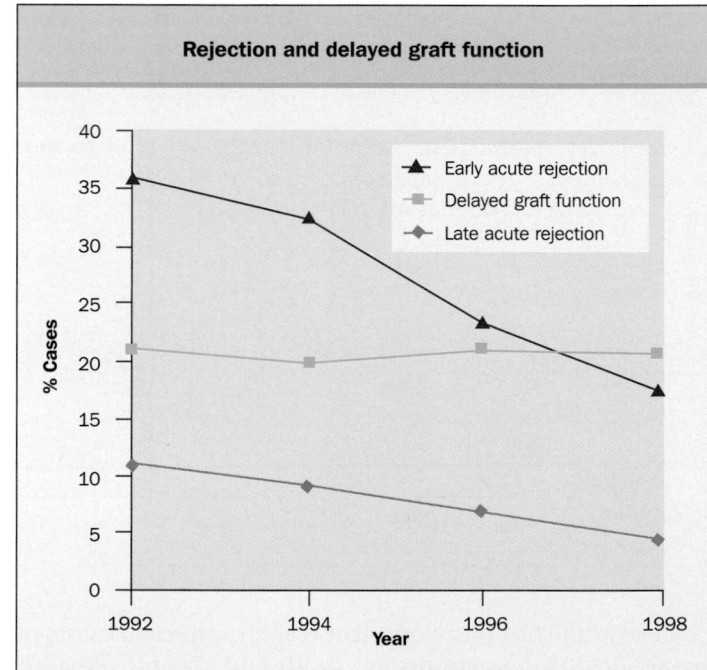

Figure 92.7 Rejection and delayed graft function. Annual incidences of early acute rejection, late acute rejection (occurring after 6 months) and delayed graft function. (Adapted, with permission, from Gjertson[7].)

immunological failures. In both the USA[9] and UK[10], there is an overall benefit from using a national strategy of preferentially performing zero HLA mismatched transplants – even though cold ischemia times may be slightly prolonged.

CMV status of donor and recipient

Registry data show a small but definite effect of donor and recipient CMV serological status on renal allograft survival.

Risk factors for delayed graft function	
Risk factor	Odds ratio
Donor age (10–40 years)	
< 10 years	1.2
41–55 years	1.7
> 55 years	2.1
Cold ischemia time (< 12 h)	
13–24 h	1.4
25–36 h	2.3
> 36 h	3.5
Recipient race (non-African American)	
African American	1.6
PRA (< 50%)	
> 50%	1.2
HLA mismatch (> 0)	
0 mismatches	0.8
Duration per dialysis	
Per year	1.1

Table 92.1 Risk factors for delayed graft function. The reference groups are in bold type. (Adapted, with permission, from Halloran and Hunsicker[6].)

Donor negative – recipient negative pairings had the best outcomes whereas donor positive – recipient positive pairings had the worst[11]. The reasons why donor positive – recipient positive pairings had worse outcomes than donor positive – recipient negative pairings are unclear. One theory is that two 'hits' with two CMV virotypes is particularly deleterious. There is also evidence that CMV infection upregulates the immune response, thereby increasing the risk of rejection.

Timing of transplantation

In the case of living donor renal transplantation, there is evidence that pre-emptive – before initiation of dialysis – transplantation is associated with a lower risk of allograft failure[12]. This, in part, reflects a higher risk of acute rejection in patients previously on long-term dialysis. Although this important study used multivariable analysis of registry data, the results may still have been influenced by unmeasured confounders such as differences in the quality of medical care and of self-care between the two patient groups. However, another multivariate analysis (of cadaveric and living donor recipients) showed that longer time on dialysis (compared with a reference group of < 12 months on dialysis) was independently associated with poorer graft survival[7]. Minimizing time on dialysis has of course many potential benefits; this strategy should thus be pursued whenever possible.

Center effect

Not surprisingly, outcomes have varied widely from transplant center to center. This reflects normal statistical variance as well as center 'expertise'. It is important to note that outcomes will be confounded by many donor and recipient factors that differ across centers. Thus, between center comparisons are difficult. Recent USRDS data suggest minimal difference in outcomes between small and large transplant centers in the USA[13].

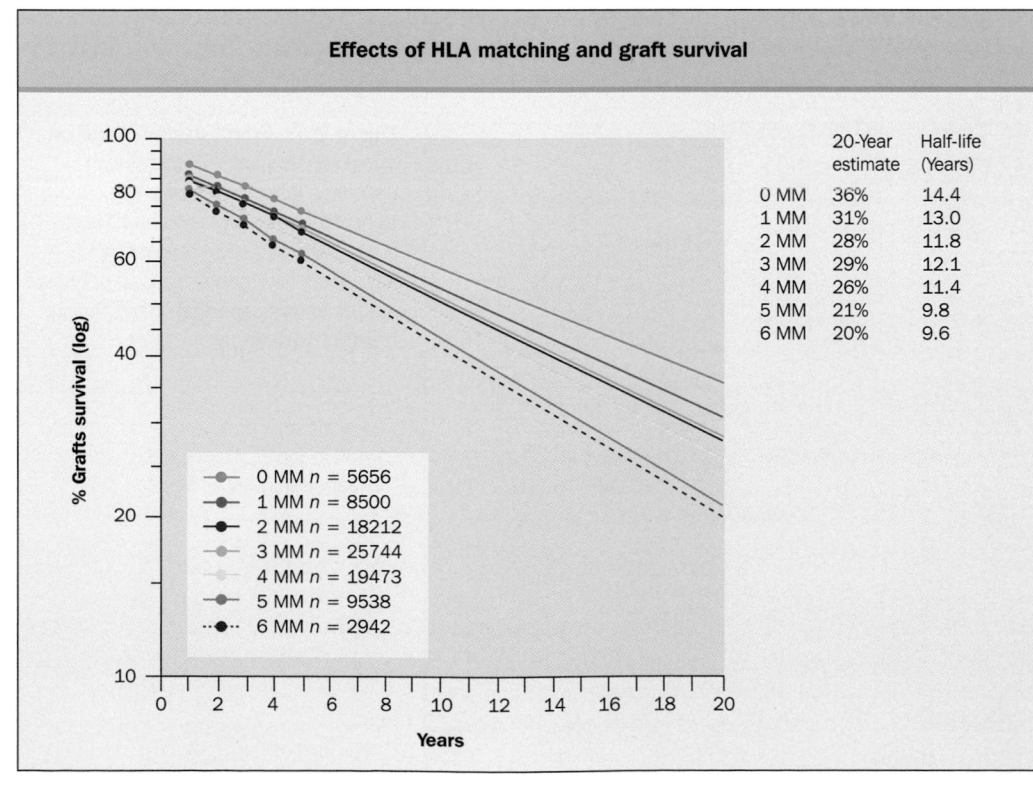

	20-Year estimate	Half-life (Years)
0 MM	36%	14.4
1 MM	31%	13.0
2 MM	28%	11.8
3 MM	29%	12.1
4 MM	26%	11.4
5 MM	21%	9.8
6 MM	20%	9.6

Legend:
- 0 MM n = 5656
- 1 MM n = 8500
- 2 MM n = 18212
- 3 MM n = 25744
- 4 MM n = 19473
- 5 MM n = 9538
- 6 MM n = 2942

Figure 92.8 Effects of HLA A, B, DR mismatches on survival of first cadaveric kidney transplants. *Source:* CTS database.

Transplantation

Year of transplant

Long-term allograft survival is slowly, but steadily increasing. This presumably reflects multiple factors, including more effective but not more toxic immunosuppressive regimens, better pretransplant and post-transplant general medical care, and more effective prevention and treatment of opportunistic infections (particularly CMV).

Genetic polymorphism

It has been hypothesized that genetic variation (with regard to the organ donor or recipient) may influence post-transplant outcomes such as susceptibility to infections, susceptibility to acute rejection and allograft survival. Candidate polymorphic genes would be those encoding cytokines, chemokines, adhesion molecules and their relevant receptors. Some studies have suggested that polymorphisms of such molecules can influence outcomes. There are many caveats with regard to the current literature on this topic: studies have been retrospective, usually single-center, have not incorporated multivariate analysis and, in some cases, have yielded contradictory results. Thus, it is premature to alter immunosuppression or other facets of post-transplant care based on the data available. It is hoped that prospective, multicenter studies will be performed to assess the clinical importance of polymorphisms of immune molecules.

Donor factors

The quality of the kidney immediately prior to transplantation has a major impact on long-term graft function and the risk of developing CAN.

Donor source: cadaver versus living donor

The donor source is one of the most important predictors of short and long-term graft outcomes. In general, living donor grafts are superior to cadaveric grafts. Figures 92.2 and 92.5

illustrate how the short and long-term survival of living-donor allografts is clearly higher than for cadaveric grafts. This benefit applies across all degrees of HLA mismatching. The better outcomes reflect several factors: healthy living donors, avoidance of ischemia-reperfusion injury, high nephron mass and probably the effects of a shorter waiting time (see above). Better compliance by the recipient may also play a role in improving outcome. Excellent results are now being demonstrated with living unrelated kidney transplantation where HLA matching is not optimum[14]. This further emphasizes the importance of the 'healthy transplant kidney' effect.

Donor age

Kidneys from those aged over 45 years, and particularly over 60 years, have poorer outcomes[2]. This effect is especially pronounced in cadaveric grafts (Fig. 92.9). These results are thought to reflect a higher incidence of delayed graft function and of nephron 'underdosing'. Grafts from older donors have fewer functioning nephrons because of the aging process and donor related conditions such as hypertension and atherosclerosis. However, because of the organ donor shortage, elderly cadaveric kidneys are being increasingly used (Fig. 92.6).

Donor age < 5 years is also associated with poorer outcomes, which likely reflects relatively high rates of technical complications and probably nephron underdosing (see below). En bloc transplants (consisting of both kidneys with a segment of aorta and inferior vena cava) from donors aged 0–5 years significantly improve survival, however.

Donor race

In the USA, the survival of cadaveric grafts obtained from black donors is poorer than grafts from white donors[5,7,15]. This effect persists even in black recipients, implying that the

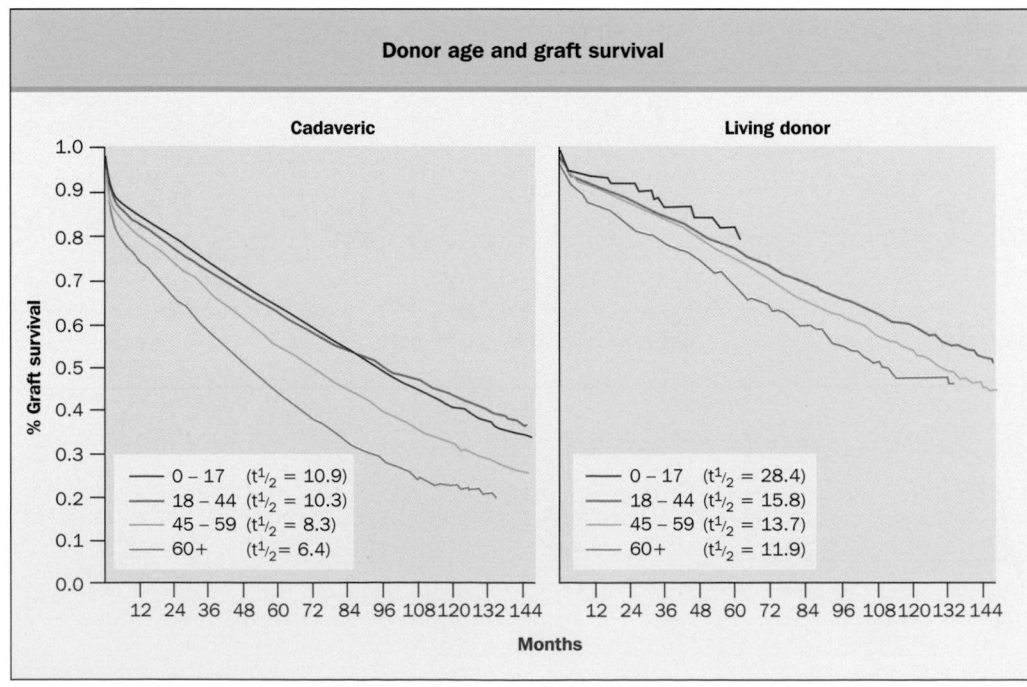

Figure 92.9 Effect of donor age on allograft survival – Kaplan-Meier estimates in recipients of a first transplant between 1988 and 1998. Note: donors aged 0–5 years are associated with poorer survival but these are not shown separately here. *Source*: USRDS 2001 Report.

poorer outcomes are not due to immunogenetic differences alone. One theory is that lower nephron number in blacks is important.

Donor sex

There is evidence that grafts from female donors have slightly poorer survival[2,15]. Again, this probably reflects a nephron 'underdosing' effect (see below), as females have smaller renal mass than males.

Donor nephron mass

An imbalance between the metabolic/excretory demands of the recipient and the functional transplant mass has been postulated to play a causative role in the development and progression of CAN. Nephron underdosing, exacerbated by perioperative ischemic damage and postoperative nephrotoxic drugs, might lead to nephron overwork and eventual failure, similar to the mechanisms occurring in native kidney disease. Thus, kidneys from small, 'marginal' donors and recipients of large body mass index would be at highest risk of this problem. There is support for this hypothesis from animal studies and retrospective human studies[15]. Prospective human trials to determine the role of inadequate nephron mass are not available, however.

Marginal donors

The issue of 'nephron dosing' has assumed greater importance because of the pressure to use cadaveric allografts from 'expanded criteria' donors. Typically, these kidneys have impaired *pretransplant* function because of advanced donor age (> 60 years) and/or donor disease such as chronic hypertension. Not surprisingly, short- and long-term outcomes with such grafts have are somewhat inferior to grafts from 'normal criteria' donors. However, it should be emphasized that transplantation with a marginal kidney confers a significant survival advantage compared to remaining on the transplant waiting list (on dialysis)[16].

Transplantation of both kidneys into one recipient would obviously double the functioning nephron number; limited medium-term data suggest outcomes of this procedure are good. However, the number of recipients is obviously halved. Halloran has argued that dual kidney transplantation should only be performed in the context of a randomized control trial comparing outcomes in recipients of two allografts to outcomes in the two recipients of single allografts. Otherwise, transplantation should be single kidney to single recipient (with informed consent), recognizing that long-term allograft function is more likely to be suboptimal[17].

Another group of marginal donors, in which there has been renewed interest, is nonheart beating donors. The use of nonheart beating donors has been controversial as short-term outcomes are inferior to those seen with heart beating cadaveric donors. This reflects the longer period of warm ischemia. Reported rates of primary nonfunction are approximately 10% and of DGF, 45–80%. There is accumulating evidence, however, that long-term graft survival is similar to heart beating cadaveric donors although renal function may be inferior[18].

Recipient factors

Recipient age

In general, graft survival rates are poorer in those at the extremes of age: < 18 and > 60 years[5]. In the young, technical causes of graft loss such as vessel thrombosis are relatively more common. Acute rejection is also a more common cause of graft loss; conversely, death with a functioning graft is relatively rare.

In most western countries, the elderly are forming an increasing percentage of the incident and prevalent ESRD population. Many of these patients have significant comorbid disease, particularly cardiovascular disease and type 2 diabetes mellitus. Nevertheless, age *per se* is not a contraindication to transplantation: among elderly patients carefully screened and deemed fit for the procedure, long-term outcomes are clearly better with transplantation than dialysis[1]. The percentage of elderly ESRD patients in the USA who have received a kidney transplant is steadily increasing: from 3.7% in 1989 to 8.4% in 1998[19]. The same benefits of living donor allografts accrue to the elderly as to younger patients. Interestingly, although matching older cadaveric kidneys to older recipients is a common practice that is performed in an attempt to allocate the best kidneys to younger recipients, recent analysis of USRDS data has shown that this does not improve *overall* graft survival[20].

Not surprisingly, compared with younger recipients, death with a functioning graft is a more common cause of graft loss (responsible for > 50% of graft failures), with most cases being secondary to cardiovascular disease, infection or neoplasia. Conversely, acute rejection is less common. Thus, although randomized controlled trials are not available, it seems reasonable to use less aggressive immunosuppression in the elderly.

Recipient race

In the USA, African American recipients have poorer cadaveric and living donor graft survival compared with Caucasians[5]. This probably reflects multiple factors including: higher incidence of DGF, higher incidence of acute and late acute rejection, stronger immune responsiveness, a predominantly Caucasian donor pool (with resultant poorer matching of HLA and non-HLA antigens), altered pharmacokinetics of immunosuppressive drugs and a higher prevalence of hypertension. Socioeconomic factors associated with inability to pay for transplant medications (an issue in the USA where universal health coverage does not exist), poorer access to high quality medical care and 'noncompliance' probably also play a role. There is some evidence to suggest that African Americans also have inferior outcomes in Europe. In the USA, Asian recipients have superior outcomes to Caucasians; the reasons for this are unknown. These interracial differences in graft survival are shown in Figure 92.10.

Strategies which should improve outcomes in African American recipients include increasing living donor transplant rates by African Americans (currently, lower than by Caucasians) and increasing cadaveric donor rates by African Americans. In randomized controlled trials of recently introduced immunosuppressive drugs, rates of acute rejection were

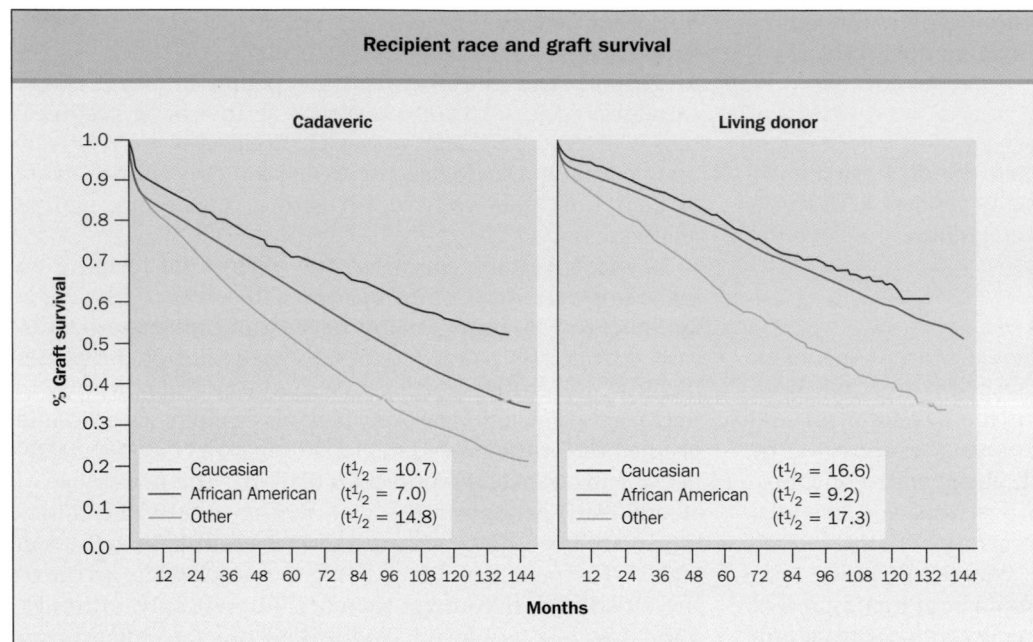

Recipient race and graft survival

Figure 92.10 Effect of recipient race on allograft survival – Kaplan-Meier estimates in recipients of a first transplant between 1988 and 1998. Note: Other includes Asian. *Source:* USRDS 2001 Report.

higher in African Americans than Caucasians. *Post-hoc* analysis of one trial showed that, in African American recipients, mycophenolate 2 g/d was only partially effective in reducing acute rejection rates (compared to azathioprine); mycophenolate 3 g/d was more effective. Conversely, mycophenolate 2 g/d was adequate in Caucasians[21]. Tacrolimus is also a very effective immunosuppressant in African Americans. Thus, many American centers routinely use more aggressive immunosuppression – incorporating tacrolimus – in African Americans recipients.

Recipient gender
The impact of gender on transplant outcomes was recently assessed in a multivariate analysis of USRDS data[22]. Overall patient and graft survival was better in females compared to males but graft survival was similar after censoring for death. Interestingly, females were at higher risk of acute rejection but at lower risk of graft loss from chronic dysfunction. The higher rate of acute rejection could reflect unmeasured sensitizing effects of prior pregnancies (adjustment was made for the status of panel of reactive antibodies (PRA)). The reasons for the lower risk of graft loss from chronic dysfunction are unknown.

Recipient sensitization
Patients who are broadly sensitized (e.g., have a PRA status > 50%) generally have poorer early and late graft survival compared to nonsensitized recipients. This is mainly related to an increased incidence of complications in the early post-transplant period such as delayed graft function and acute rejection. The principal reasons for sensitization are previous transplants, pregnancy and previous blood transfusion. Thus, allograft survival is poorer in recipients of 2nd or 3rd transplants compared to recipients of a first transplant. In the 1995–1999 cohort of USA patients, graft half-life was 13.9 years in those with PRA < 10%, but 10.7 years in those with PRA > 50%[8]. Highly sensitized patients are thus usually given more intensive immunosuppression.

Acute rejection
Acute rejection has been consistently associated with an increased risk of graft loss. This is due to actual graft destruction at the time of acute rejection and probably ongoing subclinical immune mediated injury. Such damage accentuates the effects of poor quality donor tissue, perioperative ischemic injury, nephron underdosing, etc. Acute rejection refractory to steroids, acute rejection with arteritis and late acute rejection (occurring after the first 6 months) are particularly associated with poorer graft and patient outcomes. Gjertson's recent analysis of UNOS data showed that late acute rejection had a more negative impact on graft survival than early acute rejection or delayed graft function, and was associated with a reduction in graft half-lives by approximately 50%[7]. Positive C4d staining of peritubular capillaries is also associated with poorer graft survival. Fortunately, more effective immunosuppressive regimens have steadily decreased rates of acute rejection (Fig. 92.7). This must be one of the primary reasons why early and late renal allograft survival statistics have continued to improve.

Recipient immunosuppression
Undoubtedly, the improvements in short- and long-term allograft survival reflect, in part, the effectiveness of the newer antirejection drugs such as the calcineurin inhibitors (CNIs) and mycophenolate. The contribution of long-term CNI therapy, particularly with currently used maintenance doses, to chronic renal allograft dysfunction remains controversial. Traditionally, the CNIs have been thought to have greater beneficial effects on short-term compared with long-term renal graft survival. Certainly, in non-renal transplant patients (e.g., those with cardiac allografts or autoimmune disease), prolonged intake of CNIs is associated with significant decreases in native kidney GFR and chronic histopathologic changes on biopsy. CNIs could contribute to chronic allograft dysfunction by induction of chronic renal ischemia, by stimulation of intragraft production of the fibrogenic cytokine, TGFβ and by

promotion of systemic hypertension. Balancing these effects, of course, is the high efficacy of CNIs in preventing acute rejection, which is one of the most important determinants of graft outcomes. The increases in short- and long-term graft survival in the CNI era (cyclosporine became widely used in the early 1980s) suggest that these antirejection effects override the nephrotoxic effects. Furthermore, lower dosages (< 5 mg/kg per d) have been associated with the development of CAN[23].

There is accumulating evidence that MMF improves long-term graft survival both by preventing overt acute rejection and by other mechanisms[24]. No differences in survival with MMF compared with placebo were seen in the 3 years follow-up of the USA trial; the trial was not powered to detect such differences, however.

Although antilymphocyte antibody preparations (e.g., OKT3, thymoglobulin) are widely used, particularly in the setting of DGF, their beneficial effect on long-term graft survival is controversial. Recent UNOS data suggest that antibody induction protocols slightly reduce early acute rejection episodes in recipients with DGF and slightly improve graft survival[25].

Recipient compliance

Poor compliance with the immunosuppressive regimen is known to increase the risk of acute rejection (particularly late acute rejection) and chronic allograft nephropathy. The magnitude of this problem is difficult to define.

High recipient body mass index

Overweight and obesity are the most common nutritional disorders in the USA and many western countries. It is unknown if the obese are forming an increasing percentage of the incident and prevalent ESRD population; but, because of the background increase in prevalence of obesity and because of its association with type 2 diabetes, hypertension and cardiovascular disease, this is likely to be so.

Pischon and Sharma recently reviewed the literature regarding obesity and outcomes in renal transplant recipients[26]. They concluded that obesity was associated with more transplant surgery related complications, more DGF, higher mortality (related to cardiovascular complications) and poorer graft survival. Similar evidence of poorer patient and graft outcomes were found in a multivariable analysis of USRDS data[27]. Poorer long-term graft survival probably reflects the effects of DGF, nephron overwork and more difficult dosing of immunosuppressive drugs. No data are available comparing survival outcomes of overweight dialysis patients remaining on the transplant waiting list with matched patients who receive a kidney transplant but it is probable that transplantation is overall of benefit, as seen in other patient groups[1].

Recipient hypertension: the renin–angiotensin system

Retrospective studies have shown that the degree of hypertension correlates with the rate of deterioration in graft function and the severity of histological change. Of course, hypertension could be a marker of deteriorating function rather than a cause. No prospective human studies of the effect of treating hypertension on allograft outcomes are available. Animal studies have shown that hypertension accelerates development of CAN. Common sense dictates that treatment of hypertension should be the goal, to prevent both its renal and nonrenal complications.

Multiple studies have confirmed the ability of angiotensin converting enzyme (ACE) inhibitors and angiotensin receptor antagonists (ATRA) to slow the progression of both diabetic and nondiabetic proteinuric native kidney disease. Some have argued that ACE inhibitors and ATRA should be similarly beneficial in transplant kidney disease and thus should be used more frequently. While several studies have shown that both classes of drugs are effective in treating post-transplant hypertension and in reducing proteinuria in the short term, no long-term studies of their effects on progression of transplant kidney dysfunction have been published. In one randomized controlled trial, patients randomized to nifedipine had sustained improvement in GFR up to 2 years after transplant; no improvement was seen in the lisinopril group[28]. This may reflect the ability of nifedipine to attenuate CNI-induced vasoconstriction of the afferent arteriole.

Recipient hyperlipidemia

The prominence of the vascular lesions in CAN and the similarity of these lesions to atherosclerosis, suggest that hyperlipidemia plays a role in the pathogenesis of CAN and graft failure. Some studies have suggested that hypercholesterolemia and/or hypertriglyceridemia are associated with poorer graft outcomes. Again, common sense dictates that hyperlipidemia should be treated aggressively, to prevent both its renal and nonrenal complications.

Recurrence of primary disease

Determining the incidence and prevalence of recurrent or *de novo* renal disease is difficult. The original cause of ESRD is often unknown; most relevant studies are small and retrospective with variable follow-up periods. In the 5-year interval of 1995–1999, recurrent disease was reported to cause < 5% of graft losses from 1–5 years after transplant[5]. One multivariate analysis of almost 5000 patients found a relative risk of graft failure due to recurrent and *de novo* disease of 1.9. The diseases particularly associated with poor graft survival were primary focal segmental glomerulosclerosis (RR 2.3), membranoproliferative glomerulonephritis (RR 2.4) and hemolytic uremic syndrome/thrombotic thrombocytopenic purpura (RR 5.4)[29]. It is likely that as renal allograft survival continues to improve, recurrent or *de novo* disease will be increasingly diagnosed (both clinically and histologically) and will become a more important cause of late graft loss.

To date, allograft failure from recurrence of diabetic nephropathy has not been a major problem. More important is the poor patient survival in this transplant population. It is likely that with better management of cardiovascular risk factors, overall survival for diabetic transplant recipients will improve. Thus, recurrence of clinically significant diabetic nephropathy will likely be more common. It should be emphasized that diabetic patients benefit greatly from renal transplantation[1].

Proteinuria

The degree of proteinuria correlates with poorer renal outcome in both native and transplant kidney disease. Proteinuria may simply be a marker of renal damage but there is speculation that proteinuria *per se* may accelerate allograft loss from CAN. The role of ACE inhibitors and ATRA in slowing the progression of proteinuric transplant renal diseases is discussed briefly above.

IMPROVING RENAL ALLOGRAFT OUTCOMES

Measures, which would likely further improve allograft survival, are summarized in Table 92.2. Probably the most important (in terms of achievable impact) is increased use of living kidney donors. In the UK/Ireland, for example, the percentage of living donors is increasing, but is still only about 20% of the total[30]. Ideally, most living donor kidneys would be transplanted before the recipient begins dialysis. It is critical, however, that donation should only be allowed when the risk of medical and psychological complications to the donor are minimal.

The criteria used for allocation of cadaveric allografts can have an important impact on *overall* allograft survival. A purely utilitarian approach would imply directing organs to those who possess certain demographic and clinical characteristics, are likely to live longer etc. In practice, a balance must be struck between utility and equity (ensuring that anyone medically fit for a transplant has a reasonable chance of obtaining one). In many countries, this balance is achieved by means of a points system – points being awarded for zero HLA mismatching, time on the waiting list, etc.

CONCLUSION

Improvements in short- and long-term renal allograft survival have been very encouraging. This likely reflects multiple influences including more effective immunosuppression, more use of living donors and better medical and surgical care. The focus is likely to shift somewhat to improving other post-transplant outcomes such as patient survival, complications of immunosuppression and allograft function.

Improving renal allograft survival	
Measure	**Comment**
Increased living donor donation: both related and nonrelated	Underutilized in many countries
Pre-emptive transplantation	Underutilized in many countries
Increased donation from younger, previously healthy cadaveric donors	Difficult to achieve; Spain best example of successful high donation rates
Zero mismatching of HLA antigens	Already practiced in many countries
Improved organ preservation	Controversial if machine perfusion improves long-term graft function
Faster matching and transplantation; reduced cold ischemia time	Difficult to achieve
ACE inhibitors, ATRA	No data in transplant patients *per se* showing that renal function is better preserved; reasonable to extrapolate from native kidney disease
Nephron dosing (matching of donor-recipient sex, BMI etc.)	No large RCTs; complex to administer in practice
High quality general medical care (aggressive control of hyperlipidemia, hypertension etc.)	No RCTs showing benefits in transplant patients but benefits likely

Table 92.2 Measures which should improve renal allograft survival. (RCT; randomized controlled trial).

REFERENCES

1. Wolfe RA, Ashby VB, Milford EL, et al. Comparison of mortality in all patients on dialysis, patients on dialysis awaiting transplantation, and recipients of a first cadaveric transplant. N Engl J Med. 1999;341(23):1725–30.
2. USRDS. USRDS 2001 Annual Data Report: NIH and NIDDK, Bethesda. MD: USRDS; 2002.
3. Russ GR. Transplantation. 2001 Report of the ANZDATA Registry. Transplantation: Australia and New Zealand Dialysis and Transplant Registry (ANZDATA); 2002. Accessed at www.anzdata.org.au
4. Dijk PC van, Jager KJ, Charro F de, et al. Renal replacement therapy in Europe: the results of a collaborative effort by the ERA-EDTA registry and six national or regional registries. Nephrol Dial Transplant. 2001;16(6):1120–9.
5. Cecka JM. The UNOS Scientific Renal Transplant Registry – 2000. Clin Transpl. 2000:1–18.
6. Halloran P, Hunsicker L. Delayed graft function: state of the art. Am J Transplantion. 2001;1:115–20.
7. Gjertson DW. Impact of delayed graft function and acute rejection on kidney graft survival. Clin Transpl. 2000:467–80.
8. Terasaki PI. The HLA-matching effect in different cohorts of kidney transplant recipients. Clin Transpl. 2000:497–514.
9. Takemoto SK, Terasaki PI, Gjertson DW, Cecka JM. Twelve years' experience with national sharing of HLA-matched cadaveric kidneys for transplantation. N Engl J Med. 2000;343(15): 1078–84.
10. Morris PJ, Johnson RJ, Fuggle SV, et al. Analysis of factors that affect outcome of primary cadaveric renal transplantation in the UK. HLA Task Force of the Kidney Advisory Group of the United Kingdom Transplant Support Service Authority (UKTSSA). Lancet. 1999;354(9185):1147–52.
11. Brennan DC. Cytomegalovirus in renal transplantation. J Am Soc Nephrol. 2001;12(4):848–55.
12. Mange KC, Joffe MM, Feldman HI. Effect of the use or nonuse of long-term dialysis on the subsequent survival of renal transplants from living donors. N Engl J Med. 2001;344(10):726–31.
13. Terasaki PI, Cecka JM. The center effect: is bigger better? Clin Transpl. 1999:317–24.
14. Gjertson DW, Cecka JM. Living unrelated donor kidney transplantation. Kidney Int. 2000;58(2):491–9.

15. Chertow GM, Milford EL, Mackenzie HS, Brenner BM. Antigen-independent determinants of cadaveric kidney transplant failure. JAMA. 1996; 276(21):1732–6.

16. Ojo AO, Hanson JA, Meier-Kriesche H, et al. Survival in recipients of marginal cadaveric donor kidneys compared with other recipients and wait-listed transplant candidates. J Am Soc Nephrol. 2001;12(3):589–97.

17. Halloran PF, Melk A, Barth C. Rethinking chronic allograft nephropathy: the concept of accelerated senescence. J Am Soc Nephrol. 1999;10(1):167–81.

18. Metcalfe MS, Butterworth PC, White SA, et al. A case-control comparison of the results of renal transplantation from heart-beating and non-heart-beating donors. Transplantation. 2001; 71(11):1556–9.

19. Kasiske BL, Snyder J, Matas A, Collins A. The impact of transplantation on survival with kidney failure. Clin Transpl. 2000:135–43.

20. Kasiske BL, Snyder J. Matching older kidneys with older patients docs not improve allograft survival. J Am Soc Nephrol. 2002; 13(4):1067–72.

21. Neylan JF. Immunosuppressive therapy in high-risk transplant patients: dose-dependent efficacy of mycophenolate mofetil in African-American renal allograft recipients. U.S. Renal Transplant Mycophenolate Mofetil Study Group. Transplantation. 1997; 64(9):1277–82.

22. Meier-Kriesche HU, Ojo AO, Leavey SF, et al. Gender differences in the risk for chronic renal allograft failure. Transplantation. 2001;71(3):429–32.

23. Almond PS, Matas A, Gillingham K, et al. Risk factors for chronic rejection in renal allograft recipients. Transplantation. 1993; 55(4):752–7.

24. Ojo AO, Meier-Kriesche HU, Hanson JA, et al. Mycophenolate mofetil reduces late renal allograft loss independent of acute rejection. Transplantation. 2000;69(11):2405–9.

25. Takemoto SK. Maintenance immunosuppression. Clin Transpl. 2000:481–95.

26. Pischon T, Sharma AM. Obesity as a risk factor in renal transplant patients. Nephrol Dial Transplant. 2001;16(1):14–17.

27. Meier-Kriesche HU, Arndorfer JA, Kaplan B. The impact of body mass index on renal transplant outcomes: a significant independent risk factor for graft failure and patient death. Transplantation. 2002;73(1):70–74.

28. Midtvedt K, Hartmann A, Foss A, et al. Sustained improvement of renal graft function for two years in hypertensive renal transplant recipients treated with nifedipine as compared to lisinopril. Transplantation. 2001;72(11):1787–92.

29. Hariharan S, Adams MB, Brennan DC, et al. Recurrent and de novo glomerular disease after renal transplantation: a report from Renal Allograft Disease Registry (RADR). Transplantation. 1999; 68(5):635–41.

30. UK Transplant Support Services Authority. UK Transplant Support Services Authority Annual Report 1999–2000. UK Transplant Support Services Authority; 2002. http://www.uktransplant.org.uk

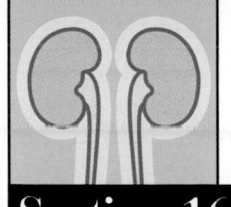

Chapter 93

Pancreas and Islet Transplantation

Ramasamy Bakthavatsalam, Connie I Davis, and Christopher Marsh

INTRODUCTION

Pancreas transplantation is performed primarily for the amelioration of insulin-requiring diabetes and is the only therapy that can render a patient euglycemic without the risk of severe hypoglycemia. Initially pancreas transplants were performed in those diabetic patients with end-stage renal disease (ESRD) who needed kidney transplants; today pancreas transplant alone or pancreas transplantation after living related or unrelated kidney transplant is increasingly common. To date, more than 15 000 pancreas transplants have been performed worldwide, 75% in the USA. In the year 1999 alone 1524 pancreas transplants were done, 25% as pancreas alone (PTA) or pancreas after kidney (PAK)[1]. (Fig. 93.1) More recently there has been an increase in the number of patients receiving islet cell transplants. As the experience in islet cell transplantation grows and demonstrates improved outcome, it may become the modality of choice. This chapter will discuss both solid organ and islet transplantation.

Patient selection criteria for pancreas or islet transplantation

Indications for pancreas transplantation include (1) insulin dependent diabetes with associated diabetic complications (nephropathy, neuropathy, retinopathy) and (2) diabetes with episodes of 'hypoglycemic unawareness'. The indications for islet transplantation are the same.

The medical evaluation for the prospective pancreas transplant candidate is similar to that for the kidney-only recipient, although the cardiac workup is more extensive (see Chapter 86). The best candidates for transplantation are under the age of 50 and lack major complications of diabetes such as vascular complications, orthostatic hypotension or severe gastroparesis, but these criteria are not uniform. The patient's cardiovascular status is the deciding factor for transplant eligibility because the surgery, infections, risk for thrombotic complications, and, until recently, rejection are more severe in the pancreas recipient, demanding that the cardiovascular system be strong enough to withstand the potential of multiple prolonged hemodynamically stressful events[2]. All patients are required to undergo a noninvasive cardiac stress evaluation (thallium, sestamibi or echo) often with pharmacologic stress because of the limited exercise capabilities of many patients. Cardiac catheterization is performed based upon the results of noninvasive testing or performed initially for high-risk patients, those over age 45, duration of diabetes of over 25 years, smoking for more than five pack-years, and/or an abnormal electrocardiogram[2]. Peripheral vascular disease is

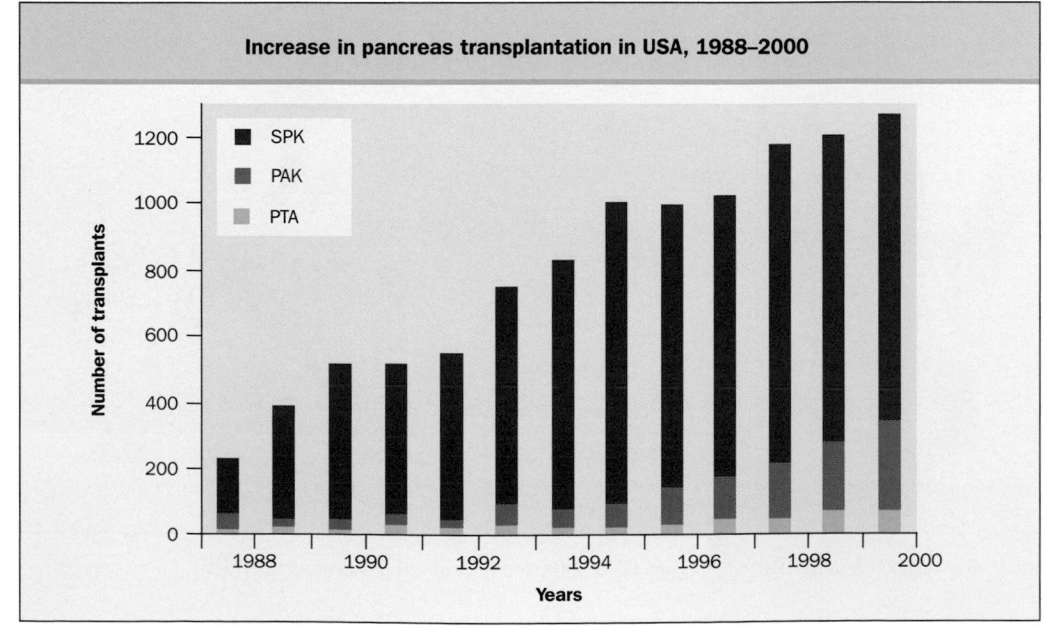

Figure 93.1 Pancreas transplantation. Catagories of pancreas transplant performed in USA 1988–2000. SPK-simultaneous pancreas and kidney transplant PAK-pancreas transplant after kidney transplant PTA-pancreas transplant alone

Transplantation

evaluated by clinical examination and frequently by arterial duplex ultrasonography. Patients with limb threatening ischemia are not good pancreas transplant candidates. Likewise those patients with marked orthostatic hypotension may have difficulties with organ perfusion and are not safe candidates. The medical evaluation for islet transplantation is similar to that for pancreas transplantation but less stringent due to fewer surgical and inflammatory risks.

Once a patient is accepted as a pancreas transplant candidate, the last criteria for transplantation are that the donor and recipient be matched for ABO blood type and the recipient sera must be cross-match negative (without preformed antibodies) against donor T cells using either the standard antiglobulin or flow cytometry cross-match.

SURGICAL PROCEDURE

Current practice is to transplant the whole pancreas with a cuff of duodenum. The duodenal cuff preserves the blood supply of the head of the pancreas and is a means to drain exocrine secretions into either the small bowel (enteric drainage) or the bladder (Figs 93.2–93.4). At present, in the USA, over 50% of the pancreas transplants are enterically drained (Figure 93.4). The pancreas graft is commonly placed in the right iliac fossa like a kidney, but intraperitoneally and vascularized from the common iliac vessels so that the insulin output enters the systemic circulation. Venous anastomosis to superior mesenteric vein of the recipient allows insulin output into the portal circulation which is more physiological[3]. Pancreas transplantation is performed in three ways: (1) simultaneous pancreas and kidney transplantation (SPK), (2) pancreas transplant after kidney transplant (PAK), and (3) pancreas transplantation alone(PTA).

The advantage of bladder drainage is the ability to monitor the trend in the urinary amylase, which is helpful in the detection of rejection. Hence, it is still the technique of choice for exocrine drainage in PAK and PTA transplants, which have poorer graft survival compared with SPK transplants. Bladder drainage also avoids the enterotomy associated risks of infection and leak. The disadvantages of bladder drainage are dehydration, metabolic acidosis, and genito-urinary tract complications. Primary enteric drainage avoids these complications and is more physiological but loses the ability to monitor the urinary amylase. Overall outcomes to date are not different whether the venous drainage is systemic or portal, although portal drainage is more physiological and avoids hyperinsulinemia, the effect of which is not well characterized[3].

PATIENT AND GRAFT SURVIVAL

Pancreatic allograft survival rates have increased as a result of improved surgical technique (described above), improvement in the composition of the preservation fluid, better patient selection, and more effective immunosuppressive treatments. Currently, the most commonly used cold storage solution is the University of Wisconsin solution (see Chapter 87), which has increased early pancreas graft function and reduced the occurrence of preservation pancreatitis. Selecting patients with minimal vascular disease, good compliance, lack of tobacco and alcohol use, good family support has been shown

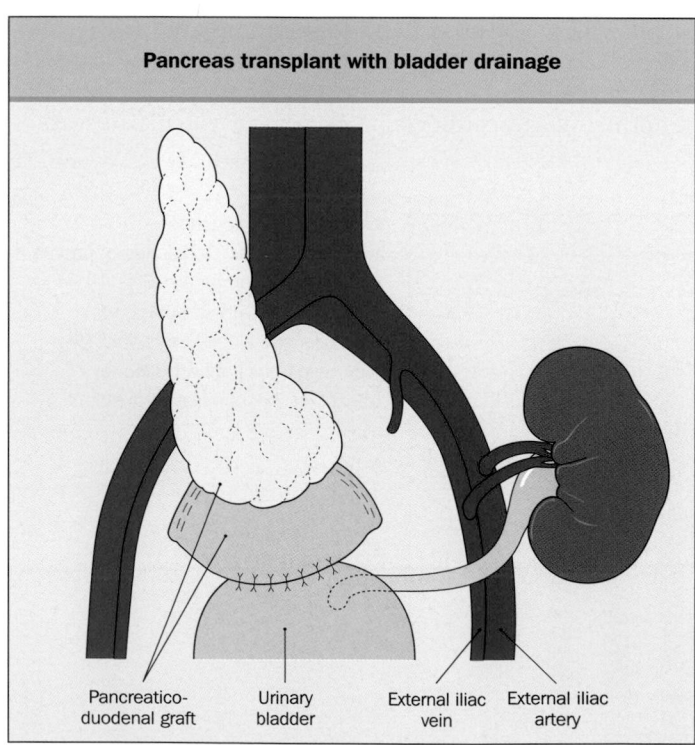

Figure 93.2 Pancreas transplant with bladder drainage. The pancreas may be placed in either intra- or extraperitonal position.

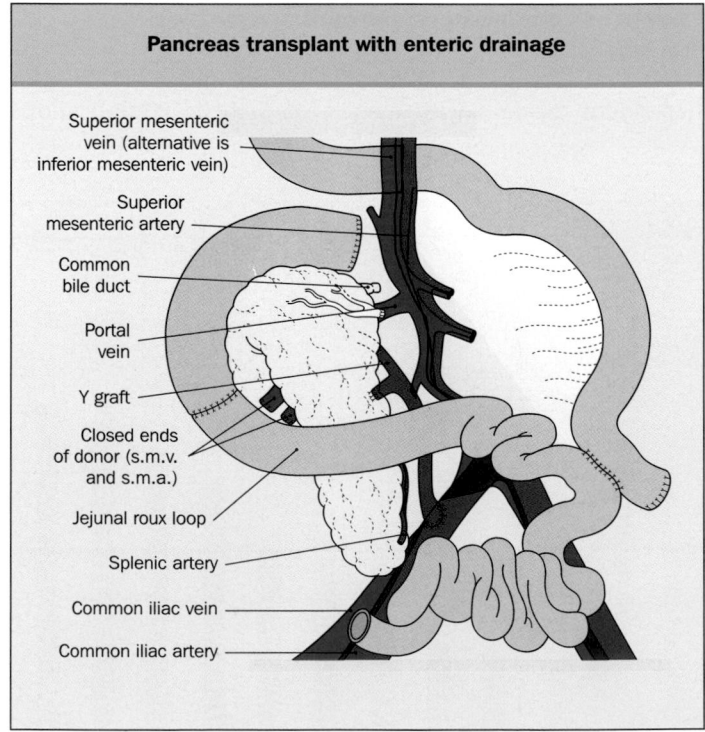

Figure 93.3 Enterically drained pancreas transplant. Portal venous drainage.

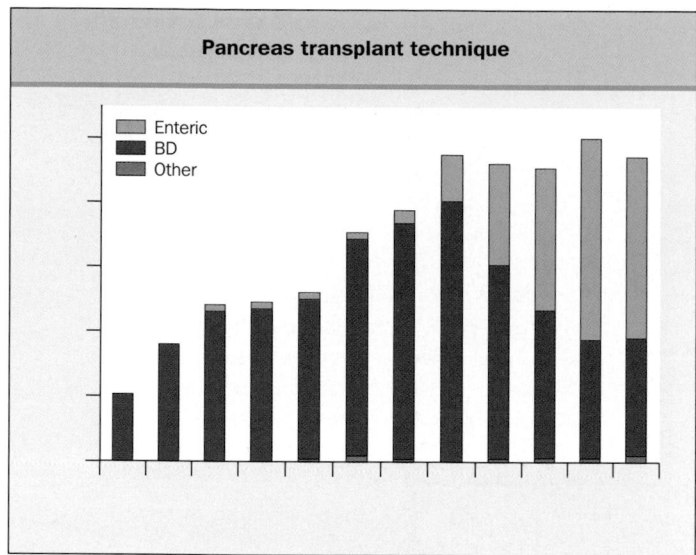

Figure 93.4 Pancreas transplant technique. There has been a shift towards performing more enterically drained transplants compared to bladder drained (BD) pancreas transplants in the last few years.

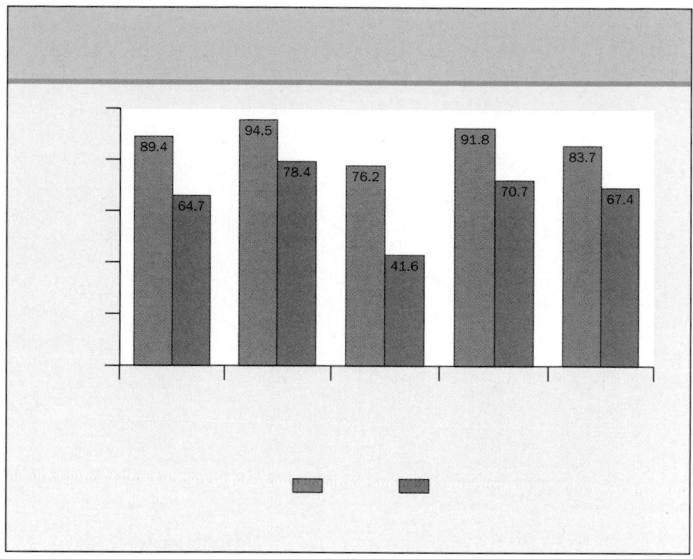

Figure 93.5 Graft Survival for kidney and pancreas transplant recipients. UNOS data: 1 year is from the 1997–1998 cohort; data from the 5 year survival rates is from the 1990–1998 cohort)

to increase graft survival. Tacrolimus in combination with mycophenolate mofetil has led to a decrease in rejection rates (20% vs. 90%) and improved 1-year pancreas survival. Finally, analysis of pancreas transplant data from UNOS registry has shown HLA matching had no effect on the outcome in SPK category while for PAK and PTA a beneficial effect was seen by matching at the A and B loci[1]. Using these techniques and criteria, the reported 1-, 3-, and 5-year patient and graft survival rates by UNOS are given in the Figures 93.5–93.7. Though pancreas transplantation is not routinely performed for type 2 diabetes mellitus because of the insulin resistance, in a retrospective review Sasaki et al. reported 13 patients who received SPK transplants and were found to be type 2 diabetics with high C-peptide level on analyzing the pre transplant

sera. With a mean follow up of 45.5 months the reported patient and pancreas graft survival were similar to the type 1 diabetic patients[4].

IMMEDIATE POSTOPERATIVE MANAGEMENT

Immunosuppression

Although immunosuppressive regimens vary, most centers currently utilize antibody induction therapy (antithymocyte globulin (ATG), thymoglobulin, or OKT3) during the first 1–2 weeks post-transplant and then continue triple drug maintenance immunosuppression with tacrolimus (or uncommonly cyclosporine), mycophenolate mofetil (or rarely azathioprine), and prednisone. Although the combination of tacrolimus,

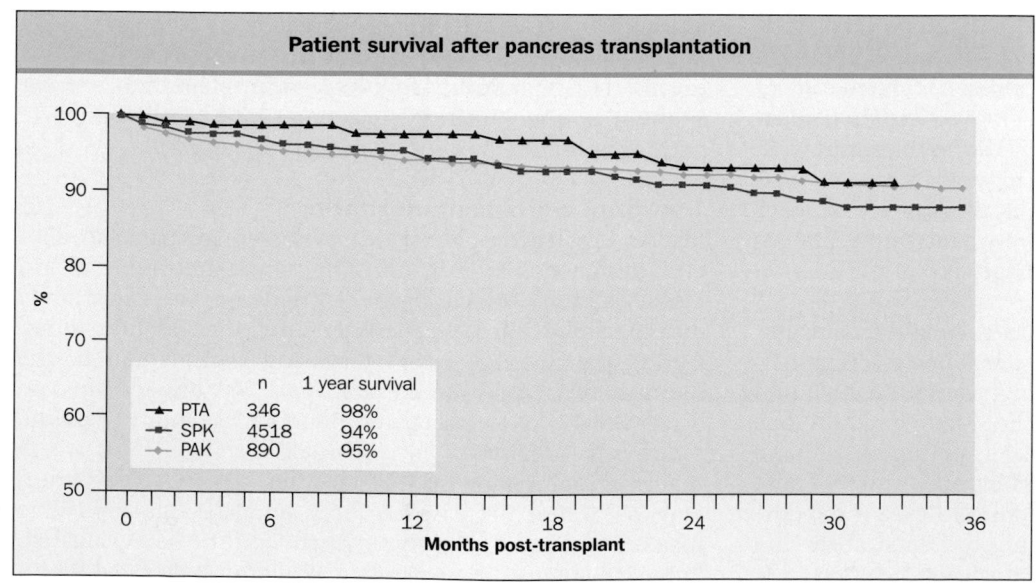

Figure 93.6 Patient survival after pancreas transplantation 1996–2001. (PTA, pancreas transplant alone; SPK, simultaneous pancreas kidney; PAK, pancreas after kidney).

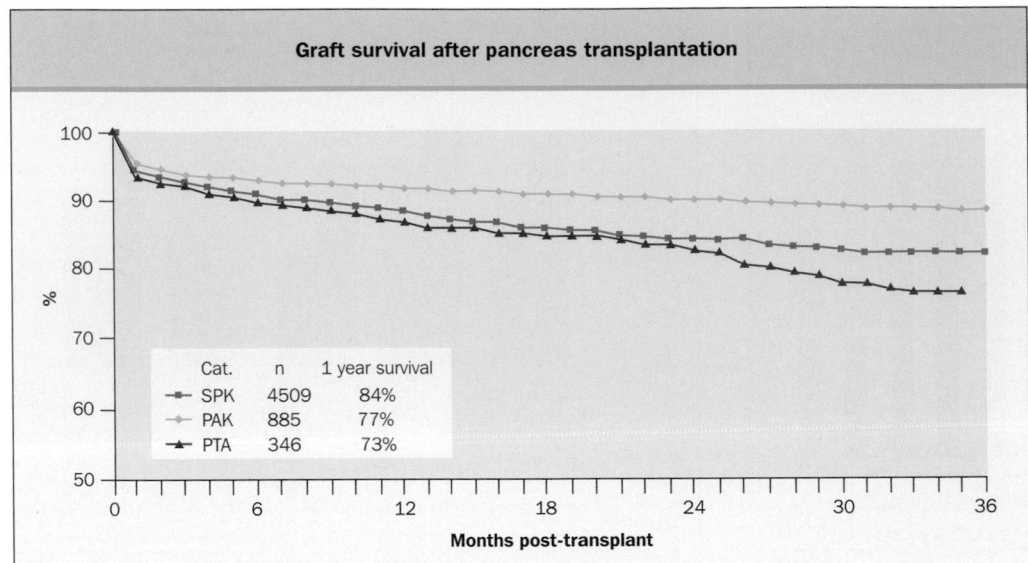

Figure 93.7 Graft survival after pancreas transplantation 1996–2001. (SPK, simultaneous pancreas and kidney; PAK, pancreas after kidney; PTA, pancreas transplant alone).

mycophenolate and prednislone is currently favored by most centers because of reduced rejection rates[5], the results of ongoing controlled trials are needed in order to determine if the benefits of decreased rejection and prolonged graft survival are not compromised by complications (infections and malignancy) resulting from this degree of immunosuppression. The use of interleukin 2 (IL-2) receptor antagonists (basiliximab, daclizumab) for induction therapy with tacrolimus, mycophenolate prednisone without antilymphocyte induction and steroid free immunosuppression using tacrolimus and sirolimus are also under evaluation[5]. During the immediate perioperative phase intravenous insulin is used to decrease the stress on the transplanted pancreas and maintain the glucose level around 100 mg/dL (5.5mmol/L). In cases of bladder drainage urinary amylase is monitored every 12 h and the trend is followed.

Pancreas allograft biopsies are now commonly performed (either cystoscopically or percutaneously), by protocol or at times of suspected dysfunction, in order to identify rejection or other causes of pancreas injury early in the process before irreversible tissue damage has occurred. The easiest approach is percutaneous biopsy using ultrasound or computed tomography scan guidance; the cystoscopic biopsy is used in bladder drained transplants in situations where the percutaneous technique is not possible because of difficult visualization or overlying bowel. The most frequent complication of percutaneous biopsy is transient hematuria, but rarely pancreatitis, arteriovenous fistula, abdominal hemorrhage, bowel perforation requiring exploration or rarely graft loss may result.

Early post-transplant, whole blood tacrolimus levels are usually maintained at 15–20 ng/mL. Cyclosporine levels are targeted around 200–250 ng/mL (by high performance liquid chromatography (HPLC) measurement). Methylprednisolone is administered intravenously immediately postoperatively and then tapered at variable rates depending upon the program. Mycophenolate is given at a standard dose of 1 g q 8 h and dose adjustments are then made according to hematologic and gastrointestinal toxicity. Mycophenolic acid levels are available by HPLC measurement but have not yet been routinely used to guide therapy. Reports of sirolimus use in pancreas recipients, notably in steroid free protocols. No guidelines for use are yet available.

Antimicrobial prophylaxis

Trimethoprim/sulfamethoxazole is given for the prevention of urinary tract infections and for *Pneumocystis*, *Legionella*, *Toxoplasma* and *Nocardia* species. It is usually given for at least 6 months following transplantation but may be administered for the lifetime of the allograft. Dosing varies from one double strength tablet per day, to one single strength tablet twice a week. Clotrimazole troches used orally, nystatin swish and swallow, or fluconazole are administered for the prevention of oral candidiasis, candidal urinary tract infections, and intra-abdominal fungal or yeast infection. Oral acyclovir (aciclovir) is given to patients with a history of herpes simplex infection and to patients who are cytomegalovirus (CMV) negative and receive CMV-negative donor organs. Valacyclovir (valaciclovir) or ganciclovir is given to all patients who are CMV-positive or who receive CMV-positive organs for 3 months following transplantation or for 3 months after treating rejection with antilymphocyte antibodies, for the prevention of CMV disease.

Transplant and patient monitoring

Bladder-drained recipients are monitored for pancreas allograft dysfunction by measuring the serum amylase level and urinary amylase excretion rate. Urinary amylase excretion is measured on 12-h collections and reported as units/hour. During the first 1–2 weeks following transplantation, the serum amylase may be elevated and the urinary amylase decreased owing to pancreatic preservation injury. Baseline serum and urinary levels are usually attained by 2 weeks following transplantation. Thereafter, an elevated serum amylase and/or decreased urinary amylase signal possible pancreas allograft injury, which must be evaluated. Enterically-drained transplants may manifest elevated serum amylase and human anodal trypsinogen levels at the time of dysfunction. The causes of pancreas allograft dysfunction and the evaluation process are shown in Tables 93.1–93.3 and Figure 93.8.

In addition to following the serum and urinary amylase, the serum creatinine, potassium, magnesium, phosphorus, and bicarbonate must be monitored closely. Hyperkalemia (secondary to calcineurin inhibitors, β-blockers, hyperglycemia) and hypomagnesemia are common and may need to be treated. Hypophosphatemia develops as a result of persistent hyperparathyroidism and/or from phosphate wasting (possibly due to the release of 'phosphatonin' (see Chapter 10)), and may require oral replacement. Of particular importance is the high urinary loss of bicarbonate in cases of bladder drainage, which may require 130 mmol daily or more replacement. Without replacement, patients develop metabolic acidosis with nausea, vomiting, and generalized fatigue and weakness, which may lead to volume loss, hypotension (exacerbated by underlying autonomic neuropathy), and graft thrombosis. Intravenous solutions of 5% dextrose in water with 50–150mmol of sodium bicarbonate may be used for repletion. Sodium bicarbonate tablets providing 8 mmol/tablet are used for oral replacement; on average four tablets four times a day are needed. Additionally, fluid intake needs to approach 2.5 to 3 L/d to accommodate pancreatic and renal fluid outputs. This volume may be difficult to consume because abdominal bloating from diabetic gastroparesis is exacerbated by large fluid intakes and the gas released from bicarbonate tablets.

Surgical complications

Pancreas transplantation may be associated with a variety of surgical complications (see Table 93.4). They are wound

Causes of pancreas graft dysfunction
Rejection
Ductal obstruction
Vascular: Arterial/venous thrombosis (Partial /complete) Arterio-venous fistula
Volume depletion
High calcineurin inhibitor levels
Graft pancreatitis (preservation, viral, bacterial, or fungal)
In cases of bladder drainage: –Reflux pancreatitis –Urinary tract infection –Anastomotic leak –Bladder outflow obstruction
In cases of enteric drainage: –Anastomotic leak –Bowel obstruction

Table 93.1 Causes of pancreas graft dysfunction.

Workup for pancreas graft dysfunction	
Assessment	Tests
Laboratory tests	Serum amylase, Blood glucose human anodal trypsinogen, Cyclosporine tacrolimus levels, C-peptide
	In bladder drained cases urinary amylase and urine culture
Doppler ultrasound	Pancreatic blood flow, peripancreatic fluid collection, pancreatic ductal dilatation
	In bladder drained cases evidence of bladder outlet obstruction
Computed tomography + cystogram	Looking for leak, and collections. This is performed by cystogram in bladder drained cases

Table 93.2 Workup for pancreatic allograft dysfunction.

Table 93.3 Diagnostic tests for pancreas transplant complications.

Diagnostic tests for pancreas transplant complications						
Tests	Leak	Rejection	Thrombosis	Obstruction	Arterio-venous fistula	Hematuria
Doppler ultrasound	+	–	+++	++	+++	+
CT cystogram (bladder drained pancreas)	+++	–	+	+	–	–
CT abdomen (bowel drained pancreas)	+++	–	++	++	±	–
Cystoscopy (bladder drained pancreas)	+	+	+	++	–	+++
Pancreas biopsy	–	+++	–	–	–	–
Magnetic resonance angiography	+	–	+++	++	++	–
Angiography	–	–	+++	–	+++	–

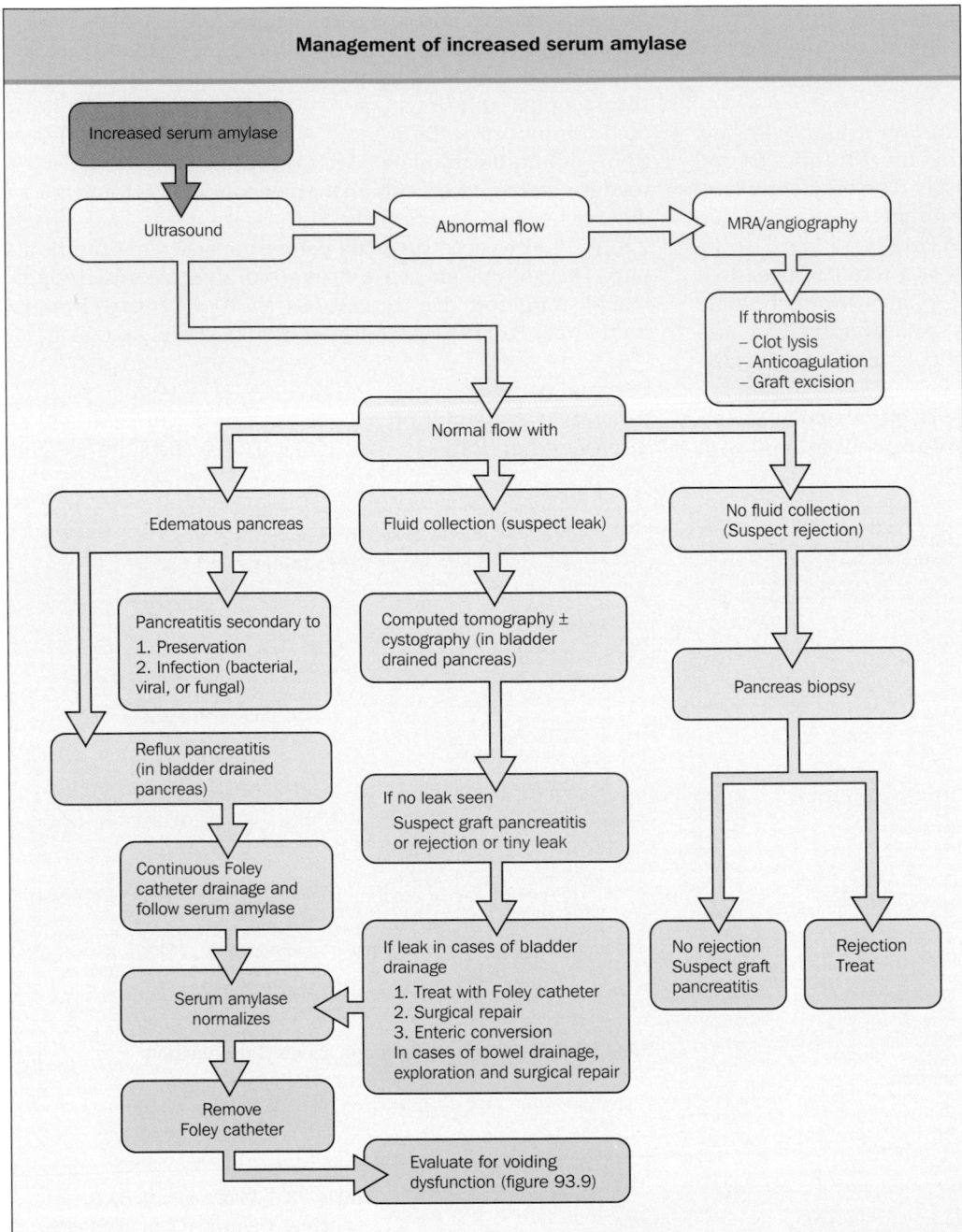

Figure 93.8 Management of increased serum amylase after pancreas transplantation.

drainage, dehiscence, superficial infections and deep-seated abscesses especially with fungi. The source of fungal contamination is thought to be the duodenal segment. Therefore, topical antibiotic solutions are used to irrigate the organ during procurement and implantation. In addition, transplant antimicrobial prophylaxis has been modified to cover possible deep-seated bacterial and fungal infections by administering up to 48 h of postoperative antibiotics and up to several months of oral fluconazole.

The causes of wound drainage are seroma, lymphocele, pancreatic fistula either from the tail or from the anastomosis to the bladder or bowel, wound dehiscence and preservation pancreatitis. Preservation pancreatitis may lead to wound drainage

of pancreatic goo, a whitish-yellow, thick, noninfectious material formed from the enzymatic digestion of tissue leading to fat necrosis and saponification; it is seen more often with the extraperitoneal placement of the pancreas and also with a fatty allograft. It is also associated with a mild increase in serum amylase, low urinary amylase excretion, and variable changes in the serum glucose.

Vascular complications occur in about 5% of patients and they include arterio-venous fistula either from the surgery or from a biopsy, venous/arterial thrombosis and rarely mycotic aneurysms. As the pancreas is a low blood flow organ, vascular thrombosis is a significant concern and hence deserves careful attempts to minimize warm and cold ischemia, procurement

Surgical complications following pancreas transplantation			
Type of complication	Presentation	Diagnostic findings and testing	Treatment options
Abscess	Fever, erythema of wound, drainage of wound	Elevated white cell count (WBC), fluid collection on CT scan, pus on aspiration	Open or percutaneous drainage
Graft pancreatitis	Pain over allograft, lower abdominal pain	Elevated serum amylase, enlarged pancreas allograft	Foley catheter if bladder drained, octreotide or somatostatin
Lymphocele	Mass on palpation, urgency if bladder compression	Fluid collection on CT scan, clear fluid on aspiration	Open or percutaneous drainage
Wound drainage	Pancreatic goo, no erythema	Culture, CT scan to rule out deep abscess	Local wound care
Dehiscence	Wound open		Wound care/surgical closure
Arterio-venous fistula	Hematuria, abdominal bleeding	Doppler ultrasound, angiography	Embolization, surgical repair
Graft thrombosis	Bloody urine if bladder drained, elevated blood sugars	Low serum and urine amylase, sepsis-like syndrome, ultrasound or magnetic resonance imaging	If partial: thrombolytic therapy or anticoagulation (high risk for bleeding), graft pancreatectomy
Pancreatic fistula/leak (bowel drained)	Pain over allograft, sepsis, peritonitis, fever	Elevated WBC, fluid collection on CT scan	Surgical drainage and repair

Table 93.4 Surgical complications following pancreas transplantation.

procedures involving a no-touch technique using the duodenum and spleen as handles, the intraoperative use of low-molecular-weight dextran and calcium channel blockers, postoperative aspirin and avoidance of hypotension. Partial thrombosis may resolve with thrombolytic therapy or anticoagulation. If the graft completely thromboses, especially in the immediate postoperative period immediate graft removal is necessary to prevent the development of a sepsis syndrome or a more diffuse hypercoagulable state, leading to further vascular thrombosis such as myocardial infarction.

Nausea and vomiting may be secondary to gastroparesis; constipation; CMV disease; medications; cholelithiasis or esophageal reflux developing from motility problems; esophagitis; or infection (see Table 93.5). Generally, regular antiemetics plus histamine H_2 blockers or proton pump inhibitors are effective therapy and are given for 2 to 3 months following transplantation. Changing the administration of mycophenolate to 500 mg q 6 h or tacrolimus to q 8 h may also decrease symptoms. Persistent symptoms may require abdominal ultrasound or endoscopy. Diarrhea can be caused by tacrolimus or mycophenolate, intrinsic gut motility problems, food intolerance, or infection. Spreading out tacrolimus and mycophenolate dosing, reviewing oral intake, and evaluating the patient for enteric pathogens or specifically for CMV may help in management. Constipation is treated with increased fluid intake, dietary modification, increased activity, and a regular low-dose schedule of stool softeners or laxatives.

Orthostatic hypotension may also occur following transplantation and is a consequence of bedrest in the presence of diabetic autonomic neuropathy; it is prevented by ensuring adequate intravenous hydration and early ambulation. Patients must not be allowed to stay in bed unless prevented by ventilatory requirements, wound complications, mental confusion, or supine hypotension.

Nausea and vomiting following pancreas transplantation	
Causes of nausea and vomiting	Treatment
Postoperative Anesthesia, pain medications, ileus, hypotension, cardiac ischemia (rarely)	Early ambulation, delay oral intake, keep nasogastic tube in place, total parenteral nutrition/hydration/bicarbonate infusion, limit pain medications, enemas, antiemetics
Gastroparesis	Metoclopramide, Ondansetron, Erythromycin i.v., hydration, limit food intake, possibly domperidone
Medications Cyclosporine and tacrolimus	Spread out dose to q6 h or q8 h
Mycophenolate mofetil	Change dosing to q6 h/decrease dose if necessary
Trimethoprim-sulfamethoxazole	Stop
Azathioprine	Look for hepatitis/pancreatitis
Metabolic acidosis: for bladder-drained pancreas recipients	Sodium bicarbonate tablets or infusion if acidemia is severe; sodium chloride tablets or infusion if volume depletion is severe
Cholelithiasis and duodenal ulcers	Ultrasound for diagnosis of gallstones and then surgery; endoscopy for diagnosis and treatment of findings
Infection Cytomegalovirus	May also cause persistent diarrhea with minimal pain, i.v. ganciclovir until antigenemia or PCR testing is negative; in recurrent disease, check for ganciclovir resistance, may administer foscarnet while monitoring serum calcium and renal function, CMV IgG(?)

Table 93.5 Postoperative and delayed nausea and vomiting following pancreas transplantation: causes and treatment.

TRANSPLANT MANAGEMENT

Maintenance immunosuppression

Targeted immunosuppressive medication levels are higher in the kidney/pancreas recipient than in patients receiving a kidney only. Whole blood cyclosporine levels for kidney/pancreas recipients are targeted around 200–250 ng/mL by 3 months, 150–200 ng/mL by 6 months, and 150 ng/mL by 1 year. Long-term goal levels are 100–125 ng/mL. Tacrolimus levels have been maintained around 15–20 ng/mL for the first post-transplant month and gradually decreased over 1–5 years to 5–10 ng/mL depending upon transplant function and symptoms of toxicity. At the higher levels of tacrolimus, patients may notice more frequent neurologic symptoms (headache, tremor) and increased blood sugar levels.

Pancreas transplant rejection

Pancreas allograft rejection in patients on cyclosporine-based immunosuppression has been found by protocol biopsy to occur in up to 46% of patients at day 21 and 56% at day 40, with a total histologic rejection rate of over 80%. With tacrolimus plus mycophenolate, this rate has dropped to about 20%. Histologically, rejection is marked by lymphocytic infiltrates of the acinar tissue and endothelitis. The islets are not infiltrated.

Markers of pancreatic rejection are an increase in the serum amylase, lipase, human anodal trypsinogen or a decrease in the urinary amylase in a bladder-drained pancreas transplant. Unfortunately, as determined by protocol biopsy studies, these tests are not sensitive early after transplantation because the same laboratory findings are present during the healing process of preservation injury. Later following transplantation, these tests are helpful for the detection of graft dysfunction but are not specific for rejection. Therefore, biopsy is suggested as a confirmatory step in the evaluation of graft dysfunction. Increased plasma glucose levels are also a marker of rejection but are a late finding in this setting. Hyperglycemia may indicate severe parenchymal loss from chronic rejection, thrombosis, or isleitis or it may result from calcineurin toxicity or insulin resistance caused by weight gain. Treatment of pancreatic rejection is similar to that used for kidney rejection and generally involves pulse steroids or antilymphocyte antibodies (see Chapter 88).

Urological complications

Urologic complications are common after bladder drainage of the pancreas allograft (Table. 93.6)[6]. Pretransplant bladder dysfunction caused by autonomic neuropathy (large capacity bladder, decreased bladder sensation, increased residual urine volume, and decreased urinary flow rates) is worsened by the 'autoaugmentation' of the bladder by the added duodenal segment and also because of poor muscle contraction and outlet dysfunction created by pelvic nerve neuropathy and weak muscle activity. However, although the preoperative

Urological complications of bladder-drained pancreas transplants				
Complication	Etiology	Presentation	Workup	Treatment options
Urinary tract infection (UTI)	Diabetic bladder dysfunction (DBD)	Asymptomatic, or dysuria, fever, sepsis	Urine culture; check postvoid residual, if elevated urodynamics	Culture-specified antibiotics, prophylactic antibiotics Female: double and timed voiding, clean intermittent catheterization (CIC) Male: α-adrenoeptor blockers to aid bladder emptying, CIC, bladder/prostate incision If treatment failure enteric conversion
Reflux pancreatitis	DBD	Asymptomatic or pain over pancreas allograft, elevated serum amylase	Check serum amylase, CT cystogram to exclude leak or duct obstruction	Foley catheter drainage If DBD: double and timed voiding, CIC, α-blockers to aid bladder emptying If multiple and symptomatic episodes: bladder/prostate incision or enteric diversion
Duodenal cystotomy leak	Ischemic injury to duodenal cuff, cytomegalovirus or other infection, rejection, DBD	Pain over allograft, or peritonitis, elevated serum amylase	Check serum amylase, elevated creatinine, leak on CT cystogram	Foley catheter, drainage, if small If early, open surgical repair with resection and closure of layers, evaluate for DBD post recovery. If late, consider enteric conversion
Urethritis/dysuria syndrome, occasional urethral disruption	UTI or DBD causing activation of pancreatic enzymes with digestion of urethral mucosa	Dysuria, urinary retention, hematuria	Check post void residual, low-grade UTI; once recovered evaluate for DBD	Foley catheter, analgesics, empiric treatment of UTI If multiple and symptomatic: enteric conversion

Table 93.6 Urological complications of bladder-drained pancreas transplants.

urodynamics are abnormal in up to 43% of patients, the urodynamic abnormalities do not predict post-transplant urologic complications such as reflux pancreatitis or infections[7].

Urine evaluation is made difficult in bladder-drained pancreas patients as it contains white cells from duodenal mucosal sloughing. This results in leukocyte esterase-positive urine without the presence of bacteriuria. Additionally, the 24-h total protein excretion is elevated to 1–3 g daily in most patients and comprises pancreatic enzymes, immunoglobulins, other globulins, albumin, and digested fragments of these proteins. Urinary albumin, if measurable in the presence of enzymatic degradation, may come from the transplanted or native kidneys.

Hematuria is seen in up to 28% of bladder-drained pancreas recipients. Early hematuria is usually related to surgical trauma to the bladder or duodenal mucosa near the cystoduodenostomy site and it usually clears with diuresis or manual bladder irrigation[6]. Caution should be exercised when using continuous bladder irrigation in pancreas recipients because the cystoduodenostomy is vulnerable to rupture if the drainage catheter becomes obstructed. Late hematuria, beyond 2–4 weeks post-transplant, can arise from anastomotic bleeding, duodenal mucosal sloughing or ulceration, reflux pancreatitis, cystitis, graft thrombosis, rarely arteriovenous fistula, and pseudoaneurysms. Evaluation should include urine culture, cystoscopy, and, possibly, bladder and/or pancreas biopsy.

Urinary tract infections

Large bladder capacity, incomplete bladder emptying, high bladder urine pH (due to pancreatic bicarbonate), bladder and urethral mucosal irritation from activated pancreatic enzymes with the loss of mucosal barrier; prolonged bladder catheterization, and immunosuppression all contribute to the increased risk of urinary tract infection following pancreatic transplantation[8]. Because of the increased risk for urinary tract infections, most centers administer oral antibacterial and antifungal prophylaxis immediately perioperatively and for up to 12 months following transplantation.

'Urinary reflux' pancreatitis, which causes pancreas allograft dysfunction, may be associated with periallograft abdominal pain and fever. It is often a result of poor bladder function. Treatment consists of bladder drainage for approximately 5–7 d with a Foley catheter and attention to the bladder dysfunction. The management of voiding dysfunction is outlined in Figure 93.9.

Pancreas recipients (2–8%) may additionally develop a urethritis dysuria syndrome caused by uroepithelial exposure to the activated pancreatic proenzymes trypsinogen, chymotrypsinogen, and procarboxypeptidase. Pancreas exocrine secretions consist of bicarbonate, amylase, lipase, and proenzymes, which are activated by the enterokinase in the allograft duodenal brush border. Increased intravesical enzyme activation occurs with low-grade urinary infections and urinary stasis. Patients develop voiding pain and/or penile, glandular, meatal or vulval ulceration. Enzyme activation may be minimized by treating even low-count bacteriuria, by markedly increasing fluid intake and by frequent voiding. In those individuals who fail to improve emptying with α-blockers, continuous Foley catheter drainage for 7–10 d has been effective. Enteric conversion is considered for recurrent or refractory episodes.

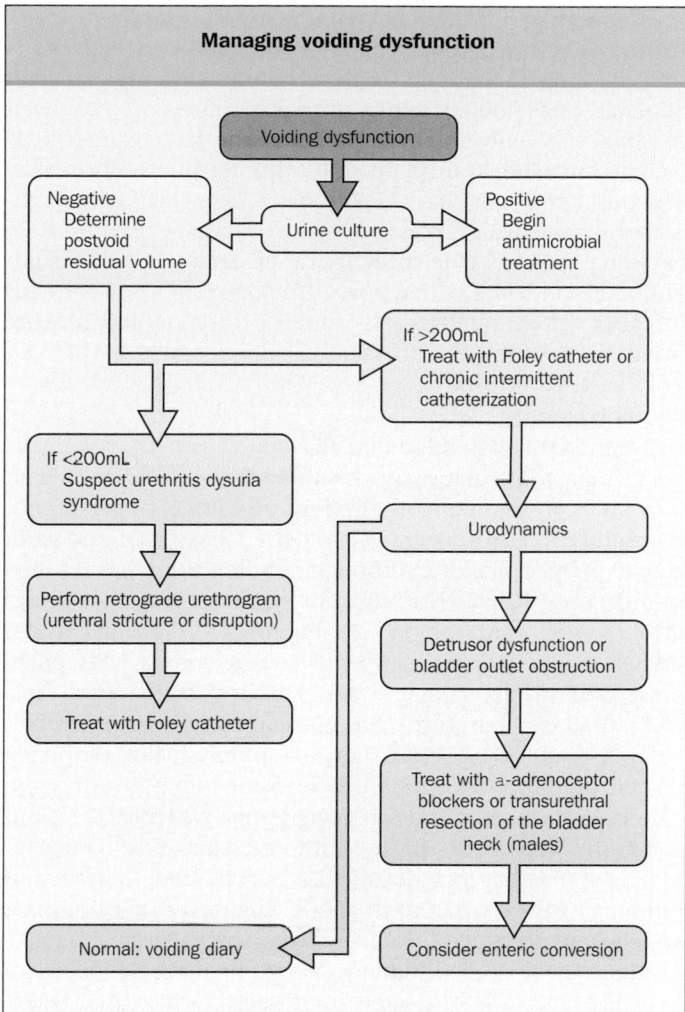

Figure 93.9 Management of post-transplant voiding abnormalities. (With permission from Kuhr et al.[6].)

Enteric conversion

This is an option for most of the chronic urologic complications associated with bladder drained pancreas transplantation. The indications are urethral disruption, recurrent urine leak, persistent bleeding, chronic UTI, dysuria, recurrent hypovolemia and metabolic acidosis. The conversion rate varies from 8–14%. It is ideal to wait until 6–12 months after transplantation, when possible, to allow monitoring of urine amylase for early rejection episodes.

THE DIABETIC CONSEQUENCES OF PANCREAS TRANSPLANTATION

Pancreatic transplantation is performed to obviate the need for exogenous insulin, eliminate the risk of severe hypoglycemic episodes, and to stop or reverse the consequences of hyperglycemia. Well-functioning pancreas transplants are found in up to 90% of patients at 1 year and result in normal fasting blood sugars, normal glycated hemoglobin levels, and only slightly abnormal oral glucose tolerance testing[9].

Hypoglycemia

Although severe hypoglycemia is rare, mild hypoglycemia may develop in patients with a well-functioning pancreas allograft once low baseline immunosuppression has been reached, especially in those patients who have gained little weight following transplant and who are physically active. The onset of hypoglycemic episodes is associated with high-carbohydrate meals, excessive intake of caffeine or alcohol, or excessive exercise. One study found evidence for anti-insulin antibodies in some patients with hypoglycemia[10]. Treatment includes eating small meals, limiting caffeine and alcohol intake, and eating prior to exercise.

Hyperglycemia

Post-transplant hyperglycemia may be caused by pancreatic graft dysfunction, inadequate insulin release secondary to high tacrolimus or, less frequently, cyclosporine levels, or a resistance to insulin effect secondary to steroid use, weight gain, and inadequate physical activity. Although tacrolimus use has resulted in a decrease in pancreas allograft rejection, it also decreases insulin gene transcription, leading to a decline in insulin mRNA production. Evaluation of hyperglycemia is as previously outlined for pancreas allograft dysfunction (see Table 93.2). If all of these studies are normal, then hyperglycemia is likely a result of decreased insulin output and/or peripheral insulin resistance, which can be identified by measuring glucose utilization rates and glucose/arginine-potentiated insulin secretion. Treatment of nonimmunologic post-transplant hyperglycemia has included dietary intervention; exercise; and minimizing the tacrolimus dose or changing it to cyclosporine, and, when necessary, insulin, or oral hypoglycemic agents. Insulin may be needed initially depending upon the degree of hyperglycemia but can often be discontinued as oral hypoglycemic agents begin to take effect. Sulfonylureas are very effective therapy. Hyperglycemia secondary to rejection is a late event and indicates the irreversible nature of the damage.

Retinopathy

In a 10-year follow-up study of SPK patients, diabetic retinopathy showed stabilization in 75%, improvement in 14% and progression in 10%[11]. Cataracts of all types increased after transplantation while visual acuity may improve. In the postoperative period patients may develop neoproliferation and retinal hemorrhages if blood glucose control is very poor at the time of surgery and blood sugars normalize rapidly following the transplant. Patients continue to remain at risk for retinal detachment because of the scarring present secondary to previous retinal damage.

Neuropathy

Sensory and motor nerve conduction velocities improve rapidly following transplantation and then stabilize[12]. The largest degree of recovery is seen in nonobese, younger, shorter patients and those not on dialysis at transplantation. The recovery of action potential amplitudes is slow, continues to improve over years, and is most notable beyond 5 years from transplantation. Recovery is more complete in sensory than in motor nerves. More improvement is noted in nonobese patients, those with better initial amplitudes, and, perhaps, with the use of nifedipine and ACE inhibitors for the treatment of hypertension[12].

Improved autonomic reactivity to changing position and respiratory rate variation in addition to stabilization or improvement in gastric emptying is noted in pancreas/kidney recipients compared with kidney-only diabetic transplant recipients[13]. However, many patients will remain orthostatic, develop progressive gastroparesis, and continue to demonstrate bladder dysfunction. If symptoms are severe at the time of pancreas transplantation, improvement is unlikely.

Nephropathy

Early diabetic nephropathy is characterized by increased glomerular basement membrane thickness and an increase in mesangial volume. Renal transplant biopsies in diabetics with kidney/pancreas and kidney-only transplants within 2.5 years of transplant show glomerular basement membrane thickness to be within the normal range[14]. After 2.5 years from transplant, 91.7% of the biopsies from the kidney/pancreas recipients have a normal glomerular basement membrane thickness compared with only 35.3% of the biopsies in the kidney-only group, while relative mesangial volume was normal in 81.8% of the biopsies from pancreas/kidney recipients compared with only 11.8% in the kidney-only recipients[15]. Therefore, concurrent pancreas transplantation decreases the occurrence of the changes of diabetic nephropathy that may result in allograft loss[14].

Vascular disease

Successful kidney pancreas transplantation results in a significant improvement in the control of hypertension compared to kidney transplant alone in type 1 diabetics[16]. Peripheral vascular disease has been reported to increase in kidney/pancreas compared with kidney-alone transplant recipients[17]. Conversely, in another study using intravital microscopic evaluation of nailbeds and conjunctival vasculature, improved vascularization (as assessed by a reduction in venular diameter, increased number of arterioles per unit area, and elevation of the perfusion capacity) was found only in the kidney/pancreas recipients[18]. Another study found a 14% incidence of peripheral vascular disease as determined by duplex Doppler ultrasonography over 1–8 years following pancreas transplant, which was comparable to the rate seen in diabetic kidney-only recipients who refused pancreas transplant for nonmedical reasons and in nondiabetic renal transplant recipients[19]. Despite reducing atherosclerotic risk factors pancreas transplantation has failed to halt the progression of macrovascular disease[20, 21].

Quality-of-life and social issues

Pancreas transplantation is a very stressful event. It taxes even the strongest of family relationships as many of the patients not only need significant postoperative care (dressing changes, catheterizations, intravenous medication administration, frequent clinic visits) but also assistance with pretransplant debilities that may be exacerbated by the surgery and immunosuppressive medications (decreased vision, neuropathy, muscle weakness, orthostatic symptoms). The presence and degree of social support must be assessed pretransplant and nurtured after, as it has been shown that those patients who smoke, drink, and are without family support do not survive as long following transplantation.

However, kidney/pancreas transplant recipients with social support and well-functioning allografts report an increased global quality of life and frequently return to work, although the number returning to work is not much different from that in those receiving a kidney transplant only[22]. They report less fatigue, nausea, and pruritus, and fewer painful joints; they also have less need for physical and emotional support.

Pregnancy following pancreas transplantation

Within 1 year of transplantation, menstruation and ovulation return in most women of childbearing age, making pregnancy possible following kidney/pancreas transplantation. National Transplantation Pregnancy Registry has reported 36 pregnancies in 27 patients[23]. The outcomes were 31 live births, therapeutic and spontaneous abortions three each (one twin reduction) and one ectopic twin pregnancy. The newborn outcomes were prematurity (24/31), low birth weight (20/31), newborn complications (17/31) and neonatal death (1/31). Six patients had rejections losing the graft (four kidneys, two pancreas and kidney) and 50% of the patients required Cesarean section. Optimal outcome was seen when the mother had a serum creatinine < 1.5 mg/dL at the beginning of pregnancy. Even with good renal function, hypertension, prematurity, pre-eclampsia, and growth retardation frequently complicated the pregnancies. Urinary tract infections occurred in up to 73% of pregnant pancreas recipients. To prevent rejection, cyclosporine levels, which often decline during pregnancy, require close monitoring. Cesarean section is the most common method of delivery although it is not mandatory; vaginal deliveries, however, must be observed for signs of allograft duodenal rupture. The average gestational period is 35 ± 2 weeks; the average birth weight is 2150 ± 680 g. To date, most children have developed normally.

Birth control, an important but rarely discussed topic, should be managed as for the renal transplant recipient. Condom use is safe; however, diaphragms, cuffs, and sponges may increase the risk for urinary tract infections. Intrauterine devices may not be effective because of the decreased inflammatory response imposed by immunosuppressive medications and is associated with an increased risk for tubal pregnancy. Hormonal therapy (pills and injections) is effective and safe even though there are theoretical risks for thrombotic complications and alterations in cyclosporine levels.

Medical issues like osteoporosis, lipoprotein abnormalities, cardiovascular complications, infections and malignancy specific to transplantation are similar in pancreas and kidney only transplant recipients. A review of these issues is in Chapter 89. However, there is an increased risk of post-transplant lymphoproliferative disorder due to the enhanced amount of the immunosuppression compared to kidney only protocols.

ISLET CELL TRANSPLANTATION

Historical perspective

Human allogeneic islet transplantation was rarely successful until recently (Fig 93.10)[24] and the recent (since 1990) successes in many instances have been only partial and associated with nonconventional immunosuppressive regimens.

Gores et al.[25] reported two successful instances of islet transplantation (out of six attempts) in type 1 diabetic recipients who received a simultaneous cadaveric kidney transplant. These patients, while euglycemic, had mildly elevated HbA1c levels. Partial success has also been demonstrated as the reduction of exogenous insulin requirements (not total independence)[26]. In patients with reduced insulin requirements, fewer episodes of hypoglycemic unawareness have been noted. Recently, reports of greater success in allogeneic islet transplantation by the Edmonton group have renewed interest in islet transplantation as a viable therapeutic option for patients with diabetes[27]. In their updated report, of the 17 preuremic diabetic patients transplanted with allogeneic islets 85% achieved insulin independence at 1 year and 80% (four out of five patients) were insulin free at 2 years[28].

A close analysis of the successes and failures in both autologous and allogeneic islet transplantation sheds light on the reasons for the unprecedented success of the Edmonton experience. The low cure rates associated with allogeneic islet transplantation were in stark contrast to the success reported with autologous islet transplantation (8% vs. 75% insulin independence at 1 year)[29]. In the autologous setting, recipient transplanted with > 250 000 islets achieved a persistent euglycemic state (70–80%) and normal HbA1c levels[30]. However, in the cadaveric setting the islet yield is lower[36] with increased immunogenicity[31] and an increased number

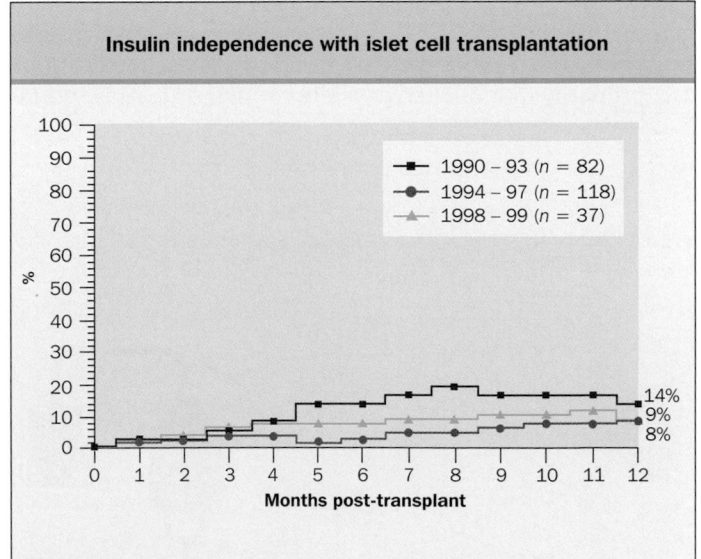

Figure 93.10 One-year insulin independence with islet cell transplantation type-1 diabetic recipients with negative C peptide levels; 1990–1999; n = 237*. (International Islet Transplant Registry Newsletter No. 9, Vol. 8 (No.1, June), 2001.

of islets per body mass are needed for success, supporting the importance of pancreas preservation, islet isolation techniques, islet toxicity of immunosuppressive drugs[32] and the immune response/ inflammation[32] in the decreased success of the allogeneic tissue. With refined islet isolation and purification methods becoming widely applicable, a considerable increase in the number and success of clinical islet transplants has occurred. The 1999, islet Transplant Registry (ITR) report[29] concluded that establishment of insulin independence after islet transplantation was associated with the following factors: (1) pancreatic preservation times ≤ 8 h, (2) islet mass transplanted is adjusted to body weight (≥ 6000 islet equivalents per kilogram of body weight (IE/kg)), (3) intrahepatic transplantation, and (4) induction with monoclonal or polyclonal T-cell antibodies. In the ITR report, one-third of islet allograft recipients with type 1 diabetes who were C-peptide–negative before transplant met all of these characteristics. A total of 48% of these patients showed basal C-peptide levels of 0.5 ng/mL, 73% had HbA1c levels ≤ 7%, and 22% were insulin independent at 1 year follow-up. Insulin independent and -dependent recipients did not differ in age, body mass index, duration of diabetes, pretransplant HbA1c level or insulin requirements, or age of the cadaveric pancreas donor.

The current technique of islet transplant involves isolation of the islets in the laboratory immediately after procurement, standardization of the islet counts, and percutaneously injecting sterile islets into the liver through the portal vein by a catheter placed under radiographic guidance. Though accessing the portal vein percutaneously is relatively invasive, the entire procedure can be performed as an outpatient (Figure 93.11).

Toxicity of standard immunosuppressive agents on islets

Tacrolimus, cyclosporine, and prednisone are clearly diabetogenic through properties that increase peripheral insulin resistance or by direct islet cell toxicity[32]. These medications are primarily administered orally, which increases portal venous drug concentrations and the possibility of significant injury to intrahepatic islet allografts. To circumvent this problem, many programs have developed steroid-free and calcineurin inhibitor-sparing protocols for islet and/or kidney recipients using different combinations of mycophenolate and sirolimus. Mycophenolate has been shown to reduce early renal and pancreas rejection rates[33]. Edmonton's success in Islet alone transplants using low dose tacrolimus, sirolimus, and daclizamab seem to confirm that low-dose immunosuppression protocols will be important in preventing islet toxicity and exhaustion[27]. Anti-T-cell therapy using ATG or OKT3 is associated with increased cytokine release which is toxic to the islets and hence the newer induction agents (anti-IL2 receptor blockers) may be particularly useful as they do not release large amounts of cytokines[34].

Impact of cytokines on islet function

Cytokines influence multiple cellular processes from cell maturation to cytotoxicity. Increased cytokine expression is associated with rejection, graft-versus-host disease, and immune-mediated islet injury. Macrophage products (IL-1, IL-6, TNF-α, and nitric oxide) have been shown to be primary mediators of transplanted islet dysfunction. During islet cell isolation procedures and subsequent implantation, cytokines (IL-1, IFN-α -gamma, and TNF-α) are released by passenger leukocytes and Kupffer cells within the liver. Interleukin-ß, IL-6, TNF-α, and C-reactive protein have been shown to be elevated after intraportal islet transplantation[35]. Furthermore, TNF-α potentiates the activity of other cytokines with regard to islet cytotoxicity. Standard T cell cytolytic immunosuppression is also associated with a 'cytokine storm' phenomenon.

Factors associated with success of the Edmonton protocol

The Edmonton protocol addresses many of the barriers discussed above[27]. Success was associated with use of a steroid-free and calcineurin inhibitor sparing immunosuppression

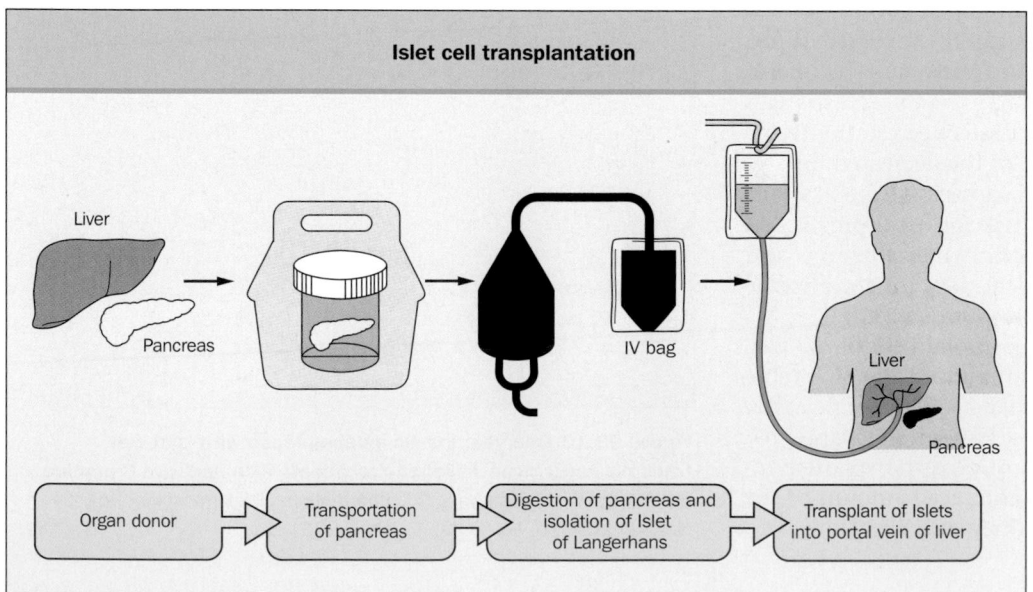

Figure 93.11 Islet cell transplantation.

Islet cell transplantation

Liver

Pancreas

IV bag

Liver

Pancreas

Organ donor → Transportation of pancreas → Digestion of pancreas and isolation of Islet of Langerhans → Transplant of Islets into portal vein of liver protocol. Induction involved use of interleukin-2 receptor antibodies. The use of experienced pancreas procurement teams, rapid pancreas processing using the Ricordi chamber, use of Librase® (an endotoxin free collagenase) all helped diminish islet preservation injury. Furthermore, transplantation of a predetermined maximal islet mass (11 547 ± 1604 IE/kg) assured adequate function to cure. Thus, a less 'islet toxic' immunosuppression protocol, in conjunction with rapid transplantation of a sufficient islet mass, can result in achievement of a persistent euglycemic state in 'ideal' diabetic recipients. However, in the Edmonton protocol, for every patient cured, usually two to three pancreases were transplanted. Furthermore, many islet isolations were unsuccessful. In contrast, pancreas transplantation requires only one donor. If an adequate number of islets per pancreas with a single processing event could enable one to donor can culminate in one successful transplant, then this procedure would surely replace pancreas transplantation. There are approximately 1 million islets per pancreas, currently pancreas preservation and islet isolation techniques enable recovery of fewer than half[29,30]. One technique that may help obviate this problem is preservation of the pancreas after retrieval with the two-layer method (TLM) prior to islet isolation. This technique provides for continued oxygenation of the pancreas by floating the organ on the interface of two fluid layers of differing density. The more dense fluid layer, perfluorocarbon, carries oxygen in solution. The less dense layer, University of Wisconsin (UW) preservation solution, is currently used for preservation of solid organs. When pancreases are preserved by the TLM before islet isolation, yields are increased when compared to storage in conventional UW solution in both canine and human 24-h preservation models[36].

Islet transplantation: current status

The Edmonton protocol has resulted in unprecedented success in which 85% of patients remain euglycemic and insulin independent at 1 year. However, this protocol has been applied to a select, relatively healthy and low weight group of patients receiving islets from a very select group of donors. Typically, candidates for pancreas or islet transplantation have progressive complications of diabetes, with proteinuria and/or deteriorating renal function or severe hypoglycemic unawareness. The Edmonton trial was successful in 'non-uremic' patients, and it is expected that variations of this strategy can also be applied to those requiring a kidney transplant or those who have had a previous kidney transplant. Clearly, we will need a better understanding of the long-term success rates donor utilization, and cost and risk to benefit ratio as compared with pancreas transplantation.

REFERENCES

1. Gruessner AC, Sutherland DE. Analysis of US and non-US pancreas transplants reported to the United network for organ sharing (UNOS) and the non-US cases reported to the international pancreas transplant registry (IPTR). Clinical Transplantation. 2001;41–72.
2. Manske DL, Thomas W, Wang Y, Wilson RF. Screening diabetic transplant candidates for coronary artery disease: identification of a low risk subgroup. Kidney Int. 1993;44:617–21.
3. Stratta RJ, Gaber O, et al. A 9-year experience with 126 pancreas transplants with portal enteric drainage. Arch Surg. 2001; 136:1141–9.
4. Sasaki TM, Gray RS, Ratner RE, et al. Successful long-term kidney–pancreas transplants in diabetic subjects with high C peptide levels. Transplantation. 1998;65(11):1510–12.
5. McAlister VC, Gao Z, Peltekian K, et al. Sirolimus-tacrolimus combination immunosuppression. Lancet. 2000;355:376–7.
6. Kuhr CS, Lin DW, Marsh CL. Pancreas transplantation and associated urologic complications. Contemp Urol. July 1998;76–84.
7. Taylor RJ, Mays SD, Grothe TJ, Stratta RJ. Correlation of preoperative urodynamic findings to postoperative complications following pancreas transplantation. J Urol. 1993;150:1185
8. Smets YF, Pijl JW van der, Dissel JT van, et al. Infectious disease complications of simultaneous pancreas kidney transplantation. Nephrol Dial Transplant. 1997;12:764–71.
9. Robertson RP, Sutherland DE, Kendall DM, et al. Metabolic characterization of long term successful pancreas transplants in type I diabetes. J Invest Med. 1996;44:549–55.
10. Tran MP, Larsen JL, Duckworth WC, et al. Anti-insulin antibodies are a cause of hypoglycemia following pancreas transplantation. Diabetes Care. 1994;17:988–93.
11. Chow VC, Pai RP, Chapman JR, et al. Diabetic retinopathy after combined kidney-pancreas transplantation. Clin Transplant. 1999; 4:356–62.
12. Allen RD, Al Harbi IS, Morris JG, et al. Diabetic neuropathy after pancreas transplantation: determinants of recovery. Transplantation. 1997;63:830–8.
13. Hathaway DK, Abell T, Cardoso S, et al. Improvement in autonomic and gastric function following pancreas-kidney versus kidney-alone transplantation and the correlation with quality of life. Transplantation. 1994;57:816–22.
14. Fioretto P, Steffes MW, Sutherland DER, et al. Reversal of lesions of diabetic nephropathy after pancreas transplantation. N Engl J Med. 1998;339:69–75.
15. Hariharan S, Smith RD, Viero R, First MR. Diabetic nephropathy after renal transplantation. Clinical and pathologic features. Transplantation. 1996;62:632–5.
16. Elliot MD, Kapoor A, Parker MA, et al. Improvement in hypertension in patients with diabetes mellitus after kidney/pancreas transplantation. Circulation. 2001;104:563–9.
17. Morrissey PE, Shaffer D, Monaco AP, Conway P, Madras PN. Peripheral vascular disease after kidney-pancreas transplantation in diabetic patients with end-stage renal disease. Arch Surg. 1997; 132:358–61.
18. Cheung AT, Chen PC, Leshchinsky TV, et al. Improvement in conjuctival microangiopathy after simultaneous pancreas-kidney transplants. Transplant Proc. 1997;29:660–1.
19. Kausz A, Brunzell J, Marcovina S, et al. Lipid profile and peripheral vascular disease among diabetic patients receiving kidney-pancreas or kidney transplants. J Am Soc Nephrol. 1998;9:A680.
20. Florina P, Rocca E La, Venturini M, et al. Effects of kidney-pancreas transplantation on atherosclerotic risk factors and endothelial function in patients with uremia and type 1 diabetes. Diabetes. 2001;50:496–501.
21. Nankivell BJ, Lau SG, Chapman JR, et al. Progression of macrovascular disease after pancreas transplantation. Transplantation. 2000;69(4):574–81.

22. Adang EM, Engel GL, Hooff JP van, Kootstra G. Comparison before and after transplantation of pancreas-kidney and pancreas-kidney with loss of pancreas: a prospective, controlled quality of life study. Transplantation. 1996;62:754–8.

23. Wilson GA. Coscia LA, McGrory CH. National Transplantation Pregnancy Registry: Postpregnancy Graft Loss among female pancreas-kidney recipients. Transpl Proc. 2001;33:1667–9.

24. International Islet transplant registry. Newsletter 9, 2001;8(1).

25. Gores PF, Najarian JS, et al. Insulin independence in type I diabetes after transplantation of unpurified islets from single donor with 15-deoxyspergualin. Lancet. 1993;341:19–21.

26. Meyer C, Hering BJ, et al. Improved glucose counterregulation and autonomic symptoms after intraportal islet transplants alone in patients with long-standing type I diabetes mellitus. Transplantation. 1998;66:233–40.

27. Shapiro AM, Lakey JR, et al. Islet transplantation in seven patients with type 1 diabetes mellitus using a glucocorticoid-free immunosuppressive regimen. N Engl J Med. 2000;343:230–8.

28. Shapiro A M, Ryan E A, Lakey J R. Diabetics islet cell transplantation. Lancet. 2001;358:S21.

29. Hering B, Brendel M, et al. International Islet Transplant Registry Newsletter 1999; 8:2–23. Giessen, Germany: Justus-Liebig University of Giessen.

30. Pyzdrowski KL, Kendall DM, et al. Preserved insulin secretion and insulin independence in recipients of islet autografts. N Engl J Med. 1992;327:220–6.

31. Takada M, Nadeau K, et al. Effects of explosive brain death on cytokine activation of peripheral organs in the rat. Transplantation. 1998;65:1533–42.

32. Drachenberg CB, Klassen DK, et al. Islet cell damage associated with tacrolimus and cyclosporine: morphological features in pancreas allograft biopsies and clinical correlation. Transplantation. 1999;68:396–402.

33. Gruessner R, Sutherland D, et al. Mycophenolate mofetil in pancreas transplantation. Transplantation. 1998;66:318–23.

34. Scoulillou J, Cantarovich D, et al. Randomized controlled trial of a monoclonal antibody against the interleukin-2 receptor (33B3.1) as compared with rabbit antithymocyte globulin for prophylaxis against rejection of renal allografts. N Engl J Med. 1990;322:1172–75.

35. Hao LM, Wang Y, et al. Role of lymphokine in islet allograft rejection. Transplantation. 1990;49:609–14.

36. Matsumoto S, Qually S, et al. Prolonged preservation of the human pancreas prior to islet isolation using the two-layer (University of Wisconsin solution (UW)/Perfluorocarbon) method. Transplantation. 2000;69:S213.

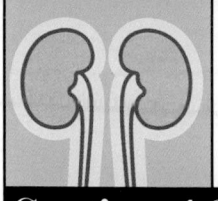

Chapter 94

Renal Disease in Liver, Cardiac, Lung, and Bone Marrow Transplantation

Connie I Davis and Michael J Ryan

LIVER TRANSPLANTATION

Renal disease before liver transplantation

Glomerular disease

Renal biopsy and autopsy studies have confirmed that many patients with end-stage liver disease (ESLD) have glomerular abnormalities (Table 94.1)[1,2]. In addition to hepatitis C virus (HCV) associated-cryoglobulinemic membranoproliferative glomerulonephritis (MPGN; see Chapter 23) and hepatitis B virus (HBV) associated-membranous nephropathy, other glomerular diseases have been reported. Patients with ESLD of any etiology may develop a lesion resembling IgA

Diseases requiring both liver and kidney transplantation	
Idiopathic or alcoholic cirrhosis Hepatic sclerosis *Infectious diseases* Hepatitis C* 　Membranoproliferative glomerulonephritis 　Membranous nephropathy 　Fibrillary glomerulonephritis 　Diabetic nephropathy 　Liver failure in HCV infected hemodialysis patients Hepatitis B 　Membranous nephropathy 　Membranoproliferative glomerulonephritis 　Polyarteritis nodosa 　Liver failure in infected hemodialysis patients Schistosomiasis *Systemic diseases* Primary biliary cirrhosis* 　Membranous nephropathy 　ANCA positive vasculitis 　Renal tubular acidosis Sarcoidosis * 　Interstitial granulomas 　Tubulointerstitial nephritis 　Nephrolithiasis 　Renal tubular acidosis Ulcerative colitis 　Membranous nephropathy 　Membranoproliferative glomerulonephritis Autoimmune hepatitis 　Membranous nephropathy 　Renal tubular acidosis	*Congenital diseases* Polycystic liver disease* 　Polycystic kidney disease Primary hyperoxaluria* 　Interstitial fibrosis Alagille's syndrome (arteriohepatic dysplasia) 　Renal dysplasia 　Mesangiolipidosis 　Cystic disease 　Tubulointerstitial nephritis 　Membranous nephropathy Alpha-1 anti-trypsinogen deficiency 　Membranoproliferative glomerulonephritis 　Antiglomerular basement membrane disease Congenital hepatic fibrosis 　Nephronopthisis 　Autosomal recessive polycystic kidney disease Cystinosis Glycogen storage disease type 1 　Focal glomerulosclerosis Tyrosinemia 　Fanconi's syndrome 　Glomerulosclerosis 　Interstitial nephritis and fibrosis Wilson's disease 　Fanconi's syndrome *Other* Pregnancy 　Toxemia 　Acute fatty liver Toxin/drug induced 　Acetaminophen 　Antineoplastic agents 　　TTP like syndrome–mitomicin C 　*Amanita phalloides* 　Carbon tetrachloride 　Elemental phosphorus 　Methoxyflurane 　Tetracyclines

*Most common.
ANCA, antineutrophil cytoplasmic antibodies.

Table 94.1 Diseases requiring both liver and kidney transplantation. Many of the liver diseases are associated with more than one renal pathological process.

nephropathy (see Chapter 24) or 'hepatic glomerulosclerosis'. The latter is a MPGN-type of lesion with splitting of the capillary basement membranes, segmental or mesangial sclerosis, occasionally with IgM and IgA deposition, and with subendothelial widening noted by electron microscopy[1]. Despite the frequency of glomerular abnormalities noted by biopsy, microscopic hematuria and low-grade proteinuria are observed in less than 20% of all patients with ESLD and less than 40% of patients with HCV-associated ESLD. The nephrotic syndrome occurs in less than 2%[3].

Acute renal failure

Patients with ESLD awaiting orthotopic liver transplantation (OLT) often have renal insufficiency usually as the result of hepatorenal syndrome (HRS) (see Chapter 16) or acute tubular necrosis (ATN). ATN may be precipitated by infection, bleeding, or radiocontrast studies and is associated with increased illness severity. HRS has been reported in 5% of children and 10–15% of adults awaiting OLT. Treatment of HRS is discussed in detail in Chapter 16. Acute renal failure (ARF) may also accompany the fulminant hepatic failure associated with ingestion of *Amanita* mushrooms carbon tetrachloride poisoning, and acetaminophen (paracetamol) overdose.

Pretransplant dialysis is required in 10 to 20% of patients with HRS; overall dialysis rates have increased from 2 to 4% due to prolonged waiting times since 1995, with some studies reporting pretransplant dialysis rates of up to 16%. Ultrafiltration is often not well tolerated because of peripheral vasodilatation and shunting caused by ESLD. Intermittent dialyses may also lead to transient increases in intracranial pressure as a result of osmotic shifts and decreased perfusion pressure. This is of most concern in patients with fulminant hepatic failure, in which intracranial pressures are often elevated. These patients are best treated with continuous slow dialysis therapies when the standard indications for dialysis are met (continuous venovenous or continuous arteriovenous hemofiltration (CVVH or CAVH) or peritoneal dialysis). In patients with fulminant hepatic failure intracranial pressure (ICP) should be monitored, and dialysis should be discontinued if the ICP increases to over 30–40 mmHg (normal ICP is < 10 mmHg). Cerebral perfusion pressures should be maintained over 60 mmHg; a head up position with less than 20° elevation and cooling by lowering the circuit temperature may help. Although patients requiring pretransplant dialysis more often require ICU care than those without renal failure, preoperative dialysis is not uniformly associated with decreased post-transplant survival[4].

Renal disease occurring early after liver transplantation

ARF within 30 days of transplantation is often seen in those with poor preoperative renal function, preoperative HRS, poor liver allograft function, induction with cyclosporine or tacrolimus, other nephrotoxin use (e.g., amphotericin B), and/or reoperation for bleeding. Between 5 and 15% of patients require dialysis for 2–6 weeks after transplantation, and this increases to 35% in those with pre-existing HRS. The requirement for dialysis increases post transplant mortality. Post-transplant CVVH is associated with higher mortality than intermittent hemodialysis likely due to patient selection[4]. Permanent end-stage renal disease (ESRD) following post-transplant ARF develops in approximately 15% of patients secondary to multiple post-transplant medical complications[4].

Avoiding early calcineurin inhibitor toxicity helps to prevent perioperative ARF. Such toxicity is minimized by withholding calcineurin inhibitors completely until renal function improves and avoiding intravenous tacrolimus. Immunosuppression is initiated with antilymphocyte products, corticosteroids, and mycophenolate mofetil. Sirolimus has also been used in this setting, although the experience is limited.

The hemolysis syndrome associated with an ABO-incompatible transplant

Hemolysis causing ARF may occur in an A or B blood group liver recipient of an O type (universal donor) organ due to passenger lymphoid tissue that is capable of producing anti-A or anti-B antibodies. Anti-A or anti-B antibodies are usually detected between 10 and 25 days after transplantation but then resolve spontaneously[5]. Treatment of hemolysis consists of plasma exchange, urinary alkalinization, and the use of type O blood for transfusion.

Patients likely to die within 24 h without transplantation may be given an ABO-incompatible liver allograft as final therapy or more often as a bridge to a permanent ABO-compatible graft. These patients may also develop ARF due to hemolysis as well as hepatic failure caused by host antibodies binding to recipient hepatocytes. Treatment consists of plasma exchange to maintain the anti-A or anti-B antibody titer at less than 1 : 8. In most patients, this is adequate to provide a safe and functioning bridge to permanent transplantation.

Renal disease occurring late after liver transplantation

Natural history of renal function

A reduction in glomerular filtration rate (GFR) to approximately 60 mL/min per 1.73 m² occurs within 3 months of transplantation and is attributed to cyclosporine or tacrolimus use[6] (Fig. 94.1). This level of renal function is maintained in most patients over the next 5 to 10 years. Patients with HRS prior to transplantation recover renal function post-transplant but require more post-transplant dialysis treatments and a longer hospitalization[6]. Up to 16% of patients requiring perioperative dialysis develop ESRD within a few years of transplantation[4]. Historically, patients with pretransplant HRS and in particular, HRS requiring dialysis within 6 weeks of OLT, have had the highest risk of long-term ESRD (11.4% HRS vs 4.4% no-HRS at 13 years)[7].

Calcineurin inhibitor toxicity

Chronic cyclosporine or tacrolimus use is the most frequent cause of long-term renal dysfunction and is associated with progressive interstitial fibrosis and arteriolar hyalinosis (see Chapter 88). In patients with cyclosporine toxicity, targeting lower calcineurin inhibitor levels (50–75 ng/mL for cyclosporine and less than 5 ng/mL for tacrolimus) coupled with increased doses of other immunosuppressive agents may be helpful. Conversion of cyclosporine to mycophenolate monotherapy is not recommended due to the increased risk

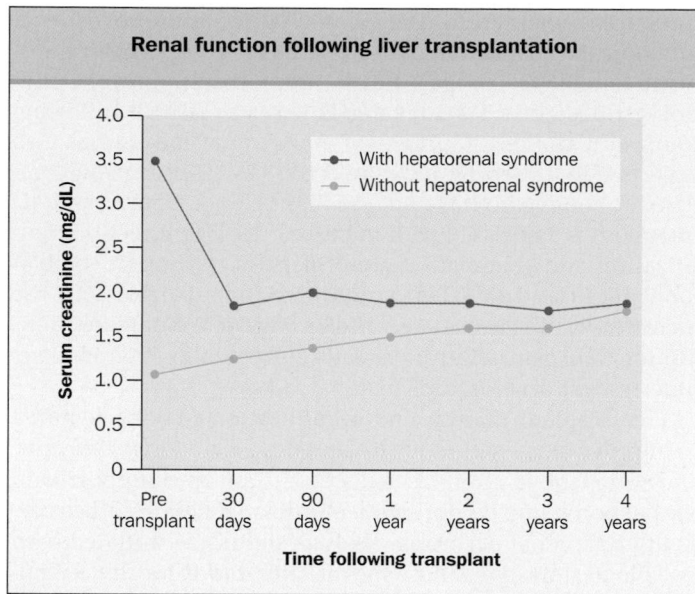

Figure 94.1 Renal function following liver transplantation in patients with or without hepatorenal syndrome.

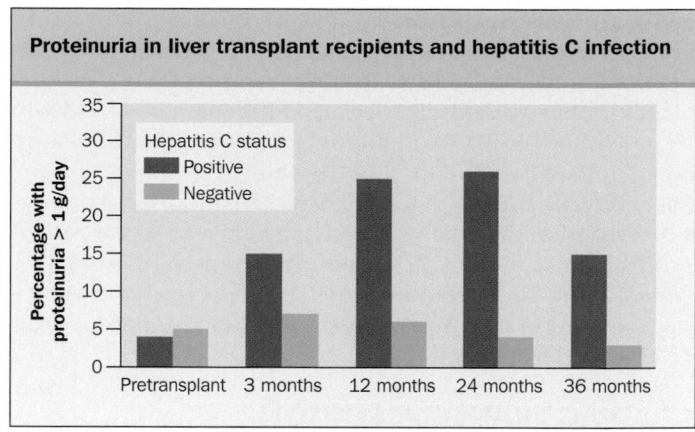

Figure 94.2 Proteinuria in liver transplant recipients and hepatitis C infection.

of hepatic rejection[8,9]. In contrast, recent studies suggest that substitution of the calcineurin inhibitor with sirolimus in conjunction with steroids and mycophenolate mofetil resulted in improved renal function[10]. Combination tacrolimus and sirolimus has also been reported to result in stable and near normal creatinine values in one study of 56 liver recipients[11]. In two patients tacrolimus was discontinued due to increasing creatinine values; these patients showed improved renal function on sirolimus and prednisone[11]. These studies suggest that combination therapy using sirolimus may be an alternative for patients who show chronic renal disease from calcineurin inhibitor toxicity.

Post-transplant glomerular disease

Patients with OLT are at increased risk for developing glomerular disease after transplantation. The greatest risk is for patients with HCV infection, which accounts for 30% of all patients undergoing OLT. Proteinuria of more than 1 g/day is seen in 3% of HCV-negative and 5% of HCV-infected patients at transplantation, increasing to a maximum of 25% in the HCV-positive and 5% in HCV-negative patients at 2 years (Fig. 94.2)[2]. Renal biopsies in HCV-infected patients usually show idiopathic or cryoglobulinemic MPGN or mesangial proliferative GN. HCV-infected patients are also more likely to develop diabetes post-transplantation (31% versus 7% in HCV-negative patients)[12].

Even though HCV-infected liver allograft recipients more frequently have proteinuria and MPGN or mesangial proliferative GN, they maintain similar levels of renal function compared with HCV-negative recipients over the first few years post-transplant[12]. Florid cryoglobulinemic disease including glomerulonephritis, pulmonary vasculitis, purpura and arthralgias may respond to interferon with or without ribavirin and plasma exchange. However, the long-term benefits of interferon on renal function and proteinuria have not been documented in the liver recipient. Although a virologic

response may be seen after treatment, relapse is the rule and treatment is often poorly tolerated.

Hemolytic–uremic syndrome or thrombotic microangiopathy

Thrombotic microangiopathy (TMA) is characterized by microangiopathic hemolysis, thrombocytopenia, and renal failure; it is seen in up to 2% of liver transplant recipients and may occur within a few months to 10 years after transplantation. Cyclosporine- or tacrolimus-induced endothelial injury has been thought to be the initiating factor. Withholding these agents and instituting plasma exchange may reduce hemolysis but renal function may not improve. Hemolysis frequently recurs with reinstitution of the same calcineurin inhibitor although this is not inevitable[13]. Utilizing low doses of cyclosporine to tacrolimus may permit continued maintenance therapy.

Combined liver–kidney transplantation

Combined disease of the liver and kidney may require transplantation of both organs. Preliminary criteria for transplantation are listed in Table 94.2. Patients with ARF and HRS are excluded from liver–kidney transplantation, although there is difficulty determining whether a patient on dialysis for more than 2 months after the onset of HRS or acute tubular necrosis has developed permanent renal failure. Some centers list such patients for both transplants, but only place the kidney if the intraoperative renal biopsy shows significant glomerulosclerosis or interstitial fibrosis. Long-term patient survival of combined transplants approaches 62% at 5 years.

Criteria for renal transplantation with liver transplant
Creatinine clearance ≤ 40 mL/min
Renal biopsy showing ≥ 40% glomerulosclerosis
Renal biopsy showing ≥ moderate interstitial fibrosis (30% of interstitial volume)
Or: On dialysis ≥ 2 months with no renal function and poor renal perfusion on duplex ultrasound or renal scan

Table 94.2 Criteria for renal transplantation with liver transplant.

ESRD after liver transplantation

Long-term patient survival is decreased in liver recipients developing ESRD[7]. By 13 years after transplantation, survival is only 28% in patients developing ESRD compared to 55% in those without ESRD. Mortality is most often due to dialysis access related sepsis. Morbidity is caused by blood pressure instability, bleeding and thrombosis. Renal transplantation is a better option than dialysis for liver recipients; 6 year patient survival on dialysis is 27% and after transplant is 71.4%[7]. Patients with HCV liver disease (*n* = 17) do well after kidney transplantation with 3-year patient and kidney graft survivals of 71 and 61%, respectively.

CARDIAC TRANSPLANTATION

Renal disease occurring pretransplant

Renal insufficiency frequently accompanies cardiac failure as a result of impairment of renal perfusion and rarely due to associated primary renal disorders. Cardiac failure causes a decrease in renal plasma flow, with a relative preservation of the GFR through an increase in efferent arteriolar pressure, which increases glomerular hydraulic pressure causing an increased filtration fraction. The increase in glomerular hydrostatic pressure may be associated with mild proteinuria (generally < 500 mg/day), as well as glomerular changes, including mesangiolysis and mesangial proliferation. Progressive cardiac dysfunction eventually is not compensated for by the kidney, resulting in renal functional impairment and volume overload.

Attempts to improve cardiac output with the use of angiotensin-converting enzyme (ACE) inhibitors, angiotensin receptor antagonists (ATRA), β-blockers, and spironolactone may be complicated by worsening renal function or hyperkalemia. Intraaortic balloon pumps may improve systemic and renal perfusion; however, they may cause renal failure due to occlusion of the renal arteries, cholesterol embolization, cortical necrosis, excessive exit site bleeding and hypotension or line sepsis. Left ventricular assist devices (LVAD) effectively increase cardiac output and are increasingly used as a bridge to cardiac transplantation. The use of LVAD's has improved renal function at transplantation in status 1 (Table 94.3) heart transplant candidates compared to inotrope therapy (serum creatinine 1.0 ± 0.1 vs 1.3 ± 0.4 mg/dL at transplant)[14]. Following transplant the development of acute renal failure has also decreased in those who have undergone LVAD placement compared to those who have not (16.7 vs 52.6%). However, LVAD treatment is associated with increased risks for infection, sensitization and coagulation abnormalities. Although the balloon pump and LVAD have improved renal perfusion, the increased waiting times (e.g., median wait of 116 days for status 1B) for transplantation increase the probability that medical illnesses will develop causing renal failure[14].

Pretransplant dialysis and ultrafiltration may be required to improve oxygenation when diuretics are no longer effective and intravenous afterload reduction, inotropic support, and the balloon pump do not augment cardiac function sufficiently to improve renal perfusion. Dialysis should be initiated with low blood flow and fluid removal rates and is ideally accomplished by continuous hemofiltration rather than intermittent dialysis therapy (see Chapter 82). Continuous dialysis with small dialyzers may also be effective with blood flow rates of 100–150 mL/min, although some patients have difficulty with hypotension, arrhythmias, and clotting.

Renal failure occurring after cardiac transplantation
Acute renal failure

ARF following cardiac transplantation is usually seen within the first 4 postoperative days and is caused by calcineurin inhibitor-induced renal vasoconstriction in combination with the effects of anesthesia, pressor support, the bypass procedure, poor allograft function and blood loss (Table 94.4). Dialysis is required in 5–15% of patients and is associated with a higher mortality rate. Treatment consists of optimizing cardiac function and reducing or withholding the calcineurin inhibitor. In patients with postoperative ARF, induction treatment utilizes antilymphocyte preparations and calcineurin inhibitors are restarted when renal function improves.

Medical urgency status codes for heart allocation

Status 1A: Adult- Registrant at least 18 years of age, admitted to listing hospital with at least one of the following: (a) mechanical circulatory support for acute hemodynamic decompensation; (b) mechanical circulatory support for more than 30 days with objective medical evidence of significant device-related complications; (c) mechanical ventilation, (d) continuous infusion of a single high-dose intravenous inotrope or multiple intravenous inotropes, in addition to continuous hemodynamic monitoring of left ventricular filling pressures, or (e) meets none of the criteria specified above but admitted to the listing hospital with a life expectancy without a heart transplant of less than 7 days.

Status 1B: Adult- A registrant who (a) has a left and/or right ventricular assist device implanted for more than 30 days; or (b) receives continuous infusion of intravenous inotropes.

Status 2: A patient of any age who does not meet the criteria for Status 1A or 1B.

Status 7: Temporarily inactive.

Table 94.3 Medical urgency status codes for heart allocation in the United States.

Acute renal failure in the cardiac allograft recipient

Poor allograft function primary non-function or delayed function

Acute allograft rejection with depressed cardiac function

Vasopressor use

Cardiopulmonary bypass

Radiocontrast administration

Nephrotoxic medications – cyclosporine, amphotericin

Medications affecting intrarenal hemodynamics i.e., ACEI, ATRA

Rhabdomyolysis

Hemolysis

Thrombotic microangiopathy

Hemorrhage

Table 94.4 Main etiologies associated with acute renal failure in the cardiac allograft recipient.

Chronic renal failure

In most patients, GFR declines to 60–65% of the preoperative value within 6 to 8 weeks of surgery and remains stable for 5 to 7 years[15]. Renal plasma flow also declines and microalbuminuria may develop. Hypertension develops in 80–90% of patients. By 10 years after surgery, approximately 10% of patients will develop ESRD; this risk is somewhat increased in the older allograft recipient[16].

The etiology of the progressive renal dysfunction is usually due to interstitial fibrosis from chronic calcineurin inhibitor exposure. Toxicity is more frequent in cardiac transplant recipients compared with liver transplant patients because higher trough and peak levels are targeted due to the increased risk for rejection. Once renal insufficiency is present, reducing or stopping calcineurin inhibitors may improve function but may not prevent ultimate renal progression. Although calcium channel blockers may acutely improve GFR and renal blood flow, no long-term benefit on renal histology or outcome has been proven.

Other etiologies of late renal failure include hemodynamic instability secondary to allograft rejection, thrombotic microangiopathy, sepsis and possibly renal viral infection. Thrombotic microangiopathy secondary to calcineurin inhibitors may require renal biopsy for diagnosis as not all patients demonstrate schistocytes or thrombocytopenia. While the hemolysis responds to discontinuation of the calcineurin inhibitor and plasma exchange, renal function may not improve[17]. Viral interstitial nephritis is a little reported complication of nonrenal transplantation. While a recent study reported the presence of urinary decoy cells and BK virus detected by polymerase chain reaction in the urine of long-term heart recipients, no evidence was found for viral-induced renal failure[18].

ESRD after cardiac transplantation

The risk for death in heart transplant recipients with ESRD is double that of patients of comparable age with ESRD without heart transplants. Cardiac transplant patients treated with peritoneal dialysis have a higher mortality risk than patients on hemodialysis. Survival rates at 2 years for cardiac transplant patients undergoing peritoneal dialysis may be as low as 25% (range 25 to 65%) whereas hemodialysis survival averages 66%. The increased mortality of peritoneal dialysis patients may be due to the selection of more patients with cardiac compromise[19]; however, cardiac allograft recipients on peritoneal dialysis also have more frequent peritonitis than nontransplant peritoneal dialysis patients[19]. Patients who undergo renal transplantation have 1-year graft survival rates of over 80% but due to increased requirements for immunosuppression may be at increased risk for malignancy.

COMBINED HEART–KIDNEY TRANSPLANTATION

Poor renal function prior to heart transplantation predicts decreased survival following transplantation. One treatment option for those with intrinsic renal disease is combined heart–kidney transplantation. The dual procedure is usually staged such that the renal transplant is placed during a second operation to allow for hemodynamic and coagulation stabilization. Renal allograft survival after combined transplantation approaches 90% at 2 years[20]. Dual transplantation should only be performed in those with fixed, irreversible renal disease. Patients who are dialysis dependent due to hemodynamic induced renal failure, as for the liver failure patients, should not receive a kidney transplant. While criteria for heart–kidney transplantation have not been formally introduced, normal kidney size, lack of significant proteinuria and lack of diseases associated with renal dysfunction should rule out combined transplantation. Ideally a renal biopsy should be performed to determine the degree of permanent renal injury prior to committing to a kidney transplant.

LUNG TRANSPLANTATION

Renal disease occurring pretransplant

Renal disease was historically a relative contraindication to lung transplantation. However, recently it has been recognized that renal blood flow may be markedly impaired in the setting of pulmonary failure and that this may improve after successful lung transplantation[21]. Furthermore, some primary pulmonary diseases such as cystic fibrosis are associated with an increased incidence of nonhemodynamically mediated renal disease. Patients with cystic fibrosis have an increased occurrence of diabetes, drug-related (aminoglycoside) renal injury, dehydration-related ARF, nephrocalcinosis (increased oxalate absorption), and urolithiasis[22].

Renal disease occurring post-transplant

Acute post-transplant

Renal function declines over the first 6 months post lung transplant to the same degree as for liver and cardiac recipients in both adults and children[23]. This acute decline, as for other allograft recipients, is largely attributed to calcineurin inhibitor nephrotoxicity.

Late post-transplant

After an initial decline, renal function usually remains stable over the next 5 years. In 19 pediatric patients with at least 3 years of follow-up (mean 5.36 years), 57% had mild chronic renal insufficiency and 5% had advanced renal failure[23]. Chronic decline in renal function resulting in ESRD typically occurs 6–7 years after transplant and is usually attributed to calcineurin inhibitor nephrotoxicity. Diabetes, which develops in 30–50% of patients with cystic fibrosis, may increase the risk for ESRD in these patients[24].

Minimizing calcineurin inhibitor toxicity in the lung transplant recipient is more difficult than other transplant patients due to the higher risk of rejection with lower long-term survival. Modification of the target calcineurin inhibitor trough levels to approximately 100–150 ng/mL for cyclosporine and 5–10 ng/mL for tacrolimus along with mycophenolate use may improve renal function substantially while limiting rejection episodes[25]. Once ESRD develops, renal transplantation provides better survival rates than dialysis[26].

RENAL DISEASE IN THE HEMATOPOIETIC CELL TRANSPLANT RECIPIENT

Approximately 12 000 bone marrow transplants (BMT) or peripheral blood progenitor cells (PBPCs) transplants (collectively known as hematopoietic cell transplants (HCT)) are performed annually in the USA, and ARF occurs in approximately 5–15% of these patients. The presence of ARF markedly affects mortality, and varies from 17% (no renal failure), 37% (renal failure not requiring dialysis) and 84% (dialysis-dependent) during the initial hospitalization[27]. Clinically, one may subdivide HCT-associated renal disease according to time of onset: immediate (within the first 5 days), early (within the first month), and late (after 1 month).

Immediate-onset renal failure

Renal failure presenting within 5 days of transplantation is usually caused by tumor lysis syndrome (TLS) or toxicity from the infused marrow. TLS refers to the metabolic derangements that occur as a result of release of tumor-derived intracellular constituents as a consequence of cytoreductive therapy. It is seen most commonly in patients with extensive, rapidly growing tumors that are very sensitive to radiation and chemotherapy. Intratubular precipitation of released intracellular constituents such as uric acid, phosphate and xanthine (which have low urinary solubilities) has been implicated as the cause of ARF[29].

Volume depletion is a major risk factor in the development of TLS. Aggressive volume repletion can often correct electrolyte disturbances, increase GFR, increase urine volume, decrease tubular precipitation of uric acid, phosphate and xanthine and hence prevent the development of ARF. Urinary alkalinization to maintain the urine pH between 6.5–7.5 increases uric acid solubility, and is also useful in the prevention of ARF in patients with hyperuricemia. Allopurinol blocks uric acid synthesis and is routinely used in the USA. Recombinant urate oxidase (uricase) (rasburicase) is also available and degrades uric acid to allantoin which is freely soluble in the urine[29]. When aggressive preventative measures are unsuccessful at preventing ARF, dialysis may be necessary (Table 94.5).

TLS is uncommon in HCT recipients because of the preventative measures that are employed. In addition, most patients who undergo transplantation do not have *de novo* disease but rather have disease in relapse, where the tumor burden is not as extreme[27]. If TLS does occur, the prognosis for recovery from ARF is excellent.

Cryopreservation is necessary for the storage and maintenance of autologous marrow used for transplantation. Dimethyl sulfoxide (DMSO) is frequently employed as a protectant. During marrow infusion, patients are exposed to toxic products of cell lysis as well as to DMSO. Hemoglobin is noted in the urine of 75–100% of patients and is possibly caused by DMSO-induced disruption of red cells in the infusate. Although hemoglobinuria is common, ARF is not, undoubtedly because a prophylactic solute and bicarbonate diuresis is routinely instituted.

Early-onset renal failure

The most common period for the development of renal failure is between 10 and 21 days after HCT (Table 94.6). During

---

Prophylaxis and treatment of tumor lysis syndrome

Prophylaxis:

1. Allopurinol, 300–600 mg/day
2. Intravenous fluids 4–5 L/24 h
3. Patients with hyperuricemia: maintain urine pH 6.5–7.5 with 5% dextrose containing 100 mmol/L $NaHCO_3$. Stop if serum HCO_3 > 30mmol/L, or uric acid normalizes
4. If uric acid is normal, use normal (0.9%) saline
5. Add diuretics if the patient is well hydrated, and urine output is not maintained.

Treatment:

1. Hemodialysis. Indications include: hyperuricemia, hyperkalemia, hyperphosphatemia, hypocalcemia, acidemia, control of uremia, volume overload
2. Dose reduction of allopurinol for renal failure
3. Treatment with recombinant uricase for markedly elevated uric acid (> 10 mg/dL)

Table 94.5 Prophylaxis and treatment of tumor lysis syndrome.

Causes of early onset acute renal failure after hematopoietic cell transplantation

1. Volume depletion (nausea, vomiting, diarrhea) caused by graft-versus-host disease or chemotherapy

2. Acute tubular necrosis: nephrotoxins (aminoglycosides, amphotericin B, ifosfamide, contrast, bisphosphonates, carboplatin), sepsis

3. Interstitial nephritis due to medications: penicillins, cephalosporins, allopurinol

4. Obstruction: fungus ball in collecting system, clot from hemorrhagic cystitis

5. Hepatorenal-like syndrome associated with bone marrow transplant

Table 94.6 Causes of early onset acute renal failure after hematopoietic cell transplantation.

---

this period, the complications of radiochemotherapy manifest, including pancytopenia, sepsis, pneumonitis, mucositis, and gastrointestinal and hepatic toxicities. This is the period when dialysis is most often required.

In spite of the multitude of medical complications and nephrotoxic drug exposures, the large majority of patients who develop early BMT-associated ARF develop a single clinical disorder that is reminiscent of HRS. Veno-occlusive disease (VOD) of the liver precedes the development of early onset ARF in approximately 90% of patients (Table 94.7). VOD is thought to result from hepatic venule endothelial cell injury caused by radiochemotherapy; endothelial injury results in thrombosis, fibrin deposition, and sinusoidal and portal hypertension[30]. Because liver biopsy is seldom performed due to thrombocytopenia and coagulopathy, the diagnosis is made clinically. The incidence of VOD in BMT recipients varies depending on the center and type of transplant, but has been reported to occur in up to 50% of patients. The incidence is probably increasing, possibly as a result of the use of more aggressive cytoreductive regimens. Approximately 25–30% of reported cases of VOD are severe, and mortality in these patients is 98% in spite of treatment. Management of VOD-associated ARF is supportive (Table 94.8).

Hepatorenal-like syndrome in bone marrow transplant recipients

Diagnosis

Hyperbilirubinemia, jaundice, hepatomegaly, right upper quadrant pain
Weight gain, edema, pulmonary vascular congestion
Relatively low blood pressure
Hyponatremia
Sodium avidity (urinary sodium < 10 mmol/L)
High BUN/creatinine ratio[30]
Normal urinary sediment

Predisposing factors

Age > 25 years
Mismatched grafts
Elevated baseline serum creatinine
Pre-existing hepatic disease
Fever during cytoreductive therapy
Use of estrogen–progestin, amphotericin B, or methotrexate

Table 94.7 Hepatorenal-like syndrome in bone marrow transplant recipients.

Treatment of acute renal failure associated with veno-occlusive disease

Maintain intravascular volume

Maintain hematocrit 38–40%

Avoid intravenous albumin (will accumulate in extravascular space)

Avoid volume overload:
  restrict sodium
  use diuretics (loop diuretics, spironolactone)
  consider renal-dose dopamine or fenoldopam (no proven value)

Paracentesis to control symptomatic ascites

Protein restriction, lactulose for encephalopathy

Hemodialysis (often necessary for volume overload/pulmonary edema)

Table 94.8 Treatment of acute renal failure associated with veno-occlusive disease.

Although hepatic endothelial injury plays a central role in early onset ARF, a superimposed clinical event usually triggers the renal failure. Sepsis is the most common event. Since fungemia is common, amphotericin B therapy is empirically initiated and is the single strongest predictor of the development of ARF[27]. The clinical characteristics of early onset ARF are the same as those seen in HRS. Histologic findings at autopsy have not shown structural changes to explain the ARF, lending further support to the assertion that hemodynamic rather than structural perturbations are the main cause of the ARF.

Because treatment of fungal infections with amphotericin B results in significant renal toxicity, other agents are being investigated for fungal prophylaxis, including fluconazole (400 mg/day) and liposomal amphotericin B. Voraconazole, a second generation triazole, was found to have fewer infusion-related side effects than liposomal amphotericin B, but may not be as effective when used as empiric therapy for fungal infections[31]. Caspofungin is a new antifungal agent that inhibits cell wall glucan synthesis and is as effective, better tolerated, and less nephrotoxic than amphotericin B for patients with Candida esophagitis[32].

A controlled trial of ursodeoxycholic acid for the prevention of VOD in allogeneic BMT patients resulted in a reduction in the incidence of VOD, and is used routinely at some centers[33]. Low-dose heparin (100 U/kg) has also shown promise in some, but not all, studies. No therapy for established VOD has been shown to be effective in a controlled study. However, defibrotide, an adenosine receptor agonist that increases levels of endogenous prostaglandins, has shown promise, and a randomized trial is underway to further evaluate this agent. The combination of tissue plasminogen activator and heparin has been shown to reduce jaundice and increase urine output, but this treatment is not routinely employed because of the high risk of bleeding complications.

Late-onset renal disease

Renal disease occurring more than 1 month after BMT is often the result of calcineurin inhibitor use to prevent graft-versus-host-disease (GVHD). The syndrome of delayed chronic renal insufficiency, anemia, and hypertension not attributable to calcineurin inhibitor is referred to as BMT nephropathy, which is thought to be a form of radiation nephropathy. This syndrome is observed in 10–25% of BMT recipients and presents 6–12 months after BMT. Some patients present with the insidious onset of renal insufficiency, hypertension and disproportionate anemia, and histologic features suggestive of TMA[36] (Figs 94.3 and 94.4). In milder cases, the hemolytic anemia and thrombocytopenia may be minimal or absent. The most severe presentation is hemolytic–uremic syndrome in which hypertension, proteinuria (average = 2 g/day), hematuria, red blood cell casts, progressive renal insufficiency, and microangiopathic hemolytic anemia are present[37]. Central nervous system abnormalities may also occur.

BMT TMA is thought to result from endothelial cell damage secondary to the total body irradiation (TBI). The conditioning regimen for BMT usually includes 8–14 Gy radiation administered in one or two fractions which provides a dose comparable to that delivered to patients who develop radiation nephropathy[35,37]. The underlying disease for which the patient received a transplant also is not a factor. Although cyclosporine may contribute to the disease, TMA has been described in patients who have not received cyclosporine treatment.

The histologic features and clinical presentation of BMT-associated TMA display a striking similarity to acute radiation nephropathy. The histopathology reveals enlarged hypocellular

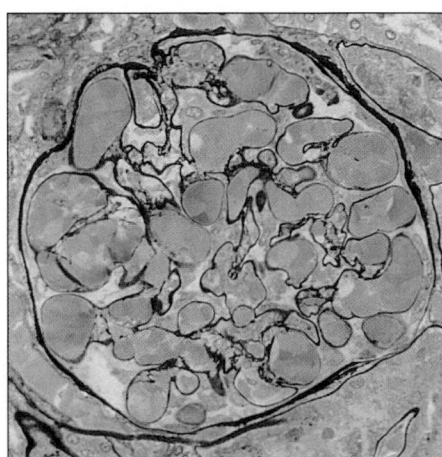

Figure 94.3 Thrombotic microangiopathy. Mesangiolysis in a patient with thrombotic microangiopathy associated with bone marrow transplantation.

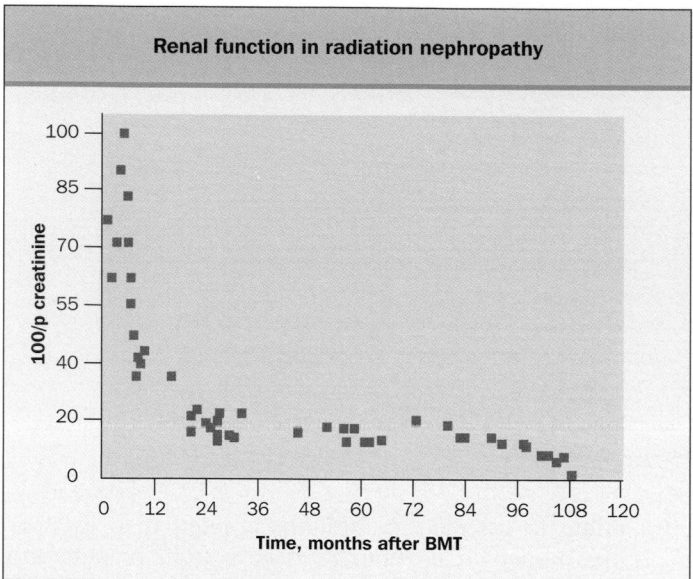

Renal function in radiation nephropathy

Figure 94.4 Renal function in radiation nephropathy. Evolution of renal function in a patient with radiation nephropathy shown here as 100/plasma creatinine versus time. There is a biphasic pattern, with an initial rapid decline, then a plateau that culminates in end-stage renal disease. (Adapted with permission from Cohen[35].)

glomeruli with mesangiolysis (Fig. 94.3). There is accumulation of spongiform material along the inner aspect of the glomerular basement membrane that extends into the glomerular capillary loops, producing a double contour appearance. There is marked narrowing of the arteriolar lumen caused by mucoid intimal thickening, which is the histologic alteration seen in radiation nephropathy[35,37].

Shielding the kidneys during TBI reduces renal injury, but the optimal treatment of established BMT-associated TMA is not known. Aggressive treatment of hypertension is important, and ACE inhibitors may be preferable to other agents in light of their proven benefit in animal models of BMT nephropathy. Plasma exchange with or without vincristine therapy has been employed successfully in some patients, but results in BMT-associated TMA have for the most part been disappointing. The role of apheresis in this setting is therefore controversial. Although it is unlikely that cyclosporine is responsible for causing BMT-associated TMA, cyclosporine has known deleterious effects on the vasculature, and the dose should be reduced whenever possible. In light of the gravity of GVHD, it may be dangerous to discontinue cyclosporine.

The natural history of patients with BMT-associated TMA is variable. While some cases spontaneously resolve, other cases experience a biphasic course, with an initial rapid loss in renal function, followed by a slower phase of deterioration (Fig. 94.4). Some patients progress to ESRD and require long-term renal replacement therapy[35,37]. Transplantation of a kidney from the bone marrow donor has been accomplished in two cases and was well tolerated because the donor marrow had previously reconstituted the patient's immune system.

Cyclosporine in combination with prednisone, methotrexate or mycophenolate is usually used in the prevention of GVHD, which if severe has a mortality of 50%. Renal insufficiency may be seen with cyclosporine use in this setting and correlates with trough levels. Cyclosporine rarely causes dialysis-requiring ARF. In patients without GVHD, full therapeutic doses are used only for a short time and chronic cyclosporine toxicity is not seen. Tacrolimus is also used for the prevention of GVHD and carries the same profile of renal impairment. There is a trend toward more chronic GVHD with peripheral blood stem cell transplantation, likely due the larger dose of mature, immunocompetent T cells[38]. As more unrelated grafts are used, it is likely that more chronic GVHD will develop and chronic cyclosporine toxicity may become more common. Rarely, patients with GVHD present with the full-blown nephrotic syndrome, including heavy proteinuria, edema, hypoalbuminemia and hyperlipidemia, and have renal biopsy findings of membranous nephropathy.

Renal transplantation for ESRD following BMT
ESRD develops in up to 10% of BMT recipients. Survival on dialysis is less than for nontransplant patients[37]. Success of renal transplantation from the BMT donor is excellent and without the requirement for immunosuppression. Cadaveric or nonbone marrow donor renal transplantation requires immunosuppression and is complicated by the increased development of infection and malignancy[39]. Furthermore, BMT recipients may be more sensitive to cytotoxic agents and careful monitoring is necessary.

STEM CELL TRANSPLANTATION

Stem cell transplantation has been employed for primary systemic amyloidosis including patients with renal involvement, and response rates are higher than for patients treated with low-dose traditional melphalan and prednisone. Complication rates are high, however due to multiorgan failure of tissues infiltrated with amyloid, especially cardiac involvement. Patients with multiple myeloma are also candidates for either autologous or allogeneic stem cell transplantation, even in the presence of pre-existing renal impairment. The allograft recipients appear to enjoy long-term disease-free survival, (most likely due to allogeneic graft-versus-myeloma effect), but transplant-related mortality is high[35].

REFERENCES

1. Crawford DH, Endre ZH, Axelsen RA, et al. Universal occurrence of glomerular abnormalities in patients receiving liver transplants. Am J Kidney Dis. 1992;19:339–44.

2. Davis CL, Gonwa TA, Wilkinson AH. Pathophysiology of renal disease associated with liver disorders: implications for liver transplantation. Liver Transpl. 2002;8:193–211.

3. Kendrick EA, McVicar JP, Kowdley KV, et al. Renal disease in hepatitis C-positive liver transplant recipients. Transplantation. 1997;63:1287–93.

4. Gonwa TA, Mai ML, Melton LB, et al. Renal replacement therapy (RRT) and orthotopic liver transplantation (OLTX): the role of continuous veno-venous hemodialysis (CVVHD). Transplantation. 2001;71:1424–8.

5. Triulzi DJ, Shirey RS, Ness PM, Klein AS. Immunohematologic complications of ABO-unmatched liver transplants. Transfusion. 1992;32:829–33.

6. Gonwa TA, Klintmalm G, Levy M, et al. Impact of pre-transplant renal function on survival after liver transplantation. Transplantation. 1995;59:361–5.

7. Gonwa TA, Mai ML, Melton LB, et al. End stage renal disease (ESRD) following orthotopic liver transplantation (OLTX) utilizing calcineurin based immunotherapy: risk of development and treatment. Transplantation. 2001;72:1934–9.

8. Stewart SF, Hudson M, Talbot D, et al. Mycophenolate mofetil monotherapy in liver transplantation. Lancet. 2001;357:609–10.

9. Schlitt HJ, Barkmann A, Boker KH, et al. Replacement of calcineurin inhibitors with mycophenolate mofetil in liver-transplant patients with renal dysfunction: a randomised controlled study. Lancet. 2001;357:587–91.

10. Chang GJ, Mahanty HD, Quan D, et al. Experience with the use of sirolimus in liver transplantation—use in patients for whom calcineurin inhibitors are contraindicated. Liver Transpl. 2000;6:734–40.

11. McAlister VC, Peltekian KM, Malatjalian DA, et al. Orthotopic liver transplantation using low-dose tacrolimus and sirolimus. Liver Transpl. 2001;7:701–8.

12. Kendrick EA, McVicar JP, Kowdley KV, et al. Renal disease in hepatitis C-positive liver transplant recipients. Transplantation. 1997;63: 1287–93.

13. Singh N, Gayowski T, Marino IR. Hemolytic uremic syndrome in solid-organ transplant recipients. Transpl Int. 1996;9:68–75.

14. Bank AJ, Mir SH, Nguyen DQ, et al. Effects of left ventricular assist devices on outcomes in patients undergoing heart transplantation. Ann Thorac Surg. 2000;69:1369–74; discussion 1375.

15. Lindelow B, Bergh CH, Herlitz H, Waagstein F. Predictors and evolution of renal function during 9 years following heart transplantation. J Am Soc Nephrol. 2000;11:951–7.

16. Goldstein DJ, Zuech N, Sehgal V, et al. Cyclosporin-associated end-stage nephropathy after cardiac transplantation: incidence and progression. Transplantation. 1997;63:664–8.

17. Mercadal L, Petitclerc T, Assogba U, et al. Hemolytic and uremic syndrome after heart transplantation. Am J Nephrol. 2000;20:418–20.

18. Etienne I, Francois A, Redonnet M, et al. Does polyomavirus infection induce renal failure in cardiac transplant recipients? Transplant Proc. 2000;32:2794–5.

19. Jayasena SD, Riaz A, Lewis CM, et al. Outcome in patients with end-stage renal disease following heart or heart–lung transplantation receiving peritoneal dialysis. Nephrol Dial Transplant. 2001;16:1681–5.

20. Blanche C, Kamlot A, Blanche DA, et al. Combined heart–kidney transplantation with single-donor allografts. J Thorac Cardiovasc Surg. 2001;122:495–500.

21. Navis G, Broekroelofs J, Mannes GP, et al. Renal hemodynamics after lung transplantation. A prospective study. Transplantation. 1996;61:1600–5.

22. Schindler R, Radke C, Paul K, Frei U. Renal problems after lung transplantation of cystic fibrosis patients. Nephrol Dial Transplant. 2001;16:1324–8.

23. Tsimaratos M, Viard L, Kreitmann B, et al. Kidney function in cyclosporine-treated paediatric pulmonary transplant recipients. Transplantation. 2000;69:2055–9.

24. Broekroelofs J, Navis G, Stegeman CA, et al. Lung transplantation. Lancet. 1998;351:1064.

25. Soccal PM, Gasche Y, Favre H, et al. Improvement of drug-induced chronic renal failure in lung transplantation. Transplantation. 1999;68:164–5.

26. Coopersmith CM, Brennan DC, Miller B, et al. Renal transplantation following previous heart, liver, and lung transplantation: an 8-year single-center experience. Surgery. 2001;130:457–62.

27. Zager RA. Acute renal failure in the setting of bone marrow transplantation. Kidney Int. 1994;46:1443–58.

28. Jeha S. Tumor lysis syndrome. Semin Hematol. 2001;38:4–8.

29. Goldman SC, Holcenberg JS, Finklestein JZ, et al. A randomized comparison between rasburicase and allopurinol in children with lymphoma or leukemia at high risk for tumor lysis. Blood. 2001;97:2998–3003.

30. McDonald GB, Hinds MS, Fisher LD, et al. Veno-occlusive disease of the liver and multiorgan failure after bone marrow transplantation: a cohort study of 355 patients. Ann Intern Med. 1993;118:255–67.

31. Walsh TJ, Pappas P, Winston DJ, et al. Voriconazole compared with liposomal amphotericin B for empirical antifungal therapy in patients with neutropenia and persistent fever. N Engl J Med. 2002;346:225–34.

32. Villanueva A, Arathoon EG, Gotuzzo E, et al. A randomized double-blind study of caspofungin versus amphotericin for the treatment of candidal esophagitis. Clin Infect Dis. 2001;33: 1529–35.

33. Essell JH, Schroeder MT, Harman GS, et al. Ursodiol prophylaxis against hepatic complications of allogeneic bone marrow transplantation. A randomized, double-blind, placebo-controlled trial. Ann Intern Med. 1998;128:975–81.

34. Bensinger WI, Maloney D, Storb R. Allogeneic hematopoietic cell transplantation for multiple myeloma. Semin Hematol. 2001;38: 243–9.

35. Cohen EP. Radiation nephropathy after bone marrow transplantation. Kidney Int. 2000;58:903–18.

36. Cruz DN, Perazella MA, Mahnensmith RL. Bone marrow transplant nephropathy: a case report and review of the literature. J Am Soc Nephrol. 1997;8:166–73.

37. Cohen EP, Piering WF, Kabler-Babbitt C, Moulder JE. End-stage renal disease (ESRD) after bone marrow transplantation: poor survival compared to other causes of ESRD. Nephron. 1998;79: 408–12.

38. Cutler C, Antin JH. Peripheral blood stem cells for allogeneic transplantation: a review. Stem Cells. 2001;19:108–17.

39. Butcher JA, Hariharan S, Adams MB, et al. Renal transplantation for end-stage renal disease following bone marrow transplantation: a report of six cases, with and without immunosuppression. Clin Transplant. 1999;13:330–5.

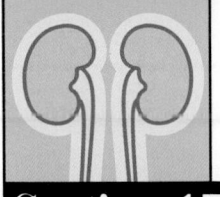

Chapter 95

Poisoning and Drug Overdose

John Feehally

POISONING THROUGH DELIBERATE OR ACCIDENTAL SELF-HARM

Poisoning may be iatrogenic through failure to appreciate the principles and practice of prescribing described in Chapter 96. Poisoning may also be caused by deliberate self-harm (attempted suicide), accidental self-harm (most commonly in children), or deliberate harm (homicide or war). It may also be caused by environmental exposure (industrial poisons or poisonous wildlife). Usually the event is acute and the presentation to hospital early, although chronic poisoning may also occur.

The nephrologist is involved in the clinical care of poisoning for several reasons:

- Iatrogenic drug nephrotoxicity may require active management.
- Acute renal failure is a common consequence of many poisonings.
- The metabolic consequences of poisoning may require intervention.
- Many agents are excreted via the kidney, and drug removal may occasionally require promotion at controlled urinary pH.
- Drug removal using extracorporeal techniques may be valuable: usually by hemodialysis or hemoperfusion.

Epidemiology of poisoning

In the developed world, deliberate self-harm is a common cause for emergency admission: about 1% of all hospital admissions. Admissions for poisoning steadily increased until the 1970s, since that time there has been a gradual decline. Deliberate self-harm has a peak incidence around 25 years of age and is more common in women; the majority of these incidents are not serious suicide intents.

In serious cases of poisoning, the individual dies before admission: this particularly includes carbon monoxide (car exhaust) poisoning, which is the most common cause of death by suicide in males age 15–44 years. After admission, 50% are discharged from the emergency room, and in-hospital mortality from poisoning is extremely low. Only 4% of all cases of self-poisoning require hospital admission, and among these mortality is only 1–2%.

One factor in the falling mortality is the changing pattern of drugs involved. Until the 1970s, barbiturates and other lipid-soluble sedatives such as glutethimide and meprobamate were widely available and frequently produced severe clinical effects in overdose. They were subsequently replaced by 'safer'

hypnotic agents such as benzodiazepines[1]. Mortality from acute sedative overdose was 45% in 1945, had fallen to 1% by the mid-1960s and was no more than 0.2% by the late-1990s. Paraquat has also been taken less commonly in overdose as other safer herbicides have come into horticultural and agricultural use. Among common drug poisonings, few require extracorporeal drug removal (Table 95.1).

Approximately 75% of accidental self-harm occurs in children under 4 years of age; this is decreasing in frequency. Only 15% have symptoms of poisoning and deaths are rare. The majority results from exposure to household commodities including alcohol and domestic cleansing agents, as well as pharmaceutical preparations.

Pattern of drug use in deliberate self-harm	
Drug	Percentage of total occurrences
Acetaminophen (paracetamol)	29
Benzodiazepines	13
Antidepressants	11
Compound analgesics (including acetaminophen)	10
NSAIDs	6
Aspirin*	6
Street drugs	5
β-blockers	2
Antibiotics	2
Anticonvulsants*	2
Household compounds	1
Theophylline*	0.7
Lithium*	0.7
Iron	0.5
Hypoglycemics	0.5
Others	10.4
*Extracorporeal drug removal may be indicated	

Table 95.1 Pattern of drug use in deliberate self-harm. Data for admissions to the emergency department at Leicester Royal Infirmary, UK in 1994. (Adapted from Macnamara et al.[1].)

In the developing world, patterns of poisoning are very different. Poisoning with animal and plant products is more common: snake bites and insect stings can be particularly devastating since their venoms may provoke hemorrhage, hemolysis, and rhabdomyolysis. Deliberate self-harm often involves hydrocarbons (especially paraffin) and agrochemicals (pesticides, herbicides, and fertilizers) because of their easy availability.

There are very large numbers of poisons for which detailed information must be readily available to influence immediate management. This information is beyond the scope of this chapter. There are published reference texts that are frequently updated[2]. Poisons information centers are freely accessible by telephone or the Internet for urgent advice. For example, in the UK there are six regional Poisons Information Centres (www.doh.gov.uk/npis.htm); in the USA there are state centers within the American Association of Poison Control Centers (www.aapcc.org), which publishes data annually[3].

MANAGEMENT OF POISONING

General management
The diagnosis of poisoning is not always straightforward, since the patient may deny intoxication or may be comatose or otherwise unable to give the necessary information. Poisoning may present as unexplained coma, unexplained acute renal failure, or as a metabolic disorder. High anion gap metabolic acidosis is a characteristic presentation of several poisonings including ethylene glycol and methanol, while salicylate poisoning may present with a mixed acid–base disorder.

The primary aim of the management of poisoning is not to retrieve the poison but to save life. The mainstay of treatment for most poisonings is supportive care while spontaneous excretion or metabolism of the drug occurs. It may include correction of fluid, electrolyte, and acid–base derangements, cardiovascular support, and respiratory support, including artificial ventilation.

Acute renal failure in poisoning
Acute renal failure may develop in poisoning (Table 95.2) as a result of circulatory collapse, or the hepatorenal syndrome when there is severe hepatic toxicity. Rhabdomyolysis may result from prolonged coma or seizures. In addition, a range of poisons are directly nephrotoxic. Acute tubular necrosis may be caused by direct toxicity or by myoglobinuria, hemoglobinuria, or crystalluria[4]. Acetone, taken itself or derived from metabolism of isopropyl alcohol ingestion, interferes with colorimetric assays for creatinine, and may produce false elevations of serum creatinine with normal blood urea.

Specific antidotes
In a small minority of poisonings, a specific antidote is available (Table 95.3) that may prevent life-threatening consequences. Antidotes are valuable when toxicity develops too rapidly and irreversibly to wait for spontaneous excretion or to introduce techniques that accelerate drug removal[5]. Most commonly this is because the poison or a metabolite fixes in tissues and does not remain in the plasma to be accessible for removal.

Prevention of drug absorption
Absorption is usually gastrointestinal following oral intoxication but other routes to consider are intravenous injection, through the skin, or by inhalation.

Gastric lavage
Gastric lavage (via an orogastric tube) is a long-established treatment to remove drug from the stomach before it is

Acute renal failure in poisoning	
Cause of acute renal failure	Drugs
Secondary to generalized effects of severe poisoning	
Hypotension	
Sepsis	
Rhabdomyolysis: prolonged coma, seizures	
Hepatorenal syndrome	Acetaminophen, *Amanita* mushroom, carbon tetrachloride
Specific nephrotoxicity	
Nephrotoxic acute tubular necrosis (ATN)	Heavy metals, acetaminophen (ATN may occur without hepatic failure), salicylate, phenoxyacetate herbicides
Myoglobinuric ATN	Amphetamines, barbiturates, cocaine, heroin, methadone, carbon monoxide, snake venoms, arthropod and insect venoms
Hemoglobinuric ATN	Copper sulfate, sodium chlorate, snake venoms, arthropod venoms
Crystalluric ATN	Ethylene glycol

Table 95.2 Acute renal failure in poisoning.

Antidotes in common causes of poisoning	
Poison	Antidote
Benzodiazepines	Flumazenil
Carbon monoxide	Oxygen
Cyanide	Amyl nitrite, sodium nitrite, sodium thiosulfate, edetate dicobalt
Digoxin	Digoxin-specific Fab antibodies
Ethylene glycol	Ethanol
Iron salts	Desferoxamine
Methanol	Ethanol
Opioids	Naloxone
Organophosphate insecticides	Atropine, pralidoxime
Acetaminophen (paracetamol)	Methionine, N-acetylcysteine

Table 95.3 Antidotes of proven value in common causes of poisoning.

absorbed. However, recent evidence indicates it is relatively ineffective at removing solid tablet accretions and may actually promote absorption by propelling some gastric contents into the duodenum. It no longer has a place in routine management[6] but is of value when the patient presents within 1 h of overdosing or when the drug taken slows gastric emptying (e.g., aspirin or tricyclic antidepressants).

Emesis by syrup of ipecacuanha no longer has a role in the management of poisoning[6]. It has been shown to be no more efficient than lavage or activated charcoal, leaving significant gastric solids behind and carries important side effects: up to 15% of those treated will have vomiting and drowsiness, which may be confused with the toxicity of the poisoning agent; aspiration pneumonitis may also occur.

Activated charcoal

Activated charcoal (50 g orally) is now the mainstay of immediate treatment for most poisoning in the emergency department[6]. The charcoal is 'activated' by exposure to gas or chemicals, which increases the internal pore structure, expanding the surface area available for adsorption. Multiple doses of activated charcoal for up to 72 h may continue to reduce absorption[7] since it decreases absorption of any residual drug in the gut (particularly relevant for slow-release formulations and drugs that delay gastric emptying). Activated charcoal also adsorbs drug secreted in the bile, interrupting intestinal reabsorption, and adsorbs any drug permeating from the circulation into the gut, thus blocking enteroenteric circulation.

TOXICOKINETICS

The great majority of poisonings require no specific removal strategies. Once absorption has been minimized, supportive treatment is given while spontaneous metabolism or excretion takes place.

However, it is necessary to be aware of factors affecting drug removal since these will influence the decision to employ additional drug-removal techniques in the small minority of patients in which they are valuable. Normal pharmacokinetics for any drug do not necessarily apply in overdose. Toxicokinetics may differ since the poison may damage an organ that contains the major route of elimination or the usual routes of excretion and metabolism may be saturable. Alternatively, in chronic overdose, clearance may be increased by enzyme induction (e.g., carbamazepine) so extracorporeal removal will not have the same value for the drug as in acute overdose.

Several toxicokinetic factors must be considered, as follows.

Time since overdose

Accidental poisoning will usually present immediately. Deliberate poisoning (suicide or homicide) may present hours or days later so irreversible organ damage may have occurred; although it may still be possible to remove toxin from blood and tissues this may be futile, having no impact on outcome.

Toxic and lethal doses

Toxic and lethal dosages are defined from previous case reports, but toxic and lethal plasma concentrations correlate better with clinical evidence of severity. The precise dose taken is often not known and will be influenced by subsequent vomiting and gastric lavage. Gastrointestinal absorption is usually rapid, but may be prolonged (e.g., by anticholinergics); the efficacy of drug removal depends on the availability of drug in the plasma in the period between absorption and redistribution.

Plasma protein binding

Protein binding limits drug removal by hemodialysis and hemofiltration, but not by hemoperfusion or plasma exchange. Protein binding is reversible, allowing distribution of drug into other compartments. Protein binding may be saturated in severe poisoning with the result that more drug than expected is available for clearance; rapid removal of unbound drug will also liberate further bound drug, making it accessible to removal.

Ionization

Nonionized (lipid-soluble) drugs redistribute easily through cell membranes; ionized drug can only redistribute slowly through membrane pores. Ionized drugs are, therefore, more susceptible to extracorporeal removal. Many drugs are weak acids and bases and their degree of ionization *in vivo* is predicted by the pK_a; for example, the weak acid diazepam (pK_a 3.3) is mostly nonionized in the circulation; as a result, it is rapidly redistributed and is a poor candidate for extracorporeal removal.

Volume of distribution and redistribution

Volume of distribution (V_D) is an imaginary space for drug distribution measured in volume per body weight units (L/kg). It is not a single space: absorbed drug moves rapidly from the blood compartment (8% of total volume) to a central compartment comprising the major organs (heart, lungs, kidneys, and liver) (7%), then slowly to the peripheral compartment comprising muscle, adipose tissue, skin, and bone (75%). At equilibration, 70% of a drug will usually be in the peripheral compartment. This pattern may vary if a toxin becomes concentrated in a specific tissue, for example, carbon monoxide in hemoglobin or paraquat in the lung. Toxins may also become concentrated in a nontoxic site. For example, lead is stored in bone where it is nontoxic, but it is toxic in soft tissues.

A large V_D will reduce clearance efficacy, for example amitriptyline, which has a volume of distribution of 20 L/kg. Extracorporeal removal will be efficient if the V_D is less than 0.5 L/kg (e.g., alcohols, lithium, salicylate, theophylline) and if rapid removal from central and peripheral compartments will allow redistribution into the 'empty' plasma compartment. Extracorporeal removal may be 'too rapid', removing toxin faster than it can be redistributed from the peripheral space; as a result it may be more effective to discontinue removal and restart later (e.g., for lithium). This additional deferred treatment will have no value if the initial distribution has produced irreversible target organ damage.

Saturation of metabolic pathways

Excretory and metabolic pathways may be saturated in overdose, which delays the proportional excretion rates.

IMPLEMENTATION OF DRUG-REMOVAL TECHNIQUES

In making a decision to use drug-removal techniques, measurements of plasma drug levels must be interpreted with the toxicokinetic factors described above in the context of clinical signs and symptoms of severity.

Early signs
Nausea and vomiting, fatigue, and grade I/II coma are not usually indications for extracorporeal treatment unless the toxin is known to have a 'silent period'.

Late signs
Grade III/IV coma, cardiorespiratory failure, and hyper- and hypothermia may be indications for extracorporeal treatment.

Irreversible late signs
Some signs and symptoms indicate irreversible damage. Extracorporeal measures are usually useless in late organ injury when tissue damage is irreversible, for example hepatic failure caused by acetaminophen (paracetamol) or the *Amanita phalloides* mushroom.

DRUG REMOVAL BY DIURESIS

Although the majority of drugs and poisons are renally excreted, enhanced diuresis only occasionally makes a worthwhile contribution to accelerated drug removal.

Forced diuresis
The provocation of a large increase in urine volumes was widely used in the past. The aim was to reduce the tubular concentration of freely filtered intact drug by increasing urine flow rate, thus reducing passive reabsorption by minimizing the increasing concentration gradient that would otherwise develop in the distal tubule. Maintaining fluid balance required vigilance, and, particularly in the elderly, pulmonary edema caused by fluid overload, hypotension caused by volume depletion, and electrolyte disturbance were not uncommon. Forced diuresis now has no place in the management of poisoning.

Diuresis at controlled pH
In some poisonings, alteration of urine pH will substantially alter the rate of excretion. Nonionized drugs are lipid soluble and will diffuse through cell membranes relatively easily, promoting passive reabsorption of filtered drug. By contrast, drug in the ionized state is very poorly reabsorbed. For weak acids and alkalis, pK_a dictates that the proportion of ionized to nonionized drug can be significantly increased within the range of urine pH.

In common practice, alkaline diuresis only applies to salicylate, phenobarbitone and phenoxyacetate herbicides. Salicylate is a weak acid (pK_a 3.5) and its urine excretion is significantly enhanced in alkaline urine (pH 8.0). Alkaline diuresis is achieved by administering isotonic sodium bicarbonate, with careful monitoring of serum potassium to avoid hypokalemia, aiming for a urine pH target of 7.5 to 8.5.

Amphetamine is a weak alkali (pK_a 9.8) and its excretion is significantly enhanced in acid urine (pH 5.0). Urine can be acidified by administration of ammonium chloride, but this approach is not used regularly since amphetamine may cause rhabdomyolysis, thus increasing the risk of acute renal failure at low urine pH.

REMOVAL OF POISONS BY EXTRACORPOREAL TREATMENT

The original description of hemodialysis by Abel, Rowntree, and Turner in 1913[8] was an attempt to remove salicylate and this was next described in the 1960s. Over the next 30 years increasing numbers of drugs were reported that could be removed by extracorporeal techniques. Since many poisons have small molecular size, they are accessible to removal from the plasma by hemodialysis or hemofiltration[9]. Many can also be removed by hemoperfusion in which the poison is adsorbed to activated charcoal in an extracorporeal circuit[9].

However, nephrologists have become less involved since the 1980s in the management of poisoning as the indications for extracorporeal drug removal have become fewer. Even for those relatively frequently encountered poisons in which it is effective, there is often no demonstrable advantage over simple supportive treatment measures combined with oral activated charcoal. Extracorporeal treatment was only used in two per 1000 of all poisonings registered by the American Association of Poisons Control Centers in the 1990s[3]. Even among those poisonings requiring admission to an intensive care unit, only 1% require extracorporeal drug removal.

No extracorporeal detoxification treatments have been the subject of prospective randomized controlled trials to test the hypothesis that they reduce morbidity and mortality. Retrospective studies have sometimes shown worse outcome in the treated groups, which is usually attributed to the selection of more severely poisoned patients[10]. The small number of appropriate cases mean that prospective randomized trials may never be performed.

Extracorporeal detoxification is only indicated if it will provide a significant addition to removal by biotransformation, renal excretion, or pulmonary excretion (Table 95.4). If extracorporeal treatment is indicated, it should be started as soon as possible provided there is sufficient cardiovascular stability. There is no absolute contraindication to extracorporeal treatment – the usual restriction is circulatory insufficiency in the severely ill patient.

Techniques of extracorporeal drug removal
Dialysis
Small molecules that are free in the plasma (i.e., not protein bound) will be removed using hemodialysis by diffusion down a concentration gradient from plasma into dialysate. Toxins of molecular mass 100–2000 Da can pass unhindered through all dialysis membranes; the cut off for high-flux membranes is above 10 000 Da. At molecular masses above 200 Da, clearance is determined by the blood flow rate provided the toxin is confined to the plasma alone.

Hemodialysis is ineffective when poisons are lipid soluble or significantly protein bound. Removal efficacy depends on the

Indications for extracorporeal detoxification
Ingestion of a dose that will cause serious toxicity or death for which supportive care is ineffective
Extracorporeal treatment known to eliminate significant amounts of drug: it is generally accepted that extracorporeal elimination is worthwhile if it increases total body clearance by 30%
Clinical evidence of severe toxicity grade IV coma, hypotension; hypothermia, respiratory depression.
Impaired clearance of the toxic compound: excretory/metabolic pathways are saturated genetic defect in metabolism coincidental hepatic or renal dysfunction (pre-existing or acute)
Undue susceptibility because of concurrent disease states or age (very young and elderly)

Table 95.4 Indications for extracorporeal detoxification.

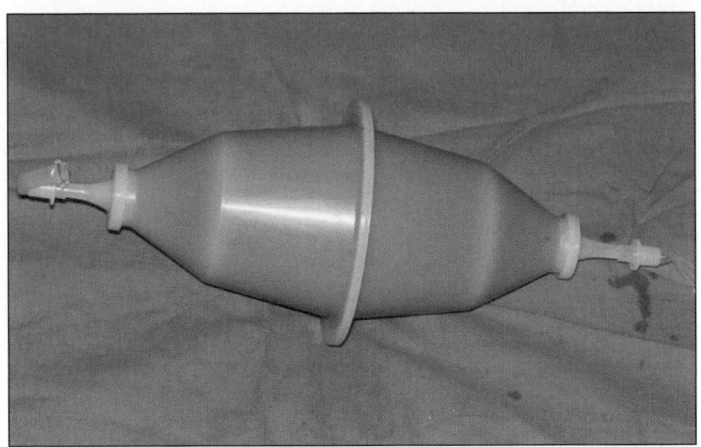

Figure 95.1 A charcoal hemoperfusion cartridge.

volume of distribution of the drug and the rate of equilibration between peripheral tissues and the plasma once removal has been started. There is no time limit to the dialysis treatment; efficiency does not lessen since fresh dialysate is continually presented and the membrane permeability is not affected. Hemodialysis may be combined with other strategies, for example with induction of alcohol dehydrogenase by ethanol or fomepizole for the treatment of ethylene glycol or methanol poisoning[11].

Hemodialysis is also indicated when acute renal failure complicates poisoning and as adjunctive therapy for the complications of poisoning, including electrolyte disturbance, acidosis, hyper- and hypothermia, pulmonary edema, and volume overload.

Peritoneal dialysis is inefficient compared with hemodialysis, achieving low mass transfer of solute relatively slowly. It should only be used in poisoning when hemodialysis is not rapidly available or is contraindicated.

Hemofiltration

Hemofiltration (see Chapters 78 and 82) generates convective transport of solute through the membrane and allows high flux up to a molecular mass of 40 000 Da. Below this cut off, removal rate is determined by blood drug concentration and is independent of molecular size. Since most poisons have molecular weights of < 1000 Da, hemofiltration offers no particular advantages over hemodialysis but is occasionally needed for larger substances, for example metal chelating complexes such as desferoxamine (desferrioxamine) and sodium edetate, and aminoglycosides.

Hemoperfusion

In hemoperfusion, blood comes into direct contact with a sorbent system by passage in the extracorporeal circuit through an adsorbent cartridge (Fig. 95.1). The first usable cartridge containing charcoal was introduced in 1954. Early use was complicated particularly by platelet depletion, which was overcome by microencapsulation of the charcoal with a polymer such as cellulose nitrate, rendering the surface biocompatible. Presently available devices use activated charcoal that adsorbs uncharged toxin molecules to carbon by van der Waals interactions (e.g., Gambro Adsorba 300

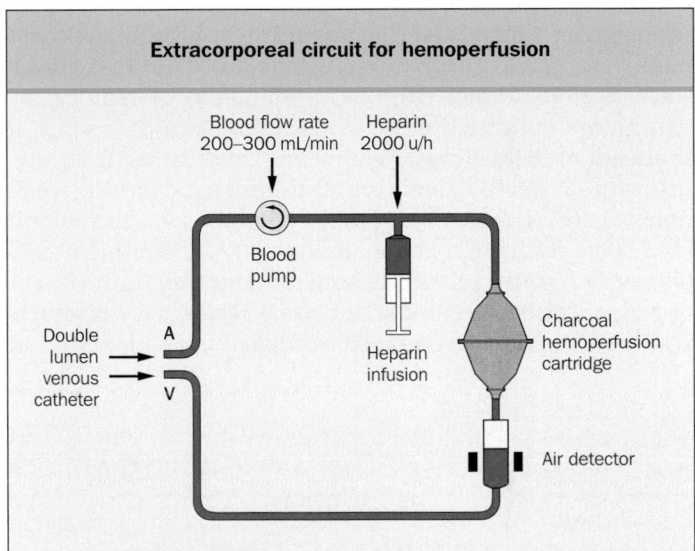

Figure 95.2 Extracorporeal circuit for hemoperfusion.

containing 300 g activated charcoal). The rate-limiting step for coated carbon is diffusion through the polymer membrane. Nonionic polystyrene exchange resins are also available (e.g., Braun Haemoresin, containing 750 g Amberlite XAD-4). Amberlite may be superior to charcoal for lipophilic molecules.

The extracorporeal circuit for hemoperfusion is shown in Figure 95.2. Hemoperfusion requires careful monitoring for, and treatment of, potential complications. The main complications are:
- mild thrombocytopenia caused by adsorption: the platelet counts usually fall by less than 30%; if the fall is greater than 30% or initial thrombocytopenia existed, prostacyclin treatment should be considered
- mild leukopenia resulting from margination owing to complement activation on surface contact
- low fibrinogen (and other coagulation factors) caused by adsorption
- hypothermia
- hypocalcemia
- hypoglycemia.

The crucial difference from hemodialysis is that hemoperfusion is time limited. After 4–8 h, the capacity of the adsorbents is exhausted because of clotting and adherence of cellular debris and plasma proteins on the adsorbent. Heparin itself is adsorbed and clotting of the cartridge is not uncommon. The heparin infusion rate should be at least 2000 U/h at a blood flow rate of 200–300 mL/min.

At one time hemoperfusion was heralded as the 'universal antidote'. But it does not remove ionized or protein-bound toxins; and although it removes many poisons, it does not offer superior clearance to hemodialysis in the great majority of circumstances. The use of hemoperfusion is now steadily declining. Although hemoperfusion can remove many poisons, in the majority of cases it has no advantage over hemodialysis, which in turn is used less and less as simpler measures are proving to be equally effective.

Hemodialysis–hemoperfusion

Although expensive, the concurrent use of hemodialysis and hemoperfusion is theoretically the treatment of first choice since it offers a very effective combination of removal by adsorption and diffusion[12]. The perfusion cartridge is placed upstream of the dialyzer. This system is very efficient for toxins with a small volume of distribution, achieving total removal in 4–6 h. For larger volumes of distribution (1–3 L/kg), it is slower and more than 10 h of treatment may be needed, with further treatment later when the toxin becomes redistributed into the plasma. There have been few systematic reports of combined hemodialysis–hemoperfusion

Kinetic characteristics that assist extracorporeal drug removal		
Hemodialysis	Hemofiltration	Hemoperfusion
Relative molecular mass <500 Da	Relative molecular mass less than cut off of filter fibers (usually 40 000 Da)	Adsorbed by activated charcoal
Water soluble		
Small volume of distribution (V_D; <1 L/kg)	Small V_D (<1 L/kg)	Small V_D (<1 L/kg)
Poorly bound to plasma proteins	Poorly bound to plasma proteins	
Single compartment kinetics	Single compartment kinetics	Single compartment kinetics
Low endogenous clearance (<4 mL/min per kg)	Low endogenous clearance (<4 mL/min per kg)	Low endogenous clearance (<4 mL/min per kg)

Table 95.5 Kinetic characteristics of drugs that assist extracorporeal drug removal.

but its effective use is described for theophylline[13,14] and *Amanita phalloides* mushroom poisoning[15].

Exchange transfusion

Exchange transfusion has a role for poisoning complicated by massive hemolysis, for example sodium chlorate or arsine,

Common poisonings for which extracorporeal removal may be indicated		
Hemodialysis	Drug level or other criterion for extracorporeal treatment	Comment
Ethanol	> 5 g/L (108 mmol/L)	
Methanol	> 50 mg/L (15 mmol/L)	Combine with fomepizole 15 mg/kg i.v. over 30 min; then 10 mg/kg 4-hourly during HD
Ethylene glycol	> 500 mg/L (8 mmol/L)	
Lithium	> 4 mmol/L 2.5 mmol/L if severe symptoms	Postdialysis rebound as intracellular lithium diffuses into ECF
Methanol	> 500 mg/L (15 mmol/L)	
Salicylate	> 800 mg/L (5.8 mmol/L)	Lower threshold if renal impairment or if fluid overload restricts treatment with sodium bicarbonate
Hemofiltration		
Aminoglycosides	Various	
Hemoperfusion		
Amanita mushroom	Clinical severity	
Barbiturates	Phenobarbitone 150 mg/L (630 mol/L)	
Carbamazepine	Clinical severity	
Paraquat	Clinical severity	
Theophylline	Acute > 100 mg/L Chronic > 40 mg/L	
Valproic acid	> 1 g/L	

Table 95.6 Common poisonings for which extracorporeal removal may be indicated.

since it will remove not only the poison but also red cell fragments and free hemoglobin. Exchange transfusion is also indicated when poisoning with hydrogen sulfide is complicated by methemoglobinemia and sulfhemoglobinemia.

Clinical decision making in poisoning

The final decision to deploy an extracorporeal drug-removal technique in any individual case requires the interpretation of the known toxicokinetics for that drug in the context of the clinical severity[16]. The kinetic characteristics of poisons that make them amenable to the different modalities of extracorporeal removal are shown in Table 95.5. The lack of controlled trials means that even the best-documented indications are still being debated.

The common poisonings for which extracorporeal removal is presently indicated are shown in Table 95.6.

REFERENCES

1. Macnamara AF, Riyat MS, Quinton DN. The changing profile of poisoning and its management. J Roy Soc Med. 1996;89:608–10.
2. Seyffart G. Poison Index: The Treatment of Acute Intoxication. Lengerich, Germany: Pabst Science; 1997.
3. Litovitz TL, Klein-Schwartz W, White S, et al. 2000 Annual report of the American Association of Poison Control Centers Toxic Exposure Surveillance System. Am J Emerg Med. 2001; 19:337–95.
4. Abuelo GJ. Renal failure caused by chemicals, foods, plants, animal venoms and misuse of drugs. Arch Intern Med. 1990; 150:505–10.
5. Lheureux P, Even-Adin D, Askenasi R. Current status of antidotal therapies in acute human intoxications. Acta Clin Belg Suppl. 1990;13:29–47.
6. Vale JA. Review in medicine. Clinical toxicology. Postgrad Med J. 1993;69:19–32.
7. Position statement and practice guidelines on the use of multi-dose activated charcoal in the treatment of acute poisoning. American Academy of Clinical Toxicology; European Association of Poisons Centres and Clinical Toxicologists. J Toxicol Clin Toxicol. 1999;37:731.
8. Abel JJ, Rowntree LG, Turner BB. On the removal of diffusible substances from the circulating blood by means of dialysis. Trans Assoc Am Physic. 1913;28:51–4.
9. Winchester JF. Active methods of detoxification. In: Haddad LM, Shannon MW, Winchester JF, ed. Clinical Management of Poisoning and Drug Overdose, 3rd edn. Philadelphia: WB Saunders; 1997:175.
10. Pond SM. Extracorporeal techniques in the treatment of poisoned patients. Med J Aust. 1991;154:617–22.
11. Brent J, McMartin K, Phillips S, et al. Fomepizole for the treatment of methanol poisoning. N Engl J Med. 2001;344:424–9.
12. Verpooten GA, Broe M de. Combined hemoperfusion-hemodialysis in severe poisoning. Kinetics of drug extraction. Resuscitation. 1984;11:275–89.
13. Higgins RM, Hearing S, Goldsmith DJA, et al. Severe theophylline poisoning: charcoal haemoperfusion or haemodialysis? Postgrad Med J. 1995;71:224–6.
14. Heath A, Knudsen K. Role of extracorporeal drug removal in acute theophylline poisoning: a review. Med Toxicol. 1987; 2:294–308.
15. Sabeel AI, Kurkus J, Lindholm T. Intensive hemodialysis and hemoperfusion treatment of Amanita mushroom poisoning. Mycopathologia. 1995;131:107–14.
16. Richlie DG, Anderson RJ. Contemporary management of salicylate poisoning: should hemodialysis and hemoperfusion be used? Sem Dial. 1996;9:257–64.

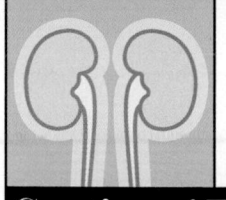

Section 17 Drugs and the Kidney

Chapter 96

Principles of Drug Dosing and Prescribing in Renal Failure

Ali J Olyaei, Angelo M de Mattos and William M Bennett

INTRODUCTION

Optimal management of patients with renal failure requires the use of pharmacotherapeutic agents for comorbid conditions. The kidney is the major organ in which drug elimination from the body occurs. Renal insufficiency and dialysis alter the pharmacokinetics and pharmacodynamics of most commonly used drugs. A recent report form the US Renal Data System (USRDS) indicates that the median number of medications prescribed in renal failure is eight different classes of drugs per patient. In comparison to the general population, patients with renal insufficiency experience significantly more adverse drug reactions. Therefore, clinicians should be familiar with the pharmacokinetic behavior of each agent and of the impact of renal failure on the drug elimination process. A particular area of concern is that patients with renal insufficiency also grow older and this also may effect drug disposition. Approximately 80% of patients with renal failure are concomitantly prescribed a phosphate binder, antihypertensive agent, iron supplement, antihypercholesteremic drug in addition to other medications. Because these patients take multiple medications, they are at a greater risk for drug–drug interactions.

This chapter highlights the commonest prescribing issues for the practicing nephrologist. It describes the principles of pharmacotherapy in patients with renal disease of varying severity and proposes prescribing guidelines for physicians who care for patients with renal impairment. This is particularly important since physiologic changes associated with chronic renal failure affect virtually every organ system in the body, and, thus, drug disposition. It is imperative that clinicians have a basic understanding of the biochemical and physiologic effects of drugs in patients with renal disease. Specific dosing guidelines and pharmacokinetic information are provided in the Appendix at the end of this chapter.

GENERAL PRINCIPLES OF DRUG PHARMACOKINETICS

Pharmacokinetics is the study of drug behavior (absorption, distribution, metabolism and elimination) in the body. The key elements of drug pharmacokinetics are shown in Figure 96.1. Following oral administration, only a certain proportion of the drug is absorbed and reaches systemic circulation (bioavailability). Drugs can be highly bound to plasma proteins or unbound. Only the free or unbound concentration of the drug interacts with specific receptors at the site of pharmacologic action. The three major processes affecting drug excretion and/or elimination from the body include metabolism by the liver, metabolism by the gastrointestinal tract (cytochrome P450 and P-glycoproteins) or elimination and metabolism by the kidney. The kidney remains the most important organ for drug elimination, both of the parent compound and of drug metabolites[1]. The liver can also metabolize drugs in the 'first pass' as the drug is absorbed into the portal circulation, or later when the drug is delivered to the liver via the systemic blood flow prior to reaching the systemic circulation. First pass metabolism can significantly reduce the rate and extent of drug absorption. Lidocaine, for example, is metabolized extensively before it reaches the systemic circulation, renal failure may decrease its biotransformation and ultimately the first pass metabolism. Changes in cardiac output in patients with renal failure may also reduce the rate and extent of drug metabolism of drugs with significant first pass metabolism. For example, increased bioavailability has been reported for propranolol and dihydrocodeine, which undergo a significant first pass metabolism in patients with renal failure. In one report, the overall drug exposure in 24 h and plasma drug concentration of dihydrocodeine was significantly higher in patients with renal failure[1].

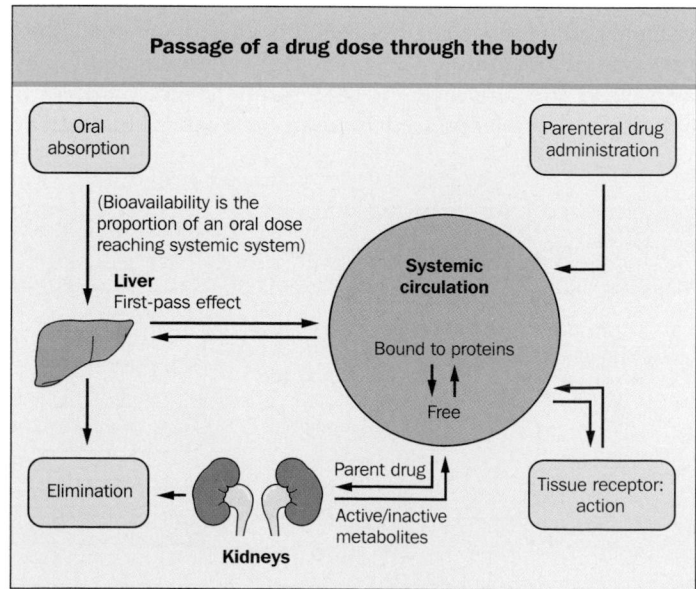

Figure 96.1 The passage of a drug through the body.

Bioavailability

The percentage of a drug dose that appears in the systemic circulation following oral administration compared with the intravenous route for the same drug defines its bioavailability. In general, drugs given by the intravenous route reach the central compartment directly and usually have a more rapid onset of action. Drugs given by other routes must pass through a series of biologic membranes before entering the systemic circulation. For many drugs, only a fraction of the administered dose may reach the circulation to exert any pharmacodynamic effect. Chronic renal failure may influence drug absorption and bioavailability. Edema of the gastrointestinal tract is a limiting factor in drug absorption. Drug absorption is particularly a problem when patients have diabetes mellitus as a cause of chronic renal insufficiency. Gastrointestinal neuropathy may decrease gastric emptying time and slow the rate and extent of drug absorption. In addition, since gastrointestinal symptoms are common in advanced renal failure of any cause, nausea and vomiting often impair drug dosing and contact time between the individual drug and the mucosa of the gastrointestinal tract. In advanced renal failure with uremia, there is an alkalinizing effect of salivary urea, which is converted to ammonia by urease. This effect decreases the absorption of drugs that are optimally absorbed in an acid milieu (see Fig. 96.2). For example, supplemental iron requires conversion by acid from the ferrous to the ferric state for absorption. The administration of histamine H_2-receptor blockers may also contribute to an alkalinizing effect and impair the absorption of iron. In addition, other drugs used as phosphate-binding agents and even dairy products themselves may decrease drug absorption by chelating and formation of nonabsorbable complexes. Hypertensive crisis has been reported following administration of the orally active lipase inhibitor, orlistat, in hypertensive patients.

Hepatic first-pass metabolism may also be altered in patients with chronic renal insufficiency. Decreased biotransformation of drugs to inactive metabolites, may lead to an increased amount of active drug reaching the systemic circulation. Some drugs have increased bioavailability in renal failure, leading to increased pharmacologic effects after a relatively small dose, for example zidovudine (AZT). The P-glycoprotein pump may also effect the drug delivery system. The P-glycoprotein is an efflux pump expressed in many tissues including the gastrointestinal tract, liver and brain. Drugs that induce P-glycoproteins may decrease drug absorption or decrease active drug moiety at the pharmacologic site[2]. Since the interactions of drug absorption and hepatic metabolism are very complex, the situation in individual patients is difficult to predict from general principles. Therefore drug bioavailability should always be considered as a factor in either increased or decreased pharmacologic effects of a given dose of drug administered to a patient with renal insufficiency[3].

Drug distribution
Volume of distribution

There is a characteristic volume of distribution (V_D) for any drug, which represents the ratio of the administered dose to the resulting plasma concentration at equilibrium. This is really an 'apparent' volume of distribution (V_D) since this mathematical construct does not correspond to a specific anatomic space but instead relates the amount of drug in the body to its plasma concentration. It is obvious that for drugs with a low plasma concentration relative to the dose, such as digoxin, this apparent V_D may exceed the total body water. Conversely, drugs that are highly protein bound and thus are restricted to the circulation have low V_D relative to the dose. The concept of V_D is useful in predicting loading doses of drugs to achieve the desired plasma concentration relative to the dose prior to drug administration. The mathematical formula relating apparent V_D to the dose and blood concentration is:

■ EQUATION 96.I

$$V_D = \frac{\text{Dose}}{\text{Blood concentration}}$$

Highly protein-bound agents or drugs that are water soluble tend to be restricted to the extracellular fluid space and have relatively small V_D while drugs that are lipid soluble penetrate body tissues and have large V_D.

Any factor that alters the V_D will alter plasma drug levels and hence their effects. Renal insufficiency may alter the apparent drug V_D. Increases in the V_D occur in massive edema or ascites, particularly for drugs that are water soluble or are ordinarily protein bound. If the usual drug doses are given to patients with hypoalbuminemia or dehydration, low plasma drug levels may result. By comparison, muscle wasting or volume depletion may decrease the apparent V_D of water-soluble drugs. In these cases, giving the usual dose may result in unexpectedly high blood concentrations of the drug[2].

Plasma protein binding

Plasma protein binding is often altered in patients with renal insufficiency and this has an important effect on the V_D of any drug. Since the quantity of drug that is free or unbound is the pharmacologically active component, this fraction determines the amount available for pharmacologic action as well as the degree to which a particular therapeutic agent will be metabolized by the liver or excreted by the kidneys. Protein-bound drugs attach reversibly to either albumin or various glycoproteins in plasma. Organic acids usually have a single binding site on albumin whereas organic bases tend to have

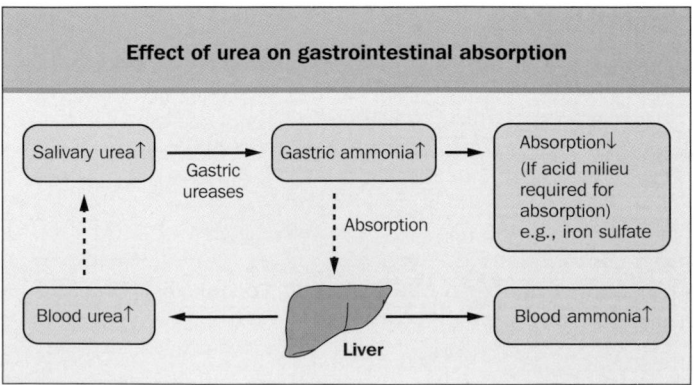

Effect of urea on gastrointestinal absorption

Figure 96.2 Effect of urea levels on gastrointestinal absorption.

multiple binding sites and their behavior in the presence of increasing renal insufficiency is less predictable. In general, acidic drugs have reduced plasma protein binding in patients with renal failure; this reduction is attributable to a combination of decreased albumin concentration and a reduction in albumin affinity, which is, in turn, influenced by either structural changes in the albumin molecule or accumulation of competing endogenous inhibitors of protein binding.

Common drugs that have plasma protein-binding changes in renal dysfunction are shown in Table 96.1. This list is clearly not complete but is chosen to represent drugs of different classes that have been studied. The consequences to the patient of impaired plasma protein binding are important since the unbound fraction of the drug may be substantially increased, resulting in toxicity. The best clinical example is phenytoin, which exhibits marked decreases in plasma protein binding with concomitant increased pharmacologic effects, particularly if plasma concentrations are assumed to be in the usual therapeutic range for the nonuremic patient. If protein binding is reduced, pharmacologic effects may be seen at lower plasma levels, particularly if such levels correspond to total drug. Furthermore, decreased protein binding may increase the apparent volume of distribution of any drug. However, predicting the clinical consequences of protein-binding abnormalities is difficult since while more free drug may be available to the site of drug action, lower plasma concentrations of the drug after a given dose can also occur. When more unbound drug is available for metabolism or renal excretion, the half-life of a drug in the body may actually be decreased rather than increased by altered protein binding. Again the clinician must be vigilant for unexpected adverse reactions and not rely on the numerical value of any plasma level but, instead, observe carefully.

Drug metabolism

The presence of progressive renal insufficiency obviously affects most body biochemical processes, and this includes drug biotransformation. In general, reduction and hydrolysis reactions are slowed, but glucuronidation, sulfation, conjugation, and microsomal oxidation reactions occur at normal rates. Since there may be significant patient variation, no prior assumptions will substitute for careful clinical evaluation. Furthermore, some drugs have pharmacologically active metabolites, which, although unimportant in patients with normal renal function, may accumulate in patients with renal insufficiency, causing adverse drug reactions. Some of these pharmacologic reactive metabolites may account for the high incidence of adverse drug reactions in patients with renal failure. Some of the best-known examples of this phenomenon are the accumulation of pharmacologically active metabolites of meperidine causing seizures, nitrofurantoin causing peripheral neuropathy, and morphine sulfate causing respiratory depression[3].

Renal handling of drugs

The renal excretion of drugs depends primarily on the glomerular filtration rate (GFR) and the balance between reabsorption and secretion of drugs in the renal tubules. In turn, the GFR of drugs depends on molecular size and protein binding of the agent. Therefore, for drugs that have decreased protein binding in renal failure, increased amounts of drug may be secreted by the renal tubule in compensation. However, when GFR is impaired by renal disease, the clearance of drugs eliminated primarily by the kidney is decreased and usually the plasma half-life of drugs is prolonged. The quantitation of drug elimination by the kidney is usually expressed as clearance, which equals the volume of blood or plasma from which the drug is cleared per unit time. This depends on renal blood flow and the ability of the kidney to extract the drug. For the total body, the clearance is expressed as the drug dose divided by the area under the drug concentration curve (AUC). For the kidney, this is the well understood clearance formula (Table 96.2). The drug half-life describes the rate of drug removal from the body related to the volume distribution and the clearance (Table 96.2). If drug half-life increases, the renal clearance is usually decreased. Occasionally there is compensation by extrarenal elimination pathways in a patient with renal failure. Clinically, it is very difficult to measure tubular function, and the secretion of drugs that are eliminated by active tubular transport systems may also be affected in patients with renal disease. For practical purposes, as the rate of creatinine clearance (C_{cr}) decreases, drugs dependent on renal tubular secretion are also excreted more slowly. Therefore, C_{cr} is a reasonable clinical estimate of GFR and the tubular capacity for drug excretion[3,4].

Pharmacokinetics

Pharamacokinetics is the study and mathematical expression of the time course of drugs in the body. Mathematical equations can explain the behavior of an individual drug with regard to its absorption, distribution, metabolism, and excretion (for both the parent drug and any metabolites). After the administration of a drug, there is a high initial plasma concentration of the drug, followed by a decrease in the drug level as the drug is distributed from the plasma into an

Plasma protein binding of drugs in renal failure			
Acidic drugs	Binding	Basic drugs	Binding
Barbiturates	D	Dapsone	N
Benzylpenicillin	D	Desmethylimipramine	N
Clofibrate	D	Diazepam	D
Dicloxacillin	D	Morphine	D
Furosemide (frusemide)	D	Propranolol	N
Indomethacin	N	Quinidine	N
Phenytoin	D	Triamterene	D
Salicylate	D	Trimethoprim	N
Warfarin	D		
D, decreased; N, normal.			

Table 96.1 Plasma protein binding of drugs in renal failure.

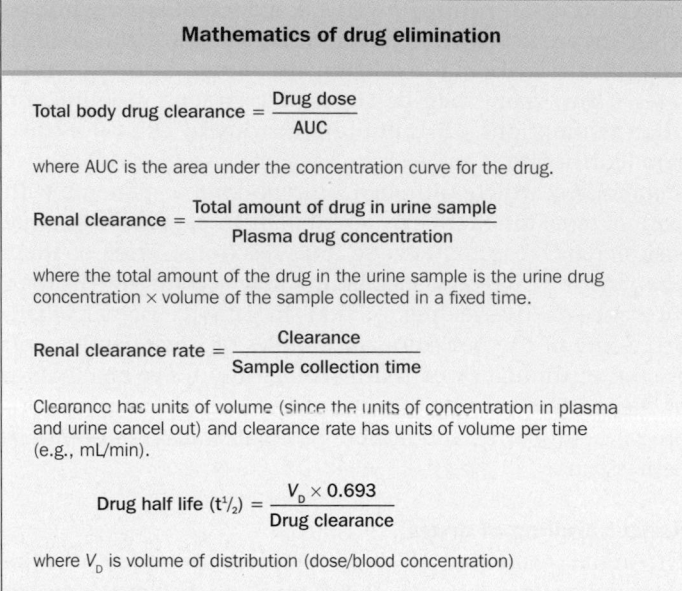

Mathematics of drug elimination

Total body drug clearance $= \dfrac{\text{Drug dose}}{\text{AUC}}$

where AUC is the area under the concentration curve for the drug.

Renal clearance $= \dfrac{\text{Total amount of drug in urine sample}}{\text{Plasma drug concentration}}$

where the total amount of the drug in the urine sample is the urine drug concentration × volume of the sample collected in a fixed time.

Renal clearance rate $= \dfrac{\text{Clearance}}{\text{Sample collection time}}$

Clearance has units of volume (since the units of concentration in plasma and urine cancel out) and clearance rate has units of volume per time (e.g., mL/min).

Drug half life $(t^{1/2}) = \dfrac{V_D \times 0.693}{\text{Drug clearance}}$

where V_D is volume of distribution (dose/blood concentration)

Table 96.2 Mathematics of drug elimination.

extravascular compartment. Along with this absorption and distribution, drug metabolism and elimination is beginning. At steady state, drug concentrations in plasma reach equilibrium with concentrations in body tissue. It is useful to determine the behavior of a given drug in patients with varying degrees of renal dysfunction. This is usually done by comparing pharmacokinetic data from individuals with normal renal function with that from patients with renal insufficiency. This is the basis for most dosage recommendations. However, individual patient factors almost always limit the utility of broad generalities when the physician is confronted with a complex, sick individual. It is here that the judgment of the physician in regard to a particular patient's ability to handle a drug or chemical substance is paramount. There is no easy substitute for knowing the pharmacology of the drug under normal circumstances, and there is no easy way to understand dosing other than to consider individual patient factors. The pharmacokinetic parameters usually used in describing drug behavior are shown in Table 96.3. These terms are utilized throughout the Appendix, which gives information on specific drug dosing[5]. The key effects of renal dysfunction on drug handling that will affect dosing are:
- accumulation of drugs normally excreted
- accumulation of 'active' drug metabolites
- changes in drug distribution: protein binding
- decreases in renal drug metabolism.

PRESCRIBING FOR THE PATIENT WITH RENAL DISEASE

The thought process that goes into prescribing drugs for patients with renal disease should be systematic and careful because of the high incidence of adverse drug reactions in this group. A stepwise approach is outlined in Figure 96.3. The goal of therapy, of course, is to maintain efficacy while avoiding drug accumulation and associated adverse reactions.

Pharmacokinetic parameters

Parameter (abbreviation)	Clinical application
Bioavailability (F)	Determines the amount of drug reaching the systemic circulation and, therefore, the amount at the site of action
Volume of distribution (V_D)	Determines the size of a loading dose
Clearance (C)	Determines the maintenance dose
Half-life ($t^{1/2}$)	Determines the amount of time needed to reach steady-state serum concentrations

Table 96.3 Pharmacokinetic parameters.

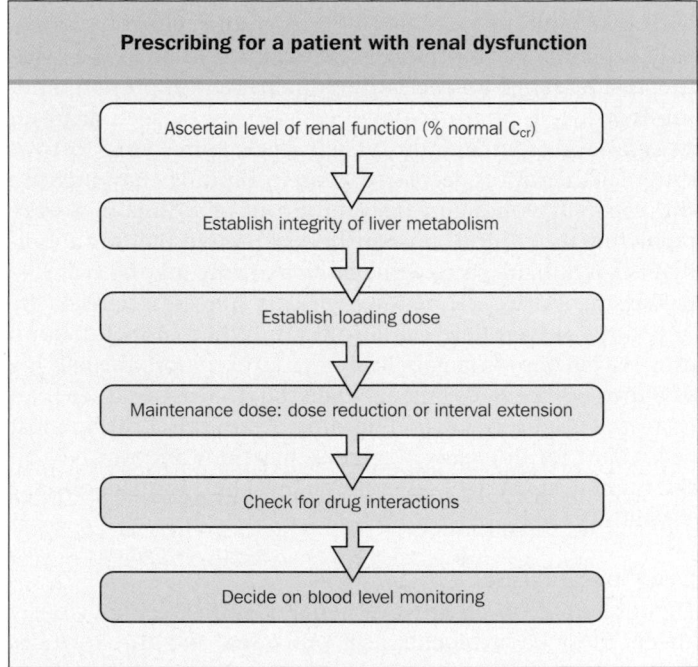

Prescribing for a patient with renal dysfunction

Ascertain level of renal function (% normal C_{cr})

↓

Establish integrity of liver metabolism

↓

Establish loading dose

↓

Maintenance dose: dose reduction or interval extension

↓

Check for drug interactions

↓

Decide on blood level monitoring

Figure 96.3 Prescribing for a patient with renal dysfunction.

Dosing for the renal patient
When the GFR is reduced, the elimination of many compounds and pharmacologically active metabolites declines proportionally. The prolongation of a drug's elimination half-life is proportional to the reduction in GFR. Although drug accumulation may occur at any level of renal insufficiency, such adverse events are relatively uncommon when the GFR remains > 50 mL/min. If dosage restrictions are excessive because of fears of toxicity, inadequate therapy may result. In acute renal failure, the decline in GFR is virtually total so patients should be dosed as if they have GFR < 10 mL/min until a steady state is reached[6,7].

Dosing of individual drugs
Patients with renal failure are heterogeneous and their responses to drug therapy are variable. Dosage nomograms, tables, and computer-assisted dosing recommendations are helpful but are not necessarily associated with better

therapeutic outcomes. Any fixed approach to dosing will probably fail because of the complexity of renal failure in patients. In the Appendix, dosing recommendations are made based on various levels of renal function, but it must be realized that these doses vary with the specific needs of each patient. It should be emphasized that physicians should use their clinical judgment to evaluate every individual situation, choose a dosage regimen based on factors present in that patient and continually re-evaluate the patient's response to therapy. The Appendix details common drugs used in patients with renal failure and is not complete. For individual drugs that are not listed in the Appendix, the reader is referred to the more encyclopedic compilations of drug information[9,10].

Initial assessment

A targeted history and physical examination constitute the first step in assessing dosage in patients with renal impairment. Previous drug toxicity or intolerance should be ascertained if possible. The patient's current medication list (both prescription and nonprescription formulations) must be reviewed to identify potential drug interactions and nephrotoxins. Physical findings suggest the patient's volume status, provide height and weight data used in calculating ideal body mass, and determine whether extrarenal disease states such as hepatic dysfunction are present, requiring additional dosage adjustment.

Estimating renal function for drug dosing

Renal function and GFR can be estimated by measuring the clearance of certain compounds (see Chapter 3). Blood urea nitrogen (BUN) and serum creatinine levels are insensitive measures of renal function. Creatinine clearance (C_{cr}) is traditionally used to approximate GFR. The fact that lean body mass and age correlate with C_{cr} directly and inversely, respectively, allows the use of serum creatinine level to estimate the C_{cr} (using the Cockcroft and Gault formula)[11].

■ EQUATION 96.2

$$\text{Calculated } C_{cr} = \frac{(140 - \text{age}) \text{ ideal body weight (kg)}}{72 \times \text{serum creatinine (mg/dL)}}$$

In women, the result is multiplied by 0.85.

It is important to remember that this formula represents only an approximation of renal function (see Chapter 3). If a patient has acute renal failure, $C_{cr} < 10$ mL/min should be assumed for purposes of drug dosage adjustment.

The loading dose

For most drugs in the setting of normal renal function, a steady-state concentration is achieved after five drug half-lives. Because renal failure may prolong an agent's half-life, simply reducing drug doses would be a therapeutic error because such a strategy would delay achievement of steady-state concentrations and therapeutic drug levels. Therefore, a loading dose needs to be given for most drugs. This dose usually does not vary much from the initial dose given to patients with normal renal function. An exception to this rule is

digoxin, for which 50–75% of the usual loading dose should be given because of its reduced V_D in renal failure. In patients with significant volume contraction superimposed on renal failure, it is prudent to lower the standard loading doses of aminoglycosides by 20–25% to avoid toxicity.

Maintenance dosing

The Appendix provides general dosing guidelines for several different classes of drugs commonly used in patients with renal failure. Patient specific factors, risk of drug–drug interactions and general risk of adverse events for a particular agent should be considered prior to starting pharmacotherapy. After a loading dose has been given, a maintenance dosing regimen should be calculated[11]. The maintenance dose may be determined by one of two methods. First, the dosing interval can be lengthened by the use of the following formula:

■ EQUATION 96.3

$$\text{Dosing interval} = \frac{\text{Normal } C_{cr}}{\text{Patient's } C_{cr}} \times \text{Normal interval}$$

Alternatively, each individual dose can be reduced and given at standard intervals:

$$\text{Dose} = \frac{\text{Patient's } C_{cr}}{\text{Normal } C_{cr}} \times \text{Normal dose}$$

The first or 'varying interval' method can potentially lead to periods of subtherapeutic drug concentrations. The latter, or 'varying dose method' allows for more constant drug levels but risks toxicity owing to higher trough levels. For these reasons, the interval method is preferable for aminoglycosides, whereas the dosage method is more applicable to anticonvulsants and antiarrhythmics. An example of calculations for dosage of aminoglycosides is shown in Figure 96.4.

Drug level monitoring

Simply varying the dose or dosing interval is usually not sufficient when adjusting drug regimens for patients with complex disease including renal failure. Monitoring drug levels when possible may be necessary to ensure therapeutic levels while avoiding toxicity[4]. Drug assays usually measure only total blood concentrations and may significantly underestimate plasma levels of the active or free form of the drug. Phenytoin represents a prototype. As a result of opposing pharmacokinetic changes in protein binding and distribution factors, no dose adjustment is generally needed. The therapeutic range, however, is reduced to 4–8 mg/L (16–32 mmol/L) from 10–20 mg/L (40–80 mmol/L), reflecting the increased proportion of active or 'free' drug present. In clinical practice, drug level monitoring is only necessary to assist prescribing in renal failure for a minority of drugs, especially those with a narrow therapeutic index. The drugs for which such monitoring is recommended are shown in Table 96.4.

Drugs in nephrotic syndrome

Drug handling in patients with heavy proteinuria and nephrotic syndrome is complex. In patients with low serum

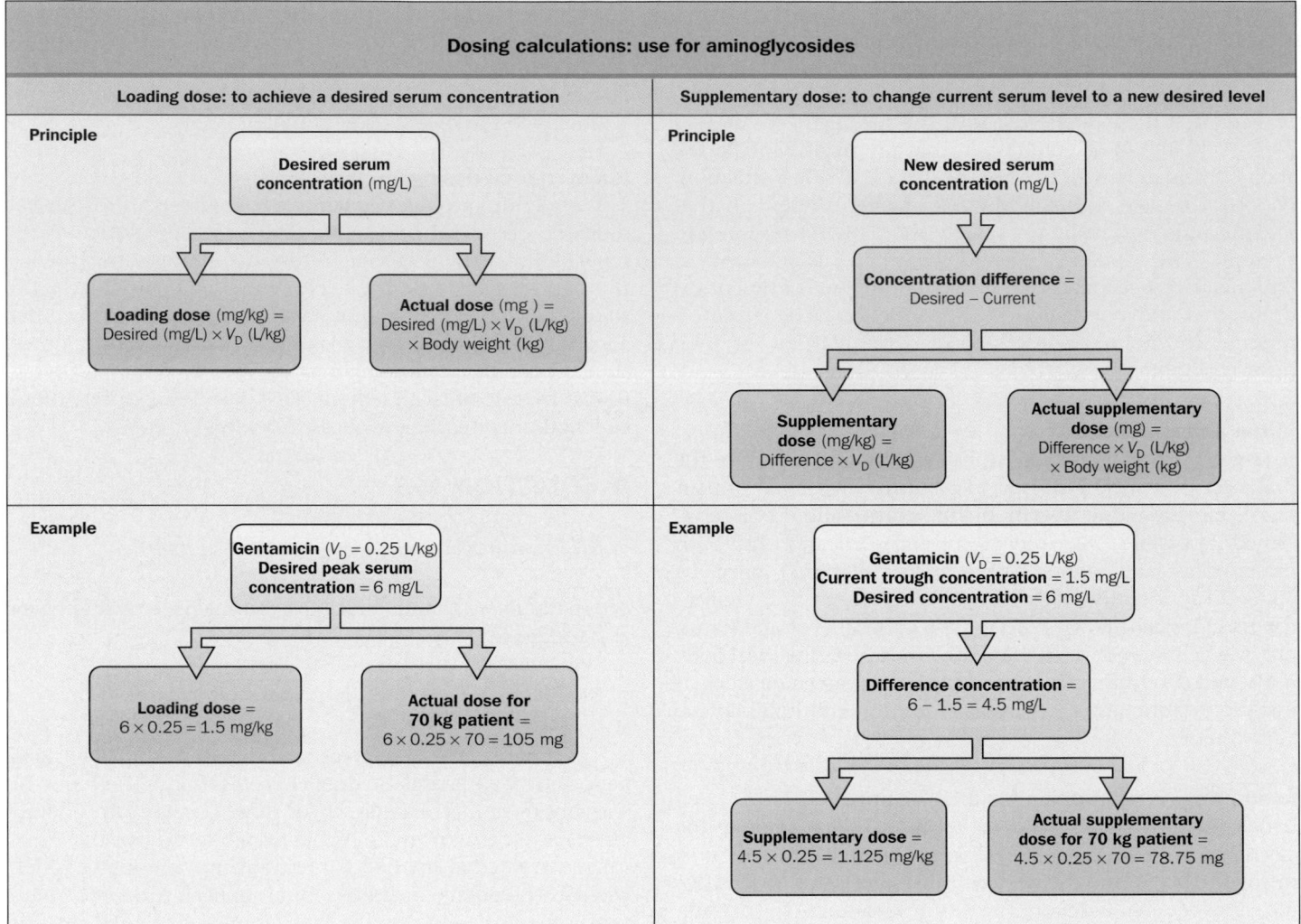

Figure 96.4 Dosage calculations.

albumin and coexisting renal dysfunction, drug binding to plasma proteins may be altered. In this case, more free drug is available for any total drug concentration; this may result in adverse effects or more rapid metabolism, depending on the clinical circumstances. Furthermore, when albumin is lost in the urine, bound drug may also be lost. This may be a partial explanation for the refractoriness of some nephrotic patients to diuretic therapy. Some drugs produce adverse effects more readily in nephrotic patients, for example clofibrate, which can provoke severe muscle necrosis; all fibrates should be used with caution in patients with nephrotic syndrome.

Extracorporeal drug losses

Hemodialysis

For patients receiving hemodialysis, attention must be paid to dose scheduling and the need to give supplemental doses to replace lost body stores. Dialysis clearance of a drug depends primarily on its molecular weight and degree of protein binding. As protein binding increases, dialysis clearance decreases. Likewise, the smaller the compound (< 500 Da), the more drug is removed during a dialysis treatment. In general, scheduled doses should be given after dialysis if possible. Additionally, if a significant portion of a drug is removed, supplemental doses should be given after each dialysis session. Commonly used drugs for which supplemental post dialysis dosing may be required are shown in Table 96.5.

Peritoneal dialysis

Many of the same properties of drugs that affect removal by hemodialysis also apply to peritoneal dialysis, but the latter treatment is very inefficient. For significant removal to occur by peritoneal dialysis, the drug must have a very low volume of distribution, low protein binding, and few other routes of drug elimination. Therefore, for most drugs in clinical use, there is little evidence of significant drug removal during chronic peritoneal dialysis[11]. It is also generally true that if hemodialysis does not remove a drug significantly, neither will peritoneal dialysis. As an example, one conventional hemodialysis treatment removes about two-thirds of the body stores of aminoglycoside antibiotics, whereas 24 h of continuous ambulatory peritoneal dialysis, will remove only 25–30% of the drug.

Drugs for which monitoring of drug levels is routinely recommended			
Drug Name	**Therapeutic range**	**When to draw sample**	**How often to check levels**
Aminoglycosides (Conventional dosing) Gentamicin Tobramycin Amikacin	**Gentamicin** and **Tobramycin:** Peak: 5–8 mg/L Trough: 0.5–2 mg/L **Amikacin:** Peak: 20–30 mg/L Trough: <10 mg/L	Trough: Immediately prior to dosing Peak: 30 min after a 30 min infusion	Check peak and trough with 3rd dose For therapy less than 72 h, levels not necessary. Repeat drug levels weekly or if renal function changes
Aminoglycosides (24 h dosing) Gentamicin Tobramycin Amikacin	0.5–3 mg/L	Obtain random drug level 12 h after dose	After initial dose. Repeat drug level in 1 week or if renal function changes
Carbamazepine	4–12 µg/mL	Trough: Immediately prior to dosing	Check 2–4 days after first dose or change in dose
Cyclosporine	150–400 ng/mL	Trough: Immediately prior to dosing	Daily for first week, then weekly
Digoxin	0.8–2.0 ng/mL	12 h after maintenance dose	5–7 days after first dose for patients with normal renal and hepatic function; 15–20 days in anephric patients
Lidocaine	1–5 µg/mL	8 h after i.v. infusion started or changed	
Lithium	Acute: 0.8–1.2 mmol/L Chronic: 0.6–0.8 mmol/L	Trough: Before a.m. dose at least 12 h since last dose	
Phenobarbital	15–40 µg/mL	Trough: Immediately prior to dosing	Check 2 weeks after first dose or change in dose. Follow-up level in 1–2 months
Phenytoin	10–20 µg/mL	Trough: Immediately prior to dosing	5–7 days after first dose or after change in dose
Free Phenytoin	1–2 µg/mL		
Procainamide	4–10 µg/mL Peak: 8 µg/mL Trough: 4 µg/mL	Trough: Immediately prior to next dose or 12–18 h after starting or changing an infusion	
NAPA (n-acetyl procainamide) a procainamide metabolite	10–30 µg/mL	With Procainamide sample	
Quinidine	1–5 µg/mL	Trough: Immediately prior to next dose	
Sirolimus	10–20 ng/dL	Trough: Immediately prior to next dose	
Tacrolimus	10–15 ng/mL	Trough: Immediately prior to next dose	
Theophylline p.o. or Aminophylline i.v.	15–20 µg/mL	Trough: Immediately prior to next dose	
Valproic acid	40–100 µg/mL	Trough: Immediately prior to next dose	Check 2–4 days after first dose or change in dose
Vancomycin	Peak: 25–40 mg/L Trough: 5–15 mg/L	Trough: Immediately prior to dose Peak: 60 min after a 60 min infusion	With 3rd dose (when initially starting therapy, or after each dosage adjustment). For therapy less than 72 h, levels not necessary. Repeat drug levels if renal function changes

Table 96.4 Therapeutic drug monitoring in renal insufficiency. Drugs for which monitoring is routinely recommended.

Continuous renal replacement therapy

Continuous therapies with arteriovenous hemofiltration or venovenous hemofiltration use relatively porous membranes with convective transport of solute. If dialysate is added, diffusion of solutes can also occur. Therefore, low-molecular-weight drugs are removed at a greater rate using these continuous techniques. The rate of removal is determined by the drug protein binding and the device filtration rate. A series of sieving coefficients is available that allows calculation of the amount of drug actually lost if the ultrafiltration flow rate is known[11]. Specialized dosage of compounds with continuous therapy is dependent on the general state of the patient. It is difficult to adjust doses except by carefully timed and interpreted blood measurements.

COMMON PRESCRIBING ISSUES IN RENAL INSUFFICIENCY

Even when the principles of drug dosing in renal failure are followed, a substantial risk remains of drug-related adverse events. If there is still residual renal function, drugs may aggravate established renal impairment. Furthermore other drugs may aggravate the metabolic problems of renal failure, or cause nervous system or other toxicities because of accumulation.

Nephrotoxicity

A wide range of drugs may cause nephrotoxicity with or without pre-existing renal insufficiency (Table 96.6).

Commonly used drugs that require replacement dosing following conventional hemodialysis					
Acebutolol	Cefazolin	Chloral hydrate	Ifosfamide	Nadolol	Vigabatrin
Acetaminophen	Cefdinir	Chloramphenicol	Imipenem	Ofloxacin	Zidovudine
Acyclovir	Cefepime	Cyclophosphamide	Iodixanol	Penicillin	
Allopurinol	Cefmenoxime	Disopyramide	Isosorbide	Piperacillin	
Amikacin	Cefmetazole	Enalapril	Lisinopril	Procainamide	
Amoxicillin	Cefotaxime	Esmolol	Lithium	Pyrazinamide	
Ampicillin	Cefotetan	Ethosuximide	Loracarbef	Sotalol	
Aspirin	Cefoxitin	Famciclovir	Meropenem	Streptomycin	
Atenolol	Cefpirome	Fluconazole	Metformin	Sulfamethoxazole	
Aztreonam	Ceftazidime	Flucytosine	Methotrexate	Sulfisoxazole	
Captopril	Ceftibuten	5-fluorouracil	Methylprednisolone	Theophylline	
Carboplatin	Ceftizoxime	Foscarnet	Metoprolol	Ticarcillin	
Cefaclor	Cefuroxime	Gabapentin	Metronidazole	Tobramycin	
Cefdroxil	Cephalexin	Ganciclovir	Mezlocillin	Trimethoprim	
Cefamandole	Cephradine	Gentamicin	Minoxidil	Valacyclovir	

Table 96.5 Commonly used drugs that require replacement dosing following conventional hemodialysis.

Idiosyncratic nephrotoxic effects are unpredictable and independent of dosage. Acute interstitial nephritis and acute tubular necrosis are both common. Chronic effects result from interstitial nephritis or glomerulonephritis, most commonly membranous nephropathy with gold or D-penicillamine.

Predictable nephrotoxic effects are dose related. The four commonest classes of drug that aggravate renal impairment are aminoglycosides, angiotensin-converting enzyme (ACE) inhibitors and AT receptor antagonists (ATRA), NSAIDs and radiologic contrast media. Other examples include vancomycin, amphotericin B, cisplatin, and cyclosporine.

Aminoglycosides

Because of a narrow therapeutic window and GFR-dependent excretion, close attention must be paid to aminoglycoside dosing regimens, drug levels, changes in renal function, and concomitant nephrotoxic drug use[25]. As aminoglycosides accumulate, the risk of nephrotoxicity and ototoxicity increases. Bactericidal efficacy of aminoglycosides correlates with therapeutic peak concentrations. Toxicity, however, corresponds to rising trough levels. Therefore, dosage adjustment for these antimicrobial agents should primarily involve the varying interval approach (Fig. 96.4). Individual dose reductions are also occasionally necessary. Assessment of peak and trough aminoglycoside serum levels as well as C_{cr} are required to monitor therapy and avoid toxicity[22]. As well as aggravating pre-existing renal impairment, aminoglycoside toxicity may cause *de novo* acute renal failure. Nephrotoxicity is usually reversible, but ototoxicity may cause irreversible vestibular damage with long-term disability. Concomitant use of loop diuretics, especially ethacrynic acid, greatly increases the risk of ototoxicity.

ACE inhibitors and ATRAs

Worsening of renal impairment or even acute oliguric renal failure may occur when prescribing an ACE inhibitor or ATRA in patients with pre-existing renal disease. Those with atherosclerotic renal artery stenosis are at greatest risk, but

Drug nephrotoxicity		
Nephrotoxicity	Type of nephritis	Drugs
Without pre-existing renal impairment		
Acute idiosyncratic	Nephrotoxic acute tubular necrosis (ATN)	Many (see Chapter 15)
	Crystalluric ATN	Many (see Chapter 15)
	Acute interstitial nephritis	Many (see Chapter 60)
	Acute interstitial nephritis with nephrotic syndrome	NSAIDs
Acute predictable, dose related	–	Aminoglycosides, amphotericin, cisplatinum, cyclosporine, vancomycin
Chronic	Interstitial nephritis	Many (see Chapter 62)
	Glomerulonephritis	Gold, D-penicillamine
With pre-existing renal impairment		Aminoglycosides, ACE inhibitors, ATRAs, NSAIDs, contrast media

Table 96.6 Patterns of drug nephrotoxicity.

these drugs may also cause deterioration of renal function in the absence of conduit artery stenosis, particularly in dehydrated patients or where renal perfusion is compromised. Monitoring renal function is necessary seven to ten days after starting therapy to ensure that there has been no precipitous decline in GFR or hyperkalemia. Renal impairment caused by ACE inhibitors is usually, but not always, reversible on withdrawal of the drug[15].

Nonsteroidal anti-inflammatory drugs

By far the commonest nephrotoxic effect of NSAIDs is an acute deterioration in renal function due to renal vasoconstriction caused by renal prostaglandin inhibition[11]. The consequent acute renal failure may be oliguric or non oliguric.

The newer cyclooxygenase II (COX II) inhibitors (celecoxib and rofecoxib) have significantly less gastrointestinal complications than conventional NSAIDs. However, the COX II enzyme is constitutively expressed and regulates important physiological functions in the kidney, and available evidence indicates COX II inhibitors are no less nephrotoxic than other NSAIDs[12-15]. The overall incidence of hypertension, edema, and cardiovascular events is significantly higher for rofecoxib compared to celecoxib. In addition, more congestive heart failure and non-fatal myocardium infarction have been reported with the use of rofecoxib compared with other NSAIDs[13]. Use of rofecoxib should be avoided in patients with recent incidence of cardiovascular events, uncontrolled hypertension and impaired renal function.

Another uncommon form of NSAID nephrotoxicity involves drug hypersensitivity, resulting in interstitial nephritis with nephrotic-range proteinuria, histology showing glomerular podocyte changes similar to minimal change nephrotic syndrome. These changes are thought to result from the effects on glomerular permeability of cytokines released from infiltrating interstitial T cells. This form of renal failure typically has a protracted course; it is insidious in onset and slow in resolution. Long-term use of NSAIDs has also been linked to the development of renal papillary necrosis.

Specific recommendations for dose reduction of NSAIDs are not well defined. In patients at risk for developing acute renal failure or worsening renal function, NSAID use should be avoided. If NSAID use is necessary, particularly on a continuous basis, close monitoring of creatinine clearance, as well as urinalysis, should be performed at regular intervals[14].

Radiologic contrast media

Worsening of renal impairment by radiologic contrast media is common, particularly if large contrast volumes are used (e.g., in vascular imaging). Nonionic contrasts are safer but do not eliminate the risk. Fluid depletion aggravates the risk. Concomitant use of metformin enhances renal toxicity and it should be withdrawn 48 h before the use of contrast if circumstances allow.

Aggravation of metabolic effects of renal impairment

A number of drugs have no direct adverse influence on renal function but when used inappropriately in patients with renal impairment will aggravate the metabolic consequences of renal failure (Table 96.7).

Hyperkalemia

As well as potassium supplements and potassium-sparing diuretics (spironolactone, amiloride), hyperkalemia may also occur with ACE inhibitors, ATRAs, NSAIDs, and potassium citrate mixture. Tetracyclines are catabolic and provoke release of intracellular potassium into the extracellular fluid; this produces significant problems in advanced renal failure.

Uremia

Protein catabolic drugs will accelerate urea production and, therefore, aggravate uremia with no change in renal excretory function. Corticosteroids will provoke a modest rise in urea whenever they are used in the context of renal impairment.

Drug aggravation of metabolic effects of pre-existing renal impairment	
Metabolic effect	Drugs
Hyperkalemia	Potassium supplements, potassium-sparing diuretics (especially combination diuretics), NSAIDs, potassium citrate, tetracyclines, ACE inhibitors, ATRAs
Uremia	Corticosteroids, tetracyclines
Sodium and water retention	Sodium chloride, sodium bicarbonate, sodium-containing antacids (e.g., Gaviscon), fludrocortisone, carbenoxolone
Metabolic acidosis	Acetazolamide, metformin
Coagulopathy	Aspirin

Table 96.7 Aggravation by drugs of the metabolic effects of pre-existing renal impairment.

Tetracyclines are extremely catabolic and may rapidly worsen uremia and produce life-threatening hyperkalemia. They are absolutely contraindicated in moderate or severe renal impairment and in end-stage renal disease (ESRD). Second-generation tetracyclines such as doxycycline and minocycline are, however, safe in this regard.

Sodium and water retention

Most patients with renal impairment are intolerant of sodium loading, which may provoke fluid overload and hypertension. All sodium-containing medications and those that promote sodium and water retention should, therefore, be used with caution. These include sodium chloride, sodium bicarbonate, sodium-containing antacids (e.g., alginate preparations such as Gaviscon), fludrocortisone, and carbenoxolone.

Acidosis

Both acetazolamide and metformin aggravate metabolic acidosis and are contraindicated in renal failure.

Coagulopathy

The platelet dysfunction of uremia may be aggravated by aspirin. Low-dose aspirin (up to 150 mg daily) is widely used, with few problems, in the management of coronary and cerebral vascular disease in renal failure. Nevertheless, there may be a major clinical bleeding problem when the uremic patient on aspirin requires surgery. Aspirin in a full anti-inflammatory dose is contraindicated in renal failure.

Drug accumulation in renal failure

Many other drugs and their metabolites accumulate in renal failure unless adequate dose reductions are made, usually by increasing dosing intervals. Fortunately, only a small minority of drugs produce clinically important adverse effects. Some important examples are aluminum (confusion and dementia), nitrofurantoin (peripheral neuropathy), acyclovir (confusional state), morphine (obtundation and coma), digoxin (cardiotoxicity), fibrates (myopathy), and allopurinol (rash). The common side effects are included in the Appendix.

REFERENCES

1. Winters ME, Basic Clinical Pharmacokinetics. Winter ME, Applied Therapeutic Inc. Vancouver, WA, 1994.
2. Zhang Y, Benet LZ. The gut as a barrier to drug absorption: combined role of cytochrome P450 3A and P-glycoprotein. Clinical Pharmacokinetics. 2001;40(3):159–68.
3. Olyaei AJ, Bennett WM. 'The effect of renal failure on drug handling', Oxford Textbook of Critical Care, 1996.
4. Benedetti P, de Lalla F. Antibiotic therapy in acute renal failure, Contributions to Nephrology, 2001;132:136–45.
5. Olyaei AJ, de Mattos AM, Bennett WM. 'Prescribing drugs in renal failure', Brenner and Rector's, eds. The Kidney, 2000.
6. Olyaei AJ, de Mattos AM, Bennett WM. 'Drug-drug interaction and most commonly used drug in transplant recipients', Primer on Transplantation, American Society of Transplantation, 2000.
7. Olyaei AJ. 'Drug dosing in renal failure'. In: Treatment Strategies In Nephrology and Hypertension. Bennett, ed. PocketMedicine.com Inc 2001; 1st edn.
8. Olyaei AJ, de Mattos AM, Bennett WM. 'Principle of drug usage in dialysis patients', Dialysis Therapy, Hanley & Belfus Inc., 2001.
9. Olyaei AJ, de Mattos AM, Bennett WM. Drug usage in dialysis patients. In: Nissenson AR, Fine RN, Gentile DE, eds. Clinical Dialysis. Norwalk, NJ: Appleton and Lange; 2001.
10. Bennett WM. Guide to drug dosage in renal failure. In: Speight TM, Holford N, eds. Avery's Drug Treatment, 4th edn. Auckland: ADIS International; 1997:1725–92.
11. Aronoff GR, Golper TA, Morrison G, et al. Drug Prescribing in Renal Failure. Philadelphia, PA: American College of Physicians; 1999.
10. Henrich WL, Agodoa LE, Barrett B, et al. Analgesics and the kidney: summary and recommendations to the Scientific Advisory Board of the National Kidney Foundation from an ad hoc committee of the National Kidney Foundation. Am J Kidney Dis. 1996;27:162–5.
11. Becker-Cohen R, Frishberg Y. Severe reversible renal failure due to naproxen-associated acute interstitial nephritis. Eur J Pediat. 2001;160(5):293–5.
12. Perazella MA, Tray K. Selective cyclooxygenase-2 inhibitors: a pattern of nephrotoxicity similar to traditional nonsteroidal anti-inflammatory drugs. Am J Med. 2001;111(1):64–7.
13. Whelton A, Fort JG, Puma JA, et al. SUCCESS VI Study Group. Cyclooxygenase-2–specific inhibitors and cardiorenal function: a randomized, controlled trial of celecoxib and rofecoxib in older hypertensive osteoarthritis patients. Am J Ther. 2001; 8(2):85–95.
14. Gault MH, Barrett BJ. Analgesic nephropathy. Am J Kidney Dis. 1998;32(3):351–60.
15. Brater DC. Effects of nonsteroidal anti-inflammatory drugs on renal function: focus on cyclooxygenase-2-selective inhibition. Am J Med. 1999;107(6A):65S–70S.
16. Pisoni R, Ruggenenti P, Remuzzi G. Renoprotective therapy in patients with nondiabetic nephropathies. Drugs. 2001;61(6): 733–45.
17. Swan SK, Brater DC. Clinical pharmacology of loop diuretics and their use in chronic renal insufficiency. J Nephrol. 1993;6: 118–23.
18. Kellum Ja VR. The role of diuretic agents in the management of acute renal failure. Contrib Nephrol. 2001;132:158–70.
19. Andreucci M, Russo D, Fuiano G, et al. Diuretics in renal failure. Miner Electrolyte Metab. 1999;25(1/2):32–8.
20. Sirivella S, Gielchinsky I, Parsonnet V. Mannitol, furosemide, and dopamine infusion in postoperative renal failure complicating cardiac surgery. Ann Thorac Surg. 2000;69(2):501–6.
21. Klinge J. Intermittent administration of furosemide or continuous infusion in critically ill infants and children: does it make a difference? Intensive Care Med. 2001;27(4):623–4.
22. Nicolau DP, Freeman CD, Belliveau PP, et al. Experience with a once-daily aminoglycoside program administered to 2,184 adult patients. Antimicrob Agent Chemother. 1995;39:650–5.
23. Bennett WM, Craven R. Ampicillin and trimethoprim-sulfamethoxazole treatment of urinary tract infections in patients with severe renal disease. JAMA. 1976;236:236–9.
24. Muther RS, Bennett WM. Cyst fluid antibiotic concentrations in polycystic kidney disease: differences between proximal and distal cysts. Kidney Int. 1981;20:519–22.
25. Elzinga LW, Golper TA, Rashad AL, et al. Ciprofloxacin activity in cyst fluid from polycystic kidneys. Antimicrob Agent Chemother. 1988;32:844–7.
26. Bennett WM, Elzinga LW, Barry JM. Polycystic kidney disease: II. Diagnosis and management. Hosp Pr. 1988;27:61–72.
27. Bennett WM, Hartnett MN, Craven R, et al. Gentamicin concentrations in blood, urine, and renal tissue of patients with end-stage renal disease. J Lab Clin Med. 1977;90: 389–93.
28. Bennett WM. Guide to drug dosage in renal failure. In: Speight TM, Holford N, eds. Avery's drug treatment, 4th edn. Auckland, New Zealand: ADIS International; 1997:1725–92.
29. Bennett WM, Aronoff GR, Golper TA et al. Drug prescribing in renal failure. Philadelphia, PA: American College of Physicians; (1994).

APPENDIX

This appendix gives drug dosing guidelines and pharmacokinetic information on agents commonly used in patients with renal failure. It is not an exhaustive compilation. Additional information can be obtained from encyclopedic published sources.

Antimicrobial agents					
Drugs normal doses		**Renal excretion (%)**	**Dosage adjustment in renal failure**		**Comments**
			GFR > 50	GFR 10–50	GFR < 10	
Antimicrobial agents						
Aminoglycoside						Nephrotoxic, ototoxic, may prolong the neuromuscular blockade effect of muscle relaxants. Check level post-HD
Gentamicin	2 mg/kg q.8 h	95	60–90% q.12 h	30–70% q.24 h	20–30% q.24 h	Peak 6–8, Trough < 2
Tobramycin	2 mg/kg q.8 h	95	60–90% q.12 h	30–70% q.24 h	20–30% q.24 h	Peak 6–8, Trough < 2
Netilmicin	2 mg/kg q.8 h	95	60–90% q.12 h	30–70% q.24 h	20–30% q.24 h	Peak 6–8, Trough < 2
Amikacin	7.5 mg/kg q.12 h	95	60–90% q.12 h	30–70% q.24 h	20–30% q.24 h	Peak 20–30, Trough < 5
Cephalosporin						Coagulation abnormalities, transitory elevation of BUN, rash and serum sickness-like syndrome.
Oral Cephalosporin						
Cefaclor	250–500 mg t.i.d.	70	100%	100%	50%	
Cefadroxil	500 to 1 g b.i.d.	80	100%	100%	50%	
Cefixime	200 to 400 mg q.12h	85	100%	100%	50%	
Cefpodoxime	200 mg q.12 h	30	100%	100%	100%	
Ceftibuten	400 mg q.24 h	70	100%	100%	50%	
Cefuroxime	250–500 mg t.i.d.	90	100%	100%	100%	
Cephalexin	250–500 mg t.i.d.	95	100%	100%	100%	
Cephradine	250–500 mg t.i.d.	100	100%	100%	50%	
i.v. Cephalosporin						
Cefamandole	1–2 g i.v. q.6–8 h	100	q.6 h	q.8 h	q.12 h	
Cefazolin	1–2 g i.v. q.8 h	80	q.8 h	q.12 h	q.12–24 h	
Cefepime	1–2 g i.v. q.8 h	85	q.8–12 h	q.12 h	q.24 h	
Cefmetazole	1–2 g i.v. q.8 h	85	q.8 h	q.12 h	q.24 h	
Cefixime	200 mg q.12hr	50	q.12 h	q.24 h	q.24 h	
Cefoperazone	1–2 g i.v. q.12 h	20	No renal adjustment is required			
Cefotaxime	1–2 g i.v. q.6–8 h	60	q.8 h	q.12 h	q.12–24 h	
Cefotetan	1–2 g i.v. q.12 h	75	q.12 h	q.12–24 h	q.24 h	
Cefoxitin	1–2 g i.v. q.6 h	80	q.6 h	q.8–12 h	q.12 h	
Cefpodoxime	200–400 mg p.o. q.12 h	30	q.12 h	q.12–24 h	q.24 h	Three times a week in dialysis patients
Ceftazidime	1–2 g i.v. q.8 h	70	q.8 h	q.12 h	q.24 h	
Ceftriaxone	1–2 g i.v. q.24 h	50	No renal adjustment is required			
Cefuroxime	750–1.5 g i.v. q.8 h	90	q.8 h	q.8–12 h	q.12–24 h	
Penicillin						Bleeding abnormalities, hypersensitivity
Oral penicillin						
Amoxicillin	500 mg p.o. t.i.d.	60	100%	100%	50–75%	
Ampicillin	500 mg p.o. q.6 h	60	100%	100%	50–75%	
Dicloxacillin	250–500 mg p.o. q.6 h	50	100%	100%	50–75%	
Penicillin V	250–500 mg p.o. q.6 h	70	100%	100%	50–75%	
IV Penicillin						
Ampicillin	1–2 g i.v. q.6 h	60	q.6 h	q.8 h	q.12 h	
Nafcillin	1–2 g i.v. q.4 h	35	No renal adjustment is required			
Penicillin G	2–3 million Units i.v. q.4 h	70	q.4–6 h	q.6 h	q.8 h	
Piperacillin	3–4 g i.v. q.4–6 h		No renal adjustment is required			
Ticarcillin/clavulanate	3.1 g i.v. q.4–6 h		100%	3.1 g q.8 h	3.1 g q.12 h	
Piperacillin/tazobactam	3.375 g i.v. q.6–8 h		100%	2.25 g q.6 h	2.25 g q.8 h	
Quinolones						Photosensitivity, food, dairy products, tube feeding and Al (OH)3 may decrease the absorption of quinolones
Ciprofloxacin	200–400 mg i.v. q.24 h	60	q.12 h	q.12–24 h	q.24 h	
Gatifloxacin	400 mg p.o./i.v. q.24 h	88	100%	50%	50%	
Levofloxacin	500 mg p.o. q.i.d.	70	100%	50%	50%	
Moxifloxacin	400 mg q.i.d.	20	No renal adjustment is required			
Norfloxacin	400 mg p.o. q.12 h	30	q.12 h	q.12–24 h	q.24 h	
Ofloxacin	200–400 mg p.o. q.12 h	70	q.12 h	q.12–24 h	q.24 h	
Miscellaneous agents						
Azithromycin	250–500 mg p.o. q.i.d.	6	No renal adjustment is required			NO drug-drug interaction with cyclosporine/tacrolimus
Clarithromycin	500 mg p.o. b.i.d.	20	No renal adjustment is required			Pseudomembranous colitis
Clindamycin	150–450 mg p.o. t.i.d.	10	No renal adjustment is required			Increase cyclosporine/tacrolimus level
Dirithromycin	500 mg p.o. q.i.d.		No renal adjustment is required			*(Cont'd.)*

Drugs and the Kidney

Antimicrobial agents (continued)					
Drugs normal doses		**Renal excretion (%)**	**Dosage adjustment in renal failure**		**Comments**
			GFR > 50	GFR 10–50	GFR < 10	
Erythromycin	250–500 mg p.o. q.i.d.	15	No renal adjustment is required			Increase cyclosporine/tacrolimus level, avoid in transplant patients
Imipenem/Cilastatin	250–500 mg i.v. q.6 h	50	500 mg q.8 h	250–500 q.8–12 h	250 mg q.12 h	Seizure
Linezolid	400–600 mg i.v./P.O. q.12 h	30	q.12 h	q.12 h	q.12 h	Thrombocytopenia
Meropenem	1 g i.v. q.8 h	65	1 g q.8 h	0.5–1 g q.12 h	0.5–1 g q.24 h	
Metronidazole	500 mg i.v. q.6 h	20	No renal adjustment is required			Peripheral neuropathy, increase LFTs, disulfiram reaction with alcoholic beverages
Pentamidine	4 mg/kg per day	5	q.24 h	q.24 h	q.48 h	Inhalation may cause bronchospasm, i.v. administration may cause hypotension, hypoglycemia and nephrotoxicity
Rifampin	300–600 mg p.o. q.i.d.	20	No renal adjustment is required			Decrease cyclosporine/tacrolimus level
Trimethoprim/Sulfamethoxazole	DS p.o. q.12 h	70	q.12 h	q.12 h	q.24 h	Increase serum creatinine
Vancomycin	1 g i.v. q.12 h	90	q.12 h	q.24–36 h	q.48–72 h	Nephrotoxic, ototoxic, may prolong the neuromuscular blockade effect of muscle relaxants. Peak 30, trough 5–10
Vancomycin oral	125–250 mg p.o. q.i.d.	0	100%	100%	100%	Oral vancomycin is indicated only for the treatment of C. diff
Antifungal agents						
Amphotericin	B 0.5 mg–1.5 mg/kg per day	< 1	No renal adjustment is required			Nephrotoxic, infusion related reactions, give 250 cc NS before each dose
Amphotec	4–6 mg/kg per day	< 1	No renal adjustment is required			
Abelcet	5 mg/kg per day	< 1	No renal adjustment is required			
AmBisome	3–5 mg/kg per day	< 1	No renal adjustment is required			Less nephrotoxic
Azoles and other antifungals						Increase cyclosporine/tacrolimus level
Fluconazole	200–800 mg i.v. q.i.d./b.i.d.	70	100%	100%	50%	
Itraconazole	200 mg q.12 h	35	100%	100%	50%	Poor oral absorption
Ketoconazole	200–400 mg p.o. q.i.d.	15	100%	100%	100%	Hepatotoxic
Miconazole	1200–3600 mg/day	1	100%	100%	100%	
Terbinafine	250 mg p.o. q.i.d.	< 1	100%	100%	100%	CHF and edema
Voriconazole	200 mg b.i.d.		100%	100%	Avoid	Ocular toxicity
Antiretroviral agents						
Abacavir	300 mg q.12 h	< 1	100%	100%	100%	
Amprenavir	1200 mg q.12 h		100%	100%	100%	
Delavirdine	400 mg q.8 h	< 5	100%	100%	100%	
Didanosine	200 q.12 h 18		100%	200 mg q.i.d.	100 mg q.i.d.	Pancreatitis
Efavirenz	600 mg q.i.d.	< 1	100%	100%	100%	
Indinavir	800 mg q.8 h	< 20	100%	100%	100%	May cause nephrolithiasis. Require adequate hydration
Lamivudine	150 mg b.i.d.	71	100%	100–150 mg q.i.d.	25–50 mg q.i.d.	
Lopinavir/ritonavir	400/100 mg q.12 h	< 3	100%	100%	100%	
Nelfinavir	750 mg q.8 h	< 1	100%	100%	100%	
Nevirapine	200 mg q.12 h	< 5	100%	100%	100%	
Ritonavir	600 mg q.12 h		100%	100%	100%	
Saquinavir	200 mg q.8hr	< 1	100%	100%	100%	Take with meals
Stavudine	40 mg q.12 h	40	100%	20 mg q.12 h	20 mg q.24 h	
Zalcitabine	0.75 mg q.8 h	70	100%	0.75 mg q.12 h	0.75 mg q.24 h	Neuropathy
Zidovudine	100 mg q.4 h	14	100%	100 mg q.6 h	100 mg q.8 h	Pancytopenia
Antiviral agents						
Amantadine	100–200 mg q.12 h	90	100%	50%	25%	
Famciclovir	250–500 mg p.o. b.i.d. to t.i.d.	60	q.8 h	q.12 h	q.24 h	VZV: 500 mg p.o. t.i.d.. HSV: 250 p.o. b.i.d.
Foscarnet	40–80 mg i.v. q.8 h	85	40–20 mg q.8–24 h according to ClCr			Nephrotoxic, neurotoxic, hypocalcemia, hypophosphatemia, hypomagnesemia and hypokalemia
Ganciclovir	i.v. 5 mg/kg q.12 h	95	q.12 h	q.24 h	2.5 mg/kg q.i.d.	Granulocytopenia and thrombocytopenia
Ganciclovir p.o.	1000 mg p.o. t.i.d.	95	1000 mg t.i.d.	1000 mg b.i.d.	1000 mg q.i.d.	Oral ganciclovir should be used ONLY for prevention of CMV infection. Always use i.v. ganciclovir for the treatment of CMV infection
Valganciclovir	450 mg p.o. b.i.d.	95	q.12 h	q.24 h	Mon, Wed and Fri	Oral ganciclovir can be use for the treatment of mild to moderate CMV infection
Lamivudine	150 mg p.o. b.i.d.	80	q.12 h	q.24 h 50 mg	q.24 h	For hepatitis B
Ribavirin	500–600 mg q.12 h	30	100%	100%	50%	Hemolytic uremic syndrome
Rimantadine	100 mg p.o. b.i.d.	25	100%	100%	50%	
Oseltamivir	75 mg p.o. b.i.d.	99	100%	100%	50%	
Valacyclovir	500–1000 mg q.8 h	50	100%	50%	25%	Thrombotic thrombocytopenic purpura/hemolytic uremic syndrome. Avoid in transplant recipients
Zanamivir	2 puffs b.i.d. × 5 d	4–17	100%	100%	100%	

Cardiovascular agents

Cardiovascular agents	Normal doses		Renal excretion (%)	Dosage adjustment in renal failure			Comments
	Starting dose	Maximum dose		GFR > 50	GFR 10–50	GFR < 10	
Ace-inhibitors							Hyperkalemia, acute renal failure, angioedema, rash, cough, anemia and liver toxicity
Benazepril	10 mg q.i.d.	80 mg q.i.d.	20	100%	75%	25–50%	
Captopril	6.25–25 mg p.o. t.i.d.	100 mg t.i.d.	35	100%	75%	50%	
Enalapril	5 mg q.i.d.	20 mg b.i.d.	45	100%	75%	50%	
Fosinopril	10 mg p.o. q.i.d.	40 mg b.i.d.	20	100%	100%	75%	
Lisinopril	2.5 mg q.i.d.	20 mg b.i.d.	80	100%	50–75%	25–50%	
Ramipril	2.5 mg q.i.d.	10 b.i.d.	15	100%	50–75%	25–50%	
Trandolapril	1–2 mg q.i.d.	4 mg q.i.d.					
Angiotensin ii receptors antagonists							Hyperkalemia, angioedema (less common than ace-inhibitors)
Losartan	50 mg q.i.d.	100 mg q.i.d.	13	100%	100%	100%	
Valsartan	80 mg q.i.d.	160 mg b.i.d.	7	100%	100%	100%	
Candesartan	16 mg q.i.d.	32 mg q.i.d.	33	100%	100%	50%	
Irbesartan	150 mg q.i.d.	300 mg q.i.d.	20	100%	100%	100%	
Beta blockers							Decrease HDL mask symptoms of hypoglycemia, bronchospasm, fatigue, insomnia, depression and sexual dysfunction
Atenolol	25 mg q.i.d.	100 mg q.i.d.	90	100%	75%	50%	
Carvedilol	3.125 mg p.o. t.i.d.	25 mg t.i.d.	2	100%	100%	100%	
Esmolol (i.v. only)	50 mcg/kg per min	300 mcg/kg per min	10	100%	100%	100%	
Labetalol	50 mg p.o. b.i.d.	400 mg b.i.d.	5	100%	100%	100%	
Nadolol	80 mg q.i.d.	160 mg q.i.d.	90	100%	50%	25%	
Propranolol	40–160 mg t.i.d.	320 mg/day	< 5	100%	100%	100%	
Sotalol	80 b.i.d.	160 mg b.i.d.	70	100%	50%	25–50%	
Calcium channel blockers							Dihydropyridine: headache, ankle edema, gingival hyperplasia and flushing. Non-dihydropyridine: bradycardia, constipation, gingival hyperplasia and av block
Amlodipine	2.5 p.o. q.i.d.	10 mg q.i.d.	10	100%	100%	100%	
Diltiazem	30 mg t.i.d.	90 mg t.i.d.	10	100%	100%	100%	
Felodipine	5 mg p.o. b.i.d.	20 mg q.i.d.	1	100%	100%	100%	
Isradipine	5 mg p.o. b.i.d.	10 mg b.i.d.	< 5	100%	100%	100%	
Nicardipine	20 mg p.o. t.i.d.	30 mg p.o. t.i.d.	< 1	100%	100%	100%	
Nifedipine	XL 30 q.i.d.	90 mg b.i.d.	10	100%	100%	100%	Avoid short-acting nifedipine formulation
Nimodipine			10	100%	100%	100%	
Nisoldipine	20 mg q.i.d.	30 mg b.i.d.	10	100%	100%	100%	
Verapamil	40 mg t.i.d.	240 mg/day	10	100%	100%	100%	
Diuretics							Hypokalemia/hyperkalemia (potassium sparing agents), hyperuricemia, hyperglycemia, hypomagnesemia, increase serum cholesterol.
Acetazolamide	125 mg p.o. t.i.d.	500 mg p.o. t.i.d.	90	100%	50%	Avoid	
Amiloride	5 mg p.o. q.i.d.	10 mg p.o. q.i.d.	50	100%	100%	Avoid	
Bumetanide	1–2 mg p.o. q.i.d.	2–4 mg p.o. q.i.d.	35	100%	100%	100%	
Ethacrynic Acid	50 mg p.o. q.i.d.	100 mg p.o. b.i.d.	20	100%	100%	100%	
Furosemide	40–80 mg p.o. q.i.d.	120 mg p.o. t.i.d.	70	100%	100%	100%	
Metolazone	2.5 mg p.o. q.i.d.	10 mg p.o. b.i.d.	70	100%	100%	100%	
Spironolactone	100 mg p.o. q.i.d.	300 mg p.o. q.i.d.	25	100%	100%	Avoid	
Torsemide	5 mg p.o. b.i.d.	20 mg q.i.d.	25	100%	100%	100%	
Miscellaneous agents							
Clonidine	0.1 p.o. b.i.d./t.i.d.	1.2 mg/day	45	100%	100%	100%	Sexual dysfunction, dizziness, postal hypotension
Digoxin	0.125 mg q.od/q.i.d.	0.25 mg p.o. q.i.d.	25	100%	100%	100%	
Hydralazine	10 mg q.i.d.	100 mg p.o. q.i.d.	25	100%	100%	100%	Lupus-like reaction
Minoxidil	2.5 mg p.o. b.i.d.	10 mg p.o. b.i.d.	20	100%	100%	100%	Pericardial effusion, fluid retention, hypertrichosis and tachycardia
Nitroprusside	1 mcg/kg per min	10 mcg/kg per min	< 10	100%	100%	100%	Cyanide toxicity
Amrinone	5 mcg/kg per min	10 mcg/kg per min	25	100%	100%	100%	
Dobutamine	2.5 mcg/kg per min	15 mcg/kg per min	10	100%	100%	100%	
Milrinone	0.375 mcg/kg per min	0.75 mcg/kg per min		100%	100%	100%	

Drugs and the Kidney

Anti-lipidemic agents							
Anti-lipidemic agent	Normal doses		Renal excretion (%)	Dosage adjustment in renal failure			Comments
	Starting dose	Maximum dose		GFR > 50	GFR 10–50	GFR < 10	
Atorvastatin	10 mg/day	80 mg/day	< 2	100%	100%	100%	Liver dysfunction, myalgia and rhabdomyolysis with cyclosporine/tacrolimus
Cholestyramine	4 g b.i.d.	24 g/day	None	100%	100%	100%	Schedule cyclosporine/tacrolimus 3 h before the dose, N/V and constipation
Colestipol	5 gmbid	30 g/day	None	100%	100%	100%	Schedule cyclosporine/tacrolimus 3 h before the dose, N/V and constipation
Fluvastatin	20 mg daily	80 mg/day	< 1	100%	100%	100%	Liver dysfunction, myalgia and rhabdomyolysis with cyclosporin/tacrolimus
Gemfibrozil	600 b.i.d.	600 b.i.d.	None	100%	100%	100%	Hyperglycemia, rhabdomyolysis, elevation of LFTs
Lovastatin	5 mg daily	20 mg/day	None	100%	100%	100%	Liver dysfunction, myalgia and rhabdomyolysis with cyclosporine/tacrolimus
Pravastatin	10–40 mg daily	80 mg/day	< 10	100%	100%	100%	Liver dysfunction, myalgia and rhabdomyolysis with cyclosporine/tacrolimus
Simvastatin	5–20 mg daily	20 mg/day	13	100%	100%	100%	Liver dysfunction, myalgia and rhabdomyolysis with cyclosporine/tacrolimus

Anti-platelet and anti-coagulant agents							
Anti-platelets and Anti-coagulation	Normal doses		Renal excretion (%)	Dosage adjustment in renal failure			Comments
	Starting dose	Maximum dose		GFR > 50	GFR 10–50	GFR < 10	
Aspirin	81 mg/day	325 mg/day	10	100%	100%	100%	GI irritation and bleeding tendency
Clopidogrel	75 mg/day	75 mg/day	50	100%	100%	100%	
Dalteparin	2,500 units Sq./day	5,000 units Sq./day	Unknown	100%	100%	100%	
Enoxaparin	20 mg/day	30 mg b.i.d.	8	100%	100%	50%	1 mg/kg q.12 h for treatment of DVT. Check anti-factor Xa activity 4 h after second dose in patients with renal dysfunction. There are some evidence of drug accumulation in renal failure
Ticlopidine	250 mg b.i.d.	250 mg b.i.d.	2	100%	100%	100%	Decrease cyclosporine level and may cause severe neutropenia and thrombocytopenia
Warfarin	5 mg/day	Adjust per INR	< 1	100%	100%	100%	Monitor INR very closely. Start at 5 mg/day. 1 mg Vit. K i.v. over 30 min or 2.5–5 mg p.o. can be used to normalize INR.

Gastrointestinal agents

Gastrointestinal agents	Normal doses		Renal excretion (%)	Dosage adjustment in renal failure			Comments
	Starting dose	Maximum dose		GFR > 50	GFR 10–50	GFR < 10	
Anti-ulcer agents							
Cimetidine	300 mg p.o. t.i.d.	800 mg p.o. b.i.d.	60	100%	75%	25%	Multiple drug-drug interactions; beta blockers, sulfonylurea, theophylline, warfarin, etc
Famotidine	20 mg p.o. b.i.d.	40 mg p.o. b.i.d.	70	100%	75%	25%	Headache, fatigue, thrombocytopenia, alopecia
Lansoprazole	15 mg p.o. q.i.d.	30 mg b.i.d.	None	100%	100%	100%	Headache, diarrhea
Nizatidine	150 mg p.o. b.i.d.	300 mg p.o. b.i.d.	20	100%	75%	25%	Headache, fatigue, thrombocytopenia, alopecia
Omeprazole	20 mg p.o. q.i.d.	40 mg p.o. b.i.d.	None	100%	100%	100%	Headache, diarrhea
Rabeprazole	20 mg p.o. q.i.d.	40 mg p.o. b.i.d.	None	100%	100%	100%	Headache, diarrhea
Pantoprazole	40 mg p.o. q.i.d.	80 mg p.o. b.i.d.	None	100%	100%	100%	Headache, diarrhea
Ranitidine	150 mg p.o. b.i.d.	300 mg p.o. b.i.d.	80	100%	75%	25%	Headache, fatigue, thrombocytopenia, alopecia
Cisapride	10 mg p.o. t.i.d.	20 mg q.i.d.	5	100%	100%	50–75%	Avoid with Azole Antifungal, Macrolide antibiotics and other P450 IIIA-4 inhibitors
Metoclopramide	10 mg p.o. t.i.d.	30 mg p.o. q.i.d.	15	100%	100%	50–75%	Increase cyclosporine/tacrolimus level. Neurotoxic
Misoprostol	100 mcg p.o. b.i.d.	200 mcg p.o. q.i.d.		100%	100%	100%	Diarrhea, N/V Abortifacient agent
Sucralfate	1 g p.o. q.i.d.	1 g p.o. q.i.d.	None	100%	100%	100%	Constipation, decrease absorption of MMF

Hypoglycemic agents

Hypoglycemic agents	Normal doses		Renal excretion (%)	Dosage adjustment in renal failure			Comments
	Starting dose	Maximum dose		GFR > 50	GFR 10–50	GFR < 10	
Acrobose	25 mg t.i.d.	100 mg t.i.d.	35	100%	50%	Avoid	Abdominal pain, N/V and flatulence
Glimepiride	1 mg q.i.d.	8 mg q.i.d.	60	100%	50%	50%	
Glipizide	5 mg q.i.d.	20 mg b.i.d.	80	100%	50%	50%	
Glyburide	2.5 mg q.i.d.	10 mg b.i.d.	50	100%	50%	Avoid	
Metformin	500 mg b.i.d.	2550 mg/day (b.i.d. or t.i.d.)	95	100%	Avoid	Avoid	Lactic acidosis
Pioglitazone	15 mg q.i.d.	45 mg q.i.d.	3	100%	100%	100%	Hepatotoxic. Edema
Repaglinide	0.5–1 mg	4 mg t.i.d.	8	100%	100%	100%	
Rosiglitazone	4 mg q.i.d.	8 mg q.i.d.	3	100%	100%	100%	Hepatotoxic. Edema, increase LDL

Index